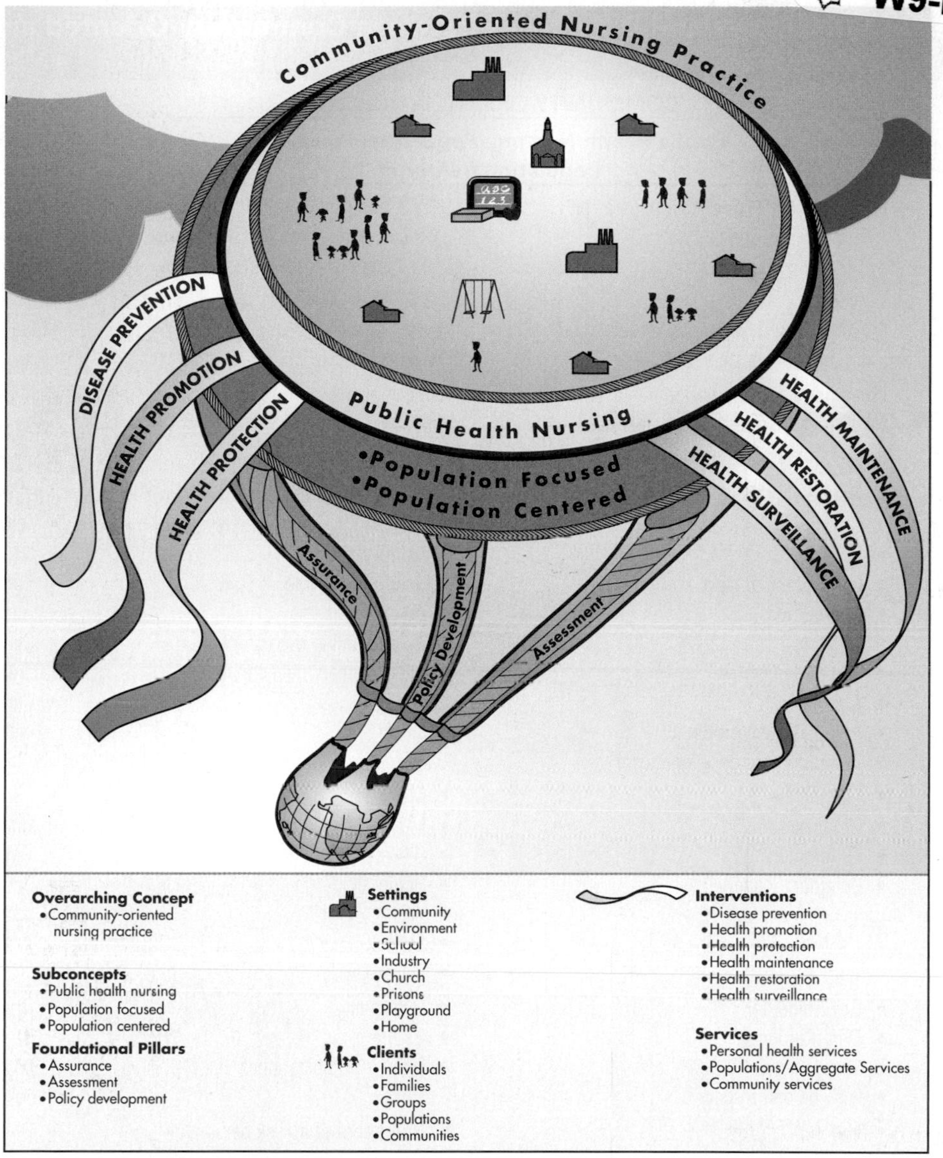

COMMUNITY NURSING DEFINITIONS

Community-Oriented Nursing Practice is a philosophy of nursing service delivery that involves the generalist or specialist public health and community health nurse providing "health care" through community diagnosis and investigation of major health and environmental problems, health surveillance, and monitoring and evaluation of community and population health status for the purposes of preventing disease and disability and promoting, protecting, and maintaining "health" in order to create conditions in which people can be healthy.

Public Health Nursing Practice is the synthesis of nursing theory and public health theory applied to promoting and preserving health of populations. The focus of practice is the community as a whole and the effect of the community's health status (resources) on the health of individuals, families, and groups. Care is provided within the context of preventing disease and disability and promoting and protecting the health of the community as a whole. Public Health Nursing is population focused, which means that the population is the center of interest for the public health nurse. *Community Health Nurse* is a term that is used interchangeably with *Public Health Nurse.*

Community-Based Nursing Practice is a setting-specific practice whereby care is provided for "sick" individuals and families where they live, work, and go to school. The emphasis of practice is acute and chronic care and the provision of comprehensive, coordinated, and continuous services. Nurses who deliver community-based care are generalists or specialists in maternal–infant, pediatric, adult, or psychiatric–mental health nursing.

Select Examples of Similarities and Differences Between Community-Oriented and Community-Based Nursing

	COMMUNITY-ORIENTED NURSING Public Health Nursing: Population Focused/ Population Centered		Community-Based Nursing
Philosophy	PRIMARY focus is on "health care" of communities and populations	SECONDARY focus is on "health care" of individuals, families, and groups in community to unserved clients by health care system	Focus is on "illness care" of individuals and families across the life span
Goal	Prevent disease; preserve, protect, promote, or maintain health	Prevent disease; preserve, protect, promote, or maintain health	Manage acute or chronic conditions
Service context	Community and population health care "the greatest good for the greatest number"	Personal health care to unserved clients	Family-centered illness care
Community type	Varied: local, state, nation, world community	Varied, usually local community	Human ecological
Client characteristics	• Nation • State • Community • Populations at risk • Aggregates • Healthy • Culturally diverse • Autonomous • Able to define problem • Client primary decision maker	• Individuals/families at risk if unserved by health care system • Usually healthy • Culturally diverse • Autonomous • Able to define own problem • Client primary decision maker	• Individuals • Families • Usually ill • Culturally diverse • Autonomous • Client able to define own problem • Client involved in decision making
Practice setting	• Community • Organization • Government • Community agencies	• May be organization • May be government • Community agencies • Home • Work • School • Playground	• Community agencies • Home • Work • School
Interaction patterns	• Governmental • Organizational • Groups • May be one-to-one	• One-to-one • Groups • May be organizational	• One-to-one
Type of service	• Indirect • May be direct care of populations	• Direct care of at-risk persons • Indirect (program management)	• Direct illness care
Emphasis on levels of prevention	• Primary	• Primary • Secondary: screening • Tertiary: maintenance and rehabilitation	• Secondary • Tertiary • May be primary

Select Examples of Similarities and Differences Between Community-Oriented and Community-Based Nursing—cont'd

	COMMUNITY-ORIENTED NURSING: Public Health Nursing: Population Focused/ Population Centered		Community-Based Nursing
Roles	**Client and delivery oriented: community/ population** • Educator • Consultant • Advocate • Planner • Collaborator • Data collector/evaluator • Health status monitor • Social engineer • Community developer/partner • Facilitator • Community care agent • Assessor • Policy developer/maker • Assuror of health care • Enforcer of laws/compliance • Disaster responder **Population oriented** • Program manager, aggregates • Health initiator • Program evaluator • Counselor • Change agent—population health • Educator • Population advocate	**Client and delivery oriented: individual, family, group** • Individual/family oriented—as needed • Caregiver • Social engineer • Educator • Counselor • Advocate • Case manager **Group Oriented** • Leader, personal health management • Change agent, screening • Community advocate • Case finder • Community care agent • Assessment • Policy developer • Assurance • Enforcer of laws/compliance	**Client and delivery oriented: individual, family** • Caregiver • Educator • Counselor • Advocate • Care manager **Group Oriented** • Leader, disease management • Change agent, managed care services
Priority of nurses' activities	**Community development** • Community assessment/monitoring • Health policy/politics • Community education • Interdisciplinary practice • Program management • Community/population advocacy	**For individual and family clients—as needed** • Case finding • Client education • Community education • Interdisciplinary practice • Case management, direct care • Program planning, implementation • Individual and family advocacy	**Care management, direct care** • Patient education • Individual and family advocacy • Interdisciplinary practice • Continuity of care provider

PUBLIC HEALTH NURSING

10

TENTH COMMEMORATIVE EDITION

Population-Centered Health Care in the Community

MARCIA **STANHOPE**
PhD, RN, FAAN

Education and Practice Consultant
and Professor Emerita
College of Nursing
University of Kentucky
Lexington, Kentucky

JEANETTE **LANCASTER**
PhD, RN, FAAN

Sadie Heath Cabiness Professor and Dean
Emerita
School of Nursing
University of Virginia
Charlottesville, Virginia
Associate, Tuft & Associates, Inc.

ELSEVIER

3251 Riverport Lane
St. Louis, Missouri 63043

PUBLIC HEALTH NURSING: POPULATION-CENTERED HEALTH CARE IN THE COMMUNITY, TENTH EDITION

ISBN: 978-0-323-58224-7

Notices

Practitioners and researchers must always rely on their own experience and knowledge in evaluating and using any information, methods, compounds or experiments described herein. Because of rapid advances in the medical sciences, in particular, independent verification of diagnoses and drug dosages should be made. To the fullest extent of the law, no responsibility is assumed by Elsevier, authors, editors or contributors for any injury and/or damage to persons or property as a matter of products liability, negligence or otherwise, or from any use or operation of any methods, products, instructions, or ideas contained in the material herein.

Previous editions copyrighted 2016, 2014, 2008, 2004, 2000, 1996, 1992, 1988, 1984.

Library of Congress Control Number: 2019946140

Senior Content Strategist: Jamie Blum
Content Development Manager: Lisa P. Newton
Senior Content Development Specialist: Tina Kaemmerer
Publishing Services Manager: Julie Eddy
Senior Project Manager: Tracey Schriefer
Designer: Amy Buxton

Printed in Canada

Last digit is the print number: 9 8 7 6 5 4 3 2 1

ABOUT THE AUTHORS

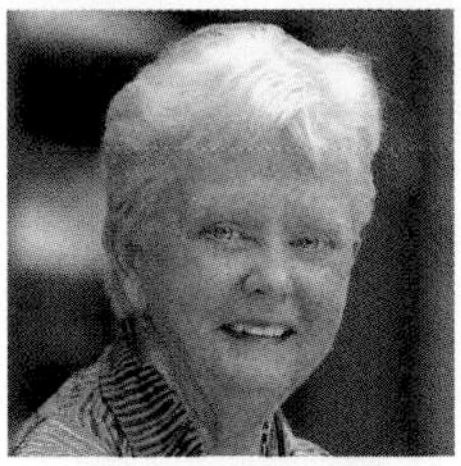

MARCIA STANHOPE, PhD, RN, FAAN

Marcia Stanhope is currently an education consultant, an Associate with Tuft and Associates Search Firm, Chicago, Illinois, and Professor Emerita from the University of Kentucky, College of Nursing, Lexington, Kentucky. In recent years she was a co-developer of the doctorate of nursing practice (DNP) program and co-director of the first DNP program nationally, which began at the University of Kentucky. While at the University of Kentucky she received the Provost Public Scholar award for contributions to the communities of Kentucky. She was also appointed to the Good Samaritan Endowed Chair in Community Health Nursing by the Good Samaritan Foundation, Lexington, Kentucky. She has practiced public health, community, and home health nursing, has served as an administrator and consultant in home health, and has been involved in the development of a number of nurse-managed centers. She has taught community health, public health, epidemiology, primary care nursing, and administration courses. Dr. Stanhope was the former Associate Dean and formerly directed the Division of Community Health Nursing and Administration at the University of Kentucky. She has been responsible for both undergraduate and graduate courses in population-centered, community-oriented nursing. She has also taught at the University of Virginia and the University of Alabama, Birmingham. Her presentations and publications have been in the areas of home health, community health, and community-focused nursing practice, nurse-managed centers, and primary care nursing. Dr. Stanhope holds a diploma in nursing from the Good Samaritan Hospital, Lexington, Kentucky, and a bachelor of science in nursing from the University of Kentucky. She has a master's degree in public health nursing from Emory University in Atlanta and a PhD in nursing from the University of Alabama, Birmingham. Dr. Stanhope is the co-author of four other Elsevier publications: *Handbook of Community-Based and Home Health Nursing Practice, Public and Community Health Nurse's Consultant, Case Studies in Community Health Nursing Practice: A Problem-Based Learning Approach,* and *Foundations of Community Health Nursing: Community-Oriented Practice.*

Recently Dr. Stanhope was inducted into the University of Kentucky College of Nursing Hall of Fame and was named an outstanding alumni of the University of Kentucky.

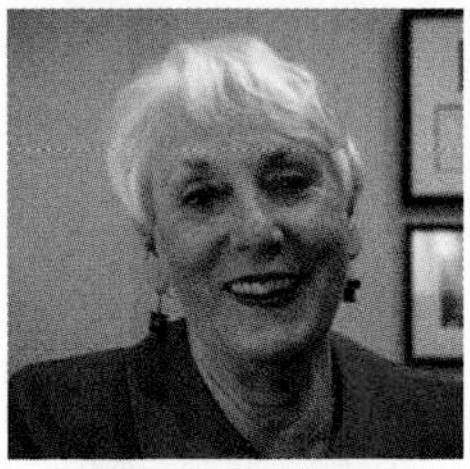

JEANETTE LANCASTER, PhD, RN, FAAN

Jeanette Lancaster is Professor and Dean Emerita at the University of Virginia School of Nursing in Charlottesville, Virginia. She served as Dean of the School of Nursing at the University of Virginia from 1989 until 2008. From 2008 to 2009 she served as a visiting professor at the University of Hong Kong, where she taught courses in public health nursing and worked with faculty to develop their scholarship programs and a doctoral program in nursing. She then taught at the University of Virginia from 2010 until 2012. She also taught at Vanderbilt University and is an Associate with Tuft & Associates, Inc., an executive search firm. She has practiced psychiatric nursing and taught both psychiatric and community health nursing. She formerly directed the master's program in community health nursing at the University of Alabama, Birmingham, and served as Dean of the School of Nursing at Wright State University in Dayton, Ohio. Her publications and presentations have been largely in the areas of community and public health nursing, leadership, change, and the significance of nurses to effective primary health care. Since 2009 she has returned to the University of Hong Kong to teach graduate courses in public health nursing, comparative health care systems, and health policy. Dr. Lancaster is a graduate of the University of Tennessee Health Science Center Memphis. She holds a master's degree in psychiatric nursing from Case Western Reserve University and a doctorate in public health from the University of Oklahoma. Dr. Lancaster is the author of another Elsevier publication, *Nursing Issues in Leading and Managing Change*, and the co-author with Dr. Marcia Stanhope of *Foundations for Population Health in Community/Public Health Nursing.*

ACKNOWLEDGMENTS

Two very important people assisted us in the editing of this edition through their research efforts.

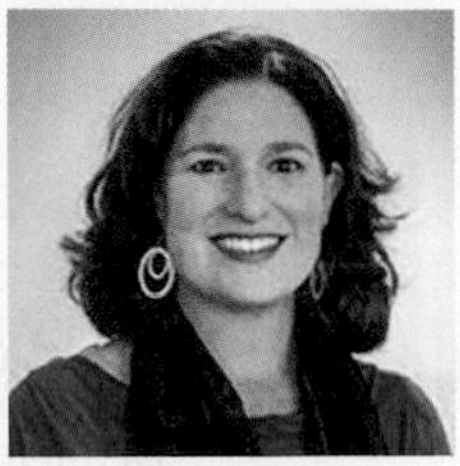

Dr. Sawin is an Associate Professor of Nursing at James Madison University, Harrisonburg, Virginia. She received her MSN from the University of Texas, Austin, and her PhD in nursing from the University of Virginia.

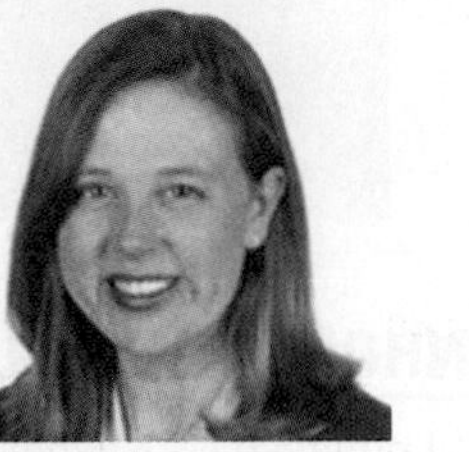

Dr. Turner is an Associate Professor at Berea College, Berea, Kentucky where she holds an endowed chair. She holds a BSN and MSN from the University of Virginia and a PhD from the University of Kentucky.

IN APPRECIATION

To the contributing authors, please accept our gratitude for helping to make this text a success over the many years of publication. While some of you contributed your expertise to one edition, many of you contributed to a number of editions. One of you contributed to all ten editions. You helped lay the foundation and made the continuation of this text possible. Whether it was one edition or ten, we thank you.

To the families of some of the authors, now deceased, we thank you for sharing them with us.

Marcia Stanhope and Jeanette Lancaster

Theresa Acquaviva
Swann Adams
Brenda Afzal
Mary Albrecht
Mollie Aleshire
Rena Alford
Jeanne Alhusen
Kacy Allen-Bryant
Debra Anderson
Sandra Anderson
Dyan Aretakis
Sidney Axson
Ellen Bailey
Julie Balzer
Amber Bang
Sara Barger
Eleanor Bauwens
Anne Belcher
Ruth Berry
Virginia T. Betts
Marjorie Glaser Bindner
Patricia Birchfield
Linda Birenbaum
Whitney Bischoff
Kathleen Blomquist
Tina Bloom
Jean Bokinskie
Christine DiMartile Bolla
Joyce Bonick
Nisha Botchwey
Kathryn Bowles
Diane Boyer
Laurel Briske
Hazel Brown
Vivienne Brown
Bonnie Brueshoff
Marjorie Buchanan
Jeanne Bucsela
Angeline Bushy
Jacquelyn Campbell
Catherine Carroca
Ann Cary
Sudruk Chitthathairatt
Laura Clayton
Ann Connor
Marcia Cowan
Erin Cruise
Lois Davis
Sharon K. Davis
Karen Dawn
Cynthia Degazon
Louise Ivanor Dennis
Edie Devers
Nancy Dickenson-Hazard
Janna Dieckmann
Diane Downing
Sadie Elizabeth
Amanda Fallin
Sharon Farra
Hartley Feld
Mary Eure Fisher
James Fletcher
Kathleen Fletcher
Beverly Flynn
Douglas Charles Forness
Sara Fry
Carol Garrison
Denise Geolot
Mary Gibson
Debra Giese
Doris Glick
Jean Goeppinger
Mary Goldschmidt
Rosa Gonzalez-Guardia
Phyllis Graves
Monty Gross
Cynthia Gustafson
Patty Hale
Melanie Gibbons Hallman
Shirley M.H. Hanson
Susan Hassmiller
Diane Hatton
Anita Heisterman
Irma Heppner
Beth Hibbs
Joanna Horn
Patricia B. Howard
Linda Hulton
Anita Hunter
Kathleen Huttlinger
Judy Igoe
Janet Ihlenfeld
L. Louise Ivanov
Gerard Jellig
Alicia Jensen
Bonnie Jerome-D'Emilia
Rosemary Johnson
Cheryl B. Jones
Kim D. Jones
Linda C. Jones
Joanna Kaakinen
Lisa Kaiser
Linda Keller
Marjorie Keller
Loren Kelly
Susan Kennel
Ellen Kent
David Kerschner
Katherine Kinsey
Thomas Kippenbrock
Sandra Kirkland
Tammy Kiser

Andrea Knopp
Joyce Krothe
Candace Kugel
Pamela Kulbok
Karen Labuhn
Shirley Laffrey
Wade Lancaster
Karen Landenburger
Peggy Lassiter
Roberta Lavin
Natasha Le
Gwendolyn Lee
Roberta "Bobbi" Lee
Sharon Lock
Jacquelyn Hurbel Logue
Susan Long-Marin
Carol Loveland-Cherry
Myra Lovvorn
Lois Lowry
Max Lum
P.J. Maddox
Karen Martin
Mary Lynn Mathre
Carol Maxwell-Thompson
Natalie McClain
Mary Ann McClellan
Beverly McElmurry
Robert McKeown
Kathleen McPhaul
DeAnne Messias
Mary Ellen Miller
Margaret Millsap
Emma Mitchell
Lillian Mood
Geneva Morris
Carole Myers
Marie Napolitano
Diane Narkunas
Victoria Niederhauser
Cynthia Northrup
Julie Novak
Lisa Onega
Charlene Ossler
Eunhee Park
Susan Patton
Bobbie Perdue
Lynelle Phillips
Paula Pointer
Demetrius Porche
Kristine Qureshi
Mary Riner
Bonnie Rogers
Molly Rose
Cynthia Rubenstein
Barbara Sattler
Erika Metzler Sawin
Linda Sawyer
Marjorie Schaffer
Jennifer Schaller-Ayers
Nancy Scheet
Cheryl Schenk
Juliann Sebastian
Cynthia Selleck
Sharon Shehan
Sallie Shipman
Maria Shirey
Linda Shortridge
George Shuster III
Mary Silva
Ann Sirles
Delois Skipwith
Rebecca Sloan
Donna E. Smith
Kellie Smith
Sherrill Smith
Jeanne Sorrell
Patricia Speck
Sudie Speer
Sharon A.R. Stanley
Patricia Starck
Sharon Strang
Sue Strohschein
Melissa Sutherland
Laura Suzuki
Susan Swider
Francisco Sy
Michele Talley
Esther Thatcher
Karen Thompson
Shirleen Trabeaux
Joan Turner
Lisa Turner
Connie Ulrich
Barbara Valanis
Doris Wagner
Heather Ward
Lynn Wasserbauer
Prapin Watanakij
Jacqueline Webb
Sally Weinrich
Cynthia Wesley
Connie White-Williams
Eileen Wiles
Carolyn A. Williams[a]
Cora Withrow
Judith Wold
Nannette Worel
Elke Jones Zchaebitz
Lisa Zerull

[a]Contributing author for 10 editions.

It has been my special privilege to be advised and mentored by a number of exemplary professionals and to be loved and supported by numerous friends, big and small. Their contributions have made significant differences to my life and career. This edition of the text is dedicated to the memory of Charlotte Denny and Lois Merrill, University of Kentucky; Mary Hall, Emory University, Atlanta; Dorothy Carter, my community partner, Pikeville, Kentucky; and Norma Mobley, University of Alabama, Birmingham; as well as to two special friends, John C. and CiCi.

Marcia Stanhope

I would like to dedicate my work on this 10th edition to my late husband, I. Wade Lancaster. He supported and encouraged me through the first nine editions of the text, and I am deeply grateful for his love, support, and encouragement.

Jeanette Lancaster

CONTRIBUTORS

Swann Arp Adams, MS, PhD
Associate Professor
College of Nursing
University of South Carolina
Columbia, South Carolina
Chapter 13: Epidemiology

Mollie E. Aleshire, DNP, MSN, FNP-BC, PPCNP-BC, FNAP
Associate Professor
School of Nursing
University of North Carolina at Greensboro
Greensboro, North Carolina;
Family and Pediatric Nurse Practitioner
Greensboro, North Carolina
Chapter 27: Family Health Risks

Jeanne L. Alhusen, PhD, CRNP, RN, FAAN
Associate Professor and Assistant Dean for Research
School of Nursing
University of Virginia
Charlottesville, Virginia
Chapter 38: Violence and Human Abuse

Kacy Allen-Bryant, PhD(c), MSN, MPH, RN
Lecturer
College of Nursing
University of Kentucky
Lexington, Kentucky
Chapter 27: Family Health Risks

Debra Gay Anderson, PhD, PHCNS-BC
Associate Dean for Research
College of Nursing
South Dakota State University
Brookings, South Dakota
Chapter 27: Family Health Risks

Sydney A. Axson, MPH, RN
Hillman Scholar in Nursing Innovation
School of Nursing
University of Pennsylvania
Philadelphia, Pennsylvania
Chapter 7: Application of Ethics in the Community

Amber M. Bang, RN, BSN
Registered Nurse
Grants Pass, Oregon
Chapter 37: Alcohol, Tobacco, and Other Drug Problems

Whitney Rogers Bischoff, DrPH, MSN, BSN
Associate Professor
Nursing
Texas Lutheran University
Seguin, Texas
Chapter 5: Economics of Health Care Delivery

Nisha D. Botchwey, PhD, MCRP, MPH
Associate Professor
City and Regional Planning
Georgia Institute of Technology
Atlanta, Georgia;
Public Health
Emory University
Atlanta, Georgia
Chapter 18: Building a Culture of Health to Influence Health Equity Within Communities

Kathryn H. Bowles, RN, PhD, FAAN
van Ameringen Professor in Nursing Excellence
School of Nursing
University of Pennsylvania
Philadelphia, Pennsylvania;
Director of the Center for Home Care Policy and Research
Visiting Nurse Service of New York
New York, New York
Chapter 41: The Nurse in Public Health, Home Health, Hospice, and Palliative Care

Hazel Brown, DNP, RN
Chief Nursing Officer
Nursing Administration
Cayman Islands Health Services Authority
George Town, Grand Cayman
Cayman Islands
Chapter 29: Major Health Issues and Chronic Disease Management of Adults Across the Life Span

Bonnie L. Brueshoff, DNP, MSN, RN, PHN
Director
Public Health
Dakota County
West St. Paul, Minnesota
Chapter 11: Population-Based Public Health Nursing Practice: The Intervention Wheel

Angeline Bushy, PhD, RN, FAAN
Professor, Bert Fish Chair
College of Nursing
University of Central Florida
Orlando, Florida
Chapter 32: Population-Centered Nursing in Rural and Urban Environments

Jacquelyn C. Campbell, PhD, RN, FAAN
Professor
Anna D. Wolf Chair
National Program Director, Robert Wood Johnson Foundation Nurse Faculty Scholars
Department of Community-Public Health
The Johns Hopkins University
Baltimore, Maryland
Chapter 38: Violence and Human Abuse

Catherine Carroca, MSN, RN
Assistant Professor
School of Nursing
Massachusetts College of Pharmacy and Health Sciences
Worcester, Massachusetts
Chapter 23: Program Management

Ann H. Cary, PhD, MPH, RN, FNAP, FAAN
Dean
School of Nursing and Health Studies
University of Missouri Kansas City
Kansas City, Missouri
Chapter 25: Case Management

Laura H. Clayton, PhD, RN, CNE
Professor
Department of Nursing Education
Shepherd University
Shepherdstown, West Virginia
Chapter 22: Public Health Surveillance and Outbreak Investigation

Erin G. Cruise, PhD, RN
Associate Professor
School of Nursing
Radford University
Radford, Virginia
Chapter 42: The Nurse in the Schools

Lois A. Davis, RN, MSN, MA
Public Health Clinical Instructor
College of Nursing
University of Kentucky
Lexington, Kentucky
Chapter 46: Public Health Nursing at Local, State, and National Levels

Sharon K. Davis, DNP, APRN, WHNP-BC
Clinical Assistant Professor
Nursing
University of Tennessee
Knoxville, Tennessee
Chapter 35: Teen Pregnancy

Karen R. Dawn, DNP, MSN, BSN
Assistant Professor
School of Nursing
George Washington University
Ashburn, Virginia
Chapter 3: Public Health, Primary Care, and Primary Health Care Systems

Cynthia E. Degazon, RN, PhD
Professor Emerita
School of Nursing
Hunter College
New York, New York
Chapter 8: Achieving Cultural Competence in Community Health Nursing

Janna Dieckmann, PhD, RN
Associate Professor
School of Nursing
University of North Carolina at Chapel Hill
Chapel Hill, North Carolina
Chapter 2: History of Public Health and Public and Community Health Nursing

Sherry L. Farra, PhD, RN, CNE, CHSE, NDHP-BC
Associate Professor
Nursing
Wright State University
Dayton, Ohio
Chapter 21: Public Health Nursing Practice and the Disaster Management Cycle

Mary E. Gibson, PhD, RN
Associate Professor
Nursing
University of Virginia
Charlottesville, Virginia
Chapter 17: Community As Client: Assessment and Analysis

Mary Kay Goldschmidt, DNP, MSN, RN, PHNA-BC
Assistant Professor
Family and Community Health
Virginia Commonwealth University School of Nursing
Richmond, Virginia;
Commissioner on Government Relations
Board member
Virginia Nurses Association
Richmond, Virginia;
Co-director
PIONEER NEPQR Grant
Health Resources and Services Administration
Washington, DC
Chapter 33: Poverty and Homelessness

Monty Gross, PhD, MSN, RN, CNE, CNL
Senior Nurse Leader for Professional Development
Nursing Administration
Health Services Authority
George Town, Grand Cayman
Cayman Islands
Chapter 29: Major Health Issues and Chronic Disease Management of Adults Across the Life Span

Melanie Gibbons Hallman, DNP, CRNP, CEN, FNP-BC, ACNP-BC, FAEN
Assistant Professor / Nurse Practitioner
Family, Community and Health Systems
University of Alabama at Birmingham School of Nursing
Birmingham, Alabama
Chapter 39: Advanced Nursing Practice in the Community

Joanna Horn, BA, MS
Senior Genetic Counselor
Center for Human Genetics
University Hospital Cleveland Medical Center
Cleveland, Ohio
Chapter 12: Genomics in Public Health Nursing

Gerard M. Jellig, EdD
School Principal/Leader
KIPP DC WILL Academy
Washington, DC
Chapter 38: Violence and Human Abuse

Tammy Kiser, DNP, RN
Assistant Professor of Nursing
School of Nursing
James Madison University
Harrisonburg, Virginia
Chapter 15: Communicable and Infectious Disease Risks

Andrea Knopp, PhD, MPH, MSN, FNP-BC
Nurse Practitioner Program Coordinator, Associate Professor
School of Nursing
James Madison University
Harrisonburg, Virginia
Chapter 29: Major Health Issues and Chronic Disease Management of Adults Across the Life Span

Candace Kugel, BA, MS, FNP, CNM
Clinical Specialist
Migrant Clinicians Network
Austin, Texas
Chapter 34: Migrant Health Issues

Pamela A. Kulbok, DNSc, RN, PHCNS-BC, FAAN
Professor Emerita
School of Nursing
University of Virginia
Charlottesville, Virginia
Chapter 18: Building a Culture of Health to Influence Health Equity Within Communities

Roberta Proffitt Lavin, PhD, FNP-BC, FAAN
Professor and Executive Associate Dean of Academic Programs
College of Nursing
University of Tennessee
Knoxville, Tennessee
Chapter 21: Public Health Nursing Practice and the Disaster Management Cycle

Natasha Le, BA, BS
Informatics and Quality Coordinator
Home Care and Hospice
Penn Care at Home
Philadelphia, Pennsylvania
Chapter 41: The Nurse in Public Health, Home Health, Hospice, and Palliative Care

Susan C. Long-Marin, DVM, MPH
Epidemiology Manager
Public Health
Mecklenburg County
Charlotte, North Carolina
Chapter 14: Infectious Disease Prevention and Control

Karen S. Martin, RN, MSN, FAAN
Health Care Consultant
Martin Associates
Omaha, Nebraska
Chapter 41: The Nurse in Public Health, Home Health, Hospice, and Palliative Care

Mary Lynn Mathre, RN, MSN, CARN
President and Co-founder
Patients Out of Time
Howardsville, Virginia
Chapter 37: Alcohol, Tobacco, and Other Drug Problems

Natalie McClain, PhD, RN, CPNP
Associate Clinical Professor Visiting Scholar
William F. Connell School of Nursing
Boston College
Chestnut Hill, Massachusetts
Chapter 44: Forensic Nursing in the Community

DeAnne K. Hilfinger Messias, PhD, RN, FAAN
Professor
College of Nursing and Women's and Gender Studies
University of South Carolina
Columbia, South Carolina
Chapter 13: Epidemiology

Emma McKim Mitchell, PhD, MSN, RN
Assistant Professor
Department of Family, Community & Mental Health Systems
University of Virginia School of Nursing
Charlottesville, Virginia
Chapter 4: Perspectives in Global Health Care

Carole R. Myers, PhD, MSN, BS
Associate Professor
College of Nursing
University of Tennessee
Knoxville, Tennessee
Chapter 31: Health Equity and Care of Vulnerable Populations

Victoria P. Niederhauser, DrPH, RN, PPCNP-BC, FAAN
Dean and Professor
College of Nursing
University of Tennessee
Knoxville, Tennessee
Chapter 19: Health Education Principles Applied in Communities, Groups, Families, and Individuals for Healthy Change

Eunhee Park, PhD, RN, APHN-BC
Assistant Professor
School of Nursing
University at Buffalo
Buffalo, New York
Chapter 18: Building a Culture of Health to Influence Health Equity Within Communities

Bobbie J. Perdue, RN, PhD
Professor Emerita
College of Human Ecology
Syracuse University
Syracuse, New York;
Adjunct faculty
Jersey College of Nursing
Tampa, Florida
Chapter 8: Achieving Cultural Competence in Community Health Nursing

Bonnie Rogers, DrPH, COHN-S, LNCC, FAAN
Professor and Director
North Carolina Occupational Safety and Health Education and Research Center
University of North Carolina
Chapel Hill, North Carolina
Chapter 43: The Nurse in Occupational Health

Cynthia Rubenstein, PhD, RN, CPNP-PC
Chair and Professor
Nursing
Randolph-Macon College
Ashland, Virginia
Chapter 28: Child and Adolescent Health

Barbara Sattler, RN, MPH, DrPH, FAAN
Professor
School of Nursing and Health Professions
University of San Francisco
San Francisco, California
Chapter 6: Environmental Health

Erika Metzler Sawin, PhD
Associate Professor
Nursing
James Madison University
Harrisonburg, Virginia
Chapter 15: Communicable and Infectious Disease Risks

Marjorie A. Schaffer, PhD, PHN, RN
Professor Emerita
Nursing
Bethel University
St. Paul, Minnesota
Chapter 11: Population-Based Public Health Nursing Practice: The Intervention Wheel

Cynthia Selleck, PhD, RN, FAAN
Adjunct Professor
University of Alabama at Birmingham School of Nursing
Birmingham, Alabama
Chapter 20: The Nurse-Led Health Center: A Model for Community Nursing Practice

Sallie J. Shipman, EdD, MSN, RN, CNL, NHDP-BC
Clinical Assistant Professor
College of Nursing
The University of Florida
Gainesville, Florida
Chapter 39: Advanced Nursing Practice in the Community

Maria R. Shirey, PhD, MBA, RN, NEA-BC, ANEF, FACHE, FNAP, FAAN
Associate Dean, Clinical and Global Partnerships
Jane H. Brock-Florence Nightingale Endowed Professor in Nursing
University of Alabama at Birmingham School of Nursing
Birmingham, Alabama
Chapter 20: The Nurse-Led Health Center: A Model for Community Nursing Practice

Donna E. Smith, MSPH
Epidemiology Specialist
Epidemiology Program
Mecklenburg County Health Department
Charlotte, North Carolina
Chapter 14: Infectious Disease Prevention and Control

Sherrill J. Smith, RN, PhD, CNE, CNL
Professor
College of Nursing and Health
Wright State University
Dayton, Ohio
Chapter 21: Public Health Nursing Practice and the Disaster Management Cycle

Patricia M. Speck, DNSc, APN, APRN, FNP-BC, DF-IAFN, FAAFS, FAFN, FAAN
Professor
Family, Community, & Health Systems
University of Alabama at Birmingham School of Nursing
Birmingham, Alabama
Chapter 39: Advanced Nursing Practice in the Community

Sue Strohschein, MS, RN/PHN, APRN, BC
Culture of Excellence Project Coordinator
University of Minnesota
School of Nursing
Minneapolis, Minnesota
Chapter 11: Population-Based Public Health Nursing Practice: The Intervention Wheel

Melissa A. Sutherland, PhD, FNP-BC
Professor
Nursing
Binghamton University
Binghamton, New York
Chapter 44: Forensic Nursing in the Community

Laura Suzuki, PhD(c), MPH, BSN, RN
Doctoral student
Connell School of Nursing
Boston College
Boston, Massachusetts
Chapter 44: Forensic Nursing in the Community

Michele H. Talley, PhD, ACNP-BC, FAANP
Assistant Professor and Assistant Dean for Graduate Clinical Education
University of Alabama at Birmingham
Birmingham, Alabama
Chapter 20: The Nurse-Led Health Center: A Model for Community Nursing Practice

Esther J. Thatcher, PhD, RN, APHN-BC
Assistant Nurse Manager
Internal Medicine
University of Virginia Health System
Charlottesville, Virginia
Chapter 17: Community As Client: Assessment and Analysis

Anita Thompson-Heisterman, MSN, PMHCNS-BC, PMHNP-BC
Assistant Professor
School of Nursing
University of Virginia
Charlottesville, Virginia
Chapter 36: Mental Health Issues

Lisa M. Turner, PhD, RN, PHCNS-BC
Associate Professor of Nursing
Department of Nursing
Berea College
Berea, Kentucky
Chapter 10: Evidence-Based Practice
Chapter 40: The Nurse Leader in the Community

Connie M. Ulrich, PhD, RN, FAAN
Professor of Nursing and Bioethics
University of Pennsylvania
Philadelphia, Pennsylvania
Chapter 7: Application of Ethics in the Community

Lynn Wasserbauer, RN, FNP, PhD
Nurse Practitioner
Strong Ties Community Support Program
University of Rochester Medical Center
Rochester, New York
Chapter 30: Disability Health Care Across the Life Span

Jacqueline Webb, DNP, FNP-BC, RN
Associate Professor
School of Nursing
Linfield College
Portland, Oregon
Chapter 26: Working With Families in the Community for Healthy Outcomes

Connie White-Williams, PhD, RN, NE-BC, FAHA, FAAN
Senior Director, Nursing
University of Alabama at Birmingham Hospital
Birmingham, Alabama;
Assistant Professor
University of Alabama at Birmingham School of Nursing
Birmingham, Alabama
Chapter 20: The Nurse-Led Health Center: A Model for Community Nursing Practice

Carolyn A. Williams, RN, PhD, FAAN
Professor and Dean Emerita
College of Nursing
University of Kentucky
Lexington, Kentucky
Chapter 1: Public Health Foundations and Population Health

Lisa M. Zerull, PhD, RN-BC
Director and Academic Liaison
Nursing
Winchester Medical Center-Valley Health System
Winchester, Virginia;
Adjunct Clinical Faculty
School of Nursing
Shenandoah University
Winchester, Virginia
Chapter 45: The Nurse in the Faith Community

Elke Jones Zschaebitz, DNP, APRN, FNP-BC
Family Nurse Practitioner
School of Nursing and Health Science
Georgetown University
Washington, DC
Chapter 12: Genomics in Public Health Nursing

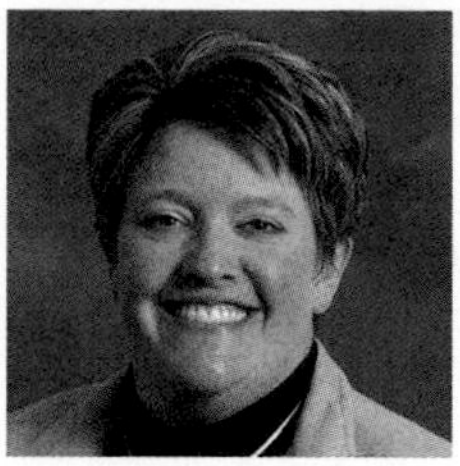

Swann Arp Adams, MS, PhD

Dr. Swann Arp Adams has over 17 years of experience in clinical epidemiology. She holds a PhD in epidemiology and an MS in biomedical sciences. Dr. Adams has previous experience in a variety of research fields, including physical activity, bone marrow transplantation, diabetes, breast cancer, and cancer disparities. She is the Associate Director of the Cancer Prevention and Control Program and is an associate professor with a joint appointment in the College of Nursing and the Department of Epidemiology and Biostatistics at the University of South Carolina. Her current research work focuses on reducing the burden of cancer disparities experienced by African Americans. Past honors include the Doctoral Achievement Award (2004) and the Gerry Sue Arnold Alumni Award (2008) from the Arnold School of Public Health of the University of South Carolina.

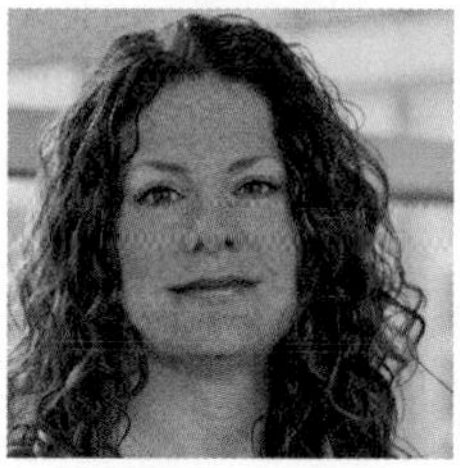

Mollie E. Aleshire, DNP, MSN, FNP-BC, PPCNP-BC, FNAP

Dr. Mollie E. Aleshire is a faculty member at the University of North Carolina Greensboro School of Nursing and is certified as a family nurse practitioner and pediatric primary care nurse practitioner. Dr. Aleshire has taught interprofessional health care systems, health promotion, and primary care prevention in both undergraduate and graduate courses. She received a master of science in nursing and a doctor of nursing practice from the University of Kentucky. Dr. Aleshire maintains an active clinical practice in a rural community health center, where she provides collaborative care for diverse patient populations across the life span. Both locally and nationally, Dr. Aleshire serves in leadership roles as well as maintaining active membership in the American Public Health Association (APHA) and its Social Justice and Diversity Committee. Dr. Aleshire's primary clinical and scholarship interests include promoting health and health care access for vulnerable and minority populations with a focus on LGBTQ* populations.

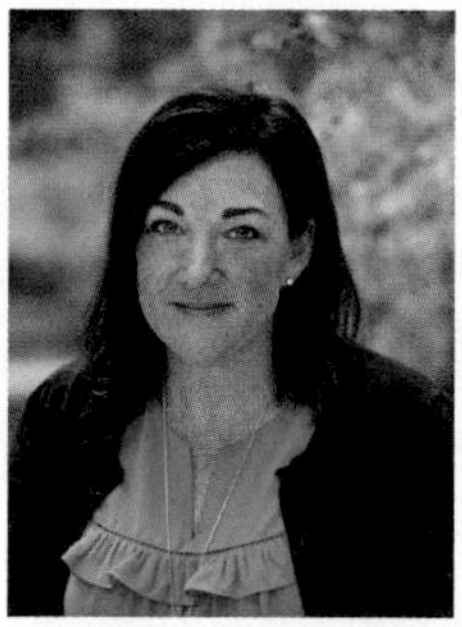

Jeanne L. Alhusen, PhD, CRNP, RN, FAAN

Jeanne L. Alhusen is an associate professor and Assistant Dean for Research at the University of Virginia School of Nursing. Her BSN, MSN, and PhD are from Villanova University, Duke University, and Johns Hopkins University. Dr. Alhusen works as a family nurse practitioner, and her research interests are in maternal mental health and early childhood outcomes, particularly among families living in poverty. She has received funding from the National Institutes of Health (NIH) to conduct research on the impact of domestic violence on early childhood outcomes.

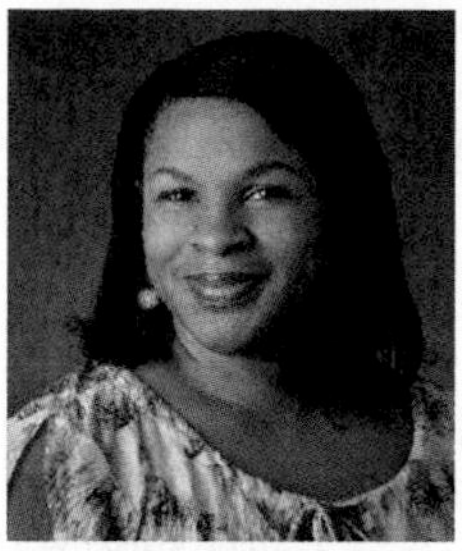

Kacy Allen-Bryant, PhD(c), MSN, MPH, RN

Kacy Allen-Bryant is a lecturer for the University of Kentucky College of Nursing. In that role, Allen-Bryant engages in community outreach to a host of organizations, including homeless shelters, day centers for those with mental illnesses, after-school programs for disadvantaged youth, and the public school system. For the past 18 years she has worked in a variety of community/public health settings such as home health, schools, and worksites. She has been a longtime member of the Lexington-Fayette County Health Department Board of Health and currently serves as its chair. During her time on the board she has been instrumental in such initiatives as the passing of a resolution to add electronic cigarettes to the Lexington-Fayette County smoking ordinance and implementation of the Needle Exchange Program. Ms. Allen-Bryant is also the Director of Occupational Health for KC WELLNESS, INC. and is currently in the University of Kentucky College of Nursing's PhD program. She received a bachelor of science degree in nursing, master of science degree in nursing, master of public health degree, and a graduate certificate in gerontology, all from the University of Kentucky. Her research interest is workplace smoking- and tobacco-related policies.

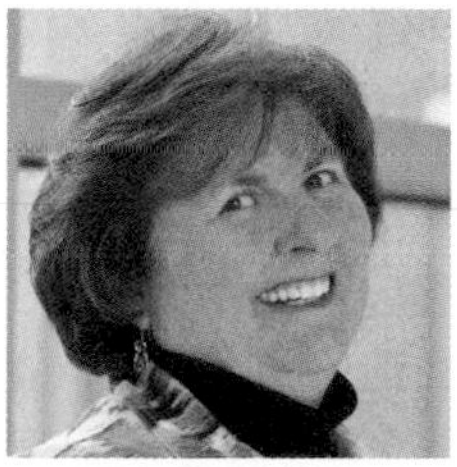

Debra Gay Anderson, PhD, PHCNS-BC

Dr. Debra Gay Anderson is the Associate Dean of Research at South Dakota State University's College of Nursing. She is certified as a clinical specialist in public/community health nursing and has provided health care for the homeless and other vulnerable populations. Dr. Anderson has taught public health, epidemiology, leadership, and research courses at both the graduate and undergraduate levels. The focus of her program of research, publications, and presentations is social justice, particularly with vulnerable populations, including women who have experienced homelessness, domestic violence, or workplace violence. Dr. Anderson completed her doctoral studies and a family nursing postdoctoral fellowship at Oregon Health Sciences University in Portland, Oregon. Dr. Anderson is an active member of the American Public Health Association (APHA) and has served in various leadership capacities, including Chair of the Public Health Nursing Section of APHA.

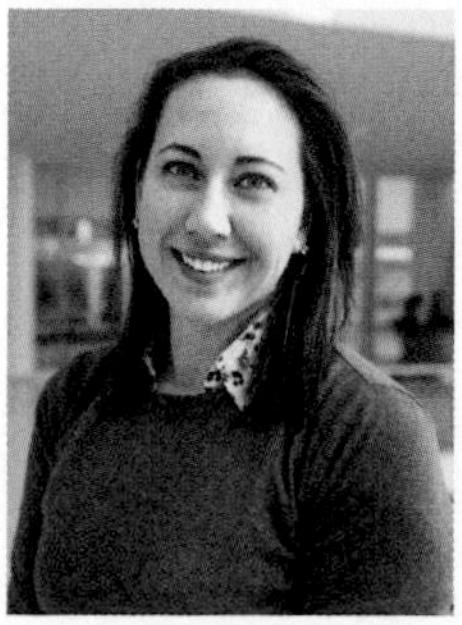

Sydney A. Axson, MPH, RN

Ms. Axson is a doctoral student and Hillman Scholar in Nursing Innovation at the University of Pennsylvania School of Nursing.

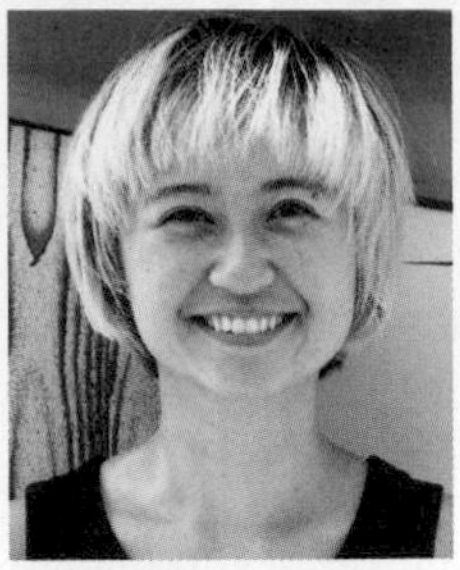

Amber M. Bang, RN, BSN

Amber Bang graduated from Reed College with a BA in biology, specializing in neuroscience. She then received her BSN at Duke University School of Nursing in 2015. She works as a community health nurse, serving largely unhoused and low-income populations. She has experience in primary care engaging with addictions treatment and currently works in a drug and alcohol detoxification center, as well as a youth correctional facility.

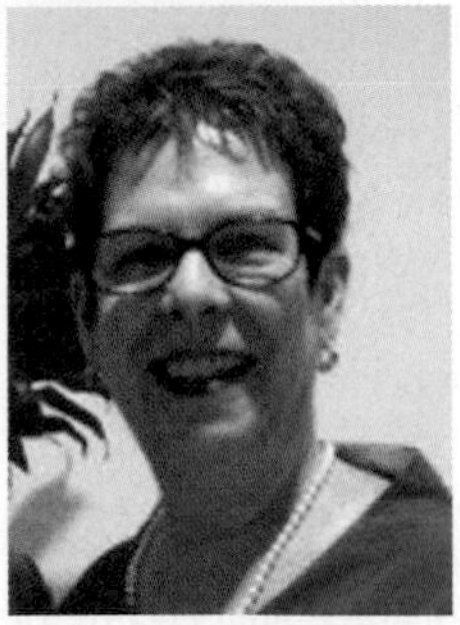

Whitney Rogers Bischoff, DrPH, MSN, BSN

Dr. Whitney Bischoff is retired from the Canseco School of Nursing at Texas A&M International University in Laredo, Texas. She has worked in hospitals, clinics, as a parish nurse, and for 20 years as a nurse educator teaching undergraduate and graduate courses in community health, research, transcultural nursing, public health, health policy, and nursing administration. She has a particular interest in financing of health care. Her presentations and publications have been in the areas of technology in education and practice.

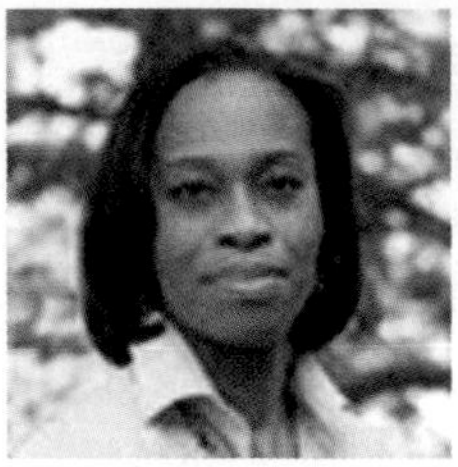

Nisha D. Botchwey, PhD, MCRP, MPH

Nisha Botchwey earned her AB from Harvard University, MCRP and PhD in City and Regional Planning from the University of Pennsylvania, and her MPH from the University of Virginia. She was on the faculty at the University of Virginia in Urban and Environmental Planning and Public Health. She is currently an Associate Professor of City and Regional Planning in the College of Design at the Georgia Institute of Technology and Professor of Public Health at Emory University's School of Public Health. Dr. Botchwey specializes in community engagement, public health, and health equity. She conducts research on healthy communities, youth engagement for health, and data dashboards for evidence-based decision. Dr. Botchwey is Director of the Healthy Places Lab that oversees the work of the Physical Activity Research Center, the Built Environment and Public Health Clearinghouse (www.bephc.gatech.edu), the Atlanta Dashboard, and the Health, Environment and Livability Platform for Fulton County. Botchwey is an NSF ADVANCE Woman of Excellence Faculty award recipient, Georgia Tech Outstanding Faculty, member of the National Academies of Science, Engineering and Medicine Committee on Summertime Experiences and Child and Adolescent Education, Health and Safety, and served on the Advisory Committee to the Director of the Centers for Disease Control and Prevention.

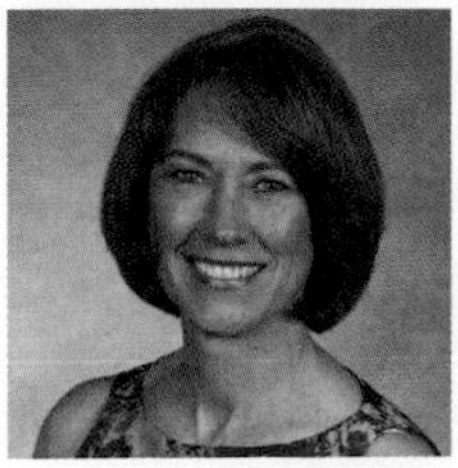

Kathryn H. Bowles, RN, PhD, FAAN

Kathryn H. Bowles is the van Ameringen Professor of Nursing Excellence at the University of Pennsylvania School of Nursing and the Vice President and Director of the Center for Home Care Policy and Research at the Visiting Nurse Service of New York. Her program of research focuses on improving the care of adults using information technology such as decision support for hospital discharge planning and referral decision making, examining the effects of early and intensive home care, as well as testing telehealth technologies in community-based settings.

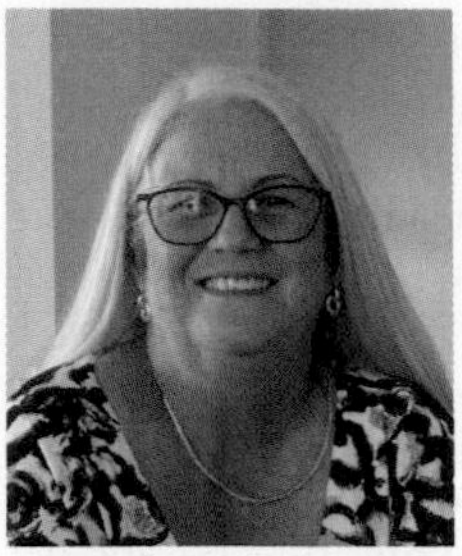

Hazel Brown, DNP, RN

Dr. Hazel Brown is Chief Nursing Officer for the Health Services Authority, Cayman Islands. She received her BSN from West Indies College in Mandeville, Jamaica, and MSN from the University of Miami, in Miami, Florida. In 2016, she completed her DNP from American Sentinel University. Her clinical background is in primary health care and her leadership expertise has been honed in over 30 years of escalating responsibility in the national health system. She is a passionate advocate of the theory of complex adaptive systems as an explanation of the context of modern health care systems and a guide for leadership development strategies. She is a Rotarian for whom the motto "Service Above Self" is a guide to daily practice and advocacy locally and regionally.

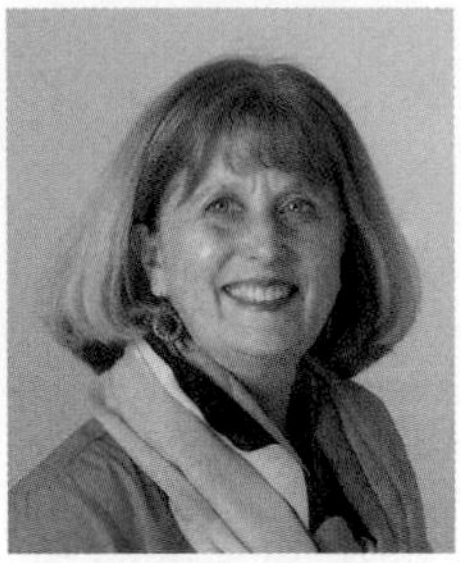

Bonnie L. Brueshoff, DNP, MSN, RN, PHN

Bonnie Brueshoff is the Director for the Dakota County Public Health Department located in West St. Paul, Minnesota. She has been in this position for the past 10 years. In her current role, Brueshoff manages and provides leadership for the public health department, including 100 staff and a budget of $10 million. Her expertise in public health has been sought out at the national, state, and regional levels, having held leadership roles with the National Association of County and City Health Officials (NACCHO) and the Minnesota Local Public Health Association.

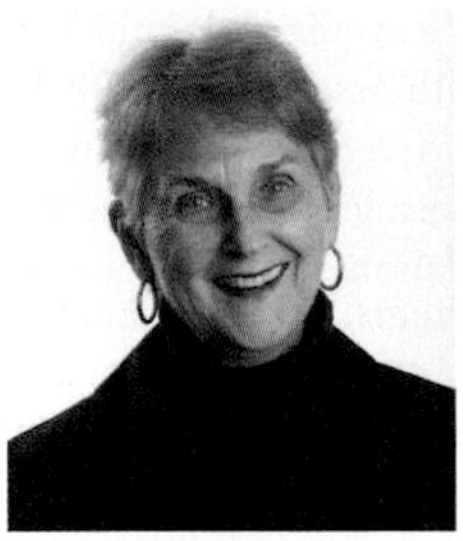

Angeline Bushy, PhD, RN, FAAN

Dr. Angeline Bushy, Professor and Bert Fish Endowed Chair at the University of Central Florida College of Nursing, holds a BSN degree from the University of Mary in Bismarck, North Dakota; an MN degree in rural community health nursing from Montana State University in Bozeman; an MEd in adult education from Northern Montana College in Havre; and a PhD in nursing from the University of Texas at Austin; and is a Fellow in the American Academy of Nursing. Dr. Bushy has worked in rural health care facilities located in the north-central and intermountain states; presented nationally and internationally on various rural nursing and rural health issues; published six textbooks and numerous articles on that topic; and is a U.S. Army Reserve Lieutenant Colonel (Ret.).

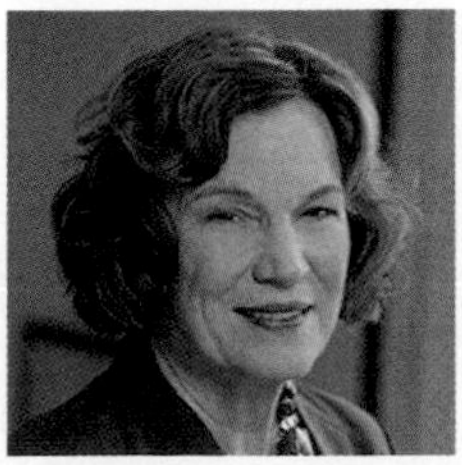

Jacquelyn C. Campbell, PhD, RN, FAAN

Jacquelyn C. Campbell is the Anna D. Wolf Chair and Professor at the Johns Hopkins University School of Nursing with a joint appointment in the Bloomberg School of Public Health. Her BSN, MSN, and PhD are, respectively, from Duke University, Wright State University, and the University of Rochester schools of nursing. Dr. Campbell has been the principal investigator on 10 major National Institutes of Health, National Institute of Justice, and Centers for Disease Control and Prevention research grants and has published more than 220 articles and seven books on this subject. She is an elected member of the National Academy of Medicine and the American Academy of Nursing, is on the Board of Directors of Futures Without Violence, and was a member of the congressionally appointed U.S. Department of Defense Task Force on Domestic Violence.

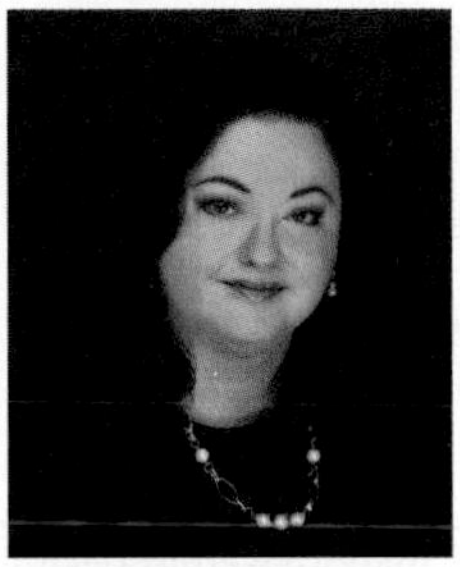

Catherine Carroca, MSN, RN

Catherine Carroca is a community health nurse and nurse educator. She received her bachelor's degree in nursing from the University of Massachusetts, Amherst, and her master's degree in nursing education from Norwich University in Vermont. She is currently an assistant professor at Massachusetts College of Pharmacy and Health Sciences in Worcester, Massachusetts, where she teaches community and home health nursing in an accelerated post-baccalaureate program. She has presented her work on simulation in community health at the St. Anselm's and the Massachusetts/Rhode Island League for Nursing (MARILN) conferences. She is currently pursuing her doctorate in global public health.

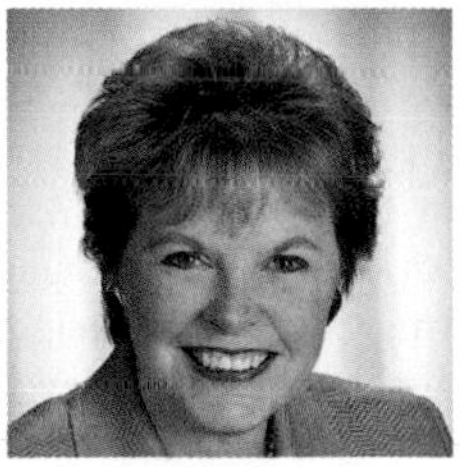

Ann H. Cary, PhD, MPH, RN, FNAP, FAAN

Dr. Ann H. Cary began practicing public health nursing as a home health nurse in New Orleans, Louisiana, where she executed case management functions daily. She has served on national workgroups to establish the standards of practice for public health nurses and case managers and organizations that created certification examinations for case managers, authored numerous articles on case management issues, taught baccalaureate and graduate-level courses in case management, and directed graduate programs in case management and continuity of care and care coordination. She is the Dean of the School of Nursing and Health Studies at the University of Missouri, Kansas City, Missouri. In Kansas City, she also serves on a variety of nonprofit and interprofessional foundation, health care systems, and community boards whose missions are to increase access, coordinated care, and quality delivery for clients and to prepare health care leaders of the future to assure population health.

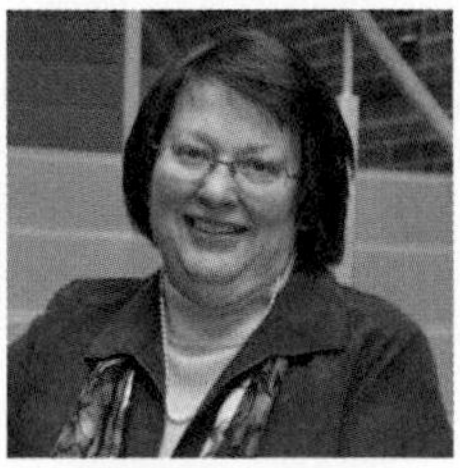

Laura H. Clayton, PhD, RN, CNE

Dr. Clayton earned her PhD from West Virginia University (WVU) in 2007, certificate in health care administration from WVU in 1998, master of science in nursing and family nurse practitioner from WVU in 1993, and bachelor of science in nursing from Alderson-Broaddus College in 1983. Dr. Clayton co-founded the Emmanuel's Table Free Clinic in Martinsburg in 2006, serves on the Eastern Panhandle Medical Reserve Corps Steering Committee, is the peer reviewer for Nursing Education Perspectives by the National League for Nursing, and is the president of the board of directors for the Shenandoah Valley Medical System. In 2010 she received the West Virginia University School of Nursing Golden Graduate Award and received the Nursing Excellence Award in Nursing Education from the West Virginia Center for Nursing in 2007. Dr. Clayton received her certification as a certified nurse educator by the National League for Nursing in 2010.

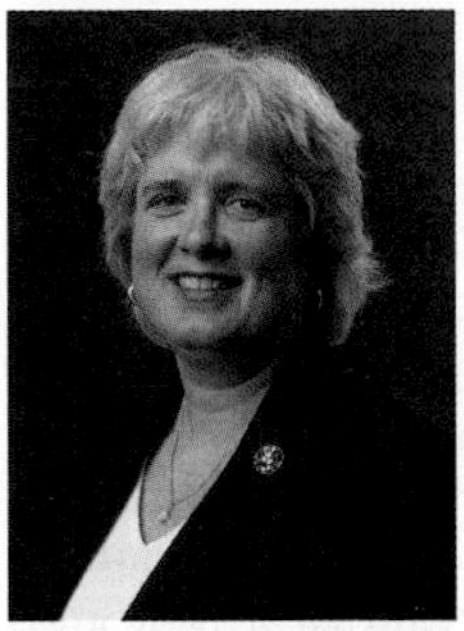

Erin G. Cruise, PhD, RN

Dr. Erin Cruise completed her BSN at Berea College in Berea, Kentucky, where she was first introduced to the concepts of community and public health nursing. Service to the community is a major focus at Berea: nursing students provide health education and screening programs to vulnerable populations, such as seniors, low-income families, and schoolchildren as part of their clinical education. Here, Dr. Cruise learned that poverty and lack of education can lead to poor health and prevent vulnerable populations from achieving their full potential. Dr. Cruise has worked in a variety of inpatient and outpatient settings, but her true passions are public health and school health. Forming relationships with community members helped her understand important influences on her clients' health, illness, or ability to access health care. She was a school nurse supervisor for many years and developed programs and policies in two counties in the Appalachian region of southwestern Virginia. Dr. Cruise completed her MSN in community/public health leadership at the University of Virginia and her PhD in health education/curriculum and instruction from Virginia Tech. Her dissertation research was in the field of school nurse education. Dr. Cruise is an associate professor at Radford University School of Nursing and leads the undergraduate community health nursing course. She also teaches health promotion to DNP students and writes and presents nationally on the subjects of health literacy and school health. Her students work with school nurses in their clinics and provide health education and screening for schoolchildren throughout the region.

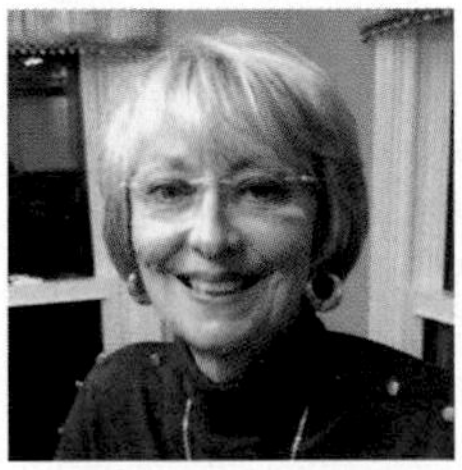

Lois A. Davis, RN, MSN, MA

Lois A. Davis began her public health career in 1977 in Eastern Kentucky with the Breathitt County Health Department, where she worked with the Appalachian population in a variety of public health preventive programs. She expanded her role in public health as a school nurse and initiated a program to reduce teen pregnancy in the Breathitt County Schools. She worked in community mental health and understands the importance of community partnerships. Lois spent three years in South America and afterwards fulfilled a desire to assist migrant health populations and the underserved. After 20 years in community/public health nursing, Lois retired in July 2016 from the Lexington–Fayette County Health Department in Lexington, Kentucky, where she served as the Maternal–Child Health Coordinator and directed several community services programs, including Health Access Nurturing Development Services (HANDS), school health, and health equity and education. She has functioned as incident commander for preparedness exercises and as the operations lead for real events, such as special needs shelters during ice storms. At the state level, Lois served on the Nurse Executive Council, where she helped define public health protocols and public health nursing competencies for local health department nurses. Lois served on the board of the Bluegrass Community Health Center, a Health Resources and Services Administration (HRSA) Federally Qualified Health Center, for 10 years. She is currently on the board of the Kentucky CancerLink, a local nonprofit that provides case management services for cancer victims. Additionally, she has served as an adjunct faculty member and on advisory boards for the University of Kentucky College of Nursing, Eastern Kentucky University, and Midway College. She has precepted numerous nursing students and is passionate about preventive health. Lois currently works as a public health clinical instructor for the University of Kentucky College of Nursing.

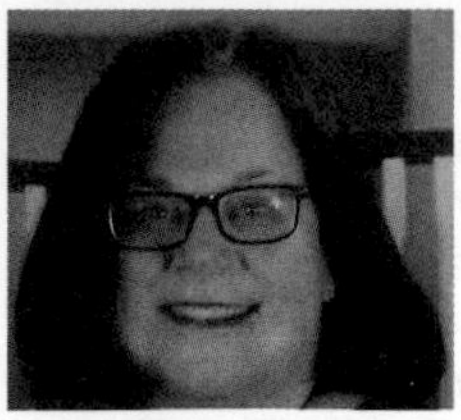

Sharon K. Davis, DNP, APRN, WHNP-BC
Sharon K. Davis earned her diploma in nursing from St. Mary's School of Nursing in Knoxville, Tennessee, BSN and MSN from the University of Tennessee, Knoxville, and DNP from the University of Tennessee, Chattanooga. She began her nursing practice in obstetrics and gynecology at a regional hospital and then transitioned to a private practice where she cared for women for over 20 years. In 2010, she entered academia, where she teaches core courses in the doctor of nursing practice program.

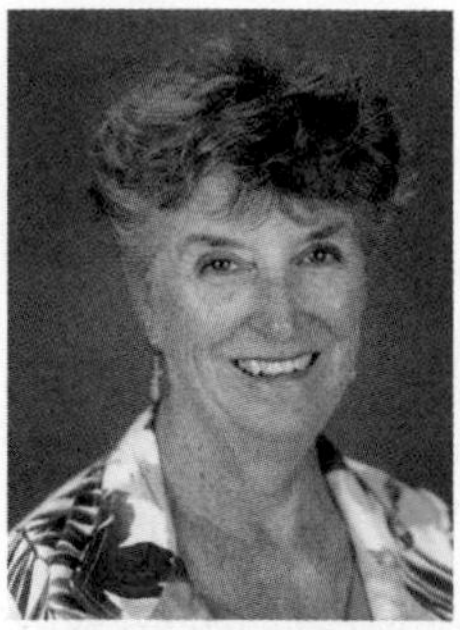

Karen R. Dawn, DNP, MSN, BSN
Karen Dawn is a registered nurse with over 30 years' experience in diabetes management, disease prevention, health promotion, and patient education. She completed a DNP from the University of Virginia School of Nursing in March 2014. She is a full-time faculty member at George Washington University school of nursing in the accelerated second-degree program focusing on public health and chronic disease prevention, specifically diabetes.

Cynthia E. Degazon, RN, PhD

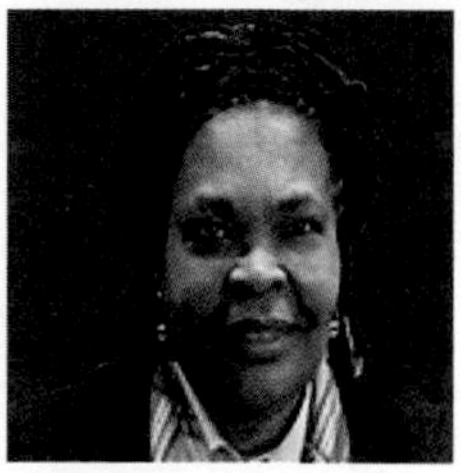

Dr. Cynthia E. Degazon is Professor Emerita at Hunter College, City University of New York. She received a BS in nursing from Long Island University and an MA in community health nursing and a PhD in nursing research and theory development from New York University. For 20 years she has prepared undergraduate and graduate nurses to provide culturally competent care to ethnically diverse populations. Dr. Degazon has given many national and international presentations and authored several scholarly publications.

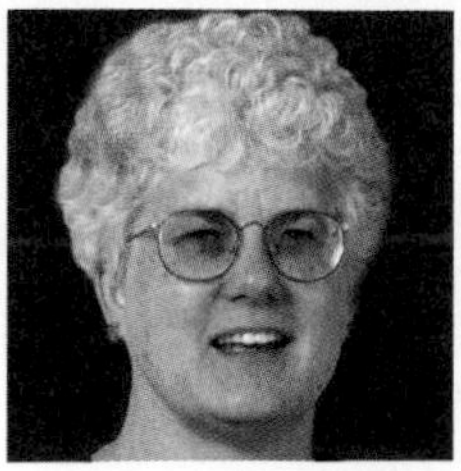

Janna Dieckmann, PhD, RN
Dr. Janna Dieckmann is an associate professor at the University of North Carolina at Chapel Hill. She received her BSN from Case Western Reserve University and her MSN in community health nursing and her PhD from the University of Pennsylvania. She has practiced as a public health nurse with both the Visiting Nurse Association of Cleveland, Ohio, and the Visiting Nurse Association of Philadelphia. She uses written and oral historical materials to research the history of public health nursing and care of the chronically ill and to comment on contemporary health policy.

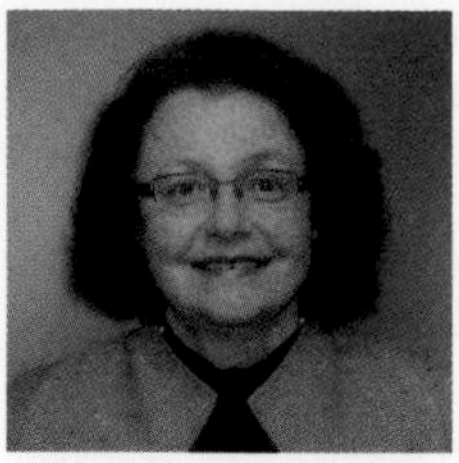

Sherry L. Farra, PhD, RN, CNE, CHSE, NDHP-BC
Dr. Sherry Farra has practiced nursing for over 30 years and is experienced in emergency and disaster preparedness, response, and recovery. She is an associate professor at Wright State University in Dayton, Ohio, where she is the Director for the National Disaster Health Consortium. Dr. Farra is the Research Consultant to the Chief Nurse of the American Red Cross. As a nurse educator, she has designed, developed, and launched disaster courses for health care providers for nurses and other allied health professionals. She is a certified disaster health care provider and has a research concentration in disaster training, including the use of virtual reality training.

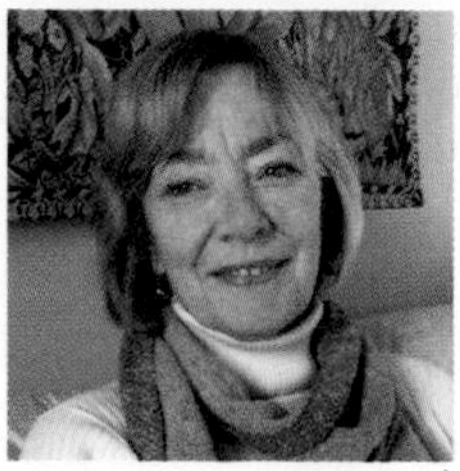

Mary E. Gibson, PhD, RN
Dr. Mary E. Gibson was a public health nurse in Albemarle County, Virginia, early in her career. Since that time, she has practiced in a variety of maternal–child health settings. Mary was involved in the Virginia Department of Health's early initiative to regionalize high-risk pregnancies and has worked as an outpatient nurse, childbirth educator, and perinatal outreach nurse, including systems work with regional hospitals and nurses, and outreach education; and as a labor and delivery and perinatal nurse. She concentrated on community health in her master's program, and her doctoral work at University of Pennsylvania focused on nursing history, and this continues to be her research focus. She currently serves as President of the American Association for the History of Nursing. At the University of Virginia, Mary serves as the Associate Director of the Bjoring Center for Nursing Historical Inquiry and her teaching experience includes graduate-level community assessment, undergraduate obstetrics and neonatal nursing, and clinical undergraduate community health nursing. She is currently a member and past chair of a local nonprofit organization's board that serves at-risk, underserved children and families.

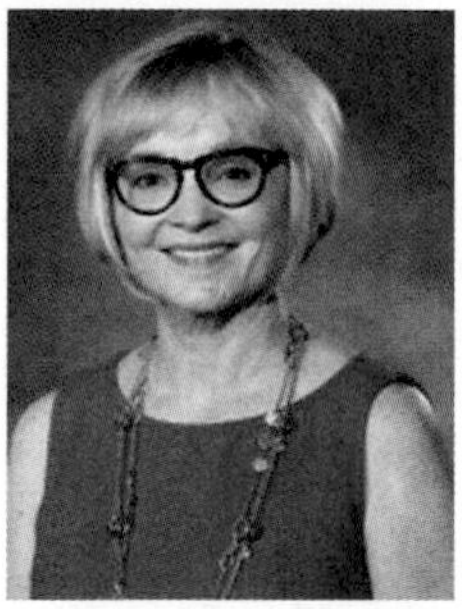

Mary Kay Goldschmidt, DNP, MSN, RN, PHNA-BC
Mary Kay Goldschmidt holds a BSN, an MSN in public health nursing leadership, and a DNP from the University of Virginia in Charlottesville and holds a certificate in advanced public health nursing. She is an assistant professor of nursing at Virginia Commonwealth University School of Nursing. Her research and clinical practice focuses on working with medically underserved populations and health policy. Dr. Goldschmidt completed a fellowship in translational research and public policy at the L. Douglas Wilder School of Government and Public Affairs at Virginia Commonwealth University and currently serves as the Commissioner on Government Relations for the Virginia Nurses Association. Dr. Goldschmidt continues to develop and advocate for health policy which supports the health and well-being of all Virginians. She is the co-director of two HRSA Nursing Education, Practice, Quality and Retention grants, which seek to increase access to health care for medically underserved populations by strengthening the nursing workforce in community-based primary care settings. Dr. Goldschmidt

serves as a volunteer with Remote Area Medical Clinics and Homeward Virginia and continues her work with vulnerable populations such as those living in multidimensional poverty, the homeless, children, and victims of natural disaster.

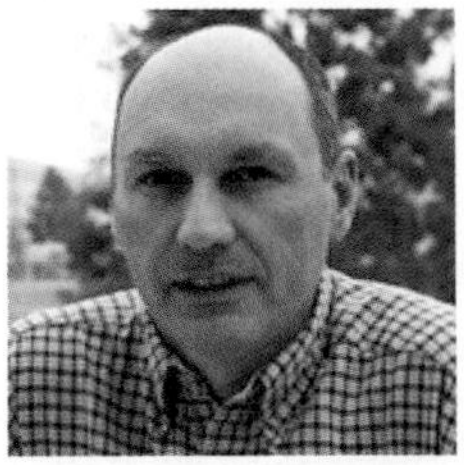

Monty Gross, PhD, MSN, RN, CNE, CNL

Dr. Monty Gross is Senior Nurse Leader for Professional Development for the Cayman Islands Health Service Authority in Grand Cayman. He received his BS in communications from Clarion University of Pennsylvania and his BSN and MSN from the University of Virginia. His PhD was awarded from Virginia Tech. He has practiced nursing in acute care, critical care, and underserved communities in Latin America. He serves as a Commission on Collegiate Nursing Education (CCNE) nursing program on-site evaluator. He has taught nursing as an associate professor at the undergraduate and graduate levels.

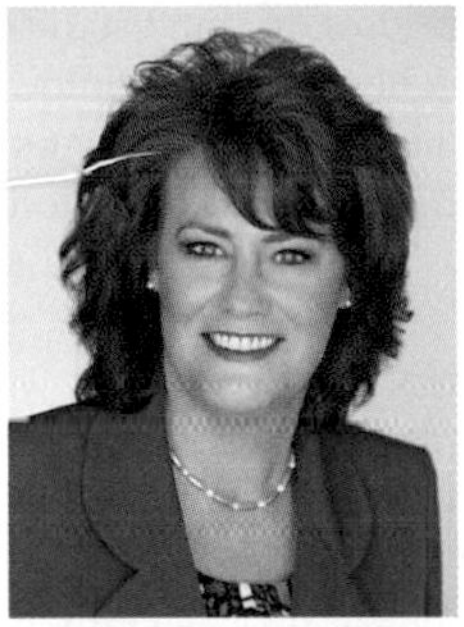

Melanie Gibbons Hallman, DNP, CRNP, CEN, FNP-BC, ACNP-BC, FAEN

Dr. Hallman is an instructor at the University of Alabama at Birmingham School of Nursing in Birmingham, Alabama. Dr. Hallman has provided prehospital and hospital emergency services for more than 39 years. She continues to provide patient care as an emergency nurse practitioner and volunteers with various organizations as a family nurse practitioner, providing access to medically underserved populations locally and internationally. Dr. Hallman has been an active member of the Emergency Nurses Association since 1988, serving in multiple leadership positions at local, state, and national levels.

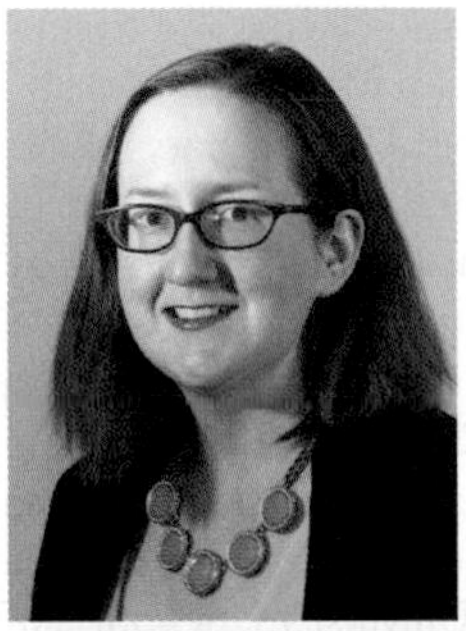

Joanna Horn, BA, MS

Joanna Horn is a senior genetic counselor in the Center for Human Genetics at University Hospital Cleveland Medical Center. She currently works with both pediatric and oncology populations but has also worked in prenatal genetics. She has over a decade of experience working in academic medical centers. She is dedicated to making the field of genetics accessible to her patients and families and working collaboratively with her health care teams.

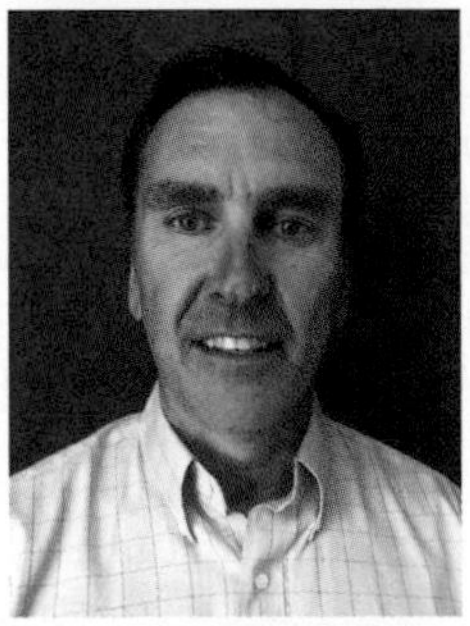

Gerard M. Jellig, EdD

Gerard M. Jellig is Head of Secondary Schools and Turnaround Principal for KIPP DC. He is a Turnaround for Children trained team member and has instituted trauma-informed teaching practices on his urban campus, reducing office referrals 80% and suspensions 99%, while dramatically increasing test scores. He has been a teacher, principal, and superintendent over 25 years in public education. Dr. Jellig has a BA in history and secondary education from Providence College, MA from Johns Hopkins University in leadership and literacy practice, and an EdD from University of Pennsylvania, where his research focused on the impact of emotional intelligence on leadership practice in diverse, challenged public schools. He's on the faculty at the University of Pennsylvania and has also taught at Johns Hopkins and Rowan University.

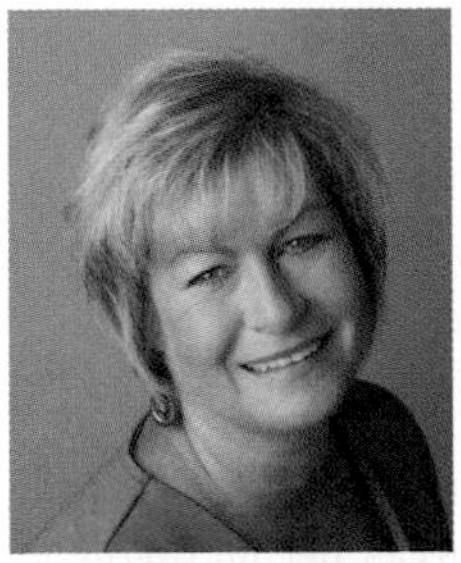

Tammy Kiser DNP, RN

Dr. Tammy Kiser is an assistant professor of nursing at James Madison University, where she teaches community health and faith community nursing courses. Her areas of research interest are vulnerable populations. Dr. Kiser has worked with several community initiatives, including working extensively with the Healthcare for the Homeless Suitcase Clinic in Harrisonburg, Virginia, both on the leadership team and in clinics, since 2009. She received her bachelor's degree in nursing from Eastern Mennonite College, master's degree in nursing from James Madison University, and an MSN certificate and DNP from the University of South Alabama in public health nursing administration.

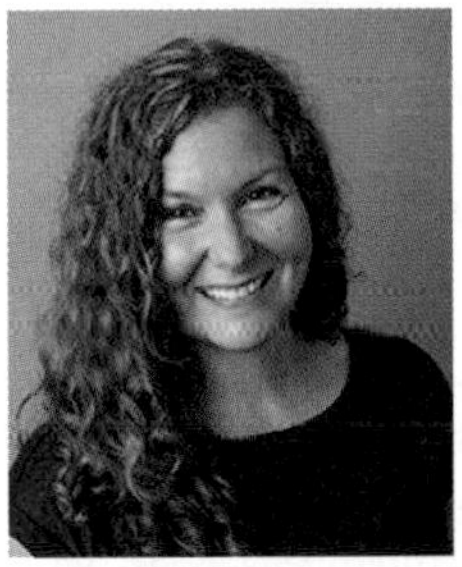

Andrea Knopp, PhD, MSN, MPH, FNP-BC

Dr. Andrea Knopp is an associate professor of nursing at James Madison University and coordinator of the nurse practitioner program. She received her BSN in nursing from the Medical College of Georgia and her master of science in nursing and master of public health from Emory University. Her PhD was awarded from the University of Virginia. Dr. Knopp stays active as a family nurse practitioner and conducts international research and domestic research focused on disadvantaged and vulnerable populations. In 2013, she received the VCNP Education Award from the Virginia Council of Nurse Practitioners and the March of Dimes Nurse of the Year Educator Award in 2017.

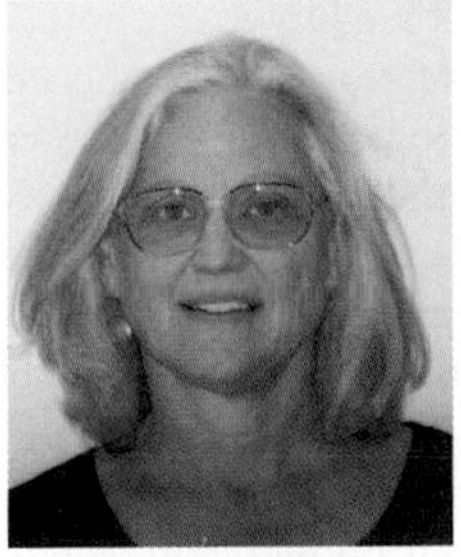

Candace Kugel, BA, MS, FNP, CNM

Ms. Candace Kugel has over 30 years' experience in health care for the underserved. She is a family nurse practitioner and certified nurse-midwife with extensive expertise in training and technical assistance to under resourced communities and working to provide health services to farmworkers, immigrant workers and families, and other underserved populations. She has worked in various clinical settings, including family planning, migrant health, community health centers, and private practice. She currently works as a clinical specialist for the Migrant Clinicians Network and as a clinical consultant for the HRSA Bureau of Primary Health Care.

Ms. Kugel has extensive experience in the United States and internationally with training of community health workers and health education using popular education methodology. She has written and provided continuing education on cultural competency, women's health access, and services in under-resourced settings.

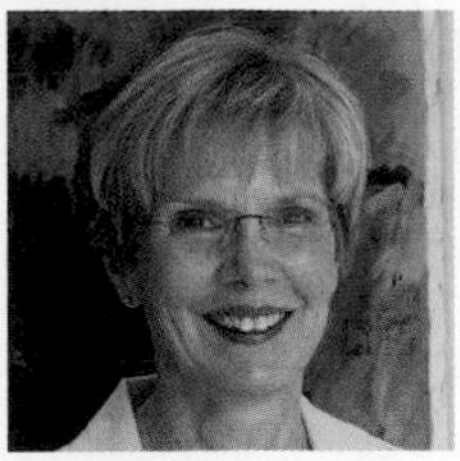

Pamela A. Kulbok, DNSc, RN, PHCNS-BC, FAAN

Pamela A. Kulbok earned her BS and MS at Boston College, her doctorate at Boston University, and did postdoctoral work in psychiatric epidemiology at Washington University in St. Louis. She was on the faculty at St. Louis University, University of Illinois at Chicago, and the Catholic University of America. She is Professor Emerita, University of Virginia School of Nursing. She has taught undergraduate and graduate courses in public health nursing, health promotion research, and nursing knowledge development. Dr. Kulbok is a Robert Wood Johnson Foundation Executive Nurse Fellow (2012 cohort). She was the principal investigator of an interprofessional, cross-institution, community-based participatory research project to design a youth substance use prevention program and of a series of studies of youth nonsmoking behavior. She was chair of the Environmental and Public Health Expert Panel, American Academy of Nursing; co-chair of the American Nurses Association workgroup that revised the Public Health Nursing: Scope and Standards of Practice (2013); a member of the American Public Health Association (APHA) PHN Section taskforce that updated the Definition of Public Health Nursing (2013); president of the Association of Community Health Nursing Educators, and chair of the Quad Council of Public Health Nursing Organizations. In 2016, she was awarded the APHA, Public Health Nursing Section's Ruth B. Freeman Distinguished Career Award.

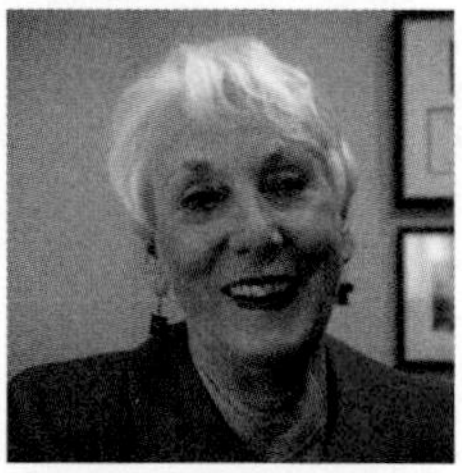

Jeanette Lancaster, PhD, RN, FAAN

Dr. Lancaster is Professor and Dean Emerita of Nursing at the University of Virginia. She has edited this book with Dr. Marcia Stanhope through its previous nine editions.

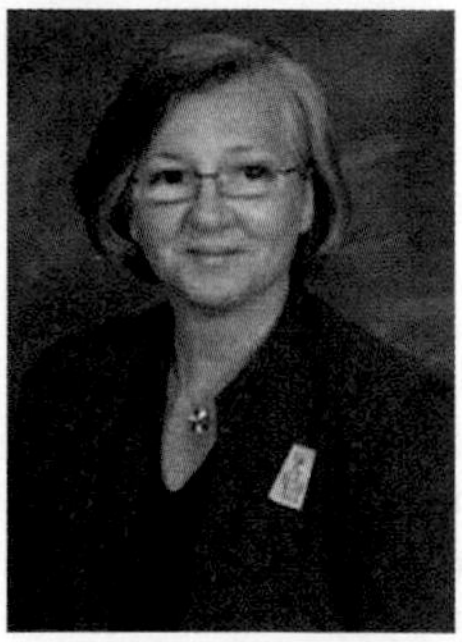

Roberta Proffitt Lavin, PhD, FNP-BC, FAAN

Roberta Lavin, Professor and Associate Dean of Academic Programs, spent 20 years as a U.S. Public Health Service (USPHS) officer. She began her career at St. Elizabeths Hospital in Washington, DC, on an acute psychiatric admission unit for those who were homeless. In her work she has coordinated mass migrations in Guatemala, managed health care in an immigration detention center in Batavia, New York, before becoming the Chief of Field Operations of the Division of Immigration Health Services, worked for the Federal Bureau of Prisons in Tucson, Arizona, and spent a few months "tooling around" the South Pacific on a National Oceanic and Atmospheric Administration research vessel. After 9/11 and the anthrax attacks she was selected to be the Director of the Secretary's Command Center for the Department of Health and Human Services and later became the Chief of Staff for the Assistant Secretary for Preparedness and Response. She ended her USPHS career again working with the poor and underserved leading the research and development for a national disaster case management program. Her current research focuses on bringing cultural competency around urban and rural communities to practicing nurses and disaster preparedness. Current projects include infusion and assessment of cultural competency in training DNP students and research of training gaps for health care primary care providers for disaster response. She is developing an interprofessional curriculum around disaster preparedness.

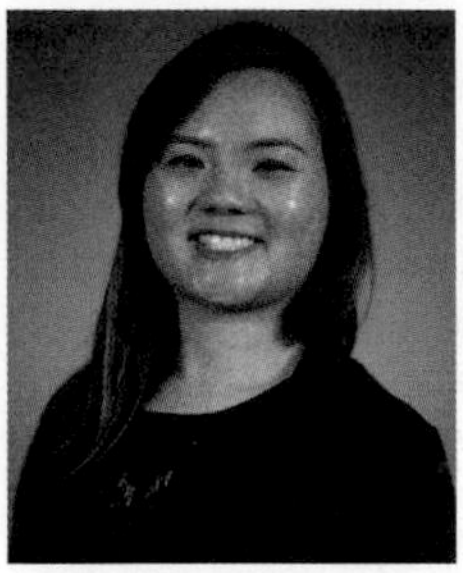

Natasha Le, BA, BS

Natasha Le is a second-degree nurse who received her first degree in public health policy at the University of California, Irvine, and her BSN at the University of Pennsylvania School of Nursing, where she is also a graduate student working towards her MSN. Presently, she works at Penn Medicine's Home Care and Hospice entity as a Quality and Informatics Coordinator and as a temporary research employee at Drexel University College of Nursing and Health Professions. Her research focuses on understanding information requirements, decision-making needs, and workflow of home care nurse in the admission and care planning processes. Of specific interest to her is examining if and how health information technology helps or hinders these needs.

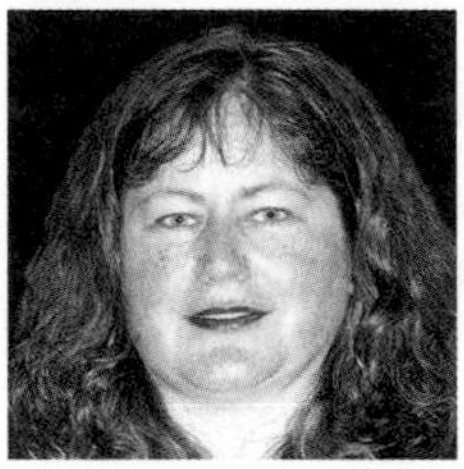

Susan C. Long-Marin, DVM, MPH

Susan Long-Marin developed an interest in infectious diseases and public health while serving as a Peace Corps Volunteer in the Philippines. Training in veterinary medicine further increased her respect for emerging infectious diseases, the ingeniousness of the microbes that cause them, and the importance of primary prevention. Today she manages the Epidemiology Program of the Mecklenburg County Health Department in Charlotte, North Carolina, which serves a rapidly growing and changing population. Dr. Long-Marin earned her doctor of veterinary medicine degree from the Virginia-Maryland College of Veterinary Medicine at Virginia Tech and her master of public health degree in epidemiology from the Norman J. Arnold School of Public Health at the University of South Carolina.

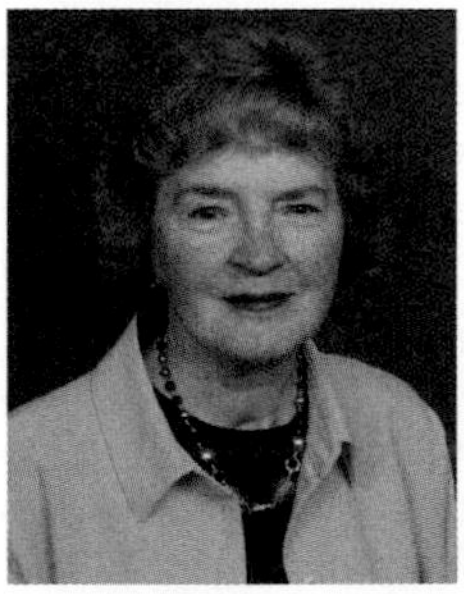

Karen S. Martin, RN, MSN, FAAN

Karen S. Martin is a health care consultant who has been in private practice since 1993. She works with clinicians, managers, administrators, educators, researchers, and software developers nationally and internationally. Her focus is evaluation and improvement of practice, documentation, and information management systems to meet quality, data exchange, and interoperability standards for electronic health records. Karen has been employed as a staff nurse, director of a combined home care/public health agency, and, from 1978 to 1993, the Director of Research of the Visiting Nurse Association of Omaha, Nebraska, where she was the principal investigator of Omaha System research.

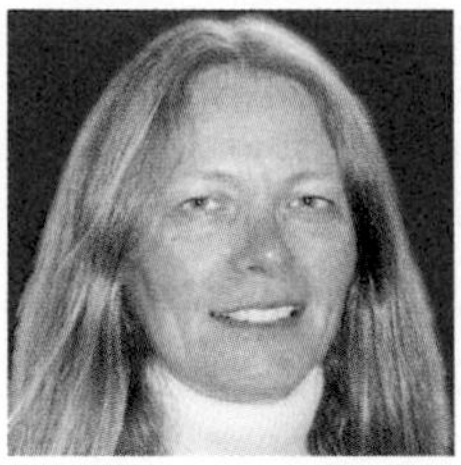

Mary Lynn Mathre, RN, MSN, CARN

Mary Lynn Mathre earned the BSN from the College of St. Teresa in Winona, Minnesota, and the MSN from the Frances Payne Bolton School of Nursing at Case Western Reserve University. She has 39 years of experience as an acute care nurse and has worked in the field of alcohol, tobacco, and other drugs for the past 25 years. From 1991 to 2003, she worked as the addictions consult nurse for the University of Virginia Health System and interacted with many community resources to provide appropriate referrals and aftercare for clients. From 2004 to 2007, she worked in an outpatient opioid treatment program as the executive director. Currently she works as an independent consultant on substance abuse prevention and brief interventions. She is an active member of the International Nurses Society on Addictions and serves on the editorial board for the *Journal of Addictions Nursing*.

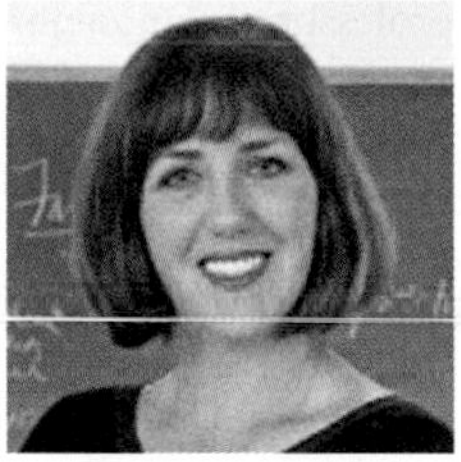

Natalie McClain, PhD, RN, CPNP

Dr. McClain earned her bachelor's and master's degrees from the University of Texas Health Sciences Center–Houston and her PhD from the University of Virginia. She has worked at the Children's Assessment Center, an advocacy center providing services for child victims of sexual abuse in Houston, Texas. At the assessment center and later in Charlottesville, Virginia, Dr. McClain performed medical forensic exams in cases of sexual assault, testified in both civil and criminal trials, and served as an expert witness for the FBI. Dr. McClain served on the 2012-2013 Committee on Commercial Sexual Exploitation and Sex Trafficking of Minors in the United States. Dr. McClain is currently a visiting scholar at Boston College William F. Connell School of Nursing in Boston, Massachusetts.

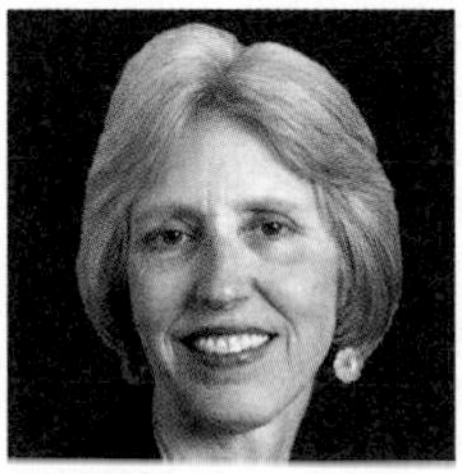

DeAnne K. Hilfinger Messias, PhD, RN, FAAN

Dr. DeAnne K. Hilfinger Messias is an international community health nurse, educator, and researcher. She spent more than two decades in Brazil, where she directed a primary health care project on the lower Amazon, taught women's health and community health nursing, and organized women's health initiatives among poor urban populations. Her research and scholarship focus on women's work and health, immigrant women's health, language access, and community empowerment. Her current research involves a community-based intervention trial of a *promotora*-delivered physical activity intervention among low-income Latinas. Dr. Messias was a fellow with the International Center for Health Leadership Development at the School of Public Health, University of Illinois at Chicago (2002–2004) and a Fulbright Senior Scholar in Global/Public Health at the Federal University of Goiás, Brazil (2005). She is the Emily Myrtle Smith Endowed Chair and Carolina Trustee Professor of the University of South Carolina College of Nursing, with a joint appointment in the Women's and Gender Studies Program.

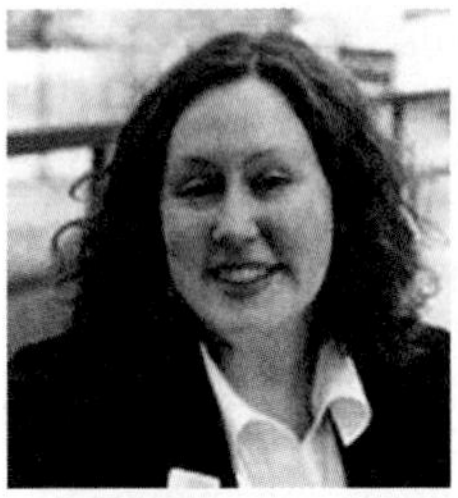

Emma McKim Mitchell, PhD, MSN, RN

Dr. Emma Mitchell is an assistant professor at the University of Virginia School of Nursing and co-directs global initiatives surrounding research, study abroad, and community-based capacity building in rural and remote settings. A public health nurse, her program of research has focused on women's health, health disparities, and particularly on the prevention of cervical cancer as a cancer of disparities globally. Her graduate work at the University of Virginia (MSN and PhD) centered on women's health in global settings. She completed her PhD in nursing at the University of Virginia, where she did extensive fieldwork in her NIH/National Institute of Nursing Research (NINR) funded ethnographic dissertation study with vulnerable women in Nicaragua. Winner of the 2017 Excellence in Education Award from the University of Virginia's Nursing Alumni Association and the 2018 University of Virginia Provost's Excellence in Education Award, Mitchell has developed innovative courses focused on women's health and social entrepreneurship in global settings. Locally, she has fostered a longtime partnership with community health workers trained in Charlottesville, Virginia, and surrounding rural areas, many of whom represent immigrant communities. Her publications support a global perspective on the need for culturally tailored nursing interventions to promote women's health and prevent cervical cancer.

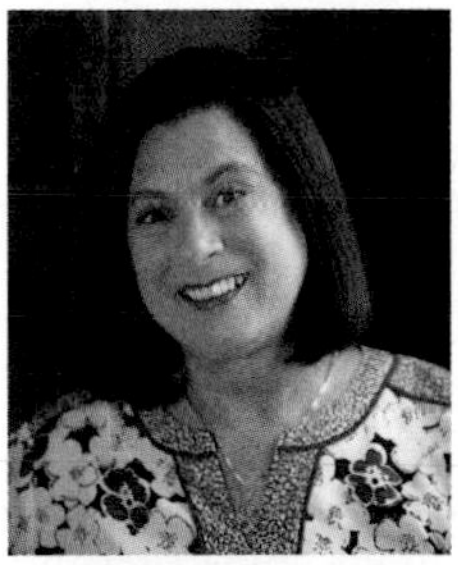

Carole R. Myers, PhD, MSN, BS

Dr. Carole R. Myers is an associate professor at the University of Tennessee with a joint appointment in the College of Nursing and Department of Public Health.

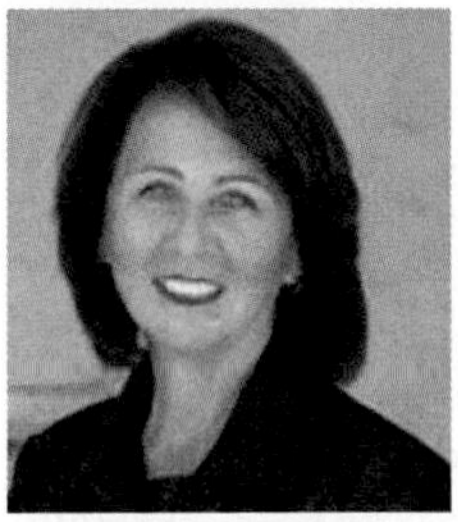

Victoria P. Niederhauser, DrPH, RN, PPCNP-BC, FAAN

Dr. Niederhauser is Professor and Dean at the University of Tennessee Knoxville College of Nursing. Dr. Niederhauser is a board-certified pediatric nurse practitioner, a Robert Wood Johnson Executive Nurse Fellow and a fellow in the American Academy of Nursing. She has received several national awards and currently serves on the board of the Beryl Institute and the National Advisory Council for Accelerating Interprofessional Community-Based Education and Practice Initiative.

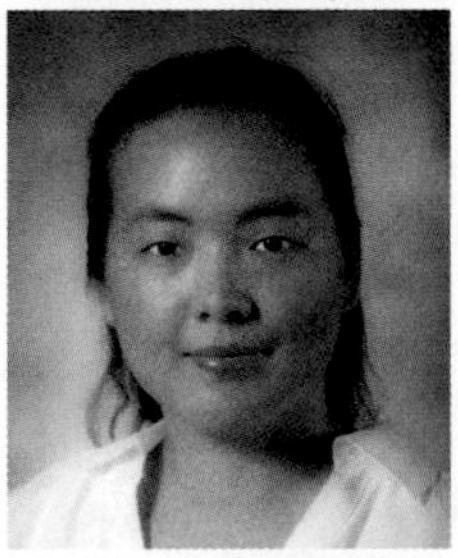

Eunhee Park, PhD, RN, APHN-BC

Eunhee Park earned her master's degree in the public health nursing leadership (PHNL) specialty track and her PhD degree at the University of Virginia. Dr. Park is an assistant professor of the School of Nursing at the University at Buffalo. With experience in a variety of community and clinical settings, she has taught undergraduate and graduate public health nursing courses, such as public health nursing practicum, health promotion and epidemiologic methods, informatics in health care, health behavior and health promotion research, nursing care in the community, public health nursing leadership, etc. Her research focus is on health promotion with the use of technology and community-based approaches to find innovative ways to promote population health particularly for adolescents and vulnerable populations. Therefore her research areas include understanding the factors of health behavior patterns and trajectory development, the development of youth health education programs utilizing interactive technology and health literacy strategies for smoking and substance use prevention, and linking individual health with the community for health promotion via the community participatory approach.

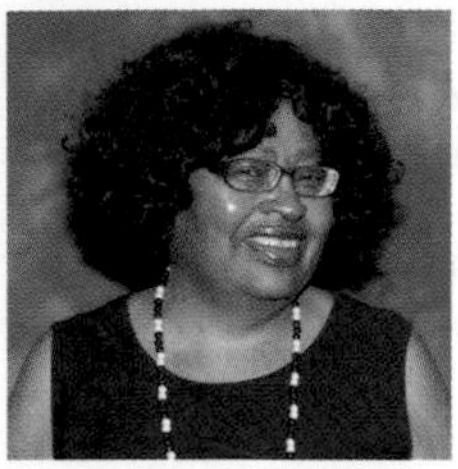

Bobbie J. Perdue, RN, PhD

Dr. Bobbie Perdue is Professor Emerita at Syracuse University. Her teaching career in nursing spans 46 years and includes the teaching of associate degree, baccalaureate, and master's degree nursing students. She received a BSN from Vanderbilt University, an MSN in child-psychiatric mental health nursing from Wayne State University, and a PhD in nursing research and theory development from New York University.

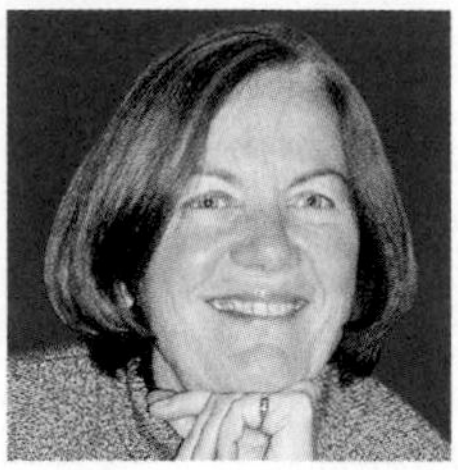

Bonnie Rogers, DrPH, COHN-S, LNCC, FAAN

Bonnie Rogers is a professor of public health and nursing and is Director of the North Carolina Occupational Safety and Health Education and Research Center and the Occupational Health Nursing Program at the University of North Carolina, School of Public Health, at Chapel Hill, North Carolina. Dr. Rogers received her diploma in nursing from the Washington Hospital Center School of Nursing, Washington, DC; her baccalaureate in nursing from George Mason University School of Nursing, Fairfax, Virginia; and her master of public health degree and doctorate in public health, the latter with a major in environmental health sciences and occupational health nursing, from the Johns Hopkins University School of Hygiene and Public Health, Baltimore, Maryland. She holds a postgraduate certificate as an adult health clinical nurse specialist. She is certified in occupational health nursing, case management, legal nurse consulting, and is a fellow in the American Academy of Nursing and the American Association of Occupational Health Nurses. Dr. Rogers completed an academic certificate program in bioethics and health policy at Loyola University, Chicago, is a nurse ethicist, and was invited to study ethics as a visiting scholar at the Hastings Center in New York. She was granted a National Institute for Occupational Safety and Health (NIOSH) career award to study ethical issues in occupational health. In addition to managerial, consultant, and educator/researcher positions, Dr. Rogers has also practiced for many years as a public health nurse, occupational health nurse, and occupational health nurse practitioner. She has published more than 200 articles and book chapters, and two books, including *Occupational and Environmental Health Nursing: Concepts and Practice* and *Occupational Health Nursing Guidelines for Primary Clinical Conditions,* in their third and fifth editions, respectively. She is a member of several editorial panels and has given nearly 500 presentations nationally and internationally on occupational health and safety issues, ethical issues in occupational health, and total worker health. Dr. Rogers has had several funded research grants on clinical issues in occupational health, health promotion, research priorities, hazards to health care workers, and ethical issues in occupational health. She is past editor for the *Journal of Legal Nurse Consulting*. Dr. Rogers is honored to serve as Chairperson of the NIOSH Board of Scientific Counselors. She was elected in 2013 as a fellow in the Collegium Ramazzini. She served two elected terms as Vice President of the International Commission on Occupational Health (ICOH) and completed two terms as Chairperson of the Scientific Committee on Education and Training in Occupational Health, ICOH. Dr. Rogers is past president of the American Association of Occupational Health Nurses and the Association of Occupational and Environmental Clinics and completed several terms as an appointed member of the National Advisory Committee on Occupational Safety and Health. She is a consultant in occupational health and ethics.

Dr. Rogers served as Chairperson of the NIOSH National Occupational Research Agenda Liaison Committee for 15 years and has served on numerous Institute of Medicine/National Academy of Medicine committees.

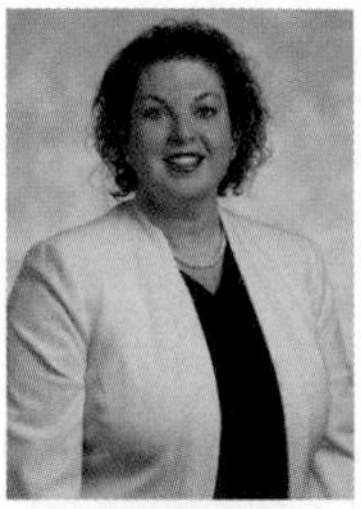

Cynthia Rubenstein, PhD, RN, CPNP-PC

Cynthia Rubenstein is currently chair of the nursing department and professor at Randolph-Macon College. She has extensive experience in pediatric nursing, including neonatal intensive care unit (NICU), emergency department (ED), home health, and primary care. She has been a practicing pediatric nurse practitioner for 20 years and has collaborated on childhood obesity prevention educational programs for Virginia's youth. She practices clinically through Remote Area Medical (www.ramusa.org) to support youth access to medical, dental, and vision care.

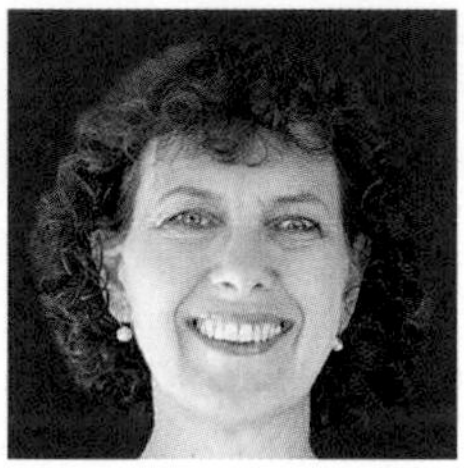

Barbara Sattler, RN, MPH, DrPH, FAAN

Dr. Barbara Sattler has a diploma in nursing from Pilgrim State Psychiatric Center School of Nursing, a BS in political science from the University of Baltimore, and the MPH and DrPH from Johns Hopkins University. She is a professor at the University of San Francisco. She is a founding member of the Alliance of Nurses for Healthy Environments (www.enviRN.org), a national network of nurses who are addressing the integration of environmental health into our nursing education, practice, research, and policy/advocacy efforts. She has been working in the area of environmental health and nursing for over three decades and has been involved in issues associated with air, water, food, and products, as well as climate change and energy policies as they relate to human health.

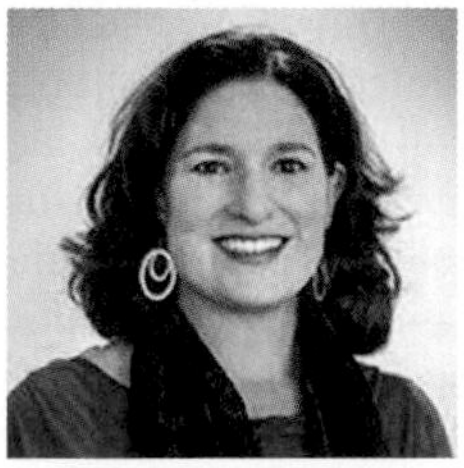

Erika Metzler Sawin, PhD

Erika Metzler Sawin is a second-degree nurse who received her master's in community health nursing from the University of Texas, Austin, and her PhD in nursing from the University of Virginia. She is an associate professor in the School of Nursing at James Madison University in Harrisonburg, Virginia, where she teaches community health nursing to BSN students. Her research interests are in the areas of domestic violence and culturally aware care. In 2015, she was a U.S. Fulbright-Nehru Scholar, teaching nursing and public health in Puducherry, India. She is currently Project Director for the HRSA NEPQR grant "Undergraduate Primary Care and Rural Education (UPCARE) Project: A Community-Based Nursing Education Collaboration" based in rural Page County, Virginia.

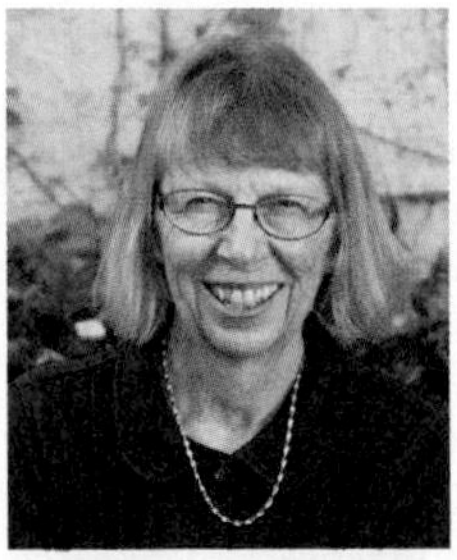

Marjorie A. Schaffer, PhD, PHN, RN
Marjorie Schaffer is Professor Emerita at Bethel University, where she taught public health nursing for 31 years. She consulted on public health nursing education during Fulbright awards in Norway and New Zealand and has published research articles on public health nursing practice and education.

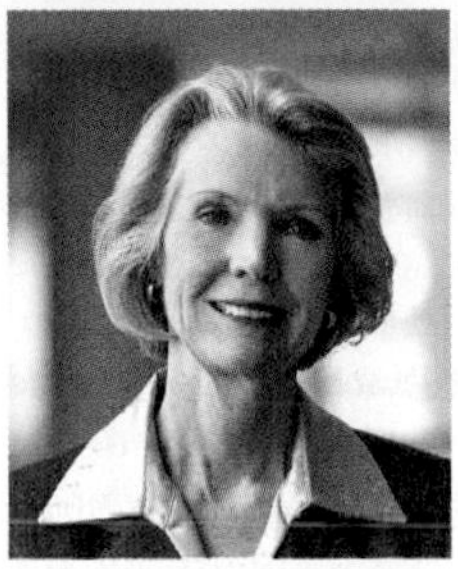

Cynthia Selleck, PhD, RN, FAAN
Dr. Cynthia Selleck is Professor and Associate Dean for Clinical and Global Partnerships at the University of Alabama at Birmingham School of Nursing. In this role, she oversees faculty practice initiatives for the School of Nursing, including the school's nurse-led clinics and Nurse-Family Partnership program. Dr. Selleck also holds an appointment as professor in the Department of Family and Community Medicine at the University of Alabama School of Medicine and serves as Director of the Alabama Statewide Area Health Education Center (AHEC) Program. She received her bachelor's in nursing from Emory University, her master's as a family nurse practitioner from Vanderbilt University, and a PhD from the University of Alabama at Birmingham School of Nursing. Her interests include care of underserved populations, health disparities, social justice issues, team-based care, and the preparation of a primary care workforce for medically needy populations.

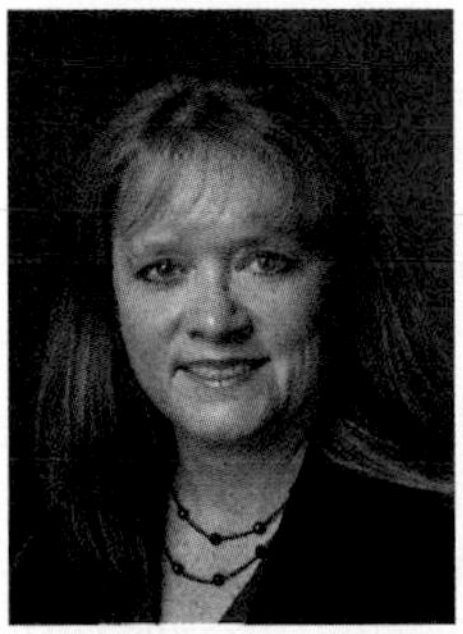

Sallie J. Shipman, EdD, MSN, RN, CNL, NHDP-BC
Sallie J. Shipman is a clinical assistant professor at the University of Florida College of Nursing in Gainesville, Florida, and teaches community/population and public health nursing in the undergraduate curriculum. She is board certified as a clinical nurse leader and national healthcare disaster professional. She has been teaching nursing since 2011 and has more than 18 years of experience as a public health nurse at the Alabama Department of Public Health (ADPH) with extensive experience in public health emergency preparedness planning, community/academic partnerships, and prenatal/perinatal outreach. She started her role at the ADPH Center for Emergency Preparedness in 2002 as an area surveillance nurse coordinator, which evolved into a state level position as a hazard vulnerability analysis nurse coordinator. Dr. Shipman serves nationally on the Practice Committee of the Society for the Advancement of Disaster Nursing.

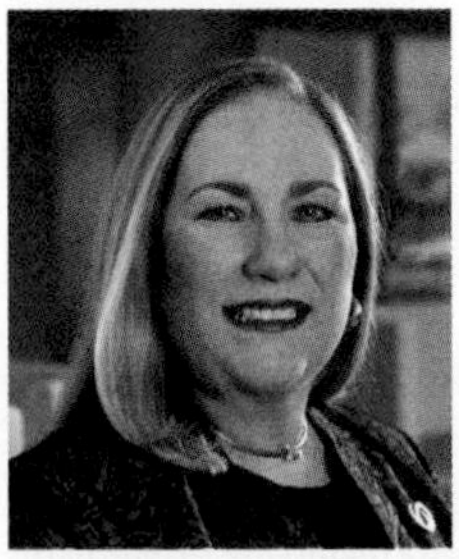

Maria R. Shirey, PhD, MBA, RN, NEA-BC, ANEF, FACHE, FNAP, FAAN
Dr. Maria R. Shirey, professor in the School of Nursing at the University of Alabama at Birmingham, teaches in both the PhD in nursing and doctor of nursing practice programs, focusing on leadership, management, health policy, and scholarly writing. Since 2003 her program of research has focused on building leadership capacity to advance quality, safety, and health care transformation. Since joining the University of Alabama at Birmingham in 2013, Dr. Shirey has extended her funded scholarly work to include leadership for population health through testing of innovative interprofessional collaborative practice (IPCP) models to impact the Quadruple Aim outcomes of enhancing the patient experience, improving population health, reducing the cost of care, and enhancing care team member well-being. As principal investigator of a $1.5 million Health Resources Services Administration grant, "Interprofessional Collaborative Practice Enhancing Transitional Care Coordination in Heart Failure Patients," Dr. Shirey led the creation and sustainability of a medical home at UAB Hospital designed to provide guideline-driven, coordinated care for an uninsured, vulnerable population. The medical home serves as a clinical training site for students (undergraduate, graduate, doctoral) from multiple health professions to engage in both interprofessional education (IPE) and IPCP. Dr. Shirey's "real world" approach to leadership over the last 40 years well integrates her extensive experience as an accomplished nurse clinician, executive, educator, researcher, and scholar.

Dr. Shirey received a bachelor of science in nursing from Florida State University, a master of science in nursing from Texas Woman's University, a master of business administration from Tulane University, and a PhD in nursing science from Indiana University. Dr. Shirey's practice expertise is in executive nursing leadership, and her broad career experience includes roles as staff nurse, clinical nurse specialist, academic faculty, nurse manager, nursing director, hospital vice-president, clinic administrator, and entrepreneur.

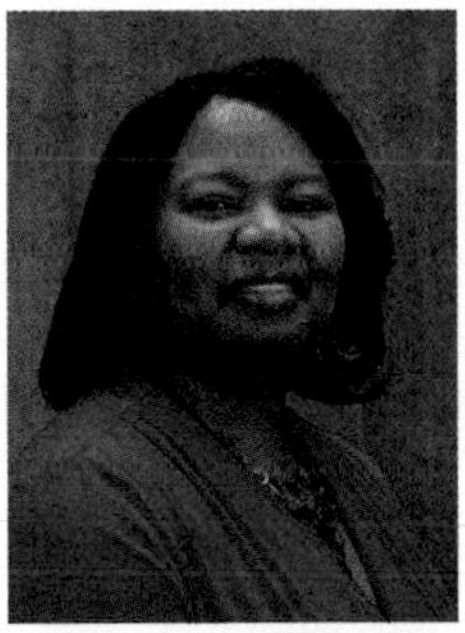

Donna E. Smith, MSPH
Donna Smith is an epidemiology specialist with the Mecklenburg County Health Department in Charlotte, North Carolina. She has expertise in the areas of human immunodeficiency virus (HIV)/acquired immunodeficiency syndrome (AIDS) research, racial and ethnic health disparities, social determinants of health, and community health assessments. Prior to her work in Charlotte, Ms. Smith served as an epidemiologist with the South Carolina Office of Minority Health, where she researched a broad range of health disparity topics impacting minority populations. She also served as a project coordinator for the South Carolina HIV/AIDS Surveillance Unit, where she led a Centers for Disease Control and Prevention (CDC)-funded initiative researching risk behaviors of persons newly reported with HIV.

Ms. Smith earned her master's degree (MSPH) in epidemiology from the Norman J. Arnold School of Public Health, University of South Carolina in Columbia.

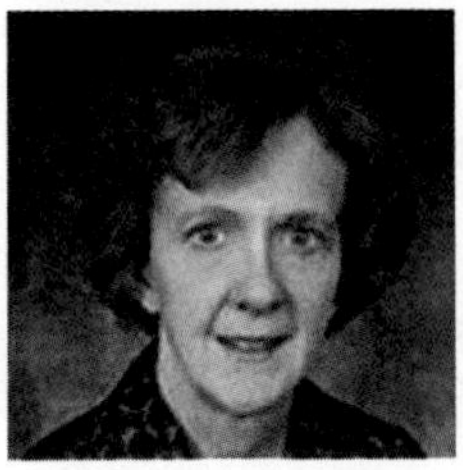

Sherrill J. Smith, RN, PhD, CNE, CNL
Dr. Sherrill Smith is a professor in the College of Nursing and Health at Wright State University in Dayton, Ohio, where she has taught full time since 2008. She served in the United States Air Force Nurse Corps for 26 years, retiring as a colonel in the Air Force Reserves in 2011. She is certified both as a nurse educator and clinical nurse leader. Her scholarship and funding is in the area of nursing education, including the use of virtual reality training for disaster training.

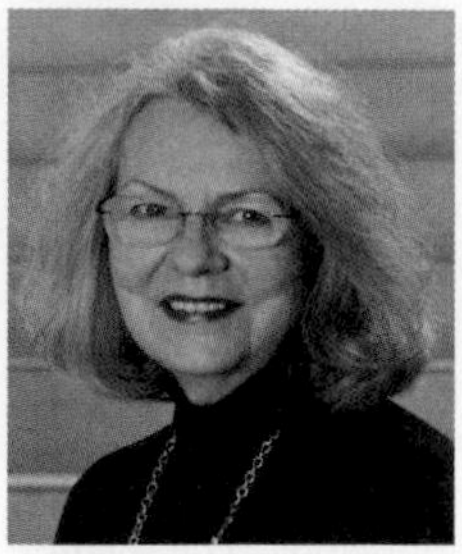

Patricia M. Speck, DNSc, APN, APRN, FNP-BC, DF-IAFN, FAAFS, FAFN, FAAN

Patricia Speck is a professor at the University of Alabama at Birmingham School of Nursing in Birmingham, Alabama, and the coordinator of the advanced forensic nursing program and internationally recognized as a board-certified family nurse practitioner (1984-present) and expert in advanced forensic nursing care of patients experiencing an intersection with the legal system. Her clinical practice with forensic populations globally spans over 35 years, consulting nationally and internationally in Africa, Eurasia, the Caribbean, and Central, South, and North America with governments, universities, institutions, and nongovernmental organizations to evaluate and implement infrastructure change in response to victims of violence. As a family nurse practitioner and forensic nursing practice expert who is a published and funded researcher, she develops policy, evaluates programs, and builds workforce capacity in rural and underserved communities through publication, education, and violence prevention initiatives. She was President of the International Association of Forensic Nurses (2003-2004) and Chair of the American Public Health Association's Family Violence Prevention Forum/Caucus (2011-2013), and her awards include fellow status from the International Association of Forensic Nurses (2001), American Academy of Forensic Sciences (2008), fellow in the Academy of Forensic Nursing (2018), and the premier American Academy of Nurses (2002). She was the first nurse to receive the Professional Impact Award from End Violence Against Women International organization in 2017.

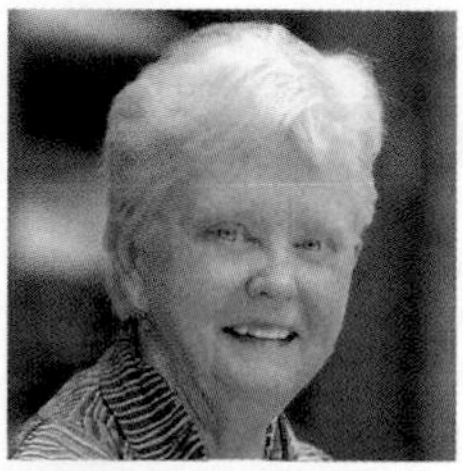

Marcia Stanhope, PhD, RN, FAAN

Dr. Marcia Stanhope is former Associate Dean and is Professor Emeritus, University of Kentucky, Lexington, Kentucky. She has edited this book with Dr. Jeanette Lancaster through its previous nine editions.

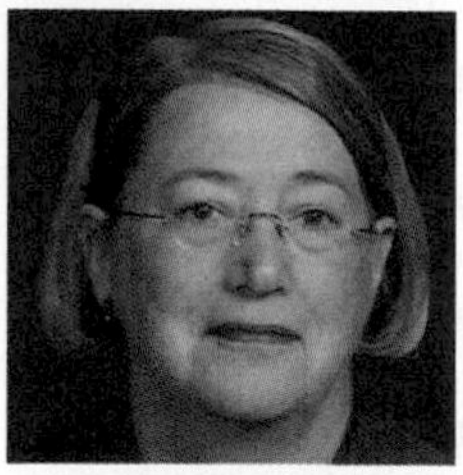

Sue Strohschein, MS, RN/PHN, APRN, BC

Sue Strohschein's public health nursing career spans more than 40 years and includes practice in both local and state health departments in Minnesota. She was a generalized public health nurse consultant for the Minnesota Department of Health for 25 years. She provided leadership in the initial development and dissemination of the Public Health Intervention Wheel.

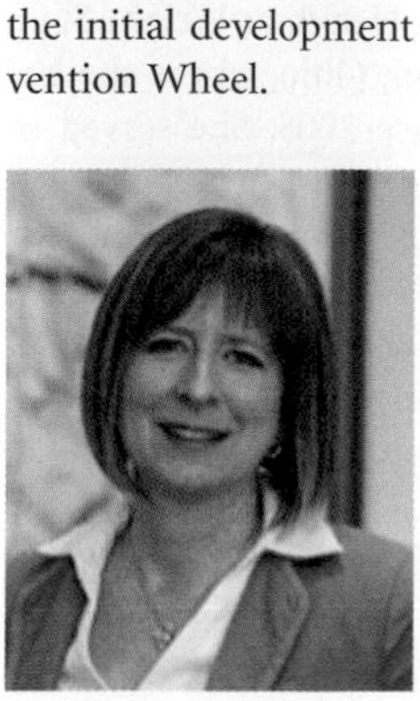

Melissa A. Sutherland, PhD, FNP-BC

Dr. Sutherland earned her bachelor's and master's degrees from Binghamton University in New York, and her PhD from the University of Virginia. She is a board-certified family nurse practitioner and a professor at the Decker School of Nursing, Binghamton University. Her major areas of research and practice are interpersonal violence and women's health. She is a member of the International Association of Forensic Nurses and the American Public Health Association.

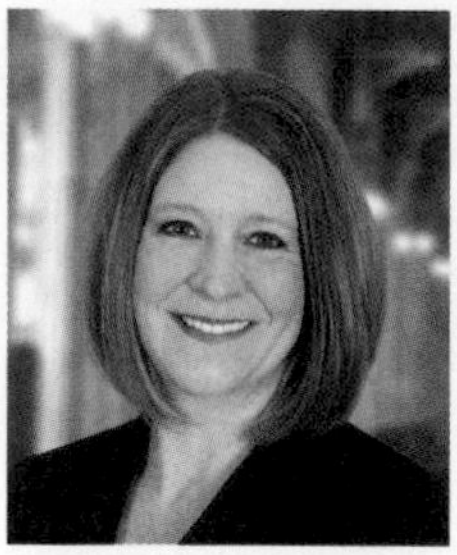

Laura Suzuki, PhD(c), MPH, BSN, RN

Laura Suzuki is a public health nurse who has spent most of her career in a large local health department managing maternal and child health services for a diverse population of vulnerable women and families. She has worked for the Centers for Disease Control and Prevention in Atlanta, Georgia, and the World Health Organization in Africa. Dr. Suzuki's practice and research efforts focus on gender-based violence among marginalized women, including immigrants and ethnic minorities. Her dissertation centers on the phenomenon of reproductive coercion and the extent of autonomy in decision making related to sexual and reproductive health among low-income Latina women. She is an active member of the American Public Health Association, Public Health Nursing Section, and serves on the APHA Gun Violence Prevention Workgroup. She is a member of the Massachusetts Public Health Association and Massachusetts Association of Public Health Nurses. She has previously served on the Maternal Child Health Advisory Committee for the National Association of County and City Health Officials (NACCHO). She earned her BSN from the University of Virginia and her MPH from Johns Hopkins University. She currently is a doctoral candidate at the William F. Connell School of Nursing, Boston College.

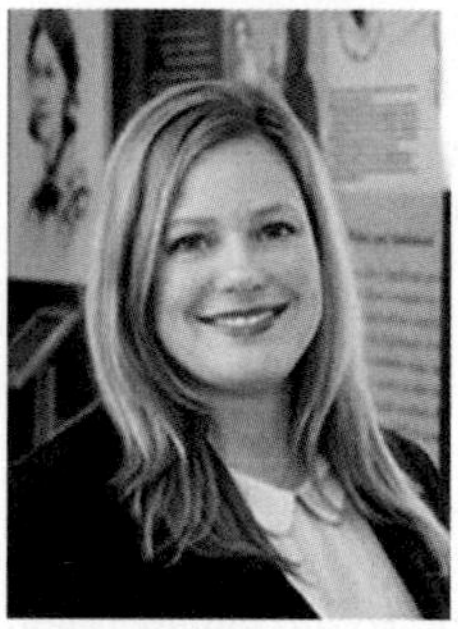

Michele H. Talley, PhD, ACNP-BC

Dr. Talley, assistant professor at the University of Alabama at Birmingham School of Nursing, serves as the clinic director for a nurse-led clinic founded by the University of Alabama at Birmingham School of Nursing in 2011. This clinic, the Providing Access to Healthcare (PATH), was opened to provide care to uninsured patients with diabetes using an interprofessional model of care delivery. Additionally, in fulfillment of the school's tripartite mission (teaching, service, and scholarship), Dr. Talley serves as an educator, a provider of diabetes care, and a nursing researcher. Currently, she also serves as the master's program director where she leads a team of faculty in 11 different specialty tracks. Likewise, Dr. Talley serves as mentor and preceptor for MSN and DNP students. In her service role, Dr. Talley shares her extensive diabetes management expertise with patients while also addressing the challenges faced by this vulnerable population. Indeed, her research efforts are focused on diabetes self-care management with vulnerable patients. Dr. Talley received her bachelor of science in nursing (BSN) from the University of Alabama Capstone College of Nursing in 1996, her master of science in nursing (MSN) (adult acute care nurse practitioner) in 2005, as well as her doctor of philosophy in nursing in 2015 from the University of Alabama at Birmingham School of Nursing.

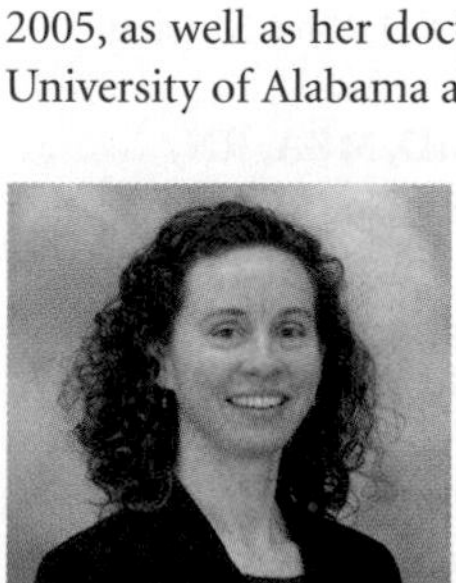

Esther J. Thatcher, PhD, RN, APHN-BC

As a BSN nursing student, Dr. Thatcher volunteered in El Salvador several times with a group called Nursing Students Without Borders. After graduating, she continued to work with Latinos as a migrant farmworker outreach nurse in rural Virginia. She then worked in adult internal medicine settings, where she became interested in preventing chronic diseases in underserved populations. Later, as a public health nurse, Dr. Thatcher reignited her interest in how community environments affect health outcomes. Her PhD research at the University of Virginia was to describe community influences on healthy food access in rural Appalachia. She completed a postdoctoral fellowship at the University of North Carolina–Chapel Hill, and now works at University of Virginia Health System.

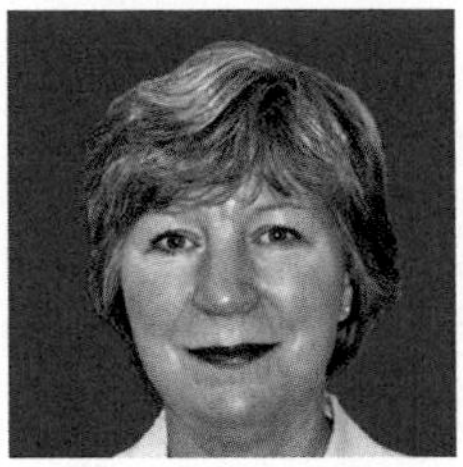

Anita Thompson-Heisterman, MSN, PMHCNS-BC, PMHNP-BC

Anita Thompson-Heisterman earned the BSN, MSN, FNP, and PMHNP degrees and certificates from the University of Virginia. She began practicing community mental health nursing in 1983 as a psychiatric nurse in a community mental health center. Her community practice has included clinical and management activities in a psychiatric home care service, a nurse-managed primary care center in public housing, and an outreach program for rural older adults. Currently she is an assistant professor and assistant department chair in the Division of Family, Community and Mental Health Systems at the University of Virginia School of Nursing and co-director of global initiatives at the school of nursing.

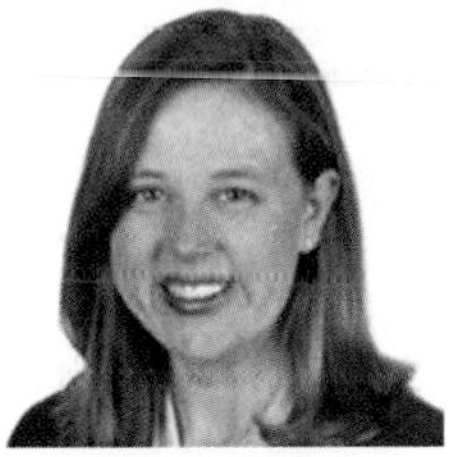

Lisa M. Turner, PhD, RN, PHCNS-BC

Lisa M. Turner felt called to the field of public and community health nursing while obtaining her BSN degree, inspired by the focus on preventing disease and helping underserved populations. Since then, she has provided care for a wide variety of vulnerable populations, including children in the schools, adults who are homeless, low-income families, and elders in long-term care facilities. She served as a nurse and clinic coordinator of the Good Samaritan Nursing Center at the University of Kentucky for 12 years. Her work at the Good Samaritan Nursing Center focused on providing school health services to underserved populations as well as developing a K-12 school health curriculum for a county in rural Kentucky. She has lectured and supervised students studying public health nursing in myriad community settings, including school clinics, homeless shelters, and free clinics for adults and children. She has contributed to several projects to evaluate school health services and has presented at national and international symposia on nursing clinics in the community. Her research interests are in the areas of vulnerable populations, access to health care, and obesity prevention. She is an active member in several nursing organizations, including leadership roles in the Association of Community Health Nurse Educators. Dr. Turner currently serves as an associate professor at Berea College, Berea, Kentucky.

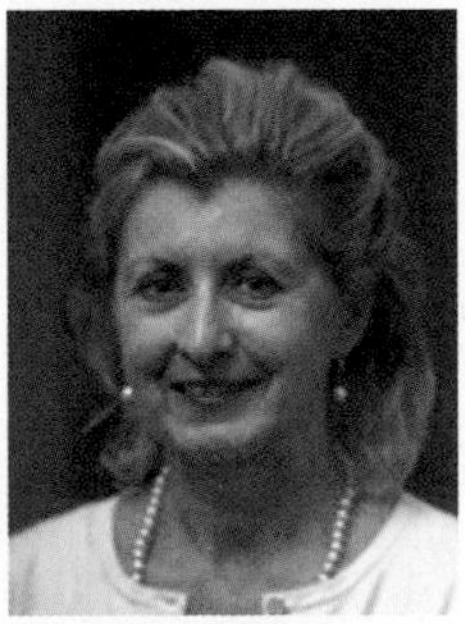

Connie M. Ulrich, PhD, RN, FAAN

Dr. Ulrich is a professor of nursing and bioethics and the Lillian S. Brunner Chair in Medical-Surgical Nursing at the University of Pennsylvania School of Nursing with a secondary appointment in the Department of Medical Ethics and Health Policy, Perelman School of Medicine.

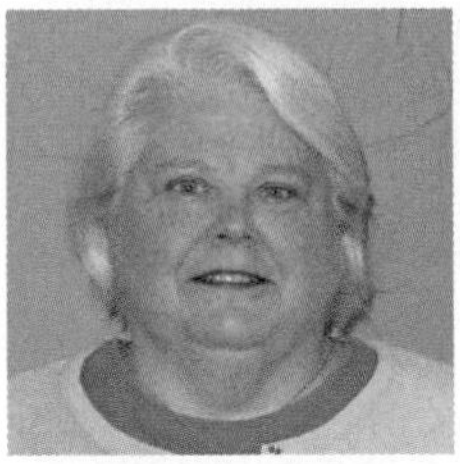

Lynn Wasserbauer, RN, FNP, PhD

Lynn Wasserbauer earned an undergraduate degree in zoology from the State University of New York, Oswego, a BS and MS in nursing from the University of Rochester, and a PhD and FNP certificate from the University of Virginia. She is a nurse practitioner at the University of Rochester Medical Center. Her current practice is in psychiatric nursing.

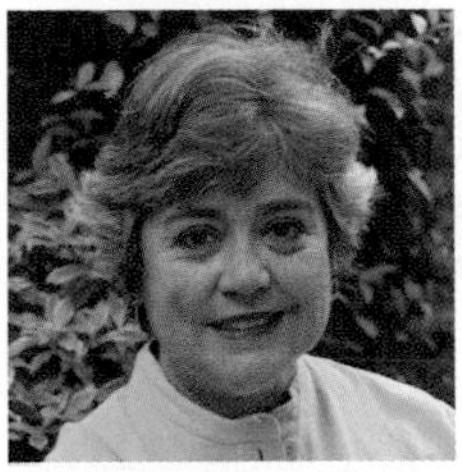

Jacqueline Webb, DNP, FNP-BC, RN

Dr. Jackie Webb has been a practicing family nurse practitioner for over 25 years, working primarily with underserved populations. She has taught nursing students both at the undergraduate and graduate levels for the past 15 years. Currently she is an associate professor at Linfield College School of Nursing in Portland, Oregon. Her research focus is on community nursing and innovative delivery health care models to deal with chronic pain and health inequities in vulnerable populations. She is the current Oregon Chapter President of the National Association of Hispanic Nurses.

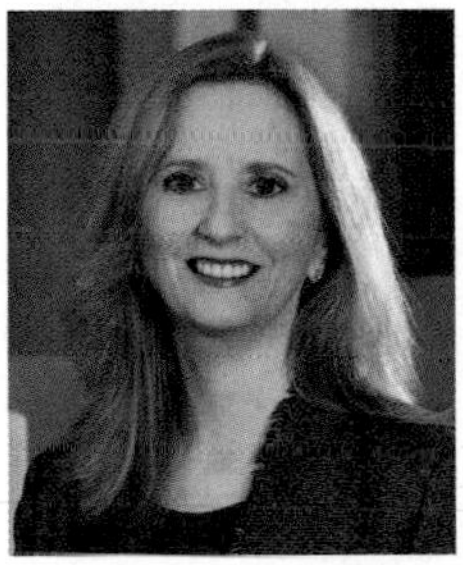

Connie White-Williams, PhD, RN, NE-BC, FAHA, FAAN

Dr. White-Williams is Senior Director of the University of Alabama Hospital Heart Failure Transitional Care Services for Adults (HRTSA) Clinic and the Center for Nursing Excellence and an assistant professor at University of Alabama School of Nursing (UABSON) in the Department of Acute, Chronic, and Continuing Care. She has extensive clinical experience in cardiovascular nursing, especially heart failure and heart transplantation. Dr. White-Williams served as the Clinical Practice Partner in the grant-funded HRSA Heart Failure Clinic for the Underserved. Dr. White-Williams received her BSN from the University of Pittsburgh in 1984, MSN in cardiovascular nursing (clinical nurse specialist) from UABSON in 1991, family nurse practitioner from UABSON in 2000, PhD in nursing from UABSON in 2009, and Post Graduate Certificate in Healthcare Quality and Safety in 2015. She also completed a Health Disparities Research Training Program in 2010 and a Hartford Geriatric Grant Writing Workshop in 2011.

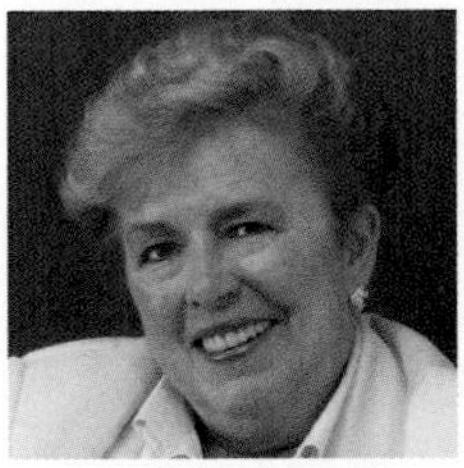

Carolyn A. Williams, RN, PhD, FAAN

Dr. Carolyn A. Williams is Professor and Dean Emerita at the College of Nursing at the University of Kentucky, Lexington, Kentucky. Dr. Williams began her career as a public health nurse. She has held many leadership roles, including President of the American Academy of Nursing; membership on the first U.S. Preventive Services Task Force, Department of Health and Human Services; and President of the American Association of Colleges of Nursing. She received the Distinguished Alumna Award from Texas Woman's University in 1983. In 2001, she was the recipient of the Mary Tolle Wright Founder's Award for Excellence in Leadership from Sigma Theta Tau International, and in 2007 she received the Bernadette Arminger Award from the American Association of Colleges of Nursing. In 2011, she was awarded an Honorary Doctorate of Public Service from the University of Portland, Portland, Oregon. In 2014, she received the honor of being inducted into the University of Kentucky College of Public Health Hall of Fame for international, national, state, and local contributions to public health and nursing, and in 2017 she was honored by the American Academy of Nursing as a Living Legend.

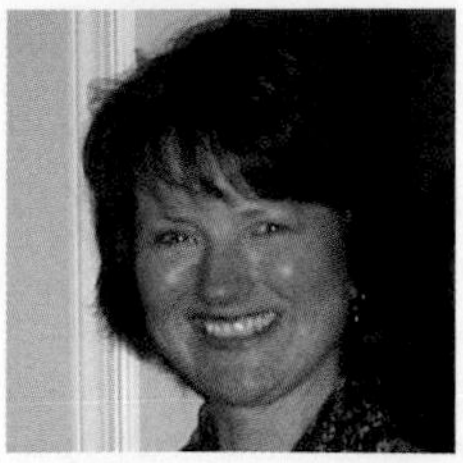

Lisa M. Zerull, PhD, RN-BC

Dr. Lisa M. Zerull provides leadership for nursing professional development and faith-based services, including faith community nursing and chaplaincy, at Valley Health System in Winchester, Virginia. She is also employed as adjunct clinical faculty at the Shenandoah University Eleanor Wade Custer School of Nursing teaching fundamentals and faith community nursing preparation courses. Since 1996, Dr. Zerull has served as a board-certified and unpaid faith community nurse in her home congregation of Grace Evangelical Lutheran Church. Currently the editor for *Perspectives*, an international publication for faith community nurses, Dr. Zerull is an author and frequent conference presenter. Her research interests include nursing history, outcome measures of faith community nursing, and youth health care career exploration.

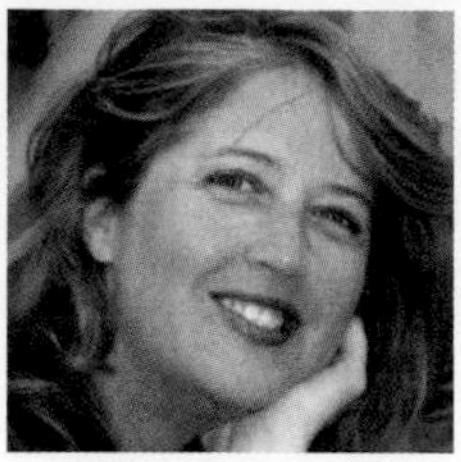

Elke Jones Zschaebitz, DNP, APRN, FNP-BC

Elke Jones Zschaebitz is a nurse practitioner who has worked in the fields of student health, pediatrics, and women's health, as well as in a telehealth practice in primary care. She received her BSN from Villanova University, her MSN-FNP from Midwestern State University in Wichita Falls, Texas, and her DNP from Duquesne University in Pittsburgh, Pennsylvania. She currently is employed full time at the University of Virginia Student Health Center in Charlottesville, Virginia, and is part-time adjunct faculty for the family nurse practitioner program at Georgetown University.

PREFACE

Since the last edition of this text, many changes have occurred in society as well as in health care. The news media daily discuss events including violence, man-made disasters, and disasters that are the result of naturally occurring events, including hurricanes, earthquakes, fires, and tornados that destroy homes, lives, businesses, and communities. Many countries around the world are engaged in health care reform, and a major driver propelling this reform is the cost of health care. The need for strong and effective public health care has grown in most countries, yet the reality has been that many countries have not prioritized public health.

A key component of public health is population health. The need for population health has not been greater than it is at present. This 10th edition of the text emphasizes population health as well as preventive services for individuals in the community. Two early and significant proponents of the importance of population health are David Kindig and Greg Stoddart. They have been writing about this concept for over 15 years. The beginning discussions of their work and of population health begin in Chapter 1 of the text. The health of a population is measured by health status indicators including social, economic, and the physical environments of a population, as well as the personal health practices of the members of the population, their biological including genetic makeup, early childhood and development throughout life, and the health care services available to the population. Populations in public health are broad and wide-ranging. They could include a population of ethnic groups or other affinity groups such as employees, disabled persons, prisoners, members of a specific religious affiliation, or those who live in a specific community (Kindig and Stoddart, 2003; Kindig, 2007).

The health outcomes of a population are influenced by a multitude of factors often described as social determinants. These determinants are discussed in chapters throughout the text. Other chapters focus on the myriad of factors that are considered social determinants of health such as economics, policy, the environment, culture, and many others. What is important is to look at population health from a multifaceted approach. Consider all factors that influence the health of a given population.

As is explained in Chapter 1 and discussed in other chapters throughout the text, there are three core functions of public health: assessment, policy development, and assurance. The Centers for Disease Control and Prevention (CDC, 2018, p. 1) has developed 10 essential public health services and aligns these services with the core functions of assessment, assurance, and policy development.

Chapters in this text include all of the critical elements of the public health services and the core functions cited above, as well as guidance in how to deal with other major issues, including the quality of care, the cost of care, and access to care. The growing shortage of nurses and other health care providers will only increase the concerns about these issues. One of the ways in which quality of care could be improved would include new uses of technology to manage an information revolution. Great improvements in quality would require a restructuring of how care is delivered, a shift in how funds are spent, changing the workplace, and using more effective ways to manage chronic illness. There will be costs associated with these quality improvements. However, the future costs of health care may be reduced as a result of improved health of populations and individuals.

The United States' health care spending has slowed in recent years due to the economy. A useful resource that describes health care systems in 19 countries around the world is *International Profiles of Health Care Systems,* edited by Mossiaios et al. and written for the Commonwealth Fund in May 2017. This monograph uses the same format to describe health care systems in large countries like Australia, Canada, India, and the United States, as well as much smaller countries, including New Zealand and Singapore.

In the past two decades, the greatest improvements in population health have come from public health achievements such as immunizations leading to eliminating and controlling infectious diseases, motor vehicle safety, safer workplaces, lifestyle improvements reducing the risk of heart disease and strokes, safer and healthier foods through improved sanitation, clean water and food fortification programs, better hygiene and nutrition to improve the health of mothers and babies, family planning, fluoride in drinking water, and recognition of tobacco as a health hazard. Continued changes in the public health system are essential if death, illness, and disability resulting from preventable problems are to continue to decline.

The need to focus attention on health promotion, lifestyle factors, and disease prevention led to the development of a major public policy about health for the nation. This policy was designed by a large number of people representing a wide range of groups interested in health. The policy, first introduced in 1979, was updated in 1990 and in 2000; it is reflected in the most recent document updated in 2010, titled *Healthy People 2020.* This document includes objectives related to population health. The newest document, *Healthy People 2030*, is being developed. These five documents have identified a set of national health promotion and disease prevention objectives for each of four decades. Examples of these objectives are highlighted in chapters throughout the text.

Healthy People 2020 emphasizes the concept of social determinants of health—that is, the belief that health is affected by many social, economic, and environmental factors that extend far beyond individual biology of disease. This means that improving health requires a broad approach to including the concept of health in all policies and creating environments where the healthy choice is the easy choice. To improve health in the United States individuals, families, communities, and populations must commit to these approaches. Also, society, through the development of health policy, must support better health care, the design of improved health education, and new ways of financing strategies to alter health status.

Some indicators have been substantially improved since the release of *Healthy People 2000*; *Healthy People 2010 and 2020* highlighted many of the original objectives and added new ones. The *Healthy People 2030* framework has as its purpose to (1) provide context and rationale for the initiative's approach, (2) communicate the principles that underlie decisions about *Healthy People 2030*, and (3) situate the initiative in the five-decade history of Healthy People. Since the framework is general, it is useful to review the foundational principles, overarching goals, and plan of action (www.healthypeople2030.gov). What does this mean for nurses who work in public health? Because people do not always know how to improve their health status, the challenge of nursing is to create change. Nursing takes place in a variety of public and private settings and includes disease prevention, health promotion, health protection, surveillance, education, maintenance, restoration, coordination, management, and evaluation of care of individuals, families, and populations, including communities.

To meet the demands of a constantly changing health care system, nurses must have vision in designing new and changing current roles and identifying their practice areas. To do so effectively, the nurse must understand concepts, theories, and the core content of public health, the changing health care system, the actual and potential roles and responsibilities of nurses and other health care providers, the importance of health promotion and disease orientation, and the necessity of involving consumers in the planning, implementation, and evaluation of health care efforts.

Since its initial publication in 1984, this text has been important in the education of nurses in baccalaureate, BSN-completion, and graduate programs. The text was written to provide nursing students and practicing nurses with a comprehensive source book that provides a foundation for designing population-focused nursing strategies. Content has been added to address the changing aspects of population health, including a section on human trafficking, the use and some cautions of genetic inquiries, and selected content about the health of veterans. There have also been changes where some of the prior appendixes and documents may be found on the book's Evolve website.

The unifying theme for the book is the integrating of health promotion and disease prevention concepts into the many roles of nurses. The prevention focus emphasizes traditional public health practice with increased attention to the effects of the internal and external environment on the health of populations and communities. The focus on interventions for the individual and family emphasizes the aspects of population-centered practice with attention to the effects of all of the determinants of health, including lifestyle, on personal health.

CONCEPTUAL APPROACH TO THIS TEXT

The term *community-oriented* has been used to reflect the orientation of nurses to the community and the public's health. In 1998, the Quad Council of Public Health Nursing composed of members from the American Nurses Association Congress on Nursing Practice, the American Public Health Association Public Health Nursing section, the Association of Community Health Nursing Educators, and the Association of State and Territorial Directors of Public Health Nursing developed a statement on the *Scope of Public Health Nursing Practice*. Through this statement, the leaders in public and community health nursing attempted to clarify the differences between public health nursing and the newest term introduced into nursing's vocabulary during health care reform of the 1990s, *community-based nursing*. The Quad Council recognized that the terms *public health nursing* and *community health nursing* have been used interchangeably since the 1980s to describe population-focused, community-oriented nursing and community-focused practice. They decided to make a clearer distinction between community-oriented and community-based nursing practice. In 2007, the definitions were further refined, and nurses once referred to as *public health nurses* and *community health nurses* are now referred to only as *public health nurses* in the revised standards of practice. The standards were again revised in 2013 by the renamed Quad Council Coalition and can be found in the appendixes of this edition of the text.

In this textbook, two different levels of care in the community are acknowledged: community-oriented care and community-based care. Two role functions for nursing practice in the community are suggested: public health nursing (community health nursing) and community-based nursing. This text focuses only on public health nursing (community health nursing), using the overarching term *community-oriented nursing*, which encompasses a focus on populations within the community context, or *population-centered nursing practice*.

For the fifth edition of this text, with consultation from C.A. Williams (author) and June Thompson (Mosby editor), Marcia Stanhope developed a conceptual model for community-oriented nursing practice. This model was influenced by a review of the history of community-oriented nursing from the 1800s to today. Marcia Stanhope studied Betty Neuman's model intensively while in school, which influenced this model.

The model itself is presented as a caricature of reality—or an abstract—with a description of the characteristics and the philosophy on which community-oriented nursing is built. The *model* is shown as a flying balloon (see inside the front cover of this book). The balloon represents community-oriented nursing and is filled with the knowledge, skills, and abilities needed in this practice to carry the world (the basket of the balloon) or the clients of the world who benefit from this practice. The *subconcepts* of public health nursing with the community and populations as the center of care are the *boundaries* of the practice. The public health foundation pillars of assurance, assessment, and policy development hold up the world of communities, where people live, work, play, go to school, and worship. The ribbons flying from the balloon indicate the interventions used by nurses. These ribbons (interventions) serve to provide lift and direction, tying the services together for the clients who are served. The intervention names and the services are listed with the balloon. The *propositions* (statements of relationship) for this model are found in the definitions of practice, public health functions, clients served, specific settings, interventions, and services. Many *assumptions* have served as the basis for the development of this model. Community-oriented nursing practice has evolved over time, becoming more complex. The practice of nursing in public health is based on a philosophy of care rather than being setting specific. It is different from community-based nursing care delivery. The development of community-oriented nursing has been influenced by public health practice, preventive medicine, community medicine, and shifts in the health care delivery system. Community-oriented nursing, whether a public health nurse or a community-based nurse, requires nurses to have specific competencies to be effective providers of care.

The definition of community-oriented nursing appears near the inside of the front cover of this book. This practice involves public health nurses. Community-based nurses differ from public health nurses in many ways. These differences are described in the table following the definitions. The differences are described as they relate to philosophy of care, goals, service, community, clients served, practice settings, ways of interacting with clients, type of services offered to clients, prevention levels used, goals, and priority of nurses' activities.

The four concepts of nursing, person (client), environment, and health are described for this model. These concepts appear in many works about nursing and in almost every educational curriculum for undergraduate students. Each of the four concepts may be defined differently in these works because of the beliefs of the persons writing the definitions.

In this text *nursing* is defined as community-oriented with a focus on providing health care through community diagnosis and investigation of major health and environmental problems. Health surveillance, monitoring, and evaluating community and population status are done to prevent disease and disability and to promote, protect, preserve, restore, and maintain health. This in turn creates conditions in which clients can be healthy. The person, or client, is the world, nation, state, community, population, aggregate, family, or individual.

The boundaries of the client *environment* may be limited by the world, nation, state, locality, home, school, work, playground, religion, or individual self. *Health*, in this model, involves a continuum of health rather than wellness, with the best health state possible as the goal. The best possible level of health is achieved through measures of prevention as practiced by the nurse.

The nurse engages in autonomous practice with the client, who is the primary decision maker about health issues. The nurse practices in a variety of environments, including, but not limited to, governments, organizations, homes, schools, churches, neighborhoods, industry, and community boards. The nurse interacts with diverse cultures, partners, other providers in teams, multiple clients, and one-to-one or aggregate relationships. Clients at risk for the development of health problems are a major focus of nursing services. Primary prevention–level strategies are the key to reducing risk of health problems. Secondary prevention is done to maintain, promote, or protect health, whereas tertiary prevention strategies are used to preserve, protect, or maintain health.

Nurses have many roles related to community clients and roles that relate specifically to practice with populations (or population-centered). Public health nurses especially engage in activities specific to community development, assessment, monitoring, health policy, politics, health education, interdisciplinary practice, program management, community/population advocacy, case finding, and delivery of personal health services when these services are otherwise unavailable in the health care system. This conceptual model is the framework for this text.

ORGANIZATION

The text is divided into eight sections:

- **Part 1, Influencing Factors in Public Health Nursing and Population Health,** describes the historical and current status of the health care delivery system and public health nursing practice, both domestically and internationally.
- **Part 2, Forces Affecting Nurses in the Delivery of Public and Population Health Care Delivery,** addresses environmental health, ethics, policy, and cultural issues that affect public health, nurses, and clients.
- **Part 3, Conceptual and Scientific Frameworks Applied to Nursing Practice,** provides conceptual models and scientific bases for public health nursing practice. Selected models from nursing and related sciences are also discussed.
- **Part 4, Community Level Interventions,** looks at promoting healthy communities, looking at the community as a client, and how principles are applied to all populations in community environments.
- **Part 5, Issues and Approaches in Population-Centered Nursing,** examines the management of health care, quality and safety, and populations in select community environments and groups, as well as issues related to managing cases, programs, and disasters.
- **Part 6, Promoting the Health of Target Populations Across the Life Span,** discusses risk factors and population-level health problems for families and individuals throughout the life span.
- **Part 7, Promoting and Protecting the Health of Vulnerable Populations,** covers specific health care needs and issues of populations at risk.
- **Part 8, Nurses' Roles and Functions in the Community,** examines diversity in the role of public health nurses and describes the rapidly changing roles, functions, and practice settings.

NEW TO THIS EDITION

New content and illustrations have been included in the 10th edition of *Public Health Nursing: Population-Centered Health Care in the Community* to ensure that the text remains a complete, current, and comprehensive resource:

- **NEW!** Each chapter has a brief box to check your practice. A brief clinical situation is provided, and the answers can be determined by content in the chapter.

PEDAGOGY

Other key features of this edition are detailed below. Each chapter is organized for easy use by students and faculty.

Additional Resources

Additional Resources listed at the beginning of each chapter direct students to chapter-related tools and resources contained in the book's Evolve website.

Objectives

Objectives open each chapter to guide student learning and alert faculty to what students should gain from the content.

Key Terms

Key Terms are identified at the beginning of the chapter and defined either within the chapter or in the glossary to assist students in understanding unfamiliar terminology.

Chapter Outline

The Chapter Outline alerts students to the structure and content of the chapter.

How To Boxes

How To boxes provide specific, application-oriented information.

Evidence-Based Practice Boxes

Evidence-Based Practice boxes in each chapter illustrate the use and application of the latest research findings in public health, community health, and community-oriented nursing.

Practice Application

At the end of each chapter a case situation helps students understand how to apply chapter content in the practice setting. Questions at the end of each case promote critical thinking while students analyze the case.

Key Points

Key Points provide a summary listing of the most important points made in the chapter.

Clinical Decision-Making Activities

Clinical Decision-Making Activities promote student learning by suggesting a variety of activities that encourage both independent and collaborative effort.

Appendixes

The **Appendixes** provide additional content resources, key information, and clinical tools and references.

EVOLVE STUDENT LEARNING RESOURCES

Additional resources designed to supplement the student learning process are available on this book's website at http://evolve.elsevier.com/Stanhope/community/, including:

- **Additional Resources for Students** in select chapters
- **Audio Glossary** with complete definitions of all key terms and other important community and public health nursing concepts
- **Review Questions** with answers
- **Student Case Studies** with questions and answers
- **Answers to Practice Application Questions**

INSTRUCTOR RESOURCES

Several supplemental ancillaries are available to assist instructors in the teaching process:

- **TEACH for Nurses lesson plans** provided for each chapter, with Nursing Curriculum Standards, Teaching Strategies and Learning Activities, Case Studies, and more
- **Test Bank** with 1200 questions and answers coded for NCLEX Client Needs category, nursing process, and cognitive level
- **PowerPoint Lecture Slides** for each chapter, with current accessibility guidelines incorporated
- **Image Collection** with illustrations from the text

REFERENCES

Centers for Disease Control and Prevention: The public health system and the 10 essential public health services. *MMWR Morb Mortal Wkly Rep* 48(12):241-243, 1999. Available at http://www.cdc.gov. Accessed June 26, 2018.

Kindig D: Understanding population health. *Milbank Q* 85(1):139-161, 2007.

Kindig D, Stoddart G: What is population health? *Am J Public Health* 93(3):380-383, 2003.

United States Department of Health and Human Services: *Healthy People 2030*. Available at www.healthypeople.gov.

CONTENTS

PART 1 Influencing Factors in Public Health Nursing and Population Health

1 Public Health Foundations and Population Health, 1
2 History of Public Health and Public and Community Health Nursing, 22
3 Public Health, Primary Care, and Primary Health Care Systems, 45
4 Perspectives in Global Health Care, 62
5 Economics of Health Care Delivery, 91

PART 2 Forces Affecting Nurses in the Delivery of Public and Population Health Care Delivery

6 Environmental Health, 121
7 Application of Ethics in the Community, 149
8 Achieving Cultural Competence in Community Health Nursing, 165
9 Public Health Policy, 196
10 Evidence-Based Practice, 218

PART 3 Conceptual and Scientific Frameworks Applied to Nursing Practice

11 Population-Based Public Health Nursing Practice: The Intervention Wheel, 231
12 Genomics in Public Health Nursing, 255
13 Epidemiology, 269
14 Infectious Disease Prevention and Control, 299
15 Communicable and Infectious Disease Risks, 333

PART 4 Community Level Interventions

16 Promoting Healthy Communities, 357
17 Community As Client: Assessment and Analysis, 370
18 Building a Culture of Health to Influence Health Equity Within Communities, 395
19 Health Education Principles Applied in Communities, Groups, Families, and Individuals for Healthy Change, 414

PART 5 Issues and Approaches in Population-Centered Nursing

20 The Nurse-Led Health Center: A Model for Community Nursing Practice, 437
21 Public Health Nursing Practice and the Disaster Management Cycle, 454
22 Public Health Surveillance and Outbreak Investigation, 481
23 Program Management, 498
24 Quality Management, 521
25 Case Management, 546

PART 6 Promoting the Health of Target Populations Across the Life Span

26 Working With Families in the Community for Healthy Outcomes, 575
27 Family Health Risks, 604
28 Child and Adolescent Health, 626
29 Major Health Issues and Chronic Disease Management of Adults Across the Life Span, 653
30 Disability Health Care Across the Life Span, 678

PART 7 Promoting and Protecting the Health of Vulnerable Populations

31 Health Equity and Care of Vulnerable Populations, 697
32 Population-Centered Nursing in Rural and Urban Environments, 716
33 Poverty and Homelessness, 735
34 Migrant Health Issues, 756
35 Teen Pregnancy, 772
36 Mental Health Issues, 789
37 Alcohol, Tobacco, and Other Drug Problems, 811
38 Violence and Human Abuse, 836

PART 8 Nurses' Roles and Functions in the Community

39 Advanced Nursing Practice in the Community, 863
40 The Nurse Leader in the Community, 880
41 The Nurse in Public Health, Home Health, Hospice, and Palliative Care, 899
42 The Nurse in the Schools, 928
43 The Nurse in Occupational Health, 957
44 Forensic Nursing in the Community, 976
45 The Nurse in the Faith Community, 989
46 Public Health Nursing at Local, State, and National Levels, 1009

APPENDIXES

Appendix A: Program Planning and Design, 1026
Appendix B: Flu Pandemics, 1029

Appendix C: Friedman Family Assessment Model (Short Form), 1031
Appendix D: Comprehensive Occupational and Environmental Health History, 1033
Appendix E: Essential Elements of Public Health Nursing, 1036
Appendix F: American Public Health Association Definition of Public Health Nursing, 1042
Appendix G: American Nurses Association Scope and Standards of Practice for Public Health Nursing, 1048
Appendix H: The Health Insurance Portability and Accountability Act (HIPAA): What Does It Mean for Public Health Nurses?, 1049

Index, 1051

1

Public Health Foundations and Population Health

Carolyn A. Williams, RN, PhD, FAAN

OBJECTIVES

After reading this chapter, the student should be able to do the following:

1. State the mission and core functions of public health, the essential public health services, and the quality performance standards program in public health.
2. Describe specialization in public health nursing and other nurse roles in the community and the practice goals of each.
3. Describe what is meant by population health.
4. Identify barriers to the practice of community and prevention oriented, population-focused practice.
5. Describe the importance of the social determinants of health to the health of a population.
6. State key opportunities for nurses to provide the leadership in implementing Public Health 3.0.

CHAPTER OUTLINE

Public Health Practice: The Foundation for Healthy Populations and Communities
Public Health Nursing as a Field of Practice: An Area of Specialization
Public Health Nursing Versus Community-Based Nursing
Roles in Public Health Nursing
Challenges for the Future

KEY TERMS

aggregate, p. 10
assessment, p. 3
assurance, p. 4
capitation, p. 17
community-based nursing, p. 15
Community Health Improvement Process (CHIP), p. 6
community health nurse, p. 15
cottage industry, p. 17
integrated systems, p. 17
levels of prevention, p. 11
policy development, p. 3
population, p. 10
population-focused practice, p. 11
population health, p. 2
population health management p. 8
public health, p. 2
Public Health 3.0, p. 8
public health core functions, p. 3
public health nursing, p. 2
Quad Council, p. 7
social determinants of health, p. 8
subpopulations, p. 11

As the United States approaches the third decade of the twenty-first century, considerable public attention is being given to issues related to the availability of affordable health insurance so individuals are assured that they can have access to health care. The central feature in the Patient Protection and Affordable Care Act (ACA) of 2010 are the mechanisms to increase the number of people with health insurance. Despite initial turbulence in implementation of the legislation, including difficulties with enrollments due to technological problems, there is good evidence that progress was made in enrolling people. The U.S. Census Bureau reported that after the first enrollment period in the fall of 2013 the number of uninsured Americans fell from 41 million to 27 million in 2017 (Berchick, 2017; Census Bureau, 2018). In 2014, Blumenthal and Collins reported that the Urban Institute projected that the proportion of uninsured adults in the United States fell from 18 percent in the third quarter of 2013 to 13.4 percent in May 2014. The latest data from the Census Bureau put the uninsured rate for the total population at 8.8 percent in 2017 (Census Bureau, 2018). However, Collins et al. reported in May 2018 that, based on the Commonwealth Fund's tracking survey, ACA gains in coverage are beginning to reverse (Commonwealth Fund, 2018). They suggested the factors likely responsible are the lack of federal legislation to improve weaknesses in the ACA and the current administration's deep cuts in advertising and outreach during the open enrollment period, a shorter enrollment period, and other administrative actions that may have confused people about the status of the law. They anticipate further erosion of coverage in 2019 due to repeal of the individual mandate penalty, which was a part of the 2017 tax law; actions to increase insurance policies that are not in compliance with the minimum benefits of the ACA; and support for Medicaid work requirements.

Before the passage of the ACA, many at the national level were seriously concerned about the growing cost of medical care as a part of federal expenditures (Orszag, 2007; Orszag & Emanuel, 2010). The concern with the cost of medical care remains a national issue, and Blumenthal and Collins (2014) argued that the sustainability of the expansions of coverage provided by the ACA will depend on whether the overall costs of care in the United States can be controlled. If costs are not controlled, the resulting increases in premiums will become increasingly difficult for all—consumers, employers, and the federal government. Other health system concerns focus on the quality and safety of services, warnings about bioterrorism, and global public health threats such as infectious diseases and contaminated foods. Because of all of these factors, the role of public health in protecting and promoting health, as well as preventing disease and disability, is extremely important.

Whereas the majority of national attention and debate surrounding national health legislation has been focused primarily on insurance issues related to medical care, there are indications of a growing concern about the overall status of the nation's health. In 2013, the Institute of Medicine (IOM) issued a report, *U.S. Health in International Perspective: Shorter Lives, Poorer Health,* which presented some sobering information. The report concluded that "Although Americans' life expectancy and health have improved over the past century, these gains have lagged behind those in other high-income countries. This health disadvantage prevails even though the United States spends far more per person on health care than any other nation." Why is this so? Bradley and Taylor (2013) undertook a study to try to answer that question and concluded that one answer could be that compared to other high-income countries the United States spends less on social services. The IOM report on Shorter Lives and Poorer Health summarizes their findings with this statement, "The U.S. health disadvantage has multiple causes and involves some combination of inadequate health care, unhealthy behaviors, adverse economic and social conditions, and environment factors, as well as public policies and social values that shape those conditions." Thus it is timely to refocus attention on public health, on the concept of population health, which is emerging as a focal point for improving the health of the population, and the opportunities for nurses to be involved in and provide leadership in population health initiatives.

This chapter and others that follow in this book will present information on many factors, perspectives, and strategies related to the protection, maintenance, and improvement of the health of populations. This chapter is focused on three broad topics: **public health** as a broad field of practice that is the backbone of the infrastructure supporting the health of a country, state, province, city, town, or community; **population health,** which can be viewed as a particularly important set of analytical strategies and approaches that was first used in public health to describe, analyze, and mobilize efforts to improve health in community-based populations and is now being used in initiatives to improve outcomes of clinical populations; and a discussion of **public health nursing** and emerging opportunities for nurses practicing in a variety of settings to be engaged in community-based, population-focused efforts to improve the health of populations.

This is a crucial time for public health nursing, a time of opportunity and challenge. The issue of growing costs together with the changing demography of the U.S. population, particularly the aging of the population, is expected to put increased demands on resources available for health care. In addition, the threats of bioterrorism, highlighted by the events of September 11, 2001, and the anthrax scares, will divert health care funds and resources from other health care programs to be spent for public safety. Also important to the public health community is the emergence of modern-day epidemics (such as the mosquito-borne West Nile virus, the H1N1 influenza virus, the opioid epidemic, and gun violence) and globally induced infectious diseases such as avian influenza and other causes of mortality, many of which affect the very young. Most of the causes of these epidemics are preventable. What has all of this to do with nursing?

Understanding the importance of community-oriented, population-focused nursing practice and developing the knowledge and skills to practice it will be critical to attaining a leadership role in health care regardless of the practice setting. The following discussion explains why those who practice community and prevention-oriented, population-focused nursing will be in a very strong position to affect the health of populations and decisions about how scarce resources will be used.

PUBLIC HEALTH PRACTICE: THE FOUNDATION FOR HEALTHY POPULATIONS AND COMMUNITIES

During the last 30 years, considerable attention has been focused on proposals to reform the American health care system. These proposals focused primarily on containing costs in medical care financing and on strategies for providing health insurance coverage to a higher proportion of the population. As discussed earlier, in the national health legislation that passed in

2010, the ACA, the majority of the provisions and the vast majority of the discussion of the bill focused on those issues. While it was important to make reforms in the medical insurance system, there is a clear understanding among those familiar with the history of public health and its impact that such reforms alone will not be adequate to improve the health of Americans.

Historically, gains in the health of populations have come largely from public health efforts. Safety and adequacy of food supplies, the provision of safe water, sewage disposal, public safety from biological threats, and personal behavioral changes, including reproductive behavior, are a few examples of public health's influence. In 2008, Fielding et al. argued that there is indisputable evidence that public health policies and programs were primarily responsible for increasing the average life span from 47 years in 1900 to 78 years in 2005, an increase of 66 percent in just a little over a century. They asserted that most of that increase was through improvements in sanitation, clean water supplies, making workplaces safer, improving food and drug safety, immunizing children, and improving nutrition, hygiene, and housing (Fielding et al., 2008).

In an effort to help the public better understand the role public health has played in increasing life expectancy and improving the nation's health, in 1999, the Centers for Disease Control and Prevention (CDC) began featuring information on the Ten Great Public Health Achievements in the 20th Century. The areas featured include Immunizations, Motor Vehicle Safety, Control of Infectious Diseases, Safer and Healthier Foods, Healthier Mothers and Babies, Family Planning, Fluoridation of Drinking Water, Tobacco as a Health Hazard, and Declines in Deaths From Heart Disease and Stroke (CDC, 2014). A case can be made that the payoff from public health activities is well beyond the resources directed to the effort. For example, data reported by the Centers for Medicare and Medicaid Services (CMS) showed that in 2012 only three percent (up from 1.5 percent in 1960) of all national expenditures supported governmental public health functions (CMS, 2012). The latest data show that in 2017 such expenditures remained at three percent (CMS, 2018).

Unfortunately, the public is largely unaware of the contributions of public health practice. After the passage of Medicare and Medicaid, federal and private monies in support of public health dwindled, public health agencies began to provide personal care services for persons who could not receive care elsewhere, and the health departments benefited by getting Medicaid and Medicare funds. The result was a shift of resources and energy away from public health's traditional and unique prevention-oriented, population-focused perspective to include a primary care focus (U.S. Department of Health and human Services [USDHHS], 2002).

Time will tell whether the gains in insurance coverage due to the ACA will stabilize or whether the reported indication of a decline mentioned above will continue. What happens will have an impact on the activities of public health organizations. If the majority of the population remains covered by insurance, public health agencies will not need to provide direct clinical services in order to ensure that those who need them can receive them. Public health organizations could refocus their efforts on the core functions and emphasize community-oriented, population-focused health promotion and preventive strategies if ways can be found to finance such efforts. An IOM report, *For the Public's Health: Investing in a Healthier Future,* released in 2012, began with a presentation of data showing that in comparison with other wealthy countries, the United States lags well behind its peers on health status while outspending every country in the world on health care. However, a key message was that health-related spending in the United States is primarily expended on clinical care costs for medical and hospital services; very little spending is for public health activities.

A central conclusion of the report was that "to improve health outcomes in the United States, there will need to be a transforming of the way the nation invests in health to pay more attention to population-based prevention efforts; remedy the dysfunctional manner in which public health funding is allocated, structured, and used; and ensure stable funding for public health departments." Further, the committee recommended that "a minimum package of public health services—those foundational and program services needed to promote and protect the public's health"—be developed. The report concluded by recommending that "Congress authorize a dedicated, stable, and long-term financing structure—a national tax on all health care transactions—to generate the enhanced federal revenue required to deliver the minimum package of public health services in every community" (IOM, 2012a). Unfortunately, the CMS data presented earlier clearly show that in the five years between 2012 and 2017 there has not been any overall increase in government funds directed to public health efforts.

Definitions in Public Health

In 1988, the IOM published a report on the future of public health, which is now seen as a classic and influential document. In the report, public health was defined as "what we, as a society, do collectively to assure the conditions in which people can be healthy" (IOM, 1988, p. 1). The committee stated that the mission of public health was "to generate organized community efforts to address the public interest in health by applying scientific and technical knowledge to prevent disease and promote health" (IOM, 1988, p. 1; Williams, 1995).

It was clearly noted that the mission could be accomplished by many groups, public and private, and by individuals. However, the government has a special function "to see to it that vital elements are in place and that the mission is adequately addressed" (IOM, 1988, p. 7). To clarify the government's role in fulfilling the mission, the report stated that assessment, policy development, and assurance are the **public health core functions** at all levels of government:

- **Assessment** refers to systematically collecting data on the population, monitoring the population's health status, and making information available about the health of the community.
- **Policy development** refers to the need to provide leadership in developing policies that support the health of the population,

including the use of the scientific knowledge base in making decisions about policy.

- **Assurance** refers to the role of public health in ensuring that essential community-oriented health services are available, which may include providing essential personal health services for those who would otherwise not receive them. Assurance also refers to making sure that a competent public health and personal health care workforce is available. Fielding, (2009) made the case that assurance also should mean that public health officials should be involved in developing and monitoring the quality of services provided.

Because of the importance of influencing a population's health and providing a strong foundation for the health care system, the U.S. Public Health Service and other groups strongly advocated a renewed emphasis on the population-focused essential public health functions and services that have been most effective in improving the health of the entire population. As part of this effort, a statement on public health in the United States was developed by a working group made up of representatives of federal agencies and organizations concerned about public health. The list of essential services presented in Fig. 1.1 represents the obligations of the public health system to implement the core functions of assessment, assurance, and policy development. The How To box further explains these essential services and lists the ways public health nurses implement them (U.S. Public Health Service, 1994 [updated 2008]; CDC, 2018)

PUBLIC HEALTH IN AMERICA

Vision:

Healthy people in healthy communities

Mission:

Promote physical and mental health and prevent disease, injury, and disability

Public health

- Prevents epidemics and the spread of disease
- Protects against environmental hazards
- Prevents injuries
- Promotes and encourages healthy behaviors
- Responds to disasters and assists communities in recovery
- Ensures the quality and accessibility of health services

Essential public health services by core function

Assessment

1. Monitor health status to identify community health problems
2. Diagnose and investigate health problems and health hazards in the community

Policy Development

3. Inform, educate, and empower people about health issues
4. Mobilize community partnerships to identify and solve health problems
5. Develop policies and plans that support individual and community health efforts

Assurance

6. Enforce laws and regulations that protect health and ensure safety
7. Link people to needed personal health services and assure the provision of health care when otherwise unavailable
8. Assure a competent public health and personal health care workforce
9. Evaluate effectiveness, accessibility, and quality of personal and population-based health services

Serving All Functions

10. Research for new insights and innovative solutions to health problems

Fig. 1.1 Public health in America. (From U.S. Public Health Service: *The core functions project.* Washington, DC, 1994/update 2000, Office of Disease Prevention and Health Promotion. Update 2008, CDC, 2018.)

HOW TO Participate, as a Public Health Nurse, in the Essential Services of Public Health

1. Monitor health status to identify community health problems.
    - Participate in community assessment.
    - Identify subpopulations at risk for disease or disability.
    - Collect information on interventions to special populations.
    - Define and evaluate effective strategies and programs.
    - Identify potential environmental hazards.
2. Diagnose and investigate health problems and hazards in the community.
    - Understand and identify determinants of health and disease.
    - Apply knowledge about environmental influences of health.
    - Recognize multiple causes or factors of health and illness.
    - Participate in case identification and treatment of persons with communicable disease.
3. Inform, educate, and empower people about health issues.
    - Develop health and educational plans for individuals and families in multiple settings.
    - Develop and implement community-based health education.
    - Provide regular reports on health status of special populations within clinic settings, community settings, and groups.
    - Advocate for and with underserved and disadvantaged populations.
    - Ensure health planning, which includes primary prevention and early intervention strategies.
    - Identify healthy population behaviors and maintain successful intervention strategies through reinforcement and continued funding.
4. Mobilize community partnerships to identify and solve health problems.
    - Interact regularly with many providers and services within each community.
    - Convene groups and providers who share common concerns and interests in special populations.
    - Provide leadership to prioritize community problems and development of interventions.
    - Explain the significance of health issues to the public, and participate in developing plans of action.
5. Develop policies and plans that support individual and community health efforts.
    - Participate in community and family decision-making processes.
    - Provide information and advocacy for consideration of the interests of special groups in program development.
    - Develop programs and services to meet the needs of high-risk populations as well as broader community members.
    - Participate in disaster planning and mobilization of community resources in emergencies.
    - Advocate for appropriate funding for services.
6. Enforce laws and regulations that protect health and ensure safety.
    - Regulate and support safe care and treatment for dependent populations such as children and frail older adults.
    - Implement ordinances and laws that protect the environment.
    - Establish procedures and processes that ensure competent implementation of treatment schedules for diseases of public health importance.
    - Participate in development of local regulations that protect communities and the environment from potential hazards and pollution.
7. Link people to needed personal health services, and ensure the provision of health care that is otherwise unavailable.
    - Provide clinical preventive services to certain high-risk populations.
    - Establish programs and services to meet special needs.
    - Recommend clinical care and other services to clients and their families in clinics, homes, and the community.
    - Provide referrals through community links to needed care.
    - Participate in community provider coalitions and meetings to educate others and to identify service centers for community populations.
    - Provide clinical surveillance and identification of communicable disease.
8. Ensure a competent public health and personal health care workforce.
    - Participate in continuing education and preparation to ensure competence.
    - Define and support proper delegation to unlicensed assistive personnel in community settings.
    - Establish standards for performance.
    - Maintain client record systems and community documents.
    - Establish and maintain procedures and protocols for client care.
    - Participate in quality assurance activities such as record audits, agency evaluation, and clinical guidelines.
9. Evaluate effectiveness, accessibility, and quality of personal and population-based health services.
    - Collect data and information related to community interventions.
    - Identify unserved and underserved populations within the community.
    - Review and analyze data on health status of the community.
    - Participate with the community in assessment of services and outcomes of care.
    - Identify and define enhanced services required to manage health status of complex populations and special risk groups.
10. Research for new insights and innovative solutions to health problems.
    - Implement nontraditional interventions and approaches to effect change in special populations.
    - Participate in the collecting of information and data to improve the surveillance and understanding of special problems.
    - Develop collegial relationships with academic institutions to explore new interventions.
    - Participate in early identification of factors that are detrimental to the community's health.
    - Formulate and use investigative tools to identify and impact care delivery and program planning.

Public Health Core Functions

The *Core Functions Project* (U.S. Public Health Service, 1994 [updated 2008]); CDC, 2018) developed a useful illustration, the Health Services Pyramid (Fig. 1.2), which shows that

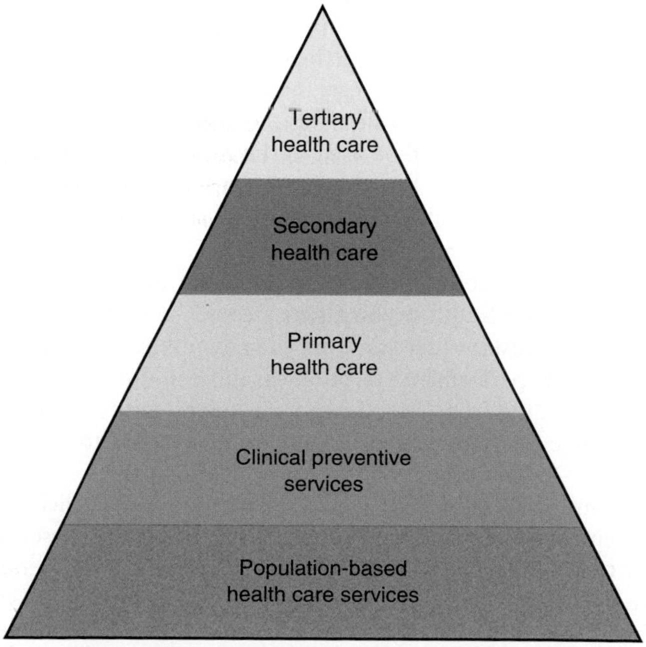

Fig. 1.2 Health Services Pyramid.

population-based public health programs support the goals of providing a foundation for clinical preventive services. These services focus on disease prevention; on health promotion and protection; and on primary, secondary, and tertiary health care services. All levels of services shown in the pyramid are important to the health of the population and thus must be part of a health care system with health as a goal. It has been said that "the greater the effectiveness of services in the lower tiers, the greater is the capability of higher tiers to contribute efficiently to health improvement" (U.S. Public Health Service, 1994 [updated 2008]). Because of the importance of the basic public health programs, members of the Core Functions Project argued that all levels of health care, including population-based public health care, must be funded or the goal of health of populations may never be reached.

Several new efforts to enable public health practitioners to be more effective in implementing the core functions of assessment, policy development, and assurance have been undertaken at the national level. In 1997, the IOM published *Improving Health in the Community: A Role for Performance Monitoring* (IOM, 1997). This monograph was the product of an interdisciplinary committee, co-chaired by a public health nursing specialist and a physician, whose purpose was to determine how a performance-monitoring system could be developed and used to improve community health.

CHECK YOUR PRACTICE

As a student you have been placed on a committee in your community to develop a community health profile. This is being done to focus the public health efforts more on the health of the population. What can you contribute to this committee? Where would you look for data that includes your county's health ranking? What would you do?

The major outcome of the committee's work was the **Community Health Improvement Process (CHIP)**, a method for improving the health of the population on a community-wide basis. The method brings together key elements of the public health and personal health care systems in one framework. A second outcome of the project was the development of a set of 25 indicators that could be used in the community assessment process (see Chapter 17) to develop a community health profile (e.g., measures of health status, functional status, quality of life, health risk factors, and health resource use) (Box 1.1). A third product of the committee's work was a set of indicators for specific public health problems that could be used by public health specialists as they carry out their assurance function and monitor the performance of public health and other agencies.

In 2000, the CDC established a Task Force on Community Preventive Services, which is in place and works to provide evidence-based findings and recommendations about a variety of community preventive services, programs, and policies to prevent morbidity and mortality (CDC, 2014b). The result is *The Community Guide: What Works to Promote Health*, a versatile set of resources available electronically at https://www.thecommunityguide.org that can be used by public health specialists and others interested in a community-level approach to health improvement and disease prevention. A particularly useful interactive Internet-based resource available on the CDC website is the *Community Health Navigator*.

The Navigator can be reached at www.gov. It is an interactive Internet-based resource that allows the user to locate

BOX 1.1 Indicators Used to Develop a Community Health Profile

Sociodemographic Characteristics
- Distribution of the population by age and race/ethnicity
- Number and proportion of persons in groups such as migrants, homeless, or the non–English speaking, for whom access to community services and resources may be a concern
- Number and proportion of persons aged 25 and older with less than a high school education
- Ratio of the number of students graduating from high school to the number of students who entered ninth grade three years previously
- Median household income
- Proportion of children less than 15 years of age living in families at or below the poverty level
- Unemployment rate
- Number and proportion of single-parent families
- Number and proportion of persons without health insurance

Health Status
- Infant death rate by race/ethnicity
- Numbers of deaths or age-adjusted death rates for motor vehicle crashes, work-related injuries, suicide, homicide, lung cancer, breast cancer, cardiovascular diseases, and all causes, by age, race, and sex as appropriate
- Reported incidence of AIDS, measles, tuberculosis, and primary and secondary syphilis, by age, race, and sex as appropriate
- Births to adolescents (ages 10 to 17) as a proportion of total live births
- Number and rate of confirmed abuse and neglect cases among children

Health Risk Factors
- Proportion of two-year-old children who have received all age-appropriate vaccines, as recommended by the Advisory Committee on Immunization Practices
- Proportion of adults aged 65 and older who have ever been immunized for pneumococcal pneumonia; proportion who have been immunized in the past 12 months for influenza
- Proportion of the population who smoke, by age, race, and sex as appropriate
- Proportion of the population aged 18 and older who are obese
- Number and type of U.S. Environmental Protection Agency air quality standards not met
- Proportion of assessed rivers, lakes, and estuaries that support beneficial uses (e.g., approved fishing and swimming)

Health Care Resource Consumption
- Per capita health care spending for Medicare beneficiaries—the Medicare adjusted average per capita cost (AAPCC)

Functional Status
- Proportion of adults reporting that their general health is good to excellent
- Average number of days (in the past 30 days) for which adults report that their physical or mental health was not good

Quality of Life
- Proportion of adults satisfied with the health care system in the community
- Proportion of persons satisfied with the quality of life in the community

AIDS, Acquired immunodeficiency syndrome.

evidence-based interventions depending on a variety of factors: type of risk factor, target population, outcome desired, intervention setting, intervention type, and assets. The information provided, which includes systematic reviews of research, can be used to help make choices about policies and programs that have been shown to be effective.

Core Competencies of Public Health Professionals

To improve the public health workforce's abilities to implement the core functions of public health and to ensure that the workforce has the necessary skills to provide the 10 essential services listed in Fig. 1.1, a coalition of representatives from 17 national public health organizations (the Council of Linkages) began working in 1992 on collaborative activities to "assure a well-trained, competent workforce and a strong, evidence-based public health infrastructure" (U.S. Public Health Service, 1994 [updated 2008]). In the spring of 2010, the Council, funded by the CDC and USDHHS, adopted an updated set of Core Competencies ("a set of skills desirable for the broad practice of public health") for all public health professionals, including nurses. In 2014, the Core Competencies were updated again (Council on Linkages, 2010/2014). The 72 Core Competencies are divided into 8 categories (Box 1.2). In addition, each competency is presented at three levels (tiers), which reflect the different stages of a career. Specifically, Tier 1 applies to entry-level public health professionals without management responsibilities. Tier 2 competencies are expected in those with management and/or supervisory responsibilities, and Tier 3 is expected of senior managers and/or leaders in public health organizations. It is recommended that these categories of competencies be used by educators for curriculum review and development and by agency administrators for workforce needs assessment, competency development, performance evaluation, hiring, and refining of the personnel system job requirements. A detailed listing of the 2014 competencies can be found at www.phf.org.

A coalition of public health nursing organizations initially called the **Quad Council** developed descriptions of skills to be attained by public health nurses for each of the public health core competencies. Skill levels are specified and have been updated for nurses by the Quad Council Coalition in three tiers: the generalist/public health staff nurse (Tier 1); the public health staff nurse with an array of program implementation, management, and supervisory responsibilities, including clinical services, home visiting, community-based, and population-focused programs (Tier 2); and the public health nurse at an executive or senior management level and leadership levels in public health or community organizations (Tier 3) (Quad Council Coalition, 2018). (See Resource Tool 45.A on the Evolve website for the Public Health Nursing Core Competencies.)

BOX 1.2 Categories of Public Health Workforce Competencies

- Analytic/assessment
- Policy development/program planning
- Communication
- Cultural competency
- Community dimensions of practice
- Basic public health sciences
- Financial planning and management
- Leadership and systems thinking

Compiled from www.phf.org

Quality Improvement Efforts in Public Health

In 2003, the IOM released a report, "Who Will Keep the Public Healthy?" that identified eight content areas in which public health workers should be educated—informatics, genomics, cultural competence, community-based participatory research, policy, law, global health, and ethics—in order to be able to address the emerging public health issues and advances in science and policy.

Two broad efforts designed to enhance quality improvement efforts in public health have been developed within the last 20 years: the National Public Health Performance Standards program and the accreditation process for local and state health departments. The National Public Health Performance Standards (NPHPS) program is a high-level partnership initiative started in 1998 and led by the Office of Chief of Public Health Practice, CDC. The collaborative partners are the American Public Health Association (APHA), Association of State and Territorial Health Officials, National Association of County and City Health Officials, National Association of Local Boards of Health, National Network of Public Health Institutes, and the Public Health Foundation. The NPHPS "provide a framework to assess capacity and performance of public health systems and public health governing bodies." The program is "to improve the practice of public health, the performance of public health systems, and the infrastructure supporting public health actions" (CDC, 2014). The performance standards, collectively developed by the participating organizations, set the bar for the level of performance that is necessary to deliver essential public health services. Four principles guided the development of the standards. First, they were developed around the 10 essential public health services (see the How To box on p. 5). Second, the standards focus on the overall public health system rather than on single organizations. Third, the standards describe an optimal level of performance. Finally, they are intended to support a process of quality improvement.

States and local communities seeking to assess their performance can access the assessment instruments developed by the program and other resources such as training workshops, on-site training, and technical assistance to work with them in conducting assessments (CDC, 2014a).

Public Health 3.0

The Public Health 3.0 initiative, which represents a call to action for public health to regenerate and refocus to meet the challenges of the twenty-first century, emerged after the growing recognition that there are troubling indicators regarding the health of Americans. For example, the CDC reported in 2014 that the historical gains in longevity had plateaued for three years in a row (Murphy et al., 2014). It is important to note that more recent data discussed by Woolf in an editorial in the *British Journal of Medicine* (2018) shows that life expectancy in the United States is actually beginning to decline. Other data have shown wide variations in life expectancy between those with the highest incomes and lowest incomes in some communities, while the variation was small in others (National Center for Health Statistics, 2016). Researchers (Chapman et al., 2015–2016) have shown that life expectancy can vary by up to 20 years in areas only a few miles apart. Such information suggests that more attention needs to be given to the environments in which people live, work, play, and age and requires community-based interventions. In discussing Public Health 3.0, DeSalvo et al. argue that in dealing with the challenges presented by such disturbing population data an approach that goes beyond health care is called for and requires community-based interventions. These factors that influence an individual's health and well-being are now commonly referred to as the **social determinants of health**. They include housing, transportation, environments that are safe, access to healthy foods, economic development, and social support.

Two other factors that have contributed to the development of Public Health 3.0 are policy changes in approaches to payment, that is, efforts to move away from the episodic nonintegrated approach to care to value-based approaches and the continuing limitations in resources available for public health initiatives and limited resources to deal with the social determinants of health. The 2008 recession resulted in reductions in many public health services at the state and local levels, and the very small governmental investment in public health discussed above along with the limited investment of the United States (as compared to other wealthy peer countries) in nonmedical determinants of health such as social services, housing, and environmental protection have created a major challenge for those who are concerned about the population's health. These circumstances make putting more emphasis on partnerships and collaborative efforts in addressing community health problems more compelling.

Public Health 3.0 as described by DeSalvo et al. (2017) represents an effort to build on the past and put forth "a new era of enhanced and broadened public health practice that goes beyond traditional public department functions and programs" (p. 4). Key features of the Public Health 3.0 agenda are to focus on prevention at the total population level or community-wide prevention; to improve the social determinants of health; and to engage multiple sectors and community partners to generate collective impact. To accomplish the stated goals a major recommendation is that "Public health leaders should embrace the role of Chief Health Strategists for their communities—working with all relevant partners so that they can drive initiatives, including those that explicitly address 'upstream' social determinants of health" (p. 4).

Population Health

Kindig and Stoddard are credited with publishing the first formal definition of population health in the *American Journal of Public Health* in 2003. Their definition is "the health outcomes of a group of individuals, including the distribution of such outcomes within the group" (p. 1).

With the growing popularity and use of the term *population health* has come confusion about the meaning of the term. Some of this confusion can be resolved by being descriptive about the type of population whose health is being considered. For example, those in public health primarily focus on community-based populations defined in geographic terms, such as those residing in a particular country, state, county, city, or a specific community. Whereas those working in a health care institution such as a hospital or health care system may define the population as those who are receiving or did receive care in their system or institution, which would constitute a clinical population. An example of a definition that focuses on a geographic population is the consensus definition developed by a group of public health and health care stakeholders convened by the Health Policy Institute of Ohio. Their definition of population health is "The distribution of health outcomes across a geographically defined group which results from the interaction between individual biology and behavior, the social, familial, cultural, economic and physical environments that support or hinder wellbeing; and the effectiveness of the public health and health care systems" (Center for Health Affairs, 2017).

Although the health of community-based populations has historically been the focus of public health practice, specifically defined populations of patients/clients, potential or actual, are increasingly becoming a focus of the "business" of managed care. As a result, managed care executives, program managers, and others associated with health care organizations are joining public health practitioners in becoming population-oriented. They and the consultants they hire are beginning to apply the biostatistical and analytical tools of the field of public health. However, their focus is on using such epidemiologic, statistical, and information science strategies to develop databases and analytical approaches to developing information useful in making decisions for defined populations enrolled in their care delivery organization or those covered by a particular insurance company or Medicare or Medicaid. This focus on clinical populations can be described as **population health management**. A population-focused approach to planning, delivering, and evaluating various interventions, whether they be community-wide or programs of care delivered by a hospital or hospital system, is increasingly being used in an effort to achieve better outcomes in the population of interest and has never been more important.

The concept of population health is relevant to populations defined in a variety of ways beyond those in a geographic jurisdiction or those receiving care from a particular care facility and can be applied to various groups such as workers/employees and students in a school setting. In order to be clear about what population is being considered by indicating that a specific population should be identified and to focus on the health of the population rather than the many factors responsible for that health, Williams proposed in a presentation at the spring 2018 meeting of the Association of Community Health Educators (ACHNE) the following definition, which is adapted from Kindig and Stoddard: "Population Health is the health status of a defined population of individuals, including the distribution of health status within the group" (Williams, 2018).

In a later discussion with doctoral students, Williams suggested that in view of all of the activity and "buzz" around the concept of population health it appears that *population health could also be seen as an emerging field within the health sciences that includes ways of defining health status, determinants of the population's health, policies and interventions that link those factors, and biostatistical and analytical strategies and approaches to describe, analyze, and mobilize collaborative, interdisciplinary, and cross-sector efforts to improve health in a defined population.*

The idea of looking at the health of populations is not new; epidemiologists have been doing this for many years, but what is different now and makes the effort much more feasible, practical, and useful is the use of technology in gathering, processing, analyzing, displaying, and sharing the data. In the not-too-distant past it was necessary to rely on very basic hand counts or paper records that were processed by hand and involved the investment of much time and a considerable lag between when the data were originally obtained and when they could be available for decision making. With the development of information technology—computers, handheld devices, and amazing software—it is now becoming increasing possible to look at population health data in ways that are practical, useful, and actionable.

Examples of Public Accessible Electronic Databases for Assessment of Population Health at the National, State, and County Level

The availability of interactive databases that has made it more feasible for public health practitioners and others to have access to population health data that they can actually use to understand what is happening in their state and community. Two such databases are Healthy People 2020 and County Health Rankings. Healthy People focuses on national level data, but for some of the areas examined state level data are available. In Healthy People 2020 (https://www.healthypeople.gov), 42 topic areas are examined—for each topic area, national objectives to be reached over the period of 10 years (from 2010 to 2020) are stated. In addition, a subset of high-priority topics/metrics referred to as leading indicators have been identified. Several of the leading indicators are infant deaths (under one year) per 1000; suicide per 100,000; obesity among adults per 100; and adolescent cigarette smoking in the past 30 days per 100. A very important part of the Healthy People initiative is the identification of recommended evidence-based interventions that can be used to address each of the objectives. The information on evidence-based recommendations and tools to assess community needs, create and implement program plans, and monitor community progress are also available on the website under the Tools and Resources tab. In January 2017, a midcourse review of data on progress toward the 2020 goals became available. Work is already under way to develop the goals and objectives for Healthy People 2030.

The County Health Rankings and Roadmaps (www.countyhealthrankings.org) is an interactive database that provides information at the state and county levels on Health Outcomes (length of life and quality of life); Health Factors (health behaviors—tobacco use, diet and exercise, alcohol and drug use, and social activity); Clinical Care (access to care and quality of care); Social and Economic Factors (education, employment, income, family and social support, and community safety); and Physical Environment (air and water quality, and housing and transit). In addition, there is a searchable database of evidence-informed policies and programs (road maps) that can make a difference. Other features are the Action Center, which helps users move from data to action at the community level; a Partner Center, which helps users identify possible partners and provides tips for engaging them; and Community Coaches, which can provide guidance to local communities to assist them in their efforts to make change. The user of the website can compare data on a given county with other counties in their state, with data at the state level, and with counties in other states. This website is a collaboration between the Robert Wood Johnson Foundation and the University of Wisconsin Population Health Institute.

PUBLIC HEALTH NURSING AS A FIELD OF PRACTICE: AN AREA OF SPECIALIZATION

Most of the preceding discussion has been about the broad field of public health. Now attention turns to **public health nursing**. What is public health nursing? Is it really a specialty, and if so, why? It can be argued that public health nursing is a specialty because it has a distinct focus and scope of practice, and it requires a special knowledge base. The following characteristics distinguish public health nursing as a specialty:

- *It is population-focused.* Primary emphasis is on populations whose members are free-living in the community as opposed to those who are institutionalized.
- *It is community-oriented.* There is concern for the connection between the health status of the population and the environment in which the population lives (physical, biological, sociocultural). There is an imperative to work with members of the community to carry out core public health functions.
- *There is a health and prevention focus.* The primary emphasis is on strategies for health promotion, health maintenance, and disease prevention, particularly primary and secondary prevention.
- *Interventions are made at the community or population level.* Target populations are defined as those living in a particular geographic area or those who have particular characteristics in common, and political processes are used as a major intervention strategy to affect public policy and achieve goals.
- *There is concern for the health of all members of the population/community, particularly vulnerable subpopulations.*

In 1981, the Public Health Nursing Section of the American Public Health Association (APHA) developed *The Definition and Role of Public Health Nursing in the Delivery of Health Care* to describe the field of specialization (APHA, 1981). This statement was reaffirmed in 1996 (APHA, 1996). In 1999, the American Nurses Association, with input from three other nursing organizations—the Public Health Nursing Section of the APHA, the Association of State and Territorial Directors of

Public Health Nursing, and the Association of Community Health Nurse Educators—published the *Scope and Standards of Public Health Nursing Practice* (Quad Council, 1999 [revised 2005]). In that document, the 1996 definition was supported. Since 1999, the scope and standards have been revised twice. In the latest version Public Health Nursing continues to be defined as "the practice of promoting and protecting the health of populations using knowledge from nursing, social, and public health sciences" (APHA, 1996; and Quad Council, 1999 [revised 2005], 2011), but the following statement was added in 2011: "Public Health Nurses engage in population-focused practice, but can and do often apply the Council of Linkages concepts at the individual and family level" (see Quad Council, 2011, p. 9). In 2018, the Quad Council Coalition (QCC) of Public Health Nursing Organizations, which is comprised of the Alliance of Nurses for Healthy Environments (AHNE), the Association of Community Health Nursing Educators (ACHNE), the Association of Public Health Nurses (APHN), and the American Public Health Association—Public Health Nursing Section (APHA-PHN), published an update of Competencies for Community/Public Health Nurses (Quad Council Coalition, 2018) and adopted the APHA-PHN's 2013 definition of Public Health Nursing, which is "the practice of promoting and protecting the health of populations using knowledge from nursing, social, and public health sciences. Public health nursing is a specialty practice within nursing and public health. It focuses on improving *population health* by emphasizing prevention and attending to multiple determinants of health. Often used interchangeably with community health nursing, this nursing practice includes advocacy, policy development, and planning, which addresses issues of social justice" (APHA-PHN, 2013).

Educational Preparation for Public Health Nursing

Targeted and specialized education for public health nursing practice has a long history. In the late 1950s and early 1960s, before the integration of public health concepts into the curriculum of baccalaureate nursing programs, special baccalaureate curricula were established in several schools of public health to prepare nurses to become public health nurses. Today it is generally assumed that a graduate of any baccalaureate nursing program has the necessary basic preparation to function as a beginning staff public health nurse.

Since the late 1960s, public health nursing leaders have agreed that a specialty in public health nursing requires a master's degree. In the future, a Doctor of Nursing Practice (DNP) degree will probably be expected, since the American Association of Colleges of Nursing has proposed that the DNP should be the expected level of education for specialization in an area of nursing practice (AACN, 2004, 2006). The educational expectations for public health nursing were highlighted at the 1984 Consensus Conference on the Essentials of Public Health Nursing Practice and Education sponsored by the USDHHS Division of Nursing. The participants agreed "that the term 'public health nurse' should be used to describe a person who has received specific educational preparation and supervised clinical practice in public health nursing" (USDHHS, 1985, p. 4). At the basic or entry level a public health nurse is one who "holds a baccalaureate degree in nursing that includes this educational preparation; this nurse may or may not practice in an official health agency but has the initial qualifications to do so" (USDHHS, 1985, p. 4). Specialists in public health nursing are defined as those who are prepared at the graduate level, with either a master's or doctoral degree, "with a focus in the public health sciences" (USDHHS, 1985, p. 4) (Box 1.3). The consensus statement specifically pointed out that the public health nursing specialist "should be able to work with population groups and to assess and intervene successfully at the aggregate level" (USDHHS, 1985, p. 11).

BOX 1.3 Areas Considered Essential for the Preparation of Specialists in Public Health Nursing

- Epidemiology
- Biostatistics
- Nursing theory
- Management theory
- Change theory
- Economics
- Politics
- Public health administration
- Community assessment
- Program planning and evaluation
- Interventions at the aggregate level
- Research
- History of public health
- Issues in public health

From *Consensus Conference on the Essentials of Public Health Nursing Practice and Education,* Rockville, MD, 1985, U.S. Department of Health and Human Services, Bureau of Health Professions, Division of Nursing.

The ACHNE reaffirmed the results of the 1984 Consensus Conference (ACHNE, 2003). The educational requirements were reaffirmed by ACHNE (2009) and in the revised *Scope and Standards of Public Health Nursing Practice* and include both clinical specialists and nurse practitioners who engage in population-focused care as advanced practice registered nurses in public health (Quad Council, 1999 [revised 2005]). The latest iteration of the *Scope and Standards of Practice for Public Health Nursing* was published by the American Nurses Association in 2013 (ANA, 2013).

Population-Focused Practice Versus Practice Focused on Individuals

A key factor that distinguishes public health nursing from other areas of nursing practice is the focus on populations, a focus historically consistent with public health philosophy and a cornerstone of population health. Box 1.4 lists principles on which public health nursing is built. Although public health nursing is based on clinical nursing practice, it also incorporates the population perspective of public health. It may be helpful here to define the term *population.*

A **population**, or **aggregate**, is a collection of individuals who have one or more personal or environmental characteristics in common. Members of a community who can be defined in terms of geography (e.g., a county, a group of counties, or a state) or in terms of a special interest or circumstance (e.g., children attending a particular school) can be seen as constituting a population.

BOX 1.4 Eight Principles of Public Health Nursing

1. The client or "unit of care" is the population.
2. The primary obligation is to achieve the greatest good for the greatest number of people or the population as a whole.
3. The processes used by public health nurses include working with the client(s) as an equal partner.
4. Primary prevention is the priority in selecting appropriate activities.
5. Selecting strategies that create healthy environmental, social, and economic conditions in which populations may thrive is the focus.
6. There is an obligation to actively reach out to all who might benefit from a specific activity or service.
7. Optimal use of available resources to assure the best overall improvement in the health of the population is a key element of the practice.
8. Collaboration with a variety of other professions, organizations, and entities is the most effective way to promote and protect the health of the people.

Quad Council of Public Health Nursing Organizations: *Scope and standards of public health nursing practice,* Washington, DC, 1999, revised 2005, 2007, 2013 with the American Nurses Association.

Often there are **subpopulations** or high-risk groups within the larger population, such as high-risk infants under the age of one year, unmarried pregnant adolescents, or individuals exposed to a particular event such as a chemical spill. In **population-focused and community-based practice**, problems are defined (by assessments or diagnoses) and solutions (interventions), such as policy development or providing a particular preventive service, are implemented for or with a defined population or subpopulation (examples are provided in the **Levels of Prevention** box). In other nursing specialties the diagnoses, interventions, and treatments are usually carried out at the individual client level. However, with the adoption of population health strategies by those working with clinical populations—population health management—this is beginning to change. Specifically, in some clinical settings population health management efforts are being developed in which patients with a common set of problems or conditions are defined as a population, and a defined set of services are offered to the entire population or a specific set of services are offered to those at varying levels of risk.

LEVELS OF PREVENTION

Examples in Public Health Nursing

Primary Prevention

Using general and specific measures in a population to promote health and prevent the development of disease (incidence) and using specific measures to prevent diseases in those who are predisposed to developing a particular condition.

Example: The public health nurse develops a health education program for a population of school-age children that teaches them about the effects of smoking on health.

Secondary Prevention

Stopping the progress of disease by early detection and treatment, thus reducing prevalence and chronicity.

Example: The public health nurse develops a program of toxin screenings for migrant workers who may be exposed to pesticides and refers for treatment those who are found to be positive for high levels.

Tertiary Prevention

Stopping deterioration in a patient, a relapse, or disability and dependency by anticipatory nursing and medical care.

Example: The public health nurse provides leadership in mobilizing a community coalition to develop a Health Maintenance and Promotion Center to be located in a neighborhood with a high density of residents with chronic illnesses and few health education and appropriate recreation resources. In addition to educational programs for nutrition and self-care, physical activity programs such as walking groups are provided.

Professional education in nursing, medicine, and other clinical disciplines focuses primarily on developing competence in decision making at the individual client level by assessing health status, making management decisions (ideally *with* the client), and evaluating the effects of care. Fig. 1.3 illustrates three levels at which problems can be identified. For example, community-based nurse clinicians, or nurse practitioners, focus on individuals they see in either a home or a clinic setting. The focus is on an individual person or an individual family in a subpopulation (the *C* arrows in Fig. 1.3). The provider's emphasis is on defining and resolving a problem for the individual; the client is an individual.

In Fig. 1.3 the individual clients are grouped into three separate subpopulations, each of which has a common characteristic (the *B* arrows in Fig. 1.3). Public health nursing specialists often define problems at the population or aggregate level as opposed to an individual level. Population-level decision making is different from decision making in clinical care. For example, in a clinical, direct care situation, the nurse may determine that a client is hypertensive and explore options for intervening. However, at the population level, the public health nursing specialist might explore the answers to the following set of questions:

1. What is the prevalence of hypertension among various age, race, and sex groups?
2. Which subpopulations have the highest rates of untreated hypertension?
3. What programs could reduce the problem of untreated hypertension and thereby lower the risk of further cardiovascular morbidity and mortality for the population as a whole?

Public health nursing specialists are usually concerned with more than one subpopulation and frequently with the health of the entire community (in Fig. 1.3, arrow *A:* the entire box containing all of the subgroups within the community). In reality, of course, there are many more subgroups than those in Fig. 1.3. Professionals concerned with the health of a whole community must consider the total population, which is made up of multiple and often overlapping subpopulations. For example, the population of adolescents at risk for unplanned pregnancies would overlap with the female population 15 to 24 years of age. A population that would overlap with infants under one year of age would be children from zero to six years of age. In addition, a population focus requires considering those who may need particular services but have not entered the health care system (e.g., children without immunizations or clients with untreated hypertension).

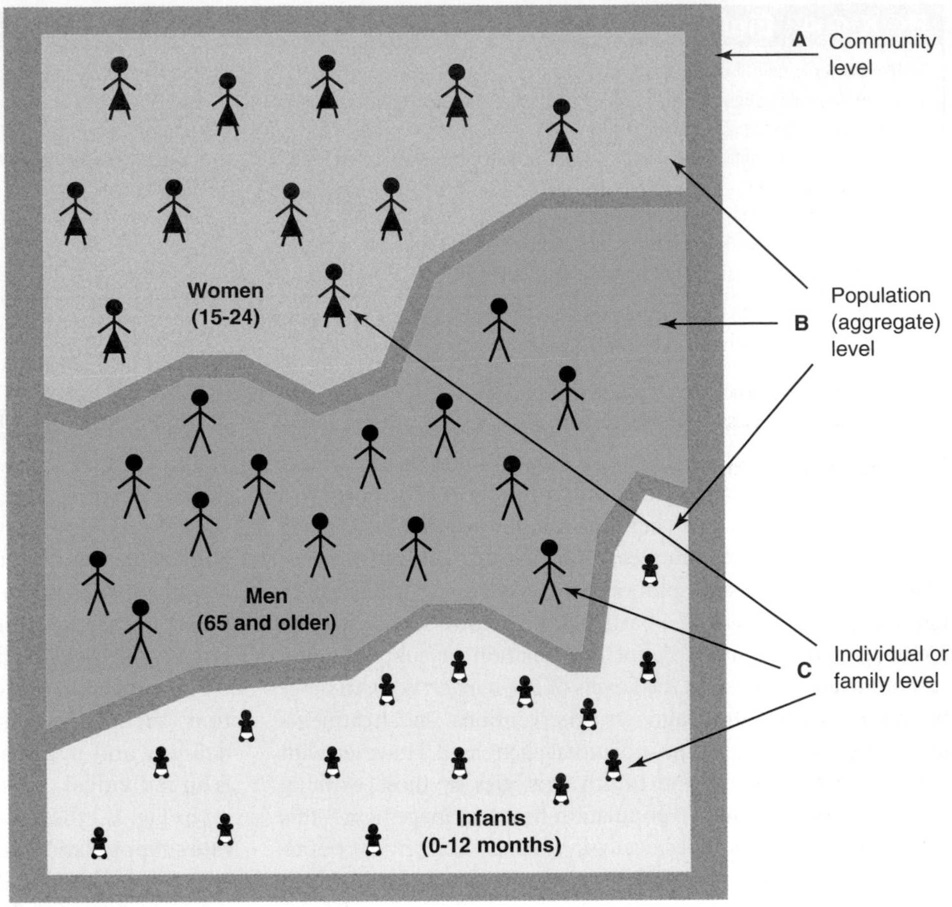

Fig. 1.3 Levels of health care practice.

Public Health Nursing Specialists and Core Public Health Functions: Selected Examples

The core public health function of *assessment* includes activities that involve collecting, analyzing, and disseminating information on both the health status and the health-related aspects of a community or a specific population. Questions such as whether the health services of the community are available to the population and are adequate to address needs are considered. Assessment also includes an ongoing effort to monitor the health status of the community or population and the services provided. As described earlier in this chapter, Healthy People is an excellent example of the efforts of the USDHHS to organize the goal setting, data collecting and analysis, and monitoring necessary to develop the series of publications describing the health status and health-related aspects of the U.S. population. These efforts began with *Healthy People: The Surgeon General's Report on Health Promotion and Disease Prevention* in 1980 and continued with *Promoting Health/Preventing Disease: Objectives for the Nation, Healthy People 2000, Healthy People 2010,* and *Healthy People 2020*, and are now moving forward into the future with *Healthy People 2030* (U.S. Department of Health, Education, and Welfare, 1979; USDHHS, 1980, 1979, 1991, 2000, 2010, 2020; *Healthy People 2030* retrieved from https://www.healthypeople.gov).

In addition to the County Health Rankings described earlier, many states and other jurisdictions have developed publications describing the health status of a defined community, a set of communities, or populations. Unfortunately, it is difficult to find published descriptions of health assessments on particular communities unless they demonstrate new methods or reveal unusual findings about a community. Such working documents and data sets should be available in specific settings, such as a county or state health department, and should be used by public health practitioners to develop services.

EVIDENCE-BASED PRACTICE

This study was a quasi-experimental pre-post design with no control group. The study sample consisted of 21 community institutions (7 hospitals, 8 YMCAs, 4 community health centers, and 2 organizations serving homeless populations). All Boston hospitals were invited to participate because they have an employee base that includes many lower-wage workers who live in the priority neighborhoods. The other settings were selected from priority neighborhoods defined as those with the highest proportion of black and Latino residents and a disproportionate chronic disease burden. The researchers estimated that about 78,000 people were reached by the intervention every week.

The goal was to reduce the percent of prepackaged foods available at the sites with greater than 200 milligrams (mg) of sodium; thus the outcome measure was the change in the percent of prepackaged foods with greater than 200 mg per serving from baseline to follow-up. The intervention consisted of education provided by registered dietitians to the food service directors at the sites, feedback on

EVIDENCE-BASED PRACTICE—cont'd

baseline assessment of levels of sodium in products available at each site and how they compared with other organizations in their sector, an action plan at each site for goal setting, technical assistance that included webinars on how they could support the desired changes, and educational materials to identify healthy, lower-sodium options and to increase consumer awareness of the health effects associated with excess sodium. The intervention period ranged from 1 to 1.5 years. Overall the percent of prepackaged products with greater than 200 mg of sodium decreased from 29.0 percent at baseline to 21.5 percent at follow-up ($P = .003$) Those changes were found to be due to improvements in the hospital cafeterias and kiosks. In the YMCA vending machines the percent of high-sodium products decreased from 27.2 percent to 11.5 percent ($P = .017$). While declines were observed in the vending machines in the community health centers and the organizations serving the homeless, they were not statistically significant due to the small sample sizes. While the study has the limitation of not having a control group, it cannot be said whether the changes were from the intervention or due to secular trends. However, the investigators had documented information that the sites made intentional decisions to produce the outcome. The study also is limited in not including any information on consumption behavior. The study provides information on the feasibility and modest effectiveness of a community-level intervention to increase the availability of lower sodium products in the food supply.

Nurse Use

This study indicates that there is potential to reduce the public's access to high-sodium products by providing options with less sodium, which can be useful in nurse-led public policy advocacy for healthier options in vending machines in schools and public buildings.

Brooks CJ, Barret J, Daly J, et al.: A community-level sodium reduction intervention, Boston, 2013-2015, *Am J Public Health* (12)107:1951-1957, 2017.

Policy development is both a core function of public health and a core intervention strategy used by public health nursing specialists. Policy development in the public arena seeks to build constituencies that can help bring about change in public policy. In an interesting case study of her experience as director of public health for the state of Oregon, Christine Gebbie (1999), a nurse, describes her experiences in developing a constituency for public health. This enabled her to mobilize efforts to develop statewide goals for *Healthy People 2000* as well as to update Oregon's disease-reporting laws. Gebbie's experiences as a state director of public health illustrate how a public health nursing specialist can provide leadership at a very broad level. Gebbie left Oregon to go to Washington, DC, to serve in the federal government as President Clinton's key official in the national effort to control acquired immunodeficiency syndrome (AIDS). Clearly, Gebbie is an example of an individual who has provided leadership in policy development at both state and national levels. Another public health nursing specialist who has provided and continues to provide strong policy leadership is Ellen Hahn, PhD, director of the Kentucky Center for Smoke Free Policy (https://www.uky.edu), which is based at the University of Kentucky's College of Nursing. This website is a treasure trove of information about reducing exposure to tobacco through advocacy and policy. There are fact sheets, videos, and research studies. Through her research Dr. Hahn has developed considerable evidence to support important policy changes (antismoking ordinances) to reduce exposure to tobacco smoke in Kentucky, a state that has a long tradition of a tobacco culture, both in production of tobacco and in use. A number of studies conducted by Hahn and her colleagues can be found on the website above.

The third core public health function, *assurance,* focuses on the responsibility of public health agencies to make certain that activities have been appropriately carried out to meet public health goals and plans. This may result in public health agencies requiring others to engage in activities to meet goals, encouraging private groups to undertake certain activities, or sometimes actually offering services directly. Assurance also includes the development of partnerships between public and private agencies to make sure that needed services are available and that assessing the quality of the activities is carried out. A report suggested that much more attention should be paid by public health officials to the quality of direct care services provided by clinicians in their communities (Fielding, 2009). It is important to point out that when personal services to individuals are offered by public health agencies to ensure that they can get care they might not receive without the intervention of the official agency, the goal is to "promote knowledge, attitudes, beliefs, practices and behaviors that support and enhance health with the ultimate goal of improving … population health" (Quad Council, 1999 [revised 2005]; and see Evidence-Based Practice box).

HEALTHY PEOPLE 2020

In 1979, the surgeon general issued a report that began a 30-year focus on promoting health and preventing disease for all Americans. The report, entitled *Healthy People,* used morbidity rates to track the health of individuals through the five major life cycles of infancy, childhood, adolescence, adulthood, and older age.

In 1989, *Healthy People 2000* became a national effort of representatives from government agencies, academia, and health organizations. Their goal was to present a strategy for improving the health of the American people. Their objectives were being used by public and community health organizations to assess current health trends, health programs, and disease prevention programs.

Throughout the 1990s, all states used *Healthy People 2000* objectives to identify emerging public health issues. The success of the program on a national level was accomplished through state and local efforts. Early in the 1990s, surveys from public health departments indicated that 8 percent of the national objectives had been met, and progress on an additional 40 percent of the objectives was noted. In the midcourse review published in 1995, it was noted that significant progress had been made toward meeting 50 percent of the objectives.

In light of the progress made in the past decade, the committee for *Healthy People 2010* proposed two goals. The hope was to reach these goals by such measures as promoting healthy behaviors, increasing access to quality health care, and strengthening community prevention.

The major premise of *Healthy People 2010* was that the health of the individual cannot be entirely separate from the health of the larger community. Therefore the vision for *Healthy People 2010* was "Healthy People in Healthy Communities."

The vision for *Healthy People 2020* is a society in which all people live long, healthy lives (https://www.healthypeople.gov).

PUBLIC HEALTH NURSING VERSUS COMMUNITY-BASED NURSING

The concept of public health should include all populations within the community, both free-living and those living in institutions. Furthermore, the public health specialist should consider the match between the health needs of the population and the health care resources in the community, including those services offered in a variety of settings. Although all direct care providers may contribute to the community's health in the broadest sense, not all are primarily concerned with the population focus—the big picture. All nurses in a given community, including those working in hospitals, physicians' offices, and health clinics, may contribute positively to the health of the community. However, the special contributions of public health nursing specialists include looking at the community or population as a whole; raising questions about its overall health status and associated factors, including environmental factors (physical, biological, and sociocultural); and *working with the community* to improve the population's health status.

Fig. 1.4 is a useful illustration of the arenas of practice. Because most nurses working in the community and many staff public health nurses, historically and at present, focus on providing direct personal care services—including health education—to persons or family units outside of institutional settings (either in the client's home or in a clinic environment), such practice falls into the upper right quadrant (section *B*) of Fig. 1.4. However, specialization in public health nursing is population-focused and focuses on clients living in the community and is represented by the box in the upper left quadrant (section *A*).

There are three reasons, in addition to the population focus, that the most important practice arena for public health nursing is represented by section *A* of Fig. 1.4, the population of free-living clients:

1. Preventive strategies can have the greatest impact on free-living populations, which usually represent the majority of a community.
2. The major interface between health status and the environment (physical, biological, sociocultural, and behavioral) occurs in the free-living population.
3. For philosophical, historical, and economic reasons, prevention-oriented, population-focused practice is most likely to flourish in organizational structures that serve free-living populations (e.g., health departments, health maintenance organizations, health centers, schools, and workplaces).

What roles in the health care system do public health nursing specialists (those in section *A* of Fig. 1.4) have? Options include director of nursing for a health department, director of the health department, state commissioner for health, director of maternal and child health services for a state or local health department, director of wellness for a business or educational organization, and director of preventive services for an integrated health system. Nurses can occupy all of these roles, but, with the exception of director of nursing for a health department, they are in the minority. Unfortunately, nurses who occupy these roles are often seen as "administrators" and not as public health nursing specialists. However, those who work in such roles have the opportunity to make decisions that affect the health of population groups and the type and quality of health services provided for various populations.

Where does the staff public health nurse or nurse working in the community fit on the diagram in Fig. 1.4? That depends on the focus of the nurse's practice. In many settings most of the staff nurse's time is spent in community-based direct care activities, where the focus is on dealing with individual clients and individual families, in which case the practice falls into section *B* of Fig. 1.4. Although a staff public health nurse or a nurse practicing in the community may not be a public health nurse specialist, this nurse may spend some time carrying out core public health functions with a population focus, and thus that part of the role would be represented in section *A* of Fig. 1.4. In summary, the field of public health nursing can be seen as primarily encompassing two groups of nurses:

- Public health nursing specialists, whose practice is community-oriented and uses population-focused strategies

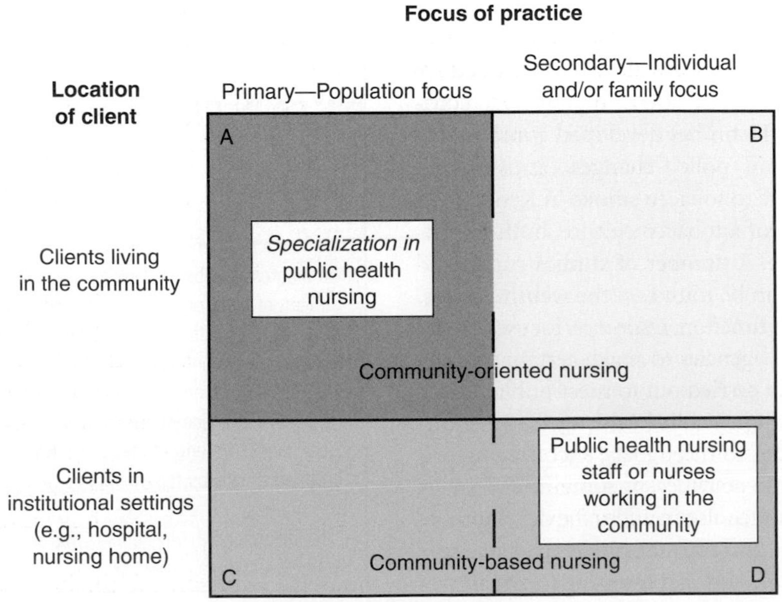

Fig. 1.4 Arenas for health care practice.

for carrying out the core public health functions (section *A* of Fig. 1.4)

- Staff public health nurses or clinical nurses working in the community nurses, who are community-based, who may be clinically oriented to the individual client, and who combine some primary preventive population-focused strategies and direct care clinical strategies in programs serving specified populations (section *B* of Fig. 1.4)

Sections *C* and *D* of Fig. 1.4 represent institutionalized populations. Nurses who provide direct care to these clients in hospital settings fall into section *D*, and those who have administrative/managerial responsibility for nursing services in institutional settings fall into section *C*.

Fig. 1.4 also shows that specialization in public health nursing, as it has been defined in this chapter, can be viewed as a specialized field of practice with certain characteristics within the broad arena of community. This view is consistent with recommendations developed at the Consensus Conference on the Essentials of Public Health Nursing Practice and Education (USDHHS, 1985). One of the outcomes of the historical conference was consensus on the use of the terms *community health nurse* and *public health nurse*. It was agreed that the term *community health nurse* could apply to all nurses who practice in the community, whether or not they have had preparation in public health nursing. Thus nurses providing secondary or tertiary care in a home setting, school nurses, and nurses in clinic settings (in fact, any nurse who does not practice in an institutional setting) could fall into the category of **community health nurse**. Nurses with a master's degree or a doctoral degree who practice in community settings could be referred to as *community health nurse specialists*, regardless of the area of nursing in which the degree was earned. According to the conference statement, "The degree could be in any area of nursing, such as maternal/child health, psychiatric/mental health, or medical-surgical nursing or some subspecialty of any clinical area" (USDHHS, 1985, p. 4). The definitions of the three areas of practice have changed, however, over time.

In 1998, the Quad Council began to develop a statement on the scope of public health nursing practice (Quad Council, 1999 [revised 2005]). The council attempted to clarify the differences between the term *public health nursing* and the term introduced into nursing's vocabulary during health care reform of the 1990s: **community-based nursing**. The authors recognized that the terms *public health nursing* and *community health nursing* had been used interchangeably since the 1980s to describe population-focused, community-oriented nursing practice and community-based practice. However, the Council decided to make a clearer distinction between community-oriented and community-based nursing practice. Community-based nursing care was described as the provision or assurance of personal illness care to individuals and families in the community, whereas community-oriented nursing was the provision of disease prevention and health promotion to populations and communities. It was suggested that there be two terms for the two levels of care in the community: *community-oriented care* and *community-based care* (see the list of definitions presented in Box 1.5).

There is a need and a place for a nursing specialty in the community; the nurse in this specialty is more than a clinical specialist with a master's degree who practices in a community-based setting, as was suggested by the Consensus Conference more than 25 years ago. Although in 1984 these nurses were referred to as community health nurses, today they are referred to as nurses in community-based practice (see definitions in the inside cover of this text). Those who provide community-oriented service to specific subpopulations in the community and who provide some clinical services to those populations may be seen as nurse specialists in the community. Although such practitioners may be community-based, they are also community-oriented as public health specialists but are usually focused on only one or two special subpopulations. Preparing for this specialty includes a master's or doctoral degree with emphasis in a direct care clinical area, such as school health or occupational health, and ideally some education in the public health sciences. Examples of roles such specialists might have in direct clinical care areas include case manager, supervisor in a home health agency, school nurse, occupational health nurse, parish nurse, and a nurse practitioner who also manages a nursing clinic.

BOX 1.5 Definitions of the Key Nursing Areas in the Community

- *Community-oriented nursing practice* is a philosophy of nursing service delivery that involves the generalist or specialist public health and community health nurse. The nurse provides health care through community diagnosis and investigation of major health and environmental problems, health surveillance, and monitoring and evaluation of community and population health status for the purposes of preventing disease and disability and promoting, protecting, and maintaining health to create conditions in which people can be healthy.
- *Community-based nursing practice* is a setting-specific practice whereby care is provided for clients and families where they live, work, and attend school. The emphasis of community-based nursing practice is acute and chronic care and the provision of comprehensive, coordinated, and continuous services. Nurses who deliver community-based care are generalists or specialists in maternal/infant, pediatric, adult, or psychiatric/mental health nursing.

ROLES IN PUBLIC HEALTH NURSING

In community-oriented nursing circles, there has been a tendency to talk about public health nursing from the point of view of a role rather than the functions related to the role. This can be limiting. In discussing such nursing roles, there is a preoccupation with the direct care provider orientation. Even in discussions about how a practice can become more population focused, the focus is frequently on how an individual practitioner, such as an agency staff nurse, can adopt a population-focused practice philosophy. Rarely is attention given to how nurse administrators in public health (one role for public health nursing specialists) might reorient their practice toward a population focus, which is particularly important and easier for an administrator to do than for the staff nurse. This is because many agencies' nursing administrators, supervisors, or others (sometimes program directors who are not nurses) make the key decisions about how staff nurses will spend their time and what types of clients will be seen and under what circumstances. Public health nursing administrators who are prepared to practice in a population-focused manner will be more effective than those who are not prepared to do so.

Although their opportunities to make decisions at the population level are limited, staff nurses benefit from having a clear understanding of population-focused practice for three reasons:

- First, it gives them professional satisfaction to see how their individual client care contributes to health at the population level.
- Second, it helps them appreciate the practice of others who are population-focused specialists.
- Third, it gives them a better foundation from which to provide clinical input into decision making at the program or agency level and thus to improve the effectiveness and efficiency of the population-focused practice.

A curriculum was proposed by representatives of key public health nursing organizations and other individuals that would prepare the staff public health nurse or generalist to function as a community-oriented practitioner (Association of State and Territorial Directors of Nursing, 2000). The AACN developed a supplement to the document "The Essentials of Baccalaureate Education for Professional Nursing Practice," which highlights this organization's recommendations for public health nursing (AACN, 2013).

Unfortunately, nursing roles as presently defined are often too limited to include population-focused practice, but it is important not to think too narrowly. Furthermore, roles that entail population-focused decision making may not be defined as nursing roles (e.g., directors of health departments, state or regional programs, and units of health planning and evaluation; directors of programs such as preventive services within a managed care organization). If population-focused public health nursing is to be taken seriously, and if strategies for assessment, policy development, and assurance are to be implemented at the population level, more consideration must be given to organized systems for assessing population needs and managing care. Clearly, public health nurse specialists must move into positions where they can influence policy formation. This means, however, that some nurses will have to assume positions that are not traditionally considered nursing. It also means that some nurses will practice in settings not traditionally considered health organizations, such as nonprofit organizations providing services such as housing, supplemental food, and access to safe physical recreation activities and socialization opportunities.

Redefining nursing roles so that population-focused decision making fits into the present structure of nursing services may be difficult in some circumstances at the present time, but future needs will require that nurses be prepared to make such decisions (IOM, 2010). At this point, it may be more useful to concentrate on identifying the skills and knowledge needed to make decisions in population-focused practice (see Appendix F.1), to define where in the health care system such decisions are made, and then to equip nurses with the knowledge, skills, and political understanding necessary for success in such positions. Although some of these positions are in nursing settings (e.g., administrator of the nursing service and top-level staff nurse supervisors), others are outside of the traditional nursing roles (e.g., director of a health department).

CHALLENGES FOR THE FUTURE

Barriers to Nurses Specializing in Leadership Roles in Population Health Initiatives

One of the most serious barriers to the development of specialists in public health nursing is the mindset of many nurses that the only role for a nurse is at the bedside or at the client's side (i.e., the direct care role). Indeed, the heart of nursing is the direct care provided in personal contacts with clients. On the other hand, two things should be clear. First, whether a nurse is able to provide direct care services to a particular client depends on decisions made by individuals within and outside of the care system. Second, nurses need to be involved in those fundamental decisions. Perhaps the one-on-one focus of nursing and the historical expectations of the "proper" role of women have influenced nurses to view other ways of contributing, such as administration, consultation, and research, less positively. Fortunately, things are changing. Within and outside of nursing, women have taken on every role imaginable. Further, the number of male nurses is steadily growing; nursing can no longer be viewed as a profession practiced by women exclusively. These two developments have opened doors to new roles that may not have been considered appropriate for nurses in the past.

A second barrier to population-focused public health nursing practice consists of the structures within which nurses work and the process of role socialization within those structures. For example, the absence of a particular role in a nursing unit may suggest that the role is undesirable or inaccessible to nurses. In another example, nurses interested in using political strategy to make changes in health-related policy—an activity clearly within the domain of public health nursing—may run into obstacles if their goals differ from those of other groups. Such groups may subtly but effectively lead nurses to conclude that their involvement in political effort takes their attention away from the client and it is not in their own or in the client's best interest to engage in such activities.

A third barrier is that few nurses receive graduate-level preparation in the concepts and strategies of the disciplines basic to public health (e.g., epidemiology, biostatistics, community development, service administration, and policy formation). As mentioned previously, master's-level programs for public health nursing do not give the in-depth attention to population assessment and management skills that other parts of the curriculum receive, such as the direct care aspects. In 1995, Josten et al. noted that, with few exceptions, graduate programs in public health nursing have not aggressively developed the population-focused skills that are needed. After many years of teaching and consulting with graduate programs in public health nursing and DNP programs, it is clear to this writer that the problem Josten et al. pointed out over 20 years ago continues to need attention. For individuals who want to specialize in public health nursing, these skills are as essential as direct care skills, and they should be given more attention in graduate programs that prepare nurses for careers in public health. There is hope. Fortunately, the curricular expectations for academic programs leading to the DNP degree include serious attention to preparing nurses to develop a population perspective as well as the analytical, policy, and leadership skills necessary to be successful as a specialist in public health nursing (AACN, 2006).

Developing Population Health Nurse Leaders

The massive organizational changes occurring in the health delivery system present a unique opportunity to establish new roles for nurse leaders who are prepared to think in population health terms. In a book that is now viewed as a classic, Starr (1982) described the trend toward the use of private capital in financing health care, particularly institution-based care and other health-related businesses. The movement can be thought of as the "industrialization" of health care, which operated very much like a **cottage industry** or a small business for a very long time. The implications and consequences of this movement are enormous. First, the goal was to provide investors a return on their investment. Other aspects included more attention to the delivery of primary and community-based care in a variety of settings; less emphasis on specialty care; the development of partnerships, alliances, and other linkages across settings in an effort to build **integrated systems**, which would provide a broad range of services for the population served; and in some situations adoption of **capitation**, a payment arrangement in which insurers agree to pay providers a fixed sum for each person per month or per year, independent of the costs actually incurred. Initially with the spread of capitation and now with the development by the CMS of value-based reimbursement, health professionals have become more interested in the concept of populations, sometimes referred to by financial officers and others as *covered lives* (i.e., individuals with insurance that pays on a capitated basis). For public health specialists, it is a new experience to see individuals involved in the business aspects of health care, and frequently employed by hospitals, thinking in population terms and taking a population approach to decision making.

This new focus on populations, coupled with the integration of acute, chronic, and primary care that is occurring in some health care systems, is likely to create new roles for individuals, including nurses, who will span inpatient and community-based settings and focus on providing a wide range of services to the population served by the system. Such a role might be director of client care services for a health care system, who would have administrative responsibility for a large program area. There will also be a demand for individuals who can design programs of preventive and clinical services to be offered to targeted subpopulations and those who can implement the services. Who will decide what services will be given to which subpopulation and by which providers? How will nurses be prepared for leadership in the emerging and future structures for health care delivery and health maintenance?

Physician leaders are recognizing that physicians need to be prepared to use population-focused methods, such as epidemiology and biostatistics, to make evidence-based decisions in the development of programs and protocols. In contrast, the attention being given to preparing nurses for administrative decision making seems to be declining. This may be a result of (1) the recent lack of federal support for preparing nurse administrators and (2) the growing popularity of nurse practitioner programs. However, it is time that nurse leaders give more attention to preparing nurses for leadership in the area of population-focused practice. Perhaps it is time to combine the specialty in public health nursing and nursing administration. As suggested some time ago by Williams (1985), some DNP programs are combining much of the preparation for specialization in public health nursing and administration into a systems-oriented curriculum with differentiation in the application to practice. This is the approach that is being taken in the DNP program in the College of Nursing at the University of Kentucky (www.uky.edu). This makes sense because regardless of how the population is defined, there will be a growing need for nurses with population-level assessment, management, and evaluation skills to assume leadership roles as urged in the IOM's report The Future of Nursing (IOM, 2010).

A primary focus of the health care system of the future will be on community-based strategies for health promotion and disease prevention and on population-focused strategies for primary and secondary care. Directing more attention to developing the specialty of public health nursing as a way to provide nursing leadership may be a good response to the health care system changes. Preparing nurses for population-focused decision making will require greater attention to developing programs at the doctoral level that have a stronger foundation in the public health sciences, while providing better preparation of baccalaureate-level nurses for community-oriented as well as community-based practice.

Some observers of public health have anticipated that if access to health care for all Americans becomes more of a reality, public health practitioners will be in a position to turn over the delivery of personal primary care services to practitioners in accountable care organizations and integrated health plans and return to the core public health functions. However, assurance (making sure that basic services are available to all) is a core function of public health. Thus even under the condition of improved access to care, there will still be a need to monitor subpopulations in the community to ensure that necessary care is available to all and that its quality is at an acceptable level. When these conditions are not met, public health practitioners are accountable for finding a solution.

Shifting Public Health Practice to Address the Social Determinates of Health and More Vigorous Policy Efforts to Create Conditions for a Healthy Population

The growing concern about the role played by the social determinants of health in contributing to negative health outcomes coupled with the Public Health 3.0 call for public health leaders to be health strategists in their communities suggests that public health leaders need to be more active in assuming community level leadership in addressing issues like homelessness, food insecurity, and unsafe physical and social environments. This translates into mobilizing various community constituencies to take collaborative action within the constraints of current policies and to mobilize for the policy changes necessary to reduce the barriers to healthy conditions. This also means that public health nurse specialists need to be health strategists in their communities.

In 2012, the IOM published a report (IOM, 2012b) on shifting public policy from a primary focus of supporting medical care to creating conditions for a healthy population. A major challenge for the future is the need for public health nursing specialists to be more aggressive in working collaboratively with various groups in the community as well as professional colleagues in institutional settings to deal with barriers to health like the social determinants discussed above. Another challenge is to be more aggressive in their practice of the core public health function of policy development, one of the major ways public health specialists intervene, with the focus on actively engaging in influencing public decisions that will create conditions for a healthy population. This is necessary at the local, state, and national levels, and encompasses a wide range of concerns from the availability of adequate nutrition to the maintenance of a healthy and safe environment in schools, to the reduction of secondhand smoke, to assuring access to needed health services. Policy development is not a solitary activity; it involves working with many groups and coalitions. Also, policy development is not just the responsibility of public health specialists; it is important that all professional nurses become more serious and adept in the process of policy development.

In the IOM's influential report, *The Future of Nursing: Leading Change, Advancing Health* (IOM, 2010), a key message is that "Nurses should be full partners, with physicians and other health professionals, in redesigning health care in the United States" (IOM, 2010, pp. 1-11). In discussing this message the report states that "to be effective in re-conceptualized roles, nurses must see policy as something they can shape rather than something that happens to them" (IOM, 2010, pp. 1-11). In other words, nurses need to be key actors. However, the report also makes clear that nurses need to be prepared for leadership in that area.

The history of public health nursing shows that a common attribute of leaders is to move forward to deal with unresolved problems in a positive, proactive way. This is the legacy of Lillian Wald at the Henry Street Settlement, the nurse who is credited with founding public health nursing, and others who have met a need by being innovative. Within the context of the core public health functions of assurance and policy making, public health nursing specialists clearly have an opportunity to affect public decisions that will help create conditions for a healthy population and influence the provision of needed health promotion and health maintenance services to populations in the community, particularly those that are most vulnerable. As a specialty, public health nursing can have a positive impact on the health status of populations, but to do so it will be necessary to have broad vision; to prepare nurses for roles in community leadership and policy making and in the design, development, management, monitoring, and evaluation of population-focused health care systems; and to develop strategies to support nurses in these roles. With the focus on quality and safety education for nurses, public health nursing education will want to reflect this renewed focus and assist nurses who are population-focused in developing the competencies noted in the QSEN box.

LINKING CONTENT TO PRACTICE

In this chapter emphasis is placed on defining and explaining public health nursing practice with populations. The three essential functions of public health and public health nursing are assessment, policy development, and assurance. The Council on Linkages' "Core Competencies for Public Health Professionals" revised in 2014 describes the skills of public health professionals, including nurses. In assessment function, one skill is assessment of the health status of populations and their related determinants of health and illness. For policy development, one of the skills is development of a plan to implement policy and programs. For the assurance function, one skill that public health nurses will need is to incorporate ethical standards of practice as the basis of all interactions with organizations, communities, and individuals. These skills can also be linked to the 10 essential services of public health nursing found in Fig. 1.1. Assessment of health status is a skill needed for implementing essential service 1, the monitoring of health status to identify community problems. Development of a plan for policy and program implementation is a skill needed for essential service 5, to support individual and community health efforts. Incorporating ethical standards is done in essential service 3 when informing, educating, and empowering people about health issues.

QSEN FOCUS ON QUALITY AND SAFETY EDUCATION IN NURSES

QSEN Competency	Competency Definition
Client-Centered Care	Recognize the client or designee as the source of control and full partner in providing compassionate and coordinated care based on respect for client preferences, values, and needs
Teamwork and Collaboration	Function effectively within nursing and interprofessional teams, fostering open communication, mutual respect, and shared decision making to achieve quality care
Evidence-Based Practice	Integrate best current evidence with clinical expertise and client/family preferences and values for delivery of optimal health care
Quality Improvement	Use data to monitor the outcomes of care processes and use improvement methods to design and test changes to continuously improve the quality and safety of health care systems
Safety	Minimize risk for harm to clients and providers through both system effectiveness and individual performance
Informatics	Use information and technology to communicate, manage knowledge, mitigate error, and support decision making

QSEN, Quality and Safety Education for Nurses.
Prepared by Gail Armstrong, PhD(c), DNP, ACNS-BC, CNE, Associate Professor, University of Colorado Denver College of Nursing.

PRACTICE APPLICATION

Population-focused nursing practice is different from clinical nursing care delivered in the community. If one accepts that the specialist in public health nursing is population-focused and has a unique body of knowledge, it is useful to debate where and how public health nursing specialists practice. How does their practice compare with that of the nurse specialist in community or community-based nursing?

A. In your public health class, debate with classmates which nurses in the following categories practice population-focused nursing and provide reasons for your choices:
  1. School nurse
  2. Staff nurse in home care
  3. Director of nursing for a home care agency
  4. Nurse practitioner in a health maintenance organization
  5. Vice president of nursing in a hospital
  6. Staff nurse in a public health clinic or community health center
  7. Director of nursing in a health department

B. Choose three categories in the preceding list, and interview at least one nurse in each of the categories. Determine the scope of practice for each nurse. Are these nurses carrying out population-focused practice? Could they? How?

Answers can be found on the Evolve site.

KEY POINTS

- Public health is what we, as a society, do collectively to ensure the conditions in which people can be healthy.
- Assessment, policy development, and assurance are the core public health functions; they are implemented at all levels of government.
- *Assessment* refers to systematically collecting data on the population, monitoring of the population's health status, and making available information about the health of the community.
- *Policy development* refers to the need to provide leadership in developing policies that support the health of the population; it involves using scientific knowledge in making decisions about policy.
- *Assurance* refers to the role of public health in making sure that essential community-wide health services are available, which may include providing essential personal health services for those who would otherwise not receive them. Assurance also refers to ensuring that a competent public health and personal health care workforce is available.
- The setting is frequently viewed as the feature that distinguishes public health nursing from other specialties. A more useful approach is to use the following characteristics: a focus on populations that are free-living in the community, an emphasis on prevention, a concern for the interface between the health status of the population and the living environment (physical, biological, sociocultural), and the use of political processes to affect public policy as a major intervention strategy for achieving goals.
- According to the 1985 Consensus Conference sponsored by the Division of Nursing of the U.S. Department of Health and Human Services, *specialists in public health nursing* are defined as those who are prepared at the graduate level, either master's or doctoral, "with a focus in the public health sciences" (USDHHS, 1985). This is still true today.
- Population-focused practice is the focus of specialists in public health nursing. This focus on populations and the emphasis on health protection, health promotion, and disease prevention are the fundamental factors that distinguish public health nursing from other nursing specialties.
- A *population* is defined as a collection of individuals who share one or more personal or environmental characteristics. The term *population* may be used interchangeably with the term *aggregate.*

CLINICAL DECISION-MAKING ACTIVITIES

1. Define the following for your personal understanding, and suggest ways to check whether your understanding is correct:
   A. Essential functions of public health
   B. Specialist in public health nursing
   C. Nurse specialist in the community
2. State your opinion about the similarities and/or differences between a clinical nursing role and the population-focused role of the public health nursing specialist. What are some of the complex issues in distinguishing between these roles?
3. Review the model of public health nursing practice of the APHA as described in this chapter. Can you elaborate on the differences between the staff nurse and the specialist nurse?
4. With three or four classmates, identify some nurses in your community who are in an administrative role and discuss with them the following:
   A. The way they define the populations they are serving
   B. Strategies they use to monitor the population's health status
   C. Strategies they use to ensure that the populations are receiving needed services
   D. Initiatives they are taking to address problems
5. Do additional questions need to be asked to determine their views on population-focused practice and the responsibilities of the staff nurse? Elaborate.

ADDITIONAL RESOURCES

EVOLVE WEBSITE

http://evolve.elsevier.com/Stanhope/community/

- Answers to Practice Application
- Case Study
- Glossary
- Review Questions

REFERENCES

American Association of Colleges of Nursing (AACN): *AACN Position Statement on the Practice Doctorate in Nursing*, Washington, DC, 2004, AACN.

American Association of Colleges of Nursing (AACN): *The Essentials of Doctoral Education for Advanced Nursing Practice*, Washington, DC, 2006, AACN.

American Association of Colleges of Nursing (AACN): Public Health: Recommended Baccalaureate Competencies and Curricular Guidelines for Public Health Nursing: A Supplement to The Essentials of Baccalaureate education for Professional Nursing Practice"? 2013. Retrieved from http://www.aacn.nche.edu.

American Nurses Association (ANA): *Public Health Nursing: Scope and Standards of Practice*, Washington, DC, 2013, ANA.

American Public Health Association (APHA): *The Definition and Role of Public Health Nursing in the Delivery of Health Care: A Statement of the Public Health Nursing Section*, Washington, DC, 1981, APHA.

American Public Health Association (APHA): *The Definition and Practice of Public Health Nursing*, 2013. Retrieved from www.apha.org.

American Public Health Association (APHA): *The Definition and Role of Public Health Nursing: A Statement of the APHA Public Health Nursing Section*, [March 1996 update]. Washington, DC, 1996, APHA.

Association of Community Health Nursing Educators (ACHNE): *Essentials of Master's Level Nursing Education for Advanced Community/Public Health Nursing Practice*, Lathrop, NY, 2003, ACHNE.

Association of Community Health Nursing Educators (ACHNE): *Essentials of Baccalaureate Nursing Education for Entry Level Community/Public Health Nursing*, Wheat Ridge, CO, 2009, ACHNE.

Association of State and Territorial Directors of Nursing (ASTDN): *Public Health Nursing: A Partner for Healthy Populations*, Washington, DC, 2000, ASTDN.

Berchick ER, Hood E, Barrett JC: *Health Insurance Coverage in the United States: 2017. Current Population Reports*, Census Bureau, 2018. Retrieved from www.census.gov.

Blumenthal D, Collins SR: Health care coverage under the Affordable Care Act—a progress report, *N Engl J Med* 371:275–281, 2014.

Bradley EH, Taylor LA: *The American Health Care Paradox: Why Spending More is Getting Us Less*, Philadelphia, PA, 2013, Public Affairs.

Brooks CJ, Barrett J, Daly J, et al: A community-level sodium reduction intervention, Boston, 2013-2015, *Am J Public Health*, 107:1951–1957, 2017.

Center for Health Affairs: *What Does Population Health Mean?* 2017. Retrieved from www.neohospitals.org.

Centers for Disease Control and Prevention (CDC): *Ten Great Public Health Achievements in the 20th Century*, 2014. Retrieved from www.cdc.gov.

Centers for Disease Control and Prevention (CDC): *National Public Health Performance Standards Program*, 2014a. Retrieved from www.phf.org.

Centers for Disease Control and Prevention (CDC): *The Community Guide: What Works to Promote Health*, 2014b. Retrieved from www.thecommunityguide.org.

Centers for Disease Control and Prevention (CDC): *The public health system and the ten essential services*, 2018, Atlanta, GA, CDC.

Centers for Medicare and Medicaid Services (CMS) Office of the Actuary, National Health Statistics Group: *The Nation's Health Dollar Calendar Year 2012: Where It Came From, Where It Went*, 2012. Retrieved from http://www.cms.gov.

Centers for Medicare and Medicaid Services (CMS) Office of the Actuary, National Health Statistics Group: *The Nation's Health Dollar Calendar Year 2017*. Retrieved from www.cms.gov.

Chapman DA, Kelley L, Woolf SH: *Mapping Life Expectancy 2015-2016. VCU Center on Society and Health*, 2016. Retrieved from http://www.societyhealth.vcu.edu.

Collins SR, Gunja MZ, Doty MM, Bhupal HK: *First Look at health Insurance Coverage in 2018 Finds ACA Gains Beginning to Reverse: Findings from the Commonwealth Fund*, 2018. Retrieved from www.commonwealthfund.org

Commonwealth Fund. *Affordable Care Act Tracking Survey*, Feb-Mar, 2018. To the Point (blog). Commonwealth Fund, May 1, 2018.

Consensus Conference on the Essentials of Public Health Nursing Practice and Education. Rockville, MD, 1985, U.S. Department of Health and Human Services, Bureau of Health Professions, Division of Nursing.

Council on Linkages between Academia and Public Health Practice: *Core Competencies for Public Health Professionals*, Washington, DC, 2010, revised 2014. Retrieved from www.phf.org.

County Health Rankings & Roadmaps: *Health is Where We Live*. Retrieved from www.countyhealthrankings.org.

DeSalvo KB, Wang YC, Harris A, Auerbach J, Koo D, O'Carroll P: *A Call to Action for Public Health to Meet the Challenges of the 21st Century. Perspectives, Discussion Paper, the National Academies*, 2017. doi:10.5888/pcd14.170017.

Fielding J: Commentary: public health and health care quality assurance—strange bedfellows? *Milbank Q* 87:581–584, 2009.

Fielding J, Tilson H, Richland J: *Medical care reform requires public health reform: expanded role for public health agencies in improving health, partnership for prevention*, 2008. Retrieved from www.prevent.org.

Gebbie K: Building a constituency for public health, *J Public Health Manag Pract* 3:1, 1999.

Institute of Medicine (IOM): *The Future of Public Health*, Washington, DC, 1988, National Academy Press.

Institute of Medicine (IOM): *Improving Health in the Community: A Role for Performance Monitoring*, Washington, DC, 1997, National Academies Press.

Institute of Medicine: Improving Health in the Community: *A Role for Performance Monitoring. Washington*, DC, 1997, National Academy Press.

Institute of Medicine (IOM): *Who Will Keep the Public Healthy?* Washington, DC, 2003, National Academies Press.

Institute of Medicine (IOM): *The Future of Nursing: Leading Change, Advancing Health*, Washington, DC, 2010, National Academies Press.

Institute of Medicine (IOM): *For the Public's Health: Investing in a Healthier Future* [Brief Report]. 2012a. Retrieved from www.iom.edu.

Institute of Medicine (IOM): *Primary Care and Public Health: Exploring Integration to Improve Population Health*, Washington, DC, 2012b, National Academies of Sciences Press.

Josten L, Clarke PN, Ostwald S, et al: Public health nursing education: back to the future for public health sciences, *Fam Community Health* 18:36, 1995.

Kentucky Center for Smoke-Free Policy: Retrieved from www.uky.edu.

Kindig D, Stoddart G: What is population health? *Am J Public Health* 93:380–383, 2003.

Murphy SL, Kochanek KD, Xu J, Arias E: Mortality in the United States 2014, *NCHS Data Brief* (229):1–8, 2015.

Orszag PR: Health Care and the Budget: Issues and Challenges for Reform *[Statement before the Committee on the Budget, U.S. Senate]*. Washington, DC, June 21, 2007, Congressional Budget Office.

Orszag PR, Emanuel EJ: Health care reform and cost control, *N Engl J Med* 363:601–603, 2010.

Patient Protection and Affordable Care Act: *Health Care and Education Affordability Reconciliation Act of 2010*, 2010. Retrieved from www.hhs.gov.

Public Health Functions Steering Committee: *Public Health in America*, 1998. Retrieved from www.health.gov.

Quad Council Coalition Competency Review Task Force: *Community/Public Health Nursing Competencies*, 2018. Retrieved from www.quadcouncilphn.org.

Quad Council of Public Health Nursing Organizations: *Scope and Standards of Public Health Nursing Practice*, Washington, DC, 1999 [revised 2005], American Nurses Association.

Quad Council of Public Health Nursing Organizations: *Competencies for Public Health Nursing Practice*, Washington, DC, 2003 [revised 2009], Association of State and Territorial Directors of Nursing.

Quad Council of Public Health Nursing Organizations: *Quad Council Competencies for Public Health Nurses*, Summer 2011. November 2014 from: www.quadcouncilphn.org.

Starr P: *The Social Transformation of American Medicine*, New York, 1982, Basic Books.

Trust for America's Health: *The Truth about the Prevention and Public Health Fund*, 2013. Retrieved from www.healthyamericans.org.

Turnock B: *Public Health: What Is It and How Does It Work*, ed 4, Boston, 2009, Jones and Bartlett.

Turnock B: *Public Health: What Is It and How Does It Work?* ed 5, Boston, 2012, Jones & Bartlett.

U.S. Department of Health, Education, and Welfare: Healthy People: *The Surgeon General's Report on Health Promotion and Disease Prevention, DHEW (PHS) Publication No. 79-55071*. Washington, DC, 1979, U.S. Government Printing Office.

U.S. Department of Health and Human Services: *Promoting Health/Preventing Disease: Objectives for the Nation*, Washington, DC, 1980, U.S. Government Printing Office.

U.S. Department of Health and Human Services (USDHHS): *Healthy People 2000: National Health Promotion and Disease Prevention Objectives, DHHS Publication No. 91-50212*. Washington, DC, 1991, U.S. Government Printing Office.

U.S. Department of Health and Human Services (USDHHS): *Healthy People 2010: Understanding and Improving Health*, ed 2, Washington, DC, 2000, U.S. Government Printing Office.

U.S. Department of Health and Human Services: *Health US: 2000*, Washington, DC, 2002, National Center for Statistics.

U.S. Department of Health and Human Services (USDHHS): *National Center for Health Statistics*, Washington, DC, 2010.

U.S. Department of Health and Human Services (USDHHS): *Healthy People 2020: The Road Ahead*, 2010. Retrieved from www.healthypeople.gov.

U.S. Department of Health and Human Services (USDHHS): *Healthy People 2020: Leading Health Indicators—Progress Update*, 2014. Retrieved from www.healthypeople.gov. [when on site click on Leading Health Indicators].

U.S. Department of Health and Human Services, Bureau of Health Professions, Division of Nursing: *Consensus Conference on the Essentials of Public Health Nursing Practice and Education* [APHA Report Series], Washington, DC, 1985, American Public Health Association.

U.S. Preventive Services Task Force: *Guide to Clinical Preventive Services*, ed 3, Baltimore, MD, 2000, Williams & Wilkins.

U.S. Public Health Service: *The Core Functions Project*, Washington, DC, 1994 [updated 2008], Office of Disease Prevention and Health Promotion.

Williams CA: Population-focused community health nursing and nursing administration: a new synthesis. In McCloskey JC, Grace HK, editors: *Current Issues in Nursing*, ed 2, Boston, 1985, Blackwell Scientific.

Williams CA: Public health nursing: does it have a future? In Aiken LH, Fagin CM, editors: *Charting Nursing's Future: Agenda for the 1990s*. Philadelphia, PA, 1992, Lippincott.

Williams CA: Beyond the Institute of Medicine report: a critical analysis and public health forecast, *Fam Community Health* 18:12, 1995.

Woolf S, Aron L: Failing health of the United States: the role of challenging life conditions and the policies behind them, *BMJ* 360:k496, 2018.

Woolf S, Aron L, editors: *US Health in International Perspective: Shorter Lives, Poorer Health. Institute of Medicine and the National Research Council*, Washington DC, The Academies Press, 2013.

2

History of Public Health and Public and Community Health Nursing

Janna Dieckmann, PhD, RN

OBJECTIVES

After reading this chapter, the student should be able to do the following:

1. Interpret the focus and roles of public health nurses through a historical approach.
2. Trace the ongoing interaction between the practice of public health and that of nursing.
3. Discuss the dynamic relationship between changes in social, political, and economic contexts and nursing practice in the community.
4. Outline the professional and practice impact of individual leaders on population-centered nursing, especially the leadership of Florence Nightingale and Lillian Wald.
5. Identify structures for delivery of nursing care in the community such as settlement houses, visiting nurse associations, official health organizations, and schools.
6. Recognize major organizations that contributed to the growth and development of population-centered nursing.

CHAPTER OUTLINE

Change and Continuity
Public Health During America's Colonial Period Across the New Republic
Nightingale and the Origins of Trained Nursing
America Needs Trained Nurses
School Nursing in America
The Profession Comes of Age
Public Health Nursing in Official Health Agencies and in World War I
Paying the Bill for Public Health Nurses
African American Nurses in Public Health Nursing
Between the Two World Wars: Economic Depression and the Rise of Hospitals
Increasing Federal Action for the Public's Health
World War II: Extension and Retrenchment in Public Health Nursing
The Rise of Chronic Illness
Declining Financial Support for Practice and Professional Organizations
Professional Nursing Education for Public Health Nursing
New Resources and New Communities: The 1960s and Nursing
Community Organization and Professional Change
Public Health Nursing From the 1970s Into the Twenty-First Century
Public Health Nursing Today

KEY TERMS

American Nurses Association, p. 35
American Public Health Association, p. 30
American Red Cross, p. 28
district nursing, p. 27
district nursing association, p. 27
Florence Nightingale, p. 26
Frontier Nursing Service, p. 31
Lillian Wald, p. 28
Metropolitan Life Insurance Company, p. 31
National League for Nursing, p. 35
National Organization for Public Health Nursing, p. 30
official health agency, p. 32
settlement houses, p. 28
Sheppard-Towner Act, p. 31
Social Security Act of 1935, p. 32
Town and Country Nursing Service, p. 29
visiting nurse, p. 28
William Rathbone, p. 27

Nurses use historical approaches to examine both the profession's present and its future. In doing so, several questions are asked: First, who is the population-centered nurse? In the past, population-centered nurses have been called public health nurses, district nurses, and visiting nurses, as well as home health care nurses, school nurses, and occupational health nurses. Second, how does the past contribute to the work of the population-centered nurse today? Next, what are the times and places in which these nurses have worked and continue to work? When a conscious process of critique and insight is used to look into past actions of the specialty, what can be discovered? Must contemporary nurses agree with or endorse past actions of the profession? How might society today review the magnitude of work that public health nurses have provided on behalf of individuals, families, groups and communities and use this information to provide support for public health nurses to continue to make these contributions to population health? And last, how might knowledge of population-centered nursing history serve both as a source of inspiration and also as a creative stimulus to solve the enduring and new problems of the current period? This chapter serves as an introduction to these questions through tracing the development and evolution of population-centered nursing.

CHANGE AND CONTINUITY

For more than 130 years, public health nurses in the United States have worked to develop strategies to respond effectively to emerging and prevailing public health problems. The history of population-centered nursing reflects changes in the specific focus of the profession while emphasizing continuity in approach and style. Nurses have worked in communities to improve the health status of individuals, families, and populations, especially those who belong to vulnerable groups. Part of the appeal of this nursing specialty has been its autonomy of practice and independence in problem solving and decision making conducted in the context of an interprofessional practice. Many varied and challenging public health nursing roles originated in the late 1800s when public health efforts focused on environmental conditions such as sanitation, control of communicable diseases, education for health, prevention of disease and disability, and care of aged and sick persons in their homes.

Although these threats to health have changed over time, the foundational principles and goals of public health nursing have remained the same. Many communicable diseases, such as diphtheria, cholera, and typhoid fever, have been largely controlled in the United States, but others continue to affect many lives across the globe, including human immunodeficiency virus (HIV), poliomyelitis, Ebola virus, and tuberculosis. Emerging and re-emerging communicable diseases with widespread impact, for example, influenza subtypes, continue to change and challenge the work of those who develop the vaccines. Even though environmental pollution in residential areas now receives increased public attention, communities continue to be threatened by overcrowded garbage dumps and pollutants affecting the air, water, and soil. The neglected presence of lead and other pollutants in household and drinking water in Flint, Michigan, beginning in 2014, suggests that advocates must remain alert and have a ready response. Natural disasters continue to challenge public health systems, and bioterrorism and other human-made disasters have the potential to overwhelm existing resources.

Research has identified means to avoid or postpone chronic disease onset, and nurses implement strategies to modify individual and community risk factors and behaviors. Finally, with the growing population percent of older adults in the United States and their preference to remain at home, additional nursing services are required to sustain the frail, the disabled, and the chronically ill in the community. Allowing people to remain in their homes when care can be provided there is far less costly than institutional care.

Contemporary nursing roles in the United States developed from several sources and are a product of various ongoing social, economic, and political forces. This chapter describes the societal circumstances that influenced nurses to establish community-based and population-centered practices. For the purposes of this chapter, the term *nurse* will be used to refer to nurses who rely heavily on public health science to complement their focus on nursing science and practice. The nation's need for community and public health nurses, the practice of population-centered nursing, and the organizations influencing public health nursing in the United States from the nineteenth century to the present are discussed.

PUBLIC HEALTH DURING AMERICA'S COLONIAL PERIOD ACROSS THE NEW REPUBLIC

Concern for the health and care of individuals in the community has characterized human existence. All people and all cultures have been concerned with the events surrounding birth, death, and illness. Human beings have sought to prevent, understand, and control disease. Their ability to preserve health and treat illness has depended on the contemporary level of science, use and availability of technologies, and degree of social organization.

In the early years of America's settlement, as in Europe, the care of the sick was usually informal and was provided by household members, almost always women. The female head of the household was responsible for caring for all household members, which meant more than nursing them in sickness and during childbirth. She was also responsible for growing or gathering healing herbs for use throughout the year. For the increasing numbers of urban residents in the early 1800s, this traditional system became insufficient.

American ideas of social welfare and community-based care of the sick were strongly influenced by the traditions of British settlers in the New World. Just as American law is based on English common law, colonial Americans established systems of care for the sick, poor, aged, mentally ill, and dependents based on England's Elizabethan Poor Law of 1601. In the United States, as in England, local poor laws guaranteed medical care for poor, blind, and "lame" individuals, even those without family. Early county or township government was responsible for the care of all dependent residents, but provided almshouse charity carefully, economically, and only for local residents. Travelers and wanderers from elsewhere were returned to their native counties for care. In 1751, Pennsylvania Hospital was founded in Philadelphia, the first hospital in what would become the United States. Yet until much later, hospitals were few and found only in large cities.

Early colonial public health efforts included the collection of vital statistics, improvements to sanitation systems, and control of communicable diseases introduced through seaports. Colonists lacked an organized and ongoing means to ensure support and enforcement of public health efforts. Communicable disease epidemics intermittently taxed the limited local organization for health during the seventeenth, eighteenth, and nineteenth centuries (Rosen, 1958).

After the American Revolution, the threat of disease, especially yellow fever epidemics, encouraged public support for new government-sponsored, official boards of health. New York City, with a population of 75,000 by 1800, established basic public health services, which included monitoring water quality, constructing sewers and a waterfront wall, draining marshes, planting trees and vegetables, and burying the dead (Rosen, 1958).

Increased urbanization and early industrialization in the new United States contributed to increased incidence of disease, including epidemics of smallpox, yellow fever, cholera, typhoid, and typhus. Tuberculosis and malaria remained endemic at a high incidence rate, and infant mortality was about 200 per 1000 live births (Pickett & Hanlon, 1990). American hospitals in the early 1800s were generally unsanitary and staffed by poorly trained workers; institutions were a place of last resort. Physicians received a limited education through proprietary schools or simple apprenticeship. Medical care was difficult to secure, although public dispensaries (similar to outpatient clinics) and private charitable efforts attempted to address gaps in the availability of sickness services, especially for the urban poor and working classes. Environmental conditions in urban neighborhoods, including inadequate housing and sanitation, were additional risks to health. Table 2.1 presents milestones of public health efforts that occurred from 1601 to the present.

TABLE 2.1 Milestones in the History of Public Health and Community Health Nursing: 1601 to 2018

Year	Milestone
1601	The Act for the Relief of the Poor (the Elizabethan Poor Law) passed
1751	Pennsylvania Hospital founded in Philadelphia
1793	Baltimore Health Department established
1798	Marine Hospital Service established; in 1912 renamed the U.S. Public Health Service
1813	Ladies' Benevolent Society of Charleston, South Carolina, founded
1815	Sisters of Mercy established in Dublin, Ireland, where nuns visited the poor
1836	Lutheran deaconess movement founded in Kaiserswerth, Germany
1851	Florence Nightingale visits Kaiserswerth for three months of nurse training
1859	District nursing established in Liverpool, England, by William Rathbone
1860	Florence Nightingale Training School for Nurses established at St. Thomas Hospital in London, England
1866	New York Metropolitan Board of Health established
1872	American Public Health Association established
1873	New York Training School opens at Bellevue Hospital, New York City, as first Nightingale-model nursing school in the United States
1877	Women's Board of the New York Mission hires nurse Frances Root to visit the sick poor
1881	Clara Barton and a circle of her acquaintances found the American Red Cross in Washington, DC, on May 21, 1881
1885	Visiting Nurse Association established in Buffalo, NY
1886	Visiting nurse agencies established in Philadelphia and Boston
1892	First organized movement against tuberculosis
1893	Lillian Wald and Mary Brewster organize a visiting nursing service for the poor of New York, which later became the famous Henry Street Settlement and the Visiting Nurse Service of New York
	Society of Superintendents of Training Schools of Nurses in the United States and Canada established (in 1912 it became known as the National League of Nursing Education)
1896	Associated Alumnae of Training Schools for Nurses established (in 1911 it became the American Nurses Association)
1902	School nursing started in New York City, by Nurse Lina Rogers of Henry Street Settlement
1903	First Nurse Practice Acts passed; began with North Carolina Nurse Registration Act
1908	National Association of Colored Graduate Nurses founded
1909	Metropolitan Life Insurance Company provides first insurance reimbursement for nursing care
1910	Public health nursing program instituted at Teachers College, Columbia University, NYC
1912	National Organization for Public Health Nursing formed; Lillian Wald is first president
1916	*Public Health Nursing* textbook by Mary Sewall Gardner published
1918	Vassar Training Camp for Nurses organized
	U.S. Public Health Service (USPHS) establishes division of public health nursing to work in the war effort
	Worldwide influenza epidemic begins
1921	Maternity and Infancy Act (Sheppard-Towner) passed
1925	Frontier Nursing Service using nurse-midwives established in Kentucky
1933	Pearl McIver is first nurse employed by the U.S. Public Health Service
1935	Social Security Act passed
	Association of State and Territorial Directors of Nursing founded
1941	United States enters World War II

TABLE 2.1 **Milestones in the History of Public Health and Community Health Nursing: 1601 to 2018—cont'd**

Year	Milestone
1943	Bolton Act provides five million dollars for nursing education; establishes Cadet Nurse Corps, with Lucille Petry as chief; 124,000 nurses graduate by 1948 when Corps ends
	USPHS Division of Nurse Education begun; becomes Division of Nursing in 1946
1944	First basic program in nursing accredited as including sufficient public health content
1946	Nurses classified as professionals by U.S. Civil Service Commission
	Hill-Burton Act approved, providing funds for hospital construction in underserved areas and requiring these hospitals to provide care for poor people
	Passage of National Mental Health Act
1950	25,091 nurses employed in public health
1951	National organizations recommend that college-based nursing education programs include public health content
1952	National Organization for Public Health Nursing merges into the new National League for Nursing
	Closure of Metropolitan Life Insurance Nursing Program
1964	Passage of Civil Rights Act and Economic Opportunity Act
	Public health nurse defined by the American Nurses Association (ANA) as a graduate of a BSN program
1965	ANA position paper recommends that nursing education take place in institutions of higher learning
1966	Medicare and Medicaid (Titles 18 and 19 of the Social Security Act) are implemented on July 1 (legislation passed in 1965)
1977	Passage of Rural Health Clinic Services Act, which provided indirect reimbursement for nurse practitioners in rural health clinics
1978	Association of Graduate Faculty in Community Health Nursing/Public Health Nursing founded (later, Association of Community Health Nursing Educators)
1979	Publication of *Healthy People: The Surgeon General's Report on Health Promotion and Disease Prevention*
1980	Medicaid amendment to the Social Security Act to provide direct reimbursement for nurse practitioners in rural health clinics
	ANA and APHA develop statements on the role and conceptual foundations of community and public health nursing, respectively
1983	Beginning of Medicare prospective payment system
1985	National Center for Nursing Research established in the National Institutes of Health
1988	Institute of Medicine reports on *The Future of Public Health*
1988	The Quad Council of Public Health Nursing Organizations (later became the Quad Council Coalition of Public Health Nursing Organizations) is founded to address priorities for public health nursing education, practice, leadership, and research, and as the voice of public health nursing.
1990	*Essentials of Baccalaureate Nursing Education,* from Association of Community Health Nursing Educators
1991	More than 60 nursing organizations join in support of health care reform; publish *Nursing's Agenda for Health Care Reform*
1993	American Health Security Act of 1993 (The Clinton Plan). Legislation for national health care reform fails; states and the private sector left to design own programs 1993-1994.
1994	National Institute of Nursing Research (previously NCNR), gained official institute status as part of the National Institutes of Health.
1996	*The Definition and Role of Public Health Nursing,* updated: Public Health Nursing Section, American Public Health Association
1998	*The Public Health Workforce: An Agenda for the 21st Century,* U.S. Public Health Service; examines current workforce in public, health, and educational needs, and the use of distance learning strategies to prepare future public health workers
1999	The Quad Council of Public Health Nursing Organizations works with American Nurses Association on new *Scope and Standards of Public Health Nursing Practice;* differentiates between community-oriented and community-based nursing practice.
2001	Public health gains a national presence in addressing concerns about biological and other terrorism following September 11 attacks
2002	Department of Homeland Security established to provide leadership to protect against intentional threats to the health of the public
2003	*Public Health Nursing Competencies* finalized by the Quad Council of Public Health Nursing Organizations
2003-2005	Multiple natural disasters, including earthquakes, tsunamis, and hurricanes, demonstrate the weak infrastructure for managing disasters in the United States and other countries, and emphasize the need for strong public health programs that included disaster management
2007	An entirely new *Public Health Nursing: Scope and Standards of Practice* is released through the ANA, reflecting the efforts of the Quad Council of Public Health Nursing Organizations
2010	The Patient Protection and Affordable Care Act is signed by President Barack Obama (March 23, 2010)
2012	The Association of State and Territorial Directors of Nursing (ASTDN), formed in (1935) became The Association of Public Health Nurses (APHN) in 2012
2013	The revised (second edition) of *Public Health Nursing: Scope and Standards of Practice,* prepared by representatives of the Quad Council of Public Health Nursing Organizations, is released by the American Nurses Association
2014	Council on Linkages Between Academia and Public Health Practice released their revised competencies, *Core Competencies for Public Health Professionals.*
2018	The Quad Council Coalition (QCC) of Public Health Nursing Organizations is composed of the Alliance of Nurses for Healthy Environments (AHNE); the Association of Community Health Nursing Educators (ACHNE); the Association of Public Health Nurses (APHN); and the American Public Health Association–Public Health Nursing Section (APHA-PHN). It provides voice and visibility for public health nurses; sets a national policy agenda on issues related to public health nursing; and advocates for excellence in public health nursing education, practice, leadership, and research. The Coalition revised their operating guidelines in 2014 and again in 2017, and in 2018 released their Community/Public Health Nursing (C/PHN) Competencies.

The federal government's early efforts for public health aimed to secure America's maritime trade and major coastal cities by providing health care for merchant seamen and by protecting seacoast cities from epidemics. The U.S. Public Health Service, still the most important federal public health agency in the twenty-first century, was established in 1798 as the Marine Hospital Service. The first Marine Hospital opened in Norfolk, Virginia, in 1800. Additional federal legislation to establish quarantine regulations for seamen and immigrants was passed in 1878.

During the early 1800s, experiments in providing nursing care at home focused on moral improvement and less on illness intervention. The Ladies' Benevolent Society of Charleston, South Carolina, provided charitable assistance to the poor and sick beginning in 1813. In Philadelphia, following a brief training program, lay nurses cared for postpartum women and newborns in their homes. In Cincinnati, Ohio, the Roman Catholic Sisters of Charity began a visiting nurse service in 1854 (Rodabaugh & Rodabaugh, 1951). Although these early programs provided services at the local level, they were not adopted elsewhere, and their influence on later public health nursing is unclear.

During the mid-nineteenth century, national interest increased for addressing public health problems and improving urban living conditions. New responsibilities for urban boards of health reflected changing ideas of public health, and these boards began to address communicable diseases and environmental hazards. Soon after it was founded in 1847, the American Medical Association (AMA) formed a hygiene committee to conduct sanitary surveys and to develop a system to collect vital statistics. The Shattuck Report, published in 1850 by the Massachusetts Sanitary Commission, called for major innovations: the establishment of a state health department and local health boards in every town; sanitary surveys and collection of vital statistics; environmental sanitation; food, drug, and communicable disease control; well-child care; health education; tobacco and alcohol control; town planning; and the teaching of preventive medicine in medical schools (Kalisch & Kalisch, 2004). However, these recommendations were not implemented even in Massachusetts until 1869, and in other states much later.

In some areas, charitable organizations addressed the gap between known communicable disease epidemics and the lack of local government resources. For example, the Howard Association of New Orleans, Louisiana, responded to periodic yellow fever epidemics between 1837 and 1878 by providing physicians, lay nurses, and medicine. The Association established infirmaries and used sophisticated outreach strategies to locate cases (Hanggi-Myers, 1995)(Fig. 2.1).

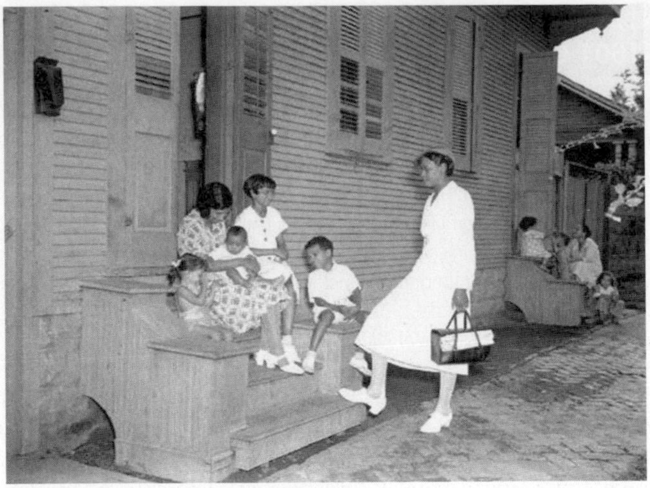

Fig. 2.1 A New Orleans nurse visiting a family on the doorstep of their home. (Courtesy the New Orleans Public Library WPA Photograph Collection.)

NIGHTINGALE AND THE ORIGINS OF TRAINED NURSING

Florence Nightingale established professional nursing in nineteenth-century Europe. With advances in transportation, communication, and other forms of technology, the Industrial Revolution led to deep social upheaval. Even with the advancement of science, medicine, and technology during the two previous centuries, nineteenth-century public health measures continued to be unsophisticated. Organization and management of cities improved slowly, and many areas lacked systems of sewage disposal and depended on private enterprise for water supply. Previous caregiving structures, which relied on the assistance of family, neighbors, and friends, became inadequate in the early nineteenth century because of human migration, urbanization, and changing demand. During this period, a few groups of Roman Catholic and Protestant women provided nursing care for the sick, poor, and neglected in institutions and sometimes in the home. For example, Mary Aikenhead, also known by her religious name Sister Mary Augustine, organized the Irish Sisters of Charity in Dublin (Ireland) in 1815. These sisters visited the poor at home and established hospitals and schools (Kalisch & Kalisch, 2004).

In nineteenth-century England, the Elizabethan Poor Law continued to guarantee medical care for all. This minimal care, provided most often in almshouses supported by local government, sought as much to regulate where the poor could live as to provide care during illness. Many women who performed nursing functions in almshouses and early hospitals in Great Britain were poorly educated, untrained, and often undependable. As the practice of medicine became more complex in the mid-1800s, hospital work required skilled caregivers. Physicians and hospital administrators sought to advance the practice of nursing. Early innovations yielded some improvement in care, but Florence Nightingale's efforts were revolutionary.

Florence Nightingale's vision for trained nurses and her model of nursing education influenced the development of professional nursing and, indirectly, public health nursing in the United States. In 1850 and 1851, Nightingale had carefully studied nursing "system and method" by visiting Pastor Theodor Fliedner at his School for Deaconesses in Kaiserswerth, Germany. Pastor Fliedner also built on the work of others, including Mennonite deaconesses in the Netherlands who were engaged in parish work for the poor and the sick, and Elizabeth Fry, the English prison reformer. Thus mid-nineteenth century efforts to reform the practice of nursing drew on a variety of interacting innovations across Europe.

The Kaiserswerth Lutheran deaconesses incorporated care of the sick in the hospital with client care in their homes, and their system of **district nursing** spread to other German cities. American requests for the deaconesses to respond to epidemics of typhus and cholera in Pittsburgh provided only temporary assistance because local women were uninterested in joining the work. The early efforts of the Lutheran deaconesses in the United States ultimately focused on developing systems of institutional care (Nutting & Dock, 1935).

Nightingale also found a way to implement her ideas about nursing practice. During the Crimean War (1854-1856) between the alliance of England and France against Russia, the British military established hospitals for sick and wounded soldiers at Scutari (now Üsküdar, a municipality of modern Istanbul). The care of sick and wounded soldiers was severely deficient, with cramped quarters, poor sanitation, lice and rats, insufficient food, and inadequate medical supplies (Kalisch & Kalisch, 2004; Palmer, 1983). When the British public demanded improved conditions, Nightingale sought and received an appointment to address the chaos. Because of her wealth, social and political connections, and knowledge of hospitals, the British government provided a staff of 40 ladies, 117 hired nurses, 15 paid servants, and extensive supplies for patient care.

In Scutari, Nightingale progressively improved soldiers' health outcomes, using a population-based approach that strengthened environmental conditions and nursing care. Using simple epidemiologic measures, she documented a decreased mortality rate from 415 per 1000 men at the beginning of the war to 11.5 per 1000 at the end (Cohen, 1984; Palmer, 1983). Paralleling Nightingale's efforts, contemporary public health nurses typically identify health care needs that affect the entire population, mobilize resources, and organize themselves and the community to meet these needs.

Nightingale's fame was established even before she returned to England in 1856 after the Crimean War. Once home, Nightingale turned her attention to reorganizing hospital nursing practice and to establishing hospital-based nursing education to replace untrained lay nurses with trained Nightingale nurses. Nightingale also emphasized public health nursing: "The health of the unity is the health of the community. Unless you have the health of the unity, there is no community health" (Nightingale, 1884/1994, p. 455). She also differentiated "sick nursing" from "health nursing." The latter emphasized that nurses should strive to promote health and prevent illness. Nightingale (1859/1946, p. v) wrote that the task of nurses is to "put the constitution in such a state as that it will have no disease, or that it can recover from disease." Proper nutrition, rest, sanitation, and hygiene were necessary for health. Nurses continue to focus on the vital role of health promotion, disease prevention, and environment in their practice with individuals, families, and communities.

Nightingale's contemporary and friend, British philanthropist **William Rathbone**, founded the first **district nursing association** in Liverpool, England. Rathbone's wife had received outstanding nursing care from a Nightingale-trained nurse during her terminal illness at home. He wanted to offer similar care to relieve the suffering of poor persons unable to afford private nurses. With Rathbone's advocacy and economic support between 1859 and 1862, the Liverpool Relief Society divided the city into nursing districts and assigned a committee of "friendly visitors" to each district to provide health care to needy people (Kalisch & Kalisch, 2004). Building on the Liverpool experience, Rathbone and Nightingale recommended steps to provide nursing in the home, leading to the organization of district nursing throughout England. Florence Sarah Lees Craven shaped the profession through her book *A Guide to District Nurses,* which highlighted, for example, that nursing care during the illness of one family member provided the nurse with influence to improve the entire family's health status (Craven, 1889/1984).

AMERICA NEEDS TRAINED NURSES

As urbanization increased during the Industrial Revolution in the 1800s, the number of occupations open to American women rapidly increased. Educated women became elementary school teachers, secretaries, or saleswomen. Less educated women worked in factories of all kinds. The idea of becoming a trained nurse increased in popularity when Nightingale's successes became known across the United States. During the 1870s, the first nursing schools based on the Nightingale model opened in the United States.

Trained nurse graduates of the early schools for nurses in the United States usually worked in private duty nursing or held the few positions as hospital administrators or instructors. Private duty nurses might live with families of clients receiving care, to be available 24 hours a day. Although the trained nurse's role in improving American hospitals was clear, the cost of private duty nursing care for the sick at home was prohibitive for all but the wealthy.

The care of the sick poor at home was made more economical by using home-visiting nurses who would attend several families in a day, rather than only one patient as the private duty nurse did. In 1877 the Women's Board of the New York City Mission hired Frances Root, a graduate of Bellevue Hospital's first nursing class, to visit sick poor persons to provide nursing care and religious instruction (Bullough & Bullough, 1964). In 1878 the Ethical Culture Society of New York hired four nurses to work in dispensaries, a type of community-based clinic. During the next few years, visiting nurse associations (VNAs) were established in Buffalo, New York (1885), Philadelphia (1886), and Boston (1886). Wealthy people interested in charitable activities funded both settlement houses and VNAs. Upper-class women, freed of some of the social restrictions that had previously limited their roles in public life, participated in the charitable work of creating, supporting, and supervising the new visiting nurses.

Public health nursing in the United States began with organizing to meet urban health care needs, especially for the disadvantaged. The public was interested in limiting disease among all classes of people, not only for religious reasons as a form of charity, but also because the middle and upper classes feared the impact of communicable diseases believed to originate in the large communities of new European immigrants. In New York City in the 1890s, about 2.3 million people lived in 90,000 tenement houses. Deplorable environmental conditions for immigrants in urban tenement houses and sweatshops were common across the northeastern United States and upper Midwest. People living in poor housing conditions were ravaged by epidemics of communicable diseases, including typhus, scarlet fever, smallpox, and typhoid fever; in the nineteenth century, tuberculosis was the leading cause of infectious disease mortality (Kalisch & Kalisch, 2004). From the beginning, nursing practice in the community included teaching and prevention.

For example, in 1886 two Boston women approached the local Women's Education Association to seek their support for district nursing. To increase the likelihood of financial support, the women used the term *instructive district nursing* to emphasize the relationship of nursing to health education. The Boston Dispensary provided support in the form of free outpatient medical care. In 1886 the first district nurse was hired, and in 1888 the Instructive District Nursing Association became incorporated as an independent voluntary agency. Sick poor persons, who paid no fees, were cared for under the direction of a trained physician (Brainard, 1922).

Nursing interventions, improved sanitation, economic improvements, and better nutrition were credited with reducing the incidence of acute communicable disease by 1910. New scientific explanations of communicable disease suggested that preventive education would reduce illness. Through home visits and well-baby clinics, the **visiting nurse** became the key to communicating this prevention campaign. Visiting nurses worked with physicians, gave selected treatments, and kept temperature and pulse records. Visiting nurses emphasized education of family members in the care of the sick and in personal and environmental prevention measures, such as hygiene and good nutrition. Most public health nursing practice in the early twentieth century was generalized practice with diverse responsibilities. Only a few public health nurses had a specialized practice, such as caring only for patients with tuberculosis or working only in an occupational health practice. Public health nurses also established **settlement houses**—neighborhood centers that became hubs for health care, education, and social welfare programs. For example, in 1893 **Lillian Wald** and Mary Brewster, both trained nurses, began visiting the poor on New York's Lower East Side. The nurses' settlement they established became the Henry Street Settlement and later the Visiting Nurse Service of New York City. By 1905 the public health nurses had provided almost 48,000 visits to more than 5000 clients (Kalisch & Kalisch, 2004). Other settlement houses influenced the growth of public health nursing, including the Richmond (Virginia) Nurses' Settlement, which became the Instructive Visiting Nurse Association; the Nurses' Settlement in Orange, New Jersey; and the College Settlement in Los Angeles, California. (See Fig. 2.2 for a photo of Lillian Wald).

Lillian Wald emerged as the key leader of public health nursing during its early decades. Wald took steps to increase access to public health nursing services nationally through insightful innovations: she persuaded the **American Red Cross** to sponsor

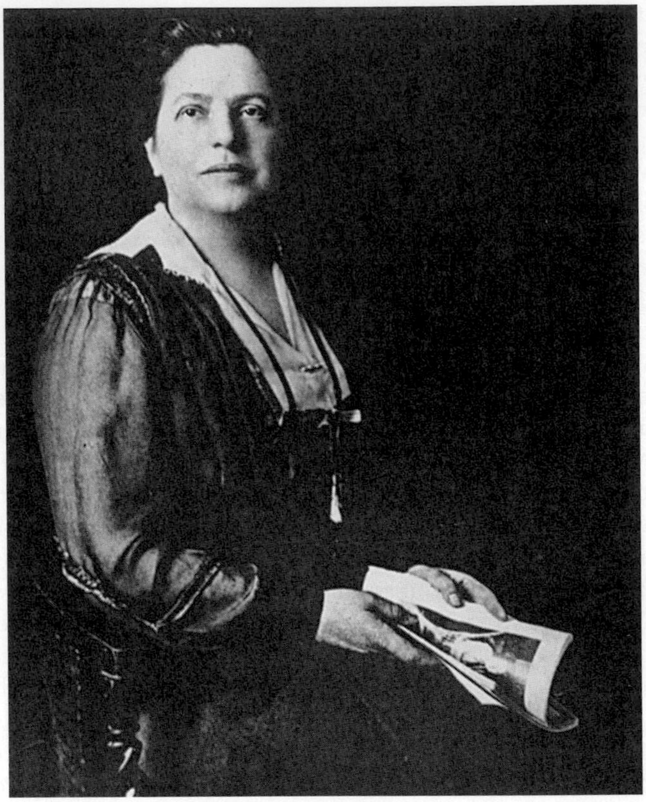

Fig. 2.2 Lillian Wald. (Courtesy the Visiting Nurse Service of New York.)

rural health nursing services across the country, which stimulated local governments to sponsor public health nursing through county health departments. Beginning in 1909, Wald worked with Dr. Lee Frankel of the Metropolitan Life Insurance Company (later, MetLife) to implement the first insurance payment for nursing services. She argued that keeping working people and their families healthier would increase their productivity. MetLife found that nursing care for communicable diseases, injuries, and mothers and children reduced mortality and saved money for this life insurance company. MetLife nursing services continued for 44 more years, with successes such as (1) providing home nursing services on a fee-for-service basis; (2) establishing an effective cost-accounting system for visiting nurses; and (3) reducing mortality from infectious diseases.

Convinced that environmental conditions as well as social conditions were the causes of ill health and poverty, Wald became actively involved in using epidemiologic methods to campaign for health-promoting social policies. She advocated for creation of the U.S. Children's Bureau as a basis for improving the health and education of children nationally. She fought for better tenement living conditions in New York City, city recreation centers, parks, pure food laws (free of contamination), graded classes for mentally handicapped children, and assistance to immigrants. She firmly believed in women's suffrage and considered its acceptance in 1917 in New York State to be a great victory. Wald supported efforts to improve race relations and championed solutions to racial injustice. She wrote *The House on Henry Street* (Wald, 1915) and *Windows on Henry Street* (Wald, 1934) to describe the diverse work of public health nursing.

Many public health nurses contributed to the development of the profession, including Jessie Sleet (Scales), a Canadian graduate of Provident Hospital School of Nursing (Chicago), who became the first African American public health nurse; Ms. Sleet was hired by the New York Charity Organization Society in 1900. At the Society in 1904 and 1905, she studied health conditions related to tuberculosis among African American residents of Manhattan, based on interviews with families and neighbors, house-to-house canvases, direct observation, and speeches at neighborhood churches. In reporting her research to the Society Board, Sleet recommended improved employment opportunities for African Americans and better prevention strategies to reduce the excess burden of tuberculosis morbidity and mortality among the African American population (Buhler-Wilkerson, 2001; Hine, 1989; Mosley, 1994; Thoms, 1929). Although it had been difficult for her to find a nursing agency willing to hire her as a district nurse, she persevered and was able to provide exceptional care for her clients until she married in 1909 and, as was common in the early twentieth century, left nursing practice.

In 1909 Yssabella Waters published her survey, *Visiting Nursing in the United States,* which documented the concentration of visiting nurse services in the northeastern quadrant of the nation (Waters, 1909). In 1901 New York City alone had 58 different organizations with 372 trained nurses providing care in the community. Despite the numbers, 68 percent of visiting nurses nationally were employed in single-nurse agencies. In addition to VNAs and settlement houses, a variety of other organizations sponsored visiting nurse work, including boards of education, boards of health, mission boards, clubs, churches, social service agencies, and tuberculosis associations. With tuberculosis then responsible for at least 10 percent of all mortality, visiting nurses contributed to its control through gaining "the personal cooperation of patients and their families" to modify the environment and individual behavior (Buhler-Wilkerson, 1987, p. 45). Most visiting nurse agencies depended financially on the philanthropy and social networks of metropolitan areas. Even today, fund-raising and service delivery in less densely populated and rural areas remains challenging.

The American Red Cross, through its Rural Nursing Service (later the **Town and Country Nursing Service**), provided a framework to initiate home nursing care in areas outside larger cities. Lillian Wald secured initial donations to support this agency, which provided care of the sick and instruction in sanitation and hygiene in rural homes. The agency also improved living conditions in villages and isolated farms. The Town and Country nurse dealt with diseases such as tuberculosis, pneumonia, and typhoid fever with a resourcefulness born of necessity. The rural nurse might use hot bricks, salt, or sandbags to substitute for hot water bottles; chairs as back-rests for the bedbound; and boards padded with quilts as stretchers (Kalisch & Kalisch, 2004). In the two years after World War I, the 100 existing Red Cross Town and Country Nursing Services expanded to 1800 programs and eventually developed almost 3000 programs in small towns and rural areas. This service demonstrated the importance and feasibility of public health nursing across the country at local and county levels. Once established, ongoing responsibilities for these new agencies were passed on to local voluntary agencies or local government support.

Occupational health nursing began as industrial nursing and was a true outgrowth of early home-visiting efforts. In 1895, Ada Mayo Stewart began work with the employees and families of the Vermont Marble Company of Proctor, Vermont. As a free service for the employees, Stewart provided obstetric care, sickness care (e.g., for typhoid cases), and some postsurgical care in workers' homes. Although her employer provided a horse and buggy, she often made home visits on a bicycle.

Unlike contemporary occupational health nurses, Stewart provided few services for work-related injuries. Before 1900 a few nurses were hired in industry, such as in department stores in Philadelphia and Brooklyn. Between 1914 and 1943, industrial nursing grew from 60 to 11,220 nurses, reflecting increased governmental and employee concerns for health and safety in the workplace (American Association of Industrial Nurses, 1976; Kalisch & Kalisch, 2004).

SCHOOL NURSING IN AMERICA

In New York City in 1902, more than 20 percent of children might be absent from school on a single day. The children suffered from the common conditions of pediculosis, ringworm, scabies, inflamed eyes, discharging ears, and infected wounds. Physicians had begun to make limited inspections of school students in 1897, but they focused on excluding sick children from school rather than on providing or obtaining medical treatment to enable children to return to school. Familiar with the limitations of this community-wide approach from her work with the Henry Street Nurses' Settlement, Lillian Wald sought to place nurses in the schools and gained consent from the city's health commissioner and the Board of Education for a one-month demonstration project.

Lina Rogers, a Henry Street Settlement resident, became the first school nurse. She worked with the children in New York City schools and made home visits to instruct parents and to follow up on children excluded or otherwise absent from school. The school nurses found that "many children were absent for lack of shoes or clothing, because of malnourishment, or because they were serving their families as babysitters" (Hawkins et al., 1994, p. 417). The school nurse experiment made such a significant and positive impact that the innovation became permanent in New York City schools, with 12 more nurses appointed one month later. School nursing was soon implemented in Los Angeles, Philadelphia, Baltimore, Boston, Chicago, and San Francisco.

THE PROFESSION COMES OF AGE

Established by the Cleveland Visiting Nurse Association in 1909, the *Visiting Nurse Quarterly* initiated a professional communication medium for clinical and organizational concerns. In 1911 a joint committee of existing nurse organizations convened to standardize nursing services outside the hospital. Under the leadership of Lillian Wald and Mary Gardner, the committee recommended forming a new organization to address public health nursing concerns. Eight hundred agencies involved in public health nursing were invited to send delegates to the June 1912 organizational meeting in Chicago. After a heated debate on its name and purpose, the delegates established the National Organization for Public Health Nursing (NOPHN) and chose Wald as its first president (Dock, 1922). Unlike other professional nursing organizations, the NOPHN membership included both nurses and their non-nurse supporters. The NOPHN sought "to improve the educational and services standards of the public health nurse, and promote public understanding of and respect for her work" (Rosen, 1958, p. 381). With greater administrative resources than other contemporary national nursing organizations, the NOPHN was soon the dominant force in public health nursing (Roberts, 1955).

The NOPHN also sought to standardize public health nursing education. Visiting nurse agencies found that hospital training school graduates were unprepared for home visiting. Hospital training schools emphasized hospital care of sick patients, but public health nurses required additional educational preparation to provide services through home-visiting and population-focused programs. In 1914, in affiliation with the Henry Street Settlement, Mary Adelaide Nutting began the first post–training-school course in public health nursing at Teachers College in New York City (Deloughery, 1977). The American Red Cross provided scholarships for graduates of nurse training schools to attend the public health nursing course. Its success encouraged the development of other programs, using curricula that might seem familiar to today's nurses. During the 1920s and 1930s, many newly hired public health nurses had to verify completion or promptly enroll in a certificate program in public health nursing. Others took leave for a year to travel to an urban center to obtain this further education.

Public health nurses were also active in the American Public Health Association (APHA), which had been established in 1872 to facilitate interprofessional efforts and to promote the "practical application of public hygiene" (Scutchfield & Keck, 1997, p. 12). The APHA targeted reform efforts toward contemporary public health issues, including sewage and garbage disposal, occupational injuries, and sexually transmitted diseases. In 1923 the Public Health Nursing Section was formed within the APHA to provide a forum for nurses to discuss their concerns and strategies within the larger APHA. The PHN Section continues to serve as a focus of leadership and policy development for public health nursing in the twenty-first century.

PUBLIC HEALTH NURSING IN OFFICIAL HEALTH AGENCIES AND IN WORLD WAR I

Public health nursing in voluntary agencies and through the Red Cross grew more quickly than public health nursing in official agencies, those sponsored by state, local, and national government. By 1900, 38 states had established state health departments; however, these early state boards of health had limited impact. Only three states—Massachusetts, Rhode Island, and Florida—annually spent more than two cents per capita for public health services (Scutchfield & Keck, 1997).

Yet, the federal role in public health gradually expanded. In 1912 the federal government redefined the role of the U.S. Public Health Service, empowering it to "investigate the causes and spread of diseases and the pollution and sanitation of navigable streams and lakes" (Scutchfield & Keck, 1997, p. 15). During World War I, the NOPHN loaned a nurse to the U.S. Public Health Service to establish a public health nursing program for military outposts. This led to the first federal government sponsorship of nurses and nursing (Shyrock, 1959; Wilner et al., 1978).

During the 1910s, public health organizations began to target infectious and parasitic diseases in rural areas. The Rockefeller Sanitary Commission, a philanthropic organization active in hookworm control in the southeastern United States, argued that concurrent efforts for all phases of public health were necessary to successfully address any individual public health problem (Pickett & Hanlon, 1990). For example, in 1911, efforts to control typhoid fever in Yakima County, Washington, and to improve health status in Guilford County, North Carolina, led to the establishment of local health units to serve local populations. As the number of local and county public health departments expanded, public health nurses became the primary staff members of local health departments. These nurses assumed a leadership role on health care issues through collaboration with local residents, nurses, and other health care providers.

The experience of Orange County, California, during the 1920s and 1930s illustrates the role of the public health nurse in these new local health departments. Following the efforts of a private physician, a Red Cross nurse, and social welfare agencies, the county board created the public health nurse's position, which began in 1922. Presented with a shining new Ford Model T automobile, which sported the bright orange seal of the county, the nurse focused on the serious communicable disease problems of diphtheria and scarlet fever. Typhoid became epidemic when a drainage pipe overflowed into a well, infecting those who drank the well water or raw milk from an infected dairy. Almost 3000 residents were immunized against typhoid. Weekly well-baby conferences provided an opportunity for mothers to learn about care of their infants, and the infants were weighed and given communicable disease immunizations. Children with orthopedic disorders and other disabilities were identified and referred for medical care in Los Angeles. At the end of a successful first year of public health nursing work, the Rockefeller Foundation and the California Health Department recognized the favorable outcomes and provided funding for more public health professionals.

The need for nurses to care for the injured and dying of World War I in Europe depleted the ranks of public health nurses in the United States. Concurrently, the NOPHN identified a need for more public health nurses within the United States. Jane Delano of the Red Cross (which was sending 100 nurses a day to the war) agreed that despite the sacrifice, the greatest patriotic duty of public health nurses was to stay at home. This proved a wise decision when, in 1918, the worldwide influenza pandemic swept the United States from coast to coast within three weeks and was met by a coalition of the NOPHN and the Red Cross. Houses, churches, and social halls were turned into hospitals for the immense numbers of sick and dying. Some of the nurse volunteers died of influenza as well (Shyrock, 1959; Wilner et al., 1978).

PAYING THE BILL FOR PUBLIC HEALTH NURSES

Inadequate funding was the major obstacle to extending nursing services in the community. Most early VNAs sought charitable contributions from wealthy and middle-class supporters. Even poor families were encouraged to pay a small fee for nursing services, reflecting social welfare concerns against promoting economic dependency by providing charity. In 1909, as a result of Wald's collaboration with Dr. Lee Frankel, the **Metropolitan Life Insurance Company** began a cooperative program with visiting nurse organizations that expanded availability of public health nursing services. The nurses assessed illness, taught health practices, and collected data from policyholders. By 1912, 589 Metropolitan Life nursing centers provided care through existing agencies or through visiting nurses hired directly by the Company. In 1918 Metropolitan Life calculated an average decline of 7 percent in the mortality rate of policyholders and almost a 20 percent decline in the mortality rate of policyholders' children under age three. The insurance company attributed this improvement and their reduced costs to the work of visiting nurses. Voluntary health insurance was still decades in the future; public and professional efforts to secure compulsory health insurance seemed promising in 1916 but had evaporated by the end of World War I.

Nursing efforts to influence public policy bridged World War I, including advocacy for the Children's Bureau and the Sheppard-Towner Program. Responding to lengthy advocacy by Lillian Wald and other nurse leaders, the Children's Bureau was established in 1912 to address national problems of maternal and child welfare. Children's Bureau experts conducted extensive scientific research on the effects of income, housing, employment, and other factors on infant and maternal mortality. Their research led to federal child labor laws and to the 1919 White House Conference on Child Health.

Problems of maternal and child morbidity and mortality spurred the passage of the Maternity and Infancy Act (often called the **Sheppard-Towner Act**) in 1921. This act provided federal matching funds to establish maternal and child health divisions in state health departments. Education during home visits by public health nurses stressed promoting the health of mother and child as well as seeking prompt medical care during pregnancy. Although credited with saving many lives, the Sheppard-Towner Program ended in 1929 in response to charges by the American Medical Association and others that the legislation gave too much power to the federal government and that it too closely resembled socialized medicine (Pickett & Hanlon, 1990). Federal funding during the 1930s and 1940s established maternal-child health programs that continued some of the successes of the Sheppard-Towner Program.

Some nursing innovations were the result of individual commitment and private financial support. In 1925 Mary Breckinridge established the **Frontier Nursing Service** (FNS), based on systems of care used in the Highlands and islands of Scotland. The unique pioneering spirit of the FNS influenced the development of public health programs geared toward improving the health care of the rural and often inaccessible populations in the Appalachian region of southeastern Kentucky (Browne, 1966; Tirpak, 1975). Breckinridge introduced the first nurse-midwives into the United States when she deployed FNS nurses trained in nursing, public health, and midwifery. Their efforts led to reduced pregnancy complications and maternal mortality and to one third fewer stillbirths and infant deaths in an area of 700 square miles (Kalisch & Kalisch, 2004). The early efforts of the FNS are recorded in the book, *Wide Neighborhoods* (Breckinridge, 1952). Today the FNS continues to provide comprehensive health and nursing services to the people of that area and sponsors Frontier Nursing University, which provides advanced practice nursing education for midwifery and other nursing specialties.

AFRICAN AMERICAN NURSES IN PUBLIC HEALTH NURSING

African American nurses seeking to work in public health nursing faced many challenges. Nursing education was absolutely segregated in the South until at least the 1960s, and elsewhere was also generally segregated or rationed until mid-century. Even public health nursing certificate and graduate education programs were segregated in the South; study outside the South for southern nurses was difficult to afford, and study leaves from the workplace were rarely granted. The situation improved somewhat in 1936, when collaboration between the U.S. Public Health Service and the Medical College of Virginia (Richmond) established a certificate program in public health nursing for African American nurses, with tuition provided by the federal government. Discrimination continued during nurses' employment: African American nurses in the American South were paid significantly lower salaries than their white counterparts for the same work. In 1925 just 435 African American public health nurses were employed in the United States, and in 1930 only 6 African American nurses held supervisory positions in public health nursing organizations (Buhler-Wilkerson, 2001; Hine, 1989; Thoms, 1929).

African American public health nurses had a significant impact on the communities they served. The National Health Circle for Colored People was organized in 1919 to promote public health work in African American communities in the South. One approach provided scholarships to assist African American nurses to pursue university-level public health nursing education. Bessie B. Hawes, the first recipient of the scholarship, completed the Columbia University program in New York City. The Circle sent Hawes to Palatka, Florida, a small, isolated lumber town. Hawes' first project recruited local school girls to promote health by dressing as nurses and marching in a parade while singing community songs. She conducted mass meetings, led mothers' clubs, provided school health education, and visited the homes of the sick. Eventually she gained the community's trust, overcame opposition, and built a health center for nursing care and treatment (Thoms, 1929).

BETWEEN THE TWO WORLD WARS: ECONOMIC DEPRESSION AND THE RISE OF HOSPITALS

The economic crisis during the Depression of the 1930s deeply influenced the development of nursing. Not only were agencies and communities unprepared to address the increased needs and numbers of the impoverished, but decreased funding for nursing services reduced the number of employed nurses in hospitals and in community agencies. The NOPHN's tenacious effort to ensure inclusion of public health nursing in federal relief programs secured success after a flurry of last-minute telegrams and lobbying efforts. Federal funding led to a wide variety of programs administered at the state level, including new public health nursing programs.

The Federal Emergency Relief Administration (FERA) supported nurse employment through increased grants-in-aid for state programs of home medical care. FERA often purchased nursing care from existing visiting nurse agencies, thus supporting more nurses and preventing agency closures. The FERA program varied among states; the state FERA program in New York emphasized bedside nursing care, whereas in North Carolina, the state FERA prioritized maternal and child health, and school nursing services. Some Depression-era federal programs built new services; public health nursing programs of the Works Progress Administration (WPA) were sometimes later incorporated into state health departments. In West Virginia, as elsewhere, the Relief Nursing Service had a dual purpose—to assist unemployed nurses and to provide nursing care for families on relief. Fundamental services included "(1) providing bedside care and health supervision for the family in the home; (2) arranging for medical and hospital care for emergency and obstetric cases; (3) supervising the health of children in emergency relief nursery schools; and (4) caring for patients with tuberculosis" (Kalisch & Kalisch, 2004, p. 283).

In another Depression-era program, more than 10,000 nurses were employed by the Civil Works Administration (CWA) and assigned to official health agencies. "While this facilitated rapid program expansion by recipient agencies and gave the nurses a taste of public health, the nurses' lack of field experience created major problems of training and supervision for the regular staff" (Roberts & Heinrich, 1985, p. 1162).

A 1932 survey of public health agencies found that only seven percent of nurses employed in public health were adequately prepared (Roberts & Heinrich, 1985). Basic nursing education focused heavily on the care of individuals, and students received limited information on groups and the community as a unit of service. Thus in the 1930s and early 1940s, new hospital training school graduates continued to be inadequately prepared to work in public health and required considerable remedial orientation and education from the hiring agencies (NOPHN, 1944).

Public health nurses continued to weigh the relative value of preventive care compared with bedside care of the sick. They also questioned whether nursing interventions should be directed toward groups and communities or toward individuals and their families. Although each nursing agency was unique and services varied from region to region, voluntary VNAs tended to emphasize care of the sick, whereas official public health agencies provided more preventive services. Compared with nursing in VNAs, nurses in official agencies may have had less control over their practice roles because physicians and politicians often determined services and personnel assignments in public health departments. See Fig. 2.1 for a photo of a nurse making a home visit to a family in New Orleans.

Not surprisingly, the conflicting visions and splintering of services between "visiting" and "public health" nurses further impeded development of comprehensive population-centered nursing services (Roberts & Heinrich, 1985). In addition, some households received services from several community nurses representing several agencies, for example, visits to the same home (1) for a postpartum woman and new baby, (2) for a child sick with scarlet fever, and (3) for an older adult sick in bed. Nurses believed that multiple caregivers and agencies confused families and duplicated scarce nursing resources. Interest grew in the "combination service"—the merger of sick care services and preventive services into one comprehensive agency, administered jointly between a voluntary agency and an **official health agency**.

INCREASING FEDERAL ACTION FOR THE PUBLIC'S HEALTH

Expansion of the federal government during the 1930s affected the structure of community health resources. Credited as "the beginning of a new era in public nursing" (Roberts & Heinrich, 1985, p. 1162), Pearl McIver in 1933 became the first nurse employed by the U.S. Public Health Service. In providing consultation services to state health departments, McIver was convinced that the strengths and abilities of each state's director of public health nursing would determine the scope and quality of local health services. Together with Naomi Deutsch, director of nursing for the federal Children's Bureau, and with the support of nursing organizations, McIver and her staff of nurse consultants influenced the direction of public health nursing. Between 1931 and 1938, greater than 40 percent of the increase in public health nurse employment was in local health agencies. Even so, nationally more than one third of all counties still lacked local public health nursing services.

The **Social Security Act of 1935** was designed to prevent reoccurrence of the problems of the Depression. Title VI of this act provided funding for expanded opportunities for health protection and promotion through education and employment of public health nurses. More than 1000 nurses completed educational programs in public health in 1936. Title VI also provided eight million dollars to assist states, counties, and medical districts in the establishment and maintenance of adequate health services, as well as two million dollars for research and investigation of disease (Buhler-Wilkerson, 1985, 1989; Kalisch & Kalisch, 2004).

A categorical approach to federal funding for public health services reflected the U.S. Congress's preference for funding specific diseases or specific groups, rather than providing dollar allocations to local agencies. In categorical funding, resources are directed toward specific priorities rather than toward a comprehensive community health program. When funding is directed by established national preferences, it becomes more difficult to respond to local and emerging problems. Even so, local health departments shaped their programs according to the pattern of available funds, including maternal and child health services and crippled children (in 1935), venereal disease control (in 1938), tuberculosis (in 1944), mental health (in 1947), industrial hygiene (in 1947), and dental health (in 1947) (Scutchfield & Keck, 1997). Categorical funding continues to be a preferred federal approach to address national health policy objectives.

WORLD WAR II: EXTENSION AND RETRENCHMENT IN PUBLIC HEALTH NURSING

The U.S. involvement in World War II in 1941 accelerated the need for nurses, both for the war effort and at home. The Nursing Council on National Defense, organized in the summer of 1940, was the coalition of the national nursing organizations that planned and coordinated activities for the war effort (How We Prepared for Defense in '41, 1942).

National interests prioritized the health of military personnel and workers in essential industries. Many nurses joined the Army and Navy Nurse Corps. Through the influence and leadership of U.S. Representative Frances Payne Bolton of Ohio, substantial funding was provided by the Bolton Act of 1943 to establish the Cadet Nurse Corps, which led to increased enrollment in schools of nursing at undergraduate and graduate levels. Under management by the U.S. Public Health Service, the Nursing Council for National Defense received one million dollars to expand facilities for nursing education. Additional programs that expanded both the total number of nurses and the number of nurses with preparation in public health nursing included the Training for Nurses for National Defense, the GI Bill, the Nurse Training Act of 1943, and Public Health and Professional Nurse Traineeships (McNeil, 1967).

As more and more nurses and physicians left civilian hospitals to meet the needs of the war, responsibility for client care was shifted to families, non-nursing personnel, and volunteers. "By the end of 1942, over 500,000 women had completed the American Red Cross home nursing course, and nearly 17,000 nurse's aides had been certified" (Roberts & Heinrich, 1985, p. 1165). By the end of 1946, more than 215,000 volunteer nurse's aides had received certificates.

In some cases, public health nursing expanded its scope of practice during World War II. For example, nurses increased their presence in rural areas, and many official agencies began to provide bedside nursing care (Buhler-Wilkerson, 1985; Kalisch & Kalisch, 2004). The federal Emergency Maternity and Infant Care Act of 1943 (EMIC) provided funding for medical, hospital, and nursing care for the wives and babies of servicemen. Health services seeking EMIC funds were required to meet the high standards of the U.S. Children's Bureau, which resulted in increased quality of care for all. In other situations, nursing roles were constrained by wartime and postwar nursing shortages. For example, the Visiting Nurse Society of Philadelphia ceased home birth services, drastically reduced industrial nursing services, and deferred care for the long-term chronically ill client.

Reflecting the complex social changes that had occurred during the war years, in the late 1940s local health departments faced sudden increases in client demand for care of emotional problems, accidents, alcoholism, and other responsibilities new to the domain of official health agencies. Changes in medical technology offered new possibilities for screening and treatment of infectious and communicable diseases, such as antibiotics to treat rheumatic fever and venereal diseases, and photofluorography for mass case finding of pulmonary tuberculosis. Local health departments expanded, both to address underserved areas and to expand types of services, and they often fared better economically than voluntary agencies.

Job opportunities for public health nurses grew because they continued to constitute a large proportion of health department personnel. Between 1950 and 1955, the proportion of U.S. counties with full-time local health services increased from 56 percent to 72 percent (Roberts & Heinrich, 1985). With more than 20,000 nurses employed in health departments, VNAs, industry, and schools, public health nurses at the middle of the twentieth century continued to have a crucial role in translating the advances of science and medicine into saving lives and improving health.

In 1946, representatives of agencies interested in community health met to improve coordination of various types of community nursing and to prevent overlap of services. The resulting guidelines proposed that a population of 50,000 be required to support a public health program and that there should be 1 nurse for every 2200 people. Nursing functions should include health teaching, disease control, and care of the sick. Communities were encouraged to adopt one of the following organizational patterns (NOPHN, 1946):

- Administration of all community health nurse services by the local health department
- Provision of preventive health care by health departments, and provision of home visiting for the sick by a cooperating voluntary agency
- A combination service jointly administered and financed by official and voluntary agencies with all services provided by one group of nurses

THE RISE OF CHRONIC ILLNESS

Between 1900 and 1955, the national crude mortality rate decreased by 47 percent. Many more Americans survived childhood and early adulthood to live into middle and older ages. Although in 1900 the leading causes of mortality were pneumonia, tuberculosis, and diarrhea/enteritis, by mid-century the leading causes had become heart disease, cancer, and cerebrovascular disease. Nurses helped to reduce communicable disease mortality through immunization campaigns, nutrition education, and provision of better hygiene and sanitation. Additional factors included improved medications, better housing, and innovative emergency and critical care services. Studies such as the National Health Survey of 1935-1936 had documented the national transition from communicable to chronic disease as the primary cause of significant illness and death. However, public policy and nursing services were diverted from addressing the emerging problem, first by the 1930s Depression and then by World War II.

As the aged population grew from 4.1 percent of the total U.S. population in 1900, to 9.2 percent in 1950, so did the prevalence of chronic illness. Faced with a client population characterized by extended life spans and increased longevity after chronic illness diagnosis, nurses addressed new challenges related to chronic illness care, long-term illness and disability, and chronic disease prevention. In official health agencies, categorical programs focusing on a single chronic disease emphasized narrowly defined services, which might be poorly coordinated with other community programs. Screening for chronic illness was a popular method of both detecting undiagnosed disease and providing individual and community education.

Some VNAs adopted coordinated home care programs to provide complex, long-term care to the chronically ill, often after long-term hospitalization. These home care programs established a multidisciplinary approach to complex client care. For example, beginning in 1949, the Visiting Nurse Society of Philadelphia provided care to clients with stroke, arthritis, cancer, and fractures using a wide range of services, including physical and occupational therapy, nutrition consultation, social services, laboratory and radiographic procedures, and transportation services. During the 1950s, often in response to family demands and the shortage of nurses, many visiting nurse agencies began experimenting with auxiliary nursing personnel, variously called housekeepers, homemakers, or home health aides. These innovative programs provided a substantial basis for an approach to bedside nursing care that would be reimbursable by commercial health insurance (such as Blue Cross), and later by Medicare and Medicaid.

The increased prevalence of chronic illness also encouraged a resurgence in combination agencies—the joint operation of official (city or county) health departments and voluntary visiting nurse agencies by a unified staff. The nursing profession preferred that services be provided in a coordinated, cost-effective manner respectful to the families served, as well as to avoid duplication of care. Where nursing services were specialized, one household might simultaneously receive care from three different agencies for postpartum and newborn care, tuberculosis follow-up, and stroke rehabilitation. In cities with combination agencies, a minimal number of nurses provided improved services, ensuring continuity of care at a cheaper price. No longer would an agency "pick up and drop a baby," but instead would follow the child through infancy, preschool, school, and into adulthood as part of one public health nursing program using one client record. The "ideal program" of the combination agency proved difficult to fund and administer, and many of the combination services implemented between 1930 and 1965 later retrenched into their former divided, public and private structures.

During the 1950s, public health nursing practice, like nursing in general, increased its focus on the psychological elements of client, family, and community care. To be more effective as helping professionals, nurses sought improved understanding of their own behavior, as well as the behavior of their clients and their coworkers. The nurse's responsibility for health and human needs expanded to include stress and anxiety reduction associated with situational or developmental stressors, such as birth, adolescence, and parenting. Public health nurses sought a comprehensive approach to mental health that avoided dividing persons into physical components and emotional components (Abramovitz, 1961). The following Evidence-Based Practice example traces the development of nursing and home health care in the United States.

EVIDENCE-BASED PRACTICE

No Place Like Home: A History of Nursing and Home Care in the United States (Buhler-Wilkerson, 2001) is a book-length analysis of the development of nursing care for those at home. Buhler-Wilkerson traces how the care of the sick moved from a domestic function to a charitable or public responsibility provided through visiting nurse associations and official health agencies. The central dilemma she raises is "why, despite its potential as a preferred, rational, and possibly cost-effective alternative to institutional care, home care remains a marginalized experiment in caregiving" (p. xi).

Buhler-Wilkerson follows the origins of home care from its beginnings in Charleston, South Carolina, to its expansion into northern cities at the end of the nineteenth century. She interprets the founding of public health nursing by Lillian Wald "as a new paradigm for community-based nursing practice within the context of social reform" (p. xii), and she particularly analyzes the effects of ethnicity, race, and social class. She traces the difficulties of organizing and financing care of the sick in the home, including the work of private duty nurses and the role of health insurance in shaping home services. The concluding section of the book highlights contemporary themes of "chronic illness, hospital dominance, financial viability, and struggles to survive" (p. xii), and projects the future of home care.

Buhler-Wilkerson brings to contemporary readers the stories of patients' needs and nurses' work against the financial challenges that have characterized home care. While focusing on one element, this book raises important questions for nurses' work across elements of community/public health nursing. Clearly identified need does not by itself open the doors to adequate financing for nursing care of the sick, for public health nursing, or for population care for health promotion.

Nurse Use

This book points out the complex issues involved in trying to provide the most effective care to patients. The needs of patients and their families may not entirely correlate with what is financially available. A lesson for each of us to learn is the following: identified need does not always influence the availability of funds to provide the desired care.

From Buhler-Wilkerson K: *No place like home: a history of nursing and home care in the United States.* Baltimore, 2001, Johns Hopkins Press.

DECLINING FINANCIAL SUPPORT FOR PRACTICE AND PROFESSIONAL ORGANIZATIONS

During the 1930s and 1940s hospitals became the preferred place for illness care and childbirth. Improved technology and the concentration of physicians' work in the acute care hospital were influential, but the development of health insurance plans such as Blue Cross provided a means for the middle class to seek care outside the traditional arena of the home. Federal health policy after World War II supported the growth of institutional care in hospitals and nursing homes rather than community-based alternatives. Fig. 2.3 depicts a public health nurse speaking with a family on their porch. Insurance companies did not consistently support the valuable care that home health care nurses provided.

Financing for voluntary nursing agencies was greatly reduced in the early 1950s when both the Metropolitan and John Hancock Life Insurance Companies ceased to fund visiting nurse services for their policyholders. The life insurance companies had found nursing services financially beneficial when communicable disease rates were high in the 1910s and 1920s, but reductions in communicable disease rates, improved infant and maternal health, and the increased prevalence of expensive chronic illnesses reduced sponsor interest in financing home visiting. The American Red Cross also discontinued its programs of direct nursing service by the mid-1950s.

The NOPHN had long sought additional approaches for funding public health nursing. Beginning in the 1930s, the NOPHN collaborated with the American Nurses Association (ANA) through the Joint Committee on Prepayment. Both organizations had identified the growth potential of early health insurance innovations. Voluntary nursing agencies developed a variety of initiatives to secure health insurance reimbursement for nursing services, including demonstration projects and educational campaigns directed toward nurses, physicians, and insurers. Blue Cross and other hospital insurance programs gradually adopted a formula that exchanged unused days of hospitalization coverage for post-discharge nursing care at home. Unlike organized medicine and hospital associations, nursing organizations contributed substantially to securing

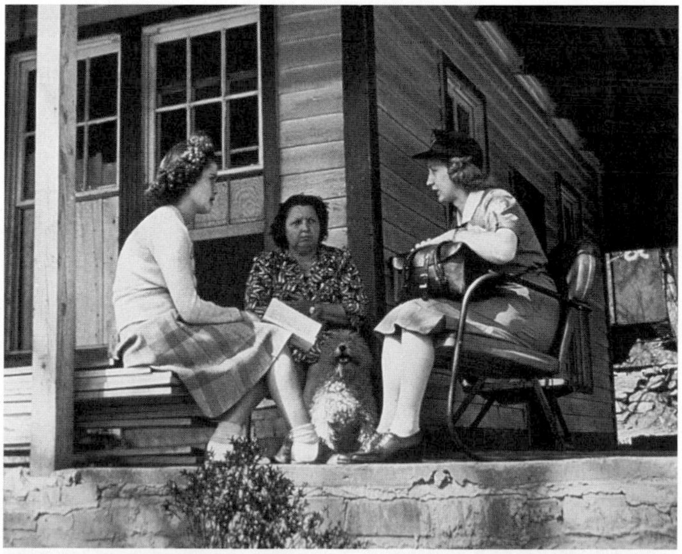

Fig. 2.3 A public health nurse talks with a young woman and her mother about childbirth, as they sit on a porch. (U.S. Public Health Service photo by Perry, Images from the History of Medicine, National Library of Medicine, Image ID 157037.)

federal medical insurance for the aged, which was implemented as the Medicare program in 1966. The support of the ANA, so integral to the passage of Medicare legislation, was publicly recognized by President Lyndon Baines Johnson at the 1965 ceremony to sign the bill.

Despite the successes and importance of the NOPHN, by the late 1940s its membership had declined and financial support was weak. At the same time, the nursing profession as a whole sought to reorganize its national organizations to improve unity, administration, and financial stability. Three existing organizations—the NOPHN, the National League for Nursing Education, and the Association of Collegiate Schools of Nursing—were dissolved in 1952. Their functions were distributed primarily to the new National League for Nursing. The American Nurses Association, which merged with the National Association of Colored Graduate Nurses, continued as the second national nursing organization. Occupational health nursing and nurse-midwifery organizations declined to join the consolidation, and both nursing specialties have continued to set their own course. School nurses also soon established a separate specialty organization. Despite the optimism of the national reorganization and its success in some areas, the subsequent loss of independent public health nursing leadership and focus resulted in a weakened specialty.

PROFESSIONAL NURSING EDUCATION FOR PUBLIC HEALTH NURSING

The National League for Nursing enthusiastically adopted the recommendations of Esther Lucile Brown's 1948 study of nursing education, reported as *Nursing for the Future* (Brown, 1948). Her recommendation to establish basic nursing preparation in colleges and universities was consistent with the NOPHN's goal of including public health nursing concepts in all basic baccalaureate programs. The NOPHN believed that this would remedy the preparation problems found among many nurses new to the practice and would thus upgrade the public health nursing profession. Unfortunately, the implementation of the plan fell short, and training programs in public health nursing for college and university faculty were very brief and inadequate. The population focus of public health nursing toward groups and the larger community was compromised and became less distinct in the hands of educators who themselves lacked education and practice in public health nursing.

During the 1950s, public health nursing educators carefully considered steps to enhance undergraduate and graduate education. Educational programs for public health nurses were then found in schools of nursing, schools of public health, and other university departments. Although all claimed legitimacy, collegiate education for nurses gradually moved completely into schools of nursing. The Haven Hill Conference (NOPHN, 1951) and Gull Lake Conference (Robeson & McNeil, 1957) clarified roles and definitions, built expectations for graduate education, and set standards for undergraduate field experiences. As public health nursing education drew closer to university schools of nursing, it adopted and applied broad principles characteristic of general nursing education. For example, rather than have the education director of the placement agency teach nursing students as done previously, collegiate programs themselves hired faculty who provided direct student supervision at community placements (NOPHN, 1951; Robeson & McNeil, 1957). The How To box describes the way to conduct an oral history interview in order to preserve vital information about public health nursing.

HOW TO Conduct an Oral History Interview

Nurse historians are increasingly using oral history methodology to uncover and preserve the history of public health nursing and individual nurses on audio files and written transcripts.

1. Identify an issue or event of interest.
2. Research the issue or event, using a variety of written and/or photographic materials.
3. Locate a potential oral history interviewee or narrator.
4. Obtain the agreement of the narrator to be interviewed. Arrange an interview appointment.
5. Research the narrator's background and the time period of interest.
6. Write an outline of questions for the narrator. Open-ended questions are especially helpful.
7. Meet with the narrator. Bring an audio recorder to the interview.
8. Interview the narrator. Ask one brief question at a time. Give the narrator time to consider your question and answer it. You can download an app on your smartphone or tablet to record the interview.
9. Ask clarifying questions. Ask for examples. Give encouragement. Allow the narrator to tell his or her story without interruption.
10. After the interview, transcribe the interview tape and prepare a written transcript (some digital programs can immediately produce a written transcript).
11. Carefully compare the written transcript with the narrator's recorded interview. It may be appropriate to have the narrator review and edit the written transcript.
12. If you have made written arrangements with the narrator, place the oral history audio and transcripts in an appropriate archive or library (highly recommended).

Keep in Mind: Oral history is a type of nursing research. Please consider that oral history interviews may require formal consent by the interviewee or narrator before the interview, as well as prior approval of the research from an institutional review board.

Consult the Literature: An example of oral history is presented in an article on the Michigan Oral History Project (Gates et al., 1994).

NEW RESOURCES AND NEW COMMUNITIES: THE 1960S AND NURSING

Beginning in earnest in the late 1940s, but on the basis of advocacy begun in the late 1910s, policymakers and social welfare representatives sought to establish national health insurance. In 1965 Congress amended the Social Security Act to include health insurance benefits for older adults (Medicare) and increased care for the poor (Medicaid). Unfortunately, the revised Social Security Act did not include coverage for preventive services, and home health care was reimbursed only when ordered by a physician. Nevertheless, this latter coverage prompted the rapid proliferation of home health care agencies, with for-profit agencies responding to new financial opportunities. Many local and state health departments rapidly changed their policies to include reimbursable home health care as bedside nursing. This could result in reduced health promotion and disease prevention activities, as funding for these activities was less stable. From 1960 to 1968, the number of official agencies providing home care services grew from 250 to 1328, and the number of for-profit agencies also continued to grow (Kalisch & Kalisch, 2004).

COMMUNITY ORGANIZATION AND PROFESSIONAL CHANGE

Social changes during the 1960s and 1970s influenced both nursing and public health. "The emerging civil rights movement shifted the paradigm from a charitable obligation to a political commitment to achieving equality and compensation for racial injustices of the past" (Scutchfield & Keck, 1997, p. 328). New programs addressed economic and racial differences in health care services and delivery. Funding was increased for maternal and child health, mental health, mental retardation, and community health training. Beginning in 1964, the federal Economic Opportunity Act provided funds for neighborhood health centers, Head Start, and other community action programs. Neighborhood health centers increased community access for health care, especially for maternal and child care. The work of Nancy Milio in Detroit, Michigan, is an example of this commitment to action, through partnering with the community. Milio built a dynamic decision-making process that included neighborhood residents, politicians, the Visiting Nurse Association and its board, civil rights activists, and church leaders. The Mom and Tots Center emerged as a neighborhood-centered service to provide maternal and child health services, as well as a daycare center. Milio (1971) recorded this story in her book, *9226 Kercheval: The Storefront That Did Not Burn*. As shown in Fig. 2.4 visiting nurses provided vital services to families.

New personnel also added to the flexibility of the public health nurse to address the needs of communities. Beginning

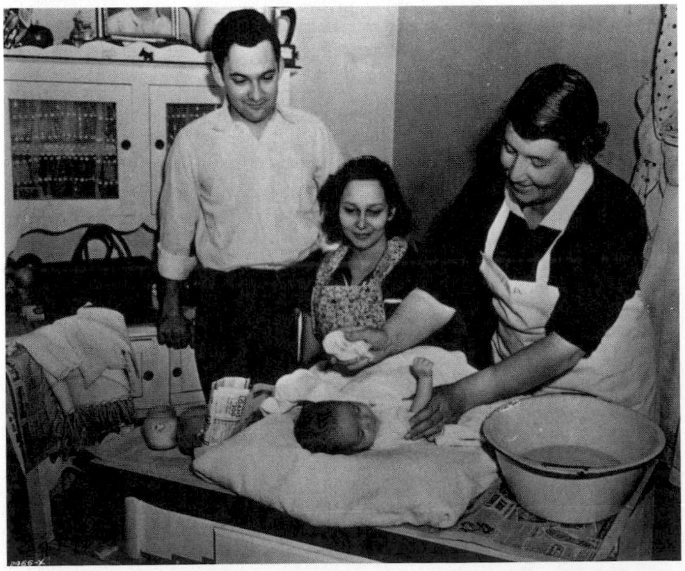

Fig. 2.4 A Visiting Nurse Association nurse demonstrates proper infant care and bathing techniques to the parents. (Images from the History of Medicine, National Library of Medicine, Image ID 144048.)

in 1965 at the University of Colorado, the nurse practitioner movement opened a new era for nursing involvement in primary care that became part of the delivery of services in community health clinics. Initially, the nurse practitioner would often be a public health nurse who had acquired additional skills in the diagnosis and treatment of common illnesses. Although some nurse practitioners chose to practice in other clinical areas, those who continued in public health settings made sustained contributions to improving access and providing primary care to people in rural areas, inner cities, and other medically underserved areas (Roberts & Heinrich, 1985). As evidence of the effectiveness of their services grew, nurse practitioners became increasingly accepted as cost-effective providers of a variety of primary care services.

PUBLIC HEALTH NURSING FROM THE 1970s INTO THE TWENTY-FIRST CENTURY

During the 1970s, nursing was viewed as a powerful force for improving the health care of communities. Nurses made significant contributions to the hospice movement, the development of birthing centers, daycare for older adult and disabled persons, drug abuse programs, and rehabilitation services in long-term care. Federal evaluation of the effectiveness of care was emphasized (Roberts & Heinrich, 1985).

By the 1980s, concern grew about the high costs of health care in the United States. Programs for health promotion and disease prevention received less priority as funding was shifted to meet the escalating costs of acute hospital care, medical procedures, and institutional long-term care. The use of ambulatory services, including health maintenance organizations, was encouraged, and the use of nurse practitioners increased. Home health care weathered several threats to adequate reimbursement and, by the end of the decade, had secured favorable legal decisions that increased its impact on the care of the sick at home. Individuals and families assumed more responsibility for their own health because health education, always a part of nursing, became increasingly popular. Advocacy groups representing both consumers and professionals urged the passage of laws to prohibit unhealthy practices in public such as smoking and driving under the influence of alcohol. Sophisticated media campaigns contributed to changing health behaviors and improving health status. As federal and state funds grew scarce, fewer nurses were employed by official public health agencies. Committed and determined to improve the health care of Americans, nurses continued to press for greater involvement in official and voluntary agencies (Kalisch & Kalisch, 2004; Roberts & Heinrich, 1985).

The National Center for Nursing Research (NCNR), established in 1985 within the federal National Institutes of Health near Washington, DC, had a major impact on promoting the work of nurses. Through research, nurses analyze the scope and quality of care provided by examining the outcomes and cost-effectiveness of nursing interventions. With the concerted efforts of many nurses, the NCNR gained official institute status within the National Institutes of Health in 1993, becoming the National Institute of Nursing Research (NINR).

By the late 1980s, public health as a whole had declined significantly in its effectiveness in accomplishing its mission and in shaping the public's health. Significant reductions in local and national political support, financing, and outcomes were vividly described in a landmark report by the Institute of Medicine, *The Future of Public Health* (Institute of Medicine [IOM], 1988). The IOM study group found America's public health system in disarray and concluded that, although there was widespread agreement about what the mission of public health should be, there was little consensus on how to translate that mission into action. Not surprisingly, the IOM reported that the mix and level of public health services varied extensively across the United States (Williams, 1995).

The Future of Public Health (IOM, 1988) determined that "contemporary public health is defined less by what public health professionals know how to do than by what the political system in a given area decides is appropriate or feasible" (p. 4). Nurses working in health departments saw underfunding reduce the breadth and depth of their role. When local public health departments provided insufficient care, voluntary agencies such as VNAs stepped in to assist vulnerable groups. However, without adequate funding for care of the poor, VNAs and other voluntary home health agencies faced hard economic choices, and some closed their doors.

America's *Healthy People* initiative has influenced goals and priority setting in both public health and nursing, beginning in 1979 (U.S. Department of Health, Education, and Welfare, 1979), with the current objectives detailed in *Healthy People 2020* (U.S. Department of Health and Human Services [USDHHS], 2010). Evidence-based practice recommendations that complement the Healthy People initiative are detailed for health promotion, disease prevention, and screening in primary care through the clinical guidelines from the U.S. Preventive Services Task Force, *Guide to Clinical Preventive Services* (2014), and for groups and communities, through *The Guide to Community Preventive Services*, now known also as *The Community Guide* (Community Preventive Services Task Force, 2014). Implementation of these strategies has influenced the work of public health nurses through their employment in health agencies and through participation in state or local health coalitions. See the Healthy People box that traces the development of this important series of documents.

HEALTHY PEOPLE 2020

History of the Development of Healthy People

In 1979 the groundbreaking *Healthy People: The Surgeon General's Report on Health Promotion and Disease Prevention* asserted that "the health of the American people has never been better" (U.S. Department of Health, Education, and Welfare [USDHEW], 1979, p. 3). But this was only the prologue to deep criticism of the status of American health care delivery. Between 1960 and 1978, health care spending increased 700 percent—without related improvements in mortality or morbidity. During the 1950s and 1960s, evidence had accumulated about chronic disease risk factors, particularly cigarette smoking, alcohol and

Continued

HEALTHY PEOPLE 2020

History of the Development of Healthy People—cont'd

drug use, occupational risks, and injuries. But these new research findings were not systematically applied to health planning and to improving population health.

In 1974 the Government of Canada published *A New Perspective on the Health of Canadians* (Lalonde, 1974), which found death and disease to have four contributing factors: inadequacies in the existing health care system, behavioral factors, environmental hazards, and human biological factors. Applying the Canadian approach, in 1976 U.S. experts analyzed the 10 leading causes of U.S. mortality and found that 50 percent of American deaths were the result of unhealthy behaviors, and only 10 percent were the result of inadequacies in health care. Rather than just spending more to improve hospital care, clearly prevention was the key to saving lives, improving the quality of life, and saving health care dollars.

A multidisciplinary group of analysts conducted a comprehensive review of prevention activities. They verified that the health of Americans could be significantly improved through "actions individuals can take for themselves" and through actions that public and private decision makers could take to "promote a safer and healthier environment" (p. 9). Similar to Canada's *New Perspectives,* America's *Healthy People* (USDHEW, 1979) identified priorities and measurable goals. *Healthy People* grouped 15 key priorities into three categories: key preventive services that could be delivered to individuals by health providers, such as timely prenatal care; measures that could be used by governmental and other agencies, as well as industry, to protect people from harm, such as reduced exposure to toxic agents; and activities that individuals and communities could use to promote healthy lifestyles, such as improved nutrition.

In the late 1980s, success in addressing these priorities and goals was evaluated, new scientific findings were analyzed, and new goals and objectives were set for the period from 1990 to 2000 through *Healthy People 2000: National Health Promotion and Disease Prevention Objectives* (U.S. Department of Health and Human Services [USDHHS], 1991). This process was repeated 10 years later to develop goals and objectives for the period 2000 to 2010 (USDHHS, 2000; (USDHHS, 2010). As the decade of 2010 to 2020 neared its end, work increased on planning and designing *Healthy People 2030.* Recognizing the continuing challenge to employ emerging scientific research to encourage modification of health behaviors and practices, as used for *Healthy People 2020,* planners for *Healthy People 2030* expect continued emphasis on health equity, elimination of health disparities, and improved health for all groups across the life span through disease prevention, improved social and physical environments, and healthy development and health behaviors (USDHHS, 2018).

Overarching Goals for *Healthy People 2020*

The goals identified for *Healthy People 2020* will be studied, revised, and updated for inclusion in *Healthy People 2030,* when *Healthy People 2030* is fully developed.

As examples, the goals for *Healthy People 2020* have included:

- Attain healthy, thriving lives and well-being, free of preventable disease, disability, injury and premature death.
- Eliminate health disparities, achieve health equity, and attain health literacy to improve the health and well-being of all.
- Create social, physical, and economic environments that promote attaining full potential for health and well-being for all.
- Promote healthy development, healthy behaviors and well-being across all life stages.
- Engage leadership, key constituents, and the public across multiple sectors to take action and design policies that improve the health and well-being of all.

Preliminary work on *Healthy People 2030* includes the vision, mission, foundational principles, and overarching goals.

Vision

A society in which all people can achieve their full potential for health and well-being across the life span.

Mission

To promote, strengthen, and evaluate the Nation's efforts to improve the health and well-being of all people.

Foundational Principles

Foundational principles explain the thinking that guides decisions about *Healthy People 2030.*

- Health and well-being of all people and communities are essential to a thriving, equitable society.
- Promoting health and well-being and preventing disease are linked efforts that encompass physical, mental, and social health dimensions.
- Investing to achieve the full potential for health and well-being for all provides valuable benefits to society.
- Achieving health and well-being requires eliminating health disparities, achieving health equity, and attaining health literacy.
- Healthy physical, social, and economic environments strengthen the potential to achieve health and well-being.
- Promoting and achieving the Nation's health and well-being is a shared responsibility that is distributed across the national, state, tribal, and community levels, including the public, private, and not-for-profit sectors.
- Working to attain the full potential for health and well-being of the population is a component of decision making and policy formulation across all sectors.

Overarching Goals

- Attain healthy, thriving lives and well-being, free of preventable disease, disability, injury, and premature death.
- Eliminate health disparities, achieve health equity, and attain health literacy to improve the health and well-being of all.
- Create social, physical, and economic environments that promote attaining full potential for health and well-being for all.
- Promote healthy development, healthy behaviors, and well-being across all life stages.
- Engage leadership, key constituents, and the public across multiple sectors to take action and design policies that improve the health and well-being of all.

Just as the public health nurse in the early twentieth century spread the "gospel of public health" to reduce communicable diseases, today's population-centered nurse uses *Healthy People* to reduce chronic and infectious diseases and injuries through health education, environmental modification, and policy development.

Data from Lalonde M: *A new perspective on the health of Canadians*, Ottawa, Canada, 1974, Department of Supply and Services. Retrieved from http://www.phac-aspc.gc.ca; U.S. Department of Health and Human Services, *Healthy People 2010: understanding and improving health*, ed. 2, Washington, DC, 2000, U.S. Government Printing Office; U. S. Department of Health and Human Services, *Healthy People 2030*.

DESIGNING HEALTH CARE FOR THE AMERICAN PEOPLE

The health care debate in the 1990s focused on cost, quality, and access to direct care services. Despite considerable interest in health care reform and securing universal health insurance coverage, the core economic debate—who will pay for what—emphasized reform of medical care rather than comprehensive changes in health promotion, disease prevention, and health care. In 1993, the American Health Security Act received insufficient Congressional support. Reflecting the weakness of public health, the aims of public health were never clearly considered in the proposed program. Proposals to reform existing services also failed to apply the lesson learned from the *Healthy People* initiative—that health promotion and disease prevention appear to yield reductions in costs and illness/injury incidence while increasing years of healthy life.

In 1991 the ANA, the American Association of Colleges of Nursing, the National League for Nursing, and more than 60 other specialty nursing organizations joined to support health care reform. The coalition of nursing organizations emphasized key health care issues of access, quality, and cost, and proposed a range of interventions designed to build a healthy nation through improved primary care and public health efforts. Professional nursing's continued support for improved health care access and reduced cost was rewarded in 2010 with the passage of the federal Patient Protection and Affordable Care Act. These successes emphasize that public health nursing must continue to advocate for extension of public health services to prevent illness, promote health, and protect the public.

The Quad Council of Public Health Nursing Organizations was founded in the early 1980s, and was composed of representatives from four organizations that include public health nurses. Current members include the Association of Community Health Nursing Educators (ACHNE, established in 1977); the Association of Public Health Nurses (APHN), which began as the Association of State & Territorial Directors of Nursing (ASTDN) in 1935; the Public Health Nursing Section of the American Public Health Association (PHN-APHA) (the Section was formed within APHA in 1923); and the Alliance of Nurses for Healthy Environments (formed in late 2008).

During the 1990s and 2000s the Quad Council of Public Health Nursing Organizations supported the efforts of its organizational members and public health organizations to establish mechanisms to improve quality of care and to advance the public health nursing profession during the twenty-first century. For example, the certification of public health nurses with graduate degrees was reinforced through collaborative agreements with the American Nurses Credentialing Center (ANCC).

The Quad Council (currently called the Quad Council Coalition of Public Health Nursing Organizations) also revised its *Competencies for Public Health Nurses* in 2011 and again in 2018. These competencies are separated into three tiers: Tier 1 for generalist public health nurses who conduct clinical, home visiting and population-based services; Tier 2 for public health nurses with management and/or supervisory responsibilities; and Tier 3 for public health nurses at executive, senior management, or leadership levels in public health nursing organizations. The 2018 revision of the *Competencies* is available at: http//www.quadcouncilphn.org.

In addition to the actions of the Quad Council itself, the four constituent members of the Council have also worked in their areas of expertise to link content to the practice of public health nursing through their development of standards and competencies that influence practice in various ways. In recent years, the name of the Quad Council has changed to the Quad Council Coalition (QCC) of Public Health Nursing Organizations and is currently comprised of representatives from APHN, ACHNE, APHA, and the Alliance of Nurses for Healthy Environments (ANHE) (Community/Public Health Nursing [C/PHN] Competencies, Quad Council 2018).

The Association of Community Health Nursing Educators developed important position papers, including *Graduation Education for Advanced Practice Public Health Nursing* (ACHNE, 2007) and *Academic Faculty Qualifications for Community/Public Health Nursing* (ACHNE, 2009). The Association of State and Territorial Directors of Nursing asserted the importance of public health nurses within public health systems through the publication of *Every State Health Department Needs a Public Health Nurse Leader* (ASTDN, 2008). And the Association of Public Health Nurses revised the ASTDN position paper on *The Role of the Public Health Nurse in Disaster Preparedness, Response, and Recovery* (APHN, 2014).

The Council on Linkages Between Academia and Public Health Practice provides exchanges and collaborations among all public health disciplines, including public health nursing. The Council's *Core Competencies for Public Health Professionals* (2014) features a core competency under the domain of public health sciences skills: "Identifies prominent events in the history of the public health profession" (p. 17).

The American Nurses Association's *Scope and Standards of Public Health Nursing Practice* (ANA, 2013) is a key guide for the practice of public health nursing. Periodically revised, the *Scope and Standards* is developed by a group of public health nursing leaders representing the major public health nursing organizations and reflects the central ideas of public health nursing. As there is substantial agreement about the characteristics and goals of public health nursing across organizations, it is not surprising that the ANA *Scope and Standards* and the Quad Council's *Public Health Nursing Competencies* both include the processes of assessment, analysis, and planning. Each also incorporates the importance of communication, cultural competency, policy, and public health skills in their recommendations for effective public health nurse practice. The Linking Content to Practice box describes how historically public health nursing journals have preserved the history of public health nursing.

LINKING CONTENT TO PRACTICE

Public Health Nursing, a major journal in the field of public health nursing, publishes articles that very broadly reflect contemporary research, practice, education, and public policy for population-based nurses. Begun in 1984, *Public Health Nursing (PHN)* was published quarterly through 1993 and has been a bimonthly journal since 1994. Patricia J. Kelly, PhD, MPH, APRN, is the journal's current editor (2019).

More than any other journal, *PHN* has assumed responsibility for preserving the history of public health nursing and for publishing new historical research on the field. The contemporary *Public Health Nursing* shares its name with the official journal of the National Organization for Public Health Nursing in the period 1931 to 1952 (earlier names were used for the official journal from 1913 to 1931, which built on the *Visiting Nurse Quarterly*, published 1909 to 1913).

The contemporary *Public Health Nursing* presents a wide variety of articles, including both new historical research and reprints of classic journal articles that deserve to be read and reapplied by modern public health nurses. One historical article reprinted in *PHN* addressed a nurse's 1931 work on county drought relief that underscores continuing professional themes of case-finding, collaboration, and partnership (Wharton, 1999). Another historical reprint recalled the important 1984 dialogue between two public health nurse leaders, Virginia A. Henderson and Sherry L. Shamansky, with an added contextual introduction from Sarah Abrams (Abrams, 2007). Original historical research presented in *PHN* is extremely varied, from public health nursing education, to public health nurse practice in Alaska's Yukon, to excerpts from the oral histories of public health nurses.

Contemporary nurses find inspiration and possibilities for modern innovations in reading the history of public health nursing in the pages of *PHN*.

Data from Abrams SE: Nursing the community, a look back at the 1984 dialogue between Virginia A. Henderson and Sherry L. Shamansky. *PHN* 24:382, 2007; reprinted from *PHN* 1:193, 1984; Wharton AL: County drought relief: a public health nurse's problem. *PHN* 16(4):307-308, 1999; reprinted from *PHN* 23, 1931.

PUBLIC HEALTH NURSING TODAY

In the last decades, new and continuing challenges have triggered growth and change in nursing. Where existing organizations have been unable to meet community and neighborhood needs, nurse-managed health centers provide a diversity of nursing services, including health promotion and disease/injury prevention. New populations in communities continue to challenge schools of nursing, health departments, rural health clinics, and migrant health services to provide the range of services to meet specific needs, including the needs of new immigrants. Transfer of official health services to private control has sometimes reduced professional flexibility and service delivery. Nurses also make the difficult choice to leave public health nursing to work in acute care, where the salaries are often higher. This is even more prominent in times of a nursing shortage. The Association of Community Health Nurse Educators calls for increased graduate programs to educate public health nurse leaders, educators, and researchers. Natural disasters (such as floods, hurricanes, and tornados) and human-made disasters (including explosions, building collapses, and airplane crashes) require innovative and time-consuming responses. Preparation for future disasters and potential bioterrorism demands the presence of well-prepared nurses. Many of these stories are detailed in the chapters that follow.

Some states have heard renewed persuasion to deploy school nurses in every school; a new recognition of the link between school success and health is again making the school nurse essential. Evidence from cost-benefit research on school nursing services underscores modern financial advantages for families and communities (Wang et al., 2014). Renewed evidence is also available from research on the use of nurses for prenatal and infant/toddler home visits to reduce "all-cause mortality among mothers and preventable-cause mortality in their first-born children living in highly disadvantaged settings" (Olds et al., 2014, p. E1). Even though both of these research inquiries have related precedents in the history of nursing, contemporary public health nurses must seek research approaches to demonstrate the outcomes of this work.

Today, public health nurses' past contributions ground twenty-first century public health nurses in a narrative that explains and gives importance to contemporary work. Nurses look to their history for inspiration, explanation, and prediction. Information and advocacy are used to promote a comprehensive approach to address the multiple needs of the diverse populations served. In the twenty-first century, public health nursing both reflects the past and builds on and beyond it.

CHECK YOUR PRACTICE

As you think about what you have read in the chapter about the rich history of public health nursing, identify what you think the ideal role for a public health nurse would be today. Assume that the federal and state governments are willing to pay for high-quality care for their citizens; how would you craft the role? Be realistic since budgets are not endless. What would be your priorities for caring for the citizens? Who would be the agencies providing the care? How interested would you be in becoming a public health nurse?

Nurses will seek to learn from the past and to avoid known pitfalls, even as they seek successful strategies to meet the complex needs of today's vulnerable populations. As plans for the future are made, and as the public health challenges that remain unmet are acknowledged, it is this vision of what nursing can accomplish that sustains these nurses. In public health nursing as in all other specialty areas, quality and safety are key issues. The box below outlines the six Quality and Safety in Nursing Education (QSEN) competencies and describes the development of these competencies.

QSEN FOCUS ON QUALITY AND SAFETY EDUCATION IN NURSES

Although the scope and responsibilities of public health nurses have changed over time, the commitment to quality and safety has remained constant. Since the beginning of population-centered nursing in the United States, the nurses who worked in this specialty have been committed to preserving health and preventing disease. They have focused on environmental conditions such as sanitation and control of communicable diseases, education for health, prevention of disease and disability, and at times care of the sick and aged in their homes. This long-standing commitment to quality and safety is consistent with the work of *Quality and Safety Education for Nurses* (QSEN), a national initiative designed to transform nursing education by including in the curriculum content and experiences related to building knowledge, skills, and attitudes for six quality and safety initiatives (Cronenwett et al., 2009). The QSEN work, led by Drs. Linda Cronenwett and Gwen Sherwood at the University of North Carolina, has made great progress in bridging the gap between quality and safety work in both practice and academic settings (Brown et al., 2010). The six QSEN competencies for Nursing are:

1. **Patient-centered care:** Recognizes the client or designee as the source of control and as a full partner in providing compassionate and coordinated care that is based on the preferences, values, and needs of the client.
2. **Teamwork and collaboration:** Refers to the ability to function effectively with nursing and interprofessional teams and to foster open communication, mutual respect, and shared decision making to provide quality client care.
3. **Evidence-based practice:** Integrates the best current clinical evidence with client and family preferences and values to provide optimal client care.
4. **Quality improvement:** Uses data to monitor the outcomes of the care processes and uses improvement methods to design and test changes to continually improve quality and safety of health care systems.
5. **Safety:** Minimizes the risk for harm to clients and provides safety through both system effectiveness and individual performance.
6. **Informatics:** Use information and technology to communicate, manage knowledge, mitigate error, and support decision making (Brown et al., 2010, p. 116).

Of the six QSEN competencies, all but safety were derived from the Institute of Medicine report, *Health Professions Education* (Greiner & Knebel, 2003). The QSEN team added safety because this competency is central to the work of nurses. Articles have been published to teach educators about QSEN, and national forums have been held. Also the American Association of Colleges of Nursing (AACN) has held faculty development institutes for faculty and academic administrators using a train-the-trainer model, and safety and quality objectives have been built in the AACN essentials for nursing education. Similarly, the National League for Nursing has incorporated the "NLN Educational Competencies Model" into their educational summits. The six QSEN competencies will be integrated in the chapters throughout the text to emphasize the importance of quality and safety in public health nursing today. *Note:* The terms *patient* and *care* will be changed to *client* and *intervention* to reflect a public health nursing approach.

Specifically related to the history of nursing, the following targeted competency can be applied:

Targeted Competency: Safety

Minimizes risk for harm to clients and providers through both system effectiveness and individual performance.

Important aspects of safety include:

- **Knowledge:** Discuss potential and actual impact of national client safety resources, initiatives and regulations
- **Skills:** Participate in analyzing errors and designing system improvements
- **Attitudes:** Value vigilance and monitoring by clients, families, and other members of the health care team

Safety Question

Updated definitions around client safety include addressing safety at the individual level and at the systems level. The history of public health nursing demonstrates the myriad ways that public health nurses have addressed client safety in their evolving practice. Public health nurses support safety through caring for individuals and providing care for communities and groups. Historically, how have public health nurses addressed safety at the individual client level? How have public health nurses addressed client safety at the systems level? How have public health nurses been involved in system improvements?

Answer

Individual level: A rich part of public health nursing's history has been the development of home visitation, in which clients are cared for in their own environment. Similarly, public health nurses have improved client outcomes by pioneering new models of interventions for maternal–child health and individuals in rural communities.

Systems level: Through their work with communities, public health nurses were an integral part of reducing the incidence of communicable diseases by the mid-twentieth century. More recently, public health nursing has contributed to health care system improvements through the development of the hospice movement, birthing centers, daycare for elderly and disabled persons, and drug-abuse and rehabilitation services. These initiatives have updated the health care system to provide targeted care for previously overlooked populations.

Prepared by Gail Armstrong, PhD, DNP, ACNS-BC, CNE, Associate Professor, University of Colorado Denver College of Nursing.

PRACTICE APPLICATION

Mary Lipsky has worked for the county health department in a major urban area for almost two years. Her nursing responsibilities include a variety of services, including consultations at a senior center, maternal/newborn home visits, and well-child clinics. As she leaves work each evening and returns to her own home, she keeps thinking about her clients. Why was it so difficult today to qualify a new mother and her baby to receive WIC (Women, Infants, and Children) nutrition services? Why must she limit the number of children screened for high lead levels, when last year the health department screened twice as many children? Several children last month seemed asymptomatic, but the laboratory found lead levels that were high enough to cause damage. One of the mothers Ms. Lipsky is acquainted with is having a difficult time emotionally. Why is it so difficult to find a behavioral health provider for her? And the health department still cannot find a new staff dentist! And families on welfare cannot find a private dentist to care for their children.

A. Why might it be difficult to solve these problems at the individual level, on a case-by-case basis?

B. What information would you need to build an understanding of the policy background for each of these various populations?

Answers can be found on the Evolve site.

KEY POINTS

- A historical approach can be used to increase understanding of public health nursing in the past, as well as its current dilemmas and future challenges.
- The history of public health nursing can be characterized by change in specific focus of the specialty but continuity in approach and style of the practice.
- Public health nursing, referred to in this text as population-centered nursing, is a product of various social, economic, and political forces; it incorporates public health science in addition to nursing science and practice.
- Federal responsibility for health care was limited until the 1930s, when the economic challenges of the Depression permitted reexamination of local responsibility for care.
- Florence Nightingale designed and implemented the first program of trained nursing, and her contemporary, William Rathbone, founded the first district nursing association in England.
- Urbanization, industrialization, and immigration in the United States increased the need for trained nurses, especially in public health nursing.
- Increasing acceptance of public roles for women permitted public health nursing employment for nurses, as well as public leadership roles for their wealthy supporters.
- In 1877 the Women's Board of the New York City Mission hired Frances Root, a trained nurse, to provide care to sick persons at home.
- The first visiting nurses' associations were founded in 1885 and 1886 in Buffalo, Philadelphia, and Boston.
- Lillian Wald established the Henry Street Settlement, which became the Visiting Nurse Service of New York City, in 1893. She played a key role in innovations that shaped public health nursing in its first decades, including school nursing, insurance payment for nursing, national organization for public health nurses, and the United States Children's Bureau.
- Founded in 1902 with the vision and support of Lillian Wald, school nursing sought to keep children in school so that they could learn.
- The Metropolitan Life Insurance Company established the first insurance-based program in 1909 to support community health nursing services.
- The National Organization for Public Health Nursing (founded in 1912) provided essential leadership and coordination of diverse public health nursing efforts; the organization merged into the National League for Nursing in 1952.
- Official health agencies slowly grew in numbers between 1900 and 1940, accompanied by a steady increase in public health nursing positions.
- The innovative Sheppard-Towner Act of 1921 expanded community health nursing roles for maternal and child health during the 1920s.
- Mary Breckinridge established the Frontier Nursing Service in 1925, which influenced provision of rural health care.
- African American nurses seeking to work in public health nursing faced many challenges, but ultimately had significant impact on the communities they served.
- The specialty of Public Health Nursing has been characterized since the 1910s by the tension between the nursing role of caring for the sick and the role of providing preventive care for individuals and families, and by the more population related tension between intervening for individuals and intervening for groups.
- As the Social Security Act attempted to remedy some of the setbacks of the Depression, it established a context in which public health nursing services expanded.
- The challenges of World War II sometimes resulted in extensions of nursing care, and sometimes in retrenchment and decreased public health nursing services.
- By the mid-twentieth century, the reduced prevalence of communicable diseases and the increased prevalence of chronic illness, accompanied by large increases in the population more than 65 years of age, led to examination of the goals and organization of public health nursing services.
- Between the 1930s and 1965, organized nursing and community health nursing agencies sought to establish health insurance reimbursement for nursing care at home.
- Implementation of Medicare and Medicaid programs in 1966 established new possibilities for supporting community-based nursing care but encouraged agencies to focus on services provided after acute care rather than on prevention.
- Efforts to reform health care organization, pushed by increased health care costs during the last 40 years, have focused on reforming acute medical care rather than on designing a comprehensive preventive approach.
- The 1988 Institute of Medicine report documented the reduced political support, financing, and impact that increasingly limited public health services at national, state, and local levels.
- In the late 1990s, federal policy changes dangerously reduced financial support for home health care services, threatening the long-term survival of visiting nurse agencies.
- *Healthy People 2000* (USDHHS, 1991), *Healthy People 2010* (USDHHS, 2000), and recent disasters and acts of terrorism have brought renewed emphasis on prevention to nursing.

CLINICAL DECISION-MAKING ACTIVITIES

1. Interview nurses at your clinical placement about the changes they have seen during their years in a population-centered nursing practice. How do these changes relate to the changing needs of the community or the population?
2. Identify the visible record of nursing agencies in your community. Note the buildings, plaques, and display cases that document the past provision of nursing care in community settings. What forces have influenced these agencies over

time? Which factors do they wish to make known publicly, and which factors are less apparent?
3. Secure a copy of your clinical agency's recent annual report. How is the history of the agency presented? How does this agency's history fit in with the points made in this chapter? What are your conclusions about how this agency's past influences its present?
4. Interview older relatives for their memories of public health nursing care received by them, their families, and their friends. When they were younger, how was the public health nurse perceived in their community? What interventions were used by the public health nurse? How was the public health nurse dressed? How has the position of the public health or community health nurse changed?
5. Of what element or aspect of the history of public health nursing would you like to learn more? At your nursing library, review a period of 10 years in one journal from the past to identify trends in how this element or aspect was addressed. What conclusions do you reach?
6. The work and impact of several nursing leaders is reviewed or noted in this chapter. Of these leaders, which one strikes you as most interesting? Why? Locate and read further articles or books about this leader. What personal strengths do you note that supported this nurse's leadership?

ADDITIONAL RESOURCES

EVOLVE WEBSITE

http://evolve.elsevier.com/Stanhope/community/

- Answers to Practice Application
- Case Study
- Glossary
- Review Questions

REFERENCES

Abramovitz AB, editor: *Emotional factors in public health nursing: a casebook*, Madison, WI, 1961, University of Wisconsin Press.

Abrams SE: Nursing the community, a look back at the 1984 dialogue between Virginia A. Henderson and Sherry L. Shamansky, *PHN* 24:382, 2007; reprinted from PHN 1:193, 1984.

American Association of Industrial Nurses (AAIN): *The nurse in industry: a history of the American Association of Industrial Nurses Inc*, New York, NY, 1976, AAIN.

American Nurses Association (ANA): *Public health nursing: scope and standards of practice*, ed 2, Washington, DC, 2013, ANA.

Association of Community Health Nursing Educators (ACHNE): *Graduate Education for Advanced Practice Public Health Nursing: At the Crossroads*, 2007. Retrieved from http://achne.org.

Association of Community Health Nursing Educators (ACHNE): *Position paper: Academic Faculty Qualifications for Community/ Public Health Nursing*, 2009. Retrieved from https://www .resourcenter.net.

Association of Public Health Nurses (APHN): *The Role of the Public Health Nurse in Disaster Preparedness, Response, and Recovery*, 2014. Retrieved from http://www.phnurse.org.

Association of State and Territorial Directors of Nursing (ASTDN): *Every State Health Department Needs a Public Health Nurse Leader*, 2008. Retrieved from http://www.phnurse.org.

Brainard A: *Evolution of public health nursing, Philadelphia*, PA. 1922, WB Saunders.

Breckinridge M: *Wide neighborhoods: a story of the frontier nursing service*, New York, NY, 1952, Harper.

Brown EL: Nursing for the Future: *A Report Prepared for the National Nursing Council*, New York, NY, 1948, Russell Sage Foundation.

Browne HE: A tribute to Mary Breckenridge, *Nurs Outlook* 14:54–55, 1966.

Brown R, Feller L, Benedict L: Reframing nursing education: the Quality and Safety Education for Nurses Initiative, *Teach Learn Nurs* 5:115–118, 2010.

Buhler-Wilkerson K: Public health nursing, in sickness or in health? *Am J Public Health* 75:1155–1161, 1985.

Buhler-Wilkerson K: Left carrying the bag: experiments in visiting nursing, 1877–1909, *Nurs Res* 36:42–45, 1987.

Buhler-Wilkerson K: False Dawn: *The Rise and Decline of Public Health Nursing, 1900–1930*, New York, NY, 1989, Garland.

Buhler-Wilkerson K: *No place like home: a history of nursing and home care in the United States*, Baltimore, MD, 2001, Johns Hopkins Press.

Bullough V, Bullough B: *The emergence of modern nursing*, New York, NY, 1964, Macmillan.

Cohen IB: Florence Nightingale, *Sci Am* 250:128–137, 1984.

Community Preventive Services Task Force: *The Community Guide*, 2014. Retrieved from http://www.thecommunityguide.org/.

Council on Linkages between Academia and Public Health Practice: *Core competencies for public health professionals*, [revised 2014]. Retrieved from http://www.phf.org.

Craven FSL: *A guide to district nurses, 1889, Reprint*, New York, NY, 1984, Garland.

Cronenwett L, Sherwood G, Gelmon SB: Improving quality and safety education: the QSEN learning collaborative, *Nurs Outlook* 57:304–312, 2009.

Deloughery GL: *History and trends of professional nursing*, ed 8, St. Louis, MO, 1977, Mosby

Dock LL: The history of public health nursing, *Public Health Nurs* 14:522, 1922.

Gates MF, Schim SS, Ostrand L: Uniting the past and the future in public health nursing: the Michigan Oral History Project, *Public Health Nurs* 11(6):371–375, 1994.

Greiner AC, Knebel E, editors: *Health professions education: a bridge to quality. Institute of Medicine, Committee on the Health Professions Education Summit*, Washington, DC, 2003, National Academies Press.

Hanggi-Myers L: The Howard Association of New Orleans: precursor to district nursing, *Public Health Nurs* 12:78–82, 1995.

Hawkins JW, Hayes ER, Corliss CP: School nursing in America: 1902–1994: a return to public health nursing, *Public Health Nurs* 11:416–425, 1994.

Hine DC: *Black women in white: racial conflict and cooperation in the nursing profession, 1890–1950*, Bloomington, IN, 1989, Indiana University Press.

How We Prepared for Defense in '41, *Am J Nurs* 42:2–4, 1942.

Institute of Medicine (IOM): *The future of public health*, Washington, DC, 1988, National Academies Press.

Kalisch PA, Kalisch BJ: *American nursing: a history*, ed 4, Philadelphia, PA, 2004, Lippincott Williams & Wilkins.

Lalonde M: *A new perspective on the health of Canadians*, Ottawa, Canada, 1974, Department of Supply and Services. Retrieved from http://www.phac-aspc.gc.ca.

McNeil EE: *Transition in public health nursing: John Sundwall Lecture*, Ann Arbor, MI, February 27, 1967, University of Michigan.

Milio N: *9226 Kercheval: the storefront that did not burn*, Ann Arbor, MI, 1971, University of Michigan Press.

Mosley MO: Jessie Sleet Scales: first black public health nurse, *ABNF J* 5:45–51, 1994.

National Organization for Public Health Nursing (NOPHN): Approval of Skidmore College of Nursing as preparing students for public health nursing, *Public Health Nurs* 36:371, 1944.

National Organization for Public Health Nursing (NOPHN): Desirable organization for public health nursing for family service, *Public Health Nurs* 38:387–389, 1946.

National Organization for Public Health Nursing (NOPHN): *Proceedings of work conference: collegiate council on public health nursing education*, New York, NY, 1951, NOPHN.

Nightingale F: *Notes on Nursing: What It Is, and What It Is Not. 1859*, Reprint, Philadelphia, PA, 1946, Lippincott.

Nightingale F: Sick nursing and health nursing. 1894. Reprint. In Billings JS, Hurd HM, editors: *Hospitals, dispensaries, and nursing*, New York, NY, 1994, Garland.

Nutting MA, Dock LL: *A history of nursing*, New York, NY, 1935, Putnam.

Olds DL, Kitzman H, Knudtson MD, et al: Effect of home visiting by nurses on maternal and child mortality: results of a 2-decade follow-up of a randomized clinical trial, *JAMA Pediatr* [serial online] 2014. Retrieved from http://www.ncbi.nlm.nih.gov.

Palmer, IS: *Florence Nightingale and the first organized delivery of nursing services*, Washington, DC, 1983, American Association of Colleges of Nursing.

Pickett G, Hanlon JJ: *Public health: administration and practice*, St. Louis, MO, 1990, Mosby.

Quad Council Coalition Competency Review Task Force: *Community/Public Health Nursing [C/PHN] Competencies*, 2018. Retrieved from http://www.quadcouncilphn.org.

Roberts M: *American nursing: history and interpretation*, New York, NY, 1955, Macmillan.

Roberts DE, Heinrich J: Public health nursing comes of age, *Am J Public Health* 75:1162–1165, 1985.

Robeson KA, McNeil EE: *Report of conference on field instruction in public health nursing*, New York, NY, 1957, National League for Nursing.

Rodabaugh JH, Rodabaugh MJ: *Nursing in Ohio: a history*, Columbus, OH, 1951, Ohio State Nurses' Association.

Rosen G: *A history of public health*, New York, NY, 1958, MD Publications.

Scutchfield FD, Keck CW: *Principles of public health practice*, Albany, NY, 1997, Delmar.

Shyrock H: *The history of nursing*, Philadelphia, PA, 1959, WB Saunders.

Thoms AB: *Pathfinders: a history of the progress of colored graduate nurses*, New York, NY, 1929, Kay Printing House.

Tirpak H: The Frontier Nursing Service: fifty years in the mountains, *Nurs Outlook* 33:308, 1975.

U.S. Department of Health, Education, and Welfare (USDHEW): *Healthy People: The Surgeon General's Report on Health Promotion and Disease Prevention.* DHEW (PHS) Publication No. 79-55071, Washington, DC, 1979, U.S. Government Printing Office.

U.S. Department of Health and Human Services (USDHHS): *Healthy People 2000: National Health Promotion and Disease Prevention Objectives.* DHHS Publication No. 91-50212, Washington, DC, 1991, U.S. Government Printing Office. Retrieved from http://odphp.osophs.dhhs.gov.

U.S. Department of Health and Human Services (USDHHS): *Healthy People 2010: understanding and improving health*, ed 2, Washington, DC, 2000, U.S. Government Printing Office.

U.S. Department of Health and Human Services (USDHHS): *Healthy People 2020: improving the health of Americans*, 2010. Retrieved from http://www.healthypeople.gov.

U.S. Department of Health and Human Services (USDHHS): *Healthy People 2030*. Retrieved November 24, 2018.

U.S. Preventive Services Task Force: *Guide to clinical preventive services*, 2014. Retrieved from http://www.ahrq.gov.

Wald LD: *The house on Henry Street*, New York, NY, 1915, Holt.

Wald LD: *Windows on Henry Street*, Boston, MA, 1934, Little, Brown.

Wang LY, Vernon-Smiley M, Gapinski MA, et al: Cost-benefit study of school nursing services, *JAMA Pediatr* 168:642–648, 2014. Retrieved from http://www.msno.org.

Waters Y: *Visiting nursing in the United States*, New York, NY, 1909, Charities Publication Committee.

Wharton AL: County drought relief: a public health nurse's problem, *PHN* 16(4):307–308, 1999; reprinted from PHN 23, 1931.

Williams CA: Beyond the Institute of Medicine report: a critical analysis and public health forecast, *Fam Community Health* 18:12, 1995.

Wilner DM, Walkey RP, O'Neill EJ: *Introduction to public health*, ed 7, New York, NY, 1978, Macmillan.

3

Public Health, Primary Care, and Primary Health Care Systems

Marcia Stanhope, PhD, RN, FAAN and Karen R. Dawn, DNP, MSN, BSN

OBJECTIVES

After reading this chapter, the student should be able to do the following:

1. Describe the events and trends that influence the status of the health care system.
2. Discuss key aspects of the private health care system.
3. Compare the public health system to primary care.
4. Explain the model of primary health care in the United States.
5. Assess the effects of health care and insurance reform on health care delivery.
6. Evaluate the changes needed in public health and primary care to have an integrated health care delivery system.

CHAPTER OUTLINE

Health Care in the United States
Forces Stimulating Change in the Demand for Health Care
Current Health Care System in the United States
Organization of the Health Care System
Forces Influencing Changes in the Health Care System
Health Care Delivery Reform Efforts—United States

KEY TERMS

advanced practice nursing (APN), p. 48
Affordable Care Act (ACA), p. 49
community participation, p. 55
Declaration of Alma-Ata, p. 45
disease prevention, p. 46
electronic health record (EHR), p. 48
health, p. 45
health promotion, p. 46
managed care, p. 50
population replacement level, p. 46
primary care, p. 50
primary health care (PHC), p. 54
public health, p. 50
quintile, p. 47
U.S. Department of Health and Human Services (USDHHS), p. 51

As is known, the U.S. government began providing public health services in the 1700s, and public health nursing was first recognized 125 years ago (see Chapter 2). Although there were physicians in England in the 1600s and 1700s and in the United States since the 1700s, official recognition of the general practitioner (GP) occurred in England only in 1844. In the 1950s and 1960s in the United States, discussions were held to elevate the GP to a specialty practice in medicine. Thus family practice medicine became a reality in the 1960s (ABFM, 2005). After this development in medicine the first nurse practitioner (NP) program was begun in 1965 (AANP, 2018). Then in September 1978 an international conference was held in the city of Alma-Ata, which at that time was the capital of the Soviet Republic of Kazakhstan. During this conference the **Declaration of Alma-Ata** and the primary health care model emerged (see Appendix A.3). This declaration states that **health** is a human right and that the health of its people should be the primary goal of every government. One of the main themes of this declaration was the involvement of community health workers and traditional healers in a new health system (World Health Organization [WHO], 1978).

It was through this conference that the concept of primary health care (PHC) was introduced, defined, and described. In 2008 the WHO renewed its call for health care improvements and reemphasized the need for public policy makers, public health officials, primary care providers, and leadership within countries to improve health care delivery. The WHO said: "Globalization is putting the social cohesion of many countries under stress, and health systems … are clearly not performing as well as they could and should. People are increasingly impatient with the inability of health services to deliver. … Few would disagree that health systems need to respond better—and faster—to the challenges of a changing world. PHC can do that" (WHO, 2008; see Chapter 4).

As defined by the WHO, PHC reflects and evolves from the economic conditions and sociocultural and political characteristics of the country and its communities and is based on the application of social, biomedical, and health services research and public health experience. It addresses the main health problems in the community, providing for **health promotion**, **disease prevention**, and curative and rehabilitative services (WHO, 1978).

Defined differently than primary care or public health, PHC promotes the integration of all health care systems within a community to come together to improve the health of the community, including primary care and public health.

HEALTH CARE IN THE UNITED STATES

Despite the fact that health care costs in the United States are the highest in the world and make up the greatest percent of the gross domestic product, the indicators of what constitutes good health do not document that Americans are really getting a good return on their investment. In the first decade of the twenty-first century there have been massive and unexpected changes to health, economic, and social conditions as a result of terrorist attacks, hurricanes, fires, floods, infectious diseases, and the 2008 economic recession. New systems have been developed to prevent and/or deal with the onslaught of these horrendous events. Not all of the systems have worked, and many are regularly criticized for their inefficiency and costliness. Simultaneously, new, nearly miraculous advances have been made in treating health-related conditions. Advances in medicine and nursing are keeping people alive who only a few years ago would have suffered and died. These advances save and prolong lives, and a number of deadly and debilitating diseases have been eliminated through effective immunizations and treatments. National and global health outcomes have improved through sanitation, clean water supplies, better nutrition, and genetic engineering.

However, attention to all of these advances may overshadow the lack of attention to public health, health promotion, and disease prevention. Several of the most destructive health conditions can be prevented through changes in lifestyle, health screenings, and/or immunizations. The increasing rates of obesity, especially among children; substance use; lack of exercise; violence; and accidents are alarmingly expensive, particularly when they lead to disruptions in health.

This chapter describes a health care system in transition as it struggles to meet evolving global and domestic needs and challenges. The overall health care and public health systems in the United States are described and differentiated, and the changing priorities are discussed. Nurses play a pivotal role in meeting these needs, and the role of the nurse is described.

FORCES STIMULATING CHANGE IN THE DEMAND FOR HEALTH CARE

In recent years, enormous changes have occurred in society, in the United States and most other countries of the world. The extent of interaction among countries is stronger than ever, and the economy of each country depends on the stability of other countries. The United States has felt the effects of rising labor costs, and many companies have shifted their production outside the United States to reduce labor costs. It is often less expensive to assemble clothes, automobile parts, and appliances, and to have call distribution centers and call service centers in a less industrialized country and pay the shipping and other charges involved than to have the items fully assembled in the United States. In recent years the vacillating cost of fuel has affected almost every area of the economy, leading to both higher costs of products and layoffs as some industries have struggled to stay solvent. This has affected the employment rate in the United States. The economic downturn of 2008 left many people unemployed, and many lost their homes because they could not pay their mortgages. When the unemployment rate is high, more people lack comprehensive insurance coverage, since in the United States this has been typically provided by employers. In 2008 the U.S. unemployment rate was 5.8 percent. In 2012 the unemployment rate had increased to 8.1 percent, close to double the rate in 2007. In 2016 the unemployment rate dropped to 4.9 percent, and in 2017, 4.4 percent (Bureau of Labor Statistics [BLS], 2018a). In addition to changes in the labor market, health care services and the ways in which they are financed changed after the implementation of the Patient Protection and Affordable Care Act (ACA, enacted in 2010). The ACA continues to be a hot topic for policy debates within the U.S. government.

Demographic Trends

The population of the world is growing as a result of changing fertility and decreased mortality rates. The greatest growth is occurring in underdeveloped countries, and this is accompanied by decreased growth in the United States and other developed countries. According to historical data of the Centers for Disease Control and Prevention (CDC), the U.S. total fertility rate has been below the replacement level in 43 of the last 45 years (2018). **Population replacement level** means that for every person who dies, another is born (Hamilton & Kirmeyer, 2017). Both the size and the characteristics of the population contribute to the changing demography.

Seventy-seven million babies were born between the years of 1946 and 1963, giving rise to the often-discussed baby boomer generation (Office for National Statistics, 2014). The oldest of these boomers reached 65 years of age in 2011, and they are expected to live longer than people born previously (see Chapter 5). The impact on the federal government's insurance program for people 65 years of age and older, Medicare, is expected to be enormous. Medicare spending is projected to grow the fastest among the major health insurance categories between 2021 and 2026, averaging 7.7 percent. Sustained Medicare growth in both enrollment and per enrollee spending contributes to the spending increase above the 5.7 percent projected for the national health spending (CMS, 2018).

In 2018 the U.S. population was 326,766,000 people, representing the third most populated country in the world, following China and India. From 1990 to 2016 the U.S. foreign-born immigrant population grew from 7.9 percent of the total population to 13.2 percent. The future growth rate is likely to be impacted by policy changes implemented at the federal level (U.S. Census Bureau, 2018).

According to the Census Bureau (2017), the United States population is made up of 76.6 percent whites, 18.1 percent

Hispanic or Latino, 13.4 percent black or African American, 5.8 percent Asian, and 2.7 percent claiming two or more races.

The composition of the U.S. household is also changing (see Chapters 26 and 27 for changes in families). From 1935 to 2016, mortality for both genders in all age groups and races declined (Heron, 2018) as a result of progress in public health initiatives, such as antismoking campaigns, acquired immunodeficiency syndrome (AIDS) prevention programs, and cancer screening programs. Over the last century the leading causes of death have shifted from infectious diseases to chronic and degenerative diseases (NCHS, 2017). The top 10 causes of death in 2016 were diseases of heart; malignant neoplasms; accidents (unintentional injuries); chronic lower respiratory diseases; cerebrovascular diseases; Alzheimer's disease; diabetes mellitus; influenza and pneumonia; nephritis, nephrotic syndrome and nephrosis; and intentional self-harm (suicide). These causes accounted for 74 percent of all deaths in the United States (Heron, 2018). New infectious diseases are emerging, based on transmission rates throughout the United States and globally. New treatments for infectious diseases have resulted in steady declines in mortality among children, as long as parents participate in immunization programs. Recent measles outbreaks throughout the United States demonstrates that continuous focus on control of infectious diseases is essential. The mortality for older Americans has also declined. However, people 50 years of age and older have higher rates of chronic and degenerative illness, and they use a larger portion of health care services than other age groups.

Social and Economic Trends

In addition to the size and changing age distribution of the population, other factors also affect the health care system. Several social trends that influence health care include changing lifestyles, a growing appreciation of the quality of life, the changing composition of families and living patterns, changing household incomes, and a revised definition of quality health care.

Americans spend considerable money on health care, nutrition, and fitness (Bureau of Labor Statistics, 2018), because health is seen as an irreplaceable commodity. To be healthy, people must take care of themselves. Many people combine traditional medical and health care practices with complementary and alternative therapies to achieve the highest level of health. Complementary therapies are those that are used in addition to traditional health care, and alternative therapies are those used instead of traditional care. Examples include acupuncture, herbal medications, and more (National Center for Complementary and Integrative Health, 2017). People often spend a considerable amount of their own money for these types of therapies because few are covered by insurance. In recent years some insurance plans have recognized the value of complementary therapies and have reimbursed for them. State offices of insurance are good sources to determine whether these services are covered and by which health insurance plans.

About 70 years ago income was distributed in such a way that a relatively small portion of households earned high incomes; families in the middle-income range made up a somewhat larger proportion, and households at the lower end of the income scale made up the largest proportion. By the 1970s, household income had risen, and income was more evenly distributed, largely as a result of dual-income families.

Since 1979 and to 2014, two trends in income distribution have emerged. The first is that the average per-person income in the United States has increased. In 2014 there were about 310 million people living in 125 million households in the United States. In total the people living in those households received about $12.7 trillion in annual income. The second trend is that income was unevenly distributed. The average income among households in the highest quintile was more than 10 times the average income of households in the lowest **quintile**. A quintile is defined as any of five equal groups into which a population can be divided according to the distribution of values of a particular variable, like income. Income within the highest quintile was also significantly skewed toward the very top. The average income among the 1.2 million households in the top one percent of the income distribution was more than 10 times the average income of households in the bottom half of the highest quintile (the 81st to 90th percentiles) (Congressional Budget Office [CBO], 2018). Chapter 5 provides a detailed discussion of the economics of health care and how financial constraints influence decisions about public health services.

Health Workforce Trends

The health care workforce ebbs and flows. The early years of the twenty-first century saw the beginning of what is expected to be a long-term and sizable nursing shortage. Similarly, most other health professionals are documenting current and future shortages. Employment of registered nurses (RNs) is projected to grow 15 percent from 2016 to 2026, much faster than the average for all occupations. This growth is due to increased focus on preventive care; growing rates of chronic conditions, including heart disease and diabetes; and the aging of America (Bureau of Labor Statistics [BLS], 2018a). Historically, nursing care has been provided in a variety of settings, primarily in the hospital. About 54 percent of all RNs continue to be employed in hospitals (BLS, 2018b). A few years ago hospitals began reducing their bed capacity as care became more community based. Hospitals have begun to expand their services, including mental health, substance abuse, and long-term care facilities. This growth is due to the factors previously discussed: the ability to treat and perhaps cure more diseases, the complexity of the care and the need for inpatient services, and the growth of the older age group.

A 2017 Healthcare Survey of Registered Nurses showed that 27 percent of RNs plan to retire within one year. In addition, 73 percent of baby boomer RNs plan to retire within three years (Sanborn, 2017). By 2026 there are expected to be 438,100 new nursing positions (BLS, 2018c).

There tend to be periodic shortages, especially in the primary care workforce in the United States, as providers choose to be specialists in fields such as medicine and nursing. Primary care providers include generalists who are skilled in preventive health care, diagnostic, and emergency services. The health care personnel trained as primary care providers include family physicians, general internists, general pediatricians, nurse practitioners (NPs), clinical nurse specialists (CNSs), physician assistants, and certified nurse-midwives (CNMs).

NPs, CNSs, and CNMs, considered advanced practice nursing (APN) specialties, are vital members of the primary care teams (see Chapter 39). Although there is a shortage of primary care physicians, NPs may or may not be able to fill the gap because of state nurse practice acts and medical practice acts, which influence the practice of both groups.

In terms of the nursing workforce, increasing the number of minority nurses remains a priority and a strategy for addressing the current nursing shortage. In 2013 minority nurses represented about 22 percent of the RN population. It is thought that increasing the minority population will help close the health disparity gap for minority populations (Phillips & Malone, 2014). For example, persons from minority groups, especially when language is a barrier, often are more comfortable with and more likely to access care from a provider from their own minority group.

Technological Trends

The development and refinement of new technologies such as telehealth have opened up new clinical opportunities for nurses and their clients, especially in the areas of managing chronic conditions, assisting persons who live in rural areas, and in providing home health care, rehabilitation, and long-term care. On the positive side, technological advances promise improved health care services, reduced costs, and more convenience in terms of time and travel for consumers (see Chapter 5). Reduced costs result from a more efficient means of delivering health care as well as automation. Telehealth also reduces paperwork; speeds transmission; gets accurate information to providers, clients, and agencies; assists with care coordination, quality, and safety; and provides direct access to health records between agencies, providers, and clients (HealthIT, 2018. The more high-technology equipment and computer programs become available, the more they are used. High-technology equipment is expensive and may quickly become outdated when newer developments occur. There are other drawbacks to new technology, particularly in the area of home health care, some of which include the effect on people's routine, alteration in face-to-face visits, cost, and the possible stigma of technology in the home (Demiris, 2015).

Advances in health care technology will continue. One example of an effective use of technology is the funding provided by the U.S. Department of Health and Human Services (HHS) and the Health Resources and Services Administration (HRSA) to health centers so they can adopt and implement electronic health records (EHR) and other health information technology (HRSA, 2008). HRSA's Office of Health Information Technology was created in 2005 to promote the effective use of health information technology (HIT) as a mechanism for responding to the needs of the uninsured, underinsured, and special-needs populations (HRSA, 2012). One innovative use of the EHR in public health is to embed reminders or guidelines into the system. For example, the CDC published health guidelines that contain clinical recommendations for screening, prevention, diagnosis, and treatment. To find and keep current on these guidelines, clinicians must visit the CDC website. The availability of an EHR system allows the embedding of reminders so that the clinician can have access to practice guidelines at the point of care. Some additional benefits in public health (and these are some of the uses health centers make of such records) include the following:

- Twenty-four–hour availability of records with downloaded laboratory results and up-to-date assessments
- Coordination of referrals and facilitation of interprofessional care in chronic disease management
- Incorporation of protocol reminders for prevention, screening, and management of chronic disease
- Improvement of quality measurement and monitoring
- Increased client safety and decline in medication errors

Three federal programs, Medicaid, the Military Health System within the Department of Defense, and the State Children's Health Insurance Program (SCHIP), have effectively used HIT in several key functions, including outreach and enrollment, service delivery, and care management, as well as communications with families and the broader goals of program planning and improvement. Consumers can develop their personalized health record, including an electronic family health history, a tool from the Surgeon General accessed at https://familyhistory.hhs.gov (National Institutes of Health [NIH], 2017). This is an easy-to-use computer application for people to keep a personal record of their family health history.

CURRENT HEALTH CARE SYSTEM IN THE UNITED STATES

Despite the many advances and the sophistication of the U.S. health care system, the system has been plagued with problems related to cost, access, and quality (see more discussion in Chapters 5, 20, and 24). These problems have been affected by the ability of individuals to obtain health insurance. The health care goals of most industrialized countries are similar: they strive for high-quality, affordable care.

Cost

Beginning in 2008 a historic weakening of the national and global economy—the "Great Recession"—led to the loss of 7 million jobs in the United States (Economic Report of the President, 2010). Even as the gross domestic product (GDP), an indicator of the economic health of a country, declined in 2009, health care spending continued to grow and reached $2.5 trillion in the same year (Truffer et al., 2010). In the years between 2017 and 2026, national health spending is expected to grow at an average annual rate of 5.5 percent, reaching $5.7 trillion by 2026, for a share of about 19.7 percent of the GDP. This translates into a projected increase in per capita spending (see Chapter 5).

In Chapter 5, additional discussion illustrates how health care dollars are spent. The largest share of health care expenditures goes to pay for acute care, with physician services being the next largest item. The amount of money that has gone to pay for public health services is much lower than for the other categories of expenditures. Other significant drivers of the increasingly high cost of health care include prescription drugs, technology, and care for chronic and degenerative diseases.

Following the Great Recession, the economic rebound will likely coincide with the burgeoning Medicare enrollment of the aging baby boomer population. It was projected that these new Medicare enrollees will increase Medicare expenditures for the foreseeable future. Medicaid recipients can be expected to decline as jobs are added to the economy, and the percent of workers covered by employer-sponsored insurance should rise to reflect that growth. Although workers' salaries have not kept pace, employer-sponsored insurance premiums had grown 119 percent since 1999 (Kaiser Family Foundation, 2009), and the inability of workers to pay this increased cost led to a rise in the percent of working families who were uninsured. It is essential to read about the changes in these facts as the American **Affordable Care Act (ACA)** has been implemented. One change with the ACA is that more individuals have been able to purchase health insurance and employers have shifted more of the cost of health insurance to the employee (KFF, 2018).

Access

Another significant problem is poor access to health care (case study in Box 3.1). The American health care system is described as a two-class system: private and public. People with insurance or those who can personally pay for health care are viewed as receiving superior care; those who receive lower quality care are (1) those whose only source of care depends on public funds or (2) the working poor, who do not qualify for public funds either because they make too much money to qualify or because they are undocumented immigrants. Employment-provided health care is tied to both the economy and to changes in health insurance premiums. In 2012, before the passing of the ACA, the total number of uninsured persons in the United States was 48 million. In 2016 it was 27.6 million. As discussed, there is a strong relationship between health insurance coverage and access to health care services. Insurance status determines the amount and kind of health care people are able to afford, as well as where they can receive care. Uninsured rates vary by state and region, with individuals living in southern or western states more likely to be uninsured. Eight out of the twelve states with the highest uninsured rates in 2016 were in the South. This is due to different economic conditions, state Medicare expansion status, availability of employer-based coverage, and demographics (Artiga & Damico, 2016).

The uninsured receive less preventive care, are diagnosed at more advanced disease states, and once diagnosed tend to receive less therapeutic care in terms of surgery and treatment options. As discussed later in this chapter, there are more than 1300 federally funded community health centers throughout the country (HRSA Health Center Program, 2018). Federally funded community health centers provide a broad range of health and social services, using NPs, RNs, physician assistants, physicians, social workers, and dentists. Community health centers serve primarily in medically underserved areas, which can be rural or urban. These centers serve people of all ages, races, and ethnicities, with or without health insurance.

BOX 3.1 Case Study

Public health nurses who worked with local Head Start programs noted that many children had untreated dental caries. Although the children qualified for Medicaid, only two dentists in the area would accept appointments from Medicaid patients. Dentists asserted that Medicaid patients frequently did not show up for their appointments and that reimbursement was too low compared with other third-party payers. They also said the children's behavior made it difficult to work with them. So the waiting list for local dental care was about six years long. Although some nurses found ways to transport clients to dentists in a city 70 miles away, it was very time consuming and was feasible for only a small fraction of the clients. When decayed teeth abscessed, it was possible to get extractions from the local medical center. The health department dentist also saw children, but he, too, was booked for years.

Created by Deborah C. Conway, Assistant Professor, University of Virginia School of Nursing.

Quality

The quality of health care leaped to the forefront of concern following the 1999 release of the Institute of Medicine (IOM) report *To Err Is Human: Building a Safer Health System* (IOM, 2000). As indicated in this groundbreaking report, as many as 98,000 deaths a year could be attributed to preventable medical errors. Some of the untoward events categorized in this report included adverse drug events and improper transfusions, surgical injuries and wrong-site surgery, suicides, restraint-related injuries or death, falls, burns, pressure ulcers, and mistaken client identities. It was further determined that high rates of errors with serious consequences were most likely to occur in intensive care units, operating rooms, and emergency departments. Beyond the cost in human lives, preventable medical errors result in the loss of several billions of dollars annually in hospitals nationwide. Categories of error include diagnostic, treatment, and prevention errors as well as failure of communication, equipment failure, and other system failures. Significant to nurses, the IOM estimated the number of lives lost to preventable errors in medication alone represented more than 7000 deaths annually, with a cost of about $2 billion nationwide.

Although the IOM report made it clear that the majority of medical errors today were not produced by provider negligence, lack of education, or lack of training, questions were raised about the nurse's role and workload and its effect on client safety. In a follow-up report, *Keeping Patients Safe: Transforming the Work Environment of Nurses,* the IOM (2003) stated that nurses' long work hours pose a serious threat to patient safety, because fatigue slows reaction time, saps energy, and diminishes attention to detail. The group called for state regulators to pass laws barring nurses from working more than 12 hours a day and 60 hours a week—even if by choice (IOM, 2003). Although this information is largely related to acute care, many of the patients who survive medical errors are later cared for in the community.

After both IOM reports the quality of health care and ways to address it have changed significantly. In 2015 the National Patient Safety Foundation (NPSF) convened an expert panel to assess patient safety and develop a 15-year strategic plan to improve quality.

The NPSF report calls for a systems approach and a culture of safety and action by government, regulators, health professionals, and others to place higher priority on patient safety science and implementation.

The report makes eight recommendations:

- Ensure that leaders establish and sustain a safety culture
- Create centralized and coordinated oversight of patient safety
- Create a common set of safety metrics that reflect meaningful outcomes
- Increase funding for research in patient safety and implementation science
- Address safety across the entire care continuum
- Support the health care workforce
- Partner with patients and families for the safest care
- Ensure that technology is safe and optimized to improve patient safety

The culture of quality improvement and safety has made providers and consumers more conscious of safety, but medical errors and untoward events continue to occur. As a means to improve consumer awareness of hospital quality, the Centers for Medicare and Medicaid Services (CMS) began publishing a database of hospital quality measures, Hospital Compare, in 2005. Hospital Compare, a consumer-oriented website that provides information on how well hospitals provide recommended care in such areas as heart attack, heart failure, and pneumonia, is available (www.medicare.gov). In a further effort the CMS in 2008 announced that it will no longer reimburse hospitals under Medicare guidelines for care provided for "preventable complications," such as hospital-acquired infections. This reimbursement policy was extended to Medicaid reimbursement in 2011 (CMS, 2009; Galewitz, 2011).

To ensure quality in public health, the accreditation process for public health was developed, through the Public Health Accreditation Board. Outcome analysis demonstrates that public health districts that are accredited have increases in multisector partnerships to promote health in communities, and it strengthens quality improvement and performance management to improve community health. The Public Health Accreditation Board has an interactive U.S. map that identifies health departments that have been accredited and can be accessed at http://www.phaboard.org (PHAB, 2018).

The ability of a public health agency or a community to respond to community disasters is one event that is monitored. In August 2018, 223 of 416 local, tribal, and state centralized integration systems and multijurisdictional health departments had received accreditation. The accredited health departments served 214 million people. The purpose of the accreditation is to:

- Assist and identify quality health departments to improve performance and quality and to develop leadership
- Improve management
- Improve community relationships (PHAB, 2018)

ORGANIZATION OF THE HEALTH CARE SYSTEM

An enormous number and range of facilities and providers make up the health care system. These include physicians' and dentists' offices, hospitals, long-term care facilities, mental health facilities, ambulatory care centers, freestanding clinics and clinics housed inside stores and drugstores, as well as free clinics, public health districts, and home health agencies. Providers include nurses, advanced practice nurses, physicians and physician assistants, dentists and dental hygienists, pharmacists, and a wide array of essential allied health providers such as physical, occupational, and recreational therapists; nutritionists; social workers; and a range of technicians. In general, however, the American health care system is divided into the following two, somewhat distinct, components: a private or personal care component and a public health component, with some overlap, as discussed in the following sections. It is important to discuss primary health care (PHC) and examine the interest in developing such a system.

Primary Care System

Primary care, the first level of the private health care system, is delivered in a variety of community settings, such as physicians' offices, urgent care centers, in-store clinics, community health centers, and community nursing centers. Near the end of the past century, in an attempt to contain costs, managed care organizations grew. **Managed care** is defined as a system in which care is delivered by a specific network of providers who agree to comply with the care approaches established through a case management approach. The key factors are a specified network of providers and the use of a gatekeeper to control access to providers and services. Managed care plans are a type of health insurance that includes contracts with health care providers and medical facilities to provide care for members at reduced costs. These providers make up the plan's network. How much health care is covered is dependent on the network's rules (MedlinePlus, 2017).

The government tried to reap the benefits of cost savings by introducing the managed care model into Medicare and Medicaid, with varying levels of success. The traditional Medicare plan involves Parts A and B. Part C, the Medicare Advantage program, incorporates private insurance plans into the Medicare program, including health maintenance organizations (HMOs) and preferred provider organizations (PPOs) managed care models and private fee-for-service plans. In addition, Medicare Part D covers prescriptions (see Chapter 5).

Public Health System

The **public health** system is mandated through laws that are developed at the national, state, or local level. Examples of public health laws instituted to protect the health of the community include a law mandating immunizations for all children entering kindergarten and a law requiring constant monitoring of the local water supply and food service inspections. The public health system is organized into many levels in the federal, state, and local systems. At the local level, health districts provide care that is mandated by state and federal regulations.

The Federal System

The U.S. Department of Health and Human Services (USDHHS, or simply HHS) is the agency most heavily involved with the health and welfare concerns of U.S. citizens. The organizational chart of the HHS (Fig. 3.1; https://www.hhs.gov.) shows the office of the secretary, 11 agencies, and an office of support services and operations (USDHHS, 2018a). Ten regional offices are maintained to provide more direct assistance to the states. Their locations are shown in Table 3.1. The HHS is charged with regulating health care and overseeing the health status of Americans. HHS administers more than 100 programs across its operating divisions. HHS goals are to protect the health of all Americans and provide essential human services, especially for those who are least able to help themselves. See Fig. 3.2 and Box 3.2 for the goals and objectives of the HHS strategic plan for fiscal years 2018–2022. The Office of Public Health Preparedness was added to assist the nation and states in preparing for bioterrorism after September 11, 2001. The goal of the Office of Global Affairs is to promote global health by coordinating HHS strategies and programs with other governments and international organizations (HHS, 2018).

The U.S. Public Health Service (USPHS, or simply PHS) is a major component of the HHS. The PHS consists of eight agencies: Agency for Healthcare Research and Quality, Agency for Toxic Substances and Diseases Registry, Centers for Disease Control and Prevention, Food and Drug Administration, Health Resources and Services Administration, Indian Health Service, National Institutes of Health, and Substance Abuse and Mental Health Services Administration. Each has a specific purpose (see Chapter 8 for relevancy of the agencies to policy and providing health care). The PHS also has the Commissioned Corps, which is a uniformed service of more than 6500 health professionals who serve in many HHS and other federal agencies. The surgeon general is head of the Commissioned Corps. The corps fills essential services for public health such as, clinical services and provides leadership within the federal government departments and agencies to support the care of the underserved and vulnerable populations. The mission of the PHS Commissioned Corps is to protect, promote, and advance the health and

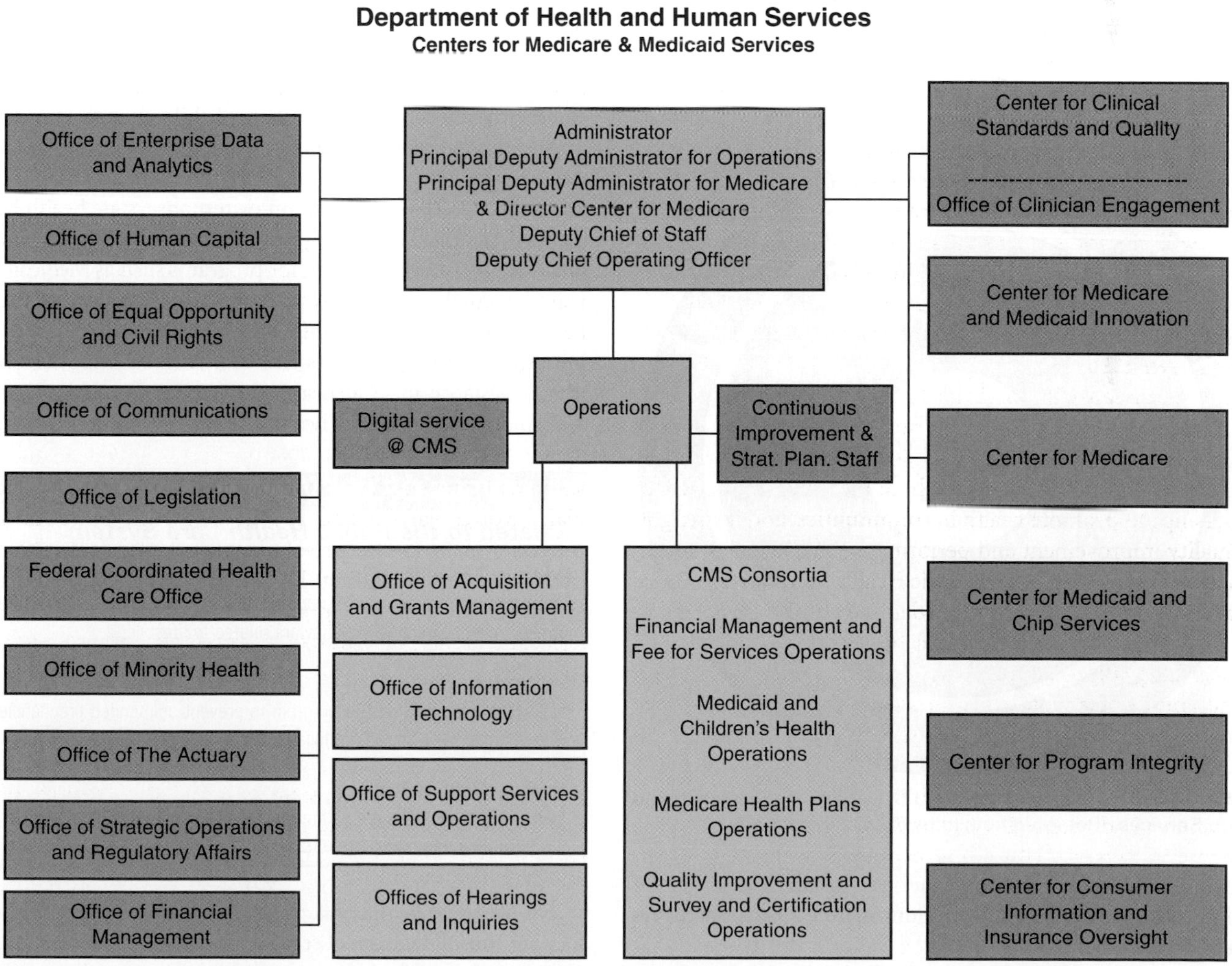

Fig. 3.1 HHS Organizational Chart. (From U.S. Department of Health and Human Services. Available at https://www.hhs.gov.)

TABLE 3.1 Regional Offices of the U.S. Department of Health and Human Services

Region	Location	Territory
1	Boston	Connecticut, Maine, Massachusetts, New Hampshire, Rhode Island, Vermont
2	New York	New Jersey, New York, Puerto Rico, Virgin Islands
3	Philadelphia	Delaware, District of Columbia, Maryland, Pennsylvania, Virginia, West Virginia
4	Atlanta	Alabama, Florida, Georgia, Kentucky, Mississippi, North Carolina, South Carolina, Tennessee
5	Chicago	Illinois, Indiana, Michigan, Minnesota, Ohio, Wisconsin
6	Dallas	Arkansas, Louisiana, New Mexico, Oklahoma, Texas
7	Kansas City	Iowa, Kansas, Missouri, Nebraska
8	Denver	Colorado, Montana, North Dakota, South Dakota, Utah, Wyoming
9	San Francisco	Arizona, California, Hawaii, Nevada, American Samoa, Commonwealth of the Northern Mariana Islands, Federated States of Micronesia, Guam, Republic of the Marshall Islands, Republic of Palau
10	Seattle	Alaska, Idaho, Oregon, Washington

From U.S. Department of Health and Human Services: *HHS regional offices*. Retrieved from www.hhs.gov.

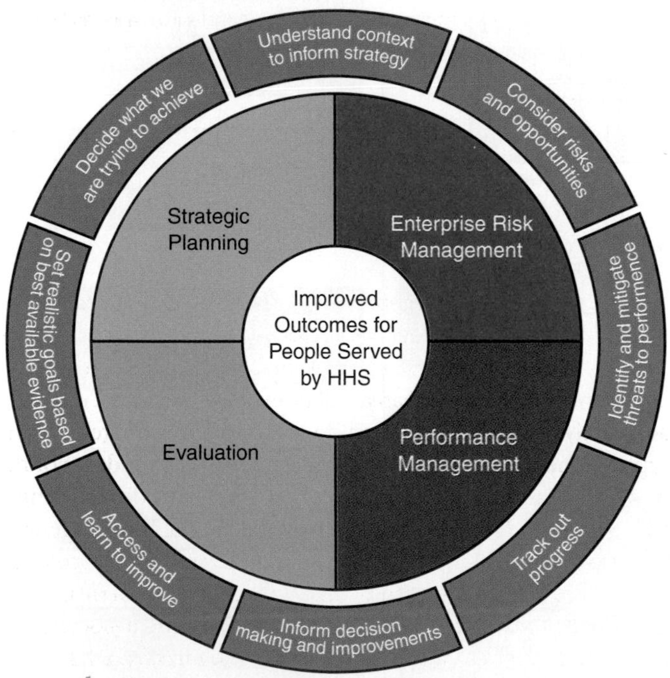

Fig. 3.2 Goals and Objective of The U.S. Department of Health and Human Services. (Retrieved from https://www.hhs.gov.)

safety of the United States. As America's uniformed service of public health professionals, the Commissioned Corps achieves its mission through:

- Rapid and effective response to public health needs
- Leadership and excellence in public health practices
- Advancement of public health science

The core values of the Commissioned Corps are leadership, service, integrity, and excellence (USPHS, 2018).

Related to public health is the U.S. Department of Homeland Security (USDHS, or simply DHS), which was created in 2003 (USDHS, 2018). The mission of the DHS is to ensure a homeland that is safe, secure, and resilient against terrorism and other hazards. The goals for the department include awareness, prevention, protection, response, and recovery. The DHS works with first responders throughout the United States, and through the development of programs such as the Community Emergency Response Team (CERT) program trains people to be better prepared to respond to emergency situations in their communities. Nurses working in state and local public health districts, as well as those employed in hospitals and other health facilities, may be called on to respond to acts of terrorism or natural disaster in the course of their careers, and the DHS, along with the Food and Drug Administration (FDA) and CDC, is developing programs to ready nurses and other health care providers for emergency response (USDHS, 2018).

The State System

When the United States faced a pandemic flu outbreak in 2009, the federal government and the public health community quickly prepared to meet the challenge of educating the public and health professionals about the H1N1 flu and making vaccinations available. In 2014 public health within the states was responding to an enterovirus affecting large numbers of children with symptoms of upper respiratory disease and weakness in arms and legs. The virus was considered life threatening (AAP, 2016). In addition to standing ready for disaster prevention or response, state health departments have other equally important functions, such as health care financing and administration for programs such as Medicaid, providing mental health and professional education, establishing health codes, licensing facilities and personnel, and regulating the insurance industry. State systems also have an important role in direct assistance to local health departments, including ongoing assessment of community health needs (see Chapter 46).

LEVELS OF PREVENTION

Related to the Public Health Care System

Primary Prevention
Implement a community-level program such as walking for exercise to assist citizens in improving health behaviors related to lifestyle.

Secondary Prevention
Implement a family-planning program to prevent unintended pregnancies for young couples who attend the local community health center.

Tertiary Prevention
Provide a self-management asthma program for children with chronic asthma to reduce their need for hospitalization.

Nurses serve in many capacities in state health departments; they are consultants, direct service providers, researchers, teachers, and supervisors. They also participate in community assessment, program development, planning, and the evaluation of health programs.

BOX 3.2 HHS Strategic Plan, Goals, and Objectives—Fiscal Years 2018-2022

Strategic Goal 1: Reform, Strengthen, and Modernize the Nation's Healthcare System
Strategic Goal 2: Protect the Health of Americans Where They Live, Learn, Work, and Play
Strategic Goal 3: Strengthen the Economic and Social Well-Being of Americans Across the Lifespan
Strategic Goal 4: Foster Sound, Sustained Advances in the Sciences
Strategic Goal 5: Promote Effective and Efficient Management and Stewardship

GOAL 1: Strengthen Health Care

Objective A Make coverage more secure for those who have insurance, and extend affordable coverage to the uninsured.
Objective B Improve health care quality and patient safety.
Objective C Emphasize primary and preventive care linked with community prevention services.
Objective D Reduce the growth of health care costs while promoting high-value, effective care.
Objective E Ensure access to quality, culturally competent care for vulnerable populations.
Objective F Promote the adoption and meaningful use of health information technology.

GOAL 2: Advance Scientific Knowledge and Innovation

Objective A Accelerate the process of scientific discovery to improve patient care.
Objective B Foster innovation to create shared solutions.
Objective C Invest in the regulatory sciences to improve food and medical product safety.
Objective D Increase our understanding of what works in public health and human service practice.

GOAL 3: Advance the Health, Safety, and Well-Being of the American People

Objective A Promote the safety, well-being, resilience, and healthy development of children and youth.
Objective B Promote economic and social well-being for individuals, families, and communities.
Objective C Improve the accessibility and quality of supportive services for people with disabilities and older adults.
Objective D Promote prevention and wellness.
Objective E Reduce the occurrence of infectious diseases.
Objective F Protect Americans' health and safety during emergencies, and foster resilience in response to emergencies.

GOAL 4: Increase Efficiency, Transparency, Accountability and Effectiveness of HHS Programs

Objective A Ensure program integrity and responsible stewardship of resources.
Objective B Fight fraud and work to eliminate improper payments.
Objective C Use HHS data to improve the health and well-being of the American people.
Objective D Improve HHS environmental, energy, and economic performance to promote sustainability.

GOAL 5: Strengthen the Nation's Health and Human Service Infrastructure and Workforce

Objective A Invest in the HHS workforce to meet America's health and human service needs today and tomorrow.
Objective B Ensure that the Nation's health care workforce can meet increased demands.
Objective C Enhance the ability of the public health workforce to improve public health at home and abroad.
Objective D Strengthen the Nation's human service workforce.
Objective E Improve national, state, local, and tribal surveillance and epidemiology capacity.

HHS, U.S. Department of Health and Human Services.
From the U.S. Department of Health and Human Services, 2018. Retrieved from https://www.hhs.gov.

The Local System

The local health district has direct responsibility to the citizens in its community or jurisdiction. Services and programs offered by local health departments vary depending on the state and local health codes that must be followed, the needs of the community, and available funding and other resources. For example, one health department might be more involved with public health education programs and environmental issues, whereas another health department might emphasize direct client care. Local health departments vary in providing sick care or even primary care (see Chapter 46). More often than at other levels of government, public health nurses at the local level provide population level or direct services. Some of these nurses deliver special or selected services, such as follow-up of contacts in cases of tuberculosis or sexually transmitted infections (STIs), or providing child immunization clinics. Others provide more general care, delivering services to families in certain geographic areas. This method of delivery of nursing services involves broader needs and a wider variety of nursing interventions. The local level often provides an opportunity for nurses to take on significant leadership roles, with many nurses serving as directors or managers.

Since the tragedy of September 11, 2001, state and local health departments have increasingly focused on emergency preparedness and response. In case of an event, state and local health departments in the affected area will be expected to collect data and accurately report the situation, to respond appropriately to any type of emergency, and to ensure the safety of the residents of the immediate area, while protecting those just outside the danger zone. This level of knowledge—to enable public health agencies to anticipate, prepare for, recognize, and respond to gun violence, terrorist threats, and natural disasters such as hurricanes or floods—has required a level of interstate and federal-local planning and cooperation. Whether participating in disaster simulations or preparing a shelter, nurses play a major role in meeting the challenge of disaster preparedness and response.

FORCES INFLUENCING CHANGES IN THE HEALTH CARE SYSTEM

Although most people are personally satisfied with their own health care provider, at present few people are satisfied with the health care system in general. Costs have been high and have continued to rise while quality and access have been uneven across the country and within communities, depending on the ability to pay. What, then, were some of the factors that might influence health care to change? First, as a nation, citizens must decide what has to be provided for all people, who will be in charge of the system, and who will pay for these services. In recent years, federal and state services have been reduced, and more responsibility for health care delivery has been moved to the private sector. Health care is big business. Health care company stocks are now traded by major stock exchanges, directors receive benefits when profits are high, and the locus of control has shifted from the provider to the payer. Many competing forces have influenced the changing design of the health care system, some of which are consumers, employers (purchasers), care delivery systems, and state and federal legislation.

First, consumers want lower costs and high-quality health care without limits and with an improved ability to choose providers and services of their choice. Second, employers (purchasers of health care) want to be able to obtain basic health care plans at reasonable costs for their business and employees. Many employers have seen their profits diminish as they put more money into providing adequate health care coverage for employees. Third, health care systems want a better balance between consumer and purchaser demands. Thus they continually watch their own budget and expenses. To maintain a profit while providing quality care, many health care delivery groups have downsized and created alliances, mergers, and other joint ventures. Finally, legislation, especially concerning access and quality, continues to be enacted, thus creating one more force helping shape a health care system. The goal of "evidence-based care" is to ensure high-quality health care.

Many have said that solving the health care crisis requires the institution of a rational health care system that balances equity, cost, and quality. The fact that millions of people have been uninsured, that wide disparities have existed in access, and that a large proportion of deaths each year seem attributable to preventable causes (health care errors as well as tobacco, substance abuse, preventable injuries, and obesity) has indicated that the U.S. health care system is currently not serving the best interests of the population. The WHO has suggested that integrating primary care and public health into a PHC system will be the basis for better health for all world citizens (WHO, 1986a).

Integration of Public Health and the Primary Care Systems

Although primary care and public health share a goal of promoting the health and well-being of all people, these two disciplines historically have operated independently of one another. Problems that stem from this separation have long been recognized, but new opportunities are emerging for bringing these systems together to promote lasting improvements in the health of individuals, communities, and populations (IOM, 2012).

In recognition of this potential, the CDC and the HRSA, both agencies of the HHS, asked the IOM to convene a committee of experts, including input from nursing, to examine the integration of primary care and public health (IOM, 2012).

To recognize the differences in these two systems, definitions were used to guide the work of the experts. Primary care was defined as "the providing of integrated, accessible health care services by clinicians who are accountable for addressing a large majority of personal health care needs, while developing partnerships with patients and practicing in the context of family and community" (IOM, 1996, p. 1). Public health was defined as "fulfilling society's interest in assuring conditions in which people can be healthy" (IOM, 1988, p. 140). The purpose of the integration is to achieve the WHO goal of PHC.

Potential Barriers to Integration

Contrasting the two systems, primary care, which can be either a public or a private entity, is person focused, provides a point of first contact for individuals to address health problems, and is considered comprehensive and provides coordination of individual care. Public health can also be delivered through public and private entities to contribute to the health of society, and local, state, and federal government plays a major role in public health. Health departments are legally bound to provide essential public health services and to work with the total community and multiple stakeholders to address community-level health problems. Public health also has specific functions of assurance, assessment, and policy development to address community-level health issues and has a charge to create healthy communities (see Chapter 1).

In addition to differing roles and functions and issues related to funding, different clients and different foci will need to be addressed to form a solid foundation for a partnership. Primary care is largely funded through health insurance, individual client payments, and sometimes through federal grants. Public health is largely funded through tax dollars, federal and state grants, and sometimes health insurance payments through Medicare and Medicaid. Primary care serves the individuals who present to the practice, while public health serves to assess the health problems of the population. Both focus on meeting the most prevalent health needs of the population. Primary care focuses more on the curative aspect of individualized care, while public health focuses more on the prevention of health problems for the population (Levesque et al., 2013).

The common goal of public health and primary care, although these systems operate independently, is to ensure a healthier population. Integration of these two systems has the potential to produce a greater impact on the health of populations than either could have working alone, said the committee of experts convened by the IOM (2012).

The Healthy People initiatives, beginning with the U.S. surgeon general's 1979 report, indicate the long-standing desire to improve population health in the United States.

Primary Health Care

Primary health care (PHC), is the first point of contact people have with the health care system. It provides comprehensive, accessible, community-based care that meets the health needs of individuals throughout their life. This includes a variety of services from prevention (vaccinations, family planning, and screenings) to management of chronic health conditions and palliative care (WHO, 2018). This system is composed of public health agencies, community-based agencies and primary care clinics, and health care providers. From a conceptual point of view, PHC is essential care made universally accessible to individuals, families, and the community. Health care is made available to them with their full participation and is provided at a cost that the individual, community, and country can afford. This care is not uniformly available and accessible to all people in many countries, including the United States. Full **community participation** means that individuals within the community help in defining health problems and in developing approaches to address the problems.

The PHC movement officially began in 1977 when the 30th WHO Health Assembly adopted a resolution accepting the goal of attaining a level of health that permitted all citizens of the world to live socially and economically productive lives. At the international conference in 1978 in Alma-Ata, in Kazakhstan, formerly a Soviet Republic, it was determined that this goal was to be met through PHC. This resolution, the Declaration of Alma-Ata, became known by the slogan "Health for All (HFA) by the Year 2000," which captured the official health target for all the member nations of the WHO. In 1998 the program was adapted to meet the needs of the new century and was deemed "Health for All in the 21st Century."

In 1981 the WHO established global indicators for monitoring and evaluating the achievement of HFA. In the *World Health Statistics Annual* (WHO, 1986b), these indicators are grouped into the following four categories: health policies, social and economic development, provision of health care, and health status. The indicators suggest that health improvements are a result of efforts in many areas, including agriculture, industry, education, housing, communications, and health care. Because PHC is as much a political statement as a system of care, each United Nations member country interprets PHC according to its own culture, health needs, resources, and system of government. Clearly, the goal of PHC has not been met in most countries, including the United States.

CHECK YOUR PRACTICE

As a senior nursing student you have been exploring options for future employment. You have developed an interest in working in the community, especially in a primary care clinic setting in a rural community. You wonder why there has not been more emphasis in your nursing program about possible jobs in primary care, and you are aware that in many clinics a medical assistant is the person who is most accessible to clients. If you are interested in finding a job in primary care, what would you do? How would you present yourself to a potential employer to show how you could benefit the practice and the clients of the practice? How can you, in a primary care position, improve the health of the population in the community?

The Changing Role of Registered Nurses in Primary Care

The ACA has brought many changes to health care, with an emphasis on primary care and reducing hospital admissions and length of stay. The role of the nurse in primary care can help achieve both of these goals through an expanded RN role and positions in primary care. RNs are well equipped and trained to coordinate client care; work with all members of the interprofessional team; manage complex comorbidities; promote healthy lifestyles; coordinate medication reconciliation and monitor effects of polypharmacy; bridge the gap between community resources and the people who need them; advocate for clients, families, and community members; and work toward local, state, and federal policy change that improves the health of the community members.

A recent study by Flinter et al. (2017) identifies the expanding role of the RN in primary care, by surveying RNs in 30 different primary care practices. Studies like this demonstrate the expanded role of nurses in primary care and help justify the cost of the care offered by nurses. The 2016 Macy Foundation's conference on *Preparing Registered Nurses for Enhanced Roles in Primary Care* recommended six domains for improving the involvement of RNs in primary care:

1. Changing the cultures in both nursing schools and practices to place greater value on primary care and the role of nurses in it
2. Redesigning practices to make full use of the expertise of nurses
3. Rebalancing nursing education to elevate primary care content
4. Promoting the career development of nurses in primary care
5. Developing primary care expertise in nursing school faculty
6. Increasing opportunities for interprofessional education and teamwork development in both education and practice (Macy Foundation, 2017)

In 2018 the USDHHS, Division of Nursing, funded grants to select schools in the United States to develop approaches to include an emphasis on primary care in their nursing curricula.

Promoting Health/Preventing Disease: Year 2020 Objectives for the Nation

As a WHO member nation, the United States has endorsed PHC as a strategy for achieving the goal of "Health for All in the 21st Century." However, the PHC emphasis on broad strategies, community participation, self-reliance, and a multidisciplinary health care delivery team is not the primary strategy for improving the health of the U.S. population. The national health plan for the United States identifies disease prevention and health promotion as the areas of most concern in the nation. Each decade since the 1980s has been measured and tracked according to health objectives set at the beginning of the decade. The PHS of the HHS publishes the objectives after gathering data from health professionals and organizations throughout the country.

Healthy People 2020, which was officially launched in December 2010 (HHS, 2010), is composed of 42 topic areas with 1200 objectives. These objectives are designed to serve as a road map for improving the health of all people in the United States during the second decade of the twenty-first century. These objectives are described by four main goals (HHS, 2018):

- Attain high-quality, longer lives free of preventable disease, disability, injury, and premature death

- Achieve health equity, eliminate disparities, and improve the health of all groups
- Create social and physical environments that promote good health for all
- Promote quality of life, healthy development, and healthy behaviors across all life stages

These goals provide the framework with which measurable health indicators can be tracked. The emphasis on the social and physical environment moves *Healthy People 2020* from the traditional disease-specific focus to a more holistic view of health consistent with a public health frame of reference (Healthy People 2020, 2012). This in turn will encourage public health nurses to broaden their scope to all aspects of their clients' lives that may need assessment and intervention, including where they live, the condition of their home, and how the appropriateness of their environment may change as the client ages. The Healthy People 2020 box presents indicators of *Healthy People 2020* related to the strengthening of the public health infrastructure. These objectives will assist nurses in having data to show that their assessments and interventions are changing practice.

HEALTHY PEOPLE 2020

Selected Objectives That Pertain to Strengthening the Public Health Infrastructure

- **PHI-7**: Increase the proportion of population-based *Healthy People 2020* objectives for which national data are available for all major population groups.
- **PHI-8:** Increase the proportion of *Healthy People 2020* objectives that are tracked regularly at the national level.

From U.S. Department of Health and Human Services: *Healthy People 2020*. Available at https://www.healthypeople.gov.

HEALTH CARE DELIVERY REFORM EFFORTS—UNITED STATES

Over the centuries, both health insurance and health care reform have been the focus of numerous discussions and political battles. As can be seen in Chapter 5, the first health insurance plan, established in about 1798 in the United States, was for the Merchant Marines to assist in treating infectious diseases and protecting the ports of entry into the United States. The United States has discussed national health care reform since the 1900s (see Chapter 5). In 1912 Theodore Roosevelt campaigned on a health insurance proposal for industry. Then in 1915 the "progressive reformers" campaigned for a state-based system of compulsory health insurance. In the 1920s the Committee on the Costs of Medical Care suggested group medicine and voluntary insurance, and this movement was labeled as promoting "socialized medicine." Since the 1930s, surveys have demonstrated that Americans have shown support of guaranteed access to health care and health insurance and a governmental role in financing of care. Some strides were made in improving access and defining the role of government financing through the passing of Medicare in 1965, with Medicaid as a part of the proposal for Social Security amendments, and the Children's Health Insurance Program (SCHIP) bill passed in 1996. Many proposals have been put forward over the decades for health care reform, as well as health insurance reform. Beginning in the 1970s Senator Ted Kennedy, President Richard Nixon, President Gerald Ford, and President Jimmy Carter all made health-related proposals, all followed by the Health Security Act of President Bill Clinton. None were accepted by Congress (KFF, 2009a). It was not until 2014 the first plan was accepted—the ACA put forth by President Obama and his team.

EVIDENCE-BASED PRACTICE

It is often said that the states are the laboratories of democracy. One state, Massachusetts, began an experiment in health reform in 2006. Two years after health reform legislation became effective, only 2.6 percent of Massachusetts residents were uninsured, the lowest percent ever recorded in any state (Dorn et al., 2009; KFF, 2012). However, the program became one of the most successful and a model for the ACA. After five years about 98 percent to 99 percent of all of the commonwealth's citizens were covered by the plan.

Although other states have experimented with various programs to decrease the number of uninsured, the Massachusetts plan has had the most success. The health reform plan rests on an individual mandate that requires everyone who can afford insurance to purchase coverage. Those unable to afford insurance receive subsidies that allow low-income individuals and families to purchase coverage. A new state-run program, Commonwealth Care (CommCare), provides benefits to adults who are not eligible for Medicaid but whose incomes fall below 300 percent of the federal poverty level.

To understand how the state was so successful in this effort toward universal coverage, a group of evaluators met with 15 key informants representing hospitals, community health centers, insurance companies, Medicaid, and CommCare. Several factors, it was found, have contributed to the historic level of coverage seen in the state. Rather than requiring consumers to complete separate applications for programs such as Medicaid, the Children's Health Insurance Program (CHIP), or CommCare, a single application system provides entry to all the state programs. If an uninsured client was admitted to a hospital or visited a community health center, his or her eligibility was automatically evaluated, and, if eligible, the client would be automatically converted to CommCare coverage, even without completing an application. A "Virtual Gateway" has been developed through which staff of community-based organizations have been trained to complete online applications on behalf of consumers and to provide education and counseling about insurance options to underserved communities. By holding back reimbursement to providers who do not help consumers sign up for one of the available insurance options, hospitals and health centers are motivated to dedicate staff to provide education and counseling to the formerly uninsured. The result is that at least half of the new enrollees in Medicaid and CommCare have been enrolled without filling out any forms on their own. In addition to these efforts, shortly after the reform legislation was enacted, the state financed a massive public education effort to inform consumers about their new options.

Nurse Use

As health reform evolves on the national level, nurses can play a crucial role in driving down the number of uninsured. Nurses should educate themselves so that they can encourage clients to apply and take advantage of all available coverage options. Taking an active role in consumer educational programs is a natural extension of a nurse's role as a client advocate. Nurses can promote legislation to simplify enrollment processes and encourage the development of shared databases for community health care providers, thus preventing consumers from a lack of care or interruption of services in our fragmented health care system.

Nurses and the American Nurses Association (ANA) have been involved in the debates about health care reform over time and developed a Healthcare System Reform Agenda. The ANA (2008) promoted a blueprint for reform that included the following:

- Health care is a basic human right, and so a restructured health care system with universal access to a standard package of essential health care services for all citizens and residents must be assured.
- The development and implementation of health policies that reflect the aims put forth by the Institute of Medicine (safe, effective, patient centered, timely, efficient, equitable) and are based on outcomes research will ultimately save money.
- The overuse of expensive, technology-driven, acute, hospital-based services must give way to a balance between high-tech treatment and community-based and preventive services, with emphasis on the latter.
- A single-payer mechanism is the most desirable option for financing a reformed health care system.

In 2010 the ACA introduced by President Obama was passed, after much debate. This act reflects many of the tenets offered by the ANA in its 2008 Health System Reform Agenda and puts into place comprehensive health insurance reforms that began in 2014. The goals of the ACA include improve quality and lower health care costs, provide access to care, and provide for consumer protection. Table 3.2 provides an overview of the key features of the act by year. The ACA has a major focus on prevention. This focus is designed to improve the health of Americans but also help to reduce health care costs and

TABLE 3.2 Overview of Key Features of the Affordable Care Act by Year

2010

New Consumer Protections

- Putting information for consumers online
- Prohibiting denying coverage of children based on preexisting conditions
- Prohibiting insurance companies from rescinding coverage
- Eliminating lifetime limits on insurance coverage
- Regulating annual limits on insurance coverage
- Establishing consumer assistance programs in the states

Improving Quality and Lowering Costs

- Providing small business health insurance tax credits
- Offering relief for 4 million seniors who hit the Medicare prescription drug "donut hole."
- Providing free preventive care
- Preventing disease and illness
- Cracking down on health care fraud

Increasing Access to Affordable Care

- Providing access to insurance for uninsured Americans with pre-existing conditions
- Extending coverage for young adults
- Expanding coverage for early retirees
- Rebuilding the primary care workforce
- Holding insurance companies accountable for unreasonable rate hikes
- Allowing states to cover more people on Medicaid
- Increasing payments for rural health care providers
- Strengthening community health centers

2011

Improving Quality and Lowering Costs

- Offering prescription drug discounts
- Providing free preventive care for seniors
- Improving health care quality and efficiency
- Improving care for seniors after they leave the hospital
- Introducing new innovations to bring down costs

Increasing Access to Affordable Care

- Increasing access to services at home and in the community

Holding Insurance Companies Accountable

- Bringing down health care premiums
- Addressing overpayments to big insurance companies and strengthening Medicare Advantage

2012

Improving Quality and Lowering Costs

- Linking payment to quality outcomes
- Encouraging integrated health systems
- Reducing paperwork and administrative costs
- Understanding and fighting health disparities

Increasing Access to Affordable Care

- Providing new, voluntary options for long-term care insurance

2013

Improving Quality and Lowering Costs

- Improving preventive health coverage
- Expanding authority to bundle payments

Increasing Access to Affordable Care

- Increasing Medicaid payments for primary care doctors
- Open enrollment in the health insurance marketplace begins

2014

New Consumer Protections

- Prohibiting discrimination due to pre-existing conditions or gender
- Eliminating annual limits on insurance coverage
- Ensuring coverage for individuals participating in clinical trials

Improving Quality and Lowering Costs

- Making care more affordable
- Establishing the health insurance marketplace
- Increasing the small business tax credit

Increasing Access to Affordable Care

- Increasing access to Medicaid
- Promoting individual responsibility

2015

Improving Quality and Lowering Costs

- Paying physicians based on value, not volume

For more detail about each of the bulleted statements please refer to HHS.gov/HealthCare (*Key features of the Affordable Care Act*, 2014. Available at http://www.hhs.gov).

improve quality of care. Through the Prevention and Public Health Fund, the ACA will address factors that influence health—housing, education, transportation, the availability of quality affordable food, and conditions in the workplace and the environment. By concentrating on the causes of chronic disease, the ACA has begun to move the nation's focus on sickness and disease to one based on wellness and prevention.

In 2016, after the ACA was implemented, ANA's Principles for Health System Transformation outlined an equitable health care system that includes:

- Universal access to a standard package of essential health care services for all citizens and residents
- Optimizing primary, community-based, and preventive services while supporting the cost-effective use of innovative, technology-driven, acute, hospital-based services
- Encouraging mechanisms to stimulate economic use of health care services while supporting those who do not have the means to share in costs
- Ensuring a sufficient supply of skilled workforce dedicated to providing high-quality health care services

Many states have opted for an expansion of Medicaid under the ACA. Research has focused on access to care and health outcomes since this expansion has taken place. The large body of evidence has demonstrated that expanded Medicaid, as a whole, has had largely positive impacts on coverage; access to care, utilization, and affordability; and economic outcomes—including impacts on state budgets, uncompensated care costs for hospitals and clinics, and employment and the labor market (Antonisse et al., 2018). Discussions and debates will continue about the impact of the ACA and the IOM's discussions of integrating public health and primary care, reducing cost, increasing quality, and access for all Americans. It is important to focus on the goal: to protect and improve the health of all populations, as well as the ANA tenets for an equitable health care system.

Recent evidence based on a national survey of 1143 public health nurses (PHNs) when asked about the ACA and its impact on their perceptions and practice, noted that they are making substantial contributions to the implementation of the ACA. These nurses have been involved in public-private partnerships, access to primary care and care coordination, client navigation, integration of primary care and public health, population health data analysis and health strategies, and community health assessments (Edmonds et al., 2017).

QSEN FOCUS ON QUALITY AND SAFETY EDUCATION IN NURSES

Targeted Competency: Informatics

Use information and technology to communicate, manage knowledge, mitigate error, and support decision making.

Important aspects of informatics include the following:

- **Knowledge:** Identify essential information that must be available in a common database to support interventions in the health care system.
- **Skills:** Use information management tools to monitor outcomes of intervention processes.
- **Attitudes:** Value technologies that support decision making, error prevention, and case coordination.

Informatics Question

Updated informatics definitions focus on having access to the necessary client and system information at the right time to make the best clinical decision. In the U.S. Department of Health and Human Services (HHS) Strategic Plan for 2018-2022, there are five overarching goals. Specifically, Goal 1: Strengthen Health Care, Objective F, focuses on promoting the adoption and meaningful use of health information technology.

Which community data would a public health nurse assess to determine the work that needs to be done in a community related to this HHS strategic goal?

Answer

To assess future work that could be done to effectively address Goal 1, Objective F, public health nurses might gather data and answer questions in the following areas:

- What are the children and adult immunization rates in the community?
- What strategies are used by the health districts and primary care providers to increase vaccine rates?
- Are there characteristics within the unvaccinated population that can be addressed on a system and community level?
- What is the best method to reach this population?
- What strategies would be implemented to educate the unvaccinated?
- Have there been infectious disease outbreaks in the community over the last three years?
- What are the rates of the most common chronic diseases in the community?
- Where are the people living who have these diseases? Is there a cluster of individuals with the chronic disease?
- What resources are available in the community for these chronic diseases?
- How are these resources shared with the population?
- How are these services financed?
- Are communicable and noncommunicable diseases disproportionately affecting a particular group within the population?
- What impact does the environment have on the development of chronic diseases in the community?

PRACTICE APPLICATION

During a well-child clinic visit, Jenna Wells, RN, met Sandra Farr and her 24-month-old daughter, Jessica. The Farrs had recently moved to the community. Mrs. Farr stated that she knew that Jessica needed the last in a series of immunizations and because they did not have health insurance, she brought her daughter to the public health clinic. On initial assessment, Mrs. Farr told the nurse that her husband would soon be employed, but the family had no health care coverage for the next 30 days. The Farrs also needed to decide which health care package they wanted. Mr. Farr's company offers a preferred provider organization (PPO), a health maintenance organization (HMO), and a community nursing clinic plan to all employees. Neither Mr. nor Mrs. Farr has ever used an HMO or a community nursing clinic, and they are not sure what services are provided.

Mrs. Farr asks Nurse Wells what she should do.

Nurse Wells should do which of the following?

A. Encourage Mrs. Farr to choose the HMO because it will pay more attention to the family's preventive needs, and direct Mrs. Farr to other sources of health care should the family need to see a provider while they are uninsured.
B. Encourage Mrs. Farr to choose the PPO because it will have a greater number of qualified providers from which to choose, and direct Mrs. Farr to other sources of health care should the family need to see a provider while they are uninsured.
C. Encourage Mrs. Farr to choose the local community nursing center because it is staffed with nurse practitioners who are well qualified to provide comprehensive health care with an emphasis on health education, and direct Mrs. Farr to other sources of health care should the family need to see a provider while they are uninsured.
D. Explain the differences between a PPO, HMO, and community nursing clinic and encourage Mrs. Farr to discuss the options with her husband about signing up for a health insurance plan under the ACA plans, and direct Mrs. Farr to other sources of health care should the family need to see a provider while they are uninsured.

Answers can be found on the Evolve site.

KEY POINTS

- Health care in the United States is made up of a personal care system and a public health system, with overlap between the two systems.
- Primary care is a personal health care system that provides for first contact and continuous, comprehensive, and coordinated care.
- Primary health care is essential care made universally accessible to individuals and families in a community. Health care is made available to them through their full participation and is provided at a cost that the community and country can afford.
- Primary care and the public health systems are part of primary health care.
- Public health refers to organized community efforts designed to prevent disease and promote health of the population.
- Important trends that affect the health care system include political, demographic, social, economic, and technological trends.
- More than 48 million people in the United States were uninsured in 2012, and this was reduced to 28 million by the end of 2016.
- With the implementation of the Affordable Care Act (ACA), by 2016 the numbers of uninsured dropped by 6.3 percent.
- Many federal agencies are involved in government health care functions. The agency most directly involved with the health and welfare of Americans is the U.S. Department of Health and Human Services (HHS).
- Most state and local jurisdictions have government activities that affect the health care field.
- Health care and insurance reform measures seek to make changes in the cost and quality of and access to the present system, such as the ACA passed in 2010.
- To achieve the specific health goals of programs such as *Healthy People 2020*, primary care and public health must work within the community for community-based care.
- The most sustainable individual and system health changes come when people who live in the community actively participate.
- Nurses are more than able to bridge the gap between individualized care and public health because they have skills in assessment, health promotion, disease and injury prevention, and disease management; knowledge of community resources; and the ability to develop relationships with community members and leaders.
- Nurses, particularly public health nurses, are important to the success of the ACA.

CLINICAL DECISION-MAKING ACTIVITIES

1. Compare local and state health services. How have they been affected by the implementation of the ACA? What changes would you recommend to your local health district to improve public health and primary care?
2. Debate the following with a classmate. The major problem with the health care system is (choose one of the following topics):
   A. Escalating costs (including those from increased technology)
   B. Fragmentation of services
   C. Limited access to care
   D. Quality of care

   Explain your choice and give examples of reasons for the choice.
3. Visit your local health department and determine how its services fit into a primary care, public health, community-based health care system. Illustrate what you mean by your answer with examples.
4. Determine whether there is a Federally Qualified Health Center in your community. Visit https://www.ruralhealthinfo.org for locations and more information. If yes, learn what services are provided. Are there services that are needed in the community that are not being provided? If so, what are they?
5. Analyze the impact of a lack of primary care on the development of both acute and chronic illnesses in a foreign-born population. What media campaign would you implement to improve access to primary care within this population? What policy changes are needed at the local and national level to improve access to primary care?

ADDITIONAL RESOURCES

EVOLVE WEBSITE

http://evolve.elsevier.com/Stanhope/community/

- Answers to Practice Application
- Case Study
- Glossary
- Review Questions

REFERENCES

American Academy of Pediatrics (AAP): *Children and Disasters, Enterovirus D68*, 2016. Retrieved from https://www.aap.org.

American Association of Nurse Practitioners (AANP): *Historical Timeline*, Austin, TX, 2018, AANP.

American Board of Family Medicine (ABFM): *History of the Specialty*, Lexington, KY, 2005, ABFM.

American Nurses Association (ANA): *Health System Reform*, Silver Spring, MD, 2008, ANA. Retrieved from https://www.nursingworld.org.

Antonisse L, Garfield R, Rudowitz R, Artiga S. *The effects of Medicaid expansion under the ACA: Updated findings from a literature review*, 2018, Kaiser Family Foundation. Retrieved from https://www.kff.org.

Artiga S, and Damico A. *Health and Health Coverage in the South: A Data Update*, 2016, Kaiser Family Foundation. Retrieved from https://kaiserfamilyfoundation.files.wordpress.com.

Bureau of Labor Statistics (BLS), U.S. Department of Labor: *Databases, Tables, and Calculators*, 2018. Retrieved from https://data.bls.gov.

Bureau of Labor Statistics (BLS), U.S. Department of Labor: *Occupational Outlook Handbook: Registered Nurses*, 2018a. Retrieved from https://www.bls.gov.

Bureau of Labor Statistics, U.S. Department of Labor: *Consumer Price Index—2018*, 2018. Retrieved from https://www.bls.gov.

Centers for Disease Control and Prevention (CDC): *Public Health Genomics: Family History Public Health Initiative*. Atlanta, GA, 2013 CDC, U.S. Department of Health & Human Services.

Centers for Medicare and Medicaid Services: *Hospital acquired conditions (present on admission)*, 2009. Retrieved from www.cms.gov.

Centers for Medicare and Medicaid Services: *National Health Expenditure Data*, 2018. Retrieved from https://www.cms.gov.

Congressional Budget Office (CBO): *Trends in the Distribution of Household Income between 1979 and 2018*, 2018, p. 9. Retrieved from https://www.cbo.gov.

Demiris G, Forum on Aging, Disability, and Independence; Board on Health Sciences Policy; Division on Behavioral and Social Sciences and Education; Institute of Medicine; National Research Council: Innovations in technology. In *The Future of Home Health Care: Workshop Summary*, Washington, DC, 2015, National Academies Press. Retrieved from https://www.ncbi.nlm.nih.gov.

Dorn S, Hill I, Hogan S: *The secrets of Massachusetts' success: why 97 percent of state residents have health coverage: state health access reform evaluation, Rommneycare-The truth about Massachusetts health care*, 2009. Accessed at mittromneycentral.com, Robert Wood Johnson Foundation. Retrieved from http://www.urban.org.

Economic Report of the President, Washington, DC, 2010, U.S. Government Printing Office. Retrieved from http://www.whitehouse.gov.

Edmonds JK, Campbell LA, Gilder RE: Public health nursing practice in the Affordable Care Act Era: A national survey, *Public Health Nurs* 34(1):50–58, 2017. Retrieved from https://onlinelibrary.wiley.com.

Flinter M, Hsu C, Cromp D, Ladden MD, Wagner EH: Registered nurses in primary care: Emerging new roles and contributions to team-based care in high-performing practices, *J Ambul Care Manage* 40(4):287–296, 2017. Retrieved from https://www.ncbi.nlm.nih.gov.

Galewitz P: Medicaid to stop paying for hospital mistakes, *Kaiser Health News*, 2011. Retrieved from http://kaiserhealthnews.org.

Hamilton BE, Kirmeyer SE, Division of Vital Statistics: Trends and variations in reproduction and intrinsic rates: United States, 1990–2014, *Natl Vital Stat Rep* 66(2), 2017. Retrieved from https://www.cdc.gov.

Health Information Technology (HealthIT): Rockville, MD, 2018, USDHHS. Retrieved from https://www.healthit.gov.

Health Resources and Services Administration (HRSA): *Affordable Care Act Helps Expand the Use of Health Information Technology*, Washington, DC, 2012, HRSA, U.S. Department of Health and Human Services. Retrieved from http://www.hrsa.gov.

Health Resources and Services Administration (HRSA): *2017 National Health Center Data*, Washington, DC, 2018, HRSA, U.S. Department of Health and Human Services. Retrieved from https://bphc.hrsa.gov.

Health Resources and Services Administration (HRSA): *HRSA Awards $18.9 Million to Expand Use of Health Information Technology at Health Centers*. Washington, DC, 2008, HRSA, U.S. Department of Health and Human Services. Retrieved from http://archive.hrsa.gov.

Healthy People 2020: *Brochure with leading health indicators*, 2012. Retrieved from www.healthypeople.gov/2020.

Heron M: Deaths: Leading causes for 2016, *Natl Vital Stat Rep* 67(6). Hyattsville, MD, 2018, National Center for Health Statistics.

Institute of Medicine (IOM): *The Future of Public Health*, Washington, DC, 1988, National Academies Press.

Institute of Medicine (IOM): *Primary Care: America's Health in a New Era*, Washington, DC, 1996, National Academies Press. Retrieved from http://www.nap.edu.

Institute of Medicine (IOM): *To Err is Human: Building a Safer Health System*, Washington, DC, 2000, National Academies Press. Retrieved from http://www.iom.edu.

Institute of Medicine (IOM): *Keeping Patients Safe: Transforming the Work Environment of Nurses*, Washington, DC, 2003, National Academies Press. Retrieved from http://www.iom.edu.

Institute of Medicine (IOM): *Primary Care and Public Health: Exploring Integration to Improve Population Health*, Washington, DC, 2012, National Academies Press.

Kaiser Family Foundation: *Focus on Health Reform Massachusetts Health Care Reform: 6 years later*, Washington DC, 2012. Retrieved from https://kaiserfamilyfoundation.files.wordpress.com.

Kaiser Family Foundation: *Kaiser/HRET Survey of Employer-Sponsored Health Benefits, 1999-2009*. 2009. Retrieved from http://facts.kff.org.

Kaiser Family Foundation: *Key Facts about the Uninsured Population*, 2018. Retrieved from https://www.kff.org.

Kaiser Family Foundation: *National Health Insurance—a Brief History of Reform Efforts in the U.S.* 2009a, Kaiser Family Foundation. Retrieved from https://kaiserfamilyfoundation.files.wordpress.com.

Levesque JF, Breton M, Senn N, et al: The interaction of public health and primary care: Functional roles and organizational models that bridge individual and population perspectives, *Public Health Rev* 35:1–27, 2013.

Macy Foundation: Registered Nurses: *Partners in Transforming Primary Care Proceedings of a conference on Preparing Registered Nurses for Enhanced Roles in Primary Care*, 2017. Retrieved from http://macyfoundation.org.

MedlinePlus. *Managed Care*, Rockville, MD, 2017, U.S. National Library of Medicine. Retrieved from https://medlineplus.gov.

Migration Policy Institute: *American Community Survey and Census Data on the Foreign Born by State*, Washington, DC, 2014, Migration Policy Institute. Retrieved from www.migrationinformation.org.

National Center for Complementary and Integrative Health, National Institutes of Health: 2017. Retrieved from https://nccih.nih.gov.

National Center for Health Statistics (NCHS). *Health, United States, 2016: With Chartbook on Long-term Trends in Health*, Hyattsville, MD, 2017, NCHS. Retrieved from https://www.cdc.gov.

National Institutes of Health (NIH): My family health portrait: a tool from the surgeon general, *NIH MedlinePlus* 5(1):4, 2010. Retrieved from http://www.nlm.nih.gov.

Office for National Statistics (ONS): *Vital statistics: population and health reference tables, annual time series data*, 2014.

Pew Research Center: *Tabulations of the 2012 American Community Surveys*, 2013. Retrieved from www.pewresearch.org.

Phillips JM, Malone B. Increasing racial/ethnic diversity in nursing to reduce health disparities and achieve health equity, *Public Health Rep* 129(Suppl 2):45–50, 2014. Retrieved from https://www.ncbi.nlm.nih.gov

Public Health Accreditation Board (PHAB): *Accredited Health Departments*, Alexandria, VA, 2014, PHAB. Retrieved from http://www.phaboard.org.

Public Health Accreditation Board: *Accreditation Standards*, 2018. Retrieved from http://www.phaboard.org.

Sanborn BJ. As baby boomer nurses retire, concern grows about national shortage. *Healthcare Finance*, 2017. Retrieved from https://www.healthcarefinancenews.com.

Truffer CJ, Keehan S, Smith S, et al.: Health spending projections through 2019: the recession's impact continues, *Health Aff (Millwood)* 29:522–529, 2010. Retrieved from http://content.healthaffairs.org.

U.S. Census Bureau: *Population*, 2018. Retrieved from https://www.census.gov.

U.S. Department of Health and Human Services (HHS): *Healthy People 2020: Improving the Health of Americans*, 2010. Retrieved from http://www.healthypeople.gov.

U.S. Department of Health and Human Services (HHS): *Healthy People 2020 Leading Health Indicators*, 2018. Retrieved from https://www.healthypeople.gov.

U.S. Department of Health and Human Services (HHS): *HHS Organizational Chart*, 2014. Retrieved from https://www.hhs.gov.

U.S. Department of Health and Human Services (HHS): *Strategic Plan: Fiscal Years 2018-2022*, 2018. Retrieved from https://www.hhs.gov.

U.S. Department of Homeland Security (USDHS): *Homeland Security*, 2014. Retrieved from http://www.dhs.gov.

U.S. Public Health Service (USPHS): *The Commissioned Corps of the PHS*, 2018. Retrieved from https://www.usphs.gov.

World Health Organization (WHO): *Primary Health Care*, 2018. Retrieved from http://www.who.int/primary-health/en.

World Health Organization (WHO): *Primary Health Care: Report of the International Conference on Primary Health Care, Alma-Ata, USSR, September 6-12*, 1978. [Health for All Series No. 1]. Geneva, 1978, WHO.

World Health Organization (WHO): *Basic Documents*, ed 36. Geneva, 1986a, WHO.

World Health Organization (WHO): *World Health Statistics Annual*. Geneva, 1986b, WHO.

World Health Organization (WHO): *The World Health Report 2008: Primary Health Care (Now More Than Ever)*. Geneva, 2008, WHO. Retrieved from http://www.who.int.

4

Perspectives in Global Health Care

Emma McKim Mitchell, PhD, MSN, RN

OBJECTIVES

After reading this chapter, the student should be able to do the following:

1. Identify the major aims and goals for global health that have been presented by the *Millennium Development Goals* and 2017 *UN Sustainable Development Goals.*
2. Identify the health priorities of Health for All in the 21st Century (HFA21) and *Healthy People 2020.*
3. Analyze the role of nursing in global health.
4. Explain the role and focus of a population-based approach for global health.
5. Discuss the many causes of global health problems.
6. Identify some sustainable solutions for at least one of these global health problems.
7. Describe how global health is related to economic, industrial, environmental, and technological development.
8. Compare and contrast the health care system in a developed country with one in a less developed country.
9. Define *burden of disease.*
10. Explain how countries can prepare for natural and man-made disasters and the role of nurses in these efforts.
11. Describe at least five organizations that are involved in global health.

CHAPTER OUTLINE

Overview and Historical Perspective of Global Health
The Role of Population Health
Primary Health Care
Nursing and Global Health
Major Global Health Organizations
Global Health and Global Development
Health Care Systems
Major Global Health Problems and the Burden of Disease

KEY TERMS

bilateral organization, p. 69
bioterrorism, p. 84
chemical emergency, p. 85
determinants of health, p. 66
developed country, p. 64
disability-adjusted life-years (DALYs), p. 75
environmental sanitation, p. 77
genocide, p. 85
global burden of disease, p. 75
global health diplomacy, p. 71
health commodification, p. 71
Health for All in the 21st Century (HFA21), p. 63
less developed country, p. 64
man-made disasters, p. 84
Millennium Development Goals, p. 65
multilateral organizations, p. 69
natural disasters, p. 83
nongovernmental organizations (NGOs), p. 69
Pan American Health Organization (PAHO), p. 70
philanthropic organizations, p. 71
population health, p. 66
primary health care, p. 67
private voluntary organizations (PVOs), p. 69
radiation poisoning, p. 85
religious organizations, p. 71
Sustainable Development Goals (SDGs), p. 65
United Nations Children's Fund (UNICEF), p. 70
World Bank, p. 70
World Health Organization (WHO), p. 69

Sincere thanks to Anita Hunter who authored several editions of this chapter.

This chapter presents an overview of the major public health problems of the world, along with a description of the role and involvement of nurses in global and community health care settings. It describes health care delivery from a global and population health perspective, illustrates how health systems operate in different countries, presents examples of organizations that address global health, and explains how economic development relates to health care throughout the world.

OVERVIEW AND HISTORICAL PERSPECTIVE OF GLOBAL HEALTH

Global warming and the melting of the polar ice caps; worldwide droughts and the natural disasters of blizzards, hurricanes, tornadoes, volcanoes, typhoons, and earthquakes; war; growing populations and the impoverished, destitute populations of the world make it imperative that nurses know about global health. Recent movements in the global arena identify the need for nurses to practice global health diplomacy, expanding beyond the tenets of health care and education we once provided (Hunter et al., 2013). Evidence indicates that contamination of water sources by heavy metals such as arsenic, copper, cadmium, mercury, and lead, to name a few, arising from the earth's crust appears to be increasing around the globe because of the changing environmental conditions (Alliance of Nurses for Healthy Environments, 2018; Bolender et al., 2012, 2013; Fernández-Luqueño et al., 2013; World Health Organization, 2018c). What once were the unique health challenges of people in less developed countries, such as loss of human rights; and lack of access to food, housing, safety, and health care are now common problems of people all over the world. Contamination of the water sources in many countries, worsening poverty, increasing global violence, the declining global economy, and the depletion of food supplies all contribute to current global health crises. See the Evidence-Based Practice box to learn how nurses are using innovative technology in Botswana to increase access to cervical cancer screening in vulnerable women.

EVIDENCE-BASED PRACTICE

A leading cause of death for women in Botswana, cervical cancer, is largely preventable through vaccination and screening/early detection. Human papillomavirus, the leading cause of cervical cancer, can be detected through DNA testing of samples. Incorporation of self-collection of HPV samples for DNA testing into large-scale screening programs can reduce barriers women experience to accessing care. Through a partnership with Jhpiego, a Johns Hopkins University–affiliated organization, nurses are promoting HPV self-collection through a clinical research trial to increase access to cervical cancer screening in vulnerable women in Botswana (Yakutchik, 2018).

Nurse Use

Being culturally sensitive and responsive means that nurses need to understand where patients come from, what barriers exist that contribute to the public health problems they develop, and what can reasonably be done to reduce the health consequences of poverty and access deprivation. Given this research study, how could you as a nurse help reduce the barriers women face in accessing cervical cancer and other types of cancer screening? One example might be to meet with a group of women who have not been screened to discuss the barriers women in their communities' face in accessing cervical cancer screening. What might be other examples?

Preventable conditions such as malaria, malnutrition, communicable diseases, chronic health problems, and conditions related to environmental pollution are taxing the health care systems of many nations. Immigrants from developing nations may have experienced a lack of access to health care services that could successfully diagnose or treat health issues in their country of origin. Understanding global health and factors that contribute to immigrants' health problems better prepares the nurse to develop interventions that are culturally congruent, culturally responsive, and culturally acceptable to the target group. The vision of the International Council of Nurses (ICN)'s Leadership for Change program is that nursing is to take a leadership role in helping achieve better health for all (International Council of Nurses, 2018). Through this program the ICN works to build leadership capacity through in-country partnerships with ministries of health and nursing associations and leadership. In June 2018, for example, the ICN Leadership for Change program (sponsored by Johnson & Johnson) trained 36 nurses from 10 provinces in China with a train-the-trainer model. Looking forward, the program aims to cover 12 provinces and support over 500 future nurse leaders (ICN, 2018).

In 1977 attendees at the annual meeting of the World Health Assembly stated that all citizens of the world should enjoy a level of health that would permit them to lead a socially and economically productive life. This goal was to have been achieved by the year 2000; however, man-made and natural disasters, political corruption, lack of infrastructure in less developed nations, and unforeseen obstacles have inhibited this goal from being achieved. The goals of Health for All by the Year 2000 (HFA2000) were extended into the next century with the document **Health for All in the 21st Century (HFA21):** http://www.euro.who.int). The four main HFA21 strategies for action to ensure that scientific, economic, social, and political sustainability were those designed as follows:

1. To tackle the determinants of health, taking into account physical, economic, social, cultural, and gender perspectives and ensuring the use of health impact assessment
2. As health-outcome-driven programs and investments for health development and clinical care
3. For integrated family- and community-oriented primary health care, supported by a flexible and responsive hospital system
4. As a participatory health development process that involves relevant partners for health at home, school, and work and at local community and country levels, and that promotes joint decision making, implementation, and accountability

HFA laid the foundation for the Healthy People agendas of *Healthy People 2020*.

HEALTHY PEOPLE 2020

Selected Objectives That Apply to Global Health Care

- **EH-4:** Increase the proportion of persons served by community water systems who receive a supply of drinking water that meets the regulations of the Safe Drinking Water Act.
- **EH-5:** Reduce waterborne disease outbreaks arising from water intended for drinking among persons served by community water systems.
- **FP-1:** Increase the proportion of pregnancies that are intended.
- **GH-1:** Reduce the number of cases of malaria reported in the United States.
- **HIV-1:** Reduce the number of new HIV diagnoses among adolescents and adults.
- **MICH-3:** Reduce the rate of child deaths.

From U.S. Department of Health and Human Services: *Healthy People: 2020 topics and objectives*. Retrieved from http://www.healthypeople.gov.

Each of the previous goals has relevance to global health. The millions of deaths related to unsafe water and poor hygiene are highest in Africa and Southeast Asia. This relates to objectives EH-4 and EH-5 (see the Healthy People 2020 box). Six in ten pregnancies in developing nations are unintended and relate to objective FP-1 (Kott, 2011). Malaria caused an estimated 445,000 deaths in 2016, with 90 percent of cases and 91 percent of mortalities in the WHO African Region (World Health Organization [WHO], 2018a), which relates to objective GH-1. The WHO African Region remains severely affected with human immunodeficiency virus (HIV)/acquired immunodeficiency syndrome (AIDS), with 27 million people in 2017 living with HIV and over two-thirds of the global total of new HIV infections (WHO, 2018b; WHO, 2014d), which relates to objective HIV-1. Last, the leading causes of death in under-five children are pneumonia, preterm birth complications, birth asphyxia, diarrhea, and malaria (WHO, 2013b; WHO, 2018c, 2018d); this relates to objective MICH-3. See the Quality and Safety Education for Nurses box for suggestions for how to deal with malaria through a team approach

QSEN FOCUS ON QUALITY AND SAFETY EDUCATION FOR NURSES

As described in earlier chapters of the text, including Chapter 2, there are six QSEN competencies for nursing. Because of the complex and multifaceted nature of providing public health nursing care in countries around the world, competency number two, teamwork and collaboration, is emphasized here.

Teamwork and collaboration refer to the ability to function effectively with nursing and interprofessional teams and to foster open communication, mutual respect, and shared decision making in order to best provide safe and quality care. One of the United Nations Millennium Development Goals is to combat HIV/AIDS, malaria, and other diseases (Box 4.1).

Quality and Safety Question

How would nurses working in a country that is plagued by malaria develop a team to help control this mosquito-borne disease?

Answer

The spread of malaria can be interrupted by prevention, treatment, and control measures such as using insecticide-treated bed nets and spraying in and near where people live, work, and go to school. Nurses would develop a team including representatives from funding agencies, environmental health, NGOs, medical practitioners, and local governments to locate funds and develop, implement, and evaluate prevention, control, and treatment measures.

Because of the ease of global travel, contagious and preventable health conditions are not endemic in just an isolated country; they are prevalent around the world. Health professionals and world leaders want to be enlightened about these health issues and want answers on how to address them, which becomes problematic in the countries most afflicted but without the technological infrastructure to help their people.

Many terms are used to describe nations that have achieved a high level of industrial and technological advancement (along with a stable market economy) and those that have not. For the purposes of this chapter, the term **developed country** refers to those countries with a stable economy and a wide range of industrial and technological development, low child mortality, high gross national income, and a high human asset index (e.g., the United States, Canada, Japan, the United Kingdom, Sweden, France, and Australia). A country that does not meet these criteria is referred to as a **less developed country** (e.g., Congo, Bangladesh, Somalia, Haiti, Guatemala, most countries in sub-Saharan Africa, and the island nation of Indonesia). Both developed and less developed countries are found in all parts of the world and in all geographic and climatic zones (UN Department of Economic and Social Affairs [DESA], 2014).

Health problems exist throughout the world, but the less developed countries often have more unusual health care problems. There are more than 6000 rare diseases (Forman et al., 2012), and in developing countries such conditions as Buruli ulcers, leishmaniasis, river blindness, schistosomiasis, brucellosis, typhus, yellow fever, scurvy, and malaria are often unknown entities in the world of Western medicine (WHO, 2018e). Ongoing health problems needing control in less developed countries include measles, mumps, rubella, and polio; the current health concerns of the more developed countries are problems such as hepatitis, infectious diseases, and new viral strains such as hantavirus, severe acute respiratory syndrome (SARS), H1N1, and avian flu. Chronic health problems such as hypertension, diabetes, cardiovascular disease, obesity, cancer, the resurgence of HIV/AIDS among adolescents and young adults, drug-resistant tuberculosis (TB); and the larger social, yet health-related, issues such as terrorism, warfare, violence, and substance abuse are now global issues (Shah, 2014). World travelers may expose themselves to diseases and environmental health hazards that are unknown or rare in their home country and may serve as hosts to various types of disease agents. Two examples of diseases that were once fairly isolated and rare but have increased in prevalence are the mosquito-borne viruses of Zika and Chikungunya (CDC, 2017, 2018)

In addition to direct health problems, increasing populations, migration between and within countries, political corruption, lack of natural resources, and natural disasters affect the health and well-being of populations. Dr. Paul Farmer in his book *Pathologies of Power* (2005) talks about the war on the poor; how many people migrate to the city to find employment, where limited employment opportunities exist. Such migration leads to the development of shanty towns often built on the outskirts of cities, on unstable ground, and in areas vulnerable to natural disasters such as hurricanes, tsunamis, and earthquakes such as those in Haiti, Chile, and Indonesia. These environments are unsanitary, unsafe, and a breeding ground for TB, dysentery, malnutrition, abuse of women and children, and mosquito and other insect- or animal-borne diseases.

Nations plagued by civil war and political corruption are faced with chronic poverty, unstable leadership, and lack of economic development. The effects of war and conflict also have devastating effects on a country and the health of its population. The wars in Afghanistan, Iraq, Syria, and the West Bank of Palestine, to name a few, have had devastating mental and physical health consequences, leaving each country and its people with few health care services or other resources to sustain life. A recent research study about the long-term effects of children exposed to war (Slone & Mann, 2016) supports the negative health consequences of such exposure. For example, changes in biomarkers can lead to future chronic health conditions such as cardiovascular and pulmonary diseases and autoimmune conditions, cancer, and mental health problems.

As countries promote the objectives of HFA21, they realize that they need to improve their economies and infrastructures. They often seek funds and technological expertise from the wealthier and more developed countries. According to the WHO Europe (2013a), HFA21 is not a single, finite goal but a strategic process that can lead to progressive improvement in the health of people. In essence it is a call for social justice and solidarity. Unfortunately, the less developed nations still lack the infrastructure necessary to achieve health promotion and healthy living conditions, as many of these countries continue to deteriorate for the poor, and environments that breed infections are the norm (Fig. 4.1).

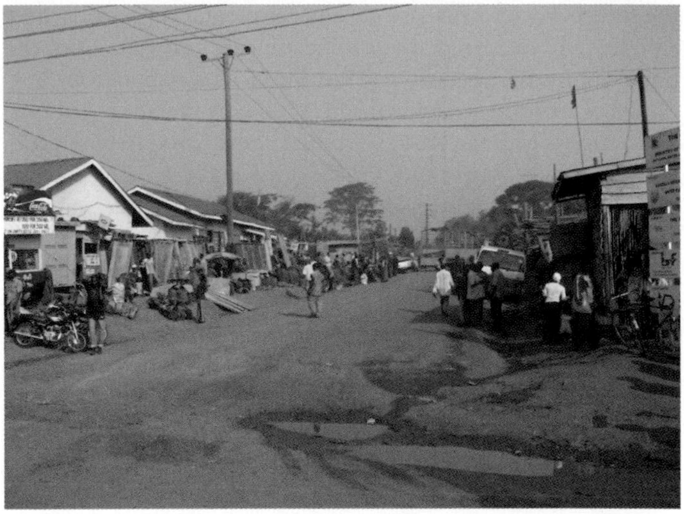

Fig. 4.1 The streets of a town in Uganda. (Courtesy A. Hunter.)

The UN **Millennium Development Goals** (MDGs) were first agreed on by world leaders at the Millennium Summit in 2000 and assessed through the 2015 Gap Finding Task Force. The MDGs were developed to relieve poor health conditions around the world and to establish positive steps to improve living conditions by the year 2015 (UN, 2013a; see goals in Box 4.1). These goals have continued to evolve as natural disasters and internal strife continue to affect the poor and the vulnerable. The Millennium Report (UN, 2015) describes the developed nations' responsibility to the betterment of those in less developed nations, as well as areas where progress is still needed. The MDGs highlight the global responsibility to eradicate poverty and hunger; achieve universal primary education for all children; promote gender equality and empower women; reduce child mortality; improve maternal health; combat HIV/AIDS, malaria, and other diseases; ensure environmental sustainability; and develop a global partnership for development.

The MDGs were updated by the United Nations (UN) and collaborative groups to reflect the **Sustainable Development Goals (SDGs)** in 2017. These are (listed in Box 4.1) designed to be a more comprehensive and detailed guide for progress into

BOX 4.1 Millennium Development Goals and Sustainable Development Goals

Millennium Development Goals

MDG 1: Eradicate extreme poverty and hunger.
MDG 2: Achieve universal primary education.
MDG 3: Promote gender equality and empower women.
MDG 4: Reduce child mortality.
MDG 5: Improve maternal health.
MDG 6: Combat HIV/AIDS, malaria, and other diseases.
MDG 7: Ensure environmental sustainability.
MDG 8: Develop a global partnership for development.

Sustainable Development Goals

SDG 1: No Poverty
SDG 2: Zero Hunger
SDG 3: Good Health and Well-Being
SDG 4: Quality Education
SDG 5: Gender Equality
SDG 6: Clean Water and Sanitation
SDG 7: Affordable and Clean Energy
SDG 8: Decent Work and Economic Growth
SDG 9: Industry, Innovation, and Infrastructure
SDG 10: Reduced Inequalities
SDG 11: Sustainable Cities and Communities
SDG 12: Responsible Consumption and Production
SDG 13: Climate Action
SDG 14: Life Below Water
SDG 15: Life on Land
SDG 16: Peace, Justice, and Strong Institutions
SDG 17: Partnerships for the Goals

From United Nations: *UN millennium development goals (MDGs)*, 2013. Available at http://www.un.org; United Nations: *UN Sustainable Development Goals (SDGs)*, 2017. Available at https://www.un.org.

the future. Focus areas include environmental concerns; gender equality and increased access to health care and education; and partnerships necessary to reach these goals collaboratively.

Other major worldwide health problems include nutritional deficiencies in all age groups, women's health and fertility problems, sexually transmitted infections (STIs), and illnesses related to HIV, malaria, drug-resistant TB, neonatal tetanus, leprosy, occupational and environmental health hazards, and abuses of tobacco, alcohol, and drugs. Because of these continuing problems, the director general of the WHO has made a commitment to renew all of the policies and actions of HFA21. The WHO Europe (2013a) continues to develop new and holistic health policies that are based on the concepts of equity and solidarity, with an emphasis on the individual's, family's, and community's responsibility for health. Strategies for achieving the continuing goals of HFA21 include building on past accomplishments and the identification of global priorities and targets for the first 20 years of the new century.

Nurses need to be informed about global health. Many of the world's health problems directly affect the health of individuals who live in the United States. For example, the One Hundred Third U.S. Congress passed the North American Free Trade Agreement (NAFTA), which opened trade borders between the United States, Canada, and Mexico in 1994 and allowed increased movement of products and people. Along the United States–Mexico border, an influx of undocumented immigrants in recent years has raised concerns for the health of people who live in this area. NAFTA has also provided an impetus and framework for the government of Mexico to modernize its medical system so that Mexico can compete and respond to the demands of more global competition. Although some improvements have been made, there is still an overriding concern that environmental and health regulations in Mexico have not kept up with the pace of increased border trade (California Department of Public Health, 2015). The Mexican National Academy of Medicine continues to make health and environmental recommendations to the government, which illustrates the beneficial interactions that are occurring between Mexico, Canada, and the United States as part of this trade agreement. Nurses play a significant role in obtaining health for the indigent and undocumented persons who live along the border regions in Texas, New Mexico, Arizona, and California. Nurses supported by private foundations and by local and state public health departments often provide critical and reliable health care in these areas. At present there is uncertainty about the future of NAFTA and the relationship between the United States and the countries that border the United States.

THE ROLE OF POPULATION HEALTH

Population health refers to the health outcomes of a group of individuals, including the distribution of such outcomes within the group, and includes health outcomes, patterns of health determinants, and policies and interventions that link these two. It is an approach and perspective that focuses on the broad range of factors and conditions that have a strong influence on the health of populations (environment, genetics, ethnicity, pollution, and physical and mental stressors affecting a community). Using epidemiologic trends, population health emphasizes health for groups at the population level rather than at the individual level and focuses on reducing inequities, improving health in these groups to reduce morbidity and mortality, and assessing emerging diseases and other health risks to a community. A population can be defined by a geographic boundary, by the common characteristics shared by a group of people such as ethnicity or religion, or by the epidemiologic and social conditions of a community.

The factors and conditions that are important considerations in population health are called **determinants of health**. Population health determinants may include income and social factors, social support networks, education, employment, working and living conditions, physical environments, social environments, biology and genetic endowment, personal health practices, coping skills, healthy child development, health services, sex, and culture (WHO, 2014a). The determinants do not work independently of each other but form a complex system of interactions.

Canada is a leader in promoting the population health approach. Canada has been implementing programs using this framework since the mid-1990s and builds on a tradition of public health and health promotion. Box 4.2 presents the development of the Healthy Cities movement in Toronto. This successful project has been adopted by the WHO and is being implemented in several countries around the world—most specifically Europe, Southeast Asia, Africa, and the Western Pacific (WHO, 2014b). A key to the success of this project has been the identification and definition of health issues and of the investment decisions within a population that were guided by evidence about what keeps people healthy. Therefore a population health approach directs investments that have the greatest potential to influence the health of that population in a positive manner. A Healthy City aims to create a health-supportive environment, achieve a good quality of life, provide basic sanitation and hygiene needs, and supply access to health care. The most successful Healthy Cities programs have a commitment of local community members, a clear vision, ownership of policies, a wide array of stakeholders, and a process for institutionalizing the program.

Integration of health determinants into public policies is apparent on the global stage. At the 2009 Nairobi Global Conference on Health Promotion, more than 600 participants representing 100 countries adopted a Call to Action on addressing population health and finding ways to promote health at the global level. Health and development today face unprecedented threats by the financial crisis, global warming and climate change, and security threats. Since 1986, with the development of the first Global Conference, until 2009, a large body of evidence and experience has accumulated about the importance of health promotion as an integrative, cost-effective strategy and as an essential component of health systems primed to respond adequately to emerging concerns (WHO, 2010a, 2018b).

As nurses work with immigrants from global arenas or become active participants in health care around the world, understanding such concepts as population health and the

BOX 4.2 Examples of the Healthy Cities Movement

Toronto, Ontario, Canada, was one of the first cities in North America to become involved in the Healthy Cities movement. Toronto began with a strategic planning committee to develop an overall strategy for health promotion. The committee conducted vision workshops in the community and a comprehensive environmental scan to help identify health needs in Toronto. The outcome was a final report outlining major issues, and it included a strategic mission, priorities, and recommendations for action. The Toronto Healthy City program involved a number of projects. One of them, the Healthiest Babies Possible project, was an intensive antenatal education and nutritional supplement program for pregnant women who were identified by health and social agencies as being at high risk. The program included intensive contact and follow-up of women, along with food supplements. It has been successful in decreasing the incidence of low-birth-weight infants.

Another example is Chengdu, China. Chengdu is located on the upper parts of the Yangtze River. It is surrounded on four sides by the Fu and Nan Rivers and was one of the most polluted cities in southwestern China. The pollution created severe environmental problems as a result of industrial waste, raw sewage, and the intensive use of fresh water. The proliferation of slum and squatter settlements exacerbated the social, economic, and environmental problems of the city. The Fu and Nan Rivers Comprehensive Revitalization Plan was started in 1993 as a Healthy Community and City initiative to deal with the growing environmental problems. The principles of participatory planning and partnership were used to raise awareness of the problem among the general public and to mobilize major stakeholders to invest in a sustainable future for Chengdu and its inhabitants. The plan resulted in providing 30,000 households living in the slum and squatter settlements with decent and affordable housing, and with projects to deal with sewage and industrial waste. In addition, the plan was able to improve parks and gardens, turning Chengdu into a clean and green city within the natural flow of its rivers.

From Flynn B, Ivanov L: Health promotion through healthy communities and cities. In *Community & public health nursing,* ed. 6, St. Louis, 2004, Mosby, pp. 396-411.

determinants of health for a population becomes more important than the most advanced acute care skills. These skills, though important, are intended to help an individual; population health skill sets can help the world.

PRIMARY HEALTH CARE

The ultimate goal of **primary health care** (PHC) is to achieve better health for all. WHO (2014c) has identified five key elements to achieving that goal:

1. Reducing exclusion and social disparities in health
2. Organizing health services around people's needs and expectations
3. Integrating health into all sectors
4. Pursuing collaborative models of policy dialogue
5. Increasing stakeholder participation

These aims continue to be reinforced and modified and were recently updated to incorporate MDGs. Such services included the following:

- An organized approach to health education that involves professional health care providers and trained community representatives
- Aggressive attention to environmental sanitation, especially food and water sources
- Involvement and training of community and village health workers in all plans and intervention programs
- Development of maternal and child health programs that include immunization and family planning
- Initiation of preventive programs that are specifically aimed at local endemic problems such as malaria and schistosomiasis in tropical regions
- Accessibility and affordability of services for the treatment of common diseases and injuries
- Availability of chemotherapeutic agents for the treatment of acute, chronic, and communicable diseases
- Development of nutrition programs
- Promotion and acceptance of traditional medicine

Global leaders have recognized the need to get nations committed to the health care agenda. An important effort is needed at the level of recruitment, education, and retention of PHC workers, including primary care nurses, family physicians, and mid-level care workers. Professional organizations, clinical agencies, universities, and other institutions for higher education should continue to demonstrate their "social accountability" by training appropriate providers.

It is well documented that PHC practiced in high-income countries exerts a positive influence on health costs, appropriateness of care, and outcomes for most of the major health indicators. PHC also has more equitable health outcomes than systems oriented toward specialty care. In low- and middle-income countries the research studies did find consistent evidence of the impact of PHC on improved health outcomes; however, there were problems with the research rigor and validity of instrumentation to make any further statement than that health outcomes did improve.

NURSING AND GLOBAL HEALTH

Nurses play a leadership role in health care throughout the world. Those with public health experience provide knowledge and skill in countries where nursing is not an organized profession, and they give guidance to the nurses as well as to the auxiliary personnel who are part of the PHC team (Bryar et al., 2012). In many areas in the developed world, nurses provide direct client care and help meet the education and health promotion needs of the community. They are viewed as strong advocates for PHC, through social commitment to equality of health care and support of the concepts that are contained in the Declaration of Alma-Ata (Bryar et al., 2012).

In the less developed countries the role and scope of practice of the nurse may be less explicitly defined, and care often depends on and is directed by physicians. Work is needed to support and promote education of nurses, as well as promote professionalization of nursing in countries where this is the case (Fig. 4.2).

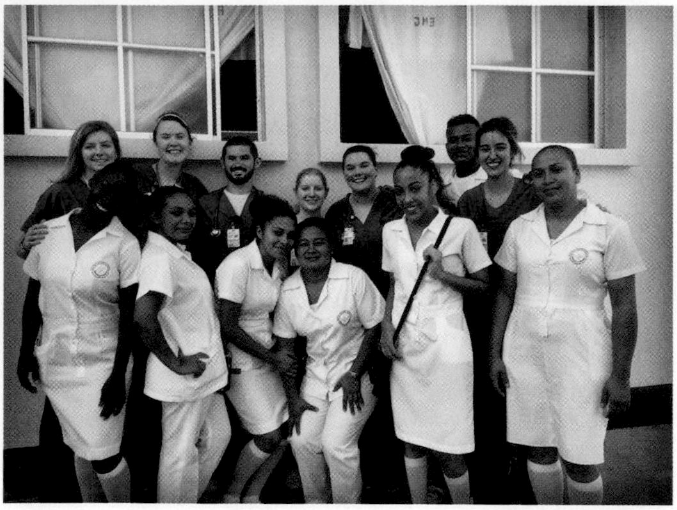

Fig. 4.2 Support for professionalization of nursing in global settings must be in the context of respectful, sustained, cultural engagement. Nursing students from the University of Virginia and the Bluefields Indian and Caribbean University in Bluefields, Nicaragua. (Courtesy E. Mitchell.)

Nurses have led in care delivery after the devastating tsunami in South Asia and after the earthquakes in Haiti and Chile in 2010. Nurses currently are leading advocacy and policy change efforts specific to climate change and extreme weather. In 2016 the Alliance of Nurses for Healthy Environments (ANHE) published a comprehensive report outlining the evidence nurses can use to lead change and promote health for vulnerable populations (ANHE, 2016). Other health interventions have been the interprofessional work of nursing and science to build and open a dedicated children's hospital in Uganda (Bolender & Hunter, 2010; Bolender et al., 2013), a nurse-led chronic illness management program in Thailand (Sindhu et al., 2010), a nurse-led mental health program for Chinese patients (Chien et al., 2012), and the nurse-led cervical cancer prevention program in the Evidence-Based Practice box; these are just a few examples of nurse-initiated health programs around the globe.

The role of nursing in China is noteworthy. Nursing in China is undergoing a dramatic change, largely because of an evolving political and economic environment. In the past, nursing was viewed as a trade, and the acquisition of nursing skills and knowledge took place in the equivalent of a middle school or junior high school in the United States. Increasing pressure on the health care system in China provided an impetus for education at the university level. In the past the Chinese government sent many nurses to the United States, Europe, and Australia to receive university-level education in nursing at the undergraduate and graduate levels in hopes that these individuals will return to China to provide the nursing and nursing education needed there. Currently, there are many nursing programs in institutions of higher learning. As of 2016 there were about 22 doctoral programs in nursing across China (Wang et al., 2016).

In some countries, the physician-to-population ratio is higher than the nurse-to-population ratio. In these cases, physicians influence nursing practice and place economic and political pressure on local, regional, and national governments to control the services that nurses provide. Often nurses feel threatened by physicians who want to remove the nurses and replace them with the more costly services of physicians. A useful source of information about health in a variety of countries can be found in the *Health at a Glance* documents published by the Organization for Economic Cooperation and Development (OECD, 2017). Another useful resource is the Mossiaios, et al. (2017) monograph that provides a review of 19 health care systems around the world. Box 4.3 describes nursing and health care efforts in Zambia.

BOX 4.3 Community Health Nursing in Zambia

The Ministry of Health, Churches Health Association, the private medical practitioners, and the traditional healer services provide health care in Zambia. By 1995 there were 86 hospitals and 1345 health centers in the country. About 60 percent of the bed capacity is provided by the government hospitals and health centers, 26 percent by mission hospitals, and 13 percent by the Zambia Consolidated Copper Mines. At the time of independence the population of Zambia was sparsely distributed, especially in the rural area, and there were inadequate health facilities. Health facilities were concentrated along the line of rail, and the provision of care was poor. This prompted the government to review the health care provision system after independence in 1964. The government then declared that health care services would be free for all, with the main health care services being curative rather than preventive. This policy was detrimental to Zambia, whose population was increasing.

In 1991 the government of the Republic of Zambia, under the leadership of the Movement for Multiparty Democracy, introduced the concept of National Health Reforms, the vision being to provide equitable access to high-quality, cost-effective health care intervention as close to the family as possible. Health reforms stress the need for families and communities to be self-reliant and to participate in their own health care provision and development. The major component of the health policy reform is the restructured primary health care (PHC) program. This has been defined as essential health care made universally accessible to individuals and families by means acceptable to them through their full participation and at a cost that the community and country can afford. The principles of PHC include community participation and intersectoral collaboration. Families are considered a unit of service, as most health care provision starts with the family setting. The Zambian government is committed to the fundamental and humane principle in the development of the health care system to provide Zambians with equity of access to cost-effective quality health care as close to the family as possible.

The National Health Reforms decentralized power to districts, and home-based care (HBC) was introduced. HBC was adopted and implemented in all districts as a way of cost sharing between the government, families, and community. HBC led to reduced congestion in hospitals, and government resources were not overstrained as families also took part in supplying the needed resources, time, and personnel (caregivers) when the clients were cared for at home.

Nurses provide about 75 percent of the health force in Zambia. The community health nursing component is one of the major components of the nursing curriculum at all levels of training. Basically, every general nurse is taught to operate as a community health nurse. However, to be registered as a public health nurse by the General Nursing Council of Zambia, one must undergo the following levels of training. The individual undergoes three years of training as a registered nurse followed by one year of training as a midwife. In the past the person

BOX 4.3 Community Health Nursing in Zambia—cont'd

would then undergo two years of training at the University of Zambia to obtain a diploma in public health nursing. This was phased out when the bachelor of science in nursing degree was initiated. At present the individual pursues the bachelor of science in nursing degree and majors in community health nursing in the final year.

The main role of the community health nurse includes competence and skill in the care of individuals, families, and communities in the following ways:

1. Critically explore and analyze current developments in community health as they relate to different populations at different levels of care.
2. Apply health promotion models and theories to community health nursing practice.
3. Design, implement, and manage community-based projects, programs, and services.
4. Integrate community-based agents into the health care system.
5. Use epidemiology concepts in the management of communicable and noncommunicable diseases.

Courtesy Prudencia Mweemba, University of Zambia, School of Medicine, Department of Post Basic Nursing, Lusaka, Zambia, 2006.

Several nursing initiatives based in the United States have been developed to help address some of these global health problems. For example, SEED Global Health is an initiative aimed at building capacity in trained health care providers, specifically nurses, in Malawi, Tanzania, Uganda, Swaziland, and Liberia (SEED Global Health, 2018).

According to Sheila Davis, ANP-BC, FAAN, Director of Global Nursing, Partners in Health, the Dana Farber Cancer Institute supported the creation of a nursing oncology partnership with Inshuti Mu Buzima (IMB) in Rwanda. Four experienced oncology nurses worked alongside local nurses and physicians at IMB for 3-month rotations to help Rwandan nurses develop the specialized skills and experience needed to raise the quality of oncology care. A new entry into this global nursing arena is the development of the Global Nursing Caucus, which seeks to "improve collaboration and information dissemination in the rapidly growing field of global health nursing" (Global Nursing Caucus [GNC], 2018). It is vitally important to the success of such initiatives to assess reciprocity and local buy-in in global partnerships to promote nursing (Leffers & Mitchell, 2011; Kulbok et al., 2012).

MAJOR GLOBAL HEALTH ORGANIZATIONS

Many international organizations have an ongoing interest in global health. Despite the presence of these well-meaning organizations, it is estimated that the less developed countries still bear most of the cost for their own health care and that contributions from major international organizations actually provide for less than five percent of needed costs. The UN Office for the Coordination of Humanitarian Affairs (OCHA) has priority areas at the population level (namely refugees and children) and also emphasizes food security and access to health care more broadly (UN OCHA, 2018). Shah (2012) reports that aid is often wasted by requiring recipients to use overpriced goods and services from donor countries; most aid does not go to the country in greatest need as aid is often used in order for the richer country to get its foot in the door of the poorer country to access its resources, and graft is still a major problem in developing countries—promised monies are funneled into the pockets of the local politicians who were chosen to help the people.

International health organizations are classified as **multilateral organizations**, bilateral organizations, or **nongovernmental organizations (NGOs)** or **private voluntary organizations (PVOs)** (including philanthropic organizations). Multilateral organizations are those that receive funding from multiple government and nongovernment sources. The major organizations are part of the UN, and they include the World Health Organization (WHO), UNICEF, the Pan American Health Organization (PAHO), and the World Bank. A **bilateral organization** is a single government agency that provides aid to less developed countries, such as the U.S. Agency for International Development (USAID). NGOs or PVOs, including the philanthropic organizations, are represented by such agencies as Oxfam, Project Hope, the International Red Cross, various professional and trade organizations, Catholic Relief Services (CRS), church-sponsored health care missionaries, and many other private groups.

Specifically, the **World Health Organization (WHO)** is a separate, autonomous organization that, by special agreement, works with the UN through its Economic and Social Council. The idea for this worldwide health organization developed from the First International Sanitary Conference in 1902, a precursor to the WHO. The WHO was created in 1946 as an outgrowth of the League of Nations and the UN charter that provided for the formation of a special health agency to address the wide scope and nature of the world's health problems. The WHO, headed by a director general and five assistant generals, has three major divisions: (1) the World Health Assembly approves the budget and makes decisions about health policies, (2) the executive board serves as the liaison between the assembly and the secretariat, and (3) the secretariat carries out the day-to-day activities of the WHO. The principal work of the WHO is to direct and coordinate international health activities and to provide technical medical assistance to countries in need. More than 1000 health-related projects are ongoing within the WHO at any one time. Requests for assistance may be made directly to the WHO by a country for a project, or the project may be part of a larger collaborative endeavor involving many countries. Examples of current collaborative, multinational projects include comprehensive family planning programs in Indonesia, Malaysia, and Thailand; applied research on communicable disease and immunization in several East African nations; and projects that investigate the viability of administering AIDS vaccines to pregnant women in South Africa and Namibia. For further information about the WHO, visit http://www.who and find the tab such as publications, countries, program, or health topics that meets your need. The WHO has supported the development of multiple health training programs for professionals in developing nations. An example of one is the Tanzania Nurse Initiative, which has been successful in strengthening nursing education in Tanzania by educating 415 nurses in HIV/AIDS prevention, care, and treatment; providing technical assistance and support on curriculum development and revision; and providing support to Tanzanian nursing schools (Global Health Workforce Alliance, 2014).

Another multilateral agency is the **United Nations Children's Fund (UNICEF)** (http://www.unicef.org). Formed shortly after World War II (WWII) to assist children in the war-ravaged countries of Europe, it is a subsidiary agency to the UN Economic and Social Council. After WWII many social agencies realized that the world's children needed medical and other kinds of support. With financial assistance from the newly formed UN General Assembly, post-WWII programs were developed to control yaws, leprosy, and TB in children. Since then, UNICEF has worked closely with the WHO as an advocate for the health needs of women and children under the age of 5. In particular there have been multinational programs aimed at the provision of safe drinking water, sanitation, education, and maternal and child health.

The **Pan American Health Organization (PAHO)** is one of the oldest continuously functioning multilateral agencies, founded in 1902, and predates the WHO. At present, PAHO serves as a regional field office for the WHO in Latin America, with a focused effort to improve the health and living standards of the Latin American countries. PAHO distributes epidemiologic information, provides technical assistance over a wide range of health and environmental issues, supports health care fellowships, and promotes health and environmentally related research, along with professional education. Focusing primarily on reaching people through their communities, PAHO works with a variety of governmental and nongovernmental entities to address the health issues of the people of the Americas. At present a primary concern of PAHO is the prevention and control of AIDS and other STIs among the most vulnerable: mothers and children, workers, the poor, older adults, refugees, and displaced persons. With the earthquakes in Haiti and Chile, and the drought and starvation in Guatemala, PAHO's attentions are being directed toward crisis intervention (http://www.paho.org). Other focused efforts include the provision of public information, the control and eradication of tropical diseases, and the development of health system infrastructure in the poorer Latin American countries. PAHO collaborates with individual countries and actively promotes multinational efforts as well. Recently PAHO has examined the effects of health care reform on nurses and midwifery in the Latin American countries and found that the reform changed the work environments, the scope of practice, and the relationship of nurses with other health care workers and providers. The role of PAHO in the development of healthy communities is discussed in Chapter 16.

The **World Bank** (http://www.worldbank.org) is another multilateral agency that is related to the UN. Although the major aim of the World Bank is to lend money to the less developed countries so that they might use it to improve the health status of their people, it has collaborated with the field offices of the WHO for various health-related projects such as the control and eradication of the tropical disease onchocerciasis in West Africa, as well as programs aimed at providing safe drinking water and affordable housing, developing sanitation systems, and encouraging family planning and childhood immunizations. The World Bank also sponsors programs to protect the environment, as reflected by the $30 million project in Brazil to protect the Amazon ecosystem and reduce the effects on the ozone layer; to support people in less developed countries to pursue careers in health care; and to improve internal infrastructure, including communication systems, roads, and electricity, all of which ultimately affect health care delivery.

Bilateral agencies operate within a single country and focus on providing direct aid to less developed countries. The USAID (http://www.usaid.gov) is the largest of these and supports long-term and equitable economic growth and advances U.S. foreign policy objectives by supporting economic growth, agriculture, and trade; global health; and democracy, conflict prevention, and humanitarian assistance. It provides assistance in five regions of the world: sub-Saharan Africa, Asia, Latin America and the Caribbean, Europe and Eurasia, and the Middle East. All bilateral organizations are influenced by political and historical agendas that determine which countries receive aid. Incentives for engaging in formal arrangements may include economic enhancements for the benefit of both countries, national defense of one or both countries, or the enhancement and protection of private investments made by individuals in these nations. Something similar is present in other developed nations around the globe. For example, the Japanese government currently has an active collaborative arrangement with Indonesia to study ways to control the spread of yellow fever and malaria. France gives most of its aid to its former colonies.

NGOs or PVOs, as well as philanthropic organizations, provide almost 20 percent of all external aid to less developed countries. NGOs and PVOs are represented by many different kinds of religious and secular groups. Representatives of these independent citizen organizations are increasingly active in policy making at the UN. These organizations are often the most effective voices for the concerns of ordinary people in the international arena. NGOs include the most outspoken advocates of human rights, the environment, social programs, women's rights, and more (Kaiser Family Foundation, 2010). An example of an NGO is Pigs for Peace (Pigs for Peace, 2016). This initiative focused on microcredit, sustainable development, and women's empowerment was developed based on collaborations from nurse scholars at Johns Hopkins University and communities in the eastern Democratic Republic of Congo (DRC). Started in 2007, it is now a Congolese-led microcredit women's empowerment initiative with a far-reaching impact: 1400 families across 25 villages have been impacted (as of December 2014).

The International Red Cross (http://www.icrc.org) is one of the best-known NGOs. Although the Red Cross is most often associated with disaster relief and emergency aid, it lays the groundwork for health intervention as a result of a country's emergency. It is a volunteer organization that consists of about 160 individual Red Cross societies around the world, and it prides itself on its neutrality and impartiality with respect to politics and history. Therefore it seeks permission from the country in which the disaster occurs before services are rendered.

Another NGO that provides health services and aid to countries experiencing warfare or disaster is *Médecins sans Frontières* (MSF) (Doctors Without Borders) (http://www.msf.org). It is an international, independent, medical humanitarian organization that delivers emergency aid to people affected by armed conflicts, epidemics, health care exclusion, and natural or man-made disasters. Unlike the Red Cross, MSF does not seek government approval to enter a country and provide aid, and it often speaks out against observed human rights abuses in the country it serves. MSF was the recipient of the Nobel Peace Prize in 1999 and the Conrad Hilton Prize in 1998.

The professional and trade organizations are PVOs that are found mostly in the more developed and industrialized countries. One of the most famous of the professional and technical organizations is the Institut Pasteur (https://www.pasteur.fr), which began in the 1880s. Its laboratories have facilitated the development of sera and vaccines for countries in need, disseminated current health information, and trained and provided fellowships for medical training and study in France. They have facilities in Africa, South and Central America, and Southeast Asia.

Religious organizations, reflecting several denominations and religious interests, support many health care programs, including hospitals in rural and urban areas, refugee centers, orphanages, and leprosy treatment centers. For example, the Maryknoll Missionaries, sponsored by the Roman Catholic Church, carry out health service projects around the world. The missionaries make up a large group of religious as well as lay people trained and educated in a variety of educational and health care professions. The Catholic Relief Services (CRS) (http://crs.org) is the official international humanitarian agency of the Catholic community in the United States. CRS alleviates suffering and provides assistance to people in need who are affected by war, starvation, famine, drought, and natural disasters, in more than 100 countries, without regard to race, religion, or nationality. Many Protestant and evangelical groups throughout the world function both as separate entities and as part of the Church World Service, which works jointly with secular organizations to improve health care, community development, and other needed projects. Other private and voluntary groups that assist with the worldwide health effort include CARE (http://www.care.org) and Oxfam (www.oxfam.org.uk).

Philanthropic organizations receive funding from private endowment funds. A few of the more active philanthropic organizations that are involved in world health care include the W. K. Kellogg Foundation, the Milbank Memorial Fund, the Pathfinder Fund, the Hewlett Foundation, the Ford Foundation, the Rockefeller Foundation, the Carnegie Foundation, and the Gates Foundation. The purpose and programmatic goals of each organization differ widely with respect to funding, and their purposes often change as their governing boards change. Some of the worldwide health care activities that have been sponsored in the past include projects in public and preventive health; vital statistics; medical, nursing, and dental education; family planning programs; economic planning and development; and the formation of laboratories to investigate communicable diseases.

Many private and commercial organizations such as Nestlé and the Johnson & Johnson Company provide financial and technical backing for investment, employment, and access to market economies and to health care. Although these organizations have been present throughout the world for more than 30 years, they have come under criticism for the promotion and marketing of infant formulas, pharmaceuticals, and medical supplies, especially to less developed countries. The intense marketing that is done in these countries is known as *commodification,* turning health care into a business with clients as consumers and health care professionals from altruistic healers to business technicians. Breast cancer awareness is the best known of these practices in the United States (http://www.theguardian.com).

There is global controversy as to the legitimacy of commodification. For example, in the sentinel article by Segal et al. (2003) the **health commodification** of pharmaceuticals in southern India was a concern because the companies gave little consideration to the cultural and social structure of the country, thus interfering with the long-standing traditional Indian medical system. In southern India, good health and prosperity are related to certain social parameters bestowed to families and communities as a result of their conformity to the socio-moral order that was established by their ancestors, gods, and patron spirits. The taking of pharmaceutical agents thus disrupts the social and cultural order of things that have been traditionally addressed by cultural practices.

Information about volunteering for many NGOs and PVOs can be obtained from the Internet websites included in the text. Nurses have developed global initiatives, participate in global health projects, and lead global health organizations such as Doctors Without Borders. Becoming a global citizen is the responsibility of all.

GLOBAL HEALTH AND GLOBAL DEVELOPMENT

Global health is not just a global public health agenda; it does not begin and end with the individual; it must consider all factors within a country that affect health, such as environment, education, national and local policies, health care and access to health care, economics (importing and exporting of goods, industry, technology), war, and public safety. This paradigm shift is called **global health diplomacy**, which refers to multilevel and multifactor negotiation processes involving environment, health, emerging diseases, and human safety. It is now recognized that to solve global health problems, one must build capacity for global health diplomacy by training public health professionals and diplomats, respectively, to prevent the imbalances that emerge between foreign policy and public health experts and the imbalances that exist in negotiating power and capacity between developed and developing nations (Hunter et al., 2013). The cutting edge of global health diplomacy raises certain cautions regarding health's role in trade and foreign policies. Unfortunately, securing health's fullest participation in foreign policy does not ensure health for all, but it supports the principle that foreign policy achievements by any country in promoting and protecting health will be of value to all (Hunter et al., 2013). Nurses cannot think in isolation about health for the global population; they must think more broadly to achieve their goals through a multidisciplinary, multilevel approach involving such dimensions as economic, industrial, and technological development.

Access to services and the removal of financial barriers alone do not account for the public's use of health services. In fact, the introduction of health care technology from developed countries to less developed countries has led to less-than-satisfactory results. The World Bank reported that during the 1980s in an eastern Mediterranean country, two thirds of the high-output X-ray machines were not in use because of a lack of qualified and trained individuals to carry out routine maintenance and repairs.

Countries devastated by war have lost their total infrastructure for food, trade, social justice, health, water, and public security as evident today in Afghanistan, the West Bank, Gaza, Darfur, Syria, and other war-torn countries. When implementing services for less developed nations, it is essential to conduct needs assessments to learn what a community has, what a community wants, and what it can sustain. Quite simply, well-intended projects can fail because first, the project served the purpose of the donors and not the needs of the people, and second, because no assessment was done to ascertain what resources the country had and what services the country could sustain.

One example is in the form of material donations. These donations often are sent to a country with the best of intentions, but there may be a gap between recipient-country identified material needs and donation-country inventory intended for donation (Compton et al., 2018). Without collaboration, well-intended material donations could end in detritus; broken parts without a plan for specialized part replacement; nonfunctional machinery without an endowment or training for specialized mechanics; and lack of a disposal plan for material/medical waste subsequent to using the material donation (Fig. 4.3). Critical examination of this phenomenon in times of crisis is even more necessary. Recipient countries may need support and plans for disposing of unnecessary or used material donations, particularly in times of added stress to health care systems. The Global Humanitarian Assistance Report (Development Initiatives, 2018) notes that in 2016 the country that received the most international humanitarian aid was Syria.

When projects are developed that pay attention to the intent of global health diplomacy, then there is improvement in the overall health status of a population, which secondarily can contribute to the economic growth of a country in several ways (WHO, 2013a):

- Reduction in production loss caused by workers who are absent from work because of illness
- Increase in the use of natural resources that, because of the presence of disease entities, might have been inaccessible
- Increase in the number of children who can attend school and eventually participate in their country's economic growth

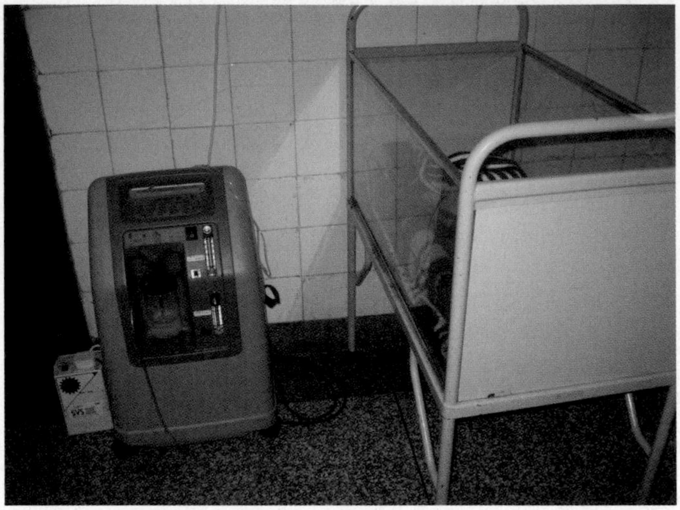

Fig. 4.3 A neonatal critical care unit in Uganda. Material donations require thoughtful plans for implementation, servicing, and disposal. (Courtesy A. Hunter.)

- Increase in monetary resources, formerly spent on treating disease and illness, now available for the economic development of the country

Because the economics of international development are complex, it is often difficult to convince governments to direct their resources away from perceived needs such as military and technology and instead place resources in health and educational programs. Ideally, the role of the more developed countries is to assist less developed countries to identify internal needs and to support cost-efficient measures and share their technology and industrial expertise. It is important that nurses who work in international communities acknowledge the importance of global health diplomacy and its various parameters: culture, politics, economics, technology, public health, social justice, foreign policy, and public safety. Provision of health services alone will not ease a country's health care plight (Fig. 4.4).

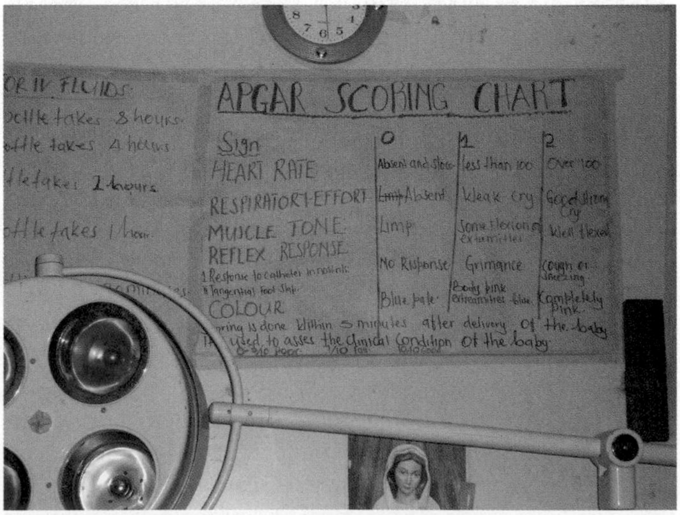
APGAR SCORING CHART
Sign
0
1
2
HEART RATE
Absent and Slow
less than 100
Over 100
RESPIRATORY EFFORT
Absent
Weak cry
MUSCLE TONE
Limp
REFLEX RESPONSE
No Response
Grimance
COLOUR
Blue pale
Completely Pink
used to asses the clinical condition of the baby

Fig. 4.4 An informational sign at a maternal/child ward in Uganda. Capacity building in nursing workforces begins with collaboration. (Courtesy A. Hunter.)

HEALTH CARE SYSTEMS

The countries of the world present many different kinds of health care systems and models for comparison. Most consist of the population to be served, health care providers, third-party payers, health care facilities, and those who control access and usability of the system (Shakarishvili et al., 2010). Understanding some of these principles is highlighted when one compares the health care systems in the Netherlands, Mexico, Uganda, Ecuador, the United Kingdom, and China. For more information on the lists of countries and the per capita expenditures on health care, please see the report at http://dpeaflcio.org and the 2017 Commonwealth Report, which can be found at https://www.commonwealthfund.org.

The Netherlands

In the Netherlands, under a health policy reform movement in 2006, residents are required to purchase health insurance, which is provided by private health insurers (for-profit or nonprofit) that compete for business. Everyone must be insured, and the insurers are required to accept every resident in their coverage area, regardless of pre-existing conditions. In 2014 less than 0.2 percent of the total population (about 30,000 people) were uninsured. Undocumented immigrants must pay for most health care services themselves. The government provides larger subsidies to insurers for participants who are sicker, are elderly, or have pre-existing conditions. Tax credits are given to low-income clients to help them purchase insurance. People under age 18 are insured at no cost. There is a separate universal national social insurance program for long-term care, known as the AWBZ, or Exceptional Medical Expenses Act. Insurers offer a choice of policies at a range of costs. In some of the plans the insurer negotiates and contracts with the health provider, whereas more costly plans allow clients to choose their health provider and be reimbursed by the insurer. The insured also pay a flat-rate premium to their insurer for a policy. Everyone with the same policy pays the same premium, and lower-income residents receive a health care allowance from the government to help make payments (Daley & Gubb, 2013, Commonwealth Fund Report, 2017).

Mexico

Mexico has a fractionalized system with a variety of public programs. There is no universal coverage, but a social security–administered system does cover those who are employed. The private insurance market is used mostly by wealthy residents. The Seguro Popular program, created in 2003, has been set up to help cover more of the uninsured population. Poor families can participate in Seguro Popular for free, and people who do not participate in the insurance program can still access services through the Ministry of Health, although sometimes with some difficulty. The different public setups and private insurers all use different systems of medical facilities and providers, with a wide range of quality reported in those services. The social security system provides broad coverage for medical services, including primary care, acute care, ambulatory and hospital care, pregnancy and childbirth, as well as prescription medications. The Seguro Popular system provides access to an established set of essential medical services and the needed drugs for those conditions, as well as 17 high-cost interventions such as breast cancer treatment. The services are provided through government, usually state-run, facilities. Out-of-pocket payments by clients represent over half of financing for the Mexican health care system, whereas the public schemes are financed through general taxes and payment from the employer and employee, determined by salary. The Seguro Popular is also funded by taxes, contributions from the state and federal government, and payments by the families, as a percent of income. Participants in Seguro Popular pay nothing at the time of delivery of the service (Puig et al., 2009).

Uganda

Uganda's health care system is a national service, meaning that health care is supposed to be free and accessible to all. There are five clinic and hospital facilities that patients can access (if they are staffed, if the staff workers are not extorting money from the people, and if they have supplies). These clinics and hospitals work on a referral basis; if a level I or II facility cannot handle a case, it refers it to a unit the next level up. Often units do not have the essential drugs, meaning the patients have to buy them from pharmacies or other drug sellers. Level I clinics do health counseling; level II can take care of common diseases such as malaria and antenatal care; level III clinics are where outpatients are seen and treated, a maternity ward exists, and minimal (screening) laboratory services are provided; level IV is a mini-hospital with the kind of services found at level III clinics, but with wards for men, women, and children who can be admitted for short stays; and level V is a tertiary hospital for patients who are trauma victims, have major health problems, or are in need of mental health, dentistry, and surgery services. Although this sounds like an excellent system, my years of experience in Uganda can attest to both its strengths and weaknesses, with the greatest weakness being the lack of health professionals and the lack of supplies—too many children die because they have no oxygen, no intravenous (IV) fluids, and no antibiotics. Other aspects of the health system in Uganda are the faith-based hospitals; private medical practices/clinics set up by individual physicians or nurses as an income generator for themselves; and the traditional healers who practice herbal therapy, magic, bloodletting, and other nontherapeutic activities that often cause more harm than good (Kamwesiga, 2011; Kelly, 2009).

Ecuador

The health system in Ecuador has both a public sector and a private sector, with the public sector providing health care services to the whole working and uninsured populations. Private insurance is for the middle- and high-income group, which includes about three percent of the population. In addition, there are about 10,000 private physicians' offices, generally equipped with basic infrastructure and technology, located in major cities, and the population tends to make direct payments out of pocket at the time they receive care. There are special government programs to provide nutrition for the poor and maternity services to ensure healthy pregnancies and deliveries (Lucio et al., 2011). Recent reports by expatriate visitors to Ecuador indicate that the greatest perk for foreign residents is the high-quality, low-cost health care. There is personal attention from medical practitioners not seen in the United States since the 1960s, and in the bigger cities, one will find hospitals with state-of-the-art equipment, as well as specialists in all fields and physicians with private clinics.

The United Kingdom

It is also useful to examine the United Kingdom, with a tax-supported health system that is owned and operated by the government (the National Health Service, or NHS). Services are available to all citizens without cost or for a small fee. Administration of health services is conducted through a system of health authorities (Trusts). Each Trust plans and provides services for 250,000 to 1 million people. The services offered by each Trust are comprehensive, in that health care is available to all who want it and covers all aspects of general medicine, disability and rehabilitation, and surgery. Although physicians are the primary providers in this system, nurses and allied health professionals are also recognized and used. Services are made available through hospitals, private physicians and allied health professional clinics, health outreach programs such as hospice, and environmental health services. Physicians are paid by the number of clients they serve and not by individual visits (Boyle, 2011).

Although the British system has come under criticism in past years, individual citizens still maintain a high level of support for government funding and control of their health services. Clients, especially the elderly and new mothers, receive assistance from the district nurses (public health nurses). One of the hallmarks of the British system is a reduction in infant mortality, from 14.3 deaths per 1000 births in 1975 to 5.4 in 2002. Overall life expectancy in Great Britain also improved during the same period (77.2 years in 2000). This has been done while holding down gross spending on health care. A 2009 report by Sutherland found that the United Kingdom has seen a significant fall in mortality rates from the major killers: cancer, coronary heart disease, and stroke. Client ratings of quality care are high all across the United Kingdom; however, there is concern about rising health expenditure over the past 10 years (Sutherland, 2009). The system provides universal care to all residents and to nonresidents with a European Health Insurance Card. Emergency services and treatment for certain infectious diseases are also free to undocumented nonresidents, though all other care they pay for. The NHS publishes an annual report on health disparities based on gender, disability, age, socioeconomic status, and ethnicity, as well as strategies implemented nationally to mitigate disparities in health outcomes (Commonwealth Fund Report, 2017).

China

China has made tremendous strides since 1949 in providing access to health care for its citizens. At present, China is a large developing country with many human resources (Yun et al., 2010). Nursing makes up a large segment of the health care workforce, yet there are too few nurses to meet the needs of the population. China, like the United States, is engaged in health care reform. China also has more physicians than nurses, which is different than in most other areas of the world. Nurse density in China is higher in urban than in rural areas, and this poses a problem in a large country in which much of the territory is rural in nature. Like many other countries, China has made public health advances by controlling contagious diseases such as cholera, typhoid, and scarlet fever and by reducing infant mortality (Yun et al., 2010). These accomplishments in public health were credited to a political system that was and is largely socialistic and features a health care system that is described in socialistic terms as collective. The Chinese collective system emphasized the common good for all people, not individuals or special groups. This system was financed through cooperative insurance plans. In 2014, 5.6 percent of the GDP in China was allocated for health care expenditures. The collective health care system was owned and controlled by the state and used "barefoot" doctors. Barefoot doctors were medical practitioners trained at the community level and could provide a minimal level of health care throughout the country. Barefoot doctors combined Western medicine with traditional techniques such as acupuncture and herbal remedies. The government focused on improving the quality of water supplies and disease prevention and implemented massive public health campaigns against sanitation problems, such as flies, mosquitoes, and the snails that spread schistosomiasis. Box 4.2 describes a Healthy Cities initiative that took place in Chengdu, China.

Today, health care in China is managed by the Ministry of Public Health, which sets national health policy. The current Chinese government continues to make health care a priority and has set goals to provide medical care to all of its citizens. The Chinese government published its health care reform plan in 2009. In developing this plan the government took into account recommendations from the WHO and the World Bank. Among the aims of the plan are to develop a system of health insurance to help people pay for catastrophic illness, to increase and improve education for nurses in order to intervene in the growing nursing shortage, and to develop urban health centers. At present a small percent of Chinese nurses work in public health, and some authors attribute this to the low pay in these settings. Hospitals and clinics are typically located in urban areas; therefore people in rural areas must travel a great distance for care, and even then, the care may be substandard and the wait time to receive care may be long. It is estimated that about 200 million people in China lack health insurance. When the State Council published its health care reform plan in April of 2009, a three-year goal of "covering 90 percent of the Chinese population by 2011 and achieving universal health care by 2020" was established. Health insurance coverage is now close to universal and has been since around 2011 (Commonwealth Fund Report, 2017).

The nursing education system in China has developed rapidly. All college-based nursing education was terminated during the period of the Cultural Revolution and began again only in the mid-1980s. At present the nursing education system includes associate degree, baccalaureate, master's degree, and doctoral programs. Interestingly, the image of nursing has improved, based on the effectiveness of nurses during recent public health crises and events that claimed international attention. Specifically, nurses played important and effective roles in caring for people during the disasters caused by the SARS virus in 2003 and the Sichuan earthquake in 2008. More recently, nurses were well recognized in China for their considerable work during the 2008 Olympic Games in Beijing (Yun et al., 2010). Unfortunately, pay and working conditions are contributing to the desire of many Chinese nurses to leave the country (Commonwealth Fund Report, 2017).

MAJOR GLOBAL HEALTH PROBLEMS AND THE BURDEN OF DISEASE

Despite the gains that have been made in improving the health of so many around the globe, the increasing population, decreasing food and water sources, and increasing poverty related to a global economic crisis are all contributing to a critical demise in health. The amount of debt incurred by less developed countries has increased steadily over the last 20 years, and money that was once used for health care has been used to pay off growing debt. Communicable diseases that are often preventable are still common throughout the world and are more common in less developed countries. Also, both developed and less developed countries are seeking ways to cope with the aging of their populations—a population that presents governments with the burden of providing care for those who become ill with more expensive noncommunicable and chronic forms of diseases and disabilities. Illnesses such as AIDS continue to raise concerns, especially in child-bearing women, adolescents, and young adults. Long-standing diseases such as TB, dysentery, and mosquito-borne diseases, especially malaria, still persist and have become drug resistant, adding to the growing burden of overextended health care delivery systems.

Mortality statistics do not adequately describe the outlook of health in the world. The WHO (2018f) has developed an indicator called the **global burden of disease** (GBD). The GBD combines losses from premature death and losses of healthy life that result from disability. Premature death is defined as the difference between the actual age at death and life expectancy at that age in a low-mortality population. People who have debilitating injuries or diseases must be cared for in some way, most often by family members, and thus they no longer can contribute to the family's or a community's economic growth. The GBD represents units of **disability-adjusted life-years (DALYs)** (WHO, 2018g) (Box 4.4). Table 4.1 reflects the top 20 conditions with the greatest impact on DALYs from 2000 to 2016 (WHO, 2018g). An interesting shift of note is that for the 2000 top 20 leading causes of DALYs globally, 35 percent were from communicable diseases, while 65 percent were from noncommunicable diseases. In 2016 there is a notable shift, with 20 percent from communicable diseases and 80 percent from noncommunicable diseases. Table 4.1 indicates that from 2000 to 2016, 56.1 percent of the DALYs were the result of the top 20 conditions. Psychiatric disorders, although traditionally not regarded as a major epidemiologic problem, are shown by consideration of DALYs to have a huge impact on population, ranking in the top 20 on the GBD index. The table indicates that 2.6 billion DALYs were lost worldwide. In 2000 there about 312,000 neonatal deaths, while in 2016 there were about 219,000. Similarly, in 2000 there was a higher maternal mortality rate globally (28,109) than in 2016 (19,217). While these reductions in maternal/child mortality can be attributed to several global factors, this demonstrates the importance of having accessible and affordable disease prevention programs for mothers and children around the world (WHO, 2018g). Infections and parasitic diseases remain a threat to the health of the majority of the world and are diseases seen in the United States. Studies demonstrate the continuing need for intervention for infectious and other kinds of communicable diseases. Conditions that contribute to one fourth of the GBD throughout the world include diarrheal disease, respiratory tract infections, worm infestations, malaria, and childhood diseases such as measles and polio. The WHO African Region in 2016 demonstrated a GBD of 61 percent DALYs lost due to communicable, maternal, perinatal, and nutritional causes of death versus the 29 percent average global DALYs lost for the same causes

BOX 4.4 Calculating Disability-Adjusted Life-Years

DALYs are composed of years lost to disability (YLDs) and years of life lost due to premature mortality (YLLs). YLDs, the morbidity component of the DALYs, are calculated as follows: YLD = ¼ Number of cases × duration till remission or death × disability weight.

Within the DALY calculation are the social weighting factors:

1. *Duration of time lost because of a death at each age:* Measurement is based on the potential limit for life, which has been set at 82.5 years for women and 80 years for men.
2. *Disability weights:* The degree of incapacity associated with various health conditions. Values range from 0 (perfect health) to 1 (death). Four prescribed points between 0 and 1 represent a set of accepted disability classes.
3. *Age-weighting function,* $Cxe^{-\beta x}$, where $C = 0.16243$ (a constant), $\beta = 0.04$ (a constant), $e = 2.71$ (a constant), and $x =$ age; this function indicates the relative importance of a healthy life at different ages.
4. *Discounting function,* $e^{-r(x-a)}$, where $r = 0.03$ (the discount rate), $e = 2.71$ (a constant), $a =$ age at onset of disease, and $x =$ age; this function indicates the value of health gains today compared with the value of health gains in the future.
5. *Health is added across individuals:* 2 people each losing 10 DALYs are treated as showing the same loss as 1 person losing 20 years.

"In summary, one DALY can be thought of as one lost year of 'healthy' life. The sum of these DALYs across the population, or the burden of disease, can be thought of as a measurement of the gap between current health status and an ideal health situation where the entire population lives to an advanced age, free of disease and disability. DALYs for a disease or health condition are calculated as the sum of the Years of Life Lost (YLL) due to premature mortality in the population and the Years Lost due to Disability (YLD) for people living with the health condition or its consequences" (see http://www.who.int).

DALY, Disability-adjusted life-year.

TABLE 4.1 Top 20 DALY Conditions 2000-2016

Rank	Cause	DALYs (000s)	% DALYs	DALYs per 100,000 Population
	All Causes	2,668,476	100.0	35,761
1	Ischaemic Heart Disease	203,700	7.6	2,730
2	Stroke	137,941	5.2	1,849
3	Lower Respiratory Infections	129,690	4.9	1,738
4	Preterm Birth Complications	101,397	3.8	1,359
5	Road Injury	82,538	3.1	1,106
6	Diarrhoeal Disease	81,743	3.1	1,095
7	Chronic Obstructive Pulmonary Disease	72,512	2.7	972
8	Diabetes Mellitus	65,666	2.5	880
9	Birth Asphyxia and Birth Trauma	63,928	2.4	857
10	Congenital Abnormalities	62,980	2.4	844
11	HIV/AIDS	59,951	2.2	803
12	Tuberculosis	51.643	1.9	692
13	Back and Neck Pain	47,515	1.8	637
14	Other Hearing Loss	47,352	1.8	635
15	Cirrhosis of the Liver	45,287	1.7	607
16	Depressive Disorders	44,175	1.7	592
17	Trachea, Bronchus, Lung Cancers	41,121	1.5	551
18	Kidney Diseases	39,079	1.5	524
19	Neonatal Sepsis and Infections	39,009	1.5	523
20	Falls	38,162	1.4	511

DALY, Disability-adjusted life-years.
Global health estimates 2016*: Disease burden by cause, age, sex, by country and by region, 2000-2016,* Geneva, 2018, World Health Organization.

(WHO, 2018g). Geographic analysis of DALYs provides important comparative data and highlights some of the needs and areas for nursing interventions globally.

According to the Global HIV/AIDS Epidemic fact sheet published by the Kaiser Family Foundation (2019a), globally about 36.9 million people are living with HIV and about 77 million people have been infected since the beginning of the epidemic, the result of continuing new infections, people living longer with HIV, and general population growth. HIV is a leading cause of death worldwide and the number one cause of death in Africa. An estimated 8 in 10 people infected with HIV do not know it. HIV has led to a resurgence of TB, particularly in Africa, and TB is a leading cause of death for people with HIV worldwide. Women represent half of all people living with HIV worldwide and more than half (60 percent) in sub-Saharan Africa. Globally, there are 1.8 million children living with HIV in 2019. Young people between 15 and 24 years make up a third of new HIV infection. Uganda's emphasis on ameliorating HIV/AIDS is a model for all African nations; however, there are still too many Ugandan children under 5 years old who are AIDS orphans. Unfortunately, despite the efforts of advocates, donors, and affected countries, there needs to be greater attention given to the long overdue effort to expand access to antiretroviral therapy (ART), which is still available to less than 10 percent of those who urgently require it (KFF, 2019a). See a later section of the chapter for a more detailed discussion of the global burden of HIV/AIDS.

Determining the total amount of loss, even using the GBD, is difficult because it does not address the many consequences of disease and injury such as post-trauma and infectious physical disabilities. Nor can it measure the short- or long-term effects of familial and marital dysfunction, family violence, or war. The following further elaborates on selected communicable diseases that still contribute substantially to the worldwide disease burden (TB, AIDS, and malaria) and other health problems such as maternal and women's health, diarrheal disease in children, nutrition, and natural and man-made disasters.

Communicable Diseases

Prevention of communicable diseases is through immunization and improving environmental conditions. One example of the long-term benefits of immunizing children against communicable diseases is the successful campaign against smallpox that the WHO conducted during the 1960s and 1970s. Smallpox has been virtually eliminated throughout the world, with only occasional and incidental reporting from laboratory accidents and inoculation complications. The systematic and planned smallpox program formed the basis for a series of worldwide efforts that are now being implemented to control and eradicate other infectious and communicable diseases.

In 1974 the WHO formed the Expanded Program on Immunization, which sought to reduce morbidity and mortality from diphtheria, pertussis, tetanus, TB, measles, and poliomyelitis throughout the world (WHO, 2010b). In the 2010 State of the World Report on immunizations and vaccines, the WHO noted that for the first time in documented history the number of children dying every year had fallen below 10 million. This appears to be the result of improved access to clean water and sanitation, increased immunization coverage, and the integrated delivery of essential health interventions. Unfortunately, almost 20 percent of the children born each year do not get the complete routine immunizations scheduled for their first year of life. This is most prevalent in developing countries and for those children born in very rural communities. In developing countries, more vaccines are available and more lives are being saved; however, death from pertussis in developing countries is 40 per 1000 infants, and 10 per 1000 in older children. It still occurs in industrialized countries but at less than 1 per 1000 cases. Although free vaccination clinics are brought to the people, they are often not used because of lack of knowledge, fear propagated by the traditional healers, and suspicion of anything offered by the government. Reaching these vulnerable children—typically in poorly served remote rural areas, deprived urban settings, fragile states, and strife-torn regions—is essential in order to meet the MDGs (United Nations, 2013b).

The WHO estimated that if all the vaccines now available against childhood diseases were widely adopted, and if countries could raise vaccine coverage to a global average of 90 percent, by 2015 an additional 2 million deaths a year could be prevented among children under age 5. This level of vaccination would have reduced child deaths by two thirds and achieved one of the MDG goals. In 2015, when the SDGs were adopted, SDG goal 3 target 3.2 was to end preventable deaths of newborns (target: reduce mortality to at least as low as 12 per 1000 live births in every country) and under-five children (target: reduce mortality to at least as low as 25 per 1000 live births in every country) by 2030. This would also greatly reduce the burden of illness and disability from vaccine-preventable diseases and contribute to improving child health and welfare, as well as reducing hospitalization costs. Of note as well, human papillomavirus (HPV) is the most common infectious disease globally, and as of 2017 80 countries had implemented national vaccination programs against high-risk strains of HPV (WHO, 2018f).

As discussed in Chapter 6, **environmental sanitation** is critical to the well-being of people around the globe. Many of the major health risks relate to interactions between people and their environment. For example, in developing nations, community drinking water sources can be contaminated by agricultural runoffs containing toxic pesticides and fertilizers, but they can also be contaminated by naturally occurring elements in the earth such as arsenic and fluoride.

In developing nations, hospitals and HIV testing centers may dump waste products into the local rivers that supply household water. Worldwide, environmental factors play a role in more than 80 percent of adverse outcomes reported by the WHO, including infectious diseases, injuries, mental retardation, and cancer, to name a few. Globalization and industrialization in the developing world have increased daily exposure to pollution and a wide array of chemicals in air, water, and food. At the same time, fecal pollution of drinking water sources caused by a lack of basic sanitation still exists. The effects of environmental risk factors are magnified by conditions often prevalent in poorer, less developed countries such as poor nutrition, poverty, lack of education about risks, and conflicts. Children are particularly susceptible to environmental risks because their systems are still developing. It is estimated that about one quarter of global disease is caused by avoidable environmental exposures; for young children in the developing world, causes of environmentally related deaths are acute respiratory infections, related to poor air quality; and diarrhea, related to poor drinking water quality. Annually, about 3 million children under the age of five die of environment-related diseases. There are projects that train and give technical assistance, data collection and analysis, laboratory analyses, research, surveillance, and emergency responses to international communities (American Society of Hematology, 2013; WHO, 2018d).

In 2016, the Centers for Disease Control and Prevention estimated that 780 million people did not have access to clean water, and their water sources are often far away, unclean, and unaffordable; 2.5 billion people or 35 percent of the world's population lack an adequate toilet or latrine (Centers for Disease Control and Prevention, 2016). Getting hold of clean water is not good enough if the water is being made dirty because there are no toilets, and toilets are not good enough if there is no hygiene promotion to persuade whole communities to change the habits of generations and use the latrines. UNICEF estimates that 2.4 billion people do not use improved sanitation and 663 million do not have access to improved water sources (UNICEF, 2010).

Tuberculosis. In 2017, according to the WHO (2017), TB was one of the top 10 leading global causes of death, with about 10.4 million people ill from TB, 1.7 million deaths from TB, and about one third of the world's population infected with TB. Ninety-five percent of TB deaths occur in low- to middle-income countries, and TB is the leading killer of HIV-positive people. Children are not immune to this bacterium, as the WHO report indicates that in 2016 more than one million children became ill with the disease, and 250,000 children died of TB. People with HIV are much more likely to develop TB, as are those infected with malaria, especially children, because of the physiological damage to the liver, spleen, and hematological systems. A child or adult with any one of the three diseases mentioned is more prone to the other two, and this triad is the new scourge of impoverished nations. The WHO estimates that more than one third of infectious disease deaths are due to this deadly triad of AIDS, TB, and malaria (WHO, 2017).

It is expected that at least one third of the world's population harbor the TB pathogen *Mycobacterium tuberculosis*. The Stop TB Partnership, engaging nearly 300 governments and agencies, has brought consensus on approaches to global control of this disease, galvanized support, and launched new support mechanisms, such as the Global TB Drug Facility, an initiative to increase access to high-quality TB drugs. The Working Group on Tuberculosis recommended seven priorities to meet the MDG targets for this disease for 2015. It has been shown that the number of people falling ill with TB each year is declining, although very slowly (TB mortality rate dropped 45 percent between 1990 and 2010, for example). The world will continue to measure progress of ending the TB epidemic by 2030 through the SDGs.

Two factors are a threat to TB control and eradication. The first is the AIDS virus. The appearance of HIV has added to the difficulty of treatment programs in both developed and less developed countries. More important, HIV-positive individuals with infectious TB have an increased likelihood of transmitting TB to their families and to the community, further increasing the prevalence of this condition.

The second is the growing multidrug resistance of the TB bacillus to isoniazid and rifampin, the two drugs used to treat it. Resistance to these drugs is already evident around the world, though the multidrug-resistant TB (MDR-TB) burden is experienced mostly in India, China, and the Russian Federation. The WHO and other organizations maintain that a high priority should be given to TB control and eradication programs around the world. In 2016 the WHO approved a rapid diagnostic test to identify patients with TB more quickly. For tertiary prevention the WHO advocates a short-term chemotherapy regimen for smear-positive clients as being one of the most cost-effective health interventions available (Forman et al., 2012; WHO, 2017).

The bacille Calmette-Guérin (BCG) vaccine, which has been available since the 1920s, was promoted as an effective vaccine to induce active immunity against TB, especially among children living in TB-endemic or high-risk TB areas that are impoverished and crowded. The BCG vaccine has a documented protective effect against meningitis and disseminated TB in children. It does not prevent primary infection and, more importantly, does not prevent reactivation of latent pulmonary infection, the principal source of bacillary spread in the community. The impact of BCG vaccination on transmission of TB is therefore limited (WHO, 2017). The standard chemotherapeutic agents used in many countries for TB are isoniazid, thioacetazone, and streptomycin, and they are effective at converting sputum-positive cases to noninfectivity. The drugs and the combinations that are used vary from country to country. To be effective, however, treatment must be carried out on a consistent basis, and many less developed countries have difficulty persuading clients to purchase the medications and to adhere to any treatment regimen. In 1990 the WHO Global Tuberculosis Program (GTB) promoted the revision of national TB programs to focus on short-course chemotherapy (SCC), with directly observed treatment (DOT). DOT programs have been successful in the United States and in several less developed countries, including Malawi, Mozambique, Nicaragua, and Tanzania, producing a cure rate of about 80 percent. The SCC program involves aggressive administration of chemotherapeutic drugs combined with short-term hospitalization. The key to the program lies in a well-managed system with a regular supply of anti-TB drugs to the treatment centers, follow-up care, and rigorous reporting and analysis of client information . More recently, as of June 2017, 35 countries in the WHO African Region and Asian Region had started using shorter MDR-TB regimens for treatment and control of the disease, and 89 countries had introduced bedaquiline for treatment. Fifty-four additional countries had introduced delamanid, both in order to promote efficacy of MDR-TB regiments (WHO, 2017).

Lasting control of AIDS, TB, and/or malaria will depend on strengthening the health, economic, political, educational, and other infrastructure necessary to sustain life and promote the well-being of the people. It will require sustained investment in physical infrastructure, drug distribution systems, management at all levels, and, most importantly, human resources such as the training and appropriate use of community health workers to deliver some essential services and education. Unfortunately, the failure of developed countries to fulfill their pledges of more development aid and the failure of developing countries themselves to invest in health are overarching barriers to health systems development. HIV/AIDS, TB, and malaria are only three of the challenges facing poor people. Only stronger, integrated health systems can provide a platform to sustain a successful fight against these diseases while advancing the other health priorities of developing countries, including child and maternal health and chronic disease.

It is important, when conducting a health assessment interview, always to ask whether the client has recently traveled out of the United States or to one of the border areas along the United States–Mexico perimeter. People who travel abroad may bring back diseases that are difficult to diagnose. In addition, people often cross the border into Mexico to fill a prescription for medicine because it is often less expensive than in the United States. Medications brought back to the United States may have been relabeled or are out of date.

Human Immunodeficiency Virus/Acquired Immunodeficiency Syndrome. As discussed in Chapter 15, AIDS remains a major cause of morbidity and mortality throughout the world. More than 70 million people have been infected with HIV since the beginning of the epidemic; about 35 million people have died of AIDS. At the end of 2017, 36.9 million people globally were living with HIV, with 59 percent of adults and 52 percent of children living with HIV receiving lifelong ART. The burden of the epidemic continues to vary considerably between countries and regions; however, the WHO African Region remains most severely affected, with 25.7 million people living with HIV, and accounts for over two thirds of global total new HIV infections (WHO, 2018b). For more information, go to http://www.who.int.

The Kaiser Family Foundation report (KFF, 2019) stated that about 36.9 million people were living with HIV and tens of millions of people have died of AIDS-related causes since the epidemic began. Many of the people living with HIV or at risk for HIV do not access to prevention, treatment and care. Currently, there is no cure so the most important issue to is prevent, treat and follow up. Although HIV testing has improved over time, about one in four people who have HIV are unaware of this. While deaths have declines due to antiretroviral treatment (ART), 940,00 people died of AIDS in 2017 (KFF, 2019).

Sub-Saharan Africa is the hardest hit area of the world in terms of HIV followed by Asia and the Pacific area. Also, the Caribbean, Eastern Europe, and Central Asia are heavily affected. For details on this epidemic from a global perspective see "The Global HIV/AIDS Epidemic," January 2019, KFF. See Chapter 15 for details on HIV/AIDS.

Worldwide prevention programs are important because failing to control this virulent disease will result in damaging and costly consequences for all countries in the future. Ideally, the goal is primary prevention of HIV. When prevention efforts fail at this level, the next goal is secondary prevention, or early diagnosis and treatment. Aggressive interventions in many African nations have begun to make a difference in the life potential for patients diagnosed with HIV. See the Levels of Prevention box to learn about prevention of HIV.

LEVELS OF PREVENTION

Global Health Care

Primary Prevention

Teach people how to avoid or change risky behaviors that might lead to contracting human immunodeficiency virus (HIV).

Secondary Prevention

Initiate screening programs for HIV.

Tertiary Prevention

Manage symptoms of HIV, provide psychosocial support, and teach clients and significant others about care and other forms of symptom management.

Malaria. Malaria affects more than 50 percent of the world's population and hits tropical Africa the hardest. However, there have been major global efforts to control and eliminate malaria. In 2016 an estimated U.S. $2.7 million was spent on malaria control and elimination. While Malaria is not a health issue in the United States, a major portion of funding comes from the United States. The areas of the world most affected by malaria are the WHO African region (74 percent), followed by WHO South-East Asia (7 percent), and then Eastern Mediterranean Europe and the Americas (6 percent each), and the Western Pacific (4 percent) (WHO, 2017, p xiii).

Malaria is caused by the *Anopheles* mosquito and is the only mosquito-borne disease that can be prevented and cured by pharmacological means. It is caused by parasitic transmission from the infected female mosquito to its host. There are four parasite species that cause malaria, the most serious being *Plasmodium falciparum,* which causes microvascular sequestration and obstruction in the brain, kidney, and liver, leading to cerebral malaria, anemia, kidney failure, hypoglycemia, disseminated intravascular coagulation (DIC), fluid-electrolyte imbalance, and death (CDC, 2013a). Symptoms vary and range from mild to severe physiological responses (mild fever and chills to temperatures of 106° F with prolonged chills, seizures, and dehydration).

A range of effective antimalarial interventions exists for the prevention, treatment, and control of malaria. These include the use of insecticide-treated bed nets (ITNs); indoor residual spraying; intermittent presumptive treatment during pregnancy; early diagnosis and prompt treatment with effective antimalarials; management of the environment to control mosquitoes; health education; and epidemic forecasting, prevention, and response (CDC, 2013a; WHO, 2018a). Methods of vector control vary widely, from using the larvae-eating fish tilapia to the use of insecticidal sprays and oils. Needless to say, the latter poses a potential threat to the environment in tropical areas where a delicate ecosystem is already threatened by other potential hazards such as lumbering and mining.

Countries that do not have strict environmental laws continue to use dichlorodiphenyltrichloroethane (DDT) sprays to control mosquito populations despite the advent of DDT-resistant mosquitoes. The non-DDT insecticide sprays, such as malathion, generally cost more, presenting an extra financial burden to less developed countries. Methods for control and eradication that are being considered by malaria-ridden countries are environmental management, reduction and control of the source, and elimination of the adult mosquito. There are significant global efforts being made to "blanket" endemic communities with insecticide-treated mosquito nets. A multitude of NGO projects are distributing ITNs to contribute to this initiative: Project Mosquito Net in Kenya (www.projectmosquitonet.org), Nothing But Nets (www.nothingbutnets.net), Global Giving for Africa (www.globalgiving.org), and Angola Mosquito Net Project (https://angolamosquitonetproject.wordpress.com) are examples of organizations actively engaged in preventing malaria and saving lives.

However, coverage levels are inadequate in endemic countries, especially in poor communities. Without adequate and predictable funding, the progress against malaria is also threatened by emerging parasite resistance to artemisinin, the core component of artemisinin-based combination therapies (ACTs), and mosquito resistance to insecticides. Artemisinin resistance has been detected in 4 countries in Southeast Asia, and insecticide resistance has been found in at least 64 countries. Children are most likely to be treated with ACTs (WHO, 2018a).

Although chemotherapeutic agents can be used for both protection and treatment of the disease, they are expensive and often cause side effects. However, evidence suggests that the *Plasmodium* sporozoites are becoming resistant to both treatment and preventive chemotherapeutic agents, especially chloroquine and its derivatives. Alternative therapies and/or combinations of medications such as sulfadoxine/pyrimethamine (Fansidar), amodiaquine, artemisinin, artemether, and atovaquone/proguanil (Malarone) are somewhat effective in treating malaria. Recent reports indicate that drug manufacturers in these endemic countries are diluting the drugs so that clients, especially children, are not receiving therapeutic levels of the medications. Many children suffer the effects of partially treated malaria, and once hospitalized, IV quinine is the drug of choice. Unfortunately, quinine has significant neurotoxic and cardiovascular side effects that need monitoring (CDC, 2013a). As discussed in Chapter 14, persons who live or travel to *Anopheles*-infested areas should protect themselves with mosquito netting, clothing that protects vulnerable parts of the body, repellents for both their bodies and their clothes, and antimalarial medications such as Malarone or doxycycline.

Diarrheal Disease

The normal intestinal tract regulates the absorption and secretion of electrolytes and water to meet the body's physiological needs. More than 98 percent of the 10 L of fluid per day entering the adult intestines is reabsorbed (Alexander and Blackburn, 2013; Bulled et al., 2014; Amour et al., 2016). The remaining stool water, related primarily to the indigestible fiber content, determines the consistency of normal feces from dry, hard pellets to mushy, bulky stools, varying from person to person, day to day, and stool to stool. This variation complicates the definition of *diarrhea.* For adults diarrhea is present when three or more liquid stools are passed in 24 hours. The frequent passage of formed stool is not diarrhea. Although young nursing infants tend to have five or more bowel movements per day, stools that are liquid without any formation and/or are more than what is normal for the child constitute diarrhea (Farthing et al., 2012). Definitions are complicated by the observable presence of blood, mucus, or parasites and the age of the affected person.

Diarrhea, one of the leading causes of illness and death in children less than five years of age throughout the world, is most prominent in the less developed countries despite recent initiatives by the WHO to correct this problem. Each year there are 760,000 diarrhea deaths in children under five; there are 1.7 billion cases of diarrheal disease every year related to unsafe water, sanitation, and hygiene; and it is the leading cause of malnutrition in children under five (WHO, Diarrhea Fact Sheet, 2013c). Causes of diarrhea are just as varied and diverse as its definitions and perceptions. Some of the causes include (1) viruses such as the rotavirus and Norwalk-like agents, (2) bacteria, including *Campylobacter jejuni, Clostridium difficile, Escherichia coli, Salmonella,* and *Shigella,* (3) environmental toxins, (4) parasites such as *Giardia lamblia* and *Cryptosporidium,* and (5) worms. Nutritional deficiencies can also cause diarrhea and are most often a result of infectious agents. Of these, the rotavirus has emerged as a major world concern, hospitalizing 55,000 American children and killing 1 million children in the world each year (Farthing et al., 2012; WHO, 2013c). Three major diarrhea syndromes exist:

- Acute watery diarrhea, which results in varying degrees of dehydration and fluid losses that quickly exceed total plasma and interstitial fluid volumes and is incompatible with life unless fluid therapy can keep up with losses. Such dramatic dehydration is usually due to rotavirus, enterotoxigenic *E. coli,* or *Vibrio cholerae* (the cause of cholera), and it is most dangerous in the very young.
- Persistent diarrhea, which lasts 14 days or longer and is manifested by malabsorption, nutrient losses, and wasting; it is typically associated with malnutrition, either preceding or resulting from the illness itself. Even though persistent diarrhea accounts for a small percent of the total number of diarrhea episodes, it is associated with a disproportionately increased risk of death.
- Bloody diarrhea, which is a sign of the intestinal damage caused by inflammation. Bloody diarrhea, defined as diarrhea with visible or microscopic blood in the stool, is associated with intestinal damage and nutritional deterioration, often with secondary sepsis. Mild dehydration and fever may be present. Bloody diarrhea should not be confused with dysentery, because dysentery is a syndrome consisting of the frequent passage of characteristic, small-volume, bloody mucoid stools, abdominal cramps, and tenesmus (a severe pain that accompanies straining to pass stool). Agents that cause bloody diarrhea or dysentery can also provoke a form of diarrhea that clinically is not bloody diarrhea, although mucosal damage and inflammation are present microscopically. The release of host-derived cytokines alters host metabolism and leads to the breakdown of body stores of protein, carbohydrate, and fat and the loss of nitrogen and other nutrients. Those losses must be replenished during the expected prolonged convalescence. For these reasons, bloody diarrhea calls for management strategies that are markedly different than those for watery or persistent diarrhea. New bouts of infection that occur before complete restoration of nutrient stores can initiate a downward spiral of nutritional status terminating in fatal protein-energy malnutrition (Farthing et al., 2012).

Diarrheal diseases are rampant among the impoverished. Poverty is associated with poor housing, crowding, dirt floors, lack of access to sufficient clean water or to sanitary disposal of fecal waste, cohabitation with domestic animals and zoonotic transmission of pathogens, and a lack of refrigerated storage for food. Unfortunately, even when the cause of the diarrhea is eliminated, poverty can restrict the ability to provide age-appropriate, nutritionally balanced diets or to modify diets so as to mitigate and repair nutrient losses. The lack of adequate, available, and affordable medical care increases the problem. Children suffer from an apparently never-ending sequence of infections and rarely receive appropriate preventive care, and too often their parents seek health care only when the children have become severely ill.

Dehydration is an immediate result of diarrhea and leads to a loss of fluid and electrolytes. The loss of up to 10 percent of the body's electrolytes can lead to shock, acidosis, stupor, and failure of the body's major organs (e.g., kidneys, heart). Persistent diarrhea often leads to loss of body protein, an increased time-limited inability to digest and absorb dairy products, and increased susceptibility to infection. Every country should have as a major aim the prevention and control of diarrheal disease, especially in infants and children. Many countries have developed diarrhea control programs that improve childhood nutrition. These programs instruct in breastfeeding and weaning practices and promote oral rehydration therapy and the use of supplementary feeding programs (Farthing et al., 2012). However, all these programs must be considered in conjunction with improving the social and economic conditions that contribute to safe environmental, sanitary, and general living conditions of populations around the world. The following How To box provides useful resources for keeping well informed about public health issues, including water quality.

HOW TO Stay Current About Global Health

One way to stay current with the world's health problems and advances is by reading the newspaper daily. Examples of newspapers that cover international health on an ongoing basis include the *Wall Street Journal, USA Today,* the *Washington Post,* and the *New York Times.* The following websites are examples of sources that pertain to international or global health:

- U.S. Department of Health and Human Services: *http://www.globalhealth.gov*
- Global Health Council: *http://www.globalhealth.org*
- Centers for Disease Control and Prevention: *http://www.cdc.gov/globalhealth*
- World Health Organization: *http://www.who.int/en*
- Pan American Health Organization: *http://new.paho.org*
- World Bank: *http://www.worldbank.org*
- Institute of Medicine: *http://www.iom.edu*
- Millennium Development Goals: *http://www.undp.org/mdg*
- *Sustainable Development Goals: https://www.un.org*

Maternal and Women's Health

Maternal health is central to the health of women, as well as the well-being of their children and families and the economic productivity of their countries. A woman's ability to survive pregnancy and childbirth is closely related to how effectively societies invest in and realize the potential of women not only as mothers, but as critical contributors to sustaining families and transforming nations. When investments in women—as mothers, as individuals, as family members, and as citizens—lag, the economic cost of maternal death and illness is enormous. The MDGs and SDGs both emphasized that women's education and empowerment results in greater household decision-making power and their children are better educated, becoming productive adults able to help build long-term economic growth. The World Bank found that during economic crises, poor families who sent women to work were better able to make ends meet.

Progress and investment in maternal health lagged far behind estimates of what was needed to achieve MDG 5, Improve Maternal Health. Progress in the last 20 years on key maternal health indicators varies by outcome and region, but it has been uneven, inequitable, and inadequate overall. Sustainable Development Goal 3 is to reduce the global maternal mortality ratio to less than 70 per 100,000 births, and globally that no country will have a maternal mortality rate of more than twice the global average. The two regions of the world with the highest maternal mortality rate—South Asia and sub-Saharan Africa—show minimal signs of improvement largely because of poverty, disempowerment of women, and overall poor health status of women in developing countries. Women's reproductive health, especially their ability to control their fertility and avoid HIV infection, is also closely associated with their health as mothers. Although maternal death and disability represent a high burden of disease in the developing world, interventions to improve maternal health are available and cost-effective (KFF, 2013c; Kott, 2011; WHO, 2018g).

The WHO and UNICEF have continued their worldwide initiatives to reform the health care received by women and children in less developed countries (WHO, 2018g). However, studies on women's health indicate that nearly 75 percent of all maternal deaths around the world are due to severe bleeding, infections, pre-eclampsia and eclampsia, complications post-delivery, and unsafe abortion. In developing nations (where the WHO notes 99 percent of maternal mortality takes place) there is a significant incidence of lack of prenatal care during pregnancy and high fertility rates, often due to a lack of access to contraception and other family planning and reproductive health services, as well as cultural belief systems that increase the lifetime risk of maternal death.

Every year more than half a million women die in pregnancy and childbirth around the world. This figure has altered little in the last 30 years. In sub-Saharan Africa a number of countries have halved their levels of maternal mortality since 1990 but not in the more impoverished nations such as the Congo, Uganda, Ghana, and others. However, between 1990 and 2010 the global maternal mortality ratio declined by only 3.1 percent per year. This is far from the annual decline of 5.5 percent required to achieve MDG 5 (WHO, 2018g).

Between 1900 and 2017, early death from enteric infection, respiratory infections and tuberculosis and maternal and neonatal disorders dropped, The greatest declines were in the least developed countries. The leading causes of death in 2017 were: ischemic heath disease, neonatal disorders, stroke, lower respiratory infections, diarrheal diseases, road injuries, COPD, NIV/AIDS, congenital birth defects, and malaria. (WHO, 2017). Specifically in sub-Saharan Africa, infectious diseases, childhood illnesses, and maternal causes of death account for as much as 70 percent of the burden of disease. By comparison, these conditions account for only one third of the burden in South Asia and Oceania and less than 20 percent in all other regions. In addition, whereas the average age of death throughout Latin America, Asia, and North Africa increased by more than 25 years between 1970 and 2010, it rose by less than 10 years in most of sub-Saharan Africa (WHO, 2017). The WHO found that some of the sociocultural factors that prevent women and girls from benefiting from quality health services and attaining the best possible level of health include the following (WHO, 2018g):

- Unequal power relationships between men and women
- Social norms that decrease education and paid employment opportunities
- An exclusive focus on women's reproductive roles
- Potential or actual experience of physical, sexual, and emotional violence

Within Africa the greatest disease burden remains from maternal health, child health, HIV, TB, and malaria; outside Africa the greatest disease burden is the rising incidence of noncommunicable diseases and rising life expectancy. Throughout the world, women between 15 and 49 years of age account for about one third of the world's disease burden, and women between 50 and 59 for one fifth of the burden. This burden is composed of diseases and conditions that are either exclusively or predominantly found in women, including maternal mortality and morbidity, cervical cancer, anemia, STIs, osteoarthritis, and breast cancer, with HIV/AIDS leading the statistics (Mathers, 2009; WHO, 2018g).

Although most of these conditions can be dealt with by cost-effective prevention and screening programs, many less developed countries have ignored women's health issues other than those directly related to pregnancy and childbirth for two major reasons: (1) women are not seen as valued members of society, and (2) most of the afflicted women are poor, malnourished, and cannot pay for health care services.

The WHO African Region accounts for the majority of the world's births. Although all countries profess to offer prenatal services and safe birthing services, most are unavailable, inaccessible, and unaffordable by women (WHO, 2018g). Of global maternal deaths, over half occur in fragile and humanitarian settings (WHO, 2018g). An African woman's risk of dying of pregnancy-related causes is 1 in 20, followed by Bangladesh, Pakistan, and India. These three countries account for nearly half of the world's maternal deaths, but only 29 percent of the world's births; they have more maternal deaths each week than Europe has in a year. Still, an accurate reporting of maternal deaths is difficult to obtain because many of the women who die are poor and live in remote areas (Mathers, 2009).

Risk factors for maternal mortality include poor nutritional status, disease conditions, high parity, and age less than 20 years and greater than 35 years. To date, little attention has been paid to the problem of maternal mortality, even though the reported incidences are high throughout the world. The WHO and the UN are addressing this problem by calling for government initiatives and actions to address maternal morbidity and mortality from obstetrical deaths as well as those that arise from indirect causes. MDG 5 aims to reduce the maternal mortality ratio by three quarters, improve the proportion of births attended by skilled health personnel, promote universal access to reproductive health, improve contraceptive rates, decrease adolescent birth rates, provide antenatal care coverage, and address the unmet need for family planning (WHO, 2018hg). In some countries it is difficult to counsel women on family planning and spacing their children so as to promote maternal and fetal health when a woman's value depends on her ability to reproduce and more than 50 percent of children die before they reach adolescence.

The result of poor maternal health accounts for the increase in premature births and the increased risk for high morbidity rates in children less than five years because of their own compromised nutritional and immune state. Low birth weight is a major risk factor for premature births, which account for more than one quarter (29 percent) of newborn deaths, followed by asphyxia (22 percent), sepsis (15 percent), pneumonia (10 percent), congenital abnormalities (7 percent), diarrhea (2 percent), and tetanus (2 percent). Undernutrition and lack of access to clean water and sanitation significantly increase children's vulnerability to death. Newborn deaths account for most child deaths (41 percent), followed by diarrhea (14 percent), pneumonia (14 percent), malaria (8 percent), injuries (3 percent), HIV/AIDS (2 percent), and other infectious or noncommunicable diseases (18 percent, including measles [1 percent]) (KFF, 2013b). In 2012 about 6.6 million children died before the age of five, which is nearly one half the number that died in 1990 but still much too high a number of deaths (World Bank, 2013b).

Even though programs in many countries have been initiated, safe motherhood initiatives are still needed throughout the world. These programs and initiatives need to include providing accessible family planning services and prenatal and postnatal health care services, ensuring access to safe abortion procedures, and improving the nutritional status of all women.

Nutrition and World Health

Many children around the world are underweight and have multiple micronutrient deficiencies such as for iron, zinc, and vitamin A. Poor nutrition by itself or that associated with infectious disease accounts for a large portion of the world's disease burden (Mathers, 2009; WHO, 2013a). Improved nutrition is related to stronger immune systems, decreased illness, better maternal and child health, longer life spans, and improved learning outcomes for children. Healthy protein balances are able to support major physiological stress with improved healing and ability to utilize protein-binding drugs; better nutrition is a prime entry point to ending poverty and a milestone to achieving better quality of life. Environmental and economic conditions related to poverty contribute to underconsumption of nutrients, especially those nutrients needed for protein building such as iodine, vitamin A, and iron. Worldwide, women and children suffer disproportionately from nutrition deficits, especially the micronutrients just mentioned (Mathers, 2009).

Poor nutrition also leads to stunting, or low height and weight for a given age. In 2014 the International Food Policy Research Institute published analysis on progress toward World Health Assembly Nutrition Targets internationally, with emphasis on the relevance of these targets within the context of the SDGs. Authors also promoted transparency in analyses through including details on the quality, year, and type of data available internationally for analysis. Indicators applied to several countries included child stunting, child obesity, availability of nutrients, benefit-cost ratios of scaling up specific interventions, and anemia indicators in reproductive aged women, among others (International Food Policy Research Institute, 2014). These indicators are important in order to track progress, particularly as authors note that at the time of this publication, several countries were not on track to meet goals.

Iron deficiencies are also common in less developed countries and severely affect women and children. When iron is low, fewer red blood cells are produced, and this reduces the capacity of the blood to transport oxygen. As a result, symptoms ranging from fatigue and inability to concentrate to impaired physical and cognitive development of children can occur. Iron deficiency anemia may also cause problems during pregnancy, particularly in developing countries, where it can increase the risk of premature delivery, as well as the risk of maternal and fetal complications and death. Inadequate iron from food is the most common reason for iron deficiency anemia, especially among infants and children. Parasites, infections, stomach and digestive diseases, and blood loss during menstruation may also worsen anemia. A deficiency of iron in the diet can reduce appetite, physical productivity, the ability to learn, and growth.

The American Society of Hematology (2013) reported that while the global prevalence of anemia decreased between 1990 and 2010 (from 40.2 percent to 32.9 percent), the disease has demonstrated an increase in global YLDs from 65.5 million to 68.4 million. The DALY burdens associated with major depression (63.2 million YLDs), chronic respiratory diseases (49.3 million YLDs), and general injuries (47.2 million YLDs) are less than the DALY burden of anemia. This is due to the increased incidence of anemia in children younger than 5 years. This age group accounted for more cases of anemia than any other age group and had the highest severity of disease in low- and middle-income regions. The data also demonstrated a widening gender gap in anemia burden over time with female prevalence rates remaining higher in most regions and age groups.

Other common dietary deficiencies include zinc, iodine, vitamin A, folic acid, and calcium. Zinc is important because it is an essential part of many enzymes and plays an important role in protein synthesis and cell division. The health consequences of zinc deficiency include poor immune system function, growth retardation, and delayed sexual maturity in children. Zinc deficiency is caused by low intake and/or low absorption of bioavailable zinc. Diets low in meat and fish increase the risk of zinc deficiency, because zinc is poorly bioavailable in cereals. Vitamin A is another essential nutrient in the human diet, contributing to the functioning of the retina, the growth of bone, and the immune response. Apart from preventable, irreversible blindness, vitamin A deficiency also causes reduced immune function, leading to an increased risk of severe infectious disease and anemia. It also increases the risk of death during pregnancy for both the mother and fetus and after birth for the newborn. An estimated 250 million preschool children in developing countries are affected by vitamin A deficiency, although severe deficiency that causes blindness is declining (KFF, 2013c; WHO, 2013d).

The impact of malnutrition and dietary deficiencies is significant. Any malnourished condition in a population can increase susceptibility to illness. For example, the principal causes of death among malnourished persons are measles, diarrheal and respiratory disease, TB, pertussis, and malaria. The loss of life from these diseases can be measured as 231 DALYs worldwide, with one fourth of the 231 being directly attributable to malnourishment and dietary deficiencies. Individual governments and organizations such as the International Red Cross, WHO, and many international religious and private foundations have been active in promoting better nutrition. Worldwide initiatives directed at overcoming nutritional deficits include the following (Global Alliance for Improved Nutrition, 2018): food fortification, food financing, improving child/adolescent nutrition, availability of nutritious foods in the workplace, and business ventures and research to support global nutrition.

Médecins sans Frontières (Doctors Without Borders) was the first to use the lifesaving supplement, invented in 2003 by a French scientist, called Plumpy'nut. Plumpy'nut requires no water preparation or refrigeration and has a two-year shelf life, making it easy to deploy in difficult conditions to treat severe acute malnutrition. It is distributed under medical supervision to humanitarian organizations for food aid distribution. The ingredients include peanut paste; vegetable oil; powered milk; powdered sugar; vitamins A, B-complex, C, D, E, and K; and minerals, including calcium, phosphorus, potassium, magnesium, zinc, copper, iron, iodine, sodium, and selenium. These are combined in a foil pouch, and each 92-g pack provides 500 kilocalories (kcal) or 2.1 megajoules (MJ).

Natural and Man-Made Disasters

As discussed in Chapter 21, earthquakes, floods, drought, and other natural hazards continue to cause tens of thousands of deaths, hundreds of thousands of injuries, and billions of dollars in economic losses each year around the world. Disasters represent a major source of risk for the poor and wipe out development gains and accumulated wealth in developing countries. In 2012 only 357 natural triggered disasters were registered; a decrease from 394 observed in the years past. However, natural disasters still killed a significant number, even though there was a decline in deaths. Contrary to other indicators, economic damages from natural disasters did show an increase to above average levels (U.S.[2012]$143 billion), with estimates placing the figure at U.S.$157 billion. Over the last decade, China, the United States, the Philippines, India, and Indonesia together constitute the top five countries that are most frequently hit by natural disasters. In 2012, China had its fourth highest number of natural disasters over the last decade with 13 floods and landslides, 8 storms, 7 earthquakes, and 1 period of extreme temperature. The single deadliest disaster in 2012 was Typhoon Bopha, which killed 1901 people in the Philippines (Guha-Sapir et al., 2013).

Natural disasters such as earthquakes, tsunamis, and floods can often come at the least expected time. Others, such as hurricanes and cyclones, are increasing in severity and destruction. Droughts are increasing as the threat of global warming rises. Typically, the poor are the worst hit, for they have the least resources to cope and rebuild. Hurricane Katrina resulted in a 90,000 square mile disaster zone, equivalent to the area of Great Britain, and more than 1800 died. The Indonesian tsunami of 2005 killed at least 230,000 people, and the livelihoods of millions were destroyed in more than 10 countries affected by the tsunami. The earthquake in Haiti in 2010 destroyed a country and crushed the hopes of thousands of Haitians. Human activity is contributing to massive extinctions, from various animal species, to forests, and the ecosystems that support marine life. The costs associated with deteriorating or vanishing ecosystems are high. The World Resources Institute reports that there is a link between biodiversity and climate change, and rapid global warming can affect an ecosystem's chance to adapt naturally (World Resources Institute, 2012). The four worst types of natural disasters are as follows:

- *Earthquakes and tsunamis:* Examples are April 25, 2015—nearly 9,000 people were killed and 22,000 injured when a 7.8-magnitude earthquake struck Nepal; January 12, 2010—more

than 230,000 people were killed when a 7.0-magnitude earthquake struck Haiti; May 12, 2008—about 70,000 people were killed and 18,000 people were reported missing after a 7.9-magnitude earthquake struck Sichuan, China.
- *Volcanic eruptions:* Examples are June 24, 2011, when Nabro Volcano erupted in Eritrea, resulting in 31 deaths, producing an ash cloud requiring large-scale evacuations; July 15, 1991, when Mount Pinatubo on Luzon Island in the Philippines erupted, blanketing 750 square kilometers with volcanic ash and more than 800 died; November 13-14, 1985, when at least 25,000 were killed near Armero, Colombia, when the Nevado del Ruiz volcano erupted, triggering mudslides.
- *Hurricanes, cyclones, and floods:* Examples are September 16-20, 2017 when Hurricane Maria, a category 5 hurricane and the deadliest storm of 2017, hit several Caribbean nations, resulting in a disputed death toll ranging from 146 to 1509. July-August 2010, when monsoon rains hit northwest Pakistan and more than one fifth of the country was under water, more than 1700 people were killed, and 17.2 million people were victims; May 3, 2008, when Cyclone Nargis, with winds that exceeded 190 km/hour and waves 6 m high, struck Myanmar, leaving as many as 100,000 dead, according to U.S. estimates; October 26-November 4, 1998, when Hurricane Mitch killed 11,000 in Honduras and Nicaragua and left 2.5 million homeless; October 1988 when Hurricane Joan hit Nicaragua.
- *Pandemics and famines:* 1900-present, malaria has been the leading cause of death in the developing world, causing severe illness in 500 million people each year and killing more than 1 million annually; 1984-1985, the Ethiopian famine that killed at least 1 million in Ethiopia; and 1980-present, the toll from AIDS worldwide is estimated at 25 million, with 40 million others infected with HIV (http://www.cbc.ca).

When poor countries face natural disasters, such as hurricanes, floods, earthquakes, and fires, the cost of rebuilding becomes even more of an issue when they are already burdened with debt. Often, poor countries suffer with many lost lives and/or livelihoods. Aid and disaster relief often do come in from international relief organizations, rich countries, and international institutions, but poor countries often pay millions of dollars a week back in the form of debt repayment.

The aftermath of a natural disaster may be as devastating as the disaster itself. Inadequate shelter, unclean water, and lack of security are some of the most commonly reported problems, even a year after the event. The physical force of a disaster not only causes immediate injury and death, but each type of disaster can result in its own combination of physical injuries. In earthquakes, buildings and the objects inside them can fall, injuring those who live or work there. Floods can result in drowning, and wildfires can cause burns and illness from smoke inhalation.

In addition to the direct injury and death caused by the disaster's force, there can be other serious adverse effects on the well-being of those living in the area. The large numbers of people who are suddenly ill or injured can exceed the capacity of the local health care system to care for them. In addition to the burden of increased numbers of clients, the system itself can become a victim of the disaster. Hospitals may be damaged, roads blocked, and personnel unable to perform their duties. The loss of these resources occurs at a time when they are most critically needed. The disaster can also hamper the ability to provide routine, nonemergency health services. Many people may be unable to obtain care and medications for their ongoing health problems. The disruption of these routine services can result in an increase in illness and death in segments of the population that might not have been directly affected by the disaster. The most serious consequences of natural disasters are related to mass population displacements, unsanitary conditions, lack of clean water, lack of nutritious foods, lack of safe housing, and the increased risk of diseases prevalent in crowded and unsanitary living conditions: typhoid fever, cholera, dysentery, TB, and infectious respiratory conditions (Petrucci, 2012).

Man-made disasters may include bioterrorism, chemical agents, pandemics and epidemics, radiation, and terrorism. The five worst man-made disasters in recent history are as follows:
- *Bhopal gas tragedy, India,* in 1984, in which more than 500,000 people were exposed to methyl isocyanine gas and other chemicals. Thousands of people died within the first hours of the leak, but over time estimates of 5000 to 16,000 deaths from the leak have been made.
- *Deepwater Horizon oil spill, Gulf of Mexico,* in 2010, which killed 11; leaked anywhere from 40,000 to 162,000 barrels of oil a day; took 47,829 people 89 days to finally cap the well; and 3500 workers and volunteers on the clean-up site are suffering liver and kidney damage from their exposure to the 1.8 million gallons of toxic oil.
- *Chernobyl meltdown, Ukraine,* in 1986. Thirty-one volunteers died trying to shut the reactor down, and nearly 4000 deaths so far have been thought to be attributable to the radiation poisoning people living near Chernobyl underwent. To this day, no one is sure what the final death toll from the Chernobyl meltdown will be.
- *Fukushima meltdown, Japan,* in 2011 with more than 100,000 people evacuated and displaced from the surrounding areas; 600 people dying during the evacuation; 300 cleanup workers receiving excessive exposure to radioactive waste; and the resulting unknown long-term health effects that could include people as far away from the meltdown as North America.
- *Global warming,* which impacts rising sea levels, desertification, animal extinction, and damage from intense superstorms such as Hurricane Katrina, Hurricane Sandy, and Typhoon Haiyan in the Philippines, has already created some of the first groups of climate-change refugees, and some estimate that number will rise to 150 million by 2050 (https://mic.com).

Other man-made disasters are the **bioterrorism** attack and the deliberate release of viruses, bacteria, or other germs (agents) used to cause illness or death of people, animals, or plants, which may lead to pandemics and epidemics (anthrax, cholera, Ebola virus, Lassa fever, plague, and smallpox, to name a few). A pandemic is an epidemic of infectious diseases that spread through human populations across a large region such as a continent or the globe (e.g., HIV/AIDS, smallpox, TB, H1N1, SARS), whereas an epidemic is when new cases of a certain disease in a given human population exceed what is expected (cancer, heart disease, seasonal flu).

These agents are typically found in nature, but it is possible that they could be changed to increase their ability to cause disease, to make them resistant to current medicines, or to increase their ability to be spread into the environment in order to threaten a government or intimidate or coerce a civilian population (CDC, 2013b; Infectious Disease, 2013). Bioterrorism is a significant public health threat that could produce widespread, devastating, and tragic consequences, and it would impose particularly heavy demands on international public health and health care systems. Nurses and other health personnel need to be aware and vigilant to the health consequences of terrorism and the potential use of biological agents to instill fear and to spread disease.

A nation's capacity to respond to the threat of bioterrorism depends in part on the ability of health care professionals and public health officials to rapidly and effectively detect, diagnose, respond, and communicate during a bioterrorism event. The national health care community—including public health agencies, emergency medical services, hospitals, and health care providers—would bear the brunt of the consequences of a biological attack. Attacks with biological agents are likely to be covert, rather than overt (CDC, 2013b). Terrorists may prefer to use biological agents because they are difficult to detect; they do not cause illness for several hours to several days.

A **chemical emergency** occurs when a hazardous chemical has been released and the release has the potential to harm people's health. Chemical releases can be unintentional, as in the case of an industrial accident, or intentional, as in the case of a terrorist attack. Sarin and ricin are the two most recent notorious chemicals used; however, mustard gas, cyanide, and tear gas have existed for decades. Agent Orange was used by the American troops in Vietnam, and mustard gas was commonly used during World War I and even during the Gulf War (https://mic.com; http://science.howstuffworks.com).

Radiation poisoning occurs when an excess amount of radiation is released to harm people's health. These may be unintentional and intentional events. Intentional terrorist events are those designed to contaminate food and water with radioactive material; spread radioactive material into the environment by using conventional explosives (e.g., dynamite), called a dirty bomb, or by using wind currents or natural traffic patterns; bomb or destroy a nuclear reactor; cause a truck or train carrying nuclear material to spill its load; or explode a nuclear weapon.

The word **genocide** was developed by a jurist named Raphael Lemkin in 1944. By combining the Greek word *genos* (race) with the Latin word *cide* (killing), genocide was defined by the UN in 1948 to mean any of the following acts committed with intent to destroy, in whole or in part, a national, ethnic, racial, or religious group, including (1) killing members of the group, (2) causing serious bodily or mental harm to members of the group, (3) deliberately inflicting on the group conditions of life calculated to bring about its physical destruction in whole or in part, (4) imposing measures intended to prevent births within the group, and (5) forcibly transferring children of the group to another group (Genocide Watch, 2013). The most notable genocides were the *Al-Anfal genocide* of the Kurds in Iraq, with more than 280,000 killed and many thousands unaccounted for; the *Rwandan genocide,* where the Hutus slaughtered hundreds of thousands (possibly 1 million) of their Tutsi relatives; the *Irish potato famine,* where more than a million Irish died because of lack of intervention by the British to feed the starving populace; the Native American genocide, with the loss of more than 1 million indigenous people to intentional infections with smallpox, war, and starvation; the *Bosnian genocide* and the annihilation of the Bosnian Muslims and Serbs to ethnically cleanse the country; and the most notable, the *Holocaust,* in which more than 6 million Jews and other ethnically disenfranchised populations were lost (http://listverse.com). Genocide continues today in Syria, Darfur, and the Central African Republic.

Following genocide, there are biopsychological changes such as physical stress reactions (cardiovascular, neurological) and mental stress responses, especially post-traumatic stress disorders and depression. Many people flee and become refugees or internationally displaced people. These refugees flee to neighboring countries, placing social, political, and economic burdens on these countries.

The biological and psychosocial effects of genocide are not exclusive to the child and adult victims, but affect the perpetrators as well. Marginalization and dehumanization place a mental toll on the victims that often results in negative cognitive, behavioral, affective, relational, and spiritual effects. Many perpetrators are forced into committing these acts, and achieving desensitization is necessary for a nonviolent person to kill or to commit violent acts. This is evident in the boy soldiers of the Lord's Resistance Army (LRA) (some as young as six years old) who are forced to kill or be killed and become desensitized through the use of alcohol, drugs, and repeated exposure to death (Vollhardt & Bilewicz, 2013).

After genocidal conflicts have ceased, restoration of a country's infrastructure, as well as reconciliation, must begin. The ramifications of genocide are widespread, and community leaders must find the most effective ways of initiating the healing process. The UN has tried to develop strategies to prevent genocide from occurring and is encouraging initiatives that include appropriate comprehensive cultural competence in the delivery of services; supporting and organizing treatment and care that is fair and just to all members of specific societies, regardless of age, gender, race, cultural beliefs, religion, sexual orientation, affiliation, and civil status; encouraging international organizations to make mental and behavioral health a priority in conflict assistance throughout the various stages of genocide; and encouraging its member organizations to emphasize the importance of social work in regard to genocide in their respective countries (Vollhardt & Bilewicz, 2013).

CHECK YOUR PRACTICE

As a nursing student you are asked to participate in a study abroad program in a less developed country. What steps or actions would you take to ensure your safety, health, and the legality of your work? Consider what evidence-based practices would guide your actions. Think also about how you could make a sustainable impact. What organizations and key leaders would you need to involve in your work?

Surveillance Systems. Surveillance systems, discussed in Chapter 22, are used to track potential risks for intentional harm to the people of the world. There are systems in place to assess the risks for man-made and natural disasters to prevent the atrocities to mankind discussed previously. These systems may be on-the-ground specialists who acquire information about the political stability of nations, or they may be satellite systems that track weather, volcanic, and earthquake activities.

How would a government find out that a deliberate outbreak had taken place? For the international system, the WHO monitors disease outbreaks through the Global Outbreak Alert and Response Network (Center for Research on the Epidemiology of Disaster, 2013; WHO, 2014e). This network, formally launched in April 2000, electronically links the expertise and skills of 72 existing networks from around the world, several of which were uniquely designed to diagnose unusual agents and handle dangerous pathogens. Its purpose is to keep the international community constantly alert to the threat of outbreaks and ready to respond. It has four primary tasks:

1. *Systematic disease intelligence and detection:* The first responsibility of the WHO network is to systematically gather global disease intelligence, drawing from a wide range of resources, both formal and informal. Ministries of health, WHO country offices, government and military centers, and academic institutions all file regular formal reports with the Global Outbreak Alert and Response Network. An informal network scours world communications for rumors of unusual health events.
2. *Outbreak verification:* Preliminary intelligence reports from all sources, both formal and informal, are reviewed and converted into meaningful intelligence by the WHO Outbreak Alert and Response Team, which makes the final determination on whether a reported event warrants cause for international concern.
3. *Immediate alert:* A large network of electronically connected WHO member nations, disease experts, health institutions, agencies, and laboratories is kept continually informed of rumored and confirmed outbreaks. The network also maintains and regularly updates an Outbreak Verification List, which provides a detailed status report on all currently verified outbreaks.
4. *Rapid response:* When the Outbreak Alert and Response Team determines that an international response is needed to contain an outbreak, it enlists the help of its partners in the global network. Specific assistance available includes targeted investigations, confirmation of diagnoses, handling of dangerous biohazards (biosafety level IV pathogens), client care management, containment, and logistical support in terms of staff and supplies.

In summary, if health care professionals and emergency responders are to be prepared to manage natural or man-made disasters, it is critical that there be cooperative efforts at the international, national, state, and local levels. Such disaster response is not the domain of any one specialty; nurses, doctors, mental health experts, first responders, emergency medical technicians, volunteers, engineers, and many more need to be part of the team that helps people overcome the physical, emotional, social, and economic devastation. Nurses need to have political, historical, social, medical, nursing, and public health knowledge in order to be more effective in finding the resources their clients need to recover successfully. See Chapter 21 for a thorough description of public health nursing practices related to disasters.

LINKING CONTENT TO PRACTICE

The role and involvement of nurses in global health relies heavily on nursing standards of practice and core competencies of both nurses and other public health professionals. The role also varies from country to country. It is not surprising to learn that nursing plays a more active role in health care delivery in the more technologically advanced countries. The more developed countries have a defined role for nurses, whereas the role is less well defined, if it is defined at all, in less developed countries. However, nurses need to remember that addressing the health of the people of the world is not restricted to meeting the physical health needs but, in order to be successful, must incorporate the concept of global health diplomacy. Physical, environmental, mental, political, fiscal, economic, safety, and educational "health" are intertwined in achieving the goals we all have for helping the people of the world obtain optimal well-being. Assessment of each of these areas is cited in standards of practice for nursing and public health professionals and is essential in the global nursing role. See the 2018 update by the Quad Council on Nursing's competencies (Swider et al., 2014; Council on Linkages, 2014; Quad Council Coalition of Nursing Organizations, 2018), which incorporate those of the Council on Linkages core competencies for public health professionals. Each set of competencies recommends analytic/assessment skills that are crucial to working in a global health arena. They also talk about the importance of cultural competence skills and communication skills that are relevant to the people with whom you are working.

During the last decade, some less developed countries have implemented PHC programs directed at prevention and management of important public health problems. With the increasing migration between and within countries because of war and famine, a greater need for nursing expertise to alleviate suffering of refugees and displaced persons has emerged. Starvation, disease, death, war, and migration underscore the need for support from the wealthier nations of the world.

More than 30 million refugees and internally displaced persons in less developed countries currently depend on international relief assistance for survival. Death rates in these populations during the acute phase of displacement have been up to 60 times the expected rates. Displaced populations in Ethiopia and southern Sudan have suffered the highest death rates. In Afghanistan and in war-torn Iraq, infectious diseases accounted for one half of all admissions to the hospital—mostly malaria and typhoid fever. The greatest death rate has been in children 1 to 14 years old. The major causes of death have been measles, diarrheal diseases,

LINKING CONTENT TO PRACTICE —cont'd

acute respiratory tract infections, and malaria. In addition, poor sanitation in many hospitals and clinics and shortages of drugs and qualified health care workers produce huge gaps for needed health care services. Continued violence accounts for a population afraid to leave home to seek medical help.

Nurses from more developed countries are recruited to combat the major mortality in refugee camps: malnutrition, measles, diarrhea, pneumonia, and malaria. Nurses, collaborating with other experts, are following the principles of PHC and are promoting adequate food intake, safe drinking water, shelter, environmental sanitation, and immunizations. These lifesaving practices have been implemented in the following countries: Thailand (Myanmar refugees), Rwanda, Zaire, Angola, Afghanistan, the Sudan, Uganda, and the former Yugoslavia. Nurses are making a difference; however, nurses involved in this work must be culturally astute and responsive, well educated about the world and well versed in the tasks required to achieve positive outcomes, able to critically reason, able to make decisions, able to identify who are appropriate team members, and able to collaborate with the team. They ought not be afraid of taking risks; they should be action-oriented, and they need to be flexible and altruistic. Global health work is a labor of love, it is a giving of self to make a difference in the lives of others less fortunate, and it is the most rewarding work in which many nurses have ever been engaged.

Council on Linkages Between Academia and Public Health Practice: *Core Competencies for Public Health Professionals,* Washington, DC, 2014, Public Health Foundation/Health Resources and Services Administration; Quad Council Coalition of Public Health Nursing Organizations: *Competencies for public health nursing practice,* Washington, DC, 2018.

PRACTICE APPLICATION

You are sent to a country ravaged by war, in which many people are refugees. You are asked to work side by side with other nurses, both foreign and native to the country.

A. What would you do first to develop this group of nurses into a functioning team?
B. Which health and environmental problems would you attempt to handle early in your work?
C. Identify second-stage interventions and prevention once the initial crisis stage is relieved.

Answers can be found on the Evolve site.

KEY POINTS

- Global health is a collective goal of nations and is promoted by the world's major health organizations.
- Global health cannot be achieved without using the constructs of global health diplomacy: addressing and finding solutions to physical, environmental, fiscal, economic, political, safety, educational, and trade issues.
- As the political and economic barriers between countries fall, the movement of people back and forth across international boundaries increases. This movement increases the spread of various diseases throughout the world.
- Nurses play an active role in the identification of potential health risks at U.S. borders, with immigrant populations throughout the United States, and as participants in global health care delivery.
- Understanding a population approach is essential for understanding the health of specific populations.
- Universal access to health care for the world's populations relies on strong primary care.
- The major organizations involved in world health are (1) multilateral, (2) bilateral and nongovernmental or private voluntary, and (3) philanthropic.
- The health status of a country is related to its economic and technical growth. More technologically and economically advanced countries are referred to as *developed,* whereas those that are striving for greater economic and technological growth are termed *less developed.* Many less developed countries shift financial resources from health and education to other internal needs, such as defense or economic development, and this shift does not help the poor.
- The global burden of disease (GBD) is a way to describe the world's health. The GBD combines losses from premature death and losses that result from disability. The GBD represents units of disability-adjusted life-years (DALYs).
- Critical global health problems still exist and include communicable diseases such as tuberculosis, measles, mumps, rubella, and polio; maternal and child health; diarrheal diseases; nutritional deficits; malaria; and AIDS.
- Natural and man-made disasters have become global health concerns.

CLINICAL DECISION-MAKING ACTIVITIES

1. In your class, divide into small groups and discuss how you might find out if there are immigrant communities in your area (you may need to contact your local health department, area social workers, or community social organizations and churches).
2. Discuss how you can gain access to one of these immigrant groups.
3. On gaining access, how would you go about determining what specific kinds of services the people need? What are their beliefs about health and health care? What customs regarding health were followed in their country of origin? How does the American health care system differ from the health care system in their country?

4. As a nurse, what kinds of interventions can you implement with immigrant populations? What special skills or knowledge do you need to provide care to immigrant populations?
5. Write to one of the major international health organizations or visit their Internet website and obtain their mission and goal statements. What is the focus of their health-related activities? Does the organization that you identified have a specific role defined for nurses? How can a nurse who is interested become involved in their programs and activities?
6. Pick a country or area of the world outside the United States that interests you. Go to the library or use the Internet to obtain information about the following:
   a. Status of health care in that country
   b. Major health concerns
   c. Global burden of disease (GBD)
   d. Whether this country is developed or less developed
   e. Which, if any, global health care organizations are involved with the delivery of health care in that country
7. Choose one or more of the following countries, and find out from your local or state health department the health risks that are involved in visiting that country: Indonesia, Zaire, Paraguay, Bangladesh, Kuwait, Kenya, Mexico, China, and Haiti.
8. Establish communication with nurses in a country of interest (via telecommunication [e.g., Internet, phone, blog]) to discuss the state of nursing in that country, their problems, and plans to overcome some of the barriers that obstruct them from achieving their professional goals.

ADDITIONAL RESOURCES

EVOLVE WEBSITE

http://evolve.elsevier.com/Stanhope/community/

- Answers to Practice Application
- Case Study
- Glossary
- Review Questions

REFERENCES

Alexander KA, Blackburn JK: Overcoming barriers in evaluating outbreaks of diarrheal disease in resource poor settings: assessment of recurrent outbreaks in Chobe District, Botswana, *BMC Public Health* 13:775, 2013.

Alliance of Nurses for Healthy Environments (ANHE): *Water and Health: Opportunities for Nursing Action*. 2018. https://envirn.org/water-and-health.

Alliance of Nurses for Healthy Environments (ANHE): *Climate Change, Health, and Nursing*. 2016. https://envirn.org/climate-change-health-and-nursing.

American Society of Hematology (ASH): *New Report Illustrates Persistent Global Burden of Anemia among High-Risk Populations Including Young Children and Women*, 2013. Retrieved from http://www.hematology.org.

Amour C, Gratz J, Mduma E, et al.: Epidemiology and impact of campylobacter infection in children in 8 low-resource settings: Results from the MAL-ED Study, *Clin Infect Dis* 63(9):1171–1179, 2016.

Bolender J, Hunter A: The Uganda project: a cross-disciplinary student-faculty research and service project to develop a sustainable community-development program, *Counc Undergrad Res Q* 30(2):1–5, 2010.

Bolender J, McDonald K, Hunter A: Arsenic contamination of the water sources in Western Uganda. Unpublished research, 2012, 2013.

Boyle S: United Kingdom (England): Health system review, *Health Syst Transit* 13(1):1–483, 2011. Retrieved from http://www.euro.who.int.

Bryar B, Kendall S, Mogotlane SM, et al.: *Reforming Primary Health Care: A Nursing Perspective,* Geneva, 2012, International Council of Nurses. Retrieved from www.ichrn.org.

Bulled N, Singer M, Dillingham R: The syndemics of childhood diarrhoea: A biosocial perspective on efforts to combat global inequities in diarrhoeal-related morbidity and mortality, *Global Public Health* 9(7):841–853, 2014.

California Department of Public Health, Office of Binational Border Health: *Border Health Status Report to the Legislature*, 2015. Retrieved from https://www.cdph.ca.gov.

Centers for Disease Control and Prevention: *About Malaria*, 2013a. Retrieved from http://www.cdc.gov.

Centers for Disease Control and Prevention. *Bioterrorism*, 2013b. Retrieved from http://www.cdc.gov.

Centers for Disease Control and Prevention. *Global WASH Fast Facts*, 2016. Retrieved from https://www.cdc.gov.

Centers for Disease Control and Prevention. *Chikungunya Virus*, 2017. Retrieved from https://www.cdc.gov.

Centers for Disease Control and Prevention. *Zika Virus*, 2018. Retrieved from https://www.cdc.gov.

Center for Research on the Epidemiology of Disaster: *Annual Disaster Statistical Review 2012: The numbers and trends*, 2013. Retrieved from http://reliefweb.int.

Chien W, Leung S, Chu C: A nurse-led, needs-based psycho-education intervention for Chinese patients with first-onset mental illness. *Contemp Nurse* 40(2):194–209, 2012. Retrieved from http://www.questia.com.

Commonwealth Fund: *International Profiles of Health Care Systems*, 2017. In Mossialos E, Djordjevic A, Osborn R, Sarnak D, editors. Retrieved from https://www.commonwealthfund.org.

Compton B, Barash DM, Farrington J, et al.: *Access to medical devices in low-income countries: Addressing sustainability challenges in medical device donations. NAM Perspectives. Discussion Paper*, Washington, DC, 2018, National Academy of Medicine. https://doi.org/10.31478/201807a.

Council on Linkages Between Academia and Public Health Practice: *Core Competencies for Public Health Professionals*, Washington, DC, 2014, Public Health Foundation/Health Resources and Services Administration.

Daley C, Gubb J: *Healthcare systems: The Netherlands*, 2013. Retrieved from http://www.digitalezorg.nl.

Development Initiatives. *Global Humanitarian Assistance Report 2018*, 2018. Retrieved from http://devinit.org.

Farmer P: Pathologies of Power: *Health, Human Rights, and the New War on the Poor*, Berkeley, CA, 2005, University of California Press.

Farthing M, Salam M, Lindberg G, et al.: Acute diarrhea in adults and children: a global perspective, *World Gastroenterol Organ Glob Guidel*, 2012. Retrieved from http://www.worldgastroenterology.org.

Fernández-Luqueño F, López-Valdez F, Gamero-Melo P, et al.: Heavy metal pollution in drinking water—a global risk for human health: A review, *Afr J Environ Sci Technol* 7(7):567–584, 2013.

Forman J, Taruscio D, Llera VA, et al.: The need for worldwide policies and action plans for rare diseases, *Acta Paediatr* 101(8):805–807, 2012.

Genocide Watch: *International Alliance to End Genocide*, 2013. Retrieved from http://www.genocidewatch.org.

Global Alliance for Improved Nutrition: *Our Programs*, 2018. Retrieved from https://www.gainhealth.org.

Global Health Workforce Alliance: *The Tanzania Nursing Initiative. The Tanzania Nursing Initiative: using the HRH Action Framework to strengthen Tanzania's healthcare workforce*, 2014. Retrieved from http://www.who.int.

Global Nursing Caucus: *About the Organization*, 2018. Retrieved from https://www.globalnursingcaucus.org.

Guha-Sapir D, Hoyois P, Below R: *Annual Disaster Statistical Review 2012: The Numbers and Trends*, Brussels, 2013, CRED.

Hunter A, Wilson L, Stanhope M, et al.: Global health diplomacy: An integrative review of the literature and implications for nursing, *Nurs Outlook* 61(2):85–92, 2013.

Infectious Disease: *Global Challenges. Bioterroism*, 2013. Retrieved from http://needtoknow.nas.edu.

Institute of Medicine: *Addressing the Threat of Drug-Resistant Tuberculosis: A Realistic Assessment of the Challenge*. Workshop Summary. 2011b. Retrieved from http://www.ncbi.nlm.nih.gov.

International Council of Nurses: *Leadership for Change*, 2018. Retrieved from http://www.icn.ch.

International Food Policy Research Institute: *Global Nutrition Report 2014: Actions and Accountability to Accelerate the World's Progress on Nutrition*, Washington, DC, 2014, International Food Policy Research Institute.

Kaiser Family Foundation: The *U.S. Government and Global Health Policy. Fact sheet December 2019.* Retrieved from http://www.kff.org.

Kaiser Family Foundation: *The global HIV/AIDS epidemic overview*, 2013a. http://www.kff.org.

Kaiser Family Foundation: *The U.S. government and global maternal, newborn & child health*, 2018b. Retrieved from http://www.kff.org.

Kaiser Family Foundation: The *U.S. government and global health fact sheet 2019: The U.S.* Retrieved from http://www.kff.org.

Kamwesiga J: *Uganda health care system*, 2011. Retrieved from https://news.mak.ac.ug.

Kelly A: Healthcare a major challenge for Uganda, *The Guardian* 2009. Retrieved from http://www.theguardian.com.

Kott A: Rates of unintended pregnancy remain high in developing regions, *Int Perspect Sex Reprod Health* 37(1):46–47, 2011. Retrieved from http://www.guttmacher.org.

Kulbok PA, Mitchell EM, Glick DF, Greiner D: International Experiences in Nursing Education: A review of the literature, *Int J Nurs Educ Scholarsh* 24(9):1–21, 2012.

Leffers J, Mitchell E: Conceptual Model for Partnership and Sustainability in Global Health, *Public Health Nurs* 28(1):91-102, 2011.

Lucio RM, Villacres N, Henriquez R: The health system of Ecuador, *Salud Pública Mex* 53(2):s177–s187, 2011. Retrieved from https://scielosp.org.

Mathers C: Global burden of disease among women, children, and adolescents. In Ehiri JE, editor: *Maternal and Child Health*. LLC, 2009, Springer Science Business Media, p. 200. Retrieved from http://citeseerx.ist.psu.edu.

Mossiaios E, Djordjevic A, Osborn R and Sarnak D: *International Profiles of Health Care Systems, The Commonwealth Fund,* New York, NY. 2017.

OECD: *Health at a glance: 2017, OCED Indicators*. Retrieved from http://www.oecd-indicators.

Petrucci O: The impact of natural disasters: simplified procedures and open problems. In *Approaches to Managing Disaster: Assessing Hazards, Emergencies and Disaster Impact*, 2012. Open Access. doi:10.5772/29147.

Pigs for Peace. 2016. Retrieved from http://www.pigsforpeace.org.

Puig A, Pagan J, Wong R: Assessing quality across health care subsystem in Mexico, *J Ambul Care Manage* 32(2):123–131, 2009. Retrieved from http://www.ncbi.nlm.nih.gov.

Quad Council of Public Health Nursing Organizations. *Competencies for Public Health Nursing Practice*, Washington, DC, 2018.

SEED Global Health: Where we work, 2018. Retrieved from http://seedglobalhealth.org.

Segal MT, Demos V, Kronenfeld JJ: *Gender Perspectives on Health and Medicine: Key Themes*, New York, NY, 2003, Elsevier.

Shah A: *Foreign aid for developing assistance*. Global Issues Social, Political, 2012, Inter Press Service: International News Agency. Retrieved from http://www.globalissues.org.

Shah A: *Global issues: Social, political, economic, and environmental issues that affect us all: Health Issue*, 2014, Inter Press Service: International News Agency. Retrieved from http://www.globalissues.org.

Shakarishvili G, Atun R, Berman P, et al.: Converging health systems frameworks: Towards a concept-to-actions roadmap for health systems strengthening in low and middle income countries, *Global Health Governance* III(2), 2010. Retrieved from http://www.ghgj.org.

Sindhu A, Pholpet C, Puttapitukpol S: Meeting the challenges of chronic illness: a nurse-led collaborative community care program in Thailand, *Collegian* 17(2):93–99, 2010.

Slone M, Mann S: Effects of War, Terrorism and armed conflict on Young Children: A systematic review, *Child Psychiatry Hum Dev* 47(6):950–965, 2016.

Sutherland K: Quality in healthcare in England, Wales, Scotland, and Northern Ireland: an intra-UK chartbook, *Quest Qual Improved Perform* 2009. Retrieved from https://www.health.org.uk.

Swider SM, Levin PF, Kulbok P: *Quad Council of Public Health Nursing Organizations Invitational Forum on the Role and Future of Nurses in Public Health: Final Report*, 2014. Retrieved from http://www.achne.org.

UNICEF: *Water, Sanitation and Hygiene*, 2010. Retrieved from http://www.unicef.org.

United Nations: *The Millennium Development Goals Report 2013: Big strides in Millennium Development Goal with more targets achievable by 2015*, 2013a. Retrieved from http://www.un.org.

United Nations: *The Millennium Development Goals Report*, 2013b. Retrieved from http://www.un.org.

United Nations: *Millennium Development Goals MDG Gap Task Force Report*, 2015. Retrieved from http://www.un.org.

United Nations, Department of Economic and Social Affairs (DESA): *World Economic Situation and Prospects*, 2014. Retrieved from http://www.un.org.

United Nations Office for the Coordination of Humanitarian Affairs (OCHA). *What we do*, 2018. Retrieved from http://www.un.org.

UN Sustainable Development Goals (SDGs). *About the Sustainable Development Goals*, 2017. Retrieved from https://www.un.org.

U.S. Department of Health and Human Services: *Healthy People: 2020 Topics and Objectives*. 2010, Retrieved from http://www.healthypeople.gov.

Vollhardt JR, Bilewicz M: After the genocide: Psychological perspectives on victim, bystander, and perpetrator groups, *J Soc Issues* 69(1):1–15, 2013.
Wang CC, Whitehead L, Bayes S: Nursing education in China: Meeting the global demand for quality healthcare, *Int J Nurs Sci* 3(1):131–136, 2016.
World Health Organization (WHO): *7th Global conference on health promotion*, 2010a. Retrieved from http://www.who.int.
World Health Organization: *State of the world's vaccines and immunization*, ed 3, Immunization, Vaccines and Biologicals, 2010b. Retrieved from http://whqlibdoc.who.int.
World Health Organization: Global burden of disease report, 2010, *The Partners Matern Newborn and Child Health*, 2018. Retrieved from http://www.who.int.
World Health Organization Europe: *European Health for All database (HFA-DB)*, 2013a. Retrieved from http://www.euro.who.int.
World Health Organization: *World malaria report 2013 shows major progress in fight against malaria, calls for sustained financing*, 2013b. Retrieved from http://www.who.int.
World Health Organization: *Fact Sheet. Diarrhoeal disease*, 2013c. Retrieved from http://www.who.int.
World Health Organization: *Global prevalence of Vitamin A deficiency micronutrient deficiency information system working paper No. 2*, 2013d. Retrieved from http://www.who.int.
World Health Organization: *Health impact assessment (HIA): The determinants of health*, 2014a. Retrieved from http://www.who.int.
World Health Organization: *Healthy settings: Healthy cities*, 2014b. Retrieved from http://www.who.int.
World Health Organization: *Primary health care*, 2014c. Retrieved from http://www.who.int.
World Health Organization: *HIV/AIDS. Global health observatory*, 2014d. Retrieved from http://www.who.int.
World Health Organization: *Global outbreak alert & response network*, 2014e. Retrieved from http://www.who.int.
World Health Organization: *Tuberculosis Key Facts*, 2017. Retrieved from http://www.who.int.
World Health Organization: *Fact sheet on malaria*, 2018a. Retrieved from http://www.who.int.
World Health Organization (WHO): *Fact sheet on global HIV/AIDS*, 2018b. Retrieved from http://www.who.int.
World Health Organization: *Children; reducing mortality*, 2018c. Retrieved from http://www.who.int.
World Health Organization: *Fact sheet on child deaths*, 2018d. Retrieved from http://www.who.int.
World Health Organization: *Neglected Tropical Diseases*, 2018e. Retrieved from http://www.who.int.
World Health Organization: *Global Burden of Disease*, 2018f. *Health stats and health information systems*. Retrieved from http://www.who.int.
World Health Organization: *Metrics: Disability-Adjusted Life Year (DALY). Health statistics and health information systems*, 2018g. Retrieved from http://www.who.int.
World Health Organization: *Maternal mortality fact sheet*, 2018h. Retrieved from http://www.who.int.
World Resources Institute: *World resource report 2010-2011*, 2012. Retrieved from http://www.wri.org.
Yakutchik M: In Botswana, nurses lead Jhpiego's life-saving efforts to screen, treat women for HPV, *Glob Health* 2018. Retrieved from https://hub.jhu.edu.
Yun H, Jie S, Anli J: Nursing shortage in China: State, causes, and strategy, *Nurs Outlook* 58(3):122–128, 2010.

5

Economics of Health Care Delivery

Whitney Rogers Bischoff, DrPH, MSN, BSN

OBJECTIVES

After reading this chapter, the student should be able to do the following:

1. Identify major factors influencing national health care spending.
2. Relate public health and economic principles to nursing and health care.
3. Describe the economic theories of microeconomics and macroeconomics.
4. Analyze the role of government and other third-party payers in public health care financing.
5. Discuss the implications of health care rationing from an economic perspective.
6. Evaluate levels of prevention as they relate to public health economics.

CHAPTER OUTLINE

Public Health and Economics
Principles of Economics—Microeconomics and Macroeconomics
Factors Affecting Resource Allocation in Health Care
Primary Prevention
The Context of the U.S. Health Care System
Trends in Health Care Spending
Factors Influencing Health Care Costs
Financing of Health Care
Health Care Payment Systems

KEY TERMS

American Health Benefit Exchanges, p. 99
American Health Care Act, p. 93
budget limits, p. 95
business cycle, p. 96
capitation, p. 116
cost-benefit analysis, p. 97
cost-effectiveness analysis, p. 97
cost-utility analysis, p. 97
demand, p. 95
diagnosis-related groups, p. 110
donut hole, p. 107
economic growth, p. 96
economics, p. 93
effectiveness, p. 96
efficiency, p. 95
fee-for-service, p. 100
gross domestic product, p. 96
gross national product, p. 96
health care rationing, p. 98
health economics, p. 93
human capital, p. 96
inflation, p. 93
intensity, p. 100
investment in public health, p. 92
macroeconomic theory, p. 96
managed care, p. 114
managed competition, p. 114
market, p. 95
means testing, p. 107
Medicaid, p. 109
medical technology, p. 101
Medicare, p. 109
microeconomic theory, p. 94
Patient Protection and Affordable Care Act, p. 93
prospective payment system, p. 110
public health economics, p. 93
public health finance, p. 93
quality-adjusted life-years, p. 97
retrospective reimbursement, p. 115
safety net providers, p. 99
supply, p. 95
third-party payer, p. 113

Health care disparities are differences among population groups in the availability, accessibility, and quality of health care services aimed at prevention, treatment, and management of diseases and their complications, including screening, diagnostic, treatment, management, and rehabilitation services (Orgera & Artiga, 2016).

In the United States, health and health care disparities are routinely seen in individuals who are marginalized because of their socioeconomic status, race, culture, primary language, sexual identity, and, in some cases, gender. How health care is financed and delivered has a direct effect on the ability of all U.S. residents to obtain timely, appropriate care that is affordable. Additionally, there is an emerging recognition that social determinants of health (SDOH) along with health behavior play a major role in the health of individuals and families (Artiga & Hinton, 2018).

There is strong evidence to suggest that poverty can be directly related to poorer health outcomes. Poorer health outcomes lead to reduced educational outcomes for children, poor nutrition, low productivity in the adult workforce, and unstable economic growth in a population, community, or nation. However, improving health status and economic health is dependent on the "degree of equality" in policies that improve living standards for all members of a population, including the poor.

To address health care disparities, two significant events occurred. In 2010 a significant health reform law, the Patient Protection and Affordable Care Act (PL 111-148) (ACA) was passed by Congress and signed into law on March 23, 2010, resulting in a greater emphasis on access to care, leading to improvements in prevention of illness, patient outcomes, and population health.

To move toward improving a population's health, it was determined that there must be an "**investment in public health**" by all levels of government. The Prevention and Public Health Fund (PPHF), which was part of the Consolidated Appropriations Act of 2016, was specifically designed to invest in public health in communities (USDHHS, 2016).

Estimates indicate that public spending on health care makes a difference, although this funding is highly variable from state to state. A baseline of prevention services should be provided to all regardless of where they live (Trust for America's Health, 2015). Several facts are known and based on the literature (Garfield et al, 2019; Barnett & Berchick, 2017; U.S. Department of Health and Human Services [USDHHS], 2016):

- In 2016 approximately 28.1 million (8.8%) of the estimated 320.3 million people in the United States were without health insurance (Barnett & Berchick, 2017). Since many provisions of the Patient Protection and Affordable Care Act (PPACA or ACA) went into effect in 2014 and some states expanded Medicaid coverage, the number of uninsured individuals has decreased from levels around 44 million people in 2013 (Kaiser Family Foundation, 2017a).
- Although the number of uninsured has decreased under ACA, 45% of uninsured adults cited the high cost of coverage as the reason they were not insured (Kaiser Family Foundation, 2017a).
- Lack of workplace insurance and failure of some states to expand Medicaid under ACA are some of the reasons given for remaining uninsured.
- For households with less than $25,000 annual income, 13.7% did not have health insurance coverage in 2016 (Barnett & Berchick, 2017).
- Adults under the age of 65 are more likely to be uninsured than children (Barnett & Berchick, 2017).
- Young adults (ages 19-25 years) were beneficiaries of the ACA provision allowing them to remain on their parent's insurance policy until age 26. This resulted in falling uninsured rates among this group from 2013 to 2016 of about 11.5% or more for each age between 21 and 28. Even with this change in policy, 17.5% of adults aged 26 were uninsured in 2016 (Barnett & Berchick, 2017).
- The uninsured rate for all children under age 19 was 5.4% in 2016. For children living in poverty the uninsured rate was 7.0%, which was higher than the rate for children not in poverty (5.0%) (Barnett & Berchick, 2017).
- Minorities are more likely to be uninsured than whites. About 16% of Hispanics, 10.5% of African Americans, and 7.6% of Asians were uninsured in 2016, compared with 6.3% of non-Hispanic whites (Barnett & Berchick, 2017). These uninsured rates are about half the uninsured rates reported in 2013 (Kaiser Family Foundation, 2017a). States that expanded Medicaid coverage to more people showed greater gains in insured population than those that did not—9,110,784 versus 4,575,853 (Kaiser Family Foundation, 2017a).
- More than 8 in 10 (80%) of the uninsured were in working families with income below 400% of poverty in 2016 (Kaiser Family Foundation, 2017a).
  - About 75% were from families with one or more full-time workers.
  - About 11% were from families with part-time workers.
- Higher level of education, higher household income, and living in a family arrangement is associated with a greater rate of health insurance coverage (Barnett & Berchick, 2017).

Previously demonstrated consequences of lack of health insurance continue to hold even as more people came under insurance coverage through the ACA (Kaiser Family Foundation, 2017a):

- Individuals without health insurance are less likely to receive preventive care and treatment for chronic diseases than those with insurance coverage (Kaiser Family Foundation, 2017a).
- Those without health insurance are more likely to be hospitalized for preventable problems and, when hospitalized, receive fewer diagnostic and therapeutic services; they also have higher mortality rates than those with insurance (Kaiser Family Foundation, 2017a).
- Adults without insurance are nearly twice as likely to report being in fair or poor health than those with private insurance (Kaiser Family Foundation, 2017a).
- Studies indicate that gaining health insurance restores access to health care considerably and reduces the adverse effects of having been uninsured (Kaiser Family Foundation, 2017a).
- The poor are more likely to receive health care through publicly funded agencies.

- An emphasis on individual health care will not guarantee improvement of a population or a community's health (see Chapter 3 for more discussion).

Approximately 97% of all health care dollars are spent for individual care, whereas only 2.5% are spent on population-level health care. The 2.5% includes monies spent by the government on public health as well as the preventive health care dollars spent by private sources. These numbers indicate that there has not been a large investment in the public's health or population health in the United States (National Center for Health Statistics [NCHS], 2017). The PPHF increased total state funding for fiscal year (FY) 2017 over FY 2016 overall, yet it does not reflect the increased need related to the opioid epidemic, growth in population, aging of the population, or emerging infectious diseases such as Zika and flea-, tick-, and mosquito-borne illnesses (Trust for America's Health, 2018).

The United States spends more on health care than any other nation. The cost of health care has been rising more than the rate of **inflation** since the mid-1960s, yet the U.S. population does not enjoy greater longevity as compared with nations that spend far less than the United States. The current health care system has been reaching the point where it is not affordable and is expected to consume 19.7% of the economy by 2026 (Turnock, 2015; Cuckler et al., 2018).

An estimated $10 per person invested in community-based prevention programs can lead to improved health status of the population and reduced health care costs (Trust for America's Health, 2016). This return on investment represents medical cost savings only and does not include the significant gains that could be achieved in worker productivity, reduced absenteeism at work and school, and enhanced quality of life. Health spending is not the only way to achieve better population health and its attendant benefits as social service spending also has benefits to health and well-being (Bradley et al., 2016).

Nurses are challenged to implement changes in practice and participate in research, evidence-based practice, and policy activities designed to provide the best return on investment of health care dollars (i.e., to design models of care at a reasonable price that improve access or quality of care). Meeting this challenge requires a basic understanding of the economics of the U.S. health care system. Nurses should be aware of the effects of nursing practice on the delivery of cost-effective care. In 2010 a significant health reform law, the ACA, was passed by Congress and signed into law on March 23, 2010, resulting in a greater emphasis on access to care, leading to improvements in prevention of illness, patient outcomes, and population health.

Although the ACA and the PPHF were showing health care improvements, gains for prevention and access were short-lived, when the new administration and the 115th U.S. Congress repeatedly attempted to repeal aspects of the ACA. Thus the **American Health Care Act** of 2017 (H.R. 1628), often shortened to the AHCA, a U.S. Congress bill introduced to partially repeal the **Patient Protection and Affordable Care Act** (ACA), was passed into law.

A survey by the Commonwealth Fund found that gains achieved under ACA were reversing as early as spring 2018 (Collins et al., 2018). For individuals living in states that did not expand Medicaid under ACA the uninsured rate rose to 21%.

PUBLIC HEALTH AND ECONOMICS

Economics is the science concerned with the use of resources, including the production, distribution, and consumption of goods and services. **Health economics** is concerned with how scarce resources affect the health care industry (McPake et al., 2018). **Public health economics**, then, focuses on the producing, distributing, and consuming of goods and services as related to public health and where limited public resources might best be spent to save lives or increase the quality of life for the population (USDHHS, 2016).

Economics provides the means to evaluate the attaining of society wants and needs in relation to limited resources. In addition to the day-to-day decision making about the use of resources, there is a focus on evaluating economics in health care (McPake et al., 2018). While in the past there has been limited focus on evaluating public health economics, it is becoming more obvious what evaluating public health and preventive care expenditures can do in terms of evaluating cost savings and, more importantly, quality of life (Trust for America's Health, 2017; Schulte et al., 2016). This type of evaluation will help to present funding proposals to public policymakers (legislators).

Public health financing often causes conflict because of the views and priorities of individuals and groups in society, which may differ from those of the public health care industry. If money is spent on public health care, then money for other public needs, such as education, transportation, recreation, and defense may be limited. When one is trying to argue that more money should be spent for population-level health care or prevention, data are becoming available that show the investment is a good one. **Public health finance** is a growing field of science and practice that involves the acquiring, managing, and using of monies to improve the health of populations through disease prevention and health promotion strategies. This field of study also focuses on evaluating the use of the money and its effect on the public health system (Meit et al., 2013).

Although the public health system had been considered for many years as involving only government public health agencies such as health departments, today the public health system is known to be much broader and includes schools, industry, media, environmental protection agencies, voluntary organizations, civic groups, local police and fire departments, religious organizations, industry/business, and private sector health care systems, including the insurance industry. All can play a key role in improving population health (Institute of Medicine, 2012; Trust for America's Health, 2017).

The goal of public health finance is to support population-focused preventive health services (Meit et al., 2013). Four principles are suggested that explain how public health financing may occur (Sturchio & Goel, 2012):

- The source and use of monies are controlled solely by the government.
- The government controls the money, but the private sector controls how the money is used.

- The private sector controls the money, but the government controls how the money is used.
- The private sector controls the money and how it is used.

When the government provides the funding and controls the use, the monies come from taxes, user fees (e.g., license fees and purchase of alcohol/cigarettes), and charges to consumers of the services.

Services offered at the federal government level include the following:

- Policy-making
- Public health protection
- Collecting and sharing information about U.S. health care and delivery systems
- Building capacity for population health
- Direct care services

Select examples of services offered at the state and local levels include the following:

- Environmental health monitoring
- Population health planning
- Disaster management
- Preventing communicable and infectious diseases
- Direct care services (see Chapter 46 for more examples)

When the government provides the money but the private sector decides how it is used, the money comes from business and individual tax savings related to private spending for illness prevention care. When a business provides disease prevention and health promotion services to its employees and sometimes families, such as immunizations, health screenings, and counseling, the business taxes owed to the government are reduced. This is considered a means by which the government provides money through tax savings to businesses to use for population health care.

When the private sector provides the money but the government decides how it is used, either voluntarily or involuntarily, the money is used for preventive care services for specific populations. A voluntary example is the private contributions made to reaching *Healthy People 2020* goals. An involuntary example is the Occupational Safety and Health Administration requiring industry to provide the financing to adhere to certain safety standards for use of machinery, air quality, ventilation, and eyewear protection to reduce disease and injury. This, for example, has the effect of reducing occupation-related injuries in the population as a whole.

When the private sector is responsible for both the money and its use of resources, the benefits incurred are many. For example, an industry may offer influenza vaccine clinics for workers and families that may lead to "herd immunity" in the community (see Chapter 13 on epidemiology). A business or community may institute a no-smoking policy that reduces the risk of smoking-related illnesses for workers, family, and the consumers of the business's services. A voluntary philanthropic organization may give a local community money to provide services for assisting low-income communities with improving their environment (Sessions et al., 2016).

These are but a few examples of how public health services and the ensuring of a healthy population are not only government related. The partnerships between government and the private sector are necessary to improve the overall health status of populations. This partnership was emphasized in the ACA enacted in 2010. A main feature of the public health ACA coverage included the "individual mandate" that all citizens acquire coverage providing the Ten Essential Health Benefits. Because all individuals were required to purchase coverage, persons previously excluded from insurance coverage were able to get coverage regardless of preexisting conditions. By requiring all people to obtain coverage, actuarial risk would be spread among all insured individuals receiving coverage; this would prevent cost shifting from the insured to the uninsured (Feldstein, 2015). This partnership between government regulating health insurance policies and the private insurance marketplace began to unravel after the 2016 presidential election with the President and Congress vowing to "repeal and replace" the ACA.

Toward the end of 2017, Congress's efforts to repeal and replace the ACA were not immediately successful, and insurance companies had to publish their policies and rates for group employers for the coming year. A pull-back in government funding for marketplace advertising and navigators to assist individuals with marketplace health insurance policies, as well as a shortened enrollment period, resulted in some eligible individuals not obtaining marketplace coverage (Jost, 2018a). During December 2017 Congress passed a tax bill that included a provision to repeal the individual mandate by removing the penalty on individuals who do not purchase health insurance. This provision was set to go into effect in 2019, and, according to a Kaiser Family Foundation poll in March 2018, it will not be a reason to drop health insurance coverage (Kaiser Family Foundation, 2018a). Without the individual mandate, costs of coverage for health insurance were expected to increase due to the pool of covered individuals being in poorer health. Individuals unable to afford insurance may not be covered, and the Ten Essential Health Benefits, which were responsible for some of the increased cost of coverage under the ACA, were no longer required, and insurance policies with fewer covered benefits were being sold (Jost, 2017, 2018b). This disproportionately affects the working poor, who may no longer be eligible for health insurance premium subsidies under the new rules.

PRINCIPLES OF ECONOMICS—MICROECONOMICS AND MACROECONOMICS

Microeconomics

Knowledge about health economics is particularly important to nurses because they are the ones who are often in a position to allocate resources to solve a problem or to design, plan, coordinate, and evaluate community-based health services and programs. Two branches of economics are important to understand for their application in health care: microeconomics and macroeconomics. **Microeconomic theory** deals with the behaviors of individuals and organizations and the effects of those behaviors on prices, costs, and the allocating and distributing of resources. Economic behaviors are based on (1) individual or organization choices and the consumer's level of satisfaction with a particular good (product) or service, or use of a service, and (2) the amount of money available to an individual or organization to spend on a particular good or service (its **budget limits**). Microeconomics applied to health care looks at the behaviors of individuals and organizations that result from tradeoffs in the use of a service and budget limits. A good example of an organization reducing services because of cost is the reduction in school health nursing services by health departments.

The microeconomic example of the industry providing preventive services to its employees represents a behavior by the industry that provides for the use of a service and helps the industry's budget by reducing health care insurance premium costs. The terms of the ACA (2010) allowed employers to provide incentive rewards to employees for participation in wellness programs with a goal of increasing worker productivity and promoting a healthier workforce, thus enhancing economic growth (Hall, 2010). Studies looking at the benefits of these wellness programs have not demonstrated the hoped-for reduction in health costs and absenteeism with individuals who do not currently have a chronic disease (Jones et al., 2018), although persons who are offered support in managing a previously diagnosed condition were demonstrated to improve (Caloyeras et al., 2014). A recent U.S. District Court decision determined that the U.S. Equal Employment Opportunity Commission's (EEOC's) wellness rules were coercive and did not comply with the generally accepted definition of "voluntary" (Sullivan, 2018). New rules for workers were scheduled to go into effect after January 1, 2019.

Because of the unique characteristics of health care, some economists believe that health care is special. There are debates about whether health care markets can ensure that health care is delivered efficiently to consumers. Cost-benefit and cost-effectiveness analyses are techniques used to judge the effect of interventions and policies on a particular outcome, such as health status (Feldstein, 2015).

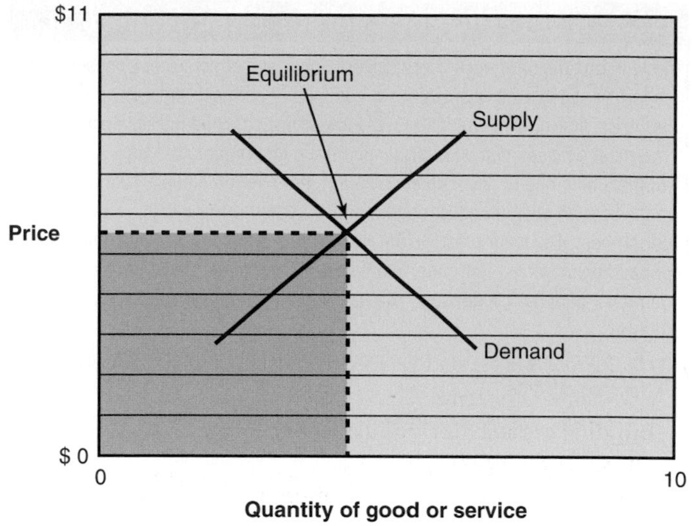

FIG. 5.1 Supply-and-demand curve.

BOX 5.1 Principles of the Laws of Supply and Demand

The Law of Supply

- At higher prices, producers are willing to offer *more* products for sale than at lower prices.
- The supply increases as prices increase and decreases as prices decrease.
- Those already in business will try to increase production as a way of increasing profits.

The Law of Demand

- People will buy more of a product at a lower price than at a higher price, if nothing changes.
- At a lower price, more people can afford to buy more goods and more of an item more frequently than they can at a higher price.
- At lower prices, people tend to buy some goods as a substitute for more expensive goods.

Data from Curriculum Link, 2010.

Supply and Demand. Two basic principles of microeconomic theory are **supply** and **demand**, both of which are affected by price. A simple illustration of the relationship between supply and demand is provided in Fig. 5.1. The upward-sloping supply curve represents the seller's side of the **market**, and the downward-sloping demand curve reflects the buyer's desire for a given product.

As shown in Fig. 5.1, suppliers are willing to offer increasing amounts of a good or service in the market for an increasing price (Colander, 2017). The demand curve represents the amount of a good or service the consumer is willing to purchase at a certain price. This curve illustrates that when few quantities of a good or service are available in the marketplace, the price tends to be higher than when larger quantities are available. The point on the curve where the supply-and-demand curves cross is the equilibrium, or the point where producer and consumer desires meet (Box 5.1). Supply-and-demand curves can shift up or down as a result of the following factors (McPake et al., 2018):

- Competition for a good or service
- An increase in the costs of materials used to make a product
- Technological advances
- A change in consumer preferences
- Shortages of goods or services

Using the example of industry-offered health care, it was not likely that an industry of fewer than 50 employees would be able to offer incentive-based on-site illness prevention services. Though the demand might be great to keep employees healthy and on the job, the supply has been limited by the cost and numbers of services available in the community. Therefore the cost is likely to be higher for the small business than for the large industry that offers its own services. The ACA required selected preventive services and screening tests be offered at no cost to the consumer; therefore they were included in the essential services covered by insurance companies because they are useful in maximizing health per dollar spent (USDHHS, 2016).

Efficiency and Effectiveness. Two other terms are related to microeconomics: efficiency and effectiveness. **Efficiency** refers

BOX 5.2 Efficiency versus Effectiveness

To illustrate the differences between efficiency and effectiveness, consider the case of a nurse who is designing a community outreach program to educate high-risk, first-time mothers about the importance of childhood immunizations. The most *efficient* method to disseminate the information to a large number of mothers might be to have the child health team from the public health department hold an evening educational session, open to the public, at the health department. The most *effective* means of offering the program might be to link public health nurses with new mothers for one-on-one, in-home counseling, demonstration, and follow-up. The goals of the program could be stated as follows:

- To change the behavior of the mothers regarding providing immunizations for their children
- To increase community mothers' knowledge and awareness of infectious diseases
- To reduce the incidence of preventable infections in the community
- To decrease the number of hospital admissions

to producing maximal output, such as a good or service, using a given set of resources (or inputs), such as labor, time, and available money. Efficiency suggests that the inputs are combined and used in such a way that there is no better way to produce the service, or output, and that no other improvements can be made. The word *efficiency* often focuses on time or speed in performing tasks and the minimizing of waste, or unused input, during production. Although these notions are true, efficiency depends on tasks as well as processes of producing a good or service and the improvements made (Feldstein, 2015).

Effectiveness, on the other hand, refers to the extent to which a health care service meets a stated goal or objective or how well a program or service achieves what is intended. For example, the effectiveness of a mass immunization program would be evaluated by the level of herd immunity developed by participants as that was the goal of the immunization program (see Chapter 13). Box 5.2 illustrates the differences between efficiency and effectiveness (Feldstein, 2015).

Macroeconomics

Microeconomics focuses on the individual or an organization, whereas **macroeconomic theory** focuses on the "big picture"—the total, or aggregate, of all individuals and organizations (e.g., behaviors such as growth, expansion, or decline of an aggregate). In macroeconomics the aggregate is usually a country or nation. Factors such as levels of income, employment, general price levels, and rate of economic growth are important. This aggregate approach reflects, for example, the contribution of all organizations and groups within health care, or all industry within the United States, including health care, on the nation's economic outlook.

When the media refer to "the economy," the phrase is typically used as a macroeconomic term to describe the wealth and financial performance of the nation as an aggregate. Health care contributes to the economy through goods and services produced and employment opportunities.

The primary focuses of macroeconomics are the **business cycle** and economic growth. Business expands and contracts in cycles. These cycles are influenced by a number of factors, such as political changes (a new president is elected), policy changes (new legislation is implemented, such as the PPACA of 2010), knowledge and technology advances (a new vaccine to treat a new strain of influenza is placed on the market), or simply the belief by a recognized business leader that the cycle is or should be shifting (e.g., when the head of the Federal Reserve Board changes interest rates).

The **human capital** approach is a measure of macroeconomic theory (Goodwin et al., 2014). In this approach, improving population qualities, such as aggregate health, are a focus for developing and spending money on goods and services because health is valued and it increases productivity, enhances the income-earning ability of people, and improves the economy. Therefore there is a positive rate of return on the "investment in human capital."

The individual, population, community, and nation all benefit. If the population is healthy, premature morbidity and mortality are reduced, chronic disease and disability are reduced, and economic losses to the nation are reduced. As an example, more people can work and be productive because they are healthy. The employing company makes more money because people are more productive. More taxes are paid into the local, state, and national economy, and more money is spent by individuals because they are productive, earning money, and taking advantage of the goods and services offered in their community.

Measures of Economic Growth

Economic growth reflects an increase in the output of a nation. Two common measures of economic growth are the **gross national product** (GNP) and the **gross domestic product** (GDP). GNP is the total market value of all goods and services produced in an economy during a period of time (e.g., quarterly or annually). GDP is the total market value of the output of labor and property located in the United States (Ockert, 2018). GDP reflects only the national U.S. output, whereas GNP reflects national output plus income earned by U.S. businesses or citizens, whether within the United States or internationally. This discussion focuses on GDP, because U.S. health care spending reports are based on GDP (NCHS, 2017).

Nurses face microeconomic and macroeconomic issues every day. For example, they are influenced by microeconomics when referring clients for services, informing clients and others of the cost of services, assessing community need for a particular service, evaluating client access to services, and determining health provider and agency response to client needs. Nurses who work with aggregates of individuals and communities are faced with macroeconomic issues, such as health policies that make the development of new programs possible; local, state, and federal budgets that support specific programs; and the total effect that services will have on improving the health of the community and reducing the poverty level of the population. In short, knowledge about health economics and the tools of economic assessment can enhance a nurse's ability to understand and argue a position for meeting population health needs.

Economic Analysis Tools

The primary methods used to assess the economics of an intervention are **cost-benefit analysis** (CBA), **cost-effectiveness analysis** (CEA), and **cost-utility analysis** (CUA). CBA is considered the best of these methods. In simple form, CBA involves listing all costs and benefits that are expected to occur from an intervention during a prescribed time. Costs and benefits are adjusted for time and inflation. If the total benefits are greater than the total costs, the intervention has a *net positive value* (NPV). Future or continued funding is given to the intervention with the highest NPV. This technique provides a way to estimate overall program and social benefits in terms of net costs. A good example of using CBA would be the cost of an influenza vaccine mass immunization program in a community. If most people in the community are vaccinated and the rate of influenza is low or decreased from past years or in relation to the national average, the benefits are many. Citizens can work, play, go to school, participate in other community activities, and, again, be productive. The community is healthy. These are but a few of the benefits of this program.

CBA requires that all costs and benefits be known and quantifiable in dollars; herein lies the major problem with its use. Although it is fairly easy to estimate the direct dollar costs of a health care program, it is often very difficult to quantify the non-dollar benefits and indirect costs. For example, benefits and costs could come in the form of increased income and expenses, which are easy to measure. More difficult to measure are benefits such as improved community welfare resulting from a particular program and the costs to the community that would result if the program did not exist. The value of *potential lives* lost because of lack of access to health care services is one example. The potential for a great number of lives saved from vaccine effectiveness against seasonal flu in 2014–2015 found the following:

- Less than 20% of "medically attended illnesses" were caused by influenza virus
- Vaccination prevented 11,000–144,000 influenza-associated hospitalizations
- Vaccination prevented 300–4000 influenza associated deaths

The effectiveness of that season's influenza vaccine saved a substantial number of lives and prevented an even greater number of hospitalizations that would have resulted in missed work/school days as well as lower productivity on the job. A side benefit was the saving of dollars for care because funds were invested in vaccines and campaigns to promote vaccination (CDC, 2018).

CEA expresses the net direct and indirect costs and cost savings in terms of a defined health outcome. The total net costs are calculated and divided by the number of health outcomes. Although the data required for CEA are the same as for CBA, CEA does not require that a dollar value be put on the outcome (e.g., on an outcome such as quality of life). CEA is best used when comparing two or more strategies or interventions that have the same health outcome in the population. Both CEA and CBA are useful to nurses as they conduct community needs analyses and develop, propose, implement, and evaluate programs to meet community health needs. In both cases the cost of a particular program or intervention is examined relative to the money spent and outcomes achieved. Using the same example of the mass immunization program, a comparison of the overall outcomes of the client visit to the clinic for vaccination in one community versus the mass immunization program at the community center in another community could be done. Outcomes could be the percentage of the population vaccinated by each method and the rate of influenza in each community. In this process, if the higher-cost program results in lower rates of illness, then that program would be considered the most effective.

An objective commonly used when CEA is performed in health care is improvement in **quality-adjusted life-years** (QALYs) for clients. QALYs are the sum of years of life multiplied by the quality of life in each of those years. The QALY assigns a value, ranging between 0 (death) and 1 (perfect health), to reflect quality of life during a given period of years (Feldstein, 2015). In conducting a CEA, the cost of a program or an intervention is compared with real or expected improvements in clients' quality of life. The How To box lists the steps involved in conducting a CEA. The QALY is often used in malpractice suits to determine money awarded to clients who have been injured by health care.

HOW TO Do a Cost-Effectiveness Analysis (CEA)

In a cost-effectiveness analysis (CEA), the outcome of the service option is measured in a natural, nonmonetary unit such as years of life gained, therapeutic successes such as reducing the numbers of influenza cases in a community, or lives saved. Results are expressed as the net cost required to produce one or each of the outcomes. The relation between cost and outcome is expressed as a ratio of cost per unit of outcome, where the numerator is a monetary value corresponding to the net expenditure of resources and the denominator is the net improvement in health expressed in nonmonetary terms. The steps for performing a simplified CEA for influenza prevention are as follows:

1. Establish a program or service goals and objectives.
2. Consider all possible alternatives to achieve the goal or objectives, which could mean comparing two different programs that are attempting to achieve the same outcome.
3. Measure net effects to reflect a change in health status or health outcome.
4. Analyze costs for each alternative or program for reducing the cases of influenza in a community, such as a mass immunization clinic for a total community population or having individuals choose to go to their private provider for the vaccine.
5. Combine CEA results with other types of information such as past results of a similar program in a different year and the change in influenza cases in the community for the year of the comparison of programs, not included in the CEA, to make the most appropriate therapeutic or policy decision.

Depending on the program or intervention goals, the most effective means of providing a service is not necessarily the least costly, particularly in the short run. This is particularly true in public health, where the cost-effectiveness of a preventive service may not be known until sometime in the future. For example, the total cost savings of a community no-smoking program might be difficult to project 10 years into the future. After 10 years the number of lung cancer cases or deaths that have occurred can be compared with those in the 10 years before the program, and the cost-effectiveness of the no-smoking program can be shown. Trust for America's Health (2018), along with several other organizations, is publishing reports that show positive results and cost savings from prevention programs. Investing just $10 per person in evidence-based community health programs to increase physical activity, improve nutrition, and reduce tobacco use could result in $16 billion each year in savings. This represents a return of $5.06 for every $1 spent on the programs (Trust for America's Health, 2018).

FACTORS AFFECTING RESOURCE ALLOCATION IN HEALTH CARE

The distribution of health care services is affected largely by the way in which health care is financed in the United States. Third-party coverage, whether public or private, greatly affects the distribution of health care. Also, socioeconomic status affects health care consumption, because it determines the ability to purchase insurance or to pay directly out-of-pocket for care. A description of the effects of barriers to health care access and the effects of **health care rationing** on the distribution of health care follow.

Early results after passage of the ACA in 2010 demonstrated that by 2016 when the major components of expanded coverage went into effect, the number of individuals with health insurance had increased (Barnett & Berchick, 2017). These increases were a result of several provisions of the ACA: (1) coverage regardless of preexisting condition, (2) young adults could retain coverage under parents until age 26, (3) voluntary expansion of Medicaid by states to include a greater percentage of the low-income population, (4) subsidies for qualifying individuals buying coverage on the marketplace, (5) availability of coverage outside of employment or government programs through the insurance marketplace, (6) mandated minimum coverage for certain conditions and prevention services, and (7) no lifetime cap on benefits (PL111-148, 2010).

By early 2018, effects of threatening the repeal of key aspects of the ACA by the president and Congress resulted in a robust enrollment in exchange policies; however, changes to the enrollment process with less marketing, fewer dollars for navigators, and a shorter window to enroll led many to fail to obtain coverage by the open enrollment deadline; enrollment in 2018 did not surpass that of 2017 (Jost, 2018a).

The Uninsured

In 1996, 68% of the total U.S. population had private health insurance. An additional 15% received insurance through public programs, and 17%, or 37 million, were uninsured. In 2008 the number of uninsured persons had increased to 47 million. By 2012 the number had grown to 48 million citizens (DeNavas-Walt et al., 2013). The uninsured landscape changed dramatically from 2013 to 2016 once the full implementation of the ACA went into effect in 2014. In 2013, 41.7 million individuals were uninsured; by 2016 there had been a steady increase in the number of individuals covered by health insurance, and the uninsured rate had dropped to 28 million individuals. The percentage of uninsured dropped from 13.3% in 2013 to 8.7% in 2016 (Barnett & Berchick, 2017).

Historically, the typical uninsured person was a member of the workforce or a dependent of this worker. Uninsured workers were likely to be in low-paying jobs, part-time or temporary jobs, or jobs at small businesses (Garfield, 2019). People of color have been more likely to be uninsured than non-Hispanic whites (Kaiser Family Foundation, 2017b). Until the ACA these uninsured workers had not been able to afford to purchase health insurance, or their employers may not have offered health insurance as a benefit. Others who were typically uninsured were young adults (especially young men), minorities, persons less than 65 years of age in good or fair health, and the poor or near poor. These individuals may have been unable to afford insurance, may have lacked access to job-based coverage, or, because of their age or good health status, may not have perceived the need for insurance. Eligibility requirements for Medicaid meant the poor were more likely to be insured than the "near poor" also called the "working poor". As changes occur in the federal support of the ACA and other health insurance initiatives, these individuals may once again find themselves uninsured (Paradise, 2017).

Socioeconomic status is inversely related to mortality and morbidity for almost every disease. Poor Americans with an income below the poverty level have a mortality rate several times greater than that of middle-income Americans, even after accounting for age, sex, race, education, and risky health behaviors (e.g., smoking, drinking, obesity, and lack of exercise) (Robert Wood Johnson Foundation, 2013; Buettgens, 2018). Historically, the link between poor health and socioeconomic status resulted from poor housing, malnutrition, inadequate sanitation, and hazardous occupations. Today, explanations include the cumulative effects of a number of characteristics that explain the concept of poverty. These characteristics include (1) low educational levels, (2) unemployment or low occupational status (blue-collar or unskilled laborer), (3) low wages, (4) being a child or an older person over the age of 65 years, or (5) being a member of a minority group (NCHS, 2012). Additionally, mental illness as a causal factor in morbidities and early mortality is a recognized mortality risk factor with the mentally ill dying 15–30 years earlier than their counterparts without mental illness (Thornicroft, 2011).

Access to Health Services

Access to health services is a public health issue (Wesson et al., 2018; AHRQ, 2017). Medicaid is intended to improve access to health care for the poor. Although persons with Medicaid have improved access to health care compared with the uninsured, Medicaid recipients have difficulty obtaining mental health services from psychiatrists and dental services when compared to the privately insured (Paradise, 2017). Uninsured individuals have far worse access and outcomes. When Medicaid covers pregnant women and children, the results are impressive and include reduced teen mortality, reduced disability, improved long-run educational attainment, and fewer emergency department and hospital visits. It remains to be seen how the proposals put forth in the American Health Care Act (AHCA) to cap Medicaid funding to states as well as impose lifetime caps on funding for services will affect individual insurance coverage and population health (Kaiser Family Foundation, 2017a).

The primary reasons for delay, difficulty, or failure to access care included the inability to afford health care as well as a variety of insurance-related reasons, including the insurer not approving, covering, or paying for care; the client having preexisting conditions; and physicians not participating in some insurance plans. Other barriers include lack of transportation, physical barriers, communication problems, child care needs, lack of time or information, and refusal of services by providers. In addition, lack of after-hours care, long office waits, and long travel distance are cited as access barriers. Community characteristics also contribute to individuals' ability to access care. For example, the limited prevalence of managed care and the limited number of safety net providers, as well as the wealth and size of the community, affect accessibility. There is an increasing awareness that culturally congruent health care providers or at least a guarantee of preferred language services are important for some individuals when accessing health care.

Because reimbursement for services provided to Medicaid recipients has been low, physicians are effectively discouraged from serving this population. Although physicians can respond to monetary incentives in client selection, emergency departments are required by law to stabilize every client regardless of ability to pay. Emergency department copayments are modest and are frequently waived if the client is unable to pay; additionally, the hours of operation are convenient for people who work during business hours. Thus low out-of-pocket costs have provided incentives for Medicaid clients and the uninsured to use emergency departments for primary care services.

Poverty level income is adjusted annually for each state by the federal government to indicate how much money an individual or families may earn to qualify for subsidies such as food stamps, Medicaid, and the Children's Health Insurance Program (CHIP). In 2018 the federal poverty level for an individual was $12,140; for a family of four the poverty level was $25,100. If, for example, an individual's income was 133% of the poverty level, then that individual earned no more than $16,146.20 (USDHHS, 2018).

Rationing Health Care

Rationing health care in any form implies reduced access to care and potential decreases in acceptable quality of services offered. For example, health providers may refuse to accept Medicare or Medicaid clients, restrict the appointments available to individuals with these forms of payment, or limit the percent of their patient panel enrolled in these benefits; all are forms of rationing. As with access to care, rationing health care is a public health issue. Where care is not provided, the public health system and nurses must ensure that essential clinical services are available. Managed care was thought to offer the possibility of more appropriate health care access and better-organized care to meet basic health care needs of the total population. A shift in the general approach to health care from a reactive, acute-care orientation toward a proactive, primary prevention orientation has been necessary for some time to achieve not only a more cost-effective but also a more equitable health care system in the United States.

The ACA, while providing coverage to more people, did not eliminate rationing because the law provided for five plans (bronze, silver, gold, platinum, and catastrophic). Each plan had different amounts and types of out-of-pocket spending such as premiums, co-pays, deductibles, and coinsurance. The state-based American Health Benefit Exchanges provided persons with differing levels of income subsidies to reduce out-of-pocket expenses based on income up to 400% of the poverty level, and some received tax credits and subsidies to assist with out-of-pocket expenses. Benefits varied by state (National Council of State Legislatures, 2014). New proposals under the American Health Care Act (AHCA) passed by Congress in 2017 offered a variety of health plans with a range of premiums. Co-pays and out-of-pocket costs will come with restricted health coverage based on individual selection and will result in its own form of rationing based on an individual's ability to pay for covered and uncovered care. This discussion has already resulted in Idaho's offering plans that do not meet ACA guidelines but do meet AHCA guidelines (Jost, 2018b).

Healthy People 2020

Healthy People 2020 goals are examples of strategies to provide better health care access for all people. The Levels of Prevention box shows the levels of economic prevention strategies.

LEVELS OF PREVENTION

Economic Prevention Strategies

Primary Prevention
Work with legislators and insurance companies to support Affordable Care Act coverage for health promotion services to reduce the risk of disease.

Secondary Prevention
Encourage clients who are pregnant to participate in prenatal care and Women, Infants, and Children (WIC) programs to increase the number of healthy babies and reduce the costs related to preterm baby care and pregnancy complications.

Tertiary Prevention
Participate in home visits to mothers who are at risk for neglecting or abusing babies to reduce the costs related to abuse and neglect by providing guidance and education on newborn and postpartum care.

PRIMARY PREVENTION

Society's investment in the health care system has been based on the premise that more health services will result in better health, but non–health care factors also have an effect. Of the major factors that affect health—personal biology and behavior (or lifestyle), environmental factors and policies (including physical, social, health, cultural, and economic environments), social networks, living and working conditions, and the health care system—medical services are said to have the least effect. Behavior and lifestyle have been shown to have the greatest effect on longevity, with the environment and biology accounting for the greatest effect on the development of all illnesses (National Prevention Council, 2011; NCHS, 2012; HP 2020, 2018).

The U.S. Department of Health and Human Services (USDHHS) has argued that a higher value should be placed on primary prevention. The goal of this approach is to preserve and maximize *human capital* by investing in primary prevention and public health efforts that reduce disease and disability (e.g., Alzheimer's disease prevention, fall prevention, promotion of breastfeeding, heart disease prevention). An emphasis on primary prevention may reduce dollars spent and increase quality of life and longevity. Funding is provided through the PPHF (USDHHS, 2016).

The return on investment in primary prevention through gains in human capital has not been acknowledged in the past, unfortunately. As a consequence, large investments in primary prevention and public health care have not been made. Reasons given for this lack of emphasis on prevention in clinical practice and lack of financial investment in prevention include the following:

- Provider uncertainty about which clients should receive services and at what intervals
- Lack of information about preventive services
- Negative attitudes about the importance of preventive care
- Lack of time for delivery of preventive services
- Delayed or absent feedback regarding success of preventive measures
- Less reimbursement for these services than curative services
- Lack of organization to deliver preventive services
- Lack of use of services by the poor and elderly
- More out-of-pocket expenses for the poor and those who lack health insurance

A focus on prevention theoretically means reducing the need for and use of medical, dental, hospital, and health provider services. Under **fee-for-service** payment arrangements, this would mean that the health care system, the largest employer in the United States, would be reduced in size and would become less profitable. However, with the increasing costs of health care and consumer demand and the changes in financing mechanisms, there is a new trend toward financing more preventive care services as was reflected in the ACA coverage for these services. This trend is based on decades of research into modifiable risks factors associated with the leading causes of death. On the other hand, the millions of Americans with chronic disease and disability are not going to disappear just because the system is more focused on prevention. It is possible that the chronically ill will benefit from a proactive emphasis on prevention, but diseases and disabilities will still have to be treated and managed.

Today, third-party payers cover preventive services, recognizing that the growth of a disease-focused health care system can no longer be supported. Under capitated health plans, health care providers are incentivized to earn money by keeping clients healthy and reducing unnecessary health care use. Through combining client interests with financial interests of the health care industry, primary prevention and public health can be raised to the status and priority currently held by acute care and chronic care. Despite difficulties, methods for determining prevention effectiveness, such as CEAs and CBAs, are becoming standard and used more widely. Two agendas for preventive services have been published that promote the disease prevention agenda:

- The U.S. Preventive Services Task Force Recommendations for Primary Care Practice (Agency for Healthcare Research and Quality [AHRQ], 2019) for clinicians in primary care, which outlines the regular screening and risk factors to identify at various ages
- *The Community Guide* (USDHHS, n.d.), which emphasizes population-level interventions to promote primary prevention

Regardless of the method, prevention-effectiveness analyses (PEAs) are outcome oriented. This area of research seeks to link interventions with health outcomes and economic outcomes and to reveal the tradeoffs between the two. In theory, support for increasing national investment in primary prevention is sound and long-standing. Since the public health movement of the mid-nineteenth century, public health officials, epidemiologists, and nurses have been working to advance the agenda of primary prevention to the forefront of the health care industry. Today, these efforts continue across several disciplines, in both the public and the private sectors, through the efforts for health care reform (Healthy People 2020 box).

HEALTHY PEOPLE 2020

Objectives Related to Access to Health Services

- **AHS-1:** Increase the proportion of persons with health insurance.
- **AHS-2:** (Developmental) Increase the proportion of insured persons with coverage for clinical preventive services.
- **AHS-6:** Reduce the proportion of individuals that experience difficulties or delays in obtaining necessary medical care, dental care, or prescription medicines.

THE CONTEXT OF THE U.S. HEALTH CARE SYSTEM

The U.S. health care system is a diverse collection of industries that are involved directly or indirectly in providing health care services. The major players in the industry are the health professionals who provide health care services, pharmacy and equipment suppliers, insurers (public/government and private), managed care plans (health maintenance organizations [HMOs], preferred provider organizations [PPOs]), and other groups, such as educational institutions, consulting and research firms, professional associations, and trade unions (see Chapter 3). Today, the health care industry is large, and its characteristics and operations differ between rural and urban geographic areas.

In the twenty-first century, health policy and national politics reflect the importance of health care delivery in the general economy. Conflicts arise between competing special-interest groups that have different goals and objectives when it comes to the producing and consuming of health services. To some degree this is caused by federal and state policy changes about how health services are financed (public and private).

Fig. 5.2 illustrates the four basic components that make up the framework of health services delivery: service needs and intensity, facilities, technology, and labor. **Intensity** is the extent of use of technologies, supplies, and health care services by or

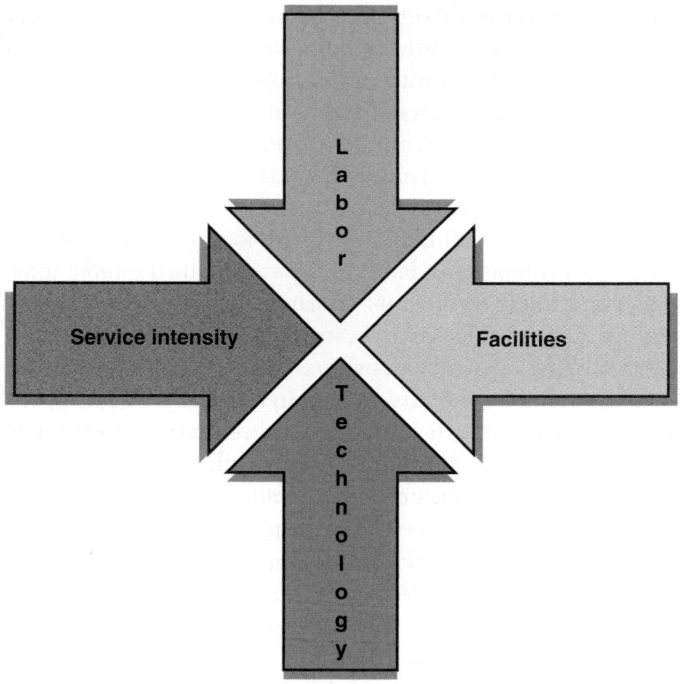

Fig. 5.2 Components of health services development.

for the client. Intensity includes and is a partial measure of the use of technology (NCHS, 2012). **Medical technology** refers to the set of techniques, drugs, equipment, and procedures used by health care professionals in delivering medical care to individuals. It also includes information technology and the system within which such care is delivered (NCHS, 2012).

Health care systems have developed in three phases from the 1700s through 2019. These developmental stages correspond to different economic conditions. Developmentally, the four components of the health services delivery framework have changed over time, reflecting macrolevel, or societal, changes in morbidity and mortality, national health policy, and economics (Fig. 5.3).

The Preindustrial Era

The first developmental era (1760s to 1880s) was characterized by epidemics of infectious diseases, such as cholera, typhoid, smallpox, influenza, malaria, and yellow fever. Health concerns of the time related to social and public health issues, including contaminated food and water supplies, inadequate sewage disposal, and poor housing conditions. The practice of medicine was unregulated and the quality uneven (Shi & Singh, 2019). Family and friends provided most health care in the home. Hospitals were few in number and suffered from overcrowding, disease, and unsanitary conditions. Sick persons who were cared for in hospitals often died as a result of these conditions. Most people avoided being cared for in a hospital unless there was no alternative. In this first developmental era, health care was paid for by individuals who could afford it, through bartering with physicians or through charity from individuals or organizations. The first county health departments were established in 1908.

Technology to aid in disease control was very basic and practical but in keeping with the knowledge of the time. The physician's "black bag" contained the few medicines and tools available for treatment. The economics of health care was influenced by the types of health care providers and the number of practitioners, and the labor force then was composed mostly of physicians and nurses who attained their skills through apprenticeships or on-the-job training. Nurses in the United States were predominantly female, and education was linked to religious orders that expected service, dedication, and charity (Young & Kroth, 2017). The focus of nursing was primarily to support physicians and assist clients with activities of daily living.

The Postindustrial Era

The second developmental era (1880s to 1980s) of U.S. health care delivery was focused on the control of acute infectious diseases. Environmental conditions influencing health began to

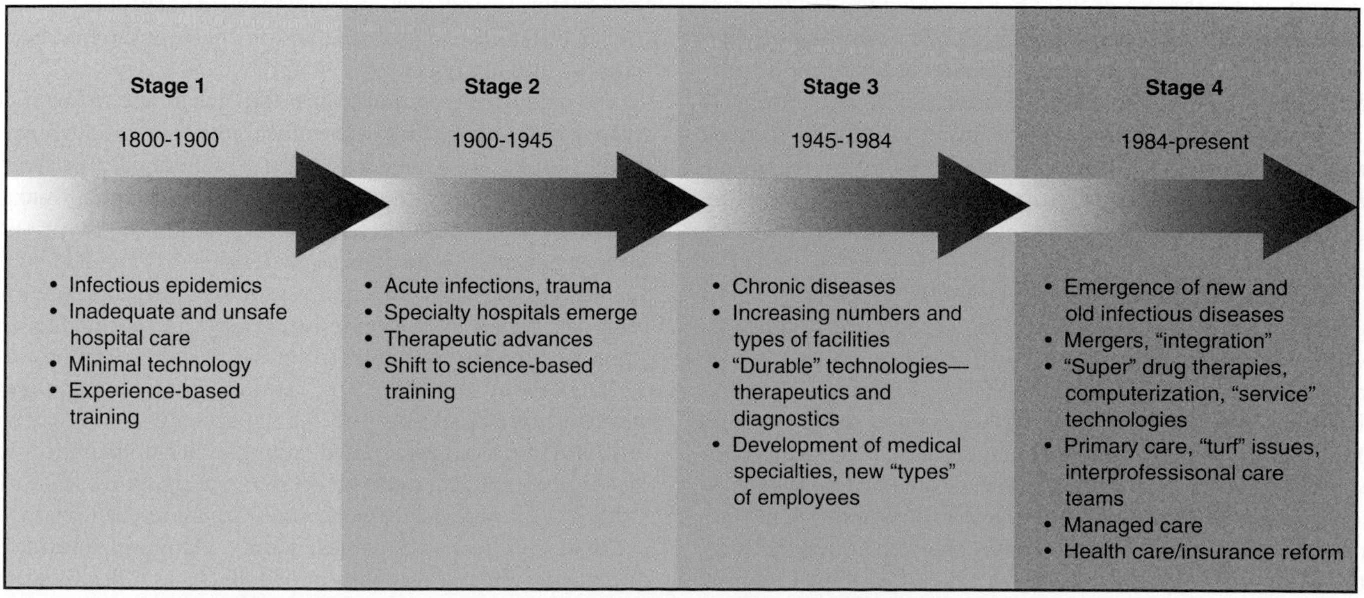

Stage 1
1800-1900
Stage 2
1900-1945
Stage 3
1945-1984
Stage 4
1984-present
• Infectious epidemics
• Inadequate and unsafe hospital care
• Minimal technology
• Experience-based training
• Acute infections, trauma
• Specialty hospitals emerge
• Therapeutic advances
• Shift to science-based training
• Chronic diseases
• Increasing numbers and types of facilities
• "Durable" technologies—therapeutics and diagnostics
• Development of medical specialties, new "types" of employees
• Emergence of new and old infectious diseases
• Mergers, "integration"
• "Super" drug therapies, computerization, "service" technologies
• Primary care, "turf" issues, interprofessisonal care teams
• Managed care
• Health care/insurance reform

Fig. 5.3 Developmental framework for health service needs and intensity, facilities, technology, and labor.

improve, with major advances in water purity, sanitary sewage disposal, milk and water quality, and urban housing quality. The health problems of this era were no longer mass epidemics but individual acute infections or traumatic episodes (Shi & Singh, 2019).

Hospitals and health departments experienced rapid growth during the late 1800s and early 1900s as technological advances in science were made (Young & Kroth, 2017). In addition to private and charitable financing of health care, city, county, and state governments were beginning to contribute by providing services for poor persons, state mental institutions, and other specialty hospitals, such as tuberculosis hospitals. Public health departments were emphasizing case finding and quarantine. Although health care was paid for primarily by individuals, the Social Security Act of 1935 signaled the federal government's increasing interest in addressing social welfare problems.

Clinical medicine entered its golden age during this period. Major technological advances in surgery and childbirth and the identification of disease processes, such as the cause of pernicious anemia, increased the ability to diagnose and treat diseases. The first serological tests used as a tool for diagnosis and control of infectious diseases were developed in 1910 to detect syphilis and gonorrhea (Shi & Singh, 2019). The first virus isolation techniques were also developed to filter yellow fever virus, for example. The discovery and development of pharmacological agents, such as insulin in 1922 for control of diabetes, sulfa drugs in 1932 for treatment of infectious diseases, and antibiotics such as penicillin in the 1940s, eradicated certain infectious diseases, increased treatment options, and decreased morbidity and mortality (Shi & Singh, 2019).

Advances in technology and knowledge shifted physician education away from apprenticeships to scientifically based college education, which occurred as a result of the *Flexner Report* in 1910. It was the beginning of medical education as it is today. Nurses were trained primarily in hospital schools of nursing, with an emphasis on following and executing physicians' orders. Nurses in training were required to be unmarried and under the age of 30. They provided the bulk of care in hospitals (Young & Kroth, 2017). Public health nurses, who tracked infectious diseases and implemented quarantine procedures, worked more collegially with physicians (Young & Kroth, 2017). In this period the university-based nursing programs were established to accommodate the expanding practice base of nursing. Client education became a nursing function early in the development of the health care delivery system.

The later part of the twentieth century ushered in a shift away from acute infectious health problems of previous stages toward chronic health problems such as heart disease, cancer, and stroke. These illnesses resulted from increasing wealth and lifestyle changes in the United States. To meet society's needs, the number and types of facilities expanded to include, for example, hospital clinics and long-term care facilities. The Joint Commission on Accreditation of Hospitals, established in 1951 and later renamed The Joint Commission on Accreditation of Healthcare Organizations (and now called The Joint Commission [TJC]), focused on the safety and protection of the public and the delivery of quality care initially in hospitals and later including home care, behavioral health, ambulatory care, and nursing homes (The Joint Commission, 2018).

Changes in the overall health of American society also shifted the focus of technology, research, and development. Major technological advances included developments in the realms of chemotherapeutic agents; immunizations; anesthesia; electrolyte and cardiopulmonary physiology; diagnostic laboratories with complex modalities such as computed tomography; organ and tissue transplants; radiation therapy; laser surgery; and specialty units for critical care, coronary care, and intensive care. The first "test-tube baby" was born via in vitro fertilization, and other fertility advances soon emerged. Negative staining techniques for screening viruses via electronic microscope became available in the 1960s (Shi & Singh, 2019).

Health care providers constituted more than 5% of the total U.S. workforce during this period. The three largest health care employers were hospitals, convalescent institutions, and physicians' offices. Between 1970 and 1984 alone, the number of persons employed in the health care industry grew by 90%. The number of personnel employed in the community also increased. The expansion of care delivery into other sites, such as community-based clinics, increased not only the number but also the types of health care employees.

Technological advances brought about increased special training for physicians and nurses, and care was organized around these specialties. The ongoing shortage of nurses throughout the century was being seen in the 1970s and early 1980s. Nursing education expanded from hospital-based diploma and university-based baccalaureate education to include associate degree programs at the entry level. As the diploma schools of nursing began closing in the early- to mid-1980s, the number of baccalaureate and associate degree programs began to increase. Graduate nursing education expanded to include the nurse practitioner (NP) and clinical nurse specialist (CNS) to meet increasing demands for the education of nurses in a specialty such as public health. The first doctoral programs in nursing were instituted to build the scientific base for nursing and to increase the number of nurse faculty members.

The role of the commercial health insurance industry increased, and a strong link between employment and the providing of health care benefits emerged. Furthermore, the federal government's role expanded through landmark policymaking that would affect health care delivery well into the twenty-first century. Specifically, the passage of Titles XVIII and XIX of the Social Security Act in 1965 created the Medicare and Medicaid programs, respectively. The health care system appeared to have access to unlimited resources for growing and expanding.

Throughout the twentieth century, many public health advances were achieved. The life expectancy of U.S. citizens increased and has been related to public health activities. The most important achievements were in vaccinations, improved motor vehicle safety, safer workplaces, safer and healthier foods, healthier mothers and babies, family planning, fluoride in drinking water, and recognition of tobacco as a health hazard (Shi & Singh, 2019).

The Corporate Era

The third era (1980s to 2019) has been a period of limited resources, with an emphasis on containing costs, restricting growth in the health care industry, and reorganizing care delivery. For example, amendments were made to the Social Security Act in 1983 that created diagnostic-related groups and a prospective system of paying for health care provided to Medicare recipients. The 1997 Balanced Budget Act legislated additional federal changes in Medicare and Medicaid. Private-sector employer concerns about the rising costs of health care for employees and fear of profit losses spurred a major change in the delivery and financing of health care. Managed care systems were developed.

This period included drastic change in the settings and organization of health care delivery. Transforming health care organizations became commonplace, and buzzwords of the period were reorganization, reengineering, restructuring, and downsizing. Organization mergers occurred at an increased rate to consolidate care, to save money, and to coordinate care across the continuum (i.e., from "cradle to grave"). Merger discussions focused on *horizontal integration,* which indicated the union of similar agencies (e.g., a merger of hospitals), and *vertical integration* between different types of organizations (e.g., an acute care hospital, long-term care institution, and a home health facility).

Initially these pressures brought about hospital closings and a shifting of care to other settings, such as ambulatory and community-based clinics and specialty diagnostic centers that offer technologies such as magnetic resonance imaging (MRI) and sonography. Rehabilitative, restorative, and palliative care, once delivered in the hospitals, was shifted to other settings, such as subacute care hospitals, specialty rehabilitation hospitals, long-term care institutions, and even individual homes. Although the location of care delivery was no longer the traditional acute care hospital, the nature of the care delivered in hospitals changed remarkably, as evidenced by the following:

- Patients admitted to hospitals were more acutely ill.
- Length of stay for patients admitted to hospitals became shorter.
- Care delivery became more intense as a result of these first two changes.
- Management of chronic illness increasingly took place in a home or community setting.

The widespread use of computers and the Internet enabled society to become increasingly sophisticated about health. The public's increasing knowledge about health care and awareness of health care advances influenced the demand for health care, such as diagnostic and therapeutic services for treatment. Furthermore, pharmaceutical companies and other technological suppliers actively marketed their products to the public through television, printed advertisements, the Internet, and other sources, so clients rapidly became aware of the new technologies.

Health professionals were increasingly dependent on technology to care for clients. Distance, as a barrier to the diagnosis and treatment of disease, was overcome through the use of telemedicine. The insurance industry became the principal buyer of technology for the client. Insurance companies often made decisions about when and if a certain technology would be used for a client problem. Nurses became dependent on technologies to monitor client progress, make decisions about care, and deliver care in innovative ways.

The shift away from traditional hospital-based care to the community, together with the need to consider new models of care, brought about an increased emphasis on providing primary care, on developing care delivery teams, and on collaborating in practice and education. The substitution of one type of health personnel for another occurred to control care delivery costs. As examples, NPs were replacing physicians as primary care providers, and unlicensed personnel were replacing staff nurses in hospitals and long-term care facilities. These replacements caused much debate, with territorial, or "turf," battles, for example, between physicians and nurses.

The increase in specialization by health professionals led to changes in certification, qualifications, education, and standards of care in health professions. These factors, in turn, caused an increase in the number and kinds of providers to meet the demands of the health care system. In the last part of the twentieth century, molecular tools were developed to provide a means of detecting and characterizing infectious disease pathogens and a new capacity to track the transmission of new threats, such as bioterrorism, and determine new ways to treat them.

The Bureau of Labor Statistics predicts that health care support and health care practitioners, as well as technical occupations, are projected to be the two fastest-growing occupational groups through 2024 (Hogan and Roberts, 2015).

Challenges for the Twenty-First Century

In the twenty-first century the emergence of new and the reemergence of old communicable and infectious diseases are occurring, as well as larger foodborne disease outbreaks and acts of terrorism. Seven out of ten of all deaths in the United States are related to chronic disease (NCHS, 2017). One in every two Americans has one or more chronic diseases. There is some concern that certain chronic diseases may be caused or intensified by infectious disease processes. Often there are complications that occur as a result of infectious disease, such as human immunodeficiency virus (HIV)/acquired immunodeficiency syndrome (AIDS) and tuberculosis, which can result in chronic lung disease and certain types of cancer because of the compromised immune system. Health behaviors and economics related to poverty are also continuing to build the path to acute and chronic health problems (e.g., the global obesity epidemic; infectious diseases related to sanitation and environmental pollution) (WHO, 2018). Those who are poor, malnourished, and live in unsanitary conditions have compromised capacity to withstand the types of bodily insults that wealthier and more robust individuals throw off with proper environment, rest, food, and health care. While some people choose to ignore behavioral factors related to obesity, such as physical activity and eating, those with insufficient income choose foods high in fat and sugar because those are the cheaper foods to obtain. They may use digital media or television as a babysitter for low-cost entertainment (Weese, 2017). The chronic disease burden is concentrated among the poor. Poor people are more vulnerable for several reasons, including increased exposure to risks and decreased access to health services. Chronic diseases can cause poverty in individuals and families and draw them into a downward spiral of worsening disease and poverty.

Investment in chronic disease prevention programs is going to be essential for many low- and middle-income countries struggling to reduce poverty. For the United States this issue was a focus of the ACA in 2010. Health promotion and protection, disease surveillance, emergency preparedness, new laboratory and epidemiologic methods, continued antimicrobial and vaccine development, and environmental health research are continuing challenges for this century. The role of technology has also intensified during this century.

Technology is now defined as the application of science to develop solutions to health problems or issues such as the prevention or delay of onset of diseases or the promotion and monitoring of good health. Examples of technology include medical and surgical procedures (e.g., angioplasty, joint replacements, organ transplants), diagnostic tests (e.g., laboratory tests, biopsies, imaging), drugs (e.g., biological agents, pharmaceuticals, vaccines), medical devices (e.g., implantable defibrillators, stents), prosthetics (e.g., artificial body parts), and new support systems (e.g., electronic health records [EHRs], e-prescribing, telemedicine, and wearable electronics for monitoring and research).

The labor force has been changing to include greater specialization in both licensed and certified providers such as radiology oncologists, geneticists, interventional radiologists, and surgical subspecialists, as well as allied and support professionals such as medical sonographers, radiation technologists, and laboratory technicians. These have all been created to support the use of specific types of technology for diagnosis and treatment (HITC, 2015).

The infrastructure necessary to support more complex technologies is also considered to be a part of health care technology. EHRs and electronic prescribing are methods for coordinating the increasingly complex array of services provided, as well as allowing for electronic checks of quality to reduce medical errors (e.g., drug interactions, best therapy for treatment based on genetics, and decision support systems). Technology applied to health and treatment is exploding whether from artificial intelligence to solve medical mysteries or 3-D printing to develop low-cost custom prosthetics, the future of technology solutions in health diagnosis, treatment, and rehabilitation is exploding (The Medical Futurist, 2017). These innovations will require different skills for the provider workforce, greater involvement of patients in their own care, and new opportunities for industry to develop, produce, and maintain these technologies.

In addition to the labor force changes just described, physicians are increasingly moving away from solo practice to group practices, selling primary care practices to hospitals, or working as hospital or corporation employees. Hospital intensivists are the standard of care in 2019, with hospitals employing physicians to be in-house and available to patients and their community physicians to cover nonurgent, urgent, and emergent care while the patient is hospitalized. More nurse practitioners and physician assistants can be found working side by side with the physician in the community and in the hospital as a member of the office, clinic team, or hospital staff. (See QSEN box about teamwork and collaboration.)

QSEN FOCUS ON QUALITY AND SAFETY EDUCATION FOR NURSES

Teamwork and Collaboration

Refers to the ability to function effectively with nursing and interprofessional teams and to foster communication, mutual respect, and shared decision making to provide quality client care.

- **Knowledge:** Identify system barriers and facilitators of effective team functioning.
- **Skill:** Participate in designing systems that support effective teamwork.
- **Attitudes:** Value the influences of systems solutions in achieving effective functioning.

Teamwork and Collaboration Question

As a strategy set forth by the ACA, a fund was established to support prevention and wellness activities within states to reduce health risks. Among the options for spending the funds was the establishment of programs and processes to reduce the rate of chronic disease.

Monies have been distributed to states to promote prevention and wellness. Find out through your state government how the money is to be used.

The Quad Council Coalition's PHN competency on community dimensions of practice indicates that beginning PHNs will collaborate with community partners to promote the health of their clients.

Have PHNs at the state level or locally in your state been involved in collaborations to determine how chronic disease rates might be reduced in your area? If yes, how? If not, can you suggest how they might be? Also, the PHN competency that addresses financial management and planning suggests that PHNs may provide input into the fiscal planning and the narrative component of proposals submitted for external funding.

Determine what the process will be for obtaining local funds for chronic disease and whether PHNs have had or will have input into the proposals.

ACA, Affordable Care Act; *PHN,* public health nurse.

Discussions are increasing regarding the integration of public health and primary care and developing the primary health care system (see Chapter 3).

Public health nurses are more involved with population-centered care, assessment of community needs, and the development or implementation of programs that meet the needs of certain populations. There is a move to provide more care to clients in the home, such as programs to provide care to new mothers and babies who are defined as at-risk. Public health nurses play key roles in developing and implementing plans for bioterrorism and natural disasters in the community.

Nursing education is seeing a dramatic change in this century. There is a recommendation to move all advanced practice nursing to the level of the doctor of nursing practice program, begun in 2000. This has the potential for closing specialist master's programs in nursing or transitioning them to postdoctorate certificate programs. This means the new bachelor of science in nursing graduate, for example, can go into a doctoral program at graduation and become an advanced public health nurse or an NP working in the community. The health care industry is one of the largest employers in the United States and, despite the economic downturn in 2008, has continued to grow. In addition, the largest number of employees in the health care industry are RNs (American Association of Colleges of Nursing, 2017; U.S. Department of Labor, 2017).

Along with other changes in health care delivery and health insurance plans, the ACA (2010) provided an emphasis on prevention and wellness by establishing the National Prevention, Health Promotion, and Public Health Council to coordinate health promotion and public health activities and the creation of the PPHF to expand and sustain these activities. It was planned that these activities will assist in the development of a national strategy to improve health, reduce chronic disease rates, and address health disparities. However, cuts to this fund through the Tax Cuts and Jobs Act on December 22, 2017, reduced $750 million from the PPHF, representing 12% of the CDC budget targeted for state and local programs (Yeager, 2018). Several states have skirted the rules of the ACA and are now marketing plans with variable coverage that do not comply with the requirements for coverage or premium parity (Jost, 2018b). A lawsuit seeking to invalidate the ACA (e.g., Texas, et al. v. United States, et al., 2018) is currently before U.S. District Court, Northern District of Texas, Fort Worth Division Court.

TRENDS IN HEALTH CARE SPENDING

Much has been written in the popular and scientific literature about the costs of U.S. health care and how society makes decisions about using available and scarce resources. Given that economics in general and health care economics in particular are concerned with resource use and decision making, any discussion of the economics of health care must consider past and current health care spending. The trends shown here reflect public and private decisions about health care and health care delivery in the past. Past spending reflects past decision making; likewise, past decisions reflect the values and beliefs held by society and policymakers that undergirded policymaking at the time.

According to the Centers for Medicare and Medicaid Services (CMS; formerly the Health Care Financing Administration), national health expenditures reached $3.3 trillion in 2016. This is compared with the $600 billion in health care dollars that were spent in 1990 (CMS, 2018a). The CMS projects total U.S. health spending in 2019 will be $3.8 trillion and $5.7 trillion in 2026 (CMS, 2018b). Health spending has outpaced increases in the gross domestic product, accounting for 17.3% of the GDP by 2009, rising to 17.9% in 2016, and projected to increase to 18.6% of the GDP in 2021. The percent of GDP can be translated into dollars per $100 spent out of pocket. In 2009 $17.30 of every $100 was spent for health care. It also means that in 2009 approximately $8100 was spent on health care for every person in the U.S. population. In 2019 it is projected that out-of-pocket costs will be approximately $20 for every $100 spent. The effect of this economic growth represents a significant increase in contrast to the approximately 13% of GDP spent between 1992 and 2001. The percent of GDP was at 17.3% in 2012 (CMS, 2017). It was projected with the implementation of the ACA that costs would actually decline due to the emphasis on prevention and early intervention in disease process. The reality after full implementation of the ACA was (1) many healthy people opted to pay the fine rather than obtain health insurance, (2) persons with poor health enrolled in health insurance coverage at a high rate, (3) the Ten Essential Services were costly to cover and resulted in higher premiums, and (4) the ACA emphasis on prevention was admirable but failed to account for all the people with chronic illnesses who expected treatment, which did not lower costs to provide care for all those covered.

Fig. 5.4 shows a breakdown of the distribution in health care expenses for 2016, and Table 5.1 shows the growth in

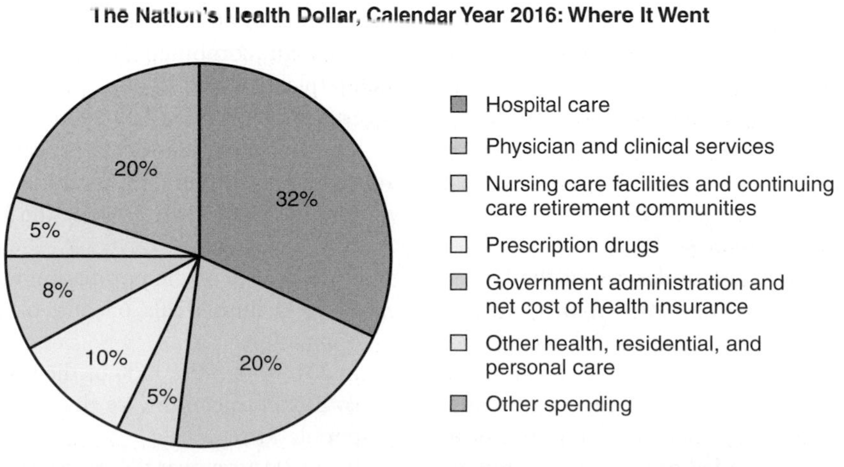

Fig. 5.4 Distribution of U.S. health care expenditures, 2016. (From National Center for Health Statistics: *National health care spending in 2016*. Available at www.cms.gov.)

TABLE 5.1 Health Care Expenditures: 1960–2026[a]

Calendar Year	Total Health Expenditures (in billions of dollars)	Total Health Expenditures per Capita per Person (in billions of dollars)	Percentage of Gross Domestic Product
1960	27.2	146	5.0
1970	74.6	355	6.9
1980	255.3	1,108	8.9
1990	721.4	2,843	12.1
2000	1,369.1	4,855	13.3
2010[b]	2,598.8	8,412	17.4
2015[b]	3,200.8	9,994	17.7
2018[a]	3,675.3	11,193	18.2
2019[a]	3,867.6	11,670	18.3
2020[a]	4,090.9	12,230	18.4
2026[a]	5,696.2	16,168	19.7

[a]Projected expenditures.

From Centers for Medicare and Medicaid Services, Office of the Actuary: *National health expenditures aggregate and per capita amounts: 1960–2016 (Historical Table 01).* U.S. Department of Health and Human Services, 2018. Available at www.cms.gov/Research-Statistics-Data-and-Systems/Statistics-Trends-and-Reports/NationalHealthExpendData/NationalHealthAccountsHistorical.html; [a,b]Centers for Medicare and Medicaid Services, Office of the Actuary: *National health expenditures and selected economic indicators: 1960–2026 (Projected Table 01 Summary),* U.S. Department of Health and Human Services, 2017. Retrieved July 5, 2018, from www.cms.gov.

U.S. health care expenditures between 1960 and 2026 (NCHS, 2018). During fiscal year 2012– 2013, the amount spent for public health activities ranged from $7.63 per person in Arizona to $144.99 per person in Hawaii (Trust for America's Health, 2014).

The largest portions of health care expenses were for hospital care and physician services, respectively, in 2011 and again in 2016. Home health care has been exceeding hospital expenditures since 2012 and is expected to rise dramatically in the coming years; it is projected to exceed physician services in terms of expenditures beginning in 2017 (NCHS, 2018).

FACTORS INFLUENCING HEALTH CARE COSTS

Health economists, providers, payers, and politicians have explored a variety of explanations for the rapid rate of increase in health expenses as compared with population growth. That individuals have, over time, consumed more health care is not an adequate explanation. The following factors are frequently cited as having caused the increases in total and per capita health care spending since 1960: inflation, changes in population demographics, and technology and intensity of services (Shi & Singh, 2019).

Demographics Affecting Health Care

Aging. A major demographic change underway in the United States is the aging of the population. Population changes are also affected by illnesses such as AIDS and by chemical dependency epidemics. These changes have implications for providers' health services, and they affect the overall costs of health care. Because the majority of older adults and other special populations receive services through publicly funded programs, the growing health needs among these populations have an effect on costs, payments, and providers associated with Medicaid and Medicare programs. The growing recognition that U.S. veterans needed more services than the U.S. Department of Veterans Affairs (VA) could provide resulted in additional funding for these individuals as well (HR 5674 VA Mission Act of 2018). As the population ages and the baby boomer generation ages and retires, federal expenditures on Social Security have increased (Congressional Budget Office [CBO], 2018a). At 78 million strong, the oldest of the baby boomers—born between 1946 and 1964—are already making demands on federal entitlement programs such as Medicare and Medicaid that will not be sustainable in their current form (see Chapter 3 for further discussion). In its *2018 Long-Term Budget Outlook* the Congressional Budget Office (CBO) reports that spending for those programs accounted for about 5% of GDP in 2017 and is projected to be 6% of GDP by 2026 (CBO, 2018b).

By 2035, in the absence of change, spending for Medicare alone (which is more likely to be affected by aging baby boomers) will be 4% of GDP, and by 2050 it will have grown to 5% in the absence of any changes to health policy (CBO, 2018b). Projections for combined Medicare, Medicaid, and CHIP plus marketplace subsidies (or whatever replaces them under AHBA) will reach 10% of GDP by 2050 (CBO, 2018b).

The aging population is expected to affect health services more than any other demographic factor:

- In 1950 more than 50% of the U.S. population was under 30 years of age.
- In 1994 50% of the population was 34 years of age or older.
- In 1990 individuals 65 and older comprised 12% of the population.
- In 2016 they were 15% of the population.
- By 2020 projections are that they will comprise 17% of the population

By 2060 those over 65 are estimated to comprise up to 25% of the population. In addition, the number of individuals 85 and older is expected to double by 2035 to 6.4 million and triple by 2060 to 19 million people because the population is living longer, healthier lives (U.S. Census Bureau, 2014, 2018).

Although many older adults are independent and active, they are likely to experience multiple chronic and degenerative conditions that may become disabling. They are admitted to hospitals more often than the general population, and their average length of stay is more than 3 days longer than the overall average. They visit physicians more often and make up a larger percentage of nursing home residents than the general population (NCHS, 2013, 2015).

Life expectancy, at an average of 78.7 years, and positive health status have been increasing in the United States. However, older adults continue to consume a large portion of financial resources. Health care providers are concerned about the growth in the older adult population because public funding sources, such as Medicare, have not been increasing their reimbursement rates sufficiently to cover inflation, and thus providers have been collecting a smaller amount for visits by older adult clients each year.

The aging of the population also spurs concerns about funding their health care because of changes in the proportion of employed individuals to fully retired individuals. Persons in the workforce pay the majority of income taxes and all Social Security payroll taxes. The funding base for Medicare decreases as the population ages, as retirement rates increase, and as the numbers in the workforce decrease. As a result, some policymakers believe that Medicare and system reforms could ensure adequate financing and delivery of health care services to an aging population (PL 111-148, 2010).

Health policy reform options being considered include increased age limits to become eligible for Medicare, **means testing** (i.e., determining financial need) for Medicare eligibility, increased coverage for long-term care insurance, increased incentives for prevention, and less expensive and more efficient delivery arrangements and care settings (e.g., managed care arrangements). One example of a policy change to reduce the Medicare program burden was the prescription plan (Medicare Part D) that was passed by Congress in 2005 and became effective in January 2006. This plan, although complicated, required most Medicare recipients to provide a copayment for prescription medications. Although controversial, the plan is thought to provide positive gains for the elderly who did not have prescription drug coverage and could not afford to pay for their prescriptions, while reducing the cost burden for those without coverage who were paying full price for prescriptions.

The ACA promised to close the "**donut hole**" coverage gap of variable prescription deductibles and co-pays for Medicare Part D participants by 2020, but Congress has accelerated the cost savings in the gap to achieve the reductions to 25% of the price of brand name and generic drugs once the deductible and the maximum out-of-pocket cost is met. Some drug plans may offer more comprehensive pharmaceutical coverage for a higher premium (CMS, 2017).

Ethnicity. Health disparities fuel some of the cost of health care in that persons who are racially, ethnically, linguistically, or gender nonconforming tend to have worse health outcomes than non-Hispanic white members of the U.S. population. The population who is two or more races is the fastest growing group followed by Asians and Hispanics; both populations are projected to double by 2060. While the multiracial and ethnically diverse groups tend to be younger, many in this category will also be aging.

- In 1900 one in eight people were a race other than white (12.5%).
- By 1990 almost one in five were a race other than white (20%).
- In the 2000s one in four people were a race other than white (25%).
- In 2060 demographers project 32% of the population will be a race other than white (U.S. Census Bureau, 2018).

This rich diversity in population will present a challenge to a health care system largely staffed with white middle class workers. To the extent that the health professions can attract persons who mirror the population they serve, health care can be provided in a way that is congruent with an individual's cultural and health beliefs (Johnson, 2018).

Technology and Intensity

The introduction of innovative technology enhances the delivery of care, but it also has the potential to increase the costs of care. As new and more complex technology is introduced into the system, the cost is typically high. However, clients often demand access to the technology, and providers want to use it. In an effort to keep health care costs down, however, payers have attempted to restrict the use of certain technologies. For example, the drug Viagra, developed for the treatment of impotence by Pfizer Pharmaceuticals, was a controversial technological advance that, as soon as it was available to the public, was in high demand and prescribed by providers. Initially use was restricted by payers because of cost. The adoption of new technology demands investment in personnel, equipment, and facilities. Furthermore, new technology adds to administrative costs, especially if the federal government provides financial coverage for the service or is involved in regulating the technology. Table 5.2 outlines federal policy that has affected technology adoption and the cost of health care over time.

Chronic Illness

Chronic illness is a factor that is driving health care spending. Chronic disease accounted for 70% of deaths in the United States (CDC, 2017) and accounted for the majority of the $2.7 trillion spent on health care in 2015 (CDC, 2017). Using Medical Expenditure Panel Survey (MEPS) 2015 data, chronic medical conditions are identified by those costing the most, the number of bed days, work-loss days, and activity impairments. Estimates are that 1% of the population ranked by health care expenditures accounted for 22.5% of all health care dollars with an annual mean expenditure of $112,395. The top 5% of population by health care expenditures accounted for 51% of health care dollars with an annual mean expenditure of $50,572. The bottom 50% of the population with low health care dollar expenditures averaged $278 per person per year. Among the top 5% of spenders the medical condition treated most often was hypertension at 53.9% (Mitchell & Machlin, 2017).

TABLE 5.2 Federal Regulations Contributing to Health Care Technology/Cost Controls

Year	Federal Regulation
1906	Prescription drug regulation: Food, Drug, and Cosmetic Act, now the U.S. Food and Drug Administration (FDA)
1935	Social Security Act (PL 74-271): Provides grants-in-aid to states for maternal and child care, aid to crippled children, and aid to the blind and aged
1938	Food, Drug, and Cosmetic Act (PL 75-540): Establishes federal FDA protection for drug safety and protection for misbranded goods, drugs, cosmetics
1946	Hill-Burton Act (PL 79-725): Enacts Hospital Survey and Construction Act providing national direct support for community hospitals; establishes rudimentary standards for construction and planning; establishes community service obligation
1954	Hill-Burton Act amended (PL 83-482): Expands scope of program for nursing homes, rehabilitation facilities, chronic disease hospitals, and diagnostic or treatment centers
1963	Community Mental Health and Mental Retardation Center Construction Act (PL 88-164)
1965	Medicare Title 18; Medicaid Title 19 (PL 89-97): Amendments to Social Security Act provide Medicare and Medicaid to support health care services for certain groups
1966	Comprehensive Health Planning Act (PL 89-749): For health services, personnel, and facilities in federal/state/local partnerships
1971	President Nixon introduces concept of HMOs as the cornerstone of his administration's national health insurance proposal
1972	Social Security Act Amendments (PL 92-603): Extend coverage to include new treatment technologies for end-stage renal disease; provide for professional standards review organizations to review appropriateness of hospital care for Medicare/Medicaid recipients
1973	HMO Act (PL 93-222): Provides assistance and expansion for HMOs
1975	National Health Planning and Resources Development Act (PL 93-641): Designates local health system areas and establishes a national certificate-of-need (CON) program to limit major health care expansion at local and state levels
1978	Medicare End-Stage Renal Disease Amendment PL 95-292: Provides payment for home dialysis and kidney transplantation
	Health Services Research, Health Statistics, and Health Care Technology Act PL 95-623 establishes national council on health care technology to develop standards for use
1981	Omnibus Budget Reconciliation Act of 1981 (PL 97-351): Consolidates 26 health programs into 4 block grants (preventives, health services, primary care, and maternal and child health)
1982	Tax Equity and Fiscal Responsibilities Act (PL 97-248): Seeks to control costs by limiting hospital costs per discharge adjusted to hospital case mix
1983	Amended Social Security Act (PL 98-21): Establishes new Medicare hospital prospective payment system based on diagnosis-related groups (DRGs)
1986	1974 Health Planning and Resource Development Act (PL 93-641): was amended and moves certificate of need program to states
1989	Omnibus Reconciliation Act of 1989 (PL 101-239): Creates physician resource–based fee schedule to be implemented by 1992, with emphasis on high-tech specialties of surgery; creates Agency for Healthcare Policy and Research to research effectiveness of medical and nursing services, interventions, and technologies
1990	Ryan White CARE Act (PL 101-381): Authorizes formula-based and competitive supplemental grants to cities and states for HIV-related outpatient medical services
	Safe Medical Devices Act (PL 101-629): Gives FDA authority to regulate medical devices and diagnostic products
1993	Omnibus Budget Reconciliation Act (OBRA 93) (PL 103-66): Cuts Medicare funding and ends ROE payments to skilled nursing facilities; provides support for immunizations for Medicaid children
1996	Health Insurance Portability and Accountability Act: Protects health insurance coverage for laid-off or displaced workers
1997	Balanced Budget Act of 1997: Creates a new program for states to offer health insurance to children in low-income and uninsured families
1998	Balanced Budget Act of 1997 (PL 105-33): Authorizes third-party reimbursement for Medicare Part B services for NPs and CNSs
2003	Medicaid Nursing Incentive Act (HR 2295): Expands direct reimbursement to all NPs and CNSs and recognizes specialized services offered by advanced practice registered nurses such as primary care case management, pain management, and mental health services
2006	Medicare Part D: Provides a plan for prescription payments
2010	Patient Protection and Affordable Care Act (PPACA): Passed and signed into law on March 23, 2010
2012	Affordable Care Act (ACA): Provides for $18 million to expand health information technology to 37 health center networks; contraceptive mandate implemented; new insurance policies must cover certain preventive services
2013	ACA: Health insurance exchanges opened to enrollment
2014	ACA: Insurers may not deny coverage based on preexisting conditions; some states expanded Medicaid eligibility; premium subsidies for qualified individuals; Congress and staff offered ACA exchange plans exclusively
2015	Physician reimbursement based on performance
2016	Veterans' health care and benefits improved
	Access to clinical trials
2017	American Health Care Act (AHCA) (HR 1628): Passed House and went to Senate for approval May 2017; sought to repeal major provisions of ACA to lower insurance coverage costs; still pending
	Tax Cuts and Jobs Act (PL 115-97): Repeals the individual mandate and turns it into a health insurance penalty fee for persons who do not obtain coverage before 2019
2018	***Proposed*** legislation related to opioid addiction and treatment: Patient access to treatment; eliminating opioid-related infectious diseases; substance use disorder workforce loan repayment; opioid crisis response

FINANCING OF HEALTH CARE

Against the backdrop of today's chronic conditions, it must be appreciated that health care financing has evolved through the twentieth and into the twenty-first century from a system supported primarily by consumers to a system financed by third-party payers (public and private). From 1980 to 2010 the percent of third-party public insurance payments (Medicaid, CHIP, and Medicare) increased from 25% to 36% of national health expenditures while the percent of out-of-pocket payments declined from 23% to 12%. For those same years, private health insurance accounted for 27% and 33% respectively. Combined state and federal governments paid the greatest percent of the health care bill (CMS, 2017).

Public Support

The U.S. federal government became involved in health care financing for population groups early in its history. In 1798 the federal government created the Marine Hospital Service to provide medical care for sick and disabled sailors and to protect the nation's borders against the importing of disease through seaports. The Marine Hospital Service is considered the first national health insurance plan in the United States. The National Health Board was established in 1879 and was later renamed the U.S. Public Health Service (PHS). Within the PHS the federal government developed a public health liaison with state and local health departments to control communicable diseases and improve sanitation. Additional health programs were also developed to meet obligations to federal workers and their families within the PHS, the Department of Defense, and the VA (see Chapter 9).

Medicare and Medicaid, two federal programs administered by the CMS, account for the majority of public health care spending. Table 5.3 compares these programs. The CMS is the federal regulatory agency within the USDHHS that is responsible for overseeing and monitoring Medicare and Medicaid spending. This agency routinely collects and reports actual health care use and spending and projects future spending trends. Through these programs the federal government purchases health care services for population groups through independent health care systems, such as managed care organizations, private practice physicians, and hospitals. Representing the shift to population health in recent years, there is a new type of provider incentivized by Medicare to be reimbursed based on achieving prevention goals and treatment targets. This shared risk group is called an accountable care organization (ACO). The members of the group agree to care for a specified panel of patients and receive reimbursement on a scale based on the number of specific metrics achieved (e.g., diabetic blood glucose checking and eye exams, flu shots, and counseling about smoking or obesity).

Medicare. The Medicare program, established in Title XVIII of the Social Security Act of 1965, provides hospital insurance and medical insurance to persons aged 65 and older, to permanently disabled persons, individuals with amyotrophic lateral sclerosis (ALS), and to persons with end-stage renal disease (ESRD)—altogether approximately 56 million people in 2016 (CMS, 2016b). Medicare has two parts: Part A (hospital insurance) covers inpatient hospital care, home health care, hospice care, and skilled nursing care (limited); Part B (noninstitutional care insurance) covers "medically necessary" services such as health care provider services, outpatient care, home health, and other medical services such as diagnostic services and physiotherapy. In 1999, Medicare Advantage plans were added to the program (Part C). This is an option that can be chosen for additional

TABLE 5.3 Comparison of Medicare and Medicaid Program Features

Feature	Medicare	Medicaid
Where to obtain information	Local Social Security Administration office or website	State Medicaid office or website
Recipients	Client is 65 years or older, is disabled, or has ALS or permanent kidney failure	Specified low-income and needy, children, aged, blind, and/or disabled; those eligible to receive federally assisted income
Type of program	Insurance	Social insurance
Government affiliation	Federal	Joint federal/state
Availability	All states	All states
Financing of hospital insurance	Medicare Trust Fund, dedicated payroll tax, trust fund interest	Federal and state governments
Financing of medical insurance	Beneficiary premium payments, general revenue, interest	Federal and state governments
Types of coverage	Part A. Inpatient, skilled nursing facilities (SNFs), home health services and hospice care Part B. Doctor's services, outpatient care, home health services, durable medical equipment, mental health services, prevention and screening services Part D. Prescription drugs from a formulary (based on plan selected)	Inpatient and outpatient hospital services; nursing facility services: home health, physician services, rural health clinic services, community health center services; laboratory and x-rays; medications as prescribed; family planning; advanced practice nurse services, free-standing birth center services; medical care transportation; tobacco cessation counseling for pregnant women; vaccines for children; many optional services are available by state's choice

ALS, Amyotrophic lateral sclerosis.
From U.S. Department of Health and Human Services, Centers for Medicare and Medicaid Services: *Medicare and you, and Medicaid benefits*, Baltimore, MD, 2017, USDHHS.

coverage. This option includes both Part A and B services. The Part C plans are coordinated care plans that include HMOs, private fee-for-service plans, and medical savings accounts (MSAs). Part C provides for all health care coverage costs after meeting deductibles, with a uniform level of premium and cost sharing resulting in lower out-of-pocket costs for beneficiaries who opt for a Medicare Advantage plan (CMS, n.d.b). An estimated 30% of Medicare beneficiaries elected Part C. New legislation in 2018 allows Part C plans to offer a wider array of services to prevent costly and avoidable procedures (e.g., allowing payment for grab bars to be installed as a way to prevent falls and broken bones), thus reducing overall health spending.

Medicare Part A is primarily financed by a federal payroll tax that is paid by employers and employees. The proceeds from this tax go to the Hospital Insurance Trust Fund, which is managed by the CMS. Part A coverage is available to all persons who are eligible to receive Medicare, with older adults making up most of these individuals. If a person did not contribute by federal payroll deductions when working, Part A can be obtained by paying a monthly premium upon reaching Medicare eligibility. There is concern about the future of the Medicare Trust Fund because projected expenses may be more than the trust fund resources. Payments to hospitals for covered services have been and continue to be higher than fund growth. Thus Medicare reimbursement policy has been changing in an attempt to control increasing hospital costs. For those with traditional Medicare, Part A requires a deductible from recipients for the first 60 days of services with a reduced deductible for 61 to 90 days of service. The deductible has increased as daily hospital costs have increased. For skilled nursing facility (SNF) care, persons pay nothing for the first 20 days and a cost per day for days 21 through 100 for an episode of care. After 100 days of care the entire cost is borne by the individual (CMS, n.d.a). Each year the deductibles must be met. The person pays zero for hospice and home health care.

The medical insurance package, Part B, is a supplemental (voluntary) program that is available to all Medicare-eligible persons for a monthly premium ($134 minimum in 2018) (CMS, n.d.b). The vast majority of Medicare-covered persons elect this coverage. Part B provides coverage for services other than hospital (physician care, outpatient hospital care, outpatient physical therapy, mental health, and home health care) that are not covered by Part A, such as laboratory services, ambulance transportation, prostheses, equipment, and some supplies. After a deductible, up to 80% of allowable charges are paid for necessary medical and other services. For mental health services, 55% of the costs are paid. Part B resembles the major medical insurance coverage of private insurance carriers. Fig. 5.5 shows the total expenses of the Medicare program from 1966 to 2016.

Since the passing of the Medicare amendments to the Social Security Act in 1965, the cost of Medicare has increased dramatically. Hospital care continues to be the major factor contributing to Medicare costs. However, because of shorter hospital stays, home health and skilled nursing facility (SNF) costs have increased dramatically. As a result of rising health costs, Congress passed a law in 1983 that radically changed Medicare's method of payment for hospital services. In 1983 federal legislation (PL 98-21) mandated an end to cost-plus reimbursement by Medicare and instituted a 3-year transition to a **prospective payment system** (PPS) for inpatient hospital services (HCFA, 1998). The purpose of the new hospital payment scheme was to shift the cost incentives away from paying for each procedure or service toward reimbursement for an episode of care. The basis for prospective reimbursement is the 468 **diagnosis-related groups** (DRGs) (see Evidence-Based Practice box). Also, the Balanced Budget Act of 1997 determined that payments to Medicare SNFs would be made on the basis of the PPS, effective July 1, 1998 (HCFA 1998). The PPS payment rates cover SNF services, including routine, ancillary, and capital-related costs (CMS, 2016a). In 2001 CMS developed a PPS for DRGs for home health with Health Insurance Prospective Payment System (HIPPS) codes. These changes in payment for services resulted in a closer attention to the cost of care provided, highlighted effective but less expensive alternatives to the usual method of care, and noted areas where higher intensity of intervention resulted in better outcomes in terms of patient function or reduced length of stay. In other words, interventions and treatment plans came under scrutiny from a cost and outcome perspective, leading to a focus on evidence-based practice.

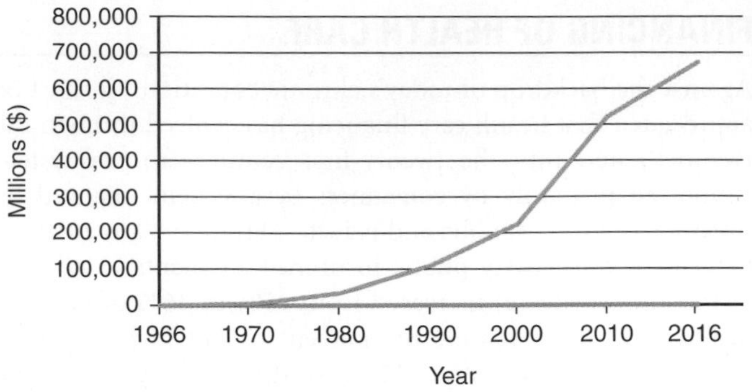

Fig. 5.5 Medicare expenditures from 1966 to 2016 (available data). (From Centers for Medicare and Medicaid Services: *National health expenditures by type of service and source of funds, CY 1960–2016.* 2018. Available at www.cms.gov.)

CHECK YOUR PRACTICE

You are walking in the hallway with a 64-year-old woman who had a myocardial infarction (MI) 3 days ago. She is scheduled to be discharged tomorrow. She is visibly anxious and irritable, ringing her hands, and talking very fast. She tells you, "My heart is pounding." You do not know if she is anxious or about to have another MI. What should you do?

EVIDENCE-BASED PRACTICE

This longitudinal cohort study followed a nationally representative sample of patients 65 years and older with and without dementia through their transitions of care from the home to the hospital and from the hospital to the nursing home. Providing effective and efficient care for this population is a priority for the United States as the disease process can be lengthy and their care needs complex as the dementia patient may have comorbidities as well as functional limitations. Transitions in care can be fraught with errors, discontinuity of care, and disorientation of the patient that result in multiple costly admissions. The study found that dementia patients experience frequent transitions between home and hospital and home and nursing home. Often (59.2%) when a dementia patient was discharged from the hospital, there were no home care services.

Nurse Use

Public health nursing initiatives, such as health education, case finding, care management, respite and other support services could significantly reduce the amount of hospital admissions in this population. Such interventions could greatly reduce the negative health effects and poor quality of life for this population. The high costs of care for the patient as well as the caregiver could be reduced with services tailored to the needs of this population and its health goals.

From Callahan, et al.: Transitions in care in a nationally representative sample of older Americans with dementia. *J Am Geriatr Soc* 63: 1495–1502, 2015.

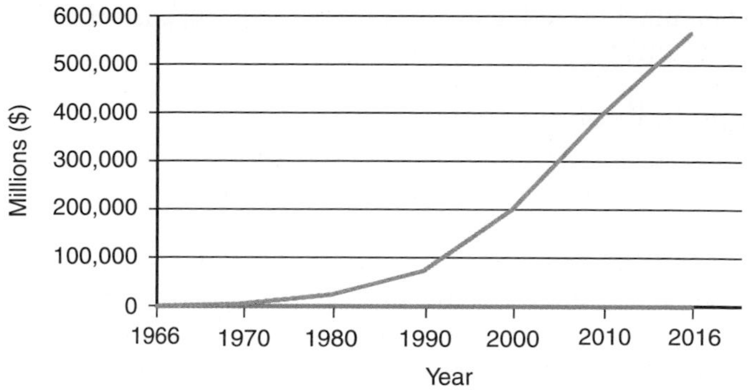

Fig. 5.6 Medicaid expenditures for 1966 to 2016 (available data). (From Centers for Medicare and Medicaid Services: *National health expenditures by type of service and source of funds, CY 1960–2016.* 2018. Available at www.cms.gov.)

In 2017 the average amount spent for services for Medicare beneficiaries was reported as $13,087 in the *2018 Annual Report of the Boards of Trustees of the Federal Hospital Insurance and Federal Supplementary Medical Insurance Trust Funds* (2018). The average out-of-pocket spending is greater for those beneficiaries who are over 85 years of age or have declining health. In 2013 Medicare beneficiaries spent 41% of their Social Security income on out-of-pocket health expenses, and this is expected to rise to 42% by 2030 (Kaiser Family Foundation, 2018b). This is because of the limits in Medicare coverage, including certain preventive care, and the limited number of physicians and agencies who accept Medicare and Medicaid payment. Older adults who do not have supplemental insurance must cover the difference between the Medicare payment and the additional costs for services.

Medicaid. The Medicaid program, Title XIX of the Social Security Act of 1965, provides financial assistance to states and counties to pay for medical services for poor older adults, the blind, the disabled, and families with dependent children. The Medicaid program is jointly sponsored and financed with matching funds from the federal and state governments. In 2018, preliminary estimates were that 73.7 million people were enrolled in Medicaid due in part to Medicaid expansion through the ACA (Medicaid.gov, 2018). Since the expansion of Medicaid under the ACA, Medicaid expansion states show a decrease in the uninsured from 2013 to 2017 that is greater than that of the nonexpansion states. Expansion resulted in a reduction in or elimination of waiting lists for home- and community-based services (Kaiser Family Foundation, 2018c).

Medicaid expenditures from 1966 to 2016 are shown in Fig. 5.6. Mandatory benefits include (Medicaid.gov, n.d.):

- Early periodic screening, diagnosis, and treatment (EPSDT) services
- Inpatient and outpatient hospital care
- Skilled nursing care at home or in a nursing home
- Rural and federally qualified health services
- Freestanding birth center services in licensed facilities
- Physician, nurse midwife, pediatric nurse practitioner (PNP), and family nurse practitioner (FNP) services
- Tobacco cessation counseling for pregnant women
- Laboratory and radiology services
- Transportation to medical care

The 1972 Social Security amendments added family planning to the list of full-pay services. States can choose to add prescriptions, dental services, eyeglasses, intermediate care facilities, and coverage for the medically indigent as program options. By law the medically indigent are required to pay a monthly premium.

Any state participating in the Medicaid program is required to provide the six basic services to persons who are below state poverty income levels. Optional programs are provided at the discretion of each state. In 1989 changes in Medicaid required states to provide care for children less than 6 years of age and to pregnant women under 133% of the poverty level. For example, if the poverty level were $12,490 (USDHHS, 2019), a pregnant woman could have a household income as high as $16,611.70 and still be eligible to receive care under Medicaid. These changes also provided for pediatric and family nurse practitioner reimbursement. States that expanded Medicaid offer premium support for individuals to purchase health coverage through American Health Benefit Exchanges.

In the 1990s states could petition the federal government for a waiver. If the waiver was approved, the states could use their Medicaid monies for programs other than the six basic services. The first waiver to be approved was given to Oregon for their health care reform plan. Other states have received waivers to develop Medicaid managed care programs for special populations. The 2010 health care reform plan provides for new approaches to offering Medicaid services and incentives for states to offer Medicaid services rather than through the waiver option as described previously (PL 111-148, 2010).

Medicaid accounts for more than half of all dollars spent on longer-term care services, which have historically been skilled nursing facility (SNF) based but are increasingly home and community based and include housing supports (Gifford et al., 2017).

Public Health

Most public government agencies operate on an annual budget, and they plan for costs by estimating salaries, expenses, and costs of services for a year. Public health agencies, such as health departments and WIC programs, receive primary funding from taxes, with additional money for select goods and services through private third-party payers. Selected public health programs receive reimbursement for services as follows: through grants given by the federal government to states for prenatal and child health; through Medicare and Medicaid for home health, nursing homes, and WIC and EPSDT programs; and through collecting of fees on a sliding scale for select client services, such as immunizations (Trust for America's Health, 2014).

In 2011 only 3% of all health care–related federal funds was expended for federal health programs such as WIC, versus 97% for other types of health and illness care (such as hospital and physician services). In addition to this 3% allotment, public health funds also come through states and territorial health agencies. State and local governments contributed 16% to public and general assistance, maternal and child health, public health activities, and other related services in 2010 (NCHS, 2013).

Other Public Support

The federal government finances health services for retired military persons and dependents through TRICARE, the VA, and the Indian Health Service (IHS). These programs are very important in providing needed health care services to these populations (see Chapter 9).

The Affordable Care Act: Public Health Support. The ACA provides for prevention and public health funds with emphasis on chronic disease. Funds are allocated to states to implement these provisions. (See Table 5.4 for more detail.) Also check the state of interest to see what that state is doing to implement this provision in ACA.

Private Support

Private health care payer sources include insurance, employers, managed care, and individuals. Although insurance and consumers have been prominent health care payment sources for some time, the role of employers, managed care, and consumers became increasingly prominent and powerful during the first decade of the twenty-first century, particularly as concerns grew about the use and changing nature of health insurance.

Evolution of Health Insurance. Insurance for health care was first offered for the private sector in 1847 by a commercial insurance company. The purpose of the insurance was to provide security and protection when health care services were needed by individuals. The idea behind insurance was that it provided security, guaranteeing (within certain limits) monies to pay for health care services to offset potential financial losses from unexpected illness or injury related to accidents, catastrophic communicable diseases (such as smallpox and scarlet fever), and recurring (but unexpected) chronic illnesses.

A comprehensive study in the 1920s by the Committee on the Costs of Medical Care showed that a small portion of the population was paying most of the costs of medical care for the majority of the people. The Depression of the 1930s, rising medical costs, and the need to spread financial risk across communities spurred the development of the third-party payment system. The system began as a major industry in the 1930s with the Blue Cross system, which initially provided prepayment for hospital care. In 1939 Blue Shield created plans to provide physician payment. The Blue Cross plans began as tax-free, nonprofit organizations established under special enabling legislation in various states.

TABLE 5.4 The Affordable Care Act's Prevention and Public Health Fund in Your State

• **Prevention and Public Health Fund** • The fund is an unprecedented investment in promoting wellness, preventing disease, and protecting against public health emergencies	• **Much of this work is done in partnership with states and communities:** • Help control the obesity epidemic • Fight health disparities • Detect and quickly respond to health threats • Reduce tobacco use • Train the nation's public health workforce • Modernize vaccine systems • Prevent the spread of HIV/AIDS • Increase public health programs' effectiveness and efficiency • Improve access to behavioral health services
• **Preventing Chronic Disease: A Smart Investment**	• **Chronic diseases: The Prevention and Public Health Fund helps states** • Tackle the leading causes of death and root causes of costly, preventable chronic disease: 1. Detect and respond rapidly to health security threats 2. Prevent accidents and injuries

AIDS, Acquired immunodeficiency syndrome; *HIV,* human immunodeficiency virus.
Since the Affordable Care Act was passed in 2010, the U.S. Department of Health and Human Services has awarded $1.25 billion in Prevention and Public Health Fund (PPHF) grants. In 2016 PPHF funding to all states totaled $624,726,012. Check your state to see what is being done to promote the public's health.

In the 1940s and 1950s, hospital and medical-surgical coverage increased. Employee group coverage appeared, and profit-making commercial insurance underwriters began offering health insurance packages with competitive premiums. The commercial insurance companies could offer lower premium rates because of the methods used to set rates. Insurance and premium setting, in general, are based on the notion of risk pooling (i.e., insurance companies were willing to risk the unlikely event that all or even a large portion of individuals covered under a plan would need payment for health services at any given time). Blue Cross used a *community rate,* establishing a similar premium rate for all subscribers regardless of illness potential. In contrast, the commercial companies used an *experience rate,* in which the premium was based on an estimate of the illness *risk* or the number of claims to be made by the subscriber (Shi & Singh, 2019).

Premium competition, the offering of health insurance as a fringe benefit, and the use of health insurance as a negotiable collective bargaining item led to an increase in covered benefits, first-dollar coverage for medical care expenses, and increased employer-paid premiums. In turn, these factors pushed up insurance premium costs and health care costs and enabled insurance plans to cover high-cost segments of the population (the aged, poor, or disabled) because of the number of low-risk enrollees.

The health needs of high-risk populations led to the passage of Medicare and Medicaid legislation. These and other national health programs targeted health care coverage for specific population groups. Because these programs directed additional money into the health care system to subsidize care, there were financial incentives to encourage the providing of services (i.e., the more services that were ordered, the greater the amount of money that would be received). Other incentives were related to the use of services by clients (i.e., the more available the payment was for services that might otherwise have gone unused, the more services that were requested).

Greater increases in health insurance premium cost as well as increasingly high deductibles have resulted in the lowest rate of coverage by workers at large employers to only 61% of those offered coverage. Cost is the often-cited factor in declining health insurance coverage. The ACA capped out-of-pocket costs for deductibles, co-pays, and coinsurance to $7150 and $14,300 in 2017 for individuals and families, respectively. Driving forces behind rising costs for care include (1) increase in the elderly population; (2) waste and duplication of services; (3) growth of technology; (4) the "health system" focus on illness treatment (more expensive) rather than health promotion (less expensive); (5) "defensive medicine," in which additional (usually unnecessary) tests may be ordered in order to cover all possible causes of a patient's complaints; (6) lack of price transparency; and (7) fragmentation of plan administration and billing (Shi & Singh, 2019).

Employers. Since the beginning of Blue Cross and Blue Shield, health insurance has been tied to employment and the business sector. This tie was strengthened during World War II to compensate, attract, and retain employees. Since that time, employers have played the major role in determining health insurance benefits. However, with the economic downturn in 2008, employers began to reduce their health insurance benefits or shift the cost of insurance to the employee. It is of interest that if a client has health insurance, the negotiated fee paid to the provider is less than the fee charged by the provider, implying that uninsured individuals pay a higher fee. Since providers are willing to accept fees lower than those charged, consumers are increasingly asking for a cash discount when an insurance company is not involved in paying for services.

In 2005 approximately 70% of the population under 65 years of age had private health insurance, most of which was obtained through the workplace (NCHS, 2005). In 2009 the percentage had decreased to about 60% (Kaiser Family Foundation, 2009). In 2005, 87% of employers paid 50% to 100% of the insurance premium (Kaiser Family Foundation, 2005). In 2009 employees paid a minimum of 26% to 36% of the health insurance premium with the employee's share of a family premium doubling in cost since 2000. For employees of small firms, the percentage of payment increased for all premiums (Kaiser Family Foundation, 2009). This substantial contribution to health care by the private business sector gave the employer considerable health care buying power in making policy about what services insurance would cover. Most older Americans were covered by Medicare; low-income children can now be covered by CHIP if enrolled by parents or guardians; and, as previously described, some low-income adults were covered by Medicaid.

After the economic downturn in 2008 employers shifted more of the cost of health care to the employees. By 2018 premiums had increased 55% since 2007 and 19% since 2012. Premiums in 2018 were projected to be an average of $6690 for single coverage and $18,764 for family coverage, 4% and 3% increases over the previous year, respectively. These increases exceed inflation, and employee wages rises are lagging behind the rise in health insurance costs (Kaiser Family Foundation, 2017a).

Before the growth of insurance (i.e., before 1930 and the beginning of Blue Cross), the health care consumer had more influence over health care costs because payment was out of pocket. Consumers made decisions about how they would spend their money, making certain tradeoffs—for example, about the type of health care they were willing to buy and how much they would pay. Entering the system was restricted in large part to those who could afford to pay for care, or to those few who could find care financed through charitable and philanthropic organizations. With the beginning of the insurance (or **third-party payer**) system, health care costs were set by payers, and they determined the type of care or service that would be offered and its price. This began to change somewhat in the 1980s with the increased use of managed care.

As the cost of health insurance has increased, some employers, in an effort to bypass the costs established by insurers, have found it more cost-effective to self-insure. The employer does this by contracting directly with providers to obtain health care services for employees rather than going through health insurance companies. Some large businesses directly employ on-site providers for care delivery or offer on-site wellness programs. These programs within the private sector offer opportunities for nurses to provide wellness programs and health assessments to screen and monitor employees and their families. This move to self-insure resulted in savings to companies and reduced overall sick-care costs (Shi & Singh, 2019).

In a truly competitive market the consumer buys goods and services at will, knowing the costs and expected value of services bought and choosing the provider of those services. In the health system where a third party pays for the services, this transaction has less meaning. The third party makes decisions about the level and type of care that will be purchased for clients and determines how payment will be made. The service provider and client have no influence on how services will be reimbursed. However, the consumer may select the payer/plan and indeed may influence the system through political channels. Increasingly, online rating scores of providers and facility statistics are available to help consumers have some information on which to base their selections.

From an economic point of view, the shift in responsibility for the cost of health insurance is not bad. In theory, this shift makes consumers more knowledgeable about (sensitive to) the price of health services. This means that they have more information for health care decision making and may consider price in making the decision to access types of health care services. Satisfaction with the quality of service rests with the person buying the insurance and receiving health care. As with employers, employees may choose health insurance voluntarily. Therefore three factors—the shifting of responsibility for health insurance premiums to employees, the changing demographics of the workforce in general, and the loss of employment due to the economic downturn—have resulted in a decline in employee enrollment in health insurance plans. Employees are choosing to use their resources to meet basic needs and are assuming the risks of having an illness for which they may have to pay. A minor health problem can lead to major medical debt for someone without health insurance (Kaiser Family Foundation, 2013). PL 111-148 includes a mandate for all citizens and legal residents to have qualifying health coverage. Employers will be required to offer coverage also, except for employers with fewer than 50 employees. These two requirements were to be in effect by 2014 unless repealed by Congress.

Given that access to health insurance is tied to employment, there was growing concern in the late 1980s and early 1990s about the employment layoffs and downsizing occurring in private business. Those who lost their jobs lost their ability to pay for health insurance and to qualify to purchase insurance privately. The Health Insurance Portability and Accountability Act of 1996 (HIPAA) was enacted to protect health insurance coverage for workers and families after a job change or loss (U. S. Department of Health and Human Services [USDHHS], 1996); Nichols and Blumberg, 1998). Although this has increased the number of people who have access to health insurance and health care, there are claims that individual premiums are high, that insurance companies have lost their ability to pool risks, and that HIPAA is just one more federal control mechanism undermining competitive market influences.

Individuals. In 2016, individuals paid approximately 28% of total health expenditures out of pocket (CMS, 2017). However, these figures do not reflect the amount of money the consumer pays in taxes to finance government-supported programs such as Medicare and Medicaid, insurance premiums, and money paid for supplemental insurance to cover the gaps in a primary health insurance policy or Medicare.

Managed Care Arrangements. Managed care is the term used for a variety of health care arrangements that integrate the financing and the delivery of health care. Managed care offers an array of services to purchasers, such as employers, Medicaid, or Medicare, for a set fee. These are called *risk-based plans*. This fee, in turn, is used to pay providers through preset arrangements for services delivered to individuals who are covered (NCHS, 2012). The concept of managed care is based on the notion that the use of costly care could be reduced if consumers had access to care and services that would prevent illness through consumer education and health maintenance. Therefore managed care employs disease prevention, health promotion, wellness, and consumer education strategies to achieve an individual's health goals (Shi & Singh, 2019). In addition to risk-based plans, wherein the managed care organization accepts a set fee to cover all costs of care for the enrollee, there are cost-based plans. An example of such a managed care organization is the primary care case management (PCCM) organization often used by Medicaid programs. These PCCMs are composed of a variety of health care providers contracted with states to locate, coordinate, and monitor covered primary care and other services on a per client case management fee payment. Whereas HMOs assume risks for the costs of care, the PCCMs do not (NCHS, 2012).

Although they seem relatively new to many clients of care, HMOs have actually been around since the 1940s. The Health Maintenance Organization Act was enacted in 1972, and since that time the number of individuals receiving care through HMOs and other types of managed care organizations has increased considerably. Managed care is based, in part, on the principles of managed competition. Managed competition was introduced in health care in the late 1980s and early 1990s to address the increasing costs of health care and to introduce quality into the forefront of discussions. Managed competition simply means that clients make decisions and choose the health care services they want on the basis of the quality or reputation of the service. To make decisions, they use knowledge and information about health care problems, care, and providers, and they look at the costs of care. However, health care is a complex market and not one in which information about health care, health problems, and the costs of care is easy to get. With the passing of the ACA (2010), accountable care organizations are being introduced as a new approach to managing care.

Health-Specific Savings Accounts. The Internal Revenue Service provides a number of ways for individuals to save or spend personal funds specifically for health care costs. The four programs are health savings accounts (HSAs), medical savings accounts (MSAs; Archer MSAs and Medicare Advantage MSAs), health flexible spending arrangements (FSAs), and health reimbursement arrangements (HRAs). These programs are designed to provide tax-advantaged monies for eligible health care costs for individuals who have specific health insurance coverage and meet certain qualifications (Internal Revenue Service [IRS], 2017). Money is contributed to an MSA by the employer, and the initial money put into an MSA does not come out of taxable income. Also, interest earned in MSAs is tax free, and unused MSA money can be held in the account from year to year until the money is used. MSAs, in theory, would allow individuals to make cost/quality trade-offs and would require that individuals become knowledgeable about health care, become involved in health care decision making, and take responsibility for the decisions made. Providers, in turn, must be willing to provide and disclose information to individuals and give up control of health care decision making. The HIPAA and MSAs are examples of health insurance reform efforts, and these efforts will very likely remain in the forefront of political discussions for some time to come, especially with the health care reform discussions.

HEALTH CARE PAYMENT SYSTEMS

Several methods have been used by public and private sources to pay health care providers for health care services. These include retrospective and prospective reimbursement for paying health care organizations, and fee-for-service and capitation for paying health care practitioners (Shi & Singh, 2019).

Paying Health Care Organizations

Retrospective reimbursement is the traditional reimbursement method, whereby fees for the delivery of health care services in an organization are set after services are delivered (Shi & Singh, 2019). In this scenario, reimbursement is based on either organization costs or charges. The cost method reimburses organizations based on cost per unit of service (e.g., home health visit, patient-day) for treatment and care. Costs include all or a percentage of added, allowable costs. Allowable costs are negotiated between the payer and provider and include items such as depreciation of building, equipment, and administrative costs, e.g., administrative salaries, utilities, and office supplies, (Shi & Singh, 2019). For example, the unit of service in home health is the visit, and the agreed-on price is a set amount of money that the home health agency will be paid for a home visit in the region of the United States in which the home care agency is located.

The *charge method* reimburses organizations on the basis of the price set by the organization for delivering a service (Shi & Singh, 2019). In this case the organization determines a charge for providing a particular service, provides the service to a client, and submits a bill to the payer; the payer in turn provides payment for the bill. With this method the charge may be greater than the actual cost to the agency to deliver the service. When the charge method is used, the client often has to pay the difference between what is paid and what is charged.

Prospective reimbursement, or payment, is a more recent method of paying an organization, whereby the third-party payer establishes the amount of money that will be paid for the delivery of a particular service before offering the services to the client (Shi & Singh, 2019). Since the establishment of prospective payment in Medicare in 1983, private insurance has followed by requiring preapprovals before clients can receive certain services, such as hospital admission or mammograms more than once a year (Kovner et al., 2011). Under this payment scheme the third-party payer reimburses an organization on the basis of the payer's prediction of the cost to deliver a particular service; these predictions vary by case mix (i.e., different types of clients, with different types, levels, and intensities of health problems), the client's diagnosis, and geographic location. This process is used in the DRG system of the hospital (Shi & Singh, 2019).

Similarly, ambulatory care services received by Medicare recipients are classified into ambulatory payment classes (APCs), which reflect the type of ambulatory clinical services received and resources required (CMS, n.d.b.). Prospective payment to SNFs is also adjusted for case mix and geographic variations (CMS, 2017).

Positive and negative incentives are built into these reimbursement schemes. The retrospective method of payment encourages organizations to inflate prices in one area to offset agency losses in another. These losses can result from providing service to nonpaying clients or from providing care to clients covered under plans that do not cover the total costs of delivering a service (Shi & Singh, 2019). The major disadvantage of this system is that little regard is given to the costs involved. This practice of charging a payer at a higher rate to cover losses in providing care is referred to as *cost-shifting.*

Prospective cost reimbursement encourages agencies to stay within budget limits and adds an incentive for providing less service to contain or reduce costs. If an organization provides care to a particular patient or group of patients and keeps the costs of delivering the service lower than the amount of reimbursement, the provider keeps the difference; however, if the provider's costs exceed the reimbursement, the provider must assume the risk and pay the difference. The major disadvantage of this method is that organizations tend to overemphasize controlling costs and sometimes compromise quality of care.

A growth in contracting, or competitive bidding, for health care services, intended to create incentives for providers to compete on price, has occurred as managed care has increased in health care markets. For example, contracting has been used by states to provide Medicaid services to eligible persons. Hospitals and other health care providers that do not have a contract with the state to provide services are not eligible to receive Medicaid payments for client care. Managed care organizations also use this approach to negotiate with health care organizations, such as hospitals, for coverage of services to be provided to covered enrollees, often called *covered lives.*

Paying Health Care Practitioners

The traditional method of paying health care practitioners is known as "fee for service" (Shi & Singh, 2019) and is like the retrospective method just described. The practitioner determines the costs of providing a service, delivers the service to a client, and submits a bill for the delivered service to a third-party payer; the payer then pays the bill. This method is based on usual, customary, and reasonable (UCR) charges for specific services in a given geographic region, determined by periodic regional evaluations of physician charges across specialties (Shi & Singh, 2019). Historically, Medicare, Medicaid, and private insurance companies have used this method of reimbursing physicians.

A major effort to regulate and control the costs of physician fees was introduced in 1990 in the Omnibus Reconciliation Act. After a study by the Physician Payment Review Commission established by Congress, the *resource-based relative value scale* (RBRVS) was established. The RBRVS method reimburses physicians for specific services provided and the amount of resources required to deliver the service. Resources are defined broadly and include not only the costs of providing the service but also the training that is required to provide a particular service and the time required to perform certain procedures, including client diagnosis and treatment. The RBRVS method of reimbursement, adopted by Medicare in 1991, acknowledges the breadth and depth of knowledge required by primary care physicians in the community to provide services aimed at prevention, health promotion, teaching, and counseling.

Preferred provider is similar to prospective reimbursement for health care organizations. Specifically, third-party payers negotiate the amount that practitioners will be paid for a unit of care, such as a client visit, before the delivery of the service, thereby placing a limit on the amount of reimbursement received per patient (Shi & Singh, 2019). In contrast to a fee-for-service arrangement, where the practitioner determines both the services that will be provided to clients and the charges for those services, practitioners being paid through preferred provider are given the rate they will be paid for a client's care, regardless of specific services provided. Therefore, for example, physicians and NPs are aware in advance of the payment they will receive to perform a routine, uncomplicated physical examination or a more complex, detailed physical examination, diagnosis, and treatment (Shi & Singh, 2019).

Capitation arrangements pay physicians and other practitioners a set amount to provide care to a given client or group of clients for a set period of time and amount of money (sometimes called per member per month rate). This arrangement, typically used by managed care organizations, is one whereby the practitioner contracts with the managed care organization to provide health care services to plan members for a preset and negotiated fee per member. The agreed-on fee is negotiated between the practitioner and the managed care organization before the delivery of services and is set at a discounted rate, and the practitioner and managed care organization come to a legal agreement or contract for the delivery and payment of services. The managed care organization pays the predetermined fee to the practitioner, often before the delivery of services, to provide care to plan members for a set period (Shi & Singh, 2019). Here the provider incentive is to treat adequately on the first patient visit to keep patients healthy and costs low.

Reimbursement for Nursing Services. Historically, practitioners eligible to receive reimbursement for health care services included physicians only. However, nurses who function in certain capacities, such as NPs, CNSs, and midwives, also provide primary care to clients and receive reimbursement for their services. Being recognized as primary care providers and eligible to receive reimbursement has not been an easy achievement. There are currently more than 250 nurse-managed clinics in the United States providing population-based preventive services, primary care, or specific wellness programs. Most are receiving financial support through Medicare, Medicaid, contracts, gifts, grants, and private donations.

Hospital nursing care costs have traditionally been included as part of the overall patient room charge and reimbursed as such. Other agencies, such as home health care agencies, include nursing care costs with administrative costs, supplies, and equipment costs. Nursing organizations, such as the American Nurses Association (ANA), have long advocated that nursing care should become a separate budget item in all organizations so that cost studies can show the efficiency and effectiveness of the nursing profession.

Spurred by efforts to control the costs of medical care, effective January 1, 1998, NPs and CNSs were granted third-party reimbursement for Medicare Part B services only under Public Law 105-33 (ANA, 1999). This new law set reimbursement for NPs and CNSs at 85% of physician rates for the same service, an extension of previous legislation that allowed the same reimbursement rate to NPs and CNSs practicing in rural areas (Buppert, 1999). This law was passed after years of work in this area, including research documenting NP and CNS contributions to health care delivery and client outcomes and after active lobbying efforts by professional nursing organizations. Reimbursement for these nurses has not changed to any extent since the 1990s.

In addition, data about the cost-to-benefit ratio, efficiency, and effectiveness of nursing care in general have been collected. Today, more than 250 nurse-managed clinics provide health care services to individuals in the United States who might not otherwise have access to health care, such as older adults, the homeless, and schoolchildren. In 2018 Medicaid reimburses for nurse midwife, PNP, and FNP care (Medicaid.gov). All of these events have moved the discipline toward more autonomy in nursing practice and are serving as a means for providing care in rural and urban areas serving our most vulnerable patients (Esperat et al., 2012; NACHC, 2013, 2016).

LINKING CONTENT TO PRACTICE

The balance of interest within society and health care will continue to shift toward a focus on quality, safety, and elimination of health disparities through public and private sector partnerships. Health care system concerns of the twenty-first century are expected to focus on examining the quality of health care relative to the costs of care delivered, reduction in disparities, access to care, and health care reform. These changes will result from continued efforts of both the public and private sectors to reform the U.S. health care system. The current era of health care delivery will be noted as a time of vast changes in all sectors of health care delivery. There will be an increased emphasis on Social Determinants of Health (SDOH) with the knowledge that 50% of health outcomes can be attributed to SDOH and health behaviors. Improving SDOH will require nurses to be involved at all levels of policymaking to advocate for education for all ages and abilities; employment; quality of the environment, including public transportation, parks, walkability, and affordable quality housing; types and quality of health services; and social support systems, including social integration and community engagement (Artiga & Hinton, 2018).

Nurses must plan for future changes in health care financing by becoming aware of the costs of nursing services, identifying aspects of care where cost savings can be safely achieved, and developing knowledge on how nursing practice affects and is affected by the principles of economics. Nursing must continue to focus on improving the overall health of the nation, defining its contribution to the health of the nation, deriving the value of nursing care, and ensuring its economic viability within the health care marketplace. Nurses must effect changes in the health care system by providing leadership in developing new models of care delivery that provide effective, high-quality care and by assuming a greater role in evaluating client care and nurse performance. It is through their leadership that nurses will contribute to improved decision making about allocating scarce health care resources and promoting primary prevention as an answer to improve many of the current population level health outcomes.

PRACTICE APPLICATION

Connie, a nursing student, has identified a caseload of five families in a chronic disease program offered by the local public health department. She is interested in assessing the costs of care to her clients and to the agency. Connie approaches the public health nurse administrator and asks the following questions:

A. How is the agency reimbursed for chronic disease management? Has the Affordable Care Act resulted in a greater number of people who can afford these services?
B. Does the client have a responsibility for paying for services?
C. Are nursing care costs known?
D. Are services rationed to clients? On what basis?
E. What effect will the chronic disease management program have on the community population?

Answers can be found on the Evolve site.

KEY POINTS

- From 1800 to 2019 the U.S. health care delivery system experienced three developmental eras, with different emphases on health care economics.
- Four basic components provide the framework for the development of delivery of health care services: service needs and intensity, facilities, technology, and labor (workforce).
- Three major factors have been associated with the growth of the health care delivery system: price inflation, changes in population demographics, and technology and service intensity.
- Chronic disease is becoming a major health factor affecting health care spending, with one in two Americans experiencing at least one chronic disease.
- Health care financing has evolved through the twentieth century from a system financed primarily by the consumer to a system financed primarily by third-party payers. In the twenty-first century the consumer is being asked to pay more.
- To solve the problems of rising health care costs, the Affordable Care Act was passed; this act also included some form of rationing.
- Excessive and inefficient use of goods and services in health care delivery has been viewed as the major cause of rising health care costs.
- Economics is concerned with use of resources, including money, to fulfill society's needs and wants.
- Health economics is concerned with the problems of producing services and programs and distributing them to clients.
- The goal of public health economics is maximal benefits from services of public health providers, leading to health and wellness of the population.
- The goal of public health is to provide the most good for the most people.
- Nurses need to understand basic economic principles to avoid contributing to rising health care costs.
- The GNP reflects the market value of goods and services produced by the United States.
- The GDP reflects the market value of the output of labor and property located in the United States.
- Microeconomic theory shows how supply and demand can be used in health care.
- Macroeconomic theory helps one look at national and community issues that affect health care.
- Social issues, economic issues, and communicable disease epidemics mark the problems of the twenty-first century.
- Medicare and Medicaid are two government-funded programs that help meet the needs of high-risk populations in the United States.

- A majority of the U.S. population has had health insurance. As of 2019 it is not mandated by law, but persons seeking insurance who have not previously been covered will pay a higher premium for their health insurance.
- The uninsured segment represents millions of people, mostly the working poor, older adults, children, and those who lost jobs in the economic downturn of 2008. Passage of the ACA in 2010 resulted in a greater number of individuals covered by health insurance.
- Efforts to repeal aspects of the ACA are underway; the impact on the number of individuals with adequate insurance is unknown.
- Poverty has a detrimental effect on health.
- Health care rationing has always been a part of the U.S. health care system and will continue to be with health care reform.
- Nurses are cost-effective providers and must be an integral part of health care delivery.
- *Healthy People 2020* is a document that has established U.S. health objectives.
- Human life is valued in health economics, as is money. An emphasis on changing lifestyles and preventive care will reduce the unnecessary years of life lost to early and preventable death.

CLINICAL DECISION-MAKING ACTIVITIES

1. Define the following terms in your own words: economics, health economics, public health economics, public health finance, gross national product, gross domestic product, consumer price index, and human capital. How do these terms relate to your work as a nurse?
2. Compare the advantages and disadvantages of applying economics to public health care issues. Be specific.
3. Compare and contrast efficiency and effectiveness of a public health program. What factors make these difficult to control?
4. Apply the concepts of supply and demand to an example from population health. Be precise in your answer.
5. Review Chapter 7. Debate in class the ethical implications of the goal of rationing. Focus your debate on the implications for nursing practice. What are some of the complexities of this question?
6. Invite a public health nurse administrator to meet with your class or clinical conference group. Ask how inflation, changes in population, and technology have changed the public health care delivery system and nursing practice. How could we check for ourselves to find the answers?

ADDITIONAL RESOURCES

EVOLVE WEBSITE

http://evolve.elsevier.com/Stanhope/community/

- Answers to Practice Application
- Case Study
- Glossary
- Review Questions

REFERENCES

Agency for Healthcare Research and Quality (AHRQ): *2016 National Healthcare Quality and Disparities Report*, AHRQ Publication No. 17-0001. Rockville, MD, 2017, AHRQ. Retrieved from www.ahrq.gov.

American Association of Colleges of Nursing (AACN): *Fact Sheet: Nursing Shortage*, 2017, AACN. Retrieved from www.aacnnursing.org.

American Nurses Association (ANA): *Medicare reimbursement for NPs and CNSs*, Silver Spring, MD, 1999, ANA.

Artiga S, Hinton E: *Beyond health care: the role of social determinants in promoting health and health equity*, 2018, Kaiser Family Foundation. Retrieved from https://www.kff.org.

Barnett JC, Berchick ER: *Current population reports, P60-260, health insurance coverage in the United States: 2016,* Washington, DC, 2017, Government Printing Office.

Bradley EH, Canavan M, Rogan E, et al.: Variation in health outcomes: the role of spending on social services, public health, and health care, 2000-09, *Health Aff (Millwood)* 35:760–768, 2016.

Buettgens M: *The implications of Medicaid Expansion in the remaining states*, 2018, Robert Wood Johnson Foundation. Retrieved from www.rwjf.org.

Buppert C: HEDIS for the primary care provider: getting an "A" on the managed care report card. *Nurse Pract* 24:84–94, 1999.

Callahan CM, Tu W, Unroe KT, LaMantia MA, Stump TE, Clark DO: Transitions in care in a nationally representative sample of older Americans with dementia, *J Am Geriatr Soc* 63:1495-1502, 2015.

Caloyeras JP, Liu H, Exum E, Broderick M, Mattke S: Managing manifest diseases, but not health risks, saved PepsiCo money over seven years. *Health Aff (Millwood)* 33:124–131, 2014.

Centers for Disease Control and Prevention (CDC): *Interim estimates of 2017-2018 seasonal influenza vaccine effectiveness—US February 2018*, 2018. Retrieved from www.cdc.gov.

Centers for Medicare and Medicaid Services (CMS): *Your Medicare coverage: skilled nursing facility (SNF) care*, n.d.a. Retrieved from https://www.medicare.gov.

Centers for Medicare and Medicaid Services (CMS): *Your Medicare Costs: Part B Costs*, n.d.b. Retrieved from https://www.medicare.gov.

Centers for Medicare and Medicaid Services (CMS): *Hospital Outpatient PPS*, 2018, U.S. Department of Health and Human Services. Retrieved from www.cms.gov.

Centers for Medicare and Medicaid Services (CMS): *Skilled nursing facility PPS*, Baltimore, MD, 2017, U.S. Department of Health and Human Services. Retrieved from http://www.cms.gov.

Centers for Medicare and Medicaid Services (CMS): *Skilled nursing facility prospective payment system*, 2016a, U.S. Department of Health and Human Services. Retrieved from www.cms.gov.

Centers for Medicare and Medicaid Services (CMS): *MDCR enroll AB 1: total Medicare enrollment*, 2016b, CMS. Retrieved from www.cms.gov.

Centers for Medicare and Medicaid Services (CMS): *Closing the coverage gap—Medicare prescription drugs are becoming more affordable, CMS Product No. 11493*, 2017, CMS. Retrieved from https://www.medicare.gov.

Centers for Medicare and Medicaid Services (CMS): *Table 01 National Health Expenditures: Aggregate and Per Capita Amounts*, 2018a, CMS. Retrieved from www.cms.gov.

Centers for Medicare and Medicaid Services (CMS): *Table 01 National Health Expenditures; aggregate and per capita amounts*, 2018b, CMS. Retrieved from https://www.cms.gov.

Colander D: *Microeconomics*, ed 10, London, UK, 2017, McGraw-Hill.

Collins SR, Gunja MZ, Doty MM, Bhupal HK: First look at health insurance coverage in 2018 finds ACA gains beginning to reverse. *To the Point: Commonwealth Fund*, 2018. Retrieved from www.commonwealthfund.org.

Congressional Budget Office (CBO): *The budget and economic outlook*, 2018a, U.S. Government Printing Office. Retrieved from https://www.cbo.gov.

Congressional Budget Office (CBO): *The 2018 long-term budget outlook*, 2018b, U.S. Government Printing Office. Retrieved from https://www.cbo.gov.

Cuckler GA, Sisko AM, Poisal JA, et al.: National Health Expenditure projections, 2017-26: Despite uncertainty, fundamentals primarily drive spending growth, *Health Aff (Millwood)* 37(3):483–493, 2018.

DeNavas-Walt C, Proctor BD, Smith JC: *U.S. Census Bureau, Current Population Reports: Income, poverty, and health insurance coverage in the United States: 2012*, 2013, U.S. Government Printing Office. Retrieved from www.census.gov.

Esperat MC, Hanson-Turton T, Richardson M, Tyree Debisette A, Rupinta C: Nurse-managed health centers: safety-net care through advanced nursing practice, *J Am Acad Nurse Pract* 24: 24–31, 2012.

Feldstein PJ: *Health policy issues: an economic perspective*, ed 6, 2015, Health Administration Press. Chicago, IL.

Flexner Report: *Birth of modern medical education*, 1910. Retrieved from MedicineNet.com.

Garfield, R., Orgera K, Damico, A: The uninsured and the ACA: a primer-key facts about health insurance and the uninsured amidst changes to the Affordable Care Act, 2019, Kaiser Family Foundation. Retrieved from www. kff.org.

Gifford K, Ellis E, Edwards BC, et al.: *Medicaid moving ahead in uncertain times: results from a 50-state Medicaid budget survey for state fiscal years 2017 and 2018*, 2017, Kaiser Family Foundation. Retrieved from https://www.kff.org

Goodwin N, Harris J, Nelson J, Brian Roach, Torras M: *Microeconomics in context*, ed 3, 2014, M.E. Sharpe, Inc. London, England.

Hall B: *A new day: what the Patient Protection and Affordable Care Act means to the incentive industry*, 2010. Retrieved from www.incentivemag.com.

Health Care Financing Administration (HCFA): *Case mix prospective payment for SNFs Balanced Budget Act of 1997*, 2018, USDHHS. Retrieved from www.cms.gov.

Health Care Financing Administration (HCFA): *HIPAA: The Health Insurance Portability and Accountability Act of 1996*, 1998, USDHHS.

Health IT Consultant Staff [HITC]: *The top 9 most in-demand medical jobs*, 2015, Health IT Consultant Staff. Retrieved from https://hitconsultant.net.

Hogan A, Roberts B: *MLR: Monthly Labor Review*, 2015, Bureau of Labor Statistics. Retrieved from www.bls.gov.

Institute of Medicine: *For the public's health: investing in a healthier future*, 2012, The National Academies Press. Retrieved from www.nap.edu.

Internal Revenue Service (IRS): *Health savings accounts and other tax-favored health plans, Publication No. 969*, 2017, Internal Revenue Service. Retrieved from www.irs.gov.

Johnson S: Can we create a fair shot at health? *Culture of health (blog)*, 2018, Robert Woods Johnson Foundation. Retrieved from www.rwjf.org.

Jost TS: ACA open enrollment starts amidst tumult, *Health Aff* 36(12): 2044–2045, 2017.

Jost TS: Mandate repeal provision ends health care calm, *Health Aff 37*(1): 13–14, 2018a.

Jost TS: Idaho's actions continue challenges for ACA, *Health Aff* 37(3): 523–524, 2018b.

Kaiser Family Foundation: *Medicare chart book*, ed 3, 2005, Kaiser Family Foundation, Menlo Park, California.

Kaiser Family Foundation: *The uninsured: a primer: key facts about Americans without health insurance*, 2009, Kaiser Commission on Medicaid and the Uninsured. Menlo Park, California.

Kaiser Family Foundation: *Employer health benefits survey*, 2013, Kaiser Family Foundation. Menlo Park, California.

Kaiser Family Foundation: *2017 Employer Health Benefits survey*, 2017a, Kaiser Family Foundation. Retrieved from www.kff.org.

Kaiser Family Foundation: *Key facts about the uninsured population*, 2017b, Kaiser Family Foundation. Retrieved from www.kff.org.

Kaiser Family Foundation: *Poll: survey of the non-group market finds most say the individual mandate was not a major reason they got coverage in 2018, and most plan to continue buying insurance despite recent repeal of the mandate penalty*, 2018a, Kaiser Family Foundation. Retrieved from www.kff.org.

Kaiser Family Foundation: *More than one-third of people with Traditional Medicare spent at least 20 percent of the total income on health care in 2013*, 2018b, Kaiser Family Foundation. Retrieved from www.kff.org.

Kaiser Family Foundation: *More than one-third of people with Traditional Medicare spent at least 20 percent of the total income on health care in 2013*, 2018b, Kaiser Family Foundation. Retrieved from www.kff.org.

Kaiser Family Foundation: *Implications of the ACA Medicaid Expansion: a look at the data and the evidence*, 2018c, Kaiser Family Foundation. Retrieved from www.kff.org.

Kaiser Family Foundation: *Beyond health care: the role of social determinants in promoting health and health equity*, 2018d, Kaiser Family Foundation. Retrieved from www.kff.org.

McCullough, JM: Return on investment of public health systems spending, Academy Health, 2018. Washington DC.

McPake B, Normand C, Smith S, Nolan A: *Health economics: an international perspective*, ed 4, New York, 2018, Routledge.

Meit M, Knudson A, Dickman I, Brown A, Hernandez N, and Kronstadt, J. *An Examination of Public Health Financing in the United States*, (Prepared by NORC at the University of Chicago.) Washington, DC, 2013, The Office of the Assistant Secretary for Planning and Evaluation.

Mitchell E, Machlin S: *Concentration of health expenditures and selected characteristics of high spenders, U.S. civilian noninstitutionalized population, 2015*, statistical brief #506, 2017, Agency for Healthcare Research and Quality. Retrieved from www.meps.ahrq.gov.

National Association of Community Health Centers: *Expanding access to primary care: the role of Nurse Practitioners, Physician Assistants, and Certified Nurse Midwives in the Health Center workforce*, 2013, National Association of Community Health Centers. Retrieved from http://www.nachc.org.

National Association of Community Health Centers: *Staffing the safety net: building the primary care workforce at America's health centers*, 2016, National Association of Community Health Centers. Retrieved from ww.nachc.org.

National Center for Health Statistics (NCHS): *Health: United States, 2005, with chartbook on trends in the health of Americans*, Hyattsville, MD, 2005, U.S. Government Printing Office.

National Center for Health Statistics (NCHS): *Health: United States, 2011 with Special Feature on Socioeconomic Status and Health*, Hyattsville, MD, 2012, U.S. Government Printing Office.

National Center for Health Statistics (NCHS): *Health, United States, 2012: with special feature on emergency care*, Hyattsville, MD, 2013, U.S. Government Printing Office.

National Center for Health Statistics (NCHS): *Health, United States, 2014: with special feature on adults aged 55-64*, Hyattsville, MD, 2015, U.S. Government Printing Office.

National Center for Health Statistics (NCHS): *Health: United States, 2016 with chartbook on long term trends in health care*, Hyattsville, MD, 2017, U.S. Government Printing Office.

National Center for Health Statistics (NCHS): *Health: United States, 2017 with special features on mortality*, Hyattsville, MD, 2018, U.S. Government Printing Office.

National Prevention Council: *National prevention strategy*, Washington, DC, 2011, USDHHS, Office of the Surgeon General. Retrieved from www.surgeongeneral.gov.

Nichols LM, Blumberg LJ: A different kind of "new federalism"? The Health Insurance Portability and Accountability Act of 1996, *Health Aff* 17:25–42, 1998.

Ockert S: *Business statistics of the United States, 2018: patterns of economic change*, ed 23, Lanham, MD, 2018, Bernan Press.

Orgera, K. & Artiga S: *Disparities in health and health care: Five key questions and answers*. Kaiser Family Foundation, 2018. Retrieved from www.kff.org.

Paradise J: *Data note: three findings about access to care and health outcomes in Medicaid*, 2017, Kaiser Family Foundation. Retrieved from www.kff.org.

Robert Wood Johnson Foundation: *Return on investments in public health: saving lives and money*, 2013, Robert Wood Johnson Foundation. Retrieved from www.rwjf.org.

Sessions K, Fortunato K, Johnson, PRS, Panek, A: Philanthropy at the intersection of health and the environment, *Health Aff* 35:2142–2147, 2016.

Schulte, T, Keating, B, Zaveri, H: *Evaluation Technical Assistance Brief: for OAH & ACYF teenage pregnancy prevention grantees*, 2016, CDC. Retrieved from www.hhs.gov.

Shi L, Singh DA: *Delivering health care in America: a systems approach*, ed 11, Sudbury, MA, 2019, Jones & Bartlett.

Sturchio JL, Goel A: *The private-sector role in public health: reflections on the new global architecture in health*, 2012, Center for Strategic and International Studies. Retrieved from www.csis.org.

Sullivan T: AARP v. EEOC: motion to vacate granted, 2018, Policy & Medicine. Retrieved from www.policymed.com.

The Boards of Trustees, Federal Hospital Insurance and Federal Supplementary Medical Insurance Trust Funds: *2018 Annual Report of the Boards of Trustees of the Federal Hospital Insurance and Federal Supplementary Medical Insurance Trust Funds*, 2018, The Boards of Trustees, Federal Hospital Insurance and Federal Supplementary Medical Insurance Trust Funds. Retrieved from www.cms.gov.

The Joint Commission: *What is accreditation?* 2018, The Joint Commission. Retrieved from www.jointcommission.org.

The Medical Futurist: *The ultimate list of what we can 3D print in medicine and healthcare!* 2017, The Medical Futurist. Retrieved from medicalfuturist.com.

Thornicroft G: Editorial: Physical health disparities and mental illness: the scandal of premature mortality, *Br J Psychiatry* 199: 441–442, 2011.

Trust for America's Health: *Key health data (by State): public health funding indicator*, 2014: Robert Wood Johnson Foundation. Retrieved from healthyamericans.org.

Trust for America's Health: *A state-by-state look at public health funding and key health facts*, 2015, Robert Wood Johnson Foundation. Retrieved from healthyamericans.org.

Trust for America's Health: *A funding crisis for public health and safety: state by state public health funding and key health facts 2017*, 2017, Robert Wood Johnson Foundation. Retrieved from healthyamericans.org.

Trust for America's Health: *A funding crisis for public health and safety: state by state public health funding and key health facts 2018*, 2018, Robert Wood Johnson Foundation. Retrieved from healthyamericans.org.

Turnock BJ: *Public health: what it is and how it works*, ed 6, Boston, 2015, Jones & Bartlett.

U.S. Census Bureau: *Fueled by aging Baby Boomers, nation's older population to nearly double in next 20 years*, Washington, DC, 2014, U.S. Census Bureau. Retrieved from www.census.gov.

U.S. Census Bureau: *Demographic turning points for the United States: population projections for 2020 to 2060 P25-1144*, Washington, DC, 2018, U.S. Census Bureau. Retrieved from www.census.go.v

U.S. Department of Health and Human Services: Health Insurance Portability and Accountability Act of 1996, Wash. DC, 1996 Retrieved from aspe.hhs.gov.

U.S. Department of Health and Human Services (USDHHS): *The ACA Prevention and Public Health Fund*, 2016. Retrieved from www.hhs.gov.

U.S. Department of Health and Human Services: The community guide, n.d. Retrieved from www.thecommunityguide.org.

U.S. Department of Health and Human Services: *Prevention and public health fund*, 2016, U.S. Department of Health and Human Services. Retrieved from https://www.hhs.gov.

U.S. Department of Health and Human Services: *Federal Register: Annual update of the HHS poverty guidelines*, Washington, DC, 2018, U.S. Department of Health and Human Services. Retrieved from www.federalregister.gov.

U.S. Department of Labor: *News release: Bureau of Labor Statistics employment projections—2016-2026*, 2017, U.S. Department of Labor. Washington, DC.

VA Maintaining Internal Systems and Strengthening Integrated Outside Networks Act of 2018. H. R. 5674 [Report No. 115–671, Part I].

Weese K: *6 things Paul Ryan doesn't understand about poverty (but I didn't, either)*, 2017. Alternet. Retrieved from www.alternet.org.

Wesson D, Kitaman H, Halloran KH, Tecson K: Innovative population health model associated with reduced emergency department use and inpatient hospitalizations, *Health Aff* 37(4):543–550, 2018. Retrieved from www.healthaffairs.org.

World Health Organization (WHO): *Global health estimates 2016: deaths by cause, age, sex, by country and region, 2000-2016*, Geneva, 2018, World Health Organization [WHO]. Retrieved from www.who.int.

Yeager A: *Cuts to Prevention and Public Health Fund puts CDC programs at risk*, 2018, The Scientist. Retrieved from www.the-scientist.com.

Young K.M., Kroth, PJ: Sultz & Young's health care USA: understanding its organization and delivery, ed 9, Jones and Bartlett Learning, 2017.

6

Environmental Health

Barbara Sattler, RN, MPH, DrPH, FAAN

"Environmental health comprises those aspects of human health, including quality of life, that are determined by physical, chemical, biological, social, and psychosocial factors in the environment. It also refers to the theory and practice of assessing, correcting, controlling, and preventing those factors in the environment that can potentially affect adversely the health of present and future generations."

United Nations University, 1993 (UNU)

OBJECTIVES

After reading this chapter, the student should be able to do the following:

1. Explain the relationship between the environment and human health and disease.
2. Understand the key disciplines that inform nurses' work in environmental health.
3. Apply the nursing process to the practice of environmental health.
4. Describe legislative and regulatory policies that have influenced the impact of the environment on health and disease patterns in communities.
5. Explain and compare the environmental health roles and skills for nurses practicing in public health, as well as those practicing in practice settings.
6. Incorporate environmental principles into practice.

CHAPTER OUTLINE

Introduction to Environmental Health
***Healthy People 2020* Objectives for Environmental Health**
Historical Context of Environmental Health and Nursing
Social Determinants of Health and Environmental Justice
Human Environmental Exposures
Environmental Health Sciences
Climate Change
Environmental Health Assessments
Environmental Exposure by Media
Right to Know
Risk Assessment
Vulnerable Populations
Precautionary Principle
Environmental Health Risk Reduction
Risk Communication
Governmental Environmental Protection
Policy and Advocacy
Environmental Justice and Environmental Health Disparities
Environmental Health Threats Associated With the Health Care Industry: New Opportunities for Practice and Advocacy
Referral Resources
Roles for Nurses in Environmental Health

KEY TERMS

agent, p. 127
bioaccumulated, p. 143
biomonitoring, p. 125
climate change, p. 129
compliance, p. 142
consumer confidence reports, p. 135
environment, p. 127
environmental justice, p. 143
environmental standards, p. 142
epidemiologic triangle, p. 127
epidemiology, p. 127
epigenetics, p. 127

Continued

KEY TERMS—cont'd

fracking, p. 127
geographic information systems, p. 127
host, p. 127
indoor air quality, p. 133
Industrial Hygiene Hierarchy of Controls, p. 139
methylmercury, p. 143
monitoring, p. 142
non–point sources, p. 132
permit, p. 141
permitting, p. 141
persistent bioaccumulative toxins, p. 143
persistent organic pollutants, p. 143
point sources, p. 132
precautionary principle, p. 138
right to know, p. 135
risk assessment, p. 135
risk communication, p. 140
risk management, p. 139
route of exposure, p. 140
toxicology, p. 125

INTRODUCTION TO ENVIRONMENTAL HEALTH

An estimated 24 percent of the global burden of disease and 23 percent of all deaths can be attributed to environmental factors (Prüss-Üstün et al., 2016). Nurses have a number of ways in which we can define our environment. Our homes, schools, workplaces, and communities are the environments in which most of us can be found at any given time. Each location holds potential health risks. As nurses, who are among the most trusted conveyors of information to the public, it is our responsibility to understand as much as possible about these risks—how to assess them, how to eliminate or reduce them, how to communicate and educate about them, and how to advocate for policies that support healthy environments.

We can also divide and examine the environment from the perspective of the media in which environmental degradation takes place: air, water, soil, food, and products. And a third approach would be to divide environmental exposures into categories: biological, chemical, and radiological. This chapter examines the environment as comprehensively as possible and considers the roles that nurses can have in assessing and addressing environmental health.

Environmental Carcinogens

Environmental exposures are rarely limited to one location or to one source. For example, the broad category of pesticides includes the insecticides used in homes, the herbicides used in gardens, the pesticide residues on fruits and vegetables, and antimicrobial soaps. Each of these forms of pesticides comes with a potential health risk. The use of pesticides has been linked to adult liver and prostate cancer (Silva et al., 2016; VoPham et al., 2017). If you have children and regularly use pesticides in your home, you increase their risk of contracting leukemia. The more you use pesticides, the greater the risk of leukemia (Chen et al., 2015; Febvey et al., 2016; Ferreira et al., 2013; Metayer et al., 2013). The childhood risk for leukemia increases if the mother was exposed during pregnancy to pesticides, including occupational exposures (Bailey et al., 2014). Many playing fields where children compete in sports are regularly sprayed with pesticides (Gilden et al., 2012). There are other chemicals like the plasticizer bisphenol A (BPA) and phthalates (commonly found in personal care products) that have non-cancer endpoints such as endocrine disruption in children (Watkins et al., 2017).

In May 2010, the President's Cancer Panel proclaimed that the contribution environmental carcinogens have made to the burden of cancer in the United States has been grossly underestimated. In addition to the main focus on chemical carcinogens, the panel noted the importance of radiation sources—ionizing and nonionizing. In a letter to President Obama, they wrote: "The Panel urges you most strongly to use the power of your office to remove the carcinogens and other toxins from our food, water, and air that needlessly increase our health care costs, cripple our Nation's productivity and devastate American lives" (President's Cancer Panel, 2010). With this call came a range of recommendations for reducing the risk of cancer, both through individual choices and through national policy.

Non-cancer Environmental Health Effects

Cancer is not the only health endpoint of environmental exposures. An estimated 64 million homes in the United States contain some lead-based paint that is associated with risks for premature births, learning disabilities in children, hypertension in adults, and many other health problems. Lead poisoning is a completely preventable disease (Fig. 6.1). This figure from the American Academy of Pediatrics describes the most common childhood lead exposures. Of the top 20 environmental pollutants that were reported to the Environmental Protection Agency (EPA), nearly three fourths were known or suspected neurotoxins. Thirty million Americans drink water that exceeds one or more of the EPA's safe drinking water standards, and 50 percent of Americans live in an area that exceeds current national ambient air quality standards. When these standards are exceeded, there is an increased risk to the public for a wide range of health effects.

Although food labeling includes nutrition information, there is no requirement to label whether pesticides are used in the food production; whether nontherapeutic antibiotics were given to the livestock, poultry, or farmed fish; the presence of genetically modified organisms (GMOs) in a product; or whether recombinant bovine growth hormone (rBGH) was given to the dairy cows. Nurses have declared that the "right to know" about potentially hazardous exposures is one of the basic principles of environmental health (Box 6.1). Nurses have an array of potential responsibilities in protecting the public from exposures and environmental health risks (ANA, 2007).

Influences including genetics, socioeconomic status, and environmental exposures impact environmental health. In evaluating

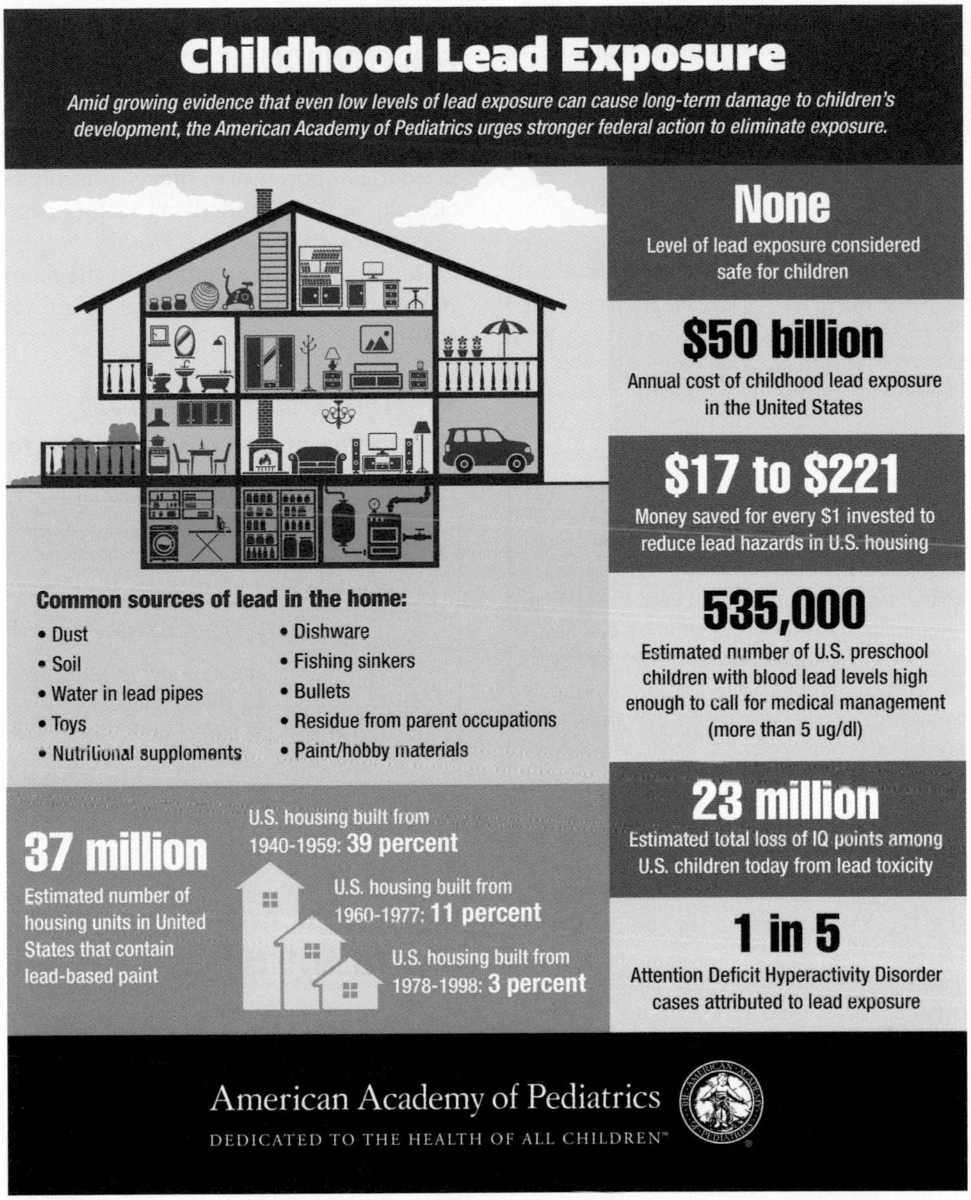
Childhood Lead Exposure
Amid growing evidence that even low levels of lead exposure can cause long-term damage to children's development, the American Academy of Pediatrics urges stronger federal action to eliminate exposure.
None
Level of lead exposure considered safe for children
$50 billion
Annual cost of childhood lead exposure in the United States
$17 to $221
Money saved for every $1 invested to reduce lead hazards in U.S. housing
535,000
Estimated number of U.S. preschool children with blood lead levels high enough to call for medical management (more than 5 ug/dl)
23 million
Estimated total loss of IQ points among U.S. children today from lead toxicity
1 in 5
Attention Deficit Hyperactivity Disorder cases attributed to lead exposure
Common sources of lead in the home:
• Dust
• Soil
• Water in lead pipes
• Toys
• Nutritional supplements
• Dishware
• Fishing sinkers
• Bullets
• Residue from parent occupations
• Paint/hobby materials
37 million
Estimated number of housing units in United States that contain lead-based paint
U.S. housing built from 1940-1959: 39 percent
U.S. housing built from 1960-1977: 11 percent
U.S. housing built from 1978-1998: 3 percent
American Academy of Pediatrics
DEDICATED TO THE HEALTH OF ALL CHILDREN™

Fig. 6.1 Although lead is no longer allowed in house paint, over 37 million homes in the United States have lead-based paint (U.S. Department of Housing and Urban Development, 2011). Pregnant women and parents who live in homes built before 1978 should be encouraged to have both their children and their homes tested for lead-based paint dust. (From American Academy of Pediatrics "Childhood Lead Exposure" Infographic [https://www.aap.org/en-us/ImagesGen/Lead_infographic.jpg]. Reproduced with permission from the American Academy of Pediatrics.)

BOX 6.1 American Nurses Association's Principles of Environmental Health for Nursing Practice

The ANA calls for all nurses to understand basic environmental health concepts, invokes the Precautionary Principle, recognizes the multidisciplinary nature of environmental health, and promotes and supports nurses' roles in developing and maintaining environmentally healthy workplaces for themselves and their patients. Principles include knowledge about environmental health and its effect on nursing practice, the Precautionary Principle, nurses' rights to work in a safe workplace and use materials, products, technology, and practices that reflect an evidence-based approach. Other principles relate to quality assessment of the environment, interdisciplinary work in environmental health, involvement in research, and support of nurses who advocate for a safe environment (ANA, 2007).

From American Nurses Association: *Principles of environmental health for nursing practice,* Silver Spring, MD, 2007.

environmental exposures in a home, nurses' assessments can begin with a set of questions: What exposures can you identify in your home? Do you use pesticides? Does your home have lead-based paint? (The age of a home is a good proxy for identifying the presence of lead-based paint because it is most likely found in homes built before 1978, when the use of lead was banned in household paint.) Is the paint chipping or peeling? Are any of your appliances or heat sources producing unhealthy levels of carbon monoxide? Have you checked your home for radon, the second largest cause of lung cancer in the United States? Do you eat fish on a regular basis? (Some fish can have unhealthy levels of mercury.) A more comprehensive home assessment tool can be found in the Resources. How about your workplace? What types of chemical, radiological, and biological exposures can be found in your work setting? An occupational exposure history should be included in an environmental health assessment.

LINKING CONTENT TO PRACTICE

The *Core Competencies for Public Health Professionals* (Council on Linkages Between Academic and Public Health Practice, 2014) is a key document that guides practice in both nursing and public health. Specifically, the core competencies of the Council on Linkages include, within the domain of public health science skills, a competency that says practitioners will apply "the basic public health sciences (including, but not limited to, environmental health sciences, health services administration, and social and behavioral health sciences) to public health policies and programs." The Quad Council Coalition of Public Health Nursing Organizations (2018) further directs this competency specifically to public health nursing practice by adding that these skills are applied to public health nursing practice, policies, and programs. In 2007, the ANA adopted 10 principles of environmental health. Although all 10 are essential, 3 are highlighted here. Nurses should know about environmental health concepts, participate in assessing the quality of the environment in which they practice, and use the precautionary principle (which is discussed later in the chapter) to guide their work. A third principle notes that healthy environments are sustained through multidisciplinary collaborations, which is a key concept discussed throughout the chapter.

In 2015, the American Nurses Association (ANA) continued to include an environmental health standard within *Nursing: Scope and Standards of Professional Practice,* which defines the profession of nursing. This means that all nurses are now expected to have knowledge of and skills associated with environmental health.

Underpinning many of these organizational decisions to include environmental health in nursing were the recommendations made in the report *Nursing, Health and Environment* (Pope et al., 1995) from the Institute of Medicine (IOM) of the National Academy of Science, which recommended that all nurses have a basic understanding of environmental health principles and integrate these principles into practice, education, advocacy, policies, and research. This chapter explores the basic competencies recommended by the IOM. Box 6.2 presents the competencies.

HEALTHY PEOPLE 2020 OBJECTIVES FOR ENVIRONMENTAL HEALTH

Environmental health is one of the priority areas of the *Healthy People 2020* objectives. The federal government has long recognized the importance of the relationship between environmental risks and the underlying factors contributing to diseases. Selected examples of the *Healthy People 2020* environmental health objectives are outlined in the following Healthy People 2020 box (U.S. Department of Health and Human Services, 2010).

HEALTHY PEOPLE 2020

Examples of Objectives Related to Environmental Health

- **EH-8.1:** Eliminate elevated blood lead levels in children.
- **EH-9:** Minimize the risks to human health and the environment posed by hazardous sites.
- **EH-10:** Reduce pesticide exposures that result in visits to the health care facility.
- **EH-11:** Reduce the amount of toxic pollutants released into the environment.
- **EH-13:** Reduce indoor allergen levels.
- **EH-18:** Decrease the number of U.S. homes that are found to have lead-based paint or related hazards.

From U.S. Department of Health and Human Services: *Healthy People 2020.* Available at http://www.healthypeople.gov.

HISTORICAL CONTEXT OF ENVIRONMENTAL HEALTH AND NURSING

Historically, nurses and physicians have been taught very little about the environment and environmental threats to health. In the nineteenth century, Florence Nightingale promoted the use of clean water and safe sanitary conditions and connected these elements to disease prevention. Early in the twentieth century, Lillian Wald, who coined the name "public health nurses," spent her life improving the environment of the Henry Street neighborhood

BOX 6.2 General Environmental Health Competencies for Nurses Recommended by the Institute of Medicine in *Nursing, Health, and the Environment*

Basic Knowledge and Concepts

All nurses should understand the scientific principles and underpinnings of the relationship between individuals or populations and the environment (including the work environment). This understanding includes the basic mechanism and pathways of exposure to environmental health hazards, basic prevention and control strategies, the interprofessional nature of effective interventions, and the role of research.

Assessment and Referral

All nurses should be able to successfully complete an environmental health history, recognize potential environmental hazards and sentinel illnesses, and make appropriate referrals for conditions with probable environmental causes. An essential component is the ability to access and provide information to clients and communities and to locate referral sources.

Advocacy, Ethics, and Risk Communication

All nurses should be able to demonstrate knowledge of the role of advocacy (case and class), ethics, and risk communication in client care and community intervention with respect to the potential adverse effects of the environment on health.

Legislation and Regulation

All nurses should understand the policy framework and major pieces of legislation and regulations related to environmental health.

From Pope AM, Snyder MA, Mood LH, editors: *Nursing, health, and environment: Strengthening the relationship to improve the public's health,* Washington, DC, 1995, Institute of Medicine, National Academy Press.

and encouraging her broad network of influential contacts to make changes in the physical environment, as well as social conditions that had direct health impacts. Modern-day nurses are recognizing their own occupational and environmental health risks and incorporating environmental health concerns into their clinical and public health practice settings.

SOCIAL DETERMINANTS OF HEALTH AND ENVIRONMENTAL JUSTICE

Increasing attention to the social determinants of health is helpful when addressing the interaction between race, economics, and environmental exposures. Poverty is highly associated with health disparities and environmental exposures. Race is also associated with disproportionately higher environmental exposures, which compound health disparities. Poverty is linked to living in substandard housing, living closer to hazardous plants and waste sites, working in more hazardous jobs, having poorer nutrition, and having less access to quality health care (particularly preventative services). The term *environmental justice* refers to the disproportionate environmental exposures that poor people and people of color experience in the United States and elsewhere, including lead exposure, the presence of pests (resulting in increased use of pesticides), and the use of supplemental heating sources that may cause dangerous carbon monoxide exposure. These combined circumstances multiply the risk for health disparities.

HUMAN ENVIRONMENTAL EXPOSURES

It is important to note how we began to understand the relationship between environmental chemical exposures and their potential for harm, referred to as their toxicity. There are several ways in which we have historically made such discoveries, for example:

- When humans present with signs and symptoms that can be clearly connected to a specific chemical exposure. This may occur with acute pesticide poisoning or carbon monoxide poisoning. It can also occur when workers are occupationally exposed. In such instances, the temporal and geographic relationships to the exposures and health effects help to identify causation (e.g., the diagnosis of mesothelioma from asbestos exposure).
- When environmental exposures occur from contaminated air, water, soil, food, or products resulting in health effects. The lead-contaminated water in Flint, Michigan, is an example of this, as were the multistate outbreaks of *Escherichia coli* infections from contaminated lettuce.
- In rare instances, when human environmental (and occupational) epidemiologic studies have been performed. Through such studies, we have learned about the health risks associated with environmental exposures.

However, the most common way in which the relationships between chemical exposures and health risks are identified is when toxicologists study the effects of chemicals on animals (or in vitro studies) and then use models to estimate what the effects might be on humans. This estimation process is called *extrapolation*. More than 84,000 man-made (synthetic) chemical compounds have been developed and introduced to our environment since World War II, and we are most often reliant on the data that are created in animal studies to warn us about their potential toxicity to humans. However, it is important to note that for many of these chemicals, no toxicity data are available nor are they required. Surprisingly, there is no current requirement for original toxicological research to be completed when a product or process is being brought to market. That is why you can find chemicals that include known carcinogens in some of your personal care products and neurotoxicants in your pet's flea soap.

Biomonitoring

We live in a radically different environment compared to a century ago. In addition to man-made pollutants contaminating our air, water, and food, many of the same pollutants are now also found in our bodies (including breast milk). In 2001, the Centers for Disease Control and Prevention began **biomonitoring**—the testing of human fluids and tissues for the presence of potentially toxic chemicals, as part of its annual National Health and Nutrition Examination Survey. They have consistently found that most Americans carry pesticides, solvents, heavy metals, and other potentially toxic chemicals in their bodies. In 2005, the Environmental Working Group (EWG), a national environmental health organization, tested the umbilical cord blood of newborn babies and found that they also contained a similar range of potentially harmful chemicals (EWG, 2005). The presence of toxic chemicals in our bodies creates a health risk, and it is also an indication that our chemical policies are inadequate. Nurses need to understand the environmental exposures and the health effects that may be associated with chemicals in order to develop assessment tools, implement hazard reduction programs, and advocate for safe and healthy chemical policies. For example, when a woman is pregnant for the first time, this is an ideal time for a nurse to help her patient assess and reduce or eliminate preventable environmental health risks in her home and workplace. A good environmental health history can help uncover a number of exposures from the products she may use, including the ways in which she addresses pests in her home and garden, to the way in which she may set up a new nursery room. It is impossible to keep track of all the health effects associated with every chemical, so nurses must learn about how to navigate the credible sources of information that will provide the evidence.

ENVIRONMENTAL HEALTH SCIENCES

Toxicology

Toxicology is the basic science that contributes to our understanding of health effects associated with chemical exposures. Historically, it was referred to as the "study of poisons." Its corollary in health care is pharmacology, the study of human health effects, both desirable and undesirable, associated with drugs. In toxicology, only the negative effects of chemical exposures are studied. However, many of the key principles of pharmacology and toxicology are the same (Table 6.1). Just as the

TABLE 6.1 Comparison of Basic Pharmacology and Toxicology Concepts and Terms

Pharmacology	Toxicology
Scientific study of origin, chemical nature, and effects of **drugs.**	Scientific investigation of the chemical nature and adverse effects of **chemicals** on health.
Dose refers to the amount of drug absorbed from administration.	**Dose** refers to the amount of a chemical introduced into a biological organism (including human).
Administration of a drug can be one time, short- or long-term.	**Exposure** is the actual contact that an organism has with a chemical which can be one time, short or long-term.
Dose-response curve graphically represents the relationship between doses of a drug and the elicited response.	**Dose-response curve** graphically represents the relationship between doses of a chemical and the adverse effect.
Distribution, Absorption, and Excretion • **Absorption** is the amount of a drug that enters the body. • **Distribution**: Organs/tissues/cells that are reached. • **Metabolism**: Chemical transformation/metabolites. • **Excretion:** Elimination/persistence.	**Distribution, Absorption, and Excretion** • **Absorption** is the amount of a toxic chemical that enters the body. • **Distribution**: Organs/tissues/cells that are reached. • **Metabolism**: Chemical transformation/metabolites. • **Excretion:** Elimination/persistence.
Routes of administration: Oral, IM, IV, inhalation, dermal, ocular, etc.	**Routes of entry:** Ingestion, inhalation, dermal absorption, ocular, etc.
In pharmacology there are therapeutic responses to drugs (desirable) and side effects (undesirable).	**In toxicology** only the negative health effects are of concern.
Potency refers to the relative amount of a drug required to produce the desired response.	The **toxicity** of a chemical refers to the relative amount it takes to elicit a toxic effect compared with other chemicals. (Toxicity is the ability to damage a cell, organ, organ system, to disrupt a biochemical process, or to disturb an enzyme/hormone system.)
Types of Effects: Additive, Antagonistic, Synergistic There is a substantial literature regarding drug interactions.	Little is known about toxic effects of multiple toxic chemicals (because they are studied one chemical at a time)
Biomonitoring may be done for drugs.	Biomonitoring may be done for chemicals.
Drugs are taken voluntarily.	Toxic chemicals are mostly non-voluntary exposures (e.g., air or water pollution).
Host factors must be considered for therapeutic drugs such as ***age, genetics, weight, drugs that a person may be taking, pregnancy status,*** and others.	**Host factors** must be considered for toxic chemicals such as ***age, genetics, weight, drugs that a person may be taking, pregnancy status,*** and others.
Therapeutic index is the dose relationship between a drug's therapeutic effect and its adverse effects.	**Threshold level** refers to the dose of a substance necessary to cause an initial toxic response in the body.
Children require lower doses of drugs to elicit desired effects.	**Children** respond to lower doses of toxic chemicals.
The **regulatory process** by which a **drug** comes to the market includes several stages of testing, including both animal and human testing.	There is **no regulatory requirement** for pre-market testing of **chemical products**. No original testing is required.

IM, Intramuscular; *IV,* intravenous.

dose of a drug makes the difference in its efficacy and its toxicity, the quantity of an air or water pollutant can determine whether or not (and the extent to which) we experience a risk of a health effect. In addition, the timing of the exposure—over the human life span—can make a difference. For example, during embryonic and fetal development, exposure to toxic chemicals can create immediate harm or, alternatively, create a critical pathway for future disease. Very young children, whose systems are still immature, are also more vulnerable to exposures (Wright, 2017). *In Harm's Way*, an online report by Physicians for Social Responsibility (with associated training materials) describes the neurological damage that several common chemicals can cause to developing children (Schettler et al., 2000). Just as is true of medications, the same dose for an adult will have a much greater effect on a child and certainly on a fetus. As we age our liver and renal functions slow, thereby creating opportunities for toxic chemicals to accumulate and thus creating higher risks for harm to older adults.

Both drugs and pollutants can enter the body from a variety of routes. Most drugs are given orally and absorbed by the gastrointestinal (GI) tract. Water- and food-associated pollutants, including pesticides and heavy metals, enter the body via the digestive tract. Some drugs are administered as inhalants, and some pollutants in the air (including indoor air) enter the body via the lungs. Some drugs are applied topically. In work settings, employees can receive dermal exposures from toxic chemicals when they immerse their unprotected hands in chemical solutions, especially solvents. Pollution can enter our bodies via the lungs (inhalation), GI tract (ingestion), skin, and even the mucous membranes (dermal absorption). Most chemicals cross the placental barrier and can directly affect the fetus, just as most chemicals cross the blood–brain barrier at any age. In addition to direct damage to cells, tissues, organs, and organ systems, there can be changes to the DNA from chemical exposures that can change gene expression, which in turn can predict disease.

This latter effect is the focus of a relatively new field of biological study: epigenetics. Scientists now understand that there are many variables that predict disease outcomes, including environmental exposures.

In the same way that we consider age, weight, other drugs taken, and underlying health status of a client when we administer drugs, we must consider that these same factors can affect an individual's response to environmental exposures. For example, children are much more vulnerable to virtually all pollutants. People who are immunosuppressed (people with human immunodeficiency virus [HIV]/acquired immunodeficiency syndrome [AIDS] or those on immunosuppressant drugs like steroids or anti-cancer medications) are especially at risk for foodborne and waterborne pathogens. Because our communities are composed of people of different ages and different health statuses, their vulnerabilities to the effects of pollution will also vary. Just as children are vulnerable because their organs and systems are still developing, the elderly can be vulnerable as their organs and systems are less effective at clearing toxic chemicals and may be more vulnerable to damage. When assessing a community's environmental health status, be sure to review the general health status of the community and to identify members who may have higher risk factors.

Chemicals that are similar are often grouped into categories or "families" so that it is possible to understand the actions and risks associated with those groupings. Examples are metals and metallic compounds (e.g., arsenic, cadmium, chromium, lead, mercury), hydrocarbons (e.g., benzene, toluene, ketones, formaldehyde, trichloroethylene), irritant gases (e.g., ammonia, hydrochloric acid, sulfur dioxide, chlorine), chemical asphyxiants (e.g., carbon monoxide, hydrogen sulfide, cyanides), and pesticides (e.g., organophosphates, carbamates, chlorinated hydrocarbons). Although some common health risks exist within these families of chemicals, the possible health risks for each chemical should be evaluated individually when a potential human exposure exists. The best source of peer-reviewed information for this is the National Library of Medicine (NLM). The NLM has a set of databases and informational sources that are focused on toxicology and environmental health called TOXNET. This is a key resource for environmental health evidence and is easily navigable. You will find the link to several of these helpful informational programs and databases in the Referral Resources.

Epidemiology

Whereas toxicology is the science that studies the poisonous effects of chemicals, epidemiology is the science that helps us understand the strength of the association between exposures and health effects. Epidemiology is often used for occupationally related illnesses but has been used less often to study environmentally related diseases. It is difficult to characterize and/or distinguish among the many exposures that we all experience, and it can be challenging to find control groups who have had no exposures, especially when the exposures are in the air, water, or food.

Epidemiologic studies have helped us to understand the association between learning disabilities and exposure to lead-based paint dust, asthma exacerbation, and air pollution (Habre et al., 2014; Smargiassi et al., 2014), and GI disease and waterborne *Cryptosporidia* (Yoder et al., 2012). Environmental surveillance, such as childhood lead registries, provides data with which to track and analyze incidence and prevalence of health outcomes. The results of such analyses can help to target scarce public health resources. Scientists are now approaching epidemiology at the molecular level, looking at gene/environment interactions. As electronic health records become universal, the inclusion of environmental exposures in patients' records will provide researchers with excellent new opportunities to explore exposure and disease relationships, which in turn will help us to develop population-based risk reduction interventions.

As described in Chapter 13, three major concepts—agent, host, and environment—form the classic epidemiologic triangle. This simple model belies the often-complex relationships between agent, which may include chemical mixtures (i.e., more than one agent); host, which may refer to a community with people of multiple ages, genders, ethnicities, diets, cultures, and disease states; and environment, which may include dynamic factors such as air, water, soil, and food, as well as electric and magnetic fields, temperature, humidity, and wind. The list of potential environmental exposures that any community might have is a particular challenge to epidemiologists. While epidemiologic studies such as occupational health studies are valuable, it is important to recognize that they are performed on healthy adult workers whose biological systems are mature and therefore difficult to generalize the results for neonates, pregnant women, children, people who are immunosuppressed, and the elderly.

Geographic Information Systems

A relatively new research tool for environmental health studies is geographic information systems (GISs), which provide a methodology for coding data so that it is related spatially to a place on Earth. By layering geographically related data, maps can be created to note where the data may be related. For instance, by taking a data set that notes geographically where children who are under 10 years old live and overlaying another data set that notes geographical areas designated by the age of housing stock, a public health nurse could see where there are the largest number of children who live in areas with older housing stock. With this information, the nurse could target a lead surveillance and educational program. Nurse researcher Mona Choi (Choi et al., 2006) used GISs to study the relationship between air pollution and emergency visits for cardiovascular and pulmonary diagnosis. Another study showed that pregnant women living in close proximity to fracking sites (natural gas extraction) had a higher risk of delivering low-birth-weight babies (Currie et al., 2017).

Community-based maps, created using GIS technologies, are helpful in educating community members and policy makers because people can easily see familiar locations and where health and environmental exposures may be the most serious. It helps to make the numbers more "real" to the viewers. Environmental health requires a combination of tried and tested nursing tools mixed with new tools, such as GISs, and the recognition that many disciplines may be involved in the identification and the resolution of environmental health issues. Sources of air and water pollution can be found using geographically oriented databases, such as EnviroFACTS.

Nurse scientists Wade Hill and Patricia Butterfield (2006) developed a model for environmental risk interventions that can be implemented by public health nurses, which improve children's health by addressing home-related sources such as lead paint, contaminated drinking water, and environmental tobacco smoke, among others. These risks can cause health effects ranging from minor learning deficiencies to serious and life-threatening diseases such as cancer. Many of the environmental risks children encountered were prevented or reduced by taking practical and affordable steps. Butterfield also developed an environmental justice framework by which to consider environmental exposures in rural areas (Butterfield & Postma, 2009).

Multidisciplinary Approaches

In addition to toxicology and epidemiology, there are a number of earth sciences that help us understand how pollutants travel in air, water, and soil. Geologists, meteorologists, physicists, and chemists all contribute information to help explain how and when humans may be exposed to hazardous chemicals, radiation (e.g., radon or exposures from cellular devices), and biological contaminants. Key public health professionals include food safety specialists, registered environmental health specialists, radiation specialists, and industrial hygienists.

The nature of environmental health demands a multidisciplinary approach to assess and reduce/eliminate environmental health risks. For instance, to assess and address a lead-based paint poisoning case we might include a housing inspector with expertise in lead-based paint or a registered environmental health specialist to assess the lead-associated health risks in the home; clinical specialists to manage the child's health needs; laboratories to assess the blood lead levels, as well as lead levels in the paint, house dust, and drinking water; and then lead-based paint remediation specialists to reduce the lead-based paint risk in the home.

A health educator and outreach worker may be helpful to educate the family and encourage compliance with a range of risk reducing behaviors and clinical treatments. And finally, it is often helpful to work with public health lawyers to address noncompliant landlords. Such combined approaches could potentially involve the local health department, the state department of environmental protection, the housing department, a primary and tertiary care setting, public or private sector laboratories, and the legal system. Nurses need to understand the roles of each respective agency and organization, know the public health laws (particularly as they pertain to lead-based paint poisoning in their communities), and work with the community to coordinate services to meet their needs. Nurses also may set up a blood lead screening program through the local health department, educate local health providers to encourage them to systematically test children for lead poisoning, and/or work with advocacy organizations to improve the condition of local housing stock. Note that although lead-based paint is no longer used in the United States, we still see lead poisoned children, and lead is still widely used in developing countries.

While all of these public health professionals and specialists involved in the lead poisoning example are providing scientifically based assessments and interventions, it is also critical to note the importance of their contributions to policy development and implementation—advocating for policies and practices that promote environmental health.

QSEN FOCUS ON QUALITY AND SAFETY EDUCATION FOR NURSES

Targeted Competency

Function effectively within nursing and interprofessional teams, fostering open communication, mutual respect, and shared decision making to achieve quality client care.

- **Knowledge:** Describe scopes of practice and roles of health care team members.
- **Skills:** Assume the role of team member or leader based on the situation.
- **Attitudes:** Value the perspectives and expertise of all health team members.

Safety Question

One of the objectives of *Healthy People 2020* related to environmental health is "Reduce pesticide exposures that result in visits to a health care facility" (EH-10). The public health nurse, who is working on a project to help mothers learn parenting skills, visits a new mother who lives and works on a large farm. When the nurse drives into the farm on her way to the housing where workers live, she sees that the fields are being sprayed with pesticides from a truck and that two young children are riding in the back of the truck. Farmworkers are also exposed to agricultural pesticides (see https://www.ewg.org/foodnews/). What action should she take?

Answer

Individual level: She should talk with the owner or manager of the farm and ask whether the person spraying the pesticides is licensed to do so (a requirement in every state). The nurse might remind the farmer or manager of the toxicity of pesticides and the danger to those in the vicinity of the spraying. She should recommend that he or she not allow anyone to ride in the open portion of the vehicle and that the driver should leave the window closed and wear an appropriate mask to protect his or her nose and mouth.

Systems level: She should identify areas where the workers on the farms congregate, such as churches, social halls, and so forth. Then she should ask if she could provide an educational program on the dangers of coming into contact with pesticides. She could distribute pamphlets about this hazard in local venues where both farm managers and workers will be able to access them, as well as providing pamphlets to local health clinics and school nurses, and to have written materials in languages understood by all of the community members.

What else might the nurse do?

CLIMATE CHANGE

Climate change is the result of the earth's warming because of the blanketing effect that is occurring from gases that are primarily man-made and collectively referred to as *greenhouse gases.* To understand the attribution of greenhouse gases, see a graphic created by using the attributions noted by the Interagency Panel on Climate Change at https://www.universityofcalifornia.edu.

For a glimpse into this blanketing effect, consider how quickly the interior of a car warms up when we leave the windows closed. On a day that is 80° outside, a car in full sun can heat up to 99° within just 10 minutes. The ever-increasing man-made gases that are now blanketing the earth's outer atmosphere are deterring the heat that is being created by the sun from being released, thus creating a "greenhouse effect." As a result, the earth is slowly warming in the same way a car warms, and this is causing our ice caps to melt, our seas to rise, and our climate to change.

Consider also what a difference a couple of degrees means to a human's health—from a body temperature of 98.6° F to 100.4° F. At 98.6° we feel fine and our body's systems are fine, not so much starting at 100.4°. This is a very narrow temperature range. Almost all living things require air, water, food, and a particular range of temperature. As the earth's temperature rises, it is placing a wide range of living organisms—from fish to the California redwoods—at risk. Historically, evolution would allow for plant and animal adaptations, but climate change is occurring so quickly that some life forms will not have time to adapt and therefore not survive the impacts of the temperature changes.

Global Climate Change

According to the World Health Organization (WHO), "**climate change** is a significant and emerging threat to public health and changes the way we must look at protecting vulnerable populations" (2014b). The 2014 report of the Intergovernmental Program on Climate Change, a WHO-related group of scientists, concludes that "climate change will act mainly, at least until the middle of this century, by exacerbating health problems that already exist, and the largest risks will apply in populations that are currently most affected by climate-related diseases" (IPCC, 2014). In the United States we are already seeing some of the earlier climate change predictions materialize: long-term warming trends, extreme weather conditions, increased fire activity, as well as disruptions in water supplies, agriculture, ecosystems, and coastal communities.

In addition, there are human health effects that are related to climate change, including increased asthma incidence; increased length of allergy seasons; expanded areas where vector-borne diseases such as malaria, Hanta virus, and Valley Fever will occur; heat-related illnesses particularly to outdoor workers like construction and farm workers; and other illnesses.

Nurses' Responses to Climate Change

In 2016, twenty nursing leaders were invited to the White House to discuss the roles for nursing regarding the developing health threats from climate change. There are three concurrent categories of roles for nurses: planning, mitigation activities, and response. We must have a comprehensive plan for climate related increased illnesses and disasters. Nurses, in all settings, should be aware of and engaged in these plans. There is still much we can do to mitigate the steep upward slope that we are now observing for temperatures, CO_2 levels, desertification, and sea water levels. Working at the individual, community, institutional (e.g., school, hospital), and governmental levels, we can help to ensure energy-conserving policies and practices, rational transportation practices, and changes in our consumption patterns.

Regarding response preparation, public health nurses must lead the development of contingencies for long-term, high-heat weather conditions, increased storm activities, more extensive fires, and the associated temporarily (and sometimes permanently) displaced populations from these various emergencies. (For more on disaster preparedness, see Chapter 21 on nurses' roles in disaster management.) Nurses should also be prepared for threats to food security from shifting weather patterns that may deter/eliminate food production and for acute shifts of populations as people flee low lying, coastal regions or other areas acutely affected. For example, in the 2018 Carr Fire in Northern California, 38,000 people were evacuated and 500 structures were lost (Vercammen et al., 2018). The cost of the Carr Fire alone is estimated at $25 million for suppression costs and $253 million in housing losses (Shoot, 2018).

In 2017, the combined cost of infrastructure damage from two major hurricanes, Irma and Harvey, was between 150 and 200 billion U.S. dollars (Allen & Davis, 2017). The cost to local, state, and federal governments of such extreme weather events impacts their total budgets, thus reducing funds that would otherwise be used for health, housing, education, transportation, and other important public needs. Helping to develop community-based and infrastructure resilience before major events can reduce the cost of destruction.

In 2018, over 130 national nurses' associations affiliated with the International Council of Nurses (ICN) approved a new position stressing the importance of climate change to nursing. It recognizes the importance of nurses keeping up with current science regarding climate change and associated predictions while we prepare for human and ecological health threats as climate change unfolds.

ENVIRONMENTAL HEALTH ASSESSMENTS

There are a number of ways to assess environmental health risks in a community. For example, risks can be assessed by medium: air, water, soil, or food. Or exposures can be listed according to urban, rural, or suburban settings, with many exposures being common to all three settings. Nurses may also divide the environment into functional locations such as home, school, workplace, and community. Each of these locations will have unique environmental exposures, as well as overlapping exposures. For instance, ethylene oxide, the toxic gas that is used in the sterilizing equipment in hospitals, is typically found only in a workplace. However, pesticides might be found in any of the four areas. When assessing environments, be sure to determine if an exposure is in the air, water, soil, and/or food and whether it is a chemical, biological, or radiological exposure.

Information Sources

The National Library of Medicine has developed some of the most useful, comprehensive, and reliable sources of environmental health information. The NLM's website for ToxTown (http://toxtown.nlm.nih.gov) is one of the best places to start when developing environmental assessment skills. Within ToxTown, there is a Household Products page where nurses can research common products such as those for personal care, cleaning, pet care, lawn care, and others to see the potential health risks that may be associated with them. Also, chemicals can be researched by brand or chemical name or by Chemical Abstracts Service number in the NLM's Hazardous Substances Data Bank. (The NLM website can be accessed at www.nlm.nih.gov; at the website, search for the environmental assessment section.)

Also within ToxTown, you can search for general environmental health risks in the "city," "town," and "farm," or even go to a "U.S.–Mexico Border Community." While in the virtual "city" you can visit places like a hair salon, hospital, or funeral home to see what kinds of environmental health risks are posed in such places. ToxTown brings together governmental and well-vetted nongovernmental sources for a rich web resource in which to learn about environmental health.

Another private database that is specific to personal care products, which includes over 73,000 products that can be searched by brand name and specific product descriptors, is the SkinDeep database (http://www.ewg.org). This database provides information with which to make decisions on how to protect your health, and the health of your families and patients, by selecting products with ingredients that have lower health risks. For example, the site points out that even top-selling brands of "natural" and "organic" products may have some toxic components. Specifically, they say that some top-selling herbal shampoos contain 1,4-dioxane, a synthetic chemical carcinogen. They also comment on the number of lipsticks that they found to contain lead. Note that in both the NLM and the Safe Cosmetics databases, the information is based on what the manufacturers place on the label as ingredients (Fig. 6.2). If the manufacturer claims that a component is a "trade secret," it will not appear on the label. Rarely are the chemicals that make up a "fragrance" listed on the label; instead, it is likely to only read "fragrance" on the label. Fragrance chemicals are associated with increased risk of asthma, allergies, and migraines, as well as being accumulated in adipose tissue and present in breast milk (Bridges, 2002). Some institutions, including hospitals and schools, have adopted fragrance-free policies.

And finally (and this is especially true with pesticides), some labels may merely say "inerts" without any further information about their chemical identity. Thus, it may be impossible to make a true assessment about the health risks based on the information provided by the manufacturer.

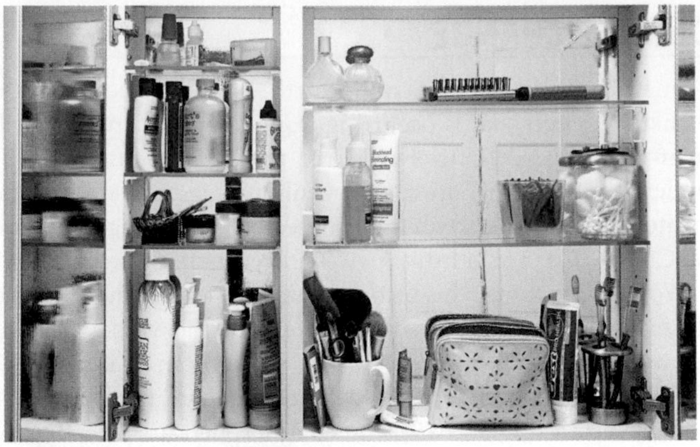

Fig. 6.2 Some of the chemicals in our personal care products can be hazardous to our health. You can look up the chemicals in your products and learn about the potential health risks by going to the SkinDeep database: http://www.ewg.org. (Copyright © Thinkstock/MargoCavin.)

One of the ANA Environmental Health Principles is the tenet of the "right to know," which promotes access to all information necessary in order for consumers to make informed decisions and protect our health. There are still a number of ways in which full disclosure of chemical exposure is lacking in terms of air and water pollution, food contents, and product ingredients. Nurses, both individually and through our professional organizations, can advocate for increasing access to information through "right to know," labeling, and other legislative and regulatory efforts.

Applying the Nursing Process to Environmental Health Assessments

If you suspect that a client's health problem is being influenced by environmental factors, follow the nursing process, and note the environmental aspects of the problem in every step of the process:

1. *Assessment.* Incorporate an occupational and environmental history into your initial assessment. Use your observational skills (e.g., windshield surveys); interview community members; ask your individual clients; and ask the families of your clients. Review web-based data on existing exposures, such as air and water pollution monitoring data, drinking water testing, and contaminated soil. The EPA's EnviroFacts provides a good start for assessing zip code-related exposures. And do not forget to ask about workplace exposures. Relate the disease and the environmental factors in the diagnosis by using them both in search terms.
2. *Planning.* Look at community policy and laws as methods to facilitate the care needs for the client; include environmental health personnel in planning.
3. *Intervention.* Coordinate medical, nursing, and public health actions to meet the client's needs. Ensure that the affected person or family is referred for appropriate clinical care, as well as agencies that are responsible for the environmental exposures.

BOX 6.3 The "I PREPARE" Mnemonic From the Agency for Toxic Substances and Disease Registry

Investigate Potential Exposures
Present Work
Residence
Environmental Concerns
Past Work
Activities
Referrals and Resources
Educate

Do an exposure history to:

- Identify current or past exposures.
- Reduce or eliminate current exposures.
- Reduce adverse health effects.

Taking an Exposure History: Questions to Consider

I—Investigate Potential Exposures

Investigate potential exposures by asking:

Have you ever felt sick after coming in contact with a chemical, such as a pesticide or other substances?

Do you have any symptoms that improve when you are away from your home or work?

P—Present Work

At your present work:

Are you exposed to solvents, dusts, fumes, radiation, pesticides, or other chemicals?

Are you exposed to loud noise?

Do you know where to find material safety data sheets for chemicals with which you work?

Do you wear personal protective equipment?

Are work clothes worn home?

Do coworkers have similar health problems?

R—Residence

When was your residence built?

What type of heating do you have?

Have you recently remodeled your home?

What chemicals are stored on your property?

Where is the source of your drinking water?

E—Environmental Concerns

Are there environmental concerns in your neighborhood (i.e., air, water, soil)?

What types of industries or farms are near your home?

Do you live near a hazardous waste site or landfill?

P—Past Work

What are your past work experiences?

What job did you have for the longest period of time? Have you ever been in the military, worked on a farm, or done volunteer or seasonal work?

A—Activities

What activities and hobbies do you and your family pursue?

Do you burn, solder, or molt any products?

Do you garden, fish, or hunt?

Do you eat what you catch or grow?

Do you use pesticides?

Do you engage in any alternative healing or cultural practices?

R—Referrals and Resources

Use these key referrals and resources:

Environmental Protection Agency (www.epa.gov)

National Library of Medicine—TOXNET Programs (www.nlm.nih.gov)

Agency for Toxic Substances and Disease Registry (www.atsdr.cdc.gov)

Association of Occupational and Environmental Clinics (www.aoec.org)

Occupational Safety and Health Administration (www.osha.gov)

EnviRN website (www.enviRN.umaryland.edu)

Local Health Department, Environmental Agency, Poison Control Center

E—Educate (A Checklist)

Are materials available to educate the client?

Are alternatives available to minimize the risk of exposure?

Have prevention strategies been discussed?

What is the plan for follow-up?

Prepared by Grace Paranzino, RN, MPH, for the Agency for Toxic Substances and Disease Registry. For more information, contact ATSDR at 1-888-42-ATSDR or visit ATSDR's website at http://www.atsdr.cdc.gov.

4. *Evaluation.* Examine criteria that include the immediate and long-term responses of the client as well as the recidivism of the problem for the client. Consider how others in the same location and/or circumstances may also be affected.

Individual Environmental Exposure History

When working with individuals, it is important to include environmental health risks as part of a client's history. Ask certain questions to assess exposures that may occur in all of the settings in which they spend time. Nurses have developed several exposure assessment tools, including forms for pregnant women, home and school assessments, community-wide assessments, and assessment tools for hospital-related exposures. The web links on the Evolve site for this book include several examples of environmental assessment tools. In addition, a helpful mnemonic was developed to assist health professionals in remembering the areas of concern when taking an environmental history: "I PREPARE." The mnemonic can be used when interviewing an individual client or when assessing a family, or it can be adapted for use with a group of community members (Box 6.3).

Community-wide Environmental Health Assessment Tools

A windshield survey is a helpful first step in understanding the potential environmental health risks in a community. If the community is urban, the age and condition of the housing stock, abandoned houses, and trash problems (and the associated pest problems) can be determined easily by driving around the neighborhood. Note proximity to factories, oil and gas operations, dump sites, major transportation routes, and other sources of pollution. In rural communities, note if and when there are aerial and other types of pesticide and herbicide spraying, if people rely on wood-burning stoves, if there are industrial-type, large scale animal feeding facilities, and/or if there are contaminated waterways. Using ToxTown can really help with identifying health risks associated with the observations from a windshield survey.

You may not be able to "see" the pollution that is in your community, but the U.S. Environmental Protection Agency's website, EnviroFACTS, can help identify air, water, and soil pollution in your area by entering your ZIP code. Nurses are often surprised to find out what is being released into their neighborhood's water and air.

The Right to Know section of this chapter contains a description of the types of information that are available to the public about air and water pollutants, drinking water quality, and other environmental sources or exposures. Armed with this information, a nurse can create a significant environmental health map of a community. There are a variety of tools on the internet that describe the process of environmental assessment. For example, see FEMA for "Guidelines for preparing an environmental assessment for FEMA" (http://www.fema.gov).

Positive Environmental Attributes in the Community

While we observe environmental health risks in our communities, it is equally important for us to identify the positive environmental contributors to our communities. Settings that connect people to nature—trees, parks, green spaces, community gardens, and beaches—are incredible assets to communities. The term *nature-deficit disorder* was coined by author Richard Louv in his book, *Last Child in the Woods,* to describe what happens to children who become disconnected from the natural world. Louv links this lack of nature to some of the most disturbing childhood trends, such as the rises in obesity, attention disorders, and depression (Louv, 2005). Policy makers, educators, and children's health advocates are considering their roles in addressing this issue. The National Park Service works to bring more people to parks—local, state, and national.

Man-made "green" spaces such as community gardens, streetscapes, bike paths, and water features can positively contribute to a community's health and sense of well-being. Recent attention has been paid to the importance of walkable communities, access to nature, and other concerns included in discussions about smart growth or sustainable communities.

Some new suburban developments are designing space for agriculture in the form of Community Sustainable Agriculture (CSA), a model of local agriculture in which community members purchase shares in the spring and receive fruits and vegetables as they are harvested. Also in this model, community members have the option to volunteer on the farm. This creative new community design addresses a number of public health issues—obesity, depression/social isolation, poor nutrition—by getting people outside and moving, creating opportunities for building supportive relationships, and providing fresh produce.

ENVIRONMENTAL EXPOSURE BY MEDIA

Many of the environmental protection regulations are based on the "medium" in which pollutants are carried—air, water, and soil. Additionally, chemical, biological, and radiological hazards can be found in food and consumer products. For air, water, and soil, the U.S. EPA and its state-level equivalents are the primary regulatory agencies. However, the EPA also regulates radon, pesticides used in agriculture, lead in paint, and other toxic products. The U.S. Department of Agriculture focuses substantially on pathogens in our food supply.

Air

Air pollution is a significant contributor to human health problems and a sign that regulatory efforts are not completely effective. Nurses can have a role in addressing both the health problems and the policies affecting the exposures. Air pollution is divided into two major categories: point source and non–point source. **Point sources** are individual, identifiable sources such as smokestacks. They are sometimes referred to as fixed sites. **Non–point sources** come from more diffuse exposures. For instance, the largest non–point source of air pollution is from mobile sources such as cars and trucks, which are the greatest single source of air pollution in the United States. The Clean Air Act regulates air pollution from point and non–point sources. Box 6.4 presents a list of the air pollutants that make up the "criteria pollutants"—a set of pollutants that the EPA uses to gauge the overall air quality. The burning of fossil fuel (e.g., diesel fuel, industrial boilers, and coal-fired power plants) and waste incineration are two other major contributors. Health effects associated with air pollution include asthma and other respiratory diseases, cardiovascular diseases (including cardiac disorders and hypertension), cancer, immunological effects, and reproductive health problems, including birth defects, infant death, and neurological problems. For children with asthma the additional insult of living near a fixed source of pollution can create additional health risks (Smargiassi et al., 2014).

The single greatest source of mercury in our air is coal-fired power plants. Many people do not know that a pea-sized amount of mercury is sufficient to contaminate a 25-acre lake and make its fish unfit to eat. Mercury, like lead, is an element, and it persists in our fresh waterways and oceans from which we continue to get our fish. We cannot readily take these elements out once they have been released into the environment; our job is to focus on policies that prevent them from being released.

BOX 6.4 U.S. EPA Criteria Air Pollutants—National Ambient Air Quality Standards (NAAQS)

Ozone (ground level)	Particulate matter
Sulfur dioxide	Carbon monoxide
Nitrogen dioxide	Lead

EPA, Environmental Protection Agency.

Indoor Air Quality. Indoor air quality (IAQ) is a growing public health concern in homes, office buildings, and schools and is reflected in the alarming rise in asthma incidence in the United States, particularly among children. Gas stoves and dryers can create risks for unhealthy carbon monoxide exposures; formaldehyde, a common ingredient in many building materials, is a known carcinogen; and fragrance devices volatilize chemicals that can create a host of health risks, including endocrine disruption.

The EPA and the American Lung Association both provide excellent materials on IAQ. The EPA has a free kit called *IAQ: Tools for Schools,* which includes a video and a number of helpful materials for people interested in improving the air quality in a school building. Radon, a naturally occurring radioactive element that is found in the earth's crust and can seep into basements and into groundwater, is the second leading cause of lung cancer in the United States, second only to smoking. Other major culprits contributing to poor indoor air are dusts, molds, pests and pets, pesticides, cleaning and personal care products (particularly aerosols), lead, and of course environmental tobacco smoke. The EPA also provides guidance to asthma-proof a home, see https://www.epa.gov and Fig. 6.3 (Air Quality Index).

Because environmental health implies a relationship between the environment and our health, we must assess both the environmental exposures and the human health status within a community. Health status is assessed by using local, state, and national health data or by collecting our own data, or a combination of the two. As we learn more about the exposures in our communities and their known or suspected health effects, we can target the health statistics we wish to review or collect.

Water

Water is necessary for all life forms, and human bodies consist of 70 percent water. Yet only 2.5 percent of the water on this planet is fresh water; the rest is salt water. Much of the fresh water is in the polar ice caps, whereas groundwater makes up most of what remains, leaving only 0.01 percent in lakes, creeks, streams, rivers, and rainfalls. People's lives are inextricably tied to safe and adequate water . Water is necessary for the production of food. In the United States, all public water suppliers must test their water in accordance with the EPA's safe drinking water standards, and they must summarize the results of their testing annually and make the summaries available to their customers—those who pay water bills. The technical term for these reports is Consumer Confidence Reports (CCR). Nurses can request these summaries from the water suppliers that serve their communities. Private wells are not regulated and need not be tested except when they are first drilled. Nurses should encourage people with private wells to have them tested annually, especially in agricultural areas where pesticides are applied.

Pollution discharges into water bodies from industries and from wastewater treatment systems can contribute to the *degradation* of water quality. An additional source of pollution in our waters is pharmaceuticals used for humans and animals. The U.S. Geological Service has found antibiotics, codeine, 17β-estradiol (an estrogen replacement hormone), and acetaminophen (Tylenol), as well as a variety of endocrine disrupting chemicals, in measurable quantities in U.S. streams and rivers.

Water quality is also affected by non–point sources of pollution, such as storm water runoff from paved roads and parking lots, soil erosion of agricultural lands and from clear-cut tracts

Air Quality Index Levels of Health Concern	Numerical Value	Meaning
Good	0 to 50	Air quality is considered satisfactory, and air pollution poses little or no risk.
Moderate	51 to 100	Air quality is acceptable; however, for some pollutants there may be a moderate health concern for a very small number of people who are unusually sensitive to air pollution.
Unhealthy for Sensitive Groups	101 to 150	Members of sensitive groups may experience health effects. The general public is not likely to be affected.
Unhealthy	151 to 200	Everyone may begin to experience health effects; members of sensitive groups may experience more serious health effects.
Very Unhealthy	201 to 300	Health alert: everyone may experience more serious health effects.
Hazardous	301 to 500	Health warnings of emergency conditions. The entire population is more likely to be affected.

Fig. 6.3 Air pollution can be categorized by health risks for the public. This color coding is used by schools, during weather reports, and other public information sources. From U.S. Environmental Protection Agency. Available at: https://airnow.gov/index.cfm?action=aqibasics.aqi

of land for timbering and mining, and runoff from chemicals added to soils such as pesticides and fertilizers. Soil erosion is another huge public health threat in the making as it is decreasing the amount of soil that can sustain agriculture and the global food supply. Eighty percent of the world's forests are gone, which is contributing to massive erosion of farmable soil and deterring the flow of and healthy biotic life in creeks and rivers.

Land and Soil

Current and past land use can affect a community's health. Local governments dictate land use through zoning laws. For instance, zoning decisions can determine if a community will have a hazardous waste site built in its neighborhood or whether the land can be used only for residential purposes (housing). Historically, communities in which poor people and people of color live have been more likely to be zoned to allow undesirable and unhealthy industries, railway lines, and hazardous waste sites. In many communities, prior use of the land has left a legacy of unhealthy contaminants. There are two designations for lands that may be contaminated: Superfund sites (highly contaminated sites, with associated health threats that are designated by the EPA) and brownfield sites (land that has been used previously, which is now slated for redevelopment, that may have contaminated soil). Public health nurses can play an important role in assessing human health threats associated with both Superfund and brownfield sites. Funds are available through both the Superfund and brownfield laws to engage the community and to do health assessments.

Food

Many health risks are associated with food and food production. In recent years, we have seen foodborne illnesses associated with *Salmonella* and *E. coli* H:0157:H7 in chicken, eggs, and meats. Good food preparation practices, such as proper washing and using adequate cooking temperatures and time, can prevent foodborne illnesses associated with most pathogens. Local health departments are responsible for monitoring food establishments (e.g., restaurants, food trucks) in the community, and the U.S. Department of Agriculture is responsible for oversight of meat, poultry, fish, and produce production.

However, there are also environmental health risks posed by the presence of pesticide residues in our food; the use of recombinant bovine growth hormone (rBGH), which is given to many dairy cows to increase milk production; the administration of antibiotics to beef cattle, pigs, and chickens at nontherapeutic doses that are given to promote growth, rather than treat an infection; and the use of genetically modified organisms (GMOs) for genetically engineered crops. There are a number of websites through which you can find out more information about food-related public health issues.

It is important that nurses understand the term *organic* regarding food labeling. If a food is labeled "USDA Certified Organic," this is a meaningful term that has a legal USDA definition. The legal definition stands for foods that have been produced without the use of pesticides, GMOs, unnecessary (nontherapeutic) use of antibiotics, and other specific practices. If a food is merely labeled "organic," without the USDA label, the consumer does not have the same guarantee for what chemicals or farming practices have been used. When purchasing foods directly from farmers through farm stands or farmers' markets, consumers can directly ask about the chemicals and farm practices. For some community members buying directly from farmers or buying USDA Certified Organic food products may not be possible. Nurses can counsel clients on how to choose the Clean 15 and avoid the Dirty Dozen foods as shown at www.ewg.org

CHECK YOUR PRACTICE

You bring your pediatric patient her lunch tray. Her mother, who is at her bedside, asks you, "Does eating organic food make any difference for children?" She goes on to say, "I don't really even know what organic means, can you tell me?"

How do you respond?

What does the literature say about the relative benefits of feeding children organic foods?

Energy

Our energy sources—coal, gas, oil, solar, and other renewable sources—can have an immense impact on the health of communities. Fossil fuels create a host of toxic exposures during their extraction, when processed in refineries, and when they are combusted for energy, such as coal-fired power plants or gasoline engines that power cars, trucks, and other vehicles. Fossil fuels are also the largest contributor to climate change. From a public health perspective, accelerating our transition to solar and other safer renewable energy choices will decrease air pollution, water pollution, and greenhouse gases. Nurses can promote energy saving practices and advocate for renewable power sources.

Electric, Magnetic, and Sound Wave Sources

Over the last several decades, new technologies have introduced levels of electric and magnetic and sound wave exposures never experienced in human history. Emerging health science is indicating that these exposures have the potential for harm, both human and ecological, but our policies and regulations do not yet reflect the emerging evidence. Most guidelines regarding exposures have not be updated since 1984. It is not unusual for policies to lag behind new scientific discoveries, but given the enormous extent that cellular technologies (cell towers and cell phones), wireless technologies (Wi-Fi access to Internet), and ultrasound technologies (tracking systems in cell phones and televisions, and new technologies in self-driving cars) are in current use, this is an important environmental health area of interest. Nurses should keep abreast of the associated science and policies.

RIGHT TO KNOW

Several environmental statutes give the public the **right to know** about hazardous chemicals in the environment. Under one of the "right to know" laws, health professionals and community members can easily access key information by ZIP code regarding major sources of pollution that are being emitted into the air or water in their community. As mentioned earlier, the EPA has an EnviroFacts section on its website that provides several sources of exposure data by ZIP code (http://www.epa.gov).

Nurses can access drinking water **consumer confidence reports**, sometimes referred to as "right to know" reports, to determine what pollutants have been found in the drinking water. If the drinking water poses an immediate health threat, the water provider must send emergency warnings out to the community via the local newspapers, radios, and television. If there is a biological hazard (microbial) in the water, the health notice may suggest boiling the water or not drinking it at all. If the hazard is chemical, boiling the water may not be helpful because that may simply concentrate the chemical. A federal law, the Freedom of Information Act, allows citizens to request many kinds of public documents, including information about environmental permits and inspections of facilities in your communities.

Employees have the right to know about the hazardous chemicals with which they work through the federal Hazard Communication Standard, which is under the purview of the Occupational Safety and Health Administration (OSHA). This standard requires employers (including hospitals) to maintain a list of all of the potentially hazardous chemicals that are used on site. Each of these chemicals should have an associated chemical information sheet known as a material safety data sheet (MSDS, now often being referred to simply as safety data sheets), which is written by the chemical manufacturer. These MSDSs are to be made available to any employee or his or her representative (e.g., a union) and should provide information about the chemicals that constitute the product, the health risks, and any special guidance on safe use or handling (e.g., requirements for protective gloves or respiratory protection). For more extensive information on workplace health and safety, see http://www.osha.gov.

RISK ASSESSMENT

Currently, the EPA uses a process referred to as "risk assessment" when they develop health-based standards. The term **risk assessment** refers to a process to determine the probability of a health threat associated with an exposure. The following are the four phases of a risk assessment:

1. Determining if a chemical is known to be associated with negative health effects (in animals or humans). For this, we rely on toxicological and/or epidemiologic data. (Remember, the available toxicological data will probably be based on animal studies, and these studies estimate the potential effects on humans by extrapolating, whereas the results of human epidemiologic studies will be for human health effects.)
2. Determining whether the chemical has been released into the environment—into the air, water, soil, or food. This is accomplished by testing for the presence of the suspected chemical in the various media (air, water, soil, food). Environmental professionals such as air and water pollution scientists, environmental engineers, meteorologists, and others might be involved in this activity. When doing a risk assessment, it is important to note if there are multiple sources of the chemical in question. For example, is lead found in the drinking water, the ambient air, *and* in the paint within the houses of a given community?
3. Estimating how much and by which route of exposure the chemical might enter the human body—inhalation, ingestion, dermally, or in utero exposure. This estimate can be based on a one-time exposure, a short-term exposure, or a projected lifetime exposure. (When federal standards are created for air, water, and other pollutants, they are based on an estimation of a lifetime exposure. However, in workplace settings the chemical exposure standards are based on an average exposure during a typical 8-hour work shift or set for a maximum exposure level that should not be exceeded.)
4. Characterizing the risk assessment process and taking into account all three of the previous steps. Is the chemical toxic? What is the source and amount of the exposure? What is the route and duration of the exposure for humans? The final synthesis attempts to predict the potential for harm based on the estimated exposure.

All science is subject to interpretation, and so is risk assessment. The reason that environmental laws are so often contentious is because there are economic interests at stake and not just public or ecological health concerns. In translating the risk assessment results for the purposes of policy development and recommendation for risk reduction activities, there are often several interpretations of each of the risk assessment steps that then result in differing recommendations for health-based standards. There are also areas of scientific uncertainty that contribute to variations in assessment of risk. It is critical to have public health voices in the debates. The American Public Health Association is actively engaged on major policy debates through the Environment Section.

VULNERABLE POPULATIONS

Many of the social determinants of health contribute to the risk levels associated with environmental exposures. Poor people who live in low-income communities are more often housed in substandard housing (with attendant risks of chipping and peeling paint, pests, and unsafe neighborhoods), live closer to pollution sources, are employed in more dangerous occupations, and have less access to healthy food options. In addition, vulnerability is variable through the human life cycle. The embryo and fetus are the most vulnerable to chemical exposures because of the rapid growth of cells and the development of tissues, organs, and organ systems. Following is a section on children's special vulnerabilities. The very young and the very old also are vulnerable because their body systems are either still developing or are less efficient, respectively. For more information about the special vulnerabilities of the elderly, see the EPA's dedicated information site on older Americans (www.epa.gov) and look at their report "Growing Smarter/Living Healthier: A Guide to Smart Growth and Active Aging. For more information on the effects of perinatal exposures, the University of California San Francisco has a Program on Reproduction and Environment that provides informational webinars, factsheets, the latest research, and policy/advocacy information available at http://www.prhe.ucsf.edu.

Children's Environmental Health

Consider some of the current childhood health statistics with which environmental factors are associated: about nine percent of American children suffer from asthma, with higher rates in African American children (CDC, 2012). About 20 percent of the world's children and adolescents suffer from a mental health problem (WHO, n.d.), and this statistic is mirrored in the United States (DHHS, 2005). The Centers for Disease Control and Prevention (CDC) monitoring system for autism spectrum disorders reports that the prevalence of autism among eight-year-olds in the United States is 1 in every 59 children (CDC, 2014a). The global prevalence of autism has increased twentyfold to thirtyfold since the earliest epidemiologic studies were conducted in the late 1960s and early 1970s with some associations to environmental exposures, particularly air pollutants (Kalkbrenner et al., 2015).

Developmental disorders and attention deficit hyperactivity disorder (ADHD) collectively are estimated to affect 17 percent of school-age children (AHRQ, 2002; Anney et al., 2006). Child obesity has doubled, and adolescent obesity has more than quadrupled in the last 30 years (CDC, 2014b). From 1975 to 2010 the incidence rates for four cancer types, acute lymphocytic leukemia, non-Hodgkin lymphoma, acute myeloid leukemia, and testicular germ cell tumors, increased in children (ACS, 2018). The most common cancers among children ages 0 through 14 are acute lymphocytic leukemia, brain and central nervous system (CNS), neuroblastoma, and non-Hodgkin lymphoma (ACS, 2018, p. 12). "All cancers involve the malfunction of genes that control cell growth and division. Only a small proportion of cancers are strongly hereditary…" (ACS, 2018, p.1). According to the American Cancer Society (ACS), about five percent of all cancers are strongly associated with heredity (ACS, 2018) The rest occur from environmental exposures, lifestyle choices (e.g., diet, smoking), and other factors during our lifetimes.

Over the past 25 years there has been great improvement in the 5-year survival rate of major childhood cancers. Nevertheless, in 2017 about 10,000 children were diagnosed with cancer in the United States (ACS, 2018). The list of possible causes of children's cancers includes the following: genetic abnormalities, ultraviolet and ionizing radiation, electromagnetic fields, viral infections, certain medications, food additives, tobacco, alcohol, and industrial and agricultural chemicals (Chen et al., 2015; Bassil et al., 2007). Clearly, the environment is playing an important role.

EVIDENCE-BASED PRACTICE

Gilden et al. examined the use of pesticides on athletic fields where children play sports. This cross-sectional descriptive study used a survey to assess playing field maintenance practices related to the use of pesticides on the field. The authors gave the survey to 33 field managers in order to assess maintenance practices. Their data were analyzed using descriptive statistics and generalized estimating equations.

They found that 65.3 percent of the managers said they applied pesticides, primarily herbicides, to the fields. They also found that managers of urban and suburban fields were less likely to apply pesticides than were managers of rural fields. The use of pesticides presents many health hazards, and the results of this study demonstrated that children who engage in sports activities on athletic fields are exposed to health hazards.

Nurse Use

Nurses can inform people such as school officials, coaches, and field managers of the dangers of using pesticides on athletic fields.

Gilden R, Friedmann E, Sattler B, et al.: Potential health effects related to pesticide use on athletic fields. *Public Health Nurs* 29(3):198–207, May/June 2012.

Children are not just little adults. They are different in many ways, particularly with regard to their exposures and responses to the environment. As nurses, we know that infants and young children breathe more rapidly than adults, and this increase in respiratory rate translates to a proportionately greater exposure to air pollutants. While infants' lungs are developing they are particularly susceptible to environmental toxicants. Although full function of the lungs is attained at about age six, changes continue to occur in the lungs through adolescence (Fudvoye et al., 2014; Hsu et al., 2015). Children are short, and, as such, their breathing zones are lower than adults, causing them to have closer contact to the chemical and biological agents that accumulate on floors and carpeting. Children of color and poor children in America are disproportionately affected by a range of environmental health threats, including lead, air pollution, pesticides, incinerator emissions, and exposures from hazardous waste sites (Landrigan et al., 2010; Suk & Davis, 2008).

Children's bodies also operate differently. Some of the protective mechanisms that are well developed in adults, like the blood–brain barrier, are immature in young children, thereby increasing their vulnerability to the effects of toxic chemicals. And finally, the kidneys of young children are less effective at filtering out undesirable toxic chemicals, and these chemicals then continue to circulate and accumulate.

Infants and young children drink more fluids per body weight than adults, thus increasing the dose of contaminants found in their drinking water, milk (hormones and antibiotics), and juices (particularly pesticides). If an adult were to drink a proportionate amount of water to an infant, the adult would have to drink about 50 glasses of water a day. Children also eat more per body weight, eat different proportions of food, and absorb food differently than adults (EPA, 2013). How many adults could eat the same amount of raisins pound-for-pound as the average two-year-old? Children consume much greater quantities of fruits and fruit juices than adults, once again adding exposure to doses of pesticide residues. The average one-year-old drinks 21 times more apple juice, 11 times more grape juice, and nearly 5 times more orange juice per unit of body weight than the average adult (Holmes et al., 2008). The Food Quality Protection Act (FQPA) was passed to specifically address the consumption patterns and special vulnerabilities of children (Box 6.5).

Toxic Exposures During Pregnancy

Toxic chemicals can have different effects depending on the timing of exposure. During fetal development, there are periods of exquisite sensitivity to the effects of toxic chemicals. During such times, even extraordinarily small exposures can prevent or change a process that may permanently affect normal development. The brain undergoes rapid structural and functional changes during late pregnancy and in the neonatal period. Therefore, it is extremely important to safeguard women's environments when they are pregnant (Table 6.2).

Alarmingly, 27 states have issued mercury contamination advisories for fish in *every* lake and river within their state's borders (EPA, 2009). According to the EPA, more than one million women in the United States of childbearing age eat sufficient amounts of mercury-contaminated fish to risk damaging brain development of their children. Nurses in all settings need to understand the implications that the fish advisories have for their clients and communities and the contribution that the

BOX 6.5 Provisions Under the Food Quality Protection Act Regarding Pesticide Exposure to Children From Multiple Sources

New provisions under the Food Quality Protection Act of 1996 related to protection of infants and children:

Health-based standard: A new standard of a reasonable certainty of "no harm" that prohibits taking into account economic considerations when children are at risk.

Additional margin of safety: Requires that the EPA use an additional 10-fold margin of safety when there are adequate data to assess prenatal and postnatal development risks.

Account for children's diet: Requires the use of age-appropriate estimates of dietary consumption in establishing allowable levels of pesticides on food to account for children's unique dietary patterns.

Account for all exposures: In establishing acceptable levels of a pesticide on food, the EPA must account for exposures that may occur through other routes, such as drinking water and residential application of the pesticide.

Cumulative impact: The EPA must consider the cumulative impact of all pesticides that may share a common mechanism of action.

Tolerance reassessments: All existing pesticide food standards must be reassessed over a 10-year period to ensure that they meet the new standards to protect children.

Endocrine disruption testing: The EPA must screen and test all pesticides and pesticide ingredients for estrogen effects and other endocrine disruptor activity.

Registration renewal: Establishes a 15-year renewal process for all pesticides to ensure that they have up-to-date science evaluations over time.

EPA, Environmental Protection Agency.
From Environmental Protection Agency: Food Quality Protection Act of 1996. Available at http://www.epa.gov.

TABLE 6.2 Workplace Hazards to Women of Reproductive Age[a]

Agent	Observed Effects	Potentially Exposed Workers
Cancer treatment drugs (e.g., methotrexate)	Infertility, miscarriage, birth defects, low birth weight	Health care workers, pharmacists
Organic solvents (e.g., toluene, xylene, formaldehyde)	Miscarriage	Health care workers, laboratory workers, print shop and manufacturing employees
Lead	Infertility, miscarriage, low birth weight, developmental disorders	Battery makers, solderers, welders, bridge repainters, firing range workers, home remodelers
Strenuous physical labor (e.g., prolonged standing, shift/night work)	Miscarriage, preterm delivery	Many types of workers
Cytomegalovirus	Birth defects, low birth weight, developmental disorders	Health care workers, workers who have contact with infants and children
Parvovirus B19	Miscarriage	Health care workers, workers who have contact with infants and children
Rubella	Birth defects, low birth weight	Health care workers, workers who have contact with infants and children
Toxoplasmosis	Miscarriage, birth defects, developmental disorders	Animal care workers, veterinarians
Varicella zoster	Birth defects, low birth weight	Health care workers, workers who have contact with infants and children

[a]This list is not complete. Information about these hazards is constantly being expanded. Readers should not assume that a substance is safe if it is missing from this list. The National Library of Medicine's Developmental and Reproductive Toxicity Database provides much more extensive information and sources: https://toxnet.nlm.nih.gov.
Data from: National Institute for Occupational Safety and Health (www.cdc.gov).

health sector has in creating this health risk, while at the same time counseling on the positive contribution of fish to a nutritionally balanced diet.

About 84,000 chemicals are used in commerce in the United States (EPA, 2014). Almost all are man-made; 15,000 of them are produced annually in quantities greater than 10,000 pounds, and 2800 of them are produced in quantities greater than 1 million pounds per year. Of the 2800, only 7 percent have been tested for developmental effects, and only 43 percent have been tested for any human health effects (Landrigan, 2016).

Companies are not required to divulge the results of their private testing. A full battery of neurotoxicity tests is not required even for pesticides that may be sprayed in nurseries and labor and delivery areas, not to mention in homes. To make things even more complicated, risks from multiple chemical exposures are rarely considered when regulations are drafted. Such an omission ignores the reality that both children and adults are exposed to many toxic chemicals, often concurrently. The only exception to this rule is in the case of regulations regarding pesticides that are used on food. See Box 6.5 for the provisions under the FQPA.

In clinical settings, there is little that can be done to address a child's body burden of toxic chemicals from air or water pollution; however, the nursing community as a profession has a weighty obligation to understand the science and risks associated with environmental pollutants and to engage in the political and economic decisions regulating the environment that have a profound effect on human health, especially the health of our children. This engagement occurs in policy-making arenas, including legislative, regulatory, and international treaties. Nurses have increasingly become involved in the policy arena. The Alliance of Nurses for Healthy Environments is actively engaging nurses in state and federal chemical policies, climate change policies, and energy policies (including fracking) as they relate to health, and policies related to sustainable foods.

PRECAUTIONARY PRINCIPLE

With thousands of chemical compounds now creating a chemical soup in our air and water (and in our bodies, in our breast milk), it is increasingly difficult to prove specific hypotheses regarding the relationship of exposure to a singular chemical and disease outcome in humans. It has been suggested that we adopt a precautionary approach when research and other indicators demonstrate a possible toxic relationship between a chemical and health. Box 6.6 presents the *Wingspread Statement on the Precautionary Principle*. This precautionary approach calls for action to reduce potentially toxic exposure to humans in light of data or other indicators, rather than delaying until more "conclusive" studies are performed. We will never have the perfect studies. Nurses, who are trained in disease prevention, appreciate and should advocate for a precautionary approach when it may prevent injuries or illnesses. The ANA has adopted the **precautionary principle** as the basic tenet on which to guide its environmental advocacy work.

BOX 6.6 Wingspread Statement on the Precautionary Principle

In 1998 an international group of health and public health professionals, scientists, government officials, lawyers, grassroots activists, and labor activists met at a conference center called Wingspread in Wisconsin to define the "precautionary principle." The group issued the following consensus statement:

> The release and use of toxic substances, the exploitation of resources, and physical alterations of the environment have had substantial unintended consequences affecting human health and the environment. Some of these concerns are high rates of learning deficiencies, asthma, cancer, birth defects and species extinctions, along with global climate change, stratospheric ozone depletion and worldwide contamination with toxic substances and nuclear materials.
>
> We believe existing environmental regulations and other decisions, particularly those based on risk assessment, have failed to protect adequately human health and the environment the larger system of which humans are but a part.
>
> We believe there is compelling evidence that damage to humans and the worldwide environment is of such magnitude and seriousness that new principles for conducting human activities are necessary.
>
> While we realize that human activities may involve hazards, people must proceed more carefully than has been the case in recent history. Corporations, government entities, organizations, communities, scientists and other individuals must adopt a precautionary approach to all human endeavors.
>
> Therefore, it is necessary to implement the Precautionary Principle: When an activity raises threats of harm to human health or the environment, precautionary measures should be taken even if some cause and effect relationships are not fully established scientifically. In this context the proponent of an activity, rather than the public, should bear the burden of proof.
>
> The process of applying the Precautionary Principle must be open, informed and democratic and must include potentially affected parties. It must also involve an examination of the full range of alternatives, including no action.

Wingspread statement on the precautionary principle, Racine, WI, 1998. Available at http://www.gdrc.org.

The bottom line is that life depends on the environment, and what humans do collectively can affect this vital resource for present and future generations. A central concept in American Indian cultures is that humans are stewards, not proprietors, of the environment. American Indians make the "Rule of Seven" central to all environmental decisions: What will be the effect on the seventh generation from now? A quote (Myths-Dreams-Symbols, 2006) attributed to Chief Seattle, a nineteenth-century American Indian, illustrates the need to think more holistically when we consider environmental impacts: "Whatever befalls the earth befalls the sons of the earth. Man did not weave the web of life; he is merely a strand in it. Whatever he does to the web, he does to himself." William McDonough suggests that, as we make policies, plans, and designs, we ask ourselves how these decision are evidence that "we love all the children of all the species for all times" (Huff, 2013).

Mary O'Brien, in her book *Making Better Environmental Decisions: An Alternative to Risk Assessment*, notes that we are repeatedly given a very short list of risk reduction choices and that the public is not effectively engaged in the decision-making process. She suggests that a broader range of options would allow us to see the possibilities for further reducing (or even eliminating) risks and that the process should be much more democratic in nature. O'Brien proposes the best approach to making effective environmental decisions is to use information, emotion, and a sense of relationship to others concurrently. By "others" she means other species, cultures, and generations (O'Brien, 2000). Her method is consistent with a nursing approach. Using her approach will require that nurses more actively engage in environmental health—assessing environmental health risks, developing risk reduction strategies, and supporting policies that embrace the precautionary principle and care for all of the children of all of the species for all times.

ENVIRONMENTAL HEALTH RISK REDUCTION

Prevention is a core goal in every public health intervention. Preventing problems is less costly whether the cost is measured in resources consumed or in human health effects. Policies, as well as practices, can promote primary prevention. After we have assessed the environmental risks in our communities, we can apply the basic principles of disease prevention when planning intervention strategies. For lead exposure, remediating a home with lead-based paint to make it lead safe applies the primary prevention strategy of removing the exposure (at least from that specific source of lead). Even good lead poisoning surveillance will not prevent lead exposure, but may help with early detection of rising blood lead levels. Such surveillance is a secondary prevention strategy. Finally, when a symptomatic child is seen, it is important to have a health care system readily available in which specialists familiar with lead poisoning will provide swift medical interventions to reduce blood lead levels, thus reducing the risk of further harm. This is a tertiary prevention response. Box 6.7 presents examples of risk reduction strategies for nurses in the health care setting.

BOX 6.7 Risk Reduction: Every Nurse's Role

In the health care setting (hospital, clinic, home health), we have many opportunities to make environmentally friendly and healthy choices:

- Shift to electronic records, thus avoiding the use of paper. When paper is a must, use products that are made from 100 percent recycled ingredients
- Recycle: paper, glass, cans, plastic, small batteries, blue wrap, electronic equipment
- Work with suppliers to get products with minimum packaging and the safest ingredients possible: "environmentally preferable purchasing"
- Promote the use of green cleaners
- Go fragrance free by using fragrance-free products in the hospital and creating a policy that requires employees to use fragrance-free personal care products (e.g., shampoos, creams)
- Turn off lights AND computers AND patient monitoring equipment when rooms are not being used
- Report leaky sinks, toilets, and other plumbing sources
- Promote the purchase of local, sustainably grown foods (with a preference for organic, no use of GMOs, no use of unnecessary antibiotics, and no pesticides)
- Start a hospital/clinic/health department garden
- Start a Green Team, or join the existing one in your institution
- Create community while doing these activities and build relationships—it makes the whole process more meaningful and fun!

GMO, Genetically modified organism.

Industrial Hygiene Hierarchy of Controls

For workplace exposures, industrial hygienists have developed a "hierarchy of control" for avoiding or minimizing employee exposures to potentially hazardous chemicals. Industrial hygienists are public health professionals who specialize in workplace exposures to hazards—physical, chemical, and biological—that create the conditions for health risks. (Box 6.8 presents the **industrial hygiene hierarchy of controls.**) Once it is established that a human health threat exists, develop a plan of action—a way of eliminating or managing (reducing) the risk. **Risk management** should be informed by the risk assessment process and involves the selection and implementation of a strategy to eliminate or reduce risks. Box 6.9 lists the three Rs for reducing environmental pollution.

Nursing interventions to reduce environmental health risks can take many forms. Education is one example of a nursing intervention. By working with a wide array of community members, nurses can help a community understand the relationship between harmful environmental exposures and human health and guide the community toward risk reduction on the basis of both individual behavior changes, as well as community-wide

BOX 6.8 Industrial Hygiene Hierarchy of Controls[a]

Eliminate unnecessary toxic chemicals.
Substitute less hazardous or nonhazardous substances (e.g., using water-based vs. solvent-based products).
Isolate the hazardous chemicals from human exposure (e.g., use closed systems).
Apply engineering controls (e.g., ventilation systems, including exhaust hoods).
Reduce the exposures through **administrative controls** (e.g., rotating employees in areas with high exposures).
Use **personal protective equipment** (e.g., gloves, respirators, protective clothing).

[a]In addition, education is a critical tool in the hierarchy of controls.
Modified from Levy B, Wegman D: *Occupational health: recognizing and preventing work-related disease and injury,* ed. 4, Philadelphia, 2000, Lippincott Williams & Wilkins.

BOX 6.9 The Three Rs for Reducing Environmental Pollution

The "three Rs" adage of the environmentalist community—*reduce, reuse,* and *recycle*—helps us consider ways to decrease our personal impact on the environment, and thereby decrease environmental health risks. These concepts can apply to our health care settings, as well as our homes. By recycling, we prevent the need to extract more resources from the earth to manufacture products. By recycling, we also prevent products from unnecessary landfilling or incineration. Choosing reusable products, versus single-use devices and products, similarly prevents the need for manufacturing more products and decreases the waste stream. Reducing our waste stream can also be accomplished generally by a reduction in consumption (buying less "stuff," as well as by reducing unnecessary packaging and other nonessential goods). The "Story of Stuff" (www.thestoryofstuff.org) provides an excellent overview of the "cradle to grave" travels of products and the full range of their human and ecological impacts.

approaches. In communities in which radon is likely to be a naturally occurring exposure, nurses can educate the community about the health risks, methods to measure radon levels in a home, and how to address unhealthy radon levels.

LEVELS OF PREVENTION

Example Applied to Lead-Based Paint Exposure

Primary Prevention

Eliminate lead-based paint and lead-based paint dust from the home.

Secondary Prevention

Provide blood lead testing of children in communities with older housing stock.

Tertiary Prevention

When a child presents with extremely elevated blood lead levels, make sure the child is being cared for by a health professional who is familiar with clinical interventions to reduce blood lead levels using clinical (chelating medications) interventions, while concurrently assuring that the child returns to a lead-safe place.

The clinical intervention is tertiary prevention. It neither prevents the exposure, nor focuses on decreasing the exposure, but rather focuses on decreasing the potential health sequelae associated with elevated lead levels.

RISK COMMUNICATION

Risk communication is both an area of practice and a skill that is a composite of two separate words: "risk" and "communication." *Risk* is a familiar term in nursing practice. It is understood in the health context when we counsel patients about the risks of pregnancy, communicable disease (especially sexually transmitted disease), unintentional injury, and risk associated with personal choices (e.g., smoking, alcohol consumption, and diet). Risk assessment in environmental health focuses on characterizing the hazard (the source), its physical and chemical properties, its toxicity, and the potential exposure pathways—**route of exposure**, defining the affected population, and determining the dose of the exposure. In their seminal work on risk communication, Sandman et al. (1991) noted that risk has traditionally been formulated as magnitude (the size, severity, extent of area, or population affected) multiplied by the probability (how likely exposure or damage is to occur) (Box 6.10). For example, an environmental risk assessment of a contaminated site would involve a calculation of the dose that might be received through all routes of exposure, the toxicity of the chemical, the size and vulnerability (age, health) of the population potentially exposed (resident, future resident, transient), and the likelihood of exposure. Sandman et al. (1991) also noted that the reaction to things that scare people and the things that kill people are often not related to the actual hazard. They have gone further to probe what is behind those differences and identified a list of "outrage factors" to explain people's responses to risk (Box 6.11). They maintain that the outrage is just as predictable and open to intervention as the science of addressing the hazard.

Communication of risk involves understanding the outrage factors relevant to the risk being addressed so they can be incorporated in the message—the information—either to create action to ensure safety or prevent harm or to reduce unnecessary fear. An example of raising outrage to produce action can be seen in the shift from emphasis on smokers (voluntary) to victims of passive smoking (involuntary) to stimulate public policy that limits or bans smoking in public places. When the emphasis on risk went from a voluntary choice of smokers to an involuntary exposure of nonsmokers, the outrage level of the nonsmoking public became high enough to result in legislation guaranteeing smoke-free public spaces (e.g., public buildings, airplanes, and restaurants).

On the other hand, outrage decreases when people receive information on the situation from a trusted source, and physicians and nurses are often cited in surveys as trusted sources of information on environmental risks (Kaiser Family Foundation, 2013). The public trust is a compelling incentive to match professional knowledge and skills to a community's expectations. The outrage factor can also be a driving force in building credibility and trustworthiness in every person whose work involves interacting with the public.

BOX 6.10 Definitions of Risk

Risk has traditionally been defined by the following equation:

$$\text{Risk} = \text{magnitude} \times \text{probability}$$

There is a growing body of literature from practitioners and researchers who have studied the human reaction to risk—real and perceived. Sandman et al. (1991) were the first to examine the "outrage" factor that can influence the way in which we perceive risk, particularly to environmental risks.

$$\text{Risk} = \text{hazard} + \text{outrage}$$

Addressing only the hazard is doing only half of the necessary work; addressing the response (outrage) is equally important.

From Sandman PM, Chess C, Hane BJ: *Improving dialogue with communities,* New Brunswick, NJ, 1991, Rutgers University.

BOX 6.11 Outrage Factors: Characteristics of Risk That Contribute to the Public's Feeling of Outrage

Safer = Less Outrage	Less Safe = More Outrage
12 Principal Outrage Components	
Voluntary	Involuntary (coerced)
Natural	Industrial (artificial)
Familiar	Exotic
Not memorable	Memorable
Not dreaded	Dreaded
Chronic	Catastrophic
Knowable (detectable)	Unknowable (undetectable)
Individually controlled	Controlled by others
Fair	Unfair
Morally irrelevant	Morally relevant
Trustworthy sources	Untrustworthy sources
Responsive process	Unresponsive process

Risk communication includes all the principles of good communication in general. It is a combination of the following:

- *The right information:* Accurate, relevant, in a language that audiences can understand. A good risk assessment is essential information for shaping the message.
- *To the right people:* Those affected and those who are worried but may not be affected. Information on the community is essential: geographic boundaries, who lives there (i.e., demographics), how they obtain information (e.g., flyers or newspapers, radio, television, word of mouth), where they congregate (e.g., school, church, community center), and who within the community can help plan the communication.
- *At the right time:* For timely action or to allay fear.

GOVERNMENTAL ENVIRONMENTAL PROTECTION

The government has a variety of tools to address environmental exposures. In addition to passing legislation, creating and enforcing standards and regulations, deciding how land should be used, providing permits, and supporting research, the government is actively engaged in educating the public. Many federal agencies are involved in environmental health regulation, such as the EPA, the FDA, and the Department of Agriculture. The Department of Health and Human Services (DHHS) has two major research institutes, the National Institute of Environmental Health Sciences (NIEHS) and the National Institute for Occupational Safety and Health (NIOSH). Within DHHS is the CDC (which includes the National Center for Environmental Health [NCEH], responsible for tracking environmental health trends, recommending clinical and public health practices, and also engaging in research). Every state has an agency responsible for environmental quality. At the city or county level, the local health department most often manages environmental health issues. However, environmental protection issues are typically directed by the state using both federal and state laws. Box 6.12 lists key environmental protection laws.

Potentially harmful pollution that cannot be prevented must be controlled. An important step in the process of controlling pollution is **permitting**, a process by which the government permits companies to pollute but places limits on the amount emitted into the air or water. A **permit** is a legally binding document.

BOX 6.12 Environmental Laws

The following are some of the major environmental laws, but it is not a fully inclusive list.

National Environmental Policy Act (NEPA)
The NEPA established the Environmental Protection Agency (EPA) and a national policy for the environment and provides for the establishment of a Council on Environmental Policy. All policies, regulations, and public laws shall be interpreted and administered in accordance with the policies set forth in this act.

Federal Insecticide, Fungicide, and Rodenticide Act (FIFRA)
FIFRA provides federal control of pesticide distribution, sale, and use. The EPA was given the authority to study the consequences of pesticide usage and requires users such as farmers and utility companies to register when using pesticides. Later amendments to the law required applicators to take certification examinations, registration of all pesticides used in the United States, and proper labeling of pesticides that, if in accordance with specifications, will cause no harm to the environment (summary from FIFRA, 1972).

Clean Water Act (CWA)
The CWA sets basic structure for regulating pollutants to U.S. waters. The law gave the EPA the authority to set effluent standards on an industry basis and continued the requirements to set water quality standards for all contaminants in surface water. The 1977 amendments focused on toxic pollutants. In 1987 the CWA was reauthorized, and again focused on toxic pollutants, authorized citizen suit provisions, and funded sewage treatment plants.

Clean Air Act (CAA)
The Clean Air Act regulates air emissions from aerial, stationary, and mobile sources. The EPA was authorized to establish National Ambient Air Quality Standards (NAAQS) to protect public health and the environment. The goal was to set and achieve the NAAQS by 1975. The law was amended in 1977 when many areas of the country failed to meet the standards. The 1990 amendments to the Clean Air Act intended to meet unaddressed or insufficiently addressed problems such as acid rain, ground level ozone, stratospheric ozone depletion, and air pollutants. Also in the 1990 reauthorization was a mandate for Chemical Risk Management Plans. This mandate requires industry to identify "worst case scenarios" regarding the hazardous chemicals that they transport, use, or discard (summary from Clean Air Act, 1970).

Occupational Safety and Health Act (OSHA)
The OSHA was passed to ensure worker and workplace safety. The goal was to make sure employers provide an employment place free of hazards to health and safety such as chemicals, excessive noise, mechanical dangers, heat or cold extremes, or unsanitary conditions. To establish standards for the workplace, the Act also created National Institute for Occupational Safety and Health (NIOSH) as the research institution for OSHA.

Safe Drinking Water Act (SDWA)
The SDWA was established to protect the quality of drinking water in the United States. The Act authorized the EPA to establish safe standards of purity and required all owners or operators of public water systems to comply with primary (health-related) standards.

Resource Conservation and Recovery Act (RCRA)
The RCRA gave the EPA the authority to control the generation, transportation, treatment, storage, and disposal of hazardous waste. The RCRA also proposed a framework to manage nonhazardous waste. The 1984 Federal Hazardous and Solid Waste Amendments to this Act required phasing out land disposal of hazardous waste. The 1986 amendments enabled the EPA to address problems from underground tanks storing petroleum and other hazardous substances.

Toxic Substances Control Act (TSCA)
The TSCA gives the EPA the ability to track the 75,000 industrial chemicals currently produced in or imported into the United States. The EPA can require reporting or testing of chemicals that may pose environmental health risks and can

Continued

BOX 6.12 Environmental Laws—cont'd

ban the manufacture and import of those chemicals that pose an unreasonable risk. TSCA supplements the Clean Air Act and the Toxic Release Inventory.

Comprehensive Environmental Response, Compensation, and Liability Act (CERCLA or Superfund)

This law created a tax on the chemical and petroleum industries and provided broad federal authority to respond directly to releases or threatened releases of hazardous substances that may endanger public health or the environment.

Superfund Amendments and Reauthorization Act (SARA)

SARA amended the Comprehensive Environmental Response, Compensation, and Liability Act with several changes and additions. These changes included increased size of the trust fund; encouragement of greater citizen participation in decision making on how sites should be cleaned up; increased state involvement in every phase of the Superfund program; increased focus on human health problems related to hazardous waste sites; new enforcement authorities and settlement tools; emphasis on the importance of permanent remedies and innovative treatment technologies in cleanup of hazardous waste sites; and Superfund actions to consider standards in other federal and state regulations. (Under Superfund legislation, the Federal Agency for Toxic Substances and Disease Registry was established.)

Emergency Planning and Community Right to Know Act (EPCRA)

The EPCRA, also known as Title III of SARA, was enacted to help local communities protect public health safety and the environment from chemical hazards. Each state was required to appoint a State Emergency Response Commission that was required to divide their state into Emergency Planning Districts and establish a Local Emergency Planning Committee (LEPC) for each district.

National Environmental Education Act

The National Environmental Education Act created a new and better coordinated environmental education emphasis at the EPA. It created the National Environmental Education and Training Foundation.

Pollution Prevention Act (PPA)

The PPA focused industry, government, and public attention on reduction of the amount of pollution through cost-effective changes in production, operation, and use of raw materials. Pollution prevention also includes other practices that increase efficient use of energy, water, and other water resources, such as recycling, source reduction, and sustainable agriculture.

Food Quality Protection Act (FQPA)

The FQPA amended the Federal Insecticide, Fungicide, and Rodenticide Act and the Federal Food, Drug, and Cosmetic Act. The Act changed the way the EPA regulates pesticides. The requirements included a new safety standard of reasonable certainty of no harm to be applied to all pesticides used on foods.

Chemical Safety Information, Site Security, and Fuels Regulatory Act (Amendment to Section 112 of Clean Air Act)

This act removed from coverage by the Risk Management Plan (RMP) any flammable fuel when used as fuel or held for sale as fuel by a retail facility (flammable fuels used as a feedstock or held for sale as a fuel at a wholesale facility are still covered). This Act required certain facilities to have in place a risk management program and submit a summary of that program, called a Risk Management Plan (RMP) to the EPA. The law has two distinct parts that pertain to flammable fuels and public access to Off-Site Consequence Analysis (OCA) data. OCA is "worst-case scenario" data.

Environmental Standards

Environmental standards may describe a permitted level of emissions, a maximum contaminant level (MCL), an action level for environmental cleanup, or a risk-based calculation; environmental standards are required to address health risks. It is the responsibility of potential polluters to operate within the regulations and standards. Compliance and enforcement are the next building blocks in controlling pollution. **Compliance** refers to the processes for ensuring that permit/standard/regulatory requirements are met. Cleanup or remediation of environmental damage is another control step. Public information and involvement processes, such as citizen advisory panels or community forums, are integral to the development of standards, ongoing **monitoring**, and remediation.

POLICY AND ADVOCACY

There are almost three million nurses in the United States today—about 1 in every 100 Americans is a registered nurse! Nurses can and should be a strong voice for a healthy environment. As informed citizens, nurses can take a variety of actions to protect the environmental health of families, clients, and communities. Nurses are perceived as trusted messengers and as reliable sources of environmental health information and as such, have a responsibility to be informed and take action in the best interest of public health. Often, legislators are called to vote on environmental legislation without a sound understanding of how the legislation may affect public health. Nurses can serve as a resource for state and federal legislators and their staff. Although every nurse may not be an expert in all aspects of environmental health, every nurse does have a basic education in human health and has a sufficient understanding of who may be most vulnerable to environmental insult. Nurses' thoughts about the potential impacts of new laws on the health of individuals and communities are valuable to legislators and other policy makers, as well as the public.

Grounded in science and using sound risk communication skills, nurses become the most credible sources of information at community gatherings, formal governmental hearings, and professional nursing forums. Nurses work as advocates for environmental justice so that all members of the community have a right to live and work in an environment that is healthy and safe (Mood, 2002).

Public health nurses also volunteer to serve on state, local, or federal commissions, and they know about zoning and permit laws that regulate the impact of industry and land use on the community. Many nurse legislators began their careers by advocating for the rights of others. Nurses must read, listen, and ask questions. Then, as informed citizens, they will be leaders, fostering community action to address environmental health threats.

In 2008 the Alliance of Nurses for Healthy Environments was created to coalesce individual nurses and nursing organizations around issues associated with the environmental exposures and human health. This organization addresses the integration of environmental health into nursing education, practice (including greening the health care sector), research, and advocacy.

ENVIRONMENTAL JUSTICE AND ENVIRONMENTAL HEALTH DISPARITIES

Some diseases differentially affect different populations. Certain environmental health risks disproportionately affect poor people and people of color in the United States. If you are a poor person of color, you are more likely to live near a hazardous waste site or an incinerator and more likely to have children who are lead poisoned. You are also more likely to have children with asthma, which has a strong association with environmental exposures. Campaigns to improve the unequal burden of environmental risks in communities of color and in poor communities are striving to achieve **environmental justice** or environmental equity.

In 1993 the Environmental Justice Act was passed, and in 1994 Executive Order 12898, "Federal Actions to Address Environmental Justice in Minority Populations," was signed. This Act and the subsequent actions created policies to more comprehensively reduce the incidence of environmental *injustice* by mandating that every federal agency act in a manner to address and prevent illnesses and injuries. Nursing interventions and involvement in environmental health policies can have a significant effect on the health disparities experienced by our most challenged communities.

ENVIRONMENTAL HEALTH THREATS ASSOCIATED WITH THE HEALTH CARE INDUSTRY: NEW OPPORTUNITIES FOR PRACTICE AND ADVOCACY

Many choices in the health care setting affect environmental health. Nurses often lead in reducing the use of mercury-containing products in hospitals. The use of mercury-containing thermometers and sphygmomanometers leads to a risk of breakage, which releases a highly toxic substance into the workplace. Further, when a hospital uses incineration to dispose of their waste, the mercury-containing products will create significant releases of mercury into the air, thus contaminating communities. This airborne mercury will be present in raindrops. When airborne mercury lands on water bodies (e.g., lakes, rivers, or oceans), it is converted by microorganisms in the water to methylmercury, which is highly toxic to humans. The **methylmercury** is then **bioaccumulated** in the fish: as larger fish eat smaller fish; the body burden of methylmercury increases significantly.

Many synthetic chemicals that contaminate the environment are referred to as **persistent bioaccumulative toxins** (PBTs) or **persistent organic pollutants** (POPs). These are chemicals that do not break down in air, water, or soil, or in the plant, animal, and human bodies in which they can be found. Ultimately, since humans are at the top of the food chain, these chemicals may come to reside in our bodies. For example, toxic flame-retardant chemicals that can be found in the cushions on our couches, adult and children's mattresses, and computers are also found in almost everyone's bodies. The adverse health effects from these ubiquitous exposures include thyroid and other endocrine disruption, impacts to the immune system, reproductive toxicity, cancer, and effects on fetal and child development and neurological disfunction. (Shaw et al., 2010) The real tragedy of this particular chemical use is that it does not retard flames when it is used in furniture cushions or mattresses.

Dioxin, another pollutant that contaminates our communities, is created, in part, by the health care industry. Dioxins are created when we manufacture or burn (incinerate) products that contain chlorine, such as bleached white paper or polyvinyl chloride (PVC) plastics. When dioxins are released into the environment and land on grasses, grains, and bodies of water they are consumed by agricultural animals (e.g., beef and dairy cows, hogs, and poultry) and fish, where they are stored in fat cells as they work their way up the food chain. This phenomenon has resulted in dioxin deposition in breast tissue and been found in both cow and human milk. Virtually all women now have dioxin in their breast tissue. Dioxin, an endocrine-disrupting chemical and a strong carcinogen, is associated with several neurodevelopmental problems, including learning disabilities, and is now in every human's body. The solution to this problem is to stop releasing dioxins into the environment. In the health care setting, one way to eliminate the creation and release of dioxins is to stop using products like PVC plastics, whenever possible, selecting safer alternatives by employing environmentally preferable purchasing policies and practices, and never sending plastic products to be incinerated.

An international campaign called Health Care Without Harm (HCWH) is working to reduce and eliminate mercury and PVC plastic in the health care industry, as well as the elimination of incineration of medical waste. The ANA was a founding member of the HCWH campaign, and nurses have taken many leadership roles in the activities in the United States and around the world. Nurse Susan Wilburn is the Director of Sustainability for Green and Global Healthy Hospitals, the international arm of HCWH, where she works with hospitals all over the world to eliminate mercury containing products, reduce waste, halt incineration, and other activities to reduce chemical exposures and air and water pollution. The HCWH website (http://www.noharm.org) provides outstanding information on greening hospitals and resources about pollution prevention in the health care sector.

REFERRAL RESOURCES

There is no one source of information about environmental health, nor is there a single resource to which a public health nurse can refer an individual or community should an environmentally related problem be suspected. As mentioned earlier, the NLM's ToxTown is a great starting place, and it allows the interested browser to dig deeply into environmental health content. TOXNET has an amalgamation of important databases and environmental health literature and additional peer-reviewed environmental health literature. The EPA is another rich source of information (www.epa.gov). Use of the Internet makes information widely accessible, but finding an actual person to assist you or the communities you serve may not be as easy. One starting point may be the poison control center, the environmental epidemiology unit or toxicology unit of your state health department, or the state department of environmental protection. The Association of Occupational and Environmental Clinics (AOEC) (http://www.aoec.org) is a national network of specialty clinics and individual practitioners available for consultation and sometimes for provision of educational programs for health professionals. Through AOEC, you can also find the Pediatric Environmental Health Specialty Units; there are 10 throughout the country. These specialty units were specifically established to provide consultation on environmental health issues. Laura Anderko at Georgetown University is the first nurse to direct a Pediatric Environmental Health Specialty Unit. Never hesitate to call people from the federal agencies such as the U.S. EPA, the CDC's National Center for Environmental Health, or the National Institute of Environmental Health Sciences. Within the CDC, there is also the Agency for Toxic Substances and Disease Registry.

Local resources include local health agencies; agricultural extension offices; and occupational and environmental departments in schools of medicine, nursing, and public health. Some local and state agencies have developed topical directories to assist in accessing the appropriate staff for specific questions. Many of the resources have websites that allow ready access through the Internet and can be located by using any of the popular search methods. Box 6.13 presents an extensive list of environmental health agency resources. The most active advocates for environmental health policies are grassroots organizations, the big environmentalist organizations, and environmental justice organizations.

BOX 6.13 Information and Guidance Sources for Referrals

Federal Agencies

Agency for Toxic Substances and Disease Registry
Centers for Disease Control and Prevention
Consumer Product Safety Commission
Environmental Protection Agency (EPA)
Office of Children's Environmental Health, EPA
Food and Drug Administration
National Institute for Occupational Safety and Health
National Institute of Environmental Health Sciences
National Institutes of Health
National Cancer Institute
National Institute of Nursing Research
Occupational Safety and Health Administration
National Library of Medicine—TOXNET

State Agencies

State Health Departments
State Environmental Protection Agencies

Nursing Organizations Focusing on Occupational and Environmental Health

Alliance of Nurses for Healthy Environments
American Association of Occupational Health Nurses

Associations and Organizations

American Association of Poison Control Centers
Association of Occupational and Environmental Clinics
Beyond Pesticides
Center for Health and Environmental Justice
Children's Environmental Health Network
Environmental Defense Fund
Environmental Working Group
Food and Water Watch
Health Care Without Harm
National Academy Press
National Environmental Education Foundation
Natural Resources Defense Council
Pediatric Environmental Health Specialty Units
Pesticide Educational Resources Collaborative
Society for Occupational and Environmental Health
University of California San Francisco Program on Reproductive Health and the Environment

ROLES FOR NURSES IN ENVIRONMENTAL HEALTH

As per the IOM recommendations, nurses should be integrating environmental health into our educational efforts and our clinical practices and greening our practice settings, our research efforts, and our advocacy and policy initiatives. Nurses who are passionate about this issue can form "green teams" at their workplaces, promote sustainable practices at their institutions, develop research expertise, teach classes, sit on commissions, write articles, and take local, state, and national leadership roles. Nurses can include and address environmental health concerns through their nursing professional associations. All nurses can include environmental exposures in their history taking; consider the environmental impacts of the products they select for their homes, clinics, hospitals, schools, and other settings; and promote reducing, recycling, and reuse of products. Each type and level of engagement is important. Starting somewhere is important. The following are some ways in which nurses can get involved both professionally and as informed citizens:

- *Community involvement/public participation.* Organizing, facilitating, and moderating; making public notices effective and public forums accessible; welcoming input. Making information exchange understandable and problem solving acceptable to culturally diverse communities are valuable assets a nurse contributes. Skills in community organizing and mobilizing can be essential for a community to have a meaningful voice in decisions that affect them.

- *Individual and population risk assessment.* Using nursing assessment skills to detect potential and actual exposure pathways and potential health effects for clients cared for in the acute, chronic, and healthy communities of practice.
- *Risk communication.* Interpreting, applying principles to practice. Nurses may serve as skilled risk communicators within health systems and agencies, working for industries, or working as independent practitioners.
- *Epidemiologic investigations.* Nurses need to have the skills to respond in scientifically sound and humanely sensitive ways to community concerns about cancer, birth defects, and stillbirths when citizens fear environmental causation.
- *Policy development.* Proposing, informing, advocating, and monitoring action from agencies, communities, and organization perspectives.

The assimilation of the concepts of environmental health into a nurse's daily practice gives new life to traditional public health values of prevention, community building, and social justice. As nurses learn more about the environment, opportunities for integration into their practice, education programs, research, advocacy, and policy work will become evident and will evolve. Opportunities abound for those pioneering spirits within the nursing profession who are dedicated to creating healthier environments for their clients and communities.

PRACTICE APPLICATION

Following are two case scenarios related to exposure pathways. The first involves lead poisoning and the second, fracking-related concerns.

At the county health department, a three-year-old boy named Billy presents with gastric upset and behavioral changes. These symptoms have persisted for several weeks. During your history taking, you discover that Billy's parents have been renovating their old home. A parent in Billy's daycare center suggested that Billy's symptoms might be associated with lead, so Billy's parents have brought him in to the clinic.

You relay this information to the primary care practitioner who, in turn, orders a blood lead level, which comes back at 45 mcg/dL. This is an extremely high value.

You research lead poisoning and discover that there are many potential health effects of lead exposure and that children are at greatest risk because their bodies, especially their nervous systems, are still developing. You also find that chronic lead poisoning may lead to long-term effects, such as developmental delays and impaired learning ability.

You let the health professional know about the lead poisoning specialists in the nearby children's hospital. On further investigation, you find that Billy's home was built before 1950 and is still under renovation. Billy should not return to the home. At this point, the registered environmental health professional from the local health department tests the dust in the home and finds high lead levels. Because of Billy's age and associated behaviors, such as hand-to-mouth activities, you determine that the lead dust in the home is the probable exposure. However, you must also consider multiple sources of exposure.

1. What other sources of exposure might exist?
2. What would you include in an assessment of this situation?
3. What prevention strategies would you use to resolve this issue? At the individual level? At the population level?

Mrs. Bell calls the local health department to report that her drinking water, from their private well, is discolored and that her son has been experiencing headaches and nose bleeds. You talk with Dan, the health department's environmental health professional, who tells you that there is new "fracking" activity on the east side of your rural county, where Mrs. Bell and her family live, and that this may be the reason for the water discoloration and the child's symptoms. You look up "fracking" and discover that the word is shorthand for hydraulic fracturing, a technique for extracting natural gas that is fraught with community and health concerns. Dan and you agree to make a site visit to the Bell's farm.

1. What will you be looking for on your visit?
2. How can you help the Bells, if any of their issues seem to be associated with the nearby fracking site?
3. What other experts are available to you and the Bells?
4. Is there a policy that could be invoked to protect the Bells and their community?

Answers can be found on the Evolve site.

KEY POINTS

- Nurses need to be informed professionals and advocates for citizens in their community regarding environmental health issues.
- Models describing the determinants of health acknowledge the role of the environment in health and disease.
- Climate change is creating profound risks to human health.
- For most chemicals in our homes, work, schools, and communities, research on their potential toxicity is not required, and for the vast majority of chemicals we lack comprehensive studies regarding health risks.
- Prevention activities include education, reduction/elimination of harmful exposures, waste minimization, sustainable energy policies, and fair and sustainable land use planning.
- Pollution control activities include elimination and reduction of the most toxic chemicals; use of technologies; environmental permitting; environmental regulations and standards, monitoring, compliance, and enforcement; and cleanup and remediation.
- Each nursing assessment should include questions and observations concerning potential and existing occupational and environmental exposures.
- Useful environmental exposure data are sometimes difficult to acquire, but those data that exist can be used to aid in the assessment, diagnosis, intervention, and evaluation of environmentally related health problems.

- Both case advocacy and class advocacy are critical skills for nurses in environmental health practice.
- Risk communication is an important skill and must be done in a culturally sensitive way and acknowledge the outrage factor experienced by communities with environmental hazards.
- Federal, state, and local laws and regulations, as well as international treaties, exist to protect the health of people from environmental hazards.
- Environmental health practice engages multiple disciplines, and nurses are important members of the environmental health team.
- Environmental health practice includes principles of health promotion, disease prevention, and health protection.
- *Healthy People 2020* objectives address both targets for the reduction of risk factors and diseases related to environmental causes.

CLINICAL DECISION-MAKING ACTIVITIES

1. Explain why the source of drinking water is important to investigate in the assessment of an unusually high number of infertility cases in a community; in increased lead levels in children from a certain school; and in an outbreak of gastrointestinal symptoms in an agricultural community.
2. Discuss the use of the epidemiologic triangle in explaining the associations between the environment and human health.
3. Discover if your jurisdiction has a law or regulation for the disclosure of lead-based paint or radon levels for personal property when an owner sells a house. If your community does not, investigate with the government officials of the community why there is not a required disclosure.

ADDITIONAL RESOURCES

EVOLVE WEBSITE

http://evolve.elsevier.com/Stanhope/community/

- Answers to Practice Application
- Case Study
- Glossary
- Review Questions

REFERENCES

Agency for Healthcare Research and Quality: *Focus on Research: Children with Chronic Illness and Disabilities, AHRQ Publication No. 02-M025*, Rockville, MD, 2002, U.S. Department of Health and Human Services, AHRQ Publications Clearing House.

Allen K, Davis M. *Hurricanes Harvey and Irma May Have Caused Up To $200 Billion in Damage, Comparable to Katrina*, 2017. Retrieved from https://abcnews.go.com.

American Cancer Society (ACS): *Cancer Facts and Figures*, 2018. Retrieved from http://www.cancer.org.

American Nurses Association: *ANA's Principles of Environmental Health in Nursing Practice with Implementation Strategies*, Silver Spring MD, 2007, Author.

Anney RJ, Hawi Z, Sheehan K, et al.: Epigenetic effects in ADHD: parent-of-origin effects in image sample, *Am J Med Genet B Neuropsychiatr Genet* 141(7):736–737, 2006.

Bassil KL, Vakil C, Sanborn M, Cole DC, Kaur JS, Kerr KJ: Cancer health effects of pesticides: systematic review, *Can Fam Physician* 53(10):1704–1711, 2007.

Bailey HD, Fritschi L, Infante-Rivard C, et al.: Parental occupational pesticide exposure and the risk of childhood leukemia in the offspring: findings from the childhood leukemia international consortium, *Int J Cancer* 135(9):2157–2172, 2014.

Bridges B: Fragrance: emerging health and environmental, *Flavour Fragr J* 17:361–371, 2002.

Butterfield P, Postma J: ERRNIE research team: The TERRA framework: conceptualizing rural environmental health inequities through an environmental justice lens, *ANS Adv Nurs Sci* 32(2):107–117, 2009.

Centers for Disease Control and Prevention (CDC): *Asthma: data and surveillance*, 2012. Retrieved from http://www.cdc.gov.

Centers for Disease Control and Prevention (CDC): Prevalence of autism spectrum disorder among children aged 8 years—Autism and Developmental Disabilities Monitoring Network, 11 sites, United States, 2010, *MMWR Surveill Summ* 63(2):1–21, 2014a.

Centers for Disease Control and Prevention (CDC): *Adolescent and school health: childhood obesity*, 2014b. facts. Retrieved from http://www.cdc.gov.

Chen M, Chang CH, Tao L, Lu C: Residential exposure to pesticide during childhood and childhood cancers: a meta-analysis, *Pediatrics* 136(4):719–729, 2015.

Choi M, Afzal B, Sattler B: Geographic information systems: a new tool for environmental health assessments, *Public Health Nurs* 23(5):381–391, 2006.

Clean Air Act: Risk management programs, Section 112(7). *Federal Register*, Part III EPA, 40 CFR, Part 68, 2014a.

Clean Air Act: 1970. Public Law 91-604. Retrieved from http://www.epa.gov.

Council on Linkages Between Academic and Public Health Practice: *Core Competencies for Public Health Professionals*, Washington DC, 2014, Public Health Foundation/Health.

Currie J, Greenstone M, Meckel K: Hydraulic fracturing and infant health: New evidence from Pennsylvania, *Sci Adv* 3(12):e1603021, 2017.

Department of Health and Human Services (DHHS): *SAMHSA: fast facts about children and mental health*, 2005. Retrieved from http://www.dbhds.virginia.gov.

Environmental Protection Agency (EPA): *America's children and the environment*, ed 3, (ACE3) 2013—Frequently asked questions, 2013. Retrieved from http://www.epa.gov.

Environmental Protection Agency: 2009. Retrieved from http://www.epa.gov.

Environmental Protection Agency: *Chemicals in commerce: TSCA Chemical Substance Inventory*, 2014 (Last updated 3/13/14). Retrieved from http://www.epa.gov.

Environmental Working Group: *Body Burden—The Pollution in Newborns: A Benchmark Investigation of Industrial Chemicals, Pollutants and Pesticides in Umbilical Cord Blood*, July 14, 2005. Found a teen body burden from 2014, a follow up from an initial 2008 study. Retrieved from: https://www.ewg.org.

Federal Insecticide, Fungicide, and Rodenticide Act: 1972. (FIFRA) Retrieved from www.epa.gov.

Febvey O, Schüz J, Bailey HD, et al.: Risk of central nervous system tumors in children related to parental occupational pesticide exposures in three European case-control studies, *J Occup Environ Med* 58(10):1046–1052, 2016.

Ferreira JD, Couto AC, Pombo-de-Oliveira MS, Koifman S: In utero pesticide exposure and leukemia in Brazilian children < 2 years of age, *Environ Health Perspect* 121(2):269–275, 2013.

Fudvoye J, Bourguignon JP, Parent AS: Endocrine-disrupting chemicals and human growth and maturation. A focus on early critical windows of exposure, *Vitam Horm* 94:1–25, 2014.

Gilden R, Friedmann E, Sattler B, Squibb K, McPhaul K: Potential health effects related to pesticide use on athletic fields, *Public Health Nurs* 29(3):198–207, 2012.

Habre R, Moshier E, Castro W, et al.: The effects of PM 2.5 and its components from indoor and outdoor sources on cough and wheeze symptoms in asthmatic children, *J Expo Sci Environ Epidemiol* 24(4):380–387, 2014.

Hill WG, Butterfield PG: Environmental risk reduction for rural children. In Lee HJ, Winters CA, editors: *Rural Nursing: Concepts, Theory, and Practice*, ed 2, New York, NY, 2006, Springer.

Holmes M, Kennedy MC, Riccio R, Hart A: Assessing the risk to U.K. children from carbendazim residues in apple products, *Int J Occup Environ Health* 14(2):86–93, 2008.

Hsu HH, Chiu YH, Coull BA, et al.: Prenatal particulate air pollution and asthma onset in urban children: identifying sensitive windows and sex differences, *Am J Respir Crit Care Med* 192(9):1052–1059, 2015.

Huff M: *Ensia Magazine Interview by Mary Huff with William McDonough*, 2013. Retrieved from http://ensia.com.

Intergovernmental Program on Climate Change: *Climate Change (IPCC) 2014: impacts, adaptation, and vulnerability, IPCC Working Group II Contribution to the 5th assessment report*, 2014. Retrieved from http://www.who.int.

Kaiser Family Foundation: *Nurses trusted source—Kaiser health tracking poll*, 2013. Retrieved from http://kff.org.

Kalkbrenner AE, Windham GC, Serre ML. Particulate matter exposure, prenatal and postnatal windows of susceptibility, and autism spectrum disorders, *Epidemiology* 26(1):30–42, 2015.

Landrigan PJ, Rauh VA, Galvez MP: Environmental justice and the health of children, *Mt Sinai J Med* 77(2):178–187, 2010.

Landrigan PJ: Children's Environmental Health: A Brief History, *Acad Pediatr* 16:1–9, 2016.

Levy B, Wegman D: *Occupational health: recognizing and preventing work-related disease and injury*, ed 4, Philadelphia, 2000, Lippincott Williams & Wilkins.

Louv R: *No Child Left Inside: Saving Our Children from Nature-Deficit Disorder*, Chapel Hill, NC, 2005, Algonquin Books.

Metayer C, Colt JS, Buffler PA, et al.: Exposure to herbicides in house dust and risk of childhood acute lymphoblastic leukemia, *J Expo Sci Environ Epidemiol* 23(4):363–370, 2013.

Mood LH: Environmental health policy: environmental justice. In Mason DJ, Leavitt JK, editors: *Policy and Politics in Nursing and Health Care*, ed 4, Philadelphia, PA, 2002, Saunders.

Myths-Dreams-Symbols: 2006. Retrieved from http://www.mythsdreamssymbols.com.

O'Brien M: *Making better environmental decisions: an alternative to risk assessment*, Cambridge, MA, 2000, MIT Press.

Pope AM, Snyder MA, Mood LH, editors: *Nursing, Health and Environment: Strengthening the Relationship to Improve the Public's Health*, Washington, DC, 1995, Institute of Medicine, National Academy Press.

President's Cancer Panel: *Reducing Environmental Cancer Risk: What Can We Do Now? NOTE: the actual quote comes from the letter transmitting the report to the President*, April 2010. Annual report 2008–2009. Released 2010. Retrieved from http://deainfo.nci.nih.gov.

Prüss-Üstün A, Wolf J, Corvalan C, Bos R, Neira M: World Health Organization: *Preventing disease through healthy environments: a global assessment of the burden of disease from environmental risks*, 2016. Retrieved from http://www.who.int.

Public Health, Environment and Social Determinants of Health (PHE): 2015. Retrieved from http://www.who.int.

Quad Council of Public Health Nursing Organizations: *Competencies for Public Health Nursing Practice*, Washington DC, 2018, ASTDN.

Sandman PM, Chess C, Hane BJ: *Improving Dialogue with Communities*, New Brunswick, NJ, 1991, Rutgers University.

Schettler T, Stein J, Reich F, et al.: *In Harm's Way: Toxic Threats to Development, a Report by Greater Boston Physicians for Social Responsibility, Prepared for a Joint Project with Clean Water*, Cambridge, MA, 2000, PSR. Retrieved from http://www.psr.org.

Shaw SD, Blum A, Weber R, et al.: Halogenated flame retardants: do the fire safety benefits justify the risks? *Rev Environ Health* 25(4):261–305, 2010.

Shoot B: *How Much the 2018 California Fires Have Cost (So Far)*, 2018. Retrieved from http://fortune.com.

Silva JF, Mattos IE, Luz LL, Carmo CN, Aydos RD: Exposure to pesticides and prostate cancer: systematic review of the literature, *Rev Environ Health* 31(3):311–327, 2016.

Smargiassi A, Goldberg MS, Wheeler AJ, et al.: Associations between personal exposure to air pollutants and lung function tests and cardiovascular indices among children with asthma living near an industrial complex and petroleum refineries, *Environ Res* 132: 38–45, 2014.

Suk WA, Davis EA: Strategies for addressing global environmental health concerns, *Ann N Y Acad Sci* 1140.40–44, 2008.

U.S. Department of Health and Human Services: *Healthy People 2020*, 2010. Retrieved from http://www.healthypeople.gov.

U.S. Department of Housing and Urban Development: *American Healthy Homes Survey, lead and arsenic findings*, April 2011, Office of Healthy Homes and Lead Hazard Control.

Watkins DJ, Sánchez BN, Téllez-Rojo MM, et al.: Impact of phthalate and BPA exposure during in utero windows of susceptibility on reproductive hormones and sexual maturation in peripubertal males, *Environ Health* 16(1):69, 2017.

Vercammen P, Chavez N, Mossburg C, Vera A: *Northern California wildfire kills two, destroys homes in redding*, 2018. Retrieved from https://www.cnn.com.

VoPham T, Bertrand KA, Hart JE, et al.: Pesticide exposure and liver cancer: a review, *Cancer Causes Control* 28(3):177–190, 2017.

Wright RO: Environment, susceptibility windows, development, and child health, *Curr Opin Pediatr*, 29(2):211-217. 2017.

United Nations University: *WHO quote found from 1993 document*, 1993. Retrieved from http://unu.edu.

Wingspread Statement on the Precautionary Principle, Racine, WI, 1998. Retrieved from http://www.gdrc.org.

U.S. Department of Housing and Urban Development: *American Healthy Homes Survey, lead and arsenic findings*, April 2011, Office of Healthy Homes and Lead Hazard Control. Retrieved from http://portal.hud.gov.

World Health Organization: *Public Health and the Environment, Public Health, Environment, and Social Determinants of Health (PHE)*, 2015. Retrieved from http://www.who.int.

World Health Organization: *Climate Change and Human Health*, 2014. Retrieved from http://www.who.int.

World Health Organization: *Fact File: 10 facts on mental health*, n.d. Retrieved from http://www.who.int.

Yoder JS, Wallace RM, Collier SA, et al.: Cryptosporidiosis surveillance—United States, 2009-2010. Centers for Disease Control and Prevention (CDC), *MMWR Surveill Summ* 61(5):1–12, 2012.

7

Application of Ethics in the Community

Sydney A. Axson, MPH, RN and Connie M. Ulrich, PhD, RN, FAAN

OBJECTIVES

After reading this chapter, the student should be able to do the following:

1. Describe a brief history of the ethics of nursing practice.
2. Analyze ethical decision-making processes.
3. Compare and contrast ethical theories and principles, virtue ethics, care ethics, and feminist ethics.
4. Comprehend the ethics inherent in the core functions of public health nursing.
5. Analyze codes of ethics for nursing and for public health.
6. Apply the ethics of advocacy to nursing in public health.

CHAPTER OUTLINE

Brief History of Ethics and Bioethics: Relationship to Nursing and Public Health
History
Ethical Decision Making
Ethical Principles and Theories as Guides to Ethical Decision Making
Principles of Bioethics
Ethics and the Core Functions of Population-Centered Nursing Practice
Nursing Code of Ethics
Public Health Code of Ethics
Advocacy and Ethics

KEY TERMS

advocacy, p. 159
assessment, p. 156
assurance, p. 157
beneficence, p. 154
bioethics, p. 150
code of ethics, p. 151
consequentialism, p. 153
deontology, p. 154
distributive justice, p. 154
ethical decision making, p. 152
ethical dilemmas, p. 152
ethical issues, p. 152
ethics, p. 150
feminist ethics, p. 156
feminists, p. 156
moral distress, p. 153
nonmaleficence, p. 154
policy development, p. 157
principlism, p. 154
respect for autonomy, p. 154
utilitarianism, p. 153
virtue ethics, p. 155
virtues, p. 155

Nurses who work in the community focus on protecting, promoting, preserving, and maintaining health while preventing disease. Working within public health settings, however, can challenge nurses in many ways. Indeed, public health nurses may be the first point of contact for patients and their families within the local community; they are in a unique position as they work to establish trusting relationships not only with their patients and families but also with a broad array of community groups that represent local interests. As health care providers, nurses navigate personal beliefs, patient and/or family wishes, and community values. And, they must do so within the parameters of community resources, organizational policies, and within the guidelines of their professional codes of conduct. This complex and challenging process has tangible ramifications.

Public health or community nurses must also be prepared for any emerging or reemerging disease that might arise within their communities. Here, they have to weigh or balance the potential benefits and risks to the patients they serve, themselves, and to the larger community. An outbreak of the Zika virus (a mosquito-borne virus), for example, presented a significant

Special thanks go to Mary Silva, James Fletcher, and Jeanne Sorrell for their valuable contributions to previous editions of this chapter.

public health threat to communities internationally and across the United States. Lucey and Gostin (2016) suggest that "training health workers to observe and report Zika-related disease and robust systems for collecting and analyzing surveillance data will complement public health strategies" (p. 865). The lead levels in the water supply in a largely minority population in Flint, Michigan, is another example of a public and community health crisis. Clean drinking water is one of public health's greatest contributions to modern life. However, despite overwhelming evidence regarding the long-term health impacts of contaminated drinking water, residents of Flint were exposed to toxic contaminants in their drinking water. Both the Zika outbreak and the Flint water crisis present numerous ethical issues rooted in social justice, respect for persons, and acting in the best interests of a community (Bellinger, 2016). Thus this chapter applies core knowledge of ethics to public health nursing. Further, characteristics unique to community health practice are explored.

BRIEF HISTORY OF ETHICS AND BIOETHICS: RELATIONSHIP TO NURSING AND PUBLIC HEALTH

Ethics is both a process for reflection and a body of knowledge that focuses on the study of morality and the moral life (Beauchamp & Childress, 2013). Stated differently, Chadwick and Gallagher (2016) explain that ethics concerns the "oughts" and "shoulds" of practice. Ethics-related questions may ask the following: How should I behave? What actions should I perform? What kind of person should I be? What are my obligations to myself and others? Ethics is important in all aspects of life and is particularly important in nursing practice. Basing actions on ethical principles and guidelines supports clinical decision making, the ethical conduct of nurses, and the care they provide within communities.

Bioethics, a multidisciplinary subfield of ethics, is the systematic study of ethical issues in research, clinical care, or other areas in the life sciences and health care using both normative and empirical methodological approaches (Jonsen, 1998; Reich, 1995). Several sentinel historical events have shaped the field of bioethics, including the well-known Nuremberg Tribunal that followed World War II. The Nuremberg Tribunal reviewed the egregious human rights abuses performed under the guise of scientific experimentation by Nazi leaders, including physicians (Grodin et al., 2018). These abuses, and the prosecution of their perpetrators, led to the development of the Nuremberg Code of 1947, "which set the standard for every subsequent attempt to regulate human experimentation." One of the most important requirements from the Nuremberg code is the voluntary nature of research (Annas, 2018). Major social movements of the 1960s and 1970s in the United States facilitated further development of the field of bioethics. Examples include the campaign for nuclear disarmament, the civil rights and peace movements, the protests against the war in Vietnam, and new medical technologies that raised challenging ethical questions about life and death (Easley & Allen, 2007). In addition, the first institution in the United States devoted to the study of bioethics was the Hastings Center, founded by Daniel Callahan, PhD, and Willard Gaylin, MD, in 1970. The Hastings Center (2019) addresses core ethical issues that arise in all areas of the life sciences and their impact on the health and well-being of individuals, communities, and societies. It remains an excellent resource in the rapidly changing health care landscape.

Despite the atrocities of Nuremberg, violation of human rights in the name of research continued, including the U.S. Public Health Service sanctioned Tuskegee syphilis study. From this the 1974 National Research Act established the National Commission for the Protection of Human Subjects of Biomedical and Behavioral Research; this commission created the seminal Belmont Report (1979). A set of guidelines differentiating clinical practice from research, the Belmont Report also outlines the ethical principles of respect for persons (informed consent and respecting autonomous decisions), beneficence (maximizing the benefits and minimizing the harms), and justice (fair subject selection in research) in the protection of human subjects who participate in research (Belmont Report, 1979).

The field of bioethics continues to evolve as a field of study and practice as ethical issues remain prevalent in clinical practice and research. For example, questions abound on how to allocate scarce resources and the benefits and harms of health technologies and research, including renal dialysis, organs for transplants, precision science, genetics and genomics, and emerging and reemerging infectious disease, among others.

HISTORY

Modern nursing has a rich heritage of ethics and morality. Florence Nightingale (1820 to 1910) is often seen as nursing's first enduring moral leader and community health nurse. Nightingale saw nursing as a call to service and thought nurses should be people of good moral character. She was a champion of primary prevention, passionate about the need to provide care to the disenfranchised, and committed to the importance of a sanitary environment, as demonstrated in her work with soldiers in the Crimean War (1854 to 1856). Her commitment to all individuals in communities, contributions to health care's body of knowledge, and established ethical tenets of clinical practice still endure today. Chapter 2 provides details about the many contributions of Nightingale to the development of the nursing profession.

In the 1960s two seminal events occurred. First, the American Nurses Association (ANA) recommended that all nursing education should occur in institutions of higher education. Before this time, many nursing programs were offered by religious institutions and had ethics embedded in their curricula. As the process of moving nursing to higher education took place, ethics, as a course, was removed from many schools of nursing. The decision to omit ethics courses was often influenced by the need to include more general education courses in the nursing curriculum. Second, because of major advances in science and technology that affected health care, the field of bioethics began to emerge and was also developing in the nursing curricula. Today, although most nursing programs integrate bioethical content into their courses or have separate courses on this topic, research suggests that about 23 percent of nurses still have no formal ethics education (Grady et al., 2008).

Nurses' codes of ethics are important in the history of public health nursing practice in the community. The *Code for Professional Nurses* was formally adopted by the ANA House of Delegates in 1950 (American Nurses Association [ANA], 1950; Fowler, 2015). It was amended and revised five more times until in 2001 the ANA House of Delegates adopted the *Code of Ethics for Nurses With Interpretive Statements* (ANA, 2001). Most recently the Code of Ethics for Nurses underwent another significant revision with approval in 2014. As stated by Marsha Fowler (2015), "the *Code of Ethics for Nurses With Interpretative Statements* is remarkable in its breadth and compass. It retains nursing's historical and ethical values, obligations, ideals, and commitments, while extending them into the ever-growing art, science, and practice of nursing in 2015" (pp. viii-ix). Importantly, the recent revision of the Code of Ethics for Nurses identifies the importance of social ethics and the role of nurses in civic engagement, deliberation, and public health. This may include running and holding political office, speaking out on gun violence, or addressing any other health-related public health concern (Fowler, 2016).

The first known international code of ethics was developed by the International Council of Nurses (ICN) in 1953 (ICN, 1953). Like the *Code of Ethics for Nurses With Interpretative Statements,* it has undergone various revisions and adoptions. The most recent version of the *ICN Code of Ethics for Nurses* was adopted in 2005, copyrighted in 2006, and revised in 2012.

As mentioned earlier in the chapter, the bioethics movement of the late 1960s influenced both nursing ethics and public health ethics. The relationship between public health and ethics has also been made explicit through the development of a code of ethics (Public Health Leadership Society, 2002). After input from many public health professionals and associations, the code of ethics for public health was approved in 2002 (Olick, 2005). This code, titled *Principles of the Ethical Practice of Public Health* defines public health in the following way: "public health not only seeks to assure the health of whole communities but also recognizes that the health of individuals is tied to their life in the community" (p. 1). It also identifies 12 guiding principles, including but not limited to respect for individuals within their communities, community engagement in policies and procedures that affect their overall health and well-being, community consent, collaborative practices that support trust within diverse communities, and upholding ethical principles of confidentiality and justice.

Professional codes are not intended to provide specific rules but rather to provide a foundation from which nurses and other public health advocates can meet their professional and moral obligations to their patients and communities. Nurses in public health have to honor their professional duties in ways that extend beyond one-on-one care, and this can present unique ethical challenges. For example, community health prevention is increasingly being informed by genomics as well as other factors. Here, nurses must become more skilled in learning how to reduce the potential impact of genetic risk factors by teaching clients how to live healthier lives. They must do this while also recognizing the potential issues of confidentiality and privacy that come with genetic information. Nurses also have to address other community health issues like the individual health effects of environmental risks within communities, such as drinking water, lead levels, air pollutants, or radiation exposure. Relevant questions for nurses that can arise regarding these issues include. Should people be held accountable for making unhealthy life choices? Should society's resources be allocated more intently at the preventive or acute care level? How do community health nurses meet the health care needs of their undocumented immigrant patients?

In addition to codes of ethics, the nursing literature and nursing associations have consistently reflected a commitment to ethics, as well as an awareness of nursing's ethical obligations to society. From the 1980s to the present, the number of centers for nursing and health care ethics has increased steadily. The majority of these centers are located in academic settings; however, in 1991 the ANA founded its Center for Ethics and Human Rights. The historical contributions of this center have affected the persistent ethicality of nursing. In 2008 the ANA published *Nursing and Health Care Ethics: A Legacy and a Vision,* which creatively assesses historical contributions of nursing scholars in ethics and explores a vision for the future scholarship of nursing ethics (Pinch & Haddad, 2008). Also in 2008 the ANA published *Guide to the Code of Ethics for Nurses: Interpretation and Application* (Fowler, 2008). Finally, in 2016 Fowler broadened the discussion on nursing's code of ethics by reinforcing its goal of social justice, calling on all nurses to be involved in civic engagement, an important goal of community health nursing.

Before discussing ethics related to nursing practice in the community, some key ethical terms are defined in Box 7.1. Other ethical terms are defined within the context of the chapter.

BOX 7.1 Key Ethical Terms

Ethics is a branch of philosophy that includes both a body of knowledge about the moral life and a process of reflection for determining what persons ought to do or be regarding this life.

Bioethics is a branch of ethics that applies the knowledge and processes of ethics to the examination of ethical problems in health care.

Moral distress is an uncontrollable state of self in which one is unable to act ethically.

Morality is shared and generational societal norms about what constitutes right or wrong conduct.

Values are beliefs about the worth or importance of what is right or esteemed.

Ethical dilemma is a puzzling moral problem in which a person, group, or community can envision morally justified reasons for both taking and not taking a certain course of action.

Codes of ethics are moral standards that delineate a profession's values, goals, and obligations.

Utilitarianism is an ethical theory based on the weighing of morally significant outcomes or consequences regarding the overall maximizing of good and minimizing of harm for the greatest number of people.

Deontology is an ethical theory that bases moral obligation on duty and claims that actions are obligatory irrespective of the good or harmful consequences that they produce. Because humans are rational, they have absolute value. Therefore persons should always be treated as ends in themselves and never as mere means.

Principlism is an approach to problem solving in bioethics that uses the principles of respect for autonomy, beneficence, nonmaleficence, and justice as the basis for organization and analysis of ethical issues and dilemmas.

Advocacy is the act of pleading for or supporting a course of action on behalf of a person, group, or community.

ETHICAL DECISION MAKING

Ethical issues are moral challenges facing all health care providers and are particularly common in community and public health nursing. Ulrich et al. state that "ethical issues can occur in any situation where profound moral questions of 'rightness' or 'wrongness' underlie professional decision-making and the beneficent care of patients" (2010b, p. 2511). A good example of an ethical issue in community or public health nursing at both the individual and community level was Ebola. One of the central ethical issues surrounding Ebola was informed consent of health care providers as well as the community regarding the risks of contracting the virus and its implications for individual and community health and well-being. From a public health perspective, other ethical issues regarding surveillance and tracking measures, availability of personal protective equipment, and quarantine and isolation procedures for hospitalized patients and American and foreign citizens who entered or re-entered the country were significant concerns. In contrast, **ethical dilemmas** are human dilemmas and puzzling moral problems in which a person, group, or community can envision morally justified reasons for both taking and not taking a certain course of action (Ulrich, 2012). With Ebola, arguments on who should receive the experimental drug ZMapp—the American health care workers who became infected or members of the African community who were dying on the front lines of the virus outbreak in Africa—was a classic example of an ethical dilemma. Here, various stakeholders presented sound arguments regarding the allocation and testing of ZMapp for each respective group.

Making ethical decisions on allocation priorities of a scarce and untested resource such as ZMapp required a systematic analysis and evaluation of the ethical issue or dilemma. Thus **ethical decision making** is the component of ethics that focuses on the process of how ethical decisions are made. Ethical theories, principles, and decision-making frameworks help us think through these issues and dilemmas. Often, ethical content is abstract, which makes decision making more difficult. Ethical decision-making frameworks use problem-solving processes and provide guides for making sound ethical decisions that can be morally justified. Some of these frameworks are presented in this chapter. The decisions we make are greatly influenced by the specifics of the situation, cultural norms and values, and more. Therefore no framework can provide a single answer for every ethical question. Nonetheless, frameworks can be useful for the ethical decision-making process. The following generic ethical decision-making framework may be useful:

1. Identify the ethical issues and dilemmas.
2. Place the ethical issues and dilemmas within a meaningful context.
3. Obtain all relevant facts.
4. Reformulate ethical issues and dilemmas, if needed.
5. Consider appropriate approaches to actions or options (such as utilitarianism, deontology, principlism, virtue ethics, care ethics, feminist ethics).
6. Make a decision and take action.
7. Evaluate the decision and the action.

TABLE 7.1 Rationale for Steps of Ethical Decision-Making Framework

Step	Rationale
1. Identify the ethical issues and dilemmas	Persons cannot make sound ethical decisions if they cannot identify ethical issues and dilemmas
2. Place them within a meaningful context	The historical, legal, sociological, cultural, psychological, economic, political, communal, environmental, and demographic contexts affect the way ethical issues and dilemmas are formulated and justified
3. Obtain all relevant facts	Facts affect the way ethical issues and dilemmas are formulated and justified
4. Reformulate ethical issues and dilemmas if needed	The initial ethical issues and dilemmas may need to be modified or changed on the basis of context and facts
5. Consider appropriate approaches to actions or options	The nature of the ethical issues and dilemmas determines the specific ethical approaches used
6. Make decisions and take action	Professional persons cannot avoid choice and action in applied ethics
7. Evaluate decisions and action	Evaluation determines whether or not the ethical decision-making framework used resulted in morally justified actions related to the ethical issues and dilemmas

The steps of a generic ethics framework are often nonlinear, and, with the exception of the ethical approach (step 5), they do not change substantially. The rationale for each of the seven steps is presented in Table 7.1. Step 5 (the one exception) lists six approaches to ethical decision-making processes; these approaches are outlined throughout the chapter in the How To boxes.

Several factors can affect the ethical decision-making process. First, we live in a multicultural society in which nurses might face ethical issues and dilemmas related to the diverse cultures, values, and beliefs of their patients, families, and communities. This at times can create conflict. Callahan (2000), cofounder of the Hastings Center, helps explain these conflicts and describes the following four situations for reflection and consideration when working with diverse communities:

1. Situations that place persons at direct risk of harm, whether psychological or physical
2. Situations in which cultural standards conflict with professional standards
3. Situations in which the greater community's values are jeopardized by values of a smaller culture within that community
4. Situations in which community customs may cause mild offense, but no major problems

Chapter 8 further discusses cultural influences on public health nursing. Applying Callahan's four standards to content in that chapter will be helpful. Callahan discusses how to consider diversity in the four situations. In situation 1, he states that "we in America imposed some standards on ourselves for important moral reasons; and there is no good reason to exempt [groups] from those standards" (p. 43). Regarding situations 2 and 3, Callahan recognizes a challenge between cultural standards of individuals, communities, and health care providers' professional standards. Within this scenario, health care providers have to recognize that some groups hold values different from those generally accepted as normative in society. Callahan notes that "in the absence of grievous harm, there is no clear moral mandate to interfere with those values" (p. 43). However, sometimes there is some degree of moral mandate pressure (not coercion) to intervene with differing values for the sake of community consensus. Finally, regarding situation 4, he notes that there is no moral mandate to intervene in non-threatening cultural traditions and values even if they create some degree of burden on others. Intervention only becomes necessary when the imposed burdens cause harm or undue hardship to other groups.

Because decision making is central to the practice of nursing, and many decisions are difficult to make, it is useful to consider experience of ethical or **moral distress**. Moral distress occurs when a person is unable to act in a way that he or she thinks is right (consistent with his or her own personal or professional values, cultural expectation, and/or religious beliefs) due to internal or external constraints (Hamric, 2014). Moral distress is different from what we may consider emotional distress because there is an ethical component associated with moral distress as well as the threat to an individual's moral integrity (Epstein & Delgado, 2010; Ulrich, Hamric, Grady, 2010a; Campbell et al., 2016). Nurses and other health care providers have experienced moral distress (Epstein & Delgado, 2010; Chen, 2009; Lomis et al., 2009; Austin et al., 2008; Førde & Aasland, 2008; Hamric & Blackhall, 2007). In a survey Ulrich et al. (2007) reported that nurses identified feeling powerless, overwhelmed, frustrated, and fatigued when they cannot resolve ethical issues they experience while working. These reported feelings are psychosocial consequences of moral distress. When this conflict occurs, it can lead to a personal sense of failure in the kind of care nurses give, subsequent performance issues, and may lead to work or career dissatisfaction. However, moral distress may be addressed in some of the following ways:

1. Identifying the type(s) of situations that lead to distress
2. Communicating that concern to your manager and examining ways to work toward addressing the stressor
3. Seeking support from colleagues
4. Seeking support from ethics committees, social workers, and pastoral care, among others
5. Being proactive and expressing one's voice on matters that are ethically concerning

Additionally, open dialogue with those in leadership positions such as nurse managers can be helpful. Collaboration like this can lead nurses to connect with other services such as ethics committees and social work, both of which have important roles in ethical practice. For those in primary community settings, speaking to the team members involved in the practice would be a starting point to address moral distress or other ethical concerns.

Two cases are presented in later sections of the chapter. Examine each using the ethical decision-making processes outlined in the How To boxes and the codes of ethics provided in the chapter. These cases provide an excellent opportunity to discuss with classmates your personal beliefs about the application of ethical processes and to assess your own thoughts, feelings, and possible actions. The cases deal with what the nursing response should be (1) when a client will not assume responsibility for his or her health, (2) when the question arises about whether a parent can adequately care for a young child, and (3) when a client is not able or willing to take personal responsibility and does not want the nurse to report the situation.

The Evidence-Based Practice box provides a summary of a research study that examined conflicting ethical concerns.

ETHICAL PRINCIPLES AND THEORIES AS GUIDES TO ETHICAL DECISION MAKING

The remainder of this section of the chapter summarizes content about ethical theories and principles. According to the American Public Health Association, public health "promotes and protects the health of people and the communities where they live, learn, work, and play" (https://www.apha.org). As you read these sections, remember that the ways ethical theories and principles are applied in the community may differ from how they are applied with individuals. To best address populations and communities, public health focuses on maximizing health benefits through a wide variety of actions: from maintaining clean water supply to facilitating community health fairs. This perspective of care may require that individuals forfeit some of their self-interests for the benefits of a safe and healthy society. For example, prohibiting people from smoking in restaurants to benefit the other people in the restaurant may inconvenience the smoker while providing a healthier environment for all people, including the smoker. Similarly, at times a person's right to privacy and confidentiality may be usurped by the public benefit of disclosure. This might take place during epidemics or other national events when contact tracing and surveillance epidemiologic measures are warranted (Gostin et al., 2003).

Utilitarianism and Deontology

At times, decisions are based on outcomes or consequences. In this approach, referred to as **consequentialism**, the right action is the one that produces the greatest amount of good or the least amount of harm in a given situation. How an end (outcome) is achieved is not as important as the final outcome. **Utilitarianism** is a well-known consequentialist ethical theory associated with outcomes or consequences in determining which choice to make. The priority of utilitarianism is to maximize benefit and minimize harm and to consider what is in the greatest good. Because the outcome is the primary concern, it can be said that the ends justify the means.

HOW TO Apply the Utilitarian Ethics Decision Process

1. Determine moral rules that are important to society and that are derived from the principle of utility.[a]
2. Identify the communities or populations that are affected or most affected by the moral rules.
3. Analyze viable alternatives for each proposed action based on the moral rules.
4. Determine the consequences or outcomes of each viable alternative on the communities or populations most affected by the decision.
5. Select the actions on the basis of the rules that produce the greatest amount of good or the least amount of harm for the communities or populations that are affected by the actions.

(Remember that the utilitarian ethics decision process is one of the approaches in step 5 of the generic ethical decision-making framework.)

[a]Moral rules of action that produce the greatest good for the greatest number of communities or populations affected by or most affected by the rules.

In other situations, nurses may conclude that the action is right or wrong in itself, regardless of the amount of good that may come from it. This is the ethical theory known as **deontology**. Coming from the Greek roots *deon* (duty) and *logos* (study of), deontology is a "theory of duty holding that some features of actions other than or in addition to consequences make actions right or wrong" (Beauchamp & Childress, 2013, p. 361). Deontological theory is often called nonconsequentialist. It is based on adhering to moral values and obligations rather than focusing on the outcomes. Here, persons should always be treated as ends in themselves and never as mere means to the ends of others.

Each theory maintains that there is a universal first principle, the principle of utility for utilitarianism and the categorical imperative for deontology, which serves as a rational norm for behavior and allows us to determine the rightness or wrongness of each individual action. Both utilitarianism and deontology also follow the lead of classic liberalism in asserting that the individual is the special center of moral concern (Steinbock et al., 2008). The focus on individual rights leads to complexities when interpreting other theories and principles as they relate to public health and nursing.

HOW TO Apply the Deontological Ethics Decision Process

1. Determine the moral rules (e.g., tell the truth) that serve as standards by which individuals can perform their moral obligations.
2. Examine personal motives for proposed actions to ensure that they are based on good intentions in accord with moral rules.
3. Determine whether the proposed actions can be generalized so that all persons in similar situations are treated similarly.
4. Select the action that treats persons as ends in themselves and never as mere means to the ends of others.

(Remember that the deontological ethics decision process is one of the approaches in step 5 of the generic ethical decision-making framework.)

PRINCIPLES OF BIOETHICS

Health professionals have specific obligations that exist because of the practices and goals of the profession. These health care obligations can be interpreted in terms of a set of principles in bioethics as outlined by Beauchamp and Childress: **respect for autonomy**, **nonmaleficence**, **beneficence**, and **distributive justice** as shown in Box 7.2. These principles are "general guidelines for the formulation of more specific rules," an approach known as **principlism** (Beauchamp & Childress, 2013, p. 13). Principlism relies on these ethical principles to guide decision making. As such, the principle of autonomy refers to self-governance. Respecting autonomy requires health care providers to understand a client's ability to decide his or her own preferences and goals (Beauchamp & Childress, 2013). Nonmaleficence is the noninfliction of harm and is often closely linked to the principle of beneficence or the duty to act in ways that will benefit others. Distributive or social justice refers to the allocation of benefits and burdens to members of society. Benefit refers to basic needs, including material and social goods, liberties, rights, and entitlements. Some benefits of society are wealth, education, and public services. Among the burdens to be shared are items such as taxes, military service, and the location of incinerators and power plants. Justice requires that the distribution of benefits and burdens in a society be fair. Although it is recognized that distribution should be based on what one needs and deserves, disagreement exists when considering what these terms mean in the context of fairness. The three primary theories of distributive justice are egalitarian, libertarian, and liberal democratic (Table 7.2).

BOX 7.2 Ethical Principles

Respect for autonomy: Based on human dignity and respect for individuals, autonomy requires that individuals be permitted to choose those actions and goals that fulfill their life plans unless those choices result in harm to another.

Nonmaleficence: Nonmaleficence requires that we do no harm. It is impossible to avoid harm entirely, but this principle requires that health care professionals act according to the standards of due care, always seeking to produce the least amount of harm possible.

Beneficence: This principle is complementary to nonmaleficence and requires that we do good. We are limited by time, place, and talents in the amount of good we can do. We have general obligations to perform those actions that maintain or enhance the dignity of other persons whenever those actions do not place an undue burden on health care providers.

Distributive justice: Distributive justice requires that there be a fair distribution of the benefits and burdens in society based on the needs and contributions of its members. This principle requires that, consistent with the dignity and worth of its members and within the limits imposed by its resources, a society must determine a minimal level of goods and services to be available to its members.[a]

[a]In public health nursing, client may be a person, group, or community.
Modified from Bateman N: *Advocacy skills for health and social care professionals,* Philadelphia, PA, 2000, Jessica Kingsley, p. 63.

HOW TO Apply the Principlism Ethics Decision Process

1. Determine the ethical principles (respect for autonomy, nonmaleficence, beneficence, justice) that are relevant to an ethical issue or dilemma.
2. Analyze the relevant principles within a meaningful context of accurate facts and other pertinent circumstances.
3. Act on the principle that provides, within the meaningful context, the strongest guide to action that can be morally justified by the tenets foundational to the principle.

(Remember that the principlism ethics decision process is one of the approaches in step 5 of the general ethical decision-making framework.)

TABLE 7.2 Three Primary Theories of Distributive Justice

Distributive Justice	Definitions
Egalitarian	• The view that everyone is entitled to equal rights and equal treatment. Ideally, each person has an equal share of the goods of society, and it is the role of government to ensure that this happens. The government has the authority to redistribute wealth if necessary to ensure equal treatment. Thus egalitarians support welfare rights—that is, the right to receive certain social goods necessary to satisfy basic needs. These include adequate food, housing, education, and police and fire protection. Both practical and theoretical weaknesses are inherent in egalitarianism.
Libertarian	• The libertarian view of justice advocates for social and economic liberty. While egalitarianism lacks incentives for individuals, libertarianism emphasizes the contribution and merit of individuals (Beauchamp & Childress, 2013). • Limited role of government
Liberal democratic	Attempts to develop a theory that values both liberty and equality. • Based on Rawl's Theory of Justice and the "veil of ignorance." Behind this veil, people (or their representatives) are unaware of social position, race, culture, doctrine, sex, endowments, or any other distinguishing circumstances (Rawls, 2001). This is known as the original position and is an exercise to address the inequalities and bargaining advantages that result from birth, natural endowments, and historical circumstances. Without these inequalities, all people are free and equal and can work together as citizens to decide what is fair and therefore just. Once impartiality is guaranteed, Rawls suggests all rational people will choose a system of justice containing the following two principles: • Each person has the same claim to a fully adequate scheme of equal basic liberties, and this scheme is compatible with the same scheme of liberties for all. • Social and economic inequalities are to satisfy two conditions: first, they are to be attached to offices and positions open all under conditions of fair equality of opportunity; and second, they are to be to the greatest benefit to the least advantaged members of society (the difference principle).

Some principles are more emphasized than others in certain conditions. For example, the principle of autonomy is arguably at the forefront of individual patient care. However, justice and beneficence tend to be the emphasis of public health. For this reason, it is useful to look at other models for ethical decision making, especially models that expand the focus of nursing beyond the individual nurse-client relationship to the social environment and systems that impact communities.

Public health ethics is based on many widely accepted norms. Bernheim and colleagues (2015, p. 21) grouped these norms into nine moral considerations: (1) producing benefits; (2) avoiding, preventing, and removing harms; (3) producing the maximal balance of benefits over harms and other costs (often called utility); (4) distributing benefits and burdens fairly (distributive justice); (5) respecting autonomous choices and actions, including liberty of actions; (6) protecting privacy and confidentiality; (7) keeping promises and commitments; (8) disclosing information as well as speaking honestly and truthfully (often grouped under transparency); and (9) building trust. These moral considerations encompass multiple principles and can be applied to individuals, populations, and providers. These public health moral considerations are also important to include in public health nursing.

Virtue, Caring, and Feminist Ethical Theories

Virtue ethics, one of the oldest ethical theories, dates back to the ancient Greek philosophers Plato and Aristotle. Rather than being concerned with actions as seen in utilitarianism and deontology, virtue ethics asks: What kind of person should I be? Virtue ethics seeks to enable persons to flourish as human beings. Not to be confused with principles, Aristotle defines **virtues** as acquired, excellent traits of character that dispose humans to act in accord with their natural good. Examples of virtues include benevolence, compassion, discernment, trustworthiness, integrity, and conscientiousness (Beauchamp & Childress, 2013). Virtue ethics emphasizes practical reasoning applied to character development rather than focusing on moral justification by relying on theories and principles. In practice, virtues in nursing shape job responsibilities and patient care. For example, the virtues listed earlier contribute to a nurse's role as one of the most trusted health professions.

HOW TO Apply the Virtue Ethics Decision Process

1. Identify communities that are relevant to the ethical dilemmas or issues.
2. Identify moral considerations that arise from a communal perspective, and apply the consideration to specific communities.
3. Identify and apply virtues that facilitate a communal perspective.
4. Modify moral considerations as needed to apply to the specific ethical dilemmas or issues.
5. Seek ethical community support to enhance character development.
6. Evaluate and modify the individual or community character traits that impede communal living.

(Remember that the virtue ethics decision process is one of the approaches in step 5 of the generic ethical decision-making framework.)

Modified from Volbrecht RM: *Nursing ethics: communities in dialogue*, Upper Saddle River, NJ, 2002, Prentice Hall, p. 138.

Care Ethics

Caring in nursing, the ethic of care, and feminist ethics are all interrelated and converged between the mid-1980s and early 1990s. Nurses have written about caring as the essence of, or the moral ideal, of nursing (e.g., Leininger, 1984; Watson, 2007). Caring and the ethic of care allows nurses to contribute to the preservation of humanity and are core values of public health nursing.

Carol Gilligan (1982) and Nell Noddings (1984) are often associated with the ethic of care. Gilligan's explorations of the psychological and moral development of women was novel. Her work emerged at a time when abilities associated with autonomous and effective decision making were considered masculine. This perpetuated a devaluing of the stereotypical feminine characteristics. Through her work Gilligan was able to accentuate the feminine experience as distinctive rather than less valuable. She formulated basic premises of responsibility, care, and relationships. In doing so, the link between caring and relationships continued to grow explicit. From this it was posited that women not only judge themselves within the context of their relationships, they also accept and are defined by the responsibility to care for others. Noddings echoed this sentiment and stated an obligation to enhance caring. The commitment that is inherent with caring facilitates ethical ideals. Gilligan and Noddings have in common a feminine ethic because they believe in the morality of responsibility in relationships that emphasize connection and caring. To them, caring is a moral imperative.

HOW TO Apply the Care Ethics Decision Process

1. Recognize that caring is a moral imperative.
2. Identify personally lived caring experiences as a basis for relating to self and others.
3. Assume responsibility and obligation to promote and enhance caring in relationships.

(Remember that the care ethics decision process is one of the approaches in step 5 of the generic ethical decision-making framework.)

HOW TO Apply the Feminist Ethics Decision Process

1. Identify the social, cultural, legal, political, economic, environmental, and professional contexts that contribute to the identified problem (e.g., underrepresentation of women in clinical trials).
2. Evaluate how the preceding contexts contribute to the oppression of women.
3. Consider how women's lives are defined by their status in subordinate social groups.
4. Analyze how social practices marginalize women.
5. Plan ways to restructure those social practices that oppress women.
6. Implement the plan.
7. Evaluate the plan, and restructure it as needed.

(Remember that the feminist ethics decision process is one of the approaches in step 5 of the generic ethical decision-making framework.)

Modified from Volbrecht RM: *Nursing ethics: communities in dialogue*, Upper Saddle River, NJ, 2002, Prentice Hall, p. 219.

Feminist Ethics

Like virtue ethics and communitarian views, **feminist ethics** rejects abstract rules and principles. According to Rogers (2006), feminist ethics is pertinent to public health because it recognizes the role of political and social structures in health. Issues of equity present major challenges in public health. Inequalities in gender, historically impacting women, gave rise to the feminist stance that devaluing and systematic oppression of women is morally wrong. Today, feminism encompasses more than just issues unique to women. Rogers says that the feminist perspective leads people to think critically about the connections among gender, disadvantage, and health, as well as the distribution of power in public health processes. **Feminists** advocate economic, social, and political equity. They pay attention to power relations that constitute, a community, to the rules that regulate it, and to who pays and who benefits from membership in the community (Rogers, 2006).

QSEN FOCUS ON QUALITY AND SAFETY EDUCATION FOR NURSES

One of the six tenets of Quality and Safety Education for Nurses (QSEN) is patient-centered care (Barton et al., 2009). This chapter has discussed many ways in which an understanding of basic principles of ethics can guide safe and effective nursing practice. Some key aspects of patient-centered care in public health nursing include being certain that the information provided to individuals, families, and communities is accurate and reflects the most current evidence and that it is presented in a timely fashion. Community health education should take into account the age, gender, and cultural and religious backgrounds of those who receive the information. Giving health information that does not meet these criteria can be unsafe and does not reflect attention to quality nursing care. One of the QSEN competencies related to patient-centered care is as follows: Recognize the patient or designee as the source of control and full partner in providing compassionate and coordinated care based on respect for patient's preferences, values, and needs. Specific aspects of patient-centered care related to communication are as follows:

- **Knowledge:** Integrate understanding of multiple dimensions of patient-centered care: information, communication, and education.
- **Skills:** Communicate patient values, preferences, and expressed needs to other members of the health care team.
- **Attitudes:** Respect and encourage individual expression of patient values, preferences, and expressed needs (Barton et al., 2009, p. 315).

Specific aspects of patient-centered care related to the public health dilemma of serving the good of the population versus serving the good of the individual are as follows:

- **Knowledge:** Explore ethical and legal implications of patient-centered care.
- **Skills:** Recognize the boundaries of therapeutic relationships (Barton et al., 2009, p. 315).
- **Attitudes:** Acknowledge the tension that may exist between patient rights and the organizational responsibility for professional ethical care.

Patient-centered ethical activity: Public health is more concerned about the good of the collective group than of the individual. In order to think more closely about quality and safety, debate with a classmate about whether children should be required to have all of the Centers for Disease Control and Prevention vaccines before they can enter school. In this scenario, pretend a parent does not want to give his or her children all the recommended immunizations because of fear of side effects of the vaccines. To support your argument see https://www.apha.org for what is required. See web articles such as www.responsibility-project.libertymutual.com for the parent's point of view.

Based on Park EJ: The development and implications of a case-based computer program to train ethical decision-making, *Nurs Ethics* 20:943–956, 2013.

ETHICS AND THE CORE FUNCTIONS OF POPULATION-CENTERED NURSING PRACTICE

In Chapter 1, the three core functions of public health nursing (i.e., assessment, policy development, and assurance) were discussed. The following discussion links these three core functions to ethics.

Assessment

"**Assessment** refers to systematically collecting data on the population, monitoring the population's health status, and making information available about the health of the community" (see Chapter 1). Two ethical tenets underlie these core functions: beneficence and nonmaleficence. The first is beneficence. "Doing good" or maximizing the benefits and minimizing the harm requires nurses' competency related to knowledge development, analysis, and dissemination. Here we can ask the following: Are the persons assigned to develop community knowledge adequately prepared to collect data on groups and populations? This question is important because the research, measurement, and analysis techniques used to gather information about groups and populations usually differ from the techniques used to assess individuals. Wrong research techniques can lead to wrong assessments, which in turn may hurt rather than help the intended group or population. Additionally, do the persons selected to develop, assess, and disseminate community knowledge possess integrity? Beauchamp and Childress (2013) define integrity as the holistic integration of moral character and "objectivity, impartiality, and fidelity in adherence to moral norms" (p. 40). It requires conscientious thought during which people reflect on the rightness or wrongness of actions. The previous discussion of virtue ethics is helpful in exploring this tenet. The importance of integrity is clear: without integrity the core function of assessment is endangered. Providers lacking integrity pose a risk for misconduct and are a threat to the goals of public health. The role of assessment is to provide information to the benefit of public health. The second ethical tenet relates to "do no harm." In any public health situation, balancing risks and benefits is essential. As discussed in the Ebola case, minimizing harm to both individuals and communities required thoughtful dialogue on personal protective equipment as well as community surveillance and monitoring measures.

Policy Development

Public health nurses are critical to the development of policies that reflect the preferences and goals of their constituents. To review, "**policy development** refers to the need to provide leadership in developing policies that support the health of the population, including the use of the scientific knowledge base in making decisions about policy" (see Chapter 1). Public health nurses are in key positions to provide leadership on the ethical issues that might arise within their communities and can use their unique training and skills to evaluate and advocate for policies and programs that reflect the health-related needs of their populations (Ivanov & Oden, 2013; Fowler, 2016; Kass, 2001). In fact, an important goal of both policy and ethics is to achieve the public good (Silva, 2002), which is part of the concept of citizenship (Denhardt & Denhardt, 2000; Rogers, 2006; Ruger, 2008). To be effective citizens, people must be both informed about policy and able and willing to do what is in the best interests of the community (Denhardt & Denhardt, 2000). Here, the voice of the community is the foundation on which policy is developed. Silva (2002) also argues service to others over self is a necessary condition of what is "good" or "right" policy (Silva, 2002).

Denhardt and Denhardt (2000) offer three perspectives on this matter:

- *Serve rather than steer.* An increasingly important role of the public servant (e.g., nurses and administrators) is to help citizens identify and meet their shared interests rather than to attempt to control or steer society in new directions (p. 553).
- *Serve citizens, not customers.* The public interest results from a dialogue about shared values rather than the aggregation of individual self-interests. Therefore public servants do not merely respond to the demands of "customers," but focus on building relationships of trust and collaboration with and among citizens (p. 555).
- *Value citizenship and public service above entrepreneurship.* The public interest is better advanced by public servants and citizens committed to making meaningful contributions to society rather than by entrepreneurial managers acting as if public money were their own (p. 556).

Service, an enduring nursing value, is at the core of these three perspectives. Service requires ethical action; therefore moral leadership from nurses is critical to the development of ethical health care policies.

Assurance

"**Assurance** refers to the role of public health in ensuring that essential community health services are available, which may include providing essential personal health services for those who would otherwise not receive them. Assurance also refers to making sure that a competent public health and personal health care workforce is available" (see Chapter 1). The ethical principle of justice can apply to this core function as follows:

1. All persons should receive essential personal health services. Put in terms of justice, "to each person a fair share" or "to all groups or populations a fair share." This does not necessarily mean that all persons in a society should share all of society's benefits equally but that they should share at least those benefits that are essential. Many individuals think basic health care for all is essential for social justice.
2. Providers of public health services should be competent and available. Although the Public Health Code of Ethics does not speak directly to workforce availability, it does speak directly to ensuring professional competency of public health employees. In addition to the Public Health Code of Ethics, the *Healthy People 2020* objectives address competencies and workforce needs.

The *Healthy People 2020* objectives address the need for all public health workers not only to have knowledge of public health, but also to have additional competencies as needed to fulfill their job responsibilities. Specific areas of knowledge include information technology, biostatistics, environmental health, cultural and linguistic competence, and genomics. The objectives also address needs of future public health leaders, who must be educated to meet new challenges in health care. Emphasis is also given to the availability and provision of lifelong learning opportunities for public health employees.

HEALTHY PEOPLE 2020

There are two new objectives outlined in *Healthy People 2020* related to access to health services:

- **AHS-1:** Increasing the proportion of persons who receive appropriate evidence-based clinical preventive services
- **AHS-4:** Increasing the proportion of practicing primary care providers, including nurse practitioners.

Both of these objectives relate to access to care and reflect important ethical considerations for nurses in community settings.

From U.S. Department of Health and Human Service, 2010, https://www.healthypeople.gov.

NURSING CODE OF ETHICS

As noted in the discussion of history earlier in this chapter, the *Code of Ethics for Nurses With Interpretive Statements* was adopted by the ANA House of Delegates in 2001 and revised in 2015. This code serves three purposes, as follows (ANA, 2015):

- "It is a succinct statement of the ethical values, obligations, duties, and professional ideals of nurses individually and collectively."
- "It is the profession's nonnegotiable ethical standard."
- "It is an expression of nursing's own understanding of its commitment to society."

These purposes are reflected in nine provisional statements of the code. The Code of Ethics for Nurses and its interpretive statements apply to nurses in public health, although the emphasis for each type of nursing sometimes varies (for the ANA Code of Ethics for Nurses, see http://www.nursingworld.org). For example, provision 1 and its interpretative statement primarily address the individual when discussing how the nurse practices with compassion and respect for the person being cared for regardless of the person's status, attributes, or the nature of the health problem. However, it is also recognized under provision 1 that there are times when individual rights may be limited because of public health concerns. The interpretive statements of provisions 2 and 8 are pertinent to public health nurses. Provision 2 states: "the nurse's primary commitment is to the patient whether an individual, family, group, community, or population." Provision 8 highlights the need for collaborative practice with other disciplines as well as the public to mitigate health disparities and promote human rights. All nurses have a responsibility to meet the obligations highlighting professional standards, active involvement in nursing, and the integrity of the profession as outlined in the code. Of note, the code also specifies that health is a universal right with economic, political, social, and cultural dimensions. (See the *Code of Ethics for Nurses With Interpretative Statements* for all provisions.) See Box 7.3 for a case study about autonomy and distributive justice.

BOX 7.3 Case Study: Autonomy and Distributive Justice

Amelia Lewis, a 31-year-old African American woman with multiple mental health diagnoses, has been monitored in the local mental health system for over 10 years. She is the mother of Tyesha, who is three years old. Multiple agencies have monitored Ms. Lewis and her little girl, who live in a sparsely furnished apartment in subsidized housing. A guardian handles all of Ms. Lewis's financial affairs. Ms. Lewis's relationship with the father of Tyesha has deteriorated, and he does not live with her.

Ms. Lewis has issues of trust, and she is often suspicious of the care providers who come to her home. She does rely on some of the professionals with whom she interacts on a weekly or biweekly basis. She is both cognitively delayed and suffers from schizophrenia. Her developmental level places her at a stage at which her own needs are her primary focus, and this is not expected to change; her interaction with Tyesha is perfunctory, involving little outward affection. She is unable to understand that Tyesha is not capable of self-care and that her three-year-old child will not always obey when Ms. Lewis instructs her to do something. Tyesha's needs, level of functioning, and cognitive development are quickly surpassing her mother's ability to cope. Frustration and misunderstanding ensue when Ms. Lewis thinks that Tyesha does not listen to her, and encouragement and parent education have done little to improve the situation as Tyesha gets older and more assertive. This has made toilet training, provision of an appropriate diet, and other aspects of child care problematic.

Many services besides those for mental health are involved to help this family of two cope. There is concern about abuse or neglect of Tyesha due to Ms. Lewis's lack of understanding of how to be a parent. Supplemental Security Income provides monetary support because of her mental disability, and they have Medicaid coverage for their health care needs, as well as food stamps and modest financial assistance through Temporary Assistance for Needy Families (TANF). Ms. Lewis cannot currently work and take care of her child due to her mental disability. Before Tyesha's birth, Ms. Lewis held a job and maintained self-care, but the care of Tyesha has precluded her managing employment at this time. Child Protective Services is also monitoring Ms. Lewis's situation to determine to what extent she can meet the needs of her child. Ms. Lewis attends a local program to complete her General Education Development (GED), which provides child care during the day. Though Ms. Lewis is not expected to complete her GED, this program provides structured time for Tyesha three times a week. The child is considered developmentally normal at this time, and an infant development program monitors her progress on developmental issues. The Child Health Partnership, an agency that addresses the needs of challenged families, provides regular visits, family support, and parenting education, and the GED teachers make regular home visits to check on Ms. Lewis and Tyesha. Ms. Lewis thinks things are going just fine.

The Child Health Partnership nurse is concerned about this family and thinks that some permanent resolution of the situation is inevitable. There is minimal coordination of services, and there is no "lead agency" in the family's care. Choose one of the ethical decision processes or one set of code of ethics discussed in the chapter, and discuss and debate these questions:

1. Should the nurse involved in the Child Health Partnership program initiate any action to try to coordinate the work of the many agencies involved with this family?
2. Who has a professional responsibility to determine when the mother can no longer cope with the developing child?
3. Whose needs, Ms. Lewis's or Tyesha's, should take precedence?
4. Using one of the ethics decision processes, analyze the role of the nurse in this situation. For example, considering the utilitarian ethics decision process, decide if it is morally right for you to take the child away from the mother. If you do this, what are the implications for the mother, the child, and the community? What would be the possible consequences of removing the child? Of not removing the child? What principles can best guide your decision making? What possible moral dilemmas will you experience?
5. Safety is a core concept of public health nursing. Using two of the six quality and safety competences (patient-centered care and safety) for nurses identified in the *Quality and Safety Education for Nurses (QSEN)* work, develop a plan of action for the nurse who is caring for this family.

Created by Mary E. Gibson, Associate Professor of Nursing, School of Nursing, University of Virginia.

The Levels of Prevention box presents actions related to ethics.

LEVELS OF PREVENTION

Ethics

Primary Prevention

Use the Code of Ethics for Nurses to guide your nursing practice.

Secondary Prevention

If you are unable to behave in accordance with the Code of Ethics for Nurses (e.g., you speak in a way that does not communicate respect for a client), take steps to correct your behavior.

Tertiary Prevention

If you have treated a client or staff member in a way that is inconsistent with ethics practices, seek guidance on other choices you could have made.

PUBLIC HEALTH CODE OF ETHICS

The Public Health Code of Ethics (PHLS, 2002) was noted in the discussion of history earlier in this chapter. Created with the assumption that all humans have the right to adequate health resources, this code consists of 12 principles related to the ethical practice of public health (Box 7.4). This code includes those values and beliefs that focus on health, community, and action and a commentary on each of the 12 principles. The preamble describes the collective and societal nature of public health to keep people healthy. In doing so, it reaffirms the World Health Organization's definition of health as "a state of complete physical, mental, and societal well-being, and not merely the absence of disease" (World Health Organization, 2006). Similar to other codes of ethics, the 12 principles of ethical public health practice incorporate the ethical tenets of preventing harm; doing no harm; promoting good; respecting both individual and community rights; respecting autonomy, diversity, and confidentiality when possible; ensuring professional competency; trustworthiness; and promoting advocacy for disenfranchised persons within a community. The code also lists values and beliefs regarding community and public health. These include the belief that collaboration is a key element of public health, that each person should have opportunities to contribute to public discourse, and that identifying and promoting requirements for health is a primary public health concern.

Commonalities exist between the *Code of Ethics for Nurses With Interpretative Statements* and the Public Health Code of Ethics. Both codes provide general ethical principles and approaches that are enduring and dynamic. They require nurses and public health personnel to think and act in accordance with the underlying ethics of their profession. Of note, they each encourage evidence-based and collaborative approaches for the betterment of health. Although the two codes do not specify (nor should they specify) details for every ethical issue, other mechanisms such as standards of practice, ethical decision-making frameworks, and ethics committees provide further guidance. Nevertheless, these two codes address most approaches to ethical justification, including traditional and emerging ethical theories and principles, humanist and feminist ethics, virtue ethics, professional-individual and/or community relationships, and advocacy. Many websites provide further information on codes of ethics and other ethical concerns in public health; all can be accessed through the WebLinks section of this book's Evolve website. Some of them are noted in the Additional Resources feature at the beginning of the chapter.

BOX 7.4 Principles of the Ethical Practice of Public Health[a]

1. Public health should address principally the fundamental causes of disease and requirements for health, aiming to prevent adverse health outcomes.
2. Public health should achieve community health in a way that respects the rights of individuals in the community.
3. Public health policies, programs, and priorities should be developed and evaluated through processes that ensure an opportunity for input from community members.
4. Public health should advocate and work for the empowerment of disenfranchised community members, aiming to ensure that the basic resources and conditions necessary for health are accessible to all.
5. Public health should seek the information needed to implement effective policies and programs that protect and promote health.
6. Public health institutions should provide communities with the information they have that is needed for decisions on policies or programs and should obtain the community's consent for their implementation.
7. Public health institutions should act in a timely manner on the information they have, within the resources and the mandate given to them by the public.
8. Public health programs and policies should incorporate a variety of approaches that anticipate and respect diverse values, beliefs, and cultures in the community.
9. Public health programs and policies should be implemented in a manner that most enhances the physical and social environment.
10. Public health institutions should protect the confidentiality of information that can bring harm to an individual or community if made public. Exceptions must be justified on the basis of the high likelihood of significant harm to the individual or others.
11. Public health institutions should ensure the professional competencies of their employees.
12. Public health institutions and their employees should engage in collaborations and affiliations in ways that build the public's trust and the institution's effectiveness.

[a]A section of the Public Health Code of Ethics is presented.
Reprinted with permission from the Public Health Leadership Society: *Public health code of ethics,* 2002, American Public Health Association (APHA). Available at http://phls.org.

ADVOCACY AND ETHICS

Advocacy is a powerful ethical concept in nursing. But what does advocacy mean? "Advocacy is the application of information and resources (including finances, effort, and votes) to effect systematic changes that shape the way people in a community live" (Christoffel, 2000, p. 722). Public health advocacy is intended "to reduce death or disability in groups of people and that is not confined to clinical settings" (p. 722). As mentioned, public health includes aggregates or populations. It also

BOX 7.5 Case Study: Applying Virtue Ethics, Truth Telling, and the Deontological Ethical Decision-Making Process

Because finding affordable housing was difficult, 26-year-old Terry White lived with her 6-month-old son, Tommy, and his father, Billy Smith, in one room of the landlord's own house. Ms. White was morbidly obese and was diagnosed with bipolar disease; Mr. Smith had served time for drug dealing and was out on parole and staying straight. Neither had finished high school. Mr. Smith's past drug use had rendered him unable to do much manual labor because of heart damage, but on occasion he would work in construction to support the family.

Public health nurse Jim Lewis had received a referral on Tommy when he was diagnosed with failure to thrive (FTT) 2 months earlier. Ms. White, who had had two children removed from her custody by Child Protective Services (CPS) in the past, and Mr. Smith seemed to adore their baby, so much so that Ms. White would hold the baby all day long. In the past two months the nurse had taught Ms. White about infant nutrition and gotten her enrolled in the Women, Infants, and Children (WIC) nutrition program; as a result, Tommy had increased his rate of physical growth and was above the five percent level of his growth percentile. Yet he was not meeting his gross motor milestones per Denver Developmental Screening Test II (DDST II) testing. Mr. Lewis thought that Tommy was not allowed to play on the floor enough to progress in sitting, pushing his shoulders up, or crawling. Most of their small room was taken up with the bed and the boxes that stored their belongings. There was not really space for "tummy time" or play. When not in the room, the family would take the bus to a discount store and spend the day walking around to get a change of scene.

One week Ms. White told the nurse she was not taking her medications for bipolar disease anymore because they caused her to gain weight. The next week she confided that Mr. Smith had had a "dirty" urine specimen check and would have to return to prison in the near future. The following week Mr. Lewis found the family living in a run-down motel since their landlord evicted them following a disagreement. Ms. White was agitated and told the nurse that they had only $100. Mr. Smith was going to have to return to prison that week, and the motel bill was already $240. Ms. White knew she would be homeless soon without Mr. Smith's support but refused to talk with her social worker about her needs. She asked the nurse not to tell anyone about her situation because she was afraid CPS would take Tommy from her. It was clear to Mr. Lewis that Ms. White might not know what would happen to Tommy after they left this motel.

1. Considering the principle of truth telling, what are Mr. Lewis's professional responsibilities to Ms. White, to Tommy, and to the social worker assigned to this family?
2. Using the generic ethical decision-making framework discussed earlier in the chapter and considering the deontological ethical decision-making process, answer the following questions:
   A. How should Mr. Lewis respond to Ms. White's request to not tell anyone about their situation?
   B. What communication, about truth telling, if any, should the nurse initiate with the social worker? With others?
   C. Consistent with the principle of truth telling, how can the nurse involve Mr. Smith in the ongoing support and involvement with his family?
3. Using virtue ethics, what actions would you take to resolve any moral dilemmas you have about the safety of Tommy in this family situation? If you do not tell anyone about the possible dangers to the child, what moral principles come into play? If you do tell the social worker about the situation and the child is removed from the mother, what moral principles come into play for you?
4. What ethical dilemmas may you experience if you are the nurse in this case? How can you deal effectively with these potential dilemmas?

Created by Deborah C. Conway, Assistant Professor of Nursing, School of Nursing, University of Virginia (retired).

encompasses both preventative and reactionary measures. Thus the problems addressed with public health advocacy affect, or have the potential to affect, a sizeable portion of a community. Several codes and standards of practice address advocacy and the various roles of nursing. Advocacy is addressed in the ANA and the Public Health Leadership Society's codes of ethics, as well as the ANA's *Public Health Nursing: Scope and Standards of Practice* (ANA, 2013). See Box 7.5 for another case study.

According to the ANA's *Code of Ethics for Nurses With Interpretive Statements,* "The nurse promotes, advocates for, and protects the rights, health, and safety of the patient" (ANA, 2015, p. 9). The focus of the interpretive statements regarding advocacy is the nurse's responsibility to take action when the client's best interests are jeopardized by questionable practice on the part of any member of the health team, the health care system, or others. However, Shannon argues that nursing does not bear the advocacy label alone. Working with communities as a public health nurse requires collaborative leadership and a team-based approach to address the needs of vulnerable patients (Shannon, 2016).

According to the Public Health Leadership Society's Public Health Code of Ethics, "Public health should advocate and work for the empowerment of disenfranchised community members, aiming to ensure that the basic resources and conditions necessary for health are accessible to all" (Public Health Leadership Society, 2002, p.1). This code elaborates on the preceding principle by addressing the following two issues: that the voice of the community should be heard and that the marginalized or underserved in a community should receive "a decent minimum" (p. 4) of health resources (Table 7.3).

TABLE 7.3 Contrast of Social Justice and Market Justice as an Advocacy Framework

Market Justice Values	Social Justice Values
Self-determination and self-discipline	Shared responsibility
Individual values and self-interest	Interconnection and cooperation among individuals in a community
Personal efforts key to desired benefits	Community shares responsibility for providing basic benefits
Limited responsibilities for good of the community	Important obligations for the collective good
Limited government intervention	Government involvement is necessary
Voluntary focus on individual moral behavior	Community well-being supersedes individual focus on well-being

Modified from Dorfman L, Wallack L, Woodruff K: More than a message: framing public health advocacy to change corporate practices, *Health Educ Behav* 32:320–336, 2005.

According to the ANA's *Public Health Nursing: Scope and Standards of Practice* (ANA, 2013), public health nurses have a moral mandate to establish ethical standards when advocating for health care policy. The preceding standards extend the prior two concepts of advocacy by moving advocacy into the policy arena, particularly health and social policy as applied to populations.

Finally, the American Public Health Association (APHA) represents a powerful voice for public health advocacy, focusing on finding ways to involve health care professionals in influencing policies related to protection of all Americans and their communities from preventable, serious health threats and helping to ensure access to health care and eliminating health disparities (APHA, 2014). The APHA notes the critical need to shift from a nation focused on treating individual illness to one that also promotes population-based health services that encourage preventive and early intervention practices.

Advocacy and Health Care Reform. The signing of the 2010 Affordable Care Act by President Obama, after many years of controversial attempts at health care reforms, provides an excellent opportunity for nurses to advocate for tying health care for all to ethics and social justice. Dr. Mary Wakefield, Acting Deputy Secretary of Health and Human Services (HHS) (2015-2017), noted that not only should nurses participate in implementing new directions for health care, but that it is important that they help to envision these new directions (Wakefield, 2008). Nurses can advocate for access to consistent, effective, efficient health care for all in our society. Wakefield points out that educating the public can be a unique challenge because clever sound bites from the popular media can lure consumers into thinking that the status quo is the best option. Nurses are an important part of the health care industry and are respected by the public; they can make meaningful contributions toward health care reform through advocating for clients and families (Box 7.6).

BOX 7.6 Ethical Principles for Effective Advocacy

1. Act in the client's best interests.
2. Act in accordance with the client's wishes and instructions.
3. Keep the client properly informed.
4. Carry out instructions with diligence and competence.
5. Act impartially, and offer frank, independent advice.
6. Maintain client confidentiality.

LINKING CONTENT TO PRACTICE

Throughout this chapter, there has been application of the content related to ethics in public health nursing and the many documents that influence the role of public health nurses. These include the ANA Scope and Standards of Public Health Nursing, the ANA Code of Ethics for Nurses, the core functions of public health as outlined by the Institute of Medicine, and the *Healthy People 2020* objectives. Ethics is also an integral part of the Core Competencies for Public Health Professionals. In the section on analytic/assessment skills, the core competencies indicate that public health professionals use "ethical principles in the collection, maintenance, use, and dissemination of data and information" and under leadership and systems thinking "incorporates ethical standards of practice as the basis of all interactions with organizations, communities, and individuals." The competencies also recognize the importance of health literacy of the populations being served, an important ethics-related component of informed consent when working with diverse populations in community settings (Council on Linkages between Academia and Public Health Practice, 2014).

PRACTICE APPLICATION

The retiring director of the division of primary care in a state health department had recently hired Ann Green, a 34-year-old nurse with a master's degree in public health, to be director of the division. Ms. Green's work involved the monitoring of millions of dollars of state and federal money as well as the supervising of the funded programs within her division.

Ms. Green received many requests for funding from a particular state agency that served a poor, large district. The poor people of the district primarily consisted of young families with children and homebound older adults with chronic illnesses. Over the past 3 years the federal government had allocated considerable money to the state agency to subsidize pediatric primary care programs, but no formal evaluation of these programs had occurred.

The director of the state agency was a physician who had been in this position for over 20 years. He was good at obtaining funding for primary care needs in his district, but the statistics related to the pediatric primary care program seemed implausible—that is, few physical examinations were performed on the children, which had resulted in extra money in the budget. This unspent federal money was being used to supplement home health care services for the indigent homebound older adults in his district. The thinking of the physician was that he was doing good by providing some needed services to both indigent groups in his district. Ms. Green felt moral discomfort because she did not have either the money or the personnel to provide both services. What should she do?

A. What facts are the most relevant in this scenario?
B. What are the ethical issues?
C. How can Ms. Green resolve the issues?

(The preceding case and answers are adapted and paraphrased from a real practice application shared by J.L. Chapin on the inappropriate distribution of primary health care funds [in Silva M, editor: *Ethical decision making in nursing administration,* Norwalk, CT, 1990, Appleton & Lange].)

Answers can be found on the Evolve site.

KEY POINTS

- Nursing has a rich heritage of ethics and morality, beginning with Florence Nightingale.
- During the late 1960s the field of bioethics began to emerge and influence nursing.
- Ethical decision making is the component of ethics that focuses on the process of how ethical decisions are made.
- Many different ethical decision-making frameworks exist; however, underlying each of them is the problem-solving process.
- Ethical decision making applies to all approaches to ethics: utilitarianism, deontology, principlism, virtue ethics, caring and the ethic of care, and feminist ethics.
- Cultural diversity makes ethical decision making more challenging.
- Moral distress can lead to a personal sense of failure in providing nursing care and may lead to work and/or career dissatisfaction.
- Classical ethical theories are utilitarianism and deontology.
- Principlism consists of respect for autonomy, nonmaleficence, beneficence, and justice.
- Other approaches to ethics include virtue ethics, caring and the ethic of care, and feminist ethics.
- The core functions of public health nursing (i.e., assessment, policy development, and assurance) are all grounded in ethics.
- *Healthy People 2020* objectives address workforce competencies, training in essential public health services, and continuing education.
- The 2015 Code of Ethics for Nurses contains nine statements that address the moral standards that delineate nursing's values, goals, and obligations.
- The 2002 Public Health Code of Ethics contains 12 statements that address the moral standards that delineate public health's values, goals, and obligations.
- Advocacy is the act of pleading for or supporting a course of action on behalf of a person, group, or community.
- Effective advocacy incorporates ethical principles and concepts.
- The Code of Ethics for Nurses, the Public Health Code of Ethics, Skills for the Ethical Practice of Public Health, and *Public Health Nursing: Scope and Standards of Practice* all address advocacy.
- Public health advocacy is composed of both products and processes.
- The products of advocacy are decreased morbidity and mortality.
- The processes of public health advocacy include, but are not limited to, identifying problems, collecting data, developing and endorsing regulations and legislation, enforcing policies, and assessing the policy process.
- Advocacy related to bioterrorism, health care reform, and ethical use of social media is important for community and public health nurses.

CLINICAL DECISION-MAKING ACTIVITIES

1. Think about the differences in duties between a nurse working in a critical care facility and a nurse working in a community care or public health setting. How might these differences lead to differences in ethical problems and decision making?
2. Interview a long-retired nurse about the most important ethical issues that this nurse faced when practicing in the community. Next, interview a nurse actively practicing in the community about the most important ethical issues that this nurse is now facing. Compare and contrast the ethical issues in the two interviews, and place each within a historical context.
3. In a local or national newspaper read one or more articles that discuss health care public policy with which you agree or disagree. Compose a letter to the editor analyzing why you agree or disagree with the policy but only after you take into account any of your own biases or vested interests.

ADDITIONAL RESOURCES

EVOLVE WEBSITE

http://evolve.elsevier.com/Stanhope/community/

- Answers to Practice Application
- Case Study
- Glossary
- Review Questions

REFERENCES

American Nurses Association: *Code for Professional Nurses*, New York, 1950, American Nursing Association.

American Nurses Association (ANA): *Code of Ethics for Nurses with Interpretive Statements*, Silver Spring, MD, 2001, American Nurses Association.

American Nurses Association (ANA): *Code of Ethics for Nurses with Interpretive Statements*, Silver Spring, MD, 2015, Nursebooks.org.

American Nurses Association (ANA): *Public Health Nursing: Scope & Standards of Practice*, Washington, DC, 2013, American Nurses Publishing.

American Public Health Association: *Advocacy and Policy*, 2014. Retrieved December 2014 from: www.apha.org/policies-and-advocacy/advocacy-for-public-health.

American Public Health Association: *What is Public Health*, 2018. Available at: https://www.apha.org/what-is-public-health.

Annas GJ: Beyond nazi war crimes experiments: The voluntary consent requirement of the Nuremberg Code at 70, *Am J Public Health* 108(1):42–46, 2018.

Austin WJ, Kagan L, Rankel M, Bergum V: The balancing act: psychiatrists' experience of moral distress, *Med Health Care Philos* 11(1):89–97, 2008.

Barton AJ, Armstrong G, Preheim G, Gelmon SB, Andrus LC: A national Delphi to determine developmental progression of

quality and safety competencies in nursing education, *Nurs Outlook* 57:313–322, 2009.
Bateman N: *Advocacy Skills for Health and Social Care Professionals*, Philadelphia, PA, 2000, Jessica Kingsley.
Beauchamp TL, Childress JF: *Principles of Biomedical Ethics*, ed 7, New York, 2013, Oxford University Press.
Bellinger DC: Lead contamination in Flint – an abject failure to protect public health, *N Engl J Med* 374(12):1101–1103, 2016.
Belmont Report: *Ethical principles and guidelines for the protection of human subjects of research,* Washington DC, 1979, Government Printing Office.
Bernheim RG, Childress JF, Bonnie RJ, et al.: *Essentials of Public Health Ethics*, Burlington, MA, 2015, Jones & Bartlett.
Callahan D: Universalism and particularism fighting to a draw, *Hastings Cent Rep* 30:37–44, 2000.
Campbell SM, Ulrich CM, Grady C: A broader understanding of moral distress, *Am J Bioeth* 16(12):2–9, 2016.
Chadwick R, Gallagher A: *Ethics and nursing practice*. London, UK, 2016, Palgrave. The UK imprint of Macmillan Publishers Limited.
Chapin JL: The inappropriate distribution of primary health care funds. In Silva M, editor: *Ethical decision making in nursing administration,* Norwalk, CT, 1990, Appelton & Lange.
Chen P: *When nurses and doctors can't do the right thing*, February 5, 2009. Retrieved from https://www.nytimes.com/2009/02/06/health/05chen.html.
Christoffel KK: Public health advocacy: process and product, *Am J Public Health* 90:722–726, 2000.
Council on Linkages between Academia and Public Health Practice: *Core Competencies for Public Health Professionals*, Washington, DC, 2014, Public Health Foundation/Health Resources and Services Administration.
Denhardt RB, Denhardt JV: The new public service: serving rather than steering, *Public Admin Rev* 60:549–552, 2000.
Dorfman L, Wallack L, Woodruff K: More than a message: framing public health advocacy to change corporate practices, *Health Educ Behav* 32:320–336, 2005.
Easley CE, Allen CE: A critical intersection: human rights, public health nursing, and nursing ethics, ANS *Adv Nurs Sci* 30:367–382, 2007.
Epstein G, Delgado S: Understanding and addressing moral distress, *Online J Issues Nurs* 15(3), manuscript 1, September 30, 2010.
Førde R, Aasland OG: Moral distress among Norwegian doctors, *J Med Ethics* 34(7):521–525, 2008.
Fowler MDM, editor: *Guide to the Code of Ethics for Nurses: Interpretation and Application*, Silver Spring, MD, 2008, American Nurses Association.
Fowler MD: Nursing's code of ethics, social ethics, and social policy. In Ulrich C, Hamric AB, Grady C, editors: *Nurses at the Table: Nursing, Ethics, and Health Policy,* special report, *Hastings Cent Rep* 46(suppl 1):S9–S12, 2016.
Fowler MDM, editor: *Guide to the Code of Ethics for Nurses: Development, Interpretation and Application*, Silver Spring, MD, 2015, American Nurses Association.
Gilligan C: *In a Different Voice: Psychological Theory and Women's Development*, Cambridge, MA, 1982, Harvard University Press.
Gostin LO, Bayer R, Fairchild AL: Ethical and legal challenges posed by severe acute respiratory syndrome: implications for the control of severe infectious disease threats, *JAMA* 290(24):3229–3237, 2003.
Grady C, Danis M, Soeken KL, et al.: Does ethics education influence the moral action of practicing nurses and social workers, *Am J Bioeth* 8(4):4–11, 2008.
Grodin MA, Miller EL, Kelly JI: The Nazi physicians as leaders in eugenics and "euthanasia": Lessons for today, *Am J Public Health* 108(1):53–57, 2018.
Hamric AB: A case study of moral distress, *J Hosp Palliat Nurs* 16(8):457–463, 2014.
Hamric AB, Blackhall LJ: Nurse-physician perspectives on the care of dying patients in intensive care units: collaboration, moral distress, and ethical climate, *Crit Care Med* 35(2):422–429, 2007.
Hastings Center: *Our Mission*, 2019. Retrieved from http://www.thehastingscenter.org/who-we-are/our-mission.
International Council of Nurses (ICN): *ICN Code of Ethics for Nurses*, Geneva, 1953, ICN.
International Council of Nurses (ICN): *ICN Code of Ethics for Nurses*, Geneva, 2012, ICN.
Ivanov LL, Oden TL: Public health nursing, ethics and human rights, *Public Health Nurs* 30(3):231–238, 2013.
Jonsen AR: *The birth of bioethics*, New York, NY, 1998, Oxford University Press.
Kass NE: An ethics framework for public health, *Am J Public Health* 91:1776–1782, 2001.
Leininger MM: Care: *The Essence of Nursing and Health*, Thorofare, NJ, 1984, Slack.
Lomis KD, Carpenter RO, Miller BM: Moral distress in the third year of medical school: a descriptive review of student case reflections, *Am J Surg* 197(1):107–112, 2009.
Lucey DR, Gostin LO: The emerging Zika pandemic: enhancing preparedness, *JAMA* 315(9):865–866, 2016.
Noddings N: *Caring: A Feminine Approach to Ethics & Moral Education*, Berkeley, CA, 1984, University of California Press.
Olick RS: From the column editor: ethics in public health, *J Public Health Manag Pract* 11:258–259, 2005.
Park EJ: The development and implications of a case-based computer program to train ethical decision-making, *Nurs Ethics* 20:943–956, 2013.
Pinch WJE, Haddad AM, editors: *Nursing and Health Care Ethics: A Legacy and a Vision*, Silver Spring, MD, 2008, American Nurses Association.
Public Health Leadership Society: Public Health Code of Ethics, *Am Public Health Assoc* 7:92:1057–1059, 2002.
Rawls J, Kelly E, editors: *Justice as Fairness: A Restatement*, Cambridge MA, 2001, Harvard University Press.
Reich WT: *Encyclopedia of bioethics*, New York, NY, 1995, Macmillan.
Rogers WA: Feminism and public health ethics, *J Med Ethics* 32(6):351–354, 2006.
Ruger JP: Ethics in American health 2. An ethical framework for health system reform, *Am J Public Health* 98:1756–1763, 2008.
Shannon SE: The nurse as the patient's advocate: A contrarian view. In Ulrich CM, Grady C, Hamric AB, Berlinger N, editors: *Nurses at the table: nursing, ethics, and health policy,* New York, 2016, Hastings Center, pp S43–S47.
Silva MC: Ethical issues in health care, public policy, and politics. In Mason D, Leavitt J, Chaffee M, editors: *Policy and Politics in Nursing and Health Care*, ed 4, Philadelphia, 2002, Saunders.
Steinbock B, Arras J, London AJ, editors: *Ethical Issues in Modern Medicine*, ed 7, Boston, 2008, McGraw-Hill.
Ulrich CM, editor. *Nursing ethics in everyday practice*, Indianapolis, 2012, Sigma Theta Tau.
Ulrich C, O'Donnell P, Taylor C, Farrar A, Danis M, Grady C: Ethical climate, ethics stress, and the job satisfaction of nurses and social workers in the United States, *Soc Sci Med* 65:1708–1719, 2007.
Ulrich CM, Hamric AB, Grady C: Moral distress: a growing problem in the health professions? *Hastings Cent Rep* 40(1):20–22, 2010a.

Ulrich CM, Taylor C, Soeken K, et al.: Everyday ethics: ethical issues and stress in nursing practice, *J Adv Nurs* 66(11):2510–2519, 2010b.

U.S. Department of Health and Human Services: *Healthy People 2020*, 2010. Retrieved from www.healthypeople.gov.

Volbrecht RM: *Nursing Ethics: Communities in Dialogue*, Upper Saddle River, NJ, 2002, Prentice Hall.

Wakefield MK: Envisioning and implementing new directions for health care, *Nurs Econ* 26:49–51, 2008.

Watson J: *Nursing: Human Science and Human Care*, revised ed, Norwalk, CT, 2007, Jones & Bartlett.

World Health Organization: *Constitution of the World Health Organization,* October 2006. Retrieved from http://www.who.int/governance/eb/who_constitution_en.pdf.

8

Achieving Cultural Competence in Community Health Nursing

Cynthia E. Degazon, RN, PhD and Bobbie J. Perdue, RN, PhD

OBJECTIVES

After reading this chapter, the student should be able to do the following:

1. Describe the role of cultural competence in achieving the public health goals of health equity.
2. Describe major facilitators and barriers to providing culturally competent health care for diverse populations.
3. Cite culturally competent nursing interventions to promote positive health outcomes for culturally diverse individuals, communities, and organizations.
4. Evaluate the role of the public health nurse in providing culturally competent nursing care.
5. Use a case scenario to chart the elements of cultural competence as described in the chapter.
6. Use electronic resources to locate current databases about culturally competent practices that increase health equity.

CHAPTER OUTLINE

Why Cultural Competence Matters
Culture, Race, and Ethnicity
Impact of Diversity on Cultural Competence
Social Issues Affecting Culturally Competent Nursing Care
Cultural Competence in Nursing
Culturally Competent Nursing Assessment of Clients
Building Culturally Competent Organizations

KEY TERMS

advocacy, p. 180
biological variations, p. 171
classism, p. 185
communication, p. 172
cultural accommodation, p. 187
cultural awareness, p. 181
cultural blindness, p. 186
cultural competence, p. 166
cultural conflict, p. 186
cultural desire, p. 183
cultural diversity, p. 170
cultural encounter, p. 183
cultural immersion, p. 184
cultural imposition, p. 186
cultural knowledge, p. 182
culturally competent nursing assessment, p. 190
cultural preservation, p. 187
cultural relativism, p. 186
cultural repatterning, p. 188
cultural skill, p. 182
cultural variations, p. 173
culture, p. 168
culture brokering, p. 188
culture shock, p. 187
discrimination, p. 185
environmental control, p. 172
ethnicity, p. 170
ethnocentrism, p. 185
foreign-born, p. 175
health equity, p. 180
health disparities, p. 179
health literacy, p. 179
immigrants, p. 174
interpreter, p. 177
lawful permanent residents, p. 175
legal immigrants, p. 175
marginalization, p. 179
non-immigrants, p. 176
nonverbal communication, p. 173
nutritional practices, p. 173
organizational cultural competence, p. 191
perception of time, p. 172
personal space, p. 171
prejudice, p. 184
quality of care, p. 168
race, p. 170
racism, p. 185
refugees, p. 176
religion, p. 174
social determinants of health, p. 178

Continued

KEY TERMS—cont'd

social justice, p. 180
social organization, p. 172
socioeconomic status, p. 178
spirituality, p. 174
stereotyping, p. 184
unauthorized immigrants, p. 176
verbal communication, p. 173

Significant milestones in public health nursing have resulted when nurses in their leadership role used culturally competent thinking interventions to resolve health problems. As early as 1893 Lillian Wald, the founder of the Visiting Nurse Service and the Henry Street Settlement, led public health nurses in New York City in providing healthful living and disease control education to inner city immigrants (Buhler-Wilkerson, 1993). These recently arrived immigrants were not from the same cultural background as the public health nurses; they could neither read nor write the English language and presented the nurses with many complex challenges previously not seen by nurses. The nurses transformed the health care system by building a culture of health for a culturally diverse society through the incorporation of health education, principles of self-care management, resource development, and shared decision making.

In 1925 Mary Breckinridge demonstrated similar leadership in caring for underserved families, women, and children in rural and remote areas of Kentucky (Jesse & Blue, 2004). With the initiation of the Frontier Nursing Service, Breckinridge started the first midwifery program in the United States, and travelled with nurses on horseback to provide holistic health care for her clients in their communities. At the end of the first five years, Breckinridge was credited with instituting culturally appropriate interventions that decreased morbidity and mortality rates to below those of the government's rates for women and children in that area.

During the mid-1900s, America's first African American public health nurse, Jessie Sleet Scales, used a strategy of persuasion with African Americans living in New York City to accept treatment for tuberculosis (Carnegie, 1991). Scales's pioneering work brought her in touch with several community health organizations, among which was the Henry Street Settlement. There she would establish Stillman House, the first health clinic for African Americans. Another pioneer Mabel Staupers, the first executive director and last president of the National Association of Colored Graduate Nurses (NACGN), is known for her ombudsman work in promoting progressive legislation advancing the role of professional African American nurses in the delivery of health care to some of the nation's most vulnerable. She actively campaigned for the dissolution of the NACGN and by 1951 had accomplished her goal to integrate African American nurses into the American Nurses Association (ANA) (Carnegie, 1991).

The cultural strategies used by these pioneering leaders were best described by Madeleine Leininger, who advanced the Culture Care Theory as a way to provide culturally congruent care to all clients and accuracy in health care outcomes (Leininger & McFarland, 2006). Since then public health nurses have become more visible leaders in developing and adopting culturally competent theories and frameworks, and they are using the theories and frameworks to deliver public health nursing care and improve the quality of life for clients: individuals, families, and communities, nationally and internationally. Today, the U.S. population reflects a greater diversity of cultures from all over the world, and ensuring that individuals from these diverse cultures receive effective and quality health care is as much a challenge for nurses as it was during Lillian Wald's and her colleagues' eras. Such assurance is viewed as a moral imperative to reduce and subsequently eliminate health disparities.

It is extensively documented in the literature that minority groups are more vulnerable, have less access to health care, receive a poorer quality of health care, have higher rates of chronic illnesses, and have shorter life expectancies than non-Hispanic white groups. Many groups other than racial and ethnic groups also differ from the expected norms relative to place of origin, sexual orientation, gender identity, literacy, income, and language. Individuals who are members of these subcultures are often disregarded by the dominant health care culture as well.

This chapter underscores the role of cultural competence in the delivery of quality nursing care. It emphasizes knowledge development in the care of clients from four culturally diverse marginalized groups: African Americans, Asian Americans, Hispanic Americans, American Indian/Alaskan Natives. Special concerns of immigrants are also discussed, as well as selected religious beliefs of people who practice Islam and how these beliefs are taken into consideration in providing care.

WHY CULTURAL COMPETENCE MATTERS

Cultural competence is one of the core competencies of public health nursing (Quad Council Coalition of Public Health Nursing Organizations, 2018). **Cultural competence** entails a combination of culturally congruent behaviors, practice attitudes, and policies that allow nurses to use interpersonal communication, relationship skills, and behavioral flexibility to work effectively in cross-cultural situations (Campinha-Bacote, 2011). Becoming culturally competent is a continuous and evolutionary process. Transcultural nursing theorists recognize and appreciate differences in health care values, beliefs, and customs and that nurses must acquire knowledge, skill, and attitudes and be committed to change to ensure positive outcomes for clients (Betancourt et al., 2003; Campinha-Bacote, 2011; Leininger & McFarland, 2006).

A number of governmental agencies such as the U.S. Department of Health and Human Services and state private and quasi-governmental regulators such as The Joint Commission and private entities have attempted to address the need for cultural competence through various standards and guidelines. For example, Culturally and Linguistically Appropriate Services (CLAS), a federal government program (https://minorityhealth.hhs.gov) ensures relevance of care with national policies and legislation. The ANA Standard 8: Culturally Congruent Practice, describes expectations for nurses in practice based on their educational preparation (Marion et al., 2017). The standards developed by the Quad Council Coalition of Public Health Nursing Organizations (2018) provide guidance to nurses in education, practice, and research, as well as to health care institutions to understand, respond to, and meet the cultural needs of diverse clients. Similarly, the American Academy of Nursing Expert Panel on Global Nursing and Health and the Transcultural Nursing Society have collaboratively advanced guidelines with nursing organizations around the world to ensure culturally competent nursing care is available to consumers (2010). These guidelines are described in Box 8.1.

Both of the accreditation bodies for nursing education, the Accreditation Commission for Education in Nursing (ACEN) and the Commission on Collegiate Nursing Education (CCNE), address the need for cultural competence as essential content in nursing education. State boards of nursing are requiring culturally competent education in nursing schools, and recent legislation in many states require cultural competency training for health care providers to receive licensure or relicensure. However, measures to determine the effectiveness of cultural competence in nursing practice remain limited (Purnell, 2016).

Cultural competence is an ongoing life process, forever growing and changing our beliefs and perceptions, in which the nurse is challenged to break with the old and engage in new ways of thinking and performing (Campinha-Bacote, 2011; Leininger & McFarland, 2006). Cultural competence allows nurses to partner with clients to deliver health promotion, disease prevention, and health restoration. Cultural competence reflects a higher level of knowledge than cultural sensitivity, which was once thought to be all that was needed for nurses to

BOX 8.1 Standards of Practice for Culturally Competent Nursing Care

Standard 1: Social Justice
Standard 2: Critical Reflection
Standard 3: Knowledge of Cultures
Standard 4: Culturally Competent Practice
Standard 5: Cultural Competence in Health Care Systems and Organizations Patient
Standard 6: Advocacy and Empowerment
Standard 7: Multicultural Workforce
Standard 8: Education and Training in Culturally Competent Care
Standard 9: Cross Cultural Communication
Standard 10: Cross Cultural Leadership
Standard 11: Policy Development
Standard 12: Evidence-Based Practice and Research

From American Academy of Nursing Expert Panel: 2010. Standards of practice for culturally competent nursing care. Available at http://www.tcns.orgfiles.

effectively care for their clients. Cultural sensitivity suggests that the nurse has basic knowledge of the client's culture but lacks the skill to use information to devise a plan of care that reflects the client's total cultural needs.

Culturally competent nurses respect individuals with values and beliefs different than their own. They understand that culturally competent care is essential to avoiding unwanted outcomes as in uncompromised patient-provider relationships and negative effects on patients' health beliefs, practices, and behaviors. Nurses know that to be successful they must have general cultural and cultural-specific information so that they know what specific questions to ask their clients (American Academy of Nursing Expert Panel, 2010). Culturally competent nurses are aware of the social determinants of health in the environment that prevent individuals from achieving optimal health.

Culturally competent nursing care is guided by the following principles:

1. Care must be client-centered, that is, designed for the specific client, family, or community.
2. Care must be based on the uniqueness of the client's culture and incorporates the cultural norms and values of the client in the management of the care plan.
3. Self-empowerment strategies of the client are identified and viewed as strengths to facilitate client decision making and self-care management in health and illness situations (American Academy of Nursing Expert Panel, 2010).

Nurses work toward becoming culturally competent for a number of reasons. First, because of differences between the nurse's cultural system and the client's own cultural system. When clients and the nurses interact, they may have different understandings about the meaning of health and different ideas about what to do to promote and protect health. Nurses who value and practice cultural competence use communication and relational strategies that respect clients' values, expectations, and goals without diminishing the nurses' own values, expectations, and goals. To illustrate, a recent Mexican immigrant who speaks little English goes to a community health center because of a urinary tract infection. The nurse understands that she must use strategies that would allow her to effectively communicate with the client and modify nursing interventions that are based upon culturally informed nursing science. The nurse also understands that the client has the right to judge whether she has received the care she wanted and to follow up with appropriate action if she did not receive that care. Clients who do not feel understood may delay seeking care or may withhold information. For example, if a client is afraid of disapproval, the client may not tell the nurse that he is using both complementary and traditional Western medicines. The two types of medicine may have conflicting effects that could be dangerous for the client.

Second, care that is not culturally competent may (1) increase barriers to access of care, (2) inhibit effective communication between the client and the nurse, (3) create obstacles in gathering assessment data, thus limiting the development and implementation of effective treatment plans, and as a consequence (4) increase the gap in racial and health disparities between minority and majority populations.

Third, culturally competent nursing practice improves the quality of care, lowers cost, and increases safety and effective outcomes. The health care industry focuses on outcomes effectiveness to balance cost and quality. Quality of care means that clients have access to care delivered by culturally competent nurses. Care that is not focused on the clients' values, expectations, and goals is likely to increase cost and diminish quality. Positive outcomes, which are indicators of quality and safety, may not be met. When quality care is compromised, additional resources that typically increase costs may be needed to achieve the desired positive health care outcomes.

Fourth, the specific *Healthy People 2020* objective for persons of different cultures needs to be met (United States Department of Health and Human Services [USDHHS], 2010). To accomplish this objective, nurses must be prepared to respond to increases in minority populations to decrease and ultimately eliminate health disparities. Clients may present their symptoms vastly differently from the way they are presented in medical and nursing textbooks; they may present with a different threshold for seeking care or expectations about their care. They may have beliefs about the origin and treatment of disease that affect their willingness to participate in the treatment plan, and they may have limited English proficiency or low health literacy. For example, American health care professionals frequently view excessive drinking as a sign of disease and alcoholism as a mental illness. However, in the American Indian/Alaskan Native culture, these behaviors signify a disharmony between the individual and the spirit world, and biomedical interventions alone may not be adequate to reduce alcoholism within this culture. While there is evidence of decline, the American Indians and Alaskan Natives continue to have an alcohol-related death rate significantly higher than it is in the overall population. This is particularly devastating among American Indian men in the 35 to 49 age group and contributes to a loss of potential life compared with those in the general population (CDC, 2008). The national goal is to reduce this disparity. However, many American Indians/Alaskan Natives view alcohol consumption as an acceptable way to participate in family celebrations and tribal ceremonies, and refusal to drink with family may be viewed as a sign of rejection. West (1993, p. 234) suggested that nurses understand the possible ramifications of not having culturally competent staff available to care for the American Indian/Alaskan Native population. She stated, "If the government sends Indians to a health clinic where personnel do not understand the holistic health practices of Indians and where young white people serve as caregivers and authority figures, failure is likely to result." To have successful outcomes, nurses who develop population-based programs to reduce alcohol-related deaths must be willing to respect the cultural uniqueness of American Indian/Alaskan Natives and explore individuals' life experiences to find the underlying causes of their behaviors and solution to the problem.

CULTURE, RACE, AND ETHNICITY

Concepts of culture, race, and ethnicity within American society pervade all aspects of life and play a strong role in understanding human behavior and health. Cultural, racial, and ethnic patterns have been developed in a socioeconomic context with historical and political underpinnings. They are equally influenced by education, income, and cross-cultural experiences and account for many of the health disparities in the United States. In everyday language, race and ethnicity are often used interchangeably, but the two concepts have different meanings. Nurses are expected to understand and appreciate the meaning of each of the concepts as they relate to providing culturally competent health care to persons from diverse cultures.

Culture

The term *culture* encompasses a broad range of concepts and is applicable to individuals, groups (majority as well as minority), systems, organizations, and a nation. Culture is an integrated pattern of thoughts, beliefs, values, communication, action, customs, and assumptions about life that are widely held among a group of people (Leininger & McFarland, 2006). It is shared worldviews, meaning, and adaptive behavior derived from simultaneous membership and participation in a variety of contexts. It is the lens by which we evaluate our environment. In response to the needs of its members and the environment, culture provides tested solutions to life's problems and a sense of predictability and belonging. For example, culture determines how information is processed, received, and distributed; how rights and protections are exercised; what is considered to be a health problem; how symptoms and concerns of problems are expressed; who provides treatment for the problem; and what type of treatment and outcomes would be accepted (Andrews & Boyle, 2016; Giger, 2017; Purnell, 2016; Spector, 2016). All cultures are equal—no one culture is better than the other. Box 8.2 summarizes factors that may influence individual differences within cultural groups.

Culture is transmitted intergenerationally and changes slowly. Each individual has membership in more than one culture and learns about culture during the process of childhood

BOX 8.2 Factors Influencing Individual Differences Within Cultural Groups

- Age
- Religion
- Dialect and language spoken
- Gender identity roles
- Socioeconomic background
- Geographic location in the country of origin
- Geographic location in the current country
- History of the subcultural group with which clients identify in their current country of residence
- History of the subcultural group with which clients identify in their country of origin
- Amount of interaction between older and younger generations
- Degree of assimilation in the current country of residence
- Immigration status*
- Conditions under which migration occurred

*Except where noted with an asterisk, from Orque M: Orque's ethnic/cultural system: a framework for ethnic nursing care. In Orque MS, Bloch B, Monrroy LSA, editors: *Ethnic nursing care: A multicultural approach*, St. Louis, 1983, Mosby.

BOX 8.3 Early Cultural Awareness

Think about the first time you had contact with someone you realized was culturally different from you.

As you reflect on that initial encounter, how culturally similar were you to them? Did you judge that culture based on the norms of your culture, or did you feel that your culture was judged based on the norms of the other culture?

Briefly describe the situation/event. How old were you? What were your feelings? What were your thoughts?

What did your parents and other significant adults say about those who were culturally different from you or your family? What adjectives were used? What attitudes were conveyed?

Did your parents or anyone in your family point out the similarities between the cultures?

Have you ever had the opportunity to be immersed in a culture other than your own?

Describe how you felt during the beginning of the experience? How did you feel at the end? If given the opportunity, would you do it again? Why or why not?

As you got older, what messages did you receive about minority groups from members of your family, school, recreational facilities, and church?

As an adult, when you hear others talk about culturally different people, what images do they conjure up for you? What knowledge source is evident in the comment of the person? Do the views of the person reinforce or contradict the views that you hold today? Give an example.

What parts of your culture make it difficult to work with clients from different cultural groups?

What parts of your culture make it easy to work with clients from similar cultural groups?

What parts of your culture facilitate your work with clients from different cultural groups?

If you are not a member of the dominant culture, were you ever imposed upon by this culture? How did this make you feel?

Modified from Randall DE: *Culturally competent HIV counseling and education,* McLean, VA, 1994, Maternal and Child Health Clearinghouse.

socialization and language development (Box 8.3). There are three ways in which culture is transferred: vertical transmission, where parents are the primary sources for the transfer of traditions and teachings; horizontal transmission, when people within the same generation (i.e., other family members) pass on the information; and oblique transmission between generations of people who are not related, such as at religious, social, and educational institutions, and among peers. Parents and family teach both explicit and implicit behaviors of the culture. The explicit behaviors, such as language, interpersonal distance, and kissing in public, can be observed and allow individuals to identify with other persons from the culture. In this way, people share the traditions, customs, and lifestyles with others. The implicit behaviors are less visible and include the way individuals perceive health and illness, body language, differences in language expressions, and the use of titles. These behaviors are subtle and may be difficult for persons to describe, yet they are part of the culture. For example, deferring to older persons when they enter the room or offering them a seat suggests a cultural value related to older people. Another example of an implicit aspect of culture is the use of language to communicate. For instance, in one culture a sign might read "No smoking is permitted." In another culture the sign might read "Thank you for not smoking." The former statement represents a culture that values directness, whereas the latter culture, indirectness (Figs. 8.1 and 8.2).

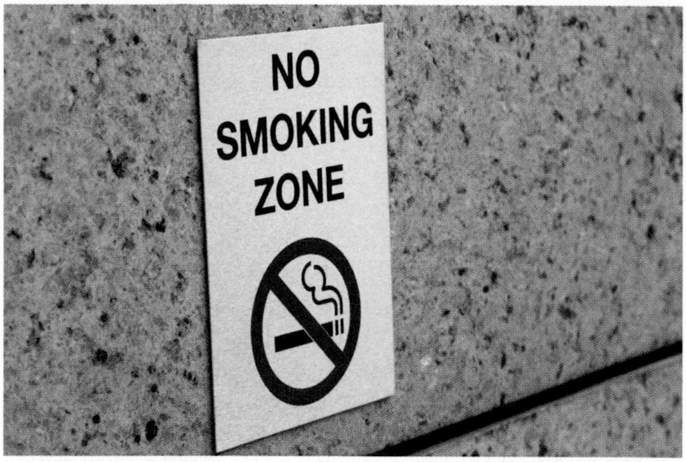
NO
SMOKING
ZONE

Fig. 8.1 The sign is from a culture that values directness in communication. (© 2012 Photos.com, a division of Getty Images. All rights reserved. Image 91883504.)

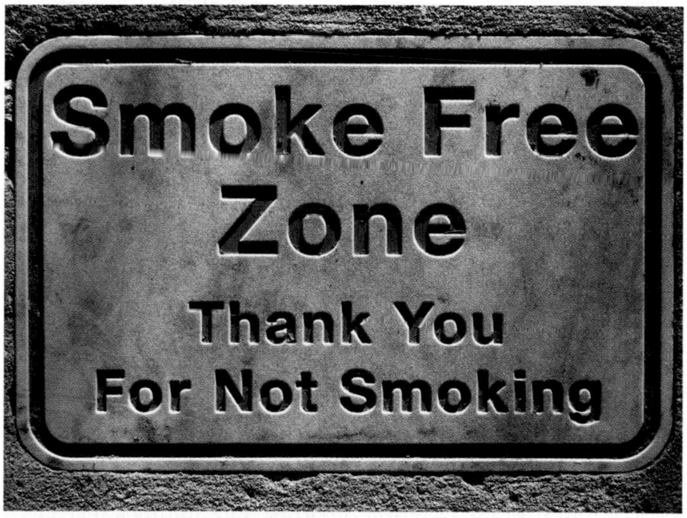
Smoke Free
Zone
Thank You
For Not Smoking

Fig. 8.2 The sign is from a culture that values indirectness in communication. (© 2012 Photos.com, a division of Getty Images. All rights reserved. Image 122153579.)

Just as all cultures are not alike, all individuals within the culture are not alike. Within a culture, often people speak different dialects, have different religions and religious practices, represent widely divergent ages, and have different socioeconomic and educational status. Also, in many countries, people who live there may be native to that country or may have immigrated there. As an immigrant, the person may continue to adhere to customs, language, and religion from his or her native country. Each person should be viewed as a unique human being with differences that are respected; for example, people in some cultures consider diseases such as cancer, mental illness, and human immunodeficiency virus (HIV) to carry a stigma.

Culture also contributes to the diversity in behaviors and attitudes that clients have about health care and the providers who care for them. As a result of this diversity, significant differences in beliefs and practices about health and illness have become apparent in health care systems. Caring for a culturally diverse population can be challenging for nurses who want to incorporate their client's beliefs of health and illness when intervening to promote and maintain wellness. In the present health care system, nurses need to understand the sociocultural views that affect perceptions, as well as the pathophysiology of an illness. Nurses have the chief responsibility for translating health information so that clients can understand it and engage in more effective strategies to achieve positive health outcomes.

Race

Race is a biological variation within population groups based on physical markers derived from genetic ancestry, such as skin color, physical features, and hair texture. It is a characteristic that allows for some groups to be separated, treated as superior, and given access to power and other valued resources, while others are treated as inferior and have limited access to power and resources. Racial differences include areas of growth and development, skin color, enzymatic differences, susceptibility to disease, and laboratory test findings. Individuals may be of the same race but of different cultures. For example, African Americans, who may have been born in Africa, the Caribbean, North America, or elsewhere, are a heterogeneous group, but they may be considered culturally homogeneous by persons who think of African Americans as one racial group. This perception can cause providers to be unaware of cultural differences of individuals who come from different countries but who share similar racial characteristics. This often blurs an understanding of this culturally diverse group. Individuals who are white also experience this same over-generalization of individuals along racial/ethnic lines.

Physical changes in biracial and multiracial generations lead to changes in the physical appearance of individuals and make race less important in ethnic identity. The findings that DNA composition for any two humans across race is 99.9 percent genetically identical and that differences between races occur in only 1 in 1000 people diminishes the ethnocentric debate about the importance of race. Another factor making race less important is the increasing number of interracial marriages that result in biracial and multiracial children whose physical and genetic pool dilute the racial characteristics of their parents (Fig. 8.3). In 1920 the "one drop rule" instituted in the United States stated that any individual with least one drop of blood from at least one ancestor of African descent is considered to be African American. Biracial babies who had one white parent were assigned the race of the nonwhite parent. In today's global village with the increased number of biracial and multiracial individuals, a new category has been added to the census that gives children from such unification the option to recognize their biracial or multiracial heritage.

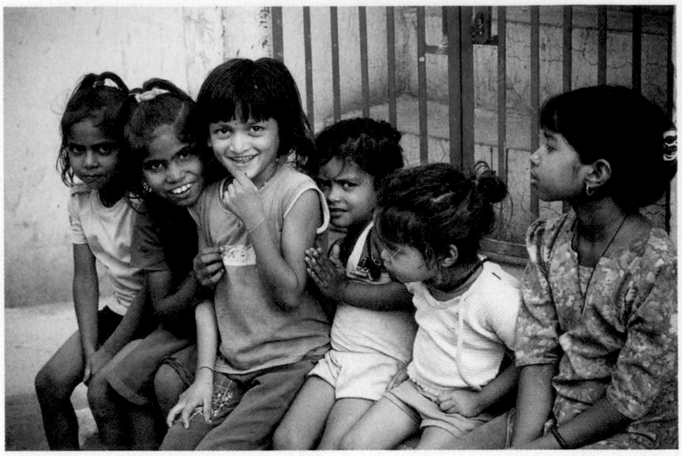

Fig. 8.3 In countries around the world there are distinct differences in people who represent the same cultural group. (Copyright © 2013 Thinkstock. All rights reserved. Image # 117003112.)

Ethnicity

Ethnicity, in contrast to race, is the shared feeling of peoplehood among a group of individuals and relates to cultural factors such as beliefs, values, language, traditions, nationality, geographic region, and ancestry (Giger, 2017). It refers to a social identity that reflects membership in a clan or group that over time creates a common history that is resistant to change. Ethnicity is influenced by education, income level, and association with people from other ethnic groups. Therefore a reciprocal relationship exists between the individual and society as members of an ethnic group give up aspects of their identity when they adopt characteristics of the group's identity. However, if the ethnic group is strong, the group maintains its values, beliefs, behaviors, practices, and ways of thinking.

IMPACT OF DIVERSITY ON CULTURAL COMPETENCE

Cultural Diversity

Cultural diversity refers to the degrees of variation that are represented among populations based on race, ethnicity, and lifestyle, across place, and place of origin across time. It also includes aspects of social class, gender identity, sexual orientation, physical abilities/disabilities, and the changing populations of the world. The United States is the most diverse nation in the world, reflecting the mixture of immigrants from various countries who have helped to shape and build America in critical ways. There are over 300 languages spoken, with English being the most frequently spoken language, followed by Spanish, Chinese, French, and German. Understanding diversity is about understanding and embracing each other's differences and similarities.

The 2017 U.S. population estimates revealed that 61.7 percent defined themselves as non-Hispanic white, 18.1 percent Hispanics, 13.4 percent African Americans, 5.8 percent Asian Americans, 1.3 percent American Indians/Alaskan Natives, 0.2 percent Native Hawaiian and other Pacific Islanders, and 2.7 percent two or more races (United States Census Bureau, 2018). The decreasing white population (72.4 percent in 2010) is attributed to a rapidly growing Hispanic population and a strong increase in the Asian population. By 2020 more than half of the nation's children will be a member of a minority or ethnic group (Vespa et al., 2018). Nonwhite ethnic groups are at greater safety risk in health care facilities as measured by their morbidity and mortality rates, premature births, and failure to access health care (United States Department of Health and Human Services, 2017). However, the nursing workforce is overwhelmingly white (83 percent), with non-Hispanic African Americans, 6 percent; Hispanics, 3 percent; Asians, 6 percent; American Indians/Alaskan Natives, 1 percent; Native Hawaiian/Pacific Islanders, 1 percent; and other nurses, 1 percent (American Association of Colleges of Nursing, 2015). One of the key recommendations from the landmark study proposed by Smedley et al. (2002) is the need to increase minority representation in the nursing workforce, have more integration of cross-cultural education into health care training, and have more advanced research activities to identify sources of disparities and interventions. Phillips and Malone (2014) report that the gap between majority and minority nurses is beginning to close as there is also a small cadre of minority students enrolled in nursing schools.

Cultural Variations Among Selected Groups

All cultures have the same organizational elements, but each cultural group has its own interpretation of the element that allows a group to differentiate itself from other groups. Organizational elements provide direction for what members of the group determine is appropriate or inappropriate behavior. The organizational elements of cultures have been described in nursing by Andrews and Boyle (2016), Giger (2017), Purnell (2016), and Spector (2016). They are biological variations, personal space, perception of time, environmental control, social organizations, and communication patterns. Nutritional and religious practices also may vary for different cultural groups. As part of the nursing process, nurses are expected to accurately assess a client's health needs based on information derived from eight primary cultural elements.

Biological Variations. Biological variations are the physical, biological, and physiological characteristics that exist between racial groups and distinguish one race from another. These characteristics occur in areas of growth and development, skin color, enzymatic differences, susceptibility to disease, and laboratory test findings (Andrews & Boyle, 2016; Giger, 2017). For example, Western-born neonates are slightly heavier at birth than those born in non-Western cultures. Variations in growth and development may be influenced by environmental conditions such as nutrition, climate, and disease. Mongolian spots are bluish discolorations that are sometimes present on the skin of African American, Asian, Hispanic, and American Indian/Alaskan Native babies. These spots may be mistaken for bruises. When nurses encounter situations involving unfamiliar biological variations, they may create embarrassing situations. Consider the following scenario: The school nurse observed a bluish discoloration on the thigh of a Filipino child that she mistook for a bruise. The nurse reported her observation to the child protective agency in her state. The mother had to disprove the allegation to the agency's social worker before her child could be released into her care. Other common and obvious variations include eye shape, hair texture, adipose tissue, shape of earlobes, thickness of lips, and body configuration.

A frequently determined enzyme deficiency which is responsible for lactose intolerance in many ethnic groups, is glucose-6-phosphate dehydrogenase (G6PD) (Giger, 2017). Differences among groups exist for drug metabolism; for example, some African Americans may experience less effectiveness than some other groups do for psychotropic, immunosuppressant, antihypertensive, cardiovascular, and antiretroviral medications.

The Levels of Prevention box gives examples of cultural strategies for primary, secondary, and tertiary levels of prevention.

LEVELS OF PREVENTION

Related to Cultural Differences (Hypertension, Stroke, and Heart Disease)

Primary Prevention

Provide health teaching about a balanced diet and exercise.

Secondary Prevention

Teach clients and/or family to monitor blood pressure. Teach about diet, keeping in mind the client's cultural preferences. Talk about health beliefs and cultural implications, such as the use of complementary and alternative therapies; make sure these therapies are compatible with any medications that may be prescribed.

Tertiary Prevention

If blood pressure cannot be controlled by diet, refer the client to a physician or nurse practitioner for medication, and advise the client to participate in a cardiac program that will oversee diet and exercise.

Personal Space. Personal space is the physical area individuals need between themselves and others to feel comfortable. When this space is violated, the client may become uncomfortable. There are four zones of interpersonal space—intimate space (direct contact to 1.5 feet), personal distance (1.5 to 4 feet), social distance (4 to 12 feet), or public distance (greater than 12 feet)—that may be observed when nurses care for clients.

To illustrate, some individuals who hold membership in Hispanic cultures tend to be comfortable with less space because these individuals like to touch some persons with whom they are speaking. Individuals in the Filipino culture may view touching strangers as inappropriate and intrusive, and people may be uncomfortable. Nurses who wish to be culturally appropriate may elect to stand farther away from Filipinos than from Hispanics. On the other hand, clients who are comfortable with closer distances may experience discomfort when nurses stand farther away, interpreting the behavior as rejecting. Nurses should take cues from clients to place themselves in the appropriate spatial zone and avoid misinterpretation of clients' behavior as they handle their health need.

Perception of Time. Perception of time refers to the duration of and period between events. Some cultures assign greater or lesser value to events that might occur in the future, are present, or have occurred. Members of cultural groups who tend to be future oriented often will delay immediate gratification until goals are accomplished. Future-oriented persons who value longevity may engage in health promotion activities to moderate their dietary intake and engage in exercise activities to minimize future health risks. In contrast, some present-oriented cultural groups may place greater emphasis on the here and now and view information about their present set of circumstances as more important than what will happen in the future—the future is unknown, but the present is known.

In the present orientation of time, how weight contributes to a client's physical characteristics may not be important; for another group the burden of excess weight and the problems it causes may be the focus. When nurses discuss health promotion and disease prevention strategies with persons from a present orientation, they should focus on the immediate benefits these clients will gain rather than emphasizing future outcomes. That is not to say that clients cannot or will not learn about preventing complications of illness, but nurses need to connect their teaching to the "here and now." It is important to listen carefully to what clients say in order to gather information about their time orientation.

In a past-oriented culture, time is viewed as being more flexible than in a present-oriented culture. It has less of a fixed point, and individuals may not be offended by being late or early for appointments. In cultures that focus on a past orientation, for example in the Vietnamese culture, individuals may focus on wishes and memories of their ancestors and look to them to provide direction for current situations (Giger, 2017). They believe that their ancestral heritage determines their current health status. Nurses socialized in the Western culture may view time as money and equate punctuality with correctness and being responsible.

Working with clients who have a different time perception than the nurse's can pose a dilemma for the nurse who wishes to be culturally competent and accountable for helping his or her client receive quality health care. Nurses should clarify the clients' perceptions to avoid misunderstanding and explain the importance of keeping appointments from the Western perspective. For example, the nurse can communicate a willingness to be flexible in scheduling appointments and explain to clients that the time will be set aside specifically for them. Nurses should incorporate issues of time in health education. For example, there are circumstances when organization's and client's perception of time differ. It is disrespectful to clients to have them wait hours beyond the scheduled appointment to be seen by a health care provider. This can result in expressions of anger and hostility, which could ultimately lead to diminished positive health outcomes for the client.

Environmental Control. Environmental control refers to the person's relationships with nature and efforts to plan and direct factors in the environment that affect them. Cultures may be distinguished based on one of three views of nature: (1) the environment has mastery over nature, (2) nature controls the environment, and (3) nature and the environment work in harmony to promote health and wellness. In cultures that perceive individuals as having mastery over the environment, nurses can expect that a client with the diagnosis of cancer will be willing to engage in rigorous treatment modalities such as chemotherapy, radiation, and laser therapy to beat the disease. Persons who value harmony with the environment (e.g., African Americans, Asians, and American Indians/Alaskan Natives) may not adhere to a cancer treatment protocol as they believe cancer is in disharmony with nature, medicine cannot cure cancer, and nothing will change. They would look to the mind, body, and spirit connection, for healing comes from within, to find treatments for the malignancy. Naturalistic solutions such as herbs, acupuncture, and hot and cold treatments would likely be their treatment of choice to resolve the suffering associated with the cancerous condition. Individuals from cultures that view the environment as dominant over nature (e.g., Hispanics) may believe that they have little or no control over the serious illness for which they have been diagnosed. Similarly, individuals who live close to coastal areas where there may be disasters such as hurricanes, and tsunamis or in other areas where there are earthquakes and volcanoes may perceive no control over the environment. These individuals are less likely to engage in illness management interventions that are harsh and that they cannot trust to yield a positive health outcome.

Social Organization. Social organization refers to the network of relationships in families, groups, and communities that allows for members to stay connected. Social organizations are structured to carry out role functions while maintaining a sense of community within the group. Members depend on the extended family and kinship networks for emotional, social, and financial support in times of crises. The significance of kinship in the formation of family relations varies across cultures. Some cultures, like the African American culture, adopt individuals who are unrelated or remotely related as family members. Some other cultures, like Hispanic and Asian, place the needs of the family above those of the individual. In the American Indian/Alaskan Native family, for example, members honor and respect their elders and look to them for leadership, believing that wisdom comes with increasing age. When working with clients who prefer family decision making over individual choice, nurses should be aware that it may be counterproductive to exclude family involvement—particularly mothers and grandmothers—in the health care decision-making process. At the same time, nurses should advocate for the individual, making sure that when families make decisions, the individual's needs have been considered.

Communication. Effective communication is consistent with Guideline 9, Cross Cultural Communication, of the Guidelines for Implementing Culturally Competent Nursing Care (American Academy of Nursing Expert Panel, 2010). Communication is about sending and receiving messages between at least two persons. Effective communication with the client or family is the most significant issue that must be addressed for the nurse to successfully help clients, solve health issues, and achieve positive health outcomes. Effective communication also helps nurses identify beliefs, values, practices, perceptions, and unique health care needs. There are two types of communication: (1) verbal communication and (2) nonverbal communication. Verbal communication is the use of words to express feelings and ideas. Nonverbal communication is the use of body language or gestures to convey a message. Aspects of nonverbal language include eye contact, gesture, touch, body posture, facial expression, and silence. For example, some Hispanic clients are reluctant to make eye contact or answer questions, and this behavior should not be viewed as rudeness. It is important to understand variations in pattern and to use words that a lay person can understand. Cultural variations are found, for example, in pronunciation, word meaning, voice quality, use of humor, and speed of talking. Many people of the United States and the United Kingdom have English as their first language. However, the word *boot* has different meanings for them. In the United States a boot typically refers to something one puts on one's feet; in the United Kingdom the boot is what Americans call the trunk of the car.

An example of nonverbal communication occurred when a nurse gave instructions to an Asian client on taking antituberculin drugs and illustrates the need to understand cultural communication. The client responded with a smile and a nod. The nurse interpreted the response to mean that the client understood the instructions and had accepted the treatment protocol. A week later, when the client returned for a follow-up visit, the nurse discovered that the medications had not been taken. The nurse knew that acceptance by and avoidance of confrontation or disagreement with those in authority are important behaviors in some Asian cultures. Interventions were adjusted accordingly: the nurse repeated the medication instructions and gave the client an opportunity to raise questions and concerns and to repeat the instructions that were given; the nurse had an opportunity to confirm understanding and correct errors and to discuss the cultural meaning and treatment of tuberculosis. Other factors influencing communication include forms of address, such as the use of first names or surnames, and whether it is polite to wait until a person finishes speaking or to talk over. It is important to respect all information that a client shares with you even when the information is in conflict with your own value system.

Communicating trust is vital to the nurse-client relationship and determines the extent to which the client will share information with the nurse. Nurses help to facilitate effective communication with their clients. Clients who view nurses as not trusting can block communication with the nurse. For example, when nurses do not create a communication system that promotes the clients as owners of their own health care and provide them with data to make good health care choices, the clients may not be receptive to health education that the nurse wants to impart.

Nutritional Practices. Nutritional practices play an integral role in understanding clients' health care issues. Nutritional practices refer to the intake of food for the purpose of providing sustenance to meet dietary requirements. For many cultures the preparation and eating of food are social activities that allow members of the group to come together to celebrate life and provide comfort for one another. Everyone has to have good nutrition to improve health, and public health nurses improve health through promoting and supporting culturally relevant nutritional practices. Knowing the client's nutritional practices enables nurses to develop dietary regimens that do not conflict with the culture and supports clients' participation in decision-making processes.

Almost all family rituals associated with birth, baptism, graduation, marriage, retirement, and death include food as part of the ceremony. The selection of many of these foods may have their origin in religion; for example, many people who subscribe to the Buddhist religion are vegetarian. Their faith teaches self-control as a means to search for happiness. The Buddhist code of morality is in their Five Moral Precepts: abstain from (1) harming living things, (2) stealing, (3) sexual misconduct, (4) lying, and (5) intoxicants such as alcohol, tobacco, or mind-altering drugs. Eating meat would conflict with both the first and fifth (i.e., meat is seen as an intoxicant). Muslims avoid pork and foods cooked with alcohol.

Box 8.4 identifies questions nurses should ask when collecting data for a dietary assessment of practices and food consumption patterns.

Health professionals need to be able to determine what is important to the culture and when necessary help clients modify their behaviors and practices. Health care teams should understand that food may be one of the last cultural practices for clients to give up and they must accommodate food practices whenever possible. For example, to prescribe an American diet to a Hispanic or an Asian client whose

BOX 8.4 Assessment of Dietary Practices and Food Consumption Patterns

1. Does the food have nutritional value based on MyPlate?
2. What is the social significance of food in the family? Has the family adopted foods from other cultural groups?
3. What foods are most frequently purchased for family consumption? Who decides and from where is the food purchased?
4. What foods, if any, are prohibited for the family?
5. What variables play a significant role in food selection (cost, variability, family rituals, religion, family tradition, celebrations)?
6. How often does the family prepare food at home? Who prepares the food? How is it prepared?
7. How much food is eaten? When is it eaten and with whom?
8. Are fresh fruits and vegetables easily accessible for purchase in the community?
9. What spices does the family's use in the preparation of the food? What are the family's favorite recipes?
10. What are the characteristics of restaurants and other eating facilities that the family uses outside of the home?

mealtime and food choices may be different from American food patterns may be negligent. When engaging in mutual goal setting with the client and a nutritionist to change harmful dietary practices, the team might need to consult culturally oriented data sources. A number of popular magazines such as *Essence*, *Ebony*, and *Latina* have created healthier dishes from revised old family recipes for Hispanic and African American families. These dishes taste good and allow those who use them to continue their food traditions. Before beginning a dietary intervention, the nurse should perform a cultural nutritional assessment to determine food preferences, rituals, and taboos and avoid conflict with cultural food preferences.

Religion. Religion plays a dominant role in protecting health and supporting healing in many cultural traditions. Religion is about the acceptance of a particular set of organized beliefs, values, and ritual practices shared by groups and communities that determines what is right and what is wrong. Religious practices include prayer, attending religious services, and being an active member of a religious community. On the other hand, spirituality serves as the connection between an individual and a higher being that guides along life's way. Spiritual practices are about meaning and purpose in life. Spirituality also includes prayer, yoga, meditation, volunteering, and contributing to community activities. The focus of spirituality is on developing awareness of who we are, what is our purpose in being, and the understanding of our connectedness with ourselves and beyond.

Among all racial groups in the United States, African Americans are most likely to report a formal religious affiliation (Pew Research Center, 2018). Many African Americans find comfort and support in their religious beliefs, believing God is responsible for health, and view health professionals as God's instruments for healing. Among Hispanics, Roman Catholic and Pentecostal beliefs and practices are prevalent. Many Jews observe Sabbath, which extends from sundown on Friday until sundown on Saturday.

Muslims are the most racially diverse group, and the religion of Islam is the second largest and fastest growing religion in the world. In the United States the majority of Muslims are white (41 percent), African American (20 percent), Asian (28 percent), and Hispanic (8 percent), and others are of mixed or more than one race (3 percent) (Pew Research Center, 2017). Muslims worship one God—Allah—and are governed by teachings as presented in the Qur'an. Some Muslims may seek a physician's care for a visible physical problem but avoid seeking help for preventive health care for problems like diabetes and hypertension. They face Mecca (which is northeast) when praying, and have their face turned toward Mecca when death is imminent. Suicide is forbidden, but do-not-resuscitate orders are acceptable. Daily prayer is a requirement, and Muslims must perform absolution before they pray. Sunni Muslims pray five times a day and Shiite Muslims pray three times a day. Muslims gather for corporate worship on Fridays. Tradition says that Muslims pray on the floor, but during illness they may pray in bed. Exceptions from traditional Muslim practices can sometimes be permitted during pregnancy, breastfeeding, illness, or travel; but the nurse should always ask the client because some Muslims may observe the practices even though they may have received permission for an exception.

Chinese and other Asian people may practice Eastern religions such as Confucianism, Buddhism, or Taoism. Confucianism emphasizes respect for the elderly and people in authority. Practitioners believe that moral conduct and maintaining harmonious relationships are the keys to life. The five most important attributes are benevolence, righteousness, loyalty, filial piety, and virtue. The Buddhist principles embrace three attributes: mercy, thriftiness, and humility. Buddhists believe that people receive good fortune for doing the right thing and misfortune for doing the wrong thing. Taoism embraces selflessness and emotional calm. The most important thing to them is to be in harmony with nature. An important element of health is outdoor exercise for peace of mind and outside air. Part of achieving good health is to adjust the thinking and the body to fit in with the natural rhythm of the universe.

Immigrant Issues. Immigrants have always been a part of the fabric of the United States, home to one fifth of the world's population, and they have a large impact on many aspects of life in the United States, from the workplace to the classroom and throughout communities (Zong et al., 2018). Immigrants to the United States are born in countries or territories external to the United States and migrate to the United States, contributing to its vast diversity. With heightened attention on the turmoil in the world and the relocation of people from different countries, there has been a shift in political views on immigration. Immigration has become increasingly controversial in recent years with increased ambivalence among people in the United States about immigrants and the laws and policies pertaining to them.

Since the events of September 11, 2001, and particularly since the inauguration of President Trump in 2017, the national debate about immigration policy has intensified, and many laws enacted reflect more difficulty for people seeking visas and more scrutiny of both visa and entry documents. For example, President Trump has (1) increased border security whether it be by sea, land, or air, and restricted entry into the United States with green cards only to spouses and minor children, (2) banned nationals from five countries, most majority-Muslim nations (Iran, Libya, Somalia, Syria, and Yemen) from entering the United States, (3) reduced refugee admission to the lowest level since the resettlement program was instituted and separated children from parents seeking asylum from some countries in Central America at border states' ports of entry, (4) cancelled the Deferred Action for Childhood Arrivals (DACA) program that gave temporarily protective status entry in the United States but was ordered by the courts to have it reinstated, (5) ended the designation of temporary protected status for nationals of Haiti, Nicaragua, and Sudan, and (6) changed the diversification program by granting visas to more persons from underrepresented nations (Pierce et al., 2018; Zong et al., 2018). These complex issues involved with the foreign-born population and health care accessibility restrict the opportunity for public health nurses to provide culturally competent care to this population. These policies may change over time and be less restrictive to foreign-born people and more culturally inclusive.

Immunizations

CHECK YOUR PRACTICE

Jorge and his mother, Cecelia, immigrated from El Salvador to the United States seeking refugee status. Before their case could be adjudicated, Cecelia was deported back to El Salvador. Cecelia left Jorge with her sister, Maria, who lives in a small rural town in Texas. As Maria was about to enroll the 5-year-old Jorge in kindergarten, she discovered that she had no record of his immunizations. Maria met with the school's secretary regarding the immunization issue who in turn consulted with the school health nurse as to the appropriate action to be taken.

What is the school health nurse's role in helping to initiate the child's immunization program? What action(s) should the school nurse recommend to the secretary?

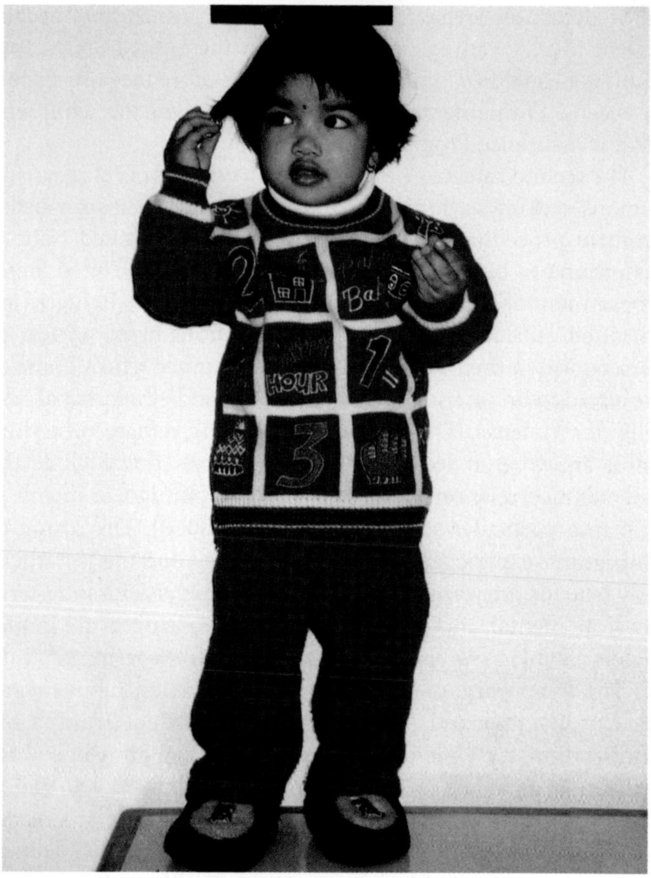

Fig. 8.4 A child from Nepal living in the United States. The child has a black dot on her forehead to protect her from the "evil eye."

Foreign-Born. Place of origin for the immigrant is distinguished from nationality, which refers to the place where the individual has or had citizenship. For example, if individuals were born in the Dominican Republic, they may be naturalized citizens, but their ethnicity is likely to be Hispanic with a Dominican place of origin. Based on 2016 data, it is estimated that the U.S. population consists of 43.7 million (foreign-born) immigrants, accounting for 13.5 percent of the total population, of which 11.4 million have illegal status (Zong et al., 2018). **Foreign-born** refers to all residents who were not U.S citizens at birth, regardless of their current legal or citizen status or those whose parents were not U.S. citizens. They carry the nationality of their home country. The majority of the foreign-born population live in or around major metropolitan areas in four states: California, Texas, New York, and Florida (Zong et al., 2018). In 2016, 46 percent of immigrants reported their race as white, 27 percent as Asian, 9 percent as African American, and 15 percent as some other race; slightly more than 2 percent reported two or more races.

Immigrants make up about 17 percent of the workforce, where slightly less than half of them are either in construction or the health care industry (Cepla, 2018), and almost 32 percent work in management, professional, and related occupations (Zong et al., 2018). With an aging American-born population, the immigrant's presence in the workforce will become even more pronounced as they are projected to replace United States-born workers when they retire from the workforce (Kosten, 2018). By 2035 all the growth in the United States workforce will be attributed to immigrants and their children.

The foreign-born are likely to be poorer than the United States-born population, 36 percent of immigrant-headed households use at least one major welfare program (primarily food assistance and Medicaid) compared to 23 percent of the United States-born population. About one third of immigrants are insured. Noncitizens are more likely to be uninsured than citizens because of higher rates of both public and private coverage. Similarly, noncitizen children and citizen children in families with mixed citizenship status are more likely to be uninsured than children of citizens (Artiga & Damico, 2017). Immigrants to the United States often bring with them unique cultural, health care, and religious practices that must be respected (Fig. 8.4). A more detailed description of the immigrant populations and what benefits they are eligible to receive can be found at https://migrationpolicy.org.

Enforcement of immigration laws often prevents many immigrants from seeking health care in a timely manner, contributing to poor health outcomes when they do seek health care services. Other factors like living in low-income and segregated neighborhoods (ethnic enclaves) and working in low-wage occupations with exposure to toxic chemicals, and poor or other unsafe working situations contribute to poor health outcomes when immigrants seek health care services (United States Department of Health and Human Services, 2018).

Types of Foreign-Born. There are four categories of foreign-born. The first category is **legal immigrants**, also known as **lawful permanent residents**. In 2016, 49 percent of this group was naturalized and had become U.S. citizens (Zong et al., 2018). Legal immigrants are not citizens but are legally allowed to live and work in the United States, usually because they fulfill labor demands or have family ties. Legal immigrants usually have a 5-year waiting period living in the United States after receiving "qualified" immigration status before they are eligible to receive entitlements such as Medicaid and the Children's Health Insurance Program (CHIP).

The second category of foreign-born consists of **refugees** and persons seeking asylum. The Refugee Act of 1980 provided a uniform procedure for refugees (based on the United Nations definition) to be admitted to the United States (United States Department of Health and Human Services, 2012). Refugees are admitted outside the usual quota restrictions based on fear of persecution in their homeland, and they cannot return home or are afraid to do so, usually because of war and ethnic, tribal, and religious violence. The grounds for seeking refugee or asylum status must be at least one of five reasons that include the person's race, religion, nationality, political opinion, or membership in a particular social group (Cepla, 2018). This group of immigrants experiences a host of difficulties, and this is particularly true for the younger children, who are at risk for long-term physical, mental, and emotional challenges. Refugees are immediately eligible to receive benefits described for legal immigrants, such as Temporary Assistance for Needy Families, Supplemental Security Income, and Medicaid. Under President Trump's administration, the United States reduced the cap on refugees' admission to its lowest in a decade, from 85,000 to 54,000, and to 45,000 in 2018 (Cepla, 2018). The Centers for Disease Control and Prevention (CDC) provides "Refugee's Health Guidelines" designed to promote and improve the health of the refugee, prevent disease, and familiarize refugees with the U.S. health system (Centers for Disease Control and Prevention, 2016).

The third category of foreign-born is **non-immigrants**; these are people admitted to the United States for a limited duration and for a specified purpose. They have a permanent residence outside the United States and include students, tourists, temporary workers, business executives, career diplomats, their spouses and children, artists, entertainers, reporters, and those wishing to receive medical treatment.

The fourth category of foreign-born is **unauthorized immigrants**, or undocumented or illegal aliens. These persons may have crossed a border into the United States illegally, or their legal permission to stay in the United States may have expired. They account for about 11 percent of the immigrant population. They are mainly from Mexico and Central America (71 percent), mostly male (54 percent) between 25 and 44 years of age (53 percent), home owners (about 33 percent), and majority employed (64 percent) but uninsured (61 percent), and slightly more than 50 percent of them live below the poverty level (Migration Policy Institute, 2018). Unauthorized immigrants are eligible to receive emergency medical services, immunizations, treatment for the symptoms of communicable diseases, and access to school lunches. They are not eligible to enroll in Medicaid, CHIP, or the Affordable Care Act (Obamacare) or purchase coverage through the Health Insurance Marketplace. This significantly reduces opportunities to have affordable health insurance and quality health care services (Artiga & Damico, 2017). Although federal funds for Medicaid are not available to the states for immigrants, six of the states and the District of Columbia have found funds to provide Medicaid health benefits to all immigrant children regardless of immigration status (Artiga & Damico, 2017).

Several misperceptions exist about the economic value of allowing immigrants to enter or to stay in the United States. Immigrants who are authorized to work in the United States pay federal, state, and local taxes. Unauthorized immigrants also pay taxes but are not entitled to benefits like Medicare and social security. It is estimated that in 2016 immigrants increased the gross domestic product to 2 trillion dollars because of their presence in the labor force and contributions in skills, education, and capital investments (Center for American Progress Team and Nicholson, 2017). Illegal immigrants contributed $11.64 billion to state and local taxes (Estrada, 2016). The dilemma for communities, however, is that immigrants typically pay federal taxes, yet the services they receive are paid for by the states and localities, and they are not entitled to tax credits. Even though noncitizens are as likely as citizens to work, they may be in jobs that do not provide health coverage for employees.

In addition to financial constraints on providing health care for immigrants, they often come to the United States with diverse health risks combined with language barriers and social, religious, and cultural backgrounds different from those of their health care providers. The use of traditional healing or complementary health care practices may be unfamiliar to U.S. health care providers, who may lack knowledge about high-risk diseases specific to particular immigrant groups for whom they care. For example, some groups are more at risk for hepatitis B (with its attendant effects on the liver), tuberculosis, intestinal parasites, and visual, hearing, and dental problems. Many of these conditions are either preventable or treatable if managed correctly. Nurses should know the major health problems and risk factors that are specific to the immigrant populations for whom they provide care and to treat them in the context of the culture from which they come.

Often children and adolescents adjust to the new culture more easily than adults. This can lead to a shift in the balance of power between adults and children, contributing to family conflict and at times violence. Inability of elders to acculturate may play a large part in their lack of adherence to health care guidelines. Nurses should be alert for warning signs of family stress and tension, remembering that older family members can help translate their culture, beliefs, religious practices, dietary habits, support systems, and risk factors for the health care provider. They can also assist with decision making and provide support to enable the individual or group seeking care to change behaviors and increase their health promotion practices.

Similarly, understanding the role of the community in the care of immigrants is important. Communities can help clients (and thus providers) with communication, crisis intervention, housing, and emotional and other forms of support. Nurses carefully assess the community and learn what strengths, resources, and talents are available; this includes the traditional practices immigrants use. Many of these practices have therapeutic value and can be blended with traditional

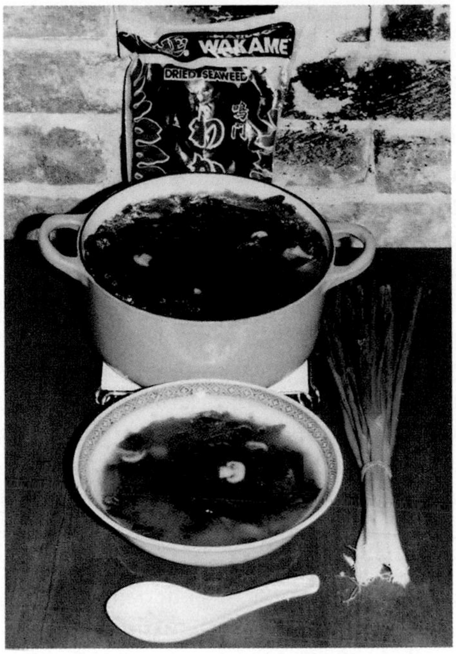

Fig. 8.5 Mi-yuk kook (seaweed soup) is a Korean dish eaten by postpartum women to stop bleeding and to cleanse body fluids. It is also eaten every birthday.

Western medicine (Fig. 8.5). The key is to know what practices are being used so the blending can be done knowledgeably. Community members are excellent sources of this information, and nurses working with immigrant populations should use the community assessment, group work, and family techniques described in other chapters to partner with immigrant clients.

The following skills are necessary for the nurse to increase authenticity, accuracy, and approachability when working with immigrant populations:

1. Self-awareness: Recognize the values, beliefs, and practices that make up your own culture. Nurses, like clients, are influenced by their culture, values, and language.
2. Identify the client's preferred or native language. When nurses do not speak or understand the client's language, they must obtain assistance from an **interpreter** to ensure that full and effective communication occurs. Health care institutions must provide clients with an interpreter. The interpreter should have knowledge of the client's culture and medical terminology. Interpreters should be trained, qualified, and hired to ensure that they have met minimum standards to provide accurate and safe interpretation. Using family members, friends, and staff who are not trained as health/medical interpreters can create errors in understanding and communicating and pose grave risks for the client and liability to the health care institution.

   While both an interpreter and a translator interpret and translate information from one language to another, there are significant differences between the two. A translator is usually associated with translating written documents such as medical records and legal documents; in contrast, the interpreter is associated with verbal communication that focuses on accurate expression of equivalent meanings rather than on word-to-word equivalence. Experiences of success that nurses report when working with an interpreter include proper use of interpreters to ensure that clients understand health care instructions; provision of linguistically appropriate educational material; ability to communicate in the client's language to provide health care instructions; and ensuring proper use of instructions. Experiences of difficulty include language barriers preventing appropriate communications; lack of available interpreters overall and for specific languages; and lack of appropriate translation by interpreters. Nurses can minimize some of these difficulties by learning basic words and sentences of the most commonly spoken languages in the community and observing client reactions when asking them questions. Also, nurses should provide written material in the client's primary language, so that family members can reinforce information when at home with the client. The How To box provides guidelines for using an interpreter.
3. Learn the health-seeking behaviors of your immigrant client and the client's family members. In asking the client about family members, you might try using a simple genogram, which places family members on a diagram. Ask who the family members are, where they live, and who is missing or deceased. You might also ask the client to talk about holiday celebrations: who comes, who is missing, what do they do?
4. Get to know the community where the immigrant client lives. Read about the culture of your clients. Take a course. Volunteer to participate in the acculturation process of the community (e.g., to give talks, hold forums with free-flowing and two-way communication), and learn who the formal and informal resources are.
5. Get to know some of the traditional practices and remedies used by families and communities. Coordinate health teaching seminars with traditional healing courses for the community so you can work with, not against, them.
6. Learn how cultural subgroups explain common illnesses or events. In cultures where the body and mind are seen as one entity or in cultures in which there is a high degree of stigma associated with mental illness, people or individuals somaticize their feelings of psychological distress. In somatization, psychological distress is experienced as a physical illness.
7. Try to see things from the viewpoint of the client, family, and community and accommodate rather than squash the client's view.
8. Conduct a cultural assessment focusing on what is working, what is not working, and changes that need to be made to accommodate cultural norms and promote positive health behaviors.

HOW TO Guidelines for Selecting and Using an Interpreter

1. The educational level and the socioeconomic status of the interpreter are important. The nurse should know that the interpreter understands the community's interpretation of the disease and understands the community's health care practices around the disease.
2. The gender and/or age of the interpreter may be of concern; in some cultures, women may prefer a female interpreter, men may prefer a male

interpreter, and older clients may want a more mature interpreter. Avoid using children as interpreters, particularly when the client is an adult.

The nurse identifies the client's country of origin and language or dialect spoken before selecting the interpreter. For example, Chinese clients speak different dialects depending on the region in which they were born.

3. The nurse evaluates the interpreter's style, approach to clients, and ability to develop a relationship of trust and respect.
4. The interpreter interprets everything that is said by all the people in the interaction and informs the public health nurse if the content might be perceived as insensitive or harmful to the dignity of the client.
5. The interpreter conveys the content, the spirit of what is said without omitting or adding.
6. The nurse makes phrase charts and picture cards available.
7. The nurse observes the client for nonverbal messages such as facial expressions, gestures, and other forms of body language. If the client's responses do not fit with the question, the nurse should check to be sure that the interpreter understood the question.
8. Increase accuracy in transmission of information by asking the interpreter to translate the client's own words and ask the client to repeat the information that was communicated.
9. The interpreter must maintain confidentiality of all information and interactions
10. At the end of the interview, the nurse reviews the material with the client and the interpreter to ensure that nothing has been missed or misunderstood

SOCIAL ISSUES AFFECTING CULTURALLY COMPETENT NURSING CARE

Social Determinants of Health

Social determinants of health are the circumstances in which all people live, learn, and work that put them at greater risk for a wide range of health functioning and quality outcomes (USDHHS, 2018). Social determinants are particularly burdensome for ethnically or culturally diverse and socially disadvantaged groups like the underserved, underrepresented, and uninsured. Regardless of genetic or biological composition, these circumstances are shaped by the distribution of money, power, and resources in homes and communities. They determine an individual's or group's morbidity and mortality. According to Healthy People 2020, the five areas of social determinants are (1) economic instability (e.g., poverty, unemployment, and housing instability), (2) education (e.g., language and literacy, graduation rates, and enrollment in higher education), (3) social environment (e.g., use of alcohol and drugs, incarceration, and civic participation), (4) health and health care (e.g., access to health and primary health care services and literacy), (5) the physical environment (e.g., safe community, crime and violence, and access to healthy foods). Social determinants are forever present, but public health nurses can work with communities to establish strategies and policies in helping people in these areas get access to safe housing, good nutrition, and after-school programs that would minimize their impact on health and primary health to ensure reducing health disparities and increasing healthy outcomes for their clients. Public health nurses should be aware of the social determinants of health in the communities in which they work that prevent individuals from achieving optimal health. For example, high school students in low-income areas play after school games in their neighborhoods that often lead them into teenage parenthood and criminal activities such as drugs, robberies, and gun violence.

Socioeconomic Status

Socioeconomic status is a measurement of an individual's, a household's, or a community's social position in relationship to others. Socioeconomic status is based on income, education, or a composite of other factors like cultural characteristics, literacy, where you live, or whether you rent or own a home. As a determinant of health, socioeconomic status influences life expectancy, infant death rates, low birth rates, access to health care, testing, and many other health measures (U.S. Census Bureau, 2017a). Educational level is key to understanding a person's economic status.

In 2016 the poverty rate in the United States was 12.7 percent. Table 8.1 indicates that there are more whites than minorities living at or below the poverty level, but minority groups have a greater concentration of poor families than the white group. For example, American Indians/Alaskan Natives and Hawaiians make up 0.09 percent and 0.02 percent, respectively, of the population; however, 27 percent and 17.6 percent, respectively, live in poverty. Minority families are disproportionately represented on the lower tiers of the socioeconomic ladder.

Low socioeconomic status refers to those who earn less than the poverty threshold calculated dollar amount based on family size and composition (U.S. Census Bureau, 2017b). Low socioeconomic status is a common characteristic found among populations at risk, such as the elderly, minorities, single-parent head of households, the homeless, migrant workers, and refugees. In 2016 the poverty rate in the United States was 12.7 percent, but there were large differences between various racial/ethnic groups.

Attributing behaviors stemming from socioeconomic deficits to behaviors embedded in cultural origins can result in misinterpretations of the client's motivation to adhere to treatment regimens. Data suggest that when nurses and clients come from the same social class, it is more likely that they operate from the same health belief model, and consequently there is less opportunity for misinterpretation and communication problems.

There is danger in believing that the use of complementary (natural and magico-religious) practices is mainly restricted to

TABLE 8.1 Estimates for 2016 Poverty Rates by Ethnic Groups

Ethnic Groups	Percent of Total Populations[a]	Percent of Poverty Rate
Non-Hispanic whites	61.0%	8.8%
Blacks	12.6%	22.0%
Asians	5.8%	10.1%
Hispanics	18.1%	19.4%
American Indian/ Alaskan Natives	0.09%	27.0%
Native Hawaiians	0.02%	17.6%

[a]The total estimate of populations does not reflect groups consisting of two or more races.

From U.S. Census Bureau: Income and poverty in the United States, 2016.

individuals on the lower socioeconomic rung. More individuals in Western cultures, including health professionals, are integrating complementary practices with the biomedical system to promote, protect, and restore their health. Acceptance of this is reflected in courses being offered in universities, the arrival of newer disciplines in health care such as homeopathic medicine, and more acceptance of traditional medicine such as acupressure and acupuncture. Nurses can consult and seek guidance from non-Western practitioners to better understand how clients and families integrate cultural concepts with other aspects of client care to meet their clients' total health care needs.

Health Literacy

Health literacy is a national public health problem affecting 90 percent of adults who enter health care institutions (Centers for Disease Control and Prevention, 2017). It is considered one of the social determinants of health. **Health literacy** is the degree to which an individual has the capacity to obtain, process, and understand basic health information. Limited health literacy negatively influences the ability to access care, share medical history with providers, complete forms and follow instructions, and know the connection between risky behaviors and health-promoting activities. Having these deficiencies places individuals at a safety risk and worsening health outcomes. Anyone may experience limited health literacy, but the elderly, minorities, immigrants, individuals with low educational skills, low socioeconomic status, and those who live in medically underserved areas are more likely to express these deficits. The pattern in which clients with limited health literacy present their illness symptomology is often different from that of persons with high literacy skills, especially when in unfamiliar places and situations.

An individual's level of health literacy changes with each health care encounter, and nurses should determine clients' health literacy to (1) assess level of understanding, (2) determine the extent to which clients are capable of making effective health care decisions, (3) provide services that are personally relevant to the client, (4) give accurate and easy-to-understand health information that includes familiar words, concepts, and images and avoids the use of jargon, (5) help clients decide on treatment options and short-term benefits as to what would work best, and (6) give reasons for taking the specific action. Public health nurses understand that they may hold a different cultural perception about the client's illness than the client, provide accurate and accessible health information, and examine available services and provider's motivation to promote and protect their clients' health. It is their responsibility to ensure that health information and services provided are understood and used by all Americans.

Public health nurses should distinguish between limited English proficiency and limited health literacy. Limited English proficiency refers to individuals who do not have English as primary language and have limited ability to read, write, speak, or understand English. Individuals with limited English proficiency include persons with hearing, other language, and or other disabilities who might require assistive services, and they too may experience poor health outcomes as a result of the limitation.

Marginalization

Marginalization occurs when a segment of the population has been excluded from the mainstream in social, economic, cultural, or political life. Those who are marginalized are systematically blocked from enjoying the same rights enjoyed by majority groups in opportunities and resources for a good education and respectable employment with the ability to become economically stable and independent of others. Marginalization is brought about by policies, practices, and programs that expose the marginalized to being devalued, rejected, and relegated to the fringe of society. Marginalized groups often internalize the untruths they have been told and behave in a powerless manner consistent with the expectations of those who have defamed them. Examples of marginalized groups include but are not limited to minorities, the homeless, immigrants with linguistic challenges, drug abusers, the economically disadvantaged, and those whose sexual orientation or gender identity differ from the expected norms. Marginalized groups are often the target of discriminatory beliefs, behaviors, and judgments from others. In some instances, *vulnerable populations* may be considered an equivalent term for *marginalization.*

Health Disparities

One of the national goals for 2020 objectives is to eliminate health disparities among groups by addressing the multiple social determinants that lead to poor health. **Health disparities** describe health differences between groups that adversely affect disadvantaged populations (National Institute of Minority Health and Health Disparities, 2018). In contrast, ethnic disparities in health care are explained largely by differences in English fluency, whereas racial disparities in health care are best explained by delayed care due to a lack of knowledge by caregivers about the client's culture and ethnic values, norms and thinking outside of their reference group, and the client's lack of insurance and transportation.

Health disparities are long-standing, persistent problems that cannot be explained by variations in health care needs, patient preferences, or treatment recommendations (Orgera & Artiga, 2018). They occur across many dimensions and are closely linked to social, economic, and environmental disadvantages. Health disparities may also arise from specific health risks that come from ongoing exposure to stigma, discrimination, and violence toward socially marginalized groups as demonstrated by unequal treatment and lack of culturally competent health care. Health disparities are expressed in at least one of the following health outcomes: (1) higher incidence and/or prevalence of specific diseases and/or disorders, (2) premature and/or excessive mortality in diseases where populations differ, (3) greater burden of disease as demonstrated with metrics such as reduced quality of life or disability-adjusted life, or (4) poorer daily functioning. Research on health disparities shows that even after controlling for socioeconomic status, insurance status, and age, racial and ethnic minority groups are disproportionately likely to have severe health problems, experience lower quality care, and have poorer health outcomes (Agency for Healthcare Research & Quality, 2014; Weirenga et al., 2017).

Health disparities have been documented for many decades. They are monitored annually by various departments within the U.S. Department of Health and Human Services as part of the national goal to achieve health equity for all within the United States (see the Healthy People 2020 box related to health disparities). The priority groups being tracked are minorities, low-income groups, women and children, older adults, and individuals with special needs (i.e., disabilities and those who need chronic or renal care).

Despite some narrowing of the gap in recent years, many disparities have persisted and, in some cases, widened (Agency for Healthcare Research & Quality, 2018). The reduction and elimination of health disparities remain a challenging issue for providers at federal, state, and local levels. For example, between 2000 and 2014, the Agency for Healthcare Research and Quality tracked access to care for African Americans, Hispanics, and whites who were living below the poverty level (2016). They reported no narrowing of the gap between the groups in many of the measurements: African Americans had worse access to care when compared to whites for 50 percent of the measures tracked; Hispanics had worse access to care for 75 percent of the measures tracked. To hasten progress in eliminating disparities, the National Quality Forum Committee (2017) has outlined a four-action performance measurements and policy implementation plan that should lead to a faster systematic reduction of health disparities. The recommended actions are (1) identifying and prioritizing health disparities, (2) implementing evidence-based interventions to reduce disparities, (3) investing in the development and use of health equity performance measures, and (4) incentivizing the reduction of health disparities and achievement of health equity. An additional force to reduce health disparities is being driven by private and public stakeholders who have linked successful patient outcomes to fee for services provided by health care organizations

HEALTHY PEOPLE 2020

Goals and Objectives of Healthy People 2020 *Related to Cultural Issues*

Goal: Eliminate health disparities among different segments of the population as defined by gender, race or ethnicity, education, income, disability, living in rural areas, and sexual orientation.

Selected Objectives

- **AHS-1:** Increase the proportion of persons with health insurance.
- **AHS-2:** Increase the proportion of insured persons with clinical preventive services coverage.
- **AHS-3:** Increase the proportion of persons with a usual primary care provider.
- **AHS-6:** Increase the proportion of persons who have a specific source of ongoing care.
- **AHS-7:** Reduce the proportion of individuals who are unable to obtain or delay in obtaining necessary medical care, dental care, or prescription medicine.

Social Justice

Social justice is the primary and overarching standard that governs all nursing practice. It is Standard 1 of the Guidelines for Implementing Culturally Competent Nursing Care (American Academy of Nursing Expert Panel, 2010). **Social justice** is concerned with values of impartiality and objectivity at a systems or governmental level and is founded on principles of fairness, equity, respect for self and human dignity, and tolerance. The need to address social justice comes from unequal distribution of wealth, opportunity, and resources globally, nationally, or at the community level. Unfair treatment is often triggered by race, culture, gender, economic status, age, sexual orientation, disability, or religion. Public health nurses advocate for social justice when they advocate for fair housing, women's rights issues, or cessation of gun violence in schools and communities. Most importantly, public health nurses work with individuals and communities to remove poverty and minimize health disparities so that all individuals and groups can enjoy optimal health regardless of ethnic-racial identification. **Advocacy** says that the public health nurse champions the causes of their clients to ensure that they have the necessary resources to enjoy a quality life. Practicing social justice is acting in accordance with fair treatment regardless of economic status, race, ethnicity, age, citizenship, disability, or sexual orientation.

Health Equity

Health equity is the principle underlying a commitment to social justice to reduce and ultimately eliminate poverty and disparities in health. Health equity is concerned with ensuring that all individuals and groups, regardless of being historically disadvantaged, are supported in achieving the highest possible quality of health. Health inequities are disparities in health and have their genesis in the structure of society (Sadana & Blas, 2013). They are attributed to the unequal life chances experienced by people of different social classes, racial/ethnic backgrounds, and other aspects of social stratification (for example gender and geography—where you live). They are systematic, avoidable, and unjust treatment between individuals or groups and are reflected in differences in access to health care, severity of disease, morbidity and mortality rates, and quality of life indicators. Achieving health equity requires giving recognition to social barriers, as well as barriers that have their origins in genetics, economics, and lifestyle factors that contribute to inequality of health. Ensuring that clients receive just and equitable care means that nurses must advocate for policies and programs that promote and protect the rights of clients to receive quality health care, education, safe water, and the right to a decent standard of living.

In addressing health inequities, government sponsored social programs such as Medicaid provides health insurance for those individuals with limited income and financial resources. It also covers children, pregnant women, parents, seniors, and individuals with disabilities who meet the state's eligibility requirements. Medicare is for those 65 years of age and older with a work history, as well as for younger people with certain disabilities or end-stage renal disease. The Affordable Care Act coverage reduces the cost of coverage for low- and moderate-income populations to increase access and eliminate health disparities.

CULTURAL COMPETENCE IN NURSING

Developing Cultural Competence

Nurses develop cultural competence through the critical reflective use of self-awareness, communications, relationship-building, and intervention skills that promote mutual respect for differences in the use of participatory decision making. In acquiring cultural competence, nurses may be guided by three principles as suggested by Campinha-Bacote (2011) and Leininger and McFarland (2006): (1) maintain a broad objective and open attitude toward individuals and their cultures, (2) avoid seeing all individuals as alike, and (3) have the desire to provide culturally competent care. Because there are varying degrees of cultural competence, not all nurses will achieve the same level of development concurrently.

In an early model developed by Orlandi (1992), three stages to acquiring cultural competence were depicted (culturally incompetent, culturally sensitive, and culturally competent). Table 8.2 shows that each stage has three dimensions—cognitive (thinking), affective (feeling), and psychomotor (doing)—that have an overall effect on nursing outcomes. The most effective outcomes are knowledgeable, committed to change, and highly skilled. The most destructive outcomes are oblivious, apathetic, and unskilled.

A widely used model to explain the process of acquiring cultural competence was created by Campinha-Bacote (2011). The most recent model depicts five interrelated constructs involved in developing cultural competence: (1) cultural awareness, (2) cultural knowledge, (3) cultural skill, (4) cultural encounter, and (5) cultural desire. Other educators (Chen, et al., 2018; Long, 2016; and Morgan & Reel, 2003) strongly recommend cultural immersion experiences, particularly for nursing students to learn from individuals about other cultures within the context of the culture and improve their cultural awareness and cultural knowledge.

Cultural Awareness

Cultural awareness is consistent with Guideline 2, Critical Reflection, of the Guidelines for Implementing Culturally Competent Nursing Care (American Academy of Nursing Expert Panel, 2010). It is an initial step that nurses take in developing cultural competence. It refers to an inward transformative and in-depth exploration of one's own cultural roots, personal biases, humanity, ethics, and professionalism that have the potential to be in conflict with the value of others. Cultural awareness is a prerequisite to understanding one's own behavioral rules and how the rules are projected onto others (Campinha-Bacote, 2011). Culturally aware nurses are conscious of culture as an influencing factor on differences between themselves and others and are receptive to learning about the cultural dimensions that define themselves as persons and others as equal partners in the nurse-client relationship. In developing cultural competence, culturally aware nurses are able to do the following:

- Learn about the cultural dimensions of clients.
- Understand their own behavior and how it helps or hinders the delivery of competent care to persons from cultures other than their own, particularly as it pertains to what is good health care, what is responsible health care, and how these are reflective in attitude and behavior. Recognize that health is expressed differently across cultures, and culture influences an individual's responses to health, illness, disease, and death.
- Recognize that health can be delivered in a variety of modes consistent with the client's health values

For example, at a community outreach program a nurse was teaching a racially mixed group the screening protocol for breast and cervical cancer detection. An African American woman in the group refused to give the return demonstration for breast self-examination. When encouraged to do so, she said, "My breasts are much larger than those on the model. Besides, the models are not like me. They are all white." After hearing the client's comments, the nurse realized that her concept was based on her own self-image and that she had a stereotypical view of breasts based on her own breast. The nurse was not aware of the significance of breasts and the size of the breast in the client's culture, and had made no reference in her talk to the influence of culture or race on screening for breast and cervical cancer.

The nurse then talked with the client, asked for her recommendations, and encouraged her to return the demonstration. The nurse coached the client through the self-examination process while pointing out that regardless of the breast size, shape, and color, the technique is the same for feeling the tissue and squeezing the nipple to make sure that there is no discharge. Because this nurse was culturally aware of the importance of understanding cultural differences, she neither became angry with herself or the client nor imposed her own values on the client. Rather, she elicited a discussion with the client about her beliefs, attitudes, and feelings about screening for breast cancer that may have been influenced by her culture. The nurse understood that she had to tailor her teaching material to the needs of diverse client groups. Subsequently, she advocated for her agency to purchase a model of an African American woman's breast to be used in future health education programs with African American women and shared her experience with her colleagues.

TABLE 8.2 The Cultural Competence Framework: Stages of Competence Development

	Culturally Incompetent	Culturally Sensitive	Culturally Competent
Cognitive	Oblivious	Aware	Knowledgeable
Affective	Apathetic	Sympathetic	Committed to change
Psychomotor (skills)	Unskilled	Lacking some skills	Highly skilled
Overall effect	Destructive	Neutral	Constructive

From Orlandi MA: Defining cultural competence: an organizing framework. In Orlandi MA, editor: *Cultural competence for evaluators*, Washington, DC, 1992, U.S. Department of Health and Human Services.

Being culturally aware, the nurse understood that her values were different from the client's own and acted in a supportive manner with the client. The interaction identified client assets and barriers, organization's barriers, and appropriate intervention strategies. A confrontation between the nurse and the client could have ensued had the nurse not recognized the need to listen to the client's concerns, express respect the client's input, and show support. Nurses should always champion the cause for clients seeking health care to have health care partners respect clients' cultural traditions. Nurses should engage in critical reflection of their own values, beliefs, and cultural heritage in order to have an awareness of how these qualities and issues can impact culturally congruent health care. Critical reflection implies that nurses examine their own values, beliefs, and cultural heritage in order to provide effective care to patients of different cultures. See Box 8.3 for questions to ask yourself about your development of cultural awareness. Campinha-Bacote (2016) has provided a list of cultural assessment instruments/tools that researchers, educators, clinicians, and students may select from to measure their level of cultural competence when caring for culturally diverse clients

Cultural Knowledge. Cultural knowledge is consistent with Guideline 3, Knowledge of Cultures, of the Guidelines for Implementing Culturally Competent Nursing Care (American Academy of Nursing Expert Panel, 2010). It refers to having a sound educational understanding about culturally diverse groups in the space of the nurse (Campinha-Bacote, 2011). Nurse have common personal and specific cultural knowledge of the populations where they mainly work. For example, if the nurses work with a large Muslim population, they need to have specific knowledge related to religion, spirituality, and cultural practices regarding nutrition, childbirth, trust, expressions of health, and death, to name a few. The emphasis is on learning about the clients' worldview from an emic (native) perspective as it pertains to health beliefs and practices, cultural values, and disease incidence and prevalence. For example, cultural knowledge indicates that Middle Eastern women might not attend prenatal classes without encouragement and support from the nurse (Meleis, 2005). The reason for this is that attending prenatal classes is about the future of the baby whereas the mother's main concern may be on the present and what is happening in the immediate environment. If nurses understand the cultural difference in this example, they can select strategies to help the mother understand the value of the classes. In contrast, specific knowledge about the Nigerian culture would help the nurse to understand that the mother might begin prenatal classes but not continue because Nigerian women often view birth as a natural process and not a process they need to attend a class to understand (Ogbu, 2005). Although the behavioral outcome of the women from these two countries may be the same, the rationale for their action is different. Nurses who have cultural knowledge are not likely to develop feelings of inadequacy and helplessness or blame clients when they do not understand the clients' health care decisions.

Although it is unrealistic to expect that nurses will have knowledge of all cultures, they should know how and where to obtain information that impacts the clients and community with whom they have frequent interaction. Developing cultural knowledge also comes from reading about, taking courses on, and discussing different cultures within multicultural settings. Students are now exposed to a variety of individuals who hold membership in cultures that are different from their own. Students therefore have greater opportunity to assess gaps in their cultural knowledge about how to care for individuals, families, and communities from diverse groups. Students also learn that clients are a rich source of information about their own culture. As leaders, nurses are expected to use leadership skills to advocate for social justice by promoting community empowerment, liberation, and relief of suffering and human oppression.

The Evidence-Based Practice box provides an example of learning how to meet the needs of a cultural group that is different from that of the nurse.

EVIDENCE-BASED PRACTICE

The purpose of this intervention study was to determine if a culturally adapted telephone-delivered smoking cessation program would be feasible and acceptable to Korean Americans. The protocol was implemented over eight weeks. It consisted of five questionnaires; counseling sessions that included explanation on the harmful effects of smoking, nicotine addiction, and high mortality rate among Koreans; nicotine replacement patches, family participation, and counseling for relapse. Recruitment of the 31 participants (29 men and 2 women) was facilitated through advertisements on a Korean-speaking radio station. The station reported on smoking-related issues and smoking cessation websites. Measures were taken at one, two, and three months post interventions. The primary outcome was for a three-month prolonged abstinence as measured by self-report of not smoking a cigarette and corroboration by a family member. The secondary outcome was seven-day point prevalence abstinence. Results were compared with the California quitline study that used the same interventions, but the cultural adaption was deeper for this study. At one month post intervention, 55 percent (17) participants reported abstinence, and at three months, 42 percent (13) participants achieved prolonged abstinence. Results showed that participants with stronger family ties were less dependent on the nicotine patches. The limitations for the study were that the sample size was small and consisted of majority of men.

Nurse Use

Results of the study underscore the importance of family in Korean culture. Nurses should be aware that there is great respect for family and in order to accomplish positive health care outcomes, they should involve the family using culturally appropriate communication. Nurses should also know that the involvement of family may vary with age, ethnic group, education, location in the country of origin, and migration history.

From Kim SS: A culturally adapted smoking cessation intervention for Korean Americans: preliminary findings. *J Transcult Nurs* 28:24–31, 2017.

Cultural Skill. Cultural skill is the third element of developing cultural competence, and it is consistent with Guideline 4, Culturally Competent Practice, of the Guidelines for Implementing Culturally Competent Nursing Care (American Academy of Nursing Expert Panel, 2010). Cultural skill refers to the ability of nurses to effectively integrate cultural awareness and cultural knowledge when conducting a cultural assessment and a culturally based physical assessment and to use these data to meet the needs of specific clients (Campinha-Bacote, 2011). Culturally skillful nurses elicit from clients their perception of the health problem, discuss treatment protocols, negotiate acceptable options, when appropriate select interventions that incorporate alternative treatment plans, and collaborate with all stakeholders. For example, culturally competent nurses use appropriate touch during conversation and modify the physical distance between themselves and others while meeting mutually agreed upon goals with the client (Fig. 8.6). To further assist in developing culturally competent skills, nurses may enroll in the e-course *Culturally Competent Nursing Care: A Cornerstone of Caring,* offered by the Office of Minority Health, U.S. Department of Health and Human Services

Cultural Encounter. Cultural encounter is the fourth and key element essential to becoming culturally competent. It has roots in the nurse-client interpersonal relationship that focuses on caring, compassion, presence, caring consciousness, and empathy. **Cultural encounter** refers to the processes that permit nurses to seek opportunities to directly engage in cross-cultural interactions with clients whose culture differs from their own to modify existing beliefs about a specific cultural group and possibly avoid stereotyping (Campinha-Bacote, 2011). These cultures can be across geographic communities, gender, religion, class, ethnicities, sexual orientation, or educational level. A cultural encounter focuses on understanding and responding to diverse needs, assessing organizational cultural diversity and competence, assessing effects of policies and programs on different populations, and taking action to support a diverse public health workforce (Quad Council of Public Health Nursing Organizations, 2018).

There are two types of cultural encounters: direct (face-to-face) and indirect. An example of a direct cultural encounter occurs when non-Hispanic nurses learn directly from their Puerto Rican clients about spicy foods that they avoid during periods of breastfeeding. Indirect cultural encounters occur when nurses share examples of culturally specific care with other nurses to help them develop their knowledge to effectively care for other Puerto Rican clients who are breastfeeding.

The most important encounters are those in which nurses share narratives about clients' life experiences and health-seeking behaviors and ways and partner with other nurses to deliver improved quality care for those in communities where they work. In some communities, nurses may have few opportunities to work directly with persons of other cultures. Thus, when nurses come in contact with clients who are culturally different from themselves, they should embrace general cultural concepts in the situation until they are able to learn directly from the clients about their culture. Research findings show that when undergraduate students are exposed to clients from multicultural backgrounds they have high cultural competence performance (Chen et al., 2018). Developing cultural competence also comes from reading about, taking courses on, and discussing different cultures within multicultural settings. Successful cultural encounters occur when nurses embrace interactions with patients from diverse backgrounds to validate, refine, or modify existing values, beliefs, and practices about a cultural group and to develop cultural awareness, cultural knowledge, cultural skill, and cultural desire (see Fig. 8.6).

Cultural Desire. **Cultural desire** is the foundation for other constructs in Campinha-Bacote's model (2011) for acquiring cultural competence. It is the nurses' willingness to learn about,

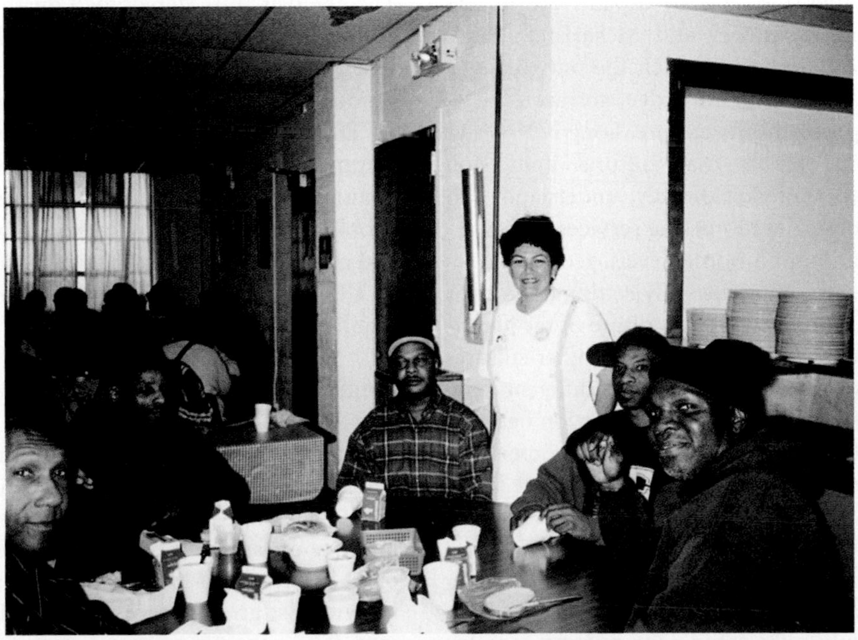

Fig. 8.6 A Hispanic nursing student interacting with African American men at a nutritional center. To interact in a culturally competent manner, the student needs to have awareness of and knowledge about the differences between her culture and the men's culture and the skill to portray this in her behavior toward them.

respect, and work with clients from different backgrounds to provide culturally competent care. Cultural desire is based on the humanistic value of caring for the individual. Nurses who wish to become culturally competent do so because they want to, rather than because they are directed to do so. They demonstrate a sense of energy and enthusiasm about the possibility of providing culturally competent nursing interventions. Unlike the other elements, cultural desire cannot be directly taught in the classroom or in other educational or work settings. Campinha-Bacote believes that having cultural desire is the motivation for nurses to seek knowledge or continuing education about different cultural groups. Nurses are more likely to demonstrate cultural desire when the environment at all levels of the organization reflects a philosophy that values ongoing learning and education in cultural competence development for all nurses to practice competently within their scope of practice. Campinha-Bacote (2011) recommends that nurses who want to acquire cultural competence should not fear making mistakes but internalize and incorporate into their own worldview selected beliefs, values, practices, lifeways, and problem-solving skills of other cultures with which they have the most frequent encounters.

Cultural Immersion. Cultural immersion is consistent with Standard 8, Education and Training in Culturally Competent Care. Once a nurse has learned the cultural norms, lifeways, values, and gained insights into circumstances and perspectives on health care of a given culture, expanding knowledge is to engage in a cultural immersion with the local people in a community of the identifying group. Cultural immersion provides the nurse with an exposure to gain in-depth insights into the nurse's own values, biases, and affective responses. This intense cultural interaction generally involves field work in which the nurse works alongside an unfamiliar population of interest to better understand how they live and to expand the nurse's intercultural competencies. Leininger and McFarland (2006) refer to this as an emic experience in which the nurse gains a deeper appreciation of the values, knowledge, and worldviews that is facilitated by the people in the culture. Long (2016) and Morgan and Reel (2003) report that cultural immersion provides an opportunity to interact directly, understand, and communicate to reduce obstacles to nursing services to distinctive groups across populations, economic levels, geographic areas, political orientation, and ethnicities. By setting aside their own cultural norms and immersing in the culture of the identified group, nurses suspend perceived barriers of other cultures and opt for the discovery of a diversity of values different from their own and discover for themselves the distinction between their culture and that of the client's. It is a contextual experience where the nurse meets and builds connections for future interaction and learns how to adapt nursing care strategies that are congruent with the clients' culture.

Barriers to Acquiring Cultural Competence

Nurses fail to provide culturally competent nursing care for a variety of reasons: they may have had minimal opportunity to learn about cross-cultural nursing, been pressured by colleagues who are not knowledgeable about cultural concepts and are offended when others use the concepts, or believe that people in the organization place greater value on productivity than on providing culturally competent care. These and other issues may result in nurses engaging in behaviors such as stereotyping, prejudice and racism, ethnocentrism, cultural imposition, cultural conflict, cultural shock, and classism.

Stereotyping. Stereotyping is an overgeneralization about a member of a particular category of people, usually referring to race, ethnicity, immigration status, or sexual orientation. Without first assessing for individual differences, the nurse ascribes to the client certain widely held beliefs and behaviors about the client's group, which is different from the nurse's. Stereotyping blocks the willingness of the nurse to be open and to learn about specific individuals or groups. Stereotypes are most often negative generalizations but can be positive. Some groups are stereotyped as "industrious and hard working," while some groups are stereotyped as "negative and noncompliant." Clients who perceive they are being stereotyped may respond with anger and hostility. This in turn perpetuates the stereotype and creates barriers to health-seeking behavior and a positive nurse-client relationship.

Many of the stereotypes about culturally diverse patient populations have not been validated through research. When data from a cultural assessment are not immediately available, it is acceptable for nurses to generalize about an individual's group behavioral pattern as a guide until they have had time to observe and assess the client's behavior. This can be a problem as it may lead to a nurse's unwillingness to incorporate new and specific data about the client in a care plan. New information may be distorted to fit with preconceived ideas. The generalizing that was a beginning point for understanding the individual becomes a final point and the basis for planned interventions. The client is thus stereotyped on the basis of the group's ascribed behavior. For many years, health diseases were classified based on factors such as income, insurance, sexual orientation, residence, gender, or ethnicity without recognition of individual differences. Factors that minimize the use of stereotypes are cultural competency training for providers, trust in effective culturally competent nursing interventions, and engaging with people and teams that nurture culturally competent discussions and understanding of ways to increase positive health outcomes for diverse populations. Change in stereotypical behavior often requires changes in social values.

Prejudice. Prejudice is the emotional manifestation of deeply held beliefs (stereotypes) about a group. These beliefs are directed toward a person who is a member of that group and who is presumed to have the qualities ascribed to the group. Prejudice is not based on reason or experience but rather on negative or favorable preconceived feelings. These feelings are often borne out of hatred and intolerance for certain kinds of individuals, groups, races, or the characteristics they represent. They are precursors for discriminatory acts based on prejudging, limited knowledge about, misinformation about, fear of, or limited contact with individuals from that group.

Discrimination is the outward manifestation of thoughts, beliefs, and attitudes put into practices and policies. Discrimination may be directed at, but not limited to, age, disability, economic level, compensation, national origin, race, religion, and sex. For example, classism is discrimination based on the individual's socioeconomic standing. Classism reflects behaviors created and maintained in a system of inequality for the purpose of benefiting those in a higher class while negatively affecting those in a lower class. Those who are prejudiced wish to deny the individuals on the basis of race, skin color, ethnicity, or social standing the opportunity to benefit fully from society's offerings of accessible health care, education, good jobs, and community activities. One way to minimize prejudice is to ask clients to share their evaluation of the health care they received, involve clients in the evaluation of their care, and ensure that their voices are heard in decision-making processes.

Racism. Racism is a form of prejudice that occurs through the exercise of power by individuals and institutions against people who are judged to be inferior on the basis of intelligence, morals, beauty, inheritance, and self-worth. Individuals may be denied certain opportunities (e.g., jobs, housing, education, and health care) typically enjoyed by the dominant group because of some characteristic over which they have no control. When racism is acted upon, it results in perceived or actual harm to the individual. Research findings give evidence of bias by health care professionals against African Americans, Hispanics, and dark-skinned people (Hall et al., 2015). Often outside of conscious awareness, providers of different specialties, levels of training, and levels of experience showed bias in patient-provider interactions, treatment decisions, treatment adherence, and patient health outcomes. The providers appeared to have had implicit bias in terms of positive attitudes toward whites and negative attitudes toward people of color.

Three types of racism exist: individual, institutional, and cultural. Individual racism refers to discriminatory behavior or acts directed toward individuals or groups because of identified characteristics, such as skin color, hair texture, and facial features. Institutional racism refers to discriminatory behavior or acts by an institution, as expressed in policies, priority setting, hiring, and resource allocation practices that are directed toward individuals and groups and restrict their access to opportunities or resources. Institutional racism provides the structure for racism at the individual level to be accepted and condoned. Cultural racism refers to discriminatory behavior or acts directed by the dominant group toward another cultural group. The cultural group is depicted in derogatory or stereotypical ways because of, for example, language or dress. All forms of racism can have individual, as well as community and population, effects. Factors such as structural inequalities and racism may have a greater impact on health disparities between particular groups than cultural differences.

The Tuskegee syphilis study is a well-known example of overt intentional racism at an institutional level (United States Public Health Service, 2017). This study was conducted by the U.S. Public Health Service to observe the effects of syphilis on African American men over a period of 40 years, beginning in 1932. When African American men with syphilis were recruited for the study, they were told that they were being treated for "bad blood," and treatment for syphilis was withheld intentionally so that the study on the deleterious effect of syphilis could be completed. As a result, hundreds of men lost their lives because of discriminatory policies that promoted substandard health care. After the study was completed the government changed its research practices to prevent a repeat of the mistakes made in Tuskegee. The consequence of such racism has contributed to the long-held beliefs by some African Americans that health research might be designed to harm them and that accessible health care for African Americans might be part of a research study, especially government-sponsored programs. In 2005 Brandon, Isaac, and LaVeist reported that a telephone survey revealed no differences by race existed between African Americans and whites in knowledge about the Tuskegee study. There were significant race differences in medical care that the researchers attributed to broader historical and personal experiences of African Americans. Perceived racism by cultural groups can have physiological and psychological negative health outcomes that include high blood pressure, stroke, engaging in risky behaviors such as smoking and substance abuse, depression, and low self-esteem. Nurses too may be recipients of prejudicial or racist acts, but they do not have to accept such behavior from clients. Rather, they should set limits, discuss the behavior with other colleagues when appropriate, and avoid personalizing the behavior.

One way to depict the effects of prejudice and racism is to use a two-dimensional matrix: overt versus covert and intentional versus unintentional. Locke and Hardaway (1992) depict four types of prejudice and racism that result from this matrix: overt intentional, covert intentional, overt unintentional, and covert unintentional (Box 8.5). Overt intentional prejudice or racism means that the behavior is both apparent and purposeful. The nurse is aware of personal biases and beliefs and integrates them into a plan of action to negatively manage client problems.

With overt unintentional the behavior is apparent but not purposeful, and no harm is intended, although harm may result. Covert intentional means that the behavior is subtle and purposeful, but the person tries to avoid being viewed as prejudicial or racist. Covert unintentional means that the person's behavior is neither apparent nor purposeful. The person is unaware of the behavior. Regardless of the type of prejudice or racism, the behavior is harmful to the client because it prevents the client from receiving or accepting necessary information to make behavioral changes. Examples of each type of prejudice and racism are presented in Box 8.5.

Ethnocentrism. Ethnocentrism is the belief that one's own cultural group is superior to all others and determines the standards by which different groups are judged. Ethnocentric nurses favor their own professional values and belief that their perspective is more important than that of the client relative to the client's illness, health-seeking behaviors, and understanding of the ways in which treatment modalities will benefit the client.

BOX 8.5 Types of Prejudice and Racist Behaviors

Overt Intentional Prejudice/Racism

Two homeless women, one African American and the other Irish, are clients at the oncology clinic at the free neighborhood health care center. Both of the women have a history of ovarian cancer and are experiencing financial difficulty from time to time due to the cost of medical care associated with the illness. Although the African American client has been homeless longer, both clients have health issues associated with diminished quality of life and functional status related to the length of the illness, the progression of the illness, and the seriousness of the illness. The nurse as case manager referred the Irish client to the social services department to inquire about available resources but did not refer the African American client. The nurse reasoned that minority clients have direct contact with some local and national government programs, know about available resources, and have experience negotiating the social system for themselves and their family. In contrast, the nurse reasoned that because the Irish woman had no prior experience negotiating government programs, she needed to advocate for her client. The nurse did not assess the health-seeking behaviors of either client before coming to these conclusions, stereotyped both women, and intentionally used her informational power to help one client while denying assistance to the other client.

Overt Unintentional Prejudice/Racism

The community health nurse was assigned to make an initial home visit to two clients recently discharged from the hospital with a diagnosis of hypertension. The nurse performed physical assessments on both clients. He developed an extensive culturally relevant teaching plan with the Filipino client that included information on sodium restriction and its effect on kidney functioning, ways to integrate cultural foods into the diet, and support in lifestyle changes. With the Puerto Rican client, the nurse performed a routine physical assessment and did not discuss the client's culturally special dietary requirements. The nurse reasoned that the Puerto Rican client was not capable of understanding such complex information and would most likely seek information from her *curandera* (a folk practitioner) to manage the hypertension. At the end of the visit, the nurse said to this client, "Take care of yourself. See you next time." This nurse did not realize that he had stereotyped the client and that his nursing interventions were minimal. He believed that he had delivered patient-centered care and the difference in his assessment and implementation approach reflected his understanding of cultural competence theory.

Covert Intentional Prejudice/Racism

An American Indian nurse works in a home-health agency that serves an ethnically diverse community. The nurse has observed that her assigned clients are always among the poorest and live in the unsafe ZIP code areas of the community. Her nonminority nurse colleagues are not assigned to clients residing in those ZIP codes. In a recent staff meeting the American Indian nurse expressed discomfort about the assignment patterns that she had observed with her nursing supervisors. Upon hearing her observations, the supervisors looked at the nurse in a surprised and skeptical manner and asked her to give a specific example. This is an example of covert racism because the nursing supervisors were aware of the informal policy that they assign minority nurses to clients residing in designated minority neighborhoods. The nursing supervisors were aware of this long-standing practice to assign minority nurses to minority clients and white nurses to white clients but would never admit to it. The supervisors thought that the best way for minority clients to be the recipients of culturally competent care was to assign a minority nurse to care for their own.

Covert Unintentional Prejudice/Racism

Ashley is the seven-year-old daughter of a lesbian middle-class couple. The school nurse is frustrated that Ashley's parents refuse to disclose the father and insist on altering the demographic form to include the two mothers as parents. Ashley frequently shows up to the nurse's office with stomach upsets, and the nurse attributes the upsets to the parents' sexual orientation. The school nurse has not conducted an in-depth assessment of the child's chief complaint. This is unusual behavior for the school nurse as she has been cited for her thorough assessments of children that have resulted in early diagnosis and treatment of disorders for this age group. This school nurse is unaware that her intolerance for the parents' sexual orientation and family's lifestyle has contributed to her decision to provide a cursory assessment for Ashley.

The nurses' refusal to own their cultural biases and to accept diverse worldviews often leads them to devalue the experiences of others, judge them to be inferior, and treat those who are different from themselves with suspicion or hostility (Andrews & Boyle, 2016).

Ethnocentrism is the reverse of cultural blindness and presents other challenges to nurses. Cultural blindness is an inability to recognize the differences between one's own cultural beliefs, values, and practices and those of the client's culture. In cultural blindness nurses employ health strategies that suggest that health care is devoid of cultural meaning and all populations interpret health care practices in the same way. Under such circumstances the tendency is to believe that the recognition of racial, ethnic, religious, or gender difference is itself prejudicial and discriminatory. Culturally competent nurses are familiar with cultural and linguistic standards, the client's health care needs, and the client's biases and that they must constantly negotiate with the client to arrive at a set of assumptions and practices that are acceptable to the client. Hence nurses who state that they treat all clients the same, regardless of culture, are demonstrating cultural blindness.

Cultural Imposition. Cultural imposition is the act of imposing culturally unacceptable and disapproving behaviors and practices on individuals and groups despite their objections. It is the belief in one's own superiority, or ethnocentrism. Nurses impose their values on clients when they forcefully promote biomedical traditions while ignoring the clients' valuing of non-Western treatments such as acupuncture, herbal therapy, or spiritualistic rituals. A goal for nurses is to develop an approach of cultural relativism, whereby they recognize that clients have different approaches to health, and that each culture should be judged based on its own merit and not on the nurse's personal beliefs.

Cultural Conflict. Cultural conflict is a perceived threat that may arise from a misunderstanding of expectations when nurses are unable to respond appropriately to another individual's cultural practice because of unfamiliarity or disagreement with the practice (Andrews & Boyle, 2016). Although cultural conflicts are unavoidable, the nursing goal is to manage conflicts so that they do not affect the delivery of culturally competent nursing care. Resolution of the conflict requires that health care providers and recipients share beliefs and practices of their culture, perceptions of diseases and their causes, and perceptions of health and illness and arrive at an acceptable approach to clients, consumers, and nurse. Being culturally competent in public health systems enables nurses to adapt their approaches to benefit individuals and groups from varying cultural backgrounds. If nurses are going to decrease conflict, they must learn the context and acknowledge that an outcome that is acceptable to both the nurse and client must be negotiated. It is important that the nurse lays the groundwork for nurse and client participation to establish equality in the discussion around areas of conflict and propose solutions that when managing conflict, all persons involved in the conflict have a way to build and "save face."

Culture Shock. Culture shock is the feeling of helplessness, discomfort, and disorientation experienced by nurses who attempt to understand or effectively adapt to a cultural group whose beliefs, values, and practices are radically different from their own. When nurses experience culture shock, it may be a normal reaction to a client's beliefs and practices that are not allowed or approved of in the nurse's own culture (Andrews & Boyle, 2016). Culture shock is brought on by anxiety that results from losing familiar signs and symbols of social interaction. As practice environments change and they leave the safety of the hospital for community settings, nurses are being confronted with ethical, moral, and behavioral dilemmas and may experience heightened discomfort and feelings of powerlessness to confront differences between themselves and clients. This is especially true when nurses have little knowledge or exposure to the culture from which the client comes. For example, nurses who are unfamiliar with "cupping" may experience culture shock when Cambodians use this practice to relieve headaches, to reduce stress and sinus tension, or to delay the onset of colds. Being aware of the clients' own cultural beliefs and having knowledge of other cultures may help nurses to be more accepting of cultural differences.

Culturally Competent Nursing Interventions. In culturally competent nursing interventions nurses integrate their professional knowledge with the client's knowledge and practices to maintain, protect, and restore culturally relevant care. Leininger and McFarland (2006) developed a nursing intervention framework to increase culturally competent care; this framework suggests three modes of action, based on compromise between the client and nurse, which guide the nurse to deliver culturally competent care: cultural preservation, cultural accommodation, and cultural repatterning. When these decisions and actions are used with cultural brokering, the nurse is able to fulfill the various roles and provide holistic care for culturally diverse clients.

Cultural Preservation. Cultural preservation means that the nurse supports and facilitates the use of scientifically supported cultural practices from a person's culture along with the biomedical health care system. The nurse helps clients of a particular culture to retain and preserve traditional values, so they can maintain, promote, and restore health. For example, acupuncture, an ancient Chinese practice of inserting needles in specific points on the skin through which life energy flows, is used to relieve pain or cure diseases by restoring balance of yin and yang (Spector, 2016). These practices are being accepted by increasing numbers of Western practitioners as a legitimate method of treatment for many health problems. It is important to know when clients are blending nontraditional health practices with those prescribed by the health care provider to make certain that they support rather than interfere with one another. The nurse should be nonjudgmental and refrain from criticizing the practice; they are providing care that is consistent with the clients' beliefs and values and helping to preserve their culture.

In another example, the nurse helps maintain cultural family values of Ms. Rodriquez, a 73-year-old Filipino woman who was discharged from hospital to home care after surgery for cancer of the large intestine. During the home visit the nurse discussed with the client and her husband about making a referral to have a home health aide assist with physical care and light housekeeping chores. The family was gracious but seemed hesitant to accept the referral. The nurse knew that in the Filipino family the older daughter is expected to be the caregiver for her mother and father. She asked the couple if they would like to discuss the situation with their daughters. Both the client and her husband seemed pleased with the idea, and the nurse promised to get back to them the next day. When the nurse returned for her visit, Ms. Rodriquez's older daughter was present and told the nurse that she would manage without additional help. The three daughters had made a schedule to take turns caring for their parents. The nurse accepted and supported the family's decision and told them that if they decided at a later time to accept the services of a home health aide, they should call the agency. The nurse then gave the family the telephone number of the agency and scheduled the next follow-up visit with them.

Cultural Accommodation. Cultural accommodation is consistent with Guideline 6, Patient Advocacy, of the Guidelines for Implementing Culturally Competent Nursing Care (American Academy of Nursing Expert Panel, 2010). Cultural accommodation means that the nurse assists, supports, facilitates, or enables clients in their use of cultural practices to achieve satisfying health care outcomes when such practices are not harmful to clients. Nurses may support and facilitate successful use of home burial of placenta alongside interventions from the biomedical health care system. For example, the delivery nurse was helpful when Ms. Sanchez asked her not to discard a piece of the amniotic sac that was present on her grandbaby's face immediately after birth. Ms. Sanchez asked the nurse to give it to her instead. The grandmother believed that being born with a piece of the amniotic sac on the face was a visible sign that something special was going to happen in the person's life. The grandmother explained that after she dried the piece of the amniotic sac, she would keep it in a safe place. She would also spend extra time protecting the baby to prevent her from being harmed. Although the delivery room nurse was not knowledgeable about this practice, she was assistive and gave the grandmother the piece of the sac as she requested. As another example using cultural accommodation, a nurse can assist older Chinese American clients to more effectively manage their hypertension by modifying their use of high-sodium soy sauce and substituting low-sodium soy sauce in their cooking. Similarly, African Americans can be guided to use more broiled and boiled foods and eat less fried foods.

In providing care to clients who practice the Islamic faith, it is important for the nurse to understand some of the key tenets of their faith. The Five Pillars of Islam define the duties that each Muslim should practice to be consistent with their faith. The second pillar, Salat, can have implications for nurses caring for these patients. Salat says that a Muslim must pray five times a day while facing Mecca, which is in an easterly direction in the United States (Koenig & Shohaib, 2014). The prayers are given in a kneeling position on a prayer mat or carpet. It is important for the agency and health care professionals to make it possible for these clients to pray at the appointed times. The Qur'an also dictates various health care choices related to contraception, birth, sanitary practices, dietary practices, and medical care concerns, to name a few.

Cultural Repatterning. Cultural repatterning means that the nurse works with clients to help them reorder, change, or modify their cultural practices when their cultural practices are harmful to them. For example, a culturally competent school nurse who works with Mexican Americans knows of the high incidence of obesity among women 20 years and older. Using this information, she developed a health education program for Mexican teenagers in the local high school. While respecting their cultural traditions, the nurse discussed weight management strategies with the teenagers. The nurse understood the teenagers' cultural issues pertaining to food and knew how to negotiate with them. She discouraged the use of fried foods (such as tortillas), sour cream, and regular cheese and encouraged and demonstrated the use of baked tortillas and salsa as dip and topping. In another example, a nurse discovered during her instructions on diabetes self-management that pregnant Haitian women were visiting an herbalist to obtain teas so they would not have to take insulin. The nurse asked for the names of the herbs in the teas that they were drinking and scheduled a conference with the pharmacist to discuss the specific ingredients in the herbs, as well as ways that they might help clients meet their cultural needs. The nurse found out that one of the herbs contributed to high blood pressure, a problem that many of the women were experiencing. She negotiated with the women not to take the tea with the specific herb. The nurse understood the importance of supernatural causes of illness in the Haitian culture and sought cooperation from the herbalist.

Culture Brokering. Culture brokering is consistent with Guideline 6, Patient Advocacy of the Guidelines for Implementing Culturally Competent Nursing Care (American Academy of Nursing expert Panel, 2010). Culture brokering means advocating, mediating, negotiating, and intervening between the client's culture and the biomedical health care culture on behalf of clients. Nurses as culture brokers act as go-betweens or advocates between groups of persons or persons of different cultural backgrounds to reduce conflict or produce change to facilitate client access to health care. As client advocates, nurse brokers are positioned to understand both cultures (the client's culture and the culture of the health care system) and resolve or lessen problems that result when individuals in either culture do not understand the other person's values. To illustrate, migrant workers tend to have high occupational mobility; many are poor and have limited formal education. They may seek health care only when they are ill and cannot work. Nurses who staff mobile health care vans often come in contact with migrant workers and usually take the opportunity to teach these individuals about prevention, health maintenance, environmental sanitation, and nutrition because it may be the only opportunity they will ever have to care for that particular migrant worker. These public health nurses also advocate for the rights of migrant workers to receive quality health care. In this instance health care nurses who provide manpower for the mobile health care van clinic may contact the migrant health services for follow-up or referral care for migrant workers who received health care from the mobile health care van.

Culturally Competent Nursing Outcomes. Nurses are uniquely positioned to make a difference in health outcomes for vulnerable populations. Nurse educators and clinicians are beginning to understand how to provide critical learning environments and workplaces for students, faculty, and practitioners to apply the concepts of cultural competence in their practice in order to improve the effectiveness of their actions. Evidenced-based cultural competence practice in nursing connecting culturally competent health care goals with the professional values of nursing and patient care outcomes and satisfaction has been the subject of recent research activity in nursing. Researchers are supporting ongoing education in cultural competence for nurses at all levels of practice. Creech et al. (2017) recommended that each undergraduate nursing course has an objective requiring that specific cultural content be integrated into teaching units and assignments with outcome measurements to help students develop cultural competence and support positive patient care outcomes

Zandee et al. (2010) described how public health nursing students used cultural competence principles to better understand the cultural background of the communities in which they were placed. By partnering with community health workers, the students were able to improve their cultural competence and provide more effective and quality care. After a service learning experience, graduate students reported feeling prepared and comfortable to care for clients who were culturally different from themselves and expressed interest in working in settings where health care professionals are underrepresented (Debonis, 2016). Debiasi and Selleck (2017) examined the effects of culturally competent training for nurse practitioners (NPs) on the delivery of culturally competent care using self-assessments, pre-training and post-training for the NPs and for client participants. NPs increased their cultural assessment documentation, were more aware of using client generalizations, and were motivated not to engage in stereotyping clients. Other outcomes indicate that increased language and communication competencies skills have led to clients' increased satisfaction and adherence to behavioral changes, as well as to higher quality of care.

Links between providing culturally effective care and improving patient health care outcomes are limited. Truong et al. (2014) conducted a systemic review of reviews and indicated moderate evidence exists that cultural competence interventions result in improvements in provider outcomes, health care access, and utilization outcomes, but less evidence exists to support the effect of cultural competence on long-term improvements in client outcomes. These reviewed studies have been mainly descriptive. Few have employed a randomized clinical trial design.

Esposito (2014) found that nurses who participated in culturally competent training state the benefits of the training cannot be sustained over time unless additional training is provided. It is important to increase dissemination of cultural competence outcomes in nursing. This can be done through public health nurses improving clinical skills in all settings where there are culturally diverse populations and attending research conferences, staff development programs, continuing education programs, and the student nursing associations conferences.

LINKING CONTENT TO PRACTICE

As has been discussed throughout the chapter, culturally competent nursing care uses many of the standards, guidelines, and competencies from key nursing and public health documents. For example, the Council on Linkages (2016) has a set of skills related to cultural competency and a set related to communication that are consistent with the information in this chapter. Likewise, the Quad Council Coalition of Public Health Nursing Organizations (2018) further develops and applies the skills of the Council on Linkages related to both cultural competency and communication to public health nursing practice. As an example, the Council on Linkages states that a necessary skill in public health is to consider "the role of cultural, social, and behavioral factors in the accessibility, availability, acceptability, and delivery of public health services." The Quad Council states that "public health nurses should consider the role of cultural, social, and behavioral factors in the accessibility, availability, acceptability, and delivery of public health nursing services." Each of the competencies in the Council on Linkages core competencies is applied directly to public health nursing practice by the Quad Council. Also, the American Academy of Nursing Expert Panel on Global Nursing and Health (2010) identifies 12 standards that serve as a resource and guide for nurses in practice, administration, education, and research by underscoring cultural competence as a priority of care for the populations that they serve.

QSEN FOCUS ON QUALITY AND SAFETY EDUCATION FOR NURSES

The six quality and safety competencies for nurses that were identified in the Quality and Safety Education for Nurses (QSEN) project are patient-centered care, teamwork and collaboration, evidence-based practice, quality improvement, safety, and informatics. While each of these is important and pertinent to the nursing actions taken with people from cultural groups other than that of the nurse, perhaps the most significant is that of patient-centered care. The chapter presents many guidelines and principles for aiding nurses in providing culturally competent care. One of the areas in which patient-centered care is lacking occurs when the nurse and the patient are not communicating effectively. The lack of communication may occur when they speak different languages, they have different cultural practices and expectations that lead them to hear messages differently, or the persons being served simply do not understand what the nurse is saying and are reluctant to acknowledge this. Nurses must observe for both verbal and nonverbal cues that a message is either understood or not understood. When the latter occurs, the nurse should clarify the message. This may include asking someone from that cultural group to assist or enlisting the aid of an interpreter. (See Issel LM, Bekemeier B, Kneipp S: A public health nursing research agenda. *Public Health Nurs* 29[4]: 330–342, 2012.)

The following applies to the QSEN competency of client-centered interventions that reflect cultural competence.

Targeted Competency: Client-Centered Intervention

Recognize the client or designee as the source of control and full partner in providing compassionate and coordinated interventions based on respect for the client's preferences, values, and needs.

Important aspects of client-centered intervention include:

- **Knowledge:** Describe strategies to empower clients or families in all aspects of the health care process.
- **Skills:** Communicate client values, preferences, and expressed needs to other members of the health care team.
- **Attitudes:** Willingly support client-centered care for individuals and groups whose values differ from your own.

Client-Centered Care Question

Competence in providing client-centered interventions involves not only effective interviewing of individual clients, but developing an awareness of their context. As a community-based clinician, it is helpful to familiarize yourself with the cultural context of your clients. Learning about community resources can sometimes be helpful in learning about the cultural context. You have just been hired as a visiting nurse in a Hispanic community. What community resources could you explore to assist you in providing effective client-centered care?

Answer

- You might explore community centers. Where are they? How well frequented are the community centers? Which programs are most popular? Which community center programs are health oriented?
- Are community members very involved with one or more churches? You might familiarize yourself with elements of this faith tradition.
- Are there community elders who are recognized as leaders in the community? Can you meet with them to understand how the community has changed and evolved over time?

Prepared by Gail Armstrong, PhD, DNP, ACNS-BC, CNE, Associate Professor, University of Colorado Denver College of Nursing.

CULTURALLY COMPETENT NURSING ASSESSMENT OF CLIENTS

A **culturally competent nursing assessment** is a systematic way to identify and document the culture care beliefs, values, meanings, and behaviors of people while considering their history, life experiences, and the social and physical environments in which they live (Leininger & McFarland, 2006). Nurses use cultural assessment data as the basis for developing culturally appropriate interventions to provide culturally competent health care to their clients. A culturally competent nursing assessment should focus on those aspects relevant to the presenting problem, such as clients' beliefs about the problem, necessary intervention, and appropriate participatory education.

Adopting a relativistic approach and using a skill set that includes understanding, eliciting, listening, explaining, acknowledging, recommending, and negotiating help nurses to use a nonjudgmental approach and focus on what matters most to the client. It is vital that nurses listen to clients' perceptions of their problem and, in turn, that nurses explain to clients their own perceptions of the problem. Nurses and clients should acknowledge and discuss similarities and differences between the two perceptions to develop recommendations and suggestions for management of issues or problems. Nurses also negotiate with clients on nursing care actions to meet the needs of clients. As part of the nursing process, nurses are expected to accurately assess a client's health needs based on information about eight primary cultural elements as discussed earlier in this chapter.

Many cultural assessment tools are available to assist nurses and nursing students in conducting cultural assessments. For example, there is the Andrews/Boyle Transcultural Nursing Assessment Guide (Andrews & Boyle, 2016), which identifies culturally appropriate areas to focus on gathering information to develop a culturally competent plan of care. The Purnell Model for Cultural Competence (2016) has several components and is flexible in its use by all health care providers and in all settings. While both of these guides are detailed and nurses may not be able to complete a thorough assessment for each client, they can select the appropriate and relevant questions that must be asked of the client.

During an initial contact with clients, nurses should perform a general cultural assessment to obtain an overview of the clients' characteristics. Nurses ask clients about their ethnic background, language, education, occupation and socioeconomic status, cultural beliefs, religious affiliation, dietary practices, family relationships, and hospital experiences. Nurses also want to know about clients' distinctive features, perceptions of the health issue, causation, treatment, anticipated results, and the impact the issue might have on the client. Such basic data help nurses understand from the client's points of view and recognize their uniqueness, thus avoiding stereotyping. The data gathered from a brief assessment will help to determine if there is need for additional information, which would be gathered during an in-depth cultural assessment.

Data for an in-depth cultural assessment should be gathered over a period of time and not be restricted to the first encounter with the client. This gives both the client and the nurse time to get to know each other, and it is especially beneficial for the client to see the nurse in a helping relationship. An in-depth assessment should be conducted in at least two phases: a data collection phase and an organization phase.

The data collection phase consists of three steps:

1. The nurse collects self-identifying data similar to those collected in the brief assessment.
2. The nurse raises a variety of questions that seek information and clarification on the clients' perception of what brings them to the health care system, health practices, the illness, and previous and anticipated treatment outcomes.
3. After the diagnosis is made, the nurse identifies cultural factors that may influence the effectiveness of nursing care actions, discusses them with the client, and negotiates a plan of interventions to ensure the best possible health outcomes for the client.

In the organization phase, data related to the client's and family's views on optimal treatment choices are routinely examined, and areas of difference between the client's cultural needs and the goals of Western medicine are identified. Nurses may use Leininger and McFarland's (2006) three actions (discussed previously in this chapter) to guide them in selecting and discussing culturally appropriate interventions with clients. The key to a successful culturally competent assessment lies in nurses being aware of their own culture and respect for the client's culture. The nurse should consider the following suggestions when eliciting cultural information. Be sensitive to the cues in the environment, and be in tune with the verbal and nonverbal communications before taking any action.

- Before beginning the assessment, know the specific areas to focus on and how to address them without offending the client.
- Know about the resources in the community such as schools, churches, hospitals, tribal councils, restaurants, taverns, and bars.
- Select a strategy for gathering the cultural data. Possible strategies include in-depth interviews, informal conversations, observations of the client's everyday activities or specific events, survey research, and a case-method approach to study certain aspects of a client.
- If the client has limited proficiency with English, select a trained interpreter.
- Identify if there is need for a confidante who will help "bridge the gap" between the client's and nurse's cultures. Be aware that in some cultures the woman's husband or a close male family friend may be the person from whom the nurse may need to obtain the cultural information.
- Interview other nurses or health care professionals who know the client, family, or community to obtain relevant information.

- Talk with formal and informal community leaders to gain a comprehensive understanding about significant aspects of community life.
- Be aware that all information has both subjective and objective aspects, and verify and cross-check the information that is collected before acting on it.
- Avoid the pitfalls that may occur when generalizations are made about a client.
- Be sincere, open, and honest with yourself and the client.

BUILDING CULTURALLY COMPETENT ORGANIZATIONS

Organizational cultural competence extends beyond competence of the individual health care provider. **Organizational cultural competence** refers to a set of congruent behaviors, attitudes, and policies that enables a system, an agency, or a group of professionals to work effectively in multicultural environments (Substance Abuse and Mental Health Services Administration, 2014). It is a term used to denote quality services specifically in meeting the needs of vulnerable populations. Organizational competence is ongoing and requires a genuine commitment to the process of evaluation and reevaluation and must be able to withstand changes in function, structure, and people. It facilitates better experiences for minority clients in relationship to nurse communication, staff responsiveness, quiet room, and pain control (Weech-Maldonado et al., 2012). Hospitals with improved cultural competence have the potential to increase positive outcomes and reduce racial/ethnic disparities for minority patients. Similarly, reduction of hospital cultural competency may adversely affect minority patients and further exacerbate the disparities between majority and minority populations.

Organizations that value cultural competence must:

1. Demonstrate values, behaviors, attitudes, policies, and structures that allow them to work effectively across cultures,
2. Value diversity, conduct self-assessment, manage the dynamics of differences, acquire and institutionalize cultural knowledge, and adapt to diversity and the cultural contexts of the communities they serve, and
3. Incorporate the above in all aspects of policy making, administration, and service delivery and systematically involve consumers and families (Substance Abuse and Mental Health Services Administration, 2014).

Researchers at the University of Kansas say that diversity is reality and that changes in one part of the world affect people everywhere (Brownlee & Lee, 2015). They cite the following steps as key to building a multicultural organization that recognizes diversity and aims to enable cultural differences to strengthen rather than weaken the organization:

- Form a cultural competence committee.
- Write a mission statement.
- Find out what similar organizations have done, and develop partnerships.
- Use free resources.
- Complete a comprehensive cultural competence assessment of your organization.
- Find out which cultural groups exist in your community and whether they access community services.
- Have a brown bag lunch to get staff involved in discussion and activities about cultural competence.
- Ask your personnel about their staff development needs.
- Assign part of your budget to staff development programing in cultural competence.
- Include a cultural competency requirement in job descriptions.
- Be sure your facility's location is accessible and respectful of difference.
- Collect resource materials on culturally diverse groups for your staff's use.
- Build a network of natural helpers, community "informants," and other "experts."

DeMeester et al. (2016) added additional steps to improve organizational cultural competence for the lesbian, gay, bisexual, and transgender (LGBT) racial and ethnic minority community. They believe that a shared decision-making model would enhance care for these individuals and proposed that institutional level interventions should focus on:

1. Establishing a work flow that includes providing private space during "check in and check out," educating and expecting all health care providers to become culturally competent, and presenting clinical results with sensitivity to identifying potential LGBT candidates for social determinants of health and treatment options;
2. Providing health information technology templates to allow for collection of data on sexual orientation and gender identity, as well as respectful and nonjudgmental language to address sexuality related issues, and engaging partners in care whenever possible;
3. Creating an organizational structure and culture that involve leadership and staff commitment to improve trust and communication, addressing quality and improving activities to reduce health and health care disparities, hiring of a diverse staff, and fostering relationships with the community;
4. Providing resources and the clinic environment to maintain a physical and welcoming environment for the community such as having forms and documents that are LGBT friendly, making referrals to organizations that are pertinent to the LGBT community, and making sure that all staff are LGBT friendly;
5. Training and education that recognize the needs of persons with limited health literacy, improving communication and trust building; and
6. Providing financial and nonfinancial incentives/disincentives such as linking financial incentives to processes that impact shared decision making, creating awards for advancing diversity and inclusion, and reducing health and health care disparities.

PRACTICE APPLICATION

Mr. Nguyen, a 64-year-old man from rural Vietnam, entered the United States with his family three years ago through the refugee program. Mr. Nguyen was a farmer in his homeland, and since his arrival he has been unable to obtain a stable job that would allow him to adequately care for his family. His financial resources are limited, and he has no insurance. He speaks enough English to interact directly with people outside his family and community. His oldest daughter, Aeyoung, is enrolled in a two-year program to become a registered nurse.

The Nguyen family attends the neighborhood church with other Vietnamese families. Mr. Nguyen has been attending the clinic at the hospital but refuses to discuss with his family, even with Aeyoung, the reason for these visits. Aeyoung became increasingly concerned as she observed her father to have insomnia, retarded motor activity, an inability to concentrate, and weight loss. However, Mr. Nguyen denied that he was not well. Aeyoung decided to discuss her concerns with a nurse, with whom she had developed an attachment, at the church. She invited the nurse to her home for lunch on a Saturday so she could meet her father and validate her impressions.

After several visits with the family, the nurse was able to establish a close enough relationship with Mr. Nguyen so that she could engage him in a discussion of his health. Because of her extensive work with other Vietnamese immigrants, the nurse was familiar with themes of loss and decided to focus her conversation with Mr. Nguyen on his adjustment to the new community living, gains and losses as a result of immigration, and coping strategies. After several discussions, Mr. Nguyen confided in the nurse that he feared that he was dying because he had been diagnosed with cancer of the small intestine. He further revealed that he had not shared the diagnosis with the family because he did not want them to know of his "bad news." Mr. Nguyen had refused treatment because he knew that people never get better when they have cancer; they always die.

A. Which of the following actions best characterize the nurse's willingness to provide culturally competent care to Mr. Nguyen and his family?
   1. Discuss with the client his understanding of his diagnosis.
   2. Discuss with the client the prognosis for a person diagnosed with cancer of the small intestine in the United States.
   3. Discuss with the client the prognosis for a person diagnosed with cancer of the small intestine in Vietnam.
   4. Discuss the medical treatment and surgical intervention for cancer of the small intestine.

B. The way in which the nurse poses questions to Mr. Nguyen is very important and determines the kind of responses the client gives to the nurse. What types of questions should the nurse pose to Mr. Nguyen to get the best responses from him?

C. Which resources should a community health agency have available to assist Mr. Nguyen with his health care concerns?

Answers can be found on the Evolve site.

KEY POINTS

- The U.S. population is culturally diverse, contributing to changes in community demographics and increased challenges for nurses to effectively communicate with their clients.
- Culture is a learned set of behaviors that are widely shared among a group of people and provides guidance for individuals in problem solving and decision-making processes. Nurses need to learn more about the culture of their clients: individuals, families, and communities and the effect culture has on the perception of health, treatment, and information to make appropriate health care decisions. Culture, race, and ethnicity are concepts often used interchangeably, but they differ. Culture is an integrated pattern of thoughts, beliefs, values, communication, action, customs, and assumptions about life that are widely held among a group of people. Race is a biological construct that includes genetic characteristics like skin color, eye color, and bone structure. Ethnicity reflects a shared history, common language, and cultural similarities within the group.
- As recommended by nursing public and private organizations, cultural competence has been identified as an essential core curricular element in undergraduate and graduate education.
- Cultural differences exist among clients and may be observed in biological variations, personal space, perception of time, environmental control, social organization, communication, nutrition, and religion.
- There are individual differences among people within a cultural group that vary with age, education, religion, and socioeconomic status.
- Cultural competence is a multifaceted concept. Nurses work to establish policies and programs to improve social and economic environments in which clients live, learn, work, and play, and the quality of relationships that would create a healthier population, society, and workforce.
- Culturally competent nurses respect individual differences and partner with clients to deliver health promotion, disease prevention, and health restoration.
- A number of professional organizations have provided standards of care to guide nurses in improving quality health care, decreasing health disparities, and achieving health equity for the clients they serve.
- Changes in immigration laws and policies have made it more difficult for people from Muslim countries to immigrate to the United States.
- When nurses do not speak or understand the client's language, interpreters should be available to assist them in communicating with clients who are linguistically challenged.
- In selecting an interpreter, nurses should consider the clients' cultural needs, as well as respecting their right to privacy.

- Members of minority groups are overrepresented on the lower tiers of the socioeconomic ladder. Poor economic achievement is also a frequent characteristic among at-risk populations such as the elderly, immigrants, homeless persons, migrant workers, and LGBT persons.
- Nurses should be able to distinguish between culture and socioeconomic class issues and not interpret behavior as having a cultural origin when in fact it is based on socioeconomic class.
- Clients who are excluded from full participation in the economic, social, and political life of the society have more complex health issues and difficulty accessing and receiving health care services.
- Social issues such as social determinants of health, socioeconomic status, limited health literacy, marginalization, health disparities, social justice, and health equity play a significant role in determining quality health outcomes for culturally diverse clients.
- The social determinants of health are the circumstances in which people are born and grow up, live, work, and age and the systems put in place to deal with illness. They are shaped by factors such as race, economics, education, the family structure, health, and access to health resources.
- Efforts to understand dietary practices should go beyond relying on the individual having membership in a specific group and should include religious requirements.
- Culturally competent nursing care is designed for a specific client, reflects the nurse's knowledge and the individual's knowledge and practices, and is implemented with care and sensitivity.
- Standards of practice, developed by the American Academy of Nursing Expert Panel in 2010, guide nurses in areas of clinical practice, research, education, and administration to deliver culturally competent nursing care. These standards have worldwide applicability.
- Nurses develop cultural competence through the critical reflective use of self-awareness, communication, relationship building, and intervention skills that promote mutual respect for difference in the use of participatory decision making.
- Culturally competent nurses are aware of differences between themselves and their clients and are motivated to select culturally appropriate interventions to care for the client holistically. Nurses must have the desire or intrinsic motivation to want to provide culturally competent nursing care and meet the needs of a diverse patient population.
- The most important aspect is a cultural encounter with the client.
- Culturally competent nurses are empowered to provide equitable nursing care that is focused on meeting the physical, physiological, social, and cultural needs of clients
- Barriers to providing culturally competent care include stereotyping, prejudice and racism, ethnocentrism, cultural imposition, cultural conflict, and culture shock.
- Culturally competent nurses may select from four action modes of interventions when providing care: cultural preservation, cultural accommodation, cultural repatterning, and culture brokering.
- Nurses perform a cultural assessment on every client with whom they interact. Cultural assessments help nurses understand clients' perspectives of health and illness and thereby guide them to develop and implement culturally competent interventions.
- Organizations, institutions, and professional associations should have policies, procedures, and practices to support a climate that values diversity in which nurses can deliver culturally competent care to the clients they serve. This should include provision for continuing education and training.

CLINICAL DECISION-MAKING ACTIVITIES

1. Select a culture that you would like to study. Go to the appropriate websites, and gather information about the cultural group. Identify the group's cultural beliefs and practices and health-seeking behaviors. Discuss this information with at least one member of that cultural group. Share what you have obtained from websites, and ask the person to evaluate the information. Compare and contrast information obtained from the two sources. Describe how you would use this information in your clinical practice.
2. Discuss how you would interview older clients who are considering giving up their independence and living in a nursing home. Prepare them for the likelihood that their health care providers are likely to be culturally diverse and may not share the same race or ethnicity. How will they engage in communication with the care provider about their health needs, family of origin, and important routine behaviors? How will they share their daily routine, dietary practices, and memories of family and friends?
3. Identify an alternative health care practitioner in the community where you have been assigned for your clinical placement. Prepare six questions, and use them as a guide to interview the alternative healer about cultural health beliefs, healing practice, and alternative biomedical explanation of illness systems.
4. Select one of the standards of practice for culturally competent care from the American Nurses Association, Expert Panel on Global Nursing and Health of the American Academy of Nursing, or the Quad Council, and determine the extent to which the public health agency in your community is compliant with the culturally competent standard that you have identified. Report your findings to a culturally competent leader in that agency.
5. On the basis of *Healthy People 2020* objectives, identify an at-risk aggregate in your community. Use the Agency for Healthcare Research and Quality website to access information for that year on the progress the community has made toward decreasing a specific health disparity. Work with the public health nurse to evaluate the effectiveness of the plan the community has developed to remedy the health disparity.

ADDITIONAL RESOURCES

EVOLVE WEBSITE

http://evolve.elsevier.com/Stanhope/community/

- Answers to Practice Application
- Case Study
- Glossary
- Review Questions

REFERENCES

Agency for Healthcare Research & Quality: *Lack of insurance and poorer health creates double jeopardy for blacks and Hispanics*, March 2014. Retrieved from http://www.ahrq.gov.

Agency for Healthcare Research & Quality: *2017 National Healthcare Quality and Disparities Report: Access and disparities in access to health care*, 2018. Retrieved from http://www.ahqr.gov.

American Academy of Nursing Expert Panel: *Standards of practice for culturally competent nursing care*, 2010. Retrieved from http://www.tcns.org.

American Association of Colleges of Nursing: *Fact sheet: enhancing diversity in the nursing workforce*, 2015. Retrieved from http://www.aacn.nursing.org.

Andrews MM, Boyle JS: *Transcultural Concepts in Nursing Care*, ed 7, Philadelphia, 2016, Lippincott Williams & Wilkins.

Artiga S, Damico A: Health coverage and care for immigrants, *Issue Brief*. July 2017, The Henry J Kaiser Foundation. Retrieved from http://www.kff.org.

Betancourt JR, Green AR, Carrillo JE, Ananeh-Firempong O: Defining cultural competence: a practical framework for addressing racial/ethnic disparities in health and health care, *Public Health Rep* 1184:293–302, 2003.

Brandon DT, Isaac LA, LaVeist TA: The legacy of Tuskegee and trust in medical care: is Tuskegee responsible for race differences in mistrust of medical care? *J Natl Med Assoc* 97:951–956, 2005.

Brownlee T, Lee K: *Building culturally competent organizations*, Lawrence, KS, 2015, Community Tool Box. University of Kansas. Retrieved from ctb.ku.edu.

Buhler-Wilkerson K: Bringing care to the people: Lilian Wald's legacy to public health nursing, *Am J Public Health* 83:1778–1786, 1993.

Campinha-Bacote J: Coming to know cultural competence: in evolutionary process, *Int J Hum Caring* 15:42–48, 2011.

Campinha-Bacote J: *The process of cultural competence in the delivery of health care services*, 2016. Retrieved from transculturalcare.net.

Carnegie ME: *The Path We Tread: Blacks in Nursing, 1854-1990*, ed 2, New York, 1991, National League for Nursing Press.

Center for American Progress Team, Nicholson MD: *The facts on immigration today: 2017 edition*, 2018. Retrieved from americanprogress.org.

Centers for Disease Control and Prevention: *Immigrant and refugee health*, 2018. Retrieved from https://www.cdc.gov.

Centers for Disease Control and Prevention: *National Action Plan to improve health literacy*, 2017. Retrieved from https://www.cdc.gov.

Centers for Disease Control and Prevention: Alcohol-attributable deaths and years of potential life lost among American Indians and Alaska Natives—United States, 2001-2005, *MMWR* 57: 938–941, 2008.

Cepla Z: *Fact sheet: U.S. refugee resettlement*, 2018, Immigration Forum. Retrieved from immigrationforum.org.

Chen HC, Jensen F, Measom G, et al.: Factors influencing the development of cultural competence in undergraduate nursing students, *J Nurs Educ* 57(1):40–43, 2018.

Council on Linkages between Academia and Public Health Practice: *Use of core competences for public health professionals for health*, 2016. Retrieved from http://www.phf.org.

Creech C, Filter M. Webbe-Alamah H, McFarland MR, Andrews M, Pryor G: An intervention to improve cultural competence in graduate nursing education, *Nurs Educ Perspect* 38(6):333–336, 2017.

Debiasi LB, Selleck CS: Cultural competence training for primary care nurse practitioners: an intervention to increase culturally competent care, *J Cult Divers* 24(2):39–45, 2017.

DeBonis R: Effects of service learning on graduate nursing students: care and advocacy for the impoverished, *J Nurs Educ* 55(1): 36–40, 2016.

DeMeester RH, Lopez FY, Moore JE, Cook SC, Chin MH: A model of organizational context and shared decision making: application to LGBT racial and ethnic minority patients, *J Gen Intern Med* 31(16):651–662, 2016.

Esposito CL: Provision of culturally competent health care: an interim status review and report, *J N Y State Nurses Assoc* 43(2):4–10, 2013.

Estrada CM: *How immigrants positively affect the business community and the U.S. economy*, 2016. Retrieved from americanprogress.org.

Giger JN: *Transcultural Nursing: Assessment and Intervention*, ed 6, St Louis, 2017, Mosby.

Hall WJ, Chapman MV, Lee KM, et al.: Implicit racial/ethnic bias among health care professionals and its influences on health care outcomes: a systematic review, *Am J Public Health* 105:e60–e75, 2015.

Issel LM, Bekemeier B, Kneipp S: A public health nursing research agenda, *Public Health Nurs* 29(4):330–342, 2012.

Jesse DE, Blue C: Mary Breckinridge meets healthy people 2010: a teaching strategy for visioning and building healthy communities, *J Midwifery Womens Health* 49(2):126–131, 2004.

Kaiser Family Foundation: *Population distribution by race/ethnicity, 2017*. Retrieved from https://www.kff.org.

Kim SS: A culturally adapted smoking cessation intervention for Korean Americans: preliminary findings, *J Transcult Nurs* 28:24–31, 2017.

Koenig HG, Shohaib SAL: *Health and well-being in Islamic societies: background, research, and applications*, 2014, Springer International Publishing Switzerland. Retrieved from https://www.springer.com.

Kosten D: *Immigrants as economic contributors: they are the new American workforce*, 2018, Immigration Forum. Retrieved from immigrationforum.org.

Leininger MM, McFarland MR: *Culture Care Diversity and Universality: A Worldwide Nursing Theory*, ed 2, Boston, 2006, Jones and Bartlett Publishers.

Locke DC, Hardaway YV: Moral perspectives in interracial settings. In Cochrane D, Manley-Casimir M, editors: *Moral Education: Practical Approaches*, New York, 1992, Praeger.

Long TB: Influence of international services learning on nursing students' self-efficacy towards cultural competence, *J Cult Divers* 23(1):28–33, 2016.

Marion L, Douglas M, Lavin MA, et al.: Implementing the new ANA Standard 8: Cultural congruent practice. 2017. Retrieved from ojin.nursingworld.org.

Meleis AI: Arabs. In Lipson JG, Dibble SL, editors: *Providing culturally appropriate care in culture and clinical care*, San Francisco, 2005, UCSF Nursing Press, pp 42–57.

Migration Policy Institute: *Profile of the unauthorized population: United States*, 2018. https://migrationpolicy.org.

Morgan LL, Reel S: Developing cultural competence in rural nursing, *Online J Rural Nurs Health Care* 3(1):28–31, 2003. Retrieved from http://rnojournal.binghamton.edu.

National Institute of Minority Health and Health Disparities: 2018. Retrieved from https://www.nimhd.nih.gov.

National Quality Forum: *A roadmap for promoting health equity and eliminating health disparities: The four I's for health equity*, 2017. Retrieved from www.qualityforum.org.

Ogbu MA: Nigerians. In Lipson JG, Dibble SL, editors: *Providing Culturally Appropriate Care in Culture and Clinical Care*, San Francisco, 2005, UCSF Nursing Press, pp. 243–259.

Orgera K, Artiga S: *Disparities in health and health care: five key questions and answers*, 2018, Kaiser Family Foundation. Retrieved from https://www.kff.org.

Orlandi MA: *Cultural Competence for Evaluators*, Washington, DC, 1992, U.S. Department of Health and Human Services.

Pew Research Center: Religion and Public Life. Demographic portrait of Muslim Americans-Pew Forum on Religion. 2017. Retrieved from www.pewforum.org.

Pew Research Center: *5 facts about blacks and religion in America*, 2018. Retrieved from http://www.pewresearch.org.

Phillips JM, Malone B: Increasing racial/ethnic diversity in nursing to reduce health disparities and achieve health equity, *Public Health Rep* 129:45–50, 2014.

Pierce S, Bolter J, Selee A: *U.S. immigration policy under Trump: deep changes and lasting impacts*, 2018, Migration Policy Institute. Retrieved from migrationpolicy.org.

Purnell LD: *Transcultural health care: a culturally competent approach*, ed 5, Philadelphia, 2016, FA Davis.

Quad Council of Public Health Nursing Organizations: *Quad Council PHN Competencies*, 2018, Quad Council Domains of Practice. Retrieved from http://www.quadcouncilphn.org.

Randall-David E: *Culturally Competent HIV Counseling and Education*, McLean, VA, 1994, Maternal and Child Health Clearinghouse.

Sadana R, Blas E: What can public health programs do to improve health equity? *Public Health Rep* 128(Suppl 3):12–20, 2013.

Smedley BD, Stith AY, Nelson AR, editors: Institute of Medicine, Committee on Understanding and Eliminating Racial and Ethnic Disparities in Health Care, Board on Health Sciences Policy. *Unequal treatment: confronting racial and ethnic disparities in health care*, Washington, DC, 2002, National Academies Press.

Spector RE: *Cultural Diversity in Health and Illness*, ed 8, Norwalk, Conn, 2016, Appleton & Lange.

Substance Abuse and Mental Health Services Administration (U.S.), Center for Substance Abuse Treatment (U.S.): *Improving Cultural Competence. Treatment Improvement Protocol (TIP) Series, No. 59*, Rockville, MD, 2014. Retrieved from https://www.ncbi.nlm.nih.gov.

Truong M, Paradies Y, Priest N: Interventions to improve cultural competency in health care organizations. A systematic review of reviews, *BMC Health Serv Res* 14:99, 2014.

United States Census Bureau: *Quick Facts*, 2017a. Retrieved from https://www.census.gov.

United States Census Bureau: *Income and poverty in the United States, 2016*, 2017b. Retrieved from https://www.census.gov.

United States Census Bureau: *Quick Facts*, 2018. Retrieved from https://www.census.gov.

United States Department of Health and Human Services, Office of Refugee Resettlement: *The Refugee Act*, 2012. Retrieved from https://www.acf.hhs.gov.

United States Department of Health and Human Services (USDHHS): *Healthy People 2020: Determinants of health*, 2018. Retrieved from https://www.healthypeople.gov.

United States Department of Health and Human Services: *Syphilis study at Tuskegee*, 2017. Retrieved from https://www.cdc.gov.

United States Department of Health and Human Services: *Healthy People 2020: Understanding and Improving Health*, Washington, DC, 2010, U.S. Government Printing Office.

Vespa J, Armstrong DM, Medina L: *Demographic turning points for the United States: population projections for 2020 to 2060*, 2018. Retrieved from https://www.census.gov.

Weech-Maldonado R, Elliott M, Pradhan R, Schiller C, Hall A, Hays RD: *Can hospital cultural competency reduce disparities in patient experiences with care*, *Med Care* 50(Suppl):S48–S55, Nov 2012.

Wierenga KL, Dekker RL, Lennie TA, Chung ML, Dracup K: African American Race is associated with poorer outcomes in heart failure patients, *West J Nurs Res* 39(4):524–538, 2017.

West EA: The cultural bridge model, *Nurs Outlook* 41:229–234, 1993.

Zandee G, Bossenbroek D, Friesen M, Blech K, Engbers R: Effectiveness of community health worker/nursing student teams as a strategy for public health nursing education, *Public Health Nurs* 27:277–284, 2010.

Zong J, Batalova J, Hallock J: Frequently requested statistics on immigrants and immigration in the United States, 2018, Migration Policy. Retrieved from https://migrationpolicy.org.

9

Public Health Policy

Marcia Stanhope, PhD, RN, FAAN

OBJECTIVES

After reading this chapter, the student should be able to do the following:

1. Discuss the structure of the U.S. government and health care roles.
2. Identify the functions of key governmental and quasi-governmental agencies that affect public health systems and nursing, both around the world and in the United States.
3. Differentiate between the primary bodies of law that affect nursing and health care.
4. Define key terms related to policy and politics.
5. State the relationships between nursing practice, health policy, and politics.
6. Develop and implement a plan to communicate with policy makers on a chosen public health issue.

CHAPTER OUTLINE

Definitions
Governmental Role in U.S. Health Care
***Healthy People 2020:* An Example of National Health Policy Guidance**
Organizations and Agencies That Influence Health
Impact of Government Health Functions and Structures on Nursing
The Law and Health Care
Laws Specific to Nursing Practice
Legal Issues Affecting Health Care Practices
The Nurse's Role in the Policy Process

KEY TERMS

advanced practice nurses, p. 209
Agency for Healthcare Research and Quality, p. 203
American Association of Colleges of Nursing, p. 213
American Nurses Association, p. 201
block grants, p. 198
boards of nursing, p. 206
categorical funding, p. 205
constitutional law, p. 206
devolution, p. 198
health policy, p. 197
judicial law, p. 206
law, p. 197
legislation, p. 206
legislative staff, p. 209
licensure, p. 208
National Institute of Nursing Research, p. 203
nurse practice act, p. 206
Occupational Safety and Health Administration, p. 201
Office of Homeland Security, p. 205
police power, p. 197
policy, p. 197
politics, p. 197
public policy, p. 197
regulations, p. 206
U.S. Department of Health and Human Services, p. 197
World Health Organization, p. 201

Nurses are an important part of the health care system and are greatly affected by governmental and legal systems. Nurses who select the community as their area of practice must be especially aware of the impact of government, law, and health policy on nursing, health, and the communities in which they practice. Insight into how government, law, and political action have changed over time is necessary to understand how the health care system has been shaped by these factors. Also, understanding how these factors have influenced the current and future roles for nurses and the public health system is critical for better health policy for the nation.

Nurses have historically viewed themselves as advocates for the health of the population. It is this heritage that has moved the discipline into the policy and political arenas. To secure a more positive health care system, nurse professionals must develop a working knowledge of government, key governmental and quasi-governmental organizations and agencies, health care law, the policy process, and the political forces that are shaping the future of health care. This knowledge and the motivation to be an agent of change in the discipline and in the community are necessary ingredients for success as a population-centered nurse.

DEFINITIONS

To understand the relationship between health policy, politics, and laws, one must first understand the definitions of the terms. **Policy** is a settled course of action, which could be a law, a regulation, or a voluntary practice to be followed by a government or institution to obtain a desired end (CDC, 2015). **Public policy** is described as all governmental activities, direct or indirect, that influence the lives of all citizens (Birkland, 2016). **Health policy**, in contrast, is a set course of action to obtain a desired health outcome for an individual, family, group, community, or society (WHO, 2018). Policies are made not only by governments, but also by such institutions as a health department or other health care agency, a family, a community, or a professional organization.

Politics plays a role in the development of such policies. Politics is found in families, professional and employing agencies, and governments. Politics determines who gets what and when and how they get it (Birkland, 2016). Politics is the art of influencing others to accept a specific course of action. Therefore political activities are used to arrive at a course of action (the policy). **Law** is a system of privileges and processes by which people solve problems based on a set of established rules; it is intended to minimize the use of force (Hill & Hill, 2018). Laws govern the relationships of individuals and organizations to other individuals and to government. Through political action, a policy may become a law, a regulation, a judicial ruling, a decision, or an order.

After a law is established, regulations further define the course of action (policy) to be taken by organizations or individuals in reaching an outcome. Government is the ultimate authority in society and is designated to enforce the policy whether it is related to health, education, economics, social welfare, or any other society issue. The following discussion explains the role of government in health policy.

GOVERNMENTAL ROLE IN U.S. HEALTH CARE

In the United States the federal and most state and local governments are composed of three branches, each of which has separate and important functions (USA.gov, 2018). The *executive branch* is composed of the president (or state governor or local mayor) along with the staff and cabinet appointed by this executive, various administrative and regulatory departments, and agencies such as the **U.S. Department of Health and Human Services** (USDHHS). The *legislative branch* (i.e., Congress at the federal level) is made up of two bodies: the Senate and the House of Representatives, whose members are elected by the citizens of particular geographic areas. There is a federal Division of Nursing and Public Health, previously known as the Division of Nursing prior to the reorganization of the Health Resources and Services Agency (HRSA) of the USDHHS. This division refines criteria for nursing education programs as funded by Congress and affirmed by the president.

The *judicial branch* is composed of a system of federal, state, and local courts guided by the opinions of the Supreme Court. Each of these branches is established by the Constitution, and each plays an important role in the development and implementation of health law and public policy.

The executive branch suggests, administers, and regulates policy. The role of the legislative branch is to identify problems and to propose, debate, pass, and modify laws to address those problems. The judicial branch interprets laws and their meaning, as in its ongoing interpretation of states' rights to define access to reproductive health services to citizens of the states.

One of the first constitutional challenges to a federal law passed by Congress was in the area of health and welfare in 1937, after the 74th Congress had established unemployment compensation and old-age benefits for U.S. citizens (U.S. Law, 1937a). Although Congress had created other health programs previously, its legal basis for doing so had never been challenged. In *Stewart Machine Co. v. Davis* (U.S. Law, 1937b), the Supreme Court (judicial branch) reviewed this legislation and determined, through interpretation of the Constitution, that such federal governmental action was within the powers of Congress to promote the general welfare. It was obvious in 2008 and beyond that unemployment benefits are important to the economy and to individuals who lose jobs during a national economic crisis (Chikhale, 2017; Rothstein & Valletta, 2017).

Most legal bases for the actions of Congress in health care are found in Article I, Section 8, of the U.S. Constitution, including the following:

1. Provide for the general welfare
2. Regulate commerce among the states
3. Raise funds to support the military
4. Provide spending power

Through a continuing number and variety of cases and controversies, these Section 8 provisions have been interpreted by the courts to appropriately include a wide variety of federal powers and activities. State power concerning health care is called **police power** (Hill & Hill, 2018). This power allows states to act to protect the health, safety, and welfare of their citizens. Such police power must be used fairly, and the state must show that it has a compelling interest in taking actions, especially actions that might infringe on individual rights. Examples of a state using its police powers include requiring immunization of children before being admitted to school and requiring case finding, reporting, treating, and follow-up care of persons with tuberculosis. These activities protect the health, safety, and welfare of state citizens.

Trends and Shifts in Governmental Roles

The government's role in health care at both the state and federal level began gradually. Wars, economic instability, and political differences between parties all shaped the government's role. The first major federal governmental action relating to health was the creation in 1798 of the Public Health Service (PHS). Then in 1890 federal laws were passed to promote the public health of merchant seamen and American Indians. In 1934 Senator Wagner of New York initiated the first national health insurance bill. The Social Security Act of 1935 was passed to provide assistance to older adults and the unemployed, and it offered survivors' insurance for widows and children. It also provided for child welfare, health department grants, and maternal and child health projects. In 1948 Congress created the National Institutes of Health (NIH), and in 1965 it passed very important health legislation creating Medicare and Medicaid to provide health care service payments for older adults, the disabled, and the categorically poor. These legislative acts by Congress created programs that were implemented by the executive branch. In March 2010 legislation was passed and signed by President Obama to improve the health of the nation and access to care; this was the health reform law, the Patient Protection and Affordable Care Act (US LAW, PL 111-148, 2010). Changes were made to the implementing of this law by the president and Congress in 2017 (Kaiser Family Foundation, 2017).

The USDHHS (known first as the Department of Health, Education, and Welfare [DHEW]) was created in 1953. The Health Care Financing Administration (HCFA) was created in 1977 as the key agency within the USDHHS to provide direction for Medicare and Medicaid. In 2002 HCFA was renamed the Centers for Medicare and Medicaid Services (CMS). During the 1980s a major effort of the Reagan administration was to shift federal government activities to the states, including federal programs for health care. The process of shifting the responsibility for planning, delivering, and financing programs from the federal level to the states is called **devolution**. Throughout the 1980s and 1990s Congress increasingly funded health programs by giving **block grants** to the states. Devolution processes, including block granting, should alert professional nurses that state and local policy has grown in importance to the health care arena. With the health reform law of 2010, stimulus grants were provided to state and local areas to improve health care access (Congressional Research Service, 2017).

The role of government in health care is shaped both by the needs and demands of its citizens and by the citizens' beliefs and values about personal responsibility and self-sufficiency. These beliefs and values often clash with society's sense of responsibility and need for equality for all citizens. A federal example of this ideological debate occurred in the 1990s over health care reform. The Democratic agenda called for a health care system that was universally accessible, with a focus on primary care and prevention. The Republican agenda supported more modest changes within the medical model of the delivery system. This agenda also supported reducing the federal government's role in health care delivery through cuts in Medicare and Medicaid benefits. The Democrats proposed the Health Security Act of 1993, which failed to gain Congress's approval. In an effort to make some incremental health care changes, both the Democrats and the Republicans in Congress passed two new laws. The Health Insurance Portability and Accountability Act (HIPAA) allows working persons to keep their employee group health insurance for up to 16 months after they leave a job (U.S. Law 107-105, 1996). The State Child Health Improvement (SCHIP) Act of 1997 provides insurance for children and families who cannot otherwise afford health insurance (U.S. Law, Title Ten SSA, BBA,1997). The program was later called simply the state Child Health Insurance Program.

With the latest health care reform, numerous debates occurred in the House of Representatives and the Senate until there was agreement that the Senate version of the bill would be passed. On March 30, 2010, President Obama signed into law the Health Care and Education Reconciliation Act of 2010, which made some changes to the comprehensive health reform law and included House amendments to the new law (Kaiser Family Foundation, 2017). In 2017 the current Congress and president made many changes to the ACA of 2010. These changes can be found at https://www.kff.org.

This discussion has focused primarily on trends in and shifts between different levels of government. An additional aspect of governmental action is the relationship between government and individuals. Freedom of individuals must be balanced with governmental powers. After the terrorist attacks on the United States in September (World Trade Center attack) and October (anthrax outbreak) of 2001, much government activity was being conducted in the name of national security.

It is interesting to note that before September 11, 2001, the Congress and president, recognizing that the public health system infrastructure needed help, passed The Public Health Threats and Emergencies Act (PL 106-505) in 2000 (U.S. Law, 2000). This law "addresses emerging threats to the public's health and authorizes the Secretary of HHS to take appropriate response actions during a public health emergency, including investigations, treatment, and prevention" (Katz et al., 2014, p. 133). This legislation is said to have signaled the beginning of renewed interest in public health as the protector for entire communities. In June 2002 the Public Health Security and Bioterrorism Preparedness and Response Act was signed into law (U.S. Law, 2002, PL 107-188), with $3 billion appropriated by Congress, to implement the following anti-bioterrorism activities:

- Improving public health capacity
- Upgrading of health professionals' ability to recognize and treat diseases caused by bioterrorism
- Speeding the development of new vaccines and other countermeasures
- Improving water and food supply protection
- Tracking and regulating the use of dangerous pathogens within the United States (Katz et al., 2014)

Yet there is considerable debate on just how much governmental intervention is necessary and effective and how much will be tolerated by citizens. For example, in 2010 about 49 percent of citizens were against the new health care reform acts, and the Republicans were seen as being obstructionists. In 2016, 52 percent of citizens were for government intervention in ensuring all Americans have health care coverage and 45 percent against (Gallup Inc, 2016).

Government Health Care Functions

Federal, state, and local governments carry out five health care functions, which fall into the general categories of direct services, financing, information, policy setting, and public protection.

Direct Services. Federal, state, and local governments provide direct health services to certain individuals and groups. For example, the federal government provides health care to members and dependents of the military, certain veterans, and federal prisoners. State and local governments employ nurses to deliver a variety of services to individuals and families, frequently on the basis of factors such as financial need or the need for a particular service, such as hypertension or tuberculosis screening, immunizations for children and older adults, and primary care for inmates in local jails or state prisons. The Evidence-Based Practice box presents a study that examined the use of a state health insurance program.

EVIDENCE-BASED PRACTICE

The purpose of this study was to determine the effects of a public health policy on meeting the primary and preventive care needs of children. A survey was used to collect data from both insured and uninsured children.

"Parents of 4142 recent enrollees and 5518 established enrollees in the CHIP program responded to the survey (response rates were 46 percent for recent enrollees and 51 percent for established enrollees)." Comparing uninsured children to CHIP enrolled children, the results of the survey indicated CHIP enrollees were more likely to have a well-child visit, receive a range of preventive care services, and have patient-centered care experiences. They were also more likely than uninsured children to have a regular source of care or provider and shorter wait times for appointments. CHIP enrollees received preventive care services at similar rates to privately insured children and were more likely to receive effective care coordination services. "However, CHIP enrollees were less likely than privately insured children to have a regular source of care or provider and nighttime and weekend access to a usual source of care." In addition to this study other outcomes are indicating that CHIP enrollees are benefiting by improved school attendance and graduations.

Nurse Use

This study supports the value of health policy and the need to evaluate the effectiveness of policy in accomplishing the purposes of the policy. The study can be used by nurses to encourage parents to enroll their children in this program and to encourage legislators to continue to support the funding of the program.

CHIP, Children's Health Insurance Program.
From Smith KV, Dye C: How well is CHIP addressing primary and preventive care needs and access for children? *Acad Pediatr* 15(3): S64–S70, 2015.

Financing. In 2016 the largest shares of total health spending were sponsored by the federal government (28.3 percent) and the households (28.1 percent). The private business share of health spending accounted for 19.9 percent of total health care spending, state and local governments accounted for 16.9 percent, while other private revenues accounted for 6.7 percent. These data are very similar from year to year with the governments at all levels and individuals sharing most of the cost burden (https://www.cms.gov).

The government also pays for training some health personnel and for biomedical and health care research (NIH, 2018). Support in these areas has greatly affected both consumers and health care providers. Federal governments finance the direct care of clients through the Medicare, Medicaid, Social Security, and SCHIP programs. State governments contribute to the costs of Medicaid and SCHIP programs. Many nurses have been educated with government funds through grants and loans, and schools of nursing in the past have been built and equipped using federal funds. Governments also have financially supported other health care providers, such as physicians, most significantly through the program of Graduate Medical Education funds.

The federal government invests in research and new program demonstration projects, with NIH receiving a large portion of the monies. The National Institute of Nursing Research (NINR) is a part of the NIH and, as such, provides a substantial sum of money to the discipline of nursing for the purpose of developing the knowledge base of nursing and promoting nursing services in health care (NINR, 2018a).

Information. All branches and levels of government collect, analyze, and disseminate data about health care and health status of the citizens. An example is the annual report *Health: United States,* compiled each year by the USDHHS (NCHS, 2017). Collecting vital statistics, including mortality and morbidity data, gathering of census data, and conducting health care status surveys are all government activities. Table 9.1

TABLE 9.1 International and National Sources of Data on the Health Status of the U.S. Population

Organization	Data Sources
International	
United Nations	http://www.un.org
	Demographic Yearbook
	Population and Vital Statistics Report
World Health Organization	http://www.who.int
	World Health Statistics Annual
Federal	
Department of Health and Human Services	http://www.hhs.gov
	Health, United States
	Healthy People
	National Health Statistics Reports
	National Vital Statistics System
	National Survey of Family Growth
	National Health Interview Survey
	National Health and Nutrition Examination Survey
	National Hospital Care Survey
	National Nursing Home Survey
	National Ambulatory Medical Care Survey
	National Morbidity Reporting System
	National Immunization Survey
	National Mental Health Services Survey
	Estimates of National Health Expenditures
	AIDS Surveillance
	Nurse Supply Estimates
Department of Commerce	http://www.commerce.gov
	U.S. Census of Population
	Current Population Survey
	Population Estimates and Projections
Department of Labor	http://www.dol.gov
	Consumer Price Index
	Employment and Earnings

lists examples of available federal and international data sources on the health status of populations in the United States and around the world. These sources are available on the Internet and in the governmental documents' section of most large libraries. This information is especially important because it can help nurses understand the major health problems in the United States and those in their own states and local communities.

Policy Setting. Policy setting is a chief governmental function. Governments at all levels and within all branches make policy decisions about health care. These health policy decisions have broad implications for financial expenses, resource use, delivery system change, and innovation in the health care field. One law that has played a very important role in the development of public health policy, public health nursing, and social welfare policy in the United States is the Sheppard-Towner Act of 1921 (U.S. Law, 1921).

The Sheppard-Towner Act made nurses available to provide health services for women and children, including well-child and child-development services; provided adequate hospital services and facilities for women and children; and provided grants-in-aid for establishing maternal and child welfare programs. The act helped set precedents and patterns for the growth of modern-day public health policy. It defined the role of the federal government in creating standards to be followed by states in conducting categorical programs such as the Women, Infants, and Children (WIC) and Early Periodic and Screening, Diagnostic and Treatment (EPSDT) programs. The act also defined the position of the consumer in influencing, formulating, and shaping public policy; the government's role in research; a system for collecting national health statistics; and the integrating of health and social services. This act established the importance of prenatal care, anticipatory guidance, client education, and nurse-client conferences, all of which are viewed today as essential nursing responsibilities.

Public Protection. The U.S. Constitution gives the federal government the authority to provide for the protection of the public's health. This function is carried out in numerous venues, such as by regulating air and water quality and protecting the borders from the influx of diseases by controlling food, drugs, and animal transportation, to name a few. The Supreme Court interprets and makes decisions related to public health, such as affirming a woman's rights to reproductive privacy (*Roe v. Wade*), requiring vaccinations, and setting conditions for states to receive public funds for highway construction/repair by requiring a minimum drinking age.

HEALTHY PEOPLE 2020: AN EXAMPLE OF NATIONAL HEALTH POLICY GUIDANCE

In 1979 the surgeon general issued a report that began a 30-year focus on promoting health and preventing disease for all Americans (DHEW, 1979). In 1989 *Healthy People 2000* became a national effort with many stakeholders representing the perspectives of government, state, and local agencies; advocacy groups; academia; and health organizations (USDHHS, 1991).

Throughout the 1990s states used *Healthy People 2000* objectives to identify emerging public health issues. The success of this national program was accomplished and measured through state and local efforts. The *Healthy People 2010* document focused on a vision of healthy people living in healthy communities (USDHHS, 2000). *Healthy People 2020* had four overarching goals, which can be found in the Healthy People 2020 box; this box compares the goals of *Healthy People* documents from 2000 to 2030.

HEALTHY PEOPLE 2020

***A Comparison of the Goals of* Healthy People 2000, Healthy People 2010, Healthy People 2020, *and* Healthy People 2030**

Healthy People 2000	Healthy People 2010	Healthy People 2020	Healthy People 2030—Preliminary Objectives
Increase the years of healthy life for Americans	Increase quality and years of healthy life	Attain high quality, longer lives free of preventable disease, disability, injury, and premature death	Attain healthy, thriving lives and well-being, free of preventable disease, disability, injury, and premature death.
Reduce health disparities among Americans	Eliminate health disparities	Achieve health equity, eliminating disparities, and improving the health of all groups	Eliminate health disparities, achieve health equity, and attain health literacy to improve the health and well-being of all.
Achieve access to preventive services for all Americans		Creating social and physical environments that promote good health for all	Create social, physical, and economic environments that promote attaining full potential for health and well-being for all.
		Promote quality of life, healthy development, and healthy behaviors across all life stages	Promote healthy development, healthy behaviors, and well-being across all life stages.
			Engage leadership, key constituents, and the public across multiple sectors to take action and design policies that improve the health and well-being of all.

From U.S. Department of Health and Human Services: *Healthy People 2000, 2010, 2020, 2030,* Washington, DC, 1991, 2000, 2010, 2020, U.S. Government Printing Office.

ORGANIZATIONS AND AGENCIES THAT INFLUENCE HEALTH

International Organizations

In June 1945, following World War II, many national governments joined together to create the United Nations (UN). By charter the aims and goals of the UN deal with human rights, world peace, international security, and the promotion of economic and social advancement of all the world's peoples. The UN, headquartered in New York City, is made up of six principal divisions, several subgroups, and many specialized agencies and autonomous organizations. With the approval and support of the UN Commission on the Status of Women, world conferences on women were held. At these conferences the health of women and children and their rights to personal, educational, and economic security as well as initiatives to achieve these goals at the country level were debated and explored, and policies were formulated (United Nations, 1975, 1980, 1985, 1995). Over a period of five years reviews were conducted of the outcomes of the four conferences. The work of the UN and the world conferences continues with agendas to include the development of human beings, eradication of poverty, protection of human rights, investment in health, education, training, trade, economic growth, reduction of disaster risk, and a continued emphasis on women (United Nations, 2000.).

One of the special autonomous organizations growing out of the UN is the World Health Organization (WHO). Established in 1946, WHO relates to the UN through the Economic and Social Council to achieve its goal to attain the highest possible level of health for all persons. "Health for All" is the creed of the WHO. Headquartered in Geneva, Switzerland, the WHO has six regional offices. The office for the Americas is located in Washington, DC, and is known as the Pan American Health Organization (PAHO).

The WHO provides services worldwide to promote health, it cooperates with member countries in promoting their health efforts, and it coordinates the collaborating efforts between countries and the disseminating of biomedical research. Its services, which benefit all countries, include a day-to-day information service on the occurrence of internationally important diseases; the publishing of the international list of causes of disease, injury, and death; monitoring of adverse reactions to drugs; and establishing of world standards for antibiotics and vaccines. Assistance available to individual countries includes support for national programs to fight disease, to train health workers, and to strengthen the delivery of health services. The World Health Assembly (WHA) is the WHO's policy-making body, and it meets annually. The WHA's health policy work provides policy options for many countries of the world in their development of in-country initiatives and priorities; however, although WHA policy statements are important everywhere, they are guides and not law. The WHA's most recent policy statement on nursing and midwifery was released in 2013 (WHO, 2013a), followed by two global meetings in 2015 (WHA, 2011; WHO, 2016). The current worldwide shortage of professional nurses is now on the WHO agenda and is being addressed by many countries (WHA, 2011; WHO, 2010; WHO, 2013a). The WHO recently released a publication on the history of nursing and midwifery (WHO, 2017), and a document discussing global and strategic directions for strengthening nursing and midwifery (WHO, 2016; WHO, 2017).

The *World Health Report,* first published in 1995, is WHO's leading publication. Each year the report combines an expert assessment of global health, including statistics relating to all countries, with a focus on a specific subject. The main purpose of the report is to provide countries, donor agencies, international organizations, and others with the information they need to help them make policy and funding decisions. In the 2010 report the WHO mapped out what countries can do to modify their financing systems so they can move more quickly toward this goal—universal coverage—and sustain the gains that have been achieved. The report builds on research and lessons learned from country experience. It provides an action agenda for countries at all stages of development and proposes ways that the international community can better support efforts in low-income countries to achieve universal coverage and improve health outcomes (WHO, 2010). The 2013 report builds on the previous research with a focus on the importance of research in advancing progress toward universal health coverage (WHO, 2013b)

The presence of nursing in international health is increasing. Besides offering direct health services in every country in the world, nurses serve as consultants, educators, and program planners and evaluators. Nurses focus their work on a variety of public health issues, including the health care workforce and education, environment, sanitation, infectious diseases, wellness promotion, maternal and child health, and primary care. Dr. Naeema Al-Gasseer of Bahrain has served as the scientist for nursing and midwifery at the WHO; Marla Salmon, former dean of nursing at the University of Washington, chaired a Global Advisory Group on Nursing and Midwifery; and Linda Tarr Whelan served as the U.S. Ambassador to the UN Commission on the Status of Women. Virginia Trotter Betts, past president of the American Nurses Association (ANA), served as a U.S. delegate to both the WHA and the Fourth World Conference on Women in Beijing in 1995, where she participated on the negotiating team of the conference to develop a platform on the health of women across the life span. Many U.S. nurse leaders, such as Dr. Carolyn Williams, current author in this book, have been WHO consultants.

Federal Health Agencies

Laws passed by Congress may be assigned to any administrative agency within the executive branch of government for implementing, supervising, regulating, and enforcing. Congress decides which agency will monitor specific laws. For example, most health care legislation is delegated to the USDHHS. However, legislation concerning the environment would most likely be implemented and monitored by the Environmental Protection Agency (EPA) and that concerning occupational health by the Occupational Safety and Health Administration (OSHA) in the U.S. Department of Labor.

U.S. Department of Health and Human Services. The USDHHS is the agency most heavily involved with the health and welfare of U.S. citizens. It touches more lives than any other federal agency. The following agencies have been selected for their relevance to this chapter.

Health Resources and Services Administration. The Health Resources and Services Administration (HRSA) has been a longstanding contributor to the improved health status of Americans through the programs of services and health professions education that it funds. The HRSA contains the Bureau of Health Workforce (BHW), which includes the Division of Nursing as well as the Divisions of Medicine and Dentistry, and Allied Health Professions. The Division of Nursing and Public Health is where the key federal focus for nursing education and practice is located. National leadership is provided to ensure an adequate supply and distribution of qualified nursing personnel to meet the health needs of the nation.

At the 122nd meeting of the Division of Nursing's National Advisory Council on Nursing Education and Practice (NACNEP), the participants discussed the role of public health nurses in participating in primary care in their communities. The speaker indicated several factors that need to be in place to support the public health nurse role:

- Baccalaureate standard for entry into practice
- Ongoing stable funding for health departments
- Competitive salaries commensurate with responsibilities
- Interventions grounded in and responsive to community needs
- Consideration of health determinants
- Experience in health promotion and prevention
- Long-term trusting relationships in the community (i.e., with clients)
- Established network of community partners
- Commitment to social justice and eliminating health disparities

In the council's 12th report to Congress (USDHHS, 2013) the council recommended further investment by the government in public health nursing, arguing the need based on system changes and the Affordable Care Act implementation, greater need to connect public health and care delivery with front-line public health nurses, plus the economic benefits of supporting this investment. Through the input of the NACNEP, the Division of Nursing sets policy for nursing nationally. The 13th report focused on incorporating interprofessional education and practice into nursing (USDHHS, 2015), and the 14th report provides recommendations for preparing nurses for new roles in population health management (USDHHS, 2016a).

Centers for disease control and prevention. The Centers for Disease Control and Prevention (CDC) serves as the national focus for developing and applying disease prevention and control, environmental health, and health promotion and education activities designed to improve the health of the people of the United States. The mission of the CDC is to protect America from health, safety, and security threats, both foreign and in the United States. Whether diseases start at home or abroad, are chronic or acute, curable or preventable, human error or deliberate attack, CDC fights disease and supports communities and citizens to do the same. As such CDC works to increase the health security of our nation (CDC, 2014a). The CDC seeks to accomplish its mission by working with partners throughout the nation and the world in the following ways:

- To provide health security
- To detect and investigate health threats
- To tackle the biggest health problems causing death and disability
- To conduct research that will enhance prevention
- To promote healthy and safe behaviors, communities, and environments
- To develop leaders and train the public health workforce, including disease detectives
- To develop and advocate sound public health policies
- To implement prevention strategies
- To promote healthy behaviors
- To foster safe and healthful environments
- To provide leadership and training

The PHS, since 1798, and the CDC, since 1941, have worked to protect the public from harm. While the Zika virus is an example of how this is done, there have been numerous examples throughout U.S. history of dangerous epidemics and the responses to these epidemics to keep the public healthy. Beginning in 1633 and through 2017 the most dangerous epidemics in the United States, in chronological order, were smallpox, yellow fever, cholera, scarlet fever, typhoid fever, influenza, diphtheria, polio, measles, water contamination, pertussis, and human immunodeficiency virus (HIV)/acquired immunodeficiency syndrome (AIDS) (CDC, 2018a).

The Zika virus outbreak of 2016 is but one example of how the CDC fulfills its mission. Zika virus disease is an arboviral disease usually causing mild illness; however, congenital infection is associated with microcephaly and other birth defects. Although most cases in residents of U.S. states were travel associated, local transmission was reported.

In 2016 a total of 5168 confirmed or probable cases of noncongenital Zika virus disease with symptom onset during January 1–December 31, 2016, were reported to ArboNET (see chapter 22) from U.S. states and the District of Columbia. Most (95 percent) cases were travel associated. Locally acquired disease accounted for four percent of cases, with transmission occurring in Florida (218) and Texas (6). Forty-seven cases (one percent) were acquired through other routes, including sexual transmission (45), laboratory transmission (1), and person-to-person through an unknown route (1).

Because of the recognized numbers of cases, states were asked to report aggregate numbers of cases twice a week along with Zika-related hospitalizations and complications. The CDC implemented an investigation to track the cases and worked with state and local health departments to perform the following:

- Detect the possible outbreak
- Define and find cases
- Generate hypotheses about the likely source
- Test the hypothesis
- Find the point of contamination
- Control the outbreak from further spread
- Decide when the outbreak is over

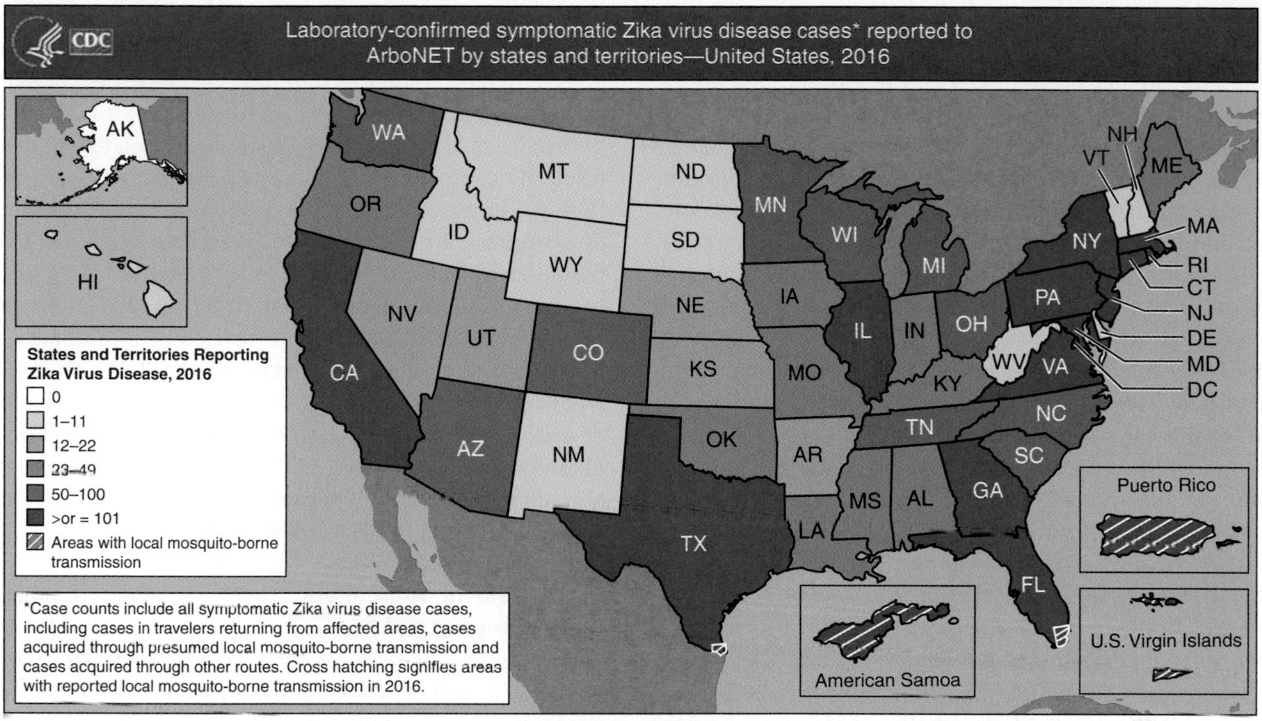

Fig. 9.1 Number of confirmed and probable Zika virus disease cases, by state of residence—50 U.S. states and the District of Columbia, January 1–December 31, 2016.

By 2017 the numbers of cases related to the Zika virus were decreasing. Although the risk for travel-associated Zika virus disease appears to be decreasing, it is important that persons traveling to areas with a risk for Zika virus transmission continue to take precautions, including using strategies to prevent mosquito bites and sexual transmission.

Fig. 9.1 presents a CDC map indicating cases per state (CDC, 2018a). All states were involved. By August 2017 the CDC determined the outbreak to be over.

National institutes of health. Founded in 1887, NIH today is one of the world's foremost biomedical research centers and the federal focus point for biomedical research in the United States. The NIH is composed of 27 separate institutes and centers. The goal of NIH research is to acquire new knowledge to help prevent, detect, diagnose, and treat disease and disability, from the rarest genetic disorder to the common cold. The NIH mission is to uncover new knowledge that will lead to better health for everyone. The NIH works toward that mission by conducting research in its own laboratories; supporting the research of nonfederal scientists in universities, medical schools, hospitals, and research institutions throughout the country and abroad; helping in the training of research investigators; and fostering communication of medical and health sciences' information (NIH, 2017).

In late 1985 Congress overrode a presidential veto, allowing the creation of the National Center for Nursing Research within the NIH. In 1993 the center became one of the divisions of the NIH and was renamed the National Institute of Nursing Research (NINR). The research and research-related training activities previously supported by the Division of Nursing were transferred to the new Institute. The NINR is the focal point of the nation's nursing research activities. It promotes the growth and quality of research in nursing and client care, provides important leadership, expands the pool of experienced nurse researchers, and serves as a point of interaction with other bases of health care research. The mission of NINR is to promote and improve the health of individuals, families, communities, and populations.

NINR supports and conducts clinical and basic research and research training on health and illness across the life span. The research focus encompasses health promotion and disease prevention, quality of life, health disparities, and end of life. NINR seeks to extend nursing science by integrating the biological and behavioral sciences, using new technologies to research questions, improving research methods, and developing the scientists of the future (NINR, 2018b).

Agency for healthcare research and quality. The Agency for Healthcare Research and Quality (AHRQ) is the lead federal agency charged with improving the quality, safety, efficiency, and effectiveness of health care for all Americans. As one of 12 agencies within the USDHHS, AHRQ supports health services research that will improve the quality of health care and promote evidence-based decision making. AHRQ is committed to improving care safety and quality by developing successful partnerships and generating the knowledge and tools required for long-term improvement. The goal of AHRQ research is to promote measurable improvements in health care in America. The outcomes are gauged in terms of improved quality of life and client outcomes, lives saved, and value gained for what we spend (AHRQ, 2018).

By examining what works and what does not work in health care, the AHRQ fulfills its missions of translating research findings into better client care and providing consumers, policy makers, and other health care leaders with information needed to make critical health care decisions. In 1999, Congress, through legislation, specifically directed AHRQ to focus on measuring and improving health care quality; promoting client safety and reducing medical errors; advancing the use of information technology for coordinating client care and conducting quality and outcomes research; and seeking to eliminate disparities in health care delivery for the priority populations of low-income groups, minorities, women, children, older adults, and individuals with special health care needs.

The AHRQ published protocols for care of clients with a variety of health problems. These protocols became the standards of health care delivery. The agency maintained a clinical practice guidelines clearinghouse for use by clinicians and others. However, after July 2018 the clearinghouse was closed due to lack of funding. Today there is a program titled the Practice-Based Research Network that rapidly develops and assesses methods and tools to ensure that new scientific evidence is incorporated into real-world practice settings (AHRQ, n.d.).

Centers for medicare and medicaid services. One of the most powerful agencies within the USDHHS is the CMS, which administers Medicare and Medicaid accounts and guides payment policy and delivery rules for services for millions of Americans (CMS, 2018). In addition to providing health insurance, CMS also performs a number of quality-focused health care or health-related activities, including regulating of laboratory testing, developing coverage policies, and improving quality of care. CMS maintains oversight of the surveying and certifying of nursing homes and continuing care providers (including home health agencies, intermediate care facilities for the developmentally disabled, and hospitals). It makes available to beneficiaries, providers, researchers, and state surveyors information about these activities and nursing home quality.

Federal Non-Health Agencies

Although the USDHHS has primary responsibility for federal health functions, several other departments of the executive branch carry out important health functions for the nation. Among these are the defense, labor, agriculture, and justice departments.

Department of Defense. The Department of Defense delivers health care to members of the military, to their dependents and survivors, to National Guard and reserve members, and to retired members and their families. The assistant secretary of defense for health affairs administers a variety of health care plans for service personnel: TriCare Prime (a managed care arrangement) and an option for fee-for-service plans called TriCare Standard, as well as TriCare Extra with many other options available. In each branch of the uniformed services, nurses of high military rank are part of the administration of these health services (U.S. Department of Defense, 2018).

Department of Labor. The Department of Labor houses OSHA, which imposes workplace requirements on industries. These requirements shape the functions of nurses and the types of health services provided to workers in the workplace. A record-keeping system required by OSHA greatly affects health records in the workplace. Each state has an agency similar to OSHA that also monitors and inspects industries, as well as the health services delivered to them by nurses.

Needlestick injuries and other sharps-related injuries that result in occupational bloodborne pathogen exposure continue to be an important public health concern, especially to health care workers. In response to this serious situation, Congress passed the Needlestick Safety and Prevention Act, which became law on November 6, 2000 (U.S. Law, 2000). To meet the requirements of this act, OSHA revised its Bloodborne Pathogen Standard to become effective on April 18, 2002. This act clarified the responsibility of employers to select safer needle devices as they become available and to involve employees in identifying and choosing the devices. The updated standard also required employers to maintain a log of injuries from contaminated sharps (OSHA, 2008, 2011).

Department of Agriculture. The Department of Agriculture houses the Food and Nutrition Service, which oversees a variety of food assistance activities. This service collaborates with state and local government welfare agencies to provide food stamps to needy persons to increase their food purchasing power. Other programs include school breakfast and lunch programs, WIC, and grants to states for nutrition education and training. WIC has provided support for up to 53% of all infants born in the United States (USDA, 2015). In 2017, 7.3 million women, infants, and children received WIC benefits, with the majority of that being infants and children (USDA, 2018). Although these programs have been successful, the increasing use of the process of giving federal block grants to states (rather than implementing national programs) may threaten the effectiveness of these programs because of differences in how decisions are made at the state level on how to spend money on nutrition (USDA, 2018).

Department of Justice. Health services to federal prisoners are administered within the Department of Justice. The Federal Bureau of Prisons is responsible for the custody and care of about 185,000 federal offenders (Bureau of Federal Prisons, 2018). The Medical and Services Division of the Bureau of Prisons includes medical, psychiatric, dental, and health support services with community standards in a correctional environment. Health promotion is emphasized through counseling during examinations, education about effects of medications, infectious disease prevention and education, and chronic care clinics for conditions such as cardiovascular disease, diabetes, and hypertension. The bureau also provides forensic services to the courts, including a range of evaluative mental health studies outlined in federal statutes. Health care for prisoners is highly regulated because of a series of court decisions on inmates' rights.

State and Local Health Departments

Depending on funding, public commitment and interest, and access to other resources, programs offered by state and local health departments vary greatly. Many state and local health officials report that employees in public health agencies lack skills in the core sciences of public health and that this has hindered their effectiveness. The lack of specialized education and skill is a significant barrier to population-based preventive care and the delivery of quality health care to the public. Public health workforce specialists report that the number of retirees expected in this decade will result in a major shortage of public health workers, including nurses. More often than at other levels of government, nurses at the local level provide direct services. Some nurses deliver special or selected services, such as follow-up of contacts in cases of tuberculosis or venereal disease or providing child immunization clinics. Other nurses have a more generalized practice, delivering services to families in certain geographic areas (APHA, 2013; Beck & Boulton, 2016; University of Michigan Center of Excellence in Public Health Workforce Studies, 2013).

At the local and state levels, coordinating health efforts between health departments and other county or city departments is essential. Gaps in community coordination are showing up in glaring ways as states and communities scramble to address bioterrorism preparedness since September 11, 2001, and since such natural disasters as Hurricane Katrina. The United States had 220,000 people lose their homes in 2013 due to extreme storms and tornadoes in Oklahoma and another 100,000 from flooding in Colorado. Health departments are on the front line in such occurrences (see Chapter 46).

IMPACT OF GOVERNMENT HEALTH FUNCTIONS AND STRUCTURES ON NURSING

The variety and range of functions of governmental agencies have had a major impact on the practice of nursing. Funding, in particular, has shaped roles and tasks of population-centered nurses. The designation of money for specific needs, or **categorical funding**, has led to special and more narrowly focused nursing roles. Examples are in emergency preparedness, school nursing, and family planning. Funds assigned to anti-bioterrorism cannot be used to support unrelated communicable disease programs or family planning.

The events of September 11, 2001, have had the public and the profession of nursing concerned about the ability of the present public health system and its workforce to deal with bioterrorism, especially outbreaks of deadly and serious communicable diseases. For example, smallpox vaccinations were stopped in 1972, but immunity lasts for only 10 years; although there have been no reported cases since the early 1970s, almost no one in the United States retains their immunity. Thus the population is vulnerable to a smallpox outbreak, and smallpox could be used as a weapon of bioterrorism. Two laboratories in the world retain a small amount of the smallpox virus. Because of these potential threats, the U.S. government began to increase production of the vaccine and currently has stockpiled enough vaccine to vaccinate the population in the event of a terrorist attack (NIH, 2014). Few public health professionals are knowledgeable of the symptoms, treatment, or mode of transmission of this disease. Most health professionals, including registered nurses (RNs), who currently work in the United States have never seen a case of anthrax, smallpox, or plague—the three major biological weapons of concern in the world today. A few have now seen the effects of the Ebola virus. The USDHHS and the federal **Office of Homeland Security** have provided funds to address this serious threat to the people of the United States.

One of the first things being done is the rebuilding of the crumbling public health infrastructures of each state to provide surveillance, intervention, and communication in the face of future bioterrorism events and natural disasters. On December 19, 2006, President George W. Bush signed the Pandemic and All-Hazards Preparedness Act (PAHPA), which was intended to improve the organization, direction, and utility of preparedness efforts (U.S. Law, 2006). PAHPA centralizes federal responsibilities, requires state-based accountability, proposes new national surveillance methods, addresses surge capacity, and facilitates the development of vaccines and other scarce resources (Morhard & Franco, 2013; USDHHS, 2014). On March 13, 2013, President Barrack Obama signed the Pandemic and All-Hazards Preparedness Reauthorization Act into law (U.S. Law, 2013). The 2013 law reauthorizes funding for public health and medical preparedness programs that enable communities to build systems to support people in need during and after disasters (USDHHS, 2016b).

THE LAW AND HEALTH CARE

The United States is a nation of laws, which are subject to the U.S. Constitution. The law is a system of privileges and processes by which people solve problems on the basis of a set of established rules. It is intended to minimize the use of force. Laws govern the relationships of individuals and organizations to other individuals and to government. After a law is established, regulations further define the course of actions to be taken by the government, organizations, or individuals in reaching an agreed-on outcome. Government and its laws are the ultimate authority in society and are designed to enforce official policy whether it is related to health, education, economics, social welfare, or any other society issue. The number and types of laws influencing health care are ever increasing. Definitions of law (Hill & Hill, 2018) include the following:

- A rule established by authority, society, or custom
- The body of rules governing the affairs of people, communities, states, corporations, and nations
- A set of rules or customs governing a discrete field or activity (e.g., criminal law, contract law)

These definitions reflect the close relationship of law to the community and to society's customs and beliefs.

The law has had a major impact on nursing practice. Although nursing emerged from individual voluntary activities, society passed laws to give formality to public health and, through legal mandates (i.e., laws), positions and functions for nurses in community settings were created. These functions in many instances carry the force of law. For example, if the nurse discovers a person with smallpox, the law directs the nurse and others in the public health community to take specific actions. In another example, in a mumps outbreak a nurse and other health professionals are required to report mumps cases. This reporting requirement helps with locating and treating cases so cases can be treated or isolated as they occur to prevent further spreading of disease. Three types of laws in the United States have particular importance.

Constitutional Law

Constitutional law derives from federal and state constitutions. It provides overall guidance for selected practice situations. For example, on what basis can the state *require* quarantine or isolation of individuals with tuberculosis? The U.S. Constitution specifies the explicit and limited functions of the federal government. All other powers and functions are left to the individual states. The major constitutional power of the states relating to population-centered nursing practice is the state's right to intervene in a reasonable manner to protect the health, safety, and welfare of its citizens. The state has *police power* to act through its public health system, but it has limits. First, it must be a "reasonable" exercise of power. Second, if the power interferes or infringes on individual rights, the state must demonstrate that there is a "compelling state interest" in exercising its power. Isolating an individual or separating someone from a community because that person has a communicable disease has been deemed an appropriate exercise of state powers. The state can isolate an individual even though it infringes on individual rights (such as freedom and autonomy), under the following conditions (Gostin & Wiley, 2016; Phua, 2013):

- There is a compelling state interest in preventing an epidemic.
- The isolation is necessary to protect the health, safety, and welfare of individuals in the community or the public as a whole.
- The isolation is done in a reasonable manner.

The legal and medical communities along with AIDS activists rejected (and made the case) that the social quarantine of individuals with AIDS was unnecessary. Thus individual freedom and autonomy of the individual come before "compelling state interest" unless science warrants another conclusion (Cole, 2014).

Legislation and Regulation

Legislation is law that comes from the legislative branches of federal, state, or local government. This is referred to as statute law because it becomes coded in the statutes of a government (Birkland, 2016). Much legislation has an effect on nursing. Regulations are specific statements of law related to defining or enacting individual pieces of legislation or statute law. For example, state legislatures enact laws (statutes) establishing boards of nursing and defining terms such as *registered nurse* and *nursing practice.* Every state has a board of nursing. The board may be found either in the department of licensing boards of the health department or in an administrative agency of the governor's office. Created by legislation known as a state nurse practice act, the board of nursing is made up of nurses and consumers. The functions of this board are described in the nurse practice act of each state and generally include licensing and examination of RNs and licensed practical nurses; licensing and/or certification of advanced practice nurses; approval of schools of nursing in the state; revocation, suspension, or denying of licenses; and writing of regulations about nursing practice and education.

The state boards of nursing operationalize, implement, and enforce the statutory law by writing explicit statements (rules) on what it means to be an RN and on the nurse's rights and responsibilities in delegating work to others and in meeting continuing education requirements.

All nurses employed in community settings are subject to legislation and regulations. For example, home health care nurses employed by private agencies must deliver care according to federal Medicare or state Medicaid legislation and regulations, so the agency can be reimbursed for those services. Private and public health care services rendered by nurses are subject to many governmental regulations for quality of care, standards of documentation, and confidentiality of client records and communications. All state health departments have a public health practice reference that governs the practice of nurses and others. Also, state public health laws define the essential public health services that must be offered in the state as well as the optional services that may also be offered.

Judicial and Common Law

Both judicial law and common law have great impact on nursing. Judicial law is based on court or jury decisions. The opinions of the courts are referred to as *case law* (Birkland, 2016). The court uses other types of laws to make its decisions, including previous court decisions or cases. Precedent is one principle of common law. This means that judges are bound by previous decisions unless they are convinced that the older law is no longer relevant or valid. This process is called *distinguishing,* and it usually involves a demonstration of how the current situation in dispute differs from the previously decided situation. Other principles of common law such as justice, fairness, respect for individual's autonomy, and self-determination are part of a court's rationale and the basis upon which to make a decision.

LAWS SPECIFIC TO NURSING PRACTICE

Despite the broad nature and varied roles of nurses in practice, two legal arenas are most applicable to nurse practice situations. The first is the statutory authority for the profession and its scope of practice, and the second is professional negligence or malpractice.

Scope of Practice

The issue of scope of practice involves defining nursing, setting its credentials, and then distinguishing between the practices of nurses, physicians, and other health care providers. The issue is especially important to nurses in community settings, who have traditionally practiced with much autonomy.

Health care practitioners are subject to the laws of the state in which they practice, and they can practice only with a license. The states' nurse practice acts differ somewhat, but they are the most important statutory laws affecting nurses. The nurse practice act of each state accomplishes at least four functions: defining the practice of professional nursing, identifying the scope of nursing practice, setting educational qualifications and other requirements for licensure, and determining the legal titles nurses may use to identify themselves. The usual and customary practice of nursing can be determined through a variety of sources, including the following:

- Content of nursing educational programs, both general and special
- Experience of other practicing nurses (peers)
- Statements and standards of nursing professional organizations
- Policies and procedures of agencies employing nurses
- Needs and interests of the community
- Updated literature, including research, books, texts, and journals
- Internet sites if it can be determined that the site is a professional source of information

All of these sources can describe, determine, and refine the scope of practice of a professional nurse. Every nurse should know and follow closely any proposed changes in the practice acts of nursing, medicine, pharmacy, and other related professions. The nurse should always examine all legislation, rules, and regulations related to nursing practice. For example, a review of the pharmacy act will let the nurse know whether to question the right to dispense medications in a family planning clinic in a local health department. Defining the scope of practice forces one to clarify independent, interdependent, and dependent nursing functions.

Just as practice acts vary by state, so do the evolving issues and tensions of scopes of practice among the health professions. In past years, several state legislatures (working closely with the National Council of State Boards of Nursing) embarked on a legislative effort to develop the interstate Nurse Licensure Compact (NLC). The compact allowed mutual recognition of generalist nursing licensure across state lines in the compact states. In 2017 the Enhanced Nurse Licensure Compact (eNLC) was implemented, replacing the original NLC. Under the eNLC, nurses in participating states are able to have one multistate license, thus able to practice in person or by telehealth within their home state and other eNLC states. As of January 2018, 29 states had adopted the eNLC (NCSBN, 2018).

Professional Negligence

Professional negligence, or *malpractice*, is defined as an act (or a failure to act) that leads to injury of a client. To recover money damages in a malpractice action, the client must prove all of the following:

1. That the nurse owed a duty to the client or was responsible for the client's care
2. That the duty to act the way a reasonable, prudent nurse would act in the same circumstances was not fulfilled
3. That the failure to act reasonably under the circumstances led to the alleged injuries
4. That the injuries provided the basis for a monetary claim from the nurse as compensation for the injury

Reported cases involving negligence and population-centered nurses are rare. However, the following is an example:

Home Nurse Fails to Properly Supervise Bottle Feeding of Child With Tracheal Tube for Oxygen—Death—$4.5 Million Verdict

The plaintiff, a child, age sixteen months, suffered insufficiency of her lungs and required a continuous supply of oxygen via a tracheal tube. She required constant supervision by a home health nurse.

In January 2008, during the day a bottle of formula was given by the nurse. The formula entered the tracheal tube and lungs. After several minutes the nurse observed that the child had stopped breathing and began cardiopulmonary resuscitation. The child did not survive. It was determined that the child had suffered asphyxiation due to ingestion of vomited material.

The plaintiff claimed that the child had choked and gagged throughout the nurse's resuscitation attempts and that CPR was not the correct method of resuscitating the child. The plaintiff claimed that the tracheal tube should have been cleared or changed.

The case was initially brought against the defendant nurse's employer, the home care agency, and the hospital which had provided the tracheal tube. The claims against the hospital were discontinued and the matter proceeded to trial against the home care agency. The defendant did not contest liability.

According to a published account a $4.5 million verdict was returned for the child's pain and suffering. A defense motion to set aside the verdict was pending.

With permission from Medical Malpractice Verdicts, Settlements & Experts; Lewis Laska, Editor, 901 Church St., Nashville, TN 37203-3411,2013 1-800-298-6288.

An integral part of all negligence actions is the question of who should be sued. When a nurse is employed and functioning within the scope of employment, the employer is responsible for the nurse's negligent actions. This is referred to as the doctrine of *respondeat superior*. By directing a nurse to carry out a particular function, the employer becomes responsible for negligence, along with the individual nurse. Because employers are usually better able to pay for the injuries suffered by clients, they are sued more often than the nurses themselves, although an increasing number of judgments include the professional nurse by name as a codefendant. In some instances, if the agency is found liable, the agency may in turn sue the nurse for negligence. At least, the nurse often loses the job.

Thus it is imperative that all nurses engaged in clinical practice carry their own professional liability insurance. Nurses may have personal immunity for particular practice areas, such as giving immunizations. In some states the legislature has granted personal immunity to nurses employed by public agencies to cover all aspects of their practice under the legal theory of *sovereign immunity* (Cherry & Jacobs, 2017).

Nursing students need to be aware that the same laws and rules that govern the professional nurse govern them. Students are expected to meet the same standard of care as that met by any licensed nurse practicing under the same or similar circumstances. Students are expected to be able to perform all tasks and make clinical decisions on the basis of the knowledge they have gained or been offered, according to their progress in their educational programs and along with adequate educational supervision.

LEGAL ISSUES AFFECTING HEALTH CARE PRACTICES

Specific legal issues of nursing vary depending on the setting where care is delivered, the clinical arena, and the nurse's functional role. The law, including legislation and judicial opinions, significantly affects each of the following areas of nursing practice. Nurses responsible for setting and implementing program priorities need to identify and monitor laws related to each special area of practice.

School and Family Health

Nurses employed by health departments or boards of education may deliver school and family health nursing. School health legislation establishes a minimum of services that must be provided to children in public and private schools. For example, most states require that children be immunized against certain communicable diseases before entering school. Children must have had a physical examination by that time, and most states require at least one physical at a later time in their schooling. Legislation also specifies when and what type of health screening will be conducted in schools (e.g., vision and hearing testing). These requirements are found in statutory laws of states. Some states are now requiring a simple dental examination in schools for the purpose of referring children to a dental health professional if needed.

Statutes addressing child abuse and neglect make a large impact on nursing practice within schools and families. Most states require nurses to notify police and/or a social service agency of any situation in which they suspect a child is being abused or neglected. This is one instance in which the law mandates that a health professional breach client confidentiality to protect someone who may be in a helpless or vulnerable position. There is *civil immunity* for such reporting, and the nurse may be called as a witness in a court hearing of the case.

Occupational health is another special area of practice that has specific legal requirements as a result of state and federal statutes. Of special concern are the state workers' compensation statutes, which provide the legal foundation for claims of workers injured on the job. Access to records, confidentiality, and the use of standing orders are legal issues that have great practice significance to nurses employed in industries.

Home Care and Hospice

Home care and hospice services rendered by nurses are shaped through state statutes and have specific nursing requirements for licensure and certification. Compliance with these laws is directly linked to the method of payment for the services. For example, a service must be licensed and certified to obtain payment for services through Medicare. Federal regulations implementing Medicare/Medicaid have an enormous effect on much of nursing practice, including how nurses record details of their visits, record time spent in care activities, and document client care and the client's status and progress.

In addition, many states have passed laws requiring nurses to report elder abuse to the proper authorities, as is done with children and youth. Laws affecting home care and hospice services have focused on such issues as the right to death with dignity, rights of residents of long-term facilities and home health clients, definitions of death, and the use of living wills and advance directives. The legal and ethical dimensions of nursing practice are particularly important. Individual rights, such as the right to refuse treatment, and nursing responsibilities, such as the legal duty to render reasonable and prudent care, may appear to be in conflict in delivering home and hospice services. Much case discussion (sometimes including outside ethics consultation) may be needed to resolve such conflicts.

Correctional Health

Correctional health nursing practice is significantly shaped by federal and state laws and regulations and by recent Supreme Court decisions. The laws and decisions primarily relate to the type and amount of services that must be provided for incarcerated individuals. For example, physical examinations are required for all prisoners after they are sentenced. Regulations specify basic levels of care that must be provided for prisoners, and access to care during illness is a particular focus. Court decisions requiring adequate health services are based on constitutional law. If minimal services are not provided, it is a violation of a prisoner's right to freedom from cruel and unusual punishment. Such decisions provide a framework that strongly influences the setting of nursing priorities. For example, providing care to the sick would take priority over wellness or health education classes.

THE NURSE'S ROLE IN THE POLICY PROCESS

The number and types of laws influencing health care are increasing. Because of this, nurses need to be involved in the policy process and understand the importance of involvement of nursing to the clients they serve.

For nurses to effectively care for their client populations and their communities in the complex U.S. health care system, professional advocacy for logical health policy that considers equality is essential. Professional nurses working in the community know all too well about the health care problems they and their clients encounter daily, and it is through policy and political activism that both big-picture and long-term solutions can be developed.

Although the term *policy* may sound rather lofty, health policy is quite simply the process of turning health problems into workable action solutions. Health policy is developed on the three-legged stool of *access, cost,* and *quality.* The policy process, which is very familiar to professional nurses, includes the following:

- Statement of a health care problem
- Statement of policy options to address the health problem
- Adoption of a particular policy option
- Implementation of the policy product (e.g., a service)
- Evaluation of the policy's intended and unintended consequences in solving the original health problem

Thus the policy process is very similar to the nursing process, but the focus is on the level of the larger society, and the adoption strategies require political action. For most professional nurses, action in the policy arena comes most easily and naturally through participation in nursing organizations such as the ANA at the state level or the Association of Community Health Nursing Educators (ACHNE) or the Association of Public Health Nurses (APHN) at the national or state level, and in certain specialty organizations like the Quad Counsel Coalition of Public Health Nursing Organizations.

CHECK YOUR PRACTICE

As a member of the National Student Nurses Association, you have been asked to participate in a write-in campaign to alert your legislator about the reduction in funding for public health efforts which keep our populations healthy. What would you do? How would you address the issue and who would you communicate with?

Legislative Action

It is often helpful to review the legislative and political processes that may have been a part of high school education. It becomes important material to remember as a professional career is embarked upon.

The people within geographic jurisdictions elect their legislative representatives and senators. An important part of the legislative process is the work of the **legislative staff**. These individuals do the legwork, research, paperwork, and other activities that move policy ideas into bills and then into law. In addition to the individual legislator's office, the congressional committee staffs are also important. They are usually experts in the content of the work of a committee, such as a health and welfare committee. Frequently, developing a working relationship with key legislative staffers can be as important to achieving a policy objective as the relationship with the policy maker (i.e., the legislator).

The legislative process begins with ideas (policy options) that are developed into bills. After a bill is drafted, it is introduced to the legislature, given a number, read, and assigned to a committee. Hearings, testimony, lobbying, education, research, and informal discussions follow. If the bill is passed from the legislative committee, the entire House of Representatives hears the bill, amends it as necessary, and votes on it. A majority vote moves the bill to Senate, where it is read and amended, and then a vote is taken. Fig. 9.2 shows the necessary formal process of the legislative pathway.

Nurses can be involved in the legislative process at any point. Many professional nursing associations have legislative committees made up of volunteers, governmental relations staff professionals, and sometimes political action committees (PACs), all engaged in efforts to monitor, analyze, and shape health policy.

Common methods of influencing health policy outcomes include face-to-face encounters, personal letters, mailgrams, electronic mail, telephone calls, testimony, petitions, reports, position papers, fact sheets, letters to the editor, news releases, speeches, coalition building, demonstrations, and lawsuits. Depending on the issue, any of these can be effective. Although most business, including politics and the policy agendas, are dependent upon the Internet today for instant communication and quick response, all of these methods continue to be of great importance in influencing policy agendas. For example, if a face-to-face encounter is used with a legislator or a staffer, these persons can put a "face on the policy" agenda, and the reality that the policy affects real persons is an important consideration when the legislator or staff pushes the policy agenda forward. Guidelines on communication are provided in the How To box. Tips on communication and visiting legislators and their staffs, as well as general tips on political action, are presented in Boxes 9.1, 9.2, and 9.3. Political activities in which nurses can and should be involved include a wide variety of activities such as being informed voters (a must!), participating in a political party, registering others to vote, getting out the vote, fundraising for candidates, building networks or communication links for issues (e.g., a phone tree or Internet distribution list), and participating in organizations to ensure their effective involvement in health policy and politics.

HOW TO Be an Effective Communicator

- Use simple communications that will be readily understood.
- Choose language that clearly conveys information to individuals of diverse cultures, different ages, and different educational backgrounds.
- Target oral or written communication to the issue, and omit jargon unique to medicine and nursing.
- State your expertise on the issue first.
- Briefly describe your education and experience.
- Identify the relevance of the issue beyond nursing.
- Provide information regarding the impact of the issue on the legislator's constituents.
- Present accurate, credible data.
- Do not oversell or give inaccurate information about the problem.
- Present information in an organized, thorough, concise form that is based on factual data (when available).
- Give examples.

The direct reimbursement of **advanced practice nurses** (APNs) in the Medicare program is one example of how nurses can use their influence. The inclusion of amendments to Medicare that authorized APN reimbursement regardless of specialty or client location in the Balanced Budget Act of 1997 (U.S. Law, 1997) required the sustained efforts of the ANA and other national nursing organizations over a long period (Phillips, 2018; USDHHS, CMS, 2016c). During that time, individual nurses provided testimony to Congress and to MEDPAC (the physicians' political action committee) on the importance of direct reimbursement to APNs. Many APNs worked closely and vigorously with their congressional representatives to lobby for this Medicare amendment. Even more wrote letters and provided position papers and fact sheets to help legislators understand the value of APNs. Although the process took more than 10 years to achieve fully, APN reimbursement in Medicare became a reality. Both the nursing profession and Medicare beneficiaries will benefit from the enhanced access of Medicare clients to APNs.

The ANA was likewise a strong supporter for the Patient Safety Act of 1997 (ANA, 1997) and the Safe Staffing for Nurse and Patient Safety Act (ANA Capitol Beat.Org, 2018). These laws required health care agencies to make public some information on nurse staff levels, staff mix, and outcomes, and it required the USDHHS to review and approve all health care acquisitions and mergers. All of these requirements are to determine any long-term effect on the health and safety of clients, communities, and staff.

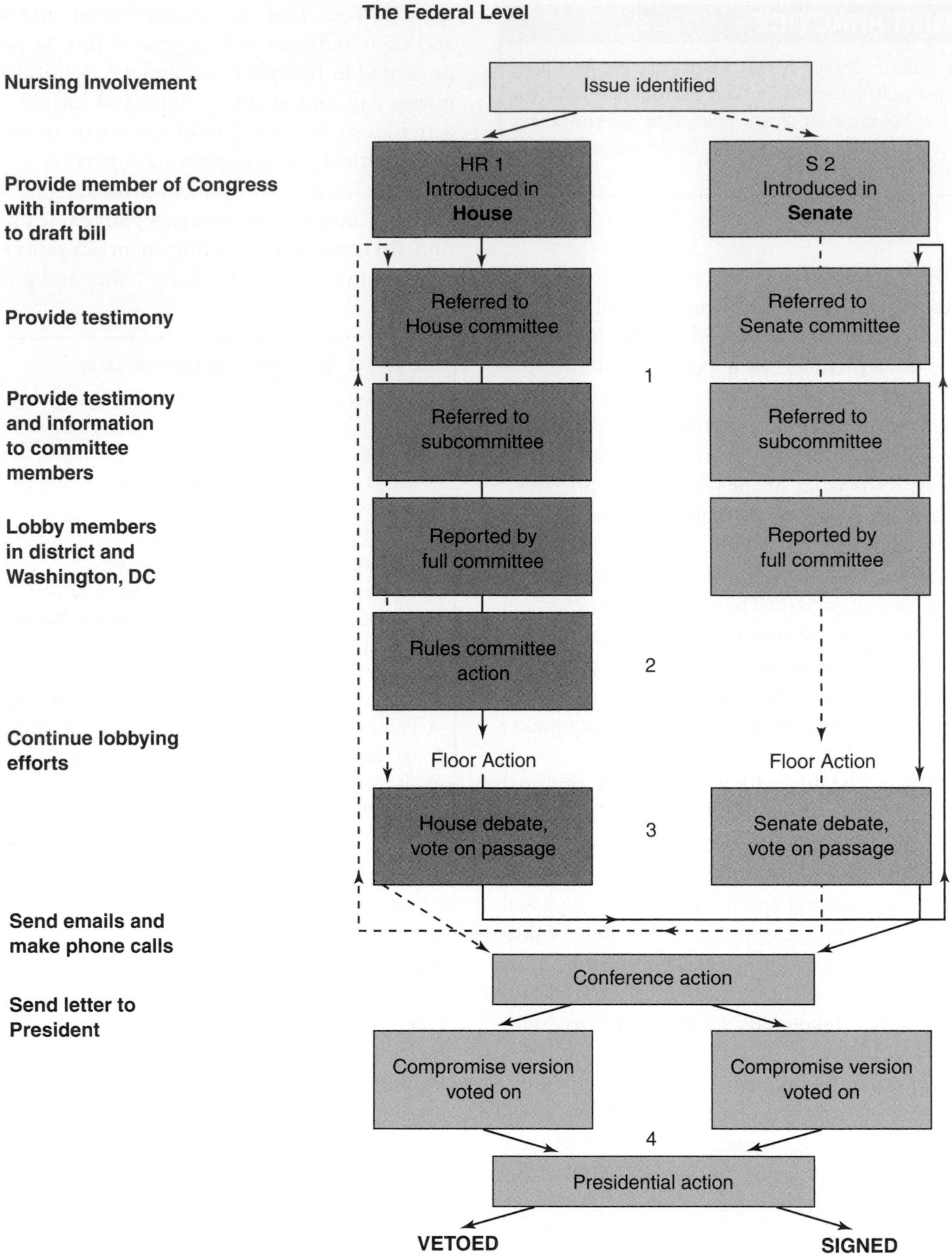

[1] A bill goes to full committee first, then to special subcommittees for hearings, debate, revisions, and approval. The same process occurs when it goes to full committee. It either dies in committee or proceeds to the next step.
[2] Only the House has a Rules Committee to set the "rule" for floor action and conditions for debate and amendments. In the Senate, the leadership schedules action.
[3] The bill is debated, amended, and passed or defeated. If passed, it goes to the other chamber and follows the same path. If each chamber passes a similar bill, both versions go to conference.
[4] The President may sign the bill into law, allow it to become law without his signature, or veto it and return it to Congress. To override the veto, both houses must approve the bill by a two-thirds majority vote.

Fig. 9.2 How a bill becomes a law. (From Mason DJ, et al.: *Policy and politics in nursing and health care*, ed. 7, St. Louis, 2016, Elsevier.)

BOX 9.1 Tips for Visits with Legislators

- Face-to-face visits are viewed as the most effective.
- Call ahead and ask how much time the staff or legislator is able to give you.
- When you arrive, ask if the appointment time is the same or if a scheduled vote on the House/Senate floor is going to need the legislator's attention.
- Engage in small talk at the beginning of the conversation only if the staff or legislator has time.
- Structure time so that the issue can be briefly presented. The visit will probably be 15 minutes or less.
- Allow an opportunity for the staff or Congress member to seek clarity or ask questions.
- Offer to provide additional information or find answers to questions asked.
- Do not assume that the legislator or the legislator's staff is well informed on the issue.
- Leave a one- or two-page fact sheet on the issue.
- Numbers count. If the views you express are shared by a local nurses' organization or by nurses employed at a health care facility, let the legislator know.
- Invite Congress members and their staffs to conferences or meetings of nurses' organizations or to tour nursing facilities to meet others interested in the same policy issues.
- If appropriate, invite the media and let the legislator know.
- Follow up with a letter of thanks to both the legislator and the staffer.

Modified from Mason DJ, et al.: *Policy and politics in nursing and health care,* ed. 7, St. Louis, 2016, Elsevier.

BOX 9.2 Tips for Written Communication with Legislators

- Communicate in writing to express opinions: letters or email.
- Identify yourself as a nurse.
- Acknowledge the Congress member's work as positive or negative, but be courteous.
- Follow up on meetings or phone calls with a letter or email.
- Share knowledge about a particular problem.
- Recommend policy solutions so the legislator or staff will know why you are writing.
- The letter should be typed, a maximum of two pages, and focused on one or two issues at most.
- The purpose of the letter should be stated at the beginning.
- Present clear and compelling rationales for your concern or position on an issue.
- If the purpose of the letter is to express disappointment regarding a stance on an issue or a vote that has been cast, the letter should be as positive as possible.
- Write letters thanking a Congress member for taking a particular position on an issue.
- A letter to the editor of the local newspaper or a nursing newsletter praising a legislator's position (with a copy forwarded to the legislator) is welcome publicity, especially during an election year.
- If you visited with the legislator or a staffer, review the major points covered in person, and answer any questions that were raised during conversation.
- Have personal business cards, and include them with letters.
- Address written correspondence as follows (the same general format applies to state and local officials):

U.S. Senator	U.S. Representative
Honorable Jane Doe	Honorable Jane Doe
United States Senate	House of Representatives
Washington, DC 20510	Washington, DC 20515
Dear Senator Doe:	Dear Representative Doe:

Modified from Mason DJ, et al.: *Policy and politics in nursing and health care,* ed. 7, St. Louis, 2016, Elsevier.

BOX 9.3 Tips for Action

- Become informed.
- Become acquainted with elected officials.
- Become involved in the state nurses association.
- Build communication and leadership skills.
- Increase your knowledge about a range of professional issues.
- Expand and strengthen your professional network.
- Build relationships within the profession and with representatives of public and private sector organizations with an interest in health care.
- Be aware of what is taking place in health care beyond the environment and the practice in which you work.
- Communicate with legislators regularly, and share expertise and perspective on issues related to health care and nursing.
- Offer your expertise to assist in developing new legislation, modifying existing legislation or regulations.
- Identify yourself as a nurse with associated education and expertise.
- Let people know that nurses are capable of functioning in many different roles and making substantial contributions.
- Be confident.
- Do not burn bridges.
- Be friendly.
- Lend a hand to other nurses. It benefits all of us.
- Find an experienced mentor to work with you if you are new to the policy arena.
- Volunteer, seek appointments, or participate in election campaigns.
- Explore opportunities for involvement through internships, fellowships, and volunteer work at all levels (local, state, and national).

Modified from previous works of Mason DJ, et al.: *Policy and politics in nursing and health care,* ed. 7, St. Louis, 2016, Elsevier.

On the state legislative level, all 50 states have passed title protection for APNs; this was achieved by individual nurses, state nurses associations, and various nursing specialty groups participating in the legislative process with the 50 state legislators. Title protection means that only certain nurses who meet state criteria can call themselves *advanced practice nurses.*

Regulatory Action

The regulatory process, although it may not be as visible a process as legislation, can also be used to shape laws and dramatically affect health policy. This process should be on the radar screen of professional nurses who wish to successfully participate in policy activity.

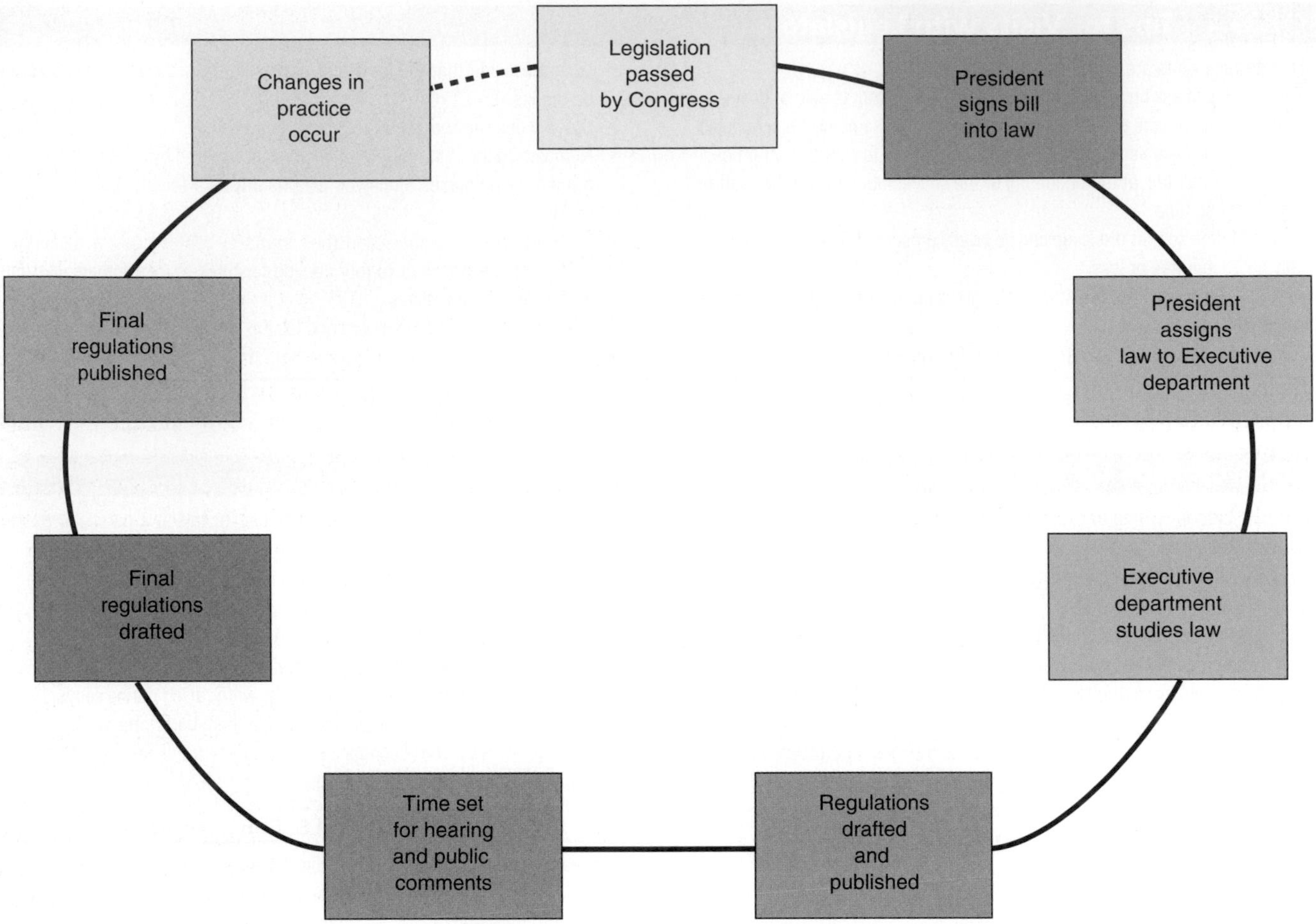

Fig. 9.3 The process of writing regulations.

At each level of government the executive branch can and, in most cases, must prepare regulations for implementing policy for new laws and new programs. These regulations are detailed, and they establish, fix, and control standards and criteria for carrying out certain laws. Fig. 9.3 shows the steps in the typical process of writing regulations. When the legislature passes a law and delegates its oversight to an agency, it gives that agency the power to make regulations. Because regulations flow from legislation, they have the force of law.

The Process of Regulation

After a law is passed the appropriate executive department begins the process of regulation by studying the topic or issue. Advisory groups or special task forces are sometimes formed to provide the content for the regulations. Nurses can influence these regulations by writing letters to the regulatory agency in charge or by speaking at open public hearings. Many letters are now accepted by Internet.

After rewriting, the proposed regulations are put into final draft form and printed in the legally required publication (e.g., at the federal level, the *Federal Register*). Similar registers exist in most states, where regulations from state executive departments, including state health departments, are published. Public comment is called for in written form or oral presentation within a given period.

Revisions made to proposed regulations are based on public comment and public hearing. Depending on the amount and content of the public reaction, final regulations are prepared or more study of the area and issues is conducted. Final published regulations carry the force of law. When regulations become effective, health care practice is changed to conform to the new regulations. Monitoring administrative regulations is essential for the professional nurse, who can influence regulations by attending the hearings, providing comments, testifying, and engaging in lobbying aimed at individuals involved in the writing of the regulations. Concrete written suggestions for revision submitted to these individuals are frequently persuasive and must be acknowledged by government in publishing the final rules. An excellent example of how nurses must continue to influence health policy outcomes, even after positive legislation has passed, occurred after the passage of the Balanced Budget Act of 1997 (BBA '97) (U.S. Law, 1997). The HCFA began to implement the BBA '97 through the publication of draft regulations seeking to define APN practice and Medicare reimbursement. The nursing community responded vigorously with negative opinions about the initial restrictive definitions and requirement. Their reactions were effective and reshaped the final regulations to recognize the state definitions for APN practice autonomy.

Final regulations, published in a *Code of Regulations* (both federal and state), usually lead to changes in practice. For example, Medicare regulations setting standards for nursing homes and home health are incorporated into these agencies' manuals. In the case of APN reimbursement, some Medicare fiscal intermediaries have had difficulty in recognizing APNs as appropriate providers, but professional nursing organization advocates have forcefully addressed these implementation barriers.

Nursing Advocacy

Advocacy begins with the art of influencing others (politics) to adopt a specific course of action (policy) to solve a societal problem. This is accomplished by building relationships with the appropriate policy makers—the individuals or groups that determine a specific course of action to be followed by a government or institution to achieve a desired end (policy outcome). Relationships for effective advocacy can be built in a number of ways.

In January 2006, Medicare Part D—the prescription drug benefits policy—became effective. Public health professionals need to continue to assist many vulnerable persons to in understanding the value of enrolling in Part D, to educate them on how to use the benefits, and to ensure that the populations who are "dually" enrolled in both Medicare and Medicaid are registered. Coordinating efforts between civic, religious, and health care agencies to provide health education is a necessity.

A letter or visit to the district, state, or national office of a legislator to discuss a particular policy or health care issue can be interesting, educational, and effective. Contributions of money, labor, expertise, or influence may also be welcomed by the policy makers involved in setting a course of action to obtain a desired health outcome for an individual, a family, a group, a community, or society (health policy). In addition, one may develop a grassroots network of community and professional friends with a mutual interest in health policy advocacy. The network may be able to promote health policy initiatives for the community. During the Obama presidential campaign, many advocacy networks were established via the Internet, and monies were solicited using this process.

Many special interest groups in health care have the potential, desire, and resources to influence the health policy process. A tremendous advantage that nursing has in advocating for issues and in influencing policy makers is the force of its numbers, since nursing is the largest of the health professions. However, nursing must organize its numbers in such a way that each nurse joins with others to speak with one voice. The greatest effect will be had when all nurses make similar demands for policy outcomes.

During 2002 the nursing profession spoke clearly, distinctly, and together on a serious problem for the health arena and for the profession: the nursing shortage. Health care facilities and employers were having ever-increasing difficulty finding experienced nurses to employ. In addition, the need for RNs was predicted to balloon in the next 20 years because of the aging of the U.S. population, technological advances, and economic factors. Demand for RNs was anticipated to increase by 22 percent by the year 2008. This increased demand for professional nurses, coupled with the expected retirement of a rapidly aging nursing workforce, placed a tremendous stress on the health care system.

Concerns regarding nursing workforce shortages continue today, anticipating a shortage of 154,018 RNs by 2020 and 510,394 RNs by 2030 (Zhang et al., 2017). Additionally, certain states and regions are expected to be impacted more than others. Predictions for 2030 anticipate both shortages and surpluses in the nursing workforce, ranging from a shortage of 44,500 full-time equivalents (FTEs) in California to a surplus of 53,700 FTEs in Florida. The states expected to have the greatest RN shortages in 2030 include California, Texas, New Jersey, and South Carolina (USDHHS, HRSA, 2017).

The workforce shortage results from a complex set of factors, such as population growth, fewer young people entering the profession, shortage of nursing school faculty, the aging of the current nurse workforce and national population, changes in health care reimbursement, and uncomfortable working conditions in which nurses felt pressured to "do more with less" (AACN, 2017; USDHHS, HRSA, 2017).

The American Association of Colleges of Nursing (AACN) remains concerned about the shortage of RNs and works with schools, policy makers, other organizations, and the media to bring attention to this health care crisis. AACN is working to enact legislation, identify strategies, and form collaborations to address the nursing shortage (AACN, 2017).

Advocacy by expert and committed health professionals can bring about positive change for the profession, the community, and the clients that nurses serve. Keeping up to date on issues within government, professional organizations, law, and public policy is vitally important. Informed activism directed toward a professional role, image, and value for professional nurses and toward a health care system in the United States that provides high-quality and affordable universal access to health care should be a lifelong commitment for all professional nurses.

LINKING CONTENT TO PRACTICE

An example of how the policy process works follows, involving a nursing organization and individual members. Whether you are a member of a group as described below or working on your own to influence health policy, the steps described here apply.

Over a 15-month time frame, the American Nurses Association (ANA) was involved in advocating for health care reform. During the presidential campaign, candidates were educated about the nursing profession and ANA's *Agenda for Health System Reform.* ANA and its members participated in national media interviews and local media events. The message was that the association and its members believed that health care is a basic right. ANA collaborated with the nursing community to outline the profession's priorities as proposals were developed in Congress. Testimony was given before three key congressional committees. ANA representatives met with White House and congressional health care reform staff and took part in two presidential press conferences at the White House.

As reported by ANA, thousands of nurses joined ANA's health care reform team, sending letters to representatives of Congress, sharing their stories, and meeting with members of Congress. They also participated in rallies and events.

For more information on ANA's health care reform work, visit http://www.rnaction.org or www.nursingworld.org.

QSEN FOCUS ON QUALITY AND SAFETY EDUCATION FOR NURSES

Targeted Competency: Quality improvement.

- **Knowledge:** Describe strategies for learning about the outcomes of care in the public setting.
- **Skills:** Seek information about outcomes of care for populations served in care settings.
- **Attitudes:** Appreciate that continuous quality improvement is an essential part of the daily work of all professionals.

Quality Improvement Question

The Quad Council competency of policy development and program planning skills indicates that the beginning public health nurse (PHN) collects information that will inform policy decisions. Also the PHN describes the legislative policy development process and identifies outcomes of current health policy relevant to PHN practice. The 2014 outbreak of the Ebola virus in the United States brought quick recognition that there was a need for improvement in policies related to infectious disease control. What were the indicators that the infection control policies in place were not sufficient to prevent the spread of disease? Describe the continuous quality improvement (CQI) data collection processes that determined the need for policy change. What role did nurses and organized nursing play in improving the infection control policy and guidelines nationally? What has been the outcome of the new policy, and how were populations affected both locally and nationally?

PRACTICE APPLICATION

Larry was in his final rotation in the Bachelor of Science in nursing program at State University. He was anxious to complete his final nursing course because upon graduation he would begin a position as a staff nurse specializing in school health at the local health department. His wife was expecting their first child, and she had been receiving prenatal care at the health department.

Larry was aware that a few years ago the federal government had, by law, provided block grants to states for primary care, maternal and child health programs, and other health care needs of states. He had read the *Federal Register* and knew that the regulations for these grants had been written through USDHHS departments. He was aware that these regulations did not require states to fund specific programs.

Larry read in the local newspaper that the health department was closing its prenatal clinic at the end of the month. When his state had received its block grant, it decided to spend the money for programs other than prenatal care. Larry found that a three-year study in his own state showed improved pregnancy outcomes as a result of prenatal care. The results were further improved when the care was delivered by population-centered nurses. After Larry's daughter was born, he read in the *Federal Register* that states could apply for federal stimulus funds and receive a grant for home visiting services to support mothers and new babies.

Larry was concerned that, as a student, he would have little influence on how such grant dollars would be spent. However, he decided to call his classmates together to plan a course of action.

What would such an action plan include?

Answers can be found on the Evolve site.

KEY POINTS

- The legal basis for most congressional action in health care can be found in Article I, Section 8, of the U.S. Constitution.
- The five major health care functions of the federal government are direct service, financing, information, policy setting, and public protection.
- The goal of the World Health Organization is the attainment by all people of the highest possible level of health.
- Many federal agencies are involved in government health care functions. The agency most directly involved with the health and welfare of Americans is the U.S. Department of Health and Human Services (USDHHS).
- Most state and local governments have activities that affect nursing practice.
- The variety and range of functions of governmental agencies have had a major impact on nursing. Funding, in particular, has shaped the role and tasks of nurses.
- The private sector (of which nurses are a part) can influence legislation in many ways, especially through the process of writing regulations.
- The number and types of laws influencing health care are increasing. Because of this, involvement in the political process is important to nurses.
- Professional negligence and the scope of practice are two legal aspects particularly relevant to nursing practice.
- Nurses must consider the legal implications of their own practice in each clinical encounter.
- The federal and most state governments are composed of three branches: the executive, the legislative, and the judicial.
- Each branch of government plays a significant role in health policy.
- The U.S. Public Health Service was created in 1798.
- The first national health insurance legislation was challenged in the Supreme Court in 1937.
- *Health: United States* (NCHS, 2017) is an important source of data about the nation's health care problems.
- In 1921 the Sheppard-Towner Act was passed, and it had an important influence on child health programs and population-centered nursing practice.
- The Division of Nursing, the National Institute of Nursing Research, and the Agency for Healthcare Quality and Research are governmental agencies important to nursing.
- Nurses, through state and local health departments, function as consultants, policy advocates, population level and direct care providers, researchers, teachers, supervisors, and program managers.

- The state governments are responsible for regulating nursing practice within the state.
- Federal and state social welfare programs have been developed to provide monetary benefits to the poor, older adults, the disabled, and the unemployed.
- Social welfare programs affect nursing practice. These programs improve the quality of life for special populations, thus making the nurse's job easier in assisting the client with health needs.
- The nurse's scope of practice is defined by legislation and by standards of practice within a specialty.

CLINICAL DECISION-MAKING ACTIVITIES

1. Conduct an interview with a local health officer. Ask for information from a 10-year period. Try to see trends in population size, health needs and corresponding roles, and activities of government that were implemented to meet these changes. What were some of the problems you identified?
2. Examine a current health department budget, and compare it with a budget from previous years. Has there been any impact on health care because of changes in government spending (especially before and after the passing of the Patient Protection and Affordable Care Act)? Give an example.
3. Locate your state register or other documents, such as newspapers, that publish proposed regulations. Select one set of proposed regulations and critique them. Submit your opinion in writing as public comment, or attend the hearing and testify on the regulations. Be sure to submit something in writing. Evaluate your participation by stating what you learned and whether the proposed regulations were changed in your favor.
4. Find and review your state nurse practice act, and define your scope of practice. Give examples of your practice boundaries.
5. Contact your local public health agency to discuss the state's official powers in regulating epidemics, such as the measles outbreak in Orange County, California (CDC, 2018b), and anthrax exposures related to bioterrorism.
6. Explore the state's right to protect the health, safety, and welfare of its citizens.
7. Ask about the conflict between the state's rights and individual rights and how such issues are resolved.
8. Ask about the standards of care that apply to this issue and how it is decided which services offered to clients should be mandatory and which should be voluntary.
9. Explore how the role of public health differs in these epidemics compared with the past epidemics of smallpox and tuberculosis. Be specific.

ADDITIONAL RESOURCES

EVOLVE WEBSITE

http://evolve.elsevier.com/Stanhope/community/

- Answers to Practice Application
- Case Study
- Glossary
- Review Questions

REFERENCES

Agency for Healthcare Research and Quality: *Profile*, Bethesda, MD, 2018, USDHHS. Retrieved from https://www.ahrq.gov.

Agency for Healthcare Research and Quality: *Practice Based Research Network*, Bethesda, MD, n.d., USDHHS. Retrieved from https://pbrn.ahrq.gov.

American Association of Colleges of Nursing: *Fact Sheet on the Nursing Shortage*, Washington, DC, 2017, AACN. Retrieved from http://www.aacnnursing.org.

American Nurses Association: *Press Release, ANA Applauds Introduction of Patient Safety Act of 1997*, 1997. Retrieved from http://www.nursingworld.org.

American Nurses Association: Introducing the Safe Staffing for Nursing and Patient Safety Act. 3-1-2018. Retrieved from https://anacapitolbeat.org.

American Public Health Association: *Strengthening public health nursing in the United States*, Policy number: 201316, 2013, APHA.

Beck AJ, Boulton ML: The public health nurse workforce in U.S. state and local health departments—2012, *Public Health Rep* 131(1): 145–152, 2016.

Birkland TA: *An Introduction to the Policy Process: Theories, Concepts and Models of Public Policy Making*, ed 4, New York, NY, 2016, Routledge, Taylor & Francis Group.

Bureau of Federal Prisons: *Population Statistics*, 2018. Retrieved from https://www.bop.gov.

Centers for Disease Control and Prevention: *Mission, role and pledge*, 2014a, USDHHS. Retrieved from https://www.cdc.gov.

Centers for Disease Control and Prevention: *Epidemiology of Escherichia Coli and Multistate Outbreak*, 2014b, USDHHS. Retrieved from www.cdc.gov.

Centers for Disease Control and Prevention: *Definition of Policy*, 2015, USDHHS, Office of the Associate Director for Policy. Retrieved from https://www.cdc.gov.

Centers for Disease Control and Prevention: *Zika Cases in the U.S.*, Atlanta, 2018a. Retrieved from www.cdc.gov.

Centers for Disease Control and Prevention: *Measles Cases and Outbreaks*, 2018b, USDHHS, Retrieved from https://www.cdc.gov.

Centers for Medicare and Medicaid Services. Home: Centers for Medicare and Medicaid Services. Washington, DC, 2018. Retrieved from https://www.cms.gov.

Cherry B, Jacobs SR: *Contemporary Nursing Issues, Trends and Management*, ed 7, St Louis, 2017, Elsevier.

Chikhale N: The importance of unemployment benefits for protecting against income drops. www.equitablegrowth.org. April 25, 2017.

Cole JP: *Federal and State Quarantine and Isolation Authority: CRS Report to Congress, Report No. 7-5700*. Washington, DC, 2014, Legislative Attorneys American Law Division. https://fas.org.

Congressional Research Service: *Appropriations and fund transfers in the Affordable Care Act, R41301*, 2017: Redhead CS. Retrieved from https://fas.org.

Department of Health, Education and Welfare: *Improving Health. Healthy People: The Surgeon General's Report on Health Promotion and Disease Prevention*, DHEW Publication No. 79-55071. Washington, DC, 1979, U.S. Government Printing Office. https://profiles.nlm.nih.gov.

Gallup Inc: *Americans still split on government healthcare role*, December 8, 2016. Retrieved from http://news.gallup.com.

Gostin LO, Wiley LF: *Public health law: power, duty, restraint*, ed 3, Oakland, 2016, University of California Press.

Hill G, Hill K: *The People's Law Dictionary*, New York, 2018, ALM media properties. https://dictionary.law.com.

Kaiser Family Foundation, Foutz J, Squires E, Garfield R, Damico A: *The uninsured: A primer – key facts about health insurance and the uninsured under the Affordable Care Act*, 2017. Retrieved from http://files.kff.org.

Katz R, Macintyre A, Barbera J: Emergency public health. In Pines JM, Abualenain J, Scott J, et al, editors: *Emergency Care and the Public's Health*, Hoboken, NJ, 2014, John Wiley and Sons, Ltd.

Mason DJ, Gardner DB, Hopkins Outlaw F, O'Grady ET: *Policy and Politics in Nursing and Health Care*, ed 7, St Louis, 2016, Elsevier.

Morhard R, Franco C: The Pandemic and All-Hazards Preparedness Act: Its contributions and new potential to increase public health preparedness. *Biosecur Bioterror* 11(2):145–152, 2013. Retrieved from http://online.liebertpub.

National Center for Health Statistics: *Health: United States, 2016*, Hyattsville, MD, 2017, U.S. Government Printing Office.

National Council of State Boards of Nursing: *Enhanced Nurse Licensure Compact (eNLC) Implementation*, 2018. Retrieved from https://www.ncsbn.org.

National Institutes of Health: *Grants and Funding, Office of Extramural Research*, 2018, USDHHS. Retrieved from https://grants.nih.gov.

National Institutes of Health: *Structure and Goals*, Bethesda, MD, 2017, USDHHS.

National Institutes of Health: *Smallpox: vaccine supply and strength*, Bethesda, MD, 2014, USDHHS.

National Institute of Nursing Research: *National Institutes of Health: Funding Opportunities*, Bethesda, MD, 2018a, USDHHS. Retrieved from https://www.ninr.nih.gov.

National Institute of Nursing Research: *National Institutes of Health: Mission and Strategic Plan*, Bethesda, MD, 2018b, USDHHS. Retrieved from https://www.ninr.nih.gov.

Occupational Safety and Health Administration: *Clarification of the Use and Selection of Blood Bourne Pathogen Safety Devices*, Washington, DC, May 5, 2008, U.S. Department of Labor. Retrieved from https://www.osha.gov.

Occupational Safety and Health Administration: *OSHA fact sheet: OSHA's bloodborne pathogen standard*, 2011. Retrieved from https://www.osha.gov.

Phillips SJ: 30th Annual APRN legislative update: improving access to healthcare one state at a time, *Nurse Pract* 43(1): 27–54, 2018.

Phua KL: Ethical dilemmas in protecting individual rights versus public protection in the case of infectious diseases, *Infect Dis* 6:1–5, 2013.

Rothstein J, Valletta RG: *Scraping by: Income and program participation after the loss of extended unemployment benefits*, Washington DC, 2017, Washington Center for Equitable Growth Working Paper Series. Retrieved from http://equitablegrowth.org.

United Nations: *Report of the World Conference of the International Women's Year, Mexico City, June 19 to July 2, Chapter I, Section A.2*, Publication No. E.76.IV.1. New York, 1975, UN.

United Nations: *Report of the World Conference of the United Nations Decade for Women: Equality, Development and Peace, Copenhagen, July 24-30, Chapter I, Section A,* Publication No. E.80.IV.3. New York, 1980, UN.

United Nations: *Report of the World Conference to Review and Appraise Achievements of the United Nations Decade for Women: Equality, Development and Peace, Nairobi, July 15-26*. New York, 1985, UN.

United Nations: *Report of the Fourth World Conference on Women, Beijing, September 4-15, Chapter I, Resolution 1, Annex I*, Publication No. E.96.IV.13. New York, 1995, UN.

United Nations: *Women 2000: Gender Equality, Development and Peace for the 21st Century, Beijing*, 23rd session of the United Nations General Assembly. New York, 2000, UN.

United Nations: *Major conferences and summits*, n.d. Retrieved from http://www.un.org.

USA.gov: *Branches of* government, 2018. Retrieved from https://www.usa.gov/branches-of-government.

U.S. Department of Agriculture: *About WIC: WIC at a glance*, Washington, DC, 2015, USDA. Retrieved from https://www.fns.usda.gov.

U.S. Department of Agriculture: *Food and Nutrition Service Overview*, Washington, DC, 2018, USDA. Retrieved from https://www.fns.usda.gov.

U.S. Department of Defense: *TRICARE: About Us*, Falls Church, VA, 2018, DOD. Retrieved from https://www.tricare.mil.

U.S. Department of Health and Human Services: *Healthy People 2000: National Health Promotion and Disease Prevention Objectives*, Rockville, MD, 1991, U.S. Government Printing Office. Retrieved from: https://www.healthypeople.gov.

U.S. Department of Health and Human Services: *Healthy People 2010: Understanding and Improving Health*, ed 2, Washington, DC, 2000, U.S. Government Printing Office. Retrieved from: https://www.healthypeople.gov.

U.S. Department of Health and Human Services: *Healthy People 2020*, Washington, DC, 2010. Retrieved from https://www.healthypeople.gov.

U.S. Department of Health and Human Services, The Division of Nursing's National Advisory Committee on Nursing Education and Practice: *Public Health Nursing: key to our nation's health*, Rockville, MD, 2013, Division of Nursing. Retrieved from https://www.hrsa.gov.

U.S. Department of Health and Human Services, Public Health Emergency: *Pandemic and All Hazards Preparedness Act*, Washington, DC, 2014. Retrieved from https://www.phe.gov.

U.S. Department of Health and Human Services, The Division of Nursing's National Advisory Committee on Nursing Education and Practice: *Incorporating interprofessional education and practice into nursing*, Rockville, MD, 2015, Division of Nursing. Retrieved from https://www.hrsa.gov.

U.S. Department of Health and Human Services, The Division of Nursing's National Advisory Committee on Nursing Education and Practice: *Preparing nurses for new roles in population health management*, Rockville, MD, 2016a, Division of Nursing. Retrieved from https://www.hrsa.gov.

U.S. Department of Health and Human Services, Public Health Emergency, *Pandemic and All Hazards Preparedness Reauthorization Act*, Washington, DC, 2016b. Retrieved from https://www.phe.gov.

U.S. Department of Health and Human Services, Centers for Medicare and Medicaid Services: *Advanced Practice Registered Nurses, Anethesiologist Assistants, and Physiciant Assistants*, 2016c. ICN 901623. Retrieved from https://www.cms.gov.

U.S. Department of Health and Human Services, Health Resources and Services Administration: *Supply and demand projections of the nursing workforce: 2014-2030*, Rockville, MD, 2017. Retrieved from https://bhw.hrsa.gov.

U.S. Law: 42 U.S.C. Section 161-175, Sheppard-Towner Maternity and Infant Protection Act. 1921.
U.S. Law: 49 Stat 622, Title II. 1937a.
U.S. Law: 42 SC 301, *Stewart Machine Co. v. Davis*. 1937b.
U.S. Law: Public Law 107-105, Health Insurance Portability and Accountability Act (HIPAA). 1996.
U.S. Law: Title XXI of the Social Security Act, BBA '97, State Child Health Improvement Act (SCHIP). 1997.
U.S. Law: Public law 105-33: Balanced Budget Act, 1997.
U.S. Law: Public Law 106-505: The Public Health Threats and Emergencies Act. 2000.
U.S. Law: Public Law 106-430: Needlestick Safety and Prevention Act. 2000.
U.S. Law: 107-188, Public Health Security and Bioterrorism and Response Act. 2002.
U.S. Law: Public Law 109-417: Pandemic and All Hazards Preparedness Act. 2006.
U.S. Law: Public Law 111-148 Patient Protection and Affordable Care Act (PPACA). 2010.
U.S. Law: Public Law 113-5: Pandemic and All-Hazards Preparedness Reauthorization Act, 2013.
University of Michigan Center of Excellence in Public Health Workforce Studies: *Enumeration and Characteristics of the Public Health Nurse Workforce: Findings of the 2012 Public Health Nurse Workforce Surveys*, Ann Arbor, MI, 2013, University of Michigan.
World Health Organization: *Health systems financing: the path to universal coverage.* The World Health Report, 2010. Retrieved from http://www.who.int.
World Health Assembly: *Strengthening nursing and midwifery*, 64th session WHA, May 24, 2011. Retrieved from http://apps.who.int.
World Health Organization: *WHO nursing and midwifery progress report: 2008-2012*, 2013a. Retrieved from http://www.who.int.
World Health Organization: *The world health report 2013: research for universal health coverage*, Geneva, Switzerland, 2013b, WHO. Retrieved from http://www.who.int.
World Health Organization: *Nursing and Midwifery in the History of the World Health Organization 1948-2017*, Geneva, Switzerland, 2017, WHO. Retrieved from http://www.who.int.
World Health Organization: *The global strategic directions for strengthening nursing and midwifery 2016-2020*, Geneva, Switzerland, 2016, WHO. Retrieved from http://www.who.int.
World Health Organization: *Health topics: Health policy*, 2018, WHO. Retrieved from http://www.who.int.
Zhang X, Tai D, Pforsich H, Lin VW: United States Registered Nurse workforce report care and shortage forecast: a revisit, *Am J Med Qual* 33(3): 229–236, 2017.

10

Evidence-Based Practice

Marcia Stanhope, PhD, RN, FAAN and
Lisa M. Turner, PhD, RN, PHCNS-BC

OBJECTIVES

After reading this chapter, the student should be able to do the following:

1. Define evidence-based practice.
2. Understand the history of evidence-based practice in health care.
3. Analyze the relationship between evidence-based practice and the practice of nursing in the community.
4. Provide examples of evidence-based practice in the community.
5. Identify barriers to evidence-based practice.
6. Apply evidence-based resources in practice.

CHAPTER OUTLINE

Definition of Evidence-Based Practice
History of Evidence-Based Practice
Paradigm Shift in Use of Evidence-Based Practice
Types of Evidence
Factors Leading to Change
Barriers to Evidence-Based Practice
Steps in the Evidence-Based Practice Process
Approaches to Implementing Evidence-Based Practice
Current Perspectives
Healthy People 2020 Objectives
Example of Application of Evidence-Based Practice to Public Health Nursing

KEY TERMS

evidence-based medicine, p. 219
evidence-based nursing, p. 219
evidence-based practice, p. 219
evidence-based public health, p. 219
grading the strength of evidence, p. 224
integrative review, p. 224
meta-analysis, p. 223
narrative review, p. 224
randomized controlled trial (RCT), p. 221
research utilization, p. 219
systematic review, p. 222

Emphasis on evidence-based practice (EBP) is a standard to be met in health care delivery in the United States. It is a relevant approach to providing the highest quality of health care in all settings, which will result in improved health outcomes. EBP is important for all professionals who work in social and health care environments, regardless of the client or the setting with which professionals are dealing, including public health nurses who work with populations. Emphasis on EBP has resulted from increased expectations of consumers, changes in health care economics, increased expectations of accountability, advancements in technology, the knowledge explosion fueled by the Internet, and the growing number of lawsuits occurring when there is injury or harm as a result of practice decisions that are not based on the best available evidence (Brower & Nemec, 2017; Makic et al., 2014). Nurses at all levels have an opportunity to improve the practice of nursing and client outcomes.

The Institute of Medicine has set a goal that by 2020 the best available evidence will be used to make 90 percent of all health care decisions, yet most nurses continue to be inconsistent in implementing EBP. An even greater concern in public health is that the field is lagging behind in developing evidence-based guidelines for the community setting. It is important to recognize that regardless of the level of education, undergraduate or graduate, nurses can be involved in the development, implementation, and evaluation of the effects of EBP (Brooke & Mallion, 2016; Davidson & Brown, 2014; Häggman-Laitila et al., 2016).

Comprehensive databases are available through various Internet sites to assist nurses in applying the most recent best evidence to their clinical practice, like the Cochrane Library Database, the Centers for Disease Control and Prevention: Guide to Community Preventive Services, and others.

DEFINITION OF EVIDENCE-BASED PRACTICE

The term *evidence-based* was first attributed to Gordon Guyatt, a Canadian physician at McMaster University in 1992 (Evidence-Based Medicine Working Group, 1992). The term was first applied in medicine to begin the development of new ways of guiding professional decision making by using the best available evidence. Because the concept was developed in medicine, some of the first definitions focused on evidence-based medicine.

The definition of **evidence-based medicine** by Sackett et al. (1996) became the industry standard. Sackett et al. (1996) defined evidence-based medicine as "the conscientious, explicit, and judicious use of current best evidence in making decisions about the care of individual clients" (p. 71). Without current best external evidence, they said, "practice risks become rapidly out of date, to the detriment of clients" (Sackett et al., 1996, p. 72). A more succinct definition was proposed as the conscientious use of the current best evidence in making decisions about patient care (Sackett et al., 2000).

Adapting the definition by Sackett et al. (1996), Rychetnik et al. (2004) defined **evidence based public health** as "a public health endeavor in which there is an informed, explicit, and judicious use of evidence that has been derived from any of a variety of science and social science research and evaluation methods" (p. 538). Brownson et al. (2009) expanded the definition of evidence-based public health to include "making decisions on the basis of the best available evidence, using data and information systems, applying program planning frameworks, engaging the community in decision making, conducting evaluations, and disseminating what has been learned" (p. 175).

In a position statement on EBP, the Honor Society of Nursing, Sigma Theta Tau International, defined **evidence-based nursing** as "an integration of the best evidence available, nursing expertise, and the values and preferences of the individuals, families, and communities who are served" (Honor Society of Nursing, Sigma Theta Tau International, 2005). The definition of EBP continues to be broadened in scope and now includes a lifelong problem-solving approach to clinical practice, integrating both external and internal evidence to answer clinical questions and to achieve desired client outcomes (Melnyk & Fineout-Overholt, 2015; Melnyk et al., 2017). *External evidence* includes research and other evidence such as reports and professional guidelines, for example, whereas *internal evidence* includes the nurse's clinical experiences and the client's preferences.

Applied to nursing, **evidence-based practice** includes the best available evidence from a variety of sources, including research studies, nursing experience and expertise, and community leaders. Culturally and financially appropriate interventions need to be identified when working with communities. The use of evidence to determine the appropriate use of interventions that are culturally sensitive and cost-effective is essential.

EVIDENCE-BASED PRACTICE

The Community Guide is a resource to public health professionals to quickly assess the evidence-based findings of public health interventions. *The Community Guide* consists of a collection of systematic reviews conducted by the Community Preventive Services Task Force (CPSTF). Vaidya et al. (2017) sought to assess the quality of practice-based evidence (PBE) and research-based evidence (RBE) within *The Community Guide*. The researchers developed operational definitions for PBE and RBE, distinguishing RBE studies as those in which there was allocation to intervention and control conditions, whereas PBE studies were studies that assessed an intervention in practice to improve health or other outcomes without allocating individuals or groups to the intervention. The investigators categorized 3656 studies in 202 reviews completed since *The Community Guide* first began. Results showed that 54 percent of the studies were PBE and 46 percent RBE. Furthermore, the researchers noted that community-based and policy reviews used more PBE, whereas health care system and programmatic reviews had more RBE. The researchers concluded that the inclusion of PBE studies in *The Community Guide* reviews indicates that adequate rigor to inform practice is being produced thus increasing stakeholders' confidence that *The Community Guide* provides recommendations with real-world relevance.

Nurse Use

Public health nurses can be assured that the systematic reviews in *The Community Guide* provide high-quality recommendations with real-world practice relevance. Nurses can continue to add to the literature through conducting evaluative population-focused intervention studies.

Data from Vaidya N, Thota AB, Proia KK, et al.: Practice-based evidence in Community Guide systematic reviews. *Am J Public Health* 107(3): 413-420, 2017.

HISTORY OF EVIDENCE-BASED PRACTICE

During the mid- to late 1970s there was growing consensus among nursing leaders that scientific knowledge should be used as a basis for nursing practice. During that time the Division of Nursing in the U.S. Public Health Service began funding research utilization projects. **Research utilization** has been defined as "the process of transforming research knowledge into practice" (Stetler, 2001, p. 272) and "the use of research to guide clinical practice" (Estabrooks et al., 2004, p. 293).

Three projects funded by the Division of Nursing received the most attention and were the most influential in shaping nursing's view of using research to guide practice: the Nursing Child Assessment Satellite Training Project (NCAST) (Barnard & Hoehn, 1978; King et al., 1981), the Western Interstate Commission for Higher Education (WICHE) Regional Program for Nursing Research Development (WICHEN) (Krueger, 1977; Krueger et al., 1978; Lindeman & Krueger, 1977), and the Conduct and Utilization of Research in Nursing Project (CURN) (Horsley et al., 1978; Horsley et al., 1983). Using very different approaches and methods, each project tested interventions to facilitate research use in practice.

Although nursing continued to focus on research utilization projects, medicine also began to call for physicians to increase their use of scientific evidence to make clinical decisions. In the late 1970s, David Sackett, a medical doctor and clinical epidemiologist at McMaster University, published a series of articles in the *Canadian Medical Association Journal* describing how to read research articles in clinical journals. The term *critical appraisal* was used to describe the process of evaluating the validity and applicability of research studies (Guyatt & Rennie, 2002). Later, Sackett proposed the phrase "bringing critical appraisal to the bedside" to describe the application of evidence from medical literature to client care. This concept was used to train resident physicians at McMaster University and evolved into a "philosophy of medical practice based on knowledge and understanding of the medical literature supporting each clinical decision" (Guyatt & Rennie, 2002, p. xiv).

With Gordon Guyatt as Residency Director of Internal Medicine at McMaster, the decision was made to change the program to focus on "this new brand of medicine" that Guyatt eventually called *evidence-based medicine* (Guyatt & Rennie, 2002, p. xiv). Guyatt and Rennie described the goal of evidence-based medicine as being "aware of the evidence on which one's practice is based, the soundness of the evidence, and the strength of inference the evidence permits" (2002, p. xiv).

PARADIGM SHIFT IN USE OF EVIDENCE-BASED PRACTICE

In 1992 the Evidence-Based Medicine Working Group published an article in the *Journal of the American Medical Association* expanding the concept of evidence-based medicine and calling it a *paradigm shift*. A paradigm shift simply means a change from old ways of knowing to new ways of knowing and practicing. Ways of knowing in nursing have included the empirical knowledge, or the science of nursing; the aesthetic knowledge, or the art of nursing; personal knowledge, or interpersonal relationships and caring; and ethical knowledge, or moral and ethical codes of conduct usually established by professional organizations (Carper, 1978). Nursing practice in the past often focused less on science and more on the other four ways of knowing described here.

According to the Working Group (Evidence-Based Medicine Working Group, 1992), the old paradigm viewed unsystematic clinical observations as a valid way for "building and maintaining" knowledge for clinical decision making (p. 2421). In addition, principles of pathophysiology were seen as a "sufficient guide for clinical practice" (p. 2421). Training, common sense, and clinical experience were considered sufficient for evaluating clinical data and developing guidelines for clinical practice. The Working Group cited developments in research over the past 30 years as providing the foundation for the paradigm shift and a "new philosophy of medical practice" (p. 2421).

The new paradigm, evidence-based medicine, acknowledged clinical experience as a crucial but insufficient part of clinical decision making. Systematic and unbiased recording of clinical observations in the form of research will increase confidence in the knowledge gained from clinical experience. Principles of pathophysiology were seen as necessary but not sufficient knowledge for making clinical decisions. The Working Group emphasized that physicians needed to be able to critically appraise the research literature in order to appropriately apply research findings in practice. Knowledge gained from authoritative figures was also deemphasized in the new paradigm (Evidence-Based Medicine Working Group, 1992).

In the years since the Working Group began, the term *evidence-based practice* has been proposed as a term to integrate all health professions. The underlying principle was that high-quality care is based on evidence rather than on tradition or intuition (Chapman, 2018).

Nurses have always used various resources for problem solving. Intuition, trial and error, tradition, authority, institutional standards, prior knowledge, and clinical experience have often been used as the basis for decision making in clinical settings. However, not all of these resources are reliable, and all have not consistently produced desired outcomes (Bower & Nemec, 2017; Weiss et al., 2018). A procedure performed based on intuition or trial and error might be performed successfully sometimes and not at other times. For example, tradition and authority, which comes from texts and policy and procedure manuals, can lead to faulty clinical decision making.

Institutional standards are developed by accrediting agencies (e.g., The Joint Commission), by licensing agencies, and by professional organizations. These standards have been developed in the past primarily by expert opinion and past experiences. The standards may not reflect the best practices in the current environment or from the literature.

Although prior knowledge gained in educational programs, through continuing education, or through experience can be a good teacher, it can also contain bias and quickly become outdated unless a nurse participates in constantly refreshing knowledge. For example, just because a nurse has experience in successfully performing an intervention a certain way today does not mean it is the best way or that it will be successful every time and in the future unless practices are changed based on the most current data.

When EBP was first emphasized in medicine, the focus was on the answer to clinical questions concerning an individual client problem in order to provide the best diagnosis to implement the best treatment. When nursing became involved in EBP, the focus seemed to shift to answering a clinical question about a health problem experienced by a group of clients (Levin et al., 2010).

The current nursing literature on EBP is primarily associated with applications in the acute and primary care settings, and little is reported about its use in community settings. However, the basic principles of EBP can be applied at the individual level or at the community level. Although definitions of EBP vary widely in the literature, the common thread across disciplines is the application of the best available evidence to improve practice (Brower & Nemec, 2017; Makic et al., 2014; Zimmerman, 2017).

EBP has been described as both a process and a product (Dang & Dearholt, 2018; Scott & McSherry, 2009; Zimmerman, 2017). The product is the use of evidence to make practice changes, whereas the process is a systematic approach to locating, critiquing, synthesizing, translating, and evaluating evidence upon which to base practice changes. Systematic reviews of research evidence can potentially assist nurses in putting evidence into practice. Systematic reviews, also known as evidence summaries, provide reliable evidence-based summaries of past research, making it easier for health care professionals to stay current on best practices without having to read a lot of research papers (Holly et al., 2016).

Scott and McSherry (2009) engaged in a process using an extensive literature review to arrive at a definition of evidence-based nursing and to differentiate the definition from evidence-based practice. Based on their review they arrived at the following definition: evidence-based nursing is a process whereby evidence, nursing theory, and the nurse's clinical expertise are evaluated and used, in conjunction with the client's involvement, to make critical decisions about the best care for the client. Continuous evaluation of the implementation of care is essential to making clinical decisions about client care for the best possible outcomes. In Chapter 11 there is extensive discussion of an example of how public health nurses have developed and used evidence on which to base population-centered nursing.

TYPES OF EVIDENCE

No matter which definition of EBP is supported, what counts as evidence has been the issue most hotly debated. A hierarchy of evidence, ranked in order of decreasing importance and use, has been accepted by many health professionals. The double-blind **randomized controlled trial (RCT)** generally ranks as the highest level of evidence followed by other RCTs, nonrandomized clinical trials, quasi-experimental studies, case-controlled reports, qualitative studies, and expert opinion (Grove et al., 2015). Some nurses would argue that this hierarchy ignores evidence gained from clinical experience. However, the definition of evidence-based nursing presented previously indicates that clinical expertise as evidence, when used with other types of evidence, is used to make clinical decisions. Also in the hierarchy of evidence, expert opinion can be gained from non-research–based published articles, professional guidelines, national guidelines, organizational opinions, and panels of experts, as well as the nurse's clinical expertise.

Because it is difficult to find or perform RCTs in the community, other types of evidence have been highlighted as the best evidence in public health literature on which to base evidence-based public health practice: scientific literature found in systematic reviews, scientific literature used or quoted in one or more journal articles, public health surveillance data, program evaluations, qualitative data obtained from community members and other stakeholders, media/marketing data such as the results of a media campaign to reduce smoking, word of mouth, and personal/professional experience (Brownson et al., 2018).

Within public health practice, guidelines for finding and using evidence include the following:

- Engaging the community in assessment and decision making
- Using data and information systems systematically
- Making decisions on the basis of the best available peer-reviewed evidence (both quantitative and qualitative)
- Applying program planning frameworks (often based in health behavior theory)
- Conducting sound evaluation
- Disseminating what is learned (Brownson et al., 2018).

FACTORS LEADING TO CHANGE

EBP represents a cultural change in practice. It provides an environment to improve both nursing practice and client outcomes. Nursing is known for providing care based on environmental and client assessments; critical observations; development of questions or hypotheses to be explored; collecting data from the environment through community or organizational assessments, or from the client through history, physical assessment, and review of past heath records; analyzing the data to develop plans of care, whether for the individual client, family, group, or community; and drawing conclusions upon which to base care for the purpose of improving client outcomes (Bowers, 2018; Melnyk et al., 2017). However, several factors have been identified in the literature that support implementation of EBP or that will need to be overcome for nursing and other disciplines to successfully implement EBP. These factors include the following:

- Knowledge of research and current evidence
- Ability to interpret the meaning of the evidence
- Individual professional's characteristics, such as a willingness to change, or personal viewpoints about the quality and credibility of evidence
- Commitment of the time needed to implement EBP and to engage in education and directed practice
- The hierarchy of the practice environment and the level of support of managers and the ability to engage in autonomous practice
- The philosophy of the practice environment and the willingness to embrace EBP
- The resources available to engage in EBP, such as amount of work, proper equipment, computer-based EBP programs, and information systems
- The practice characteristics, such as leadership and colleague attitudes
- Links to outside supports such as teaching facilities like a teaching health department or a university
- Political constraints and the lack of relevant and timely public health practice research (Bowers, 2018; Duncombe, 2018; Kristensen et al., 2016; Melnyk et al., 2017; Pereira et al., 2018; Schaefer & Welton, 2018).

BARRIERS TO EVIDENCE-BASED PRACTICE

Although a community agency may subscribe in theory to the use of EBP, actual implementation may be affected by the realities of the practice setting. Community-focused nursing agencies may lack the resources needed for its implementation in the clinical setting, such as time, funding, computer resources, and knowledge. Nurses may be reluctant to accept findings and feel threatened when long-established practices are questioned. Cost can also be a barrier if the clinical decision or change will require more funds than the agency has available. Compliance can be a barrier if the client will not follow the recommended intervention. Public health departments are moving toward EBP and are seeking accreditation through the national public health accreditation board. The accreditation process began in 2011. As of August 2018, 235 health departments and 1 statewide integrated local public health department system had achieved national accreditation (Public Health Accreditation Board, 2018).

STEPS IN THE EVIDENCE-BASED PRACTICE PROCESS

EBP is a philosophy of practice that respects client values (Melnyk et al., 2010). The seven-step EBP process was described as follows:

0. Cultivating a spirit of inquiry
1. Asking clinical questions
2. Searching for the best evidence
3. Critically appraising the evidence
4. Integrating the evidence with clinical expertise and client preferences and values
5. Evaluating the outcomes of the practice decisions or changes based on evidence
6. Disseminating EBP results (Melnyk & Fineout-Overholt, 2015)

Yes, their first step is step 0. This process was initially described as a five-step process by others (Dawes et al., 2004; Dicenso et al., 2005). The unique features of the Melnyk et al. (2010) model are the emphasis on the spirit of inquiry and the sharing of the results of the process (Melnyk & Fineout-Overholt, 2015).

Step 0 involves a curiosity about the interventions that are being applied. Do they work, or is there a better approach? In public health nursing, for example, are there better parenting outcomes if the parents attend classes at the health department? Or are home visits to new mothers and babies more effective for achieving a healthy baby? Step 1 requires asking questions in a "PICOT" format.

Although Melnyk et al. (2010) developed a specific process for the PICOT, the process was first described by Sackett (1996), who discussed the need to define the *(P)opulation* of interest, the *(I)ntervention* or practice strategy in question, the population or intervention to be used for *(C)omparision*, the *(O)utcome* desired, and the *(T)ime frame.* Step 2 involves searching for the best evidence to answer the question. This step involves searching the literature. In the case of the previous example, a literature search would focus on a search of key terms like *public health nursing, parenting of new babies, parenting classes,* and *home visits.* Step 3 requires a critical appraisal of the evidence found in step 2.

To appraise the literature found, Melnyk and Fineout-Overholt (2015) suggest asking three questions about each of the articles found in the literature search: (1) the validity, (2) the importance, and (3) whether or not the results of the article will help you as a nurse provide quality care for your clients. Step 4 is the step in which the evidence found is integrated with clinical expertise and client values. Institutional standards and practice guidelines, as well as cost of care and support of the health care environment to implement the findings, are all factors considered in this step. Step 5 requires an evaluation of the outcomes of practice decisions and changes that were based on the answers to the first four steps. The goal in evaluation is a positive change in quality of care and health care outcomes. For example, in a randomized controlled study evaluating the effects of a home visit program on asthma outcomes and costs for children with uncontrolled asthma, researchers noted the program improved health outcomes and reduced urgent care use and costs (Campbell et al., 2015).

Step 6 is disseminating outcomes of the results to others, to colleagues, to the employing agency's administration, to faculty and other students, and through a poster or podium presentation of student nurse organizations or professional organizations. Professional organizations often sponsor student presentations for undergraduates as well as graduate students. Sharing of information is most important because it prevents each individual nurse from trying to find the best answer to the same question answered by someone else, and it gives us the basis for asking new questions. Sharing makes practice more efficient and improves quality and health care outcomes.

In a busy community practice setting it is often difficult for nurses to access evidence-based resources. Using evidence-based clinical practice guidelines is one way for nurses to provide evidence-based nursing care in an efficient manner. Clinical practice guidelines are usually developed by a group of experts in the field who have reviewed the evidence and made recommendations based on the best available evidence. The recommendations are usually graded according to the quality and quantity of the evidence.

Approaches to Finding Evidence

Returning to the previous example, the clinical question has been stated, and the population has been defined as new mothers and babies. Two interventions will be compared. The outcome is stated as healthy babies, and the time frame may be 6 months or 1 year or another time at which the outcomes of the interventions will be evaluated.

Four approaches are described that allow the nurse to read research/nonresearch evidence in a condensed format. The first, a **systematic review**, is "a method of identifying, appraising, and synthesizing research evidence. The aim is to evaluate and interpret all available research that is relevant to a particular research question" (Cochrane Library, 2018). A systematic review is usually done by more than one person and describes the methods used to search for and evaluate the evidence. Systematic reviews can be accessed from most databases, such as Medline and CINAHL.

The Cochrane Library is an electronic database that contains regularly updated evidence-based health care databases maintained by the Cochrane Collaboration, a not-for-profit organization (http://www.cochrane.org). The Cochrane Library is composed of three main branches: systematic reviews, trials register, and methodology database. The Cochrane Library publishes systematic reviews on a wide variety of topics. Systematic reviews differ from traditional literature review publications in that systematic reviews require more rigor and contain less opinion of the author. Systematic reviews for public health can be found in the Guide to Community Preventive Services, the Cochrane Public Health Group, the Centre for Reviews and Dissemination, and the Campbell Collaboration (Box 10.1).

BOX 10.1 Resources for Implementing Evidence-Based Practice

The following resources can assist nurses in developing evidence-based nursing practice:

1. *PubMed* (http://www.pubmed.gov/) is a bibliographical database developed and maintained by the National Library of Medicine. Bibliographical information from Medline is covered in PubMed and includes references for nursing, medicine, dentistry, the health care system, and preclinical sciences. Full texts of referenced articles are often included. Searches can be limited to type of evidence (e.g., diagnosis, therapy) and systematic reviews.
2. The *Cochrane Database of Systematic Reviews* is a collection of more than 1000 systematic reviews of effects in health care internationally. These reviews are accessible at a cost via the website (http://www.cochrane.org). Nurses may also have free access from a medical library.
3. The *Evidence-Based Nursing Journal* (http://ebn.bmjjournals.com/) is published quarterly. The purpose of the journal is to select articles reporting studies and reviews from health-related literature that warrant immediate attention by nurses attempting to keep pace with advances in their profession. Using predefined criteria, the best quantitative and qualitative original articles are abstracted in a structured format, commented on by clinical experts, and shared in a timely fashion. The research questions, methods, results, and evidence-based conclusions are reported. The website for the journal is http://www.evidencebasednursing.com.
4. The Honor Society of Nursing, Sigma Theta Tau International, sponsors the online peer-reviewed journal *Worldviews on Evidence-Based Nursing* that publishes systematic reviews and research articles on best evidence that supports nursing practice globally. The journal is available by subscription (https://www.sigmanursing.org/).
5. The *Community Preventive Services Task Force* is an independent, nonfederal task force appointed by the director of the Centers for Disease Control and Prevention (CDC). Information about the Task Force may be found at the website http://www.thecommunityguide.org. The Task Force is charged with determining the topics to be addressed by *The Community Guide* and the most appropriate means to assess evidence regarding population-based interventions. The Task Force reviews and assesses the quality of available evidence on the effects of essential community preventive services. The multidisciplinary Task Force determines the scope of *The Community Guide,* which will be used by health departments and agencies to determine best practices for preventive health in populations.
6. The *U.S. Preventive Services Task Force (USPSTF)* is an independent panel of private-sector experts in prevention and primary care. The USPSTF conducts rigorous, impartial assessments of the scientific evidence for the effectiveness of a broad range of clinical preventive services, including screening, counseling, and preventive medications. Its recommendations are considered the "gold standard" for clinical preventive services. The mission of the USPSTF is to evaluate the benefits of individual services based on age, gender, and risk factors for disease; make recommendations about which preventive services should be incorporated routinely into primary medical care and for which populations; and identify a research agenda for clinical preventive care. Recommendations of the USPSTF are published as the *Guide to Clinical Preventive Services.* The guide is available online at https://www.ahrq.gov.
7. The *Centers for Disease Control and Prevention* (https://www.cdc.gov) publishes guidelines on immunizations and sexually transmitted diseases. Guidelines are developed by experts in the field appointed by the U.S. Department of Health and Human Services and the CDC.
8. *Cochrane Public Health Review Group (PHRG),* formerly the health promotion and public health field, aims to work with contributors to produce and publish Cochrane reviews of the effects of population-level public health interventions. The PHRG undertakes systematic reviews of the effects of public health interventions to improve health and other outcomes at the population level, not those targeted at individuals. Thus it covers interventions seeking to address macroenvironmental and distal social environmental factors that influence health. In line with the underlying principles of public health, these reviews seek to have a significant focus on equity and aim to build the evidence to address the social determinants of health. (Visit http://www.ph.cochrane.org/.)
9. *Centre for Reviews and Dissemination (CRD)* is part of the National Institute for Health Research and is a department of the University of York. CRD, which was established in 1994, is one of the largest groups in the world engaged exclusively in evidence synthesis in the health field. CRD undertakes systematic reviews evaluating the research evidence on health and public health questions of national and international importance. (Visit http://www.york.ac.uk.)
10. *Campbell Collaboration,* named after Donald Campbell, was founded on the principle that systematic reviews on the effects of interventions will inform and help improve policy and services. The collaboration strives to make the best social science research available and accessible. Campbell reviews provide high-quality evidence of what works to meet the needs of service providers, policy makers, educators and their students, professional researchers, and the general public. Areas of interest include crime, justice, education, and social welfare. (Visit http://www.campbellcollaboration.org/.)
11. The *Putting Public Health Evidence in Action Training Workshop* is an interactive training curriculum created by the Cancer Prevention and Control Research Network to support program planners and health educators in using evidence-based approaches. (Visit http://cpcrn.org.)

HOW TO Develop an Evidence-Based Practice Guide for a Community Preventive Service

- Form a coordination team to guide the review process
- Develop a conceptual framework, called a logic model for the review
- Identify and select interventions that the review will cover
- Define and develop a conceptual approach for evaluating the interventions, called an analytic framework
- Identify criteria for including and excluding studies
- Use the criteria to search for, retrieve, and screen abstracts
- Review the full text of every study and code the data from each using *The Community Guide* abstraction form
- Assess the quality of each study
- Summarize all of the evidence found, called the body of evidence
- Identify issues of applicability and barriers to implementation (when available) for recommended interventions
- Summarize information about other benefits or harms that might result from the interventions
- Identify and summarize evidence gaps
- Develop recommendations and findings
- Conduct an economic evaluation of the interventions found to be effective

From Community Preventive Services Task Force: *Our methodology: what are the steps in The Community Guide review process,* 2018. Available at https://www.thecommunityguide.org.

The second approach, **meta-analysis**, is a specific method of statistical synthesis used in some systematic reviews, where the results from several studies are quantitatively combined and summarized (Grove, et al., 2015). A well-designed systematic review or meta-analysis can provide stronger evidence than a single randomized controlled trial.

The integrative review is a form of a systematic review that does not have the summary statistics found in the meta-analysis because of the limitations of the studies that are reviewed (e.g., small sample size of the population). Narrative review is a review done on published papers that support the reviewer's particular point of view or opinion and is used to provide a general discussion of the topic reviewed. This review does not often include an explicit or systematic review process.

Undergraduate students often perform narrative reviews. However, it is important to learn the process for systematic reviews, especially the use of the results of systematic reviews. Reading systematic reviews that have been completed is helpful in answering the question related to the EBP process (Pierce, 2018).

What counts as evidence has also been argued in the public health literature (Brownson et al., 2018). RCTs, which are the highest level of evidence used to make clinical decisions, are appropriate for evaluating many interventions in medicine but are often inappropriate for evaluating public health interventions. For example, an RCT can be designed ethically to test a new medication for diabetes, but not for a smoking cessation intervention. In a smoking cessation intervention, subjects could not be assigned randomly to smoking or nonsmoking groups because a smoking cessation intervention is not appropriate for someone who does not smoke. In this situation, a case-control study would be most appropriate (see Chapter13). Today there are many community-based clinical trials assisting in finding answers to the questions of which population-level intervention has the best outcomes. (Visit the CDC website to review these trials.)

HOW TO Develop an Evidence-Based Protocol

Evidence-based protocols are a recognized approach to providing quality client care. Such protocols enhance the abilities of providers and can reduce health care errors. The following are steps to developing a protocol:

- Enlist committed leadership support that ensures consistent staff participation in the EBP process.
- Develop a committed team that works together for a set time period (e.g., 1 year) to discuss and evaluate practice protocols.
- Identify a clinical issue.
- Identify current policies, protocols, and resources related to the clinical issue.
- Recognize current practices, identifying gaps and additional resources needed to follow best-practice guidelines.
- Develop a protocol that logically follows the flow of patient care and coincides with the caregivers' thought processes.
- Align patient education materials with the new protocol.
- Develop effective dissemination methods, such as providing education and reminders of new protocol, role-modeling changes, and gathering feedback from clinicians.
- Implement the protocol.
- Establish evaluation and sustainability practices for the new protocol, such as through use of a checklist to monitor adherence and identify additional education needs.

From Dols JD, Muñoz LR, Martinez SS, et al.: Developing policies and protocols in the age of evidence-based practice. *J Contin Educ Nurs* 48(2):87-92, 2017.

Approaches to Evaluating Evidence

One approach used in evaluating evidence is grading the strength of evidence. When evidence is graded, the evidence is assigned a "grade" based on the number and type of well-designed studies and the presence of similar findings in all of the studies. Grading evidence has been debated so strongly that in 2002 the Agency for Healthcare Research and Quality (AHRQ) commissioned a study to describe existing systems used to evaluate the usefulness of studies and strength of evidence. The report reviewed 40 systems and identified three domains for evaluating systems for the grading of evidence: quality, quantity, and consistency (West et al., 2002). The *quality* of a study refers to the extent to which bias is minimized. *Quantity* refers to the number of studies, the magnitude of the effect, and the sample size. *Consistency* refers to studies that have similar findings, using similar and different study designs (Haine-Schlagel et al., 2014).

As indicated, many frameworks exist for evaluating the strength and the usefulness of the evidence found in the literature and other sources, such as professional standards. A popular framework was developed by the Agency for Healthcare Quality. Fineout-Overholt et al. (2010) have also developed an approach for evaluating evidence. Although these approaches vary in the factors they evaluate, the best approach to choose is one that evaluates not only the strength but also the usefulness of the evidence. Table 10.1 provides an example of an approach for evaluating evidence.

The strength of the literature is measured by the type of evidence it represents. For example, the RCT is the evidence that has the greatest strength upon which to make a clinical decision. In contrast, opinion articles, descriptive studies, and professional reports of expert committees have less strength. The usefulness of the evidence is measured by whether the evidence is valid, whether it is important, and whether it can be used to assist in making practice decisions or changes in the community environment and with the population of interest to improve outcomes (Melnyk et al., 2017).

The best RCT conducted in a hospital setting on using an intervention to prevent falls may not be applicable at all in a community setting. Therefore although it may be a strong study with outcomes that improve health, it may not have the usefulness for applicability in the community because of the setting in which it was conducted.

Shaughnessy et al. (1994) proposed criteria for evaluating the usefulness of evidence, calling the process *patient-oriented evidence that matters* (POEM). In general, the reader should ask the following questions: "What are the results? (Are they important?) Are the results valid? How can the results be applied to client care?" (p. 489). POEMs research summaries can be found at https://www.essentialevidenceplus.com (Essential Evidence Plus, 2018). Brownson et al. (2009) proposed that the following questions be asked for EBP (plus suggested application examples):

- What is the size of the public health problem? What is the need for improved health outcomes for new mothers and babies in our community?
- Can interventions be found in the literature to address the problem (e.g., home visits or parenting classes)?

TABLE 10.1 Typology for Classifying Interventions by Level of Scientific Evidence

Type/Category	Strength/How Established	Considerations for the Level of Scientific Evidence—Quality	Quantity/Consistency Data Source Examples
Evidence-based I	Peer review via systematic or narrative review	Based on study design and execution External validity Potential side benefits or harms Costs and cost-effectiveness	*Community Guide to Clinical Preventive Services* Cochrane reviews Narrative reviews based on published literature
Effective II	Peer review	Based on study design and execution External validity Potential side benefits or harms Costs and cost-effectiveness	Articles in the scientific literature Research-tested intervention programs (123) Technical reports with peer review
Promising III	Written program evaluation without formal peer review	Summative evidence of effectiveness Formative evaluation data Theory-consistent, plausible, potentially high-reach, low-cost, replicable	State or federal government reports (without peer review) Conference presentations
Emerging IV	Ongoing work, practice-based summaries, or evaluation works in progress	Formative evaluation data Theory-consistent, plausible, potentially high-reaching, low-cost, replicable Face validity	Evaluability assessments Pilot studies NIH CRISP database Projects funded by health foundations

CRISP, The Computer Retrieval of Information on Scientific Projects *NIH,* National Institutes of Health.
From Brownson RC, Fielding JE, Maylahn CM: Evidence-based public health: a fundamental concept for public health practice. *Annu Rev Public Health* 30:175-201, 2009.

- Is the intervention useful in this community, with this population, or with populations at risk (e.g., the low income or uninsured)?
- Is the intervention the best one, or are there other ways to address the problem considering cost and potential health outcomes for the population? (Assess cost and health outcomes of both of the interventions before choosing, including the nurses available to make home visits or who have the skills to teach the parenting class.)

Multiple variables are considered important in determining the quality of evidence used to make clinical decisions (Polit and Beck, 2017):

- *Sample selection:* Sample selection should be as unbiased as possible. For example, a sample is randomly selected when each subject has an equal chance of being selected from the population of interest. Random selection offers the least bias of any type of sample selection. Other types of sample selection such as convenience sampling contain researcher or evaluator bias.
- *Randomization:* When testing an intervention, randomly assign participants to either the intervention or control group. This type of assignment is less biased than if participants are allowed to choose the group they want to join.
- *Blinding:* The researcher or evaluator should not know which participants are in the experimental (treatment) group or which are in the control group. The researcher or evaluator is "blinded" as to who is receiving the treatment and who is not receiving the treatment.
- *Sample size:* The sample size should be large enough to show an effect of the intervention. In general, the larger the sample size, the better.
- *Description of intervention:* The intervention should be described in detail and explicitly enough that another person could duplicate the study if desired.
- *Outcomes:* The outcomes should be measured accurately.
- *Length of follow-up:* Depending on the intervention, the participants should be followed for a long enough period of time to determine if the intervention continued to work or if the results just happened by chance.
- *Attrition:* Few subjects should have dropped out of the study.
- *Confounding variables:* Variables that could affect the outcome should be accounted for either by statistical methods or by study measurements.
- *Statistical analysis:* Statistical analysis should be appropriate to determine the desired outcome.

CHECK YOUR PRACTICE

Exploring the Evidence

You are the chief public health nurse for the local health department in a community with a high rate of sexually transmitted infections (STIs) among the adolescent population.

There is a law in your state requiring abstinence-only education in public schools.

The board of education approaches you, questioning why the rate is high, what is being done to reduce the rate, and how the public school system might help in reducing the rate. WHAT WOULD YOU DO?

- What data would you need to investigate the high STI rate?
- What evidence-based interventions could you recommend to the school board? Is abstinence-only education a recommended evidence-based intervention to reduce STI risk?

APPROACHES TO IMPLEMENTING EVIDENCE-BASED PRACTICE

The first step toward implementing EBP in nursing is recognizing the current status of one's own practice and believing

QSEN FOCUS ON QUALITY AND SAFETY EDUCATION FOR NURSES

Targeted Competency: Evidence-Based Practice

Integrate best current evidence with clinical expertise and client and family preferences and values for delivery of optimal interventions.

Important aspects of EBP include:

- **Knowledge:** Describe EBP to include the components of research evidence, clinical expertise, and client and family values.
- **Skills:** Locate evidence reports related to clinical practice topics and guidelines.
- **Attitudes:** Value the need for continuous improvement in clinical practice based on new knowledge.

Evidence-Based Practice Question

As a nurse in the community, you are working within a Hispanic community that has a high prevalence of gestational diabetes. You decide to initiate a focus group with clients who attend the obstetrics and gynecology clinic at the health department to explore potential gestational diabetes intervention for this community.

1. Go to *The Community Guide* website at https://www.thecommunityguide.org. This website is a collection of evidence-based findings from the Community Preventive Services Task Force (CPSTF).
2. On the home page, click on the "topics" drop-down menu and select "diabetes."
3. Click on the "Diabetes Prevention: Lifestyle Interventions to Reduce Risk of Gestation Diabetes" 2017 systematic review.
4. Review and summarize the CPSTF findings and considerations for implementation.
5. What baseline data might you gather from your focus group participants to be best informed in how to tailor the evidence-based recommendations for this community?

Answer

- The CPSTF findings indicate strong evidence for lifestyle interventions that provide supervised exercise classes, either alone or in combination with other components, and sufficient evidence for lifestyle interventions that provide education and counseling for diet or physical activity, diet activities, or a combination of these components
- Understanding the common facilitators and barriers to the recommended lifestyle interventions for this community is a good starting place. How many participants are able to get the recommended about of exercise each week? What helps those who are able to exercise (e.g., childcare, affordable classes, accessible classes)? For those unable to exercise, what stands in their way (e.g., time, money, lack of social support)? What types of food do they eat? How do these lifestyle behaviors compare to the recommendations in *The Community Guide*?
- Developing an intervention with assistance from leaders in the community would be a helpful strategy. It will likely be more accepted and impactful if the EBP guidelines are tailored to the specific needs of the community.

Originally prepared by Gail Armstrong, PhD(c), DNP, ACNS-BC, CNE, Associate Professor, University of Colorado Denver College of Nursing. Updated in 2018 by Lisa Turner, PhD, RN, PHCNS-BC, Associate Professor, Berea College.

that care based on the best evidence will lead to improved client outcomes (Melnyk et al., 2010; Melnyk & Fineout-Overholt, 2015; Melnyk et al., 2017). Since EBP is a relatively new concept, many practicing nurses are not familiar with the application of EBP and may lack computer and Internet skills necessary to implement EBP. Also, implementation will be successful only when nurses practice in an environment that supports evidence-based care. Public health nurses consider EBP a process to improve practice and outcomes and use the evidence to influence policies that will improve the health of communities.

CURRENT PERSPECTIVES

Cost Versus Quality

Much of the pressure to use EBP comes from third-party payers and is a response to the need to contain costs and reduce legal liability. Nurses must question whether the current agenda to contain health care costs creates pressure to focus on those research results that favor cost saving at the expense of quality outcomes for clients. Outcomes include client and community satisfaction and the safety of care. Costs can be weighed against outcomes when EBP is used to show the best practices available to reduce possible harm to clients (Makic et al., 2014; Melnyk, 2017).

Individual Differences

EBP cannot be applied as a universal remedy without attention to client differences. When EBP is applied at the community level, best evidence may point to a solution that is not sensitive to cultural issues and distinctions and thus may not be acceptable to the community. Ethical practice in communities requires attention to community differences.

LEVELS OF PREVENTION

Using Evidence-Based Practice

According to evidence collected by the Community Preventive Services Task Force, the following are interventions supported by the literature at each level of prevention:

Primary Prevention

Extended and extensive mass media campaigns reduce youth initiation of tobacco use.

Secondary Prevention

Client reminders and recalls via mail, telephone, e-mail, or a combination of these strategies are effective in increasing compliance with screening activities, such as those for colorectal and breast cancer.

Tertiary Prevention

Diabetes self-management education in community gathering places improves glycemic control.

From Community Preventive Services Task Force: *The Community Guide*. Available at https://www.thecommunityguide.org; https://www.cdc.gov.

Appropriate Evidence-Based Practice Methods for Population-Centered Nursing Practice. Gaining a number of perspectives in a situated community is important for nurses using EBP. Nursing has a legitimate role to play in interprofessional community-focused practice and can contribute to its

LINKING CONTENT TO PRACTICE

It is important for nurses to acknowledge and understand EBP. They can participate by applying EBP or they can add to the research base for public health through active programs of research, participating in systematic reviews, or reviewing the best evidence available to them by reading published systematic reviews. Nurses can demonstrate leadership in supporting EBP by becoming change agents, fostering a cultural change in the practice environment, and assisting nurses who do not know how to use EBP to make a difference in practice.

For example, nurses who have recently graduated are knowledgeable about the use of evidence in practice. The new nurses can assist nurses who have been out of school for a while to find sources of evidence upon which to base their practice, such as referring them to *The Community Guide*. Using evidence in practice will demonstrate its value, but implementation can be difficult because of the sheer volume of evidence and increasing population needs. Sharing knowledge and engaging in teamwork can help overcome these barriers.

Nurses have an important role to play in developing and using clinical guidelines for community practices. Use of a community development model and engaging in community partnerships will ensure that the community's perspective is included (see Chapter 17).

Nurses active in EBP can devote attention to understanding how best to incorporate the guidelines into practice demonstrating practice excellence. EBP offers the opportunity for shared decision making because it can help nurses focus their thinking, observe process outcomes, and thus improve care for clients by communicating with leaders and other nurses what they have observed. Participation in EBP offers continuing professional growth and a feeling of value, recognition for contributions, and respect from peers and administrators (Dols et al., 2017; Melnyk et al., 2017).

From Dols JD, Munoz LR, Martinez SS, et al.: Developing policies and protocols in the age of evidence-based practice, *J Contin Educ Nurs* 48(2):87-92, 2017; Melnyk BM, Gallager-Ford L, Fineout-Overholt E: *Implementing the evidence-based practice competencies in healthcare—a practical guide for improving quality, safety, & outcomes*, Indianapolis, IN, 2017, Sigma Theta Tau International.

evidence base. Nurses are obliged to ensure that the evidence applied to practice is acceptable to the community. Establishing an EBP culture depends on the use of both qualitative and quantitative research approaches or the best evidence available at the time. For example, a quantitative research study of a community health center could provide information about patterns of client use, the cost of various services, and the use of different health care providers. However, when quantitative research is combined with qualitative research, the nurse can gain an understanding of *why* clients use or do not use the services and help the health center be both clinically effective and cost-effective. Evidence from multiple research methods has the potential to enrich the application of evidence and improve nursing practice (Weiss et al., 2018).

The rising cost of health care will demand a more critical look at the benefits and costs of EBP. Finding resources to implement EBP will continue to be a challenge requiring creative strategies. An emphasis on quality care, equal distribution of health care resources, and cost control will continue. Implementing EBP can assist nurses in addressing these issues in the clinical setting. However, EBP can save money by providing the best care possible.

As nurses implement EBP in an environment focused on cost savings, the potential for governments, managed care organizations, or other health care agencies to endorse reimbursement of health care options solely on the basis of cost, without allowing for individual variation or considering environmental issues, will continue to be a concern. Nurses must use caution in adopting EBP in a prescriptive manner in different community environments. One aspect of the Affordable Care Act (PL 111-148) addresses the development of task forces on preventive services and community preventive services to develop, update, and disseminate EBP recommendations on the use of community preventive services. In addition, grant programs to support EBP delivery in the community are addressed in the Affordable Care Act of 2010.

Although the Internet is one source of evidence data (see Box 10.1), there may be a lack of quality indicators to evaluate the myriad websites claiming to contain evidence-based information. It is essential to evaluate the quantity of the information on the website, whether it comes from a reputable agency or scholar, and whether the source of the website has a financial interest in the acceptance of the evidence presented. (Refer to Chapter 19 on health education, which discusses the Internet as a source of data and how to evaluate its usefulness and reliability.)

HEALTHY PEOPLE 2020 OBJECTIVES

Healthy People 2020 objectives offer a systematic approach to health improvement. See the Healthy People 2020 box for the most recent objectives to improve clients' understanding of EBP and how they can contribute to health care decisions.

HEALTHY PEOPLE 2020

Information access is important to assure clients and communities have the correct information to make EBP health care decisions. The *Healthy People 2020* objectives related to providing resources are as follows:

- **HC/HIT-6.3:** Increase the proportion of persons who use electronic personal health management tools.
- **HC/HIT-4:** Increase the proportion of patients whose doctor recommends personalized health information resources to help them manage their health.
- **HC/HIT-12:** Increase the proportion of crisis and emergency risk messages, intended to protect the public's health, that demonstrate the use of best practices.
- **HC/HIT-11:** Increase the proportion of meaningful users of health information technology.
- **HC/HIT-13:** Increase the social marketing in health promotion and disease prevention.

From U.S. Department of Health and Human Services: *Healthy People 2020: roadmap to improving all Americans' health,* Washington, DC, 2010, U.S. Government Printing Office.

EXAMPLE OF APPLICATION OF EVIDENCE-BASED PRACTICE TO PUBLIC HEALTH NURSING

Chapter 11 describes the Intervention Wheel, a population-based practice model for public health nursing. The model consists of three levels of practice at the community, systems, and individual/family levels. It also consists of 17 public health interventions for improving population health. The model was originally developed using a qualitative grounded theory process but did not include a systematic review of evidence to support the interventions or their application to practice. Initially, the model was developed from an extensive analysis of the actual work of 200 practicing public health nurses working in a variety of settings. The 17 interventions grew out of this analysis, as did the three levels of practice. The authors indicated that the original intent was to provide a description of the scope and breadth of public health nursing practice.

Because of the positive response to the Intervention Wheel, the decision was made to complete a systematic review of the evidence supporting the use of the Intervention Wheel. The goal was to examine the evidence underlying the interventions and the levels of practice. The systematic review involved answering six questions, a comprehensive search of literature, a survey of 51 bachelor of science in nursing (BSN) programs in 5 states, and a critique (by 5 graduate students) of the 665 pieces of evidence found in the literature review for rigor (strength and usefulness). After limiting the final review to 221 sources of evidence, each source was independently rated by at least 2 members of a 42-member panel of practicing public health nurses and educators. The 42-member panel met to reach consensus on the outcomes of the reviews. The outcomes were field-tested with 150 practicing nurses and then critiqued by a national panel of 20 experts.

TABLE 10.2 Core Public Health Functions and Related Evidence-Based Nursing Interventions

Core Functions	Related Nursing Interventions
Assessment	Diagnose and investigate health problems and hazards in the community.
	Mobilize community partnerships to identify and solve health problems.
	Link people to needed health services.
	Use evidence-based practice for new insights and innovative solutions to health problems.
Policy development	Inform, educate, and empower communities about health issues.
	Develop policies and plans using evidence-based practice that supports individual and community health efforts.
Assurance	Monitor health status to identify community health problems.
	Enforce laws and regulations that protect health and ensure safety.
	Ensure the provision of health care that is otherwise unavailable.
	Ensure a competent public health and personal health care workforce.
	Use evidence-based practice to evaluate effectiveness, accessibility, and quality of personal and population-based services.

The Intervention Wheel presented in Chapter 11 is the result of this systematic review and critique (Keller et al., 2004). Although this critique may appear overwhelming, the undergraduate or graduate student may be involved in such a systematic critique as one of many participants contributing to the outcome of such a review. Table 10.2 applies some of the interventions to the core functions of public health.

PRACTICE APPLICATION

A nurse who is the director of a public health clinic is in the process of analyzing how best to expand services to operate as a full-time clinic in the most cost-effective and clinically effective manner. The director gathers evidence from the literature on public health clinics in rural settings to evaluate cost and clinical effectiveness of various models. The nurse also considers evidence from the following sources in the decision-making process: client satisfaction research data, knowledge of clinic staff, expert opinion of community advisory board members, evidence from community partners, and data on service needs in the state. Having examined the evidence, the nurse decides that incremental (step-by-step) growth toward full-time status is warranted. Evidence of needs in the community and analysis of statistical data indicate that the addition of wellness services for children is a priority, and a pediatric nurse practitioner is hired as a first step to assist the public health nurses while planning for full-time status continues.

A. Evaluation of the evidence gathered demonstrates which of the following?

1. Effectiveness of the intervention in communities
2. Application of the data to populations and communities
3. Existence of positive or negative health outcomes
4. Economic consequences of the intervention
5. Barriers to implementation of the interventions in communities

B. Explain how this example applies principles of EBP.

Answers can be found on the Evolve site.

KEY POINTS

- Evidence-based practice(EBP) was developed in other countries before its use in the United States.
- The Institute of Medicine has indicated that by 2020, 90 percent of all health care should be evidence based.
- EBP is a paradigm shift in health care and nursing.
- EBP is both a process and a product.
- Application of EBP in relation to clinical decision making in population-centered nursing concentrates on interventions and strategies geared to communities and populations rather than to individuals.
- Nurses at all levels have an opportunity to improve the practice of nursing and client outcomes.
- The EBP process has seven steps.
- Approaches to EBP include systematic review, meta-analysis, integrative review, and narrative review.
- Evaluating the strength and usefulness of evidence is essential to finding the best evidence on which to make practice decisions.
- Cost and quality of care are issues in EBP.
- EBP includes interventions based on theory, expert opinions, provider knowledge, and research.
- Use of a community development model and community partnership model involves community leaders in making decisions about best practices in their community.
- The Intervention Wheel is an example of a result of EBP.
- Health care reform supports EBP.

CLINICAL DECISION-MAKING ACTIVITIES

1. Give an example of how undergraduates can be involved in EBP.
2. Explain how the nurse's knowledge of the community relates to EBP. Give examples.
3. What are the barriers to implementing EBP? How can these barriers be resolved?
4. Is the cost or quality of care more important in EBP? Debate this issue with classmates.
5. When working with a community to improve its health, is it more important to consider the perspectives of the community or those of the provider when defining health problems? Elaborate.
6. Invite the director of nursing from the local health department to speak to your class. Ask if evidence is used to develop nursing policies and practice guidelines. If not, why not?
7. Explain how you can apply evidence to your practice.

ADDITIONAL RESOURCES

EVOLVE WEBSITE

http://evolve.elsevier.com/Stanhope/community/

- Answers to Practice Application
- Case Study
- Glossary
- Review Questions

REFERENCES

Barnard K, Hoehn R: *Nursing Child Assessment Satellite Training: Final Report*, Hyattsville, MD, 1978, DHEW, Division of Nursing.

Bowers B: Evidence-based practice in community nursing, *Br J Community Nurs* 23(7): 336–337, 2018.

Brooke JM, Mallion J: Implementation of evidence-based practice by nurses working in community settings and their strategies to mentor student nurses to develop evidence-based practice: a qualitative study, *Int J Nurs Pract* 22(4):339–347, 2016.

Brower EJ, Nemec R: Origins of evidence-based practices and what it means for nurses, *Int J of Childbirth Educ 32*(2):14–18, 2017.

Brownson RC, Baker EA, Deshpande AD, Gillespie KN: *Evidence-based public health*, ed 3, New York, 2018, Oxford University Press.

Brownson RC, Fielding JE, Maylahn CM: Evidence-based public health: a fundamental concept for public health practice, *Annu Rev Public Health* 30:175–202, 2009.

Campbell JD, Brooks M, Hosokawa P, Robinson J, Song L, Krieger J: Community health worker home visits for Medicaid-enrolled children with asthma: effects on asthma outcomes and costs, *Am J Public Health* 105(11):2366–2372, 2015.

Carper BA: Fundamental patterns of knowing in nursing, *ANS Adv Nurs Sci* 1(1):13–23, 1978.

Chapman A: Evidence based practice and public health, *HLG Nursing Bulletin* 37(3/4):90–93, 2018.

Community Preventive Services Task Force (CPSTF): *The Community Guide*, 2018. Retrieved from http://www.thecommunityguide.org.

Cochrane Library: *Cochrane handbook for systematic reviews of interventions*, 2018. Retrieved from www.cochrane.org.

Dang D, Dearholt SL: *Johns Hopkins nursing evidence-based practice*, ed 3, Indianapolis, IN, 2018, Sigma Theta Tau International.

Davidson JE, Brown C: Evaluation of nurse engagement in evidence-based practice, *AACN Adv Crit Care* 25(1):43–55, 2014.

Dawes M, Davies P, Gray A, et al: *Evidence-Based Practice: a Primer for Health Care Professionals*, ed 2, London, 2004, Churchill Livingstone Elsevier.

Dicenso A, Guyatt G, Ciliska D, editors: *Evidence-Based Nursing: a Guide to Clinical Practice*, St. Louis, MO, 2005, Elsevier Mosby.

Duncombe DC: A multi-institutional study of the perceived barriers and facilitators to implementing evidence-based practice, *J Clin Nurs* 27(5/6):1216–1226, 2018.

Essential Evidence Plus: *POEMs research summaries*, 2018. Retrieved from https://www.essentialevidenceplus.com.

Estabrooks CA, Winther C, Derksen L: Mapping the field: a bibliometric analysis of the research utilization literature in nursing, *Nurs Res* 53:293–303, 2004.

Evidence-Based Medicine Working Group: Evidence-based medicine: a new approach to teaching the practice of medicine, *JAMA* 268:2420–2425, 1992.

Fineout-Overholt E, Melnyk B, Stillwell SB, Williamson KM: Critical appraisal of the evidence: part 1: an introduction to gathering, evaluating, and recording the evidence, *Am J Nurs* 110(7):47–52, 2010.

Grove SK; Burns NA, Gray J: *Understanding nursing research – building an evidence-based practice*, ed 6, St. Louis, MO, 2015, Elsevier Saunders.

Guyatt G, Rennie D, editors: *Users' guides to the medical literature: a manual for evidence-based clinical practice*, Chicago, 2002, AMA.

Häggman-Laitila A, Mattila LR, Melender HL: A systematic review of journal clubs for nurses, *Worldviews Evid Based Nurs* 13(2): 163–171, 2016.

Haine-Schlagel R, Fettes DL, Garcia AR, Brookman-Frazee L, Garland AF: Consistency with evidence-based treatments and perceived effectiveness of children's community-based care, *Community Ment Health J* 50(2):158–163, 2014.

Holly C, Salmond S, Saimbert M: *Comprehensive Systematic Review for Advanced Nursing Practice*, ed 2, New York, 2016, Springer Publishing Company.

Honor Society of Nursing, Sigma Theta Tau International: *Evidence-based nursing position statement,* 2005. Retrieved from http://www.nursingsociety.org.

Horsley JA, Crane J, Bingle J: Research utilization as an organizational process, *J Nurs Admin* 8:4–6, 1978.

Horsley JA, Crane J, Crabtree MK, et al: *Using Research to Improve Nursing Practice: A Guide*, San Francisco, 1983, Grune & Stratton.

Keller LO, Strohschein S, Lia-Hoagberg B, Schaffer MA: Population-based public health interventions: practice-based and evidence-supported. Part I, *Public Health Nurs* 21(5):453–468, 2004.

King D, Barnard KE, Hoehn R: Disseminating the results of nursing research, *Nurs Outlook* 29:164–169, 1981.

Kristensen N, Nymann C, Konradsen H: Implementing research results in clinical practice—the experiences of healthcare professional, *BMC Health Serv Res* 16:48, 2016.

Krueger JC: Utilizing clinical nursing research findings in practice: a structured approach, *Commun Nurs Res* 9:381–394, 1977.

Krueger JC, Nelson AH, Wolanin MO: *Nursing Research: Development, Collaboration and Utilization*, Germantown, MD, 1978, Aspen.

Levin RF, Keefer JM, Marren J, Vetter M, Lauder B, Sobolewski S: Evidence-based practice improvement: merging 2 paradigms, *J Nurs Care Qual* 25(2):117–126, 2010.

Lindeman CA, Krueger JC: Increasing the quality, quantity, and use of nursing research, *Nurs Outlook* 25:450–454, 1977.

Makic MB, Rauen C, Watson R, Poteet AW: Examining the evidence to guide practice—challenging practice habits, *Crit Care Nurse* 34(2):28–46, 2014.

Melnyk BM, Gallager-Ford L, Fineout-Overholt E: *Implementing the evidence-based practice competencies in healthcare—a practical guide for improving quality, safety, & outcomes*, Indianapolis, IN, 2017, Sigma Theta Tau International.

Melnyk BM, Fineout-Overholt E, Stillwell SB, Williamson KM: Evidence-based practice: step by step: the seven steps of evidence-based practice, *Am J Nurs* 110(1):51–53, 2010.

Melnyk BM, Fineout-Overholt E: *Evidence-Based Practice in Nursing and Healthcare: A Guide to Best Practice*, ed 3. Philadelphia, 2015, Wolters Kluwer Health.

Pereira F, Pellaux V, Verloo H: Beliefs and implementation of evidence-based practice among community health nurses: a cross-sectional descriptive study, *J Clin Nurs* 27(9/10): 2052-2061, 2018.

Pierce LL, Reuille KM: Instructor-created activities to engage undergraduate nursing research students, *J Nurs Educ* 57(3): 174–177, 2018.

Polit DF, Beck CT: *Nursing Research: Generating and Assessing Evidence for Nursing Practice*, ed 10, China, 2017, Wolters Kluwer.

Public Health Accreditation Board: *Accredited health departments*, 2018. Retrieved from http://www.phaboard.org.

Rychetnik L, Hawe P, Waters E, Barratt A, Frommer M: A glossary for evidence based public health, *J Epidemiol Community Health* 58(7):538–545, 2004.

Sackett DL, Rosenberg WMC, Gray J, et al: Evidence-based medicine: what it is and what it isn't, *BMJ* 312:71–72, 1996.

Sackett DL, Straus SE, Richardson WS, et al: *Evidence-Based Medicine: How to Practice and Teach EBM*, London, 2000, Churchill Livingstone.

Schaefer JD, Welton JM: Evidence based practice readiness: a concept analysis, *J Nurs Manag* 26(6):621–629, 2018.

Scott K, McSherry R: Evidence-based nursing: clarifying the concepts for nurses in practice, *J Clin Nurs* 18:1085–1095, 2009.

Shaughnessy AF, Slawson DC, Bennett JA: Becoming an information master: a guidebook to the medical information jungles, *J Fam Pract* 39:489–499, 1994.

Stetler CB: Updating the Stetler model of research utilization to facilitate evidence-based practice, *Nurs Outlook* 49:272–279, 2001.

U.S. Department of Health and Human Services: *Healthy People 2020: Roadmap to Improving All Americans' Health*, Washington, DC, 2010, U.S. Government Printing Office.

Vaidya N, Thota AB, Proia KK, et al: Practice-based evidence in Community Guide systematic reviews, *Am J Public Health* 107(3): 413–420, 2017.

Weiss ME, Bobay KL, Johantgen M, Shirey MR: Aligning evidence-based practice with translational research: opportunities for clinical practice research, *J Nurs Adm* 48(9):425–431, 2018.

West S, King V, Carey TS, Lohr KN, McKoy N, Sutton SF, Lux L: *Systems to rate the strength of scientific evidence: summary*, Rockville MD, 2002, Agency for Healthcare Research and Quality.

Zimmerman K: Essentials of evidence based practice, *Int J Childbirth Educ* 32(2):37–43, 2017.

11

Population-Based Public Health Nursing Practice: The Intervention Wheel

Marjorie A. Schaffer, PhD, PHN, RN, Bonnie L. Brueshoff, DNP, MSN, RN, PHN, and Sue Strohschein, MS, RN/PHN, APRN, BC

OBJECTIVES

After reading this chapter, the student should be able to do the following:

1. Identify the components of the Intervention Wheel.
2. Describe the assumptions underlying the Intervention Wheel.
3. Define the wedges and interventions of the Intervention Wheel.
4. Differentiate among three levels of practice (community, systems, and individual/family).
5. Apply the nursing process at three levels of practice.

CHAPTER OUTLINE

The Intervention Wheel Origins and Evolution
Assumptions Underlying the Intervention Wheel
Using the Intervention Wheel in Public Health Nursing Practice
Components of the Model
Adoption of the Intervention Wheel in Practice, Education, and Management
Healthy People 2020
Applying the Nursing Process in Public Health Nursing Practice
Applying the Process at the Individual/Family Level
Applying the Public Health Nursing Process to the Community Level of Practice Scenario
Applying the Public Health Nursing Process to a Systems Level of Practice Scenario

KEY TERMS

advocacy, p. 245
case finding, p. 244
case management, p. 244
coalition building, p. 245
collaboration, p. 244
community, p. 235
community-level practice, p. 236
community organizing, p. 245
consultation, p. 244
counseling, p. 244
delegated functions, p. 244
determinants of health, p. 235
disease and other health event investigation, p. 244
health teaching, p. 244
individual-level practice, p. 236
intermediate goals, p. 249
interventions, p. 236
levels of practice, p. 233
outcome health status indicators, p. 249
outreach, p. 244
policy development, p. 245
policy enforcement, p. 245
population, p. 234
population of interest, p. 234
population at risk, p. 234
prevention, p. 235
primary prevention, p. 236
public health nursing (PHN), p. 234
referral and follow-up, p. 244
screening, p. 244
secondary prevention, p. 236
social marketing, p. 245
surveillance, p. 241
systems-level practice, p. 236
tertiary prevention, p. 235
wedges, p. 238

In these times of change, the public health system is constantly challenged to keep focused on the health of populations. The Intervention Wheel is a conceptual framework that has proved to be a useful model in defining population-based practice and explaining how it contributes to improving population health.

The Intervention Wheel provides a graphic illustration of population-based public health practice (Keller et al., 1998, 2004a, 2004b). It was previously introduced as the Public Health Intervention Model and was known nationally as the "Minnesota Model"; it is now often simply referred to as the "Wheel." The Wheel depicts how public health improves population health through interventions with communities, the individuals and families that make up communities, and the systems that impact the health of communities (Fig. 11.1). The Wheel was derived from the practice of public health nurses (PHNs) and is intended to support their work. It gives PHNs a means to describe the full scope and breadth of their practice.

This chapter applies the Intervention Wheel framework to public health nursing practice. However, it is important to note that other public health members of the interprofessional team such as nutritionists, health educators, planners, physicians, and epidemiologists also use these interventions.

THE INTERVENTION WHEEL ORIGINS AND EVOLUTION

The original version of the Wheel resulted from a grounded theory process carried out by public health nurse consultants (PHN consultants) at the Minnesota Department of Health in the mid-1990s. This was a period of relentless change and considerable uncertainty for Minnesota's public health nursing community. Debates about health care reform and its impact on the role of local public health departments created confusion about the contributions of public health nursing to population-level health improvement. In response to the uncertainty the consultant group presented a series of workshops across the state highlighting the core functions of public health nursing practice (see Chapter 1 for a description of these core functions). A workshop activity required participants to describe the actions they undertook to carry out their work. The consultant group analyzed 200 practice scenarios developed at the workshops that ranged from home care and school health to home visiting and correctional health. In the final analysis 17 actions common to the work of PHNs regardless of their practice setting were identified. The analysis also demonstrated that most of these interventions were implemented at three levels: (1) with individuals, either singly or in groups, and with families; (2) with communities as a whole;

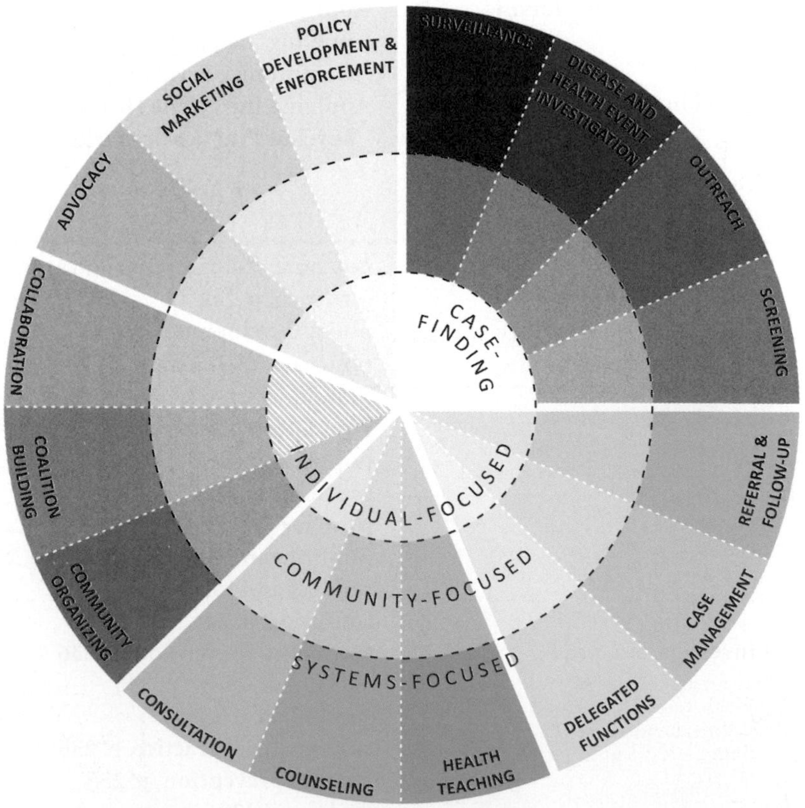

Fig. 11.1 The Intervention Wheel. (Used with permission from Keller LO, Strohschein S, Lia-Hoagberg B, et al.: Population-based public health interventions: practice-based and evidence-supported, part I. *Public Health Nurs* 21:453–468, 2004.)

and (3) with systems that impact the health of communities. A wheel-shaped graphic was developed to illustrate the set of interventions and the **levels of practice** (see Fig. 11.1).

The interventions were subjected to an extensive review of supporting evidence in the literature through a grant from the federal Division of Nursing awarded to the Minnesota Department of Health in the 1990s. In 1999 the PHN consultant group at the Minnesota Department of Health designed and implemented a systematic process identifying more than 600 items from supporting evidence in the literature. These items were rated for their quality and relevancy by a group of graduate nursing students. The resulting subset of 221 items was further analyzed by two expert panels. One panel was composed of public health nursing educators and expert practitioners from five states (Iowa, Minnesota, North Dakota, South Dakota, and Wisconsin). The other panel was a similarly composed national panel. The result was a slightly modified set of 17 interventions. Fig. 11.2 graphically illustrates the systematic critique. Each intervention was defined at multiple levels of practice; each was accompanied by a set of basic steps for applying the framework and recommendations for best practices.

Adoption of the model was rapid and worldwide. Since its first publication in 1998 the Intervention Wheel has been incorporated into the public/community health coursework of numerous undergraduate and graduate curricula. The Wheel serves as a model for practice in many state and local health departments and has been presented in Mexico, New Zealand, Norway, Poland, Hungary, Namibia, Kazakhstan, and Japan. It has served as an organizing framework for inquiry for topics such as school nursing practice (Schaffer et al., 2016; Anderson et al., 2017), nursing curriculum reviews (Schoneman et al., 2014), and building breast cancer screening coalitions to name

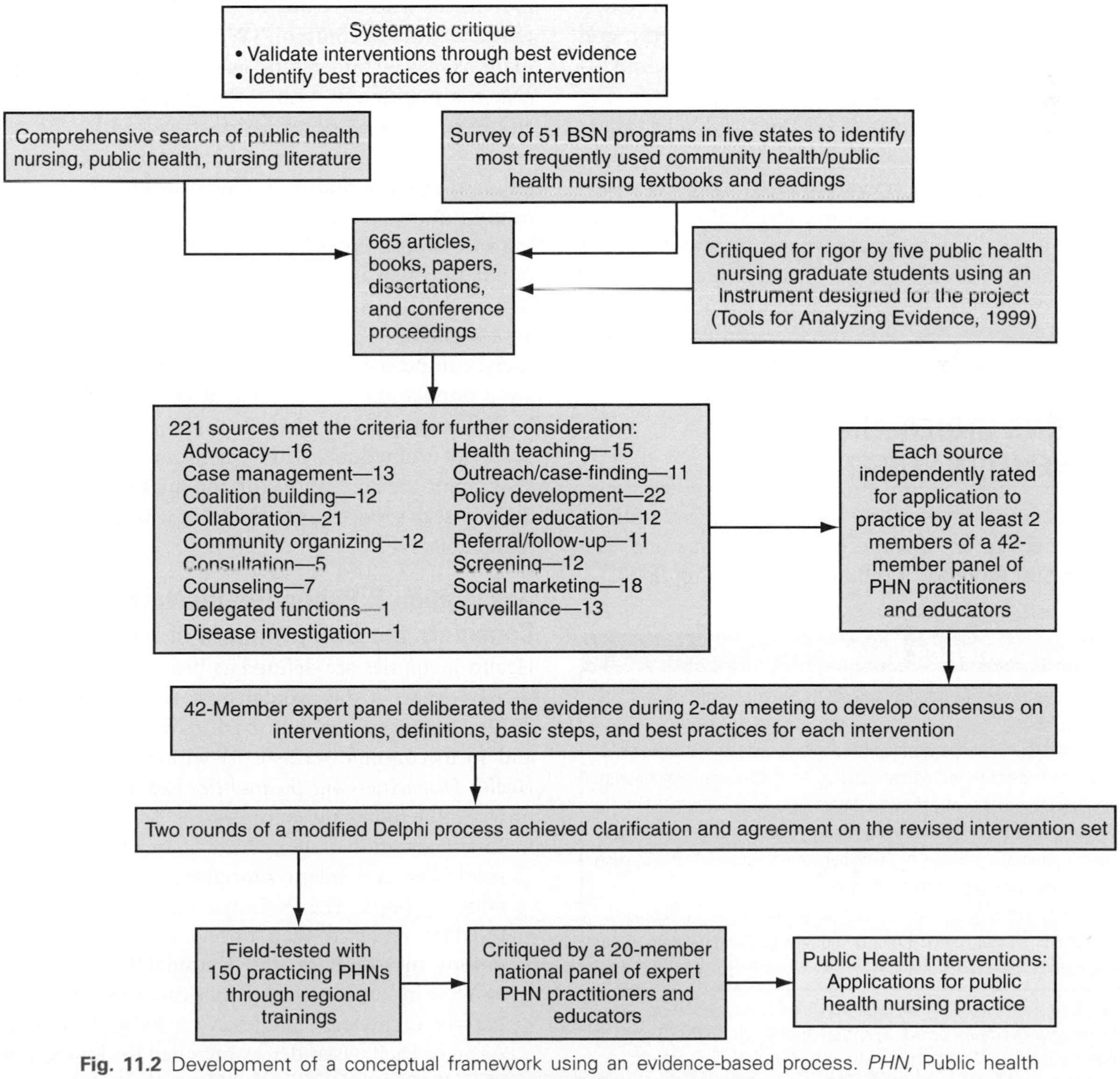

Fig. 11.2 Development of a conceptual framework using an evidence-based process. *PHN,* Public health nurse. (Used with permission from Keller LO, Strohschein S, Lia-Hoagberg B, et al.: Population-based public health interventions: practice-based and evidence-supported, part I. *Public Health Nurs* 21:459, 2004.)

a few (Depke & Onitilo, 2011). The Wheel's strength comes from the common language it affords PHNs to discuss their work (Keller et al., 1998).

In 2017 the Minnesota Department of Health (MDH) requested an update on the evidence supporting the Wheel. CINAHL was the primary database used to search for evidence on public health Wheel interventions from 2000 to 2018. Searches for evidence combined the name of the intervention with other terms, such as public health, public health nursing, intervention, community, and nursing. For some interventions, alternative terms yielded additional articles. One example is the use of health education for health teaching. Journals that yielded a high number of articles addressing public health interventions included *Public Health Nursing, Journal of Community Health Nursing, Journal of School Nursing, American Journal of Public Health*, and the *Journal of Public Health Management and Practice.*

Searches of government health-related websites, also a source of evidence, included Centers for Disease Control and Prevention (CDC), National Association of County and City Health Officials (NACCHO), World Health Organization (WHO), U.S. Department of Health and Human Services (USDHHS), and state health departments. In addition, classic texts on some interventions provided evidence for intervention basic steps. The Johns Hopkins Nursing Evidence-Based Practice Model (Dang & Dearholt, 2018) provided guidance for determining strength of evidence. Box 11.1 specifies evidence levels assigned to updated Wheel evidence. Although all five levels of evidence are represented in the evidence update, many interventions are supported primarily by level 4 and 5 evidence, which are lower-strength evidence levels. The evidence update also provides "evidence-based practice tips" and specifies evidence levels of sources of each practice tip.

ASSUMPTIONS UNDERLYING THE INTERVENTION WHEEL

As with all conceptual frameworks and models, assumptions are made that help to explain the model or framework. The Intervention Wheel framework is based on 10 assumptions.

BOX 11.1 Evidence Levels

Level 1: Experimental studies (randomized controlled trials or RCTs); systematic reviews of RCTs

Level 2: Studies with quasi-experimental designs; systematic reviews of mixed RCTs and quasi-experimental studies or only quasi-experimental studies; includes pretest-posttest evaluations

Level 3: Studies with nonexperimental designs; includes qualitative studies and surveys; systematic reviews of nonexperimental studies that may also include RCTs and quasi-experimental studies

Level 4: Clinical practice guidelines; consensus panels; position statement

Level 5: Literature reviews; quality improvement evaluation; program evaluation; case reports; expert opinion

From Dang D, Dearholt SL: *Johns Hopkins nursing evidence-based practice: model and guidelines*, ed. 3, Indianapolis, IN, 2018, Sigma Theta Tau International. ©The Johns Hopkins Hospital/The Johns Hopkins University.

Assumption 1: Public Health Nursing Practice Requires Knowledge and Skills in Both Nursing and Public Health

Public health nursing is defined as "the practice of promoting and protecting the health of populations using knowledge from nursing, social, and public health sciences" (APHA, 2013, p. 2). The title *public health nurse* designates a registered nurse with educational preparation in both public health and nursing. The primary focus of **public health nursing** is to promote health and prevent disease for entire population groups. This is done by working with individuals, families, communities, and/or systems.

Assumption 2: Public Health Nursing Practice Focuses on Populations

The focus on populations as opposed to individuals is a key characteristic that differentiates public health nursing from other areas of nursing practice. A **population** is a collection of individuals who have one or more personal or environmental characteristics in common (Williams & Highriter, 1978). Populations may be understood as two categories. A **population at risk** is a population with a common identified risk factor or risk exposure that poses a threat to health. For example, all adults who are overweight and hypertensive constitute a population at risk for cardiovascular disease. All underimmunized or unimmunized children are a population at risk for contracting vaccine-preventable diseases. A **population of interest** is a population that is essentially healthy but that could improve factors that promote or protect health. For instance, healthy adolescents are a population of interest that could benefit from social competency training. All first-time parents of newborns are a population of interest that could benefit from a public health nursing home visit. Populations include everyone in a group of individuals with a common characteristic such as geographic area or risk factor and are not limited to individuals who seek services or individuals who are poor or otherwise vulnerable.

Assumption 3: Public Health Nursing Practice Considers the Determinants of Health

Health inequities are defined as health status inequalities that society deems to be avoidable or unnecessary (Bleich et al., 2012). Significant health disparities related to race, gender, age, and socioeconomic status exist within the United States. The *Health Disparities and Inequalities Reports of the United States* provides the following examples:

- Infant gestational age, which is an important predictor of morbidity and infant mortality, differs among racial and ethnic groups. The National Center for Health Statistics (NCHS) reported that among the five racial and ethnic groups measured by the National Vital Statistics System (NVSS) in 2014, African American women had the highest percent of preterm singleton births at 11.1 percent, while Asian or Pacific Islander women had the lowest at 6.8 percent (NCHS, 2016). Within the Hispanic ethnic group, there is considerable variation in health outcomes based on country of origin. For example, the 2014 NVSS findings revealed that Puerto Rican mothers had the highest percent of preterm singleton births at 9.1 percent, and Cuban mothers the lowest at 7.2 percent (NCHS, 2016).

- While national infant mortality rates decreased overall by 14 percent from 2004 to 2014, disparities among racial and ethnic groups persisted (NCHS, 2016). For indigenous populations, infant mortality rates are staggering. American Indians and Alaska Natives have an infant mortality rate that is 60 percent higher than the rate for their white counterparts (HHS, 2014). In 2013, infants born to African American mothers experienced the highest rates of infant mortality (11.11 infant deaths per 1000 births), and infants born to Asian or Pacific Islander mothers experienced the lowest rates (3.90 infant deaths per 1000 births) (NCHS, 2016). In 2015 the percent of low-birth-weight infants rose for the first time in 7 years. For white infants the rate of low-birth-weight infants was essentially unchanged, but for African American and Hispanic infants the rate increased (Hamilton et al., 2016).
- Disparities in life expectancy exist between gender and race. In 2014 the gender gap was 4.8 years, with men and women expected to live on average 76.4 and 81.2 years, respectively. Furthermore, the life expectancy at birth for African American populations in the United States was 72.0 years for African American males and for African American females was 78.4 years compared to 78.4 years for white males and 81.4 for white females in 2015 (CDC, 2016c)

What are the factors driving these differences? Factors that influence health status across the life cycle are known as the **determinants of health**. They include income, education, employment, social support, biology and genetics, physical environment, housing, transportation, and personal health practices.

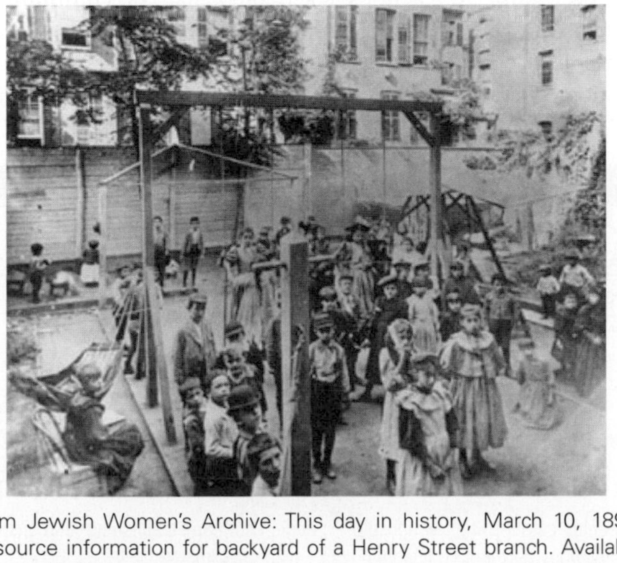

From Jewish Women's Archive: This day in history, March 10, 1893, Resource information for backyard of a Henry Street branch. Available at https://jwa.org/womenofvalor.

Resolving health inequities and addressing the determinants of health are key distinguishing characteristics of public health nursing. For example, historically, Lillian Wald's Henry Street Settlement House offered numerous social programs, including drama and theater productions, vocational training for boys and girls, three kindergartens, summer camps for children, two large scholarship funds, study rooms staffed with people to help children with their homework, playgrounds for children, a neighborhood library, and classes in carpentry, sewing, art, diction, music, and dance. The following photo shows the settlement house's backyard playground.

Recently a province-wide public health initiative in Ontario, Canada, resulted in the development and implementation of a new role for PHNs titled "Social Determinants of Health Public Health Nurse (SDH-PHN). PHNs in this role provide leadership in implementing strategies that promote health equity (McPherson et al., 2016).

Assumption 4: Public Health Nursing Practice Is Guided by Priorities Identified Through an Assessment of Community Health

In the context of the Intervention Wheel, a **community** is defined as "a group of people who share common culture, values and/or interests, based on social identity and/or territory, and who have some means of recognizing, and (inter) acting upon, these commonalities" (Gregory et al., 2009, p. 103).

Assessing the health status of the populations that make up the community requires ongoing collection and analysis of relevant quantitative and qualitative data. Community assessment includes a comprehensive assessment of the determinants of health. Data analysis identifies deviations from expected or acceptable rates of disease, injury, death, or disability, as well as risk and protective factors. Community assessment generally results in a lengthy list of community problems and issues. However, communities rarely possess sufficient resources to address the entire list. This gap between needs and resources necessitates a systematic priority-setting process. Although data analysis provides direction for priority setting, the community's beliefs, attitudes, and opinions, as well as the community's readiness for change, must be assessed. PHNs, with their extensive knowledge about the communities in which they work, provide important information and insights during the priority-setting process.

Assumption 5: Public Health Nursing Practice Emphasizes Prevention

Prevention is "anticipatory action taken to prevent the occurrence of an event or to minimize its effect after it has occurred" (Turnock, 2015). Prevention is customarily described as a continuum moving from primary to **tertiary prevention** (Leavell & Clark, 1965; Shi & Johnson, 2014; Turnock, 2015). The Levels of Prevention box provides definitions and examples of the levels of prevention.

LEVELS OF PREVENTION

Examples of Interventions Applied to Definition of Prevention

Primary Prevention

Primary prevention promotes health and protects against threats to health. It keeps problems from occurring in the first place. It promotes resiliency and protective factors or reduces susceptibility and exposure to risk factors. Primary prevention is implemented before a problem develops. It targets essentially well populations. Immunizing against a vaccine-preventable disease is an example of reducing susceptibility; building developmental assets in young persons to promote health is an example of promoting resiliency and protective factors.

Secondary Prevention

Secondary prevention detects and treats problems in their early stages. It keeps problems from causing serious or long-term effects or from affecting others. It identifies risk or hazards and modifies, removes, or treats them before a problem becomes more serious. Secondary prevention is implemented after a problem has begun but before signs and symptoms appear. It targets populations that have risk factors in common. Programs that screen populations for hypertension, obesity, hyperglycemia, hypercholesterolemia, and other chronic disease risk factors are examples of secondary prevention.

Tertiary Prevention

Tertiary prevention limits further negative effects from a problem. It keeps existing problems from getting worse. It alleviates the effects of disease and injury and restores individuals to their optimal level of functioning. Tertiary prevention is implemented after a disease or injury has occurred. It targets populations who have experienced disease or injury. Provision of directly observed therapy (DOT) to clients with active tuberculosis to ensure compliance with a medication regimen is an example of tertiary prevention.

A hallmark of public health nursing practice is a focus on health promotion and disease prevention, emphasizing primary prevention whenever possible. Although not every event is preventable, every event has a preventable component.

Assumption 6: Public Health Nurses Intervene at All Levels of Practice

To improve population health, the work of PHNs is often carried out sequentially and/or simultaneously at three levels of prevention (see Levels of Prevention box).

Community-level practice changes community norms, community attitudes, community awareness, community practices, and community behaviors. It is directed toward entire populations within the community or occasionally toward populations at risk or populations of interest. An example of community-level practice is a social marketing campaign to promote a community norm that serving alcohol to underaged youth at high school graduation parties is unacceptable. This is a community-level primary prevention strategy.

Systems-level practice changes organizations, policies, laws, and power structures within communities. The focus is on the systems that impact health, not directly on individuals and communities. Conducting compliance checks to ensure that bars and liquor stores do not serve minors or sell to individuals who supply alcohol to minors is an example of a systems-level secondary prevention strategy practice.

Individual-level practice changes knowledge, attitudes, beliefs, practices, and behaviors of individuals. This practice level is directed at individuals, alone or as part of a family, class, or group. Even though families, classes, and groups are composed of more than one individual, the focus is still on individual change. Teaching effective refusal skills to groups of adolescents is an example of individual secondary prevention strategy level of practice.

Assumption 7: Public Health Nursing Practice Uses the Nursing Process at All Levels of Practice

Although the components of the nursing process (assessment, diagnosis, planning, implementation, and evaluation) are integral to all nursing practice, PHNs must customize the process to the three levels of practice. Table 11.1 outlines the nursing process at the community, systems, and individual/family levels of practice.

Assumption 8: Public Health Nursing Practice Uses a Common Set of Interventions Regardless of Practice Setting

Interventions are "actions taken on behalf of communities, systems, individuals, and families to improve or protect health status" (ANA, 2013). The Intervention Wheel encompasses 17 interventions: surveillance, disease and other health event investigation,

TABLE 11.1 Public Health Nursing Process

Public Health Nursing Process	Systems Level	Community Level	Individual/Family Level
Recruit additional partners.	Recruit additional partners (local, regional, state, national) from systems that are key to impacting and/or who have an interest in the health issue/problem.	Recruit community organizations, services, and citizens who are part of the community intervention that have an interest in this health issue/problem.	
Identify population of interest.	Identify those systems for which change is desired.	Identify the population of interest at risk for the problem.	Identify new and current clients in caseload who are at risk for the priority problem.
Establish relationship.	Begin/continue establishing relationship with system partners.	Begin/continue establishing relationship with community partners and population of interest.	Begin/continue establishing relationship with the family.

TABLE 11.1 Public Health Nursing Process—cont'd

Public Health Nursing Process	Systems Level	Community Level	Individual/Family Level
Assess priority.	Assess the impact and interrelationships of the various systems on the development and extent of the health issue/problem.	Assess the health issue/problem (demographics, health determinants, past and current efforts). Identify the particular strengths, health risks, and health influences of the population of interest.	Identify the particular strengths, health risks, social supports, and other factors influencing the health of the family and each family member.
Elicit perceptions.	Develop a common consensus among system partners of the health issue/problem and the desired changes.	Elicit the population of interest's perception of their strengths, problems, and health influences.	Elicit family's perception of their strengths, problems, and other factors influencing their health.
Set goals.	In conjunction with system partners, develop system goals to be achieved.	In conjunction with the population of interest, negotiate and come to agreement on community-focused goals.	In conjunction with the family, negotiate and come to agreement on meaningful, achievable, measurable goals.
Select health status indicators.	Based on systems goals, select meaningful, measurable health status indicators that will be used to measure success.	Based on the refined community goal/problem, select meaningful, measurable health status indicators that will be used to measure success.	Select meaningful, measurable health status indicators that will be used to measure success.
Select interventions.	Select system-level interventions considering evidence of effectiveness, political support, acceptability to community, cost-effectiveness, legality, ethics, greatest potential for successful outcome, nonduplicative, levels of prevention.	Select community-level interventions considering evidence of effectiveness, acceptability to community, cost-effectiveness, legality, ethics, nonduplicative, greatest potential for successful outcome.	Select interventions considering evidence of effectiveness, acceptability to family, cost-effectiveness, legality, ethics, greatest potential for successful outcome.
Select intermediate outcome indicators.	Determine measurable, meaningful intermediate outcome indicators.	Determine measurable and meaningful intermediate outcome indicators.	Determine measurable, meaningful intermediate outcome indicators.
Determine strategy frequency and intensity.	Using best practices, determine intensity, sequencing, frequency of interventions considering urgency, political will, resources.	Using best practices, determine intensity, sequencing, frequency of interventions.	Using best practices, determine intensity, sequencing, frequency of interventions.
Determine evaluation methods.	Determine evaluation methods for measuring process, intermediate, and outcome indicators.	Determine evaluation methods for measuring process, intermediate, and outcome indicators.	Determine evaluation methods for measuring process, intermediate, and outcome indicators.
Implement the interventions.	Implement the interventions.	Implement the interventions.	Implement the interventions.
Regularly reassess interventions.	Regularly reassess the system's response to the interventions, and modify plan as indicated.	Reassess the population of interest's response to the interventions on an ongoing basis, and modify plan as indicated.	Reassess and modify plan at each contact as necessary.
Adjust interventions.	Adjust the frequency and intensity of the interventions according to the needs and resources of the community.	Adjust the frequency and intensity of the interventions accordingly.	Adjust the frequency and intensity of the interventions according to the needs and resources of the family.
Provide feedback.	Provide feedback to system's representatives.	Provide feedback to the population of interest and informal and formal organizational representatives.	Provide regular feedback to family on progress (or lack thereof) of client goals.
Collect evaluation.	Regularly and systematically collect evaluation information.	Regularly and systematically collect evaluation information.	Regularly and systematically collect evaluation information.
Compare results to plan.	Compare actual results with planned indicators.	Compare actual results with planned indicators.	Compare actual results with planned indicators.
Identify differences.	Identify and analyze differences in those systems that achieved outcomes compared with those that did not.	Identify and analyze differences in those in the population of interest who achieved outcomes compared with those who did not.	Identify and analyze differences in services received by families who achieved outcomes compared with those who did not.
Apply results to practice.	Apply results to identify needed system changes. Depending on readiness of the system to accept the results, present results to decision makers and the general population.	Apply results to modify community interventions. Present results to community for policy considerations as appropriate.	Report results to supervisor and other service providers as appropriate. Apply results to personal practice and agency for policy considerations as appropriate.

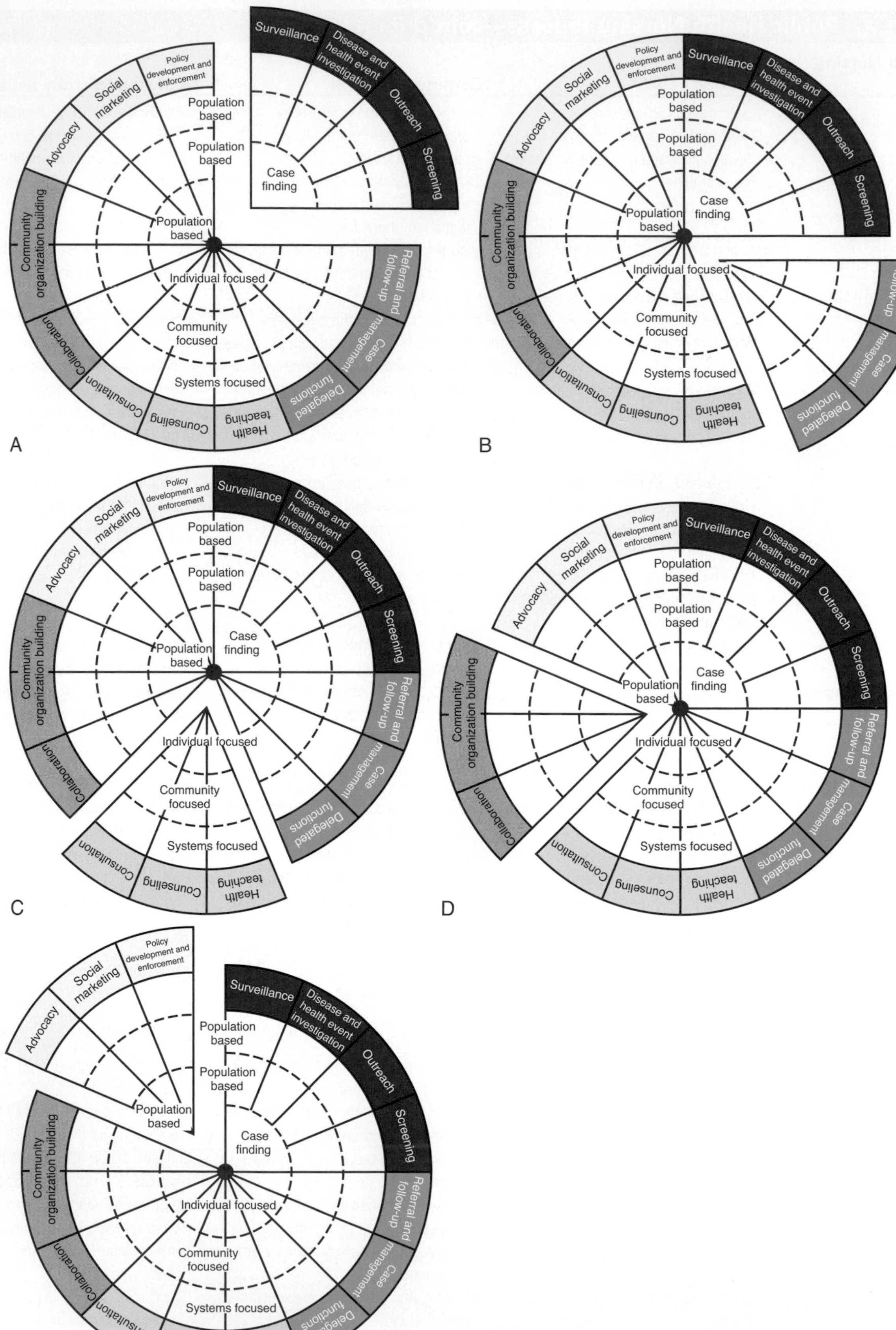

Fig. 11.3 The Intervention Wheel components (A to E). (Used with permission from Keller LO, Strohschein S, Lia-Hoagberg B, et al.: Population-based public health interventions: practice-based and evidence-supported, part I. *Public Health Nurs* 21:453–468, 2004.)

outreach, screening, case finding, referral and follow-up, case management, delegated functions, health teaching, consultation, counseling, collaboration, coalition building, community organizing, advocacy, social marketing, and policy development and enforcement.

The interventions are grouped with related interventions; these **wedges** are color coordinated to make them more recognizable (Fig. 11.3). For instance, the five interventions in the *red wedge* (Fig 11.3A) are frequently implemented in conjunction with one another. Surveillance is often paired with disease and health event investigation, even though either can be implemented independently. Screening frequently follows either surveillance or disease and health event investigation and is often preceded by outreach activities to maximize the number of those at risk who actually get screened. Most often, screening leads to case finding, but this intervention can also be carried out independently.

The green wedge consists of referral and follow-up, case management, and delegated functions—three interventions that, in practice, are often implemented together (see Fig. 11.3B).

Similarly, health teaching, counseling, and consultation—the blue wedge—are more similar than they are different; health teaching and counseling are especially often paired (see Fig. 11.3C).

The interventions in the orange wedge—collaboration, coalition building, and community organizing—although distinct, are grouped together because they are all types of collective action and are most often carried out at systems or community levels of practice (see Fig. 11.3D).

Similarly, advocacy, social marketing, and policy development and enforcement the yellow wedge—are often interrelated when implemented (see Fig. 11.3E). In fact, advocacy is often viewed as a precursor to policy development; social marketing is seen by some as a method of carrying out advocacy

The interventions on the right side of the Wheel (i.e., the red, green, and blue wedges) are most commonly used by PHNs who focus their work more on individuals, families, classes, and groups and to a lesser extent on work with systems and communities. The orange and yellow wedges, on the other hand, are more commonly used by PHNs who focus their work on affecting systems and communities. However, a PHN may use any or all of the interventions. No single PHN is expected to perform every intervention at all three levels of practice. From a management perspective, however, it is useful to ensure that a public health workforce has the capacity to implement all 17 interventions at all three practice levels.

Assumption 9: Public Health Nursing Practice Contributes to the Achievement of the 10 Essential Services

Implementing the interventions ultimately contributes to the achievement of the 10 essential public health services (see Chapter 1). The 10 essential public health services describe *what* the public health system does to protect and promote the health of the public. Interventions are the means through which public health practitioners implement the 10 essential services. Interventions are the *how* of public health practice (CDC, 2018).

BOX 11.2 Cornerstones of Public Health Nursing

Public Health Nursing Practice

- Focuses on the health of entire populations
- Reflects community priorities and needs
- Establishes caring relationships with the communities, families, individuals, and systems that constitute the populations PHNs serve
- Encompasses the mental, physical, emotional, social, spiritual, and environmental aspects of health
- Promotes health through strategies driven by epidemiological evidence
- Collaborates with community resources to achieve those strategies but can and will work alone if necessary
- Derives its authority for independent action from the nurse practice act

Cornerstones From Public Health	Cornerstones From Nursing
Population-based/focused	Relationship-based
Grounded in social justice	Grounded in an ethic of caring
Focus on greater good	Sensitivity to diversity
Focus on health promotion and disease prevention	Holistic focus
	Respect for the worth of all
Does what others cannot or will not	Independent practice
Driven by the science of epidemiology	Long-term commitment to the community
Organizes community resources	

PHN, Public health nurse.

Assumption 10: Public Health Nursing Practice is Grounded in a Set of Values and Beliefs

The Cornerstones of Public Health Nursing (Box 11.2) were developed as a companion document to the Intervention Wheel. The Wheel defines the "what and how" of public health nursing practice; the Cornerstones define the "why." The Cornerstones synthesize foundational values and beliefs from both public health and nursing. They inspire, guide, direct, and challenge public health nursing practice (Keller et al., 2011).

USING THE INTERVENTION WHEEL IN PUBLIC HEALTH NURSING PRACTICE

The Wheel is a conceptual model. It was conceived as a common language or catalog of general actions used by PHNs across all practice settings. When those actions are placed within the context of a set of associated assumptions or relations among concepts, the Intervention Wheel serves as a conceptual model for public health nursing practice (Fawcett & DeSanto-Madeya, 2013). It creates a structure for identifying and documenting interventions performed by PHNs and captures the nature of their work. The Intervention Wheel provides a framework, a way of thinking about public health nursing practice. The *Public Health Nursing: Scope and Standards of Practice* includes the Intervention Wheel as one of several public health nursing frameworks used in practice today (ANA, 2013).

COMPONENTS OF THE MODEL

As depicted in Fig. 11.1, the model has three components: a population basis, three levels of practice, and 17 interventions.

Component 1: The Model Is Population Based

All levels of practice (community, systems, and individual/family) illustrated in the Wheel are population based. Public health nursing practice identifies a focus on populations of interest or populations at risk through an assessment of community health status and an assignment of priorities. Services to individuals and families are population focused only if they meet the following criteria: (1) individuals receive services because they are members of an identified population, and (2) services to individuals clearly contribute to improving the overall health status of the identified population.

A national health and nutrition survey revealed that 23 percent of children aged two to five years had dental caries in their primary teeth (CDC, 2015). As one of the most chronic health problems in children in the United States, untreated tooth decay may lead to problems that interfere with eating, speaking, playing, and learning (CDC, 2014). In 2014 only 39 percent of children ages three to five enrolled in Medical Assistance (Medicaid) in Dakota County in Minnesota had a preventive dental visit (Dakota County Public Health Department, 2016). To respond to the problem of lack of access to dental resources, Dakota County initiated an oral health project through the Healthy Baby-Healthy Teeth Initiative to focus on at-risk populations of children zero to three years, pregnant women, and uninsured/underinsured families (Minnesota Department of Health, 2016; Schoon, 2018a).

Public health nursing students contributed to this population-focused project by surveying 42 dental clinics in the county. The survey identified a number of barriers that contribute to access problems for dental services, including lack of public transportation, interpreter services, and arrangements for dental care during school days; limited availability of dental care on evenings and weekends; and few clinics that accepted Medicaid patients (Schoon, 2018a). Public health nursing students, supervised by a nursing educator, provided oral health outreach through Women, Infants, and Children (WIC) and Head Start. They partnered with the program Child and Teen Checkup, PHNs, and health educators (Schoon, 2018b). The population reached through the project included parents, children ages zero to three years, persons living in poverty, children on Medical Assistance, recent immigrants, and members of a community of color. With expansion of the oral health population-focused project to an additional four counties, overall, students provided interventions to promote dental health and access for over 500 families and distributed an estimated 275 oral hygiene kits.

Component 2: The Model Encompasses Three Levels of Practice

Public health nursing practice intervenes with communities, the individuals and families that make up the communities, and the systems that impact the health of communities. Interventions at each level of practice contribute to the overall goal of improving population health. The work of PHNs is accomplished at all levels. No one level of practice is more important than another; in fact, many public health priorities are addressed simultaneously at all three levels.

One public health priority that almost every PHN will encounter is the potential for the occurrence of vaccine-preventable disease because of delayed or missing immunizations. A recent task analysis of 60 PHNs from 29 states revealed that 93 percent of all PHNs participated in immunization activities (Schaffer et al., 2015). This held true regardless of the PHN's work setting (e.g., home, clinic, school, correctional facility, childcare center) or the population focus (e.g., maternal–child health, elderly chronic disease management, refugee health, disease prevention and control).

Vaccine-preventable diseases, or diseases that may be prevented through recommended immunizations, include diphtheria, pertussis, tetanus, polio, mumps, measles, rubella, hepatitis A, hepatitis B, varicella, meningitis, *Haemophilus influenzae* type b (Hib), pneumococcal pneumonia, rotavirus, human papillomavirus (HPV), herpes zoster, and seasonal influenza (CDC, 2016a).

The following section illustrates strategies for reducing the occurrence of vaccine-preventable diseases at all three levels of practice. These are only selected examples of strategies to improve immunization rates; it is not an inclusive list.

Community Level of Practice. The goal of community-level practice is to increase the knowledge and attitude of the entire community about the importance of immunization and the consequences of not being immunized. These strategies will lead to an increase in the percent of people who obtain recommended immunizations for themselves and their children.

At the community level, PHNs work with health educators on public awareness campaigns. They perform outreach at schools, senior centers, county fairs, community festivals, and neighborhood laundromats.

PHNs conduct or coordinate audits of immunization records of all children in schools and childcare centers to identify children who are underimmunized. The PHNs refer them to their medical providers or administer the immunizations through health department clinics.

When a confirmed case of a vaccine-preventable disease occurs, PHNs work with epidemiologists to identify and locate everyone exposed to the index case. PHNs assess the immunization status of people who were exposed and ensure appropriate treatment.

In the event of an outbreak in the community, all PHNs have a role and ethical responsibility to take part in mass dispensing clinics. Mass dispensing clinics disperse immunizations or medications to specific populations at risk. For example, clinics may be held in response to an epidemic of mumps, a case of hepatitis A attributable to a foodborne exposure in a restaurant, or an influenza pandemic in the general population.

Systems Level of Practice. The goal of systems-level practice is to change the laws, policies, and practices that influence immunization rates, such as promoting population-based immunization registries and improving clinic and provider practices.

PHNs work with schools, clinics, health plans, and parents to develop population-based immunization registries. Registries, known officially by the CDC as "Immunization Information Systems," combine immunization information from different sources into a single electronic record. A registry provides official immunization records for schools, daycare centers, health departments, and clinics. Registries track immunizations and remind families when an immunization is due or has been missed.

PHNs conduct audits of records in clinics that participate in the federal vaccine program. PHNs ascertain if a clinic is following recommended immunization standards for vaccine handling and storage, documentation, and adherence to best practices. PHNs also provide feedback and guidance to clinicians and office staff for quality improvement.

PHNs also work with health care providers in the community to ensure that providers accurately report vaccine-preventable diseases as legally required by state statute.

Individual/Family Level of Practice. The goal of individual/family-level strategies is to identify individuals who are not appropriately immunized, identify the barriers to immunization, and ensure that the individual's immunizations are brought up to date.

At the individual level of practice, PHNs conduct health department immunization clinics. Unlike mass dispensing clinics, immunization clinics are generally available to anyone who needs an immunization and do not target a specific population. These clinics often provide an important service to individuals without access to affordable health care.

PHNs use the registry to identify children with delayed or missing immunizations. They contact families by phone or through a home visit. The PHNs assess for barriers and consult with the family to develop a plan to obtain immunizations either through a medical clinic or from a health department clinic. The PHN follows up at a later date to ensure that the child was actually immunized.

PHNs routinely assess the immunization status for clients in all public health programs, such as well-child clinics, family planning clinics, maternal–child health home visits, or case management of elderly and disabled populations, and they ensure that immunizations are up to date.

Component 3: The Model Identifies and Defines 17 Public Health Interventions

The Intervention Wheel encompasses 17 interventions: surveillance, disease and other health event investigation, outreach, screening, case finding, referral and follow-up, case management, delegated functions, health teaching, consultation, counseling, collaboration, coalition building, community organizing, advocacy, social marketing, and policy development and enforcement.

All interventions, except case finding, coalition building, and community organizing, are applicable at all three levels of practice. Community organizing and coalition building cannot occur at the individual level. Case finding is the individual level of surveillance, disease and other health event investigation, outreach, and screening. Altogether, a PHN selects from among 43 different intervention-level actions.

Table 11.2 provides examples of the intervention at the three levels of practice for each of the 17 interventions.

- **Surveillance** is "an ongoing, systematic collection, analysis and interpretation of health-related data essential to the planning, implementation, and evaluation of public health practice" (World Health Organization, 2018).

TABLE 11.2 Examples of 17 Interventions at Three Levels of Practice

Interventions	Systems	Community	Individual
Surveillance	PHNs assigned to communicable disease control programs in local and state health departments monitor data from outpatient and hospital laboratories to detect presence of the influenza virus in the area for evidence of outbreaks, which would indicate a need for increased dissemination of information on prevention to the public.	Nurses in Ontario, Canada, staffed a telephone health helpline to recruit and monitor participants with influenza-like symptoms. Participants obtained a nasal specimen through self-swabbing and submitted it for testing and laboratory confirmation (McGolrick et al., 2016).	Surveillance at the individual level is case finding (see case finding intervention).
Disease and other health event investigation	PHNs contributed to local health department prevention and response actions to Zika virus infections: information to travelers (94 percent), outreach and communication to clinicians (90 percent), laboratory testing (83 percent), maternal–child health surveillance (72 percent), and rapid detection and follow-up of birth defects (47 percent) (NACCHO, 2018).	PHNs communicated with other providers in the community to create public awareness about transmission of disease (including Zika) from mosquitoes. They shared the CDC (2018) website that offers information about mosquito surveillance; removing places where mosquitoes lay eggs; control of larvae, pupae, and adult mosquitoes; and many resources that provide instructions on mosquito control strategies.	Disease and other health event investigation at the individual level is case finding (see case finding intervention).
Outreach	In response to the rising chlamydia rate, the PHN accesses a toolkit on the Minnesota Department of Health website to address chlamydia in the community and promotes use of the toolkit to health care providers and agencies.	A county health department reaches a typically hard-to-reach population (youth ages 15 to 24) by offering a community-based screening program for chlamydia and gonorrhea in public libraries (Delair et al., 2016).	Outreach at the individual level is case finding (see case finding intervention).

Continued

TABLE 11.2 Examples of 17 Interventions at Three Levels of Practice—cont'd

Interventions	Systems	Community	Individual
Screening	The Pediatric Public Health Initiative was established to mitigate the effects of the Flint, Michigan, water crisis. This initiative provides PHNs with a wealth of resources for connecting families to additional child development screening, maternal–infant support programs, universal home-based early intervention, early childhood education, and parenting support programs (Hanna-Attisha et al., 2016).	The Michigan Department of Community Health created a checklist titled "Finding a Healthy Home," which PHNs can use to assist families in screening a potential new home for safety and findings resources that promote lead-safe homes.	Screening at the individual level is case finding (see case finding intervention).
Case finding	Does not apply at this practice level.	Does not apply at this practice level.	PHNs routinely inquire about flu-like symptoms with the individuals, families, and groups and colleagues with whom they work. When providing services to women of childbearing age, PHNs inquire about symptoms of infection in women and their partners and history of travel or residence in environments where mosquitoes infected with the Zika virus may be present. A rural "street nurse" provided outreach in British Columbia to a marginalized population. Services offered include testing for STIs, chlamydia treatment, pregnancy testing, emergency contraception, and help with completing forms for financial support (Self & Peters, 2005). For families with young children, PHNs use a lead screening questionnaire to determine risk status and need for referral.
Case management	The school nurse (SN) engages the school board's School Health Advisory Committee to develop a comprehensive set of asthma-related policies.	SNs developed a plan to hold a series of "asthma update" meetings for parents in conjunction with the local chapter of the American Lung Association and a pediatric nurse practitioner specializing in asthma management.	For a newly enrolled child in school, the SN follows up with the provider and the parent to develop the child's Asthma Action Plan, which includes a list of environmental triggers to be avoided. The SN meets with the child's teacher to explain the plan and assists in problem solving the implications for classroom, playground, and physical education class management.
Delegated functions	SNs in the school district work with administrators to develop delegation policies and guidelines for implementation of medication administration by unlicensed assistive personnel (UAP) across all schools.	The SN develops training and supervision for the UAP to provide medication administration in school.	The SN responsible for health services in elementary schools in the district provides training and supervision on medication administration for a new UAP recently hired by the school district.
Health teaching	A PHN provides an in-service training to physicians, midwives, and family-planning specialists highlighting new research findings on the effect of alcohol on pregnancy.	A PHN participates in a county task force that aims to reduce alcohol use by women during preconceptual and child-bearing years. The group develops a series of posters and distributes them to bars, restaurants, other establishments serving alcoholic beverages, and liquor retailers.	The PHN incorporates information on the impact of alcohol use on fetal development into the reproductive health class that the PHN teaches to high school and community college students.
Counseling	The PHN partners with social workers, school service providers, and community clubs to design a teen suicide community response plan to prevent repeats of a teen suicide cluster.	PHNs partner with the mental health center, schools, and faith community to raise community awareness about depression in teens. They use billboards, radio spots, movie trailers, and social media to disseminate the message.	The PHN facilitates a support group for families coping with the loss of a member through suicide.

TABLE 11.2 **Examples of 17 Interventions at Three Levels of Practice—cont'd**

Interventions	Systems	Community	Individual
Consultation	The PHN meets with childcare staff to discuss actions they can take to prevent an outbreak of measles at a childcare center.	The PHN organizes a meeting in the community to answer questions about risks of measles and prevention for parents who have concerns about the immunization.	On a home visit the PHN assists the parent in contacting the medical clinic and mutually develops a plan with the mother of young children on the steps she can take to prevent other family members from getting measles, which has been diagnosed in her youngest child.
Collaboration	A PHN collaborates on an initiative to prevent falls in older adults. Collaborative partners in the community include the ambulance service, fire department, senior centers, the university's extension services, and several hospital departments (emergency, pharmacy, rehabilitation services, physical therapy, and home care). One of the project goals is to change how providers approach seniors and their potential for falls.	A PHN joins forces with older adults at the local senior center to plan a program to change the community perception that falling is inevitable as a person ages.	Together the PHN and the older adult make a plan to remove/reduce injury risks. This includes a review of medications that may affect balance; home modifications to reduce fall hazards, such as installing grab bars, improving lighting, and removing items that may cause tripping; and exercise to improve strength, balance, and coordination.
Coalition building	A coalition worked with a faith-based organization to obtain a grant for hiring a coordinator to continue a community garden project in a refugee community.	PHNs who provided services for the community brought together agencies and advocates with similar missions and complementary skill sets to form a coalition to implement a community garden project in a refugee community (Eggert et al., 2015).	Coalition building is not implemented at the individual level of practice.
Community organizing	The state passed legislation that addressed youth violence. The city partnered with a national organization to respond to the problem of youth violence. The national organization sponsors conferences, develops tools and information, and conducts networking activities across the United States.	A PHN in a leadership role at the city health department met with community leaders, elected officials, and the police department to develop a public health response to the increasing incidence of community violence among youth.	Community organizing is not implemented at the individual level of practice
Advocacy	A citywide coalition expanded its strategies to increase awareness of and response to Adverse Childhood Experiences (ACEs) in service and professional education systems. Its goals included working to understand interventions in Philadelphia that addressed childhood adversity and trauma; and integrating ACEs into medical, nursing, allied health, and human services curricula (Pachter et al., 2017).	The coalition collaborated with community organizations to use a framework of ACEs and resiliency (Pachter et al., 2017). The coalition identified a major focus area as educating the community about ACEs.	Through the Nurse Family Partnership Program, PHNs provide home visits to pregnant and parenting mothers until their children are two years old. The PHNs develop trusting relationships and provide support that helps mothers take control of their lives, nurture their children, and build strong families (Nurse Family Partnership, 2018).
Social marketing	Stopbullying.gov is a systems-level strategy that provides communities and organizations with ideas for social marketing strategies to address bullying and cyberbullying prevention and resources. A school nurse convened a school task group, including student representatives, to determine how they could use the website in antibullying programming.	A school district worked together with students and the community to create bully-free zones. A public service announcement at a school-sponsored bully prevention event featured a video with a bullying prevention message.	School nurses market bullying prevention messages to adolescents, their families, and school staff through posters, online communication, newsletters, or classroom presentations.
Policy development and enforcement	A state program, funded by the legislature provided funding for programs that aim to reduce risk factors for chronic disease. The school district received funding for creating a program to encourage students to eat a variety of fruits and vegetables.	SNs contributed to policy development and implementation in order to encourage students to try new foods and inform parents about the benefits of new fruits and vegetables.	The SN worked with classroom teachers to determine the best way to enforce the policy placing a limitation on bringing unhealthy snacks to school to share.

Continued

TABLE 11.2 Examples of 17 Interventions at Three Levels of Practice—cont'd

Interventions	Systems	Community	Individual
Referral and follow-up	PHNs providing health services to inmates in a county jail noticed that individuals with mental health issues, chronic health concerns, chemical dependency issues, or homelessness frequently returned to jail. Few of these issues were typically addressed prior the inmates' release.	PHNs often serve as community resource directories. PHNs are known by community members for their extensive knowledge of whom or where to call for a variety of problems or issues.	A PHN received a referral on a mentally ill young man from a small town. He needed regular injections to prevent rehospitalization. When the PHN was unable to locate this client at home, she found him at his regular "hangout"—the local bar—where he only drank soda pop. While creatively maintaining confidentiality, the PHN worked with the bartender in this establishment to set up regular appointment times for the client.
	The PHNs initiated RAPP (Release Advance Planning Program), a voluntary "discharge planning" process through which referrals and other arrangements with community resources could be made prior to the inmates returning to the community. Recidivism rates decreased by 57 percent by the third year of the program's operation.	For example, PHNs in a rural health department responded to calls ranging from rats to cockroaches to bedbugs, from septic tank failures to peeling paint, and from air quality to blue-green algae. The PHNs often followed up with community members to ensure that their issues were resolved.	

PHN, Public health nurse; *STI,* sexually transmitted infection.

- **Disease and other health event investigation** systematically gathers and analyzes data regarding threats to the health of populations, ascertains the source of the threat, identifies cases and others at risk, and determines control measures.
- **Outreach** locates populations of interest or populations at risk and provides information about the nature of the concern, what can be done about it, and how services can be obtained.
- **Screening** identifies individuals with unrecognized health risk factors or asymptomatic disease conditions in populations (Box 11.3).
- **Case finding** locates individuals and families with identified risk factors and connects them with resources.

BOX 11.3 Screening

PHNs work with families to assess the growth and development of children. Minnesota offers a free, voluntary program called Follow Along to help parents track a child's development. The Follow Along Program helps identify infants and children (birth to four years old) who are at risk for falling behind in normal growth and development. The Follow Along Program uses validated screening tools to identify children with developmental and social delays before they enter school. Intervention before kindergarten has important academic, social, and economic benefits.

In Dakota County, PHNs assist getting families enrolled in the Follow Along Program. Families who decide to enroll are sent screening tools called Ages and Stages Questionnaires at key age milestones: 4, 8, 12, 16, 20, 24, 36, 42, and 48 months. These questionnaires assess the development of infants and children in communication, gross motor, fine motor, personal/social, and problem solving and social emotional behaviors. The results are shared with parents, and if there are concerns, a public health nurse contacts the parents to discuss further evaluation or early intervention services available in the local school district. In 2016, 594 children participated, including 194 newly enrolled children.

PHN, Public health nurse.

- **Referral and follow-up** assists individuals, families, groups, organizations, and/or communities with identifying and accessing necessary resources in order to prevent or resolve problems or concerns.
- **Case management** is a collaborative process of assessment, planning, facilitation, care coordination, evaluation, and advocacy for options and services to meet individual and family comprehensive health needs through communication and available resources to promote patient safety, quality of care, and cost-effective outcomes.
- **Delegated functions** are (1) direct care tasks a registered professional nurse carries out under the authority of a health care practitioner, as allowed by law, and (2) direct care tasks that a registered professional nurse entrusts to other appropriate personnel to perform.
- **Health teaching** involves sharing information and experiences through educational activities designed to improve health knowledge, attitudes, behaviors, and skills (Friedman et al., 2011).
- **Counseling** establishes an interpersonal relationship with a community, system, family, or individual intended to increase or enhance their capacity for self-care and coping. Counseling engages the community, system, family, or individual at an emotional level.
- **Consultation** seeks information and generates optional solutions to perceived problems or issues through interactive problem solving with a community, system, family, or individual. The community, system, family, or individual selects and acts on the option best meeting the circumstances.
- **Collaboration** is the action of enhancing the capacity of the other partners (communities, systems, or individuals) to promote and protect health for mutual benefit and a common

purpose. Collaboration involves the exchange of information, harmonized activities, and shared resources (National Business Coalition on Health, 2009).

- **Coalition building** promotes and develops alliances among organizations or constituencies for a common purpose. It builds linkages, solves problems, and/or enhances local leadership to address health concerns.
- **Community organizing** is the "process by which people come together to identify common problems or goals, mobilize resources, and develop and implement strategies for reaching the objectives they want to accomplish" (Center for Community Health and Development at the University of Kansas, 2017).
- **Advocacy** is the act of promoting and protecting the health of individuals and communities "by collaborating with relevant stakeholders, facilitating access to health and social services, and actively engaging key decision makers to support and enact policies to improve community health outcomes" (Ezeonwu, 2015, p. 123).
- **Social marketing** is "a process that uses marketing principles and techniques to change target audience behaviors to benefit society as well as the individual" (Lee & Kotler, 2016, p. 9).
- **Policy development** places health issues on decision makers' agendas, acquires a plan of resolution, and determines needed resources. Policy development results in laws, rules, regulations, ordinances, and policies. **Policy enforcement** compels others to comply with the laws, rules, regulations, ordinances, and policies created in conjunction with policy development.

CHECK YOUR PRACTICE

You are aware of children in a local school district who are behind on immunizations required for school entry.

You have experience working with area school nurses on addressing immunization needs. School nurses have asked if the health department can help with vaccinating children.

What are steps that need to be taken to hold an immunization clinic in the school setting?

Who would you collaborate with to plan the immunization clinic?

What other health-related activities could be offered during the immunization clinics to focus on health promotion and disease prevention (e.g., dental varnishing)?

BOX 11.4 Basic Steps for the Intervention of Counseling

- Establish a therapeutic relationship with the client (community, systems, or individual).
- Maintain professional boundaries.
- Self-monitor the counseling relationship.
- The PHN selects from a variety of effective counseling strategies, which can be tailored to address a specific health concern, for example, individual, group, telephone, email, or computer-based sessions.
- Use a behavior change model to organize the counseling intervention. The Five As model and motivational interviewing are useful frameworks for behavior change counseling.
- Identify and address possible client barriers to behavior change.
- Avoid actions in counseling, such as arguing, telling the client how to change, warning, convincing the client that he or she has a problem, and interpreting client's problem or behavior.
- Take cues from client perspectives when implementing counseling.

PHN, Public health nurse.

BOX 11.5 Examples of Evidence-Based Practice Tips for the Intervention of Referral and Follow-up

1. Take the time to develop relationships with resources that will likely be receiving referrals from PHNs (e.g., primary care providers, community clinics, income support services, housing resources, early childhood resources, daycare) to ensure that those who are referred will be well received.
   Evidence: Brega et al., 2015 (level 4); Cooper & Zimmerman, 2017 (level 2); Ezeonwu & Berkowitz, 2014 (level 5); Strass & Billay, 2008 (level 2).
2. When the PHN is the recipient of a referral, the immediacy of the PHN contacting the client increases the likelihood of client acceptance.
   Evidence: Flaten, 2011 (level 2).
3. Client receptiveness toward a referral and acting on it is more likely when the PHN:
   - Assesses client readiness to change
   - Assists client with seeing discrepancies between current and desired state
   - Listens reflectively
   - Asks open-ended questions
   - Refrains from directly countering statements of resistance
   - Restates positive or motivating statements made by client
   - Acknowledges client as an active participant in the referral process

   Evidence: APHA, 2008 (level 4).

APHA, American Public Health Association; *PHN,* public health nurse.

In addition to the definition and examples, each intervention has basic steps for implementation at each of the three levels (i.e., community, systems, and individual/family) as well as a listing of evidence tips for each intervention. The basic steps are intended as a guide for the novice PHN or the experienced PHN wishing to review his or her effectiveness. Box 11.4 describes the basic steps of the counseling intervention. Box 11.5 provides examples of evidence–based practice tips for referral and follow-up.

ADOPTION OF THE INTERVENTION WHEEL IN PRACTICE, EDUCATION, AND MANAGEMENT

The speed at which the Intervention Wheel was adopted may be attributed to the balance between its practice base and its evidence-based support. The Intervention Wheel has led to numerous innovations in practice and education since it was first published in 1998 (Keller et al., 2004a). Further dissemination of the model has occurred through the hundreds of graduate and undergraduate schools of nursing that use the Intervention Wheel as a framework for teaching public health nursing.

The Intervention Wheel has been widely adopted as a framework for public health nursing practice:

- In 2007, the American Nurses Association officially recognized the Intervention Wheel as a framework in *Public Health Nursing: Scope and Standards of Practice* (ANA, 2007, 2013).
- The County of Los Angeles Department of Public Health used the Intervention Wheel in their initiative to reinvigorate

public health nursing practice—orientation, practice standards, documentation, recruitment, and retention (County of Los Angeles Department of Public Health Nursing Administration, 2007; Avila & Smith, 2003; Smith & Bazini-Barakat, 2003).

- The Massachusetts Association of Public Health Nurses used the Intervention Wheel as the framework for their state *Leadership Guide and Resource Manual* (Massachusetts Association of Public Health Nurses, 2009).
- PHNs in the Shiprock Service Unit of the Indian Health Service use the Wheel in their practice and adapted it to reflect the Navajo culture. The Navajo Intervention Wheel (Fig. 11.4) is presented as a Navajo basket and uses the traditional colors of the Navajo nation.
- From 2001 to 2005 the Intervention Wheel served as the framework for a Division of Nursing grant that successfully brought together education and practice communities to collaboratively redesign the public health nursing student's clinical experience. Several of these collaboratives remain viable and active.
- PHN consultants at the Wisconsin Department of Health used the Intervention Wheel to differentiate levels of nursing practice in local health departments related to educational preparation and to outline the role of the associate degree and diploma nurse in public health. (Although the baccalaureate degree is the accepted standard for entry to public health nursing practice, shortages of baccalaureate prepared nurses sometimes result in health departments employing associate degree and diploma nurses.)

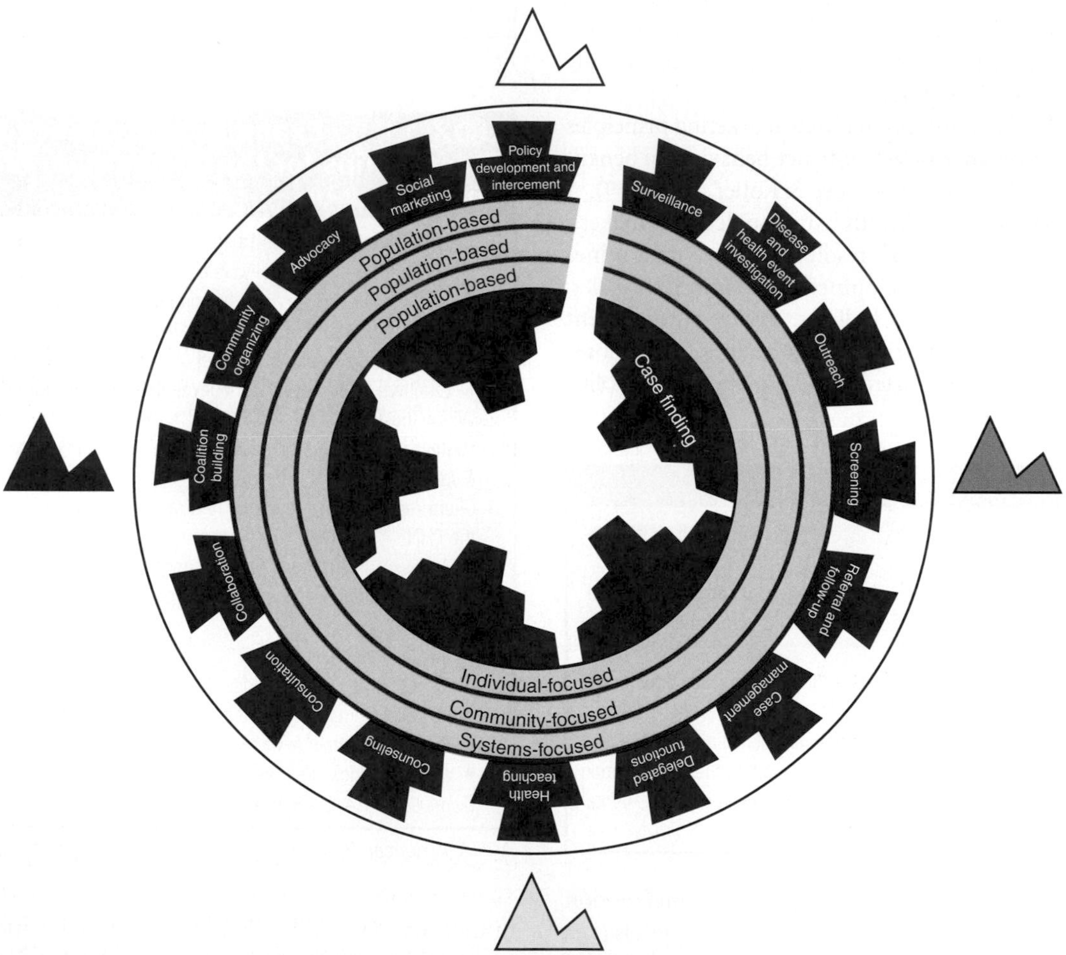

The Navajo basket represents mother earth (the tan area), the black design represents the four sacred mountains that surround the Navajo Nation, and the red area represents the rainbow, which symbolizes harmony. In Navajo philosophy, one should not enclose oneself without an opening. Therefore, the basket has an opening, or doorway, to receive all that is good/positive, and allow all the bad/negative to exit.

Neva Kayaani

Fig. 11.4 Navajo Wheel. (Courtesy Shiprock Service Unit, Shiprock, NM, Indian Health Service.)

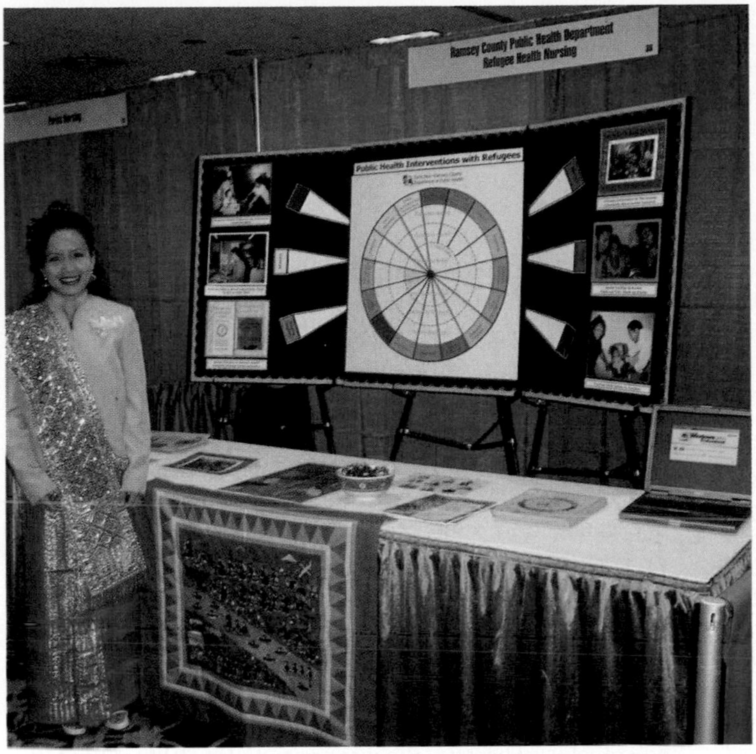

Fig. 11.5 St. Paul-Ramsey County Public Health Family Health International Team. (Courtesy Sophia Emang, Public Health Nurse, St. Paul-Ramsey.)

- PHNs at the St. Paul-Ramsey County (MN) Department of Health used the Intervention Wheel to illustrate the activities of their refugee health program. Their display (Fig. 11.5) identified the most common interventions implemented with the refugee population and illustrated each intervention with a photograph.

The Wheel provides a meaningful frame of reference and common language for staff to communicate about the nature of their work and is used in orientation programs in several states.

The concepts of the model have also been used internationally. The Intervention Wheel was used in public health nursing projects in New Zealand and Ireland. PHNs in Ireland validated the 17 Wheel interventions for public health nursing practice in their country (McDonald et al., 2015). The significance of the contributions of the Intervention Wheel has been recognized by the nursing community. The authors of the Intervention Wheel received Sigma Theta Tau International and National Pinnacle Awards for Research Dissemination and a Creative Achievement Award from the American Public Health Association, Section of Public Health Nursing.

HEALTHY PEOPLE 2020

The objectives chosen to be highlighted in this chapter show how many of the interventions from the Wheel are applied in the *Healthy People 2020* document. It further indicates how appropriate these interventions are to improving the health of individuals, populations, and communities, thus improving the health of the nation.

EVIDENCE-BASED PRACTICE

Nursing informatics is relatively new for many public health departments in the United States. Community health nurses typically use the Omaha System to document their practice; however, this system is used by various disciplines working in public health. The Omaha System taxonomy is the conceptual framework for the Automated Community Health Information System (ACHIS), which is the long-standing electronic data system used to document nursing practice in community nursing centers. However, researchers identified a gap in the Omaha System and ACHIS in that both were better at capturing individual-level interventions than community- and system-level interventions. Therefore researchers in this study incorporated interventions from the Intervention Wheel into the existing electronic record system in hopes that community- and system-level activities could be documented better. Nine Wheel interventions were added to the ACHIS: policy development, social marketing, advocacy, community organizing, coalition building, collaboration, consultation, screening, and outreach. The newly expanded system was piloted by two community/public health nurses, and the data indicated the system was successful in capturing a broad scope of the nurses' practice. The researchers documented their methodology so that other administrators in public health may replicate the adaptation of the electronic health record for community nursing practice.

Nurse Use

By having a systematic data collection method, better evaluation of processes and outcomes of public health nursing and other public health professionals would be possible. Such data would also aid in providing evidence-based decision support for public health practice that could be used for quality improvement, funding proposals, and policy decisions.

Baisch MJ: A systematic method to document population-level nursing interventions in an electronic health system. *Public Health Nurs* 29(4): 352–360, 2012.

HEALTHY PEOPLE 2020

Healthy People 2020 identifies action steps for 38 health priorities that the United States must take to achieve better population health by the year 2020. The 500 recommended objectives offer numerous opportunities for public health nurses to contribute through implementing interventions at any or all of the levels. Here are a few examples:

- **AH-8**: Adolescent Health Objective: *Increase the proportion of adolescents who have had a wellness checkup in the past 12 months.* PHNs who provide well-child screening services in school settings or local health departments will need well-designed outreach interventions to convince teens that even healthy kids can benefit from checkups. This will require consulting with parents and groups of teens themselves to identify what "benefits" would attract them and incorporating them into the outreach design. PHNs will also need to collaborate with other health care providers in the community to ensure that diagnostic and treatment services are available for teens who require additional services.
- **ECBP-10**: Education and Community-Based Programs Objective: *Increase the number of community-based organizations providing population-based primary prevention services in the following areas: injury, violence, mental illness, tobacco use, substance abuse, unintended pregnancy, chronic disease programs, nutrition, and physical activity.* PHNs may convene coalitions to address an issue or serve as facilitators or participants of coalitions already organized. For instance, PHNs with expertise in substance use prevention might offer health teaching and consultation to a coalition organized to find ways to reduce substance use during pregnancy. It could also mean the establishment of a new screening and referral system among providers to identify early pregnant women and their partners struggling with drug or alcohol use and link with resources for treatment.
- **EH-8.1**: Environmental Health Objective: *Eliminate elevated blood lead levels in children.* PHNs providing services to families with young children assess (surveillance) the living conditions for lead. Housing constructed before 1978, the year lead-based paint for residential use was banned, is particularly suspect. Depending on the community's housing and lead-abatement codes, PHNs may provide health teaching and counseling to the families regarding the dangers of lead exposure to small children or provide advocacy on their behalf with housing authorities.

APPLYING THE NURSING PROCESS IN PUBLIC HEALTH NURSING PRACTICE

PHNs use the nursing process at all levels of practice. PHNs must customize the components of the nursing process (assessment, diagnosis, planning, implementation, evaluation) to the three levels of practice. See Table 11.1 for an outline of the nursing process at the community, systems, and individual/family levels of practice.

APPLYING THE NURSING PROCESS AT THE INDIVIDUAL/FAMILY LEVEL

Community Assessment

During a health department's community assessment process, information on the health status of children was obtained from the following:

- Staff PHNs who worked with families in clinics, schools, and homes
- Community partners who worked with families, including health care providers, mental health workers, social workers, and school personnel
- Preschool screening program data on the number of young children with developmental delays and problems for the past 5 years
- Data from the county social services department on the number of substantiated child maltreatment and neglect cases for the past 5 years

PHNs participated in the community meeting that prioritized the long list of issues identified in the community assessment. One of the top community priorities that emerged was the following: *Decreasing numbers of children at risk for delayed development, injury, and disease because of inadequate parenting by parents experiencing mental health problems.*

The community health plan developed a goal to decrease the number of children with delayed development, injury, and disease attributable to inadequate parenting. The local health department, with the support of community partners, decided they would address this priority through a home visiting strategy. Home visiting enhances a child's environment and increases the capacity of parents to behave appropriately. Although parental mental health problems are a major source of stress for children, this vulnerability can be tempered through support from others and a caring environment.

Home visiting to families is an example of practice at the individual level because the interventions are delivered to families with the goal of changing parental knowledge, attitudes, practices, and behaviors.

Public Health Nursing Process: Assessment of a Family

A PHN received a referral on Tyler, age three. He was the only child of Ashley, a 19-year-old single mother with severe depression. Ashley lived in an old rented house in the small town where she grew up. She had a boyfriend who was not Tyler's biological father. Ashley survived on limited public assistance and occasional help from her mom.

The PHN assessed the resilience, assets, and protective factors as well as the problems, deficits, and health risks of this family. The PHN also tried to elicit Ashley's perception of her situation, which was difficult because of her depressed state. This step is important because often a client's perception of their problems or strengths may not align with the PHN's professional assessment.

All public health nursing practice is relationship based, regardless of level of practice. An established trust relationship increases the likelihood of a successful outcome. One of the PHN's main priorities was to establish a trusting relationship with Ashley. This was difficult because Ashley was seldom out of bed when the PHN arrived, but the PHN persisted and eventually developed the relationship.

Public Health Nursing Process: Diagnosis

- *Diagnosis:* Increased risk for delayed development, injury, and disease because of inadequate parenting by a primary parent experiencing depression
- *Population at risk:* Young children who are being parented by a primary parent who is experiencing mental health problems

- *Prevention level:* Secondary prevention, because the families have an identified risk

Public Health Nursing Process: Planning (Including Selection of Interventions)

Based on the assessment of this family, the PHN negotiated with Ashley to establish meaningful, measurable, achievable **intermediate goals**. In families experiencing mental illness (actually, in most families), behavior change occurs in very small steps. For this family, client goals included the following outcomes:

- Ashley will get out of bed at least three days in the week.
- Tyler will be dressed when the PHN arrives.
- Tyler will get to the bus on time three days in a row.
- The clutter will be cleaned off the steps.
- Ashley will call to make a doctor's appointment for Tyler's well-child check.
- Ashley will use "time-outs" instead of spanking.
- Ashley will read a story to Tyler twice a week.

(The above are examples of intermediate indicators at the individual level of practice, which are aimed at changing an individual's knowledge, attitudes, motivation, beliefs, values, skills, practices, and behavior that lead to desired changes in health status.)

The PHN also selected meaningful, measurable **outcome health status indicators** to measure the impact of the interventions on population health. Examples include no signs or reports of child maltreatment; child regularly attends preschool; child receives well-child examinations according to recommended schedule; child's immunizations are up to date; the family seeks medical care for acute illness as needed and does not seek medical care inappropriately; and child falls within normal limits on developmental tests.

The PHN selected the interventions, which included collaboration, case management, health teaching, delegated functions, and referral and follow-up. In selecting these interventions, the PHN considered evidence of effectiveness, political support, acceptability to the family, cost-effectiveness, legality, ethics, greatest potential for successful outcome, and level of prevention.

Public Health Nursing Process: Implementation

The PHN determined the sequence and frequency of her home visits based on her assessment of each family. Some families received home visits once a week, some twice a week, and others twice a month. The PHN visited this family weekly in the beginning and then spaced the home visits farther apart. She used the following interventions.

Collaboration. The PHN identified and involved as many alternative caregivers in Tyler's care as possible, including Tyler's biological father, aunt and uncle, and grandparents, as well as Ashley's boyfriend.

Case Management. The PHN arranged childcare services and coordinated transportation for Tyler to spend significant portions of his day outside of the home.

Health Teaching. The PHN provided information on child growth and development, nutrition, immunizations, safety, medical and dental care, and discipline to Ashley and the alternative caregivers.

Delegated Functions (Public Health Nurse to Community Health Worker). The PHN placed a community health worker (CHW) in the home to provide role modeling for Ashley. As part of this intervention, the PHN monitored and supervised the CHW.

Referral and Follow-up. Based on the assessment, the PHN referred Ashley to community resources and services that included early childhood services, legal aid, food stamps, mental health counselors, and transportation.

Public Health Nursing Process: Evaluation

The PHN reassessed and modified her plan at each home visit. She provided regular feedback to Ashley and the other caregivers on their progress. The PHN documented her results and compared them with the selected indicators. After six months of home visits, Ashley got out of bed most days of the week but rarely got dressed. Ashley was more successful in getting Tyler to the bus and to preschool. The CHW helped Ashley clean the clutter off the steps. Ashley scheduled a doctor's appointment for Tyler's well-child visit but failed to get him to the appointment. Ashley was successful in learning to substitute "time outs" for spanking, with the help of the CHW. Tyler exhibited no signs of child maltreatment. He attended preschool regularly. Tyler was still behind on his immunizations because of the missed appointment. All of Tyler's developmental tests were within normal limits.

The PHN reported her results to her supervisor during their regular supervisory meetings. The PHN also talked with other PHNs who worked with similar families about common issues and best practices and applied what she had learned to her practice.

APPLYING THE PUBLIC HEALTH NURSING PROCESS TO THE COMMUNITY LEVEL OF PRACTICE SCENARIO

Note: At the community level of practice, the community assessment, program planning, and evaluation process is the public health nursing process.

Community Assessment (Public Health Nursing Process: Assessment)

Childhood obesity is a serious problem in the United States putting children and adolescents at risk for poor health. Obesity prevalence, defined by a body mass index (BMI) at or above the 95th percentile (based on CDC growth charts) among children is still too high. The 2015-2016 National Health and Nutrition Examination Survey data estimated that 13.9 percent of children aged two to five were obese in the United States. Among children aged 6 to 11 years the percent was 18.4 percent. There was no significant difference in the prevalence of obesity between boys and girls by age group (CDC, 2018). Childhood obesity and hyperplasia of adipose cells are linked to obesity later in life.

A health department recognized the well-established association between overweight and obesity in childhood and the development of both continuing overweight/obesity as adults and a host of chronic diseases (CDC, 2016b). In response the public health nursing director of a health department convened a childhood obesity prevention summit. Over 80 participants representing area health care providers, schools, childcare, and governmental and community-based health organizations met for an entire day to discuss the problem and frame solutions.

Community Diagnosis (Public Health Nursing Process: Diagnosis)

The percent of children aged 2 to 11 who are overweight or obese is unacceptable and threatens the future health status of the community.

- *Population of interest:* Children aged 2 to 11
- *Level of prevention:* Primary prevention

Community Action Plan (Public Health Nursing Process: Planning, Including Selection of Interventions)

At the conclusion of the summit each organization represented committed to promoting healthy eating and physical activity habits for all residents, with an emphasis on parents of young children. The health department recognized that a substantial portion of a child's caloric intake occurs at childcare.

Based on its assessment of the community, the health department initiated a 24-week evidence-based program that promotes the consumption of fruits and vegetables by young children through intervention with licensed home childcare providers. "LANA the Iguana" (Learning About Nutrition Through Activities) encourages eating eight targeted fruits and vegetables: broccoli, sweet red pepper, cherry tomatoes, apricots, sugar snap peas, kiwi, sweet potatoes, and strawberries (Fig. 11.6). These fruits and vegetables were featured in activities throughout the program related to menu changes, classroom activities, and family involvement.

Menu Changes. Home childcare providers increased opportunities for children to eat more fruits and vegetables by serving the targeted fruits and vegetables on the menu, alternating four for one week and four the next. Fruits and vegetables were served as the morning and afternoon snack every day.

Classroom Activities. Home childcare providers increased children's preference for and knowledge of fruits and vegetables by featuring one of the targeted fruits and vegetables each week throughout the program. During that week, the featured fruit or vegetable was the focus of tasting and cooking activities as well as the topic of stories and games.

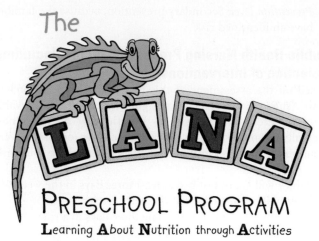

Fig. 11.6 LANA the Iguana. (Used with permission from Minnesota Department of Health, Center for Health Promotion.)

Family Involvement. Home childcare providers gave families information about the program and activities to do at home. These included quick and easy kid-tested recipes and take-home fruit/vegetable tasting kits.

The PHNs selected their interventions, which included consultation, health teaching, social marketing, collaboration, and surveillance. In selecting these interventions, the PHNs considered evidence of effectiveness, acceptability to community, cost-effectiveness, legality, ethics, and greatest potential for successful outcome.

Community Implementation Plan (Public Health Nursing Process: Implementation)

- *Social marketing:* LANA the Iguana was a social marketing program. It incorporated a range of age-appropriate social marketing techniques, including iguana puppets and storybooks, recipe cards, and activities. The PHNs promoted retention by providing home childcare providers with incentives, including two grocery store gift cards and plastic fruit/vegetable toys for the children. They worked with librarians to place LANA the Iguana kits (composed of iguana puppets, activities, and storybooks) in the local library for parents to check out. PHNs also donned the LANA the Iguana costume to implement the curriculum directly to children, as well as train the home childcare providers and parents.
- *Health teaching:* The PHNs trained the home childcare providers on the LANA curriculum to ensure fidelity to the program.
- *Consultation:* The PHNs consulted with home childcare providers about the program on a regular and ongoing basis.
- *Collaboration:* PHNs collaborated with health educators to develop and distribute LANA materials, including a curriculum guide, recipe books, storybooks, parent newsletters, and LANA the Iguana puppets. They also collaborated with public health nursing students to collect program evaluation data.
- *Surveillance:* The PHNs collected data on the consumption of fruits and vegetables in the home childcare setting.

Community Evaluation (Public Health Nursing Process: Evaluation)

Follow-up surveys with the county's 75 licensed home childcare providers, who served about 500 children, found that 67 percent of children were more or much more likely to eat fruits and 78 percent were more likely to eat vegetables; 92 percent of children were more likely to try new foods; and 76 percent of providers offered fruits and vegetables more often at snack time (Dakota County, 2010). Establishing healthy eating habits among young children will lead to reduced levels of obesity. The success in promoting healthy eating through the LANA program continues to be demonstrated in both licensed home childcare providers and daycare centers (Dakota County, 2017).

APPLYING THE PUBLIC HEALTH NURSING PROCESS TO A SYSTEMS LEVEL OF PRACTICE SCENARIO

Health departments conduct assessments of community health status, a core function of public health, on an ongoing basis. The identification of some community problems emerges out of practice, rather than through a formal community assessment. This scenario is such an example.

Public Health Nursing Process: Assessment

For several years PHNs had been very concerned about the poor living conditions in an apartment complex in which many of their clients lived. The walls were moldy, the carpet was unclean and deteriorated, and closet doors had fallen off their runners and struck children living in the apartment. The PHNs were suspicious of the required cash payments that the manager required for repairs, extra security deposits, and increased rent after the birth of a baby.

Many of the tenants were undocumented Latinos and tried not to create problems. Most could not speak or read English well and often signed lease agreements without taking note of damage or existing problems in the apartment and were therefore blamed for them. In addition, the manager blamed the tenants for the mold on the walls, implying that their cooking created too much humidity. Citing these "problems," the manager often gave bad references for the tenants, which made it difficult for them to move.

Over the years the PHNs had diligently worked with their clients to correct these problems, but with little success. When the PHNs met with the manager to discuss the issues, he became angry. As a result, the manager had the PHNs' cars towed whenever he saw them in the parking lot. The PHNs also had sought help from city officials, but the officials had no legal recourse to remedy the situation.

Finally, several events occurred that spurred the PHNs to action. One of the PHNs found a nonfunctioning smoke detector in an apartment during a home safety check. The family reported that the apartment manager had dismantled the smoke detector and left it that way. At the same time, another PHN was working with a family that was trying to move to a new, safer, cleaner apartment. The family had found a new apartment but could not move because the manager gave them a bad (although false) reference. The family no longer had a lease, but the manager said they could not move. The PHNs realized that there were many complex legal issues related to the living conditions of their clients.

Public Health Nursing Process: Diagnosis

- *Diagnosis:* Families at risk of illness and injury because of hazardous housing and abuse of legal rights
- *Population at risk:* Families living in hazardous housing in an apartment complex
- *Prevention level:* Secondary, because families are at risk for injury and illness

Public Health Nursing Process: Planning (Including Selection of Interventions)

At the systems level of practice the goal is to change policies, laws, and structures. The PHNs' goals were to enforce the tenants' legal rights and improve the living conditions in the apartment complex. Their plan was to seek advice from a housing advocate service and connect their clients with legal counsel. Before they could pursue this plan, the PHNs consulted with their supervisor. Their supervisor supported their decision but also had to clear the plan with the health department director and the city manager.

The PHNs selected their interventions, which included consultation, referral and follow-up, advocacy, policy development, and surveillance. In selecting these interventions the PHNs considered evidence of effectiveness, political support, acceptability to the family, cost-effectiveness, legality, ethics, the potential for a successful outcome, nonduplication, and level of prevention.

Public Health Nursing Process: Implementation

The PHNs worked with the tenants and the housing advocacy service to implement the following interventions.

Consultation. The PHNs consulted with attorneys at a housing advocate service.

Referral and Follow-up. The attorneys informed the PHNs that they needed to hear directly from the tenants in order to proceed. The PHNs set up a meeting time between the tenants and the attorneys from the housing advocate service.

Advocacy. The PHNs arranged for their public health interpreter to go door to door with an advocate from the housing service to invite tenants to the meeting. They also arranged for the interpreter to attend the meeting to interpret each family's concerns. The PHNs strongly encouraged all of the tenants to attend.

Policy Development. The PHNs worked with the attorneys from the housing advocate service to develop the meeting agenda.

Surveillance. The PHNs continued to conduct ongoing monitoring of living conditions in the apartment complex.

Public Health Nursing Process: Evaluation

Many of the tenants attended the meeting. As a result of the meeting, the attorney chose to have the rent paid to the court and put in escrow until a legal determination could be made. During this process the apartment owner became aware of these issues and dismissed the manager, who was discovered to have been acting fraudulently. A new manager was employed who worked to improve the living conditions of the apartments.

LINKING CONTENT TO PRACTICE

The discussions of the application of the nursing process to a variety of clients beginning on page 234 and Tables 11.1 and 11.2 provide numerous examples of how the content in this chapter is applied in practice. Please review these for examples of how you may apply this model in your practice.

PRACTICE APPLICATION

Outreach locates populations of interest or populations at risk and provides information about the nature of the concern, what can be done about it, and how services can be obtained. Outreach activities may be directed at whole communities, at targeted populations within those communities, and/or at systems that impact the community's health. Outreach success is determined by the proportion of those considered at risk that receive the information and act on it.

The chance of a 20-year-old woman developing breast cancer within the next 10 years is 1 in 1681. At age 30, a woman's chance of developing breast cancer within the next 10 years is 1 in 225; at age 40, it is 1 in 69; at age 50, it is 1 in 44; at age 60, it is 1 in 29; and at age 70, it is 1 in 26 (Susan G. Komen Foundation, 2016).

A health system decided to offer free mammograms in recognition of National Breast Cancer Month. They sponsored a mobile mammography van at a large shopping mall every Saturday in October. The van offered mammograms to everyone, regardless of age. The health system advertised the service by placing windshield flyers on all the cars in the shopping mall parking lot. The van provided 180 mammograms, mostly to women in their 30s who had health insurance that covered preventive services.

A. What is the population most at risk of breast cancer?

B. Did the mammograms in the parking lot reach this population?

C. What types of outreach would PHNs conduct to reach the population at risk?

Answers can be found on the Evolve site.

KEY POINTS

- In these times of change the public health system is constantly challenged to keep focused on the health of populations.
- The Intervention Wheel is a conceptual framework that has proved to be a useful model in defining population-based practice and explaining how it contributes to improving population health.
- The Wheel depicts how public health improves population health through interventions with communities, the individuals and families that make up communities, and the systems that impact the health of communities.
- The Wheel serves as a model for practice in many state and local health departments.
- The Wheel is based on 10 assumptions.
- The Intervention Wheel encompasses 17 interventions.
- Other public health members of the interprofessional team such as nutritionists, health educators, planners, physicians, and epidemiologists also use these interventions.
- Implementing the interventions ultimately contributes to the achievement of the 10 essential public health services.
- The Cornerstones of Public Health Nursing was developed as a companion document to the Intervention Wheel.
- The original version of the Wheel resulted from a grounded theory process carried out by public health nurse consultants at the Minnesota Department of Health in the mid-1990s.
- The interventions were subjected to an extensive review of supporting evidence in the literature.
- The Wheel is a conceptual model. It was conceived as a common language or catalog of general actions used by public health nurses across all practice settings.
- The Intervention Wheel serves as a conceptual model for public health nursing practice and creates a structure for identifying and documenting interventions performed by public health nurses and captures the nature of their work.
- The Wheel has three main components: a population basis, three levels of practice, and 17 interventions.
- The Wheel has led to numerous innovations in practice and education since the original Intervention Wheel was first published in 1998.
- Public health nurses in the Shiprock Service Unit of the Indian Health Service adapted the Intervention Wheel to reflect the Navajo culture.
- Numerous graduate and undergraduate schools of nursing throughout the United States have adopted the Intervention Wheel as a framework for teaching public health nursing practice.

CLINICAL DECISION-MAKING ACTIVITIES

1. Describe the three components of the Intervention Wheel. How do the components relate to each other? Explain how you can apply them to your clinical practice.
2. Go to Chapter 1 and reread the definitions of the core functions of public health practice and look at the 10 essential services. How does the Wheel address the core functions? How does it relate to the 10 essential services?
3. Go to the Minnesota Department of Health website and locate the Wheel document. Choose one of the 17 interventions to explore. Read about the recommended strategies to use when intervening with a client. Explain the level of practice and how you can apply the intervention. Give a concrete example.

ADDITIONAL RESOURCES

EVOLVE WEBSITE

http://evolve.elsevier.com/Stanhope/community/

- Answers to Practice Application
- Case Study
- Glossary
- Review Questions

REFERENCES

American Nurses Association: *Public health nursing: scope and standards of practice*, Silver Spring, MD, 2007, ANA. Retrieved from: http://www.nursesbooks.org.

American Nurses Association: *Public health nursing: scope and standards of practice*, ed 2, Silver Spring, MD, 2013, ANA, Nurses Publishing. Retrieved from http://www.nursesbooks.org.

American Public Health Association, Public Health Nursing Section: *Definition and role of public health nursing*, Washington, DC, 2013, APHA. Retrieved from https://apha.org.

Anderson, LJW, Schaffer, MA, Hiltz, C, O'Leary SA, Luehr RE, Yoney EL: Public health interventions: School nurse practice stories, *J Sch Nurs* 34(3):192–202, 2017.

Avila M, Smith K: The reinvigoration of public health nursing: methods and innovations, *J Public Health Manag Pract* 9:16–24, 2003.

Bastable S: *Essentials of patient education*, Burlington, MA, 2017, Jones & Bartlett Learning.

Bleich SN, Jarlenski MP, Bell CN, LaVeist TA: Health inequalities—trends, progress, and policy, *Annu Rev Public Health* 33:7–40, 2012.

Brega AG, Barnard J, Mabachi NM, et al.: Tool 21: Make referrals easy. In Agency for Health Research and Quality, *Health Literacy Universal Precautions Toolkit, Second Edition*, AHRQ Publication No. 15-0023-EF, Rockville, MD, 2015, Agency for Healthcare Research and Quality. Retrieved from https://www.ahrq.gov.

Center for Community Health and Development at the University of Kansas: *Strategies for Community Change and Improvement: An Overview*, 2017, Community Toolbox. Retrieved from https://ctb.ku.edu.

Centers for Disease Control and Prevention: *Children's oral health*, 2014. Retrieved from https://www.cdc.gov.

Centers for Disease Control and Prevention: *Dental caries and sealant prevalence in children and adolescents in the United States, 2011–2012*, NCHS Data Brief No. 191, 2015. Retrieved from https://www.cdc.gov.

Centers for Disease Control and Prevention: *Vaccines and preventable diseases*, 2016a. Retrieved from https://www.cdc.gov.

Centers for Disease Control and Prevention: *Childhood obesity causes and consequences*, 2016b. Retrieved from https://www.cdc.gov.

Centers for Disease Control and Prevention: *Deaths: Final data for 2014*, National Vital Statistics Reports, 65(4). Hyattsville, MD, 2016c, National Center for Health Statistics. Retrieved October 10, 2018 from: https://www.cdc.gov.

Centers for Disease Control and Prevention: *The Public health system and the 10 essential services*, 2018. Retrieved from https://www.cdc.gov.

Centers for Disease Control and Prevention, National Center for Health Statistics (NCHS): Prevalence of Obesity Among Adults and Youth: United States, 2015–2016. Data brief, no. 288, 2017. Retrieved from https://www.cdc.gov.

Cooper J, Zimmerman W: The effect of a faith community nurse network and public health collaboration on hypertension prevention and control. *Public Health Nurs* 34:444–453, 2017.

County of Los Angeles Department of Public Health Nursing Administration: Public Health Nursing: *Public health nursing practice model*, 2007. Retrieved from http://publichealth.lacounty.gov.

Dakota County Public Health Department: *Factsheet: tackling childhood obesity with Lana the Iguana*, 2010. Retrieved from http://www.co.dakota.mn.us.

Dakota County Public Health Department: *Access and quality of health care*, 2016. Retrieved from https://www.co.dakota.mn.us.

Dakota County Public Health Department: *Improving food choices in child care settings*, 2017. Retrieved from https://www.co.dakota.mn.us.

Dang D, Dearholt SL: *Johns Hopkins nursing evidence-based practice: Model and guidelines*, 3rd ed, Indianapolis, IN, 2018, Sigma Theta Tau International.

Delair SF, Lyden ER, O'Keefe AL, et al.: A novel library-based sexually transmitted infection screening program for younger high-risk groups in Omaha, Nebraska, USA, *J Community Health* 41: 289–295, 2016.

Depke JL, Onitilo AA: Coalition building and the Intervention Wheel to address breast cancer screening in Hmong women, *Clin Med Res* 9(1):1–6, 2011.

Eggert LL, Blood-Siegried J, Champagne M, Al-Jumaily M, Biederman DJ: Coalition building for health: A community garden pilot project with apartment dwelling refugees, *J Community Health Nurs* 32:141–150, 2015.

Ezeonwu MC: Community health nursing advocacy: A concept analysis, *J Community Health Nurs* 32(2):115–128, 2015.

Ezeonwu, M., Berkowitz, B. (2014). A collaborative community wide health fair: The process and impact on the community. *Journal of Community Health Nursing*, 31:118-129.

Fawcett J, DeSanto-Madeya S: *Contemporary Nursing Knowledge: Analysis and Evaluation of Nursing Models and Theories*, ed 3, Philadelphia, 2013, FA Davis.

Flaten C: Connecting antepartum teens from a federal food program to a public health nursing agency: a process-improvement project, *West J Nurs Res* 33(1):144–145, 2011.

Friedman AJ, Cosby R, Boyko S, Hatton-Bauer J, Turnbull G: Effective teaching strategies and methods of delivery for patient education: A systematic review and practice guideline recommendations, *J Cancer Educ* 26:12–21, 2011.

Gregory D, Johnston R, Pratt G, et al, editors: *The Dictionary of Human Geography*, ed 5, Oxford, England, 2009, Blackwell, pp. 103–104.

Hamilton BE, Martin JA, Osterman MJK: Births: Preliminary data for 2015, *Natl Vital Stat Rep* 65(3):1–15, June 2, 2016. http://www.cdc.gov.

Hanna-Attisha M, LaChance J, Sadler RC, Champney Schnepp A: Elevated blood lead levels in children associated with the Flint drinking water crisis: A spatial analysis of risk and public health response, *Am J Public Health* 106:283–290, 2016.

Infant mortality disparities fact sheets. 2014. [October 21, 2016]. http://minorityhealth.hhs.gov.

Jewish Women's Archive: *Lillian Wald: Backyard of a Henry Street Branch*, 1915. Retrieved from https://jwa.org.

Keller LO, Strohschein S, Lia-Hoagberg B, Schaffer M: Population-based public health nursing interventions: a model from practice, *Public Health Nurs* 15:207–215, 1998.

Keller LO, Schaffer MA, Strohschein S, Lia-Hoagberg B: Assessment, program planning, and evaluation in population-based public health practice, *J Public Health Manag Pract* 8:30–43, 2002.

Keller LO, Strohschein S, Lia-Hoagberg B, Schaffer MA: Population-based public health interventions: practice-based and evidence-supported, part I, *Public Health Nurs* 21:453–468, 2004a.

Keller LO, Strohschein S, Schaffer MA, Lia-Hoagberg B: Population-based public health interventions: innovations in practice, teaching, and management, part II, *Public Health Nurs* 21:469–487, 2004b.

Keller LO, Strohschein S, Schaffer MA: Cornerstones of public health nursing, *Public Health Nurs* 28(3):249–260, 2011.

Leavell HR, Clark EG: *Preventive Medicine for the Doctor in His Community*, ed 3, New York, 1965, McGraw-Hill.

Lee NR, Kotler P: *Social marketing: influencing behaviors for good*, Thousand Oaks, CA, 2016, Sage Publications, Inc.

Massachusetts Association of Public Health Nurses: *Leadership guide and resource manual*, 2009. Retrieved from www.maphn.org.

McDonald A, Frazer K, Duignan C, et al.: Validating the 'Intervention Wheel' in the context of Irish public health nursing, *Br J Community Nurs* 20(3):140–145, 2015.

McGolrick D, Belanger P, Richardson H, Moore K, Maier A, Majury A: Evaluation of self-swabbing coupled with a telephone health helpline as an adjunct tool for surveillance of influenza viruses in Ontario, *BMC Public Health* 16:1–9, 2016.

McPherson C, Ndumbe-Eyoh S, Betker C, Oickle D, Peroff-Johnston N: Swimming against the tide: A Canadian qualitative study examining the implementation of a province-wide public health initiative to address health equity, *Int J Equity Health* 15(1): 129, 2016.

Minnesota Department of Health: *Healthy Teeth–Healthy Baby*, 2016. Retrieved from http://www.health.state.mn.us.

National Association of County and City Health Officials (NACCHO): *Maternal child health capacity for Zika response*, 2018. Retrieved from https://www.naccho.org.

National Business Coalition on Health: *Community health partnerships: tools and information for development and support*, 2009. Retrieved from https://stacks.cdc.gov.

National Center for Health Statistics (NCHS): *Health, United States, 2015: With special feature on racial and ethnic health disparities*, Hyattsville, MD, 2016, National Center for Health Statistics.

Nurse Family Partnership: *A young family's bright future begins with a great nurse*, 2018. Retrieved from https://www.nursefamilypartnership.org.

Pachter LM, Lieberman L, Bloom SL, Fein JA: Developing a community-wide initiative to address childhood adversity and toxic stress: A case study of the Philadelphia ACE Task Force, *Acad Pediatr* 17(7 Suppl):S130–S135, 2017.

Schaffer MA, Keller LO, Reckinger D: Public health nursing activities: Visible or invisible? *Public Health Nurs* 32(6):711–720, 2015.

Schaffer MA, Anderson LJW, Rising S: Public health interventions for school nursing practice, *J Sch Nurs* 32(3):195–208, 2016.

Schoneman D, Simandl G, Hansen JM, Garrett S: Competency-based project to review community/public health curricula, *Public Health Nurs* 31(4):373–383, 2014.

Schoon PM: *Asset-based dental resources*, PowerPoint presentation for Minnesota Department of Health "Healthy Teeth–Healthy Baby" Lunch and Learn on March 16, 2018, 2018a. St. Paul, MN.

Schoon PM: *Henry Street Consortium innovative teaching/leaning experience description: Oral health outreach and education*, 2018b. Retrieved from http://www.henrystreetconsortium.org.

Self B, Peters H: Street outreach with no streets, *Can Nurse* 101(1):20–24, 2005.

Shi L, Johnson JA: *Novick & Morrow's Public Health Administration: Principles for Population-Based Management*, ed 3, Gaithersburg, MD, 2014, Aspen.

Smith K, Bazini-Barakat N: A public health nursing practice model: melding public health principles with the nursing process, *Public Health Nurs* 20:42–48, 2003.

Strass P, Billay E: A public health nursing initiative to promote antenatal health, *Can Nurse* 104(2):29–33, 2008.

Susan G, Komen Foundation: *Breast cancer risk factors factsheet*, 2016. Retrieved from http://ww5.komen.org.

Turnock BJ: *Public Health: What It Is and How It Works*, ed 5, Gaithersburg, MD, 2015, Aspen Publishers.

Williams CA, Highriter ME: Community health nursing: population focus and evaluation, *Public Health Rev* 7:197–221, 1978.

World Health Organization: *Public health surveillance*, 2018. Retrieved from http://www.who.int.

12

Genomics in Public Health Nursing

Elke Jones Zschaebitz, DNP, APRN, FNP-BC, Joanna Horn, BA, MS, and Jeanette Lancaster, PhD, RN, FAAN

"Maps are a timeless resource—you don't have to visit every part of them at once for them to be of value. It's worth knowing that Oxford is south of Birmingham and west of London, even if you don't plan to visit any of the places tomorrow. The same is true of the Human Genome Project—it will guide researches for centuries, even if every inch isn't explored or used tomorrow."

T. Michael Dexter, Director of Wellcome Trust and contributor to the Sanger Center for the Human Genome Project

OBJECTIVES

After reading this chapter, the student should be able to do the following:

1. Define key terms related to genetics and genomics.
2. Discuss the history of genomics and its integration into public health nursing.
3. Describe the relationship between genomics, genetics, and nursing.
4. Explain the core competencies related to genomics that nurses and selected other public health professionals should integrate into their practice.
5. Describe at least three potential implications of persons knowing their genetic information on clients, families, and communities.

CHAPTER OUTLINE

The Human Genome and Its Transforming Effect on Public Health
A Brief History of the Science
DNA and Its Relationship to Genomics and Genetics
Current Issues in Genomics and Genetics
Personalized Health Care
Genomic Competencies for Nurses
Incorporating Genomics and Genetics Into Public Health Nursing Practice
Application and Practice: Mapping Out a Pedigree
The Future

KEY TERMS

DNA, p. 257
epigenetics, p. 266
family health history, p. 257
genes, p. 257
genetics, p. 256
genetic susceptibility, p. 267
genome, p. 255
genomics, p. 256
Human Genome Project, p. 256
multifactorial diseases, p. 266
mutagen, p. 258
mutations, p. 257
pedigree, p. 264

THE HUMAN GENOME AND ITS TRANSFORMING EFFECT ON PUBLIC HEALTH

The mapping of the human genome was a strategic inflection point in the history of health care that created a massive shift in how health professionals provide care and approach public health. April 2018 marked the 15th anniversary of the completion of the Human Genome Project and the ongoing scientific investigation into how genetics and genomics influence the practice of public health nurses in the twenty-first century. This influence is still an evolving phase, although the rate of new knowledge is continuous. This chapter discusses the history of the field of genetics and genomics, what we know about genetics and genomics currently in this evolving field, their impact on current nursing practice, and the prospects for significant changes in how nursing care is delivered. Clearly, our nursing discipline is being dramatically altered by ongoing discoveries in molecular genetics. Examples of the effect on nursing include the following principles: (1) how nursing students are educated, (2) how nurses collect and use health histories, (3) how nurses learn and apply innovative biotechnology, (4) what role genetics and genomics will continue to play in traditional nursing arenas such as prevention and health education, (5) how nurses keep abreast of innovative and evolving therapies, (6) how nurses integrate the role of epigenetics in current research of disease, and (7) how nurses view public health debates, including the moral, ethical, legal, and social issues around this evolving field of knowledge.

The discipline of nursing has historically sought to keep up with the changes in health care delivery and with medical science. Therefore it is important while reading this chapter to recognize that the fields of genetics and genomics are continuously evolving, extremely complex, and involve personal health and ethical dilemmas surrounding the emergence of personal DNA discoveries. The science applications of genetics and genomics have enormous implications for the detection, prevention, and treatment of human disease, not to mention educational and economic development. Learning about genomics and genetics opens many new possibilities, such as in the prevention and treatment of human maladies ranging from cancer to cystic fibrosis and from autism to Alzheimer's disease. To understand the effects of this knowledge in public health and in nursing, it is important to pull key snapshots from this highly detailed landscape in order to begin to describe this new territory that nursing practice occupies. This chapter provides a general overview of the history of the development of this new science and briefly discusses the current state of the science of genetics and genomics in relation to the role of the nurse and the future implications for care of individuals, families, and populations. What is clear is that every nurse needs to become knowledgeable about concepts of genetics and genomics and to keep current with ongoing discoveries regarding them and their effects on populations.

In this chapter the term **genetics** refers to the study of the function and effect of single genes that are *inherited by children from their parents*. The central term of genetics, *the gene*, can no longer be defined in simple terms; however, for the purposes of this chapter we will simplify and use this definition in context for educational purposes (Portin & Wilkins, 2017). **Genomics** is the study of all of a person's genes, including their interaction with one another as well as the interaction of a person's genes with the environment. Individuals involved with the field of genomics examine the molecular mechanisms and the interplay of genetic and environmental, and of cultural and psychosocial, factors in disease. The field of genomics deals with the functions and interactions of all genes in an organism and is the study of the total DNA structure (National Human Genome Research Institute [NHGRI], 2015a).

A BRIEF HISTORY OF THE SCIENCE

It is important to understand the evolution of genetic and genomic knowledge. The concept of this hereditary information began with agriculture in the eighteenth century by Gregor Mendel, an Austrian monk who is usually considered to be the father of genetics. At about the same time, Charles Darwin expounded on the theories of evolution, and Darwin's cousin, Francis Galton, performed family studies using twins in an effort to understand the influence of heredity on various human characteristics. The word *gene* was not used until the Danish botanist Wilhelm Johannsen created it in 1909, but it quickly was adopted into the science of genetics and biology. At this time the term was used as a mere abstraction, but by the second decade in the twentieth century, a number of genes had been localized to specific positions on chromosomes, and groups of genes that showed some degree of coinheritance could be categorically placed in groups. In the early 1930s, genes were considered indivisible units of inheritance and were defined in terms of their function/behavior in four criteria: (1) hereditary transmission, (2) genetic recombination, (3) mutation, and (4) gene function (Portin & Wilkins, 2017).

A major breakthrough occurred on February 28, 1953, in Cambridge, England, when James Watson and Francis Crick announced that they had figured out the structure of deoxyribonucleic acid (DNA), and that this double-helix structure could unzip to make copies of itself—thus confirming that DNA carries life's hereditary information, or the secret to life (Science History Institute, 2017). Genetic diseases and their mode of inherited anomalies such as phenylketonuria (PKU), sickle cell disease, Huntington's disease, and cystic fibrosis were discovered. In the same decade that Watson and Crick unveiled the mystery of DNA, the correct number of human chromosomes was determined. Because of this 1956 discovery, one of the new findings in genetics included the discovery in 1959 that Down syndrome is caused by an extra copy of chromosome 21. The scientific revolution was propelled forward.

To date, the **Human Genome Project** (HGP), an international research project funded by the U.S. Congress in 1988 and completed in 2003, has mapped all of the approximately 25,000 genes in human DNA. This enormous project reflects the work of scientists from 20 research centers in six countries: China, France, Germany, Japan, the United Kingdom, and the United States (NHGRI, 2015b).

The stated goals of the HGP were *determining* the sequences of the 3 billion chemical base pairs that make up human DNA; *storing* this information in databases; *improving* tools for data analysis; *transferring* related technologies to the private sector; and *addressing* the ethical, legal, and social issues that may arise.

Many implications for health care have emerged from this project, including ethical and moral dilemmas that continue to be challenging. As health information advances, genomics has influenced the availability of genetic tests. Clinical tests and home testing kits such as 23andMe, a direct-to-consumer personal genome service, are giving individuals and families information regarding ancestry. Some of these direct-to-consumer tests promise medical information as well as ancestry, but the medical information to be gleaned from such tests is controversial at worst, limited at best (Centers for Disease Control and Prevention [CDC], 2017a).

Many genetic tests have implications for families, and it is important for nurses to help individuals and communities understand the purpose, limitations, potential benefits, and potential risks of a test before submitting samples for analysis. The controversies surrounding the information derived from tests, particularly home testing, include the trust and decisions individuals might make depending on the information derived and the uses of the genetic material and what the public understands about sharing their genetic information. The Food and Drug Administration (FDA) has urged the medical community to focus on educating health care providers and patients about the benefits—and limitations—of genetic testing (U.S. Department of Health and Human Services, 2017). The issues of genetic screening and prophylactic treatments alone are staggering and will require the full resources of the nursing profession to find answers. The following case illustrates many of the complex issues in genetics and genomics.

CHECK YOUR PRACTICE

Screening for Breast or Ovarian Cancer Risk

Ms. Brown, a 37-year old Medicaid patient, was referred by her primary care provider to the High-Risk Breast and Ovarian Cancer Clinic, a specialty clinic. During an initial visit she reports that she had found a mass during a self-breast examination. She subsequently had the mass inspected by a clinician and underwent a mammogram, which showed a suspicious finding. A breast core biopsy was performed, and the pathology report indicated that she had atypical ductal hyperplasia. Ms. Brown then had a breast lumpectomy, and the final pathology findings were benign. Later she had a total abdominal hysterectomy and bilateral salpingo-oophorectomy for endometriosis. Ms. Brown briefly took hormone replacement therapy but stopped in 2017 when the breast mass was identified. She began Evista/raloxifene therapy as a breast cancer reduction measure, but after 6 months she stopped the medication because of the side effects. Ms. Brown reports that she is not entirely opposed to considering using raloxifene again. Her family history indicated that a paternal grandmother likely had a type of "female cancer." This grandmother died in her middle 30s to early 40s. There were also three cousins on the paternal side of the family who had unilateral breast cancer when they were in their 30s and 40s.

On the maternal side of the family, her grandmother was diagnosed with breast cancer when she was in her 40s. She is alive and doing well at age 72. One of the grandmother's sisters had lymphoma and died in her late 60s. A maternal great-aunt who was a sister to her maternal grandfather, not maternal grandmother, died in her 70s of ovarian cancer. A sister to her maternal great-aunt (another maternal great-aunt) died in her 70s or 80s of a primary brain cancer.

Genetic testing for hereditary breast and ovarian cancer (HBOC) for the *BRCA1* and *BRCA2* genes is available. Ms. Brown may want to consider genetic testing for this to better define her future cancer risk, as well as the cancer risks for family members.

Reflect on the following questions, and see what implications they have for nursing action and for public health concerns:

1. What are some possible issues that could arise if Ms. Brown has positive test results? What legal and ethical issues would you consider? What considerations would you take into account if she has a teenage daughter?
2. What effect would the client's literacy level have on how you would handle this case?
3. What if Ms. Brown's Medicaid insurance would not pay for this costly test?
4. If you were caring for a family with multiple family members who obtain genetic testing and some members are found to be genetic mutation carriers while others are not, what would you anticipate might occur in relation to family dynamics? What actions might you take? Consider the referrals you might make.

Over 266,120 women in 2018 were diagnosed with new cases of invasive breast cancer, as well as an estimated 63,960 cases of in situ breast cancer (American Cancer Society, 2018).

Epidemiological studies have established that **family health history** is an important risk factor for both breast and ovarian cancer; therefore it is important for the nurse to take a brief family pedigree as done in the Check Your Practice box to identify inherited risk factors. If Ms. Brown were to have had a *BRCA1* or *BRCA2* mutation, many more implications for decision making would arise, including prophylactic surgery for prevention of breast and/or ovarian cancer. Hereditary breast and ovarian cancer (HBOC) is associated with mutations in the *BRCA1* and *BRCA2* genes, which cause an increased risk for a number of different cancers. For women, both *BRCA1* and *BRCA2* mutation carriers have the greatest risk for breast and ovarian cancer. Men have a significantly increased risk for prostate cancer if they carry a *BRCA1* or *BRCA2* mutation, as well as for male breast cancer (much higher risk for *BRCA2* mutation carriers). Both men and women have an increased risk for pancreatic cancer, especially *BRCA2* mutation carriers. Other cancers have also been associated with HBOC.

DNA AND ITS RELATIONSHIP TO GENOMICS AND GENETICS

"We are more than just our genes. We may be no stronger, or inherently more intelligent, than our cave man ancestors. But what distinguishes us from them, is the knowledge that we have accumulated over the last ten thousand years, and particularly, over the last three hundred. I think it is legitimate to take a broader view, and include externally transmitted information, as well as DNA, in the evolution of the human race."

Stephen Hawking,* George and the Unbreakable Code *(2014, p. 311).

At the core of the issues related to genetics and genomics is DNA. DNA is the chemical inside the nucleus of a cell that has the genetic instructions for making living organisms. DNA can be compared to long-term storage or a blueprint or code to construct other components of cells such as proteins and ribonucleic acid (RNA) molecules. The DNA segments that carry the genetic information are called genes. Within cells, DNA is organized into long structures called chromosomes. These chromosomes are duplicated before cells divide, in a process called DNA replication. **DNA** is composed of four bases: adenine (A), guanine (G), cytosine (C), and thymine (T). **Genes** are composed of specific sequences of these bases.

Alterations in the usual sequence of bases that form a gene or changes in DNA or chromosomal structures are called **mutations**. A large number of agents are known to cause mutations. These mutations, which are attributed to known environmental causes, can be contrasted with spontaneous mutations, which arise naturally during the process of DNA replication. Approximately 3 billion DNA base pairs must be replicated in each cell division, and considering the large number of mutagens to which we are exposed, DNA replication is fascinatingly accurate. A key reason for this accuracy is a mechanism called DNA repair, which occurs in all normal cells of higher organisms. It is estimated that repair mechanisms correct at least 99.9% of initial errors (NHGRI, 2018a).

Chemicals produced in industry are now known to be mutagenic in laboratory animals. A **mutagen** is a chemical or physical phenomenon that promotes errors in DNA replication Among these are nitrogen mustard, vinyl chloride, alkylating agents, formaldehyde, sodium nitrite, and saccharin. In addition, ionizing radiation, such as those produced by x-rays and from nuclear fallout, can promote chemical reactions that change DNA bases or break the bonds of double-stranded DNA (NHGRI, 2018b).

How does an understanding of DNA and the science of genetics relate to public health nursing? In essence, this brief history of the field of genetics shows that human disease comes from the collision between genetic variations and environmental factors. While we cannot change the genes of our fellow human beings, nurses in public health are uniquely poised to advocate for environmental changes (for example, advocating for colorectal cancer screening for those with a family history of colorectal cancer) that can impact the wider health of humankind. As knowledge has evolved with the mapping of the human genome, our understanding of this interaction continues to advance. This has increased knowledge about disease prevention and new methodologies for the practice of public health. We are learning to integrate more effectively our understanding of biological determinism within a social context affecting the delivery of health care.

We know currently that 80% of cancers are sporadic, meaning that there is no germline mutation or inherited gene that is causing the cancer. Ten to 15% of cancers are familial, meaning that they occur in families and need a gene-environment interaction or both genetic variations and environmental factors to cause cancer. Five to 10% of cancers are inherited cancers, and a patient's risk is increased if the patient carries this gene mutation (NHGRI, 2016).

Most hereditary cancer syndromes are inherited in an autosomal dominant pattern with variable expression and incomplete penetrance, which means:

- Genes exist as pairs.
- A gene pair member can occur as either the normal, unaltered form or as a mutation.
- A mutation in one member of the pair is associated with an increased risk for developing certain types of cancer. If a person has a mutation in a hereditary cancer syndrome—related gene, he or she has both a normal form and an altered form of that gene in each of the cells.
- Both men and women carry, pass on to children, and inherit these mutations.
- For mutation carriers the hereditary cancer syndrome can be mild or more severe.
- Whether or not cancer ever develops, the site at which it develops, or the seriousness of the cancer can vary among different people with the same mutation, even within the same family (National Institutes of Health, 2013).

The Challenges of Genetic and DNA Testing

Tests are now available to evaluate more than 1600 genetic disorders ranging from single-gene disorders, such as cystic fibrosis, to more complex disorders, such as diabetes (CDC, 2018a).

As will be discussed in a later section of the chapter, taking a family history is a useful place to begin when considering a genetic connection and before the onset of testing. Furthermore, improved technology has made DNA testing more accessible, including at-home testing. These advances in genetics/genomics necessitate that nurses continue to learn about this area of science in order to respond effectively to the challenges of this new knowledge.

An example of this challenge is that of genetic testing for mutations associated with hereditary disease. The best way to identify whether there is a mutation in a family where a hereditary disease is suspected is to test the person who displays the most evidence of being a mutation carrier. In the setting of a family history of cancer, for example, this is usually a relative who has had a cancer that occurs typically as part of the hereditary cancer syndrome (e.g., breast or ovarian) that is suspected in the family.

The previous example could present a difficulty because family members who have had cancer may not agree to being tested for genetic mutations or may be deceased and be unavailable for testing. The unavailability of the ideal relative for testing presents challenges to the person who desires information that might affect decision making and his or her health. An additional ethical challenge encountered involves individuals without an insurance carrier that reimburses for genetic testing or who may have a high deductible in the insurance policy. Some individuals also think that testing will decrease the quality of their life and make them anxious about the future if they were to discover they have a mutation. Other people fear a positive test result may lead to feelings of guilt about passing along a disease to children and grandchildren. Additionally, some individuals are concerned about their ability to maintain insurance coverage, for health, life, or long-term disability policies. Thankfully, the Genetic Information Nondiscrimination Act (GINA, 2018) offers some reprieve for these worries, at least for health insurance.

Case Example 1. K.N. is a 42-year-old mother with three daughters, ages 16, 18, and 22. She has an extensive family history of ovarian cancer. She is aware that there is currently no good screening for ovarian cancer and regularly worries about her ovarian cancer risk. K.N.'s mother, who was diagnosed with ovarian cancer at age 55, underwent genetic testing and was discovered to be a carrier of the *BRCA2* gene mutation predisposing to breast and ovarian cancer. Several of K.N.'s aunts have died of ovarian cancer at an early age. K.N.'s husband wants her to be tested for the *BRCA2* gene and, if results are positive, has encouraged her to undergo a prophylactic salpingo-oophorectomy. K.N. is concerned that a positive genetic test result may result in loss of insurance coverage. She is also concerned that this will have a negative psychological impact on her children.

Joan Akins is a public health nurse at the county health department serving the area where K.N. resides. Ms. Akins has recently conducted a cancer awareness campaign that included public health education on hereditary cancer syndromes. K.N. contacts Ms. Akins to request advice on whether to undergo genetic testing. Ms. Akins actively listens to K.N.'s concerns and provides general information on genetic testing and the implications of the test results for K.N. and for her children. She also discusses GINA (see the earlier information), which protects the public from genetic discrimination by employers and insurers. Ms. Akins encourages K.N. to talk with her gynecologist about her concerns and to make an appointment for genetic counseling, providing names and contact information for local genetic counselors who specialize in cancer genetics.

As mentioned, genetic testing decisions are personal and complex and can be controversial, leading to dissonance in families. It is important for public health nurses to respect individuals' and family members' decision-making processes. They must, at the same time, be well informed about genetic testing to provide accurate education to members of the public in order to support appropriate decision making.

Also, current methods of testing do not detect all of the mutations that can occur in some diseases, including hereditary cancer syndrome–related genes. If a mutation is detected during DNA testing, this would not predict a future diagnosis of cancer, but rather would indicate that a person is at increased risk for developing the cancers that are part of the particular hereditary cancer syndrome and may need high-risk management. Such a finding has implications for family members who might have inherited the same mutation, enabling them to undergo DNA testing specific to the identified mutation. Such focused testing is more accurate and cost-effective than testing for multiple potential mutations (National Cancer Institute, 2018). In contrast, if DNA testing results in a cancer-affected relative are negative, this does not indicate family members are not at risk. There might be a mutation in a different hereditary cancer syndrome gene than those tested. It is important to remember that many mutations associated with cancer susceptibility and familial syndromes have yet to be identified.

For these reasons, family history must also be considered. However, caution is needed in interpreting family history for several reasons: an inherited syndrome may not be evident for someone with a small family; not everyone is informed of their family's history of disease; death of a family member may be unrelated to cancer, such as early accidental death; or members may have been adopted, and this may not be known to others in the family. Finally, because most cancers are not hereditary, family history should be accompanied by assessment of shared familial environments.

Case Example 2. Sickle cell anemia is an autosomal recessive disease in which a gene mutation results in the production of structurally abnormal hemoglobin called hemoglobin S. Gene carriers have one normal form of the hemoglobin gene and one mutation, a condition called sickle cell trait. The highest rates of disease are among African Americans, with sickle cell anemia affecting approximately 1 in 500 African Americans and 8% of the population being carriers (National Center for Biotechnology Information, 2018).

Chris Covington is a public health nurse employed by a nonprofit, community-based organization that provides health care education and outreach services to members of the African American community in a large metropolitan area. The rate of sickle cell anemia among members of the community is higher than the national average. In response, Chris has implemented a program with the projected outcome to reduce disease rates among African Americans in the community. The program objectives are to (1) increase awareness of the disease in the community and (2) increase rates of carrier testing to support informed decision making regarding childbearing. To meet these objectives, Chris has initiated monthly educational sessions on sickle cell anemia and sickle cell trait at community centers throughout the area. Chris has also collaborated with a local hospital system to provide free biannual genetic counseling sessions with optional carrier screening at community health clinics.

Continuing education is important for public health nurses during this time of rapid integration of new genetic tests into health care practice. Only through ongoing education will public health nurses have the basis from which to appropriately educate the public regarding genetic testing. In addition, recognition of the role of gene-environment interactions in susceptibility to cancer and many other diseases underscores the importance of assessing risk from an environmental perspective. Public health nurses offer this perspective as part of the larger interprofessional team needed to address the complex issues involved in genetic testing.

CURRENT ISSUES IN GENOMICS AND GENETICS

"Translating the knowledge we are gaining from gene discoveries into practical clinical and public health applications will be critical for realizing the potential of personalized health care and improving the health of the nation."

Muin J. Khoury, MD, PhD, Director, CDC Office of Public Health Genomics, (CDC, 2017b)

Many issues are now involved in the growing field of genetics/genomics, including but are not limited to issues such as cloning, epigenomics, fertility, and manipulation of heritable disease traits. Selected current issues specific to nursing are discussed in this section, and others are available in fact sheets through the National Human Genome Research Institute (2015c).

Some of the current issues includes *genetic discrimination* and *privacy in genomics*. The daunting navigation of individualized health care of patients and families in the health system includes learning the importance of knowing their family medical history. Some health care providers are unclear about how to accurately interpret the family history of a client who has had the initiative to collect it. Moreover, many clients are reluctant to disclose this family history for fear that it will affect their health insurance status or eligibility despite current laws in place designed to protect these clients (National Human Genome Research Institute, 2018c).

Nurses can play a key role, and positive impacts that have emerged in the current health environment include not only assisting patients with obtaining their personal family history but also helping patients and families navigate through the disclosure process and uncovering their personal and family health history and understanding specific genetic tests and the costs of these tests. In addition, if patients are willing to make lifestyle changes or health decisions, the appropriate psychosocial support and education can be provided to clients and their families. Nurses play an important role in answering questions and assisting in challenges these clients and families face with making decisions when there is any suspicion of increased risk for genetically based diseases.

Another crucial issue that has emerged currently includes *regulation* of genetic tests. To make things more confusing for patients and families, companies now market their tests and advertise directly to the public. For example, *23andMe*, a private genetics company offering genetic testing services for both ancestry and personalized genetic health information, received FDA approval in 2018 to be able to offer *BRCA1* and *BRCA2* genetic testing; however, they are testing only for mutations found most commonly in those of Ashkenazi Jewish ancestry (U.S. Department of Health and Human Services, 2018). Mass public marketing has implications for nurses and other health care providers who need to provide the appropriate counseling about the implications and indications for such testing. For example, marketing on the Internet complicates client decision making since it can provide consumers with easy access to genetic tests without involving a health care professional in the testing process. Even the clinically available genetic tests, which may provide legitimate test results, are difficult to interpret without genetic counseling. Or, even if the results provided are legitimate, they may not be the test actually needed (as with the 23andMe testing).

Recently the American Academy of Nursing (AAN) issued a policy brief that asserts that public health nurses not only must be well positioned to incorporate evolving knowledge into practice but to advocate for the rights of the consumer with the current use of laboratory and direct-to-consumer genetic testing that is offered, for example, in the 23andMe package. With genetic testing offered at home the AAN released a policy brief that recommends actions be taken to increase the regulation of these tests with regard to data storage, testing standards, false-positive results, and for consumers understanding the true meaning of a test within the context of risk factors (Starkweather et al., 2018).

Currently, there is considerable discussion about the benefits and liabilities of popular sites to verify one's heritage. The nursing care here is to advise clients to carefully research any DNA testing site or facility they might choose. Also, they need to be aware that they may learn things about their heritage that they simply do not want to know. Some new information will come as a big surprise. According to Kelly (2018) individuals should be aware of a few myths and facts before they take a home DNA test.

- Myth 1: My risk of getting a disease will come in the home report.
  False: The genetic DNA overview shows trends compared to other people but they do not tell you if or when you would be likely to end up with a health condition.
- Myth 2: If no genetic mutations or disease conditions were noted on my home DNA test, then chances are I will not get a condition in the future.
  False: Lifestyle habits play a major role in health conditions (such as smoking, poor eating habits, etc.).
- Myth 3: My siblings and I will share 50% of each other's DNA if we have the same parents.
  False: The DNA in each half can be slightly different. It is possible that you received more of your father's European DNA, and your sibling received more of your mother's DNA profile from East Asia. Identical twins DO have identical DNA because they came from the SAME fertilized egg. Fraternal twins each have their own DNA.
- Myth 4: Insurance laws are in place to protect you from being denied health insurance or charged more for it.
  False: Those laws do not apply to life insurance, disability insurance, or long-term care insurance. Your information could be used by companies if the company testing you sells the results of your information to them.
- Myth 5: Harmless fun: It is exciting and entertaining to learn more about ourselves.
  Fact: Sometime genetic tests can reveal surprises in a family.
- Surprise! DNA case example: Misty, a 40 year old female was excited to share the information from her results with her siblings so they could discuss the interesting facts they found out about their heritage as their mother died when they were young and they do not know a lot about her side of the family. When her family received their results, they found out their older brother did not share the paternal line of DNA in the report, leading to many other questions that couldn't be answered. This caused stress and anger between the siblings. They were unsure whether to discuss the results with their father, who was experiencing dementia.

Currently the Centers for Disease Control and Prevention (CDC), the Centers for Medicare and Medicaid Services (CMS), and the FDA have oversight of genetic tests and products, whereas the Federal Trade Commission (FTC) has oversight of the advertising of these tests and products. The National Institutes of Health (NIH), Health Resources and Services Administration (HRSA), and Agency for Healthcare Research and Quality (AHRQ) support research related to genetic tests and products (National Human Genome Research Institute, 2018c).

Moreover, keeping current with the changes in this scientific field with many complex systems in place is a challenging task. The National Human Genome Research Institute (NHGRI) of the NIH provides reliable, up-to-date genetics and genomics information related to patient management, curricular resources, new NIH and NHGRI research activities, and ethical, legal, and social issues. Additionally, the CDC provides a weekly "Genomics & Health Impact Update" on their website for public use (CDC, 2018b). To date, the CDC continually offers a "Genomic Applications Toolkit for Public Health Departments," which is available online for download: https://www.cdc.gov/genomics/implementation/toolkit/ (CDC, 2014).

Helping patients and families understand genetic predisposition to disease versus normal population risk and the impact of lifestyle and environment on health is another role for public health nurses. The Office of Disease Prevention and Health Promotion (ODPHP) in their publication *HealthyPeople 2020* (2018) notes that genomics plays a role in 9 of the 10 leading causes of death in the United Sates, most notably chronic diseases such as cancer and heart disease. There are multifactorial influences acting together to influence disease risk, physiological and mental health conditions, pathogenic DNA, and the therapies used to treat disease. The issue of multifactorial interactions that lead to disease is becomingly increasingly recognized in occupational health, and public health nurses can play a part in educating patients and their families about avoidance of known factors that play a role, for example, in congenital disease states.

In occupational and environmental health, key issues relate to genetic changes that are *acquired during a lifetime* as a result of exposures and the interaction between genes and environmental factors. However, the use of genetic information in occupational safety and health research and practice presents both potential benefits and concerns and raises medical, ethical, legal, and social issues that are emerging in policy and procedure and have an impact on society and individuals (CDC, 2018c).

One example of this phenomenon is cleft lip and palate, a common congenital malformation that results from multifactorial inheritance, a combination of genetic *and* environmental factors, which has ongoing clinical research investigating possible causality (University of Virginia School of Medicine: Department of Pediatrics, 2018). Box 12.1 presents examples of *multifactorial diseases,* or those caused by gene and environment interaction.

Ethical and Legal Considerations

Discoveries in genetics, including those associated with the HGP, present complicated ethical issues for consumers, providers, and health care policy makers. All humans have a right to be concerned about genetic science and its effect on their well-being. Therefore, in the face of this biotechnological revolution, nurses need to carefully review the ethical and legal implications of genetic science, as well as the information used in decision making and interpretation of results, including at-home genetic tests. Ethical considerations include coverage and access to reimbursement for genetic tests through health insurance as well as ensuring that all populations benefit from the advances of genomics research. Other ethical considerations include genetic discrimination against preexisting conditions based on genetic profiling and intellectual property and genomics, as well as ensuring privacy of the genetic information obtained.

BOX 12.1 Examples of Multifactorial Disorders

Autism (strong genetic basis)	Multiple sclerosis
Neural tube disorders	Asthma
Cleft lip, palate	Allergies
Congenital heart disease	Autoimmune disorders
Coronary artery disease	Bipolar disorder
Type 1 diabetes	Schizophrenia
Type 2 diabetes	Epilepsy
Breast cancer	Gallstones
Colon cancer	Obesity
Lung cancer	Peptic ulcer disease
Rheumatic heart disease	Ischemic heart disease
Alcoholism	Pyloric stenosis

A code of ethics was developed by both the International Council of Nurses and the American Nurses Association to emphasize the responsibility of nurses to work with other health care professionals to meet such social and health care needs of the public. They include in this mandate the right that people have to seek and receive genomic health care that is nondiscriminatory, confidential, accessible, and private and that enables patients to make informed decisions. The code is regularly updated to reflect changes in health care structure, financing, and delivery (ANA, 2008). Similarly, the International Society of Nurses in Genetics (ISONG) (2018) is an organization that offers nurses genomic health care opportunities for education and leadership, as well as a place for advocacy and community. ISONG further postulates that the genetic nurse at the basic level of preparation identifies genetic risk factors, provides nursing interventions, makes referrals, and advocates on behalf of patients in ethical standard policy making. Logan Karns, a certified genetic counselor working in the prenatal genetics department at the University of Virginia Health System, describes many ethical dilemmas as medical science moves forward: "Our technological advances have always outpaced our ethical thinking about the consequences of what we're doing. We need to have a measured thoughtfulness about everything." She describes genetic knowledge as unique: "a window from the past and a glimpse into the future" (Karns, 2010).

Ethical Protections in Health Care

On November 21, 2009, the Genetic Information Nondiscrimination Act (GINA) took effect through an act of the U.S. Congress. It was designed to prohibit the improper use of genetic information in health insurance and employment. This act prevents group health plans and health insurers from denying coverage to a healthy individual or charging higher premiums based solely on genetic predisposition to disease. This legislation also prohibits employers with 15 or more employees from using individuals' genetic information when making hiring, firing, job placement, or promotion decisions.

GINA does the following: (1) prohibits employers from discriminating against an employee based on genetic information, (2) places broad restrictions on an employer's deliberate acquisition of genetic information, (3) mandates confidentiality for genetic information that employers lawfully collect, (4) strictly limits disclosure of such information, and (5) prohibits retaliation against employees who complain about genetic discrimination (U.S. Equal Employment Opportunity Commission, 2008).

In accordance with GINA, genetic information is defined as information about the following:

- An individual's genetic tests (including genetic tests done as part of a research study)
- Genetic tests of an individual's family members (defined as dependents and up to and including fourth-degree relatives)

- Genetic tests of any fetus of an individual or family member who is a pregnant woman and genetic tests of any embryo legally held by an individual or family member using assisted reproductive technology
- The manifestation of a disease or disorder in an individual's family members (family history)
- Any request for, or receipt of, genetic services or participation in clinical research that includes genetic services (genetic testing, counseling, or education) by an individual or an individual's family members

While genetic discrimination in the setting of health insurance has not really borne out, and both health insurance and employment are protected by GINA, a new risk for genetic discrimination is emerging in the setting of employer-based voluntary wellness programs. Such programs, which are deemed voluntary, offer financial or other incentives to employees in exchange for health, and potentially, genetic information. Although voluntary, one can imagine that an employee of lower pay and lower socioeconomic status would find these programs to be compulsory, even when they are not legally so.

PERSONALIZED HEALTH CARE

The importance of genetic developments to public health nursing practice is underscored by initiatives between the private sector and the public sector to improve population health through the use of genetic and genomic information. These included the initial goals for the Personalized Health Care Initiative instituted by the U.S. Department of Health and Human Services. Now policy makers and scientists agree that there are many factors involved in bringing new genomic technologies into the marketplace, and consideration of these factors is paramount. Ensuring that new technologies are accessible is of particular concern. Policies and practices for large genomic databases still need to be developed (National Cancer Institute, 2017) (see the Focus on Quality and Safety Education for Nurses box).

Despite the need for ongoing policy and practice development, however, continual integration of genetics into public health remains the objective for *Healthy People 2020.* Screening and genetic testing for specific groups of individuals remain as the standard of practice, while other routine screenings or tests are questioned for their impact on morbidity and mortality. Women with certain high-risk family health history patterns for breast and ovarian cancer, for example, could benefit from receiving genetic counseling to learn about genetic testing for *BRCA1* and *BRCA2* mutations. Surgery for women with these gene mutations could reduce the risk of breast and ovarian cancer by 85% or more.

The Evaluation of Genomic Applications in Practice and Prevention (EGAPP) Working Group supports the development of a systematic process for assessing the available

QSEN FOCUS ON QUALITY AND SAFETY EDUCATION FOR NURSES

Case 3

A role for the public health nurse in genetics: Julie is a public health nurse with the state health department, and her role is to coordinate the follow-up for positive newborn screening results. Every baby born in the state has the heel-prick test (for more information on newborn screening, visit https://www.babysfirsttest.org). This test screens for a number of health conditions, from PKU and sickle cell anemia to congenital hypothyroidism. Many of these conditions are treatable, and often heritable. Since this is a screening test, this means that some babies will have an abnormal test result but will not actually have the condition. Follow-up on the part of the baby's pediatrician and geneticist/metabolic physician is required. Further blood tests are usually necessary to determine which babies are actually affected with the disorder and which are not. Due to the nature of screening tests, false positives are common. Julie's role is to collect the follow-up information on the babies who screen positive, from biochemical and genetic test results to physician notes. It is her job to ensure that all babies who screened positive received the appropriate follow-up tests and to determine which results were true positives and which were false negatives. She then works with the state newborn screening laboratory to aid them in improving their test results.

Targeted Competency: Client-Centered Care

Recognize the client or designee as the source of control and full partner in providing compassionate and coordinated care based on respect for the client's preferences, values, and needs.

Important aspects of client-centered care include:

- **Knowledge:** Describe strategies to empower patients or families in all aspects of the health care process
- **Skills:** Assess level of patient's decisional conflict, and provide access to resources
- **Attitudes:** Appreciate shared decision making with empowered patients and families, even when conflicts occur

Client-Centered Care Question

As the study of genomics becomes more integrated in health care through the rapid growth of personalized medicine, public health nurses may be required to provide the rationale behind the value of population-based health initiatives. The following client-centered scenario speaks to this tension.

You are providing home care to a healthy newborn baby and mother. The baby is 3 weeks old, and this is your first visit. Part of your education for the mother is to review the newborn's vaccination schedule. Upon review of the baby's next needed vaccinations, the mother states that she is interested in the baby's care being based on the baby's genetics, and that she wants her baby to receive personalized medicine. The mother states that she has read an article about individualized approaches to vaccines. "What is recommended for the whole population might not be good for my baby."

- What probing questions might you ask to further understand this mother's position?
- How do you address this mother's concern about the lack of individual consideration in population-based vaccination recommendations?
- What information about personalized medicine will be helpful to this mother?
- What information about vaccines and vaccination schedules will be helpful to this mother?
- What Internet resources do you share with her, to address her questions and concerns?
- What conversation will you be ready to have in your second home visit with this mother?

Prepared by Gail Armstrong, PhD, DNP, ACNS-BC, CNE, Associate Professor, University of Colorado Denver, College of Nursing.

evidence regarding the validity and utility of rapidly emerging genetic tests for clinical practice. This independent, multidisciplinary panel prioritizes and selects tests, reviews CDC-commissioned evidence reports and other contextual factors, highlights critical knowledge gaps, and provides guidance on appropriate use of genetic tests in specific clinical scenarios (EGAPP, 2016).

HEALTHY PEOPLE 2020

The objectives for *Healthy People 2020* include two new objectives that relate to genomics:

- **G-2:** (Developmental) Increase the proportion of persons with newly diagnosed colorectal cancer who receive genetic testing to identify Lynch syndrome (or familial colorectal cancer syndromes).
- **G-1:** Increase the proportion of women with a family history of breast and/or ovarian cancer who receive genetic counseling (ODPHP, 2017).

GENOMIC COMPETENCIES FOR NURSES

Similar to EGAPP, the Essential Nursing Competencies and Curricula Guidelines for Genetics and Genomics was an initiative funded by the NIH, NHGRI, and Office of Rare Disease in collaboration with the American Nurses Association (CDC, 2018d). The competencies developed reflect a consensus and are not from any federal agency or single nursing organization; they are intended to incorporate the genetic and genomic perspective into all nursing education and practice. The guidelines can be found the *Essentials of Genetic and Genomic Nursing: Competencies, Curricula Guidelines, and Outcome Indicators,* second edition (ANA, 2008).

Furthermore, the CDC's contention is that all public health workers need to be aware of the advances in the science of genomics and incorporate the appropriate competencies into their work. They developed seven sets of competencies that related to the work of the individual public health worker. The competencies discussed here are those designed for *all* public health professionals and are to be used in educational and training programs for public health professionals. Currently a public health worker should be able to perform the following:

- Demonstrate basic knowledge of the role genomics plays in the development of disease
- Identify limits of his or her genomic expertise

Similar to the set of competencies developed by the CDC are those developed by the National Coalition for Health Professional Education in Genetics (NCHPEG) to be included in all health professional education (National Human Genome Research Institute, 2017).

The competency and curricular resources are readily available and recommend that at a minimum health care professionals should be able to do the following:

1. Examine their competence of practice regularly to identify areas of strength and areas where professional development related to genetics and genomics would be helpful.
2. Understand that health-related genetic information can have social and psychological implications for individuals and families.
3. Know how and when to make a referral to a genetics professional.

It is well established that new health technologies driven by the knowledge of human genetics can improve the safety, quality, and effectiveness of health care for every client in the United States (Thimbleby, 2013). This perspective on health care is proactive, focused on wellness by managing gene-based information to understand each individual's requirements for the maintenance of his or her health, prevention of disease, and therapy tailored to each individual's genetic uniqueness. An approach to health care that includes a genetic profile of each individual enables nurses and other health care professionals to design care highly customized to match individual needs. A continuing approach to health care built on the knowledge of continual scientific discovery of the health applications from genetics and genomics can help improve health outcomes for individuals and families. An incorporated knowledge of environment, health-related behaviors, culture, values, and the impact of social conditions such as poverty will provide additional arms of assessment when caring for patients. Genetic science emphasizes a fundamental public health nursing issue: the importance of understanding both biological predisposition to disease and the impact of behavior and social conditions on overall community health and well-being.

INCORPORATING GENOMICS AND GENETICS INTO PUBLIC HEALTH NURSING PRACTICE

Public health nursing has long been concerned with environmental or social determinants of health and disease and has only recently become engaged in genomic variations within populations. The advances brought about by genomics, however, are dynamically changing our perceptions, as advancing knowledge enables health promotion and disease prevention programs to be specifically directed at susceptible individuals and families or at subgroups of the population, based on their unique genomic risk profile. Personalized health care based on a broad cultural and social context, a core value of public health nursing, will continue to be more predictive and preventive in nature. The public is beginning to expect that all nurses will use emerging genetic information and technology in their practice, in research, and in all forms of health education.

Professional Practice Domain: Nursing Assessment: Applying/Integrating Genetic and Genomic Knowledge

The registered nurse:

- Demonstrates an understanding of the relationship of genetics and genomics to health, prevention, screening, diagnostics, prognostics, selection of treatment, and monitoring of treatment effectiveness

- Demonstrates ability to elicit a minimum of three-generation family health history
- Constructs a pedigree from collected family history information using standardized symbols and terminology
- Collects personal, health, and developmental histories that consider genetic, environmental, and genomic influences and risks
- Critically analyzes the history and physical assessment findings for genetic, environmental, and genomic influences and risk factors
- Assesses clients' knowledge, perceptions, and responses to genetic and genomic information
- Develops a plan of care that incorporates genetic and genomic assessment information

Identification

The registered nurse:

- Identifies clients who may benefit from specific genetic and genomic information and/or services based on assessment data
- Identifies credible, accurate, appropriate, and current genetic and genomic information, resources, services, and/or technologies specific to given clients
- Identifies ethical, ethnic/ancestral, cultural, religious, legal, fiscal, and societal issues related to genetic and genomic information and technologies
- Defines issues that undermine the rights of all clients for autonomous, informed genetic- and genomic-related decision making and voluntary action

Referral

The registered nurse:

- Facilitates referral for specialized genetic and genomic services for clients as needed

Provision of Education, Care, and Support

The registered nurse:

- Provides clients with interpretation of selective genetic and genomic information or services
- Provides clients with credible, accurate, appropriate, and current genetic and genomic information, resources, services, and/or technologies that facilitate decision making
- Uses health promotion/disease prevention practices that:
  - Consider genetic and genomic influences on personal and environmental risk factors
  - Incorporate knowledge of genetic and/or genomic risk factors (e.g., a client with a genetic predisposition for high cholesterol who can benefit from a change in lifestyle that will decrease the likelihood that the genetic risk will be expressed)
  - Uses genetic- and genomic-based interventions and information to improve clients' outcomes
  - Collaborates with health care providers in providing genetic and genomic health care
  - Collaborates with insurance providers/payers to facilitate reimbursement for genetic and genomic health care services
  - Performs interventions/treatments appropriate to clients' genetic and genomic health care needs
  - Evaluates impact and effectiveness of genetic and genomic technology, information, interventions, and treatments on clients' outcome (ANA, 2008)

HOW TO Help Families Complete a Health History

1. Inform the family that a family health history is a written or graphic record of diseases or health conditions present in their biological family.
2. Encourage the family to develop a three-generation history of biological relatives, their age of diagnosis of a chronic disease, and the age and cause of death of any deceased family members.
3. Explain to the family that this type of history is a useful tool to help them know about their health risks and to prevent disease in themselves and their close relatives.
4. Tell the family that the health history is not a one-time document, but rather one that should be updated periodically.
5. Suggest that the family consider using the CDC online tool "My Family Health Portrait" to collect and organize their family health history. The tool is available free at https://familyhistory.hhs.gov/FHH/html/index.html in both English and Spanish.

From National Institutes of Health: Center for BioMedical Informatics and Information Technology: *My family health portrait*, 2017. Available at https://familyhistory.hhs.gov/FHH/html/index.html.

APPLICATION AND PRACTICE: MAPPING OUT A PEDIGREE

A **pedigree** is a drawing of a family tree used by medical professionals and genetic counselors to assess families and try to spot patterns or indications that may be helpful in diagnosing or managing an individual's health. The pedigree symbols are used globally (see example from the National Society of Genetic Counselors).

Step 1: Talk to the client and/or family, and ask questions and collect all information, including biological parents, brothers and sisters including half-siblings, children, grandparents, aunts and uncles, cousins, nieces and nephews, and include the family giving the history.

Step 2: Draw a basic outline of the family tree using pedigree symbols (see symbols used in Fig. 12.1).

Step 3: Next to each family member's name, write down everything you know about his or her health and medical history. You can also ask family members if you are uncertain. If a family member is adopted, you can possibly collect information on either or both the adopted and birth families.

Include the following information: (1) age or date of birth, (2) age or date of death and cause of death for family members who have passed away, (3) medical conditions and how old the person was when diagnosed with the condition, and (4) where each side of the family comes from originally and pertinent cultural heritage (e.g., England, Iceland, Mexico, Ashkenazi or Eastern European Jewish) (Fig. 12.2).

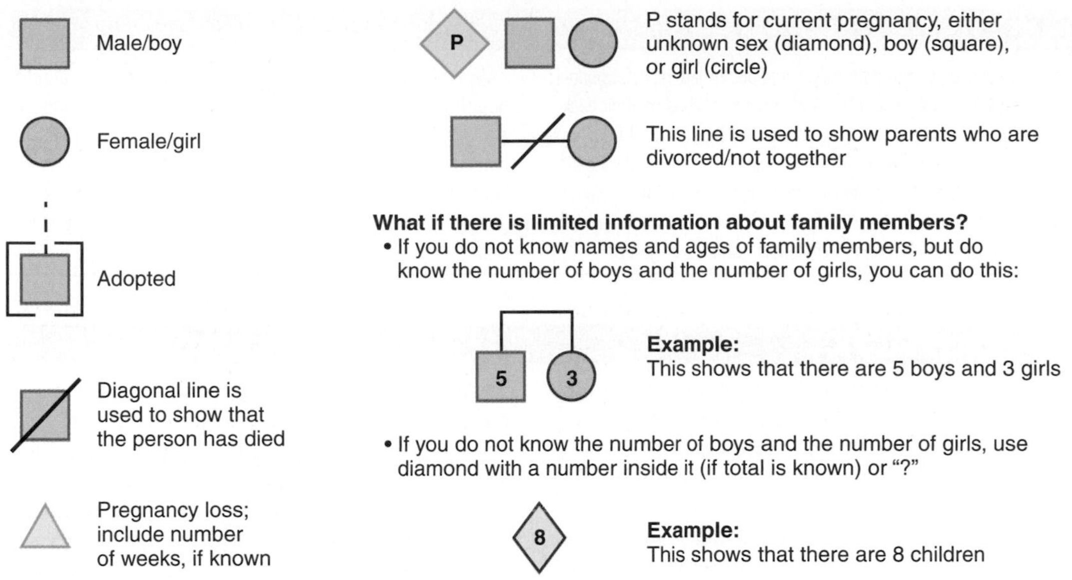

Fig. 12.1 Figures to use in a family pedigree. (National Society of Genetic Counselors, 2014.)

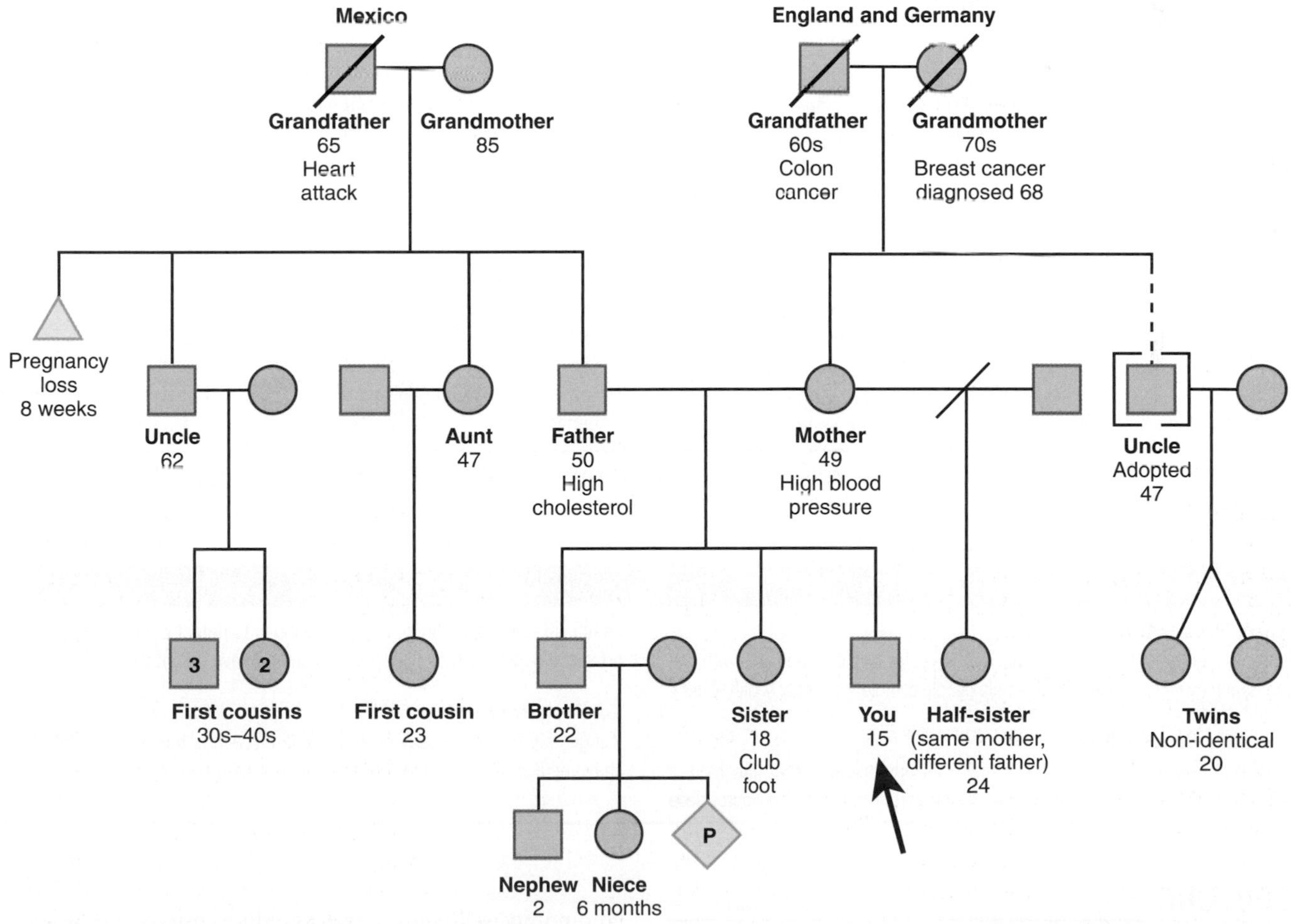

Fig. 12.2 An example of a family pedigree for four generations. (National Society of Genetic Counselors, 2014.)

LINKING CONTENT TO PRACTICE

Organizations previously discussed state that all nurses and public health professionals should have some level of competence in genetics and genomics based on their backgrounds, job duties, and years of experience. In addition, the Quad Council Coalition Competencies, which build on those of the Council on Linkages of the Public Health Foundation, state that the Tier 1 Core Competencies that apply to generalist community/public health nurses (C/PHN) who carry out day-to-day functions in community organizations include the following in relation to individuals, families, or groups:

Working with at-risk-populations for genetic conditions, carrying out health promotion programs at all levels of prevention, basic data collection and analysis, field work, program planning, outreach activities, programmatic support, and other organizational tasks (Quad Council Coalition, 2018). Nurses also promote assurance and advocacy for access to care, including genetic screening, privacy of health information, and certainty that no discrimination will be allowed.

EVIDENCE-BASED PRACTICE

The term **epigenetics** within the context of the field of genomics refers to heritable changes in gene expression that do not involve changes to the underlying DNA sequence: a change in phenotype without a change in genotype. Chemical modification is made to single genes that then affects the expression of the gene. This chemical modification is heritable but does not change the DNA sequence. Epigenetic approaches in research examine complex, **multifactorial diseases** (e.g., cancer, pain, cardiovascular disease), as well as other health conditions and therapies such as pregnancy, childbirth, and immunotherapy that have an environmental component associated with the condition. Research in epigenetics can also include previous cohorts of populations in order to identify environmental factors affecting disease states and that impact one generation to the next. Epigenetic inheritance is an unconventional finding. It goes against the idea that inheritance happens only through the DNA code that passes from parent to offspring. It proposes that a parent's experiences, in the form of epigenetic tags, can be passed down to future generations (Deans & Maggert, 2015).

Epigenetic changes are regular and natural and can be influenced by several factors, including age, the environment/lifestyle, and physical state. Many diseases and conditions that affect a population have a genetic/genomic element that is influenced by these factors. Epigenetic-related diseases have the following characteristics: (1) a heritability that cannot be fully explained by genetic inheritance patterns found in testing; (2) evidence of the influence of imprinting due to environmental exposure (e.g., maternal diet or other in utero exposure to toxins, pathogens, or drugs), which could influence the development of the disease in the offspring even into adulthood; and (3) increase in prevalence of these changes with aging. Environmental factors in epigenetic changes are extremely complex and can be examined using large cohort studies. An example of epigenetic research includes hypertension and metabolic studies to determine the impact of racial disparities, socioeconomic status, preterm birth, education stress, and health behaviors, including diet and smoking, on African Americans (Akinyemiju et al., 2018). A better understanding of the role of nursing in epigenetics and an overview of how epigenetic research relates to nursing practice, as well recommendations and online epigenetic resources that will be useful for future nursing research, is provided in the article *An Overview of Epigenetics in Nursing* (Clark et al., 2013).

Nurse Use

Tips for risk assessment related to genetics when interpreting information in family histories can be noted when evaluating patients and families. These tips can serve as a guide to help nurses provide careful and consistent assessments. The "genetic red flags" that were originally developed by the National Coalition for Health Professional Education in Genetics provide an excellent tool to determine if an individual or family might be at risk. The group says that the primary red flag for most common diseases is a large number of affected relatives who are closely related. Some of the red flags include the following:

1. Family history of multiple affected family members with the same or related disorders, which may or may not follow an identifiable pattern in the family
2. Onset at an earlier age than expected; condition occurrence in the gender that is least expected to have it
3. Disease occurrence in the absence of known risk factors
4. Ethnic predisposition to certain genetic disorders
5. Close biological relationship existing between parents
6. Levels of Prevention Applying the Three Levels of Prevention to Genetics and Genomics

American Academy of Pediatrics: *Genetic red flags*, 2018. Available at https://www.aap.org/en-us/advocacy-and-policy/aap-health-initiatives/genetics-in-primary-care/Genetics-in-Your-Practice/Pages/Genetic-Red-Flag.aspx.

LEVELS OF PREVENTION

Primary Prevention

Since family members share genes, behaviors, lifestyles, and environments with one another that may influence their health, help people complete a family health history.

Secondary Prevention

When you review the health history, observe for any diseases that may have a genetic basis; if found, immediately refer the person or family to the appropriate health care provider. The goal of screening is to detect or define risk in low-risk groups and identify those people who should have diagnostic testing.

Tertiary Prevention

If a genetic link to an early or a probable disease is found, guide the family in changing any behaviors in order to minimize the effect of the disease.

THE FUTURE

At a time of rapid discoveries in genetics and epigenetics, nurses need to be current with the ongoing discoveries and new literature surrounding these discoveries in order to help clients make effective decisions. Knowing which populations have genetic risk for various diseases will lead nursing science to develop and apply public health interventions that will improve health outcomes and community well-being as well as reduce costs. Nurses will increasingly provide guidance on policy discussions affecting health and decisions to ensure confidentiality, provide protection against discrimination based on genetic information, and regulate commercialized genetics products and services. As noted earlier in the chapter, the rate of personal genetic data from at-home kits is expanding in the private sector. However, a patient needs to understand that currently GINA laws cover only health insurance and some forms of employment discrimination. It can be rare that there is protection for disability insurance, long-term care insurance, or even life insurance protections (Williams, 2017).

PRACTICE APPLICATION

T.S., a 4-year-old with hemophilia B, is attending his Head Start program this fall. His mother brought all of his medical supplies and needles so that staff could start an emergency intravenous (IV) infusion if the need arose. The possibility of needing to start an IV concerned the staff, who were teachers, not health care workers. The mother was also anxious about her son being away from home and attending preschool for the first time. As the public health nurse who is responsible for providing health care for Head Start programs in your community, how do you manage the health care for this child while also ensuring safety and making sure that adequate plans are in place for this facility?

A. Let T.S.'s mother know that she needs a note from T.S.'s physician before he can bring any medications to the facility.

B. Notify all of the students' parents/guardians of T.S.'s condition in order to set the guidelines and prevent possible bleeds. The children at the center should be aware of the condition, and the parents also need to educate their children to ensure extra precaution around T.S.

C. Organize a meeting between staff, educators, and parents of T.S. to educate about hemophilia. The aim is to educate key people to ensure T.S.'s safety while at Head Start.

Answers can be found on the Evolve site.

KEY POINTS

- Genetics is the study of the function and effect of single genes that are inherited by children from their parents. Genomics is the study of individual genes in order to understand the interplay of genetic, environmental, cultural, and psychosocial factors in disease.
- DNA is a nucleic acid that contains genetic information called genes.
- Genetic mutations can be caused by the environment or can be spontaneous and arise naturally during the process of DNA replication.
- Human disease comes from the collision between genetic variations and environmental factors.
- Genetic testing decisions are personal and complex, and can be controversial, leading to challenging situations in families.
- The Genetic Information Nondiscrimination Act (GINA) of 2008 was designed to prohibit the improper use of genetic information in health insurance and employment.
- The use of genomics and how it relates to drug treatment will enable personalized health care and medicine to be tailored to each person's needs; health therefore can be predictive and preventive in nature.
- According to the International Society of Nurses in Genetics (ISONG), the genetic nurse carries out the responsibility for identifying genetic risk factors, providing nursing interventions, making referrals, and providing health promotion education. The advanced practice nurse can provide genetic counseling or refer to a genetic counselor and act as case manager for a person with or at risk for a disease that arises from a **genetic susceptibility**.
- Nurses can promote assurance for access to care, including genetic screening, the privacy of health information, and certainty that no discrimination will be allowed in treatment or screening for disease.
- The field of genetics/genomics is growing rapidly and will require nurses to continue to learn and to be aware of advances in research in this area.
- Genomics affects individuals, families, and communities.
- Epigenetics is the study of heritable changes in gene activity that are *not* caused by changes in the DNA sequence; it also can be used to describe the study of stable, long-term alterations in the transcriptional potential of a cell that are not necessarily heritable. Unlike simple genetics based on changes to the DNA sequence (the genotype), the changes in gene expression or cellular phenotype of epigenetics have other causes.

CLINICAL DECISION-MAKING ACTIVITIES

1. Choose a disorder that has a genetic basis. Look at three sites on the Internet to see what information is available for clients, families, and health professionals. Then evaluate the sites according to the following criteria:
   - Who wrote the information on the site? Is it written by a health professional? Is it sponsored by a government organization that is a reliable source of health information such as the CDC? Is it peer reviewed?
   - Is the information written at the literacy level that a client could understand?
   - How would you improve the usefulness of these three sites based on the clients, families, and communities with whom you work?
2. Since public health nurses often identify groups within a community who are considered high risk for illness and then provide care to them as individuals, or to their families or in groups, choose a group in your community. Then develop a plan of care, including appropriate referrals to other agencies and a comprehensive plan for follow-up.
3. Identify parent support groups in your community, and inquire about attending a meeting.

ADDITIONAL RESOURCES

EVOLVE WEBSITE

http://evolve.elsevier.com/Stanhope/community/
- Answers to Practice Application
- Case Study
- Glossary
- Review Questions

REFERENCES

Akiinyemiju T, Do AN, Patki A, et al.: Epigenome-wide association study of metabolic syndrome in African-American adults, *Clin Epigenetics* 10:49, 2018. Retrieved from https://clinicalepigenetics journal.biomedcentral.com.

American Academy of Pediatrics: *Genetic Red Flags*, 2018. Retrieved from https://www.aap.org.

American Cancer Society: *How common is breast cancer*? 2018. Retrieved from https://www.cancer.org.

American Nurses Association: *Essential of genetic and genomic nursing: Competencies, curricula guidelines, and outcome indicators*, 2 ed, 2008. Retrieved from https://www.genome.gov.

Centers for Disease Control and Prevention: *Genetics Implementation: Tier 1 Genomic Applications Toolkit for Public Health Departments*, 2014. Retrieved from https://www.cdc.gov.

Centers for Disease Control and Prevention: *Direct to consumer genetic testing: Think before you spit, 2017 edition!* 2017a. Retrieved from https://blogs.cdc.gov.

Centers for Disease Control and Prevention: *Muin J. Khoury, MD, PhD*, 2017b. Retrieved from https://www.cdc.gov.

Centers for Disease Control and Prevention: *Genetic testing*, 2018a. Retrieved from https://www.cdc.gov.

Centers for Disease Control and Prevention: *Genomics and health impact weekly update*, July 9, 2018b. Retrieved from https://www.cdc.gov.

Centers for Disease Control and Prevention: *National center for environmental health*, 2018c. Retrieved from https://www.cdc.gov.

Centers for Disease Control and Prevention: *Genomics and population health action: The collaboration continues*! 2018d. Retrieved from https://www.ncbi.nlm.nih.gov.

Clark A, Adamian M, Taylor J: An overview of epigenetics in nursing, *Nurs Clin North Am* 48(4):649–659, 2013.

Deans C, Maggert K: What do you mean, "epigenetic"? *Genetics* 199(4):887–896, 2015.

Evaluation of Genomic Applications in Practice and Prevention: *About EGAPP*, 2016. Retrieved from https://www.cdc.gov.

Hawking S, Hawking L: *George and the Unbreakable Code*, New York, NY, 2014, Simon and Schuster.

International Society of Nurses in Genetics: 2018. Retrieved from https://www.isong.org.

Karns L: *Genetics Counselor UVA Health System*, 2010. Interview by E. J. Zschaebitz (phone interview).

Kelly H: (June 22, 2018). 5 Things to Know Before you Take a Home DNA Test. California State University. Retrieved from https://www2.calstate.edu.

National Cancer Institute: *The genetics of cancer*, 2017. Retrieved from https://www.cancer.gov.

National Cancer Institute: *Genetics of breast and gynecological cancers (PDQ): Health Professional Version*, 2018. Retrieved from http://www.cancer.gov.

National Center for Biotechnology Information. *Anemia, sickle cell*, n.d. Retrieved from http://www.ncbi.nlm.nih.gov.

National Human Genome Research Institute: *A brief guide to genomics: DNA, Genes and Genomes*, 2015a. Retrieved from https://www.genome.gov.

National Human Genome Research Institute: *All about the human genome project (HGP)*, 2015b. Retrieved from https://www.genome.gov.

National Human Genome Research Institute: *Fact sheets on science, research, ethics and the Institute*, 2015c. Retrieved from https://www.genome.gov.

National Human Genome Research Institute: Transcript presentation: *Felicitas Lacbawaan: NGS Panel for Hereditary Cancer Syndromes and Cancer Targeted Therapy*, 2016. Retrieved from https://www.genome.gov.

National Human Genome Research Institute: *Competencies and curricular resources*, 2017. Retrieved from https://www.genome.gov.

National Human Genome Research Institute: *Specific genetic disorders*, 2018a. Retrieved from https://www.genome.gov.

National Human Genome Research Institute: *Genetic terms: Mutagen*, 2018b. Retrieved from https://www.genome.gov.

National Human Genome Research Institute: *Regulation of genetic tests*, 2018c. Retrieved from https://www.genome.gov.

National Institutes of Health: *Genetic testing for hereditary cancer syndromes*, 2013. Retrieved from https://www.cancer.gov.

National Institutes of Health, Center for BioMedical Informatics and Information Technology: *My Family Health Portrait*, 2017. Retrieved from https://familyhistory.hhs.gov.

Office of Disease Prevention and Health Promotion: *Genomics*, 2017. Retrieved from https://www.healthypeople.gov.

Office of Disease Prevention and Health Promotion: *HealthyPeople.gov: Genomics*, 2018. Retrieved from https://www.healthypeople.gov.

Portin P, Wilkins A: The evolving definition of the term "gene", *Genetics* 205(3):1353–1363, 2017. Retrieved from http://www.genetics.org.

Quad Council of Public Health Nursing Organizations: *Community/Public Health Nursing (C/PHN) Competencies*, 2018. Retrieved from http://www.quadcouncilphn.org.

Science History Institute: *James Watson, Francis Crick, Maurice Wilkins, and Rosalind Franklin*, 2017. Retrieved from https://www.sciencehistory.org.

Starkweather AR, Coleman B, Barcelona de Mendoza V, et al.: Strengthen federal regulation of laboratory-developed and direct-to-consumer genetic testing, *Nurs Outlook* 66(1):101–104, 2018.

Thimbleby H: Technology and the future of healthcare, *J Public Health Res* Dec 1 2(3): e28, December 1, 2013.

University of Virginia School of Medicine, Department of Pediatrics: *Causes of cleft lip & palate*, 2018. Retrieved from https://med.virginia.edu.

U.S. Department of Health and Human Services: *FDA allows marketing of first direct- to-consumer tests that provide genetic risk information for certain conditions*, 2017. Retrieved from https://www.fda.gov.

U.S. Department of Health and Human Services: *News release: FDA authorizes, with special controls, direct-to-consumer test that reports three mutations in the BRCA breast cancer genes*, March 6, 2018. Retrieved from https://www.fda.gov.

U.S. Equal Employment Opportunity Commission: *The genetic information nondiscrimination act of 2008*, 2008. Retrieved from https://www.eeoc.gov.

U.S. Genetic Information Nondiscrimination Act: *What is GINA*? 2018. Retrieved from http://ginahelp.org.

Wellcome Trust, Sanger Institute: *Human Genome Project shows the wonder and mystery of humankind*, 2001. Quoting Michael Dexter. Retrieved from https://www.sanger.ac.uk.

Williams R: *Should healthy people have their exomes sequenced*? 2017. Retrieved from https://www.the-scientist.com.

13

Epidemiology

Swann Arp Adams, MS, PhD and
DeAnne K. Hilfinger Messias, PhD, RN, FAAN

OBJECTIVES

After reading this chapter, the student should be able to do the following:

1. Define epidemiology and describe its essential elements and approach.
2. Describe current and historical contexts of the development of the field of epidemiology.
3. Identify key elements of the epidemiologic triangle and the ecological model and describe the interactions among these elements in both models.
4. Explain the relationship of the natural history of disease to the three levels of prevention and to the design and implementation of community interventions.
5. Interpret basic epidemiologic measures of morbidity (disease) and mortality (death).
6. Discuss descriptive epidemiologic parameters of person, place, and time.
7. Describe the key features of common epidemiologic study designs.
8. Describe essential characteristics and methods of evaluating a screening program.
9. Identify the most common sources of bias in epidemiologic studies.
10. Evaluate epidemiologic research and apply findings to nursing practice.
11. Discuss the role of the nurse in epidemiologic surveillance and primary, secondary, and tertiary prevention.

CHAPTER OUTLINE

Definitions of Health and Public Health
Definitions and Descriptions of Epidemiology
Historical Perspectives
Basic Concepts in Epidemiology
Screening
Surveillance
Basic Methods in Epidemiology
Descriptive Epidemiology
Analytic Epidemiology
Experimental Studies
Causality
Applications of Epidemiology in Nursing

KEY TERMS

agent, p. 278
analytic epidemiology, p. 271
attack rate, p. 277
bias, p. 293
case-control design, p. 290
case-control study, p. 290
case fatality rate (CFR), p. 278
cohort study, p. 288
cross-sectional study, p. 291
cumulative incidence rate, p. 275
descriptive epidemiology, p. 271
determinants, p. 271
distribution, p. 271
ecological fallacy, p. 291
ecological model, p. 273
ecological study, p. 291
environment, p. 278
epidemic, p. 271
epidemiologic triangle, p. 278
epidemiology, p. 271
health, p. 270
host, p. 278
incidence proportion, p. 275
incidence rate, p. 275
levels of prevention, p. 280
mortality rates, p. 277
natural history of disease, p. 280
negative predictive value, p. 284
point epidemic, p. 288
popular epidemiology, p. 294

The authors acknowledge the contribution of Robert E. McKeown, PhD, FACE, to previous editions of this chapter.

KEY TERMS—cont'd

positive predictive value, p. 284
prevalence proportion, p. 276
proportion, p. 274
proportionate mortality ratio (PMR), p. 278
public health, p. 268
rate, p. 274
relative risk, p. 275
reliability, p. 283
risk, p. 275
screening, p. 282
secular trends, p. 287
sensitivity, p. 283
social epidemiology, p. 279
specificity, p. 283
surveillance, p. 284
validity, p. 283
web of causality, p. 278

Epidemiology is the basic science of public health. Like public health nursing, epidemiology is a complex and continually evolving field with a common focus: the optimal health for all members of all communities, local and global. Nurses use epidemiologic frameworks, methods, and data in order to understand factors that contribute to health and disease; to develop health promotion and disease prevention interventions and measures; to identify the presence of infectious agents in individuals and groups; to design, implement, and evaluate community health programs; and to develop and evaluate public health policies. Since nurses care for individuals and families, it is important that they consider the broader context in which these individuals live and the complex interplay of social and environmental factors that affect individual and collective well-being. Basic knowledge of epidemiology is essential to the practice of nursing across all settings and populations.

DEFINITIONS OF HEALTH AND PUBLIC HEALTH

Health is the core concept in nursing and epidemiology. In 1978 the World Health Organization (WHO) affirmed that "health, which is a state of complete physical, mental and social well-being, and not merely the absence of disease or infirmity, is a fundamental human right and the attainment of the highest possible level of health is a most important world-wide social goal" (WHO, 1978, p. 1). As defined by the American Nurses Association (ANA), "Nursing is the protection, promotion, and optimization of health and abilities, prevention of illness and injury, alleviation of suffering through the diagnosis and treatment of human response, and advocacy in the care of individuals, families, communities, and populations" (ANA, 2012). This definition reflects the WHO goal and coincides with epidemiologic principles. A holistic approach to health, including the incorporation of epidemiologic principles, is particularly appropriate for nurses. Nurses incorporate concepts of health into their nursing practice on a daily basis.

Public health is described as the health status of the public; a system and social enterprise; a profession; a collection of methods, knowledge, and techniques; and governmental health services, especially medical care for the poor and underserved (Turnock, 2016). In the early twentieth century, C.E.A. Winslow defined public health as "the science and art of preventing disease, prolonging life and promoting physical health and efficiency through organized community effort." The Institute of Medicine (IOM) report *The Future of Public Health* drew on Winslow's definition in stating the mission of public health is to fulfill "society's interest in assuring conditions in which people can be healthy" (IOM, 1988, p. 40). This mission statement clearly indicates a societal interest in the health of all its members. More specifically, the mission of the public health enterprise is to *ensure conditions* that promote health and well-being. From both public health and nursing perspectives, *health* encompasses much more than the presence or absence of a physical disease or disability; it involves optimal functioning across a broad range of systems—physiological, somatic, psychological, social, and environmental. The authors of the 1988 IOM report caution that this broad view of health and the role of public health professionals and agencies forces "practitioners to make difficult choices about where to focus their energies and raises the possibility that public health could be so broadly defined so as to lose distinctive meaning" (IOM, 1988, p. 40). Nurses are especially well suited to address this concern because of their holistic view of health and broad, interprofessional approach to intervention.

The practice of public health nursing is based on definitions of health and public health that go beyond a narrow biomedical model of individual health. Ensuring the public's health includes delivery of specific services to individuals, but also includes the establishment and implementation of public policies and programs. Public health and public health nursing activities focus on community prevention, disease control, and personal and community health services. The IOM report, *The Future of the Public's Health in the 21st Century* (IOM, 2002) highlights the importance of intersectional collaborations to accomplish the mission of public health. There is further emphasis on an ecological approach to research and practice (discussed later). Interprofessional collaboration between nurses and other health professionals, including epidemiologists, is critical to efforts to create and sustain the conditions necessary for health promotion, health maintenance, and overall improvements in public health (Baldwin, 2007).

HEALTHY PEOPLE 2020

***Examples of New Epidemiologic Objectives Included in* Healthy People 2020**

- **AH-2:** Increase the percent of adolescents who participate in extracurricular and out-of-school activities.
- **AOCBC-4:** Reduce the proportion of adults with doctor-diagnosed arthritis who find it "very difficult" to perform specific joint-related activities.
- **C-9:** Reduce invasive colorectal cancer.
- **D-16:** Increase preventive behaviors among individuals at high risk for diabetes with pre-diabetes.
- **FS-5:** Increase the proportion of consumers who follow key food safety practices.
- **HAI-2:** Reduce invasive methicillin-resistant *Staphylococcus aureus* (MRSA) infections.

DEFINITIONS AND DESCRIPTIONS OF EPIDEMIOLOGY

Epidemiology has been defined as "the study of the occurrence and distribution of health-related states or events in specified populations, including the study of the determinants influencing such states, and the application of this knowledge to control the health problems" (Porta, 2014). The word *epidemiology* comes from the Greek words *epi* (upon), *demos* (people), and *logos* (thought), and it originally referred to the spread of diseases of infectious origin. In the past century the definition and scope of epidemiology have broadened and now include the examination of the occurrence of chronic diseases, such as cancer and cardiovascular disease; mental health and health-related events, such as accidents, injuries, and violence; occupational and environmental exposures and their effects; and positive health states.

Epidemiologists investigate the **distribution** or patterns of health events in populations in order to characterize health outcomes in terms of *what, who, where, when, how,* and *why*: What is the outcome? Who is affected? Where are they? When do events occur? This focus is called **descriptive epidemiology** because it seeks to describe the occurrence of a disease in terms of person, place, and time (Koepsell & Weiss, 2014). The *how* and *why*, or **determinants** of health events, are those factors, exposures, characteristics, behaviors, and contexts that determine (or influence) the patterns: How does it occur? Why are some individuals and groups affected more than others? Determinants may be individual, relational or social, communal, or environmental. This focus on investigation of causes and associations is called **analytic epidemiology**, in reference to the goal of understanding the etiology (or origins and causal factors) of disease; the broad consideration of many levels of potential determinants is called the *ecological approach* (IOM, 2002). The results of these investigations are used to guide or evaluate policies and programs that improve the health of the community. The differentiation between *descriptive* and *analytic* epidemiologic studies is not clear-cut: analytic studies rely on descriptive comparisons, and descriptive comparisons shed light on determinants.

LINKING CONTENT TO PRACTICE

It is important that nurses understand the relationship between population health concepts and clinical practice. Within the field of epidemiology, the definition of *population* is not necessarily confined to large groups of people, such as the population of the United States. Population health concepts also apply to other types of groups, such as the collective group of clients at a specific clinical practice site. In this case, the clinical epidemiologic application of population health concepts is evident in these types of questions: What are the factors that contribute to the health and illness issues among clients that I see in my clinic? Why do some of my clients fare better than others who have the same disease conditions? What alternative clinical practices might positively impact the health of my clients? All of these very clinical questions incorporate epidemiologic concepts of describing the *burden of disease* in a population, identifying and understanding *determinants of health,* and examining possible *root causes* of health outcomes. Two important nursing documents recently highlighted ways in which epidemiologic knowledge and skills are essential to nursing practice. *The Council on Linkages Between Academic and Public Health Practice* (2014) outlined essential analytic/assessment and public health science skills, and *The Quad Council Coalition of Public Health Nursing Organizations* (2018) provided details and examples of ways to implement these skill sets in nursing practice.

The first step in the epidemiologic process is to answer the "what" question by defining a health outcome. The case definition usually refers to cases of disease, but also may include instances of injuries, accidents, or even wellness (Koepsell & Weiss, 2014). Epidemiology has played an important role in the refinement of the case definition for acquired immunodeficiency syndrome (AIDS) and other emerging infectious diseases and in the development of more precise diagnostic criteria for psychiatric disorders. Epidemiologic methods are used to quantify the frequency of occurrence and characterize both the case group and the population from which they come. The aim is to describe the distribution (i.e., determine who has the disease and where and when the disease occurs) and to search for factors that explain the pattern or risk of occurrence (i.e., answer the questions of why and how the disease occurs).

An **epidemic** occurs when the rate of disease, injury, or other condition exceeds the usual (endemic) level of that condition. There is no specific incidence threshold that indicates the existence of an epidemic. Because of the virtual eradication of smallpox globally, any occurrence of smallpox could be considered an epidemic. In contrast, given the high rates of ischemic heart disease in the United States, a very large increase in number of cases would be necessary to be considered an epidemic. Some would argue the current high rates compared with earlier periods already indicate an epidemic. The rising rates of obesity in the United States have led the Centers for Disease Control and Prevention (CDC) to consider adult obesity as an epidemic (CDC, 2013). Recent epidemiologic data show that 35.7 percent of U.S. adults 20 years of age and older—more than 78 million people—are obese. About 19 percent of the population ages 6 to 11 and 20.6 percent of those 12 to 19 years old are considered obese (CDC, 2018). Obesity contributes to increased risk for heart disease, hypertension, diabetes, arthritis-related disabilities, and certain cancers.

Epidemiology builds on and draws from other disciplines and methods, including clinical medicine and laboratory sciences, social sciences, quantitative methods (especially biostatistics), and public health policy, among others. Epidemiology differs from clinical medicine, which focuses on the diagnosis and treatment of disease in individuals. Epidemiology is the study of populations in order to (1) monitor the health of the population, (2) understand the determinants of health and disease in communities, and (3) investigate and evaluate interventions to prevent disease and maintain health. Effective nursing practice bridges the disciplines of clinical medicine and epidemiology, incorporating a focus on both individual and collective strategies. Nurses working in the community provide clinical services to individuals as they also tend to the broader context in which these individuals live and the complex interplay of social and environmental factors that affect their well-being. Nurses apply epidemiologic methods in their daily practice, as they note trends in specific illnesses (e.g., sexually transmitted infections) or conditions (e.g., accidents) and in designing, implementing, and evaluating community health programs. The AIDS epidemic was first identified because clinicians, using basic epidemiology methods, realized that much higher numbers of *Pneumocystis jiroveci* (*Pneumocystis carinii pneumonia*) were being diagnosed than had ever been seen previously.

HISTORICAL PERSPECTIVES

The roots of epidemiology trace back to ancient Greece (Merrill & Timmreck, 2006). In the fourth century BC, Hippocrates maintained that to understand health and disease in a community, one should look to geographic and climatic factors, the seasons of the year, the food and water consumed, and the habits and behaviors of the people. Yet modern epidemiology did not emerge until the nineteenth century, and it was only in the twentieth century that the field developed as a discipline with a distinctive identity (Susser, 1985).

Two refinements in research methods in the eighteenth and nineteenth centuries were critical for the formation of epidemiologic methods: (1) use of a comparison group and (2) the development of quantitative techniques (numerical measurements, or counts). One of the most famous studies using a comparison group is the pivotal mid-nineteenth century investigation of cholera by John Snow, often credited as being the "father of epidemiology" (Merrill & Timmreck, 2017). By mapping cases that clustered around a single public water pump in one London cholera outbreak, Snow demonstrated a connection between water supply and cholera. He later observed that cholera rates were higher among households supplied by water companies whose water intakes were downstream from the city than among households whose water came from further upstream, where it was subject to less contamination (Table 13.1). Snow realized that his investigation was an example of what epidemiologists call a *natural experiment*, and his findings added credibility to his argument that foul water was the vehicle for transmission of the agent that caused cholera (Gordis, 2013; Koepsell & Weiss, 2014).

Development and application of epidemiologic methods in the twentieth century were stimulated by dramatic changes in society and population dynamics (the combined effects of birth rates, death rates, life expectancy, and patterns of illness and causes of death) (McKeown, 2009). Contributing factors included improved nutrition, new vaccines, better sanitation, the advent of antibiotics and chemotherapies, and declining infant and child mortality and birth rates. Societal changes also resulted from large-scale events, including the Great Depression and World War II, followed by a rising standard of living for many but continued deep poverty for others. These changes led to increasing longevity and significant shifts in the age distribution of the population, resulting in increases in age-related diseases, such as coronary heart disease (CHD), stroke, cancer, and senile dementia (IOM, 2002; Susser, 1985). However, disparities remain among population subgroups in life expectancy and risk of many acute and chronic diseases. Fig. 13.1 shows the 10 leading causes of death in the United States in 1900, 1950, and 2010, with the percent of all deaths attributed to each cause. The leading two causes of death have not changed since 1950, whereas the composition of the remaining eight leading causes *has* changed.

TABLE 13.1 Household Cholera Death Rates by Source of Water Supply in John Snow's 1853 Investigation

Company	No. of Houses	Deaths From Cholera	Deaths per 10,000 Households
Southwark and Vauxhall	40,046	1263	315
Lambeth	26,107	98	37
Rest of London	256,423	1422	59

From Snow J: On the mode of communication of cholera. In *Snow on cholera,* New York, 1855, The Commonwealth Fund.

With the increase in chronic disease, epidemiologists realized the necessity of looking beyond single agents (e.g., the infectious agent that causes cholera) toward a multifactorial etiology (i.e., many factors or combinations and levels of factors contributing to disease, such as the complex set of factors that cause cardiovascular disease), referred to as an **ecological model** (IOM, 2002). Researchers and practitioners also recognized the contribution of behavioral and environmental causes to some chronic conditions formerly considered as degenerative diseases of aging. This understanding prompted new thinking about the possibility of preventing or delaying the onset of certain chronic diseases (Susser, 1985). In addition, the development of genetic and molecular techniques (such as genetic markers for increased risk of breast cancer and sophisticated tests for antibodies to infectious agents or for other biological markers of exposures to environmental toxins, such as lead or pesticides) has increased the ability to identify and classify persons in terms of exposures or inherent susceptibility to disease.

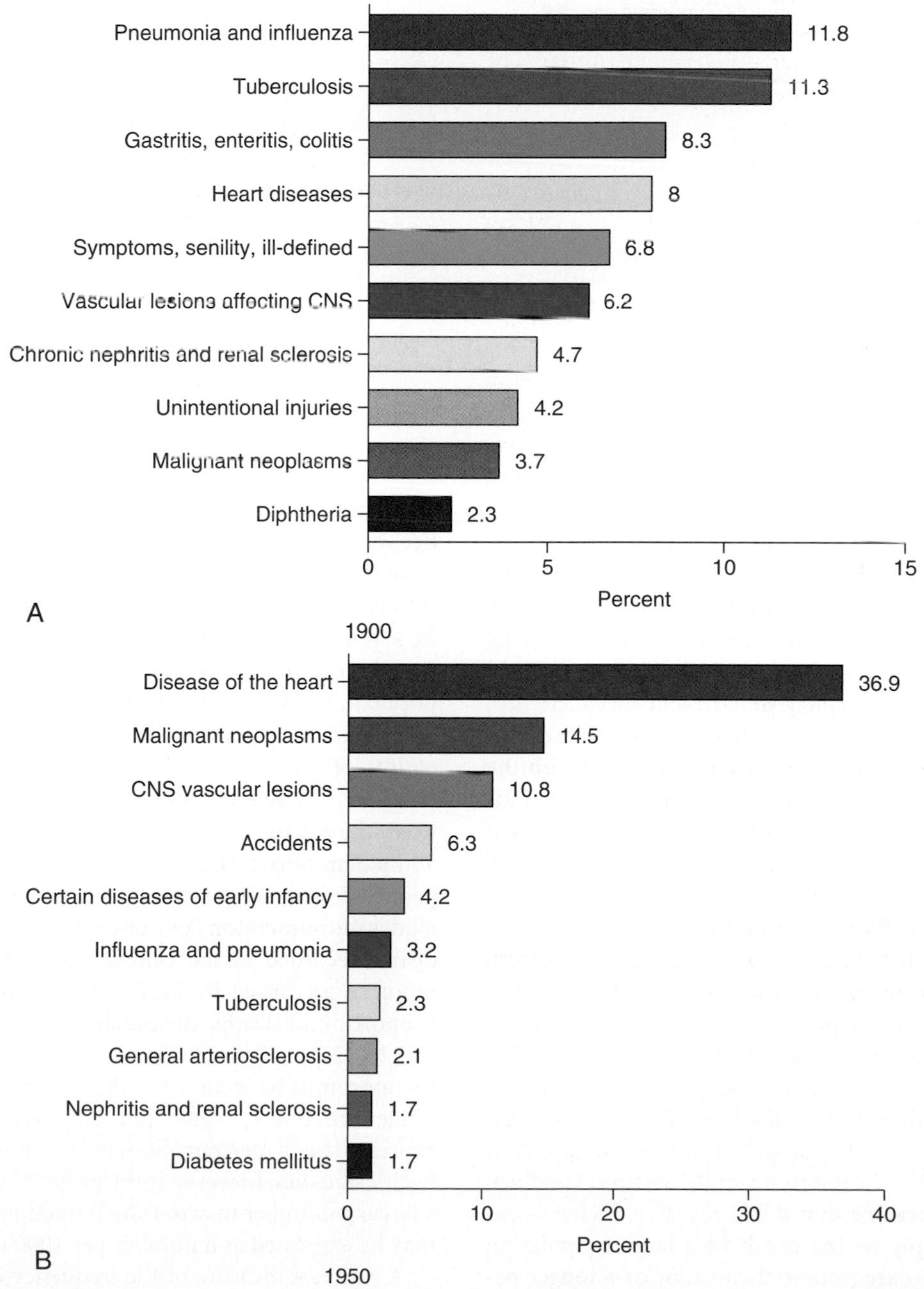

Fig. 13.1 Ten leading causes of death as a percent of all deaths, United States. **A,** 1900. **B,** 1950.

Continued

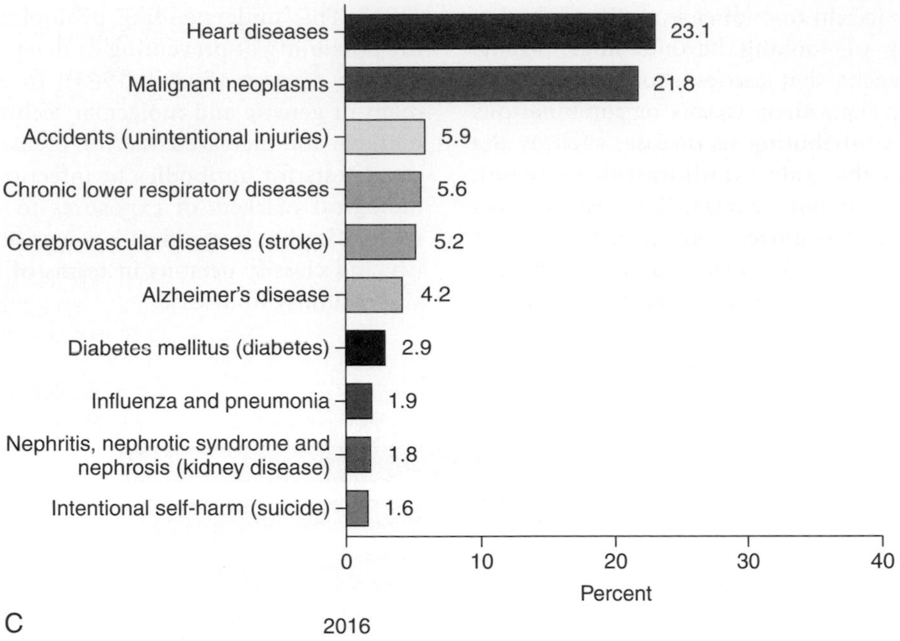

Fig. 13.1, cont'd C, 2016. *CNS,* Central nervous system. (B, Data from Anderson RN: Deaths: leading causes for 2000. *Natl Vital Stat Rep* 50:16, 2002; Brownson RC, Remington PL, Davis JR: *Chronic disease epidemiology and control,* ed. 2, Washington, DC, 1998, APHA; U.S. Department of Health, Education, and Welfare: *Vital statistics of the United States: 1950,* vol. 1, Washington, DC, 1954, USDHEW, Public Health Service. C, Data from Xu J, Murphy SL, Kochanek, MA, Bastian BS, Arias E: Deaths: final data for 2016. *Natl Vital Stat Rep* 67(5): 1, 2018.)

BASIC CONCEPTS IN EPIDEMIOLOGY

Epidemiologic concepts and data are used in ongoing assessments of both community and individual health problems. An initial component of a community health assessment is the collection of incidence, morbidity, and mortality rates for specific diseases. Health service data, such as immunization rates, causes of hospitalization, and emergency department visits, are also obtained. Individual health problems should incorporate evaluations of health risk based on lifestyle patterns along with the standard history and clinical examinations. The next sections highlight how to accomplish this community health assessment using basic epidemiologic measures.

Measures of Morbidity and Mortality

Proportions, Rates, and Risk. The distribution of health states and events is an important focus of epidemiology. Because people differ in their probability or risk of disease, a primary concern is the identification of how they differ. Today, epidemiologists use tools such as geographic information systems (GISs) to study health-related events to identify disease distribution patterns, similar to John Snow's mapping of cholera cases in London in the nineteenth century. However, mapping cases is limited in what it can reveal. A higher number of cases may simply be the result of a larger population with more people who are potential cases, or of a longer period of observation. Any description of disease patterns should take into account the size of the population at risk for the disease. That is, we should look not only at the numerator (the number of cases) but also at the denominator (the number of people in the population at risk) and at the length of time the population was observed. For example, 50 cases of influenza in a month could be considered a serious epidemic in a population of 250 but would indicate a low rate in a population of 250,000. On the other hand, even in a small population, one might observe 50 cases over a period of several years. Using rates and proportions instead of simple counts of cases takes the size of the population at risk into account (Koepsell & Weiss, 2014). Depending on the measure used, the consideration of time differs.

Epidemiologic studies rely on proportions and rates. A **proportion** is a type of ratio in which the denominator includes the numerator. For example, in 2016 there were 2,744,278 deaths recorded in the United States, of which 635,260 were reported as caused by heart disease (Xu et al., 2018); so the proportion of deaths attributable to heart disease in 2016 was 635,260/2,744,278 = 0.231, or 23.1 percent. Because the numerator must be included in the denominator, proportions can range from 0 to 1. Proportions are often multiplied by 100 and expressed as a percent, literally meaning per 100. In public health statistics, however, if the proportion is very small, we use a larger multiplier to avoid small fractions; thus the proportion may be expressed as a number per 1000 or per 100,000.

A **rate** is a measure of the frequency of a health event in "a defined population, usually in a specified period of time" (Porta, 2014). A rate is a ratio, but it is not a proportion because the denominator is a function of both the population size and the dimension of time, whereas the numerator is the number of events (Gordis, 2013; Koepsell & Weiss, 2014; Rothman, 2012). Furthermore, depending on the units of time and the frequency of events, a rate may exceed 1. As its name suggests, a rate is a measure of how rapidly something is happening: how rapidly a disease is developing in a population or how rapidly people are dying. Conceptually, a rate is the instantaneous change in a continuous process. Notice the use of the words *event* and *happening*. Rates deal with change over time, as individuals move from one state of being to another (e.g., from well to ill, alive to dead, or ill to cured). In observing a population over time to observe such changes in status, we typically exclude from the population being followed those persons who have already experienced the event.

Using the same health event of death from heart disease detailed earlier, we can also compute a rate. To calculate the death rate, the denominator will be the number of individuals in the population *during the year in which the deaths occurred*, rather than total number of deaths. For example, in 2016, the U.S. population estimate was 323,127,513. Since rates are commonly expressed per 100,000 or per 1000, we will divide this total population figure by 100,000, to get 3231.27513. The resulting calculation of the rate of death from heart disease in the United States in 2016 would be 635,260/3231.27513 = 196.6 per 100,000.

Risk refers to the probability that an event will occur within a specified period of time. A population at risk is the population of persons for whom there is some finite probability (even if small) of that event. For example, although the risk of breast cancer in men is small, a few men do develop breast cancer and therefore could be considered part of the population at risk. There are some outcomes for which certain people would never be at risk (e.g., men cannot be at risk of ovarian cancer, nor can women be at risk of testicular cancer). A high-risk population, on the other hand, would include those persons who, because of exposure, lifestyle, family history, social or environmental context, or other factors, are at greater risk for disease than the population at large. Although anyone may be susceptible to human immunodeficiency virus (HIV) infection, the degree of susceptibility does vary. Everyone in the population is at risk for HIV and AIDS, but persons who have multiple sexual partners without adequate protection or who use intravenous drugs are in the high-risk population for HIV infection. However, others who do not fit these categories may unknowingly be at high risk. An example of high risk is women who consider themselves to be in monogamous relationships but who are unaware that their partners have sexual relations with other women or men. As proportions, risk estimates have no dimensions, but they are a function of the length of time of observation. Given a continuous rate, increasing time will mean that a larger proportion of the population will eventually become ill.

Epidemiologists and other health professionals are interested in measures of morbidity, especially incidence proportions, incidence rates, and prevalence proportions (Gordis, 2013). These measures provide information about the risk of disease, the rate of disease development, and the levels of existing disease in a population, respectively.

> **HOW TO Quantify a Health Problem in the Community**
>
> Planning for resources and personnel often requires quantifying the level of a problem in a community. For example, to know how different districts compare in the rates of very-low-birth-weight (VLBW) infants, one would calculate the prevalence of VLBW births in each district:
>
> 1. Determine the number of live births in each district from birth certificate data obtained from the vital records division of the health department.
> 2. Use the birth weight information from the birth certificate data to determine the number of infants born weighing less than 1500 g in each district.
> 3. Calculate the prevalence of VLBW births by district as the number of infants weighing less than 1500 g at birth divided by the total number of live births.
> 4. If the number of VLBW births in each district is small, use several recent years of data to obtain a more stable estimate.

Measures of Incidence. Measures of incidence reflect the number of *new* cases or events in a population at risk during a specified time. An **incidence rate** quantifies the rate of development of new cases in a population at risk, whereas an **incidence proportion** indicates the proportion of the population at risk who experience the event over some period of time, for example, the proportion of the population who develop influenza during a given year (Rothman, 2012). The population at risk is considered to be persons without the event or outcome of interest but who are at risk of experiencing it. Note that existing (or prevalent) cases are excluded from the population at risk for this definition, since they already have the condition and are no longer at risk of developing it. The incidence proportion is also referred to as the **cumulative incidence rate** (and erroneously simply as the incidence rate) because it reflects the cumulative effect of the incidence rate over the time period, whether it is a month, a year, or several years. A constant incidence rate operating over a period of time results in an increasing proportion of the population being affected, that is, the incidence rate may stay constant while the cumulative incidence rate increases with time because the pool of people who have the disease is becoming larger. An incidence proportion can be interpreted as an estimate of risk of disease in that population over that period. An example of this might be the incidence proportion for cancer. Using statistics published for a five-year time period, one could calculate that 20 of 200 individuals were newly diagnosed with cancer (hypothetical example). The incidence proportion would then be 20/200 = 0.10 or 10 percent. This could be interpreted that over a five-year time period, the risk of cancer in the population was 10 percent. The risk of disease is a function of both the rate of new disease development and the length of time the population is at risk. The interpretation can be for an individual (i.e., the probability that the person will become ill) or for a population (i.e., the proportion of a population expected to become ill over the specified period). For further examples of these calculations as it relates to mortality, see Table 13.2.

Another common risk measure used by both the science and general community is **relative risk**. Essentially, the relative risk compares the incidence of disease in an "exposed" population to the incidence of disease in an "unexposed" population. In this way, the relative risk is based on the calculations that are

TABLE 13.2 Common Mortality Rates

Rate/Ratio	Definition and Example
Crude mortality rate	Usually an annual rate that represents the proportion of a population who die from any cause during the period, using the midyear population as the denominator Example: In 2016 there were 2,744,248 deaths in a total population of 323,127,513, or 849.3 per 100,000: $\frac{2,744,248}{323,127,513} = 849.3$ per 100,000
Age-specific rate	Number of deaths among persons of given age group per midyear population of that age group Example: 2016 age-specific mortality rate for 20- to 24-year-olds: $\frac{21,763}{22,381,028} = 97.2$ per 100,000
Cause-specific rate	Number of deaths from a specific cause per midyear population Example: 2016 cause-specific rate for accidents: $\frac{161,374}{323,127,513} = 5.9$ per 100,000
Case-fatality rate	Number of deaths from a specific disease in a given period divided by number of persons diagnosed with that disease Example: If 87 of every 100 persons diagnosed with lung cancer die within five years, the five-year case fatality rate is 87 percent. The five-year survival rate is 13 percent.
Proportionate mortality ratio	Number of deaths from a specific disease per total number of deaths in the same period Example: In 2016 there were 635,260 deaths from diseases of the heart, and 2,744,248 deaths from all causes: $\frac{635,260}{2,744,248} = 0.231$ or 23%
Infant mortality rate	Number of infant deaths before one year of age in a year per number of live births in the same year Example: In 2016 there were 23,161 infant deaths and 3,945,875 live births: $\frac{23,161}{3,945,875} = 286.97$ per 100,000 live births or 5.87 per 1,000 live births
Neonatal mortality rate	Number of infant deaths under 28 days of age in a year per number of live births in the same year Example: In 2016 there were 15,282 neonatal deaths and 3,945,875 live births: $\frac{15,282}{3,945,875} = 3.87$ per 1,000 live births
Postneonatal mortality rate	Number of infant deaths from 28 days to 1 year in a year per number of live births in the same year Example: In 2016 there were 7,879 postneonatal deaths and 3,945,875 live births: $\frac{7,879}{3,945,875} = 2.00$ per 1,000 live births

From Xu JQ et al. Deaths: leading causes for 2016. *Natl Vital Stat Rep* 67(5), 2018; Martin JA et al.: Births: final data for 2016, *Natl Vital Stat Rep* 67(1), Hyattsville, MD: National Center for Health Statistics, 2018.

performed for the cumulative incidence rate. As an example, one could conceptualize the exposure as "taking hormone replacement therapy" and the outcome as breast cancer. In this case, we would identify a group of women who would be of an age to take hormone replacement therapy. Next, we would categorize these women into two groups—those women not taking hormone replacement therapy and those who are taking hormone replacement. Within these two groups, then we would calculate the *cumulative incidence rate for each group*. The *relative risk* would then be expressed as the cumulative incidence rate of breast cancer among women taking hormone replacement therapy divided by the cumulative incidence rate of breast cancer among those *not* taking hormone replacement therapy.

Since the relative risk is based on a ratio, the actual value can range anywhere from > 0 to infinity (theoretically). When the cumulative incidence rates are exactly equal, the relative risk is 1.00. This is often termed the "null value" indicating that the exposure of interest has no effect on the outcome of interest. This is the statistic most frequently cited in media releases regarding scientific studies. Using the hormone replacement therapy and breast cancer example, a research study that indicated a relative risk of 1.75 can be interpreted to indicate that the risk of developing breast cancer among those women taking hormone replacement therapy is 75 percent times the risk of developing breast cancer among women not taking hormone replacement therapy. This is also the statistic nurses can use to estimate the probability of disease among their patients. This concept is discussed in more detail later in this chapter in the section Prospective Cohort Studies.

Prevalence Proportion. The prevalence proportion is a measure of existing disease in a population at a particular time (i.e., the number of existing cases divided by the current population). We can also calculate the prevalence of a specific risk factor or exposure. When used alone, the term *prevalence* typically refers to the *prevalence proportion*, although the term sometimes refers to the count of existing cases (i.e., the numerator of the prevalence proportion). For example, consider the following data from a breast cancer screening program that had reached 8000. Among these 8000 women, if 35 previously had been diagnosed with breast cancer and an additional 20 cases of breast cancer were identified as a result of the screening program, the prevalence proportion of current and past breast cancer events in this population would be 55 out of 8000, expressed as a rate of 687.5 per 100,000.

It is important to note that a prevalence proportion is not an estimate of the risk of developing disease. The prevalence proportion is a function of both the rate at which new cases of the disease develop and how long these cases remain in the population. To illustrate this point, consider the prevalence of prostate cancer. The number of people with prostate cancer at any given time reflects both the number of new cases diagnosed at that specific point in time and the number of previously diagnosed men currently living with the diagnosis of prostate cancer. The duration of a specific disease is affected by both case fatality and cure. For example, a disease with a short duration (e.g., an intestinal virus) may not have a high prevalence proportion, even if the rate of new cases is high, because cases do not accumulate (see Point Epidemic later in this chapter). A disease with a long course (e.g., Crohn's disease) will have a higher prevalence proportion than a rapidly fatal disease that has the same rate of new cases.

Comparing Prevalence and Incidence. The prevalence proportion measures existing cases of disease and is affected by factors that influence risk (incidence) and by factors that influence survival or recovery (duration). Prevalence proportions are useful in planning health care services because they indicate the level of disease existing in the population and therefore the size of the population in need of services. However, prevalence measures are less useful when we are looking for factors related to disease etiology. Because prevalence proportions reflect duration in addition to the risk of getting the disease, it is difficult to sort out what factors are related to risk and what factors are related to survival or recovery.

For example, the five-year survival rate for breast cancer is about 85 percent, but the five-year survival rate for lung cancer in women is only about 15 percent. Even if the incidence rates of breast and lung cancer were the same in women (and they are not), the prevalence proportions would differ because, on average, women live longer after a diagnosis of breast cancer than do women diagnosed with lung cancer. In other words, the duration of breast cancer is longer.

The measures of choice in studying disease etiology are incidence rates and incidence proportions, because incidence is affected only by factors related to the risk of developing disease and not to survival or cure. At the level of a local health department, epidemiologists and nurses would rely on both incidence and prevalence data in planning services focused on the prevention and control of tuberculosis (TB). They would examine the existing level of TB within the community (prevalence) to plan services and direct prevention and control measures, and they would take into consideration the rate of new TB cases (incidence) to study risk factors and evaluate the effectiveness of prevention and control programs.

HOW TO Assess Health Problems in a Community

1. Examine local epidemiologic data (e.g., incidence, morbidity, and mortality rates) to identify major health problems.
2. Examine local health services data to identify major causes of hospitalizations and emergency department visits. Consult with key community leaders (e.g., political, religious, business, educational, health, and cultural leaders) about their perceptions of identified community health problems.
3. Mobilize community groups to elicit discussions and identify perceived health priorities within the community (e.g., focus groups, neighborhood forums, or community-wide forums).
4. Analyze community environmental health hazards and pollutants (e.g., water, sewage, air, toxic waste).
5. Examine indicators of community knowledge and practices of preventive health behaviors (e.g., use of infant car seats, safe playgrounds, lighted streets, seat belt use, designated driver programs).
6. Identify cultural priorities and beliefs about health among different social, cultural, racial, or national origin groups.
7. Assess community members' interpretations of and degrees of trust in federal, state, and local assistance programs.
8. Engage community members in conducting surveys to assess specific health problems.

For Further *Note:* This process is very similar to the intake/assessment process familiar to nurses, that includes obtaining medical and family history (analogous to #1 and #2 above), identifying health concerns of the patient (analogous to #3 and #5 above), performing clinical exam (analogous to #4 above), and evaluating patient knowledge, beliefs, and personal risk (analogous to #5-#8).

Attack Rate. Another measure of morbidity, often used in infectious disease investigations, is the **attack rate**. This form of incidence proportion is defined as the proportion of persons who are exposed to an agent and develop the disease. Attack rates are often specific to an exposure; food-specific attack rates, for example, are the proportion of persons becoming ill after eating a specific food item.

Mortality Rates. **Mortality rates** are key epidemiologic indicators of interest to nurses (see Table 13.2). Although measures of mortality reflect serious health problems and changing patterns of disease, they are limited in their usefulness. Mortality rates are informative only for fatal diseases and do not provide direct information about either the level of existing disease in the population or the risk of contracting any particular disease. Furthermore, it is not uncommon for a person who has one disease (e.g., prostate cancer) to die from a different cause (e.g., stroke).

Note that many commonly used mortality rates in Table 13.2 are in fact proportions, not true rates (Gordis, 2013; Rothman, 2012). Because the population changes during the course of a year, we typically take an estimate of the population at midyear as the denominator for annual rates, because the midyear population approximates the amount of person-time contributed by the population during a given year. Using the approximation noted previously for small rates when the period of observation is a single unit of time, the annual mortality rate is an estimate of the risk of death in a given population for that year. These rates are multiplied by a scaling factor (usually 100,000) to avoid small fractions. The result is then expressed as the number of deaths per 100,000 persons. Although a crude mortality rate is easy to calculate and represents the actual death rate for the total population, it has certain limitations. It does not reveal specific causes of death, which change in relative importance over time (see Fig. 13.1). It also is affected by the age distribution of the population because older people are at much greater risk of death than younger people. Mortality rates also are calculated for specific groups (e.g., age-, sex-, or race-specific rates). In these instances, the number of deaths occurring in the specified group is divided by the population at risk, now restricted to the number of persons in that group. This rate may be interpreted as the risk of death for persons in the specified group during the period of observation.

The cause-specific mortality rate is an estimate of the risk of death from some specific disease in a population. It is the number of deaths from a specific cause divided by the total population at risk, usually multiplied by 100,000. Two related measures should be distinguished from the cause-specific mortality rate. The **case fatality rate (CFR)** is usually a proportion: the proportion of persons diagnosed with a particular disorder (i.e., cases) that die within a specified period of time. The CFR may be interpreted as an estimate of the risk of death within that period for a person newly diagnosed with the disease (e.g., the proportion of persons with breast cancer who die within five years). Because the CFR is the proportion of diagnosed persons who die within the period, 1 minus the CFR yields the survival rate. For example, if the five-year CFR for lung cancer is 86 percent, then the five-year survival rate is only 14 percent (Remington et al., 2016). Persons diagnosed with a particular disease often want to know the probability of survival. These rates provide an estimate of that probability.

The second measure to be distinguished from the cause-specific mortality rate is the **proportionate mortality ratio (PMR)**—the proportion of all deaths that are attributable to a specific cause. The denominator is not the population at risk of death but the total number of deaths in the population; therefore the PMR is not a rate nor does it estimate the risk of death. The magnitude of the PMR is a function of both the number of deaths from the cause of interest and the number of deaths from other causes. If deaths from certain causes decline over time, the PMR for deaths from other causes that remain relatively constant (in absolute numbers) may increase. For example, accidents (unintentional injuries) accounted for 4.1 deaths per 100,000 persons 10 to 14 years of age in the United States in 2016, which is 28.1 percent of all deaths in this age group (the PMR). By comparison, accidents (unintentional injuries) caused 49.1 deaths per 100,000 persons 65 to 74 years of age in 2016, which was less than 2.7 percent of all deaths in this older age group (Heron, 2018). This demonstrates that, although the risk of death from a motor vehicle accident was almost 12 times greater in the older group (based on the rates), such accidents accounted for a far greater proportion of all deaths in the younger group (based on the PMR). The reason is that there is a much greater risk of death from other causes in the older group.

Around the world, measures of infant mortality are an indicator of overall population health and availability of health care services. The most common measure, the infant mortality rate (IMR), is the number of deaths to infants in the first year of life divided by the total number of live births. Because the risk of death declines rather dramatically during the first year of life, neonatal and postneonatal mortality rates are also of interest (see Table 13.2). To effectively plan and evaluate community health interventions, nurses need to be able to understand and interpret these key epidemiologic indicators. One of the benefits of epidemiologic studies is that the results may demonstrate which disease prevention and control interventions are more useful and effective.

Epidemiologic Triangle, Web of Causality, and the Ecological Model

Epidemiologists understand that disease results from complex relationships among causal agents, susceptible persons, and environmental factors. These three elements—**agent**, **host**, and **environment**—are traditionally referred to as the **epidemiologic triangle** (Fig. 13.2A). This model originally was developed as a way of identifying causative factors, transmission, and risk related to infectious diseases. Changes in one of the elements of the triangle can influence the occurrence of disease by increasing or decreasing a person's risk for disease. As illustrated in Fig. 13.2B, specific characteristics of agent and host, as well as the interactions between agent and host, are influenced by the environmental context in which they exist, and may in turn influence the environment. Box 13.1 provides examples of these three components.

Although the interactions of host, environment, and agent are clearly key elements in disease causation, causal relationships are often more complex than implied by the concept of the epidemiologic triangle. The concept of a **web of causality** reflects the more complex interrelationships among the numerous factors interacting, sometimes in subtle ways, to increase (or decrease) risk of disease. Furthermore, associations are sometimes mutual, with lines of causality going in both directions. More recently, some epidemiologic researchers have advocated a new paradigm that goes beyond the two-dimensional causal web to consider multiple levels of factors that affect health and disease (Krieger, 1994; Macintyre & Ellaway, 2000). Krieger (1994) suggested that in addition to researching the relationships within the web, it is important to look for "the spider"—that is, focus on those larger factors and contexts that influence or create the causal web itself.

With this shift in the scientific thinking, practitioners and researchers are thinking more broadly about the multiple underlying determinants of health. There is increasing recognition of the widespread and profound influence of external factors on the health of individuals, communities, and populations. This is consistent with the ecological model for population

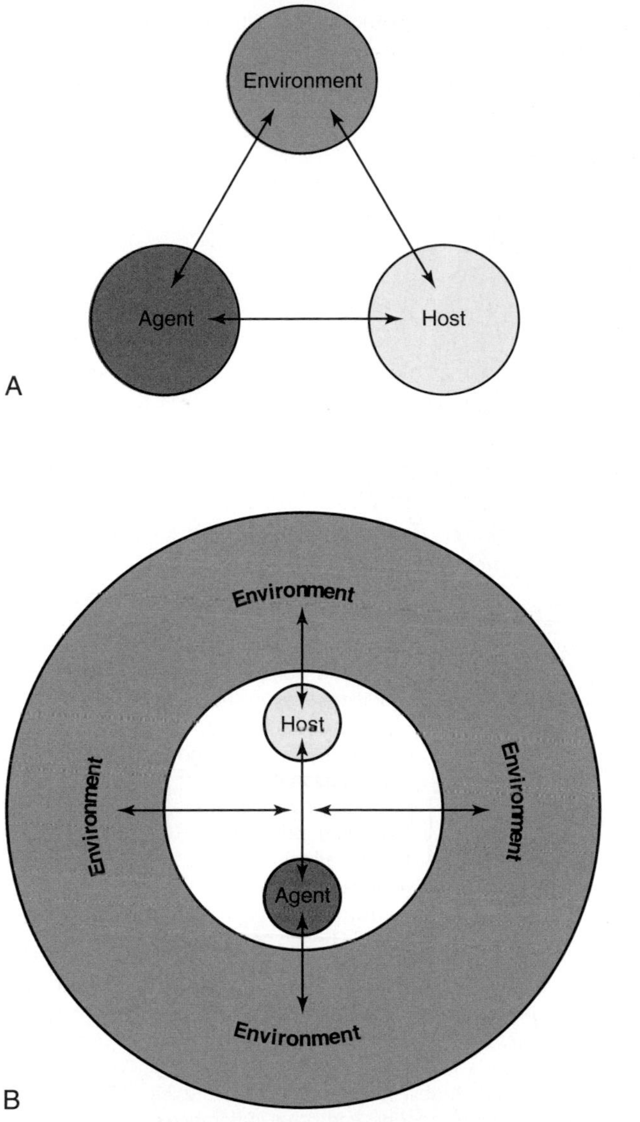

Fig. 13.2 **A** and **B**, Two models of the agent-host-environment interaction (the epidemiologic triangle).

BOX 13.1 Examples of Agent, Host, and Environmental Factors in the Epidemiologic Triangle

Agent
Infectious agents (e.g., bacteria, viruses, fungi, parasites)
Chemical agents (e.g., heavy metals, toxic chemicals, pesticides)
Physical agents (e.g., radiation, heat, cold, machinery)

Host
Genetic susceptibility
Immutable characteristics (e.g., age, sex)
Acquired characteristics (e.g., immunological status)
Lifestyle factors (e.g., diet and exercise)

Environment
Climate (e.g., temperature, rainfall)
Plant and animal life (e.g., agents or reservoirs or habitats for agents)
Human population distribution (e.g., crowding, social support)
Socioeconomic factors (e.g., education, resources, access to care)
Working conditions (e.g., levels of stress, noise, satisfaction)

health illustrated in Fig. 13.3. This approach expands epidemiologic studies both upward to broader contexts (such as neighborhood characteristics and social context) and downward to the genetic and molecular level. It is evident that the relative impact of the various factors depicted in this figure is not fixed and would vary across different populations, contexts, and settings. However, the model provides a useful guide for considering the potential relative impact for intervention across various sectors.

Similar to the web of causality model, the ecological model recognizes multiple determinants of health and treats them as interrelated and acting synergistically (or antagonistically), rather than as a list of discrete factors. The ecological model spans a broader spectrum of systems and etiological factors than the web of causality model and encompasses determinants at many levels: biological, mental, behavioral, social, and environmental factors, including policy, culture, and economic environments. Another way of thinking of this is that the ecological model moves from a two-dimensional perspective to a multidimensional perspective. Nurses have a significant role in shaping the health of the population and need to be mindful of the many environmental factors that may contribute to health behaviors and health outcomes. In addressing health behavior change, nurses often focus on patient education (within the domain of "individual behaviors" in Fig. 13.3). However, lack of attention to other environmental and social issues (i.e., lack of transportation, lack of adequate childcare arrangements, financial constraints, inadequate housing) may mean that the patient is unable to access or respond appropriately to the health education efforts.

Social Epidemiology

The renewed interest in social epidemiology is attributed in part to the recognition of persistent social inequalities in health. **Social epidemiology** is the branch of epidemiology that studies the social distribution and social determinants of health and disease (Berkman & Kawachi, 2014; Kawachi & Berkman, 2003; Krieger, 2000). Social epidemiologists focus on the roles and mechanisms of specific social phenomena (e.g., socioeconomic stratification, social networks and support, discrimination, work and employment demands) in the production of health and disease states. Social epidemiologists examine social inequalities and data related to neighborhoods, communities, employment, and family conditions in order to analyze health issues and design appropriate and feasible public health interventions. Public health professionals are concerned with relationships between social conditions and patterns of health and disease in individuals, families, groups, and populations.

Increasingly, the lens of epidemiology is applied to the analysis of the complex social, economic, and environmental factors that influence or lead to social inequalities in health. Berkman and Kawachi (2014) identified several key concepts within the subfield of social epidemiology. These include a population perspective (IOM, 2002), the social context of behavior, contextual and multilevel analysis (Diez-Roux, 2002; Sampson, et al., 1997), a developmental and life-course perspective, and general susceptibility to disease. The aim of social

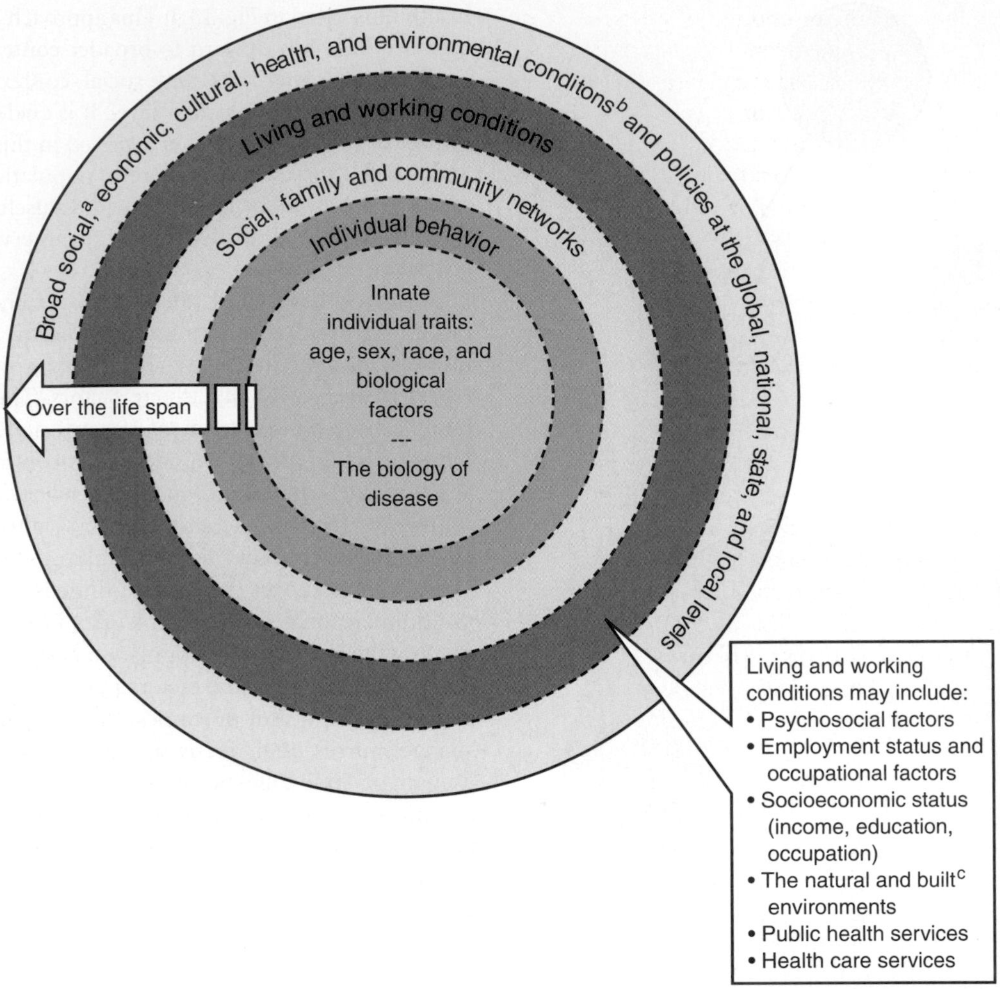

Fig. 13.3 Determinants of population health. This is a guide to thinking about the determinants of population health. (Reprinted with permission from *The Future of the Public's Health in the 21st Century,* Copyright 2002 by the National Academy of Sciences, courtesy the National Academies Press, Washington, DC.) [a]Social conditions include, but are not limited to: economic inequality, urbanization, mobility, cultural values, attitudes and policies related to discrimination and intolerance on the basis of race, gender, and other differences. [b]Other conditions at the national level might include major sociopolitical shifts, such as recession, war, major environmental disasters, and governmental collapse. [c]The built environment includes transportation, water and sanitation, housing, and other dimensions of urban planning.

epidemiology is to identify ways in which the structure of society influences the public's health, through the interactions of social context, environmental factors, biological mechanisms, and the timing and accumulation of risk, as represented by the ecological model and the life span perspective. Social epidemiologists have called for further research to examine the impact of extra-individual factors (institutions, communities, macroeconomic conditions, and economic and social policy) on exposure to resources (Kawachi & Berkman, 2014).

Levels of Preventive Interventions

The goal of epidemiology is to identify and understand the causal factors and mechanisms of disease, disability, and injuries in order to implement effective interventions to prevent the occurrence of these adverse processes before they begin or before they progress. The **natural history of disease** is the course of the disease process from onset to resolution (Porta, 2014). The three levels of prevention provide a framework commonly used in public health practice (see the Levels of Prevention box later in the chapter). As practicing epidemiologists, nurses working in the community are involved in primary, secondary, and tertiary prevention of communicable and noncommunicable diseases.

Primary Prevention. In their daily practice, nurses are often involved in activities related to all three **levels of prevention** (see Levels of Prevention box). Primary prevention refers to interventions aimed at preventing the occurrence of disease, injury, or disability. Interventions at this level of prevention are aimed at individuals and groups who are susceptible to disease but have no discernible pathology (i.e., they are in a state of pre-pathogenesis). This first level of prevention includes broad efforts such as health promotion, environmental protection, and specific protection. Health promotion includes nutrition education and counseling and the promotion of physical activity. Environmental protection ranges from basic sanitation and food safety, to home and workplace safety plans, to air quality control. Examples of specific protection against disease or injury include immunizations, proper use of seat belts and infants' car seats, preconception folic acid supplementation to prevent neural tube defects, fluoridation of water supplies to prevent dental caries, and actions taken to reduce human exposure to agents that may cause cancer. Primary prevention occurs in homes, in community settings, and at the primary level of health care (e.g., in public health clinics, physicians' offices, community health centers, and rural health clinics).

Examples of nurses' involvement in primary prevention include health education and promotion programs, such as nutrition education and counseling, sex education, and family planning services. Primary prevention efforts focus on both the general population and on specific vulnerable groups (e.g., the homeless, HIV-positive persons, certain immigrant or refugee groups) to improve the general health status and to reduce the incidence of specific diseases such as TB. An example of a primary prevention intervention is the provision of health education and training for daycare workers regarding health and hygiene issues, such as proper hand hygiene, diapering, and food preparation and storage. Immunizations are another example of primary prevention. In terms of environmental protection, nurses work proactively to develop and advocate for policies and legislation that lead to prevention of environmental hazards. They can also provide consultation to industries, local governments, and groups of concerned citizens as well as public education for a wide range of preventable environmental health problems.

LEVELS OF PREVENTION

Examples Related to Cardiovascular Disease

Primary Prevention

Counsel clients about low-fat diet and regular physical exercise.

Secondary Prevention

Implement blood pressure and cholesterol screening; give treadmill stress test.

Tertiary Prevention

Provide cardiac rehabilitation, medication, surgery.

Secondary Prevention. Secondary prevention encompasses interventions designed to increase the probability that a person with a disease will have that condition diagnosed at a stage when treatment is likely to result in cure. Health screenings are the mainstay of secondary prevention. Early and periodic screenings are critical for diseases for which there are few specific primary prevention strategies, such as breast cancer. (Screening programs are discussed in more detail later in the chapter.) As noted earlier, primary prevention is a major focus of health education. However, nurses often use health education interventions when caring for individuals with a diagnosed health problem with the aim of preventing further complications or exacerbations. For example, at the individual and family levels, teaching the asthmatic child to recognize and avoid exposure to potential asthma triggers and helping the family implement specific protection strategies, such as replacing carpets, keeping air systems clean and free of mold, and avoiding contact with household pets and second hand smoke could be considered secondary prevention.

Interventions at the secondary level of prevention may occur in community settings as well as within primary and secondary levels of health care services. Oral rehydration therapy (ORT) for infant diarrheal disease is an excellent example of secondary prevention in the community. Particularly in developing countries, when safe drinking water is available, ORT is a low-cost and effective way to treat infant diarrheal disease. When mothers identify the early signs of infant dehydration and administer a homemade ORT solution of water, sugar, and salt, they are putting secondary prevention into practice. When taking a health history with clients, nurses can integrate secondary prevention into practice by asking about family history of cancer, heart disease, diabetes, and mental illness, and then providing follow-up education about appropriate screening procedures. Other examples of secondary prevention interventions include screening tests to detect breast cancer (i.e., mammography), prenatal screening of pregnant women to detect gestational diabetes, routine tuberculin testing of specific groups (e.g., health care providers, childcare workers), and identification and screening of persons who have had contact with an individual known to have TB. In all these examples, the aim of secondary prevention is to identify the presence of a disease or condition at an early stage and begin necessary treatment early to increase the likelihood of cure or to prevent further complications.

Tertiary Prevention. Tertiary prevention includes interventions aimed at disability limitation and rehabilitation from disease, injury, or disability. Tertiary prevention interventions occur most often at secondary and tertiary levels of care (e.g., specialized clinics, hospitals, rehabilitation centers) but may also occur in community and primary care settings. Medical treatment, physical and occupational therapy, and rehabilitation are interventions characterized as tertiary prevention. With the emergence of new drug-resistant strains of TB, nurses now face the challenge of designing and implementing programs to increase long-term compliance and provide aftercare for clients in a variety of community settings. An example of tertiary prevention is a public health nurse providing directly observed treatment (DOT) to individuals diagnosed with active TB.

Depending on the community and clinical contexts and settings, primary, secondary, and tertiary prevention interventions may not be mutually exclusive categories, depending on their implementation and context at the clinical or community level. For example, conducting Pap smears and colonoscopies in primary health care settings are considered primary prevention efforts for cervical and colon cancer, aimed at identification of pre-malignant lesions, and thus preventing the development of cancer. However, at the broader community level and context, these procedures are not an example of primary prevention, as they still identify an abnormality (pre-malignant) that is not present in completely healthy individuals.

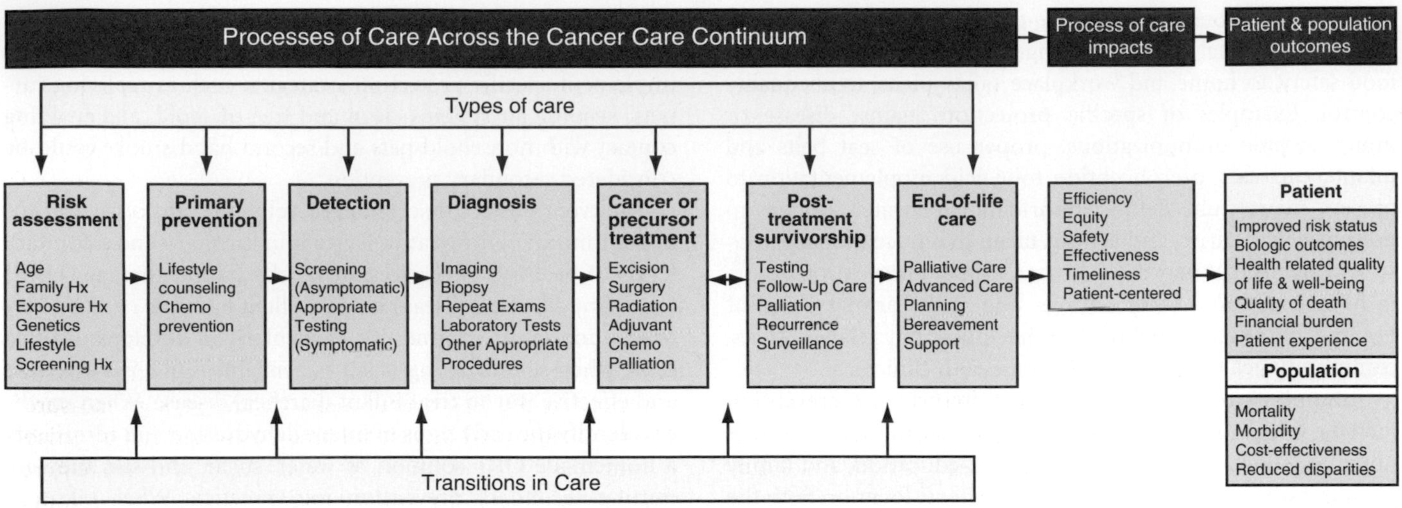

Fig. 13.4 Health intervention spectrum. (From Taplin SH, Price RA, Edwards HM, et al: Introduction: Understanding and Influencing Multilevel Factors Across the Cancer Care Continuum. *J Natl Cancer Inst Monogr* (44): 2-10, 2012. Oxford University Press.) *Hx,* History.

An Intervention Spectrum. The standard classification of preventive measures in public health is composed of the primary, secondary, and tertiary levels of prevention. However, recent revisions to these standard classifications aim to refine and tailor the application to diverse settings and health issues. For example, in the field of cancer, this potential for preventive intervention is conceptualized across the entire continuum of care (Fig. 13.4). Given that cancer is a disease that often has a relatively long period of development, the timeline for potential intervention is extended. For example, family history of breast cancer is known to be a significant risk factor among specific subgroups of women. With this information, when counseling a patient, the nurse may both encourage healthy lifestyle choices and advocate for genetic testing. In patients diagnosed with hormone positive breast cancer, the nurse can counsel and facilitate treatment adherence for the woman to her hormonal therapy (third intervention point). Other interventions would include facilitating communication with patients and their families in order to expedite the treatment trajectory from the point of diagnosis to the scheduled surgery (fourth intervention point). Clearly, nurses have critical roles in prevention at all points across the intervention spectrum.

SCREENING

Screening, a key component of many secondary prevention interventions, involves the testing of groups of individuals who are at risk for a certain condition but are not yet symptomatic. The purpose is to classify these individuals with respect to the likelihood of having the disease. From a clinical perspective, the aim of screening is early detection and treatment when these result in a more favorable prognosis. From a public health perspective, the objective is to sort out efficiently and effectively those who probably have the disease from those who probably do not, again to detect early cases for treatment or begin public health prevention and control programs. A screening test is *not* a diagnostic test. Effective screening programs must have built-in referral mechanisms for subsequent diagnostic evaluation for those who screen positive, to determine if they actually have the disease and need treatment, and there must be effective protocols in place for referral to accessible and appropriate follow-up care and treatment. If there is no effective treatment, or if the individuals or groups targeted for screening experience considerable barriers in accessing appropriate treatment, the justification of the screening program must be assessed ethically as well as epidemiologically (Childress et al., 2002).

As public health advocates, nurses are responsible for planning and implementing screening and prevention programs targeted to the at-risk populations. Nurses working in schools, worksites, primary care facilities, and public health agencies may work together to target at-risk populations on the basis of occupational and environmental risks. Successful screening programs have several characteristics related to both the tests and the target population (Box 13.2). In planning screening programs for a specific population (e.g., school, workplace,

BOX 13.2 Characteristics of a Successful Screening Program

1. *Valid (accurate):* A high probability of correct classification of persons tested
2. *Reliable (precise):* Results consistent from place to place, time to time, and person to person
3. *Capable of large group administration:*
   a. Fast in both the administration of the test and the procurement of results
   b. Inexpensive in both personnel required and materials and procedures used
4. *Innocuous:* Few, if any, side effects; minimally invasive test
5. *High yield:* Able to detect enough new cases to warrant the effort and expense (*yield* defined as the amount of previously unrecognized disease that is diagnosed and treated as a result of screening)
6. *Ethical and effective:* Meets the desired public health goal with health benefits that outweigh any moral or ethical infringements

community), nurses need to take into consideration various factors. These include the characteristics of the health problem, the screening tests available, and the population (Noonan, 2017). Screening is recommended for health problems that have a high prevalence, are relatively serious, can be detected in early states, and for which effective treatment is available. The population should be easily identifiable and assessable, amenable to screening, and willing and able to seek treatment or follow-up procedures. Criteria for evaluating the suitability of screening tests include cost-effectiveness, ease and safety of administration, availability of treatment, ethics of administration or widespread implementation, sensitivity, specificity, validity, and reliability (Gordis, 2013; McKeown & Learner, 2009).

Screening procedures exist for a wide range of health conditions, including cancer (e.g., breast, cervical, testicular, colon, rectal, and skin), diabetes, hypertension, TB, lead poisoning, hearing loss, and sexually transmitted diseases (e.g., gonorrhea, chlamydia, syphilis). Nurses must keep abreast of recommended screening guidelines, which are reviewed regularly and revised based on findings from epidemiologic research. For example, the latest U.S. Preventive Services Task Force guidelines (USPSTF, 2008) strongly recommend routine screening for lipid disorders in men 35 years and older and women 45 years and older. Screening for younger adults (men ages 20 to 35 and women ages 20 to 45) is recommended when any of the following risk factors are present: diabetes, family history of cardiovascular disease before age 50 in men or age 60 in women, family history suggestive of familial hyperlipidemia, or multiple coronary heart disease risk factors (e.g., tobacco use, hypertension). The Task Force also noted that regardless of lipid levels, all clients should receive education and counseling about the benefits of a diet low in saturated fat and high in fruits and vegetables, regular physical activity, avoidance of tobacco, and maintenance of healthy weight.

The rationale for the current lipid screening guidelines is as follows. The clearest benefit of lipid screening is identifying individuals whose near-term risk of coronary heart disease is sufficiently high to justify drug therapy or other intensive lifestyle interventions to lower cholesterol levels. Screening men older than age 35 years and women older than age 45 years will identify nearly all individuals whose risk of coronary heart disease is as high as that of the subjects in the existing primary prevention trials. Younger people typically have a substantially lower risk, unless they have other important risk factors for coronary heart disease or familial hyperlipidemia. The primary goal of screening younger people is to promote lifestyle changes, which may provide long-term benefits later in life. The average effect of diet interventions is small, and screening is not needed to advise young adults about the benefits of a healthy diet and regular exercise because this advice is considered useful for all age groups. Although universal screening may detect some clients with familial hyperlipidemia earlier than selective screening, it has yet to be determined if universal screening would lead to significant reductions in coronary events (USPSTF, 2008).

Reliability and Validity

Reliability. The precision, or reliability, of the measure (i.e., its consistency or repeatability) and its validity or accuracy (i.e., whether it really measures what we think it is measuring, and how exact the measurement is) are important considerations for any measurement. For example, suppose you are planning to conduct a blood pressure screening in a community setting. You will probably be taking blood pressure measurements on a large number of people and then following up with repeated measures for individuals identified as having higher levels of blood pressure. If the sphygmomanometer used for the blood pressure screening varies in its measurement so that it does not record a similar reading for the same person twice in a row, it lacks precision (or reliability). The instrument would be unreliable even if the overall mean of repeated measurements was close to the true overall mean for the persons measured. The problem would be that the readings would not be reliable for any individual, which is what a screening program requires. On the other hand, suppose the readings are reliably reproducible, yet unknown to you, they tend to be about 10 mm Hg too high. This instrument is producing precise readings, but the uncorrected (or uncalibrated) instrument lacks accuracy (or validity). In short, a measure can be *consistent* without producing *valid* results.

Three major sources of error can affect the reliability of measurement:

- Variation inherent in the trait being measured (e.g., blood pressure changes with time of day, activity, level of stress, and other factors)
- Observer variation, which can be divided into intraobserver reliability (the level of consistency by the same observer) and interobserver reliability (the level of consistency from one observer to another)
- Inconsistency in the instrument, which includes the internal consistency of the instrument (e.g., whether all items in a questionnaire measure the same thing) and the stability (or test-retest reliability) of the instrument over time

Validity: Sensitivity and Specificity. Validity in a screening test is measured by sensitivity and specificity. Sensitivity quantifies how accurately the test identifies those *with* the condition or trait. In other words, sensitivity represents the proportion of persons with the disease whom the test correctly identifies as positive (true positives). High sensitivity is needed when early treatment is important and when identification of every case is important.

Specificity indicates how accurately the test identifies those *without* the condition or trait—in other words, the proportion of persons whom the test correctly identifies as negative for the disease (true negatives). High specificity is needed when rescreening is impractical and when reduction of false positives is important. The sensitivity and specificity of a test are determined by comparing the results from the screening test with results from a definitive diagnostic procedure (sometimes called the gold standard). For example, the Pap smear is used frequently to screen for cervical dysplasia and carcinoma. The definitive diagnosis of cervical cancer requires a biopsy with histological confirmation of malignant cells.

The ideal for a screening test is 100 percent sensitivity and 100 percent specificity. That is, the test is positive for 100 percent

TABLE 13.3 Classification of Subjects According to True Disease State and Screening Test Results for Calculation of Indices of Validity

Result of Screening Test	Disease	No Disease
Positive	True positive (TP)	False positive (FP)
Negative	False negative (FN)	True negative (TN)

Sensitivity = TP/(TP + FN); Specificity = TN/(TN + FP); False-negative "rate" = 1 − sensitivity = FN/(FN + TP); False-positive "rate" = 1 − specificity = FP/(TN + FP); Positive predictive value = TP/(TP + FP); often multiplied by 100 and expressed as a percent.

of those who actually have the disease, and it is negative for all those who do not have the disease. In practice, sensitivity and specificity are often inversely related. That is, if the test results are such that one can choose some point beyond which a person is considered positive (a "cutpoint"), as in a blood pressure reading to screen for hypertension or a serum glucose reading to screen for diabetes, then moving that critical point to improve the sensitivity of the test will result in a decrease in specificity. In other words, an improvement in specificity can be made only at the expense of sensitivity. Table 13.3 shows how to calculate sensitivity and specificity. Some authors refer to a false-positive rate, which is 1 minus the specificity, and a false-negative rate, or 1 minus the sensitivity. These "rates" are simply the proportions of subjects incorrectly labeled as *non-diseased* and *diseased*, respectively.

A third measure associated with sensitivity and specificity is the predictive value of the test. The **positive predictive value** (also called predictive value positive) is the proportion of persons with a positive test who actually have the disease, interpreted as the probability that an individual with a positive test has the disease. The **negative predictive value** (or predictive value negative) is the proportion of persons with a negative test who are actually disease free. Although sensitivity and specificity are relatively independent of the prevalence of disease, predictive values are affected by the level of disease in the screened population and by the sensitivity and specificity of the test. When the prevalence is very low, the positive predictive value will be low, even with tests that are sensitive and specific. In addition, lower specificity produces lower positive predictive values because of the increase in the proportion of false-positive results.

In setting cut points, it is necessary to consider the potential human and economic costs of missing true cases by lowering the sensitivity versus the cost of falsely classifying non-cases by lowering the specificity. In making such decisions, factors to be considered include the importance of capturing all cases, the likelihood that the population will be rescreened, the interval between screenings relative to the rate of disease development, and the prevalence of the disease. A low prevalence typically requires a test with high specificity; otherwise, the screening will produce too many false positives in the largely non-diseased population. On the other hand, a disease with a high prevalence usually requires high sensitivity; otherwise, too many of the real cases will be missed by the screening (false negatives).

Two or more tests can be combined, in series or in parallel, to enhance sensitivity or specificity. In series testing, the final result is considered positive only if all tests in the series were positive, and it is considered negative if any test was negative. For example, in screening a blood sample for HIV, a positive enzyme-linked immunosorbent assay (ELISA) might be followed up with a Western blot, and the sample would be considered positive only if both tests were positive. Series testing enhances specificity, producing fewer false positives, but sensitivity will be lower. In series testing, sequence is important; a very sensitive test often is used first to pick up all cases including false positives, and then a second, very specific test is used to eliminate the false positives. In parallel testing, the final result is considered positive if *any* test was positive and negative only if all tests were negative. To return to the example of a blood sample being tested for HIV, a blood bank might consider a sample positive if a positive result was found on either the ELISA or the Western blot. Parallel testing enhances sensitivity, leaving fewer false negatives, but specificity will be lower.

SURVEILLANCE

Surveillance involves the systematic collection, analysis, and interpretation of data related to the occurrence of disease and the health status of a given population. Surveillance systems are often classified as either active or passive (Teutsch & Churchill, 2010). Passive surveillance is the more common form used by most local and state health departments. Health care providers in the community report cases of notifiable diseases to public health authorities through the use of standardized reports. Passive surveillance is relatively inexpensive but is limited by variability and incompleteness in provider reporting practices. Active surveillance is the purposeful, ongoing search for new cases of disease by public health personnel, through personal or telephone contacts or the review of laboratory reports or hospital or clinic records. Because active surveillance is costly, its use is often limited to brief periods for specific purposes as in the emergence of a newly identified disease, a particularly severe disease, or the reemergence of a previously eradicated disease. In situations that do not require ongoing active surveillance, or where it may not be feasible to maintain a surveillance system across larger geographic areas, sentinel surveillance systems may be instituted. Representative populations may be selected and sentinel providers identified to provide information on specific diseases or conditions. Nurses engage in surveillance activities as they monitor the health status of individuals, families, and groups in their care. They use surveillance data to assess and prioritize the health needs of populations, design public health and clinical services to address those needs, and evaluate the effectiveness of public health programs.

BASIC METHODS IN EPIDEMIOLOGY

Sources of Data

One of the first issues to address in any epidemiologic study is how to obtain the data (Gordis, 2013, Koepsell & Weiss, 2014).

There are three major categories of data sources commonly used in epidemiologic investigations:

1. Routinely collected data, such as census data, vital records (birth and death certificates), and surveillance data as carried out by the CDC.
2. Data collected for other purposes but useful for epidemiologic research, such as medical, health department, and insurance records.
3. Original data collected for specific epidemiologic studies.

The first two types of data are often referred to as *secondary data,* and the third type is commonly considered *primary data.*

Routinely Collected Data. Vital records are the primary source of birth and mortality statistics. Although registration of births and deaths is mandated in most countries, thus providing one of the most complete sources of health-related data, the quality of specific information varies. On birth certificates, for example, sex and date of birth are fairly reliable, but gestational age, level of prenatal care, and smoking habits of the mother during pregnancy are less reliable. On death certificates, the quality of the cause of death information varies over time and from place to place, depending on diagnostic capabilities and custom. Vital records, readily available in most areas, are inexpensive and convenient and allow study of long-term trends. Mortality data, however, are informative only for fatal diseases or events.

Since 1790, there has been a U.S. Census conducted every 10 years. The U.S. Census provides population data, including demographic distribution (e.g., age, race/ethnicity, sex), geographic distribution, and additional information about economic status, housing, and education. Census data serve as denominators for various rates. The American Community Survey is an ongoing survey also conducted by the U.S. Census Bureau. Data from these surveys provide important information on the status of the population and for public health planning and evaluation activities.

Data Collected for Other Purposes. Hospital, physician, health department, laboratory, and insurance records provide information on morbidity, as do surveillance systems, such as cancer registries and health department reporting systems, which solicit reports of all cases of a particular disease within a geographic region. Other information, such as occupational exposures, may be available from employer records. School and employment attendance and absenteeism records are another potential source of data that may be used in epidemiologic investigations.

Epidemiologic Data. The National Center for Health Statistics (NCHS) sponsors periodic health surveys and examinations in carefully drawn samples of the U.S. population. Examples are the National Health and Nutrition Examination Survey (NHANES), the National Health Interview Survey (NHIS), and several National Health Care Surveys, including the National Hospital Discharge Survey (NHDS), the National Ambulatory Medical Care Survey (NAMCS), and the National Nursing Home Survey (NNHS). The CDC also conducts or contracts for surveys such as the Youth Risk Behavior Survey (YRBS), the Pregnancy Risk Assessment Monitoring System (PRAMS), and the Behavioral Risk Factor Surveillance System (BRFSS). These surveys provide information on the health status and behaviors of the population. For many studies, however, the only way to obtain the needed information is to collect the required data in a study specifically designed to investigate a particular question. The design of such studies is discussed later.

With the National Institutes of Health's recent emphasis on transdisciplinary approaches to science, disciplines that have not traditionally partnered together are beginning to realize the benefits and advantage of combining methodologies to tackle public health problems. An example of this is the increase in collaborative research between public health professionals and geographers, aimed at furthering understanding of the influence of place on health outcomes. Within the field of geography, Geographic Information System (GIS; often termed ArcGIS after the software utilized) allows for mapping data to the exact location of specific occurrences or events (e.g., a family residence, the location where they receive medical care, or the number of fast food restaurants within a 1-mile radius of the residence).

This type of integrated geographic and public health data mapping allows researchers and public health professionals to conduct more detailed assessments of the environments of individuals, families, and communities. With the technological advances available through GIS, the use of cartographic data for epidemiologic studies is becoming more widespread. For example, GIS systems are now an integral component of malaria vector control in Mexico and Central America (Najera-Aguilar et al., 2005). Local health professionals and authorities who survey their communities to identify mosquito-breeding sites now use global positioning system (GPS) and GIS technology to display and analyze their data. The resulting GIS maps are graphic illustrations of their communities, including buildings, streets, rivers, mosquito-breeding sites, and dwellings where individuals with malaria live. These maps allow the calculation of preventive treatments for dwellings located inside various radiuses, from 50 to 250 meters, around the houses with malaria cases. The standardization and integration of cartographic data collection in countries with endemic malaria are part of coordinated international efforts to strengthen malaria control. Researchers have employed GIS technology to examine other health issues, such as access to prenatal care (Auchincloss, 2012). McLafferty and Grady (2005) compared levels of geographic access to prenatal clinics among immigrants groups in Brooklyn, New York. They used kernel estimation, a technique to depict the density of points (in this case, prenatal clinics) as a spatially continuous variable that can be represented as a smooth contour map. Then, using birth record data for the year 2000, which included the mother's country of birth, they compared clinic density levels among different immigrant groups. The authors noted the usefulness of these methods for public health departments in exploring demographic transitions and developing health service networks that are responsive to immigrant populations. GIS technology is applicable across a wide range of contexts, including mapping the distribution of health exposures or outcomes, linking data with geo-coded addresses of individuals to sources of potentially toxic exposures, and mapping water quality measures in sensitive ecosystems.

Rate Adjustment

Rates, which are of central importance in epidemiologic studies, can be misleading when compared across different populations. For example, the risk of death increases rather dramatically after 40 years of age; therefore a higher crude death rate is expected in a population of older people compared with a population of younger people (Gordis, 2013; Koepsell & Weiss, 2014; Rothman, 2012). Because the direct comparison of the overall mortality rate in an area with a large population of older adults to the mortality rate in an area with a much younger population would be misleading, there are methods that adjust for such differences in populations. Age adjustment is based on the assumption that a population's overall mortality rate is a function of the age distribution of the population and the age-specific mortality rates. Rates for any outcome can be adjusted by the methods described here, but we focus our discussion on age adjustment of death rates because it is most common. As previously noted, as the population ages, the risk of death increases.

Age adjustment can be performed by direct or indirect methods. Both methods require a *standard population,* which can be an external population, such as the U.S. population for a given year; a combined population of the groups under study; or some other standard chosen for relevance or convenience. A direct age-adjusted rate applies the age-specific death rates from the study population to the age distribution of the standard population. The result is the (hypothetical) death rate of the study population if it had the same age distribution as the standard population.

The indirect method, as the name suggests, is more complicated. The age-specific death rates of the standard population applied to the study population's age distribution produce an index rate that is used with the crude rates of both the study and standard populations to produce the final indirect adjusted rate, which is also hypothetical. The indirect method may be required when the age-specific death rates for the study population are unknown or unstable (e.g., based on relatively small numbers). Often, instead of an indirect adjusted rate, a standardized mortality ratio (SMR) is calculated. This is the number of observed deaths in the study population divided by the number of deaths expected on the basis of the age-specific rates in the standard population and the age distribution of the study population (Gordis, 2013; Szklo & Nieto, 2018).

Although the focus of this discussion has been age adjustment, the process can be used to adjust for any factor that may vary from one population to another. For example, to compare infant mortality rates across populations with different birth weight distributions, these methods may be used to produce birth weight–adjusted infant mortality rates. Note that all adjusted rates are fictitious rates. They may resemble crude rates if the distribution of the study sample is similar to the distribution of the standard population. The magnitude of adjusted rates depends on the standard population used. The choice of a different standard would produce a different adjusted rate. The change from the 1940 U.S. population to the 2000 U.S. population as the standard for age-adjusted rates from the NCHS demonstrates the difference a change in standard population can make (Xu, 2018).

Comparison Groups

The use of comparison groups is at the heart of the epidemiologic approach. In order to identify or further understand clues about factors influencing the distribution of disease (i.e., disease determinants or risk factors), it is necessary to compare the incidence or prevalence measures in groups that differ on important characteristics. Observing the rate of disease only among persons exposed to a suspected risk factor will not show clearly that the exposure is associated with increased risk until the rate observed in the exposed group is compared with the rate in a group of comparable unexposed persons. For example, one might investigate the effect of smoking during pregnancy on the rate of birth of low-birth-weight infants by calculating the rate of low-birth-weight infants born to women who smoked during their pregnancy. However, the hypothesis that smoking during pregnancy is a risk factor for low birth weight is supported only when the low-birth-weight rate among smoking women is compared with the (lower) rate of low-birth-weight infants born to nonsmoking women.

The ideal approach would be to compare one group of people who all have a certain characteristic, exposure, or behavior with a group of people *exactly* like them except they all *lack* that characteristic, exposure, or behavior. When this ideal approach is not possible, researchers either randomize people to exposure or treatment groups in experimental studies, or they select comparison groups that are comparable in observational studies. Advances in statistical techniques now make it possible to control for differences between groups, but these advanced techniques are effective only in reducing the bias that results from confounding by variables we have measured.

DESCRIPTIVE EPIDEMIOLOGY

Descriptive epidemiology describes the distribution of disease, death, and other health outcomes in the population according to person, place, and time, providing a picture of how things are or have been—the who, where, and when of disease patterns. Analytic epidemiology, on the other hand, searches for the determinants of the patterns observed—the how and why. That is, epidemiologic concepts and methods are used to identify what factors, characteristics, exposures, or behaviors might account for differences in the observed patterns of disease occurrence. Descriptive and analytic studies are observational, meaning the investigator observes events as they are or have been and does not intervene to change anything or introduce a new factor. Experimental or intervention studies, however, include interventions to test preventive or treatment measures, techniques, materials, policies, or drugs.

Person

Personal characteristics of interest in epidemiology include race, ethnicity, sex, age, education, occupation, income (and related socioeconomic status), and marital status. As noted previously, the most important predictor of overall mortality is age. The mortality curve by age drops sharply during and after the first year of life to a low point in childhood, then it begins to increase through adolescence and young adulthood, and after that it increases sharply (exponentially) through middle and older ages (Gordis, 2013).

There are also substantial differences in mortality and morbidity rates by sex. Female infants have a lower mortality rate than comparable male infants, and the survival advantage continues throughout life (Xu, 2018). However, patterns for specific diseases vary. For example, women have lower rates of CHD until menopause, after which the gap narrows. For rheumatoid arthritis, the prevalence among women is greater than among men (Remington et al., 2016).

Although the concept of race as a variable for public health research has come under scrutiny (CDC, 1993; Fullilove, 1998), there are clear differences in morbidity and mortality rates by race in the United States (Kochanek, 2017). According to the Office of Minority Health (OMH, 2015), racial and ethnic minority groups are among the fastest-growing populations in the United States, yet they have poorer health and remain chronically underserved by the health care system. Data in the OMH report *HHS Action Plan to Reduce Racial and Ethnic Health Disparities Implementation Progress Report* highlighted some of the significant health disparities within the leading categories of death in the United States. For example, in 2016 the overall infant mortality rate (IMR) was 5.87 deaths per 1000 live births, but the IMR among African Americans was 11.76 per 1000 live births (Xu, 2018), and the gap has been widening in recent years. Racial and ethnic health disparities have been observed in a wide range of diseases and health behaviors, from infant mortality to diabetes, heart disease, cancer, and HIV. Although there has been some progress toward meeting the goal of eliminating racial/ethnic disparities, with improvement in rates for most health status indicators across all racial/ethnic groups, the improvements have not been uniform across groups and "substantial differences among racial/ethnic groups persist" (USDHHS, OMH, 2015). Among American Indians and Alaska Natives, several health indicators actually worsened from 1990 to 1998. The IMR declined in all groups, but it remains 2.3 times higher for infants born to non-Hispanic African American mothers than for those born to white non-Hispanic mothers. Similarly, the overall age-adjusted mortality rate was 22 percent higher in the African American population than in the white population in 2006, and it was higher for 10 of the 15 leading causes of death (Xu et al., 2018). Although individual characteristics such as race, gender, and immigration status are of interest to epidemiologists, there has been increasing focus on social, economic, and cultural contexts and processes underlying racial and ethnic inequalities in health, such as discrimination (Fuller et al., 2005; Matoba et al., 2017).

Place

When considering the distribution of a disease, geographic patterns come to mind: Does the rate of disease differ from place to place (e.g., with local environment)? If geography had no effect on disease occurrence, random geographic patterns might be seen, but that is often not the case. For example, at high altitudes there is lower oxygen surface tension, which might result in smaller babies. Other diseases reflect distinctive geographic patterns. For example, Lyme disease is transmitted from animal reservoirs to humans by a tick vector. Thus the disease is more likely to be found in areas where there are animals carrying the disease, a large tick population for transmission to humans, and contact between the human population and the tick vectors (Heymann, 2014). The influence of place on disease may certainly be related to geographic variations in the chemical, physical, or biological environment. However, variations by place also may result from differences in population densities, or in customary patterns of behavior and lifestyle, or in other personal characteristics. For example, geographic variations might occur because of high concentrations of a religious, cultural, or ethnic group who practice certain health-related behaviors. The high rates of stroke found in the southeastern United States are likely to be the result of a number of social, economic, cultural, and personal factors that have little to do with geographic features per se. Recent epidemiologic research has also focused on neighborhood-level variables, such as unemployment and crime rate, social cohesion, educational levels, racial segregation, and access to important services (Fuller et al., 2005; Patel, 2015). For example, recent research on adolescent injection drug users (IDUs) found that African American IDUs from neighborhoods with a large percent of minority residents and low adult educational levels were more likely to initiate injection use during adolescence than white IDUs from neighborhoods with a low percent of minority residents and high adult education levels. Nurses need to pay attention to this wide range of community-level variables as they assess the health of communities.

Time

Time is the third component of descriptive epidemiology. In relation to time, epidemiologists ask these questions: Is there an increase or decrease in the frequency of the disease over time? Are other temporal (and spatial) patterns evident? Temporal patterns of interest to epidemiologists include secular trends, point epidemic, cyclical patterns, and event-related clusters.

Secular Trends. Long-term patterns of morbidity or mortality rates (i.e., over years or decades) are called secular trends. Secular trends may reflect changes in social behavior or health practices. For example, the increased lung cancer mortality rates among men and women in recent years reflect a delayed effect of increased smoking in prior years. Similarly, the decline in cervical cancer deaths is primarily attributable to widespread screening with the Pap test (Remington et al., 2016). Some secular trends may result from increased diagnostic capability or changes in survival (or case fatality) rather than in incidence. For example, case fatality from breast cancer has decreased in recent years, although the incidence of breast cancer has increased. Some, though not all, of the increased incidence is a result of improved diagnostic capability. These two trends result in a breast cancer mortality curve that is flatter than the incidence curve (Remington et al., 2016). Mortality data alone do not accurately reflect the true situation. For example, changes in case definition or revisions in the coding of a disease according to the International Classification of Diseases (ICD) can produce an artificial change in mortality rates.

Point Epidemic. One temporal and spatial pattern of disease distribution is the point epidemic. This time-and-space–related pattern is important in infectious disease investigations and is a significant indicator for toxic exposures in environmental epidemiology. A point epidemic is most clearly seen when the frequency of cases is plotted against time. The sharp peak characteristic of such graphs indicates a concentration of cases in some short interval of time. The peak often indicates the response of the population to a common source of infection or contamination to which they were all simultaneously exposed. Knowledge of the incubation or latency period (the time between exposure and development of signs and symptoms) for the specific disease entity can help determine the probable time of exposure. A common example of a point epidemic is an outbreak of gastrointestinal illness from a foodborne pathogen. Nurses who are alert to a sudden increase in the number of cases of a disease can chart the outbreak, determine the probable time of exposure, and, by careful investigation, isolate the probable source of the agent.

Cyclical Patterns. In addition to secular trends and point epidemics, there are also cyclical time patterns of disease. One common type of cyclical variation is the seasonal fluctuation seen in a number of infectious illnesses. Seasonal changes may be influenced by changes in the agent itself, changes in population densities or behaviors of animal reservoirs or vectors, or changes in human behavior that result in changing exposures (e.g., being outdoors in warmer weather and indoors in colder months). There may also be artificial seasons created by calendar events (e.g., holidays and tax-filing deadlines) that may be associated with patterns of stress-related illness. Patterns of accidents and injuries may also be seasonal, reflecting differing employment and recreational patterns. Some disease cycles, such as influenza, have patterns of smaller epidemics every few years, depending on strain, with major pandemics occurring at longer intervals (Heymann, 2014). Workers in public health can prepare to meet increased demands on resources by careful attention to these cyclical patterns.

Event-Related Clusters. A fourth type of temporal pattern is non-simultaneous, event-related clusters. These are patterns in which time is not measured from fixed dates on the calendar but from the point of some exposure or event, presumably experienced in common by affected persons, although not occurring at the same time. An example would be natural disasters such as hurricanes and their impact on public health. Often after hurricanes, particularly those causing significant damage to natural resources, an increase in acute infectious diseases will be seen due to lack of safe water, adequate hygiene, and sanitation. After Hurricane Maria passed through Puerto Rico on September 20, 2017, officials reported a significant increase in cases of leptospirosis (bacterial infection that can lead to kidney damage, meningitis, brain damage, liver failure, and even death). By October 2017, officials had 121 confirmed cases of leptospirosis compared to 60 in a usual year (Henry J. Kaiser Family Foundation, 2018).

ANALYTIC EPIDEMIOLOGY

Descriptive epidemiology deals with the distribution of health outcomes, whereas analytic epidemiology seeks to discover the determinants of outcomes, or the how and the why (i.e., the factors that influence observed patterns of health and disease and increase or decrease the risk of adverse outcomes). This section deals with analytic study designs and the related measures of association derived from them. Table 13.4 summarizes the advantages and disadvantages of each design.

Cohort Studies

The cohort study is the standard for observational epidemiologic studies, coming closest to the ideal of a natural experiment (Rothman, 2012). In epidemiology, the term *cohort* is used to describe a group of persons who are born at about the same time. In analytic studies, a cohort refers to a group of persons (generally sharing some characteristic of interest) enrolled in a study and followed over a period of time to observe some health outcome (Porta, 2014). Because they enable us to observe the development of new cases of disease, cohort study designs allow calculation of incidence rates and therefore estimates of disease risk. Cohort studies may be prospective or retrospective (Gordis, 2013; Rothman, 2012; Szklo & Nieto, 2018;).

Prospective Cohort Studies. In a prospective cohort study (also called a longitudinal or follow-up study), subjects determined to be free of the outcome under investigation are classified on the basis of the exposure of interest at the beginning of the follow-up period. The different exposure groups constitute the comparison groups for the study. The subjects are then followed for some period of time to determine the occurrence of disease in each group. The question is the following: "Do persons with the factor (or exposure) of interest develop (or avoid) the outcome more frequently than those without the factor (or exposure)?"

For example, one might recruit a cohort of subjects classified as physically active ("exposed") or sedentary ("not exposed"). One might further quantify the amount of the "exposure" if there is sufficient information. These subjects would then be followed over time to determine the development of CHD. This study design avoids the problem of selective survival that sometimes affects other study designs (Fig. 13.5). Because persons initially without the disease are followed over time, this design allows estimation of both incidence rates and incidence proportions. The cohort study can also estimate the relative risk of acquiring disease for those who are exposed compared with those who are unexposed (or less exposed). This ratio of incidence proportions is called the risk ratio (or relative risk), and a ratio incidence rate is called the rate ratio. For example, if the risk of CHD in smokers is twice as high as the risk among nonsmokers, the risk ratio would be 2. If a factor is unrelated to the

TABLE 13.4 Comparison of Major Epidemiologic Study Designs

Study Design	Advantages	Disadvantages
Ecological	Quick, easy, and inexpensive first study Uses readily available existing data May prompt further investigation or suggest other/new hypotheses May provide information about contextual factors not accounted for by individual characteristics	Ecological fallacy: associations observed may not hold true for individuals Problems in interpreting temporal sequence (cause and effect) More difficult to control for confounding and "mixed" models (ecological and individual data); more complex statistically
Cross-sectional	Gives general description of scope of problem; provides prevalence estimates Often based on population (or community) sample, not just those who sought care Useful in health service evaluation and planning Data obtained at once; less expensive and quicker than cohort because no follow-up Baseline for prospective study or to identify cases and controls for case-control study	No calculation of risk; prevalence, not incidence Temporal sequence unclear Not good for rare disease or rare exposure unless large sample size or stratified sampling Selective survival can be major source of selection bias; surviving subjects may differ from those who are not included (e.g., death, institutionalization) Selective recall or lack of past exposure information can create bias
Case-control (retrospective, case comparison)	Less expensive than cohort; smaller sample required Quicker than cohort; no follow-up Can investigate more than one exposure Best design for rare diseases If well designed, can be important tool for etiological investigation Best suited to disease with relatively clear onset (timing of onset can be established so that incident cases can be included)	Greater susceptibility than cohort studies to various types of bias (selective survival, recall bias, selection bias on choice of both cases and controls) Information on other risk factors may not be available, resulting in confounding Antecedent-consequence (temporal sequence) not as certain as in cohort Not well suited to rare exposures Gives only an indirect estimate of risk Limited to a single outcome because of sampling on disease status
Prospective cohort (concurrent cohort, longitudinal, follow-up)	Best estimate of disease incidence Best estimate of risk Fewer problems with selective survival and selective recall Temporal sequence more clearly established Broader range of options for exposure assessment	Expensive in time and money More difficult organizationally Not good for rare diseases Attrition of participants can bias estimate Latency period may be very long; may miss cases May be difficult to examine several exposures
Retrospective cohort (nonconcurrent cohort)	Combines advantages of both prospective cohort and case-control Shorter time (even if follow-up into future) than prospective cohort Less expensive than prospective cohort because reliant on existing data Temporal sequence may be clearer than case-control	Shares some disadvantages with both prospective cohort and case-control Subject to attrition (loss to follow-up) Relies on existing records that may result in misclassification of both exposure and outcome May have to rely on surrogate measure of exposure (e.g., job title) and vital records information on cause of death

	CHD	CHD	
Physically active	48 (a)	952 (b)	1000
Sedentary	120 (c)	880 (d)	1000

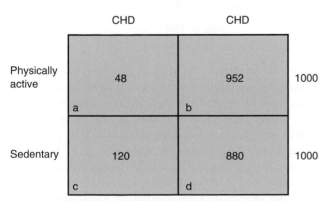

Fig. 13.5 Cohort study. *CHD,* Coronary heart disease.

risk of a disease, the risk ratio will be close to 1. A value less than 1 may suggest a protective association. For example, the risk of CHD is lower among those who are physically active than among sedentary persons, so the risk ratio for the association between physical activity and CHD should be less than 1.

Suppose 1000 physically active and 1000 sedentary middle-aged men and women enroll in a prospective cohort study. All are free of CHD at enrollment. Over a five-year follow-up period, regular examinations detect CHD in 120 of the sedentary men and women and in 48 of the active men and women. Assuming no other deaths or losses to follow-up, the data could be presented as shown in Fig. 13.5.

The incidence proportion of CHD in the active group is a/(a + b), or 48/1000, and the incidence of CHD in the sedentary group is c/(c + d), or 120/1000. The risk ratio is as follows:

$$\left(\frac{48}{1000}\right) \div \left(\frac{120}{1000}\right) = 0.4$$

Because physical activity is protective for CHD, the risk ratio is less than 1. The interpretation for this hypothetical example is that, over a five-year period, the risk of CHD in persons who are physically active is about 0.4 as great as the risk among sedentary persons. If the risk was greater for those exposed, the risk ratio would be greater than 1. For example, if the risk ratio of CHD for overweight persons compared with normal weight is 3.5, it would be interpreted to mean that the risk of CHD among overweight persons is 3.5 times the risk of those with normal weight. The null value indicating no association is 1, because the incidence proportion and thus the risk would be equal in the two groups if there were no association. This same statistic can also be expressed (and indeed is more commonly used in the media) as a percent increase or decrease in risk. For a relative risk of 0.40, it also can be expressed as a "a 60 percent decreased risk (1.0 − 0.4 = 60 percent reduction from 1.0)." Likewise, a relative risk of 1.4 could be expressed as a "40 percent increase in risk."

Because subjects are enrolled before onset of disease, using the cohort design allows us to study more than one outcome, calculate incidence rates and proportions, estimate risk, and establish the temporal sequence of exposure and outcome with greater clarity and certainty. Use of the cohort design also may avoid many of the problems of the other study designs with selective survival or exposure misclassification (discussed later). On the other hand, large samples are often necessary to ensure that enough cases are observed to provide enough statistical power to detect meaningful differences between groups. This is complicated by the long period required for some diseases to develop (the latency period). In addition, the number of subjects required to observe sufficient cases makes longitudinal studies unsuitable for very rare diseases unless they are part of a larger study of a number of outcomes.

Retrospective Cohort Studies. Retrospective cohort studies combine some of the advantages and some of the disadvantages of both case-control studies and prospective cohort studies. In these studies, the epidemiologist relies on existing records, such as employment, insurance, or hospital records, to define a cohort, whose members are classified according to exposure status at some time in the past. The cohort is followed over time using the records to determine if the outcome occurred. Retrospective cohort (also called historical cohort) studies may be conducted entirely using past records or may include current assessment or additional follow-up time after study initiation. The obvious advantage of this approach is the time savings, because one does not have to wait for new cases of disease to develop. The disadvantages are largely related to the reliance on existing historical records. Retrospective cohort studies are frequently used in occupational epidemiology where industrial records are available to investigate work-related exposures and health outcomes.

Case-Control Studies

The case-control design can be viewed against the background of an underlying cohort. The design uses a sample from the cohort rather than following the entire cohort over time. Because it uses only samples of cases and non-cases, it is a more efficient design, although it is subject to certain types of bias (Rothman, 2012). In the case-control study, participants are enrolled because they are known to have the outcome of interest (cases) or they are known *not* to have the outcome of interest (controls). Case-control status is verified using a clear case definition and some previously determined method or protocol (e.g., by an examination, laboratory test, or medical chart review). Information is then collected on the exposures or characteristics of interest, frequently from existing sources, subject interview, or questionnaire (Rothman, 2012; Szklo & Nieto, 2018). The question in a case-control study is the following: "Do persons with the outcome of interest (cases) have the exposure characteristic (or a history of the exposure) more frequently than those without the outcome (controls)?"

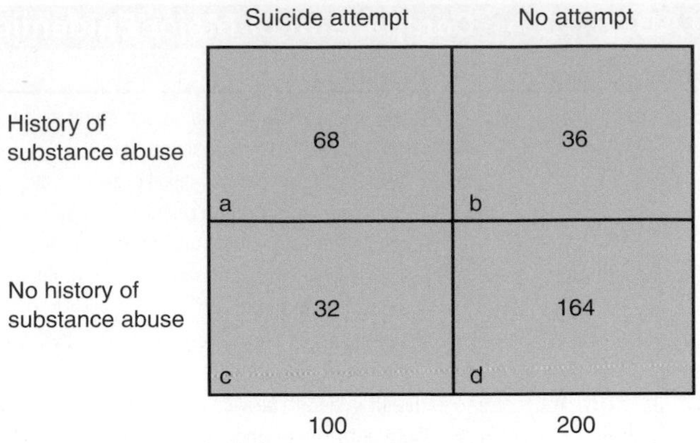

Fig. 13.6 Case-control study.

Suppose a research group wanted to study risk factors for suicide attempts among adolescents. They were able to enroll 100 adolescents who had attempted suicide, and they selected 200 adolescents from the same community with no history of suicide attempt. One of the factors they wanted to investigate is a history of substance abuse. Through a questionnaire and other medical records, they determine that 68 of the 100 adolescents who had attempted suicide had a history of substance abuse, whereas 36 of the 200 adolescents with no suicide attempt had such a history. The information could be presented as shown in Fig. 13.6. The odds of a positive history of substance abuse among adolescents who attempt suicide is a/c, or 68/32, whereas the odds of substance abuse among controls (no suicide attempts) is b/d, or 36/164. The odds ratio (equivalent to ad/bc) is as follows:

$$\frac{(68 \times 164)}{(36 \times 32)} = 9.68$$

This would be interpreted to mean that the odds of a history of substance abuse are about 10 times greater among adolescents who have attempted suicide than among adolescents who have not attempted suicide. Note that, as with the risk ratio, an odds ratio of 1 is indicative of no association (i.e., the odds of exposure are similar for cases and controls). An odds ratio less than 1 suggests a protective association (cases are less likely to have been exposed than controls).

Given the way subjects are selected for a case-control study, neither incidence nor prevalence measures can be calculated directly. However, if newly diagnosed cases are enrolled as they are found, and if case ascertainment is fairly complete and the source population well defined, an estimate of incidence may be obtained. In a case-control study, an odds ratio tells how much more or less likely the exposure is to be found among cases than among controls. The odds of exposure among cases (a/c in Fig. 13.6) are compared with the odds of exposure among controls (b/d in Fig. 13.6). Under certain conditions, the ratio of these two odds provides an estimate of the risk ratio or rate ratio.

Because the number of cases is known or actively sought out, case-control studies do not demand large samples or the long follow-up time that is often required for prospective cohort studies. Thus many of the influential cancer studies are of the case-control design.

Case-control studies are, however, prone to a number of biases (see further discussion under Bias later in this chapter). Because these studies begin with existing cases, differential survival can produce biased results. The use of recently diagnosed, or "incident," cases may reduce this bias. Also, exposure information is obtained from subject recall or past records, and there may be errors in exposure assessment or misclassification. Because participants are selected precisely because they do or do not have a specific health outcome, case-control studies are limited to a single outcome, although they may investigate a number of potential risk factors.

Cross-Sectional Studies

The cross-sectional study provides a snapshot, or cross-section, of a population or group (Gordis, 2013). Information is collected on current health status, personal characteristics, and potential risk factors or exposures all at once. The cross-sectional study is characterized by the simultaneous collection of information necessary for the classification of exposure and outcome status, although there may be historical information collected (e.g., on past diet or history of radiation exposure). Surveys are one common type of data collection for cross-sectional studies. They may be administered in person, over the phone, by mail, or, increasingly, on websites or through personal electronic devices. Each form of administration has its advantages and disadvantages, as does the use of surveys for epidemiologic studies, but a complete discussion of survey methodology is beyond the scope of this chapter.

Cross-sectional studies are sometimes called prevalence studies because they provide the frequency of existing cases of a disease in a population. One way cross-sectional studies evaluate the association of a factor with a health problem is by comparing the prevalence of the disease in those who have the factor (or exposure) with the prevalence in the unexposed. The ratio of the two prevalence proportions indicates an association between the factor and the outcome. If the prevalence of CHD in smokers was twice as high as the prevalence among nonsmokers, the prevalence ratio would be 2. If a factor is unrelated to the prevalence of a disease, the prevalence ratio will be close to 1. A value less than 1 may suggest a protective association. For example, the prevalence of CHD is lower among those who are physically active than among sedentary persons, so the prevalence ratio for the association between physical activity and CHD should be less than 1. Prevalence ratios require caution in interpretation because the prevalence measure is affected by cure, survival, and migration and does not estimate the risk of getting the disease.

Cross-sectional studies are subject to bias resulting from selective survival (i.e., people who have survived to be in the study may be different from people diagnosed about the same time who have died and are not available for inclusion). Suppose that physical activity not only reduced the risk of CHD but also markedly improved survival among those with CHD. Sedentary persons with CHD would then have higher fatality rates than physically active persons who did develop CHD. One might observe higher rates of physical activity in a group of persons surviving with CHD than in a general population without CHD, both because of the survival advantage of those who previously were active and because of increased participation of other survivors in cardiac rehabilitation programs. It could erroneously appear that physical activity was a risk factor for CHD.

Ecological Studies

An epidemiologic study that is a bridge between descriptive epidemiology and analytic epidemiology is the ecological study. The descriptive component involves examining variations in disease rates by person, place, or time. The analytic component lies in the effort to determine if there is a relationship between disease rates and variations in rates for possible risk (or protective) factors. The identifying characteristic of ecological studies is that only aggregate data, such as population rates, are used rather than data on individuals' exposures, characteristics, and outcomes. For example, information on per capita cigarette consumption might be examined in relation to lung cancer mortality rates in several countries, in several groups of people, or in the same population at different times. Other examples include comparisons of rates of breastfeeding and breast cancer, average dietary fat content and rates of CHD, or unemployment rates and levels of psychiatric disorders.

Ecological studies are attractive because they often make use of existing, readily available rates and are therefore quick and inexpensive to conduct. They are subject, however, to ecological fallacy (i.e., associations observed at the group level may not hold true for the individuals that make up the groups, or associations that actually exist may be masked in the grouped data). This may be the result of other factors operating in these populations for which the ecological correlations do not account. For that reason, ecological studies may be suggestive but require confirmation in studies using individual data (Gordis, 2013; Koepsell & Weiss, 2014;). However, it has been shown that ecological data can add important information to analyses even when individual-level data are available (Adams, 2015a; Adams, 2015b; Choi, 2015). Uncertainty concerning the temporal sequence of events is a disadvantage that ecological studies share with cross-sectional study designs. For example, in the study of unemployment rates and psychiatric disorders, it is unclear whether unemployed persons are at higher risk for psychiatric problems or whether persons with existing psychiatric problems are more likely to be unemployed. Although determining whether one event precedes or succeeds another may seem at first to be a simple matter, in practice it may be difficult to confirm.

EXPERIMENTAL STUDIES

The study designs discussed so far are called observational studies because the investigator observes the association between exposures and outcomes as they exist but does not intervene to alter the presence or level of any exposure or behavior. Studies in which the investigator initiates some treatment or intervention that may influence the risk or course of disease are called *intervention*, or *experimental, studies*. Such studies test whether interventions are effective in preventing disease or improving health. Like observational studies, experimental studies generally use comparison (or control) groups, but unlike observational studies, they are subject to the consequences of randomly allocating persons to a particular intervention group and determining the type or level of the "exposure" (the treatment or intervention). Intervention studies are of two general types: clinical trials and community trials.

Clinical Trials

In clinical trials, the research issue is generally the efficacy of a medical treatment for disease, such as a new drug or an existing drug used in a new or different way, a surgical technique, or another treatment. The preferred method of subject allocation in clinical trials is randomization (i.e., assigning treatments to clients so that all possible treatment assignments have a predetermined probability but neither subject nor investigator determines the actual assignment of any participant). Randomization avoids the bias that may result if subjects self-select into one group or the other or if the investigator or clinician chooses subjects for each group. A second aspect of treatment allocation is the use of masking, or "blinding," treatment assignments. The optimal design for most situations is the double-blind study in which neither the subject nor the investigator knows who is receiving which treatment. The aim of blinding is to reduce the bias from overestimating therapeutic benefit for the experimental treatment when it is known who is receiving it.

Clinical trials are generally thought to provide the best evidence of causality because of the assignment of treatment and the greater control over other factors that could influence outcome. Like cohort studies, clinical trials are prospective in direction and provide the clearest evidence of temporal sequence. However, clinical trials are generally conducted in a contrived situation, under controlled conditions, and with select client populations. That means that the treatment may be less effective when it is applied under more realistic clinical or community conditions in a more diverse client population. There are also ethical considerations in experimental studies that go beyond those that apply to observational studies. Also, clinical trials tend to be costly in time, personnel, facilities, and other factors.

Community Trials

Community trials are similar to clinical trials in that an investigator determines the exposure or intervention, but in this case the issue is often health promotion and disease prevention rather than treatment of existing disease. The intervention is usually undertaken on a large scale, with the unit of treatment allocation being a community, region, or group rather than individuals. Although a pharmaceutical product may be involved in a community trial (e.g., fluoridation of water or mass immunizations), community trials often involve educational, programmatic, or policy interventions. An example of community intervention is providing exercise programs and facilities and increasing the availability of healthy, fresh foods to study the effect on diabetes rates.

Although community trials provide the best means of testing whether changes in knowledge or behavior, policy, programs, or other mass interventions are effective, they are not without problems. For many interventions, it may take years for the effectiveness of the intervention to be evident. In the meantime, other factors may also influence the outcome, either positively (making the intervention look more effective than it really is) or negatively (making the intervention look less effective than it really is). Comparable community populations without similar interventions for comparative analysis are often difficult to determine. Even when comparable comparison communities are available, especially when the intervention is intended to improve knowledge or change behavior, it is difficult and unethical to prevent the control communities from making use of generally available information. Exposure to this information, however, may have the effect of making control communities more like the intervention communities. Also, because community trials are often undertaken on a large scale and over long periods, they can be expensive, requiring large staff, complicated logistics, and extensive communication resources. Although the randomized trial is often considered the "gold standard" of medical and public health research, because of the limitations noted earlier, there is clearly a need for other types of research designs to complement randomized control trials (Victora et al., 2004).

CAUSALITY

In a previous section, we introduced the concept of the *web of causation*. This is a useful analogy in considering causal agents at a population level and how these multiple factors are related to each other. This next section will focus on causality within the context of the individual study or series of studies (as with a body of evidence). This is quite different from the web analogy that was used previously because it only focuses on the relationship between a single exposure and outcome measure. It may be useful to think of the web of causation as those factors that play out at the macroscopic level, in contrast to focusing efforts to identify and prove causality at a microscopic level.

Statistical Associations

One of the first steps in assessing the relationship of some factor with a health outcome is determining whether a statistical association exists. If the probability of disease seems unaffected by the presence or level of the factor, no association is apparent. If, on the other hand, the probability of disease does vary according to whether the factor is present, there is a statistical association. The earlier discussion of null values is pertinent at this point. When an observed measure of association (such as a risk ratio) does not differ from the null value, it may not be assumed that there is an association between the factor and the outcome under investigation.

In many studies, a great deal of emphasis is placed on tests of statistical significance. This is a judgment that the observed results are or are not likely to be attributable to chance at some predetermined level of probability (usually 0.05). However, many epidemiologists contend that much more information is provided by an estimate of the association (the ratio or difference in rates or risks) and a confidence interval that indicates the precision of the estimate (Rothman, 2012). Note that statistical significance is determined by sample size, the amount of difference between groups, and the variance in the estimates.

Bias

Although statistical testing and estimation are critical, it is important to remember that statistical testing and interval estimation generally assume that deviations from the true value are the result of chance. However, estimates may appear to be greater or less than they really are because of **bias**, a systematic error resulting from the study design, execution, or confounding. For example, if there were a gumball machine with colors randomly mixed and three red ones in a row came out, that would be a result of chance. If, however, the person loading the gumball machine had poured in a bag of red ones first, then green ones, and then yellow, it would not be surprising to get three red ones in a row because of the way the machine was loaded. In epidemiologic studies, results are sometimes biased because of the way the study was "loaded" (i.e., the way the study was designed, subjects were selected, information was collected, or subjects were classified). Three generally recognized categories are selection, classification, and confounding bias (Rothman, 2012).

Bias attributable to the way subjects enter a study is called selection bias. It has to do with selection procedures and the population from which subjects are drawn. It may involve self-selection factors as well. For example, are teenagers who agree to complete a questionnaire on alcohol, tobacco, and other drug use representative of the total teenage population?

Bias attributable to misclassification of subjects once they are in the study is information, or classification (or misclassification), bias. It is related to how information is collected, including the information that subjects supply or how subjects are classified.

Bias resulting from the relationship of the outcome and study factor with some third factor not accounted for is called *confounding*. For example, there is a well-known association between maternal smoking during pregnancy and low-birth-weight babies. There is also an association between alcohol consumption and smoking that is not attributable to chance, nor is it causal (i.e., drinking alcohol does not cause a person to smoke, nor does smoking cause a person to drink alcohol). If one were to investigate the association of alcohol consumption and low birth weight, smoking would be a confounder because it is related to both alcohol consumption and low birth weight. Failure to account for smoking in the analysis would bias the observed association between alcohol use and low birth weight. In practice, one can often identify potentially confounding variables and adjust for them in analysis.

Assessing for Causality

The existence of a statistical association does not necessarily mean that there is a causal relationship or that causality is present (Susser, 1973). As noted previously, the observed association may be a random event (caused by chance) or may be attributable to bias from confounding or from flaws in the study design or execution. Statistical associations, although necessary to an argument for causality, are not sufficient proof. Some epidemiologists refer to *criteria for causality*, a term originally established to evaluate the link between an infectious agent and a disease but revised and elaborated to also apply to other outcomes. Although various lists of criteria have been proposed, the seven criteria listed in Box 13.3 are fairly commonly cited (Gordis, 2013; Koepsell & Weiss, 2014). Some have questioned the use of lists of criteria as misleading, especially because only temporal sequence is necessary, and none of the others really is a criterion (Rothman, 2012). Although no single epidemiologic study can satisfy all criteria, public health practitioners rely on the accumulation of evidence and the strength of individual studies to provide a basis for effective public health interventions and policies.

BOX 13.3 Criteria for Causality

1. *Strength of association:* A strong association between a potential risk factor and an outcome supports a causal hypothesis (e.g., a relative risk of 7 provides stronger evidence of a causal association than a relative risk of 1.5).
2. *Consistency of findings:* Repeated findings of an association with different study designs and in different populations strengthen causal inference.
3. *Biological plausibility:* Demonstration of a physiological mechanism by which the risk factor acts to cause disease enhances the causal hypothesis. Conversely, an association that does not initially seem biologically defensible later may be discovered to be so.
4. *Demonstration of correct temporal sequence:* For a risk factor to cause an outcome, it must precede the onset of the outcome. (See Prospective Cohort Studies and Table 13.4.)
5. *Dose–response relationship:* The risk of developing an outcome should increase with increasing exposure (either in duration or in quantity) to the risk factor of interest. For example, studies have shown that the more a woman smokes during pregnancy, the greater the risk of delivering a low-birth-weight infant.
6. *Specificity of the association:* The presence of a one-to-one relationship between an agent and a disease (i.e., the idea that a disease is caused by only one agent and that agent results in only one disease lends support to a causal hypothesis, but its absence does not rule out causality). This criterion is cultivated from the infectious disease model, where it is more often, although not always, satisfied and is less applicable in chronic diseases.
7. *Experimental evidence:* Experimental designs provide the strongest epidemiologic evidence for causal associations, but they are not feasible or ethical to conduct for many risk factor–disease associations.

APPLICATIONS OF EPIDEMIOLOGY IN NURSING

Both knowledge and practical application of epidemiology are essential competencies for nurses. Nurses incorporate epidemiology into their practices and take on a variety of epidemiologic roles. Nurses in diverse settings are involved in the collection, reporting, analysis, interpretation, and communication of epidemiologic data as part of their daily practice. As nurses care for persons with communicable diseases, they are implementing epidemiologic practices as they identify, report, treat, and provide follow-up on cases and contacts of TB, gonorrhea, and gastroenteritis. School nurses also function as epidemiologists, collecting data on the incidence and prevalence of accidents, injuries, and illnesses in the school population. They are also key players in the detection and control of local epidemics, such as outbreaks of lice. As described earlier in this chapter, nurses across practice settings are actively involved in activities related to primary, secondary, and tertiary prevention (see Levels of Prevention box).

CHECK YOUR PRACTICE

As a nurse working in an elementary school, you notice that following a school-sponsored picnic several students in grades three through five are absent. In order to determine what might be precipitating these absences you contact a sample of parents in each grade.

What questions would you ask to identify the cause of the absences?

Some nursing job descriptions are specifically based in epidemiologic practice. These include hospital infection control nurses, nurse epidemiologists, and nurse environmental risk communicators employed by local health departments. Nurses are key members of local fetal and infant mortality review boards, which examine cases of newborn deaths for identifiable risk factors and quality of care measures. Members of these review boards may include public health and maternal child nurses as well as representatives from hospital labor and delivery and neonatal intensive care units.

Nursing documentation on client charts and records is an important source of data for epidemiologic reviews. Client demographics and health histories are often collected or verified by nurses. As nurses collect and document client information, they might not be thinking about the epidemiologic connection. However, the reliability and validity of such data can be a key factor in the quality of future epidemiologic studies. An excellent resource for the application of epidemiologic concepts and methods in practice settings can be found in Brownson and Petitti (2006).

Community-Oriented Epidemiology

Nurses are often involved in environmental health issues, where they play important roles not only as epidemiologists but also as community liaisons (Mood, 2000). Nurses serve as important professional contacts and liaisons for people in the community who are actively investigating or concerned about the health and illness issue, such as an increase in the number of cases of cancer, asthma, or traffic accidents. The role of community liaison involves observation, data collection, consultation, and interpretation. By talking and listening to community members around their kitchen tables, at local gathering places, or at community meetings, nurses gather information from the citizens' perspectives. They can also interpret scientific information for lay persons. The liaison role also involves consultation with public health and environmental professionals and participation in environmental inspections and investigations.

Lillian Mood is a public health nurse with more than 20 years of experience in South Carolina working with communities to detect and explain the causes of illness and disability. In describing her involvement with specific communities, Mood noted that the contact often began with a telephone call of concern about a planned or existing industrial facility or a firsthand observation of illness, expressed in lay terms as "too many cases of cancer," "several people have had miscarriages," or "more respiratory problems." The citizen's reasoning behind these observations is that "'If I am seeing more health problems in my community, I ask what they have in common. The common factor may be where we live. So it must be the air or the water.' This is basic epidemiologic thinking, not irrational fear. Citizens try to make sense of what they are seeing, and they want professional help to unravel the pattern of illness" (Mood, 2000, p. 24).

Popular Epidemiology

In health departments and hospitals, nurses frequently work with other professionals who have training in epidemiology. However, in the community they may encounter citizens engaged in the practice of popular epidemiology (Brown & Ferguson, 1995; Brown & Masterson-Allen, 1994). **Popular epidemiology** is a

QSEN FOCUS ON QUALITY AND SAFETY EDUCATION FOR NURSES

Targeted Competency: Informatics

Use information and technology to communicate, manage knowledge, mitigate error, and support decision making.

Important aspects of informatics include:

- **Knowledge:** Identify essential information that must be available in a common database to support client care.
- **Skills:** Use information management tools to monitor outcomes of care processes.
- **Attitudes:** Value nurses' involvement in design, selection, implementation, and evaluation of information technologies to support client care.

Informatics Question: Determine if a Health Problem Exists in the Community

Nurses are involved in the surveillance and monitoring of health phenomena. Planning for resources and personnel often requires quantifying the level of a problem in the community. For example, to know how different districts compare in the rates of very-low-birth-weight infants, you would calculate the prevalence of very-low-birth-weight infants in each district:

1. Determine the number of live births in each district from birth certificate data obtained from the vital records division of the health department.
2. Use the birth weight information from the birth certificate data to determine the number of infants born weighing less than 1500 g in each district.
3. Calculate the prevalence of very-low-birth-weight births by district as the number of infants weighing less than 1500 g at birth divided by the total number of live births.
4. If the number of very-low-birth-weight births in each district is small, use several years of data to obtain a more stable estimate.

Prepared by Gail Armstrong, PhD, DNP, ACNS-BC, CNE, Associate Professor, University of Colorado Denver College of Nursing.

form of epidemiology in which lay people gather scientific data as well as mobilize knowledge and resources of experts to understand the occurrence and distribution of a disease or injury. Popular epidemiology is more than just adding public participation to traditional epidemiology; it also includes an emphasis on social structural factors as a component of disease etiology, as well as the involvement of social movements, political and judicial approaches to remedies, and challenges to basic assumptions of traditional epidemiology, risk assessment, and public health regulation (Brown & Ferguson, 1995, p. 149). Popular epidemiology considers the physiological, psychological, and social effects of environmental hazards and attempts to show how racial, class, and gender differences are evident in the health effects of environmental toxic exposure. In contrast, many standard environmental health assessments are not designed to understand local cultures, traditions, or ethnic backgrounds (Powers, 2015). This lack of cultural competency can render assessment tools ineffective in terms of the ability to identify potential routes of toxic exposure.

Toxic waste activists are often women living in the community who have firsthand contact with toxic hazards and therefore have experiences and access to data that would otherwise be inaccessible to scientists (Brown & Ferguson, 1995). Community toxic waste activists engage in a process of linking traditional scientific practices with more narrative approaches. Their health surveys often make use of sampling techniques, laboratory testing, and mapping of suspected pollutants together with experiential narratives of the effects of toxic pollutants on the body and on their local environments (DiChiro, 1997). The information gathered can be used by community activists and health professionals to lobby for health services; advocate for policy development at local, state, and federal levels; establish preventive programs; educate medical professionals about environmental illness; and work with other agencies and community groups to reduce or eliminate toxic exposures.

EVIDENCE-BASED PRACTICE

The Epidemiologic Basis for Community Health Interventions

Queso fresco, a popular Latin American fresh cheese often made from raw milk, has been implicated as a source of *Salmonella typhimurium* definitive type (DT) 104 in the United States. From 1992 to 1996, the annual incidence of *S. typhimurium* DT104 infections in Yakima County, Washington, increased from 5.4 to 29.7 cases per 100,000 population, making it one of the highest rates in the country. Between January and May 1997, 89 cases of *S. typhimurium* were reported in the county, of which 54 were culture-confirmed as DT104, a strain that is resistant to five major antibiotics. The median age of infected persons was four years, and 90 percent of the clients had Spanish surnames. A case-control investigation conducted by the CDC indicated that the most probable source of the outbreak was raw-milk *queso fresco.* The CDC investigation also indicated that street vendors were the most frequent source (70 percent) of *queso fresco* among those who developed the illness.

In response to the outbreak, a multiagency intervention was initiated with the goal of reducing the incidence of *S. typhimurium* infections resulting from consumption of raw-milk *queso fresco* while maintaining the traditional, nutritious food in the local Hispanic diet. A pasteurized-milk *queso fresco* recipe developed by a local Hispanic woman was modified by dairy scientists at Washington State University to inhibit undesirable microbial growth, increase shelf life, and improve ease of preparation. The new recipe was tested by local Hispanic persons and adjusted until flavor and texture were satisfactory.

A pre-intervention survey was conducted to gather background information for use in planning the multipronged intervention, which featured safe-cheese workshops introducing the new pasteurized-milk recipe, a mass media campaign about the risk of raw-milk cheese, and newsletter articles warning dairy farmers about the risks of selling or giving away raw milk. The safe-cheese workshops were conducted by older Hispanic women (*abuelas*, or grandmothers), who were recruited from the community and trained to make the new *queso fresco* recipe from pasteurized milk. Following the training, each abuela educator signed a contract indicating her willingness to teach at least 15 additional members of the community how to safely make *queso fresco* with pasteurized milk. They followed through on their commitment, which included returning surveys completed by the women they taught.

The incidence of *S. typhimurium* infection in Yakima County decreased rapidly to below pre-1992 levels after the multilevel intervention was initiated. Between June and December 1997, only 16 cases were reported, of which 2 were associated with consumption of *queso fresco;* in 1998 there were 18 reported cases, none of which were associated with *queso fresco.* Postintervention surveys of Hispanic area residents who did not participate in the workshops indicated that consumption of *queso fresco* did not decrease as a result of the intervention.

Nurse Use

The *Abuela Project* is an example of a successful combination of applied epidemiology and community-based, culturally appropriate public health interventions. This activity clearly falls within the scope of good public health nursing. To be successful in seeing correlations, nurses must be vigilant, have an inquiring mind, and be able to make associations between events and characteristics (e.g., the associations between how and by whom the cheese was being made, and by whom it was being eaten). Project designed by DeAnne Messias.

PRACTICE APPLICATION

You are a nurse providing health screenings at a health fair at a local community center. Mr. Greer, a 32-year-old African American man, stops by your station and requests that you check his blood pressure. His blood pressure measurement is 135/85 mm Hg. In conducting a brief health history, you learn that Mr. Greer is single, works part time at a convenience store, often eats at fast-food establishments, and has been a smoker since age 17. His father died of a heart attack at age 48; his mother has diabetes. He does not have health insurance at this time. Which of the following would be your best choice in providing Mr. Greer recommendations related to his need for lipid disorder screening, based on the U.S. Preventive Services Task Force guidelines?

A. Do not discuss lipid screening with Mr. Greer, because he is under 35 years of age and routine screening is not recommended.

B. Suggest that Mr. Greer stop smoking and make modifications in his diet to reduce his consumption of saturated fats. Guide him to the information on local community-based resources for tobacco cessation and healthy diet programs at the health fair.

C. Discuss with Mr. Greer his increased risk for heart disease, based on his family history and status as a smoker. Provide a referral for Mr. Greer for a lipid screening, including measurement of total cholesterol and high-density lipoprotein cholesterol (HDL-C), being offered by the local hospital at the health fair.

Answers can be found on the Evolve site.

KEY POINTS

- Epidemiology is the study of the distribution and determinants of health-related events in human populations and the application of this knowledge to improving the health of communities.
- Epidemiology is a multidisciplinary enterprise that recognizes the complex interrelationships of factors that influence disease and health at both the individual level and the community level; it provides the basic tools for the study of health and disease in communities.
- Epidemiologic methods are used to describe health and disease phenomena and to investigate the factors that promote health or influence the risk or distribution of disease. This knowledge can be useful in planning and evaluating programs, policies, and services, as well as in clinical decision making.
- Epidemiologic models explain the interrelationships between agent, host, and environment (the *epidemiologic triangle)* and the interactions of multilevel factors, exposures, and characteristics (causal web) affecting risk of disease.
- A key concept in epidemiology is that of the levels of prevention, based on the stages in the natural history of disease.
- Primary prevention involves interventions to reduce the incidence of disease by promoting health and preventing disease processes from developing.
- Secondary prevention includes programs (such as screening) designed to detect disease in the early stages, before signs and symptoms are clinically evident, to intervene with early diagnosis and treatment.
- Tertiary prevention provides treatments and other interventions directed toward persons with clinically apparent disease, with the aim of lessening the course of disease, reducing disability, or rehabilitating.
- Epidemiologic methods are also used in the planning and design of community health promotion (primary prevention) strategies and screening (secondary prevention) activities, and in the evaluation of the effectiveness of these interventions.
- Basic epidemiologic methods include the use of existing data sources to study health outcomes and related factors and the use of comparison groups to assess the association between exposures or characteristics and health outcomes.
- Epidemiologists rely on rates and proportions to quantify levels of morbidity and mortality. Prevalence proportions provide a picture of the level of existing cases in a population at a given time. Incidence rates and proportions measure the rate of new case development in a population and provide an estimate of the risk of disease.
- Descriptive epidemiologic studies provide information on the distribution of disease and health states according to personal characteristics, geographic region, and time. This knowledge enables practitioners to target programs and allocate resources more effectively and provides a basis for further study.
- Analytic epidemiologic studies investigate associations between exposures or characteristics and health or disease outcomes, with a goal of understanding the etiology of disease. Analytic studies provide the foundation for understanding disease causality and for developing effective intervention strategies aimed at primary, secondary, and tertiary prevention.

CLINICAL DECISION-MAKING ACTIVITIES

1. Identify a current health issue in your local community (e.g., childhood lead poisoning, diabetes, HIV/AIDS).
   A. Describe primary, secondary, and tertiary prevention interventions related to this health issue.
   B. How could nurses improve the effectiveness of their prevention activities related to this health issue?
2. Identify existing inequalities among the counties in your state, using infant mortality data.
   A. Describe the distribution of infant mortality in your state (by county), using rate ratio and population attributable risk data.
   B. Compare the infant mortality rates in your state with national and international data.
   C. Compare the characteristics of the counties (e.g., urban, rural, racial/ethnic distribution, economic indicators, distribution of health care facilities) with the highest and lowest infant mortality rates.
   D. Identify local, state, and national initiatives that are addressing infant mortality.
3. Examine the leading causes of infant death in the United States.
   A. What differences in intervention approaches are suggested by the various causes of death?
   B. How would you design an epidemiologic study to examine risk factors for specific causes of neonatal and postneonatal death? What types of epidemiologic measures would be useful? What study design(s) would be appropriate?
   C. How would you use the information from your study to develop an intervention program and to define the target population for your intervention?
4. Find a report of an epidemiologic study in one of the major public health, nursing, or epidemiology journals. How do the findings of this study, if valid, affect your nursing practice? How do you incorporate the results of epidemiologic research into your nursing practice?

ADDITIONAL RESOURCES

EVOLVE WEBSITE

http://evolve.elsevier.com/Stanhope/community/

- Answers to Practice Application
- Case Study
- Glossary
- Review Questions

REFERENCES

Adams SA, Choi SK, Eberth JM, et al: Is availability of mammography services at federally qualified health centers associated with breast cancer mortality-to-incidence ratios? An ecological analysis, *J Womens Health (Larchmt)* 24(11):916–923, 2015a. doi:10.1089/jwh.2014.5114.

Adams SA, Choi SK, Khang L, et al: Decreased cancer mortality-to-incidence ratios with increased accessibility of federally qualified health centers, *J Community Health* 40(4):633–641, 2015b. doi:10.1007/s10900-014-9978-8.

American Nurses Association (ANA): *The Essential Guide to Nursing Practice: Applying ANA's Scope and Standards of Practice and Education*, Washington, DC, 2012, ANA.

Anderson RN: Deaths: leading causes for 2000, *Natl Vital Stat Rep* 50:1–85, 2002.

Auchincloss AH, Gebreab SY, Mair C, Diez Roux AV: A review of spatial methods in epidemiology, 2000-2010, *Annu Rev Public Health* 33:107–122, 2012. doi:10.1146/annurev-publhealth-031811-124655.

Baldwin DC Jr: Some historical notes on interdisciplinary and interprofessional education and practice in health care in the USA. 1996, *J Interprof Care* 21:23–37, 2007.

Berkman LF, Kawachi I: A historical framework for social epidemiology. In Berkman LF, Kawachi I, Glymour MM, editors: *Social Epidemiology*, New York, 2014, Oxford University Press.

Brown P, Ferguson FIT: "Making a big stink": women's work, women's relationships, and toxic waste activism, *Gender Society* 9:145–172, 1995.

Brown P, Masterson-Allen S: Citizen action on toxic waste contamination: a new type of social movement, *Soc Natural Res* 7:269–286, 1994.

Brownson RC, Petitti DB, editors: *Applied Epidemiology: Theory to Practice*, ed 2, New York, 2006, Oxford University Press.

Centers for Disease Control and Prevention (CDC): Use of race and ethnicity in public health surveillance: summary of the DC/ATSDR workshop, *MMWR Morb Mortal Wkly Rep* 42(RR-10):1–16, 1993.

Centers for Disease Control and Prevention (CDC): Obesity — United States, 1999–2010, *MMWR Morb Mortal Wkly Rep* 62(3):120–128, 2013.

Centers for Disease Control and Prevention (CDC): *Childhood Obesity Facts,* 2018. Retrieved from https://www.cdc.gov/obesity/data/childhood.html.

Childress JF, Faden RR, Gaare RD, et al: Public health ethics: mapping the terrain, *J Law Med Ethics* 30:170–178, 2002.

Choi SK, Adams SA, Eberth JM, et al: Medicaid coverage expansion and implications for cancer disparities, *Am J Public Health* 105(Suppl 5):S706–S712, 2015. doi:10.2105/AJPH.2015.302876.

Council on Linkages Between Academic and Public Health Practice: *Core Competencies for Public Health Professionals*, Washington DC, 2014, Public Health Foundation/Health Resources and Services Administration.

DiChiro G: Local actions, global visions: remaking environmental expertise, *Frontiers* 18:203, 1997.

Diez-Roux AV: A glossary for multilevel analysis, *J Epidemiol Community Health* 56:588–594, 2002.

Fuller CM, Borrell LN, Latkin CA, et al: Effects of race, neighborhood, and social network on age at initiation of injection drug use, *Am J Public Health* 95:689–695, 2005.

Fullilove MT: Comment: abandoning "race" as a variable in public health research–an idea whose time has come, *Am J Public Health* 88:1297–1298, 1998.

Gordis L: *Epidemiology*, ed 5, Philadelphia, PA, 2013, Saunders.

Henry J. Kaiser Family Foundation. Retrieved from https://www.kff.org.

Heron M. *Deaths: Leading Causes for 2016*, National Vital Statistics Reports vol 67 no 6. Hyattsville, MD: 2018, National Center for Health Statistics.

Heymann DL, editor: *Control of Communicable Diseases Manual*, ed 20, Washington, DC, 2014, American Public Health Association.

Institute of Medicine (IOM): *The Future of Public Health*, Washington, DC, 1988, National Academy Press.

Institute of Medicine (IOM): *The future of the public's health in the 21st century,* Washington, DC, 2002, NAP, Retrieved from http://www.iom.edu/Reports/2002/The-Future-of-the-Publics-Health-in-the-21st-Century.aspx.

Kawachi I, Berkman LF: *Neighborhoods and Health*, New York, 2003, Oxford University Press.

Kochanek KD, Murphy SL, Xu JQ, Arias, E: *Mortality in the United States, 2016*, NCHS Data Brief, no 293, Hyattsville, MD, 2017, National Center for Health Statistics.

Koepsell TD, Weiss NS: *Epidemiologic Methods: Studying the Occurrence of Illness*, New York, 2014, Oxford University Press.

Krieger N: Epidemiology and the web of causation: has anyone seen the spider? *Soc Sci Med* 39:887–903, 1994.

Krieger N: Discrimination and health. In Berkman LF, Kawachi I, editors: *Social Epidemiology*, Oxford, 2000, Oxford University Press, pp 36–75.

Kawachi I, Berkman LF: Social capital, social cohesion, and health. In Berkman LF, Kawachi I, Glymour MM, editors: *Social Epidemiology*, New York, 2014, Oxford University Press, pp 13–35.

Matoba N, Collins JW Jr: Racial disparity in infant mortality, *Semin Perinatol* 41(6):354–359, 2017. doi:10.1053/j.semperi.2017.07.003.

Martin JA, Hamilton BE, Sutton PD, et al: Births, final data for 2006, *Natl Vital Stat Rep* 57:7, 2009.

McKeown RE: The epidemiologic transition: changing patterns of mortality and population dynamics, *Am J Lifestyle Med* 3(Suppl 1): 19S–26S, 2009.

McKeown RE, Learner RM: Ethics in public health practice. In Coughlin S, Beauchamp T, Weed D, editors: *Ethics and Epidemiology, ed 2*, New York, 2009, Oxford University Press, pp 147–181.

McLafferty S, Grady S: Immigration and geographic access to prenatal clinics in Brooklyn, NY: a geographic information systems analysis, *Am J Public Health* 95:638–640, 2005.

Merrill RM, Timmreck TC: *Introduction to Epidemiology*, ed 7, Burlington, MA, 2017, Jones & Bartlett.

Mood L: Toxic waste: deep in the roots of nursing comes a search for harmful sources, *Reflect Nurs Leadersh* 26:21–25, 2000.

Najera-Aguilar P, Martinez-Piedra R, Vidaurre-Arenas M: From sketch to digital maps: a geographic information system (GIS) model and application for malaria control without the use of pesticides, *Pan Am Health Org Epidemiol Bull* 26:11, 2005.

Noonan M, Galvin R, Doody O, Jomeen J: A qualitative meta-synthesis: public health nurses role in the identification and management of perinatal mental health problems, *J Adv Nurs* 73(3):545–557, 2017. doi:10.1111/jan.13155

U.S. Dept. of Health and Human Services, Office of the Secretary, Office of the Assistant Secretary for Planning and Evaluation and

Office of Minority Health (USDHHS, OMH): *HHS Action Plan to Reduce Racial and Ethnic Health Disparities Implementation Progress Report*, Washington, DC, 2015, Office of the Assistant Secretary for Planning and Evaluation.

Patel RC, Baek J, Smith MA, Morgenstern LB, Lisabeth LD: Residential ethnic segregation and stroke risk in Mexican Americans: the Brain Attack Surveillance in Corpus Christi project, *Ethn Dis* 25(1):11–18, 2015.

Porta M: *A Dictionary of Epidemiology*, ed 6, New York, 2014, Oxford University Press.

Powers M, Saberi P, Pepino R, Strupp E, Bugos E, Cannuscio CC: Popular epidemiology and "fracking": citizens' concerns regarding the economic, environmental, health and social impacts of unconventional natural gas drilling operations, *J Community Health* 40(3):534–541, 2015. doi:10.1007/s10900-014-9968-x.

Quad Council Coalition of Public Health Nursing Organizations (QCC): Community/Public Health Nursing Competences, 2018.

Remington PL, Brownson RC, Wegner MV: *Chronic Disease Epidemiology and Control*, ed 4, Washington, DC, 2016, American Public Health Association.

Rothman KJ: *Epidemiology: an Introduction*, ed 2, New York, 2012, Oxford University Press.

Sampson RJ, Raudenbush SW, Earls F: Neighborhoods and violent crime: a multilevel study of collective efficacy, *Science* 277:918–924, 1997.

Snow J: *On the Mode of Communication of Cholera. In Snow on Cholera*, New York, 1855, The Commonwealth Fund.

Susser M: *Causal Thinking in the Health Sciences*, New York, 1973, Oxford University Press.

Susser M: Epidemiology in the United States after World War II: the evolution of technique, *Epidemiol Rev* 7:147–177, 1985.

Szklo M, Nieto FJ: *Epidemiology: Beyond the Basics*, ed 4, Boston, 2018, Jones & Bartlett.

Teutsch SM, Churchill RE: *Principles and Practice of Public Health Surveillance*, ed 3, New York, 2010, Oxford.

Turnock BJ: *Public Health: What It Is and How It Works*, ed 6, Gaithersburg, MD, 2016, Aspen.

U.S. Department of Health and Human Services: *Healthy People 2010: Understanding and Improving Health*, ed 2, Washington, DC, 2000, U.S. Government Printing Office.

U.S. Preventive Services Task Force (USPSTF): *Screening for Lipid Disorders in Adults: U.S. Preventive Services Task Force Recommendation Statement*, Rockville, MD, 2008, Agency for Healthcare Research and Quality.

Victora CG, Habicht JP, Bryce J: Evidence-based public health: moving beyond randomized trials, *Am J Public Health* 94(3): 400–405, 2004.

World Health Organization (WHO): *Declaration of Alma-Ata: International Conference on Primary Health Care*, Geneva, Switzerland, 1978, WHO, p 1.

Xu JQ, Murphy SL Kochanek KD, et al: *Deaths: Leading Causes for 2015,* National vital statistics reports; vol 66 no 6. Hyattsville, MD: 2017, National Center for Health Statistics.

Xu JQ, Murphy SL, Kochanek KD, Bastian B, Arias E. *Deaths: Final Data for 2016*, National Vital Statistics Reports; vol 67 no 5. Hyattsville, MD, 2018, National Center for Health Statistics.

14

Infectious Disease Prevention and Control

Susan C. Long-Marin, DVM, MPH and Donna E. Smith, MSPH

OBJECTIVES

After reading this chapter, the student should be able to do the following:

1. Discuss the current impact and threats of infectious diseases on society.
2. Explain how the elements of the epidemiologic triangle interact to cause infectious diseases.
3. Provide examples of infectious disease control interventions at the three levels of public health prevention.
4. Discuss the factors contributing to newly emerging or re-emerging infectious diseases.
5. Explain the multisystem approach to control of communicable diseases.
6. Explain universal precautions.

CHAPTER OUTLINE

Historical and Current Perspectives
Burden and Financial Impact of Infectious Diseases
Transmission of Communicable Diseases
Surveillance of Communicable Diseases
Emerging Infectious Diseases
Prevention and Control of Infectious Disease
Agents of Bioterrorism
Vaccine-Preventable Diseases
Foodborne and Waterborne Diseases
Vector-borne Diseases
Diseases of Travelers
Zoonoses
Parasitic Diseases
Health Care-Associated Infections

KEY TERMS

acquired immunity, p. 303
active immunization, p. 303
agent, p. 302
common vehicle, p. 304
communicable diseases, p. 299
communicable period, p. 304
disease, p. 304
elimination, p. 308
emerging infectious diseases, p. 306
endemic, p. 304
environment, p. 302
epidemic, p. 304
epidemiologic triangle, p. 302
eradication, p. 308
health care-associated infection, p. 327
herd immunity, p. 303
horizontal transmission, p. 304
host, p. 302
incubation period, p. 304
infection, p. 304
infectiousness, p. 303
natural immunity, p. 303
pandemic, p. 304
passive immunization, p. 303
resistance, p. 303
surveillance, p. 304
universal precautions, p. 328
vectors, p. 304
vertical transmission, p. 304

The topic of infectious diseases includes the discussion of a wide and complex variety of organisms; the pathology they may cause; and their diagnosis, treatment, prevention, and control. This chapter presents an overview of the **communicable diseases** that nurses encounter most often. Diseases are grouped according to descriptive category (by mode of transmission or means of prevention) rather than by individual organism (e.g., *Escherichia coli*) or taxonomic group (e.g., viral, parasitic). Detailed discussion of sexually transmitted infections, human immunodeficiency virus (HIV), acquired immunodeficiency syndrome (AIDS), viral hepatitis, and tuberculosis (TB) is provided in Chapter 15. Although not all infectious diseases are directly communicable from person to person, the terms *infectious disease* and *communicable disease* are used interchangeably throughout this chapter.

HISTORICAL AND CURRENT PERSPECTIVES

In the United States, at the beginning of the twentieth century, infectious diseases were the leading cause of death. By 2000 improvements in nutrition and sanitation, the discovery of antibiotics, and the development of vaccines had put an end to infectious disease epidemics like diphtheria and typhoid fever that once ravaged entire populations. In 1900 respiratory and diarrheal diseases were major killers. For example, TB led to over 11 percent of all deaths in the United States and was the second leading cause of death; in 2015, 470 deaths or 0.02 percent of all deaths were attributed to this once frequently fatal disease (CDC, 2017a). As individuals live longer, chronic diseases—heart disease, cancer, and stroke—have replaced infectious diseases as the leading causes of death.

Infectious diseases, however, have by no means vanished, and they remain a continuing cause for concern. They persist as the leading cause of death for children and adolescents worldwide, especially those in low-income countries, killing an estimated 6 million people a year (WHO, 2018a). In the United States, the downward trend in mortality from infectious diseases, seen since 1900—with the exception of the 1918 influenza pandemic—reversed itself in the 1980s, with the emergence of new entities such as HIV disease and the increasing development of antibiotic resistance. Respiratory diseases in the form of pneumonias and influenza remain among the 10 leading causes of death, and new strains, such as novel influenza A H1N1 and avian influenza A H5N1, test our disease control abilities and consume resources. Previously unknown causal connections between infectious organisms and chronic diseases have been recognized, such as *Helicobacter pylori* and peptic ulcer disease, and human papillomaviruses (HPVs) and cervical cancer. Also, in the twenty-first century, infectious diseases have become a means of terrorism, as illustrated by the anthrax letters of 2001.

New killers emerge and old familiar diseases take on different, more virulent characteristics. Consider the following developments from the past 40 years. HIV disease reminds us of plagues from the past and although first being recognized in the early 1980s continues to challenge our ability to control and contain infection like no other disease in recent history. Because effective drugs have been developed to slow the progression but there is no cure, this initially infectious disease is now a chronic condition. Work continues on vaccine development, and pre-exposure prophylaxis (PrEP) drugs offer a new prevention tool. Legionnaires' disease and toxic shock syndrome, unknown at mid-twentieth century, have become part of common vocabulary. The identification of infectious agents causing Lyme disease and ehrlichiosis provided two new tick-borne diseases to worry about. And, in the summer of 1993 in the southwestern United States, healthy young adults were stricken with a mysterious and unknown but often fatal respiratory disease that is now known as hantavirus pulmonary syndrome. The summer of 1994 brought public attention to a severe, invasive strain of *Streptococcus pyogenes* group A, referred to by the press as the "flesh-eating" bacteria.

In the 1990s the transmission of infectious disease through the food supply became a newsworthy concern when the consumption of improperly cooked hamburgers and unpasteurized apple juice contaminated with a highly toxic strain of *E. coli* (*E. coli* 0157:H7) caused illness and death in children across the country. In 1996 multiple states reported outbreaks of diarrheal disease traced to imported fresh berries; the implicated organism in these outbreaks, *Cyclospora cayetanensis* (a coccidian parasite), was only first diagnosed in humans in 1977. Also, in 1996, the fear that "mad cow disease" (bovine spongiform encephalopathy [BSE]) could be transferred to humans through beef consumption led to the slaughter of thousands of British cattle and a ban on the international sale of British beef. Initially seen only in Europe and Japan as well as Great Britain, the first case of BSE was diagnosed in the United States in 2003. Variant Creutzfeldt-Jakob disease (vCJD), which attacks the brain with fatal results, is the human disease thought to result from eating beef infected with the transmissible agent causing BSE; only four acquired cases of vCJD have been seen in the United States, but these individuals were born outside of the United States and resided extensively in other countries, many of which were known for diagnoses of vCJD (CDC, 2017b).

In 1997 vancomycin-resistant *Staphylococcus aureus* (VRSA) was first reported; previously, vancomycin had been considered the only effective antibiotic against methicillin-resistant *S. aureus* (MRSA). Although MRSA is still largely a health care-associated infection, community-associated disease is becoming more common with outbreaks frequently associated with school athletic programs and prison populations. Also, in 1997, the first reported outbreak of avian flu affecting humans occurred in Hong Kong. No subsequent reports suggested an isolated incident, but in 2004, avian influenza A H5N1 again emerged in Southeast Asia with resulting human cases. This virus has now infected avian populations in Asia, Europe, the Near East, and North Africa, and it continues to cause sporadic human cases, especially in Southeast Asia and Egypt. Human cases are determined to largely spread through direct contact with infected poultry or infected surfaces, with human to human transmission largely ineffective and only a few rare cases thought to have occurred. The first report of human H5N1 in the Americas came from Canada in 2014 in an individual who had recently traveled from China. In 1999 the first Western Hemisphere activity of West Nile virus (WNV), a mosquito-transmitted illness that can affect livestock, birds, and humans, occurred in New York City. By 2002 WNV, thought to be carried by infected birds and possibly mosquitoes in cargo containers, had spread across the United States as far west as California and was reported in Canada and Central America as well.

The viral hemorrhagic fevers (VHFs) Ebola and Marburg, unknown to most people 40 years ago, have become the premise of movies and books. Although caused by different viruses within the *Filoviridae* family, these sporadically occurring but lethal killers have similar clinical presentations. The largest reported outbreak of Ebola VHF began in the spring of 2014 in

Guinea, West Africa, spreading to neighboring Sierra Leone and Liberia and by March of 2016 had infected over 28,600 people, killing more than 11,300, (CDC, 2016a). This outbreak in West Africa led to cases acquired through travel being diagnosed and treated in Europe and the United States, challenging our ability to respond quickly on a national and local level to an unfamiliar highly infectious disease. The reservoir host of Ebola viruses remains unknown, but there is an association with non-human primates, and evidence is beginning to point toward a fruit bat reservoir. While there is no licensed vaccine or treatment, both are in development and were employed in outbreaks of Ebola in the Democratic Republic of the Congo in 2018 (WHO, 2018b; WHO, 2018c). Marburg VHF virus had only been reported five times since its recognition in 1967 before a major outbreak in Angola occurred during 2004 and 2005, affecting more than 350 people with a fatality rate of close to 90 percent. Since then, much smaller outbreaks have occurred in Uganda in 2007 and 2012. In 2014, one fatal case of Marburg virus was reported in a health care worker in Uganda; no source was identified. The reservoir host of Marburg virus is the African fruit bat, *Rousettus aegyptiacus* (CDC, 2017c).

Severe acute respiratory syndrome (SARS) was first recognized in China in February 2003. And as if in a bestselling thriller, this newly emerging infectious disease quickly achieved pandemic proportions. By the summer of 2003, major outbreaks had occurred in Hong Kong, Taiwan, Vietnam, Singapore, and Canada. Three months after the first official news of SARS, over 8000 cases with more than 700 deaths had been reported to the World Health Organization (WHO) from 28 countries. Played out on television in pictures of people wearing face masks for protection, the rapid spread of a previously unknown disease with an initially unknown cause and no definitive treatment contributed to the creation of a perception of risk of infection far greater than actually existed. Frightened Americans canceled trips to China and Hong Kong and avoided people who had recently returned from Asia. Then, as suddenly as it began, the pandemic subsided. SARS was found to be caused by a new strain of *Coronavirus,* but since 2003, only a few cases, largely associated with laboratory workers, have been reported. A large number of individuals infected by SARS could be traced back to unrecognized cases in hospitals, suggesting that prompt identification and isolation of symptomatic people is the key to interrupting transmission. No new cases of SARS have been reported since 2004. Global efforts continue to clarify the epidemiology of this disease as well as develop a reliable diagnostic test and vaccine. In 2012, SARS coronavirus was officially declared a select agent—a bacterium, virus or toxin that has the potential to pose a severe threat to public health and safety. Additional information on SARS can be obtained at the Centers for Disease Control and Prevention (CDC) archived SARS website, http://www.cdc.gov.

In the first decades of the twenty-first century, foodborne infections again have made headlines as *E. coli*-infected spinach sickened and killed individuals across the United States. In 2008, tomatoes were blamed for a nationwide outbreak of salmonellosis but were ruled innocent when the green chilies that accompanied them in salsa were found to be the actual culprit. *Salmonella* again made the news as contaminated peanut butter forced recalls across the United States, caused hundreds of illnesses, and resulted in several deaths. Even chocolate chip cookie dough was not safe; a national recall in 2009 followed the discovery that people had been sickened after eating raw dough contaminated by *E. coli.* One of the nation's most deadly foodborne outbreaks occurred in 2012 when cantaloupes contaminated by *Listeria* resulted in 147 reported illnesses and 33 deaths. In 2015, 907 illnesses across 40 states as well as 3 deaths were attributed to *Salmonella* found in imported cucumbers. Most recently, in 2018, a nationwide outbreak of *E. coli* was linked to romaine lettuce. Read more about foodborne outbreaks by year at the CDC Foodborne Outbreaks website https://www.cdc.gov.

Perhaps the most publicized infectious disease event of 2009 was the advent of a new strain of flu, novel influenza A H1N1. First reported from Mexico and rapidly acquired by travelers to that country, H1N1 spread quickly across the world, causing the WHO to declare a pandemic and stimulate the race for a vaccine. While H1N1 did not become the major killer it was feared to, it did disproportionately result in hospitalizations and deaths in younger- and middle-aged adults. H1N1 did not disappear after this pandemic and has been included in the seasonal influenza vaccine since 2009. During the 2013-2014 flu season in the United States, H1N1 once more became the predominant circulating strain and once more hit hardest the younger- and middle-aged.

The year 2012 brought the first reports of another novel coronavirus that, like SARS, results in acute respiratory distress with a high mortality rate. Middle Eastern Respiratory Syndrome Coronavirus, or MERS-CoV, has only been seen in individuals living in or who have traveled to countries in the Arabian Peninsula, or have come into close contact with an ill traveler or a confirmed case. It seems to spread by close contact, and many of the cases have been in health care workers. The reservoir is unknown, but there appears to be an association with camels. The first cases of MERS-CoV in the United States were reported in 2014 in individuals who had traveled from Saudi Arabia. Read more about MERS-CoV at http://www.cdc.gov.

Previously seen in other parts of the world, 2013 brought the first case of chikungunya virus reported from the Americas. Transmitted by mosquitos, chikungunya most commonly involves fever and, sometimes severe, joint pain as well as headache, muscle pain, conjunctivitis, and rash. For most people the disease is mild and self-limiting, although joint pain may persist for some time. There is neither a specific treatment nor vaccine. Primates and humans are thought to be the main reservoirs and person-to-mosquito-to person transmission can occur. Cases in the United States have so far only involved travelers to infected areas outside the country. Another mosquito-borne virus, Zika, made major news in 2015 with an initial widespread outbreak in Brazil. First identified in 1947, Zika, seemingly a mild-mannered disease, was only reported in a handful of cases across equatorial Africa and Asia until outbreaks in 2007 and 2013 in the Pacific islands revealed a more aggressive virus causing large outbreaks and resulting in neurological conditions such as microencephaly and Guillain-Barré syndrome. In Brazil, as in the outbreaks in the Pacific islands with no immunity among the population, Zika spread throughout the country and to surrounding countries, leaving in its wake thousands of children with neurological birth defects, devasted families, and an economic impact that will last for decades as the cost of raising these medically fragile children mounts. At the beginning of 2016, the WHO declared a Public Health Emergency of International Concern (PHEIC), a status previously reserved for the likes of Ebola and polio, which was not lifted until the end of the year. Women were advised to delay pregnancy and, in the United States, pregnant women were warned to avoid mosquitos and traveling to infected areas. Some fans and athletes chose not to attend the 2016 Summer Olympics in Rio de Janeiro. Refraining from sexual activity with travelers from infected areas was also added to warnings when it was discovered that Zika could be transmitted sexually. As of 2018, Zika is considered endemic in much of Latin America and as a result of developed immunity, the number of newborns affected by Zika has decreased drastically. No local mosquito transmission of Zika has been documented in the United States with all identified cases associated with travel to endemic areas. Testing has been developed, and work on a vaccine continues. Read more about Zika at the WHO Zika Timeline website, http://www.who.int.

BURDEN AND FINANCIAL IMPACT OF INFECTIOUS DISEASES

Worldwide, infectious diseases are the leading killer of children and are responsible for almost half of all deaths in low-income countries. Of these infectious disease deaths, the majority results from five causes: acute lower respiratory infections, diarrheal diseases, TB, HIV disease, and malaria. The WHO reports that in 2016 lower respiratory diseases such as pneumonia and influenza killed an estimated 3.5 million people, diarrheal diseases 1.4 million, and TB 1.3 million. The CDC calculates 2016 malaria deaths at around 445,000. In 2017, the WHO estimates that 36.9 million people were living with HIV disease worldwide, and while deaths from HIV disease were no longer in the top 10 causes of death, 940,000 people died of HIV-related illnesses. The WHO also reports that pneumonia is the leading cause of infectious disease death in children, killing over 900,000 children under five annually and that diarrheal diseases are the leading cause of malnutrition and the second leading cause of death in children worldwide (WHO, 2018a).

The diversity of infectious diseases, the need for prevention and control, and challenges such as antibiotic resistance or no identified vaccine and treatment place a tremendous economic burden on both public health and the health care system. For example, the estimate for public health annual expenditures on rabies disease diagnostics, prevention, and control in the United States ranges from $245 million to $510 million (CDC, 2015). A case of multidrug-resistant TB can cost $294,00 to treat compared to $46,000 for a non-resistant case (CDC, 2017d). The United States Department of Agriculture (USDA) estimates that in the United States, foodborne illnesses cost more than $15.6 billion each year (CDC, 2018a), and the annual cost to the U.S. health care system for almost 20 million new sexually transmitted disease (STD) infections each year is thought to be almost $16 billion (CDC, 2017e).

Because of the morbidity, mortality, and associated cost of infectious diseases, the national health promotion and disease prevention goals outlined in *Healthy People 2020* list a number of objectives for reducing the incidence of these illnesses in a variety of the sections, including Immunization & Infectious Disease. Objectives for reducing salmonellosis and other foodborne infections are found in the section on Food Safety, an objective for reducing malaria cases reported in the United States may be seen under Global Health, there is a section on Sexually Transmitted Diseases, and there are objectives related to Healthcare-Associated Infections (see the *Healthy People 2020* box for examples). Although infectious diseases are not currently the leading causes of death in the United States, they continue to present varied, multiple, and complex challenges to all health care providers. Nurses must know about these diseases to effectively participate in diagnosis, treatment, prevention, and control.

HEALTHY PEOPLE 2020

Selected Objectives Related to Infectious Diseases

- **IID-1:** Reduce, eliminate, or maintain elimination of cases of vaccine-preventable diseases.
- **IID-12:** Increase the percent of children and adults who are vaccinated against seasonal influenza.
- **FS-1:** Reduce infections caused by key pathogens transmitted commonly through food.
- **HAI-2:** Reduce invasive health care-associated methicillin-resistant *Staphylococcal aureus* (MRSA) infections.

TRANSMISSION OF COMMUNICABLE DISEASES

Agent, Host, and Environment

The transmission of communicable diseases depends on the successful interaction of the infectious **agent**, the **host**, and the **environment**. These three factors make up the **epidemiologic triangle** (Fig. 14.1) as discussed in Chapter 13. Changes in the characteristics of any of the factors may result in disease transmission. Consider the following examples. Antibiotic therapy not only may eliminate a specific pathological agent, but also alter the balance of normally occurring organisms in the body. As a result, one of these agents overruns another, and disease, such as a yeast infection, occurs. HIV performs its deadly work not by directly poisoning the host but by destroying the host's immune reaction to other disease-producing agents. Individuals living in the temperate climate of the United States do not normally contract malaria at home, but they may become infected if they change their environment by traveling to a climate where malaria-carrying mosquitoes thrive. As these examples illustrate, the balance among agent, host, and environment is often precarious and may be unintentionally disrupted. At present, the potential results of such disturbance require attention as advances in science and technology, destruction of natural

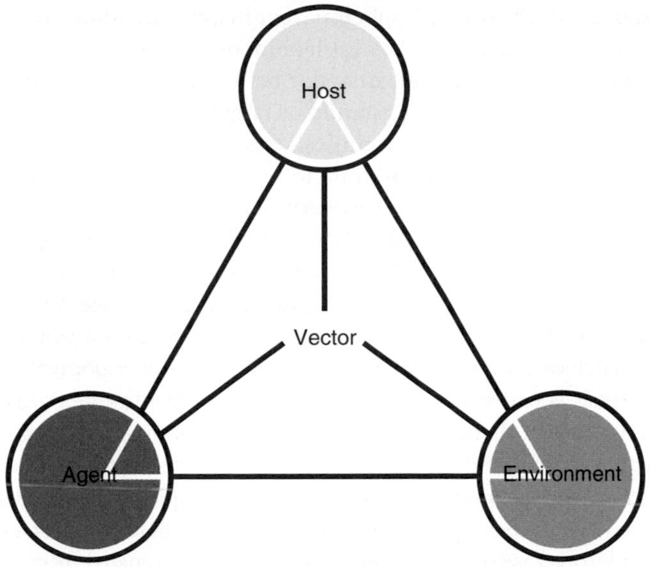

Fig. 14.1 The epidemiologic triangle of a disease. (Redrawn from the Centers for Disease Control and Prevention: Principles of epidemiology in public health practice, 2012. Available at https://www.cdc.gov.)

habitats, population growth, political instability, and a worldwide transportation network combine to alter the balance among the environment, people, and the agents that produce disease.

Agent Factor. Four major categories of agents cause most infections and infectious disease: bacteria (e.g., *Salmonella* and *E. coli*), fungi (e.g., *Aspergillus* spp. and *Candida* spp.), parasites (e.g., helminths and protozoa), and viruses (e.g., hepatitis A and B and HIV). Less commonly seen is the prion, a transmissible agent that causes abnormal folding of normal cellular prion proteins in the brain, resulting in a family of rare progressive neurodegenerative disorders that affect both humans and animals. Variant Creutzfeldt-Jakob disease and kuru are examples of prion diseases. The individual agent may be described by its ability to cause disease and by the nature and the severity of the disease. *Infectivity, pathogenicity, virulence, toxicity, invasiveness,* and *antigenicity,* terms commonly used to characterize infectious agents, are defined in Box 14.1.

Host Factor. A human or animal host can harbor an infectious agent. The characteristics of the host that may influence the spread of disease are host resistance, immunity, herd immunity,

BOX 14.1 Six Characteristics of an Infectious Agent

- *Infectivity:* The ability to enter and multiply in the host
- *Pathogenicity:* The ability to produce a specific clinical reaction after infection occurs
- *Virulence:* The ability to produce a severe pathological reaction
- *Toxicity:* The ability to produce a poisonous reaction
- *Invasiveness:* The ability to penetrate and spread throughout a tissue
- *Antigenicity:* The ability to stimulate an immunological response

and infectiousness of the host. **Resistance** is the ability of the host to withstand infection, and it may involve natural or acquired immunity.

Natural immunity refers to species-determined, innate resistance to an infectious agent. For example, opossums rarely contract rabies. **Acquired immunity** is the resistance acquired by a host as a result of previous natural exposure to an infectious agent. Having measles once protects against future infection. Acquired immunity may be induced by active or passive immunization. **Active immunization** refers to the immunization of an individual by administration of an antigen (infectious agent or vaccine) and is usually characterized by the presence of an antibody produced by the individual host. Vaccinating children against childhood diseases is an example of inducing active immunity. **Passive immunization** refers to immunization through the transfer of a specific antibody from an immunized individual to a non-immunized individual, such as the transfer of antibody from mother to infant or by administration of an antibody-containing preparation (immunoglobulin or antiserum). Passive immunity from immunoglobulin is almost immediate but short lived. It is often induced as a stopgap measure until active immunity has time to develop after vaccination. Examples of commonly used immunoglobulins include those for hepatitis A, rabies, and tetanus.

Herd immunity refers to the immunity of a group or community. It is the resistance of a group of people to invasion and spread of an infectious agent. Herd immunity is based on the resistance of a high proportion of individual members of a group to infection. It is the basis for increasing immunization coverage for vaccine-preventable diseases. Through studies, experts determine what percent coverage (e.g., >90 percent) of a specified group of people (e.g., children entering school) by a specified vaccine (e.g., two doses of measles vaccine) is necessary to ensure adequate protection for the entire community against a given disease and target immunization campaigns and initiatives to meet that goal. The higher the immunization coverage, the greater the herd immunity.

Infectiousness is a measure of the potential ability of an infected host to transmit the infection to other hosts. It reflects the relative ease with which the infectious agent is transmitted to others. Individuals with measles are extremely infectious; the virus spreads readily on airborne droplets. A person with Lyme disease cannot spread the disease to other people (although the infected tick can).

Environment Factor. The environment refers to everything that is external to the human host, including physical, biological, social, and cultural factors. These environmental factors facilitate the transmission of an infectious agent from an infected host to other susceptible hosts. Reduction in communicable disease risk can be achieved by altering these environmental factors. Using mosquito nets and repellants to avoid bug bites, installing sewage systems to prevent fecal contamination of water supplies, and washing utensils after contact with raw meat to reduce bacterial contamination are all examples of altering the environment to prevent disease.

Modes of Transmission

Infectious diseases can be transmitted horizontally or vertically. **Vertical transmission** is the passing of the infection from parent to offspring via sperm, placenta, milk, or contact in the vaginal canal at birth. Examples of vertical transmission are transplacental transmission of HIV and syphilis. **Horizontal transmission** is the person-to-person spread of infection through one or more of the following four routes: direct/indirect contact, common vehicle, airborne, or vector-borne. Most sexually transmitted infections are spread by direct sexual contact. Enterobiasis, or pinworm infection, can be acquired through direct contact or indirect contact with contaminated objects such as toys, clothing, and bedding. **Common vehicle** refers to transportation of the infectious agent from an infected host to a susceptible host via food, water, milk, blood, serum, saliva, or plasma. Hepatitis A can be transmitted through contaminated food and water, and hepatitis B through contaminated blood. Legionellosis and TB are both spread via contaminated droplets in the air. **Vectors** are arthropods such as ticks and mosquitoes or other invertebrates such as snails that transmit the infectious agent by biting or depositing the infective material near the host. Vectors may be necessary to the life cycle of the organism (e.g., mosquitoes and malaria) or may act as mechanical transmitters (e.g., flies and food).

Disease Development

Exposure to an infectious agent does not always lead to an infection. Similarly, infection does not always lead to disease. Infection depends on the infective dose, the infectivity of the infectious agent and the immunocompetence of the host. It is important to differentiate infection and disease, as clearly illustrated by the HIV disease epidemic. **Infection** refers to the entry, development, and multiplication of the infectious agent in the susceptible host. **Disease** is one of the possible outcomes of infection, and it may indicate a physiological dysfunction or pathological reaction. An individual who tests positive for HIV is infected, but if that person shows no clinical signs, the individual is not diseased. Similarly, if an individual tests positive for HIV and also exhibits clinical signs consistent with AIDS (HIV stage III), that individual is both infected and diseased.

Incubation period and communicable period are not synonymous. The **incubation period** is the time interval between invasion by an infectious agent and the first appearance of signs and symptoms of the disease. The incubation periods of infectious diseases vary from between 2 and 4 hours for staphylococcal food poisoning to between 10 and 15 years for AIDS (HIV stage III). The **communicable period** is the interval during which an infectious agent may be transferred directly or indirectly from an infected person to another person. The period of communicability for influenza is 3 to 5 days after the clinical onset of symptoms. Hepatitis B–infected persons are infectious many weeks before the onset of the first symptoms and remain infective during the acute phase and chronic carrier state, which may persist for life.

Disease Spectrum

Persons with infectious diseases may exhibit a broad spectrum of disease that ranges from subclinical infection to severe and fatal disease. Those with subclinical or inapparent infections are important from the public health point of view because they are a source of infection but may not be receiving care like those with clinical disease. They should be targeted for early diagnosis and treatment. Those with clinical disease may exhibit localized or systemic symptoms and mild to severe illness. The final outcome of a disease may be recovery, death, or something in between, including a carrier state, complications requiring extended hospital stay, or disability requiring rehabilitation.

At the community level, the disease may occur in endemic, epidemic, or pandemic proportion. **Endemic** refers to the constant presence of a disease within a geographic area or a population. Pertussis is endemic in the United States. **Epidemic** refers to the occurrence of disease in a community or region in excess of normal expectancy. Although people tend to associate large numbers with epidemics, even one case can be termed epidemic if the disease is considered previously eliminated from that area. For example, one case of polio, a disease considered eliminated from the United States, would be considered epidemic. **Pandemic** refers to an epidemic occurring worldwide and affecting large populations. HIV disease is both epidemic and pandemic, as the number of cases continues to grow across various regions of the world as well as in the United States. Zika and novel influenza A H1N1 are both recent emerging infectious diseases responsible for pandemics.

SURVEILLANCE OF COMMUNICABLE DISEASES

During the first half of the twentieth century, the weekly publication of national morbidity statistics by the U.S. Surgeon General's Office was accompanied by the statement, "No health department, state or local, can effectively prevent or control disease without knowledge of when, where, and under what conditions cases are occurring" (CDC, 1996). **Surveillance** gathers the "who, when, where, and what"; these elements are then used to answer "why." A good surveillance system systematically collects, organizes, and analyzes current, accurate, and complete data for a defined disease condition. The resulting information is promptly released to those who need it for effective planning, implementation, and evaluation of disease prevention and control programs.

Elements of Surveillance

Infectious disease surveillance incorporates and analyzes data from a variety of sources. Box 14.2 lists 10 commonly used data elements.

Surveillance for Agents of Bioterrorism

Since September 11, 2001, increased emphasis has been placed on surveillance for any disease that might be associated with the intentional release of a biological agent. The concern is, because of the interval between exposure and disease, that a covert release may go unrecognized and without response for some time if the resulting outbreak closely resembles a naturally occurring one. Health care providers are asked to be alert to: (1) temporal or geographic clustering of illnesses (people who attended the same public gathering or visited the same

BOX 14.2 Ten Basic Data Elements of Surveillance

1. Mortality registration
2. Morbidity reporting
3. Epidemic reporting
4. Epidemic field investigation
5. Case investigation
6. Laboratory reporting
7. Surveys
8. Use of biological agents and drugs
9. Distribution of animal reservoirs and vectors
10. Demographic and environmental data

location), especially those with clinical signs that resemble an infectious disease outbreak—previously healthy people with unexplained fever accompanied by sepsis, pneumonia, rash, or flaccid paralysis, and (2) an unusual age distribution for a common disease (e.g., chickenpox-like disease in adults without a child source case).

Because of the heightened concern about possible bioterrorist attacks, various sorts of syndromic surveillance systems were developed by public health agencies across the country. These systems incorporate factors such as the previously mentioned temporal and geographic clustering and unusual age distributions with groups of disease symptoms or syndromes (e.g., flaccid paralysis, respiratory signs, skin rashes, gastrointestinal symptoms) with the goal of detecting early signs of diseases that could result from a bioterrorism-related attack. Syndromic surveillance systems may include tracking emergency department, urgent care, ambulatory care, and hospitalization patient encounter data by syndrome symptoms. Other indicators may include laboratory and pharmacy data as well as poison control calls, school absenteeism, and environmental incidents. CDC currently uses the National Syndromic Surveillance Program, a collaboration among public health agencies and partners for timely exchange of syndromic data. Although more active infectious disease surveillance was developed because of the potential for bioterrorism, the positive benefit is increased surveillance for other hazardous events and communicable diseases outbreaks. This heightened surveillance has proved valuable in recognizing and monitoring environmental and health concerns such as H1N1 influenza, *Norovirus*, Zika virus, ciguatera fish poisoning, and the Deepwater Horizon oil spill. For additional information on preparedness surveillance, see the CDC website at https://www.cdc.gov.

Nurses are frequently involved at different levels of the surveillance system. They play important roles in collecting data, making diagnoses, investigating and reporting cases, and providing information to the general public. Examples of possible activities include investigating sources and contacts in outbreaks of pertussis in school settings or shigellosis in daycare; performing TB testing and contact tracing; collecting and reporting information pertaining to notifiable communicable diseases; performing infection control in hospitals; and providing morbidity and mortality statistics to those who request them, including the media, the public, service planners, and grant writers.

List of Reportable Diseases (L 2)

"A notifiable disease is one for which regular, frequent, and timely information regarding individual cases is considered necessary for the prevention and control of the disease" (CDC, 2013). Requirements for disease reporting in the United States are mandated by state rather than federal law and, as such, vary slightly from state to state. State health departments, on a voluntary basis, report cases of selected diseases to the CDC through the National Notifiable Diseases Surveillance System (NNDSS). State public health officials collaborate with the CDC to determine which diseases should be nationally notifiable. The list of nationally notifiable diseases may be revised as new diseases emerge or disease incidence declines. The conditions designated as notifiable at the national level and reported in 2018 are listed in Box 14.3. The NNDSS data are collated and published weekly in the *Morbidity and Mortality Weekly Report* (MMWR). Since

BOX 14.3 Nationally Notifiable Conditions—United States, 2018

1. Anthrax
2. Arboviral diseases, neuroinvasive and non-neuroinvasive
3. California serogroup virus diseases
4. Chikungunya virus disease
5. Eastern equine encephalitis virus disease
6. Powassan virus disease
7. St. Louis encephalitis virus disease
8. West Nile virus disease
9. Western equine encephalitis virus disease
10. Babesiosis
11. Botulism
12. Botulism, foodborne
13. Botulism, infant
14. Botulism, wound
15. Botulism, other
16. Brucellosis
17. Campylobacteriosis
18. Cancer
19. Carbapenemase Producing Carbapenem-Resistant *Enterobacteriaceae* (CP-CRE)
20. CP-CRE, *Enterobacter* spp.
21. CP-CRE, *Escherichia coli (E. coli)*
22. CP-CRE, *Klebsiella* spp.
23. Carbon monoxide poisoning
24. Chancroid
25. *Chlamydia trachomatis* infection
26. Cholera
27. Coccidioidomycosis
28. Congenital syphilis
29. Syphilitic stillbirth
30. Cryptosporidiosis
31. Cyclosporiasis
32. Dengue virus infections
33. Dengue
34. Dengue-like illness
35. Severe dengue

Continued

BOX 14.3 Nationally Notifiable Conditions—United States 2018—cont'd

36. Diphtheria
37. Ehrlichiosis and anaplasmosis
38. *Anaplasma phagocytophilum* infection
39. *Ehrlichia chaffeensis* infection
40. *Ehrlichia ewingii* infection
41. Undetermined human ehrlichiosis/anaplasmosis
42. Foodborne Disease Outbreak
43. Giardiasis
44. Gonorrhea
45. *Haemophilus influenzae*, invasive disease
46. Hansen's disease
47. Hantavirus infection, non-Hantavirus pulmonary syndrome
48. Hantavirus pulmonary syndrome
49. Hemolytic uremic syndrome, post-diarrheal
50. Hepatitis A, acute
51. Hepatitis B, acute
52. Hepatitis B, chronic
53. Hepatitis B, perinatal virus infection
54. Hepatitis C, acute
55. Hepatitis C, chronic
56. Hepatitis C, perinatal infection
57. HIV infection (AIDS has been reclassified as HIV Stage III)
58. Influenza-associated pediatric mortality
59. Invasive pneumococcal disease
60. Latent TB Infection (TB Infection)
61. Lead, elevated blood levels
62. Lead, elevated blood levels, children (<16 Years)
63. Lead, elevated blood levels, adult (≥16 Years)
64. Legionellosis
65. Leptospirosis
66. Listeriosis
67. Lyme disease
68. Malaria
69. Measles
70. Meningococcal disease
71. Mumps
72. Novel influenza A virus infections
73. Pertussis
74. Pesticide-related illness and injury, acute
75. Plague
76. Poliomyelitis, paralytic
77. Poliovirus infection, nonparalytic
78. Psittacosis
79. Q fever
80. Q fever, acute
81. Q fever, chronic
82. Rabies, animal
83. Rabies, human
84. Rubella
85. Rubella, congenital syndrome
86. Salmonellosis
87. Severe acute respiratory syndrome-associated coronavirus disease
88. Shiga toxin-producing *Escherichia coli*
89. Shigellosis
90. Silicosis
91. Smallpox
92. Spotted fever rickettsiosis
93. Streptococcal toxic shock syndrome
94. Syphilis
95. Syphilis, primary
96. Syphilis, secondary
97. Syphilis, early non-primary non-secondary
98. Syphilis, unknown duration or late
99. Tetanus
100. Toxic shock syndrome (other than streptococcal)
101. Trichinellosis
102. Tuberculosis
103. Tularemia
104. Typhoid fever
105. Vancomycin-intermediate *Staphylococcus aureus* and Vancomycin-resistant *Staphylococcus aureus*
106. Varicella
107. Varicella deaths
108. Vibriosis
109. Viral hemorrhagic fever
110. Crimean-Congo hemorrhagic fever virus
111. Ebola virus
112. Lassa virus
113. Lujo virus
114. Marburg virus
115. New World arenavirus – Guanarito virus
116. New World arenavirus – Junin virus
117. New World arenavirus – Machupo virus
118. New World arenavirus – Sabia virus
119. Waterborne Disease Outbreak
120. Yellow fever
121. Zika virus disease and Zika virus infection
122. Zika virus disease, congenital
123. Zika virus disease, non-congenital
124. Zika virus infection, congenital
125. Zika virus infection, non-congenital

AIDS, Acquired immunodeficiency syndrome; *HIV,* human immunodeficiency virus; *TB,* tuberculosis.
From Centers for Disease Control and Prevention: National Notifiable Disease Surveillance System (NNDSS)—2018 National Notifiable Conditions, 2018. Available at https://www.cdc.gov.

2016, Summary of Notifiable Infectious Diseases reports are published annually on the CDC MMWR website at https://www.cdc.gov. The CDC has launched the NNDSS Modernization Initiative to improve surveillance at the national, state, and local levels using electronic networks, information technology (IT) tools, and other advancements to make surveillance faster, more sensitive, and less expensive. Learn more about the NNDSS at the CDC website at http://www.cdc.gov. A brief history of the reporting of nationally notifiable infectious diseases in the United States is available at http://www.cdc.gov.

EMERGING INFECTIOUS DISEASES

Emergence Factors

Emerging infectious diseases are those in which the incidence has actually increased in the past several decades or has the potential to increase in the near future. These emerging diseases may include new or known infectious diseases and in our very connected world may travel quickly from one continent to another. Consider the following selected examples. Identified only in 1976 when sporadic outbreaks occurred in Sudan and Zaire, Ebola virus is a mysterious killer with a frightening mortality rate that sometimes reaches 90 percent, has no licensed vaccine or treatment, and has no recognized reservoir in nature. It appears to be transmitted through direct contact with bodily secretions and as such can be contained once cases are identified. Why outbreaks occur is not understood, although index cases have been associated with the handling of wild primates and evidence is increasing for a bat reservoir as is the case for its fellow virus Marburg. Ebola and Marburg are examples of new viruses that appear as civilization intrudes farther and farther into previously uninhabited natural environments, changing the landscape and disturbing ecological balances that may have existed unaltered for hundreds of years. Read more about the viral hemorrhagic viruses Ebola and Marburg at the CDC's viral special pathogens website: http://www.cdc.gov.

Hantavirus pulmonary syndrome was first detected in 1993 in the Four Corners area of Arizona and New Mexico, when young, previously healthy American Indians fell ill with a mysterious and deadly respiratory disease. The illness was soon discovered to be a variant of, but to exhibit different pathology from, a rodent-borne virus previously known only in Europe and Asia. Transmission is thought to occur through aerosolization of rodent excrement. One explanation for the outbreak in the Southwest is that an unseasonably mild winter led to an unusual increase in the rodent population; more people than usual were exposed to a virus that had until that point gone unrecognized in this country. Infection in American Indians first brought attention to hantavirus pulmonary syndrome because of a cluster of cases in a small geographic area, but no evidence suggests that any ethnic group is particularly susceptible to this disease. Hantavirus pulmonary syndrome has now been diagnosed in sites across the United States. The best protection against this virus seems to be avoiding rodent-infested environments.

Not only is HIV disease relatively new, but the resultant immunocompromise gave rise to previously rare opportunistic infections such as cryptosporidiosis, toxoplasmosis, and *Pneumocystis* pneumonia (PCP). HIV may have existed in isolated parts of sub-Saharan Africa for years and emerged, only recently, into the rest of the world as the result of a combination of factors, including new roads, increased commerce, and prostitution.

Escherichia coli 0157:H7 and other Shiga toxin-producing *E. coli* show a more virulent nature than strains of the past. TB is another familiar face turned newly aggressive. After years of decline, it has resurged as a result of infection resulting from HIV disease and the development of multidrug resistance. New influenza viruses like A H1N1 and A H5N1 challenge scientists to rapidly develop vaccines to protect a world population with little or no immunity.

West Nile virus (WNV), a mosquito-borne seasonal disease, was first identified in Uganda in 1937 and first detected in the United States in 1999. How WNV arrived in the United States may never be known, but the answer most likely involves infected birds or mosquitoes. Because the virus was new in this country and the outbreak of 2002 caused numerous deaths, WNV garnered a great deal of media attention. However, for the majority of people, infection with WNV results in no clinical signs (about 80 percent) or only mild flu-like symptoms. In a small percent of individuals, about 1 of 150 cases, a more severe, potentially fatal neuroinvasive form may develop, which may leave permanent neurological deficits for those who survive. The incidence of neuroinvasive disease increases with age with the highest rates in those 70 years and older.

After first appearing in New York City in 1999, the virus spent several years quietly spreading up and down the East Coast without remarkable morbidity or mortality. This situation changed abruptly in the summer of 2002 when it began moving across the country, accompanied by significant avian, equine, and human mortality. WNV has now been reported in every state except Hawaii and Alaska and is the most common neuroinvasive arbovirus disease (virus carried by arthropods, usually mosquitos and ticks) in the country. The CDC estimates that during its introduction into the United States, between 1999 and 2008, WNV led to almost 30,000 confirmed and probable cases and over 1000 deaths. From 2013 to 2017, confirmed and probable cases averaged 2200 with an average 220 reported deaths. WNV is reported through CDC ArboNET, a national surveillance system. Because ArboNET uses passive surveillance dependent on reporting from the medical community, it most likely greatly underestimates the number of non-neuroinvasive cases since many mildly affected individuals may not seek care.

While outbreaks of WNV may be influenced by multiple factors, weather patterns—dry periods after extensive rain which favors mosquito reproduction—seem to play a role. Mosquitoes become infected with WNV when they feed on infected birds. Infected mosquitoes then spread West Nile virus to people and other animals by biting them. Until a human vaccine is developed (a vaccine for horses does exist), preventing human infection is dependent on mosquito control and preventing mosquito bites. Rarely, WNV has been transmitted through blood transfusions, in utero exposure, and possibly breastfeeding (CDC, 2010a; CDC, 2018b). Learn more about WNV and view maps of recent activity at the CDC website: https://www.cdc.gov.

Other examples of emerging pathogens newly recognized or newly active include the viruses Australian bat lyssavirus, Hendra or equine morbilli virus, and Nipah virus, all transmitted by bats; and chikungunya and Zika viruses, transmitted by mosquitos. Newly recognized bacterial pathogens include *Bartonella henselae* (cat scratch fever), and *Ehrlichia* spp. (ehrlichiosis), and *Borrelia burgdorferi* (Lyme disease), transmitted by ticks. Emerging parasitic pathogens include *Babesia microti* (babesiosis), *Acanthamoeba*, and *Naegleria fowleri*, commonly referred to as the "brain-eating amoeba." These two amoebae are commonly found in soil and fresh water. *Acanthamoeba* infection may result in an ocular keratitis largely associated with wearing contact lenses and coming into contact with water or cleaning solution containing *Acanthamoeba*. Infection with *Naegleria* results in primary amoebic meningoencephalitis, or

PAM. When water containing *Naegleria* enters the nose, the amoebae can travel to the brain, causing devastating disease. The major risk factor for PAM is swimming in warm, fresh water like that found in ponds and lakes in the southern United States. PAM has also been associated with contaminated nasal rinses. Swallowing water is not a risk factor.

Several factors, operating singly or in combination, can influence the emergence of these diseases (Table 14.1) (CDC, 1994). Except for microbial adaptation and changes made by the infectious agent, such as those likely in the emergence of *E. coli* 0157:H7, H1N1, and perhaps Zika, most of the emergence factors are consequences of activities and behaviors of the human host and of environmental changes such as deforestation, urbanization, and industrialization. The rise in households with two working parents has increased the number of children in daycare, and with this shift has come an increase in diarrheal diseases such as shigellosis. Changing sexual behaviors and illegal drug use influence the spread of HIV disease as well as other sexually transmitted infections. Before the use of large air-conditioning systems with cooling towers, legionellosis was virtually unknown. Changing environmental temperatures may result in habitat change for arthropod vectors. Modern transportation systems closely and quickly connect regions of the world that for centuries had little contact. Insects and animals as well as humans may carry disease between continents on ships and planes. Immigrants, both legal and undocumented, as well as travelers bring with them a variety of known and potentially unknown diseases.

TABLE 14.1 Factors That Can Influence the Emergence of New Infectious Diseases

Categories	Specific Examples
Societal events	Economic impoverishment, war or civil conflict, population growth and migration, urban decay
Health care	New medical devices, organ or tissue transplantation, drugs causing immunosuppression, widespread use of antibiotics
Food production	Globalization of food supplies, changes in food processing and packaging
Human behavior	Sexual behavior, drug use, travel, diet, outdoor recreation, use of childcare facilities
Environmental	Deforestation/reforestation, changes in water ecosystems, flood/drought, famine, global changes (e.g., warming)
Public health	Curtailment or reduction in prevention programs, inadequate communicable disease infrastructure surveillance, lack of trained personnel (epidemiologists, laboratory scientists, vector and rodent control specialists)
Microbial adaptation	Changes in virulence and toxin production, development of drug resistance, microbes as co-factors in chronic diseases

From the Centers for Disease Control and Prevention: Addressing emerging infectious disease threats: a prevention strategy for the U.S., Atlanta, 1994, CDC.

Examples of Emerging Infectious Diseases

Selected emerging infectious diseases, including a brief description of the diseases and symptoms they cause, their modes of transmission, and causes of emergence, are listed in Table 14.2 and Fig. 14.2. Progress in addressing emerging infectious disease as well as current findings and topics can be found in the CDC journal *Emerging Infectious Diseases.* The journal is published monthly and is available online at http://wwwnc.cdc.gov.

PREVENTION AND CONTROL OF INFECTIOUS DISEASE

In 2011, the CDC published *A CDC Framework for Preventing Infectious Disease: Sustaining the Essentials and Innovating for the Future,* a plan for preventing and controlling infectious threats through a "strengthened, adaptable, and multi-purpose U.S. public health system." Updating the 1998 plan *Preventing Emerging Infectious Diseases: A Strategy for the 21st Century* and reflecting technological advances of the past decade, the plan places a heavy emphasis on the role of technology in surveillance, detection, and control. Three elements for action are identified: (1) strengthen public health fundamentals, including infectious disease surveillance, laboratory detection, and epidemiologic investigation; (2) identify and implement high-impact public health interventions to reduce infectious diseases; and (3) develop and advance policies to prevent, detect, and control infectious diseases. It also discusses linkages between infectious and chronic disease and identifies infectious disease issues of special concern: (1) antimicrobial resistance, (2) chronic viral hepatitis, (3) food safety, (4) health care-associated infections, (5) HIV/AIDS, (6) respiratory infections, (7) safe water, and (8) zoonotic and vector-borne diseases (CDC, 2011). This plan remains current and may be viewed at http://www.cdc.gov.

Infectious disease can be prevented and controlled. The goal of prevention and control programs is to reduce the prevalence of a disease to a level at which it no longer poses a major public health problem. In some cases, diseases may even be eliminated or eradicated. The goal of **elimination** is to remove a disease from a large geographic area such as a country or region of the world. **Eradication** is removing a disease worldwide by ending all transmission of infection through the complete extermination of the infectious agent. The WHO officially declared the global eradication of smallpox on May 8, 1980 (Evans, 1985). After the successful eradication of smallpox, the eradication of other communicable diseases became a realistic challenge, and in 1987 the WHO adopted resolutions for eradication of paralytic poliomyelitis and dracunculiasis (guinea worm infection) from the world by the year 2000.

These eradication goals were not reached in 2000, but substantial progress has been made. When the resolution was made in 1987 for the eradication of guinea worm disease, there were an estimated 3.5 million cases a year in 20 countries in Asia and Africa, and 120 million people were at risk for the disease. In 2016, only 25 cases were reported worldwide, making the goal of global eradication appear within reach (CDC, 2017f). Read more about guinea worm disease eradication at https://www.cdc.gov.

TABLE 14.2 Examples of Emerging Infectious Diseases

Infectious Agent	Diseases/Symptoms	Mode of Transmission	Causes of Emergence
Borrelia burgdorferi	Lyme disease: rash, fever, arthritis, neurological and cardiac abnormalities	Bite of infective *Ixodes* tick	Increase in deer and human populations in wooded areas
Cryptosporidium	Cryptosporidiosis; infection of epithelial cells in gastrointestinal and respiratory tracts	Fecal-oral, person-to-person, waterborne	Development near watershed areas; immunosuppression
Ebola-Marburg viruses	Fulminant, high mortality, hemorrhagic fever	Direct contact with infected blood, organs, secretions, and semen	Unknown, likely human invasion of virus ecological niche
Escherichia coli 0157:H7	Hemorrhagic colitis; thrombocytopenia; hemolytic uremic syndrome	Ingestion of contaminated food, especially undercooked beef and raw milk	Likely caused by a new pathogen
Hantavirus	Hemorrhagic fever with renal syndrome; pulmonary syndrome	Inhalation of aerosolized rodent urine and feces	Human invasion of virus ecological niche
Human immunodeficiency virus (HIV-1)	HIV infection; AIDS (HIV stage III); severe immune dysfunction, opportunistic infections	Sexual contact with or exposure to blood or tissues of infected persons; perinatal	Urbanization; lifestyle changes; drug use; international travel; transfusions; transplant
Human papillomavirus (HPV)	Skin and mucous membrane lesions (warts); strongly linked to cancer of the cervix and penis	Direct sexual contact, contact with contaminated surfaces	Newly recognized; changes in sexual lifestyle
Influenza A H1N1 virus (novel, pandemic)	Influenza: fever, cough, headache, myalgia, prostration, possibly GI signs	Person-to-person, airborne (droplet), and contact (direct and indirect)	Antigenic shift
Influenza A H5N1 virus (novel, avian)	Influenza: fever, cough, headache, myalgia, prostration	Direct contact with infected poultry or birds; limited person-to-person transmission	Antigenic shift
Legionella pneumophila	Legionnaires' disease: malaise, myalgia, fever, headache, respiratory illness	Air cooling systems, water supplies	Recognition in an epidemic situation
Pneumocystis jiroveci	Acute pneumonia	Unknown; possibly airborne or reactivation of latent infection	Immunosuppression
SARS coronavirus	Severe and acute pneumonia	Person-to-person, airborne (droplet), and direct and indirect contact with respiratory secretions and other bodily fluid	Unknown; newly recognized coronavirus; possible animal transmission into Chinese population
West Nile virus	No clinical signs to mild flu-like symptoms to fatal neuroinvasive disease	Bite of infected mosquitoes; infected birds serve as reservoirs	International travel and commerce
Zika virus	No clinical signs to mild flu-like symptoms with rash to neurological conditions such as microencephaly and Guillain-Barré syndrome	Bite of infected mosquitoes; in utero transmission; sexual transmission; blood transfusion	International travel and commerce; lack of immunity in populations outside of Africa and Asia; possibly previous under reporting

AIDS, Acquired immunodeficiency syndrome; *GI,* gastrointestinal; *SARS,* severe acute respiratory syndrome.
Based on information from Heymann DL, editor: *Control of communicable diseases manual,* ed. 20, Washington, DC, 2015, American Public Health Association; World Health Organization: History of the Zika virus, 2018. Available at http://www.who.int.

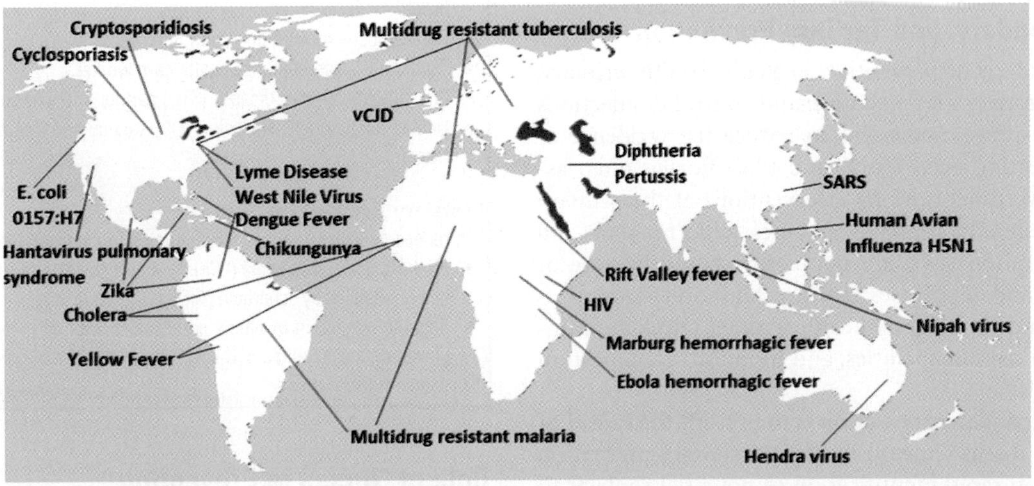

Fig. 14.2 Examples of recent emerging and re-emerging infectious diseases. *HIV,* Human immunodeficiency virus; *SARS,* severe acute respiratory syndrome; *vCJD,* variant Creutzfeldt-Jakob disease. (Based on the concept from the Institute of Medicine: *Microbial threats to health: emergence, detection, and response,* Washington, DC, 2003, National Academy Press.)

With the Global Polio Eradication Initiative, the WHO partnered with national governments, Rotary International, the CDC, and UNICEF in what has been called the largest public health initiative the world has ever known. Since 1988, over 2 billion children around the world have been immunized against polio through the cooperation of more than 200 countries and 20 million volunteers, supported by an international investment of over $3 billion. At the end of 2008, the WHO reviewed the progress of the initiative with two independent outside agencies and concluded that the remaining technical and operational challenges to eradication could be overcome in each of the polio-endemic countries by ensuring the political commitment of all polio-affected countries to attain the highest possible coverage and enhancing routine vaccination and surveillance (CDC, 2009).

As a result of the Global Polio Eradication Initiative launch in 1988, the number of polio-endemic countries has decreased from 125 to 3 (Afghanistan, Nigeria, and Pakistan); 4 of the 6 regions of the WHO are certified polio free—the Americas, Europe, Southeast Asia, and the Western Pacific; and the number of worldwide wild poliovirus cases has fallen from an estimated 350,000 to 21 in 2017. The focus now is to vaccinate every child in the three remaining endemic countries to totally interrupt transmission. In the meantime, importation of cases resulting from the ease of worldwide travel or breakdowns in coverage in a neighboring country can to lead to outbreaks in non-endemic countries without strong coverage. Challenges to maintaining coverage include political instability and sporadic violence, cultural beliefs about immunization, religious fears, and distrust of immunization. With the potential for eradication so close, in May of 2014, the WHO declared the recent international spread of wild poliovirus a Public Health Emergency of International Concern (PHEIC) and issued Temporary Recommendations under the International Health Regulations to prevent further spread of the disease and to be reviewed every three months (WHO, 2016). The PHEIC remains in place as of 2018. Read more about global polio eradication efforts at http://www.polioeradication.org.

Primary, Secondary, and Tertiary Prevention

There are three levels of prevention in public health: primary, secondary, and tertiary. In prevention and control of infectious disease, primary prevention seeks to reduce the incidence of disease by preventing occurrence, and this effort is often assisted by the government. Many interventions at the primary level, such as federally supplied vaccines and "no shots, no school" immunization laws, are population based because of public health mandate. Nurses deliver childhood immunizations in public and community health settings, check immunization records in daycare facilities, and monitor immunization records in schools.

The goal of secondary prevention is to prevent the spread of infection and/or disease once it occurs. Secondary prevention activities center on rapid identification of potential contacts to a reported case. Contacts may be (1) identified as new cases and treated, or (2) determined to be possibly exposed but not diseased and appropriately treated with prophylaxis. Public health disease control laws also assist in secondary prevention because they require investigation and prevention measures for individuals affected by a communicable disease report or outbreak. These laws can extend to the entire community if the exposure potential is deemed great enough, as could happen with an outbreak of smallpox or epidemic influenza. Nurses perform much of the communicable disease surveillance and control work in this country.

While many infections are acute, with either recovery or death occurring in the short term, some exhibit chronic courses (AIDS/HIV stage III) or disabling sequelae (leprosy/Hansen's disease). Tertiary prevention works to reduce complications and disabilities through treatment and rehabilitation. The Levels of Prevention box has examples of communicable disease prevention and control interventions at the three levels of prevention.

LEVELS OF PREVENTION

Examples of Infectious Disease Interventions

Primary Prevention

To prevent the occurrence of disease:

- Responsible sexual behavior
- Malaria chemoprophylaxis
- Tetanus boosters, flu shots
- Rabies pre-exposure immunization
- Safe food-handling practices in the home
- Repellants for preventing vector-borne disease
- Following childhood immunizations recommendations, and "no shots, no school" laws
- Regulated and inspected municipal water supplies
- Bloodborne pathogen regulations
- Restaurant inspections
- Federal regulations protecting American cattle from exposure to bovine spongiform encephalopathy (BSE)

Secondary Prevention

To prevent the spread of disease:

- Immunoglobulin after hepatitis A exposure
- Immunization and chemoprophylaxis as appropriate in meningococcal outbreak
- Rabies post-exposure immunization
- Tuberculosis screening for health care workers
- Sexually transmitted disease (STD) partner notification
- Human immunodeficiency virus (HIV) testing and treatment
- Quarantine

Tertiary Prevention

To reduce complications and disabilities through treatment and rehabilitation:

- *Pneumocystis* pneumonia (PCP) chemoprophylaxis for people with acquired immunodeficiency syndrome (AIDS)/HIV stage III
- Regular inspection of hands and feet as well as protective footwear and gloves to avoid trauma and infection for leprosy clients who have lost sensation in those areas

Role of Nurses in Prevention

Prevention is at the center of public health, and nurses perform much of this work. Examples include immunizations for vaccine-preventable disease, especially childhood immunization and the

TABLE 14.3 A Multisystem Approach to Communicable Disease Prevention and Control

System Goal	Factors Contributing to the Goal
Host resistance to infectious agents and other environmental hazards	Individual choice of hygiene, nutrition, and physical fitness; increased immunization coverage; drugs for prevention and treatment; stress control and improved mental health
Safe environment	Sanitation, clean water and air; access to healthy food and food security; proper cooking and storage of food; control of vectors and animal reservoir hosts
Strong public health systems	Increased access to health care; appropriate health education; improved surveillance and response systems; multisectoral collaborations to address health disparities and social determinants of health
Social and political change to ensure better health for all people	Individual, organizational, and community action to build political and economic stability and to foster a culture of health; legislation to protect workers, the environment, and assure health care

Based on information from Wenzel RP: The control of communicable diseases. In Last JM, Wallace R, editors: *Public health and preventive medicine,* ed. 13, Norwalk, CT, 1991, Appleton & Lange.

monitoring of immunization status in clinic, daycare, school, and home settings. Nurses work in communicable disease surveillance and control, teach and monitor bloodborne pathogen control, and advise on prevention of vector-borne diseases. They teach methods for responsible sexual behavior, screen for sexually transmitted infection, and provide HIV disease counseling and testing. They screen for TB, identify TB contacts, and deliver directly observed TB treatment in the community.

A Multisystem Approach to Communicable Disease Prevention and Control

Because illness from communicable disease represents an imbalance in the host-environment-agent relationship, any approach to controlling infection must consider multiple systems, including enhancing host resistance, improving safety of the environment, strengthening public health systems, and facilitating social and political change to support a culture of health for all. Table 14.3 provides examples of the factors that make up these multiple systems of engagement (Wenzel, 1991).

AGENTS OF BIOTERRORISM

September 11, 2001, made real the specter of terrorism on American soil. The anthrax attacks that followed further highlighted the possibilities for the intentional release of a biological agent, or bioterrorism. The CDC suggests that the agents most likely to be used in a bioterrorist attack are those having both the potential for high mortality and easy dissemination—factors most likely to result in major public panic and social disruption. Six infectious agents are considered of highest concern: anthrax (*Bacillus anthracis*), plague (*Yersinia pestis*), smallpox (variola major), botulism (*Clostridium botulinum*), tularemia (*Francisella tularensis*), and selected hemorrhagic viruses (filoviruses such as Ebola and Marburg; arenaviruses such as Lassa fever, Junin virus, and related viruses). The CDC urges health care providers to be familiar with the epidemiology of these diseases as well as illness patterns, possibly indicating an unusual infectious disease outbreak associated with the intentional release of a biological agent. More information on recognition of illness associated with the intentional release of a biological agent as well as possible agents may be found at the CDC Emergency Preparedness and Response website: https://emergency.cdc.gov.

Anthrax

Until the fall of 2001, anthrax was more commonly a concern of veterinarians and military strategists than the general public. After September 11th, the news of deaths caused by letters deliberately contaminated with anthrax and transmitted through the postal service profoundly changed our view of this infectious disease. Anthrax is an acute disease caused by the spore-forming bacterium *B. anthracis.* It is thought that anthrax may have caused the biblical fifth and sixth plagues of Exodus as well as the Black Bane of Europe in the 1600s. In 1881 anthrax became the first bacterial disease for which immunization was available. More commonly seen in cattle, sheep, and goats, anthrax in modern times has rarely and sporadically affected humans, usually through the handling or consumption of infected animal products (Cieslak & Eitzen, 1999).

Anthrax is a clever organism that perpetuates itself by forming spores. When animals dying from anthrax suffer terminal hemorrhage and infected blood comes into contact with the air, the bacillus organism sporulates. These spores are highly resistant to disinfection and environmental destruction and may remain in contaminated soil for many years. In the United States, anthrax zones are said to follow the cattle drive trails of the 1800s. Sometimes referred to as wool handler's disease, anthrax in the United States has commonly posed the greatest risk to people who work directly with dying animals, such as veterinarians, or those who handle infected animal products such as hair, wool, and bone or bone meal or products made from these materials such as rugs and drums. Products made from infected materials may transmit this disease around the world. In areas of the world where anthrax is common in animals, the disease is endemic. Outbreaks from handling and consuming meat from infected animals have been reported from Africa, Asia and Eastern Europe. Person-to-person transmission is rare.

Anthrax disease may manifest in one of four syndromes: cutaneous, gastrointestinal, respiratory or inhalational, and injection. Cutaneous anthrax, the form most commonly seen, occurs when spores come in contact with abraded skin surfaces. Itching is followed in 2 to 6 days by the development of a characteristic black eschar, usually surrounded by some degree of edema and possibly secondary infection. The lesion itself is usually not painful. If untreated, infection may spread to the regional lymph nodes and bloodstream, resulting in septicemia and death. The fatality rate for untreated cutaneous anthrax is between 5 percent and 20 percent, but if appropriately treated, death seldom occurs. Gastrointestinal anthrax is considered very rare and occurs from eating undercooked, contaminated meat. Inhalational anthrax is also considered rare, typically seen in occupations with exposure to hide tanning or bone processing. Initially, symptoms are mild and non-specific and may include fever, malaise, mild cough, or chest pain. These symptoms are followed three to five days later, often after an apparent improvement, by fever and shock, rapid deterioration, and death. Untreated cases of inhalational anthrax are fatal; treated cases may show as high as a 95 percent fatality rate if treatment is initiated after 48 hours from the onset of symptoms. Injection anthrax, a relative newcomer to anthrax syndromes, has largely been seen in heroin users in northern Europe. No cases have been reported in the United States. Cases frequently do not show symptoms consistent with the classic forms of anthrax, although presentations may vary. Localized soft tissue infections with considerable edema are most common (Heymann, 2015).

Because of factors such as the ability for aerosolization, the resistance to environmental degradation, and a high fatality rate, inhalational anthrax has long been considered to have an extremely high potential for being the single greatest biological warfare threat (Cieslak & Eitzen, 1999). An accidental release from a biological research institute in Sverdlovsk, Russia, in 1979 resulted in the documented death of 66 individuals and demonstrated the capacity of this organism as a weapon. Manufacture and delivery of the spores have been considered a challenge because of a tendency for the spores to clump. During 1998 in the United States, more than two dozen anthrax threats (letters purporting to be carrying anthrax) were made. None of them were real. The events of the fall of 2001, when 11 people were sickened and 5 died from deliberate exposure, have shown that the threat of anthrax as a weapon of bioterror is all too real.

Any threat of anthrax should be reported to the Federal Bureau of Investigation and to local and state health departments. Anthrax is sensitive to a variety of antibiotics, including the penicillins, chloramphenicol, doxycycline, meropenem, and the fluoroquinolones. Initial treatment of all forms of anthrax, other than localized cutaneous, should include intravenous therapy with two or more antimicrobial agents known to be effective against *B. anthracis*, with the first choice being ciprofloxacin or an equivalent. In cases of possible bioterrorism activity, individuals with a credible threat of exposure, with confirmed exposure, or at high risk of exposure are immediately started on antibiotic prophylaxis. Immunization is recommended as well. People who have been exposed are not contagious, so quarantine is not appropriate (Heymann, 2015).

Since 2001, no more deliberate acts of anthrax-associated bioterrorism have been reported, Cases of gastrointestinal anthrax continue to be reported from areas of the world where undercooked, contaminated meat is consumed. England and the United States have seen rare cases of cutaneous, inhalational, and gastrointestinal anthrax associated with drumming circles using drums covered with imported animal hides. In 2009-2010, anthrax was identified in over a hundred heroin users in Scotland, leading to a new clinical manifestation known as injectional anthrax. Since then sporadic cases have been reported from across Europe believed to be linked to contaminated batches of heroin. How the heroin is contaminated is not clear (ECDC, 2017).

Smallpox

Smallpox is exclusively a human disease with no known animal or environmental reservoirs. Formerly a disease found worldwide, smallpox has been considered eradicated since 1979. The last known natural case in the United States was in 1949. The last known natural case of smallpox worldwide occurred in Somalia in 1977. The United States stopped routinely immunizing for smallpox in 1982. The only documented existing virus sources are located in freezers at the CDC in Atlanta and a research institute in Novosibirsk, Russia. Controversy exists over the destruction of these viral stocks but scientists and public health officials continue to maintain there is still a need to perform research using the variola virus to be prepared in the event of an accidental or intentional exposure. Smallpox research is overseen by the WHO.

Smallpox has been identified as one of the leading candidate agents for bioterrorism. Susceptibility is 100 percent in the unvaccinated (those vaccinated before 1982 are not considered protected, although they may have some immunity), and the fatality rate is estimated at 20 percent to 40 percent or higher. Immunization with a vaccinia vaccine, the immunizing agent for smallpox, can be protective even after exposure. The WHO does not recommend vaccination of the general public because currently the risk of death (one per one million doses) or serious side effects is greater than that of acquiring the disease. Those who routinely are exposed to smallpox virus such as laboratory workers should be vaccinated. Because of the potential for bioterrorism and the fact that many health care providers have never seen this disease, it is important to become familiar with the clinical and epidemiologic features of smallpox and how it is differentiated from chickenpox (see the How To box). Should a non-varicella, small pox–like disease be detected, immediate contact with local and national health authorities is obligatory (Heymann, 2015).

HOW TO Distinguish Chickenpox From Smallpox

Despite the availability of a vaccine, chickenpox is still a common disease of childhood and may be seen in susceptible adults as well. Although many health care providers are familiar with chickenpox, most have never seen a case of smallpox. Because of the potential for smallpox to be used as a bioweapon, the CDC suggests that nurses and other practitioners familiarize themselves with the differences in presentation between the two diseases. The rash pattern for each disease is distinctive, but in the first two to three days of development, the two may be indistinguishable. Infectious disease texts and posters provide a pictorial description. If a smallpox infection is suspected, the local health department should be notified immediately.

Chickenpox (Varicella)	Smallpox (Historical Variola Major)
Sudden onset with slight fever and mild constitutional symptoms (both may be more severe in adults)	Sudden onset of fever, prostration, severe body aches, and occasional abdominal pain and vomiting, as in influenza
Rash is present at onset	Clear-cut prodromal illness, rash follows two to four days after fever begins decreasing

Rash progression is maculopapular for a few hours, vesicular for three to four days, followed by granular scabs	Progression is macular, papular, vesicular, and pustular, followed by crusted scabs that fall off after three to four weeks if client survives
Rash is "centrifugal" with lesions most abundant on the trunk or areas of the body usually covered by clothing	Rash is "centripetal" with lesions most abundant on the face and extremities
Lesions appear in "crops" and can be at various stages in the same area of the body	Lesions are all at same stage in all areas
Vesicles are superficial and collapse on puncture; mild scarring may occur	Vesicles are deep-seated and do not collapse on puncture; pitting and scarring are common

Plague

Plague is a vector-borne disease transmitted by rodent fleas carrying the bacterium *Y. pestis.* Portrayed vividly in the Bible and events throughout history, plague is believed responsible for the epidemic of Black Death that killed over a quarter of the population of Europe during the Middle Ages. The disease is endemic in much of South Asia, parts of South America, and the western United States, but the majority of outbreaks and cases today are reported from Africa, especially from the Democratic Republic of the Congo. Plague arrived in the United States as a consequence of a pandemic that began in China during the late 1800s and spread to the West Coast via shipboard rats. Although resulting plague in cities was largely controlled, the disease spread to and became enzootic in wild rodents. The current primary vertebrate reservoirs in the United States are usually ground squirrels rather than rats, rabbits, wild carnivores, and in some cases cats. Human plague in the western United States occurs infrequently and sporadically with fewer than 20 cases reported a year since 1970. Veterinarians have contracted the disease from infected cats. People with regular outdoor exposure such as hunters, trappers, and those living in rural areas as well as cat owners are at highest risk for natural transmission (Heymann, 2015).

Initial signs and symptoms of plague are non-specific and include myalgia, malaise, fever, chills, sore throat, and headache. As the disease progresses, lymphadenitis commonly develops in the lymph nodes draining the area nearest the bite. This swollen node, or bubo, most frequently seen in the inguinal area, gives rise to the name bubonic plague. Whether lymphadenitis is present or not, bubonic plague may progress to septicemic plague and secondary pneumonic plague. Secondary pneumonic plague can spread through respiratory droplets, resulting in primary pneumonic plague and human-to-human outbreaks. No such transmission has been reported in the United States since 1924, but several cases of primary pneumonic plague have developed from exposure to infected cats.

Untreated cases of primary septicemic and pneumonic plague are most often fatal; the case fatality rate for untreated bubonic plague is 50 percent to 60 percent. Streptomycin is the treatment of choice; gentamicin, tetracyclines, and chloramphenicol are alternatives. Immunization may confer some protection against bubonic plague but not pneumonic. Commercial plague vaccine is no longer available in the United States. Naturally acquired plague is usually bubonic. Plague used as a means of a terrorist attack would most likely be aerosolized, resulting in pneumonic disease and human-to-human transmission (Heymann, 2015). Read more about plague at the CDC website: http://www.cdc.gov.

VACCINE-PREVENTABLE DISEASES

Vaccines are one of the most effective methods of preventing and controlling communicable diseases. The smallpox vaccine, which left distinctive scars on so many shoulders, is no longer in general use because the smallpox virus has been declared eradicated from the world's population. Despite threats of bioterrorism, there are no plans to reintroduce universal smallpox immunization because of potential side effects. Diseases such as polio, diphtheria, pertussis, and measles, which previously occurred in epidemic proportions, are now controlled by routine childhood immunization. They have not, however, been eradicated, so children need to be immunized against them. In the United States, "no shots, no school" legislation has resulted in the immunization of most children by the time they enter school. However, many infants and toddlers, the group most vulnerable to these potentially severe diseases, do not receive scheduled immunizations despite the availability of free vaccines. And infants less than six months of age who are not yet fully immunized may be susceptible to infections in unimmunized individuals around them (see the Evidence-Based Practice box). Surveys show inner-city children from minority and ethnic groups are particularly at risk for incomplete immunization, and children from religious communities whose beliefs prohibit immunization and children with parents who have philosophical objections to immunization may receive no protection at all. Studies also show low levels of vaccination against pneumonia in senior citizens and lower levels of influenza coverage in adults from minority and ethnic groups. *Healthy People 2020* includes several objectives about obtaining and maintaining appropriate levels of immunization in all age groups. (Additional information on vaccine-preventable diseases may be found at the CDC website: http://www.cdc.gov.)

EVIDENCE-BASED PRACTICE

Infants under six months of age are at greatest risk for complications and death from pertussis because they are too young to be fully immunized. The CDC has recommended since 2012 that pregnant women be vaccinated with Tdap (tetanus, reduced diphtheria, acellular pertussis) between 27 and 36 weeks' gestation to allow for a transfer of maternal antibodies, offering protection to the infant until its first pertussis vaccination at age two months. However, despite evidence that this practice does offer protection, uptake of Tdap has been slow, with the CDC reporting 48.8 percent coverage in 2016. In this study, the University of Kansas Medical Center created a pop-up message for the electronic medical record system in their obstetrics clinic to provide a reminder of the CDC

Continued

EVIDENCE-BASED PRACTICE—cont'd

recommendation. The physician could then choose to order the vaccine directly from the message screen or note the reason for not doing so (patient declines, other with comment, not indicated). While the pop-up could be ignored, unless the physician selected one of the options, it would continue to appear at every visit for the patient between 27 and 36 weeks of pregnancy. Nurses could also view the pop-up when checking clients in, allowing them to introduce the topic of Tdap before it was broached by the physician. A comparison of the same four-month period pre- and post-intervention showed a statistically significant 15.7 percent increase in coverage, moving from 44.6 percent of 531 patients to 60.3 percent of 574 patients ($P < .0001$). No differences were noted in the characteristics of the women who did and did not receive the vaccine. This simple medical records alert resulted in increasing uptake of Tdap among pregnant women at this clinic by over a third.

Nurse Use

The adult public has been slow to embrace Tdap. One reason may be lack of awareness of the availability of the vaccine and/or of the importance it plays in keeping infants safe. There are a variety of ways to approach this issue, starting with consumer awareness and provider education and advocacy. This study shows how a change in standard practice within an institution had a dramatic effect on Tdap immunization in pregnant mothers. Whether Tdap or other issues that require attention, nurses manage clinics and take leadership roles in hospitals, physicians' offices, health departments, and safety-net health services, which puts them in a position to both assess where there are opportunities for intervention and to change practice in order to address important public health concerns.

American College of Obstetricians and Gynecologists (ACOG): 2018 Annual Meeting, Abstract 8L, Simple alert increases prenatal uptake of Tdap vaccine. *Medscape Medical News*, April 29, 2018. Available at https://www.medscape.com.

Because many children receive their vaccinations at public health departments, nurses play a major role in increasing immunization coverage of infants and toddlers. Nurses track children known to be at risk for under immunization and call or send reminders to their parents. They help avoid missed immunization opportunities by checking the immunization status of every young child encountered, whether or not the clinic or home visit is related to immunization. In addition, they organize immunization outreach activities in the community; provide answers to parents' questions and concerns about immunization; and educate parents about why immunizations are needed, inappropriate contraindications to immunization, and the importance of completing the immunization schedule on time.

Routine Childhood Immunization Schedule

The 2018 recommended immunization schedule for children and adolescents in the United States includes routine immunization against the following 16 diseases: hepatitis B, diphtheria, pertussis, tetanus, measles, mumps, rubella, polio, *Haemophilus influenzae* type B meningitis, *Varicella* (chickenpox), *Streptococcus pneumoniae*–related illnesses, rotavirus, hepatitis A, influenza, HPV, and meningococcal disease (CDC, 2018c). The vaccine schedule is a rather complex and frequently changing document that makes continuing adjustments for the latest research and recommendations and is issued annually by the Advisory Committee on Immunization Practices (ACIP). More recent additions to the schedule include hepatitis A, rotavirus, seasonal influenza for all children ages 6 months through 18 years, and Tdap (the tetanus, reduced-strength diphtheria, and acellular pertussis vaccine licensed for older children, adolescents, and adults). Because many of these vaccines require three to four doses, the schedule begins at birth with succeeding staggered vaccinations designed to achieve recommended immunization levels by two years of age. Additional doses may be required before a child enters school and at adolescence or on entering college. The ACIP, the American Academy of Pediatrics, and the American Academy of Family Physicians regularly update recommended immunization schedules. The ACIP also issues a recommended adult immunization schedule for those over 18 years old, by age group and immune status. The 2018 schedule includes, as appropriate, HPV, varicella, measles, mumps and rubella, pneumococcus, zoster to prevent shingles, and tetanus every 10 years with one dose given as Tdap. Other immunizations available in special circumstances include, but are not limited to, rabies, yellow fever, typhoid, smallpox, and anthrax. (Recommended vaccine schedules may be viewed at http://www.cdc.gov.)

Measles

Measles is an acute, highly contagious disease that, although considered a childhood illness, may be seen in the United States in adolescents and young adults. Symptoms include fever, sneezing and coughing, conjunctivitis, small white spots on the inside of the cheek (Koplik's spots), and a red, blotchy rash beginning several days after the respiratory signs. Measles is caused by the rubeola virus and is transmitted by inhalation of infected aerosol droplets or by direct contact with infected nasal or throat secretions or with articles freshly contaminated with the same nasal or throat secretions. A very contagious nature, combined with the fact that people are most contagious before they are aware they are infected, makes measles a disease that can spread rapidly through the population. Infection with measles confers lifelong immunity (Heymann, 2015).

Measles and malnutrition form a deadly combination for many children in the developing world with about 19 million cases a year. Despite the introduction in 1963 of a live attenuated measles vaccine that is safe, effective, and widely available, measles is still endemic in many countries and a leading killer of children under five. Much of this mortality is preventable by immunizing all infants. The good news is that with the launch of the Measles and Rubella Initiative in 2001, global measles deaths have decreased 84 percent, from 550,100 to 89,780 in 2016 (CDC, 2017g).

Immunization has dramatically decreased measles cases in the United States to the point that, in March 2000, a panel of experts declared measles no longer endemic in the United States. Before introduction of the vaccine in 1963, 200,000 to 500,000 cases of measles were reported yearly, but by 1983 reported cases had fallen to an all-time low of less than 1500. In the late 1980s, the incidence of measles began to climb again, with more than 55,000 cases reported between 1989 and 1991. This increase resulted from low immunization rates among preschool children and was countered with efforts to increase immunization rates and the routine use of two doses of measles vaccine for all children. Except for outbreaks in 1994 that occurred predominantly among high school and college-age persons, many of whom had not received two doses of measles vaccine, reported measles cases dropped continuously from 1991 to 2004 when only 37 confirmed cases were reported to the CDC—the lowest number since measles became a nationally reportable disease in 1912.

Since measles elimination was documented in the United States in 2000, annual reported cases have ranged from the low of 37 in 2004 to a high of 667 in 2014. In 2017, 118 cases were reported. Years with high numbers of reports are driven by outbreaks related to imported and import associated cases, usually in unvaccinated individuals. In 2011, 229 cases largely resulted from cases imported from a sizeable outbreak in France. In 2014, 23 outbreaks occurred, including a large outbreak of 383 cases, mostly among unvaccinated Amish communities in Ohio. Many of the cases in 2014 were associated with cases brought in from the Philippines, which was experiencing a large measles outbreak. In 2015, a large, multistate outbreak was linked to an amusement park in California. While the outbreak likely began with a traveler who became infected abroad and then visited the park while infectious, no source case was identified. However, CDC analysis showed that the virus type in this outbreak was identical to the type that caused the large outbreak in the Philippines in 2014. Most U.S. cases occur in unvaccinated individuals (CDC, 2018d).

These recent outbreaks in the United States highlight the ongoing risk of measles importation from other countries by people who travel and the vulnerability of groups who do not routinely accept immunization, such as people with religious or philosophical objections, students in schools that do not require two doses of vaccine, and infants in areas where immunization coverage is low. The exposure of these groups to an imported case can result in an outbreak of associated cases as in the 2017 outbreak in Hennepin County, Minnesota, among the Somali-American community. A concern about measles immunization linked to autism, a claim without documentation, has resulted in decreasing coverage rates in the United States and abroad, and in this case in conjunction with concern over the autism rates in this community, resulted in dropping immunization rates among children in the Minnesota Somali community. Coverage fell from greater than 90 percent in two-year-olds born in 2004 to 36 percent in those born in 2014. "This outbreak demonstrates the challenge of combating misinformation about MMR vaccine and the importance of creating long-term, trusted relationships with communities to disseminate scientific information in a culturally appropriate and effective manner" (CDC, 2017h).

Healthy People 2020 calls for the reduction, elimination, or maintained elimination of vaccine-preventable diseases, including the reduction of indigenous measles cases. Efforts to meet this goal will require (1) rapid detection of cases and implementation of appropriate outbreak control measures, (2) achievement and maintenance of high levels of vaccination coverage among preschool-age children in all geographic regions, (3) continued implementation and enforcement of the two-dose schedule among young adults, (4) the determination of the source of all outbreaks and sporadic infections, and (5) cooperation among countries in measles control efforts. Nurses receive reports of cases, investigate them, and initiate control measures for outbreaks. They use every opportunity to immunize adolescents and young adults who lack documentation of two doses of measles vaccine. Nurses who work in regions where undocumented residents are common, where groups obtain exemption from immunization on religious grounds or who choose not to vaccinate for philosophical reasons, where preschool coverage is low, and/or where international visitors are frequent need to be especially alert for measles cases and the necessity of prompt outbreak control among particularly susceptible populations.

Rubella

The rubella virus (German measles) causes a mild febrile disease with enlarged lymph nodes and a fine, pink rash that is often difficult to distinguish from measles or scarlet fever. In contrast to measles, rubella is only a moderately contagious illness. Transmission is through inhalation of or direct contact with infected droplets from the respiratory secretions of infected persons. Children may show few or no constitutional symptoms, whereas adults usually experience several days of low-grade fever, headache, malaise, runny nose, and conjunctivitis before the rash appears. Many infections occur without a rash (Heymann, 2015).

For many years, because it caused only a mild illness, rubella was considered to be of minor importance. Then, in 1941 the link between maternal rubella and poor pregnancy outcomes was recognized, and the disease suddenly assumed major public health significance. Rubella infection, in addition to causing intrauterine death and spontaneous abortion, may result in anomalies referred to as congenital rubella syndrome (CRS), affecting single or multiple organ systems. Defects include cataracts, congenital glaucoma, deafness, microcephaly, mental retardation, cardiac abnormalities, and diabetes mellitus. CRS occurs in up to 90 percent of infants born to women who are infected with rubella during the first trimester of pregnancy (Heymann, 2015). During the 1962 to 1965 rubella pandemic, an estimated 12.5 million cases of rubella occurred in the United States, resulting in 2000 cases of encephalitis, 11,250 fetal deaths, 2100 neonatal deaths, and 20,000 infants born with CRS. The economic impact of this epidemic was estimated at $1.5 billion (CDC, 2005).

The United States has established and achieved the goal of eliminating indigenous rubella transmission and CRS. Rubella elimination is defined as the absence of continuous endemic transmission lasting ≥12 months. With the introduction of a vaccine in 1969, cases of rubella in the United States fell precipitously from 57,686 to currently less than 10 cases per year with a large percent of the cases imported or import-linked. Rubella has not been considered endemic in the United States since 2004. All rubella cases have occurred in individuals infected when living or traveling outside the country since 2012. Between 2005 and 2015, only eight babies with CRS have been reported. To maintain rubella elimination, it is important that children and women of childbearing age are vaccinated against rubella (CDC, 2017i).

Rubella remains endemic in many parts of the world and because of international travel and countries without routine rubella vaccination, imported cases of rubella and CRS cases are possible. In 2016, the WHO estimated 22,361 cases in 165 countries, many of them in Asia and Africa where vaccination coverage is lowest, down from the estimated 110,000 in 2012. The WHO also reports that intensive and widespread rubella vaccination efforts have largely eliminated rubella and CRS in many developed and in some developing countries. The WHO Region of the Americas has had no endemic (naturally transmitted) cases of rubella infection since 2009 (WHO, 2018d).

Unimmunized immigrants do not necessarily import disease, but their unimmunized status may leave them vulnerable to infection once they arrive. In addition to a focus on identifying and vaccinating foreign-born adults, the continued elimination of rubella and CRS in the United States will require (1) maintaining high immunization rates among children, (2) ensuring vaccination among women of childbearing age, especially those who are foreign-born, (3) continuing aggressive surveillance, and (4) responding rapidly to any outbreak.

Pertussis

Pertussis (whooping cough) begins as a mild upper respiratory tract infection progressing to an irritating cough that within one to two weeks may become paroxysmal (a series of repeated violent coughs). The repeated coughs occur without intervening breaths and can be followed by a characteristic inspiratory "whoop." Pertussis is caused by the bacterium *Bordetella pertussis* and is transmitted via an airborne route through contact with infected droplets. It is highly contagious and considered endemic in the United States. Infants too young to be immunized and the elderly are the most likely to experience serious disease and death. Vaccination against pertussis, delivered in combination with diphtheria and tetanus, is a part of the routine childhood immunization schedule. Treatment of infected individuals with antibiotics such as erythromycin may shorten the period of communicability but does not relieve symptoms unless given early in the course of the infection. Prophylactic treatment with antibiotics is recommended for family members and close contacts of infected individuals, regardless of immunization status and age, if there is a child in the house under the age of one year or a woman in the last three weeks of pregnancy, or to prevent ongoing transmission within the family. Infection with pertussis does not offer permanent immunity (Heymann, 2015).

Before the development of a whole-cell vaccine, DTP (diphtheria, tetanus, pertussis) in the 1940s, pertussis led to hundreds of thousands of cases and thousands of deaths per year, the majority in children younger than 5 years. After vaccine licensure and the introduction of universal vaccination, reported cases in the United States steadily declined, hitting a record low of just over 1000 in 1976. However, beginning in the early 1980s, pertussis cases began to show cyclical increases, peaking every three to five years with the peaks getting higher and reported cases going up. In 2012, over 48,000 cases were reported, the highest number since 1955 (CDC, 2018e). By 2017, the number of pertussis cases reported had fallen to less than 16,000 with almost half occurring in youth ages 7-19 years (CDC 2018f).

In the mid-2000s the epidemiology of pertussis appears to have changed with incidence increasing in children 7-10 years old, many of whom had been fully vaccinated, suggesting that the acellular vaccine DTaP, introduced in 1997 for the entire childhood series in response to concerns over serious side effects in some children after DTP, may not offer the duration of protection seen with the whole-cell vaccine. Tdap (tetanus, reduced strength diphtheria, acellular pertussis) was licensed in 2005 as a booster for adults in place of their next tetanus vaccination and adolescents, with routine recommendation for immunization at 11-12 years. The reduction in rates in pre-teens 11-12 years old demonstrated immediate protection from Tdap, but increasing incidence in those 13-14 years old suggested waning immunity with no durable protection. While waning immunity may not be completely protective, evidence indicates that boostered individuals when infected will experience milder disease. The downside of mild disease is that this lack of symptoms may have the unintended consequence of making these people excellent inapparent-carriers (CDC, 2012a). Nonetheless, vaccination with DTaP and Tdap continues to be recommended as the single most effective strategy in reducing illness and death from pertussis. Pregnant women and close contacts to their babies are especially encouraged to be vaccinated in an effort to prevent disease in infants, the group most likely to experience severe complications and death. In addition to maintaining high rates of immunization, prevention efforts also included publicizing Tdap, increasing awareness of pertussis in adolescents and adults among providers, and promptly implementing treatment and control in the face of outbreaks (CDC, 2017j).

Since pertussis does have a cyclical pattern with periodic outbreaks, it is important for nurses to work with the community to maintain the highest possible levels of immunization coverage to minimize these occurrences. Because of the contagious nature of pertussis, nurses play a major role in limiting transmission during outbreaks by ensuring appropriate treatment of family members and close contacts.

QSEN FOCUS ON QUALITY AND SAFETY EDUCATION FOR NURSES

Targeted Competency: Safety

Minimizes risk for harm to clients and providers through both system effectiveness and individual performance. Important aspects of safety include the following:

- **Knowledge:** Discuss potential and actual impact of national client safety resources, initiatives, and regulations.
- **Skills:** Use national client safety resources for own professional development and to focus attention on safety in care settings.
- **Attitudes:** Value the relationship between national safety campaigns and implementation to local practices and practice settings.

Safety Question

Pertussis has become an increasing infectious disease concern.

1. Look into local statistics around pertussis occurrence. Has there been an increased occurrence of pertussis over the past 5 years?
2. How do your local statistics compare to national statistics for pertussis from the Centers for Disease Control and Prevention?
3. What might be some system approaches to educating your community about the risk of pertussis?
4. What might be some system approaches to providing pertussis vaccinations to the appropriate populations?
5. What data points will you want to track to assess whether your interventions have been effective?

Prepared by Gail Armstrong, PhD, DNP, ACNS-BC, CNE

Influenza

Influenza is a viral respiratory tract infection often indistinguishable from the common cold or other respiratory diseases. Transmission is airborne and through direct contact with infected droplets. Unlike many viruses that do not survive long in the environment, the flu virus is thought to exist for many hours in dried mucus. Outbreaks are common in the winter and early spring in areas where people gather indoors such as in schools and nursing homes. Gastrointestinal and respiratory symptoms are common. Because symptoms do not always follow a characteristic pattern, many viral diseases that are not influenza are often called flu. The most important factors to note about influenza are its epidemic nature and the mortality that may result from pulmonary complications, especially in older adults and children less than two years of age (Heymann, 2015).

There are four types of influenza viruses: A, B, C, and D. Type A is usually responsible for large epidemics, whereas outbreaks from type B are more regionalized; type C epidemics are sporadic, less common, and usually result in only mild illness. Influenza D is seen primarily in cattle and not known to infect people. Influenza viruses often change in the nature of their surface appearance or their antigenic makeup. Types B and C are fairly stable viruses, but type A changes constantly. Minor antigenic changes are referred to as antigenic drift, and they result in yearly epidemics and regional outbreaks. Major changes such as the emergence of new subtypes are called antigenic shift; these occur only with type A viruses. Antigenic shift and drift lead to epidemic outbreaks every few years and pandemic outbreaks every 10 to 40 years as seen with novel influenza A H1N1 in 2009. Mortality rates associated with epidemics may or may not be higher than those in non-epidemic situations.

The preparation of influenza vaccine each year is based on the best possible prediction of what type and variant of virus will be most prevalent that year. Because of the changing nature of the virus, yearly immunization is necessary and in the United States is given in early fall before the flu season begins. In recent history, if vaccine were available, immunization for seasonal flu was particularly recommended for children ages 6 months up to 19 years, pregnant women, people 50 years of age and older, people of any age with certain chronic medical conditions, people who live in nursing homes and other long-term care facilities, and people who live with or care for those at risk for complications from flu. During the 2009-2010 influenza season, pandemic novel influenza A H1N1 replaced other seasonal flu viruses as the predominant circulating virus, and the recommended priority groups shifted from seniors to the young; high school students and pregnant women seemed particularly hard hit, whereas those over 65 appeared to perhaps have some degree of protection. For the 2010-2011 flu season, novel influenza A H1N1 was added to the vaccine, and the ACIP recommended universal coverage for everyone ages six months and older, a recommendation that continues (CDC, 2018g).

Flu immunizations, when matched appropriately with circulating virus strains, are estimated to provide 70 percent to 90 percent protection against infection in healthy young adults; although they do not always prevent infection, they do result in milder disease symptoms. There are now a variety of trivalent and quadrivalent vaccines available, including one that is not grown in eggs for those with egg sensitivity and a high-dose one approved for people 65 and over. Although influenza is often self-limiting in the healthy population, serious complications, particularly viral and bacterial pneumonias, can be deadly to older adults, children under two years of age, and those debilitated by chronic disease. When appropriate, it is important to couple influenza immunization of this population with immunization against pneumococcal pneumonia.

The use of influenza antiviral drugs should be considered in the non-immunized or groups at high risk for complications. Evidence also suggests that antivirals can decrease the number of deaths in hospitalized influenza patients. The neuraminidase inhibitors (oseltamivir, zanamivir) have activity against influenza A and B viruses. The adamantanes (amantadine, rimantadine) have activity only against influenza A viruses and are not recommended for use at this time in the United States because of resistance. There have been incidences, worldwide and in the United States, of H1N1 virus resistance to oseltamivir. Current guidelines indicate antiviral treatment should be guided by surveillance data on circulating viruses and confirmatory testing of viral subgroups. CDC annually publishes *Recommendations for Influenza Antiviral Medications* (CDC, 2018h). Read more about influenza at http://www.cdc.gov.

Healthy People 2020 targets increasing the proportion of the population vaccinated annually against influenza and pneumococcal disease. Nurses often spearhead influenza immunization campaigns that target older adults. Examples include conducting flu clinics at polling places during elections or at community centers and churches during "senior vaccination Sundays." Inhabitants of residences and nursing homes for older adults are at risk, since influenza can spread rapidly with severe consequences through such living arrangements. As with children, nurses should check immunization history and encourage immunization for every older adult encountered in a clinic or home visit.

But while children, the elderly and those with health conditions that put them at high risk for complications have traditionally been targets for immunizations, new strains of influenza such as H1N1 have more seriously affected young adults, leading to the recommendation that everyone over six months of age receive flu immunization. Nurses not only can promote this message, they can provide an example by choosing immunization as well. The CDC estimates that in the flu season of 2015-2016, 79 percent of health care providers were immunized against flu, and while this is higher than the general population who were at closer to 40 percent, it is far from the *Healthy People 2020* goal of 90 percent. When nurses get immunized against influenza, they are protecting not only themselves but their patients (CDC, 2016b).

Pandemic Novel Influenza A (H1N1). Novel influenza A H1N1, a new flu virus that quickly reached pandemic proportions, was first recognized in Mexico and the United States in the spring of 2009. Originally called swine flu, the virus is of swine origins but does not spread from swine to people. Instead, it is transmitted rapidly and easily from person to person and in some cases is suspected to have spread from humans to swine as well as other animals such as dogs, cats, and ferrets. Because the virus was new, the population lacked immunity, and visitors to Mexico quickly became infected and carried it to people around the globe. By June of 2009 more than 70 countries had reported cases of novel H1N1 infection, and ongoing community level outbreaks of novel H1N1 occurred in multiple parts of the world, prompting the WHO to declare a global pandemic. This action reflected the spread of the new H1N1 virus, not the severity of illness caused by the virus.

Although novel H1N1 appeared to spread in the same manner as seasonal influenza viruses, the groups most affected were children, young adults (especially those with underlying chronic disease), and pregnant women, as opposed to seniors who are the usual targets of seasonal flu but were thought in this case to perhaps have some degree of immunity. Initial reports made it appear that the virus inflicted a high case fatality rate, but as surveillance strengthened and expanded, this did not prove to be the case; however, by the end of the year, pediatric deaths were higher than in previous years and pediatric hospitalizations higher than other age groups. The majority of 2009 novel H1N1 deaths occurred in people between the ages of 50 and 64 years of age, 80 percent of whom had an underlying health condition (CDC, 2010b).

With the identification of the virus, the scramble was on for a vaccine, which became available in the fall of 2009 in limited doses and was initially targeted to priority groups, including those 6 months to 24 years of age, caretakers, infants less than 6 months of age, pregnant women, adults 25 to 64 years of age with chronic conditions, health care providers, and first responders. Initial demand for vaccine was high, but since the virus did not appear to prove overall any more frightening than seasonal flu and more vaccine came on the market, the available supply was more than enough for anyone who wished to be immunized. The delivery of the vaccine, in addition to seasonal flu vaccine, proved a planning and logistical challenge to the public health system, demanded considerable resources, and provided a valuable exercise in implementation of preparedness strategies. Nurses were at the forefront of this expansive operation by planning for, scheduling, and immunizing—in a variety of community settings, schools, and clinics—a large portion of the population, including two doses to children. During the summer of 2009, novel H1N1 outbreaks extended the normal flu season far beyond the usual period and dominated reported circulating flu viruses from the Southern Hemisphere as well. Activity peaked at the end of October in the United States, but novel H1N1 continued into 2010 as the dominant circulating strain. Resistance to antiviral neuraminidase inhibitors was reported but remained low, and the vast majority of 2009 H1N1 viruses tested did not appear to change significantly, remaining related to the A/California/7/2009 H1N1 reference virus selected by the WHO as the 2009 H1N1 vaccine virus. An H1N1 component was included in the 2010 seasonal vaccine (CDC, 2010c). H1N1 returned as the predominant strain seen during the 2013-2014 and 2015-2016 flu seasons.

Avian Influenza A (H5N1 and H7N9). Disease caused by influenza type A viruses in birds is referred to as avian flu. Naturally occurring in wild aquatic birds worldwide, these viruses can infect domestic poultry and other bird and animal species. Avian flu viruses do not normally infect humans. However, sporadic human infections with avian flu viruses have occurred. In 1997 in Hong Kong, the first known cases of human illness associated with an avian influenza type A virus H5N1 were reported. Referred to in the press as Hong Kong bird flu, this virus appeared to have been transmitted to people through contact with infected poultry. As a result of this association, Hong Kong officials ordered the slaughter of all chickens in and around Hong Kong with a resulting halt in the spread of disease. No cases were reported outside Hong Kong and, despite recurring outbreaks of avian flu in poultry, no further H5N1 virus activity in humans was reported (CDC, 1998). This situation changed dramatically in late 2003 and early 2004 when H5N1 outbreaks occurred among poultry, people, and, in some cases, other animals in nine Asian countries. And unlike the earlier situation in Hong Kong, these outbreaks have not disappeared but only subsided to again reappear. As of the beginning of 2018, human infections with H5N1 have been reported from 16 different countries with some fatality rates as high as 70 percent. The largest numbers have been reported from Indonesia, Egypt, and Vietnam. Canada has reported one case. To date, there have been no reports of highly pathogenic avian influenza H5N1 virus infections among wild birds, poultry, other animals, or humans in the United States (WHO, 2018e).

An unanswered question is whether there are actually many more unidentified human cases because of symptoms not severe enough to recognize. Most of the reported cases have resulted from contact with infected poultry, but it is believed that a few limited cases of human-to-human transmission have occurred. So far, the documented spread from human to human has been rare and not sustained, but because influenza viruses have the ability to change, concern exists among scientists that H5N1 may modify to the point where people could easily infect each other; also, because H5N1 does not usually infect humans, they would have little immune protection. Such a change could give rise to pandemic influenza with a virus that appears to exact a high toll in human lives. Given this possibility, surveillance becomes of utmost importance, and close attention is paid to H5N1 virus activity among poultry and humans in Asia, Europe, and North Africa. Vaccine development efforts are under way and, although licensed in some countries, are not yet generally available (CDC, 2018i).

Human infections with Asian lineage avian influenza A H7N9 were first reported from China in March 2013, and annual epidemics of sporadic H7N9 human infections in China have been reported since that time. China is currently experiencing its sixth epidemic of Asian H7N9 human infections with only one reported human infection since October 1, 2017. During the fifth epidemic, from October 1, 2016, through September 30, 2017, 766 human infections were reported, making it the largest H7N9 epidemic to date. As of December 7, 2017, 1565 total human infections with Asian lineage H7N9 had been reported by the WHO since 2013. About 39 percent of people confirmed with the H7N9 infection died. Like influenza A H5N1, most of the reported cases have been associated with contact with infected poultry, but a few cases of limited human-to-human transmission have occurred (CDC, 2018j).

Along with seasonal and novel influenza viruses, CDC works with global and domestic partners to improve control and prevention of avian influenza viruses and to improve influenza pandemic preparedness and response. The response focuses on (1) building surveillance and response capacity; (2) monitoring and assessing viruses and illness; (3) improving vaccines and other interventions; and (4) applying research to enhance prevention and control policies and programs. Read more about avian influenza A viruses at the CDC website: https://www.cdc.gov.

FOODBORNE AND WATERBORNE DISEASES

In recent years the headlines have been full of stories related to foodborne illness associated with peanut butter, cookie dough, spinach, lettuce, tomatoes, chili peppers, strawberries, raspberries, oysters, uncooked eggs, poultry and hamburger, raw milk, unpasteurized apple cider, and so forth. Cans of beef stew suspected to be contaminated with botulism have been pulled off grocery store shelves, and the term *mad cow disease* has entered the popular vocabulary. Recalls of food products have become a common occurrence. Highly centralized production and processing systems using food produced in far-reaching areas and marketed through widespread distribution networks increase the potential for any contamination to result in large-scale, multistate outbreaks. One incident of contamination may affect hundreds of people across the country and result in numerous deaths. Anyone can acquire foodborne illness, regardless of socioeconomic status, race, sex, age, occupation, education, or area of residence, but the very young, old, and debilitated are most susceptible and bear the highest burden of morbidity and mortality.

In 2010, the CDC developed new lower than previously estimated but more precise estimates for foodborne illness suggesting that in the United States, as many as 1 in 6 Americans (or 48 million people) gets sick, 128,000 are hospitalized, and 3000 die from foodborne illnesses each year, most the result of unidentified agents (Scallen et al., 2011). These estimates were the first since 1999 and are currently in use (CDC, 2016c). Known pathogens cause an estimated 9.4 million foodborne illnesses annually in the United States. Because their presentations are often not clinically distinctive and frequently self-limiting, single cases of foodborne illness may be difficult to identify. Affected individuals in single cases or in outbreak situations may not see a physician or are treated presumptively and not tested. In either case, the illness goes unreported, resulting in statistics that underestimate the true magnitude of the problem.

The Foodborne Diseases Active Surveillance Network (FoodNet) is a CDC sentinel surveillance system targeting 10 sites across the country and collecting information from laboratories on disease caused by nine enteric pathogens transmitted commonly through food. It is a collaborative effort among the CDC, the USDA, and the FDA. FoodNet is the principal foodborne disease component of CDC's Emerging Infections Program. In 2017, FoodNet received reports of 24,484 illnesses, 5677 hospitalizations, and 122 deaths, largely caused by *Salmonella* and *Campylobacter* (CDC, 2018k).

Confirmed foodborne outbreaks are reported by states to the CDC through the Foodborne Disease Outbreak Surveillance System. In 2015, there were 902 foodborne disease outbreaks reported, resulting in 15,202 illnesses, 950 hospitalizations, 15 deaths, and 20 food product recalls. Of single-etiology outbreaks, norovirus was the most common cause, resulting in 164 (37 percent) outbreaks and 3893 (39 percent) illnesses. *Salmonella* was the second most common cause, accounting for 149 (34 percent) outbreaks and 3944 (39 percent) illnesses, followed by Shiga toxin-producing *E. coli*, which led to 27 (6 percent) confirmed outbreaks and 302 (3 percent) illnesses. Fish (34 outbreaks), chicken (22), and pork (19) were the most common single food categories implicated. The most outbreak-associated illnesses were from seeded vegetables (e.g., cucumbers or tomatoes, 1121 illnesses), pork (924), and leafy vegetables (383). Of outbreaks reporting a single location of preparation (469/60 percent), restaurants, most commonly those with sit-down dining (373/48 percent) were the most frequently reported locations of food preparation associated with outbreaks (CDC, 2017k). Learn more about the Foodborne Disease Outbreak Surveillance System at http://www.cdc.gov.

The ability to identify multistate outbreaks has been greatly enhanced through technology now routinely used in public health laboratories (serotyping and pulsed-field gel electrophoresis) and the rapid sharing of this information among public health officials through PulseNet, the national molecular subtyping network for foodborne disease surveillance. Since 1996, this DNA finger printing has allowed the detection of thousands of individual and multistate outbreaks, including people sickened from eating *Salmonella* contaminated peanut butter, tomatoes, and cantaloupes, *E. coli* in leafy vegetables, and *Vibrio parahaemolyticus* in oysters. Learn more about PulseNet at http://www.cdc.gov.

The CDC recommends three goals in achieving food safety: (1) control or eliminate pathogens in domestic and imported food, (2) reduce or prevent contamination during growing, harvesting, and processing, and (3) continue the education of restaurant workers and consumers about risks and prevention measures. Also noted is the need for continued efforts to understand how contamination of fresh produce and processed foods occurs and to develop and implement measures that reduce it.

Foodborne illness, or "food poisoning," as it is erroneously but commonly called, is often categorized as either infection or intoxication. Food infection results from bacterial, viral, or parasitic infection of food by pathogens such as *Salmonella, Campylobacter,* hepatitis A, *Toxoplasma,* and *Trichinella.* Food intoxication is caused by toxins produced by bacterial growth, chemical contaminants (heavy metals), and a variety of disease-producing substances found naturally in certain foods such as mushrooms and some seafood. Examples of food intoxications are botulism, mercury poisoning, and paralytic shellfish poisoning. Table 14.4 presents some of the most common agents of food intoxication and their incubation period, source, symptoms, and pathology. Although it is not a hard-and-fast rule, food infections are associated with incubation periods of 12 hours to several days after ingestion of the infected food, whereas intoxications become obvious within minutes to hours after ingestion. Botulism is a clear exception to this rule, with an incubation period up to several days or more in adults. Possessing a potent preformed toxin, capable of producing severe intoxication resulting in flaccid paralysis and death if not identified and treated early, *C. botulinum* is one of the organisms considered a strong candidate for a weapon of bioterrorism (Heymann, 2015).

The Role of Safe Food Preparation

Protecting the nation's food supply from contamination by virulent microbes is a multifaceted issue that is and will continue to be incredibly costly, controversial, and time consuming to address. The specter of terrorist threats to the food supply adds an additional layer of complexity. However, much foodborne illness, regardless of causal organism, can easily be prevented through simple changes in food preparation, handling, and storage. Common errors include (1) cross-contamination of food during preparation, (2) insufficient cooking or reheating temperatures, (3) holding cooked food or storing food at temperatures that promote growth of pathogens and/or formation of toxins, and (4) poor personal hygiene. Because these measures are so important in preventing foodborne disease, *Healthy People 2020* has continued to include an objective directed toward them. The CDC food safety campaign reduces keeping food at home safe to four, easy to remember, steps: clean, separate, cook, and chill, presented in Box 14.4. Read more about preventing foodborne illness at the CDC website on Food Safety at https://www.cdc.gov.

TABLE 14.4 Commonly Encountered Food Intoxications

Causal Agent	Incubation Period	Duration	Clinical Presentation	Associated Food
Staphylococcus aureus	30 min to 7 hr	1-2 days	Sudden onset of nausea, cramps, vomiting, and prostration, often accompanied by diarrhea; rarely fatal	All foods, especially those likely to come into contact with food-handlers' hands that may be contaminated from infections of the eyes and skin
Clostridium perfringens (strain A)	6-24 hr	1 day or less	Sudden onset of colic and diarrhea, maybe nausea; vomiting and fever unusual; rarely fatal	Inadequately heated meats or stews; food contaminated by soil or feces becomes infective when improper storage or reheating allows multiplication of organism
Vibrio parahaemolyticus	4-96 hr	1-7 days	Watery diarrhea and abdominal cramps; sometimes nausea, vomiting, fever, headache; rarely fatal	Raw or inadequately cooked seafood; period of time at room temperature usually required for multiplication of organism
Clostridium botulinum	12-36 hr, sometimes days	Slow recovery, maybe months	Central nervous system signs; blurred vision, difficulty in swallowing and dry mouth, followed by descending symmetrical flaccid paralysis in an alert person; "floppy baby" in infant; fatality <15 percent with antitoxin and respiratory support	Home-canned fruits and vegetables that have not been preserved with adequate heating; infants have become infected from ingesting honey

Based on information from Heymann DL, editor: *Control of communicable diseases manual,* ed. 20, Washington, DC, 2015, American Public Health Association.

BOX 14.4 CDC Four Steps to Food Safety

1. CLEAN: Wash your hands and surfaces often.
2. SEPARATE: Don't cross-contaminate.
3. COOK: To the right temperature.
4. CHILL: Refrigerate promptly.

CDC, Centers for Disease Control and Prevention.
From Centers for Disease Control and Prevention: Four steps to food safety, 2018. Available at https://wwwn.cdc.gov.

Salmonellosis

Salmonellosis is a bacterial disease characterized by sudden onset of headache, abdominal pain, diarrhea, nausea, sometimes vomiting, and almost always fever. Onset is typically within 48 hours of ingestion, but the clinical signs are impossible to distinguish from other causes of gastrointestinal distress. Diarrhea and lack of appetite may persist for several days, and dehydration may be severe. Although morbidity can be significant, death is uncommon except among infants, older adults, and the debilitated. The rate of infection is highest among infants and small children. It is estimated that only a small proportion of cases are recognized clinically and that only one percent of clinical cases are reported. The number of *Salmonella* infections yearly may actually be in the millions (Heymann, 2015).

Salmonella outbreaks occur commonly in restaurants, hospitals, nursing homes, and institutions for children. The transmission route is eating food derived from an infected animal or contaminated by feces of an infected animal or person. Unchlorinated municipal water supplies have also been implicated in *Salmonella* outbreaks. Raw or undercooked meat and meat products; raw or undercooked poultry; uncooked eggs; unpasteurized milk and dairy products; and contaminated produce are the foods most often associated with salmonellosis. Recent large outbreaks have been linked with eating tomatoes, cucumbers, jalapeño peppers, and peanut butter. Meat and poultry may be contaminated during preparation or cross-contaminate food being prepared with them. Improper food preparation temperatures (cooking and holding) and cross-contamination appear to be the biggest risk factors for food-associated outbreaks. Animals are the common reservoir for the various *Salmonella* serotypes, although infected humans may also fill this role. Animals are more likely to be chronic carriers. Reptiles such as iguanas have been implicated as *Salmonella* carriers along with pet turtles, poultry, cattle, swine, rodents, dogs, and cats. People have also been infected by handling *Salmonella*-contaminated dry dog food and treats. Person-to-person transmission is an important consideration in daycare and institutional settings (Heymann, 2015).

Enterohemorrhagic *Escherichia coli* (EHEC or *E. coli* 0157:H7)

Escherichia coli 0157:H7 belongs to the enterohemorrhagic category of *E. coli* serotypes producing a strong cytotoxin called a Shiga toxin and are collectively known as Shiga toxin–producing *E. coli* (STEC). *E. coli* serotypes in this group can cause a potentially fatal hemorrhagic colitis. This pathogen was first widely described in humans in 1992 following the investigation of two outbreaks of illness associated with consumption of hamburger from a fast-food restaurant chain. Transmission is through ingestion of food contaminated by infected feces. Ruminants, particularly cattle, are the most important reservoir, although humans may also serve as a source for person-to-person transmission. Undercooked hamburger has been implicated in several outbreaks, as have flour, alfalfa sprouts, melons, lettuce, uncooked spinach, unpasteurized milk and apple cider, municipal water, and person-to-person transmission in daycare centers, homes, and institutions. Recent large outbreaks have been associated with romaine lettuce, flour, and petting zoos. Infection with *E. coli* 0157:H7 causes bloody diarrhea, abdominal cramps, and, infrequently, fever. Children and older adults are at highest risk for clinical disease and complications. Hemolytic uremic syndrome (HUS) is seen in about 15 percent of cases among children and a smaller number of adults and may result in acute renal failure. The case fatality rate for infection that results in HUS can be as great as five percent (Heymann, 2015).

Hamburger often appears to be involved in outbreaks because the grinding process exposes pathogens on the surface of the whole meat to the interior of the ground meat, effectively mixing the once-exterior bacteria thoroughly throughout the hamburger so that searing the surface no longer suffices to kill all bacteria. Tracking the contamination is complicated by the fact that hamburger is often made of meat ground from several sources. The best protection against this pathogen, as with most foodborne agents, is to thoroughly cook food before eating it.

Waterborne Disease Outbreaks and Pathogens

Provision of safe water in the United States is vital to protecting public health. The delivery of clean drinking water via municipal water supply was one of the major public health achievements of the twentieth century. Waterborne pathogens may enter water supplies through animal or human fecal contamination and frequently cause enteric disease. They include viruses, bacteria, and protozoans. Hepatitis A virus is probably the most publicized waterborne viral agent, although other viruses may also be transmitted by this route (enteroviruses, rotaviruses, and paramyxoviruses). In countries without well-functioning municipal and community water systems, the most important waterborne bacterial diseases are cholera, typhoid fever, and bacillary dysentery. Other *Salmonella* spp. as well as *Shigella, Vibrio,* and *Campylobacter* species and various coliform bacteria, including *E. coli* 0157:H7 may be transmitted in the same manner along with waterborne protozoans such as *Entamoeba histolytica* (amoebic dysentery) and *Giardia lamblia.* Drinking water also may be contaminated by chemicals or toxins such as those seen with algae bloom.

In the United States in recent years, species of the bacteria *Legionella* and the one-celled parasite *Cryptosporidium parvum* have frequently been implicated in drinking water outbreaks. In 1993, a diarrheal outbreak crippled the city of Milwaukee and pushed *Cryptosporidium* into the debate over how to best safeguard municipal water supplies. Protozoans do not respond to traditional chlorine treatment as do enteric and coliform bacteria, and their small size requires special filtration. During 2013-2014, 42 drinking water outbreaks were reported, resulting in at least 1006 cases of illness, 124 hospitalizations, and 13 deaths. *Legionella* was associated with 57 percent of these outbreaks and all of the deaths. Sixty-nine percent of the reported illnesses occurred in four outbreaks of which the cause was determined to be either a chemical or toxin or the parasite *Cryptosporidium* (CDC, 2017l).

The CDC defines a waterborne disease and outbreak (WBDO) as an incident in which two or more persons experience similar illness after consuming water that epidemiologic evidence implicates as the source of that illness. Recreational water and other water not intended for drinking as well as drinking water may be involved in waterborne outbreaks. Facilities with inadequate chlorination and pools allowing diapered children pose particular risk for infection, as does drinking water without adequate disinfection while hiking and camping in the backcountry.

Since 1971, the CDC, the U.S. Environmental Protection Agency (EPA), and the Council of State and Territorial Epidemiologists have maintained a collaborative Waterborne Disease and Outbreaks Surveillance System (WDOSS) for collecting and reporting data related to occurrences and causes of WBDOs. This surveillance system is the primary source of data concerning the scope and effects of WBDOs in the United States. In 2009, the CDC and the EPA, in collaboration with public health jurisdictions, implemented electronic reporting through the National Outbreak Reporting System (NORS).

VECTOR-BORNE DISEASES

Vector-borne diseases refer to illnesses for which the infectious agent is transmitted by a carrier, or vector, which is usually an arthropod (mosquito, tick, fly), either biologically or mechanically. With biological transmission, the vector is necessary for the developmental stage of the infectious agent. Examples include the mosquitoes that carry Zika virus and the fleas that transmit plague. Mechanical transmission occurs when an insect simply contacts the infectious agent with its legs or mouth parts and carries it to the host. For example, flies and cockroaches may contaminate food or cooking utensils. Most vector-borne diseases involve zoonotic cycles requiring some sort of animal host or reservoir.

Diseases from mosquito and tick bites occur in every state. Disease cases from mosquito, tick, and flea bites tripled in the United States from 2004 to 2016 with more than 640,000 cases reported. During this same period, diseases caused by nine new organisms spread by bites from infected mosquitoes and ticks were discovered or introduced into the United States, including Zika, chikungunya, and Heartland virus. Reasons for the increase are not clear as the life cycles of these organisms are very complex but may include improved reporting and warmer temperatures. The CDC finds that the recent outbreaks of Zika, chikungunya, and West Nile viruses and the increase in Lyme disease cases illustrate the need at both the state and local levels to build comprehensive vector-borne disease prevention and control programs equipped with better tools and staffed by those with greater expertise (CDC, 2018l).

Vector-borne diseases commonly encountered in the United States are those associated with ticks, such as Lyme disease *(B. burgdorferi)*, Rocky Mountain spotted fever (RMSF; *Rickettsia rickettsii*), ehrlichiosis *(Ehrlichia* spp.*)*, and anaplasmosis *(Anaplasma phagocytophilum)*, formerly known as human granulocytic ehrlichiosis. Other more rarely seen tick-associated diseases include babesiosis (*B. microti*), tularemia (*F. tularensis*), Q fever (*Coxiella burnetii*), and Southern tick-associated rash illness (STARI), a recently described illness for which the causative organism has not been determined. Nurses who work with large immigrant populations or with international travelers may encounter along with Zika and chikungunya, malaria and dengue fever, all carried by mosquitos but rarely transmitted in the United States. West Nile virus is an example of the endemic mosquito-borne viruses that include St. Louis, La Crosse, and western and eastern equine encephalitis. Plague (*Y. pestis*) is carried by fleas of wild rodents.

Lyme Disease

Parents in Lyme, CT, concerned about the unusual incidence of juvenile rheumatoid arthritis in their children, were the first to bring attention to this tick-borne infection that now bears their town's name. First described in 1975, Lyme disease became a nationally notifiable disease in 1991 and is now the most commonly reported vector-borne disease in the United States, with over 36,000 confirmed and probable cases reported to CDC in 2016. However, studies based on positive laboratory reports and insurance claims suggest that the actual number of diagnosed cases may be around 300,000, making Lyme disease a major public health problem with an urgent need for improved prevention (Kuehn, 2013). The causative agent, the spirochete *B. burgdorferi*, was identified in 1982. Lyme disease is transmitted by ixodid ticks that are associated with white-tailed deer *(Odocoileus virginianus)* and the white-footed mouse *(Peromyscus leucopus)*. Lyme disease usually occurs in summer during tick season, and it has been reported throughout the United States, with 95 percent of cases concentrated in rural and suburban areas of the northeast, mid-Atlantic, and north-central states, particularly Wisconsin and Minnesota.

The clinical spectrum of Lyme disease can be divided into three stages. Stage I is characterized by erythema chronicum migrans, a distinctive skin lesion often called a bull's-eye lesion because it begins as a red area at the site of the tick attachment that spreads outward in a ring-like fashion as the center clears. About 50 percent to 70 percent of infected persons develop this lesion 3 to 30 days after a tick bite. The skin lesion may be accompanied or preceded by fever, fatigue, malaise, headache, muscle pains, and a stiff neck, as well as tender and enlarged lymph nodes and migratory joint pain. Most clients diagnosed in this early stage respond well to 10 to 14 days of amoxicillin or doxycycline.

If not treated during this first stage, Lyme disease can progress to stage II, which may include additional skin lesions, headache, and neurological and cardiac abnormalities. Clients who progress to stage III have recurrent attacks of arthritis and arthralgia, especially in the knees, which may begin months to years after the initial lesion. The clinical diagnosis of classic Lyme disease with the distinctive skin lesion is straightforward. Illness without the lesion is more difficult to diagnose, because serological tests are more accurate in stages II and III than in stage I (Heymann, 2015).

Rocky Mountain Spotted Fever

RMSF has been a nationally notifiable condition since the 1920s. As of January 1, 2010, cases of RMSF are reported under a new category called Spotted Fever Rickettsiosis (SFR). This category captures cases of RMSF, *Rickettsia parkeri*, rickettsiosis, Pacific Coast tick fever, and rickettsialpox. The change reflects the inability to differentiate between spotted fever group Rickettsia species using commonly available serological tests. Contrary to its name, RMSF is seldom seen in the Rocky Mountains, and over 60 percent of cases are reported from five states: North Carolina, Oklahoma, Arkansas, Tennessee, and Missouri. The infectious agent is *R. rickettsii*. The tick vector varies according to geographic region. The dog tick, *Dermacentor variabilis,* is the vector in the eastern and southern United States.

RMSF is not transmitted from person to person. It is thought that one attack confers lifelong immunity. Clinical signs include sudden onset of moderate to high fever, severe headache, chills, deep muscle pain, and malaise. About 50 percent of cases experience a rash on the extremities that spreads to most of the body. Many cases of what has been referred to as "spotless" RMSF may actually be caused by recently identified forms of human ehrlichiosis, another tick-borne infection. RMSF responds readily to treatment with tetracyclines. Definitive diagnosis can be made with paired serum titers. Because early treatment is important in decreasing morbidity and mortality, treatment should be started in response to clinical and epidemiologic considerations rather than waiting for laboratory confirmation. Doxycycline is the recommended antibiotic treatment for RMSF in adults and children of all ages (Heymann, 2015).

Prevention and Control of Tick-Borne Diseases

In *Healthy People 2020,* the *HP2010* objective for reducing Lyme disease has been archived because of lack of proven interventions to prevent transmission. A vaccine for Lyme disease, recommended for use by persons living in high-risk areas, was licensed in 1998; however, in 2002 the manufacturer withdrew it from the commercial market because of low demand and sales. Measures for preventing exposure to ticks include reducing tick populations, avoiding tick-infested areas, wearing protective clothing when outdoors (long sleeves and long pants tucked into socks), using repellants, and immediately inspecting for and removing ticks when returning indoors. The CDC reports that landscaping modifications such as removing brush and leaf litter or creating a buffer zone of wood chips or gravel between yard and forest may reduce exposure to ticks as well as appropriate pesticide application to lawns. Ticks require a prolonged period of attachment (6-48 hours) before they start blood-feeding on the host; prompt tick discovery and removal can help prevent transmission of disease. Ticks should be removed with steady, gentle traction on tweezers applied to the head parts of the tick. The tick's body should not be squeezed during the removal process to avoid infection that could be transmitted from resultant tick feces and tissue juices (Heymann, 2015). When outdoors, permethrin sprayed on clothing and tick repellents on bare skin containing 20 percent to 30 percent diethyltoluamide (DEET) can offer effective protection; use of DEET should be avoided on children less than two years of age because of reports of significant toxicity, including skin irritation, anaphylaxis, and seizures. Read more about tick-associated diseases and the prevention of tick-associated diseases on the Lyme Disease Resources CDC website, https://www.cdc.gov.

DISEASES OF TRAVELERS

Individuals traveling outside the United States need to be aware of and take precautions against potential diseases to which they may be exposed. Which diseases and what precautions depend on the individual's health status, the destination, the reason for travel, and the length of travel. Persons who plan to travel in remote regions for an extended period may need to consider rare diseases and take special precautions that would not apply to the average traveler. Consultation with public health officials can provide specific health information and recommendations for a given situation. Nurses often staff public health travel clinics and provide this information based on CDC recommendations. The CDC offers a wide variety of information for both medical professionals and travelers at their Travelers' Health webpage, including the Yellow Book, *CDC Health Information for International Travel,* which in addition to being available online, can be ordered in hard copy or accessed from mobile devices. To read more about travelers' health, consult the CDC website https://wwwnc.cdc.gov.

On return from visiting exotic places, travelers may bring back with them an unplanned souvenir in the form of disease. Therefore, in a presenting client, it is important to ask about a history of travel. Even the apparently healthy returned traveler, especially one who was in a tropical country for some time, should undergo routine screening to rule out acquired infections. Likewise, refugees and immigrants may arrive with infectious disease problems ranging from helminthic infections to diseases of major public health significance, such as TB, malaria, Zika virus, cholera, HIV disease, and hepatitis. Nurses may find themselves dealing with these diseases, since refugees and immigrants, especially the undocumented, are often treated through the public health system.

CHECK YOUR PRACTICE

Zika Virus and Pregnancy

A pregnant woman visits your clinic for her regular prenatal visit. She mentions to you that her husband has just returned from visiting with his family in South America for several weeks. What should you do?

Malaria

Caused by the bloodborne parasite *Plasmodium,* malaria is a potentially fatal disease characterized by regular cycles of fever and chills. Transmission is through the bite of an infected *Anopheles* mosquito. The word *malaria* is based on an association between the illness and the "bad air" of the marshes where the mosquitoes breed. Malaria is an old disease that appears in recorded history in 2700 BC China. Although no longer endemic in most temperate countries, worldwide, malaria is the most prevalent vector-borne disease, occurring in over 100 countries and territories. Half of the world's population is considered at risk; 90 percent of cases occur in Africa. Malaria is the fifth-leading cause of infectious disease death worldwide and the second-leading cause of infectious disease death (after HIV disease) in Africa. Currently, there is no vaccine available to prevent malaria, although several are in development. Mosquirix, an injectable vaccine that provides partial protection against malaria in young children will begin piloting in three countries in sub-Saharan Africa in 2018. If successful, this immunization would become a complementary malaria control tool that potentially could be added to, not replace, the core package of WHO-recommended preventive, diagnostic, and treatment measures (WHO, 2018f).

The decline in malaria cases and deaths seen since 2000 is considered a major public health achievement. However, in 2016, 91 countries reported a total of 216 million cases of malaria, an increase of 5 million cases over the previous year, and 445,000 deaths, about the same number reported in 2015. In the 2017 World Malaria Report, WHO officials voice concern that the once steady decline in cases has stalled and even reversed in some regions since 2014, with a similar pattern seen in mortality rates. Challenges included drug resistance, funding, access to care, and insecticide resistance (WHO, 2017).

Malaria prevention depends largely on protection against mosquitoes and appropriate chemoprophylaxis. The best means of protection for travelers is antimalarial medication. Drug resistance is an increasing problem in combating malaria. Of the five *Plasmodium* species causing human malaria, *P. vivax*, the predominant strain in Asia and Latin America is increasingly drug resistant, and *P. falciparum*, the predominant strain seen in Africa and which causes the most serious disease, is highly drug resistant. Decisions about antimalarial drugs must be tailored individually on the basis of the type of malaria in the specific area of the country to be visited, the purpose of the trip, and the length of the visit. The CDC and the WHO publish guides on the status of malaria and recommendations for prophylaxis on a country-by-country basis. At this time, there is no one drug or drug combination known to be safe and efficacious in preventing all types of malaria. Antimalarials are generally started a week to several weeks before leaving the country and are continued for four to six weeks after returning.

Despite appropriate prophylaxis, malaria may still be contracted. Travelers should be advised of this fact and urged to seek immediate medical care if they exhibit symptoms of cyclical fever and chills up to one year after returning home. Immigrants and visitors from areas where malaria is endemic may become clinically ill after entering the United States. About 1500 cases of malaria in travelers and immigrants are reported in the United States every year. And while malaria is eliminated from the United States, the *Anopheles* mosquito vector in southern states is not, so local cases can still occur if these vector mosquitoes bite people infected outside the country. The last outbreak of locally transmitted malaria involved eight individuals in Florida in 2003 (CDC, 2018m). For more information about malaria in the United States as well as worldwide, visit the malaria homepage at the CDC website: http://www.cdc.gov.

Foodborne and Waterborne Diseases

As in the United States, much foodborne disease abroad can be avoided if the traveler eats thoroughly cooked foods prepared with reasonable hygiene; eating foods from street vendors may not be a good idea. Trichinosis, tapeworms, and fluke infections, as well as bacterial infections, result from eating raw or undercooked meats. Raw vegetables may act as a source of bacterial, viral, helminthic, or protozoal infection if they have been grown with or washed in contaminated water. Fruits that can be peeled immediately before eating, such as bananas, are less likely to be a source of infection. Dairy products should be pasteurized and appropriately refrigerated.

Water in many areas of the world is not potable (safe to drink), and drinking this water can lead to infection with a variety of protozoal, viral, and bacterial agents, including amoebae, *Giardia, Cryptosporidium,* hepatitis, cholera, and various coliform bacteria. Unless traveling in an area where the piped water is known to be safe, only boiled water (boiled for 1 minute), bottled water, or water purified with iodine or chlorine compounds should be consumed. Ice should be avoided since freezing does not inactivate these agents. If the water is questionable, choose coffee or tea made with boiled water, carbonated beverages without ice, beer, wine, or canned fruit juices. Chapter 2 in the CDC Yellow Book offers useful information on food and water consumption for travelers and can be found at https://www.cdc.gov.

Diarrheal Diseases

Travelers often suffer from diarrhea, so much so that colorful names, such as Montezuma's revenge, turista, and Colorado quickstep, exist in our vocabulary to describe these bouts of intestinal upset. Some of these diarrheas do not have infectious causes; they result from stress, fatigue, schedule changes, and eating unfamiliar foods. Acute infectious diarrheas are usually of viral or bacterial origin. *E. coli* probably causes more cases of traveler's diarrhea than all other infective agents combined. Protozoan-induced diarrheas such as those resulting from *Entamoeba* and *Giardia* are less likely to be acute, and they more commonly present once the traveler returns home. Travelers need to pay special attention to what they eat and drink. Read more about travelers' health at the CDC website: http://www.cdc.gov.

ZOONOSES

A zoonosis is an infection transmitted from a vertebrate animal to a human under natural conditions. The agents that cause zoonoses do not need humans to maintain their life cycles; infected humans have simply managed somehow to get in their way. Means of transmission include animal bites (bats and rabies), inhalation (rodent excrement and hantavirus), ingestion (milk and listeriosis), direct contact (rabbit carcasses and tularemia), and arthropod intermediates. This last transmission route means that many vector-borne diseases are also zoonoses. For example, white-tailed deer harbor ticks that can carry Lyme disease, and rats and ground squirrels may be infested with fleas capable of transmitting plague. Other than vector-borne diseases, some of the more common zoonoses in the United States include toxoplasmosis *(Toxoplasma gondii)*, cat-scratch disease *(Bartonella henselae)*, brucellosis (*Brucella* species), leptospirosis *(Leptospira interrogans)*, listeriosis *(Listeria monocytogenes)*, salmonellosis (*Salmonella* serotypes), and rabies (family Rhabdoviridae, genus *Lyssavirus*). Many of the emerging infectious diseases such as avian influenza A H5N1, WNV, monkey pox, hantavirus pulmonary syndrome, and vCJD are examples of zoonoses. Also, among the diseases considered best candidates for weapons of bioterrorism, anthrax, plague, tularemia, and some of the hemorrhagic fever viruses (e.g., Lassa) are all zoonoses. The CDC estimates that 75 percent of recently emerging infectious diseases affecting humans are diseases of animal origin and that about 60 percent of all human pathogens are zoonotic.

Rabies (Hydrophobia)

Rabies is transmitted to humans by introducing virus-carrying saliva into the body, usually via an animal bite or scratch. Transmission may also occur if infected saliva comes into contact with a fresh cut or intact mucous membranes. Rabies is found in neural tissue and is not transmitted via blood, urine, or feces. Airborne transmission has been documented in caves with infected bat colonies. Transmission from human to human is theoretically possible but has not been documented except through transplant organs harvested from individuals who died of undiagnosed rabies. Guidelines for organ donation exist to minimize this possibility (Heymann, 2015).

One of the most feared of human diseases, rabies has the highest case fatality rate of any known human infection, essentially 100 percent. Despite the availability of intensive medical care, only a handful of individuals have been known to recover after the onset of rabies, three in the United States (CDC, 2012b). A significant public health problem worldwide with as many as 59,000 deaths a year, mostly in Asia and Africa, human rabies in the United States has become a rare event due to the widespread vaccination of dogs begun in the 1950s. Canine rabies virus is considered eliminated in the United States, and the current carriers of rabies are wild animals—raccoons, skunks, foxes, coyotes, and bats. Dogs and cats diagnosed with rabies are infected by a variant virus from these wild carriers. Small rodents, rabbits and hares, and opossums rarely carry rabies. Epidemiologic information should be consulted for information on the potential carriers for a given geographic region. Whereas once in the United States, 100 or more cases of human rabies were reported a year, today 1-3 cases are reported annually. Of the 23 human rabies cases reported from 2008 through 2017, 8 (35 percent) were acquired outside the United States; all but 1 resulted from the bites of infected dogs. Domestically acquired cases were largely associated with insectivorous bats (11.73 percent). Two were associated with raccoons, one with a mongoose, and one was unknown. One of the domestic cases occurred not through direct contact but as the result of organ transplant (CDC, 2017m).

The best protection against rabies remains vaccinating domestic animals—dogs, cats, cattle, and horses. If a person is bitten, the bite wound should be thoroughly cleaned with soap and water, and a physician consulted immediately. Be suspicious of bites from a wild animal or an unprovoked attack from a domestic animal. Even when there is no suspicion of rabies, contact a physician since tetanus or antibiotic prophylaxis may be needed. An estimated 40,000-50,000 Americans per year receive post-exposure prophylaxis (PEP) after being in contact with potentially rabid animals. No successful treatment exists for rabies once symptoms appear, but if given promptly and as directed, PEP with human rabies immunoglobulin (RIG) and rabies vaccine can prevent the development of the disease. Two products are available for use as rabies vaccine in the United States: human diploid cell vaccine (HDCV) and purified chick embryo cell culture vaccine (PCECV) (CDC, 2008). In 2010, the previously recommended series of five 1-mL doses of vaccine injected into the deltoid muscle was changed to four (CDC, 2010d). Reactions to the vaccine are fewer and less serious than with previously used vaccines. Individuals who deal frequently with animals, such as zookeepers, laboratory workers, and veterinarians, may choose to receive the vaccine as pre-exposure prophylaxis. The decision to administer the vaccine to a bite victim depends on the circumstances of the bite and is made on an individual basis.

Recommendations for prevention of and vaccination for rabies in animals are found in the Compendium of Animal Rabies Prevention and Control compiled by the National Association of State Public Health Veterinarians, Inc. (Brown et al., 2016). Recommendations for administering PEP are provided by the Advisory Committee for Recommendations on Immunization Practices and are available through local public health officials or the CDC (CDC, 2010c). Decisions on whether an exposure has occurred requiring the use of PEP may not always be straightforward, and public health officials are helpful in making these treatment decisions.

PARASITIC DISEASES

Parasites are organisms that depend on a host to survive. Endoparasites, those that live within the body, are classified into four major groups: nematodes (roundworms), cestodes (tapeworms), trematodes (flukes), and protozoa (single-celled animals). Nematodes, cestodes, and trematodes are all referred to as helminths along with acanthocephalans or thorny-headed worms, which are not as commonly involved in human infections. Table 14.5 presents examples of relatively common diseases caused by parasites from these groups. Ectoparasites remain on the surface of a host's body to feed. Examples are ticks, fleas, lice, and mites that attach or burrow into the skin. Many parasitic infections are vector-borne and/or zoonotic.

TABLE 14.5 Examples of Diseases Resulting From Endoparasitic Infection by Category

Category	Parasite	Disease
Cestodes	*Taenia saginata, Taenia solium*	Beef tapeworm, pork tapeworm
Nematodes	*Ancylostoma, Necator*	Ancylostomiasis, necatoriasis (hookworm)
Intestinal	*Ascaris, Toxocara*	Ascariasis, toxocariasis (roundworm)
	Enterobius vermicularis	Enterobiasis (pinworm)
	Trichuris trichiura	Trichuriasis (whipworm)
Blood/Tissue	*Drancunculis medinensis*	Guinea worm
	Onchocerca volvulus	Onchocerciasis (river blindness)
	Wuchereria bancrofti	Lymphatic filariasis (elephantiasis)
Trematodes	*Schistosoma* sp.	Schistosomiasis (snail fever)
Protozoans	*Entamoeba histolytica*	Amebiasis
	Giardia lamblia	Giardiasis
	Leishmania spp.	Leishmaniasis
	Plasmodium spp.	Malaria
	Toxoplasma gondii	Toxoplasmosis
	Trichomonas vaginalis	Trichomoniasis
	Trypanosoma spp.	African sleeping sickness, Chagas' disease

Based on information from Heymann DL, editor: *Control of communicable diseases manual,* ed. 20, Washington, DC, 2015, American Public Health Association.

Parasitic diseases are more prevalent in rural areas of low-income countries than in the United States. Contributing factors are tropical climate and inadequate prevention and control measures. Poor sanitation, a lack of cheap and effective drugs, and a scarcity of funding lead to high reinfection rates even when control programs are attempted. Parasitic organisms result in a wide spectrum of diseases, including leading causes of death and disability in Africa, Asia, Central America, and South America. Examples include malaria, schistosomiasis, guinea worm disease, river blindness (onchocerciasis), leishmaniasis, amoebiasis, African sleeping sickness, Chagas' disease, and lymphatic filariasis. These parasitic diseases not only cause major mortality in endemic regions but also tremendous morbidity. Debilitation from infection may result in an inability to attend school or work as well as growth retardation, developmental disabilities, and cognitive impairment in young children, all which contribute to significant economic burden for the countries affected.

Neglected Parasitic Infections

Parasitic infections also affect persons living in developed countries. New technology for recognizing protozoan parasites, the ease of international travel, immigration from developing countries, and immunocompromise from diseases like HIV all contribute to rising reports of and a greater attention to parasitic diseases in the United States. The CDC has targeted for action in the United States a group of five "neglected" parasitic infections (NPIs), defined as diseases that disproportionately affect people in poverty, infect a significant number of people, and receive limited attention in surveillance, prevention, and treatment. These NPIs include Chagas' disease, neurocysticercosis, toxocariasis, toxoplasmosis, and trichomoniasis. These diseases vary greatly in their presentations and routes of transmission. For example, Chagas' disease causes cardiomyopathy and results from the bite of a triatomine bug carrying *Trypanosoma cruzi,* whereas neurocysticercosis affects the brain through cyst formation by larvae formed after the ingestion of eggs from the pork tapeworm, *Taenia solium.* Trichomoniasis is a common sexually transmitted disease, easily treated with antibiotics, caused by the parasite *Trichomonas vaginalis.* About 3.7 million people are estimated to be infected with this parasite, but only 30 percent may show symptoms (CDC, 2017n). In order to ensure an accurate diagnosis, nurses and other health professionals need to familiarize themselves with the clinical presentations and risk factors associated with these parasitic diseases.

Intestinal Parasitic Infections

Common helminths infections in humans result from tapeworms, flukes, and roundworms. They frequently live in the digestive tract of their hosts but are also capable of aberrant migration to other organs, including the eyes and brain. Although intestinal parasites are major contributors to morbidity and mortality in low-income countries, climate, improved sanitary conditions, and effective drug therapy have served to greatly reduce widespread indigenous transmission in the United States, so much so that surveillance for many of these organisms is not widely practiced. A study using 1988-1994 National Health and Nutrition Examination Survey (NHANES) III data reported that 14 percent of Americans have antibodies to *Toxocara*, a roundworm carried by dogs and cats that can be passed to humans. While this suggests that tens of millions of Americans have been exposed, it does not show how many are actually infected (Won et al., 2008). Although most people show no signs of infection, this parasite can cause systemic illness and blindness. Toxocariasis is not reportable.

Enterobiasis (pinworm) is the most common helminthic infection in the United States Pinworm infection is seen most often among school-age children and is most prevalent in crowded and institutional settings. Transmission is via consumption of infected eggs found in soil contaminated by human feces. Pinworms resemble small pieces of white thread and can be seen with the naked eye. Diagnosis is usually accomplished by pressing cellophane tape to the perianal region early in the morning. Treatment with oral vermicides and concurrent disinfection is highly effective (Heymann, 2015).

Opportunistic Parasitic Infections

Opportunistic infections (OIs) are those more frequent or more severe in individuals immunocompromised by HIV infection. Before the introduction of routine prophylactic treatment and potent-combination, highly active antiretroviral therapies (ARTs) in the 1990s, OIs were the leading cause of illness and death in this group. Some of the protozoan parasitic OIs seen in clients with HIV disease and others who are immunocompromised include PCP; cryptosporidiosis, microsporidiosis, and isosporiasis, all producing diarrheal disease and transmitted by fecal-oral contact; and toxoplasmosis. With the advent of ARTs, the incidence of OIs in American HIV disease clients has dropped dramatically. Isosporiasis was always rare, but the rates for cryptosporidiosis and microsporidiosis have also declined markedly. Although no longer seen with the frequency of the past, toxoplasmosis and PCP have not disappeared. OIs are more likely to appear in individuals unaware of their HIV disease or without good access to health care. Guidelines for prevention and treatment of OIs are now regularly updated by the Panel on Opportunistic Infections in HIV-Infected Adults and Adolescents, representing opinion from the CDC, the National Institutes of Health, and the HIV Medicine Association of the Infectious Diseases Society of America. Because of rapid evolution in HIV management, the Panel makes the most recent information readily available on the AIDSinfo website at http://aidsinfo.nih.gov.

Toxoplasma gondii is a coccidial organism harbored by cats infected by eating other infected animals. While rodents, ruminants, swine, poultry, and other birds may have infective organisms in their muscle tissue, only cats carry this parasite in their intestinal tract, allowing the excretion of infected eggs. People contract the disease through contact with infected cat feces or eating improperly cooked meat. In most healthy people, toxoplasmosis produces a mild to inapparent infection, but in immunodeficient individuals, the disease may, in addition to rash and skeletal muscle involvement, result in cerebritis, pneumonia, chorioretinitis, myocarditis, and/or death. Infection early in pregnancy may cause fetal death or deformity. Central nervous system (CNS) infection is common with HIV disease. Because toxoplasmosis is not a nationally reportable disease, reliable case numbers are not readily available. On their website, CDC estimates there are over 800,000 new *Toxoplasma* infections and 300 to 4000 cases of congenital toxoplasmosis in the United States each year; an estimated 3600 people experience ocular involvement as part of infection; and toxoplasmosis is a leading cause of foodborne illnesses deaths, resulting in hundreds of deaths and thousands of hospitalizations per year (CDC, 2017p).

Protozoan Parasites Causing Foodborne and Waterborne Diarrheal Disease

In the United States protozoan organisms frequently cause foodborne and waterborne diarrheal illness *(Giardia, Cryptosporidium, Cyclospora)*. Giardiasis is a diarrheal illness caused by the parasite *Giardia intestinalis*. It is the most common intestinal parasitic infection in the United States, causing a reported 16,310 cases in 2016 (CDC, 2017o). Giardiasis became a nationally notifiable disease in 2002.

Cryptosporidiosis is also a diarrheal disease caused by the microscopic parasite *Cryptosporidium*. Because *Cryptosporidium* possesses an outer shell, allowing it to survive outside the body for extended periods of time and tolerate low levels of chlorine disinfection, it is a frequent cause of water-related disease outbreaks in swimming pools and splash parks. In the United States "crypto" is a common cause of both foodborne and waterborne disease resulting in an estimated 740,000 cases each year (Scallan, 2011). Cryptosporidiosis became a nationally notifiable disease in 1995.

Cyclospora cayetanensis is another single-celled parasite that causes an intestinal infection called cyclosporiasis. Only identified in humans in 1977, *Cyclospora* first gained attention in the United States when an outbreak of cyclosporiasis sickened almost 1500 people in the United States and Canada; the outbreak would eventually be linked to imported raspberries. Since then *Cyclospora* outbreaks have been linked to various types of imported fresh produce, including raspberries, snow peas, mesclun lettuce, and herbs like basil and cilantro. In 2017 over 1000 cases were reported with none of them linked to a particular outbreak or food item. In the summer of 2018, separate outbreaks involved packaged salad mix used by a fast-food outlet and several retail grocers and pre-cut vegetable trays sold through grocers affected over 600 people, (CDC, 2018n). Cyclosporiasis became a nationally notifiable disease in 1999.

Control and Prevention of Parasitic Infections

Correct diagnosis by nurses and other health care workers allows the provision of early and appropriate treatment and client education for preventing and controlling parasitic infections. Diagnosis of parasitic diseases is based on history, including travel, characteristic clinical signs and symptoms, and the use of appropriate laboratory tests to confirm the clinical diagnosis. Knowing what specimens to collect, how and when to collect, and what laboratory techniques to use are all important in establishing a correct diagnosis. Effective drug treatment is available for most parasitic diseases. The high cost of the drugs, drug resistance, and toxicity are some of the common therapeutic problems. Measures for prevention and control of parasitic diseases include early diagnosis and treatment, improved personal hygiene, safer sex practices, community health education, vector control, and improvements in sanitary control of food, water, and waste disposal.

HEALTH CARE-ASSOCIATED INFECTIONS

Previously referred to as nosocomial infections and hospital-acquired infections, **health care-associated infections** (HAIs) are, as the name implies, those transmitted during hospitalization or developed within a hospital or other health care setting. They may involve clients, health care workers, visitors, or anyone who has contact with a hospital or doctor's office. Invasive diagnostic and surgical procedures, broad-spectrum antibiotics, and immunosuppressive drugs, along with the original underlying illness, leave hospitalized clients particularly vulnerable to exposure to virulent infectious agents from other clients and indigenous hospital flora from health care staff. In this setting, the simple act of performing hand hygiene before approaching every client becomes critical. A CDC prevalence survey of U.S. acute care hospitals in 2011 estimated 722,000 HAIs annually, suggesting that on any given day, 1 in 25 hospital patients has at least one health care-associated infection. An estimated 75,000 hospital patients with HAIs died during their hospitalizations. More than half of all HAIs occurred outside of the intensive care unit (Magill et al., 2014). A 2013 report estimated total annual costs for five major HAIs at $9.8 billion, with surgical site infections contributing the most to overall costs (Zimlichman et al., 2013). In addition, HAIs have a high likelihood of involving and contributing to antibiotic resistance.

CDC publishes yearly reports to help each state better understand their progress and target areas that need assistance. The data used in these reports comes from two complementary HAI surveillance systems, the National Healthcare Safety Network (NHSN) and the Emerging Infections Program Healthcare-Associated Infections Community-Interface (EIP HAIC), voluntary, Internet-based surveillance systems that provide national data on the epidemiology of HAIs in the United Sates. Pulling from this information, the report *Healthcare-Associated Infections in the United States, 2006-2016* presents progress in addressing five HAI measures (central line-associated blood infection, catheter-associated urinary tract infection, surgical site infection, methicillin-resistant *Staphylococcus aureus* (MRSA) bacteremia, and *Clostridium difficile* infection) and can be found with other information on preventing health care-associated infections and antibiotic resistance at the CDC HAI website: http://www.cdc.gov.

Infection control practitioners play a key role in hospital infection surveillance and control programs. Without a qualified and well-trained person in this position, the infection control program is ineffective. Many infection control practitioners are nurses. Their common job titles are infection control nurse, infection control coordinator, and nurse epidemiologist.

Universal Precautions

In 1985, in response to concerns regarding the transmission of HIV infection during health care procedures, the CDC recommended a **universal precautions** policy for all health care settings. This strategy requires that blood and body fluids from *all clients* be handled as if infected with HIV or other bloodborne pathogens. When in a situation where potential contact with blood or other body fluids exists, health care workers must always perform hand hygiene and wear gloves, masks, protective clothing, and other indicated personal protective barriers. Needles and sharp instruments must be used and disposed of properly (CDC, 1989). The CDC also made recommendations for preventing transmission of HIV and hepatitis B during medical, surgical, and dental procedures (CDC, 1991). Updated guidelines and recommendations for preventing HAIs, including universal precautions, were published in 2007 (Siegel et al., 2017). Today the Healthcare Infection Control Practices and Advisory Committee is charged with providing guidance on hospital infection control and developing strategies for surveillance, prevention, and control of HAIs. The most recent guidance may be found on the Guidelines and Recommendations page of the CDC's Infection Control web pages at https://www.cdc.gov.

LINKING CONTENT TO PRACTICE

Public health involves the prevention of disease, promotion of health, and protection against hazards that threaten the health of the community as reflected in the public health logo and summed up in the mission "assuring conditions in which people can be healthy." The three core functions of public health in achieving this mission as defined in 1988 by the Institute of Medicine in Recommendations for the Future of Public Health are *Assessment, Policy Development,* and *Assurance.* These three have been further divided into the "10 Essential Services of Public Health" as a means of evaluating the effectiveness of public health efforts.

This chapter presents communicable diseases that commonly challenge the health of a community as well as prevention and control roles for public health nurses. Examples of some of the "Essential Services" under which these roles fall are presented by core function.

Assessment: (1) Monitor health/identify problems, and (2) Diagnose and investigate health problems. Examples include surveillance, investigation, and identification of reportable communicable disease cases. **Policy Development:** (3) Inform, educate, and empower, and (4) Mobilize community partnerships. Examples include evaluating immunization status, explaining the reason for immunizations and how to comply with the immunization schedule, organizing community partners to provide immunizations and documentation through a registry, and mounting a community campaign to inform the community of the importance of age-appropriate immunization. **Assurance:** (5) Enforce laws and regulations, and (6) Link to services and provide care. Examples include assuring compliance with communicable disease control laws through treatment or prophylaxis for exposure to reportable diseases; excluding diseased students from daycare or school; linking individuals without insurance to follow-up care for communicable disease treatment or exposure.

PRACTICE APPLICATION

The rising numbers of foreign-born residents in communities that did not previously have large immigrant populations provides a challenge to those involved with communicable disease control, especially in outbreak situations. Language barriers, specific cultural practices, and undocumented status all contribute to opportunities for infection as well as presenting obstacles to prevention and control. Diseases such as TB, brucellosis, measles, hepatitis B, and parasitic infections often originate in other countries and are diagnosed only after the individual arrives in the United States. People coming from countries without, with newly established, or with poorly enforced vaccination programs may be unimmunized. These people are particularly susceptible to infection in outbreak situations. For example, many people coming from Latin America have not been immunized against rubella. Differences in cultural practices can lead to outbreaks of foodborne illness. Listeriosis outbreaks have been traced to the use of unpasteurized milk in cottage industry cheese production.

In the face of a single infectious disease report or an outbreak situation, when working with communities whose members speak limited English, it is vital: (1) to have a means of communication, (2) to be able to provide a culturally appropriate message, and (3) to have an established level of trust. Ideally, these requirements are addressed before an outbreak occurs, allowing a prompt and efficient response when immediate action is needed.

A. What would be a useful first step in building trust with a largely non–English-speaking immigrant community?
  1. Hold a health fair in the community.
  2. Provide incentives to use health department services.
  3. Identify trusted community leaders such as religious leaders and ask their help in developing a plan.
  4. Distribute a brochure in the target community language.

B. What might best encourage undocumented residents to respond to a request to be immunized during an outbreak situation?
  1. Using an already established public health program to provide interpreter services, making it clear that proof of immigration status is not required for services
  2. Printing a request in the newspaper in the language of the targeted individuals
  3. Involving trusted community leaders in making the request
  4. Emphasizing to the individuals the severity of the consequences if immunization does not occur

C. What means of communication would work best when targeting largely non–English-speaking communities of recent immigrants?
  1. Newspaper articles in target language
  2. Radio announcements in target language
  3. Fliers in target language posted in the community
  4. Announcements from trusted community leaders

D. How would public health officials best undertake the development of information to effectively reach a largely non–English-speaking community of recent immigrants?
  1. Use the services of the local university communications department.
  2. Ask community leaders to work with translators and prevention specialists to develop messages using their own words.
  3. Hire a professional to translate an existing well-developed English-language brochure.
  4. Use brochures provided by the state health department.

Answers can be found on the Evolve site.

KEY POINTS

- The burden of infectious diseases is high in both human and economic terms. Preventing these diseases must be given high priority in our present health care system.
- The successful interaction of the infectious agent, host, and environment is necessary for disease transmission. Knowledge of the characteristics of each of these three factors is important in understanding the transmission, prevention, and control of these diseases.
- Effective intervention measures at the individual and community levels must be aimed at breaking the chain linking the agent, host, and environment. An integrated approach focused on all three factors simultaneously is an ideal goal to strive for but may not be feasible for all diseases.
- Health care professionals must constantly be aware of vulnerability to threats posed by emerging infectious diseases. Most of the factors causing the emergence of these diseases are influenced by human activities and behavior.
- Communicable diseases are preventable. Avoiding infection through primary prevention activities is the most cost-effective public health strategy.
- Health care professionals must always apply infection control principles and procedures in the work environment. They should strictly adhere to universal blood and body fluid precautions to prevent transmission of HIV and other bloodborne pathogens.
- Effective control of communicable diseases requires the use of a multisystem approach focusing on enhancing host resistance, improving safety of the environment, improving public health systems, and facilitating social and political changes to ensure health for all people.
- Communicable disease prevention and control programs must move beyond providing drug treatment and vaccines. Health promotion and education aimed at changing individual and community behavior must be emphasized.

- Nurses play a key role in all aspects of prevention and control of communicable diseases. Close cooperation with other members of the interprofessional health care team must be maintained. Mobilizing community participation is essential to successful implementation of programs.
- The successful global eradication of smallpox proved the feasibility of eradication of selected communicable diseases. As professionals and concerned citizens of the global village, health care workers must support the current global eradication campaigns against poliomyelitis and dracunculiasis.

CLINICAL DECISION-MAKING ACTIVITIES

1. Accompany a nurse who makes home visits. Discuss living situations and other risk factors that may contribute to the development of infectious diseases, as well as possible points at which the nurse may intervene to help prevent these diseases, such as checking the immunization status of all individuals in the household. What are realistic interventions and how much responsibility should a nurse take in attempting to affect the living situation?
2. To become familiar with the reportable diseases that are a problem in your community, look at how many cases have been reported during the past month, six months, and year. Contrast these numbers with national and state statistics. How is your county or city different from or similar to these larger jurisdictions? If different, what environmental, political, or demographic features may contribute to this difference?
3. Spend time with the persons who are responsible for reporting and investigating communicable disease in your community. Discuss types of surveillance conducted and outbreak procedures that may accompany the reporting of some of these diseases. If possible, attend an outbreak investigation. Would the existing surveillance systems and outbreak control policies be sufficient in the case of a bioterrorism event?
4. Review the demographic profile of your community, including trends from the past 10 years and projections for the next decade. Pay special attention to growth patterns of particular populations such as racial and ethnic groups or specific age groups (e.g., children under 18, adults 65 and older). How do changes in these populations affect the delivery of interventions for infectious disease control such as immunization?
5. Visit a clinic that serves a refugee, immigrant, or migrant labor population to observe the infectious diseases commonly seen in these groups. Compare and contrast this visit with a visit to a clinic that serves an inner-city population and a visit to a clinic that serves a rural population. How are the infectious disease control issues different and/or similar for these varied populations?
6. Sit in a clinic waiting room for immunization services and talk with parents about their concerns and the barriers they may perceive in obtaining immunizations for their children. How can this information be used to better facilitate immunization services?
7. Spend time with a school nurse to see what infectious diseases are routinely encountered in the educational setting. Discuss risk factors for disease in school-age youths and the strategies used to prevent infectious diseases in this age group. Do school policies support the strategies needed for the prevention of infectious diseases in students?
8. Visit a daycare center. Observe potential situations for the communication of infectious diseases, and discuss with the director the steps taken to prevent and control infection, including immunization requirements and procedures for hand hygiene and food preparation. Does the center have specific infection control policies and procedures, and does the staff appear to be following them?

ADDITIONAL RESOURCES

EVOLVE WEBSITE

http://evolve.elsevier.com/Stanhope/community/

- Answers to Practice Application
- Case Study
- Glossary
- Review Questions

REFERENCES

American College of Obstetricians and Gynecologists (ACOG): 2018 Annual Meeting, Abstract 8L, Simple alert increases prenatal uptake of Tdap vaccine, *Medscape Medical News*, April 29, 2018. Retrieved from https://www.medscape.com.

Brown CM, Slavinski S, Ettestad P, Sidwa TJ, Sorhage FE: Compendium of Animal Rabies Prevention and Control, 2016, *J Am Vet Med Assoc* 248(5):505–517, 2016

Centers for Disease Control and Prevention (CDC): Guidelines for prevention of transmission of HIV and hepatitis B virus to health care and public safety workers, *MMWR Morb Mortal Wkly Rep* 38(6):1–37, 1989.

Centers for Disease Control and Prevention (CDC): Recommendations for preventing transmission of HIV and hepatitis B virus to patients during exposure-prone invasive procedures, *MMWR Morb Mortal Wkly Rep* 40(RR-8):1, 1991.

Centers for Disease Control and Prevention (CDC): Addressing emerging infectious disease threats: a prevention strategy for the U.S, 1994, *MMWR Morb Mortal Wkly Rep* 43(RR-5):1–18, 1994.

Centers for Disease Control and Prevention (CDC): Notifiable disease surveillance and notifiable disease statistics—United States, June 1946 and June 1996, *MMWR Morb Mortal Wkly Rep* 45:530–536, 1996.

Centers for Disease Control and Prevention (CDC): Update: isolation of avian influenza A (H5N1) viruses from humans—Hong Kong, 1997–1998, *MMWR Morb Mortal Wkly Rep* 46:1245–1247, 1998.

Centers for Disease Control and Prevention (CDC): Achievements in Public Health: Elimination of Rubella and Congenital Rubella

Syndrome—United States, 1969–2004, *MMWR Morb Mortal Wkly Rep* 4(11):279–282, 2005.
Centers for Disease Control and Prevention (CDC): Update: Measles—United States, January–July 2008, *MMWR Morb Mortal Wkly Rep* 57(33):893, 2008.
Centers for Disease Control and Prevention (CDC): Progress toward interruption of wild poliovirus transmission—worldwide, 2008, *MMWR Morb Mortal Wkly Rep* 58(12):308–312, 2009.
Centers for Disease Control and Prevention (CDC): Surveillance for human West Nile virus disease—United States, 1999–2008, *MMWR Morb Mortal Wkly Rep* 59(2):1–17, 2010a.
Centers for Disease Control and Prevention (CDC): Update: Influenza Activity—United States, August 30, 2009–January 9, 2010, *MMWR Morbid Mortal Wkly Rep* 59(2):38–43, 2010b.
Centers for Disease Control and Prevention (CDC): *CDC's Advisory Committee on Immunization Practices (ACIP) recommends universal annual influenza vaccination, Media Advisory*, CDC, 2010c. Retrieved from http://www.cdc.gov.
Centers for Disease Control and Prevention (CDC): Use of a reduced (4-dose) vaccine schedule for postexposure prophylaxis to prevent human rabies, recommendations of the Advisory Committee on Immunization Practices, *MMWR Morb Mortal Wkly Rep Recomm Rep* 59(2):1–9, 2010d.
Centers for Disease Control and Prevention (CDC): *A CDC Framework for Preventing Infectious Diseases: Sustaining the Essential and Innovating for the Future*, 2011. Retrieved from http://www.cdc.gov.
Centers for Disease Control and Prevention (CDC): Pertussis Epidemic—Washington 2012, *MMWR Morb Mortal Wkly Rep* 61(28):517–522, 2012a.
Centers for Disease Control and Prevention (CDC): Recovery of a Patient from Clinical Rabies—California, 2011, *MMWR Morb Mortal Wkly Rep* 61(04):61–65, 2012b.
Centers for Disease Control and Prevention (CDC): Summary of notifiable diseases—United States 2011, *MMWR Morb Mortal Wkly Rep* 60(53):1–117, 2013.
Centers for Disease Control and Prevention (CDC): *Cost of Rabies Prevention*, 2015. Retrieved from https://www.cdc.gov.
Centers for Disease Control and Prevention (CDC): Overview, Control Strategies, and Lessons Learned in the CDC Response to the 2014–2016 Ebola Epidemic, *MMWR Morbid Mortal Wkly Rep* 65(Suppl 3):4–11, 2016a.
Centers for Disease Control and Prevention (CDC): Influenza Vaccination Coverage Among Health Care Personnel—United States, 2015–16 Influenza Season, *MMWR Morbid Mortal Wkly Rep* 65(38):1026–1031, 2016b.
Centers for Disease Control and Prevention (CDC): *Burden of Foodborne Illness: Methods and Data Sources*, 2016c. Retrieved from https://www.cdc.gov.
Centers for Disease Control and Prevention (CDC): *Reported Tuberculosis in the United States, 2016*, Atlanta, GA, U.S. Department of Health and Human Services, CDC, 2017a.
Centers for Disease Control and Prevention (CDC): *Variant Creutzfeldt-Jacob disease*, 2017b. Retrieved from https://www.cdc.gov.
Centers for Disease Control and Prevention (CDC): Isolated Case of Marburg Virus Disease, Kampala, Uganda, 2014, *Emerg Infect Dis* 23(6):1001–1004, 2017c.
Centers for Disease Control and Prevention (CDC): *CDC Fact Sheet: The Costly Burden of Drug-Resistant TB in the U.S.*, 2017d. Retrieved from https://www.cdc.gov.
Centers for Disease Control and Prevention (CDC): *CDC Fact Sheet: Reported STDs in the United States, 2016 High Burden of STDs Threaten Millions of Americans*, 2017e. Retrieved from https://www.cdc.gov.
Centers for Disease Control and Prevention (CDC): *Parasites—Guinea Worm, Eradication Program*, 2017f. Retrieved from https://www.cdc.gov.
Centers for Disease Control and Prevention (CDC): Progress Toward Regional Measles Elimination—Worldwide, 2000–2016, *MMWR Morbid Mortal Wkly Rep* 66(42):1148–1153, 2017g.
Centers for Disease Control and Prevention (CDC): Measles Outbreak—Minnesota April–May 2017, *MMWR Morbid Mortal Wkly Rep* 66(27):713–717, 2017h.
Centers for Disease Control and Prevention (CDC): *Rubella in the US*, 2017i. Retrieved from https://www.cdc.gov.
Centers for Disease Control and Prevention (CDC): *Pertussis Vaccination*, 2017j. Retrieved from https://www.cdc.gov.
Centers for Disease Control and Prevention (CDC): *Surveillance for Foodborne Disease Outbreaks, United States, 2015: Annual Report*, Atlanta, Georgia, US Department of Health and Human Services, CDC, 2017k.
Centers for Disease Control and Prevention (CDC): Surveillance for Waterborne Disease Outbreaks Associated with Drinking Water—United States, 2013–2014, *MMWR Morbid Mortal Wkly Rep* 66(44):1216–1221, 2017l.
Centers for Disease Control and Prevention (CDC): *Human Rabies*, 2017m. Retrieved from https://www.cdc.gov.
Centers for Disease Control and Prevention (CDC): *Trichomoniasis—CDC Fact Sheet*, 2017n. Retrieved from https://www.cdc.gov.
Centers for Disease Control and Prevention (CDC): *National Notifiable Diseases Surveillance System, 2016 Annual Tables of Infectious Disease Data*, 2017o. Retrieved from https://www.cdc.gov.
Centers for Disease Control and Prevention (CDC): *Neglected Parasitic Infections in the United States Toxoplasmosis*, 2017p. Retrieved from http://www.cdc.gov.
Centers for Disease Control and Prevention (CDC): *Food Safety*, 2018a. Retrieved from https://www.cdc.gov.
Centers for Disease Control and Prevention (CDC): West Nile Virus and Other Nationally Notifiable Arboviral Diseases—United States, 2016, *MMWR Morbid Mortal Wkly Rep* 67(1):13–17, 2018b.
Centers for Disease Control and Prevention (CDC): *2018 Immunization Schedules*, 2018c. Retrieved from https://www.cdc.gov.
Centers for Disease Control and Prevention (CDC): *Measles Control and Outbreaks*, 2018d. Retrieved from https://www.cdc.gov.
Centers for Disease Control and Prevention (CDC): *Pertussis Surveillance and Reporting*, 2018e. Retrieved from https://www.cdc.gov.
Centers for Disease Control and Prevention (CDC): *2017 Final Pertussis Surveillance Report*, 2018f. Retrieved from https://www.cdc.gov.
Centers for Disease Control and Prevention (CDC): Prevention and Control of Seasonal Influenza with Vaccines: Recommendations of the Advisory Committee on Immunization Practices—United States, 2018–19 Influenza Season, *MMWR Morbid Mortal Wkly Rep* Recomm Rep 67(3):1–20, 2018g.
Centers for Disease Control and Prevention (CDC): *Influenza Antiviral Medications: Summary for Clinicians*, 2018h. Retrieved from https://www.cdc.gov.
Centers for Disease Control and Prevention (CDC): *Highly Pathogenic Asian Avian Influenza A (H5N1) Virus*, 2018i. Retrieved from https://www.cdc.gov.
Centers for Disease Control and Prevention (CDC): *Asian Lineage Avian Influenza A (H7N9) Virus*, 2018j. Retrieved from https://www.cdc.gov.
Centers for Disease Control and Prevention (CDC): Preliminary Incidence and Trends of Infections with Pathogens Transmitted

Commonly Through Food—Foodborne Diseases Active Surveillance Network, 10 U.S. Sites, 2006–2017, *MMWR Morbid Mortal Wkly Rep* 67(11):324–328, 2018k.

Centers for Disease Control and Prevention (CDC): Vital Signs: Trends in Reported Vectorborne Disease Cases—United States and Territories, 2004–2016, *MMWR Morbid Mortal Wkly Rep* 67(17):496–501, 2018l.

Centers for Disease Control and Prevention (CDC): Malaria Surveillance—United States, 2015, *MMWR Morbid Mortal Wkly Rep Surv Summ* 2018, 67(7):1–28, 2018m.

Centers for Disease Control and Prevention (CDC): *Parasites—Cyclosporiasis, Outbreak Investigations and Updates*, 2018n. Retrieved from https://www.cdc.gov.

Centers for Disease Control and Prevention (CDC): *National Notifiable Disease Surveillance System (NNDSS)—2018 National Notifiable Conditions*, 2018o. Retrieved from https://wwwn.cdc.gov.

Centers for Disease Control and Prevention (CDC): *Four Steps to Food Safety*, 2018p. Retrieved from https://www.cdc.gov.

Cieslak TJ, Eitzen EM Jr: Clinical and epidemiologic principles of anthrax, *Emerg Infect Dis* 5:552–555, 1999.

European Centre for Disease Prevention and Control (ECDC): *Annual Epidemiological Report 2016—Anthrax*, Stockholm, ECDC, 2017. Retrieved from https://ecdc.europa.eu.

Evans AS: The eradication of communicable diseases: myth or reality? *Am J Epidemiol* 122:199–207, 1985.

Heymann DL, editor: *Control of communicable diseases manual*, ed 20, Washington, DC, 2015, American Public Health Association.

Kuehn, BM: CDC estimates 300,000 U.S. cases of Lyme disease annually, *JAMA* 310(11):1110, 2013.

Magill SS, Edwards JR, Bamberg W, et al.: Multistate point-prevalence survey of health care-associated infections, *N Engl J Med* 370:1198–1208, 2014.

Scallan E, Hoekstra RM, Angulo FJ, et al.: Foodborne illness acquired in the United States—major pathogens, *Emerg Infect Dis* 17(1): 7–15, 2011.

Scallan E, Griffin PM, Angulo FJ, Tauxe RV, Hoekstra RM: Foodborne illness acquired in the United States—unspecified agents, *Emerg Infect Dis* 17(1):16–22, 2011.

Siegel JD, Rhinehart E, Jackson M, Chiarello L: Healthcare Infection Control Practices Advisory Committee 2007: *Guidelines for isolation precautions: preventing transmission of infectious agents in healthcare settings*, 2017. Retrieved from https://www.cdc.gov.

U.S. Department of Health and Human Services: *Healthy People 2020*, 2010, Office of Disease Prevention and Health Promotion, Washington, DC, USDHHS. Retrieved from https://www.healthypeople.gov.

Wenzel RP: The Control of Communicable Diseases. In Last JM, Wallace R, editors: *Public Health and Preventive Medicine*, ed 13, Norwalk, Conn, Appleton & Lange, 1991.

Won KY, Kruszon-Moran D, Schantz PM, Jones JL: National seroprevalence and risk factors for zoonotic toxocara spp, infection, *Am J Trop Med Hyg* 79(4):552–557, 2008.

World Health Organization (WHO): *WHO response on the meeting of the International Health Regulations Emergency Committee concerning the international spread of wild poliovirus, Press Release*, Geneva, WHO Media Centre, 2016. Retrieved from http://www.who.int.

World Health Organization (WHO): *World Malaria Report 2017*, Geneva, World Health Organization, 2017.

World Health Organization (WHO): *The top 10 causes of death, Fact sheet*, WHO News, 2018a. Retrieved from http://www.who.int.

World Health Organization (WHO): *WHO supports Ebola vaccination of high risk populations in the Democratic Republic of the Congo, WHO News Release*, Geneva, WHO News, 2018b. Retrieved from http://www.who.int.

World Health Organization (WHO): *Ebola treatments approved for compassionate use in current outbreak*, Ebola Virus, 2018c. Retrieved from http://www.who.int.

World Health Organization (WHO): *Rubella Fact Sheet*, 2018d. Retrieved from http://www.who.int..

World Health Organization (WHO): *Cumulative number of confirmed human cases for avian influenza A(H5N1) reported to WHO, 2003–2018*, 2018e. Retrieved from http://www.who.int.

World Health Organization (WHO): *Malaria Fact Sheet*, 2018f. Retrieved from http://www.who.int.

World Health Organization (WHO): *History of the Zika Virus*, 2018g. Retrieved from http://www.who.int.

Zimlichman E, Henderson D, Tamir O, et al.: Health care-associated infections: A meta-analysis of costs and financial impact on the US health care system, *JAMA Intern Med* 173(22):2039–2046, 2013.

15

Communicable and Infectious Disease Risks

Erika Metzler Sawin, PhD and Tammy Kiser, DNP, RN

OBJECTIVES

After reading this chapter, the student should be able to do the following:

1. Describe the natural history of human immunodeficiency virus (HIV) infection and appropriate client education at each stage.
2. Explain the clinical signs of selected communicable diseases.
3. Evaluate the trends in incidence of HIV, sexually transmitted diseases, hepatitis, and tuberculosis, and identify groups that are at greatest risk.
4. Analyze behaviors that place people at risk of contracting selected communicable diseases.
5. Evaluate nursing activities to prevent and control selected communicable diseases.
6. Explain the various roles of nurses in providing care for those with selected communicable diseases.

CHAPTER OUTLINE

Human Immunodeficiency Virus Infection
Sexually Transmitted Diseases
Hepatitis
Tuberculosis
Nurse's Role in Providing Preventive Care for Communicable Diseases

KEY TERMS

acquired immunodeficiency syndrome, p. 334
chlamydia, p. 342
directly observed therapy, p. 352
genital herpes, p. 343
genital warts, p. 343
gonorrhea, p. 339
hepatitis A virus, p. 344
hepatitis B virus, p. 345
hepatitis C virus, p. 345
highly active antiretroviral therapy, p. 334
HIV antibody test, p. 335
HIV infection, p. 334
human immunodeficiency virus, p. 334
human papillomavirus, p. 343
incidence, p. 339
incubation, p. 334
injection drug use, p. 336
non-gonococcal urethritis, p. 342
partner notification, p. 348
pelvic inflammatory disease, p. 339
perinatal HIV transmission, p. 336
prevalence, p. 336
sexually transmitted diseases, p. 333
syphilis, p. 342
tuberculosis, p. 346

Knowledge about the risk of communicable diseases has changed dramatically in recent years. For example, in the decades following the development of antibiotics in the 1940s, **sexually transmitted diseases** (STDs) were considered to be a problem of the past. The recent emergence of new viral STDs and antibiotic-resistant strains of bacterial STDs has posed new challenges. Left unchecked, STDs can cause poor pregnancy outcomes, infertility, and cervical cancers. There is also the problem of coinfection, with one STD increasing the susceptibility to other STDs, such as human immunodeficiency virus (HIV). STDs are also called sexually transmitted infections (STIs) because many times the infections are asymptomatic. In this chapter the term *STDs* will be used.

This concern about infectious diseases has prompted the development of standards for STDs, HIV, and acquired immunodeficiency syndrome (AIDS), hepatitis, and tuberculosis (TB) in the *Healthy People 2020* report. The Healthy People 2020 box shows some objectives used to evaluate progress toward decreasing communicable diseases by the year 2020.

HEALTHY PEOPLE 2020

The following selected objectives pertain to the communicable diseases discussed in this chapter:

- **HIV-3**: Reduce the rate of HIV transmission among adults and adolescents.
- **STD-8**: Reduce congenital syphilis.
- **IID-26**: Reduce new hepatitis C infections.
- **STD-1**: Reduce the proportion of adolescents and young adults with *Chlamydia trachomatis* infections.

From U.S. Department of Health and Human Services: *Healthy People 2020 objectives*, Washington, DC, 2010, Office of Disease Prevention and Health Promotion, USDHHS.

Several communicable diseases and all STDs are acquired through behaviors that can be avoided or changed, and thus intervention efforts by nurses have focused on disease prevention. Prevention can take the form of vaccine administration (as with hepatitis A and hepatitis B), early detection (of infections like TB, for example), or instruction of clients about abstinence or safer sex. Individuals who live with chronic infections can transmit them to others.

This chapter describes selected communicable diseases and their nursing management. It concludes with implications for nursing care in primary, secondary, and tertiary prevention.

HUMAN IMMUNODEFICIENCY VIRUS INFECTION

Human immunodeficiency virus (HIV) infection has had an enormous political and social impact on society. Controversies have arisen over many aspects of HIV. Fears about HIV may lead to attitudes of blaming clients for their infections and to discrimination. These beliefs are magnified by the fact that this disease has commonly afflicted two groups who have been largely scorned by society: homosexuals and injection drug users (Hall et al., 2017). Debates have arisen over how to control disease transmission and how to pay for related health services. An ongoing debate involves whether clean needles should be distributed to injection drug users to prevent the spread of HIV.

An estimated 1.1 million individuals 13 years or older were living with HIV infection at the end of 2015 in the United States. Of that number, 162,500 had not received a diagnosis (CDC, 2018e). In 2016, 21% of new HIV infections occurred in the 13- to 24-year-old age-group (CDC, 2018e). Medicaid and Medicare primarily support the health care delivery costs of those infected. Many people with HIV qualify for Medicaid or Medicare because they are indigent or fall into poverty when paying for health care over the course of the illness. The lifetime cost of HIV care for one client infected with HIV at the mean age of 35 is $326,500 (Schackman et al., 2015). The Ryan White HIV/AIDS Program, through the Ryan White HIV/AIDS Treatment Extension Act of 2009, provides care for persons with HIV infection (USDHHS, 2019). This program provides funds for health care in the geographic areas with the largest number of AIDS cases. Health services that are covered include emergency services, services for early intervention and care (sometimes including coverage of health insurance), and drug reimbursement programs for HIV-infected individuals. The AIDS Drug Assistance Programs (ADAPs) are awards that pay for medications on the basis of the estimated number of persons living with AIDS in the individual state (USDHHS, 2019).

Natural History of HIV

The natural history of HIV includes three stages: the primary infection (within about 1 month of contracting the virus), followed by a period when the body shows no symptoms (clinical latency), and then a final stage of symptomatic disease (Buttaro et al., 2017). When HIV enters the body, a person may experience a mononucleosis-like syndrome, referred to as a primary infection, which lasts for a few weeks. This may go unrecognized. The body's CD4 white blood cell count drops for a brief time when the virus is most plentiful in the body. The immune system increases antibody production in response to this initial infection, which is a self-limiting illness. Symptoms include lymphadenopathy, myalgia, sore throat, lethargy, rash, and fever (CDC, 2018a). Even if the client seeks medical care at this time, the antibody test at this stage is usually negative, so it is often not recognized as HIV.

After a variable period of time, commonly from 6 weeks to 3 months, HIV antibodies appear in the blood. Although most antibodies serve a protective role, HIV antibodies do not. However, their presence helps in the detection of **HIV infection** because screening tests show their presence in the bloodstream.

HIV-infected persons live several years before developing symptomatic disease. During this prolonged **incubation** period, clients have a gradual deterioration of the immune system and can transmit the virus to others. The use of **highly active antiretroviral therapy** (HAART) has greatly increased the survival time of persons with HIV/AIDS.

Acquired immunodeficiency syndrome (AIDS, a.k.a. HIV stage 3) is the last stage in the long continuum of HIV infection and may result from damage caused by HIV, secondary cancers, or opportunistic organisms. AIDS is defined as a disabling or life-threatening illness caused by HIV; it is diagnosed in a person with a CD4 T-lymphocyte count of less than 200/mL with documented HIV infection (Schneider et al., 2008).

Many of the AIDS-related opportunistic infections are caused by microorganisms that are commonly present in healthy individuals but do not cause disease in persons with an intact immune system. These microorganisms proliferate in persons with HIV/AIDS because of a weakened immune system. Opportunistic infections may be caused by bacteria, fungi, viruses, or protozoa. The most common opportunistic diseases are *Pneumocystis jiroveci (carinii)* pneumonia and oral candidiasis, but they also include pulmonary TB, invasive cervical cancer, or recurrent pneumonia.

In 2008 the case definition for HIV infection was revised to include the HIV classification/staging system based on the number of CD4+ T-lymphocytes. Criteria for defining HIV infection include a positive result from the antibody screening test or a positive result from a nucleic acid test (DNA or RNA). In situations where the mother of a newborn is HIV infected, the HIV nucleic acid test (DNA or RNA) is used to identify HIV/AIDS in infants (Schneider et al., 2008). In 2014, the CDC and the Council of State and territorial Epidemiologists

QSEN FOCUS ON QUALITY AND SAFETY EDUCATION IN NURSES

Sexually Transmitted Diseases

Targeted Competency

Evidence-based practice (EBP): Integrate best current evidence with clinical expertise and client/family preferences and values for delivery of optimal care.

- **Knowledge:** Explain the role of evidence in determining best clinical practice.
- **Skills:** Locate evidence reports related to clinical practice topics and guidelines
- **Attitudes:** Value the concept of EBP as integral to determining best clinical practice.

Client-Centered Care Question

Evidence supports the fact that some medications previously effective in treating STDs no longer are effective. If you learned that a colleague was planning to use a treatment that is no longer considered effective to treat a specific STD, what would you do to ensure that the care the client receives is based on current evidence?

Answer: With your colleague collect current treatment guidelines information about that specific STD. The first place that you might look would be the Centers for Disease Control and Prevention guidelines for that disease. For example, you might look at "HIV treatment guidelines for adults and adolescents updated" at the following website to find out what is the most effective antiretroviral therapy (ART) for the treatment of HIV infection. (See Panel on Antiretroviral Guidelines for Adults and Adolescents: Guidelines for the use of antiretroviral agents in adults and adolescents living with HIV, Department of Health and Human Services. Available at http://www.aidsinfo.nih.gov/ContentFiles/AdultandAdolescentGL.pdf.)

revised and combined the surveillance case definitions for HIV into a single definition of persons of all ages. A confirmed case can be classified in one of five HIV infection stages (0, 1, 2, 3, or unknown). Early infection, recognized by a negative HIV test within 6 months of HIV diagnosis is stage 0 and AIDS is stage 3 (Selik, Mokotoff, Branson, et al, 2014).

TB, an infection that is becoming more prevalent because of HIV infection, can spread rapidly among immunosuppressed individuals. Thus HIV-infected individuals who live in close proximity to one another, such as in long-term care facilities, prisons, drug treatment facilities, or other settings, must be carefully screened and in some instances deemed noninfectious before admission to such settings. TB is covered in more depth later in this chapter. See the QSEN box for suggestions about implementing quality and safety in the care of patients with HIV and other communicable and infectious diseases.

Transmission

HIV is transmitted through exposure to blood, semen, transplanted organs, vaginal secretions, and breast milk (Heymann, 2014). Persons who had blood exposure or sexual or needle-sharing contact with an HIV-infected person are at risk for contracting the virus. The virus is not transmitted through casual contact such as touching or hugging someone who has HIV infection or through mosquitoes or other insects. Although HIV has been found in saliva and tears in some instances, there are no reports of transmission through contact with these body fluids (Heymann, 2014). The modes of transmission are listed in Box 15.1, and the exposure categories of HIV are shown in Fig. 15.1.

Potential donors of blood and tissues are screened through interviews to assess for a history of high-risk activities and screened with the HIV antibody test. Blood or tissue is not used from individuals with a history of high-risk behavior or who are HIV infected. In addition to being screened, coagulation factors used to treat hemophilia and other blood disorders are made safe through heat treatments to inactivate the virus. Screening has significantly reduced the risk of transmission of HIV by blood products and organ donations.

When a person has an STD infection such as chlamydia or gonorrhea, the risk of HIV infection increases, and HIV may also increase the risk for other STDs. This may result from any of the following: open lesions providing a portal of entry for pathogens; STDs decreasing the host's immune status, resulting in a rapid progression of HIV infection; and HIV changing the natural history of STDs or the effectiveness of medications used in treating STDs (Heymann, 2014).

The nurse serves both as an educator about the modes of transmission and as a role model for how to behave toward and provide supportive care for those with HIV infection. An understanding of how transmission does and does not occur will help family and community members feel more comfortable in relating to and caring for persons with HIV (see Box 15.1).

Epidemiology of HIV/AIDS

Worldwide 36.7 million persons live with HIV infection. Sub-Saharan Africa accounts for more than 50% of all HIV infections (UNAIDS, 2018). The epidemic is also growing in Eastern Europe, the Middle East, and central Asia (UNAIDS, 2018). Women are at highest risk for infection because of unprotected sex with infected partners. However, there is some evidence that

BOX 15.1 Modes of Transmission of Human Immunodeficiency Virus (HIV)

HIV can be transmitted in the following ways:

- Sexual contact, involving the exchange of body fluids, with an infected person
- Sharing or reusing needles, syringes, or other equipment used to prepare injectable drugs
- Perinatal transmission from an infected mother to her fetus during pregnancy or delivery, or to an infant when breastfeeding
- Transfusions or other exposure to HIV-contaminated blood or blood products, organs, or semen

From Heymann D: *Control of communicable diseases manual,* ed. 20, Washington, DC, 2014, American Public Health Association.

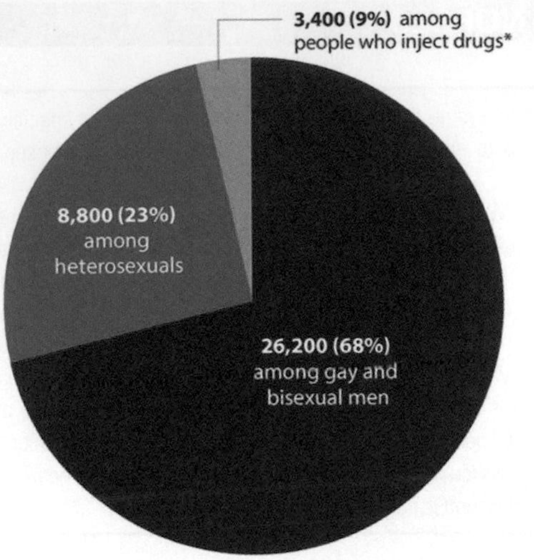

Fig. 15.1 Estimated numbers of cases of HIV by exposure category in 2015 United States. (Data from Centers for Disease Control and Prevention: *HIV surveillance report: diagnoses of HIV infection and AIDS in the United States and dependent areas, 2016*, vol. 28. Available at http://www.cdc.gov. Published November 2017.)

HIV prevention programs may be changing risk behavior in southern Africa. Worldwide, the treatment of HIV infection has been given higher priority, and the use of HAART is at 53% for those who need it (UNAIDS, 2018).

Nurses must identify the trends of HIV infection in the populations they serve so that they can screen clients who may be at risk and can adequately plan prevention programs and illness care resources. For example, knowing that AIDS disproportionately affects minorities helps nurses set priorities and plan services for these groups. Factors such as geographic location, age, and ethnic distribution are tracked to more effectively target programs. It is important to identify persons infected with HIV before symptomatic AIDS develops so that treatment can begin as early as needed. It is estimated that about 1.1 million people in the United States are infected with HIV, but 15% (one in seven people) are not aware of their infection (CDC, 2018a). Since the first cases of AIDS were identified in 1981, the total reported number of persons diagnosed with AIDS in the United States is 1,232,246 (HIV.gov, 2018). In 2016, 18,160 people received an AIDS diagnosis (CDC, 2017a). This number reflects only those people who are living; it does not include those who have died. The estimated number of annual HIV infections in the United States declined 8% from 2010 to 2015 (HIV.gov, 2018). The **prevalence** of AIDS has increased from 2010 to 2015, reflecting increased life expectancy from the use of antiretroviral therapy (HIV.gov, 2018).

Fig. 15.1 shows the exposure categories for persons with HIV in 2015 Men who have sex with men (MSM) make up the largest group with HIV in the United States, and the number of persons contracting HIV through heterosexual transmission is the second largest group. Heterosexual transmission has surpassed **injection drug use** (IDU) as the primary mode of HIV transmission in women (CDC, 2017a).

The distribution of pediatric HIV infection has fallen dramatically as a result of prenatal care that includes HIV testing, antiretroviral therapy for the mother, and cesarean delivery. **Perinatal HIV transmission** has declined, and two-thirds of pediatric HIV infection from perinatal exposure (CDC, 2017a).

As seen in Table 15.1, HIV has disproportionately affected minority groups. African Americans have the largest HIV disease burden of any racial/ethnic group in the United States; African American rates of new HIV infection are 8 times higher than in whites, the highest prevalence of those living with HIV is in the African American community, and the highest proportions of people diagnosed with HIV stage 3 (AIDS) are African American (CDC, 2017a). This overrepresentation is associated with poverty, since African Americans have a higher poverty rate than other groups do. This reflects decreased access to prevention and treatment and lack of awareness of HIV infection. Stigma, fear, and homophobia play a role as well (CDC, 2017a). Transgender people are also at high risk, particularly transgender women. Because of data collection limitations, it is difficult to estimate HIV prevalence in transgender communities. However, data from countries that collect data for transgender women separately from MSM indicate that HIV prevalence is

TABLE 15.1 Estimated Numbers of New HIV Infections and Stage 3 (AIDS) Infections in Adults and Adolescents, 2016 (50 States, the District of Columbia, and 6 U.S. Dependent Areas)

Race/Ethnicity	HIV Infection	Rate Per 100,000	Rate, Males	Rate, Females	Stage 3 (AIDS)
Black, African American	17,528	43.6	82.8	26.2	8504
White	10,345	5.2	10.6	1.7	4443
Hispanic/Latino	9,766	17	38.8	5.3	4350
Asian	977	5.5	11.6	1.8	336
American Indian/Alaska Native	243	10.2	20.9	4.5	102
Native Hawaiian/Pacific Islander	48	8.5	16.8	3.9	20
Multiple races	875	12.9	33.8	6.7	654
Total	39,782	12.3	24.3	5.4	18,409

AIDS, Acquired immunodeficiency syndrome; *HIV,* Human immunodeficiency virus.
Data from Centers for Disease Control and Prevention: *HIV surveillance report: diagnoses of HIV infection and AIDS in the United States and dependent areas, 2016*, vol. 28. Available at http://www.cdc.gov. Published November 2017.

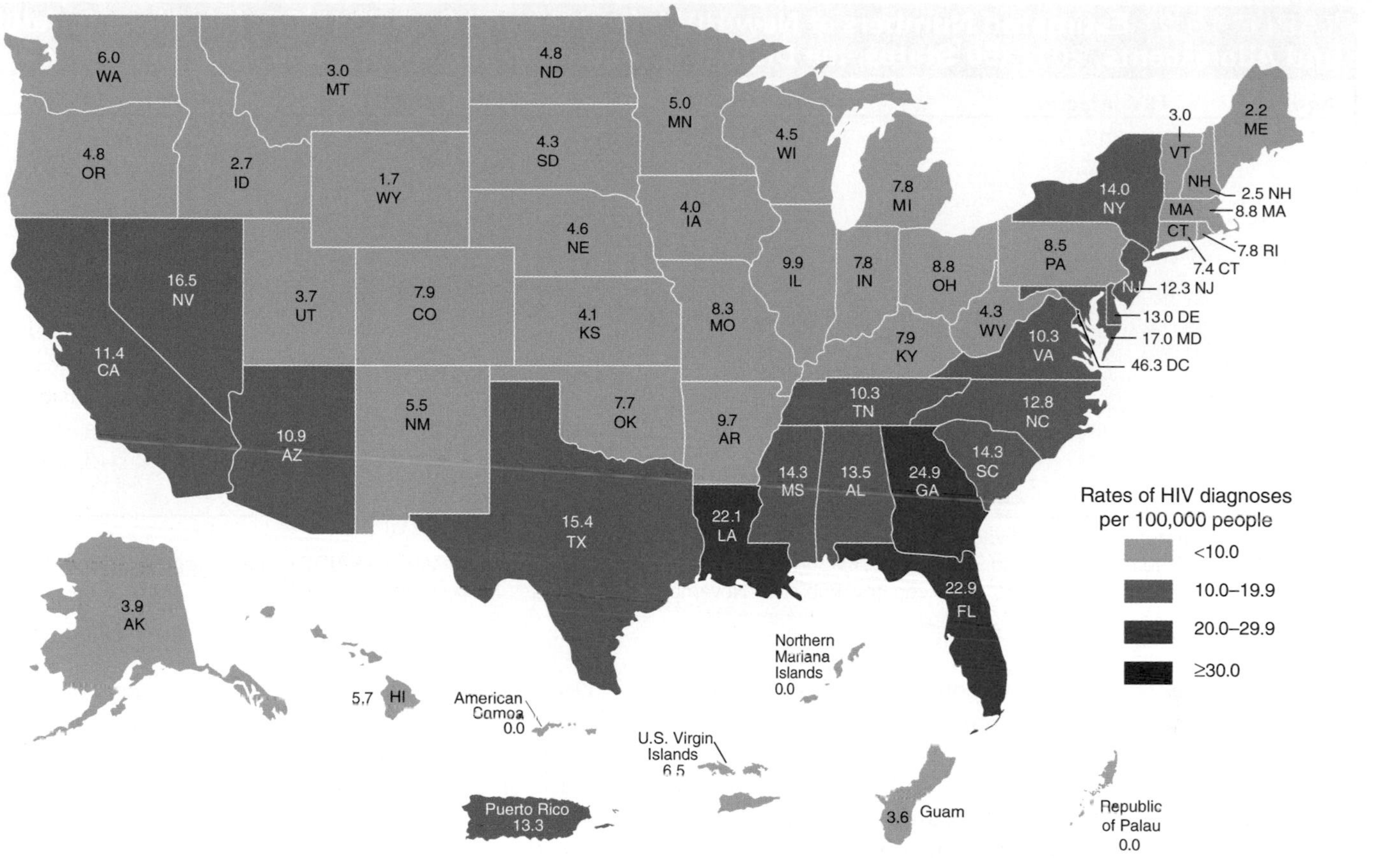

Fig. 15.2 Map of rates of diagnosis of HIV infection among adults and adolescents, 2017, in the United States and six dependent areas. (Data from Centers for Disease Control and Prevention: *HIV surveillance report: diagnoses of HIV infection and AIDS in the United States and dependent areas, 2018,* vol. 29. Available at https://www.cdc.gov. Published November 2018.

nearly 50 times higher than for other adults of reproductive age (UNAIDS, 2018).

As seen in Fig. 15.2, the geographic distribution of HIV infection is clustered in urban areas. Regionally, the southern United States and Puerto Rico report the highest rates (CDC, 2017b, 2018f, 2018g, 2018q). African Americans are disproportionately affected in all geographic regions (CDC, 2017b, 2018g). Both HIV and HIV stage 3 (AIDS) affect people across the life span, with 21% of new diagnoses occurring in youth ages 13-24, most of whom are gay or bisexual men (CDC 2018m). Peak HIV stage 3 (AIDS) rates occur in individuals age 35-39 (Table 15.2).

HIV Surveillance

A study of diagnosed cases of AIDS does not reveal current HIV infection patterns because of the interval between infection with HIV and the onset of clinical disease. Moreover, the effectiveness of antiretroviral drugs given early in the HIV infection before symptoms start provides impetus for early identification of infection. Thus in 2008 confidential laboratory reporting of HIV-positive status by name was required in all 50 states and the District of Columbia (CDC, 2017a), although not all states require viral load and CD4 counts (CDC, 2017a).

HIV Testing

The HIV antibody test is the most commonly used screening test for determining infection. This test does just as its name implies: it does not reveal whether an individual has symptomatic AIDS, nor does it isolate the virus. It does indicate the presence of the antibody to HIV. The most commonly used form of this test is the enzyme-linked immunosorbent assay (EIA). The EIA effectively screens blood and other donor products. To minimize false-positive results, a confirmatory test, the Western blot, is used to verify the results. False-negative results may also occur after infection and before antibodies are produced. Sometimes referred to as the window period, this can last from 6 weeks to 3 months.

Rapid HIV antibody testing using oral fluid samples (e.g., OraQuick, Home Access HIV-1 Test System) is 99.5% accurate and provides results within 20 minutes, allowing immediate results to be given (CDC, 2018p). In addition to the rapid results, this test may appeal to persons who fear having their blood drawn. If the test is positive, it requires a second specific confirmatory test.

Routine voluntary HIV testing is recommended for adults ages 13 to 64 (CDC, 2018p). Voluntary screening programs for HIV may be either confidential or anonymous; the process for each is unique. Confidential testing involves reporting by

TABLE 15.2 Estimated Numbers of New HIV Infections and Stage 3 (AIDS) Infections in Adults and Adolescents, 2011 (50 States, the District of Columbia, and 6 U.S. Dependent Areas) by Age

Age	HIV Infection	Rate per 100,000	Stage 3 (AIDS)	Rate per 100,000
<13	122	0.2	38	0.1
13–14	23	0.3	12	0.1
15–19	1665	7.8	209	1.
20–24	6848	30.2	1252	5.6
25–29	8030	34.7	2426	10.6
30–34	5766	26.2	2384	10.9
35–39	4312	20.5	2308	11.1
40–44	3391	17.	2049	10.4
45–49	3214	15.2	2152	10.3
50–54	3009	13.6	2165	9.9
55–59	1971	8.9	1499	6.8
60–64	1114	5.7	913	4.7
≥65	859	1.7	753	1.5

AIDS, Acquired immunodeficiency syndrome; *HIV,* Human immunodeficiency virus.
From Centers for Disease Control and Prevention: *HIV surveillance report: diagnoses of HIV infection and AIDS in the United States and dependent areas, 2016,* vol. 28. Available at http://www.cdc.gov. Published November 2017.

identifying the person's name and other identifying information; this information is considered protected by confidentiality. With anonymous testing, the client is given an identification code number that is attached to all records of the test results and is not linked to the person's name and address (CDC, 2018p). Demographic data such as the person's sex, age, and race may be collected, but there is no record of the client's name and associated identifying information. An advantage of anonymous testing may be that it increases the number of people who are willing to be tested, because many of those at risk are engaged in illegal activities. The anonymity eliminates their concern about the possibility of arrest or discrimination. However, anonymous testing does not allow for follow-up if the test results are positive because the client's name and address are not available.

Perinatal and Pediatric HIV Infection

Perinatal transmission accounts for nearly all HIV infection in children and can occur during pregnancy, labor and delivery, or breastfeeding. The effectiveness of antiretroviral therapy in pregnant women and newborns in preventing transmission from mother to fetus or infant has made pediatric HIV rates decline sharply. On the basis of the effectiveness of antiviral therapy, it is recommended that HIV testing be a routine part of prenatal care and that all pregnant women be tested for HIV—even a mother who presents in labor who is untested and whose HIV status is not known (CDC, 2018a). Rapid testing allows rapid results in women who are giving birth but have not been previously tested for HIV. HIV prevention in women must remain the primary focus of efforts to reduce pediatric HIV infection.

If left untreated, the clinical picture of pediatric HIV infection involves a shorter incubation period than in adults, and symptoms may occur within the first year of life. The physical signs and symptoms in children include failure to thrive, unexplained persistent diarrhea, developmental delays, and bacterial infections such as TB and severe pneumonia (WHO, 2017).

Detection of HIV infection in infants of infected mothers is made through different tests from those used in children over 18 months. Virologic assays that directly detect HIV (e.g., nucleic acid amplification tests [NAATs] such as HIV DNA, RNA polymerase chain reaction [PCR] assays, and related RNA qualitative or quantitative assays) must be used (AIDSinfo, 2018). The EIA test is not valid because it tests for antibodies, which in the infant reflect passively acquired maternal antibodies.

Despite having an HIV-infected mother, many children do not acquire HIV. However, one or both parents may die from HIV infection. The families of many children with AIDS are impoverished, with limited financial, emotional, social, and health care resources. The added strain of this illness makes many individuals and families unable to provide for the emotional, physical, and developmental needs of affected children.

HIV Stage 3 (AIDS) in the Community

AIDS is a chronic disease, so individuals continue to live and work in the community. Persons with AIDS have bouts of illness interspersed with periods of wellness when they are able to return to school or work. When ill, much of their care is provided in the home. The nurse teaches families and significant others about personal care and hygiene, medication administration, standard precautions to ensure infection control, and healthy lifestyle behaviors such as adequate rest, balanced nutrition, and exercise.

Adherence to HAART is critical for clients because administration must be consistent to be effective (CDC, 2016c). It is important for nurses to educate clients about accurate medication administration. Peer advocates and persons living with HIV infection who are trained to work with infected persons play a vital role in advocacy and teaching self-care management.

The Americans with Disabilities Act of 1990 and other laws protect persons with asymptomatic HIV infection and AIDS against discrimination in housing, at work, and in other public situations (HIV.gov, 2017). Policies regarding school and worksite attendance have been developed by most states and localities on the basis of these laws. These policies provide direction for the community's response when a person develops HIV infection. The nurse can identify resources such as social and financial support services and interpret school and work policies.

Mental health issues such as depression, substance abuse, and bipolar disorder are often present in someone newly diagnosed with HIV. These conditions must be addressed before or simultaneously with HIV treatment to be effective. It is vitally important that a variety of health and social services be available to support persons with HIV (CDC, 2018a).

Nurses can assist employers by educating managers about how to deal with ill or infected workers to reduce the risk of breaching confidentiality or wrongful actions such as termination. Disclosing a worker's infection to other workers, terminating employment, and isolating an infected worker are examples of situations that have led to litigation between employees and employers. The CDC supports workplace issues through programs offered by its Business and Labor Resource Service .

HIV-infected children should attend school because the benefit of attendance far outweighs the risk of transmitting or acquiring infections. None of the cases of HIV infection in the United States have been transmitted in a school setting. An interprofessional team that includes the child's physician, the nurse, and the child's parent or guardian should make decisions about educational and care needs.

Because of impaired immunity, children with HIV infection are more likely to get childhood diseases and suffer serious sequelae. Therefore DPT (diphtheria, pertussis, tetanus), IPV (inactivated polio virus), and MMR (measles, mumps, rubella) vaccines should be given at regularly scheduled times for children infected with HIV. Hib (*Haemophilus influenzae* type b), hepatitis B, pneumococcus, and influenza vaccines may be recommended after medical evaluation (USDHHS, 2013) Additionally the Panel on Opportunistic Infections in HIV-Exposed and HIV-Infected Children guidelines (Public Health Foundation, 2014) recommends meningococcal disease vaccination, as well as hepatitis A and varicella vaccination, provided that the infant or child is not severely immunocompromised.

Individual decisions about risk to the infected child or others should be based on the behavior, neurological development, and physical condition of the child. Attendance may be inadvisable in the presence of cases of childhood infections, such as chickenpox or measles, within the school because the immunosuppressed child is at greater risk of suffering complications. Alternative arrangements, such as homebound instruction, might be instituted if a child is unable to control body secretions or displays biting behavior.

Resources

As the number of individuals with HIV/AIDS has increased, services to meet these needs have grown. Voluntary and faith-based service organizations, such as community-based organizations or AIDS support organizations, have developed in many localities to address these needs. These services may include counseling, support groups, legal aid, personal care services, housing programs, and community education programs. Nurses collaborate with workers from community-based organizations in the client's home and may advise these groups in their supportive work. The federal government and many organizations have established toll-free numbers and websites to provide information, as noted on the Evolve website at http://evolve.elsevier.com/Stanhope.

SEXUALLY TRANSMITTED DISEASES

The number of new cases (the **incidence**) of STDs such as gonorrhea, herpes simplex virus, human papillomavirus (HPV), and chlamydia continues to increase. Chlamydia is the most commonly reported infectious disease; gonorrhea is the second most common. Because of the impact of STDs on long-term health and the emergence of eight new STDs since 1980, continued attention to their prevention and treatment is vital.

The common STDs listed in Table 15.3 are categorized by cause, either viral or bacterial. The bacterial infections include gonorrhea, syphilis, and chlamydia. Most of these are curable with antibiotics, with the exception of the newly emerging antibiotic-resistant strains of gonorrhea.

STDs caused by viruses cannot be cured. These are chronic diseases resulting in a lifetime of symptom management and infection control. The viral infections include herpes simplex virus, HIV, and HPV, also referred to as genital warts. The hepatitis A, B, and C viruses, which may also be transmitted via sexual activity, are discussed later in this chapter.

Gonorrhea

Neisseria gonorrhoeae is a gram-negative intracellular diplococcal bacterium that infects the mucous membranes of the genitourinary tract, rectum, and pharynx. It is transmitted through genital-genital contact, oral-genital contact, and anal-genital contact.

Gonorrhea is identified as either uncomplicated or complicated. Uncomplicated gonorrhea refers to limited cervical or urethral infection. Complicated gonorrhea includes salpingitis, epididymitis, systemic gonococcal infection, and gonococcal meningitis. The signs and symptoms of infection in males are purulent and copious urethral discharge and dysuria. Symptoms in males are usually sufficient to seek treatment. Gonococcal infection in women however, is commonly asymptomatic, and treatment may not be sought. The disease will continue to be spread to others through sexual activity and may not be recognized until **pelvic inflammatory disease** (PID) occurs (CDC, 2015b).

Some individuals may continue to be sexually active and infect others while symptomatic. Coinfection with gonorrhea and chlamydia is common; therefore treatment containing ceftriaxone combined with azithromycin is recommended (CDC, 2015b).

Reported gonorrhea rates are on the rise again after a long period of decline, particularly in the Northeast, Midwest, and West, although overall rates are still highest in the South (CDC, 2017e). The reported number of cases in the United States in 2016 was 468,514, for a rate of 145.8 cases per 100,000 population, an increase of 18.5% from 2015 (CDC,

TABLE 15.3 **Summary of Sexually Transmitted Diseases**

Disease/ Pathogen	Incubation	Signs and Symptoms	Diagnosis	Treatment	Nursing Implications
Bacterial					
Chlamydia: *Chlamydia trachomatis*	Poorly defined—probably 7-14 days or longer	*Man:* None or nongonococcal urethritis (NGU); painful urination and urethral discharge; epididymitis *Woman:* None or mucopurulent cervicitis (MPC), vaginal discharge; if untreated, progresses to symptoms of PID: diffuse abdominal pain, fever, chills	Nucleic acid amplification test (NAAT) of male urine and female endocervix	One of following treatments: Doxycycline 100 mg orally bid × 7 days; Azithromycin 1 g orally × 1 Alternative regimens: Erythromycin base 500 mg orally qid × 7 days; Erythromycin ethylsuccinate 800 mg orally qid × 7 days; Levofloxacin 500 mg orally, daily × 7 days Ofloxacin 300 mg orally bid × 7 days *Notes:* Doxycycline is effective and cheap. Azithromycin is good because single dose is sufficient.	Refer partners of past 60 days; counsel client to use condoms and to avoid sex for 7 days after start of therapy and until symptoms are gone in both client and partners; medication teaching Annual screening recommended for all sexually active women under 25, and women over 25 with new or multiple sexual partners
Gonorrhea: *Neisseria gonorrhoeae*	1-14 days, can be longer	Man: Urethritis, purulent discharge, painful urination, urinary frequency; epididymitis Woman: None, or symptoms of PID	Gram stain of discharge, culture on selective media, or NAAT	For uncomplicated gonorrhea: Ceftriaxone 250 mg IM PLUS Azithromycin 1 gm orally × 1 *Notes:* If ceftriaxone not readily available, oral cefixime may be used in combination with azithromycin, but patient should return at 1 week for a test-of-cure at the site of infection	Refer partners of past 60 days; return for evaluation if symptoms persist; counsel client to use therapy until complete and symptoms are gone in both client and partners; medication teaching
Syphilis: *Treponema pallidum*	10-90 days, usually 3 weeks. Stages are generally diagnosed by appearance of hallmark symptoms	Primary: usually single, painless chancre; if untreated, heals in few weeks Secondary: low-grade fever, malaise, sore throat, headache, lymphadenopathy, and rash Early latency: Asymptomatic, infectious lesions may recur Late latency: Asymptomatic, noninfectious except to fetus of pregnant women Gummas of skin, bone, mucous membranes, heart, liver CNS involvement: Paresis, optic atrophy Cardiovascular involvement: Aortic aneurysm, aortic value insufficiency	Nontreponemal serological test such as the rapid plasma reagin. If that is positive, then confirm with a treponemal serological test. Early in the disease, these test results may be negative. Examine smears of lesion exudate using dark -field microscopic examination or PCR or lesion biopsy. For patients with neurologic abnormalities, consider neurosyphilis, diagnosed by CSF cell testing.	For primary, secondary, or early latent < 1 year: benzathine penicillin G 2.4 million units, IM once If penicillin allergy: Doxycycline 100 mg orally bid × 14 days, Tetracycline 500 mg four times daily × 14 days Tetracycline should not be administered to pregnant women or those with neurosyphilis or congenital syphilis Latent > 1 year or latent of unknown duration: Benzathine penicillin G 7.2 million units total in three doses of 2.4 million units IM at 1-week intervals. *Notes:* See CDC treatment guidelines for treatment of syphilis in children or pregnancy, neurosyphilis, and congenital syphilis.	Counsel to be tested for HIV and other STIs; screen all partners of past 3 months; reexamine client at 3 and 6 months. Universal precautions should be used with all syphilis patients.

TABLE 15.3 Summary of Sexually Transmitted Diseases—cont'd

Disease/ Pathogen	Incubation	Signs and Symptoms	Diagnosis	Treatment	Nursing Implications
Viral					
Human immunodeficiency virus (HIV)	4-6 weeks *Seroconversion:* 6 weeks to 3 months *AIDS:* month to years (average, 11 years)	*Possible:* Acute mononucleosis-like illness (lymphadenopathy, fever, rash, joint and muscle pain, sore throat) Appearance of HIV antibody *Opportunistic diseases:* Most commonly *Pneumocystis jiroveci* pneumonia, oral candidiasis, Kaposi's sarcoma	*HIV antibody test:* EIA or Western blot test; OraSure (SmithKline Beecham) is an oral HIV-1 antibody testing system, test results in about 3 days CD4+ T-lymphocyte count of less than 200/µl with documented HIV infection, or diagnosis with clinical manifestation of AIDS as defined by CDC	Prophylactic administration of zidovudine (ZDV) immediately after exposure may prevent seroconversion Postexposure prophylaxis (PEP) should begin as soon as possible. Choice of antiviral drug therapy is made based on toxicity and drug resistance. Combinations of drugs are considered such as zidovudine (ZDV) and 3TC. Drug selection is complicated and evolving. Preexposure prophylaxis (PrEP) was approved in 2012, consisting of daily tenofovir disoproxil fumarate plus emtricitabine (TDF/FTC), for use among sexually active, at-risk adults.	HIV education and counseling; partner referral for evaluation; medication education; assessment and referral Men who have sex with men should be tested annually for HIV, chlamydia, syphilis, and gonorrhea.
Genital warts: human papillomavirus (HPV)	2-3 months; range is 1-20 months	Often asymptomatic or subclinical infection; painless lesions near vaginal openings, anus, shaft of penis, vagina, cervix, with less common sites being throat, respiratory tract, mouth, or conjunctiva; lesions are textured, cauliflower appearance; may remain unchanged over time	Visual inspection for lesions; Pap smear	Prevention: Gardasil vaccine No cure; one-third of lesions will disappear without topical treatment Client-applied: topical podofilox 0.5%, or imiquimod 3.75% or 5% cream, or sinecatechins 15% ointment. Provider-administered: or trichloroacetic acid or bichloroacetic acid 80%–90%; cryotherapy, or surgical removal	Education about HPV vaccine. Warts and surrounding tissues contain HPV, so removal of warts does not completely eradicate virus; examination of partners not necessary, since treatment is only symptomatic; condom use may reduce transmission; medication application
Genital herpes simplex virus (HSV)	2-12 days	Vesicles, painful ulceration of penis, vagina, labia, perineum, or anus; lesions last 5–6 weeks and recurrence is common; may be asymptomatic	Presence of vesicles; viral culture (obtained only when lesions present and before they have scabbed over) HSV DNA detection by PCR, HSV antigen detection by EIA or direct fluorescent antibody (DFA).	No cure; treatment may be episodic or suppressive for frequent recurrence *Episodic treatment:* acyclovir 400 mg orally tid, 7-10 days; OR Acyclovir 200 mg orally five times a day × 7-10 days; OR famciclovir 250 mg orally tid 7-10 days; or valacyclovir 1 g orally bid × 7-10 days. See CDC guidelines for recurrent infection, treatment for persons with HIV infection, and daily suppressive therapy.	Refer partners for evaluation; teach client about likelihood of recurrent episodes and ability to transmit to others even if asymptomatic; condom use; annual Pap smear. Health care providers should wear gloves when in direct contact with possible infectious lesions or mucous membranes.

AIDS, Acquired immunodeficiency syndrome; *CDC,* Centers for Disease Control and Prevention; *CNS,* central nervous system; *CSF,* cerebrospinal fluid; *EIA,* enzyme-linked immunosorbent assay; *IM,* intramuscular; *PCR,* polymerase chain reaction; *PID,* pelvic inflammatory disease; *STI,* sexually transmitted infection.

From Centers for Disease Control and Prevention: Sexually transmitted diseases treatment guidelines, 2015. *MMWR Morb Mortal Wkly Rep,* 64(3). Retrieved from https://www.cdc.gov; Heymann D: *Control of communicable diseases manual,* ed. 20, Washington, DC, 2014, American Public Health Association.

2017e). The difference between the actual cases and reported cases occurs because gonorrhea may be unreported by health care providers and because clients who are asymptomatic do not seek treatment and are therefore not identified. Groups with the highest incidence of gonorrhea are African Americans, persons living in the southern United States, and women 20 to 24 years of age, although the rates of gonorrhea are rising in the West and among men (CDC, 2017e).

The number of antibiotic-resistant cases of gonorrhea in the United States has risen at an alarming rate. Penicillin-resistant gonorrhea was first identified in 1976 when 15 cases were reported (Phillips, 1976). Antibiotic-resistant *N. gonorrhoeae* has continued to develop exponentially, making it one of the greatest threats in the nation (CDC, 2018d). In 2006 there were five treatment options for gonorrhea, but at this time there is only one remaining treatment option (CDC, 2018d), which is injected ceftriaxone combined with oral azithromycin, both in single doses, simultaneously and under direct observation (CDC, 2018h).

The increase in antibiotic-resistant infections is partially attributed to the indiscriminate or illicit use of antibiotics as a prophylactic measure by persons with multiple sexual partners. To ensure proper treatment and cure, those diagnosed with gonorrheal infection should return for health care if symptoms persist, have all partners evaluated for infection and treated if necessary, and remain sexually abstinent for 77 days (CDC, 2018h).

The development of PID is a risk for women who remain asymptomatic and do not seek treatment. PID is a serious infection involving the fallopian tubes (salpingitis) and is the most common complication of gonorrhea but may also result from chlamydia infection. Its symptoms include fever, abnormal menses, and lower abdominal pain, but PID may not be recognized because the symptoms vary among women. PID can result in ectopic pregnancy and infertility related to fallopian tube scarring and occlusion. It may also cause stillbirths and premature labor (CDC, 2017b).

Syphilis

Syphilis is caused by a member of the treponemal group of spirochetes called *Treponema pallidum*. It infects moist mucous or cutaneous membranes and is spread through direct contact, usually by sexual contact or from mother to fetus. Transmission via blood transfusion may occur if the donor is in the early stages of disease (Heymann, 2014).

Syphilis rates in the United States declined between 1990 and 2001 but have been steadily increasing since then, with last reported rates of primary and secondary syphilis rates at 8.7 cases per 100,000 people, a rate increase of 14.7% among men and 35.7% among women (CDC, 2017e). The highest rates are among MSM, but in recent years the number of infected women has increased (CDC, 2017e).

The clinical signs of syphilis are divided into primary, secondary, and tertiary infections. Latency, a period when an individual is free of symptoms but has serological evidence, may occur early or late in the infection. All cases of syphilis that are untreated progress to latent infection. During early latency, skin and mucous membrane lesions may be apparent (Heymann, 2014).

Primary Syphilis. When syphilis is acquired sexually, the bacteria produce infection in the form of a chancre at the site of entry. The lesion begins as a macula, progresses to a papule, and later ulcerates. If left untreated, this chancre persists for 3 to 6 weeks and then in most cases disappears (Heymann, 2014).

Secondary Syphilis. Secondary syphilis occurs when the organism enters the lymph system and spreads throughout the body. Signs include rash, lymphadenopathy, and mucosal ulceration. Symptoms of secondary syphilis may include skin rash, lymphadenopathy, and lesions of the mucous membranes (Heymann, 2014).

Tertiary Syphilis. About one-third of untreated syphilis patients will demonstrate signs and symptoms of tertiary syphilis (Heymann, 2014). Tertiary syphilis can lead to blindness, congenital damage, cardiovascular damage, or syphilitic psychoses. A further complication can be the development of lesions of the bones, skin, and mucous membranes, known as gummatous lesions. Tertiary syphilis usually occurs several years after initial infection and is rare in the United States because the disease is usually cured in its early stages with antibiotics. Tertiary syphilis is a major problem in developing countries.

Congenital Syphilis. When primary and secondary syphilis rates increase, so do the rates of congenital syphilis (CS), which increased to its highest rate seen in over a decade in 2014 (Bowen et al., 2015). Syphilis is transmitted transplacentally and, if untreated, can cause premature stillbirth, blindness, deafness, facial abnormalities, crippling, or death. Signs include jaundice, skin rash, hepatosplenomegaly, or pseudoparalysis of an extremity. Preferred treatment is penicillin G administered parenterally (CDC, 2015b).

Chlamydia

Chlamydia infection results from the bacterium *Chlamydia trachomatis.* It infects the genitourinary tract and rectum of adults and causes conjunctivitis and pneumonia in neonates. Transmission occurs when mucopurulent discharge from infected sites, such as the cervix or urethra, comes into contact with the mucous membranes of a noninfected person. Like gonorrhea, the infection is often asymptomatic in women; up to 70% may experience no symptoms (Heymann, 2014). If left untreated, chlamydia can result in PID. When symptoms of chlamydial infection are present in women, they include dysuria, urinary frequency, and purulent vaginal discharge. In men the urethra is the most common site of infection, resulting in **non-gonococcal urethritis** (NGU). The symptoms of NGU are dysuria and urethral discharge. Epididymitis is a possible complication (Heymann, 2014). The Centers for Disease Control and Prevention (CDC) recommends annual chlamydial screening of all sexually active women less than 25 years of age (CDC, 2015b). Older women with new partners and/or more than one sex partner and all pregnant women should also be tested (CDC, 2017e).

Chlamydia is the most common reportable condition in the United States, and in 2016 a total of 1,598,354 cases of genital chlamydial infection were reported (CDC, 2017e). Between 2000 and 2011 the rate of reported chlamydia infection increased from 251.4 to 453.4 per 100,000 population, reflecting increased screening rates, an emphasis on case reporting, and more sensitive testing (CDC, 2017e). After a brief decrease, chlamydia is on the rise again, increasing to a 2016 rate of 493.3 cases per 100,000 (CDC, 2017e). Prevention is important because chlamydia can cause PID, ectopic pregnancy, infertility, and neonatal complications. Women under 25 years of age are the most commonly infected with chlamydial infection because of inconsistent use of barrier contraceptives, multiple sexual partners, and a history of infection with other STDs (CDC, 2017e). The high frequency of other STIs in individuals diagnosed with chlamydia requires testing for HIV, syphilis, and gonorrhea (CDC, 2015b).

Herpes Simplex Virus (Genital Herpes)

Two types of herpes simplex viruses (HSV-1 and HSV-2) cause **genital herpes**. The majority of genital herpes infections are caused by HSV-2, and these herpes infections are more likely to be recurrent (CDC, 2015b). However, an increasing number of genital herpes infections are caused by HSV-1; these infections are more common in young women and MSM (CDC, 2015b).

As is true for other viral STDs, there is no cure for herpes infection, and it is considered a chronic disease. The virus is transmitted through direct exposure and infects the genitalia and surrounding skin. After the initial infection the virus remains latent in the sacral nerve of the central nervous system and may reactivate periodically with or without visible vesicles.

Signs and symptoms of herpes simplex virus (HSV) infection include the presence of painful lesions that begin as vesicles and ulcerate and crust within 1 to 4 days. The first episode is typically longer and is usually characterized by more lesions than seen in subsequent infections. Lesions may occur on the vulva, vagina, upper thighs, buttocks, and penis and have an average duration of 11 days (Fig. 15.3). The vesicles can cause itching and pain and may be accompanied by dysuria or rectal pain. Although the ability to pass the infection to others is higher with active lesions, some individuals can spread the virus even when they are asymptomatic. There can be a prodromal phase before lesions develop that includes tingling and paresthesia at the site (Heymann, 2014).

HSV-2 seroprevalence is decreasing. However, this prevalence is likely underrated because HSV-1 infections are rising, and a large number of people have no symptoms; thus HSV is difficult to identify and diagnose. Also, HSV is not nationally reportable. The majority of people with HSV-2 have never been told that they have it (CDC, 2017e). The consequences of genital herpes are of particular concern for women and their children. HSV-2 infection is linked with the development of cervical cancer. There is also an increased risk of fatal newborn infection during vaginal delivery with active lesions (Heymann, 2014). A pregnant woman who has active lesions at the time of giving birth should have a cesarean delivery before the rupture of amniotic membranes to avoid fetal contact with the herpetic lesions, whereas those who have no clinical evidence of herpes lesions should be delivered vaginally. A small number of infants are infected in utero. The clinical infection in infants may present as liver disease, encephalitis, or infection limited to the skin, eyes, or mouth (Heymann, 2014).

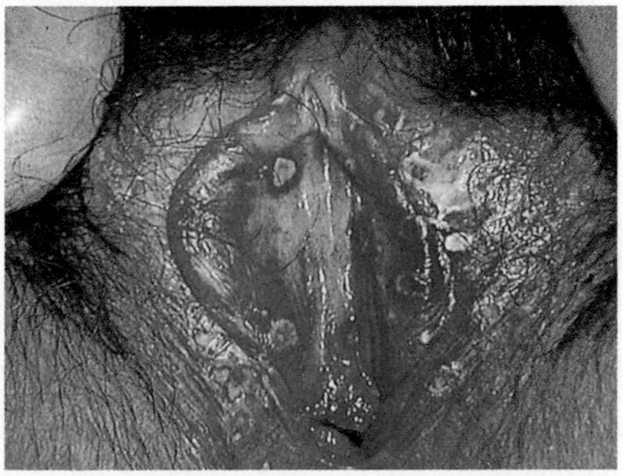

Fig. 15.3 Herpes genitalis. (From Habif TP: *Clinical dermatology: a color guide to diagnosis and therapy,* ed. 5, St. Louis, 2010, Mosby.)

Human Papillomavirus Infection

Human papillomavirus (HPV) results in **genital warts**. Two specific types of HPV (HPV 16 and HPV 18) cause cervical cancer, accounting for 70% of cervical cancer cases (Heymann, 2014). HPV is the most common STD in the United States, although it is not reportable (CDC, 2017e). Transmission of HPV occurs through direct contact with warts that result from HPV and can infect the mouth, genitals, and anus. Genital warts are most commonly found on the penis and scrotum in men, and on the vulva, labia, vagina, and cervix in women. They appear as textured surface lesions, with what is sometimes described as a cauliflower appearance. The warts are usually multiple and vary between 1 mm and 1 cm in diameter. They may be difficult to visualize, so careful examination is required (Buttaro et al., 2017).

As of 2016 there is one Food and Drug Administration (FDA)-licensed HPV vaccine available, the 9-valent HPV vaccine, which is given in a two- or three-dose schedule, depending on patient age (CDC, 2018c). The recommended age for vaccination in both girls and boys is 11 to 12 years old, but it is also recommended for females aged 13 to 26 years old, males 13 to 21, transgender people, bisexual people, and MSM, as well as for people who have certain immunocompromising conditions (CDC, 2018c). The vaccine can be given as early as 9 years of age (CDC, 2018c). Complete vaccination coverage is an issue, however. Experts recommend several strategies to increase vaccination rates in adolescent girls and boys, such as a reminder/recall system to increase vaccination rates and consideration of use of schools as a vaccination site. The two-dose schedule is now recommended for cost saving and efficacy, when initiated before the age of 15 (CDC, 2018c).

Once HPV infection occurs, the goal of therapy is to eliminate the warts. Genital warts spontaneously disappear over time, as do skin warts. However, because the condition is worrisome for the client and HPV may lead to the development of cervical neoplasia, treatment of the warts through surgical removal, laser therapy, or cytotoxic agents is often done (Buttaro et al., 2017).

Complications of HPV infection may be especially serious for women. The link between HPV infection and cervical cancer has been established and is associated with specific types of the virus (CDC 2018b). Other cancers attributed to HPV include vaginal, penile, anal, and oropharyngeal; the latter are more common in men (CDC, 2016a, 2018b). Pap smears are vitally important because they allow for microscopic examination of cells to detect HPV, which can be surgically removed if detected early (Heymann, 2014). If the Pap test findings are unclear, the HPV test can be used for diagnosis (CDC, 2016a). Infection is exacerbated in both pregnancy and immune-related disorders, which are believed to result from a decrease in cell-mediated immune functioning. HPV may infect the fetus during pregnancy and can result in a laryngeal papilloma that can obstruct the infant's airway. Genital warts may enlarge and become friable during pregnancy, and therefore surgical removal may be recommended. One challenge of HPV prevention is that condoms do not necessarily prevent infection. Warts may grow where barriers, such as condoms, do not cover, and skin-to-skin contact may occur.

HEPATITIS

Viral hepatitis refers to a group of infections that primarily affect the liver. These infections have similar clinical presentations but different causes and characteristics. Brief profiles of the types of hepatitis are presented in Table 15.4.

Hepatitis A Virus

Hepatitis A virus (HAV) is most commonly transmitted through the fecal-oral route. Sources may be water, food, feces, or sexual contact. The virus level in the feces appears to peak 1 to 2 weeks before symptoms appear, making individuals highly contagious before they realize they are ill (Heymann, 2014).

The vaccine for hepatitis A infection has been available since 1995, and since that time the incidence has steadily declined in general, with the exception of several recent imported food–related outbreaks (CDC, 2018s). Since 2006 the hepatitis A vaccine has been recommended for children greater than 1 year old, but the immunization rate remains low (CDC, 2018s). The vaccine makes HAV a completely preventable disease. Persons most at risk for HAV infection are travelers to countries with high rates of the disease, children living in areas with high rates of HAV infection, injection drug users, MSM, and persons with clotting disorders or chronic liver disease. In 2016 there were an estimated 4000 cases of HAV (CDC, 2018s).

Hepatitis A is found worldwide. In developing countries where sanitation is inadequate, epidemics are not common because most adults are immune from childhood infection. In countries with improved sanitation, outbreaks are common in daycare centers whose staff must change diapers, among household and sexual contacts of infected individuals, and among travelers to countries where hepatitis A is endemic. In many outbreaks, one individual is the source of an infection that may spread in the community. In other cases, hepatitis A is spread through food contaminated by an infected food handler, contaminated produce, or contaminated water. The source of infection may never be identified in many outbreaks (Heymann, 2014; CDC, 2018r).

TABLE 15.4 Viral Hepatitis Profiles

	Hepatitis A	Hepatitis B	Hepatitis C
Incubation period	Average, 28 days; range, 15-50 days	Average, 90 days; range, 60-150 days	Average, 45 days; range, 14-180 days
Mode of transmission	Fecal-oral, contaminated food/water, sexual	Bloodborne, sexual, perinatal	Primarily bloodborne; also sexual and perinatal
Incidence	Estimated number of new infections: 4000 in 2016 in the United States. Reported in the United States in 2016: 2007	Acute HBV: Estimated 20,900 cases/yr in United States in 2016. Reported in the United States in 2016: 3218. Chronic HBV: 14,847 reported cases in 2016. Estimated number of cases in 2016: 847,000.	Acute HCV: Estimated 41,200 cases/yr in United States in 2016. Reported in the United States in 2016: 2967. Chronic HCV: Estimated 3.5 million cases in 2016. Reported in the United States in 2016: 148,932
Chronic carrier state?	No	Yes, 5% of adult cases; 90% of infants; 25%-50% of children aged 1–5 years	Yes, 75%-85% or more of cases
Diagnosis	Serological test (anti-HAV), viral isolation	Serological tests (e.g., HBsAg), viral isolation	Serological tests (anti-HCV)
Sequelae	No chronic infection	Chronic liver disease; liver cancer	Chronic liver disease; liver cancer
Vaccine availability	Yes, vaccination of all children at 1 year, children in areas of high disease rates recommended; travelers to endemic regions; men who have sex with men; injection and non-injection drug users.	Yes, vaccination of infants recommended; all children who have not been already immunized; individuals with exposure risks; men who have sex with men; people with end-stage renal disease, people with HIV infection	No
Control and prevention	Good hygiene (e.g., hand washing); proper sanitation	Preexposure vaccination; reduce exposure risk behaviors	Screening of blood/organ donors; reduce exposure risk behaviors

HAV, Hepatitis A virus; *HBsAg,* hepatitis B surface antigen; *HBV,* hepatitis B virus; *HCV,* hepatitis C virus; *HIV,* human immunodeficiency virus.
From Centers for Disease Control and Prevention: U.S. 2016 surveillance data for viral hepatitis. Retrieved from https://www.cdc.gov.

The clinical course of hepatitis A ranges from mild to severe and often requires prolonged convalescence. Onset is usually acute, with fever, nausea, lack of appetite, malaise, and abdominal discomfort followed by jaundice after several days.

Vaccination and appropriate sanitation and personal hygiene remain the best means of preventing infection. The HAV vaccine is recommended for those who travel frequently or who spend long periods in countries where the disease is endemic. In cases of exposure through close contact with an infected individual or contaminated food or water, an injection of prophylactic immunoglobulin (Ig) is indicated. Ig should be given as soon as possible but can be given within 2 weeks of exposure. Candidates for hepatitis A vaccine or Ig are listed in Box 15.2 (CDC, 2017f).

Hepatitis B Virus

The number of new cases of **hepatitis B virus** (HBV) has steadily declined in general since HBV vaccination became available (CDC, 2018s). In 2016 a total of 3218 acute hepatitis B cases were reported, down 4.5% from 2015; however, there has been no consistent trend in acute HBV cases since 2012 (CDC, 2018s). The groups with the highest prevalence are users of injection drugs, persons with STDs or multiple sex partners, immigrants and refugees and their descendants who came from areas where there is a high endemic rate of HBV, health care workers, clients on hemodialysis, and inmates of long-term correctional institutions (Buttaro et al., 2017).

The HBV is spread through blood and body fluids and, like HIV, is a blood-borne pathogen. It has the same transmission properties as HIV, and thus individuals should take the same precautions to prevent spread of both HIV and HBV. A major difference is that HBV remains alive outside the body for a longer time than does HIV and thus has greater infectivity. The virus can survive for at least 1 week dried at room temperature on environmental surfaces, and thus infection control measures are paramount in preventing transmission from client to client (Heymann, 2014).

Infection with HBV results in either acute or chronic HBV infection. The acute infection is self-limited, and individuals develop an antibody to the virus and successfully eliminate the virus from the body. They subsequently have lifelong immunity against the virus. Symptoms range from mild, flu-like symptoms to a more severe response that includes jaundice, extreme lethargy, nausea, fever, and joint pain. Any of these more severe symptoms may result in hospitalization. A second possible outcome from infection is chronic HBV infection, which more likely occurs in persons with immunodeficiency (Heymann, 2014). Chronically infected individuals are unable to rid their bodies of the virus and remain lifelong carriers of the hepatitis B surface antigen (HBsAg). As carriers, they are able to transmit the HBV to others. They may develop hepatic carcinoma or chronic active hepatitis. The signs and symptoms of chronic hepatitis B include anorexia, fatigue, abdominal discomfort, hepatomegaly, and jaundice (Heymann, 2014).

Strategies for preventing HBV infection include immunization, prevention of nosocomial occupational exposure, and prevention of sexual and injection drug–use exposure. Vaccination is recommended for persons with occupational risk, such as health care workers, and for infants. The series of vaccines required for protection from HBV consists of three intramuscular injections, with the second and third doses administered 1 and 6 months after the first (CDC, 2018i, 2018j). Pregnant women should be tested for HBsAg; if the mother is positive, newborns require hepatitis B immune globulin in addition to the hepatitis B vaccine within 12 hours of birth, and then at 1 and 6 months thereafter (Schillie et al., 2018). In instances in which the individual is not protected by vaccination and exposure to HBV occurs, hepatitis B immune globulin is given as soon as possible (within 24 hours is optimal) and the hepatitis B vaccine given (Schillie et al., 2018).

OSHA Regulations. The Occupational Safety and Health Administration (OSHA) mandates specific activities to protect workers from HBV and other bloodborne pathogens. Potential exposures for health care workers are needlestick injuries and mucous membrane splashes. The OSHA standard requires employers to identify the risk of blood exposure to various employees. If employees perform work that involves a potential exposure to others' body fluids, employers are mandated to offer the HBV vaccine to the employee at the employer's expense and to offer annual educational programs on preventing HBV and HIV exposure in the workplace. Employees have the right to refuse the vaccine. Employees may decline the vaccine for a variety of reasons, including thinking they are not at risk since they are married or in a monogamous relationship, that the vaccine is too new to have adequate information about it, or that there may be side effects to the vaccine (Schillie et al., 2013).

BOX 15.2 Recommendations for Administration of Hepatitis A Vaccine or Ig After Exposure

- All household or sexual contacts of persons with HAV
- Persons who have shared illicit drugs with someone with HAV
- All staff and attendees of daycare centers if a case of HAV occurs among children or staff
- Household members whose children attend a daycare center where two or more families are infected
- Food handlers who have a coworker infected with HAV; patrons in unhygienic situations or involvement where food is not heated

HAV, Hepatitis A virus.
From Centers for Disease Control and Prevention. Vaccine information statement: hepatitis A, 2017. Retrieved from https://www.cdc.gov.

Hepatitis C Virus

Hepatitis C virus (HCV) infection is the most common chronic bloodborne infection in the United States (USPSTF, 2016). The HCV is transmitted when blood or body fluids of an infected person enter an uninfected person. Those groups at highest risk include health care workers and emergency personnel who are accidentally exposed through needlestick injuries, infants who are born to infected mothers, those born between 1945 and 1965, and one-time or chronic injection drug users, particularly those who share needles or other drug-use equipment (CDC,

2018s). Others at risk include hemodialysis patients (from dialysis equipment shared with infected persons) and recipients of donor organs and blood products before 1992 (USPSTF, 2016). The greatest risk factor is past or current IDU, with a hepatitis C prevalence rate of 50% (USPSTF, 2016).

During the 1980s HCV spread rapidly. It is estimated that 3.5 million people are chronically infected in the United States, and they are often unaware that they have hepatitis C (CDC, 2018s). However, that number is decreasing due to treatment and mortality (CDC, 2018s). People born between 1945 and 1965 account for a disproportionate 75% of all hepatitis C cases in the United States (CDC, 2017c). Chronic liver disease from hepatitis C is the most common indication for liver transplants, representing 30% of all transplants (USPSTF, 2016). Acute hepatitis C cases are increasing, from 0.8 per 100,000 population to 1.0 per 100,000 population between 2015 and 2016 (CDC, 2018s).

The clinical signs of hepatitis C may be so mild that an infected individual does not seek medical attention. The incubation period ranges from 2 weeks to 6 months. Clients may experience fatigue and other nonspecific symptoms. Although some have spontaneous resolution of the infection, 50% to 80% develop chronic liver disease. HCV infection may lead to cirrhosis or hepatocellular carcinoma (Heymann, 2014). Hepatitis C infection is related to about half of hepatocellular carcinoma cases, which have been increasing in incidence (USPSTF, 2016).

Primary prevention of HCV infection includes screening of blood products and donor organs and tissue; risk reduction counseling and services, including obtaining IDU history; and infection control practices. Secondary prevention strategies include testing of high-risk individuals, including those who seek HIV testing, and appropriate medical follow-up of infected clients. HCV testing should be offered to persons who received blood or an organ transplant before 1992; persons who have been on dialysis for many years; persons with signs and symptoms of liver disease; persons born between 1945 and 1965; and persons who received clotting factor before 1987. Routine testing for HCV is not recommended for health care workers, pregnant women, household contacts of HCV-positive persons, or the general population (CDC, 2018s).

Non-ABC Hepatitis

Hepatitis viruses exist that are structurally unrelated to hepatitis A, B, or C. All are very uncommon in the United States, representing less than 5% of total cases (CDC, 2015a). Hepatitis D virus (HDV), called delta hepatitis, can be acute or chronic and can only exist in people who are already infected with hepatitis B, either as a coinfection or as a superinfection. In the United States between 1.5% and 7.2% of HBV cases had serologic evidence of HDV coinfection (CDC, 2015a). It is possible to become a chronic carrier in 70% to 80% of cases. Although there is no vaccination for HDV, infection can be prevented by being vaccinated for HBV (CDC, 2018k).

Hepatitis E virus (HEV) is an acute hepatitis infection that is transmitted through the fecal-oral route. It is common in the developing world, but many people in the United States have HEV antibodies. Because it is not a chronic infection, one cannot become a chronic carrier for HEV. Although there is no hepatitis E vaccination approved for use in the United States, HEV can be prevented by protecting water systems from fecal contamination and boosting sanitation efforts (CDC, 2018l).

Another type of hepatitis virus is hepatitis G (GB virus C). This type of virus has been isolated from patients with post-transfusion hepatitis but has not been found to be the cause of either acute or chronic hepatitis (CDC, 2015a).

TUBERCULOSIS

Tuberculosis is a mycobacterial disease caused by *Mycobacterium tuberculosis.* Transmission usually occurs through exposure to the tubercle bacilli in airborne droplets from persons with pulmonary tuberculosis who talk, cough, or sneeze. Common symptoms are cough, fever, hemoptysis, chest pains, fatigue, and weight loss. The incubation period is 4 to 12 weeks. The most critical period for development of clinical disease is the first 6 to 12 months after infection. About 5% of those initially infected may develop pulmonary tuberculosis or extrapulmonary involvement. The infection in about 95% of those initially infected becomes latent, but in about 10% of otherwise healthy individuals it may be reactivated later in life. The chance of reactivation of latent infections increases in immunocompromised persons, substance abusers, underweight and undernourished persons, and persons with diabetes, silicosis, or gastrectomies (Heymann, 2014).

Epidemiology

The World Health Organization (WHO) (2017) reported 6.3 million new cases of TB worldwide in 2016 and 1.7 million deaths due to TB. Prevalence is more difficult to determine, but WHO has reported 12 million cases in 2012, a number that has fallen dramatically since 1990. Worldwide, seven countries account for 64% of the total number of cases, with India leading the count, followed by Indonesia, China, Philippines, Pakistan, Nigeria, and South Africa (WHO, 2017). In 2016 worldwide, 40% of HIV deaths were due to TB (WHO, 2017). In the United States the incidence of TB increased between 1985 and 1991 but demonstrated a steady rate of decline until 2015, when the incidence increased (CDC, 2018r). Of the new cases, 66% are foreign-born persons living in the United States, with Asians and Hispanics being the most common ethnic groups, representing 30% and 28%, respectively, of national TB cases. Half of all new cases are concentrated in four states: New York, Florida, Texas, and California (CDC, 2016b). Table 15.5 shows TB case rates in the United States by race/ethnicity and sex.

Worldwide, TB drug resistance is a significant issue. Resistance can be caused by people not completing the full course of treatment, provider prescription error, poor quality drugs, or lack of TB drug availability. Types of drug-resistant TB include multidrug resistant TB (MDRTB), defined by resistance to rifampin and isoniazid, and extremely drug-resistant TB (XDRTB), which is MDRTB plus added resistance to fluoroquinolones and at least

TABLE 15.5 U.S. Tuberculosis (TB) Case Rates by Ethnicity and Sex, 2016

Ethnicity/Sex	Number of Cases	TB Case Rate Per 100,000
Asian	3195	18
Native Hawaiian/other Pacific Islander	79	13.9
Black/African American	1975	4.9
Hispanic/Latino	2601	4.5
American Indian/Alaska Native	112	1.2
White	1208	0.6
Multiple race	64	0.9
Female	3633	2.2
Male	5639	3.5
Total population	9272	2.9

From Centers for Disease Control and Prevention (CDC). *Reported tuberculosis in the United States, 2016.* Atlanta, GA, 2017, U.S. Department of Health and Human Services, CDC. Available at https://www.cdc.gov.

three injectable second-line drugs (e.g., amikacin, kanamycin, and capreomycin) (WHO, 2017). Drug-resistant TB is a significant concern to people with weak immune systems, such as HIV-infected individuals.

To prevent TB the CDC works with public health agencies in other countries to improve screening and reporting of cases and to improve treatment strategies. This includes coordination of treatment for infected individuals who migrate to the United States. This coordination is particularly significant between Mexico and the United States (WHO, 2017).

Diagnosis and Treatment

The standard and preferred TB screening test is the Mantoux tuberculin skin test (TST) (CDC, 2018r). The TST, previously referred to as the purified protein derivative (PPD) test, is used for initial screening. It can be followed by chest radiography for persons with a positive skin reaction and pulmonary symptoms. Persons who are immunosuppressed by drugs or who have diseases such as advanced tuberculosis, measles, or chicken pox may not have the ability to mount an immune response to the TST, so the result may be a false-negative skin test reaction resulting from cutaneous anergy (nonreaction due to weakened immune system). A second issue with the TST is that a positive result may come from an earlier TST or bacille Calmette-Guérin (BCG) vaccination boosting one's ability to respond to the infection, and not reflecting a recent infection. Therefore it is difficult to determine if the infection is old or recent. A blood test (interferon-gamma release assays or IGRA) is available and is increasingly used for providing clinical care in lieu of the TST (CDC, 2018r). One example is the QuantiFeron-TB blood test to detect *M. tuberculosis* infection. Diagnosis can also be made through stained sputum smears and other body fluids to determine the presence of acid-fast bacilli (for presumptive diagnosis), and culture of the tubercle bacilli for definitive diagnosis. The following How To box describes how to read a TST.

HOW TO Perform a Tuberculin Skin Test (TST)

Apply and Read the TST

- For the Mantoux test, inject 0.1 mL containing 5 tuberculin units of purified protein derivative (PPD) tuberculin.
- Read the reaction 48 to 72 hours after injection.
- Measure only induration, not redness.
- Record results in millimeters.

Interpret the TST (Buttaro et al., 2017)

Test is positive if the induration is greater than or equal to 5 mm in the following:

- Immunosuppressed clients
- Persons known to have HIV infection
- Persons whose chest radiograph is suggestive of previous TB that was untreated
- Close contacts of a person with infectious TB
- Organ transplant recipients

Test is positive if the induration is greater than or equal to 10 mm in the following:

- Persons with certain medical conditions, such as diabetes, alcoholism, or drug abuse
- Persons who inject drugs (if HIV negative)
- Foreign-born persons from areas where TB is common
- Children under 4 years old
- Residents and staff of long-term care facilities, jails, and prisons

Test is positive if the induration is greater than or equal to 15 mm in the following:

- All persons more than 4 years of age with no risk factors for TB (Buttaro et al., 2017)

Clients with TB should be treated promptly with the appropriate combination of multiple antimicrobial drugs. Effective drug regimens used in the United States include isoniazid and in some instances, rifampin. Treatment regimens for persons with active symptomatic infection may be different from the regimens used for persons with latent TB infection or with HIV (Buttaro et al., 2017). Treatment failure may be due to clients' poor adherence in taking the medication, which can result in drug resistance. Nurses usually administer TSTs and provide education on the importance of compliance to long-term therapy. They may also be involved in directly observed therapy (DOT) and contact investigations of cases in the community.

NURSE'S ROLE IN PROVIDING PREVENTIVE CARE FOR COMMUNICABLE DISEASES

From prevention to treatment, the nurse functions as a counselor, educator, advocate, case manager, and primary care provider. Appropriate interventions for primary, secondary, and tertiary prevention are reviewed in the following sections (see Levels of Prevention box). In the following discussion of primary prevention, the nursing process is applied to the care of clients with communicable diseases. Nurses are in an ideal position to affect the outcomes of communicable diseases, and their influence begins with primary prevention.

LEVELS OF PREVENTION

Primary Prevention

- Provide community education about communicable disease prevention to well populations.
- Vaccinate for hepatitis A virus (HAV) or hepatitis B virus (HBV).
- Provide community outreach for education and needle exchange.

Secondary Prevention

- Administer tuberculin skin test (TST).
- Test and counsel for human immunodeficiency virus (HIV).
- Notify partners and trace contacts.

Tertiary Prevention

- Educate caregivers of persons with HIV about standard precautions.
- Maintain long-term directly observed therapy (DOT) for tuberculosis treatment.
- Identify community resources for providing supportive care (e.g., funds for purchasing medications).
- Set up support groups for persons with genital herpes.

HIV, Human immunodeficiency virus.

Primary Prevention

Primary prevention consists mainly of activities to keep people healthy before the onset of disease. This begins with assessing for risk behavior and providing relevant intervention through education on how to avoid infection, mostly through healthy behaviors.

Assessment. To assess the risk of acquiring an infection, the nurse takes a history that focuses on risk behaviors and potential exposure, which varies with the specific organism by its mode of transmission. The specific questions that must be asked can be especially challenging when STDs are the object of the study. In these situations the nurse should obtain a sexual and IDU history for clients and their partners. The sexual history provides information that leads to the need for specific diagnostic tests, treatment modalities, and **partner notification**. It also facilitates evaluation of risk factors and is necessary for the nurse to be able to provide relevant education for the client's lifestyle.

Assessing a client's risk of acquiring an STD should be done with all sexually active individuals. Such risk assessments should be included as baseline assessment data for those attending all clinics and those who receive school health, occupational health, public health, and home nursing services.

A thorough sexual history requires obtaining personal and sensitive information. It includes information about the types of relationships, the number of sexual partners and encounters, and the types of sexual behaviors practiced. The confidential nature of the information and how it will be used should be shared with the client to establish open communication and goal-directed interaction. Most clients feel uneasy disclosing such personal information. The nurse can ease this discomfort by remaining supportive and open during the interview to facilitate honesty about intimate activities. The nurse serves as a model for discussing sensitive information in a candid manner. When discussing precautions, direct and simple language should be used to describe specific behaviors. This encourages the client to openly discuss sexuality during this interaction and with future partners.

EVIDENCE-BASED PRACTICE

This descriptive study asked 93 largely low-income HIV-infected Latino men about their sexual practices, substance use history, and HIV disclosure patterns. A complicated picture emerged, indicating that presentation and reporting of sexual preference and behavior did not necessarily match actual orientation and behavior. This is important because the HIV rate in the Latino community is increasing, and careful history taking and question asking can help nurses to better understand the range of sexual practices and communication behaviors of their patients, hopefully leading to a better understanding of HIV disclosure patterns.

In this sample, many of the HIV-infected men also had a high rate of substance use, including 56% of the men reporting alcohol use in the past 3 months, 87.4% using marijuana, 71.9% using crack cocaine, 40.4% using IV drugs, and 35.6% reporting sharing needles. Latino men who identified as straight engaged in risky practices such as sharing needles (56%) or having sex with a partner who uses needles (54.3%) at higher rates than gay or bisexual men in this sample. Additionally, HIV testing (and therefore perceived susceptibility to contracting HIV) was typically associated with sexual orientation in this study, meaning that men who identified as straight or bisexual received testing at lower rates than gay men. HIV disclosure to partners varied among groups as well, with gay men (67.5%) most frequently disclosing their HIV-positive status to a partner than straight (57.6%) or bisexual (50%) men.

Results indicate that public health interventions for Latino straight men in particular should identify and focus on IV drug use, needle sharing, and unprotected sex as high-risk behaviors that lead to contracting HIV. Clinicians should also be aware that there is much diversity in sexual behavior for straight, gay, and bisexual people and to be aware of this when discussing self-care, risk, and protective factors with clients. For instance, gay does not always equal same-sex sexual practices, and straight does not always indicate heterosexual sex.

Nurse Use

This study highlights the importance of a nuanced history taking in terms of sexual history and substance use as an important part of maximizing public health interventions. Nurses can play a large role in open and honest HIV disclosure behavior by carefully addressing a range of risk behaviors and possible barriers to testing, indicated by this sample of HIV-positive ethnic minority men.

From Champion JD, Szlachta A: Self-identified sexual orientation and sexual risk behavior among HIV-infected Latino males. *J Assoc Nurses AIDS Care* 27(5):285–294, 2016. Retrieved from http://dx.doi.org/10.1016/j.jana.2016.03.004.

Nurses who are uncomfortable discussing topics such as sexual behavior or sexual orientation are likely to avoid assessing risk behaviors with the client. They will consequently be ineffective in identifying risks and helping clients modify risky behaviors. Nurses need to be adept at helping clients prevent and control STDs. Nurses can gain confidence in conducting sexual risk assessments by understanding their own values and feelings about sexuality and realizing that the purpose of the interaction is to improve the client's health. The nurse's comfort in discussing sexual behavior can be improved by using role playing to practice assessments of sexual and IDU behavior and by contracting with clients to make behavior changes.

Identifying the number of sexual and injection drug–using partners and the number of contacts with these partners provides information about the client's risk. The chance of exposure decreases as the number of partners decreases, so people in mutually monogamous relationships are at low risk for acquiring STDs. You can gather this information by asking, "How many sex (or drug) partners have you had over the past six months?" Try to avoid basing assumptions about the sexual partner or partners on the client's sex, age, ethnicity, or any other factor. Stereotypes and assumptions about who people are and what they do are common problems that keep interviewers from asking the questions that lead to obtaining useful information. For example, it should not be taken for granted that a homosexual man always has more than one partner. Be aware also that the long incubation of HIV and the subclinical phase of many STDs lead some monogamous individuals to assume erroneously that they are not at risk.

It is important to identify whether the person has sexual contact with men, women, or both. This information can be obtained by simply asking, "Do you have sex with men, women, or both?" This lets the client know that the nurse is open to hearing about these behaviors, and thus the nurse is more likely to obtain information that is relevant to sexual practices and risk. Women who are exclusively lesbian are at low risk for acquiring STDs, but bisexual women may transmit STDs between male and female partners. In addition, it is possible for men to have sexual contact with other men and not label themselves as homosexual. Therefore, education to reduce risk that is aimed at homosexual men will not be heeded by men who do not see themselves as homosexual. In such situations the nurse can ask, "When was the last time you had sex with another man?"

Certain sexual practices are more likely to result in exposure to and transmission of STDs. Dangerous sexual activities include all unprotected intercourse (anal, oral, or vaginal), oral-anal contact, and insertion of finger or fist into the rectum. These practices introduce a high risk of transmission of enteric organisms or result in physical trauma during sexual encounters. The nurse can obtain information about sexual encounters by asking, "Can you tell me the kinds of sexual practices in which you engage? This will help determine what risks you may have and the type of tests we should do." Clients who engage in genital-anal, oral-anal, or oral-genital contact will need throat and rectal cultures for some STDs as well as cervical and urethral cultures.

HOW TO Effectively Obtain a Client's Sexual History

To be most effective, the nurse obtaining a client's sexual history should do the following:

- Remain supportive and open to facilitate honesty.
- Use terms the client will understand (be prepared to suggest multiple terms).
- Speak candidly so the client will feel comfortable talking.
- Ask open-ended questions in a nonthreatening and nonjudgmental manner.
- Acknowledge that many people are uneasy disclosing personal information.
- Use the Five Ps Approach (CDC, 2015b). Sample questions in each category are:
  - Partners: "In the past 2 months, how many partners have you had sex with?"
- Prevention of pregnancy: "What are you doing to prevent pregnancy?"
- Protection from STDs: "What do you do to protect yourself from STDs and HIV?"
- Practices: "To understand your risk for STDs, I need to understand the kind of sex you've had recently."
- Past history of STDs: "Have you ever had an STD?"

Drug use is linked to STD transmission in several ways. Drugs such as alcohol put people at risk because they can lower inhibitions and impair judgment about engaging in risky behaviors. Addictions to drugs may cause individuals to acquire the drug or money to purchase the drug through sexual favors. This increases both the frequency of sexual contacts and the chances of contracting STDs. Thus the nurse should obtain information on the type and frequency of drug use and the presence of risk behaviors.

The administration of immunizations is another example of primary prevention, because they prevent infection. Of the diseases presented here, vaccines are available for HPV and hepatitis A and B.

Interventions. Interventions to prevent infection are aimed at preventing specific infections. These interventions can take several forms and include things such as education on how to prevent infection or the availability of vaccines. For example, on the basis of the information obtained in the sexual history and risk assessment just described, the nurse can identify specific education and counseling needs of the client. The nursing interventions focus on contracting with clients to change behavior and reduce their risk in regard to sexual practice.

Sexual Behavior. Sexual abstinence is the best way to prevent STDs. However, for many people, sexual abstinence is not realistic, and providing instruction about how to make sexual behavior safer is critical. Safer sexual behavior includes masturbation, dry kissing, touching, fantasy, and vaginal and oral sex with a condom.

If used correctly and consistently, properly fitted condoms can prevent both pregnancy and most STDs because they prevent the exchange of body fluids during sexual activity. Condom failure may occur from incorrect use rather than condom failure. Thus information about proper use and how to communicate about them with a partner is also necessary. The nurse has many opportunities to convey this information during counseling. Most agency protocols recommend the use of latex condoms. Some may be lubricated with nonoxynol-9, a spermicide. If used frequently, nonoxynol-9 may result in genital lesions, which may provide openings for viruses to enter the body.

Condom use may be viewed as inconvenient, messy, or decreasing sensation. Moreover, alcohol consumption may accompany sexual activity, which may also decrease condom use. The nurse can help clients become more skilled in discussing safer sex through role modeling and practicing communication skills through role play. Role-playing scenarios with partners who are reluctant to use condoms can help individuals prepare for situations before they occur.

Female condoms are a barrier to body fluid contact and therefore protect against pregnancy and STDs. The main advantage of the female condom is that its use is controlled by the woman. The FC2 Female Condom is the only female condom that is FDA approved for use in the United States. Since it is made of nitrile it is also useful if a latex sensitivity develops to male condoms. Symptoms of latex allergy include penile, vaginal, or rectal itching or swelling after use of a male condom or diaphragm. The female condom consists of a sheath over two rings, with one closed end that fits over the cervix. The condoms are often free at public health clinics or can be purchased in boxes of multiple condoms, making the overall cost per condom about $1.50 each. Fig. 15.4 provides instructions on its insertion.

Clients should understand the importance of knowing the risk behavior of their sexual partners, including a history of IDU and STDs, sexual preference, and any current symptoms. Each sexual partner is potentially exposed to all the STDs of all the persons with whom the other partner has been sexually active.

Drug Use. IDU is risky because the potential for injecting bloodborne pathogens, such as HIV, HBV, and HCV exists when needles and syringes are shared. During IDU small quantities of drugs are repeatedly injected. Blood is withdrawn into the syringe and is then injected back into the user's vein. Individuals should be advised against using injectable drugs and sharing needles, syringes, or other drug paraphernalia (a.k.a. works) (CDC, 2018p). Many communities have syringe services programs (SSPs), which can also assist with substance abuse treatment referrals and screening for IDU-related diseases (CDC, 2018n).

People who inject drugs are difficult to reach for health care services. Effective outreach programs include using community peers, increasing accessibility of drug treatment programs combined with HIV testing and counseling, and encouraging long-term repeat contacts after completion of the program.

Community Outreach. Because of the illegal nature of injectable drugs and the poverty associated with HIV, many people at risk have neither the inclination nor the resources to seek health care. Nurses may work to establish programs within communities because the opportunities for counseling on the prevention of HIV and other STDs are increased by bringing services into the neighborhoods of those at risk. Workers go into communities to disseminate information on safer sex, drug treatment

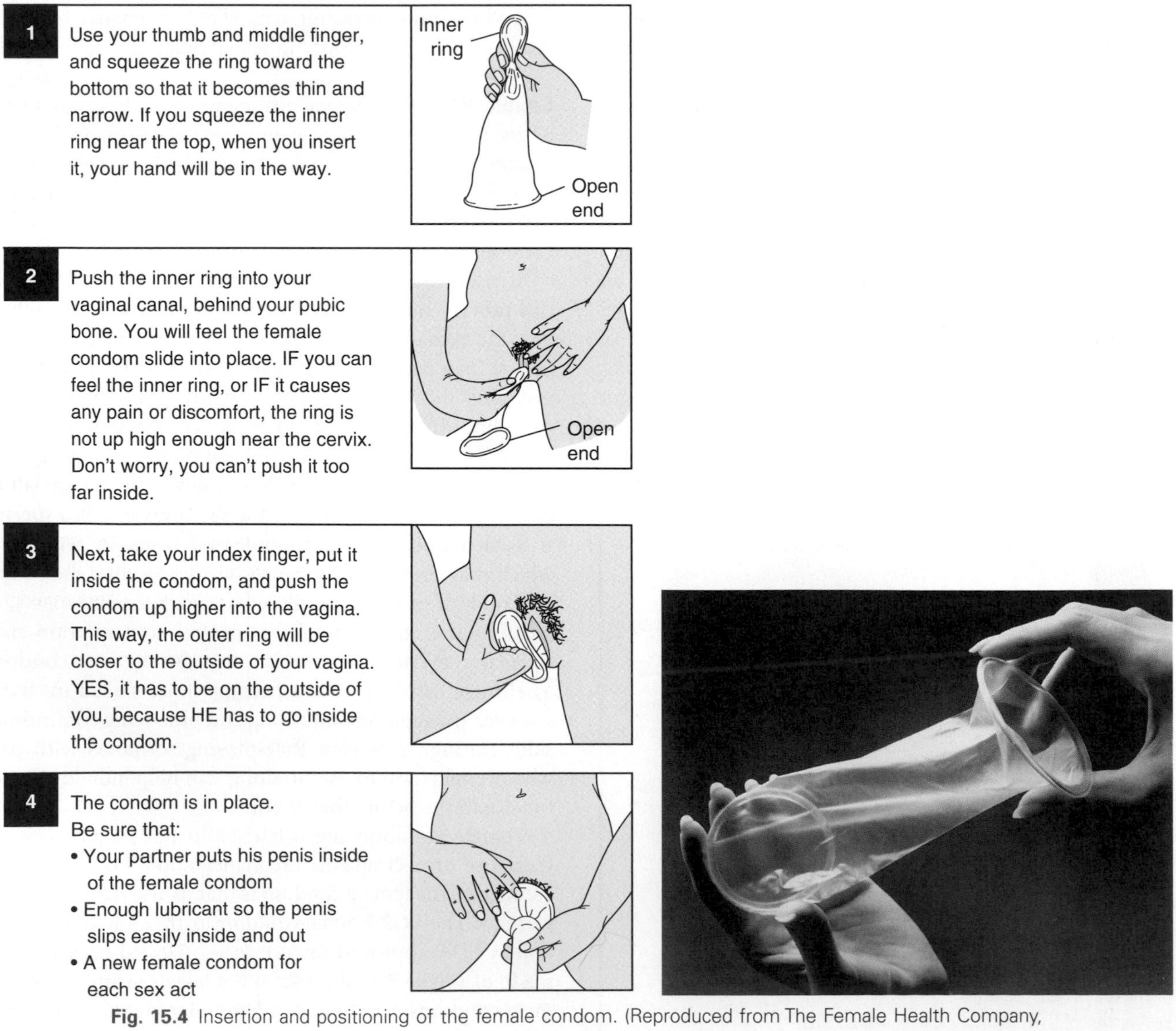
1
Use your thumb and middle finger, and squeeze the ring toward the bottom so that it becomes thin and narrow. If you squeeze the inner ring near the top, when you insert it, your hand will be in the way.
Inner ring
Open end
2
Push the inner ring into your vaginal canal, behind your pubic bone. You will feel the female condom slide into place. IF you can feel the inner ring, or IF it causes any pain or discomfort, the ring is not up high enough near the cervix. Don't worry, you can't push it too far inside.
Open end
3
Next, take your index finger, put it inside the condom, and push the condom up higher into the vagina. This way, the outer ring will be closer to the outside of your vagina. YES, it has to be on the outside of you, because HE has to go inside the condom.
4
The condom is in place.
Be sure that:
• Your partner puts his penis inside of the female condom
• Enough lubricant so the penis slips easily inside and out
• A new female condom for each sex act

Fig. 15.4 Insertion and positioning of the female condom. (Reproduced from The Female Health Company, Chicago, IL.)

programs, and discontinuation of drug use or safer drug use practices (e.g., using new needles and syringes with each injection). Some programs provide sterile needles and syringes, condoms, and literature about testing services.

Community Education. Education of well populations about prevention of communicable diseases by a nurse educator is an example of primary prevention. Relevant information about the modes of transmission, testing, availability of vaccines, and early symptoms can be provided to groups in the community. Providing accurate health information to large numbers of people is vital for preventing the spread of STDs. Nurses can provide educational sessions to community groups about HIV and other STDs. Such educational sessions are most effective in settings where groups normally meet and may include schools, businesses, and churches.

When addressing groups about HIV infection, it is important to discuss the number of people infected with HIV, the number of people living with AIDS, modes of transmission of the virus, how to prevent infection, testing services, common symptoms of illness, the need for a compassionate response to those afflicted, and available community resources. Teaching about other STDs can be incorporated into these presentations because the mode of transmission (sexual contact) is the same. Other information on these diseases can include the distribution and incidence in society and the consequences of the infection for individuals and families.

BOX 15.3 Who Should Be Advised to Receive HIV Testing and Counseling?

For clients in all health care settings:

- HIV screening is recommended for clients in all health care settings after the client is notified that testing will be performed unless the patient declines (opt-out screening).
- Persons at high risk for HIV infection should be screened for HIV at least annually.
- Separate written consent for HIV testing should not be required; general consent for medical care should be considered sufficient to encompass consent for HIV testing.
- Prevention counseling should not be required with HIV diagnostic testing or as part of HIV screening programs in health care settings.

For pregnant women:

- HIV screening should be included in the routine panel of prenatal screening tests for all pregnant women.
- HIV screening is recommended after the client is notified that testing will be performed unless the client declines (opt-out screening).
- Separate written consent for HIV testing should not be required; general consent for medical care should be considered sufficient to encompass consent for HIV testing.
- Repeat screening in the third trimester is recommended in certain jurisdictions with elevated rates of HIV infection among pregnant women.

HIV, Human immunodeficiency virus.
From Branson BB, Handsfield HH, Lampe M, et al.: Revised recommendations for HIV testing of adults, adolescents, and pregnant women in health-care settings. *MMWR Morb Mortal Wkly Rep* 55(RR14), 1–17, 2006. Retrieved from https://www.cdc.gov.

Evaluation. Evaluation is based on the extent of vaccination within a population, whether risky behavior has changed to safe behavior, and, ultimately, whether illness is prevented. Condom use can be evaluated for consistency of use if the client is sexually active. Other behaviors, such as abstinence or monogamy, can be evaluated for their implementation. At the community level, behavioral surveys can be done to measure reported condom use and condom sales, and measures of disease incidence and prevalence can be calculated to evaluate the effectiveness of intervention.

Secondary Prevention

Secondary prevention includes screening for diseases to ensure their early identification, treatment, and follow-up with contacts to prevent further spread. In general, client teaching and counseling should include education about avoiding self-reinfection, managing symptoms, and preventing the infection of others.

Testing and Counseling for HIV

Universal testing for HIV infection should be routine for all clients aged 13 to 64 years (CDC, 2018a). Younger adolescents and older adults who are at increased risk should be screened as well (CDC, 2018a, 2018m). Therefore routine HIV testing should be a part of all annual physicals, laboratory tests for every pregnancy, and all hospital visits, without securing special permission. Clients can decline or "opt out" of HIV testing, but the benefits of testing are considerable. For persons who have engaged in high-risk behavior, the nurse should recommend annual HIV testing (Box 15.3). Individuals with the following characteristics are considered at risk and should be offered HIV testing: those with a history of STDs (which are transmitted through the same behavior and may decrease immune functioning), multiple sex partners, or IDU; those who have unprotected intercourse (i.e., without using a condom or preexposure prophylaxis [PrEP]) (CDC, 2018a, 2018o); those who have intercourse with someone who has another partner and those who have had sex with a prostitute; men with a history of homosexual or bisexual activity; and those who have been a sexual partner to anyone in one of these groups.

Testing enables clients to benefit from early detection and treatment, as well as risk reduction education. If HIV infection is discovered before the onset of symptoms, early monitoring of the disease process and CD4 lymphocyte counts or viral loads is indicated. In addition, prophylactic therapy with antiretroviral therapy and/or antibiotics may begin in order to delay the onset of symptomatic illness.

Posttest counseling. Persons who negative test results should be counseled about risk reduction activities to prevent any future transmission. Clients should understand that the test results may not be truly negative because the test does not reveal infections that may have been acquired within the several weeks before the test. Evidence of HIV antibody takes from 6 to 12 weeks to develop. Newer immunoassay tests can produce results in as little as 3 weeks (CDC, 2018a). Clients must be aware of the ways viral transmission occurs and how to avoid infection. All clients who are antibody positive should be counseled about the need to reduce their risks and notify partners. If

BOX 15.4 Responsibilities of Persons Who Are HIV Infected

- Have regular medical evaluations and follow-ups.
- Do not donate blood, plasma, body organs, other tissues, or sperm.
- Take precautions against exchanging body fluids during sexual activity.
- Inform sexual or injection drug–using partners of the potential exposure to HIV or arrange for notification through the health department.
- Inform health care providers of the HIV infection.
- Consider the risk of perinatal transmission and follow up with contraceptive use.

HIV, Human immunodeficiency virus.

the client is unwilling or hesitant to notify past partners, the nurse will do partner notification (or contact tracing), as described later in this chapter. Clients should seek treatment from their primary health care provider so physical evaluation can be performed and, if indicated, antiviral or other therapies begun. Box 15.4 describes the responsibilities of individuals who are HIV positive.

Psychosocial counseling is indicated when positive HIV test results precipitate acute anxiety, depression, or suicidal ideation. The client should be informed about available counseling services. The person should be cautioned to consider carefully who should be informed of the test results. Many individuals have told others about their HIV-positive test, only to experience isolation and discrimination. Plans for the future should be explored, and clients should be advised to avoid stress, drugs, and infections in order to maintain optimal health.

LINKING CONTENT TO PRACTICE

This chapter emphasizes the epidemiology and prevention of selected communicable diseases, as well as the public health nursing services provided to clients (Public Health Foundation, 2014). Domains and core competencies are addressed through activities in caring for clients with communicable diseases. Examples of how these eight domains are used in providing nursing care to clients with communicable disease are as follows:

Domain #1, Analytic/Assessment Skills, is achieved through the review of the incidence and prevalence rates of communicable diseases to determine population health status.

Domain #3, Communication Skills, is applied when PHNs teach how to prevent and treat infections.

Domain #4, Cultural Competency Skills, is met through understanding the various social and behavioral factors that make health care acceptable to diverse populations (groups of people who are diverse in terms of culture, socioeconomic status, education level, race, gender, age, ethnicity, sexual orientation, profession, religious affiliation, and mental/physical capability).

From Public Health Foundation, Council on Linkages: *Core competencies for public health professionals,* 2014. Available at http://www.phf.org/link/corecompetencies.htm.

Partner Notification and Contact Tracing. Partner notification, also known as contact tracing or disclosure, is an example of a population-level intervention aimed at controlling communicable diseases. Partner notification programs usually occur in conjunction with reportable disease requirements and are carried out by most health departments. It involves confidentially identifying and notifying exposed individuals of clients who are found to have reportable diseases, especially STDs.

Individuals diagnosed with a reportable STD are asked to provide the names and locations of all partners so that these individuals can be informed of their exposure, receive counseling, and obtain the necessary referral and/or treatment. The originally diagnosed (index case) clients may be encouraged to notify their partners (can be sexual and/or injection drug partners) and to encourage them to seek treatment. If the client agrees to do so, suggestions on how to inform their partners and how to deal with possible reactions may be explored. In some instances, clients may feel more comfortable if the nurse notifies those who are exposed. If clients contact their partners about possible infection, the nurse contacts health care providers or clinics to verify positive test results or microscopic findings and treatment of the index case.

If the originally diagnosed client prefers not to participate in notifying partners, the public health nurse contacts the partners by phone, certified delivery letter, or home visit, depending on the nature of the individual circumstances, and counsels them to seek evaluation and treatment. Many times the client is treated for the sexually transmitted infection at the health department. At this appointment the client is offered literature regarding the STD for which they need treatment, receives risk-reduction counseling, and is offered testing for the other STDs. The identity of the infected client who names sexual and injection drug–using partners cannot be revealed. Maintaining confidentiality is critical with all STDs.

CHECK YOUR PRACTICE

You are working in the clinic with James, a young university student who went to a party last weekend and had unprotected sex with another student, named Rodrigo. Thanks to encouragement from a friend, he came to the clinic and got tested for chlamydia, gonorrhea, HIV, and syphilis. James's gonorrhea test came back positive. James does not think Rodrigo is having any symptoms. He also does not want Rodrigo to be angry with him.

What will you tell James about his treatment? What will you teach him about precautions? How will you respond to his reluctance to talk with Rodrigo?

Tertiary Prevention

Tertiary prevention can apply to many of the chronic viral STDs and TB. For viral STDs, much of this effort focuses on managing symptoms and maintaining psychosocial support. Many clients report feeling contaminated and thus feel lower self-worth. Support groups may be available to help clients cope with chronic STDs, such as genital herpes or genital warts.

Directly Observed Therapy. In directly observed therapy (DOT) programs for TB medication, nurses observe and document individual clients taking their TB drugs. When clients prematurely stop taking TB medications, there is a risk of the TB becoming resistant to the medications. This can affect an entire community of people who are susceptible to this airborne disease. Health professionals share in the responsibility of adhering to treatment, and DOT ensures that TB-infected clients have adequate medication. Thus DOT programs are aimed at the population level to prevent antibiotic resistance in the community and to ensure effective treatment at the individual level. Many health departments have DOT home health programs to ensure adequate treatment (CDC, 2018r). Directly observed therapy, short course (DOTS) is a variation applied worldwide to combat multidrug-resistant TB (WHO, 2017).

The management of AIDS in the home may include monitoring physical status and referring the family to additional care services for maintaining the client in the home. Case management is important in all phases of HIV infection. It is especially important to ensure that clients have adequate services to meet their needs. This may include ensuring that medication can be obtained through identifying funding resources, maintaining infection control standards, reducing risk behaviors, identifying sources of respite care for caretakers, or referring clients for home or hospice care. Nursing interventions include teaching families about managing symptomatic illness by preventing deteriorating conditions such as diarrhea, skin breakdown, and inadequate nutrition.

Standard Precautions. It is important to teach caregivers about infection control in the home. Clients, families, friends, and others may express concerns about the transmission of HIV. Whereas fear may be expressed by some, others who are caring for loved ones with HIV may not take adequate precautions, such as glove wearing, because of concern about appearing as though they do not want to touch a loved one. Others may believe myths that suggest they cannot be infected by someone they love.

Standard precautions must be taught to caregivers in the home setting. All blood and articles soiled with body fluids must be handled as if they were infectious or contaminated by bloodborne pathogens. Gloves should be worn whenever hands might touch nonintact skin, mucous membranes, blood, or other fluids. A mask, goggles, and gown should also be worn if there is potential for splashing or spraying of infectious material during any care. All protective equipment should be worn only once and then disposed of. If the skin or mucous membranes of the caregiver come in contact with body fluids, the skin should be washed with soap and water, and the mucous membranes should be flushed with water as soon as possible after the exposure. Thorough hand washing with soap and water—a major infection control measure—should be conducted whenever hands become contaminated and whenever gloves or other protective equipment (e.g., mask, gown) is removed. Soiled clothing or linen should be washed in a washing machine filled with hot water using bleach as an additive and dried on a hot-air cycle of a dryer.

PRACTICE APPLICATION

Yvonne Jackson is a 20-year-old woman who visits the Hopetown City Health Department's maternity clinic. Examination reveals she is at 14 weeks' gestation. She is single but has been in a steady relationship for the past 6 months with Ramón. She states that she has no other children. A routine test taken during the initial prenatal visit is an HIV test; the results are positive.

Ms. Jackson is shocked and emotionally distraught about the positive test results. Understanding that the client will not be able to concentrate on all of the questions and information that need to be covered, the nurse prioritizes essential information to obtain and provide during this visit.

A. List the relevant factors to consider on the basis of this information.
B. What questions do you need to ask with regard to controlling the spread of HIV to others?
C. What information is most important to give to Ms. Jackson at this time?
D. What follow-up does the nurse need to arrange for this client?

Answers can be found on the Evolve site.

KEY POINTS

- Nearly all communicable diseases discussed in this chapter are preventable because they are transmitted through specific, known behaviors.
- STDs are among the most serious public health problems in the United States. Not only is there an increased incidence of drug-resistant gonococcal infection, but other STDs, such as HPV (genital warts), HIV, and HSV (genital herpes), are associated with cancer.
- STDs affect certain groups in greater numbers. Factors associated with risk include being less than 25 years of age, being a member of a minority group, living in an urban setting, being poor, and using crack cocaine.
- The increasing incidence, morbidity, and mortality of specific communicable diseases highlight the need for nurses to educate clients about ways to prevent communicable diseases.
- Many STDs do not produce symptoms in clients.
- Aside from death, the most serious complications caused by STDs are pelvic inflammatory disease, infertility, ectopic pregnancy, neonatal morbidity and mortality, and neoplasia.
- Hepatitis A is often silent in children, and children are a significant source of infection to others; thus the use of the vaccination in children has caused a reduction in the number of cases.
- Hepatitis C is the most common bloodborne pathogen in the United States.
- The emergence of multidrug-resistant TB has prompted the use of directly observed therapy (DOT) to ensure adherence with drug treatment regimens.
- Early detection of communicable diseases is important because it results in early treatment and prevention of additional transmission to others. Treatment includes effective medications, stress reduction, and proper nutrition.

- Partner notification, or contact tracing, is done by identifying, contacting, and ensuring evaluation and treatment of persons exposed to sexual and injectable drug-using partners. Contact tracing is also conducted with TB and HAV.
- HIV infection has created an entirely new group of people needing health care. This rapidly growing population is straining a health care system that is already unable to meet the needs of many.
- Most of the care (both home and outpatient) that is provided for HIV is done within the community setting, which reduces direct health care costs but increases the need for financial support of home and community health services.

CLINICAL DECISION-MAKING ACTIVITIES

1. Identify sources of TB treatment in your community. Is there a DOT program available through the health department or home health agency? What factors make TB infection a difficult problem?
2. To whom does one report communicable diseases, such as HAV, in your community? How is this information given?
3. Identify the number of reported cases of AIDS and the number of reported cases of HIV infection within your state and locale (if reportable in your state). How are the cases distributed by age, sex, geographic location, and ethnicity?
4. Identify the location(s) of HIV testing services in your community. Are the test results anonymous or confidential? Describe how and to whom the results are reported.
5. Form small groups, and role play a nurse-client interaction involving risk assessment and counseling regarding safer sex and injection drug-using practices.

ADDITIONAL RESOURCES

EVOLVE WEBSITE

http://evolve.elsevier.com/Stanhope/community/
- Answers to Practice Application
- Case Study
- Glossary
- Review Questions

REFERENCES

AIDSinfo: *What's new in the guidelines pediatric ARV*, 2018. Retrieved from https://aidsinfo.nih.gov/guidelines/html/2/pediatric-arv/45/whats-new-in-the-guidelines.

Bowen V, Su J, Torrone E, Kidd S, Weinstock H: Increase in incidence of congenital syphilis—United States, 2012–2014, *MMWR Morb Mortal Wkly Rep* 64(44):1241–1245, 2015. Retrieved from https://www.cdc.gov/mmwr/preview/mmwrhtml/mm6444a3.htm#Tab1.

Branson BM, Handsfield HH, Lampe MA, et al.: Revised recommendations for HIV testing of adults, adolescents, and pregnant women in health-care settings, *MMWR Recomm Rep* 55(RR14): 1–17, 2006. Retrieved from https://www.cdc.gov/mmwr/preview/mmwrhtml/rr5514a1.htm.

Buttaro TM, Trybulski J, Polgar-Bailey P, Sandberg-Cook J: *Primary care: A collaborative practice*, ed 5, St. Louis, MO, 2017, Elsevier.

Centers for Disease Control and Prevention: *Guidelines for viral hepatitis surveillance and case management*, 2015a. Retrieved from https://www.cdc.gov/hepatitis/statistics/surveillanceguidelines.htm.

Centers for Disease Control and Prevention: Sexually transmitted diseases treatment guidelines, 2015. *MMWR Recomm Rep* 64(3):1–137, 2015b. Retrieved from https://www.cdc.gov/std/tg2015/default.htm.

Centers for Disease Control and Prevention: *Preventing HPV-associated cancers*, 2016a. Retrieved from https://www.cdc.gov/cancer/hpv/basic_info/prevention.htm.

Centers for Disease Control and Prevention: *Reported tuberculosis in the United States, 2015*, 2016b. Retrieved from https://www.cdc.gov/tb/statistics/reports/2015/pdfs/2015_Surveillance_Report_FullReport.pdf

Centers for Disease Control and Prevention: *Understand how HIV treatment works and stay in care*, 2016c. Retrieved from http://www.cdc.gov/actagainstaids/campaigns/hivtreatmentworks/stayincare/index.html.

Centers for Disease Control and Prevention: *HIV Surveillance Report: Diagnoses of HIV Infection and AIDS in the United States and Dependent Areas, 2016*, vol 28, 2017a. Retrieved from http://www.cdc.gov/hiv/topics/surveillance/resources/reports.

Centers for Disease Control and Prevention: *Pelvic inflammatory disease—CDC fact sheet*, 2017b. Retrieved from https://www.cdc.gov/std/pid/stdfact-pid.htm.

Centers for Disease Control and Prevention: *People born 1945–1965*, 2017c. Retrieved from https://www.cdc.gov/hepatitis/populations/1945-1965.htm.

Centers for Disease Control and Prevention: *Reported tuberculosis in the United States, 2016*, Atlanta, GA, 2017d, U.S. Department of Health and Human Services, CDC. Retrieved from https://www.cdc.gov/tb/statistics/reports/2016/pdfs/2016_Surveillance_FullReport.pdf.

Centers for Disease Control and Prevention: *Sexually transmitted disease surveillance 2016*, Atlanta, 2017e, U.S. Department of Health and Human Services. Retrieved from https://www.cdc.gov/std/stats16/CDC_2016_STDS_Report-for508WebSep21_2017_1644.pdf.

Centers for Disease Control and Prevention: *Vaccine information statement: hepatitis A*, 2017f. Retrieved from https://www.cdc.gov/vaccines/hcp/vis/vis-statements/hep-a.html.

Centers for Disease Control and Prevention: *About HIV/AIDS*, 2018a. Retrieved from https://www.cdc.gov/hiv/basics/whatishiv.html.

Centers for Disease Control and Prevention: *CDC—human papillomavirus (HPV) and cancer*, 2018b. Retrieved from https://www.cdc.gov/cancer/hpv/index.htm.

Centers for Disease Control and Prevention: *Clinician factsheets and guidance*, 2018c. Retrieved from https://www.cdc.gov/hpv/hcp/clinician-factsheet.html.

Centers for Disease Control and Prevention: *Combating the threat of antibiotic-resistant gonorrhea*, 2018d. Retrieved from https://www.cdc.gov/std/gonorrhea/arg/carb.htm.

Centers for Disease Control and Prevention: *Data and statistics*, 2018e. Retrieved from https://www.cdc.gov/tb/statistics/default.htm.

Centers for Disease Control and Prevention: Diagnoses of HIV infection among adults and adolescents in metropolitan statistical areas—United States and Puerto Rico, 2016, *HIV Surveillance Supplemental Report* 23(2), 2018f. Retrieved from https://www.cdc.gov/hiv/pdf/library/reports/surveillance/cdc-hiv-surveillance-supplemental-report-vol-23-2.pdf.

Centers for Disease Control and Prevention: *Geographic distribution*, 2018g. Retrieved from https://www.cdc.gov/hiv/statistics/overview/geographicdistribution.html.

Centers for Disease Control and Prevention: *Gonococcal infections—2015 STD treatment guidelines*, 2018h. Retrieved from https://www.cdc.gov/std/tg2015/gonorrhea.htm.

Centers for Disease Control and Prevention: *HBV FAQs for health professionals*, 2018i. Retrieved from https://www.cdc.gov/hepatitis/hbv/hbvfaq.htm

Centers for Disease Control and Prevention: *Hepatitis B vaccination of infants, children, and adolescents*, 2018j. Retrieved from https://www.cdc.gov/hepatitis/hbv/vaccchildren.htm.

Centers for Disease Control and Prevention: *Hepatitis D information for health professionals*, 2018k. Retrieved from https://www.cdc.gov/hepatitis/hdv/index.htm.

Centers for Disease Control and Prevention: *Hepatitis E questions and answers for health professionals*, 2018l. Retrieved from https://www.cdc.gov/hepatitis/hev/hevfaq.htm.

Centers for Disease Control and Prevention: *HIV among youth*, 2018m. Retrieved from https://www.cdc.gov/hiv/group/age/youth/index.html.

Centers for Disease Control and Prevention: *Injection drug use and HIV risk*, 2018n. Retrieved from https://www.cdc.gov/hiv/risk/idu.html.

Centers for Disease Control and Prevention: *PrEP*, 2018o. Retrieved from https://www.cdc.gov/hiv/basics/prep.html.

Centers for Disease Control and Prevention: *Prevention: HIV basics*, 2018p. Retrieved from https://www.cdc.gov/hiv/basics/prevention.html.

Centers for Disease Control and Prevention: *Statistics overview*, 2018q. Retrieved from https://www.cdc.gov/hiv/statistics/overview/index.html.

Centers for Disease Control and Prevention: *TB incidence in the U.S.*, 2018r. Retrieved from https://www.cdc.gov/tb/statistics/tbcases.htm.

Centers for Disease Control and Prevention: *U.S. 2016 surveillance data for viral hepatitis*, 2018s. Retrieved from https://www.cdc.gov/hepatitis/statistics/2016surveillance/index.htm.

Champion JD, Szlachta A: Self-identified sexual orientation and sexual risk behavior among HIV-infected Latino males, *J Assoc Nurses AIDS Care* 27(5):585–594. Retrieved from http://dx.doi.org/10.1016/j.jana.2016.03.004.

Hall HI, Song R, Tang T, et al.: HIV trends in the United States: Diagnoses and estimated incidence, *JMIR Public Health Surveill* 3(1):e8, 2017. Retrieved from https://www.ncbi.nlm.nih.gov/pmc/articles/PMC5315764/.

Heymann D: *Control of communicable diseases manual*, ed 20, Washington, DC, 2014, American Public Health Association.

HIV.gov: *Workplace rights*, 2017. Retrieved from https://www.hiv.gov/hiv-basics/living-well-with-hiv/your-legal-rights/workplace-rights.

HIV.gov: *U.S. statistics*, 2018. Retrieved from https://www.hiv.gov/hiv-basics/overview/data-and-trends/statistics.

Panel on Antiretroviral Guidelines for Adults and Adolescents: *Guidelines for the Use of Antiretroviral Agents in Adults and Adolescents Living with HIV*, 2018, Department of Health and Human Services. Retrieved from http://www.aidsinfo.nih.gov/ContentFiles/AdultandAdolescentGL.pdf.

Phillips I: Beta-lactamase producing penicillin-resistant gonococcus; *Lancet* 2:656, 1976.

Public Health Foundation: *The council on linkages between academia and public health practice: Core competencies for public health professionals*, 2014. Retrieved from http://www.phf.org/programs/corecompetencies/Pages/About_the_Core_Competencies_for_Public_Health_Professionals.aspx.

Schackman BR, Fleishman JA, Su AE, et al.: The lifetime medical cost savings from preventing HIV in the United States, *Med Care* 53(4):293–301, 2015. Retrieved from https://www.ncbi.nlm.nih.gov/pubmed/25710311.

Schillie S, Murphy T, Sawyer M, et al.: CDC guidance for evaluating health-care personnel for hepatitis B virus protection and for administering postexposure management, *MMWR Recomm Rep* 62(RR10):1–19, 2013. Retrieved from https://www.cdc.gov/mmwr/preview/mmwrhtml/rr6210a1.htm.

Schillie S, Vellozzi C, Reingold A, et al.: Prevention of hepatitis B virus infection in the United States: Recommendations of the advisory committee on immunization practices, *MMWR. Recomm Rep* 67:1–31, 2018. Retrieved from https://www.cdc.gov/mmwr/volumes/67/rr/rr6701a1.htm.

Schneider E, Whitmore S, Glynn KM, et al.: Revised surveillance case definitions for HIV infection among adults, adolescents, and children aged, *MMWR Recomm Rep* 2008; 57:1–12, 2008.

Sellik RM, Mokotoff ED, Branson B, et al.: Revised surveillance case definition for HIV infection—United States, 2014, MMWR Weekly Report, April 11, 2014, 63(RR03); 1–10.

UNAIDS: *Fact sheet—latest statistics on the status of the AIDS epidemic*, 2018. Retrieved from http://www.unaids.org/en/resources/fact-sheet.

United States Department of Health and Human Services (USDHHS): *Healthy people 2020 objectives*, 2010. Retrieved from https://www.healthypeople.gov/.

United States Department of Health and Human Services (USDHHS): *Figure 1. recommended immunization schedule for HIV-infected children aged 0–6 years—United States, 2013 figures pediatric opportunistic infection*, 2013a. Retrieved from https://aidsinfo.nih.gov/guidelines/html/5/pediatric-opportunistic-infection/431/figure-1—recommended-immunization-schedule-for-hiv-infected-children-aged-0–6-years—united-states—2013.

United States Department of Health and Human Services (USDHHS): *About the Ryan White HIV/AIDS program*, 2019. Retrieved from https://hab.hrsa.gov/about-ryan-white-hivaids-program/about-ryan-white-hivaids-program.

United States Prevention Services Task Force (USPSTF): *Final recommendation statement: Hepatitis C: Screening*, 2016. Retrieved from https://www.uspreventiveservicestaskforce.org/Page/Document/RecommendationStatementFinal/hepatitis-c-screening.

World Health Organization (WHO): *Global tuberculosis report 2017*, 2017. Retrieved from http://www.who.int/tb/publications/global_report/en/.

16

Promoting Healthy Communities

Marcia Stanhope, PhD, RN, FAAN

OBJECTIVES

After reading this chapter, the student should be able to do the following:

1. Discuss the history of the Healthy Communities movement.
2. Discuss the Centers for Disease Control and Prevention Healthy Communities Program.
3. Describe the core concepts and principles that guide the development of a healthy community program.
4. Describe the steps used when working with communities in the Healthy Communities process.
5. Apply the steps in working with Healthy Communities to the concepts of health promotion.
6. Explain the role nurses can assume in working with Healthy Communities.

CHAPTER OUTLINE

History of the Healthy Communities
Definition of Terms
Assumptions About Community Practice
Healthy Communities in the United States
Healthy Communities Around the World: Selected Examples
Developing a Healthy Community
Models for Developing a Healthy Community

KEY TERMS

appropriate technology, p. 359
Community Health Promotion Model, p. 365
community participation, p. 359
equity, p. 359
health promotion, p. 359
Healthy Communities, p. 357
healthy public policy, p. 361
international cooperation, p. 359
multisectoral cooperation, p. 359
primary health care, p. 359

This chapter provides an introduction to the history of the healthy communities movement and to the basic terminology related to the movement. It describes various models in which communities have structured their programs both in the United States and selected other countries. Key facilitators and barriers to the Healthy Communities process are discussed, as is the role for nurses in supporting the development and sustainment of healthy communities.

HISTORY OF THE HEALTHY COMMUNITIES

When the healthy communities initiative began it was known as the **Healthy Communities** and **Cities (HCC)** initiative, or movement. It began with the World Health Organization (WHO) in 1986 with the signing of the Ottawa Charter for Health Promotion. The initiative grew and has changed since 1986. This initiative, originally called *Healthy Cities,* assumed a healthy communities focus. In the past some locales used the term *healthy communities and cities,* whereas other locales talked about *healthy municipalities and cities,* and still others used the term *healthy communities.* The Centers for Disease Control and Prevention (CDC) in the United States initiated work in this area in 2003 and called their program the *steps program.* The CDC program was called *Healthy Communities.* The term *healthy communities* is used in this chapter; however,

The author wishes to acknowledge the assistance of Cynthia Collins, PhD, APRN, ANP-BC, GNP, Associate Professor and the Director of Curricular Innovation and Accreditation at Barry University in Miami, Florida.
A special thanks to Dr. Jeanette Lancaster and Loren Kelly for their work in previous editions of the text.

reference is made to other terms in order to describe the history of the movement and to refer to specific programs that use a term other than *healthy communities*. The goal of this movement was to promote health through community engagement and collaboration to activate and diffuse local changes that support good health. The premise was that community members must be involved in identifying the need for health programs and in developing programs to meet those needs. Building healthy communities relied on broad-based participation to make systems change in communities that can improve the health of the residents. The overall goals were to build community capacity, prevent chronic diseases, reduce health risk factors, and attain health equity (CDC, 2014).

HCC was found in many regions of the world. The movement began in 1986 when the WHO's Ottawa Charter became the first worldwide action plan for health promotion. At that time, the delegates to the conference declared that the following broad categories were prerequisites to health: peace, shelter, education, food, income, a stable ecosystem, sustainable resources, social justice, and equity. This is a much different approach to viewing health than the individualistic approach that holds that each person is responsible for his or her own health. Although 1986 seems to be in the distant past, the areas for action that were determined by the *Ottawa Charter for Health Promotion* are highly relevant today (WHO, 1986). They are as follows:

- *Building healthy public policy:* Many countries around the world have begun to recognize the need to integrate health considerations into policy making and programming across sectors to achieve better health and health equity. One example of this is the Health in All Policies (HiAP) approach to improve population health. What this means is that health and equity must be embedded into governmental decision making at local, state, and national levels for collaboration across all of the sectors that influence health. Intersectoral collaboration includes policies in the areas of education, housing, transportation, land use, and neighborhood safety to promote health equity.
- *Creating supportive environments:* For example, when communities are being revitalized or developed, places should be designated as "green areas" and made accessible to the public with parks, walking or bike paths, and fitness facilities. Both work and leisure should be a source of health for people.
- *Strengthening community action:* The Ottawa Charter states (and this continues to hold true) that health promotion is most effective in communities when residents are fully engaged in the development and implementation of programs. This requires a "tried and true" public health approach in which nurses *listen to and respond to the needs* of the community. Community members need to be involved in setting priorities, making decisions, planning strategies, and implementing them in order to attain better health.
- *Developing personal skills:* This includes providing information and teaching people the skills that they need in order to be healthy, such as regular and competent hand washing, choosing the right foods, engaging in regular age-appropriate exercise, and learning to avoid risk factors and increase their protective factors. This step increases the options available to people so they can have more control over their own health and their environments.
- *Reorienting health services:* This involves health care systems emphasizing health promotion and prevention, beyond providing clinical and curative services. Individuals, community groups, health practitioners, health care institutions, and the government share responsibility for health promotion (WHO, 2010).

The following Focus on Quality and Safety Education for Nurses box describes the importance of safety in community care.

QSEN FOCUS ON QUALITY AND SAFETY EDUCATION FOR NURSES

There are six Quality and Safety Education for Nurses competencies. All of the competencies could easily apply to Healthy Communities and Cities. However, safety is especially important for a healthy community program. Safety is an important competency for public health nurses who work in rural, suburban, and urban areas, and for nurses who care for clients and communities in developed and less developed countries. Aspects of community safety include but are not limited to the following:

- **Knowledge:** Learn about the potential threats to safety from the physical and social environments, including those at home, school, and at worksites.
- **Skills:** If a safety threat is identified, such as toxic materials from a factory being channeled into a water source, organize appropriate community leaders, workers, and volunteers to work toward reducing the pollution.
- **Attitudes:** Be aware of the various conflicting points of view and goals in a situation in which industrial pollution affects the health of the community.

Safety Question

If you think that a particular industry is emitting noxious chemicals into the air or water of the community, how do you get specific information to inform your actions?

Answer

Start by going to the Environmental Protection Agency (EPA) website (http://www.epa.gov) and search for pollutants by categories, including ZIP code, address, or facility name. See Envirofacts Multisystem Search User Guide at http://www.epa.gov.

Health promotion is a process designed to help people increase control over, and improve, their health. Health promotion is not just the responsibility of the health sector but rather includes individuals, families, groups, and communities. Strategies and programs should be customized to meet local needs and take into account different cultural needs, economies, customs, resources, and priorities. The original goals of the Ottawa Conference continue to be areas of concern, and work must continue to achieve the goals. From a global health perspective, a healthy community approach in selected countries around the world is needed

HCC began in the United States in 1988, with Healthy Cities Indiana and the California Healthy Cities project. Healthy Cities Indiana adapted the European experiences to the American context. The concept of Healthy Communities was used to include localities that were not cities but rather smaller communities such as towns or counties. In recent years, many U.S. communities initiated the HCC process with the result that thousands of communities have taken local action to promote health. Several of these communities are featured in the chapter as examples of what a focus on health promotion at the community level would look like.

In other parts of the world, HCC has different names, including Healthy Islands, Healthy Villages, and, in Latin America, Healthy Municipalities and Communities. In addition, national networks developed in Australia, Canada, Costa Rica, Iran, and Egypt. Other regional networks have developed in Francophone Africa, Latin America, Southeast Asia, and the western Pacific. Particular attention is given later in the chapter to Healthy Municipalities and Communities in the Pan American Health Organization (PAHO) region, since PAHO's work is long-standing and well developed and has demonstrated effective results.

Some claim that the concept of a healthy community or city is not new (Hancock, 1993). It is based on the belief that the health of the community is largely influenced by the environment in which people live and that health problems have multiple causes: social, economic, political, environmental, and behavioral. The HCC process has been applied to rural and metropolitan areas. The HCC process engaged local residents in action and was based on the premise that when people had the opportunity to work out their own locally defined health problems they would find sustainable solutions to those problems. This concept continues to be integral to good public health practice, which is to engage those for whom programs are being developed in the identification of need for, planning, implementing, and evaluating the programs. The *Healthy People 2020* process is consistent with the way healthy communities and cities have developed their priorities and plans. One of the four goals of *Healthy People 2020* is to create physical and social environments that promote good health for all. This goal relies on an ecologic perspective that says that health and health behaviors are determined by many influences, including personal, organizational, environmental, and policy factors. Many of the goals of *Healthy People 2020* are challenging to meet in light of the poor economic conditions in the United States and many other countries. For example, it is difficult to increase the income of low-income persons in an era in which people continue to lose their jobs and where unemployment, especially unemployment of youth, is high. See the Healthy People 2020 box for objectives that relate to healthy communities and cities.

HEALTHY PEOPLE 2020

Selected Goals That Pertain to Healthy Communities

- **ECBP-8:** Increase the proportion of worksites that offer a comprehensive employee health promotion program to their employees.
- **ECBP-9:** Increase the proportion of employees who participate in employer-sponsored health promotion activities.
- **ECBP-11:** Increase the proportion of local health departments that have established culturally appropriate and linguistically competent community health promotion and disease prevention programs.

From U.S. Department of Health and Human Services: *Healthy People 2020*, Washington, DC, 2010, U.S. Government Printing Office.

DEFINITION OF TERMS

There are many definitions of a healthy community. The *Healthy People 2010* document described a healthy community as one that included those elements that enable people to maintain a high quality of life and productivity (USDHHS, 2000). To expand on this definition, consider what was stated in the document *Healthy People in Healthy Communities: A Community Planning Guide Using Healthy People 2010:* that a healthy community would include access to health care services that include both treatment and prevention for all community members; the community would be safe; there would be adequate roads, schools, playgrounds, and other services to meet the needs of the people in the community; and that the environment would be healthy and safe (USDHHS, 2001).

The CDC defines a healthy place as one that is "designed and built to improve the quality of life for all people who live, work, worship, learn, and play within their borders—where every person is free to make choices amid a variety of healthy, available, accessible, and affordable options" (CDC, 2014, p. 201). The CDC also points out that a healthy community is one that continuously creates and improves both the physical and social environments and expands community resources to enable people to mutually support each other in carrying out essential life functions as well as in developing to their maximum potential. A healthy community seeks to improve the quality of life of its people and does this through collaboration, partnerships, diverse and extensive citizen ownership, and partnership in the process.

The principles of primary health care (WHO & UNICEF, 1978) and the Ottawa Charter for Health Promotion (WHO, 1986) were instrumental in the development of the Healthy Communities movement. **Primary health care** refers to meeting the basic health needs of a community by providing readily accessible health services. Because health problems transcend international borders, **international cooperation** is important to ensure health. The principles of primary health care include equity, health promotion, community participation, multisectoral cooperation, appropriate technology, and international cooperation.

Equity implies providing accessible services to promote the health of populations most at risk for health problems (e.g., the poor, the young, older adults, minorities, the homeless, and immigrants and refugees). **Health promotion** and disease prevention focus on providing community members with a positive sense of health that strengthens their physical, mental, and emotional capacities. Individuals within communities become involved in health promotion through **community participation**, whereby well-informed and motivated community members participate in planning, implementing, and evaluating health programs. **Multisectoral cooperation** is the coordinated action by all parts of a community, from local government officials to grassroots community members. **Appropriate technology** refers to affordable social, biomedical, and health services that are relevant and acceptable to individuals' health, needs, and concerns.

ASSUMPTIONS ABOUT COMMUNITY PRACTICE

There are different models of community practice, and the assumptions that professionals have about communities shape the implementation of the process. The classic work of Rothman and Tropman (1987) describing these different models and some of the key assumptions continues to be relevant today, as shown in the examples used in this chapter. The key models for community practice include the following:

1. Locality development is a process-oriented model that emphasizes consensus, cooperation, and building group identity and a sense of community.
2. Social planning stresses rational-empirical problem solving, usually by outside professional experts. Social planning does not focus on building community capacity or fostering fundamental social change.
3. Social action, on the other hand, aims to increase the problem-solving ability of the community with concrete actions that attempt to correct the imbalance of power and privilege of an oppressed or disadvantaged group in the community.

Effective models of community practice use a partnership between citizens and professionals in which there is delegated power and citizen control (Rothman & Tropman, 1987). A partnership approach, considered a bottom-up approach, incorporates the concepts of a multisectoral approach as well as community participation. A partnership approach prevents the top-down approaches in which professionals and experts tell the citizens what to do rather than involve and ask them.

HEALTHY COMMUNITIES IN THE UNITED STATES

In the following paragraphs, healthy communities initiatives in various regions of the United States are discussed. These examples show the different models of community practice that are being implemented. Specifically, the CDC's Healthy Communities Program emphasized policy, systems, and environmental changes that focus on chronic diseases and that encourage people to be more physically active, eat a healthy diet, and not use tobacco. The rationale was based on the fact that about 60 percent of Americans are affected by chronic disease, and these diseases account for 7 of the 10 leading causes of death in the country. Also, there are many direct and indirect costs associated with being obese and overweight. Many chronic diseases are preventable. By preventing a chronic disease from occurring, people can enjoy a higher quality of life, communities have a decreased burden of illness, and both the state and federal governments are able to reduce the amount they spend on health care (CDC, 2017). Some examples of chronic diseases cited by the CDC include heart disease, cancer, chronic lower respiratory diseases, stroke, Alzheimer's disease, diabetes, and chronic kidney diseases. The CDC said also that more than half of all adults fail to meet recommendations for aerobic physical activity; that tobacco is the single most preventable cause of disease, disability, and death; and that excessive alcohol use is the third leading cause of death related to lifestyle (CDC, 2017).

These chronic disease facts support the priority that the CDC has placed on funding projects that will interrupt chronic diseases in communities around the country. Beginning in 2003 and through 2014, the CDC's Healthy Communities Program funded more than 330 rural, urban, and tribal communities to support their goals. Specifically, their programs included Strategic Alliances for Health Communities, ACHIEVE (Action Communities for Health, Innovation, and EnVironmental ChangE), and REACH U.S. (Racial and Ethnic Approaches to Community Health) pioneering Healthy Communities (in collaboration with the YMCA of the USA), and Steps Communities (CDC, 2014). Also, Communities Putting Prevention to Work (CPPW) was a locally driven program that supported 50 communities as they tackled obesity and tobacco use. The CDC (2014) said that over 50 million people, or one in six Americans, lived in a city, town, county, or tribal community that benefited from these programs.

The CDC also developed a set of five "tools for community action" that could be used in developing healthy communities. The tools are no longer available, but given the usefulness of the CDC *tools for community action,* further discussion is warranted here. The recommendations for the five guides that the CDC chose came from the Community Preventive Services Task Force (CPSTF, 2018). The handbooks primarily target public health professionals but also can be used by community leaders. The Community Preventive Services Task Force continually updates its recommendations (see www.thecommunityguide.org). Also there is the current task force called the U.S. Preventive Services Task Force (USPSTF, 2018). The community guide provides health professionals with an authoritative source for making decisions about preventive services for individuals. Using the *five tools* relies on the same process used in the assessment of a community. In other words, before deciding the target in your work, follow these steps:

1. Conduct a needs assessment and set health priorities.
2. Find out what social and environmental factors may affect each health priority as well as what options are available for dealing with the chosen health priorities.
3. Think about the acceptability (to the community) and the feasibility (e.g., are resources available) to implement the project(s).

As you work with the five tools, remember to take small steps and do first things first; involve the appropriate people, and do not be reluctant to make changes as you go based on what you learn and the outcomes you have (Partnership for Prevention, 2018).

As is often true, the government will lay the groundwork for the development of health care and systems initiatives. While the government will eventually reduce or stop funding certain programs, these programs often continue with private or independent organizations. Examples are *The Community Guide,* the Community Preventive Services Task Force guide to services for individuals. Currently the U.S. Clinical Preventive Services Task Force recommends the use of *The Community Guide, Healthy People 2020,* and *Putting Prevention Into Practice* guides.

HEALTHY COMMUNITIES AROUND THE WORLD: SELECTED EXAMPLES

As mentioned earlier, PAHO in collaboration with the WHO has a long-standing involvement in developing healthy communities that they call the Healthy Municipalities and Communities movement. The mission of this movement is to "strengthen the implementation of health promotion activities at the local level, making health promotion a high priority of the political agenda; fostering the involvement of government authorities and the active participation of the community, supporting dialogue, sharing knowledge and experiences and stimulating collaboration among municipalities and countries" (PAHO, 2012). Other key concepts in their approach include multisectoral partnerships to improve social and health conditions and advocacy for developing **healthy public policy**, maintaining healthy environments, and promoting healthy lifestyles. PAHO believes that creating a healthy municipality involves a process that relies on strong political commitment and support that is aligned with equally strong communities who are determined to achieve their goals and who participate actively in the process of goal achievement (PAHO, 2012).

PAHO recommends a participatory development framework to gain commitment from the mayor, local government (all sectors), and representatives of community groups and organizations. PAHO has found this process to be the most effective in the Americas. The phases are as follows:

1. Aspects in the initial phase of the process
   - Meet with local government authorities and community leaders to gain their perspectives about such things as healthy spaces and health promotion and to request that they make a public statement as well as a joint declaration of their commitment.
   - Create an intersectoral, community planning committee.
   - Conduct a needs assessment including analysis of problems and needs.
   - Build consensus and decide on priorities for action.
2. Steps in the planning process
   - Train the committee and task forces to ensure that they understand the concept of healthy community, the settings approach to health promotion, and participatory methods including needs assessment, planning, evaluation, and health education.
   - Develop an action plan.
   - Mobilize resources needed to implement the plan and develop a detailed work plan.
3. Moments in the consolidation phase of the process
   - Implement activities that are included in the plan. Examples might be establishing health-promoting schools, workplaces, markets, hospitals, and other healthy environments.
   - Evaluate the results as well as the quality of participation.
   - Share knowledge and experiences with others.

PAHO notes that the steps that work in its region may be somewhat different from those that have been successful in Canada, the United States, and Europe. Later in this chapter, the 20 steps that PAHO says have been used by these other countries are cited as a way for nurses and other public health workers to develop a healthy community strategy. Interestingly, PAHO has found that it must start its process by gaining support from the mayor of the community and from other community leaders. These individuals must understand the concept of health promotion and the healthy municipalities process before they will offer their support. PAHO has also found that it must have a strong and knowledgeable support group who can envision a healthy municipality and convey that vision to opinion leaders (PAHO, 2012).

There are many excellent examples of Healthy Communities around the world. PAHO says that in some countries in their region, such as Mexico, Costa Rica, Chile, and Cuba, national networks have been established and have been producing good results for many years (PAHO, n.d.). A few examples are highlighted here with information on how to locate their websites and learn more about the work being done around the world.

- *Ontario (Canada) Healthy Communities Coalition:* They focus on "what makes a healthy community." Their website, www.ohcc-ccso.ca, is filled with useful resources.
- *Horsens, Denmark:* One of their key foci is on "safe community Horsens." Their website, www.horsenssundby.dk, is in Danish, but the button to choose English is clearly marked and they provide an overview of the work they are doing.
- *Community Builders of New South Wales, Australia:* They have an interactive electronic clearinghouse for persons involved in community level, social, economic, and environmental renewal, including community leaders, community and government workers, volunteers, program managers, academics, policy makers, youth, and seniors. They include rural and regional communities (www.communitybuilders.nsw.gov.au).
- *Association for Community Health Improvements:* This organization's website includes many healthy community tools and organizations in the United States and internationally. Similarly, www.healthycommunities.org hosts a website with valuable information about healthy communities and extensive links to other sites.

Selected examples of healthy communities in the United States are discussed later in this chapter.

DEVELOPING A HEALTHY COMMUNITY

What do people want from a healthy community? We know that each community is different and its challenges, goals, resources, competencies, problem-solving skills, and practices are different. As discussed throughout the chapter, many organizations in the United States and other countries have worked to help communities become healthier (Fig. 16.1). One of these organizations in the United States is the National Civic League (see www.communitycommons.org.) In 2014, the National Civic League partnered with Community Commons to celebrate 25 years of Healthy Communities and to spread the ideas and insights in published and new online media (National Civic League, 2018). They emphasize the complexity of developing

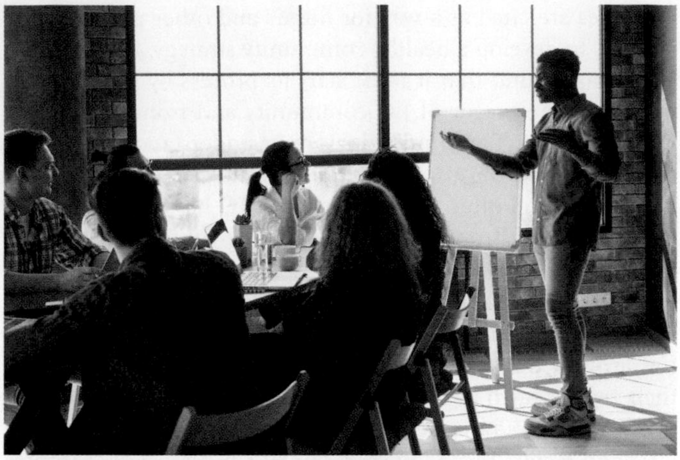

Fig. 16.1 Community participation for developing a healthy community involves a representative community planning committee. (Copyright © Milkos/iStock/Thinkstock.)

healthy communities and have identified five principles that they think should be applied in community work if the goal is to find solutions using a broad-based inclusive process. These principles are as follows:

1. A broad definition of health that goes beyond the absence of disease to address the root problems in communities and includes economy, education, parks and recreation, arts, mental health, and community spirit and unity.
2. A collaborative, consensus-based approach to problem solving that involves a diverse group of citizens from the community.
3. An assets-based approach to problem solving that defines people and relationships by their skills and abilities rather than their needs and deficits.
4. Addressing challenges at a systems level in the community rather than implementing another short-term, low-impact project.
5. Creating a shared vision for the future that captures the hopes and dreams of the community and that guides collaborative work.

Other principles will guide the development and implementation of a healthy community. Examples of useful principles include the following:

- The whole is greater than the sum of the parts; in other words, most communities have limited resources, and no one agency can do all that is needed. However, if agencies work together, the outcome of the whole can be much bigger than the outcome of the aid provided by one agency.
- A change in one part of the system affects the others. For example, if the public transportation workers in a large city go on strike and there is no public transportation for many days, many areas of the community will be affected.
- Collaboration is central to the development of a healthy community.
- All systems have feedback loops whereby information from one area is fed back to the whole and provides an opportunity for change or "course correction." For example, you might establish a helping program for dependent older adults where daycare is provided at low cost. This would enable the family members with whom the elder lives to provide safe care while they worked. However, if the family has no transportation of their own and the facility is not accessible by public transportation, the program would not be as helpful as hoped.

BOX 16.1 What Is a Healthy Community?

- A clean and safe environment
- A diverse and vibrant economy
- Good housing for all
- Good roads and good public transportation
- Parks, playgrounds, and recreational facilities
- People who respect and support each other
- A place that promotes and celebrates its cultural and historical heritage
- A place where citizens and government share power and where citizens feel a sense of belonging
- A place that has affordable health care for all
- A place that has good schools
- A place that has and supports strong families

The National Civic League also asked hundreds of communities across the country "What would your community look like if it were a really healthy place to live?" You might ask yourself that same question before looking at Box 16.1 and see how close your replies are to those of the respondents.

This chapter indicates that a healthy community has involvement, inclusiveness, cooperation, and collaboration, among other qualities. Collaboration can help make the best use of resources, reduce duplication and competition, increase effectiveness, and develop more sustainable resources. It is like a recipe in that each agency in the collaboration brings one or more ingredients to the product. Putting all the ingredients together leads to a better product. Collaboration involves doing things differently than in the past and developing different kinds of partnerships and relationships. Organizations that work together effectively have generally achieved three things:

1. High levels of trust
2. Serious time commitment from the partners
3. A diminished need to protect their own turf (Torres & Margolin, 2010)

Collaboration requires the same mix of behaviors and goals as those associated with the development of a healthy community—that is, a group of participants including those who are paid and volunteers who bring different skills and talents to the process and who work together to do the following:

1. Address a specific problem or opportunity
2. Work on a broad agenda of mutually beneficial goals
3. Provide a forum to discuss and respond to community concerns, interests, and resources
4. Recognize that there are roles in a partnership and they will be different from the role the person had in the parent organization.

EVIDENCE-BASED PRACTICE

This case study examines how lack of access to basic health care affects the health of poor, rural people in Gambia and what strategies, including extensive use of nurses, can help alleviate some of the health problems. Although this study was carried out in an African country, the information learned by the researchers has applications in any country in which people live in rural areas and have difficulty accessing health care. The authors point out that poor people in developing countries tend to suffer "from a phenomenon known as the poverty penalty (the additional cost paid for goods and services by the poor relative to the more affluent)" (Sanneh et al., 2013, p. 126).

Sub-Saharan Africa, including Gambia, has a higher under-five mortality rate than anywhere else in the world. The 2007-2020 National Health Policy Framework of Gambia, entitled "Health Is Wealth" aimed to address health issues through both preventive and curative services. They developed a health pyramid that placed primary care (village health services) at the base; secondary care (minor and major health centers) as the next two types of care delivery moving up the pyramid; and tertiary care (hospitals) at the peak of the pyramid.

Their case study took place in Kiang West, in the Lower River Region of Gambia, which has a 50 percent poverty rate among its population ratio of 30,000 people per primary health care facility. Roads are not well developed, and there is little economic activity. This was the work of a multi-stakeholder group including representatives from the government, Medical Research Council, World Health Organization, and the United Nations International Children's Emergency Fund. The representatives of the health sector and a range of stakeholders initiated various activities to improve care, including improving staffing at the Karantaba Health Centre with more traditional birth attendants and village health workers who worked with the community health nurses to provide primary health care. They expanded programs for immunizations, providing children with two high doses of vitamin A (which is critical to child health and immune function), surveillance of infectious disease, and midwifery services. Nurses play a key role in health care in this country. They documented improvements in the primary care services that they increased.

Nurse Use

What the collaborators in the multi-stakeholder group learned is that "no single organization, sector, nor approach can provide answers for underdevelopment, poverty, and ill health." They noted that "the importance of cooperation, both within a specific sector and across sectors, cannot be stressed enough."

Sanneh EJ, Hu AH, Njai M, et al.: Making basic health care accessible to rural communities: a case study of Kiang West District in rural Gambia. *Public Health Nurs* 31(2):126–133, 2013.

As mentioned earlier, Indiana and California have the longest history of Healthy Communities and Cities in the United States. Healthy Cities Indiana began as a pilot program in 1988 with a grant from the W.K. Kellogg Foundation as a collaborative effort among Indiana University School of Nursing, Indiana Public Health Association, and six Indiana cities. On the basis of this project's success, the W.K. Kellogg Foundation funded the dissemination phase, called CITYNET-Healthy Cities, in cooperation with the National League of Cities through their network of 19,000 local officials (Flynn et al., 1991). This was an extensive project that initially involved six cities (Gary, Fort Wayne, New Castle, Indianapolis, Seymour, and Jeffersonville). Activities in these cities focused on problems of diverse populations. For example, actions were consistent with local priorities that included problems of children, teen parents, the homeless, access to health care, crime and violence, and older adults. Action was also taken on the broader environmental policy issues, including management of solid waste and promotion of air quality. For each of these projects, the Community Health Promotion process was followed, thereby providing a broad base of community participation at all stages of community planning. This was a process developed at Indiana University School of Nursing, and it was consistent with many of the other U.S. and international processes for implementing healthy community initiatives.

An early example of the use of the Community Health Promotion process was the New Castle Healthy City community assessment. The community committee found that there were high death rates in the community from cancer, chronic obstructive pulmonary disease, and heart disease. The committee asked the following questions: Why were rates higher in this area than in the state and the nation? What were the lifestyle choices of people in the community? What in the environment supported or inhibited healthy choices?

The committee worked with the staff at Indiana University School of Nursing to develop a survey to obtain baseline data on health behaviors in the community. Staff at the University trained local volunteers in survey data collection. They distributed 1000 door-to-door surveys using a system that ensured appropriate geographic coverage in the community. The response rate of 50 percent demonstrated the community's interest in health concerns. They then compared their findings with the national health objectives (USDHHS, 1991). They found high levels of unhealthy behaviors, such as cigarette smoking and inadequate exercise, compared with the *Healthy People 2000* national objectives.

They used the survey results to determine the focus of their Healthy City initiatives. Using the data, they testified before the county commissioners about the need for health education and to support the employment of a health educator in the local health department. The cigarette smoking results were used by the committee to testify before the city council in support of an ordinance banning smoking in city buildings. The committee also sponsored community health awareness programs, including a family fitness walk, safety checks of bicycles, and presentations on healthy food preparation emphasizing reduced fat and salt in meals.

New Castle has expanded its focus and is now known as Healthy Communities of Henry County. They focused on developing a network of walking trails throughout the county on the Trans-Indiana National Road Heritage Trail (NRHT) (Fig. 16.2). Their 18th Annual Raintree Ride was held in September 2018. (See www.hchcin.org for more details on this worthy project and the implied enthusiasm for its accomplishment.) The process for the walking trails initiative, which began in 2002, is consistent with that of other successful healthy community projects. Specifically, consultants worked with the committee to conduct a feasibility study and write a grant. Over the years, the committee obtained broad community support and cooperation, not only in defining local problems, but also in setting priorities and implementing their initiatives. Their interventions integrated individual lifestyle changes and policy

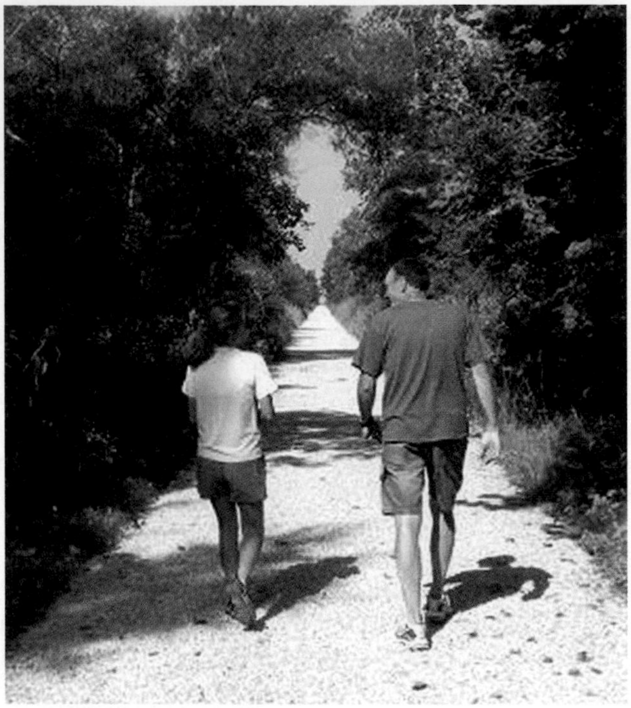

Fig. 16.2 Walking trails in Indiana help people engage in health-promoting exercise. (From indianatrails.org, 2010. Courtesy Beverly Matthews. Available at http://www.indianatrails.org.)

changes aimed at promoting supportive environments for health.

Another example in Indiana is the Healthy Communities Initiative in Bartholomew County. The Initiative began in 1994 with a goal of improving health and quality of life for residents of the county. They have remained true to their original concept of collaboration across the community. Their Guiding Principles are as follows:

- Collaboration
- Community Ownership
- Inclusive/Broad Based
- Benchmark & Measure Outcomes
- Long-Term Commitment
- Continuous Learning
- Positive Motivation

The current collaboration is between Columbus Regional Hospital, schools, businesses, local government, churches, and others working together to address identified health needs. See more at http://www.crh.org. They have action teams in community medication assistance, caring parents, domestic violence, Proyecto Salud, healthy lifestyles, tobacco awareness, volunteers in the medicine clinic, and a breast feeding coalition (Columbus Regional Hospital, 2016).

The second state to be featured is California. The California Healthy Cities and Communities (CHCC) is a program of the Center for Civic Partnerships, a part of the Public Health Institute. For over 25 years, the Center has assisted and supported over 100 cities and communities in the state to develop community health improvement initiatives (Center for Civic Partnerships, 2016). They work with communities of varying sizes and have developed strategies to curtail exposure to tobacco, increase opportunities for physical activity, encourage better nutrition, and improve public safety. This network is built on the premise of shared responsibility among community members, local officials, and the private sector. Community participation is the cornerstone of the projects, and the mission is to reduce inequities in health status that exist among diverse populations in communities (http://www.civicpartnerships.org).

In 1989 Pasadena became a charter city of the California Healthy Cities and Communities project and produced a quality-of-life index with extensive input from residents, technical panels, and neighborhood groups. The index included over 50 indicators affecting community life, such as safety, education, substance abuse, recreation, economy, and housing. The index guided policy development in tobacco control, alcohol availability, and infant health education. It also assisted city and community agencies in planning, priority setting, resource development, and budgeting. In 2008, Pasadena engaged a consulting group to help them update these indicators so they might continue their growth as a healthy city.

Another example of California Healthy Cities and Communities is in Chico. A Healthy Chico Kids 2000 community-wide initiative was started, focusing on nutrition and health promotion. Nutrition education was provided for students in kindergarten through sixth grade. A dietary assessment was conducted that led the school district to reduce fat calories in school lunches. The initiative was expanded to increase awareness of cardiovascular risk factors among elementary school students, and the work is ongoing.

In California, Building Healthy Communities is a 10-year comprehensive community effort to help Californians think about and support the health of the community. This work is funded by the California Endowment Building Healthy Communities fund. The Endowment distributed $1.7 billion in its first decade of operations. The Endowment thinks that a specific focus helps them have a great impact, and they are focusing on healthy community building. Specifically, they are targeting "a nexus of community, health, and poverty to advance a 'prevention movement' in California" (California Endowment, 2018, p. 1). The Endowment plans to focus on this area for the next decade to develop "places where children and youth are healthy, safe and ready to learn" (California Endowment, 2018, p. 2). They think that the health of children is a primary indicator of the health of its communities (Fig. 16.3). For news and information about Building Healthy Communities, see www.calendow.org.

There are thousands of Healthy Communities and Cities programs in the United States seeking local solutions to complex problems. Nurses often play key roles in the work of Healthy Communities and Cities programs.

In recent years the Robert Wood Johnson Foundation has developed several initiatives that emphasize improvement of health for all. The Foundation is working to "build a culture of health" within communities and across the nation by focusing on changing community environments for healthful living, highlighting disease prevention and health promotion approaches,

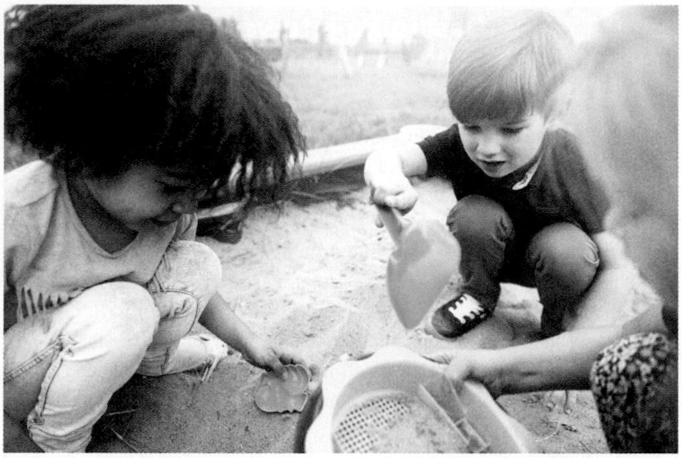

Fig. 16.3 Supportive communities provide playgrounds where children can play and exercise in a safe location. (Copyright © gpointstudio/iStock/Thinkstock.)

focusing on health disparities, and addressing the social determinants of health.

Recently, the National Civic League (NCL) joined with the Robert Woods Johnson Foundation (RWJF) to honor individuals and groups who have successfully implemented changes within their communities that have aimed at reducing health disparities in one or more of the following areas: access to quality health care, education, employment, income, community environment, housing, and public safety. The 2018 NCL-RWJF Health Equity Award winners were two citizens of Providence, Rhode Island. Entitled "The Sankofa Initiative," the project jointly led by a resident champion and a community developer, has created not only a culture of health in the community, but additionally resulted in a culture of prosperity and neighborhood pride. This project addresses multiple social determinants of health as it tackles the following:

- Urban blight
- Food scarcity
- The failing local economy
- A program that has the capacity to produce systemic, long-term growth. (Read more about this work at www.rwjf.org.)

MODELS FOR DEVELOPING A HEALTHY COMMUNITY

There are many models to guide the development of a healthy community. The models have a considerable amount of commonality. This section discusses how a nurse could either lead or be part of a team responsible for designing, implementing, and evaluating a healthy community. As has been seen, most of the successful healthy communities or cities establish priorities that are identified after careful assessment and enormous amounts of community involvement. Nearly 20 years ago, faculty at the Indiana University School of Nursing under the leadership of Beverly Flynn developed a **Community Health Promotion Model** by adapting the European model of cities to the United States. This section discusses the key steps needed to develop a healthy community and compares them to the model developed at Indiana University. The steps of a general model that PAHO described as common to models in the United States, Canada, and Europe are as follows (PAHO, 2018):

1. Build a local support group
2. Know about the Healthy Communities idea
3. Know the city or community
4. Gain financial support
5. Decide where the organization for the project will be located
6. Develop the proposal
7. Appoint a project steering committee
8. Analyze the environment in which the project will take place
9. Define clearly the work of the project
10. Set up the project office
11. Plan a long-term strategy
12. Build project capacity
13. Establish accountability mechanisms

Compare the previous 13-step model to the 9 steps in the Community Health Promotion Model (produced by the Institute for Action Research for Community Health/Indiana University, 1994 [Flynn, 1997]) below:

1. Orient the community to the idea of community health promotion. For example, meet with formal and informal leaders to identify persons in the community who have an interest in and the capability to support the community development process. You could hold an informational community forum, or establish a task force to plan. The key is to find people who are committed to the process.
2. Build the partnership. Learn who the formal and informal community leaders are so you know who is listened to in the community. Be sure to have broad-based representation on your planning committee. Remember that people participate when they think there is a need, feel a sense of community, see their involvement as helpful and worth their time, and think the benefits outweigh possible costs. Box 16.2 describes principles of community engagement that need to be considered in the community engagement process.
3. Develop a structure in the community for health promotion. This step is similar to the PAHO stage of assembling a steering committee that will plan and coordinate the work. Some ways to collaborate and get the work done that support the Healthy Communities (HC) process are (1) the whole local partnership deliberates and shares information, but subgroups make decisions and implement them; (2) the local partnership serves as a single advisory board for multiple agencies; and (3) the whole local partnership makes decisions, but subgroups take action together (PAHO 2018). The steering group might develop and communicate a clear vision and mission that is broadly understood by all participants and not just by health professionals. The mission should define the problem and acceptable solutions in such a way as to engage (not blame) those community members most affected and not to limit the strategies and environmental changes needed to address the community-identified concern. Ongoing action planning should identify specific community and system changes that can lead to widespread behavior change and community health improvement. The

BOX 16.2 Principles of Community Engagement

Before starting a community engagement effort:

- Be clear about the purposes or goals of the engagement effort, and the populations and/or communities you want to engage.
- Become knowledgeable about the community in terms of its economic conditions, political structures, norms and values, demographic trends, history, and experience with engagement efforts. Learn about the community's perceptions of those initiating the engagement activities.

For engagement to occur, it is necessary to:

- Go into the community, establish relationships, build trust, work with the formal and informal leadership, and seek commitment from community organizations and leaders to create processes for mobilizing the community.
- Remember and accept that community self-determination is the responsibility and right of all people who comprise a community. No external entity should assume it can bestow on a community the power to act in its own self-interest.

For engagement to succeed, you need to:

- Partner with the community to create change and improve health.
- Recognize and appreciate all aspects of community engagement and respect community diversity. In order to effectively design and implement approaches for community engagement, be aware of the various cultures and other areas of diversity of a community.
- Realize that you can only sustain community engagement by identifying and mobilizing community assets, and by developing capacities and resources for community health decisions and action.
- Be prepared to turn over control of actions or interventions to the community, and be flexible enough to meet the changing needs of the community.
- Make a long-term commitment to the engaging organization and its partners.

From Agency for Toxic Substances and Disease Registry (ATSDR): Principles of Community Engagement, ed 2, Atlanta, 2015. Available at https://www.atsdr.cdc.gov/communityengagement/pce_principles_occur.html.

committee should develop widespread leadership, engaging a broad group of members and allies in the work of the community organization, mobilization, and change. The membership of the working group should be diverse and clearly reflect the community's composition.

4. Determine who will lead the health promotion work. You may need to provide some leadership development work at this stage, such as sending members to conferences or workshops or using consultants or online training programs.
5. Assess the community. The steps here follow those in the chapter on community assessment. Start by clarifying the purpose of the assessment and what you will do with the data you collect. The assessment provides the frame of reference for identifying the community's strengths, needs, and resources.
6. Plan for community-wide health. Many of the skills for working with groups that are discussed in Chapter 19 will be used in this step of the process, as will models for planning in Chapter 23 that discusses program management.
7. Develop community action for health. The interventions at this stage should be designed to achieve the outcomes cited in Box 16.3. These nine areas can guide the selection of actions and provide a focus for the evaluation.

BOX 16.3 Designing Interventions and Evaluating Results of Healthy Municipalities and Cities

- **Health education:** Health knowledge, attitudes, motivation, intentions, behavior, personal skills, and effectiveness
- **Influence and social action:** Community participation, community empowerment, social standards, and public opinion
- **Healthy public policies and organizational practices:** Political statutes, legislation, and regulation; location of resources; organization practices, culture, and behavior
- **Healthy living conditions and lifestyles:** Use of tobacco, availability of food and food choices, physical activity, consumption of alcohol and drugs, relationship between protective factors and risk factors in the physical and social environment
- **Effectiveness of health services:** Delivery of preventive services, access to the health services, and quality of services
- **Healthy environments and spaces:** Restricted sale of tobacco and alcohol; restrictions on illicit drug use; positive environments for children, young people, and older adults; and sanctions for abuse and violence
- **Social results:** Quality of life, social support networks, positive discrimination, equity, development of life skills
- **Health outcomes:** Reduction of morbidity and mortality, disability, and avoidable mortality; psychosocial and life skills
- **Capacity building and development:** Measures of sustainability, community participation and empowerment, human-resources development

From Pan American Health Organization: *Healthy municipalities and communities: mayor's guide for promoting quality of life*, Washington, DC, n.d., World Health Organization, p. 24. Available at http://www.paho.org.

8. Provide information based on data to policy makers. Effective development of public policy relies on dialogue between those making the policies and the members of the public who will be affected by them. The aim is to link policy makers, professionals, and citizens together to achieve commonly agreed on health goals. Examples of healthy public policies include seat belt legislation, no-smoking policies, motorcycle helmet laws, handgun laws, and immunization policies for school-age children. Providing information is a way to serve as an advocate. Nurses may be asked to testify or assist others with preparing testimony that will give the city council, county commissioners, or other members of planning groups the information they need to promote the development of healthy public policy.
9. Monitor and evaluate the progress. This step is similar in all problem-solving processes. You must watch the progress, make sure you stay on track, or make a course correction if needed, and then evaluate the outcome.

CHECK YOUR PRACTICE

You have asked to suggest an approach to developing a healthy community. What would you do? Which approach would you recommend?

As can be seen, both models use a problem-solving approach, and the latter is clearly similar to the use of the nursing process in the community with a goal of promoting health. In the following box a brief case illustrates how a model such as the ones listed previously are used to guide the development of a healthy community.

HOW TO Work With a Healthy Community Initiative: A Case Example

The Crooked Creek Quality of Life Initiative (CC QOLI): A Community Development Experience took place in Indianapolis, Indiana. The purpose of the initiative was to improve the quality of life of residents of a geographically defined neighborhood in a Midwestern city in the United States. An advisory board provided oversight for a comprehensive assessment conducted by nursing students. The assessment results were used for developing a proposal that funded an advisory group appointed by the mayor of the city. The PAHO Healthy Municipalities and Communities model was used to bring diverse sectors of the community together to collaborate in order to address the conditions responsible for health and well-being. Organizations involved included a hospital, social service agency, housing development agency, and university.

The goal of the CC QOLI was to improve the quality of life of Crooked Creek residents through:

1. Revitalization of built environments (such as in commercial and community buildings, housing, roads, and sidewalks)
2. New collaborations among health, education, and social service organizations
3. Engagement of the residents in community improvement

Initiatives implemented to achieve these goals were investment in a housing program for low- and moderate-income residents; construction of a Family Pavilion to address the civic, social, intergenerational, cultural, and recreational needs of Crooked Creek individuals and families; and a School Health Program for area students.

Results Achieved

The Fay Biccard Glick Family Pavilion at Crooked Creek was constructed and now provides a wonderful space for community gatherings, youth and family activities, recreation, and an affordable venue for wedding receptions, family reunions, graduation ceremonies, open houses, and religious services. The School Health Program moved health care delivery beyond traditional hospital walls and is now part of a broader vision to build healthier communities. School corporations have adopted healthier school policies and are able to address chronic issues of asthma, obesity, and absenteeism. Investments in housing have resulted in completion of three congregate living homes providing a home for 12 disabled residents, and the most recent home uses "green" building practices. Additional results have been the provision of costly repairs to the homes of 33 elderly homeowners; education of 60 potential homebuyers about the home-buying process; and down payment assistance for 12 first-time buyers who purchased homes in Crooked Creek.

Factors Affecting and/or Hindering Success

A major barrier occurred when the contractor for the Family Pavilion project walked off the job midway through the project, resulting in an eight-month delay and cost overruns. Another contractor was hired, and funds were raised to complete the project. The School Health Program became more complex when partners realized that the unique nature of each school required that interventions be tailored for each particular school's student population. The investments in housing programs found the cost of projects were sustainable only to the degree that the organization continued to successfully compete for public and private funds to underwrite projects.

Summing Up

Lessons learned across initiatives include:

1. Collaboration makes individual organizations stronger—a new organization without a track record benefits from partnering with an established organization, which gives others "permission" to be supportive. Established organizations benefit from the energy and entrepreneurial aspects of start-ups.
2. Having a good plan based on good data is crucial to securing funding and support.
3. Program operators need to ensure that senior leaders (senior executives and board members) stay informed and engaged over time in order to sustain initiatives over the long term. Otherwise they risk being replaced by the next new (and not necessarily better) thing.

Authors: Alicia Chadwick with Crooked Creek Northwest Community Development Corporation, Helen Lands with Fay Biccard Glick Neighborhood Center, Mary Beth Riner with Indiana University School of Nursing, and Marty Rugh with St. Vincent Health.

Because nurses naturally work with community people from different walks of life and are respected health professionals in the community, they are well suited to promote HC. Look for opportunities within existing community partnerships that you work with and that are also interested in promoting the community's health. Plan how to introduce them to the HC process, and work together to find ways to initiate the process with your combined network of contacts to develop activities that support improved health.

Nurses may work with the healthy community process in a variety of ways and in many stages. It is important to remember that evaluation and research are important parts of the process. Specifically, nurses may initiate, coordinate, or be part of a research team conducting program evaluation research. Providing data relevant to changes in health status through short-term impact evaluation and long-term outcome evaluation is valuable in creating the knowledge base for validating the field of community health promotion. The following How To box describes the steps to use in organizing a community meeting to plan a healthy community.

The Linking Content to Practice box applies many of the key public health documents to the work of developing a healthy community. Remember that the ultimate goal is to promote the community's own leadership for health. In other words, the nurse must not do for the community what it can do for itself. The role of the nurse and of other health professionals in Healthy Communities is to work in partnership with community leaders. The role of health professionals in Healthy Communities is being available to help and not being a director of the work. The Levels of Prevention box provides suggestions for how to foster community education and action.

LINKING CONTENT TO PRACTICE

Health promotion using the healthy community model relies on key public health skills and core competencies. Such an approach includes the core functions of assessment, policy development, and assurance, which is making sure that there is a competent workforce available to meet the needs of the community. See Chapter 1 for details on the public health core functions.

Specifically, the *Public Health Nursing: Scope and Standards* DOCUMENT uses a community-focused problem-solving process that is consistent with the steps in developing a healthy community (ANA, 2013). Throughout the Quad Council Coalition Public Health Nursing Competencies document are competencies that also fit this process. For example, in many of the domains, there is an emphasis on collaboration with others for determining health priorities and in using the policy-making process to achieve health goals (Quad Council, 2018). Also, the steps in healthy community development are congruent with the Intervention Wheel discussed in Chapter 11.

LEVELS OF PREVENTION

Healthy Communities

Primary Prevention

Develop a community forum to initiate communication about health promotion.

Secondary Prevention

Assess needs and strengths in the community to detect ways to address health problems.

Tertiary Prevention

Initiate community action when problems have occurred, and evaluate and monitor progress of programs and policies.

HOW TO Organize a Community Meeting About Healthy Communities

1. Identify who should be included in the community meeting. It is critical that all sectors and population groups in the community be involved.
2. How will they be invited to the meeting? Who will invite them? Allow at least two weeks so people can arrange their schedules.
3. Who will convene the meeting?
4. Set the date and time for the meeting, and arrange for a neutral meeting place.
5. Plan the meeting agenda:
   a. Introduction of participants
   b. Introduction to Healthy Communities (HC)
   c. Identification of community people who should be there ("Whom did we miss?")
   d. Questions and discussion about HC and about community issues that are important
   e. Commitment to the HC process
   f. Formation of the HC committee (obtain names and addresses of those interested)
   g. Other suggestions

PRACTICE APPLICATION

Because nurses work in partnership with the community in Healthy Communities, the examples of outcomes of HC initiatives reflect that partnership rather than a specific nursing intervention. An example of an outcome of a HC initiative that used the Community Health Promotion process is Fort Wayne, Indiana, Healthy City.

Committee members of the Fort Wayne, Indiana, Healthy City project collaborated in a community-wide program to address the fact that only 65 percent of Fort Wayne preschool children were immunized. Access to immunization services was expanded to five sites throughout the city at three different times in a program called Super-Shot Saturday.

A nurse, along with other members of the Fort Wayne, Indiana, HC committee, would be using which of the following principles of health promotion to provide access to immunizations for preschool children?

A. Promoting healthy public policy
B. Creating supportive environments
C. Strengthening community action
D. Reorienting health services
E. Improving personal skills

Answers can be found on the Evolve site.

KEY POINTS

- Although Healthy Cities began in 1986 in Europe, it is now an international movement of communities focused on mobilizing local resources and political, professional, and community members to improve the health of the community.
- The principles of primary health care and health promotion guide the Healthy Communities movements.
- The name used for the Healthy Community activity varies from one locale to another.
- The model of community practice most frequently found in the Healthy Communities movement is that of working with the local people to plan via community partnerships that will best meet their needs.
- Community participation can be gained in many ways; it is often helpful to have a local person on the planning committee to advise on how to best enlist the aid and support of the residents.
- The CDC became involved in the Healthy Communities work in its efforts to reduce the amount of chronic illness.
- The CDC developed a wide range of tools to help communities improve their health; these tools are being recommended by the U.S. Preventive Services Task Force.
- The concept of healthy communities is used in the United States as well as in many other nations. One region that has a well-developed set of programs is that covered by the Pan American Health Organization (PAHO). The steps that are used in PAHO countries are included in the chapter.
- The steps for developing a healthy community, including the use of the PAHO model or the Community Health Promotion Model developed at Indiana University School of Nursing, can be used by nurses working with communities to improve their health capacity.
- The first two states to develop Healthy Community projects were Indiana and California. These two states have ongoing active and responsive programs; some are discussed in the chapter.
- The *Healthy People 2020* objectives incorporate many of the key concepts of healthy communities, including providing access to health services; combating chronic illnesses; and providing safe food, a safe and healthy environment, opportunities for fitness, immunizations, and reduction in injuries and violence, to name a few.

CLINICAL DECISION-MAKING ACTIVITIES

1. In collaboration with a community group, conduct a community assessment. Identify the community's assets and problems.
2. Evaluate the effectiveness of a current approach to a health problem in your community (e.g., teen pregnancy). Describe how the approach would change if you were to use the steps in developing a healthy community such as the Community Health Promotion process.
3. Discuss the role of the nurse in health promotion within a healthy community model.

4. Identify city council members, the president of the chamber of commerce, the director of family services, the mayor, a religious leader, and other community leaders who are the "movers and shakers" in getting things done. Generate a list of questions that will help these leaders describe the major assets and problems of the community. Interview several local leaders and summarize their responses.
5. You are asked by the health commissioner to organize a community coalition for orientation to the Healthy Communities process. Outline the steps you would take.
6. Describe your philosophy of community leadership development for health promotion.
7. Discuss ways in which the *Healthy People 2020* objectives can incorporate community participation. Select one topic area within *Healthy People 2020,* and outline a community inclusive approach that you could use.

ADDITIONAL RESOURCES

EVOLVE WEBSITE

http://evolve.elsevier.com/Stanhope/community/

- Answers to Practice Application
- Case Study
- Glossary
- Review Questions

REFERENCES

American Nurses Association (ANA): *Scope & Standards of Practice*, ed 2, Silver Springs, MD, 2013, Public Health Nursing, ANA.

California Endowment: *Overview Strategic Vision* 2010-2020: Building Healthy Communities, 2018, Author. Retrieved from www.calendow.org.

Center for Civic Partnerships: *CA Healthy Cities and Communities Program*, 2016. Retrieved from http://www.civicpartnerships.org.

Centers for Disease Control and Prevention (CDC): *Healthy communities: Preventing chronic disease by activating grassroots change: at a glance*, 2017. Retrieved from www.cdc.gov.

Centers for Disease Control and Prevention (CDC): *About healthy places*, 2014. Retrieved from www.cdc.gov.

Columbus Regional Hospital: *Healthy communities initiative*, 2016. Retrieved from www.crh.org.

Flynn BC: Partnerships in healthy cities and communities: a social commitment for advanced practice nurses, *Adv Pract Nurs Q* 2: 1–6, 1997.

Flynn BC, Rider M, Ray DW: Healthy Cities: the Indiana model of community development in public health, *Health Educ Q* 18: 331–347, 1991.

Hancock T: The evolution, impact, and significance of the healthy cities/healthy communities movement, *J Public Health Policy* 14:5–18, 1993.

National Civic League: *Healthy Communities Initiatives*, Denver CO, 2018, Author.

Pan American Health Organization (PAHO): *Healthy Municipalities & Communities: Mayors' Guide for Promoting Quality of Life.* Washington, DC, n.d., PAHO. Retrieved from http://www.paho.org.

Pan American Health Organization (PAHO): Healthy Municipalities and Communities. Washington, DC, 2012, PAHO. Retrieved from http://www.paho.org.

Partnership for Prevention: *The Community Health Promotion Handbook: Action Guides to Improve Community Health*, Washington, DC, 2018, Partnership for Prevention.

Quad Council Coalition of Public Health Nursing Organizations: *Public Health Nursing Competencies*, Wheat Ridge, CO, 2018, Author.

Rothman J, Tropman JE: Models of community organization and macro practice: their mixing and phasing. In Cox FM, Tropman ME, Rothman J, et al, editors: *Strategies of Community Organization*, ed 4, Itasca, IL, 1987, Peacock.

Sanneh EJ, Hu AH, Njai M, Ceesay OM, Manjang B: Making basic health care accessible to rural communities: A case study of Kiang West District in rural Gambia, *Public Health Nurs* 31(2):126–133, 2013.

Task Force on Community Preventive Services: *The guide to community preventive services: Social environment and health*, 2018. Retrieved from http://www.thecommunityguide.org.

Torres GW, Margolin FS: Collaboration Primer: *Proven Strategies, Consideration, and Tools to Get You Started*, Chicago, 2010, Health Research & Educational Trust. Retrieved from www.hret.org.

U.S. Department of Health and Human Services (USDHHS): *Healthy People 2020: National Health Promotion and Disease Prevention Objectives*, Washington, DC, 2010, USDHHS.

U.S. Department of Health and Human Services (USDHHS): *Healthy People in Healthy Communities 2010*, Atlanta, 2000, USDHHS, Centers for Disease Control and Prevention, National Center for Chronic Disease Prevention and Health Promotion (electronic version). Retrieved from http://www.healthypeople.gov.

U.S. Department of Health and Human Services (USDHHS): *Healthy People in Healthy Communities: A Community Planning Guide Using Healthy People 2010*, Washington, DC, February 2001, U.S. Government Printing Office.

U.S. Preventive Services Task Force: *The Guide to Clinical Preventive Services*, 2018. Recommendations of the U.S. Preventive Services Task Force. Retrieved from http://www.uspreventiveservices taskforce.org.

World Health Organization (WHO): *Ottawa Charter for Health Promotion*, Copenhagen, Denmark, 1986, WHO Regional Office for Europe.

World Health Organization (WHO): About WHO. *Ottawa Charter for Health Promotion, 1986*, Copenhagen, Denmark, 2010, WHO Regional Office for Europe.

17

Community As Client: Assessment and Analysis

Mary E. Gibson, PhD, RN and Esther J. Thatcher, PhD, RN, APHN-BC

"I believe that the community—in the fullest sense: a place and all its creatures—is the smallest unit of health and that to speak of the health of an isolated individual is a contradiction in terms."

Wendell Berry

OBJECTIVES

After reading this chapter, the student should be able to do the following:

1. Analyze the importance of community assessment in nursing practice.
2. Select and utilize a method and model for assessment of a community.
3. Appraise various online data sources for reliability and accuracy of information.
4. Utilize the nursing process to create a community assessment for a selected community.
5. Interpret concepts basic to community nursing practice: community, community client, community health, and partnership for health.
6. Develop a prioritized community problem list and nursing diagnosis, and a care plan for a community.

CHAPTER OUTLINE

Introduction
Community Defined
Community As Client
Community Assessment
Community As Partner
How to Conduct a Community Assessment

KEY TERMS

active participation, p. 373
aggregate, p. 371
coalitions, p. 373
community, p. 371
community as client, p. 371
community as partner, p. 380
community health, p. 372
community health workers, p. 374
Community/Public Health Nursing Competencies, p. 375
demographic data, p. 388
distributive justice, p. 372
focus group, p. 379
gatekeepers, p. 374
geographic information system (GIS), p. 380
health indicators, p. 377
key informant, p. 378
Mobilizing for Action through Planning and Partnerships (MAPP), p. 373
morbidity, p. 389
mortality, p. 389
NANDA, p. 391
Omaha System, p. 391
participant observation, p. 378
partnership, p. 373
passive participation, p. 373
Photovoice, p. 379
population-centered practice, p. 372
primary data, p. 374
secondary data, p. 374
social justice, p. 372
socio-ecological model, p. 372
spatial data, p. 380
stakeholders, p. 377
ten essential public health services, p. 372
utilitarianism, p. 372
windshield surveys, p. 381

A special thanks to George Shuster for his contributions to this chapter through many editions of this text.

INTRODUCTION

Communities are the environments where we live and work. Naturally, the community's ability to serve the needs of its members determines key aspects in the health of the community. The public health nurse (PHN) is in an ideal position to view the "community as client," and to begin to identify and harness the strengths present to meet the challenges faced by the community. Health is an interdependent concept. As defined by the World Health Organization, "Health is a state of complete physical, mental and social well-being and not merely the absence of disease or infirmity" (WHO, 1948). The influences of environment, public services and policies along with economics play a large role in the health of the community. For example, in a sophisticated community analysis of Santa Cruz, California, the authors note:

The health of Santa Cruz County residents does not begin at the doctor's office, but at their home, school, workplace, neighborhood, and in their community. In part, health is determined by the opportunities, both social and economic, that are afforded to residents throughout their lifetime. Disparities that arise as a consequence of these opportunities, or lack thereof, offer context to why some in our county thrive while others only survive (Applied Survey Research, 2017, p. 2).

As PHNs, we use the nursing process from assessment through evaluation to promote a community's health. This process begins with community assessment (sometimes called community needs assessment)—one of the core functions of public health nursing—which involves getting to know the community inside and out. It is a logical, systematic approach to identifying community needs, clarifying problems, and identifying community strengths and resources. In this chapter we will clarify specific community concepts including community as client, provide a snapshot of the nurse's role in communities, and outline the process for undertaking a comprehensive community assessment using a hybrid of the nursing process.

COMMUNITY DEFINED

Throughout history, humans have formed cooperative social groups that enhanced the survival chances of individual group members. Even today, communities that rally together in solidarity tend to recover faster after a disaster or other event (Boyd & Richerson, 2009; Mercy Corps, 2017). Each generation defines and seeks community in different ways; the "Millennial" generation of young adults has received much interest in how their definitions of community influence their work, housing, social, and political lives (Feldman et al., 2017). But what do we mean by *community,* and how might being part of a community influence a person's health?

There are many definitions of community. At its simplest, a **community** is a group of people that share something in common, such as geographic location, interests, or values (MacQueen et al., 2001; The Community Guide, n.d.). The World Health Organization defines community as "a group of people, often living in a defined geographical area, who may share a common culture, values and norms, and are arranged in a social structure according to relationships which the community has developed over a period of time" (WHO, 2004, p. 16). One study that aimed to define community among a diverse U.S. population reached the consensus definition of "a group of people with diverse characteristics who are linked by social ties, share common perspectives, and engage in joint action in geographical locations or settings" (MacQueen et al., 2001).

A community is a system, not just the sum of the characteristics of its inhabitants. In most definitions, the community includes three factors: people, place, and function. *People* are the community members or residents. An **aggregate** is a population or group of individuals who share common personal or environmental characteristics. *Place* can be a geographic location or other shared spaces such as the Internet. *Function* refers to the aims and activities of the community.

Community is a concept rather than simply a specific place, and individuals living in the same place may describe their community differently. When an organization asks a nurse to perform a community assessment, community usually refers to a specific population, an aggregate with specific characteristics that lives within the area that an organization serves, such as a school district, or a geographic area such as a county. However, it is important to remember that individuals within this defined area could view the community through a different lens. Understanding the many identities of community is part of the community assessment and is best done through talking with residents and stakeholders.

COMMUNITY AS CLIENT

Nursing Care of the Community As Client

Population-focused health care is highly relevant in the current health care environment, and the community as client is important to nursing practice for several reasons. The community is the client when the nursing focus is on the collective or common good of the population, instead of only on individual health. When focusing on the **community as client**, direct clinical care can be a part of population-focused community health practice (Fawcett & Ellenbecker, 2015). For example, sometimes direct nursing care is provided to individuals and family members because their health needs are common community-related problems. Changes in individual health will ultimately affect the health of the community.

Improved health of the community remains the overall goal of nursing intervention. This is often accomplished through individual treatment; for example, addressing intimate partner violence, child or elder abuse is intended primarily to impact the effects of abuse on society and ultimately on the population as a whole. Similarly, treating a client for tuberculosis reduces the risk to other community members, thereby reducing the risk of an epidemic in the community. Since 1965, large-scale campaigns to encourage smoking reduction or cessation among groups and individuals and laws that prohibit smoking in specific public spaces have resulted in significantly lower smoking rates in the adult population (42 percent in 1965 compared to 15.5 percent in 2016) (CDC, 2018b).

Focusing on the community client highlights the complexity of the change process. Change for the benefit of the community client must often occur at several levels, ranging from the individual to society as a whole. For example, health problems caused by lifestyle, such as lack of exercise, overeating, and speeding, cannot be solved simply by asking individuals to choose health-promoting habits. Society must also provide healthy choices. Most individuals find changing their habits independently extremely difficult; indeed, sometimes impossible. The support of family members, friends, community health care systems, and relevant social policies are necessary for success. Individuals who have lifestyle health problems are often blamed for their illness because of their choices (e.g., to smoke), often referred to as "blaming the victim." In his classic work, Ryan (1976) points out that the "victim" cannot always be blamed and expected to correct the problem without changes also being made in the helping professions and public policy. Fig. 17.1 illustrates the continuum of care from the individual to global health.

Commitment to the health of the community client requires a process of change at each appropriate level on the continuum. One nursing role emphasizes individual and direct personal care skills, another nursing role focuses on the family as the unit of service, and a third centers on the community. The most successful change processes often arise from collaborative practice models that involve the community and nurses in joint decision making (Joyce et al., 2015). Nurses must remember that collaboration means shared roles and a cooperative effort in which participants want to work together. Participants must see themselves as part of a group effort and share in the process, beginning with planning and including decision making. This means sharing not only the power but also the responsibility for the outcomes of the intervention. Viewing the community as client and thus as the target of service means a commitment to two key concepts: (1) community health and (2) partnership. These two concepts form not only the *goal* (community health), but also the *means* of population-centered practice (partnership).

Community As Client

Population-centered practice seeks healthful change for the whole community's benefit (Fawcett et al., 2015). Although the nurse may work with individuals, families or other groups, aggregates, or institutions, the resulting changes are intended to affect the whole community. For example, an occupational health nurse's target typically includes preventing illness and injury and maintaining or promoting the health of an entire company workforce. Because of this focus, the nurse might help an individual disabled worker become independent in activities of daily living. The nurse could also take action to make the whole community better able to support persons with disabilities.

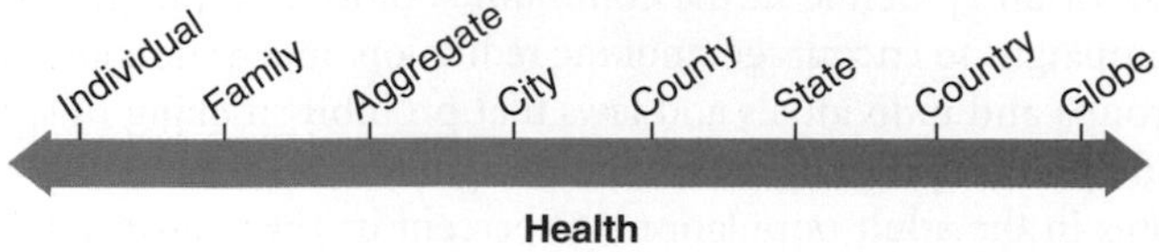

Fig. 17.1 Health on a population continuum.

These actions might include promoting vocational rehabilitation services in the community and advocating for local policies that improve equal opportunities for disabled workers.

Community health nurses join professionals from many other fields in fulfilling the core functions of assessment, assurance, and policy development for **ten essential public health services** (CDC, 2018c). The community assessment process described in this chapter is a key role of PHNs. The findings of the assessment process guide actions of *assurance,* or ensuring that all community members have access to high-quality health services. *Policy development* includes informing and mobilizing community members to advocate for business and government policies that improve health.

The community as client perspective guides decisions about allocation of resources and services to create the greatest benefit for the community. Sometimes this means spreading the benefit to as many people as possible in the community. For example, clean air and water are resources needed by everyone in a community. At other times, the community will experience the greatest benefit if resources are prioritized for groups within the community who are in high-risk categories. For example, supplies of vaccine for the 2009 H1N1 influenza pandemic were limited at first. Public health officials vaccinated population groups at highest risk for complications from the disease before making the vaccine available to the general population (Shim et al., 2011).

Two main ethical concepts that guide the community as client perspective are utilitarianism and justice. **Utilitarianism** means doing the greatest good for the greatest number of people. **Distributive justice** means treating people fairly, and distributing resources and burdens equitably among the members of a society. **Social justice** means ensuring that vulnerable groups are included in equitable distribution of resources. The outcome of social justice should be a reduction in health disparities between privileged and marginalized social groups. Nurses can use these concepts to carefully consider how to best allocate scarce resources, such as health services and funding, in ways that benefit the whole community. More information on ethics in community practice is found in other chapters of this book.

Community Health

Community health is reflected in the health behaviors and subsequent outcomes of its residents and also by the ability of the community as a system to support healthy individuals. The **socio-ecological model** views individuals as having dynamic interactions with social and environmental features of communities, for example, social networks, organizations such as schools and businesses, media, government policies, and natural and built environments (Schölmerich & Kawachi, 2016). Nurses caring for the community as the client identify effects that these complex community parts have on individuals' health; they work with all parts of a community to achieve the goal of a healthy community. Betty Neuman's Health Care Systems Model illustrates this system well (Beckman & Fawcett, 2017).

Neuman's model views systems as greater than the sum of their parts; the strength of each part of a community and the synergy between these parts contribute to the ability of its residents to be healthy. Community systems provide stability and protection from chronic or sudden stressors such as homelessness, health declines, disease outbreaks, or disasters. Another community model, Community-As-Partner, identifies major community systems as physical environment, health and social services, economy, transportation and safety, politics and government, communication, education, and recreation (Anderson & McFarlane, 2015).

The World Health Organization's (WHO) Healthy Cities program is an international leader in promoting health through community systems. It defines a healthy community as "one that is continually creating and improving those physical and social environments and expanding those community resources which enable people to mutually support each other in performing all the functions of life and developing to their maximum potential" (WHO, 2014). The WHO describes four aims of healthy communities as (1) supporting individual health, (2) promoting quality of life, (3) distributing the resources needed for basic sanitation and hygiene, and (4) creating accessible health care services.

Community Partnerships for Assessment

Partnering with community members is a key element of a successful community health program or intervention. Involving community members not only in the data collection process, but in all phases of the assessment, ensures that the data collected are more accurate and more relevant to the concerns of the community. Partnerships also promote community members' investment in the success of the assessment and in the resulting projects to improve community health. Therefore, successful strategies for improving community health must include community partnerships as the basic means or key for improvement. Some community assessment models feature community partnerships as a central activity, such as **Mobilizing for Action through Planning and Partnerships (MAPP)** (NACCHO, 2016).

Nurse-community partnerships can take many forms. A successful democratic partnership requires hard work from all parties and is usually achieved only through a long-term commitment to the process, wherein diverse community members and health care professionals share all resources and work equitably. **Coalitions** are formal partnerships in which individuals and organizations serve in defined capacities such as steering committees, advisory committees, and work groups. Coalitions are *active partnerships*, in which all participants share leadership and decision making to some degree. Unfortunately, some community health efforts view community residents only as sources of information and receivers of interventions; this limits residents to *passive participation*. **Passive participation** is the antithesis of the partnership approach most valued in nurse-community partnerships, in which all partners are actively involved in and share power in assessing, planning, and implementing needed community changes (Ocloo & Matthews, 2016).

Community members who are recognized as community leaders (whether professionals, pastors, government officials, or

BOX 17.1 Partnerships

The three main characteristics of a successful partnership are the following:

- *Being informed.* Community member and professional partners must be aware of their own and others' perceptions, rights, and responsibilities.
- *Flexibility and acceptance.* Community member and professional partners must recognize the unique contributions that each can make to a given situation. For example, professionals often contribute important knowledge and skills that laypersons lack. On the other hand, laypersons' definitions of community health problems are often more accurate than those of professionals.
- *Negotiation.* Because contributions vary and each situation is different, the distribution of power must be negotiated at every stage of the change process.

Data from Jackson EJ, Parks CP: Recruitment and training issues from selected lay health advisor programs among African Americans: a 20-year perspective [review], *Health Educ Behav* 24:418–431, 1997.

interested citizens) possess credibility and skills that health professionals often lack. The community member–professional partnership approach specifically emphasizes **active participation** of the community or its representatives in healthy change (Jagosh et al., 2015). For example, a partnership between rural community members and academic researchers ensured the development of an effective ongoing program to increase rates of colorectal cancer screening (Preston et al., 2018) (Box 17.1).

Partnership, as defined here, is an essential concept for nurses to know and use, as are the concepts of community, community as client, and community health. Experienced nurses know that partnership is important because health is not a static reality but is continuously generated through new and increasingly effective means of community member–professional collaboration. Other active professional service providers such as school teachers, public safety officers, and agricultural extension agents play a large part in the overall health of the community. Partnership in identifying strengths and problems and in setting goals is especially important because it brings commitment from all persons involved, an essential component of successful change.

Partnerships involving nurses working with community organizations offer one of the most effective means for interventions because they actively involve the community and build on existing community strengths. Nurses working with community groups and organizations can fulfill many different roles, including media advocacy, political action, community-based health communication, social marketing, and outreach facilitation. Regardless of what roles nurses fulfill as their contribution to the partnership, they must remember to "start where the people are" (Severance & Zinnah, 2009).

Kaiser and colleagues (2017) looked at the challenges and possible solutions in developing partnerships with communities. Community partnerships involve both influence and power. Nurses must focus on where and how health professionals and the community can work together, respecting voices of all community members. This approach requires nurses to do *with* rather than *to* the partner, while the partner's role throughout the process is active and empowered, not passive. Mutually determined goals and plans of action, and the assignment of roles and responsibilities, are negotiated. Through this model, community partners become more effective at working independently to solve their own problems and make their own decisions.

Prioritizing the problems through the lens of the participants may not match the identified priorities defined by other sources of data. In the language of community empowerment advocates, community participants must have an active role in the change process. The PHNs must work hard to include members of a setting, neighborhood, or organization while developing trust and providing the community with a central role throughout the process.

One historical example of a nurse-community partnership remains an inspiring story of this important work. Nancy Milio was a young, white PHN when she began working with an inner-city African American community in Detroit during the 1960s. Together, she and community members identified needs and designed a program to meet them. Milio's painstaking process of working *with* the community to create a Mom's and Tot's Center where mothers and children could access primary health care and childcare is a sentinel example of community partnership. The true value of this partnership was demonstrated when the Detroit riots occurred in 1967, and the storefront where the clinic was located remained intact while surrounding structures burned; the local rioters had spared the clinic because it "belonged to the people" (DeGuzman & Keeling, 2011; Milio, 2000). Thus, working within the community to develop priorities and to create programs promotes long-standing ownership and at the same time assures the probability for sustainability.

The Nurse's Role in the Community

The nurse's ability to establish credibility and trust in the community is important in doing a thorough community assessment. The nurse may be considered to be an *insider* if he or she grew up in the community, has personal ties to the people there, or comes from a similar cultural or ethnic background. This insider status may increase community members' willingness to speak openly and partner with the nurse. However, sometimes this insider status can be a disadvantage if it compromises the nurse's impartiality or objectivity. Nurses who are new to the community or have few insider connections can increase their familiarity with the community and its residents through taking part in informal community activities, such as shopping, attending church, or participating in organizations. They can also partner with trusted insiders in the community, such as *gatekeepers* and *community health workers.*

Gatekeepers are formal or informal community leaders who create opportunities for nurses to meet diverse members of the community (Kaiser et al., 2017). Gatekeepers can confer credibility to the nurse. For example, a church pastor may act as a gatekeeper by introducing a nurse to the congregation, thus increasing the likelihood that the church members will trust the nurse enough to provide information or to serve as partners in the assessment and throughout any program planning, intervention, and evaluation.

Community health workers (CHWs) are not professional or licensed health care providers but are community members from diverse backgrounds who receive training to do health outreach work. CHWs can assist nurses in doing community health assessments in several ways. They extend the reach of the nurse by being able to do many activities that are part of the community assessment process. They can also serve as gatekeepers, using their own insider status to engage community members in the assessment process (Olaniran et al., 2017).

CHECK YOUR PRACTICE

As a senior nursing student you have been asked by the local health department to conduct a community assessment of the central district of the city. What would you do? How would you approach this assignment?

COMMUNITY ASSESSMENT

Community assessment put quite simply is taking detailed stock of a community both from the outside in and from the inside out for the purpose of identifying and analyzing conditions therein. Community assessment, sometimes called community needs assessment, is one of three core functions of public health. This process requires clinical judgment and critical appraisal of multiple types of data from a variety of sources, and it requires a clear knowledge and understanding of the community as client. People, place, and function are the foundational dimensions of a community and need to be defined as part of the assessment process. These dimensions guide the gathering of data. Data can be primary or secondary. **Primary data** are collected directly through interaction with community members, which may include community leaders or interested stakeholders. **Secondary data** are obtained through existing reports on the community, including census, vital statistics, and numerical reports (e.g., morbidity and mortality information) or information from reference books.

There might be many reasons for conducting a community assessment, but for public health nursing the purpose is usually to identify community health needs and to develop strategies to address them. The purpose of this section is to provide a clear method for completing a comprehensive community assessment, using the tools of the nursing process adapted to communities. The Centers for Disease Control and Prevention (CDC, 2015a) offers a clear set of common elements that constitute a community assessment (Box 17.2). An example of Santa Cruz's very comprehensive and ongoing community assessment (2017) can be accessed at https://www.appliedsurveyresearch.org.

Why Community Assessment?

Community assessments may be done for various reasons. For example, a PHN in a community may want to conduct an assessment to learn more about community needs or strengths, or may want to locate confirmation data to address a recognized community problem. Assessments may also focus on setting priorities to address health issues in communities. Organizations may also be required to complete community assessments

BOX 17.2 Common Elements of Assessment and Planning Frameworks

Organize and plan
Engage the community
Develop a goal or vision
Conduct community health assessment(s)
Prioritize health issues
Develop community health improvement plan [in this case Nursing Diagnosis]
Implement and monitor community health improvement plan
Evaluate process and outcomes

From Centers for Disease Control and Prevention: *Assessment and planning models, frameworks and tools*, 2015b, www.cdc.gov.

for regulatory or accreditation standards. For example, the Affordable Care Act (ACA) directed nonprofit hospitals to perform community health needs assessments. In some cases administrators will perform these assessments, but PHNs are ideal choices to lead the community in this required activity. Public health personnel are the recognized experts in this arena. The recent formation of the Public Health Department Accreditation Board placed responsibility to implement standards for uniform performance with health departments in the United States. These standards include enhanced surveillance of community health services through regularly conducted community assessments (Swider et al., 2017).

Assessment is one of the three core functions of public health (CDC, 2011). Public health nursing places assessment at the forefront of PHN competencies. The Quad Council of Public Health Nursing Organizations is a coalition that includes the Association of Community Health Nursing Educators (ACHNE), the Association of Public Health Nurses (APHN), the American Public Health Association—Public Health Nursing (APHA-PHN) section, and the American Nurses Association's (ANA) Congress on Nursing Practice and Economics (ANA). The **Community/Public Health Nursing Competencies** include eight major domains: analytic and assessment skills, policy development/program planning skills, communication skills, cultural competency skills, community dimensions of practice skills, public health sciences skills, financial management and planning skills, and leadership and systems thinking skills. The domain of analytic and assessment skills (Table 17.1) details the competencies specific to community assessment across all tiers of public health nursing practice.

Assessing the health of the community requires a broad definition of health, including consideration of the economic,

TABLE 17.1 Community/Public Health Nursing Competencies, Domain 1: Analytic and Assessment Skills

Tier 1	Tier 2	Tier 3
A1. Assess the health status and health literacy of individuals and families, including determinants of health, using multiple sources of data.	B1. Assess the health status and health literacy of populations and their related determinants of health across the lifespan and wellness continuum.	C1. Apply appropriate comprehensive, in-depth system/organizational assessments and analyses as it relates to *population health*.
A2a. Use an *ecological perspective* and epidemiological data to identify health risks for a population. A2b. Identify individual and family assets, needs, values, beliefs, resources and relevant environmental factors.	B2. Develop *public health nursing diagnoses* and program implementation plans utilizing an *ecological perspective* and epidemiological data for individuals, families, communities, and populations.	C2a. Apply organizational and other theories to guide the development of system-wide approaches to reduce population-level health risks. C2b. Design systems that identify population assets and resources and relevant social, economic, and environmental factors.
A3. Select variables that measure health and public health conditions.	B3. Use a comprehensive set of relevant variables within and across systems to measure health and public health conditions.	C3. Adapt a comprehensive set of relevant variables within and across systems to measure health and public health conditions.
A4. Use a data collection plan that incorporates valid and reliable methods and instruments for collection of qualitative and quantitative data to inform the service for individuals, families, and a community.	B4. Use steps of program planning incorporating socio-behavioral and epidemiological models and principles to collect quality quantitative and qualitative data.	C4a. Design systems that support the collection of valid and reliable quantitative and qualitative data on individuals, families, and populations. C4b. Design systems to improve and assure the optimal validity, reliability, and comparability of data.
A5. Interpret valid and reliable data that impacts the health of individuals, families, and communities to make comparisons that are understandable to all who were involved in the assessment process.	B5. Use multiple methods and sources of data for concise and comprehensive community/population assessment that can be documented and interpreted in terms that are understandable to all who were involved in the process, including communities.	C5a. Design systems to assure that assessments are documented and interpreted in terms that are understandable to all partners/stakeholders. C5b. Design data collection system that uses multiple methods and sources when collecting and analyzing data to ensure a comprehensive assessment process.
A6. Compare appropriate data sources in a community.	B6a. Address gaps and redundancies in data sources used in a comprehensive community/population assessment. B6b. Examine the effect of gaps in data on Public Health practice and program planning.	C6a. Recognize gaps and redundancies in sources of data used in a comprehensive system/organizational assessment. C6b. Strategize plan with appropriate team members to address data gaps.

Continued

TABLE 17.1 Community/Public Health Nursing Competencies, Domain 1: Analytic and Assessment Skills—cont'd

Tier 1	Tier 2	Tier 3
A7. Contribute to comprehensive community health assessments through the application of quantitative and qualitative public health nursing data.	B7a. Synthesize qualitative and quantitative data during data analysis for a comprehensive community/population assessment. B7b. Use various data collection methods and qualitative and quantitative data sources to conduct a comprehensive community/population assessment.	C7a. Evaluate qualitative and quantitative data during data analysis for a comprehensive system/ organizational assessment. C7b. Use multiple methods and qualitative and quantitative data sources for a comprehensive system/ organizational assessment.
A8. Apply ethical, legal, and policy guidelines and principles in the collection, maintenance, use, and dissemination of data and information.	B8. Maximize the application of ethical, legal, and policy guidelines and principles in the collection, maintenance, use, and dissemination of data and information.	C8a. Evaluate information disseminated to ensure it is understandable by the community and stakeholders. C8b. Create systems that incorporate ethical, legal, and policy guidelines and principles into the collection, maintenance, use, and dissemination of data and information.
A9. Use varied approaches in the identification of community needs (i.e., focus groups, multisector collaboration, SWOT analysis).	B9. Assess the quality of various data collection methods used to conduct a comprehensive community/population assessment.	C9. Evaluate the quality of various data collection methods used to conduct a comprehensive community/population or system/organizational assessment.
A10. Use *information technology* effectively to collect, analyze, store, and retrieve data related to public health nursing services for individuals, families, and groups.	B10. Identify *information technology* to effectively collect, analyze, store, and retrieve data related to planning and evaluating public health nursing services for communities and populations.	C10a. Maximize *information technology* resources and collaboration with others in the design of data collection processes. C10b. Facilitate the collection, use, storage, and retrieval of data.
A11. Use evidence-based strategies or promising practices from across disciplines to promote health in communities and populations.	B11a. Integrate current evidence- based strategies or promising practices that address scientific, political, ethical and social issues to promote improvement in health care systems and populations. B11b. Use evidence-based strategies or promising practices that address scientific, political, ethical, and social public health issues to create and modify systems of care.	C11a. Evaluate evidence- based data, programs, and strategies or promising practices to create and modify systems of care and to support strategies that address scientific, political, ethical, and social public health issues. C11b. Promote research and evidence-based environments.
A12. Use available data and resources related to the determinants of health when planning services for individuals, families, and groups.	B12. Use data related to the determinants of health and community resources to plan for, analyze, and evaluate community- oriented and population-level programs.	C12a. Evaluate organization/system capacity to analyze the health status of the community/ population effectively. C12b. Determine the allocation of organization/system resources to support the effective analysis of the health status of the community/population.

SWOT, Strengths, weaknesses, opportunities, threats.
From Quad Council Coalition Competency Review Task Force: *Community/public health nursing competencies,* 2018. Available at http://www.quadcouncilphn.org.

social, physical, and mental health of the population. Access to resources that provide for these broad needs and services will be part of the assessment process.

The PHN should place the assessment of community strengths as high on the list as recognized problems in the development of an assessment plan. It is important to value both strengths and problems in the assessment, planning, implementation, and evaluation process.

> *Communities are better served by assets-oriented methods than by standard "problem-focused" or "needs-based" approaches. An assets orientation allows community members to identify, support and mobilize existing community resources to create a shared vision of change, and encourages greater creativity when community members do address problems and obstacles* (Oklahoma Cooperative Extension Service, 2018).

Communities have both resources and needs. We recommend a balanced approach to the assessment, highlighting community assets as well as problems to identify the community vehicles already present for positive change. Community strengths can later be called upon in the planning and intervention phases of the process to address the challenges the community faces. This strength-based approach may be better received by communities and funders and promotes the inclusion of key informants and interested stakeholders; it can make strategic planning a part of the process.

Data Sources

Health Status Indicators. Measures of health status take more than one form. Numerical data put out by a recognized agency (such as the U.S. Census Bureau or CDC, or Robert Woods Johnson Foundation) are referred to as *secondary* data (collected by someone else). Information that is gleaned from telephone surveys, personal interviews, or focus groups conducted by those who are assessing the community—any data derived from personal connections or key informants—are considered *primary* data (collected by the assessor[s]). Community Assessment requires both types of data for the community assessment, and both types of data will be included when analyzing the assessment data.

Secondary Sources of Data. Even before setting foot in the community it is possible to learn a great deal about its residents' health status. Health indicators are numerical measures of health outcomes, such as morbidity and mortality, as well as determinants of health and population characteristics. Generally, these data are from *secondary* sources such as websites or printed materials. Table 17.2 lists several of these sources.

Creation of a set of health indicator data during a community health assessment serves several purposes. First, it creates a "snapshot" of health conditions that can guide the assessment team during the analysis and problem prioritization phases. Second, it is an important and easily comprehensible means of communicating the results of the assessment to the larger community. Third, it is an effective way to compare the current health status in the community with the same community at different time points, with other communities, or with larger populations such as state or national data. Table 17.3 lists health indicators that are frequently included in community health assessments.

There are two important considerations for selecting which indicators to include in an assessment: the priorities of the community and comparability to other data. Ideally, diverse community stakeholders should participate in identifying health indicators that address their interests or concerns. Stakeholders include anyone with a personal or occupational interest or concern in a community's life. If the health indicators will be compared with other assessments, then use similar measures when possible. For example, the total number of deaths in a community is different from the annual rate of deaths per 100,000 population. The box below gives additional tips on obtaining high-quality data.

Secondary Source Data

Questions to ask about data from secondary sources:

- How current is the reported information?
- When was the site last updated?
- How credible is the data source?
- Is an author identified?
- Are demographic data reported about the people?
- Are data reported about different community systems?
- Is there any obvious bias in the reporting of data?
- Are community voices represented?

Healthy People 2020 and County Health Rankings are useful resources for health indicators. *Healthy People 2020* identifies national health priorities, providing baseline data as well as health indicator goals. For example, the U.S. baseline rate of injury-related mortality was 59.7 deaths per 100,000 population in 2007, and the *Healthy People 2020* goal rate is 53.7 deaths per 100,000 population (www.healthypeople.gov). The County Health Rankings report is updated annually and provides county-level data for a wide variety of health indicators and also compares county rankings within and across states (www.countyhealthrankings.org).

Primary Sources of Data. Primary data involve the researcher or community members at the community level. Various methods can be used to collect the data, such as participant observation, key informant interviews, surveys, town hall meetings, focus groups, Photovoice, spatial data, or windshield

TABLE 17.2 Frequently Used Secondary Sources for Health Indicator Data

Behavioral Risk Factors Surveillance Survey (BRFSS)	http://www.cdc.gov	Wide variety of data on individuals' health status, health behaviors, and preventive health services
CDC Social Determinants of Health	https://www.cdc.gov	CDC-supported data on income, education level, employment, social vulnerability, and health conditions
CDC Wonder	http://wonder.cdc.gov/	Public health data on births, mortality, infectious diseases, cancer, and environment
County Health Rankings	http://www.countyhealthrankings.org	Collates county-level data on a wide range of health outcomes and health determinants
Dartmouth Atlas of Health Care	http://www.dartmouthatlas.org	Distribution and outcomes of health care services, in chart and map formats
Local advocacy organizations		Organizations that specialize in social issues such as homelessness, child abuse, or domestic violence
National Center for Health Statistics: FastStats	https://www.cdc.gov	U.S. government website that gathers data from multiple sources and provides an extensive topic index
State Cancer Profile	http://statecancerprofiles.cancer.gov	Incidence of cancer types by race/ethnicity, sex, and geography
State Health Access Data Assistance Center (SHADAC)	http://statehealthcompare.shadac.org	Provides access to data about health statistics by demographic breakdown. Statistics can be compared state to state.
U.S. Census	http://www.census.gov	Demographic and economic data

CDC, Centers for Disease Control and Prevention.

TABLE 17.3 Health Status Indicators: Frequently Recommended Health Metrics

HEALTH OUTCOME METRICS		HEALTH DETERMINANT AND CORRELATE METRICS			
Mortality	**Morbidity**	**Health Care (Access & Quality)**	**Health Behaviors**	**Demographics & Social Environment**	**Physical Environment**
Suggested Data Sources					
• CDC Wonder • National Center for Health Statistics (NCHS)	• BRFSS • County Health Rankings • State Cancer Profiles • BRFSS • CDC Wonder	• County Health Rankings • NCHS • U.S. Census • Dartmouth Atlas • State Health Access Data Assistance Center (SHADAC)	• BRFSS • County Health Rankings • NCHS • SHADAC	• U.S. Census • County Health Rankings • CDC Social Determinants of Health • NCHS • SHADAC	• County Health Rankings • U.S. Census • CDC Wonder
Mortality: Leading Causes of Death	Obesity	Health Insurance Coverage	Tobacco Use/Smoking	Age	Air Quality
Infant Mortality	Low Birth Weight	Provider Rates (PCPs, Dentists)	Physical Activity	Sex	Water Quality
Injury-related Mortality	Hospital Utilization	Asthma-Related Hospitalization	Nutrition	Race/Ethnicity	Housing
Motor Vehicle Mortality	Cancer Rates		Unsafe Sex	Income	
Suicide	Motor Vehicle Injury		Alcohol Use	Poverty Level	
Homicide	Overall Health Status		Seatbelt Use	Educational Attainment	
	STDs (chlamydia, gonorrhea, syphilis)		Immunizations and Screenings	Employment Status	
				Foreign-Born	
	AIDS			Homelessness	
	Tuberculosis			Language Spoken at Home	
				Marital Status	
				Domestic Violence and Child Abuse	
				Violence and Crime	
				Social Capital/Social Support	

AIDS, Acquired immunodeficiency syndrome; *BRFSS,* Behavioral Risk Factors Surveillance Survey; *CDC,* Centers for Disease Control and Prevention; *PCP,* primary care physician; *STD,* sexually transmitted disease.
Modified from Centers for Disease Control and Prevention: *Community health assessment for population health improvement: resource of most frequently recommended health outcomes and determinants,* 2013. Retrieved Sept. 3, 2018, from http://c.ymcdn.com/sites/www.cste.org.

surveys. The researcher or the community members experience the events or interact directly with the community as a group, with individuals, or by observation.

Participant observation refers to the deliberate sharing in the life of a community, for example, participating in a local fair or festival or attending a political or social event. Just as you would assess a hospital patient's room upon entering and note details about the environment (family members, emotional tone, patient's level of consciousness, intravenous access or vital signs, cleanliness, organization), visiting or attending an event can be a window through which to view the community. In addition, participant observation can be a fun way to experience community events.

Key informants can be identified through formal or informal channels in the community. They might be leaders in a sector of the community such as a church congregation, civic club, governmental body, or neighborhood. They need not hold any formal title, but are generally viewed as community leaders by other community members and often have a long history in the community. Meeting with key informants and identifying local issues, strengths, and concerns from their viewpoint constitutes an important component of the overall assessment. See How To box for more information.

HOW TO Identify a Key Informant

- Talking to key informants is a critical part of the community assessment.
- Key informants are not always people who have a formal title or position.
- Key informants often have an informal role within the community.
- County health department nurses and church leaders are often key informants. They also know many community members and can identify other key informants.

Town hall meetings are opportunities for local constituents to come together, usually to discuss a particular issue or proposal that influences all members of the community. Many town hall meetings have been held recently, for example, to address the issue of health care reform. The following photo represents one town hall meeting held for that purpose in Hartford, Connecticut, in 2009. Political rallies and delegate forums are often held in this format.

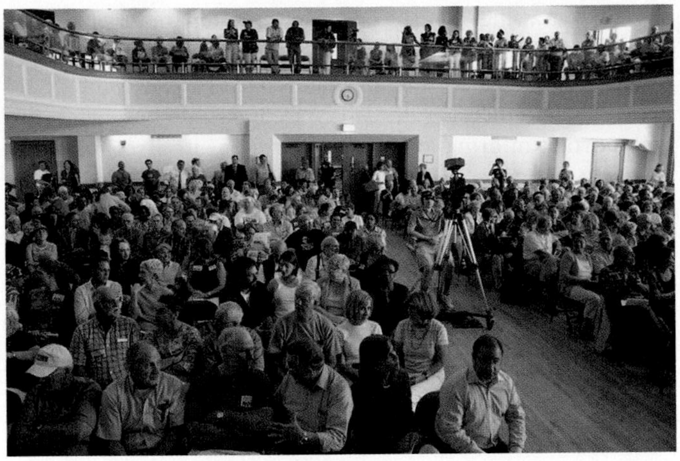

A focus group is similar to an interview, in that it collects data mainly through asking open-ended questions to participants but to a small group rather than an individual. Focus groups are useful for situations where the interaction between participants is likely to prompt discussions or generate ideas that individual interviews might not. Focus groups work well when the topic is not a sensitive one and participants feel comfortable speaking out about the issue with the group.

Focus groups should be structured to balance a diversity of perspectives with opportunities for in-depth understanding of the chosen topics. The design of the question guide should address the goals for the data: for example, do you want to generate a free-flowing discussion of ideas or obtain specific information from each participant? Participants should be recruited through community channels such as churches, associations, and other places where people gather. An ideal number of participants is between six and eight, though smaller or larger groups can work in different circumstances (Guest et al., 2017).

Each focus group should be organized so that its participants are fairly homogenous in key characteristics. For example, in a study on brain health in older adults living with HIV, focus groups were divided by gender and race (Vance et al., 2017). A typical format for a focus group is that one moderator leads the discussion, while an assistant takes written notes, and the session is often audio recorded. The recording is then transcribed and included in the analysis.

Photovoice. Photovoice, also called photo elicitation, is a community assessment technique in which community members take photos to represent a topic or theme about community health. For example, women living with human immunodeficiency virus (HIV) took photos to describe their experiences and challenges of living with the disease (Lennon-Dearing & Price, 2018). Photovoice has been used with many types of community participants, but can be especially useful in working with groups that may be marginalized or have little power such as youths, the elderly, individuals living in poverty, or those involved in substance abuse. Photovoice is a way for participants to communicate powerful messages about their experiences, without the need for words.

Photography is a relatively easy group activity because devices to take photos are relatively common and inexpensive. Disposable cameras and the participants' cell phones are examples of devices with minimal added cost. Video, sound recording, and other forms of media can also be used in ways similar to Photovoice. For example, a group of New Orleans residents used Videovoice to create their own documentary to advocate for housing, education, and economic development after Hurricane Katrina (Catalani et al., 2013).

The basic process to incorporate Photovoice into a community assessment is as follows:

1. **Train participants:** Participants receive training in Photovoice methods, including the topic of interest, basic photography techniques, and ethical and safety issues. Participants may need to learn how to obtain written consent before photographing people, businesses, or other identifiable subjects. Training is especially important when the topic of interest is sensitive or illegal, such as substance abuse.
2. **Take photos:** Participants take the cameras into their communities and take photographs that reflect the topic. Equipment should be modified to fit the participants. For example, adolescents may be very comfortable with a variety of mobile devices, whereas older adults may prefer simpler cameras with modifications for low vision or manual dexterity (Novek et al., 2012).
3. **Display photos:** The photos are collected from the participants, and then printed or digitally projected for group participants, and sometimes members of the public, to view them.
4. **Discuss photos:** Viewing the photos is meant to spark discussions that provide additional information about the topic of interest. These discussions may take place as focus groups with the Photovoice participants. If the photos are displayed in public, the aim may be to raise awareness and to start conversations among diverse stakeholders.
5. **Analyze and report results:** The information gathered through these discussions, as well as the photos themselves, can be included in the data analysis phase. The photos can also be part of the report to the community about the findings of the community assessment (Florian et al., 2016). Photovoice can be useful at different stages of a community assessment, but may be especially useful in the early stages of data collection. The "insider" knowledge gained through this type of activity can guide subsequent community assessment activities. For example, if the Photovoice topic is "barriers to healthy lifestyles" and the majority of photos focus on places that make pedestrian or bike travel difficult, then the later stages of the assessment should give additional attention to walkability and transportation.

Spatial Data.

Everything is related to everything else, but near things are more related than distant things.

Tobler's First Law of Geography (Sui, 2004)

Most of the information gathered in a community assessment has a spatial component: it is located somewhere in the community. The location of places like health care services, food stores, schools, bus routes, factories, highways, bodies of water, and parks can affect residents' access to health benefits or exposure to health threats. Demographic data can also be spatial. We can look at a neighborhood or other area and learn about its residents, such as age, racial or ethnic background, health characteristics, income, home value, and crime rates. Having this information can be very helpful for assessing health resources and risks for specific neighborhoods. By assessing the spatial distribution of health resources and disparities, we can place programs in neighborhoods where the impact will be greatest.

Maps have several uses in community assessments. Maps are a place to compile **spatial data** from primary or secondary sources. During the problem analysis and prioritization phases, these maps can support decision making about community health priorities. Later, maps can be used to plan programs and interventions. Like the idea that "a picture is worth a thousand words," a map can also be an effective means of communicating the findings of a community health assessment to a wide range of stakeholders, and encouraging their participation in discussions about the findings.

Map making is very flexible, depending on the resources that are available. A map can be as simple as a hand-drawn sketch of features in a community or neighborhood. Drawings or graphics can be added to commercially produced paper or online maps. A **geographic information system (GIS)** is a set of software and technology that can create maps electronically. The amount of training to use GIS software varies. Some free websites allow users to build GIS maps without any prior training. For example, www.communitycommons.org has demographic, health, and economic data that can be used to build a map of a specific place. More powerful software, such as ESRI ArcGIS, can analyze spatial data and display it using a variety of visual options. This type of software is sometimes expensive and time-consuming to learn, but is very useful for those who want to use maps regularly in their work.

During a community assessment spatial data can be collected in several ways. One low-tech approach is to note the address or nearest street intersection of a place and later draw it onto a map. A higher-tech approach can involve a smart phone or other mobile device that has *global positioning system (GPS)* capabilities. While walking around a community, these devices can be used to note locations by recording the latitude and longitude coordinates. Some smart phones and other devices can take photographs that store the GPS location. These photos can later be incorporated into GIS maps as images or hotlinks.

GIS can pull together multiple types of assessment data that, when viewed on a map, can identify areas of a community with a particular set of characteristics. For example, a public health study analyzed geographic data for demographic patterns of poor birth outcomes in an urban area (MacQuillan et al., 2017). They found that children living near a major roadway were much more likely to experience hospital admissions for asthma.

Using Primary Data. Informant interviews, focus groups, and participant observation are good ways to generate information about a community's unique beliefs, norms, values, power and influence structures, and problem-solving processes. These primary data can be time-consuming and challenging to collate and interpret. However, it is worthwhile to make the effort to systematically collect primary data in the community and to avoid drawing conclusions from limited observations or unconfirmed intuitions.

Contradictions within the data collected are common. If there are disconnects or the two types of data do not match, this is important information to consider for your assessment and program planning. Reports from different members of a community may not agree. Information from primary data should be compared to secondary data which can provide context about a community's assets and needs. What is important is that the voice of the informant or group is heard and that the assessor in the community takes all information into account at the time of data analysis. In addition, the priorities of the community members must be included in any planning or implementation of interventions.

Community Health Assessment Models

There are many existing models of community health assessment, making it possible to conduct an assessment without the need to design the process from scratch. Table 17.4 provides examples of commonly used models that assess for a broad array of community health concerns. The WHO's Healthy Cities initiative offers another approach to population-centered health assessment. An example of the assessment data that support this approach is found at http://www.healthycity.org. For additional information on Healthy Communities see Chapter 16.

Other assessment models focus on specific topics. For example, the CDC (2018a) developed the Community Assessment for Public Health Emergency Response (CASPER) toolkit for rapid needs assessment of communities affected by disasters or other emergencies. Another example is the Built Environment Assessment Tool Manual, a toolkit to assess the human-built features of a community that affect physical activity, nutrition, and other aspects of health (physical and social aspects of a community related to walking and bicycling) (CDC, 2017).

Selecting an assessment model or designing your own can be guided by several criteria. What are your goals for the assessment? What are the resources available for the assessment project, such as time, people, budget, and access to the community? Is there an existing model that aligns with your goals, and is feasible in terms of your available resources? (See Chapter 23 for how to develop a program. This can be applied to the assessment of the community).

COMMUNITY AS PARTNER

The **community-as-partner** model is based on nursing processes and theories and emphasizes the dynamic nature of community systems as integral to the health of residents (Anderson & McFarlane, 2015). A key feature of this model is its division of the community structure into subsystems that can serve as an organizational structure for community health assessments. The subsystems of the community structure consist of physical environment, health and social services, economy, transportation and safety, politics and government, communication, education, and recreation. Each of these subsystems represents distinct functions and organizations within the community that can be assessed separately. However, they also interact to create the complex community environment in which people

TABLE 17.4 Interprofessional Community Health Assessment Models

Assessment Model	Example
Health Impact Assessment (HIA) is a process to predict the effects on health from projects or policies such as land use, community design, transportation, or industrial facilities. The outcome of an HIA is to provide recommendations to minimize negative health impacts, and monitor results. *Learn more at https://www.naccho.org.*	Community officials in East Aldine District, a suburb of Houston, Texas, worked with health researchers to perform a HIA on a proposed town center development for this previously rural area. The HIA found positive health impacts such as better access to healthy food retailers and health care facilities, and enhanced opportunities for physical activity and active transport. These were predicted to improve health of economically vulnerable residents, such as those without cars and the elderly (Cummings et al., 2016).
Mobilizing for Action through Planning and Partnerships (MAPP) is a strategic planning process to select high-priority public health issues and to match them with resources. Public health agencies lead the MAPP, but participation of community members and agencies is a major focus. *Learn more at https://www.naccho.org.*	A public health department in Virginia assessed the five counties and independent city in its district to identify top health issues needing action. Through partnerships with 61 agencies and gathering data from more than 2000 residents, the MAPP process selected top priorities as obesity, mental health and substance abuse, pregnancy outcomes, and tobacco use (Thomas Jefferson Health District, 2016).
Community Health Assessment and Group Evaluation (CHANGE) is a tool to help communities annually gather and organize data about community health, plan programs, and monitor changes over time. Five community sectors are assessed: community at large, community institution/organization, health care, school, and work site. *Learn more at https://www.cdc.gov* (CDC, 2018a).	Researchers in a rural Missouri county used the CHANGE tool to assess why rates of chronic disease were high. Through interviews with representatives from each of the five sectors, they identified challenges, assets, and potential partnerships for addressing chronic disease (Stewart et al., 2013).
Community Health Needs Assessment (CHNA) is a set of guidelines for nonprofit hospitals to assess the communities they serve and is a requirement under the Patient Protection and Affordable Care Act (ACA). Community input and other sources provide data on priority health problems, barriers to health care access, and vulnerable populations. *Learn more at http://www.cdc.gov* (Rosenbaum, 2013).	Nursing students partnered with a hospital in rural Minnesota to complete the CHNA. They gathered data through surveys and interviews with residents and organizational leaders. They identified three priority health problems, and differentiated assets and barriers to addressing these problems in different community institutions serving vulnerable populations (Madelía Community Hospital & Clinic, 2013).

live and function. Each subsystem may protect the health of community members by addressing a particular need. Understanding the relative success of each of these subsystems in promoting health and safety can provide important insights about the community's ability to respond to health problems

HOW TO CONDUCT A COMMUNITY ASSESSMENT

Getting Started

In the previous section several models of community assessment are outlined. This section will offer a step-by-step method to complete a community assessment. In beginning the assessment, the nurse should identify one model that will guide the assessment. The steps for the assessment are in Fig. 17.2, but this process can be adapted to any model used.

The community assessor(s) should plan to visit and interact in the community and collect data about *people, place,* and *function* over a month or more to get a feel for the community and create as full a picture as possible. A "feet on the ground" approach will yield rich data, and visiting the community and interacting with its members is essential to the process. Very comprehensive assessments will require community coalitions and inclusion of key stakeholders, such as those included in MAPP assessments; expanding the participant group may extend this stage over many months or years (NACCHO: www.naccho.org). See Box 17.3 for information on personal safety while assessing communities.

Windshield Survey

Windshield surveys are a method of simple observation. They provide a quick overview of a community and can be used along with photographs and interviews to get a general overall sense of the community (Table 17.5). This can be the first step in the process of generating data that help to identify the community, trends, stability, and changes that all serve to define the health of the community (Stanhope & Knollmueller, 2000). The nurse riding in a vehicle can observe many dimensions of a community's life and environment through the windshield, but walking the streets can also provide similar information. Under those circumstances, one can readily observe common characteristics of people in the community, neighborhood gathering places, the rhythm of community life, housing quality, and geographic boundaries (see How To box and Table 17.5). A windshield survey can be used by itself for a short and simple assessment. However, it is used here as one part of the longer, more complex comprehensive community assessment.

HOW TO Obtain a Quick Assessment of a Community

- One way to get a quick, initial sense of the community is to do a windshield assessment using a format like the example provided in Table 17.5.
- Nurses interested in conducting a windshield assessment need to take public transportation, have someone else drive while they take notes, or plan to stop frequently to write down what they see.
- The windshield survey example is organized into 15 elements with specific questions related to each element.
- Nurses who use this approach will have an initial descriptive assessment of the community when they are finished.
- If interventions are planned, the more thorough and more comprehensive process described in this chapter will be necessary.

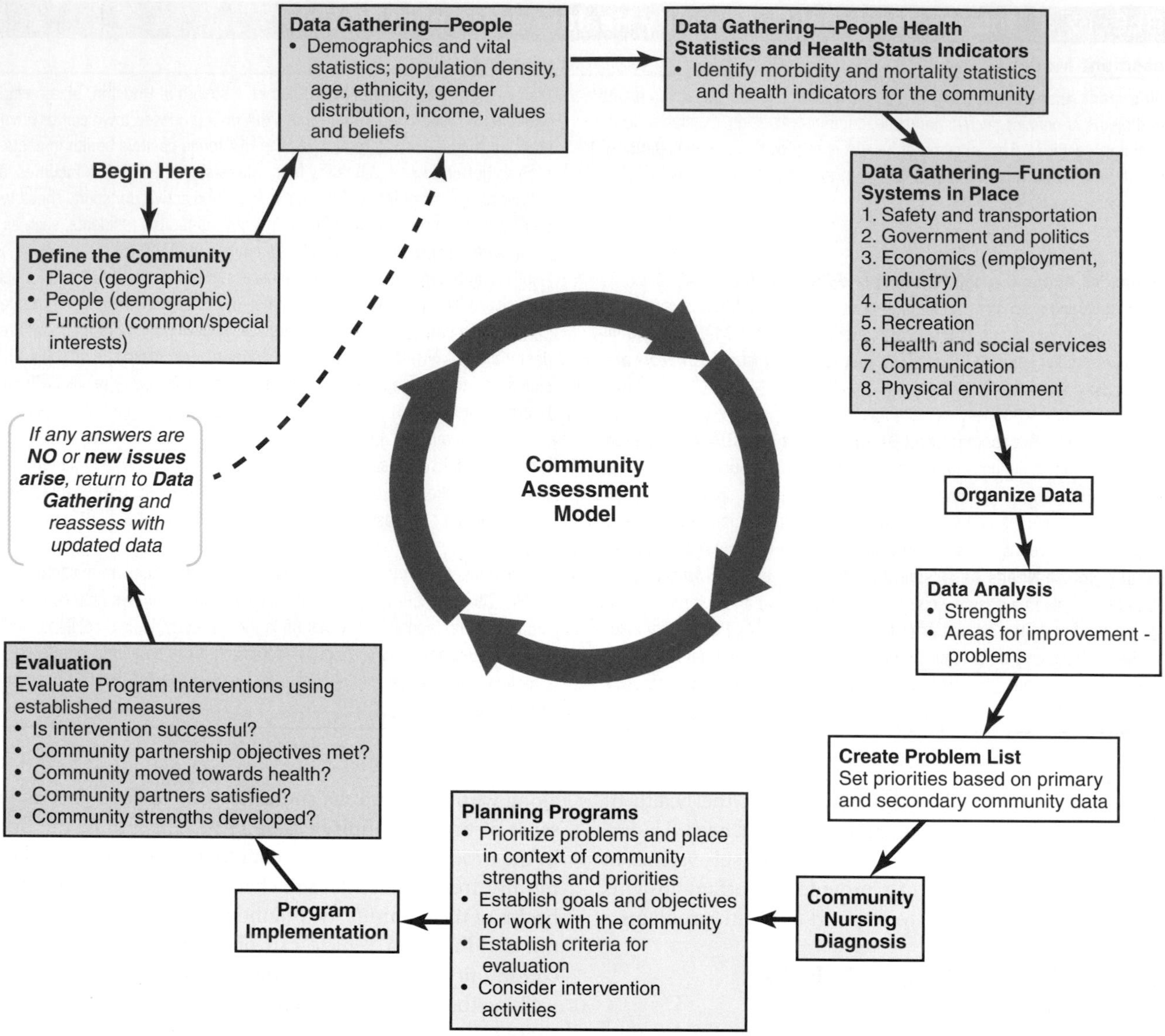
Data Gathering—People
• Demographics and vital statistics; population density, age, ethnicity, gender distribution, income, values and beliefs
Data Gathering—People Health Statistics and Health Status Indicators
• Identify morbidity and mortality statistics and health indicators for the community
Data Gathering—Function Systems in Place
1. Safety and transportation
2. Government and politics
3. Economics (employment, industry)
4. Education
5. Recreation
6. Health and social services
7. Communication
8. Physical environment
Begin Here
Define the Community
• Place (geographic)
• People (demographic)
• Function (common/special interests)
If any answers are NO or new issues arise, return to Data Gathering and reassess with updated data
Community Assessment Model
Organize Data
Data Analysis
• Strengths
• Areas for improvement - problems
Create Problem List
Set priorities based on primary and secondary community data
Community Nursing Diagnosis
Planning Programs
• Prioritize problems and place in context of community strengths and priorities
• Establish goals and objectives for work with the community
• Establish criteria for evaluation
• Consider intervention activities
Program Implementation
Evaluation
Evaluate Program Interventions using established measures
• Is intervention successful?
• Community partnership objectives met?
• Community moved towards health?
• Community partners satisfied?
• Community strengths developed?

Fig. 17.2 Community assessment model.

BOX 17.3 Personal Safety in Community Practice

Effective nursing practice starts with personal safety, and this remains important throughout the community assessment process. An awareness of the community and common sense are the two best guidelines for judgment. For example, common sense suggests not leaving anything valuable on a car seat and not leaving your car unlocked. Similar guidelines apply to the use of public transportation. Calling ahead to clients to schedule meetings will help prevent delays or confusion, and it gives the nurse an opportunity to lay the groundwork for the meeting. If there is no telephone and no access to a neighbor's telephone, plan to establish a time for any future meetings during the initial visit. Regardless of whether there has been telephone contact, there are rare situations when a meeting is postponed because the nurse arrives at a location where people are unexpectedly loitering by the entrance and the nurse has concerns about personal safety.

For nurses who either are just beginning their careers in the community or are just starting a new position, three clear sources of information will help answer many questions about personal safety:

- *Other nurses, social workers, or health care providers who are familiar with the dynamics of a given community:* They can provide valuable insights into when to visit, how to get there, and what to expect, because they function in the community themselves.
- *Community members:* The best sources of information about the community are the community members themselves, and one benefit of developing an active partnership with community members is their willingness to share their insight about day-to-day community life.
- *The nurse's own observations:* Knowledge gained during the data collection phase of the process should provide a solid basis for an awareness of day-to-day community activity. Nurses with experience practicing in the community generally agree that if they feel uncomfortable in a situation, they should trust their instincts and leave.

TABLE 17.5 Windshield Survey Guidelines (Adapted)

Each community has its own characteristics. These characteristics along with demographic data provide valuable information in understanding the population that lives within the community and the health status, strengths/limitations, risks and vulnerabilities unique to the "population of interest." Once you have defined a "community of interest" to assess, a ***windshield survey*** is the equivalent of a community head-to-toe assessment. The best way to conduct a windshield survey is with more than one person, allowing for one to observe and take notes. Having one pair of eyes on the road, you can benefit from having other individuals notice the unique characteristics of the community; a shared experience provides additional insight. As you analyze your findings, it may be necessary to make a second tour to fill in any blanks. Many of us take these characteristics for granted in our own community, but they provide a rich context for understanding communities and populations and often have significant impact on the health status of the community in general.

Elements	Description
Boundaries	What defines the boundary? Roads, water, railroads? Does the area have a name? A nickname?
Housing and zoning	What is the age of the houses? What kind of materials are used in the construction? Describe the housing including space between them, general appearance and condition, and presence of central heating, air conditioning, and modern plumbing.
Open space	Describe the amount, condition, use of open space. How is the space used? Is it safe? Attractive?
Commons	Where do people in the neighborhood hang out? Who hangs out there and at what hours during the day?
Transportation	How do people get from one place to another? If they use public transportation, what kind and how effective is it: How timely? Personal autos? Bikes, etc.? Are there pedestrians? Does the area appear to be safe?
Social service centers	Do you see evidence of recreation centers, parks, social services, offices of doctors, dentists, pharmacies?
Stores	Where do residents shop? How do they get to the shops? Do they have groceries or sources of fresh produce? Is this a "food desert"?
Street people and animals	Who do you see on the streets during the day? Besides the people, do you see animals? Are they loose or contained?
Condition of the area	Is the area well-kept or is there evidence of trash, abandoned cars or houses? What kind of information is provided on the signs in the area?
Race and ethnicity	What is the racial mix of the people you see? What do you see about indices of ethnicity? Places of worship, food stores, restaurants? Are signs in English or other languages? (If the latter, which ones)?
Religion	What indications do you see about the types of religion residents practice?
Health indicators	Do you see evidence of clinics, hospitals, mental illness, and/or substance abuse?
Politics	What indicators do you see about politics? Posters, headquarters?
Media	Do you see indicators of what people read? If they watch television? Listen to the radio? Can you tell if residents use social media? Availability of Internet?
Business & industry	What type of business climate exists? Manufacturers? Light or heavy industry? Large employers? Small business owners? Retail? Hospitality industry? Military installation? Do people have to seek employment elsewhere?

Adapted and revised in 2008 by M. Gibson & J. Lancaster from: Mizrahi TM: School of Social Work, Virginia Commonwealth University, Richmond, VA, September 1992; Stanhope MS, Knollmueller RN: *Public and community health nurse's consultant: a health promotion guide*, St. Louis, 1997, Mosby.

Community "Place" and "People" Identified

Using Fig. 17.2, the first step of the community assessment is to define the community. To do this, geographic boundaries, the population within the boundaries, the purpose of the assessment, and a data collection plan will be identified. Census blocks or tracts and geopolitical boundaries such as city or county lines will allow for collection of consistent data about the region under study. Included in "place" is the type of terrain or environment, the climate, the history of the area, and its size. The population is the next identifier. How does your assessment define those within the community? Are they members of a specific group or the population in general? What data are available for the assessment and where will you seek your sources? In essence, the community's members are the "client" within these boundaries.

What is the local history? Who were the original settlers and how has the community developed over time? Is it an area of growth or decline? Are original families still living in the area or has the early population been replaced? History can reveal a lot about customs and mores that could influence the health of the community.

Place. To define "place" identify:

- Boundaries
- Environment
- Size
- Climate
- History
- Population

People. Those inhabiting the community are a primary focus of the assessment. Various strategies can be used to identify this central core of the community. The first step often involves the use of secondary data. Using census data clarifies the population density and the demographics of the population under study. Suggested websites for the collection of these data are provided in Table 17.2. Some demographic measures include the population composition—racial and ethnic groups present, ages, socioeconomic status and poverty rates as related to geographical area; educational attainment; and the distribution of the population over census areas. Next, review this information in the context of previous census data (e.g., look back 20 years) to demonstrate how age groups are shifting. For example, if particular age groups are increasing in numbers, that can help to predict needs; if the area is shrinking or growing in population, that will predict different needs.

For quick information estimates on a specific area, consult American FactFinder (http://factfinder.census.gov). Perhaps one racial or ethnic group inhabits a particular area of the community. Census data will help identify this information. That may be important later in the PHN's assessment process for understanding morbidity and mortality data. Many states have websites that can help to predict population projections for localities. In Virginia, for example, one can visit www.virginialmi.com to see projections and historical census data for each county or independent city, helping to visualize trends.

As a next step, the PHN will identify formal and informal structures within the community. What formal and informal groups exist in the community? What structures are present that unite or separate people in the society? This will require interviews and delving into the community. For example, local government, schools, churches, and health care organizations may represent formal structures. Clubs (e.g., Rotary Club, garden clubs, country club, YWCA, neighborhood associations, or libraries) may reflect formal or informal groups, where an informal leader could be the advisor to that group on matters of all kinds, including housing, health, or legal matters. These informal leaders can be identified through interaction with the community members and by visiting community agencies. There are likely crossovers between formal and informal groups. Pay attention to advocacy groups and those that have goals of improving the community or some subset of the community in some way. This can help to identify community assets.

Carefully examine the formal and informal structures that exist and consider if they unite the population of the community or support only a specific portion of the population. Who are the leaders? For example, a private school might support only a more prosperous portion of the community or the school might reach out into the community to offer scholarships for those in different socioeconomic strata. Public schools might have broad support and funding or garner limited resources from local coffers. Some of this information may be evident but some may require deeper investigation and interviews with key informants. Leaders of formal groups may be key informants, but leaders of informal groups should be considered key informants as well.

The assessment would not be complete without an inventory of the community belief systems in place, including identifying places of worship. This could be accomplished through both primary and secondary data, by speaking to community members, or by looking in the phone book, local publications, or on the Internet. Traditions and values of the community may be classified according to portions of the community if it is heterogeneous, or in general if it is more homogenous. How the religious climate in the town might influence other goods or services should be investigated. For example, a community may have a religiously conservative population that could influence the availability or access to abortion counseling or certain birth control services for residents. When assessing the community "people" identify the:

- Size and density of population
- Demographic structure of population (e.g., race, ethnic groups, gender, and age) currently and in historical context
- Educational attainment
- Informal groups
- Formal groups
- Linking structures
- Schools
- Neighborhood associations
- Civic clubs
- Values and beliefs
- Churches
- Synagogues
- Mosques
- Political affiliations

Community Systems in Place. Using a systems approach, the PHN can explore the organizing structures in place within the community that may serve the needs of the people. Community systems contributing to community function or dysfunction include safety and transportation; politics and government; economics (including industry, employment, and commerce); education; recreation; health and social services; communication; and physical environment (Anderson & McFarlane, 2015). Each of these functional systems influences the health of the community and requires full assessment.

Safety and Transportation. Safety requires a broad assessment. Road maintenance and presence of interstate highways or curvy mountain roads will influence the safety of the community. The PHN should identify statistics on highway safety and find information about motor vehicle fatalities and moving violations, seatbelt use, and child safety seat use in the area. For example, in Virginia one can go to the state Division of Motor Vehicles site and locate the sites of most frequent motor vehicle accidents according to cause and location (http://www.dmv.state.va.us). Likewise, many county websites have information about motor vehicle accidents or fatalities in their jurisdictions. Safety also includes crime rates, issues such as sidewalks or guard rails along roadsides, crosswalks in intersections, safe playgrounds and bike paths. Police, fire protection, and emergency services also fall under the umbrella of safety, as do laws requiring helmets for motorcyclists.

Following the crime statistics for the area or individual neighborhoods in your community can provide good evidence of the effectiveness of the police force and an overall measure of citizen safety. In addition, qualitative information gained from speaking to locals and service providers can add valuable perspectives about their experience with community safety.

Community residents frequently depend on public transportation to access community services. When doing a community assessment, the PHN should survey the availability of affordable community transportation for all income levels. To do this, one should look at whether transportation options such as buses, commuter trains or cabs are present to allow access to central places in the community. What percent of the population have cars? It is also helpful to know if there are railroads and airlines available to connect to more regional or national sites. This can provide insight on potential community permeability to outside influences or community isolation.

Politics and Government. The PHN will need to identify the type of government structures in place in the geographic area. Many communities have websites that will help clarify this community governance. Is there a mayor or board of supervisors? Who are the identified formal leaders in the government? A visit to the community's office building will provide a perspective on the accessibility of the governing body. Political affiliation in the community may be relevant to certain priorities, so identifying the mix of party allegiance in past presidential, state, or local elections is a useful measure to obtain.

Government buy-in to community needs is essential for health progress to occur. For example, what dollar amount does the community spend on child health or elderly care? Take a look at the most recent budget of the community. How does that compare with other regions of the state or United States? For example, are government-supported programs in place to enhance early childhood education or elder care? There may be overlaps with economic systems of the area as well, which affect taxation and community wealth.

Economics. Regional economic prosperity frequently influences all citizens in the population. The existing jobs, the unemployment rates, and the types of industry in the community are all important. Identify the average income and wages for types of jobs available and identify the industries that operate within the community and what percent of skilled and unskilled jobs exist.

In an optimal community, the jobs that are available and the educational level needed for those jobs should mesh. Frequently, community colleges identify community employment needs and promote educational programs to meet the needs of the local job market. Virginia's Labor Market Information (www.virginialmi.com) website, for example, provides detailed data on unemployment and economic indicators for each county. Data can relate directly to where your assessment is taking place.

The state of the job markets in the community could influence the availability of health insurance associated with employment, and the need for assistance in registering for health insurance through ACA-created exchanges. If there are migrant workers in the community you are assessing, the issue of immigration is likely to be present. If so, what local programs or services are available for these legal or illegal immigrant workers within the community?

Education. When considering the educational systems in the community, the PHN should first identify all the schools in the area, including preschools, school readiness programs, primary and secondary schools and, if possible, visit some or all of them to observe the condition of the buildings and the children at recess or at the end of the day. What resources for nutrition, physical activity, and health care do the schools have? What percent of the children receive free or reduced cost meals? Are there Head Start or sponsored preschool programs available for lower-income families? Are there measures in place to identify school readiness? If different ethnic groups are part of the community, what is the language literacy? Coordinating this information with government spending on education in the locality will help to clarify the value that the community places on education.

The educational attainment of the population is relevant to the type of educational programs that are present in the community. Examining the high school dropout rates, standardized testing results, and the pupil/teacher ratios within the locality will help to evaluate the quality of the schools within the district. General Educational Development (GED) classes for students who need a high school diploma and adult literacy programs in place would indicate that the community places a high value on the education of its citizens. Higher education institutions, such as community colleges, four-year colleges, professional and technical schools, and universities will also influence the overall educational level of the community, which ultimately influences the economic prosperity of the citizens.

Recreation. Safe indoor or outdoor recreation areas for children and adults can provide the community access to healthy exercise. State, city or county parks, their condition and use, along with organized sports teams, bike paths or public gymnasiums would be indicators of public promotion of physical activities, and the importance of those to the community. If the community has hiking trails, are they well maintained? Are swimming pools open to the public? If there are lakes or rivers nearby, do they provide guarded beaches or lifeguards? Part of the assessment of recreation addresses for whom it is available.

Identifying how the residents spend their leisure time will help to clarify recreational opportunities. Local youth and adult sports teams, movie theaters, availability of cable TV or Internet, bowling alleys, prevalence of X-rated book stores, and local statistics on drug use will contribute to the information obtained on the community.

Health and Social Services. Location of and population access to health services in the form of health care providers, emergency services, hospitals, and hospice programs are key elements in the assessment of community health. The proportion of providers who accept Medicaid or Medicare, or proportion of services available to immigrants influences the access of certain populations to services. Number and type of medical practices available can identify gaps or gluts in services for the population when compared with age groups in the community. For example, the proportions of pediatricians, obstetricians, and geriatricians should somewhat mirror the related population's age groups. Private versus nonprofit hospitals, insurance coverage (and affordability of the ACA insurance exchanges), sliding scale payments, and means to reach services (proximity and transportation) all influence how health services might be used in a community. While in some communities abundant resources may be present, access to the services may be inhibited by hours of operation or limited provision of services through insurance or payment restrictions.

Number of hospitals, clinics, offices, and mental health facilities are important, but how the community uses them is a critical element in the success of health care delivery. Health care in vulnerable populations often requires care coordination, which may include home visiting, appointment arranging and transportation along with access to (and use of) a medical home. Note the availability of processes or agencies that provide introduction of vulnerable families to resources, including early childhood education, child or elder abuse prevention, and family support services. Social services in the form of community programs and state or local agencies such as community action coalitions or social service departments should be assessed. The presence of these types of services in a community would reflect positive inclinations toward holistic health for that community. Gaps in certain services represent an opportunity for program development.

Physical Environment. The climate and overall geographic description of the community contributes to health and well-being. Tendencies toward flooding, drought or hurricanes, and mountainous, ocean or waterside locations will carry concurrent health consequences. The availability of good water and air supplies and locally produced food are positive indicators for health and should be explored within your community. Industries with poorly managed runoff of chemicals, unsafe dams or chemical waste would provide negative health indicators. Environmental pollution of any kind requires further assessment. The Environmental Protection Agency (EPA) lists information about Superfund sites throughout the country on its website (https://www.epa.gov). Scorecard (http://scorecard.goodguide.com) compares localities in terms of pollutants.

The built environment, including housing and neighborhoods, provides a potential health indicator. What is the condition and age of local housing? Does the area seem prosperous? While new and energy efficient housing, including housing for low-income families, can imply a positive indicator of health, older, less efficient homes appearing run down may be an indicator of less positive neighborhood conditions. For example, houses built before 1978 can contain lead paint, which represents a significant health risk for young children (Fig. 17.3).

An additional important element related to housing is the average cost of owning or renting a home in the area. This information can identify housing availability and affordability for community members.

Communication. Communication in the United States has become intricately tied to Internet availability. Identifying the methods of communication within the community you are assessing will help to articulate the information available to the public and how they receive it. At which sites within the community is Internet available? Local libraries and certain businesses often provide free Internet access. Are there Internet providers for the community? Rural areas can sometimes have limited Internet access, thereby restricting communication with those inside or outside their locality through email or Internet-based social media.

The cell phone has become a primary source of communication. Once again, looking at the availability of cell phone coverage in the community may help reveal access to those outside and within the community. While landlines are almost universally available and can provide communication within and outside of communities, young members of the community rely heavily on social media and texting for communication with their peers. Those sources of communication require both Internet and cell phone coverage in many cases. Today one can hardly imagine limitations on these methods, yet there are rural areas that still do not have good access to them.

Cell phones and mobile devices such as tablets, iPads, and laptops are vehicles for health messages, advertising, and political messages. While in 2004 only 66 percent of adults had cell phones, now the number exceeds 95 percent. In addition, many homes in areas of good cell coverage have disconnected their landlines and use cell coverage for all phone communication (Pew Internet, 2013 & 2018). Fig. 17.4 illustrates rates of cell phone ownership in the United States between 2004 and 2013. A later survey indicates that the cell phone ownership trends were expected to continue beyond 2018. In areas where tornadoes or hurricanes are prevalent, individual communities may have systems in place for communicating early warning of weather events. Such systems usually include a siren that is tested at a regular time each week and otherwise sounds only when the threat is imminent. If your community is in a high-risk weather or topographic area, knowing the disaster plan is helpful in understanding the community's preparedness.

Radio or television can also provide information about imminent events. Radio or television also may provide news and advertise events to the local community. Local news can clue the community assessor into pertinent current events or community issues that are at the forefront. Newspapers (online or in print) can also provide interesting insights into the

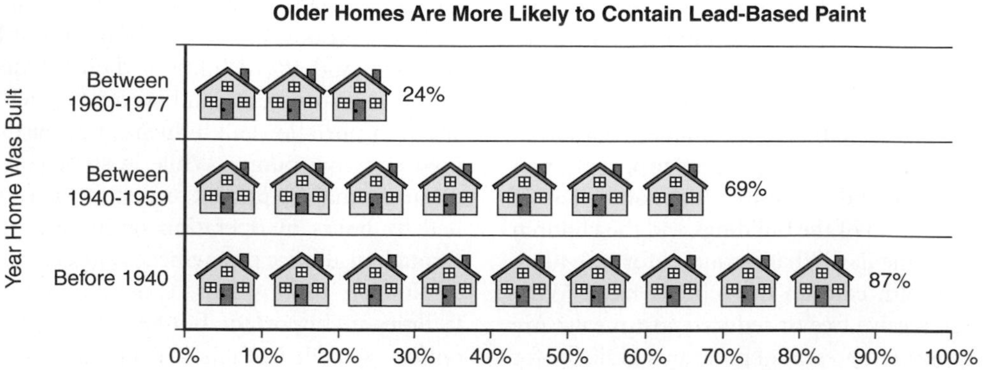

Fig. 17.3 Older homes are more likely to contain lead-based paint.

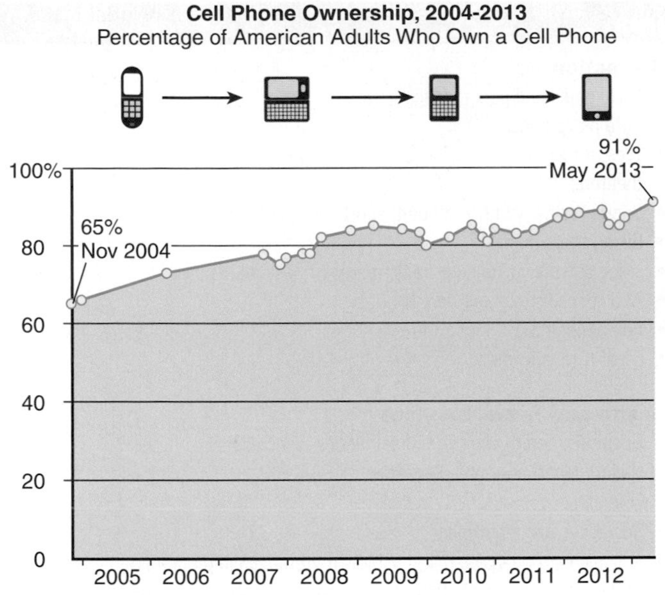

Fig. 17.4 Cell phone ownership. (Data from Pew Internet: *Mobile Fact Sheet*, Feb 5, 2018. Pew Research Center's Internet and American Life Project, April 17-May 19, 2013.)

community's current events or issues. Some communities have numerous news outlets (or papers) reflecting different political viewpoints or may target certain subsystems or aggregates in the community. They may be issued on a daily or weekly basis.

Informal methods of communication, such as signs and bulletin boards (online or in strategic locations), may offer some means of transferring information in communities. Churches, local stores, and government offices such as the post office or town hall, may continue to be relevant communication hubs in small or rural communities. The U.S. Postal Service, Fed Ex, and other carriers are common links to outside sources of goods and services for communities.

When a community's systems are robust, they afford degrees of protection for the community and its health. Weaknesses in the systems may permit health threats to enter the community. For example, a lack of sidewalks on a main street could result in pedestrian injuries or fatalities. The stronger and more focused the services/systems in place are toward individual community needs, the stronger the community resilience will be against outside threats to optimal health (Fig. 17.5). Assessing the strength of systems can be a measure of the strengths of the community. When the systems are not intact or are insufficient to meet the needs of the community, the possibility of poorer overall health of the community increases. The systems in place may act as protective factors against negative outside forces that could threaten the community. For example, a strong school immunization program could offset a measles epidemic. Box 17.4 provides more information on assessing these systems.

The Seven "A's"

Once the PHN has identified and cataloged the systems of the community, then it is most helpful to measure their effectiveness. One method that can be used to evaluate adequacy of services or systems in a community is the seven "A's" (Truglio-Londrigan & Gallagher, 2003). A series of queries about a service or system's effectiveness in reaching the community can be used with any of the above listed community components.

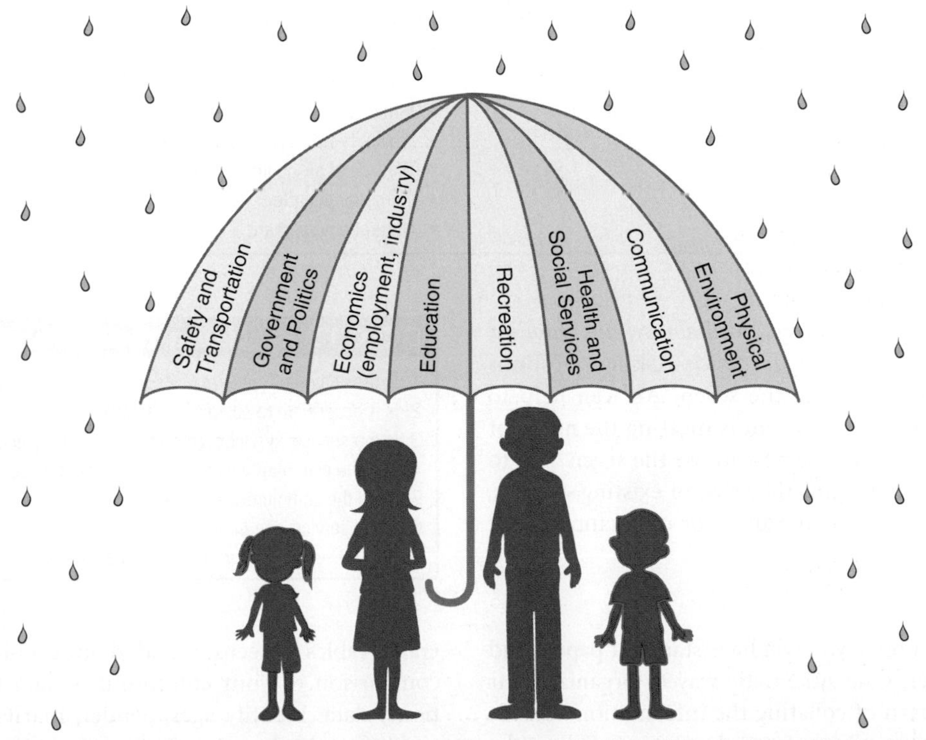

Fig. 17.5 Optimal community systems in place to protect the public. (Data from Anderson ET, MacFarlane J: *Community as partner: theory and practice in nursing*, ed. 6, Philadelphia, 2011, Lippincott Williams & Wilkins.)

BOX 17.4 Community Systems: Potential Measures

Safety and Transportation
- Crime rates and trends
- Traffic accidents and fatalities
- Fire stations and emergency responders and response times; publicly paid or volunteer?
- Police protection and public perception thereof
- Highway system and road conditions
- Availability of public transportation in, out of, and around the community
- Commuters to and from the community and methods of commute
- Child car seat assistance

Politics and Government
- Type of local government
- Budgets for public services/systems
- Diversity in government offices match to community diversity (e.g., mayor, board of supervisors)
- Local tax base and taxes levied
- Political party affiliation of county majority
- Website for locality

Economics
- Average income
- Percent of families who own their homes
- Automobile ownership
- Number of children eligible for free lunches
- Unemployment figures/types of jobs available
- Families on unemployment compensation
- Percent of food stamp recipients
- Poverty statistics
- Industries in place/largest employers/size of most businesses
- Available childcare

Education
- Number and types of primary and secondary schools (public vs. private)
- Number and access to community and four-year colleges or universities
- Preschool classes available
- Early intervention home visiting programs
- Average educational achievement of population
- Primary and additional languages of community

Recreation
- Local parks and park management
- Safe playgrounds
- Type of recreational businesses (e.g., bowling alleys, adult bookstores, movie theaters)
- Sports teams, youth and adult; sports arenas/fields
- Biking trails/lanes
- Track or walking/running trails, tennis or basketball courts
- Activity clubs (e.g., garden, hiking)
- Senior center(s)
- Local festivals/fairs

Health and Social Services
- Hospitals, health clinics/medical offices, specialists
- Health department and programs
- Free clinic
- Social service department
- In home care provision (i.e., hospice, maternal child programs)
- Statistics on child and elder abuse, sexual assault
- Immunization status of community members
- Home health care team
- Percent of Medicaid families in community
- Percent of population on disability and ages of those disabled
- Obesity rate: adults and children
- Mental health clinic(s)

Communication
- Newspapers
- Cell phone carriers and availability of service
- Internet connections
- Radio and TV stations
- Community bulletin boards (check post offices and central places)
- Informal sources of information and communication

Physical Environment
- Age and condition of housing
- Physical terrain and potential for environmental disaster (e.g., hurricanes, tornadoes)
- Proximity to Superfund sites (pollution)
- Water and air quality
- Industrial pollution
- Natural environment

The seven "A's" are *awareness, access, availability, affordability, acceptability, appropriateness,* and *adequacy*. Asking questions about an agency or service using the seven "A's" can help to identify how well the service or system is meeting the needs of the community. Box 17.5 explains how to use the seven "A's" to craft questions to assist in gauging the value of existing services, or in identifying assets in the community or opportunities for improvement.

BOX 17.5 Using the Seven "A's"

1. Is the community *aware* of its needs and of the service?
2. Is it *accessible* to community members?
3. Is the service *available* when the community needs it?
4. Can the community members *afford* the service?
5. Does the community find the service *acceptable*?
6. Is the service *adequate* to meet the needs of the community?
7. Are the services *appropriate* to meet the needs of the community?

Data Analysis

Once the data are assembled, you will have stacks of papers and multiple computer files. One systematic way to organize your data is to follow a pattern of collating the information according to the section of the assessment and the systems. Follow the model that you have chosen to order your information. You can create tables of census and **demographic data**, indicating a comparison of your community's data to state data and national data. Identify ages, gender, marital information, births and infant deaths, race or ethnicity, and density of the population and assemble the information into a table. This helps you to see the information at a glance. Identify whether the population in your community is on the rise or declining and which age and ethnic/racial groups are increasing or decreasing. How many families live below the poverty level? These items of information can pinpoint areas where needs may be increasing. Census data provide rich information about how many people live in your community and historic data about population size, composition, and income. Be sure that your data are the most recent and that when you compare data that you are comparing data reported in the same format and from a reliable source.

Next, organize all data, primary and secondary, related to each of the systems. You may decide to make tables about these data and make a report on the data available for each system. An example of this type of table, indicating whether trends are positive or negative, is in Fig. 17.6, from the Santa Cruz Community Assessment, 2017 (Applied Survey Research, 2017). Using benchmarks such as *Healthy People 2020* (https://www.healthypeople.gov) can assist in measuring the locality's needs. Be sure to include the community assets you have identified for each system, as well as any observed deficiencies. Do the perceived issues of the community match your secondary data? Synthesize the data into a coherent report based on each system (see QSEN box).

QSEN FOCUS ON QUALITY AND SAFETY EDUCATION FOR NURSES

Targeted Competency: Client-Centered Care

Recognizes the client or designee as the source of control and as a full partner in providing compassionate and coordinated care that is based on the preferences, values and needs of the client

- **Knowledge:** Understanding of multiple dimensions of client-centered care
- **Skill:** For individual, family, aggregate, or community elicits values, preferences, and expressed needs as part of clinical interview
- **Attitude:** Support care for each client level whose values differ from one's own

Question

The Quad Council core competency of analytic and assessment skills indicates the beginning PHN should collect data, both quantitative and qualitative, to be used in community assessment. The PHN then assesses data collected as part of the community assessment process to make inferences about clients (values, culture, preferences for health care)

In order to develop, revise, or even improve community health care delivery, how would the PHN use the outcomes of the community assessment? What steps would the nurse take to make change based on client choice?

Morbidity and mortality data should be tabulated identifying the top three causes of morbidity and mortality and also comparing the local data to the state, national, and previous years' local data. Are there conditions in the causes of illness or death that are rising or declining according to past data? Looking at this information and linking with the information derived from primary data will help focus priorities. Identifying health indicators such as obesity rates, smoking rates, and causes of morbidity and mortality can clarify the needs of the community.

Identification of Health Assets and Challenges. Once you have pulled together your data into an organized format, the community problems and strengths should emerge. Using a targeted layout like Santa Cruz County's "snapshot" (see Fig. 17.6) will help you to summarize these in a clear way. With the resulting "list" of identified problems and assets, you will be ready to prioritize your results.

Prioritizing. Once the data are collated and clarified on paper, the themes can be placed in the context of the earlier identified community priorities reflected in your primary data. In this way, community involvement and input in the assessment process will make your assessment and planning relevant to the community and create the opportunity to meet the community's identified needs. At the same time, try to identify within your secondary data a rationale for the community's identified need. In other words, you might compromise. Attempting to implement programs that are not recognized as most relevant by the community can result in lack of community buy-in and ultimate program failure.

For example, though secondary data may document that increased mortality due to heart disease should be the community's highest priority, as evidenced by higher than average mortality from heart disease, the community might see a different need, such as elder care or childcare, as the highest priority. There is no clear guide in this prioritizing process, but testing ideas about perceived need and actual data-driven information with community stakeholders and key informants helps the PHN come to an optimal way to prioritize problems and identify target areas for improvement. Just as in the hospital setting, make the patient (in this case the community) the center of your focus. Box 17.6 can assist you in steps to prioritize the community problem list. Identifying the top three community problems or needs should then lead to creating the priority nursing diagnoses (see Secondary Sources of Data).

The ethical concepts of utilitarianism and justice can help you navigate the negotiations and advocacy inherent in prioritizing one health problem over another. Utilitarianism means doing the most good for the most people, so a priority problem would ideally be one that affects a large proportion of the community. However, justice focuses on the fair distribution of resources among all people. Social justice means advocating for the most vulnerable populations in a community, to ensure that their problems receive higher priority than the problems found throughout the general population. For example, secondary data might find that infant mortality occurs rarely in the community; but if there is a wide disparity among racial groups in infant mortality rates, social justice would call for this problem to be given higher priority in order to address underlying determinants of health that may cause the disparity.

Community Nursing Diagnosis

The community health nursing diagnosis in this phase of the process helps clarify the prioritized problems and is an important first step to planning. Community diagnoses clarify the target population for care and identify the factors contributing to the identified problem. As the analysis of the data proceeds,

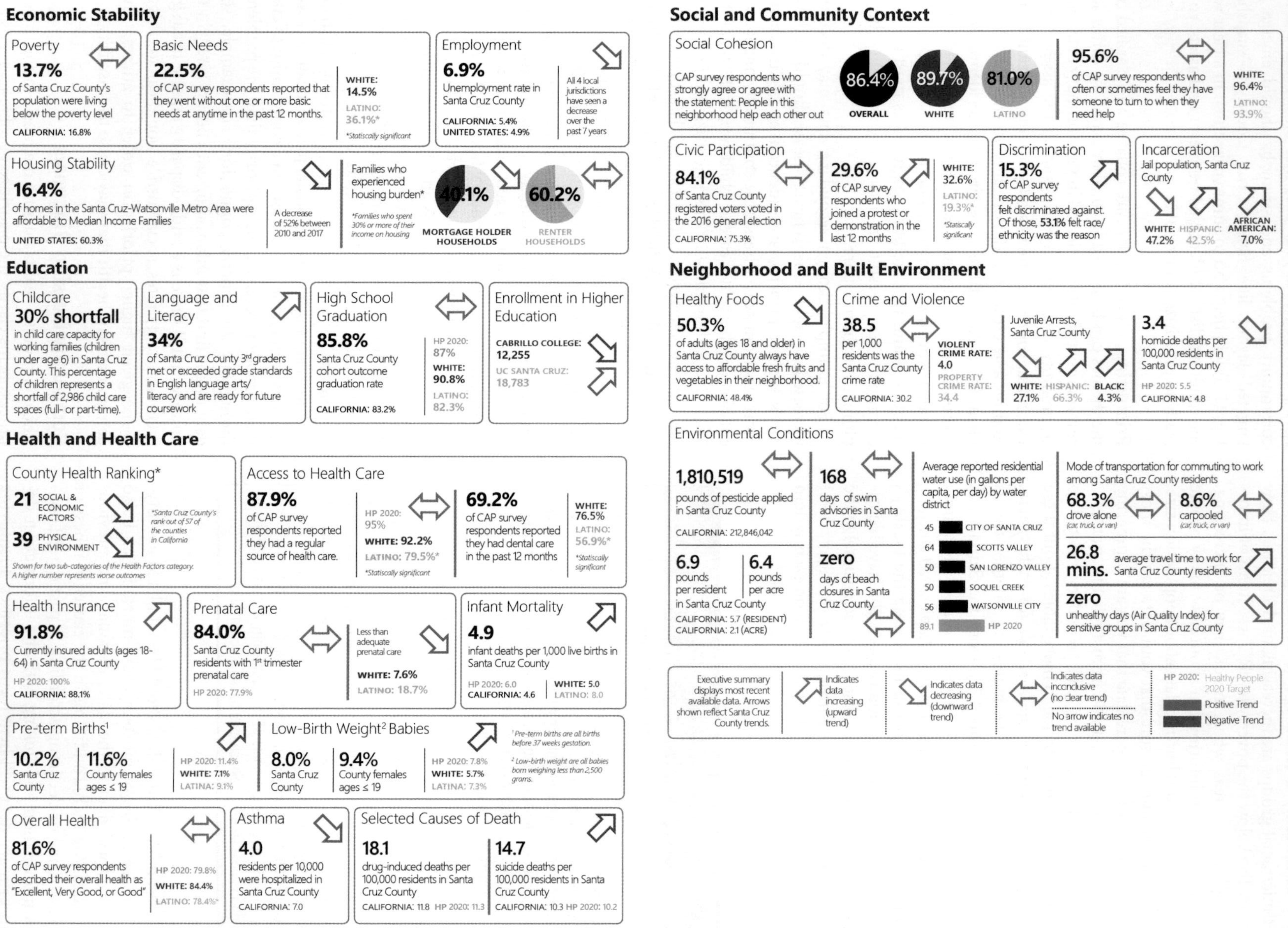

Fig. 17.6 Snapshot of Santa Cruz County (https://www.appliedsurveyresearch.org).

BOX 17.6 Problem Priority Criteria

Criteria that have been helpful in ranking identified problems include the following:

- Community awareness of the problem
- Community motivation to resolve or better manage the problem
- Nurse's ability to influence problem solution
- Availability of expertise to solve the problem
- Severity of the outcomes if the problem is unresolved
- Speed with which the problem can be solved

the nursing care plan can be formed. In the planning phase, the PHN identifies community-focused interventions, along with ways to measure outcomes. At this point in the analysis of data, collaborating with community partners and colleagues will assist in the objectivity of the analysis and uncover potentially diverse data interpretations (Anderson & McFarlane, 2015). Community diagnoses should consider the community's strengths and assets. There are several standardized classification systems to accommodate this diagnosis formation. The Omaha System and NANDA International are two prominent systems of classification. The **Omaha System** includes domains and problem classifications that are specific to community health. The Omaha System was developed by visiting nurses and expands beyond the physiological domain and includes environmental, psychosocial, and health-related behaviors domains. In addition to the problem, the Omaha System addresses the intervention scheme and the problem rating scale for outcomes. Omaha-based computer software applications are available to streamline electronic records (Omaha System, 2018). The Omaha System website, http://www.omahasystem.org, contains case studies and full explanation of the use of its standardized taxonomy and problem-oriented approach.

NANDA includes several community diagnoses and health-seeking behaviors that can apply to communities, though certain diagnoses may require some adaptation to the community (Herdman & Kamitsuru, 2014). The NANDA system provides a useful format for the diagnosis statement, but is confining in its strict parameters mostly limited to individual and family systems. This format includes:

- Identification of the problem;
- Its relation to factors, stressors or health issues; and
- The supporting data that document the problem.

We recommend the use of this problem layout. For example, a diagnosis statement might read:

> *Increased level of infant mortality in Community X related to inadequate access to prenatal care, high teen birth rate and few obstetrical providers in city; as evidenced by infant mortality rate of 8 infant deaths per 1000 live births, a preterm birth rate of 15 percent, teen birth rate of 75/1000 females, and 3 obstetrical providers for a population of 30,000.*

Community nursing diagnosis language must describe at the aggregate level—in other words, the community level—responses to actual and potential illnesses and life processes. This also means that the defining characteristics for community diagnoses must be observable and measurable at the aggregate level. To do this, community-level data must be used. Epidemiological supporting data or community survey data are two examples of community-level data. The comparison of local data with state, regional, or national data, as rates and across multiple years, is one key means of identifying community-level problems, as well as patterns and trends.

The community nursing diagnosis, no matter which classification system the PHN uses, then leads to expected outcomes and evidence-based health promotion strategies to address and improve the problem identified in the diagnosis. This becomes the nursing care plan. The expected outcomes and evaluations derived from the nursing diagnosis systems suggest subsequent evaluation measures for identified needs or problems. Just as problems are recognized and prioritized, so can strengths be identified that may offer avenues through which the PHN can address existing challenges facing the community.

LINKING CONTENT TO PRACTICE

In this chapter, the focus is placed on the partnership between the public health nurse and the community throughout the process of community assessment, problem identification, planning, intervention, and evaluation. One of the Institute of Medicine's (IOM) three core functions of public health is assessment. The process of community assessment outlined and described in this chapter closely follows The Council on Linkages' *Core Competencies for Public Health* (adopted June 26, 2014). This includes the need for public health nurses to "maintain relationships that improve health in a community." Among other identified competencies for public health providers, including public health nurses, is that one "assesses community health status and factors influencing health in a community (e.g., quality, availability, accessibility, and use of health services; access to affordable housing)." This chapter presents the means by which public health nurses can construct a composite database containing assessment data from a wide variety of sources. This initial community assessment phase also directly links with The Quad Council Domains of Public Health Practice: Domain #1: Assessment and Analytic Skills; Domain #5: Community Dimensions of Practice Skills; and Domain #6: Public Health Sciences Skills. The Council on Linkages' *Core Competencies for Public Health* also emphasizes the public health nurse's ability to develop "community health assessments using information about health status, factors influencing health, and assets and resources." Development of goals and objectives along with their problem correlates as part of the community health assessment directly relates to this competency; whereas another Council on Linkages competency—"Recommends policies, programs, and services for implementation"—directly relates to the development of intervention actions described in this chapter.

Program Planning, Implementation, and Evaluation

Once interventions and evaluation measures are identified through the nursing diagnosis framework, the PHN arrives at a new step in the nursing process—the program planning phase. This includes analyzing and establishing priorities among community health problems already identified through nursing diagnosis, establishing goals and objectives, and identifying intervention activities that will accomplish the objectives. These interventions must be clearly supported by the community stakeholders in order for the community to buy in to the identified program plans. Intervention activities, the means by which objectives are met, are the strategies that clarify what must be done to achieve the objectives or the ways change will be effected. The next phase of the nursing process is program implementation. This involves enacting the plan for improved community health using the identified goals and objectives.

Finally, upon implementation of the program and by using the established evaluation measures, the PHN can measure the success of the program and determine community satisfaction with the outcome. These evaluation criteria will already be identified through the nursing diagnosis format chosen.

Program planning and implementation should be based on the community's problems AND its strengths, as well as the priorities of the community members. If the identified problem is not resolved to the satisfaction of the community at large following program implementation, the PHN will return to the data-gathering phase and begin the process again using the updated data. As shown in Fig. 17.2, this can be an ongoing, circular process, just like the nursing process. Program management, encompassing program planning, implementation, and evaluation, is discussed in detail in Chapter 23.

PRACTICE APPLICATION

Lily, a nurse in a small city, became aware of the increased incidence of respiratory diseases through contact with families in the community and the local chapter of the American Lung Association. During family visits, Lily noticed that many of the parents were smokers. Because most of the families Lily visited had small children, she became concerned about the effects of secondhand smoke on the health of the infants and children in her family caseload.

Further assessment of this community indicated that the community recognized several problems, including school safety and the risk of water pollution, in addition to the smoking problem that Lily had identified during her family visits. Talks with different community members revealed that they wanted each of these identified problems "fixed," although these same community members were uncertain about how to start. In deciding which of the three identified problems to address first, which criterion would be most important for Lily to consider?

A. The amount of money available
B. The level of community motivation to "fix" one of the three identified problems
C. The number of people in the community who expressed a concern about each of the three identified problems
D. How much control she would have in the process

Answers can be found on the Evolve site.

KEY POINTS

- Most definitions of community include three dimensions: (1) networks of interpersonal relationships that provide friendship and support to members, (2) residence in a common locality, and (3) shared values, interests, or concerns.
- A community is defined as a locality-based entity, composed of systems of formal organizations reflecting societal institutions, informal groups, and aggregates that are interdependent and whose function or expressed intent is to meet a wide variety of collective needs.
- A community practice setting is insufficient reason for stating that practice is oriented toward the community client. When the location of the practice is in the community but the focus of the practice is the individual or family, the nursing client remains the individual or family, not the whole community.
- Population-centered practice is targeted to the community—the population group in which healthful change is sought.
- Community health as used in this chapter is defined as the meeting of collective needs through identification of problems and management of behaviors within the community itself and between the community and the larger society.
- Most changes aimed at improving community health involve, out of necessity, partnerships among community residents and health workers from a variety of disciplines.
- Assessing community health requires gathering existing data and interpreting the database.
- Five methods of collecting data useful to the nurse are analysis of existing secondary data, and primary data collection through informant interviews, participant observation, surveys, and windshield surveys.
- Nurses should identify and partner with gatekeepers, formal or informal community leaders, to gain entry or acceptance into the community.
- The planning phase includes analyzing and establishing priorities among community health problems already identified, establishing goals and objectives, and identifying intervention activities that will accomplish the objectives.
- Once high-priority problems are identified, broad relevant goals and objectives are developed; the goal is generally a broad statement of the desired outcome while the objectives are precise statements of the desired outcome.
- Intervention activities, the means by which objectives are met, are the strategies that clarify what must be done to achieve the objectives, the ways change will be effected, and the way the problem will be interpreted.
- Implementation, the next phase of the nursing process, means transforming a plan for improved community health into achieving goals and objectives. This essentially is the implementation of the program.
- Simply defined, evaluation is the appraisal of the effects of some organized activity.

CLINICAL DECISION-MAKING ACTIVITIES

1. Observe an occupational health nurse or public health nurse, school nurse, family nurse practitioner, or emergency department nurse for several hours. Determine which of the nurse's activities are population centered. Give specific examples and present your reasons for considering them population centered.
2. Using your own community as a frame of reference, develop examples illustrating the concepts of community, community client, community health, and partnership for health. What are some of the complexities of this question?
3. Read your local newspaper and identify articles illustrating the concepts of community, community client, community health, and partnership for health. How does your article specifically relate to the concept?
4. Using any two of the conditions of community competence given in the chapter, briefly analyze your own community. Give examples of each condition.
5. Search the Washtenaw County, Michigan, website (http://www.ewashtenaw.org) for information about "county conversations." Identify which issues are being addressed, and read the local newspaper for additional information. Did you find other countywide issues when you read the newspaper? Are there positions on the issues that are not presented?

ADDITIONAL RESOURCES

EVOLVE WEBSITE

http://evolve.elsevier.com/Stanhope/community/

- Answers to Practice Application
- Case Study
- Glossary
- Review Questions

REFERENCES

Anderson ET, McFarlane J: *Community as Partner: Theory and Practice in Nursing*, ed 6, Philadelphia, PA, 2015, Lippincott Williams & Wilkins.

Applied Survey Research: *Santa Cruz County Community Assessment Project*, 2017. Retrieved from https://www.appliedsurveyresearch.org.

Beckman S, Fawcett J: *Neuman Systems Model: Celebrating Academic-Practice Partnerships, IPFW eBooks*, 2017. Retrieved from https://opus.ipfw.edu.

Boyd R, Richerson PJ: Culture and the evolution of human cooperation, *Philos Trans R Soc Lond B Biol Sci* 364(1533): 3281–3288, 2009.

Catalani CE, Veneziale A, Campbell L, et al.: Videovoice: community assessment in post-Katrina New Orleans, *Health Promotion Pract* 13:18–28, 2013.

Centers for Disease Control and Prevention (CDC): *Common Elements of Assessment and Planning Frameworks*, 2015a. Retrieved from www.cdc.gov.

Centers for Disease Control and Prevention (CDC): *Assessment & Planning Models, Frameworks & Tools*, 2015b. Retrieved from http://www.cdc.gov.

Centers for Disease Control and Prevention (CDC): *Core Functions of Public Health and How they Relate to the 10 Essential Services*, 2011. Retrieved from https://www.cdc.gov

Centers for Disease Control and Prevention (CDC): *The Built Environment Assessment Tool Manual*, 2017. Retrieved from https://www.cdc.gov.

Centers for Disease Control and Prevention (CDC): *Preparedness and Response for Public Health Disasters: Community Assessment for Public Health Emergency Response (CASPER)*, 2018a. Retrieved from https://www.cdc.

Centers for Disease Control and Prevention (CDC): *Trends in Current Cigarette Smoking among Adults, United States*, 2018b. Retrieved from http://www.cdc.gov.

Centers for Disease Control and Prevention (CDC): *Ten essential public health services and how they include addressing social determinants of health inequities*, 2018c. Retrieved from https://www.cdc.gov.

Cummings PL, Schwaller E, Wesely S, et al.: *East Aldine District's Town Center Development: A Health Impact Assessment in Harris County, Texas*, 2016. Retrieved from http://www.pewtrusts.org.

DeGuzman PB, Keeling AW: Addressing disparities in access to care: lessons from the Kercheval Street Clinic in the 1960s, *Policy Polit Nurs Pract* 12(4):199–207, 2011.

Fawcett J, Ellenbecker CH: A proposed conceptual model of nursing and population health, *Nursing Outlook* 63(3):288–298, 2015.

Feldman D, Thayer A, Wall M, et al.: *The 2017 Millennial Impact Report: An Invigorated Generation for Causes and Social Issues*, 2017. Retrieved from http://www.themillennialimpact.com.

Healthy People 2020: *Injury and Violence*. Retrieved from http://healthypeople.gov.

Florian J, Roy NM, Quintiliani LM, et al. Using Photovoice and Asset Mapping to Inform a Community-Based Diabetes Intervention, Boston, Massachusetts, 2015, *Prev Chronic Dis* 13:E107, 2016.

Gibson M & Lancaster J: *School of Social Work*, Virginia Commonwealth University, Richmond VA, 1992.

Guest G, Namey E, McKenna K: How many focus groups are enough? Building an evidence base for nonprobability sample sizes, *Field Methods* 29(1):3–22, 2017.

Herdman TH, Kamitsuru S, editors: *NANDA International Nursing Diagnoses: Definitions & Classification, 2015-2017*, Oxford, UK, 2014, Wiley-Blackwell.

Jagosh J, Bush PL, Salsberg J, et al.: A realist evaluation of community-based participatory research: partnership synergy, trust building and related ripple effects, *BMC Public Health* 15(1):725, 2015.

Joyce BL, Harmon MJ, Pilling LB, Johnson RH, Hicks VL, Brown-Schott N: The preparation of community/public health nurses: Amplifying the impact, *Public Health Nurs* 32(6):595–597, 2015.

Kaiser BL, Thomas GR, Bowers BJ: A case study of engaging hard-to-reach participants in the research process: Community Advisors on Research Design and Strategies (CARDS)®, *Res Nurs Health* 40(1):70–79, 2017.

Lennon-Dearing R, Price J: Women living with HIV tell their stories with Photovoice, *J Hum Behav Soc Environ* 28(5):588–601, 2018.

MacQueen KM, McLellan E, Metzger DS, et al.: What is community? An evidence-based definition for participatory public health, *Am J Public Health* 91(12):1929–1938, 2001.
MacQuillan EL, Curtis AB, Baker KM, Paul R, Back YO: Using GIS mapping to target public health interventions: examining birth outcomes across GIS techniques, *J Community Health* 42(4): 633–638, 2017.
Madelía Community Hospital & Clinic: *Community Health Dialogue*, 2013. Retrieved from http://www.mchospital.org.
Mercy Corps: *Driving resilience: Market approaches to disaster recovery*, Portland Oregon, 2017, Mercy Corps.
Milio N: *9226 Kercheval: The Storefront that Did Not Burn*, Ann Arbor, MI, 2000, University of Michigan.
National Association of County and City Health Officials (NACCHO): *Mobilizing for Action through Planning and Partnerships (MAPP)*, 2016. Retrieved from http://www.naccho.org.
Novek S, Morris-Oswald T, Menec V: Using photovoice with older adults: some methodological strengths and issues, *Ageing Soc* 32(3):451–470, 2012.
Ocloo J, Matthews R: From tokenism to empowerment: progressing patient and public involvement in healthcare improvement, *BMJ Qual Saf* 25(8):626–632, 2016.
Oklahoma Cooperative Extension Service: *Fact Sheet-Three examples of Asset Oriented Community Assessment Tools*, 2018. Retrieved from factsheets.okstate.edu.
Olaniran A, Smith H, Unkels R, Bar-Zeev S, van den Broek N: *Who is a community health worker? – a systematic review of definitions*, 8600 Rockville Pike, Bethesda MD, 20894 USA, 2017, National Center for Biotechnology Information, U.S. National Library of Medicine.
Omaha System: *Solving the Clinical Data-Information Puzzle*, 2018. Retrieved from www.omahasystem.org.
Pew Internet: *Mobile Fact Sheet*, Feb 5, 2018. Pew Research Center's Internet and American Life Project, April 17–May 19, 2013.
Preston MA, Glover-Collins K, Ross L, et al.: Colorectal cancer screening in rural and poor-resourced communities, *Am J Surg* 216(2):245–250, 2018.
Quad Council Coalition Competency Review Task Force: *Community/Public Health Nursing Competencies*, 2018. Retrieved from http://www.quadcouncilphn.org.
Rosenbaum S: *Principles to Consider for the Implementation of a Community Health Needs Assessment Process*, 2013. Retrieved from http://nnphi.org.
Ryan W, editor: *Blaming the victim*, New York, NY, 1976, Free Press.
Schölmerich VL, Kawachi I: Translating the socio-ecological perspective into multilevel interventions: gaps between theory and practice, *Health Educ Behav* 43(1):17–20, 2016.
Severance JH, Zinnah SL: Community-based perceptions of neighborhood health in urban neighborhoods, *J Community Health Nurs* 26(1):14–23, 2009.
Shim E, Meyers LA, Galvani AP: Optimal H1N1 vaccination strategies based on self-interest versus group interest, *BMC Public Health* 11(Suppl 1):S4, 2011.
Stanhope MS, Knollmueller RN: *Public and Community Health Nurse's Consultant: a Health Promotion Guide*, St. Louis, MO, 1997, Mosby.
Stanhope MS, Knollmueller RN, editors: *Handbook of Community-Based and Home Health Nursing Practice*, ed 3, St Louis, MO, 2000, Mosby.
Stewart M, Visker JD, Cox CC: Community health policy assessment of a rural northeast Missouri County using the Centers for Disease Control and Prevention's CHANGE tool, *Health Promot Perspect* 3(1):1–10, 2013.
Sui DZ: Tobler's first law of geography: a big idea for a small world, *Ann Assoc Am Geogr* 94(2):269–277, 2004.
Swider SM, Berkowitz B, Valentine-Maher S, Zenk SN, Bekemeier B: Engaging communities in creating health: leveraging community benefit, *Nurs Outlook* 65(5):657–660, 2017.
The Community Guide: *The Guide to community preventive services*. n. d. CDC, Atlanta GA. Retrieved from http://www.thecommunityguide.org.
Thomas Jefferson Health District: *Mobilizing for Action Through Planning and Partnerships: MAPP2Health*, 2016. Retrieved from http://www.vdh.virginia.gov.
Truglio-Londrigan, M. Gallagher, LP: Using the Seven "A's to determine older adults community resource needs. *Home Healthc Nurse* 21: 827-831, 2003.
Vance DE, Gakumo CA, Childs GD, et al.: Perceptions of brain health and cognition in older African Americans and Caucasians with HIV: a focus group study, *J Assoc Nurses AIDS Care* 28(6):862–876, 2017.
Windshield Survey Lancaster J, Mizrahi TM: *School of Social Work*, Richmond VA, 1992, Virginia Commonwealth University.
World Health Organization (WHO): A glossary of terms for community health care and services for older persons. In Centre for Health Development, *Ageing Health Tech Rep*, 5, 2004. Retrieved from http://www.who.int.
World Health Organization (WHO): *Preamble to the Constitution of the World Health Organization as adopted by the International Health Conference*, New York, 19-22 June, 1946; signed on 22 July 1946 by the representatives of 61 States (Official Records of the World Health Organization, no. 2, p. 100) and entered into force on 7 April 1948. Retrieved from http://www.who.int.
World Health Organization (WHO): *Types of healthy settings*, 2014. Retrieved from http://www.who.int.

18

Building a Culture of Health to Influence Health Equity Within Communities

Nisha D. Botchwey, PhD, MCRP, MPH, Eunhee Park, PhD, RN, APHN-BC, and Pamela A. Kulbok, DNSc, RN, PHCNS-BC, FAAN

OBJECTIVES

After reading this chapter, the student should be able to do the following:

1. Describe a culture of health and community health promotion in the context of health equity, the ecological model, and social determinants of health (SDOH).
2. Analyze participatory approaches and the interrelationships among communities, populations, and interprofessional health care providers in the application of community health promotion strategies.
3. Describe evidence-based practice using the integrative model of community health promotion at multiple levels of the client system: individual, family, aggregate, and community.
4. Analyze nursing and interprofessional roles that are essential to building a culture of health through promotion of health equity.

CHAPTER OUTLINE

Introduction
Definitions, Historical Perspectives, and Methods
Community Health Promotion Models and Frameworks
The Ecological Approach to Community Health Promotion and Health Equity
An Integrative Model for Community Health Promotion
Interprofessional Application to Nursing and Public Health
Application of the Integrative Model for Health Equity Promotion Within Communities

KEY TERMS

built environment, p. 405
client system, p. 407
community, p. 400
community-based participatory research (CBPR), p. 406
community health promotion, p. 401
culture of health, p. 395
disease-oriented perspective, p. 400
ecosocial or social-ecological, p. 397
focus of care, p. 407
health, p. 397
health belief model (HBM), p. 403
health disparities, p. 396
health equity, p. 396
health-oriented perspective, p. 400
health promotion, p. 399
illness care, p. 408
multilevel interventions, p. 402
National Prevention Strategy (NPS), p. 398
Photovoice, p. 406
population health, p. 396
social cognitive theory (SCT), p. 404
social determinants of health (SDOH), p. 398
social-ecological model, p. 404
transtheoretical model (TTM) or stages of change (SOC), p. 403
vulnerable populations, p. 397

INTRODUCTION

The Robert Wood Johnson Foundation (RWJF) introduced the **culture of health** in 2013 with an emphasis on working with other sectors to "build a national Culture of Health where everyone has the opportunity to live a healthier life." Health, equity, and well-being were core to this vision then and are even more solidified now. The public health and health care sectors are important collaborators in realizing this outcome. Health and health care remain in the forefront of national debate and dialogue about health reform; nurses and other providers are questioning the foundation of our health care system, the rules that govern what they are able to do, and how they can better contribute to a healthier nation. There is a significant shift away from acceptance of the status quo and toward building a culture of health. Such a shift puts emphasis on the pursuit of long, healthy lives for all Americans and is consistent with the national health vision and health equity goals proposed in *Healthy People 2030* (U.S. Department of Health and Human Services [USDHHS], 2018a) and the National Prevention Strategy (National Prevention Council [NPC], 2011). The RWJF notes that "[g]ood health enhances every aspect of our nation, from our economic vitality to our national security. It is key to our children's futures. Yet too often, the prospects for good health are limited by where people live, how much money they make, or barriers imposed by discrimination based on race, gender, income, and many other factors. RWJF is committed to working alongside others with respect, inclusion, and intentionality to build a Culture of Health that provides everyone with a fair and just opportunity for well-being" (2018). While most people recognize the need to exercise regularly, maintain their weight at recommended levels, and manage stress in their lives, modifiable health behaviors remain the major contributors to deaths in the United States (Centers For Disease Control and Prevention [CDC], 2014). For example, tobacco use remains the leading cause of premature deaths in the United States, with 480,000 deaths annually attributed to cigarette smoking (CDC, 2018). While the national prevalence of adult smoking continues to decline (15.5 percent) and is lower for Hispanics (10.7 percent), prevalence is double for American Indian/Alaska Natives (non-Hispanic) (31.8 percent), higher for populations with less than high school or General Educational Development (GED) educational levels (24.1-40.6 percent), and higher for populations below the poverty level (25.3 percent). This unequal distribution of cigarette smoking has cascading impacts on the annual deaths. Nurses, other health professionals, and the public recognize that initiating and maintaining a healthy lifestyle and overcoming major disparities and inequities is difficult and requires different approaches directed toward individuals, families, communities, populations, and the environments in which they live.

In this chapter the emphasis is on historical underpinnings of health and health equity within communities, including the concepts of community and social determinants of health (SDOH). In addition, community health promotion models and frameworks, including those specific to public health nursing (PHN), and health promotion models from the social sciences are discussed. These concepts and models and the ways they are related are critical to building a culture of health and determine the nature of nursing practice with communities and populations. An ecological approach to community health promotion and population health is emphasized, which integrates multilevel interventions to promote the health of the public. The integrative model of community health promotion (Laffrey & Kulbok, 1999) can help nurses plan care for clients, including communities and populations. The chapter describes studies that illustrate community-based participatory research (CBPR) and multilevel interventions. Applications of the integrative model of community health promotion show that the way nurses view these concepts is important in their approach to practice.

DEFINITIONS, HISTORICAL PERSPECTIVES, AND METHODS

Definitions: Health, Population Health, Health Equity, Health Disparities

The World Health Organization (WHO) (1948) reflected a holistic perspective in its classic definition of health as a state of complete physical, mental, and social well-being, and not merely the absence of disease and infirmity. Terris expanded the WHO definition: "Health is a state of physical, mental and social well-being and the ability to function and not merely the absence of illness and infirmity" (Terris, 1975, p. 1038). By deleting "complete" and adding "ability to function," Terris placed the WHO definition in a realistic context, providing a useful framework for health promotion.

Smith (1981), a nursing scholar, suggested that the "idea of health" directs nursing practice, education, and research. She defined health along a continuum, allowing for "more" or "less" health. Smith proposed four models of health, ordered from narrow and concrete to broad and abstract: clinical health, or absence of disease; role performance health, or ability to perform one's social roles satisfactorily; adaptive health, or flexible adaptation to the environment; and eudaemonistic health, or self-actualization and attainment of one's human potential.

Population health is a term widely used in several Institute of Medicine (IOM) reports and in contemporary health care policy. The IOM Roundtable on Population Health Improvement offered a seminal definition of population health as "the health outcomes of a group of individuals, including the distribution of such outcomes within the group" (Kindig & Stoddart, 2003, p. 381). Though not a part of the definition itself, population health outcomes are the product of multiple determinants of health, including genetics, behaviors, public health, medical care, and environmental and social factors (Adler et al., 2013; IOM, 2014).

While the history of health equity dates back to the mid-nineteenth century (Fee & Gonzalez, 2017), as indicated in our introduction, health equity is core to the current national health vision and goals of *Healthy People 2030 (2018)*. **Health equity** is the attainment of the highest level of health for all people. Achieving health equity requires valuing everyone equally with focused and ongoing societal efforts to address avoidable inequalities, historical and contemporary injustices, and the elimination of health and health care disparities. **Health disparities** on the other hand, are particular types of *health difference* that is closely linked with social or economic disadvantage. Health disparities adversely affect groups of people who have systematically experienced greater social and/or economic obstacles to health and/or a clean environment based on their racial or ethnic group; religion; socioeconomic status; gender; age; mental health; cognitive, sensory, or physical disability; sexual orientation; geographic location; or other characteristics historically linked to discrimination or exclusion. As

Benjamin Marsh, an early city planning leader, stated, "No city is more healthy than the highest death rates in any ward or block" (Coburn, 2007).

Vulnerability can be created by:

- the *presence* of a risk factor or
- the *absence* of a needed resource.

Vulnerable populations are those made vulnerable by financial circumstances, place of residence, health, age, or functional/developmental status; ability to communicate effectively; or presence of chronic or terminal illness or disability (Agency for Health Care Policy and Research, 1998).

CHECK YOUR PRACTICE

You have been asked by the public health nurse educator to seek data about the health disparities in your community and to seek assistance at the health department to find out how these disparities are being addressed. What would you do? How would you approach this assignment?

It is important for nurses and health care providers to reflect on their own definition of health and recognize how their definition influences the care they provide. Likewise, it is equally important for nurses to assess clients' personal health definitions. Only through knowledge of their own health definition, together with assessment of clients' health definitions, can nurses create interventions tailored to achieve the clients' health goals. Nurses and health care providers who emphasize health promotion and population health that is congruent with the beliefs, health definitions, and goals of the population also acknowledge the importance of illness prevention. Nurses must strive to understand health policies and the consequences of these policies on vulnerable populations whose living conditions may include few determinants of good health.

Historical Perspectives

Health is the key term in the process of building a culture of health through community health promotion. Beginning with Nightingale's efforts to discover and use the laws of nature to enhance humanity, nursing has taken an active role in promoting the health of communities and populations. The way one defines health shapes the process of nursing and health care, including making decisions about what to assess, with what level of client, and how to evaluate the outcomes of care. For example, health from a medical perspective as alleviating an individual's illness symptoms involves assessment of the duration, intensity, and frequency of specific symptoms. Intervention focuses on symptom relief and treatment of the cause of symptoms. Evaluation consists of determining the extent of symptom alleviation. On the other hand, health defined from an ecological or environmental perspective as maximizing a community's physical recreation opportunities, may involve assessment of existing recreation facilities, accessibility to the population, and beliefs and knowledge related to recreation and land use in the community as resources for healthy living.

The holistic or ecological view of health is not new. The ancient Greeks viewed health as the influence of environmental forces on human well-being and healing from illness. Scientific medicine emerged slowly, and in the twentieth century, professional care took precedence over self-care. During the last five decades the concept of self-care as derived from a positive idea of health has reemerged to compete with professional care. Some proponents of self-care emphasize lay diagnosis and self-treatment, whereas others focus on teaching people how to work with their health care providers. As a result, health care system changes include the renegotiation of roles and emphasize collaboration between consumers and providers, as well as recognition of the health impact of the conditions in which people live.

Many health professionals believe that individuals are in a position to produce health. This idea is not new. In 1974 Fuchs suggested that the "greatest potential for improving health lies in what we do and don't do for and to ourselves" (p. 55). In the political arena LaLonde introduced a similar idea in *A New Perspective on the Health of Canadians* (1974). LaLonde identified four major determinants of health: human biology, environment, lifestyle, and health care. In 1976 policy makers in the United States reinforced these determinants of health and supported efforts to improve health habits and the environment as the best hope of achieving any significant extension of life expectancy (U.S. Department of Health, Education and Welfare [USDHEW], 1976, p. 69). The fundamental ideas of these landmark documents about the determinants of health emerged during the era of social ecology (Bronfenbrenner, 1977, 1979). Box 18.1 lists some landmark initiatives in health promotion and disease prevention.

The **ecosocial or social-ecological** perspective, initially presented by Bronfenbrenner in 1977, described human-environment

BOX 18.1 Landmark Health Promotion/Disease Prevention Initiatives

1974—LaLonde's *A New Perspective on the Health of Canadians*
1976—Forward Plan for Health, FY 1978-1982
1979—*Healthy People: The Surgeon General's Report on Health Promotion and Disease Prevention*
1989—Guide to Clinical Preventive Services (USPSTF, 1989)
1990—*Healthy People 2000*
1994—Put Prevention Into Practice (PPIP)
2000—*Healthy People 2010: Understanding and Improving Health and Objectives for Improving Health,* ed. 2 (supersedes Jan 2000 conference edition)
2002—Progress reviews of *Healthy People 2010* initiated
2005—*Guide to Community Preventive Services: What Works to Promote Health?* (TFCPS, 2005)
2009—*Healthy People 2020* Framework
2010—*Healthy People 2020* Objectives
2012—Guide to Clinical Preventive Services (USPSTF, 2011)
2018—*Healthy People 2030* Framework

Data from Task Force on Community Preventive Services: *The guide to community preventive services—what works to promote health?* New York, 2005, Oxford University Press; U.S. Preventive Services Task Force: *Guide to clinical preventive services: report of the U.S. Preventive Services Task Force,* Baltimore, 1989, Lippincott, Williams & Wilkins; U.S. Preventive Services Task Force: *Guide to clinical preventive services, 2012: recommendations of the U.S. Preventive Services Task Force,* October 2011, Agency for Healthcare Research and Quality, Rockville, MD. Available at http://www.ahrq.gov.

interaction and health outcomes over a life span. The environments are described as the micro-, meso-, and macro-system levels. McLeroy et al. (1988) translated these levels of the ecological model to actionable layers of influence that include intrapersonal (characteristics of the individual), interpersonal (formal and informal social networks and social support systems), institutional (social institutions), community (mediating institutions, relationships, and power), and public policy (multilevel laws and policies).

The U.S. Public Health Service established the first national objectives involving disease prevention, health protection, and health promotion strategies in the surgeon general's *Healthy People* report. Disease prevention strategies focus on services such as family planning and immunizations delivered in clinical settings. Health protection strategies include environmental measures to improve health and quality of life. Health promotion strategies focus on achieving well-being through community and individual lifestyle change measures (USDHEW, 1979).

The current health objectives for the nation outlined in *Healthy People 2020* (USDHHS, 2018b) build on initiatives that have been pursued since 1979, as discussed in a number of chapters. Designed for use by individuals, communities, states, and professional organizations, these health objectives provided a guide for community and population programs to improve health. The release of *Healthy People 2030* will include a national vision, mission, and overarching goals. The five goals emphasized prevention, health equity, environments conducive to health for all, healthy development across the life span, and leadership for actions and policies. Information on *Healthy People 2030* objectives and action plans (USDHHS, 2018a) is available at https://www.healthypeople.gov.

The **National Prevention Strategy (NPS)** published through the U.S. Surgeon General's Office by the National Prevention Council (NPC, 2011) sought to "improve the health and quality of life for individuals, families, and communities by moving the nation from a focus on sickness and disease to one based on prevention and wellness" (NPC, 2011, p. 7). To realize this vision for children, youth, adults and the elderly, the NPS targets interventions in multiple settings. These include healthy and safe community environments, clinical and community preventive services, empowered people, and elimination of health disparities. A focus on safe and healthy communities recognizes the power of the social, economic, and environmental factors that have a stronger influence on health and well-being than does the health care setting (see Fig. 18.1 for NPS).

This idea that the health of communities and populations is shaped by multiple determinants has been reinforced in the national (Institute of Medicine [IOM], 2003) and international (World Health Organization [WHO], 2014a) health policy literature. The current focus is on determinants of population health (Fig. 18.2), which include genes and biology, health behaviors, medical care, total ecology, and social/societal characteristics (Centers for Disease Control and Prevention [CDC], 2014a; IOM, 2006). In Fig. 18.2, genes, biology, and health behavioral choices account for 25 percent of population health; and **social determinants of health (SDOH)**, including medical care and the physical and social environment, account for the remaining

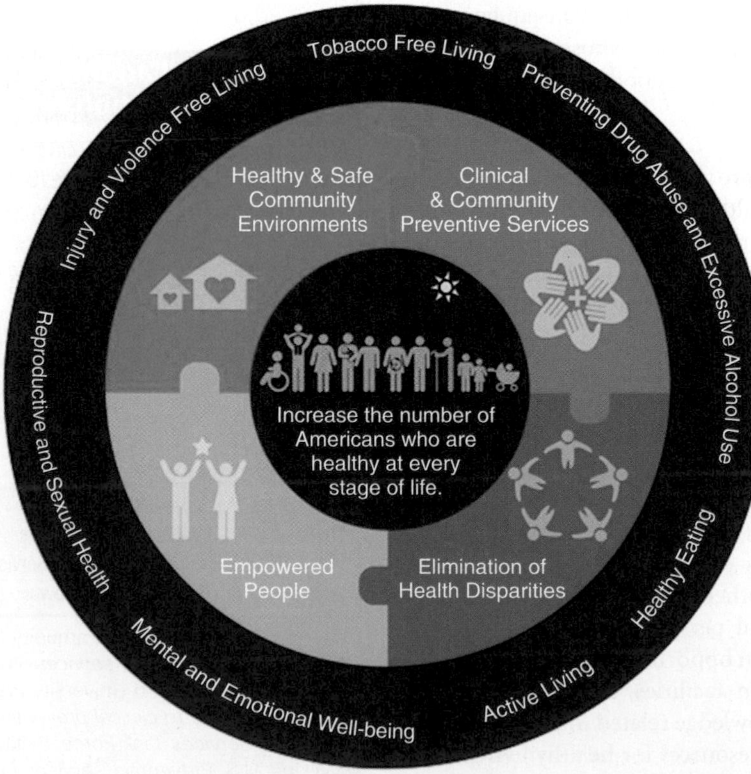

Fig. 18.1 National Prevention Strategy. (From National Prevention Council, *National Prevention Strategy*, Washington, DC, 2011, U.S. Department of Health and Human Services, Office of the Surgeon General. Available at http://www.surgeongeneral.gov.)

DETERMINANTS OF POPULATION HEALTH

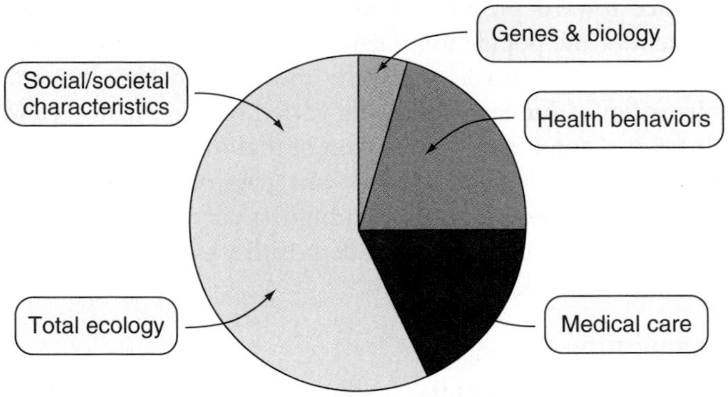

Fig. 18.2 Determinants of population health. (From Centers for Disease Control and Prevention: *Social determinants of health*. Available at http://www.cdc.gov.)

75 percent. Although recent trends reveal improvement in determinants of population health such as healthier living conditions and a decrease in smoking, these positive trends are associated with persistent socioeconomic disparities worldwide (WHO, 2014a) (see Healthy People 2020 box).

HEALTHY PEOPLE 2020

Tobacco Use

Selected objectives from *Healthy People 2020* that pertain to tobacco use:

- **TU-1**: Reduce tobacco use by adults.
- **TU-2**: Reduce tobacco use by adolescents.
- **TU-3**: Reduce the initiation of tobacco use among children, adolescents, and young adults.
- **TU-6**: Increase smoking cessation during pregnancies.
- **TU-7**: Increase smoking cessation by adolescent smokers.
- **TU-11**: Reduce the proportion of nonsmokers exposed to secondhand smoke.

From U.S. Department of Health and Human Services: *Healthy People 2020*. Available at http://www.healthypeople.gov.

Definitions of Health Promotion. Health promotion is an aim of nursing and health care, although explicit definition of health promotion and differentiation from disease prevention or health maintenance is rare. Leavell and Clark (1965) strongly influenced the evolution of health promotion and disease prevention strategies through their classic definitions of primary, secondary, and tertiary levels of prevention that were rooted in the biomedical model of health and epidemiology. The application of preventive measures, according to Leavell and Clark, corresponds to the natural history or stages of disease (see Chapter 13). Primary preventive measures apply to "well" individuals in the prepathogenesis period to promote their health and to provide specific protection from disease. Secondary preventive measures apply to diagnosis or to treatment of individuals in the period of disease pathogenesis. Tertiary prevention addresses rehabilitation and the return of people with chronic illness to a maximal ability to function (see Levels of Prevention box).

LEVELS OF PREVENTION

Substance Use

Primary Prevention

The goal for primary prevention is to prevent people from starting to use substances and to promote the nonuse of substances. Universal prevention programs including education need to be provided. In addition, vulnerable groups with risk factors for substance use can be identified, and active education can be proactively provided.

Secondary Prevention

Secondary prevention focuses on assessing people who have substance use problems and early detection of people who have used substances. Through this effort we must help people who have used substances from developing further problems with addiction.

Tertiary Prevention

For a person diagnosed with substance use and abuse, we need to provide appropriate interventions for managing symptoms and treating complications of addictive symptoms. Appropriate rehabilitation treatment must be provided as tertiary prevention.

Even though primary, secondary, and tertiary levels of prevention had their origins in the medical model, Leavell and Clark (1965) moved beyond the medical model. They conceptualized primary prevention as having two distinct components: health promotion and specific protection. Health promotion focuses on positive measures such as education for healthy living and promotion of favorable environmental conditions, as well as periodic examinations including, for example, well-child developmental assessment and health education. Specific protection includes measures to reduce the threat of specific diseases or injury, such as hygiene, immunizations, use of seat belts, and the elimination of workplace hazards.

Health promotion and specific protection, when used as subconcepts of primary prevention, stem from a definition of health as the absence of disease. However, health promotion and specific protection strategies are not the same. Some terms used to describe health promotion are linked to a positive view of health (e.g., *health habits* or *health practices*), whereas other terms are linked to the negative view of the absence of disease (e.g., *disease* or *illness prevention*). Using the terms *health promotion, health protection,* and *disease prevention* interchangeably, as indicators of preventive behavior, leads to confusion (Kulbok et al., 1997). Interestingly, similar confusion exists today in the field of health education regarding definition of the terms *health behavior*, *health education*, and *health promotion* (Simons-Morton, 2013). As interprofessional practice opportunities increase, public health nurses need to have clear definitions in mind when they use terms associated with community health promotion.

The WHO described health promotion as a process that enables individuals to increase control over and improve their health (WHO, 2014b). According to the 1986 Ottawa Charter, health promotion combines both individual- and community-level strategies to build healthful public policy, create supportive environments, strengthen community action, develop personal skills, and reorient health services. Health is a resource for daily living. For individuals or communities to realize physical, mental, and social well-being, they must become aware of and learn to use the social and personal resources available within their environment. However, resources are not equally distributed across environments; thus even this approach can lead to inequities.

There is considerable evidence supporting a positive view of health underlying health promotion activities directed toward individuals, communities, and populations. The WHO's definition of health promotion as a process and the current focus on an ecological approach to determinants of population health are grounded in the perspective of positive health. These approaches view health promotion in the context of a holistic healthy lifestyle, as well as involving simultaneous interaction with the social and physical environments. Clearly, health promotion and population health are consistent with the goals of public health nursing.

Disease-Oriented Versus Process and Environmentally Oriented Health and Health Promotion. Nurses have long recognized the importance of an emphasis on wellness and health promotion in health care. In PHN practice it is clear that many factors, beyond illness, affect the health of individuals, communities, and populations. The biomedical model, in which health is defined as absence of disease, does not explain why some populations exposed to illness-producing stressors remain healthy, whereas others, who appear to be in health-enhancing situations, become ill. Viewing clients from the perspective of the biomedical model alone makes it difficult to identify health potential beyond the absence of disease in the individual. For example, most at-risk populations such as the frail elderly have at least one diagnosed chronic disease. Limiting the definition of health potential to the absence of disease, nurses would never perceive this population as healthy. Defining health as the absence of disease is a pessimistic and individual-level definition; nursing actions can help older, chronically ill, and vulnerable persons become healthier if a broader definition of health is used.

Laffrey et al. (1986) describe two perspectives from which the key concepts of nursing science (e.g., person, health, environment) and nursing can be viewed. The first is the **disease-oriented perspective** that views health objectively and defines it as the absence of disease as discussed previously. This perspective assumes that humans are composed of organ systems and cells; in this instance, health care focuses on identifying what is not working properly with a given system and repairing it. In this context, health behavior begins with patient compliance with health professionals' recommendations. The second perspective defines health subjectively as a process, not as a presence or absence. In this **health-oriented perspective**, humans are complex and ever-changing systems and are interconnected with others and the environment. Health behavior within this latter health-oriented perspective involves a holistic view of lifestyle and interaction with the environment and not simply compliance with a prescribed regimen. It allows nurses to begin to see the sources of health disparities across populations.

Both perspectives support the aims and processes of population-focused nursing. The disease-oriented approach directs nursing toward illness prevention, risk appraisal, risk reduction, prompt treatment, and disease management of individuals. However, the health-oriented approach directs nursing practice toward promotion of positive health for a larger segment of the population. Defining health broadly as the life process, taking into account the mutual and simultaneous interaction of humans and their varied environments, views illness as a potential manifestation of that interaction. Because positive health does not exclude any part of the life process (it includes illness prevention and illness care), it goes beyond the disease perspective to include positive and holistic health (Laffrey & Kulbok, 1999).

Community

Another concept essential to building a culture of health through community health promotion is **community**. The emphasis on community as the target of practice gained increased attention since the mid-1970s when the U.S. and Canadian governments and health researchers attributed declining mortality and morbidity rates to better standards of living, such as sanitation, clean air and water, and wider availability of healthy foods. Again, these approaches were consistent with emerging ideas about social ecology during the same period. Notably, these approaches are also consistent with the current emphasis on health equity for all. The IOM's seminal report on the future of public health highlighted the importance of community in its statement that the "mission of public health is to assure conditions in which people can be healthy by generating organized community effort to prevent disease and promote health" (National Research Council [NRC], 1988, p. 7). (See Chapter 17 for more on the concept of community.)

As discussed previously, national health goals emphasize that environment and community are central to achieving health. *Healthy People in Healthy Communities: A Community Planning Guide Based on Healthy People 2010* (USDHHS, 2001) (Box 18.2) outlines practical recommendations for coalition building, creating a vision, and measuring outcomes to improve

BOX 18.2 Healthy People 2010

A Strategy for Creating a Healthy Community

To achieve the goal of improving health, a community must develop a strategy supported by many individuals who are working together. The MAP-IT technique helps you to map out the path toward the change you want to see in your community. This guide recommends that you MAP-IT—that is, ***m***obilize, ***a***ssess, ***p***lan, ***i***mplement, and ***t***rack.

Mobilize individuals and organizations that care about the health of your community into a coalition.

Assess the areas of greatest need in your community, as well as the resources and other strengths that you can tap into to address those areas.

Plan your approach: start with a vision of where you want to be as a community; then add strategies and action steps to help you achieve that vision.

Implement your plan using concrete action steps that can be monitored and will make a difference.

Track your progress over time.

Modified from Milio N: A framework for prevention: changing health damaging to health-generating life patterns. *Am J Public Health* 66:435, 1976.

the health of communities. Communities can tailor these recommendations to their own local needs, and health professionals in public and private organizations can work together with community members to develop programs that fit the needs and resources of their own communities and thus target strategies to address areas of greatest need. The NPS also offers recommendations on what can be done to improve population health in specified contexts and across goal areas (NPC, 2011). Nurses participate in this collaborative and interprofessional process through community assessments, community development activities, and identification of key persons in the community with whom to build partnerships for health programs. Nurses working with nonprofit hospitals can also directly engage in improving health of communities through completion of a Community Health Needs Assessment (CHNA) as required under the Affordable Care Act (Rosenbaum, 2013).

One of the four overarching goals of the *Healthy People 2020* Framework is to create social and physical environments that promote good health for all (USDHHS, 2014d). Community-wide program planning provides a strategy to achieve this goal. *Healthy People 2020* highlighted a community framework called MAP-IT (USDHHS, 2018c) as a guide to using *Healthy People 2020* in a local community (see http://healthypeople.gov). MAP-IT stands for Mobilize, Assess, Plan, Implement, and Track; communities can use the guide to evaluate public health interventions designed to implement the goals of *Healthy People 2020.*

Nurses and interprofessional health care providers have many opportunities to participate in community-wide health care. To address community problems, these professionals need to integrate concepts of health and illness, individual and population, public health and health care, health promotion and disease prevention, and ecology and environmental health. This integration means that nurses must consider the complex relationship between personal and environmental forces that affect health. Over 40 years ago Milio (1976) offered a set of propositions for improving health behavior by considering personal choices in the context of available societal resources. These propositions (Box 18.3) remain relevant today. They constitute a fitting model for health promotion that addresses both personal and societal resources for this and future decades.

BOX 18.3 Milio's Propositions for Improving Health Behavior

- Health status of populations is a function of the lack or excess of health-sustaining resources.
- Behavior patterns of populations are related to habits of choice from actual or perceived limited resources and related attitudes.
- Organizational decisions determine the range of personal resources available.
- Individual health-related decisions are influenced by efforts to maximize valued resources in both the personal and societal domains.
- Social change is reflective of a change in population behavior patterns.
- Health education will impact behavior patterns minimally without new health-promoting options for investing personal resources.

From U.S. Department of Health and Human Services: A strategy for creating a healthy community: MAP-IT. In *Healthy people in healthy communities: a community planning guide using Healthy People 2010,* Washington, DC, 2001, U.S. Government Printing Office.

COMMUNITY HEALTH PROMOTION MODELS AND FRAMEWORKS

Numerous models and frameworks have **community health promotion** as the goal. The following sections provide brief descriptions of models specific to community and/or health promotion that are useful to public health nurses practicing at a basic or advanced level. In this section public health nursing community models and frameworks and general health promotion models and frameworks will be introduced. These models can be the basis for addressing community health issues and will furthermore contribute to addressing health equity at the community level.

Public Health Nursing Community Models and Frameworks

Although theoretical frameworks developed within nursing and other health disciplines are traditionally oriented toward individuals, there is increasing recognition of the importance of community and person–environment interactions that go beyond social cognitive theory and other interpersonal frameworks (USDHHS, 2005; Bigbee & Issel, 2012) in promoting health. Particularly, public health nurses realize that the community is more than the sum of the individuals, families, aggregates, and organizations within it and that interaction is essential for any real change to occur. PHN defined community as "... persons in interaction, being and experiencing together, who may or may not share a sense of common purpose" (ANA, 2013, p. 65). The following are examples of PHN models focused on interventions with communities or populations.

Chopoorian (1986) was among the first to acknowledge that nurses could strengthen their position with communities by focusing on the social, economic, and political structures that make up the community, as well as the social relations and patterns of everyday life in the community. Within this perspective, interventions targeted to public health policy can have far-reaching health benefits. Shuster and Goeppinger (2012) asserted that definitions of *community* vary widely and that nurses working with communities learn quickly that there are many different aspects to define community. Shuster and Goeppinger highlighted the importance of person, place, and function, as well as interaction among systems within a community. Nurses must examine the complexity and dynamic nature inherent in the process of community building, rather than viewing the community as a geographic, racial, or cultural group that is static.

Despite the ideal, it is not easy to integrate the concept of the community as client into practice. Consequently, the provision of care to individuals *in the community* may still overshadow nursing practice and health promotion directed *to the community.* Bekemeier and Jones (2010), in a study of local public health agency (LPHA) functions, leadership, and staffing, reported that the proportion of nursing staff in an LPHA related strongly to provision of services involving individual-level care.

They found that the staff nurses were most likely to perform individual-family interventions, and that both the staff nurses and the managers rated individual-family interventions as more important than community- or system-level interventions. These findings suggest that there is an ongoing need to expand "... education and outreach to nurses regarding their roles and responsibilities to assure environmental health protection, community assessment, and health improvement planning" (Bekemeier & Jones, 2010, p. E16).

Kuehnert introduced a model to treat the community as a client in PHN (Kuehnert, 1995). The interactive and organizational model of community as client emphasized addressing the organizational context of individual, family, and community as the main focus of PHN. In this way the community can be treated as a major client.

Anderson and McFarlane (1988, 2011) and Salmon (1993, 2009) developed system models based on the assumption that assessing the various components of the system (i.e., individual, family, community, and society) facilitates a healthy community. Anderson and McFarlane's community-as-partner model includes eight major community subsystems. The basic core of the community, according to these authors, is its people, described by their demographic characteristics and their values, beliefs, culture, religion, laws, and more. Within the community system the people interact with the other subsystems. A community health assessment must include information about the subsystems and the pattern of interactions among the subsystems and of the total community with the systems external to it.

Salmon's model (1993, 2009) focused on the public health mission of organized efforts to protect, promote, and restore health. It embraces multiple determinants of health and is consistent with the IOM's perspective on population health (IOM, 2014). According to Salmon's model, nursing includes health promotion, illness prevention, and health protection strategies. Systems models provide important guidance for assessing communities and populations and indicate that system-level interventions require participation with relevant subsystems. However, systems models may not provide the guidance needed for intervention development.

Keller et al. (1998, 2004) proposed a population-based intervention model based on the scope of PHN practice that crosses multiple levels of care; this model defines the population-focused underpinning of PHN practice and provides guidance for PHN interventions at the individual, community, and system levels. The model was later termed the *Intervention Wheel* (Keller et al., 2004, p. 453). The Intervention Wheel includes community, systems, and individual/family levels of practice. (See Chapter 11 for information and updates on the Intervention Wheel.) It is population based and identifies 17 public health interventions.

A comprehensive multilevel nursing practice model (May et al., 2003) was developed based on the PHN practice model and community-based action research framework. This model focuses on public health nurses' roles by integrating general nurses' roles and unique care for the community. Thus this model emphasizes community-based interventions using community empowerment in addition to personal preventive nursing and organized indigenous caregiving. Community empowerment is an important part of this model to address community health issues with community-based participatory approaches, such as organized social action, community building, and mobilizing community resources.

The models proposed by Anderson and McFarlane (1998, 2011), Salmon (1993, 2009), Kuehnert (1995), Keller et al. (1998, 2004), and May et al. (2003) focus on stability and equilibrium. In the past the models were used to emphasize protecting the community from specific disease risks in most cases; less attention is directed toward factors that promote an optimally healthy community. A few of the classic community-wide epidemiologic studies focused on **multilevel interventions** or community health promotion are described next.

Influential Multilevel Community Studies. Two significant community studies of health risks, morbidity, and mortality are the Framingham Heart Study, initiated in 1949, and the Human Population Laboratory's longitudinal survey in Alameda County, California, initiated in the early 1970s. The Framingham Heart Study followed 5209 adults over their life span to identify factors contributing to coronary heart disease (CHD). Collecting periodic health assessments and morbidity and mortality data, the study identified major risk factors associated with CHD mortality (e.g., elevated systolic blood pressure, elevated serum cholesterol level, and cigarette smoking). The investigators used health risk appraisals to relate the risk factors in well individuals to the probability of future cardiovascular disease (Lieb et al., 2009). The Framingham study celebrated 70 years of research in 2018 and continues today (see http://www.framinghamheartstudy.org/).

The Alameda County study measured the relationships of health and social behaviors to mortality in a community sample of 6928 individuals over 4 years. The behaviors included eating three meals daily, eating breakfast, sleeping 7 to 8 hours a night, using alcohol moderately, exercising regularly, not smoking, maintaining a desirable weight-to-height ratio, and maintaining social networks. There was a positive relationship between smoking and excessive alcohol use and mortality. There was an inverse relationship between physical exercise, 7 to 8 hours of sleep, optimal weight in relation to height, and social networks and mortality (Berkman & Breslow, 1983). These findings led to the emphasis on social and environmental variables, in addition to personal behaviors, in strategies for community health promotion.

Findings from these early large-scale surveys prompted a number of public health multilevel intervention programs. Examples include the Stanford Five-City Heart Disease Prevention program (Farquhar et al., 1990), the North Karelia study (Puska et al., 1983), the Pawtucket Heart Health program (Lasater et al., 1984), the Minnesota Heart Health program (Luepker et al., 1994), and the Dutch Heart Health Community Intervention (Ronda et al., 2005). These programs provided beginning scientific evidence for the implementation of community-level risk reduction programs, although the results were modest and often not statistically significant. These studies were major contributions to theory and practice in building community partnerships, establishing social marketing, developing behavior change strategies, and evaluating health programs. Results of these studies make it clear that multiple levels of intervention are necessary to reach the community in a meaningful way. Nurses have close relationships with individuals; families; high-risk groups; organizations such as schools, congregations, and workplaces; and other health care professionals. Nurses can contribute to health promotion and health equity by participating in community projects such as the ones described here. It is important that nurses develop health programs that focus on health equity and document improved outcomes for communities and vulnerable populations with whom they interact.

Health Promotion Models and Frameworks

There are a variety of theoretical approaches that can be used to help public health nurses design and implement health promotion programs for individuals and communities. The National Cancer Institute's seminal document, *Theory at a Glance* (USDHHS, 2005), organized these health promotion models and frameworks into three levels, which are consistent with the ecological perspective used in this chapter. The first level is intrapersonal or individual, including models focused on knowledge, attitudes, personal beliefs and values. The second level is interpersonal, including models that emphasize processes and groups such as family, friends, and peers who may provide support. The third level is community, which includes institutional structures and policies that may enhance or inhibit health behavior. Brief descriptions of selected models and frameworks are provided in the following sections. While this multilevel approach to health promotion did not explicitly address health equity, the goal of health promotion is consistent with the goal of equity—to provide opportunities for all people "to attain their full health potential regardless of demographic, social, economic or geographic strata" (WHO, 2018).

Individual Health Promotion Models. There are several intrapersonal or individual level models, including the health belief model, the theory of reasoned action and the theory of planned behavior, the stages of change or transtheoretical model, and the precaution adoption process model (Edberg, 2013). The **health belief model (HBM)** can be used to plan programs to increase an individual's motivation to take a positive health action. The HBM was one of the first theories of health behavior; it began in the 1950s, when the U.S. Public Health Service sent mobile units to communities to provide chest x-rays as a way to screen for tuberculosis (Rosenstock, 1974). The chest x-rays were free, convenient, and painless, yet people did not take advantage of the service. A group of social psychologists tried to explain the failure to use this screening and to determine what would motivate people to seek health care.

The HBM includes six components that attempt to determine what motivates an individual to adopt a health behavior. These components are (1) perceived susceptibility ("Will something happen to me?"); (2) perceived severity ("If something does happen to me, will it be a big problem?"); (3) perceived benefits ("If I do what is suggested, will it really help me?"); (4) perceived barriers ("If I do what is suggested, will there be barriers that will be unpleasant or costly?"); (5) cues to action ("What might motivate me to take the recommended action?"); and (6) self-efficacy ("Can I really do this?"). This model provides guidance in planning health promotion programs because it reminds nurses to think carefully about what motivates people to change. To understand motivation, it is important to learn (1) how people involved feel about the health problem, (2) whether they think the problem is serious, (3) whether they think that action on their part will make a difference, and (4) whether they think they can both manage the barriers and actually perform the action (Edberg, 2013; USDHHS, 2005).

The **transtheoretical model (TTM) or stages of change (SOC)** and the precaution adoption process model (PAPM) are discussed together because they both deal with the process of change that occurs in stages and over time. The TTM or SOC has six stages:

1. **Precontemplation,** in which the person does not plan to change; this may be because the person does not know there is a problem or does not want to do anything about it. For example, a person may not know that potential exposure to radon, a cancer-causing radioactive gas that he cannot see, smell, or taste in his home, is a health risk.
2. **Contemplation,** in which the person begins thinking about making a change in the future and examines the pros and cons of doing so. The person may have heard about home radon exposure on the local news and is considering whether his home may have unsafe levels of radon and whether he should test for radon.
3. **Preparation,** in which the person intends to do something. In the example about radon exposure, the person might contact the environmental office of the local health department for advice about radon testing.
4. **Action** occurs when the person actually buys a radon-testing kit and uses it in his home.
5. **Maintenance** is when the person decides to test for radon and to take measures to reduce radon to acceptable levels.
6. **Termination** is when the person has adopted and sustained the behavior change process. For most behaviors this stage is rarely accomplished, and individuals stay in the maintenance stage (Edberg, 2013; USDHHS, 2005).

Although the terms used are slightly different, the intent of the PAPM is similar to the TTM or SOC. The stages are (1) unaware of the issue, (2) unengaged by the issue, (3) deciding about acting, (4) deciding not to act, (5) deciding to act, (6) acting, and (7) maintenance. You can apply the cooking example later in this chapter to these stages as well (Edberg, 2013).

Interpersonal Health Promotion Models. Interpersonal-level models generally involve interaction between individuals and the social environment. These models focus on the reciprocal or mutual nature of interaction; that is, the person's thoughts, feelings, or actions are influenced by and also exert influence on his or her immediate environment. The social environment typically involves family, friends, peers, co-workers, health providers, and others (USDHHS, 2005). Social learning theory, social cognitive theory, social network theory, and social support (Edberg, 2013) are examples of interpersonal-level frameworks that are useful for health promotion. Social cognitive theory (SCT) is one of the commonly used interpersonal theories. It evolved from Bandura's social learning theory (SLT), which proposed that individuals learned from their own behaviors and from observations of the behaviors of others and the benefits of those behaviors. Bandura expanded SLT by adding the construct of self-efficacy, which addresses the degree of confidence individuals have in their ability to perform a behavior (Edberg, 2013; USDHHS, 2005).

Continuing with the example of radon exposure, an individual would need to believe that he was capable of obtaining a radon test kit, understanding the directions for radon testing, and using it properly to test radon levels in his home. Note that there are incremental, small steps involved in a behavior seemingly as simple as using a radon testing kit. Bandura stressed the importance of understanding the target behavior in order to plan potential strategies to assist an individual in the process of behavior change. In addition to understanding the target behavior, change strategies based on SCT include (1) verbal persuasion, (2) role modeling, (3) positive affective response, and (4) positive reinforcement of the behavior. Strategies that public health nurses can use to change behavior include (1) communication skills to persuade a person to test his home for radon, (2) modeling the radon testing behavior, (3) emphasizing the positive emotional response associated with reducing the health risk for his family, and (4) providing positive encouragement and affirmation when the person has completed the radon testing in his home.

Community Level Health Promotion Models. The social-ecological model is a model used to guide PHN interventions for community health promotion (USDHHS, 2005; Edberg, 2013). The social-ecological model (SEM) guides health promotion as well as illness prevention interventions. According to this model, health care and health-related behavior are a function of individual, interpersonal, organizational, community, and population factors. Thus interventions are specific to each of these levels. In one of the first comprehensive studies using the SEM to assess factors related to the uptake of influenza vaccine, researchers examined vaccine uptake during the 2009 H1N1 pandemic. Of the 2079 adults surveyed, only 18.4 percent reported that they received the 2009 H1N1 vaccine. The results indicated that variables at all SEM levels influenced acquiring the vaccination: intrapersonal level explained 53 percent; interpersonal explained 47 percent; institutional level explained 34 percent; and the policy and community levels each explained eight percent of the variance related to influenza vaccine uptake. Together the SEM levels explained 65 percent of the variance in vaccine uptake. These data indicated that interventions aimed at multiple levels might be more effective than those targeting a single level (Kumar et al., 2013) (see Evidence-Based Practice box).

EVIDENCE-BASED PRACTICE

A study of leisure time physical activity (LTPA) in African American adults, which used the social-ecological model, helped to clarify relationships between LTPA and social-ecological factors such as self-efficacy, self-regulation, social support, outcome expectations, and policy beliefs (Li et al., 2012). The results suggested that self-regulation and intention to organize personal time for routine PA may yield successful results and that a PA intervention may succeed if participants in the intervention include people in their close network who support each other. In addition, the results suggested that planning policies to enhance the built environment and satisfy the community have the potential for wide reaching effect on PA levels of African Americans. Several other major community-wide studies have drawn on concepts such as those presented in these models.

Nurse Use

As the nurse works with a population in a community, identify persons in a close network and develop approaches to improving the health of that network that can be regulated by the individuals in the network and are flexible.

THE ECOLOGICAL APPROACH TO COMMUNITY HEALTH PROMOTION AND HEALTH EQUITY

Ecological Perspectives on Community Health Promotion and Population Health

Community health promotion and population health can be achieved with ecological perspectives. However, because individuals ultimately make decisions to engage in healthy or risky behaviors, lifestyle improvement efforts have focused typically on the individual as the target of care. Following the HBM (Rosenstock, 1974), individuals generally concentrate on immediate personal rewards or threats when deciding whether to engage in specific behaviors; in this context they may convince themselves that their immediate personal risks from certain behaviors such as smoking are low, or that the immediate rewards outweigh the risks. However, from a public health perspective, smoking in the United States has resulted in more than 480,000 deaths annually (CDC, 2018). Though still alarming, the percent of American adults who smoked in 2016 was 15.5 percent, down from 43 percent in 1964. However, inequities are apparent as rates remain higher for non-Hispanic American Indians/Alaska Natives (31.8 percent), non-Hispanic multi-race individuals (25.2 percent), and non-Hispanic African Americans (16.6 percent) (CDC, 2018). Moreover, we continue to increase spending on smoking-related medical care for adults, nearly $170 billion in 2016, and more than $156 billion in worker productivity costs due to premature death and second-hand smoke exposure (CDC, 2018; Xu et al., 2015). Therefore, it is clear that health behaviors extend beyond the individual or the intrapersonal and the interpersonal levels, having multiple determinants both internal and external to individuals and communities, as well as determinants within the society. These determinants of health inequity include demographic, economic, social, and geographic factors.

For example, adolescents' decisions not to smoke are associated with their individual attributes (e.g., positive self-image), family characteristics (e.g., parent-child connectedness), aggregate characteristics (e.g., peer influence), and community factors (e.g., living in a tobacco-growing region) (Kulbok et al., 2008a). As a result, interventions to initiate or maintain healthy behaviors have greater potential for success when directed systematically toward the multiple targets of the individual, family, group, community, and society—that is, when they use an ecological approach to community health promotion.

Farley and Cohen (2005) give an example of how to apply the ecological model to population-level health issues. They introduced the curve-shifting principle. This principle complements the ecological model and calls for targeting health interventions at the population level. They built on representations of the relationship between individual and group behavior (Rose, 1992), with individual behavior being the foundation of the total population distribution. The median of this normal distribution represents prevailing social norms that govern health behavior. Traditional approaches to health behavior interventions for public health problems like obesity focus on the intrapersonal and interpersonal levels for high-risk populations—people at the extremes of the population curve. Although treating high-risk populations may be effective for selected individuals and may move them closer to the center or the prevailing social norm, this approach does little to prevent others from becoming the extremes of the distribution. Therefore a focus on the total population, not just the high-risk group, with efforts to change the social norm so that everyone is consuming less sugar or participating in more hours of moderate to vigorous physical activity, exemplifies the curve-shifting principle.

Ecological Perspectives on Social Determinants of Health

Current trends in public health and health promotion emphasize the ecological perspective on interaction between individuals and the environment. Thus the ecological approach also addresses the SDOH and achieves health equity (McQueen, 2009) through social networks, organizations, neighborhoods, and communities (Navarro et al., 2007; Gorin et al., 2012; Paskett et al., 2016). According to the WHO, SDOH "are the conditions in which people are born, grow up, live, work and age, including their health. These circumstances are in turn shaped by a wider set of forces: economics, social policies, and politics" (2010, p. 1). The WHO is an important contributor to defining and developing strategies to address the SDOH and has outlined 10 components of SDOH (Box 18.4).

There is increasing awareness that to achieve lasting gains in population health, assessments and interventions must be directed to multiple levels of the client system like those outlined in the SDOH. For example, a multilevel analysis of depressive symptoms in a national sample of 18,473 adolescents in the United States (Wight et al., 2005) showed that individual, family, aggregate, and community characteristics accounted for significant differences in adolescent depression. The American Academy of Pediatrics (2005) issued a statement urging pediatricians to increase their partnerships with communities in developing programs to improve child health. Examples of pediatrician-community partnerships (Sanders et al., 2005) include establishing a child health consultant program, working with a community to repair and fund sites to facilitate safe physical activity for children, developing dance programs for overweight and obese adolescent girls, and arranging a program for community leaders to learn about the Medicaid enrollment process. Traditional interventions that target only an individual's risk or illness are not as effective as interventions and programs developed using an ecological approach that can affect all levels of the client system that contribute to good or ill health (Navarro et al., 2007).

BOX 18.4 The Social Determinants of Health

1. *The Social Gradient:* Life expectancy is shorter and most diseases are more common further down the social ladder in each society.
2. *Stress:* Stressful circumstances—making people feel worried, anxious, and unable to cope—are damaging to health and may lead to premature death.
3. *Early Life:* The health impact of early development and education lasts a lifetime.
4. *Social Exclusion:* Hardship and resentment, poverty, social exclusion, and discrimination cost lives.
5. *Work:* Stress in the workplace increases the risk of disease. People who have more control over their work have better health.
6. *Unemployment:* Job security increases health, well-being, and job satisfaction. Higher rates of unemployment cause more illness and premature death.
7. *Social Support:* Friendship, good social relations, and strong supportive networks improve health at home, at work, and in the community.
8. *Addiction:* Individuals turn to alcohol, drugs, and tobacco and suffer from their use, but use is influenced by the wider social setting.
9. *Food:* Because global market forces control the food supply, healthy food is a political issue.
10. *Transport:* Healthy transport means less driving and more walking and cycling, backed up by better public transport.

From World Health Organization. *Social determinants of health*, 2010, Geneva. Available at https://www.who.int.

Consider another example of addressing the SDOH using an ecological perspective. According to *Healthy People 2020*, the neighborhood and the built environment are one of the five key elements of SDOH (USDHH, 2018d). The **built environment** includes the physical parts of the environment where we live and work (e.g., homes, buildings, streets, open spaces, and infrastructure) and sources of access to foods, quality of housing, and crime and violence (CDC, 2013; USDHHS, 2018d). Thus the built environment is related to issues, particularly health disparities (Gordon-Larsen et al., 2006). For example, Prentice and Jebb (1995) were among the first to report the association between obesity and the built environment by measuring inactivity, car ownership, and television viewing.

To address health disparity issues related to the built environment, a multilevel approach with an ecological perspective is needed. For example, instead of simply teaching children the importance of walking and biking to school, the Safe Routes to Schools initiative improved the environment and the walkability of areas near schools, which correlates with increased walking among residents (Owen et al., 2004). Increased walking among local adult residents is evidence that "... increasing neighborhood walkability may affect people in the larger community, not just schoolchildren" (Watson et al., 2008, p. 5). As a result, the population living nearest to walkable areas will walk more, thereby shifting the population social norms about walking and biking, including to school. People's behavior will change based on targeted interventions to the environment in which they live, a concept advanced by B.F. Skinner (1978), a behavioral psychologist in the 1950s. These multilevel approaches with the ecological perspectives of health promotion and illness prevention show how to address health equity in those issues in order to shift social norms governing health behavior and ultimately health outcomes.

Community-Based Participatory Research

The aim of PHN is to create equal partnerships with individuals, families, groups, and communities to promote their health. **Community-based participatory research (CBPR)**, grounded in epistemology and critical social theories (Minkler & Wallerstein, 2008), provides the philosophical and theoretical basis for forming partnerships and for collaboration with the community. Researchers have used CBPR to conduct ecological, community, and environmental assessments. This approach to community assessment allows understanding of sociocultural contexts, systems, and meaning through a collaborative research process that allows for more equitable treatment. In CBPR, partnerships are active, and community members are authentically involved in assessing, planning, implementing, and evaluating change. Both professionals and community residents determine health needs and plan interventions. As residents increase their awareness, they are better able to articulate what they want for themselves, their families, and their community, and they are more likely to take leadership roles in program development, using health professionals as consultants. It is important that the health professional determine the capacity of the community in CBPR so their contributions can be maximized and supported for future action.

Just as early PHN roles extended beyond disease prevention and illness care to encompass advocacy, community organizing, health education, and political and social reform (Kulbok & Glick, 2014), contemporary PHN roles emphasize collaboration with community organizations and community members. Kulbok et al. (2012) examined emerging PHN roles that address complex, multicausal, community problems. They used a community participatory and ethnographic community assessment model and provided a PHN exemplar from their CBPR project, Youth Substance Use Prevention in a Rural County. The project involved an interprofessional team (i.e., the community participatory research team [CPRT]), including an advanced practice public health nurse, a human development specialist, a psychologist, an architecture and urban planning specialist, a nurse anthropologist, graduate students, and youths, parents, and leaders from the rural community. The CPRT used community participatory strategies, geographic information systems (GIS) mapping, and Photovoice to design a substance use prevention program in a rural tobacco-growing county in the South. The CPRT completed a comprehensive community and environmental assessment of the county, its rural ecology, context, demographics, history and culture, and reviewed evidence-based prevention programs as the foundation for designing and implementing a targeted youth substance use prevention program that was acceptable, effective, relevant, and sustainable by the rural county.

In another example of a CBPR project, the community residents of the East Side Village Health Worker Partnership (ESVHWP) on Detroit's East Side developed a community-based program titled Healthy Eating and Exercising to Reduce Diabetes (HEED) (Schulz et al., 2005). The purpose was to increase community awareness about diabetes and prevention. Community groups and individuals with expertise in diabetes served as the project steering committee. They developed training protocols and recruited and trained community advocates. After training completion the HEED advocates developed activities to promote healthy diets and physical activity. The advocates and other community residents identified important barriers to healthy dietary choices, such as lack of access to grocery stores and fresh produce. Members of the HEED project established a monthly mini-market at a community site with a few retail outlets carrying high-quality produce. The project was successful in fostering a strong interest among participants in healthy cooking demonstrations and cooking techniques. Subsequently the HEED project joined forces with another community initiative to obtain funding to expand the mini-markets and food demonstrations.

The Physical Activity and Neighborhood Resources in High School Girls study (Pate et al., 2008) followed an ecological model based on the social cognitive theory for adolescent females in urban, suburban, and rural communities. Researchers hypothesized that physical activity is influenced by a comprehensive set of personal, social, and physical environmental factors. Using GIS mapping, mixed regression models on body mass index (BMI) and environmental variables, as well as 3-day physical activity recall, they found that the physical environment explained less than five percent of the variance in physical activity among adolescent girls. However, after adjusting for race, BMI, socioeconomic status (SES), and household income, there was an association between churches and vigorous physical activity. An additional study by Botchwey (2007) showed that up to 80 percent of congregations and faith-based organizations offer health services to their community, with a greater variety of offerings than secular nonprofit organizations. Therefore, as nurses work with communities, it is important to consider the social and physical components of the environment, especially those actively engaged in health promotion.

Photovoice Method and Projects

Photovoice is a novel method used in CBPR projects that integrates the strengths of social support and engagement, building local capacity to identify and address community concerns. Wang and Burris (1997) developed this methodology in 1997 by expanding the use of "photo novella" (Wang & Burris, 1994) as a means to empower vulnerable and disenfranchised communities while gathering qualitative data. It is a grassroots community method of gathering information by using photography. By using Photovoice participants photograph, contemplate, and then verbalize stories or simple descriptions about their photo(s) taken in response to a particular prompt, thereby allowing their voices to be heard. This process prevents written text from hindering communication and is effective in a society that uses oral tradition to preserve its culture (Riley & Manias, 2004) or with groups that are drawn to photos for communication. Health care researchers have used Photovoice as an assessment tool (Lacson, 2007; Strecher, 2004; Thompson et al., 2008).

This study by Kulbok et al. (2008b) addressed gaps in the youth tobacco prevention literature. The purpose was to identify attitudes, beliefs, values, strategies, and shared meanings associated with tobacco-free behaviors of rural-dwelling male adolescents and their parents. The study examined differences in the meaning attached to nonsmoking and nonuse of smokeless tobacco among groups of African American and white male adolescents and their parents from two tobacco-growing counties in Virginia. In addition, the study assessed whether a modified Photovoice method would enhance the contribution of male adolescent participants and parents in individual and group interviews. Photovoice is a qualitative approach that uses images to promote effective ways of sharing beliefs about a specific topic. Researchers have used Photovoice to facilitate group conversations and to encourage participants to share their thoughts among themselves. In this study, Photovoice was a concrete way for youth and parents to express their perceptions about being tobacco-free, amplified through photographs that respond to questions about this topic. This approach was particularly effective with the male adolescents, who were hesitant to share their thoughts and feelings and had a hard time articulating their views.

The Ngudo Nga Zwinepe (NNZ) Learning Through Photos projects use Photovoice to understand water perceptions and innovations as well as health in the Limpopo Province of rural South Africa, where water resources are scarce and frequently contaminated (Cunningham et al., 2009). In one Photovoice project, community members took pictures documenting their perception of water and their water system. In contrast to the researchers' expectations, there was little mention of the deleterious health effects of contaminated water. Instead, the participants listed infrastructure/storage, community, money, and food as their top priorities; health/hygiene ranked fifth overall. Photovoice provided data to characterize the water priorities of this community and to implement an intervention that meets the community's primary concerns in the shorter term while developing educational strategies regarding the health risks of contaminated water.

The projects described in the previous paragraphs show the importance of multiple approaches to reaching the target population. In multilevel intervention approaches to community-oriented programs, it is important to pay attention to all client levels (i.e., individual, family, aggregate, and community). For example, in nutritional programs it is important to address the individual, the household, grocery store accessibility and environment, the community, and the food environment. No one individual can address all of these levels, but there is increasing emphasis on working in teams and in developing partnerships consisting of residents, health providers, and other professionals outside the health field as specified through the National Prevention Strategy. In addition, it is important to frame and initiate interventions based on participants' priorities, not the priorities of experts. This approach promotes increased buy-in to more equitable projects and the necessary compliance by community participants to adhere to healthy behaviors. Nurses have many opportunities to work with and to lead these multidisciplinary teams to conduct assessments, develop strategies with the community and its populations, and facilitate the empowerment of a cross-section of community residents and recommended targeted change. It is increasingly important that nurses integrate these intervention strategies with the epidemiologic evidence base for practice.

AN INTEGRATIVE MODEL FOR COMMUNITY HEALTH PROMOTION

Laffrey and Kulbok (1999) developed an integrative model for community health promotion to guide nursing and health care. The model assists nurses with seeing the continuity of care at multiple levels. Second, it helps nurses describe their own areas of expertise within the complex health care system. Third, the model provides a basis for collaboration and partnership among nurses, other health care providers, and the population. Each of these collaborators brings expertise to the client system. Important assumptions underlying the model include the need for integration of care in the complex health care system; the inseparable nature of individuals, families, aggregates, and community systems; and the maximization of health potential through health promotion interventions. In addition, the model builds upon complementary health and disease perspectives described previously (see Fig. 18.1). The health perspective focuses on promoting health as a dynamic and positive quality of life and includes the promotion of physical, mental, emotional, functional, spiritual, and social well-being considered in the context of ecological and environmental factors. The disease perspective includes both the care and prevention of illness (disease and disability) and focuses on reducing risks and threats to health.

The integrative model (Laffrey & Kulbok, 1999) includes two dimensions: **client system** and **focus of care**. The client system is multidimensional with nursing and health care targeting the multiple levels of clients. The simplest level of the client system is its most delimited target, the individual. When the individual is the client, the environment includes the family, the broader aggregate, and the community of which the individual is a part. The nurse and health care provider are concerned with how these environments affect the individual's health.

Each succeeding level of the client system is more complex, since the client can also be the family, an aggregate, or the community. The aggregate and community make up the environment for the family, and the community is the environment for the aggregate. The integrative model of community health promotion is consistent with the ecological approach described earlier, which addresses social networks, organizations, neighborhoods, and communities (Navarro et al., 2007).

Focus of care in the integrative model includes health promotion, illness (disease or disability) prevention, and illness care (health care). Each focus is appropriate for some aspects of nursing and health care. It is even more important to remember that the goal of health care is a healthier community, achieved through health promotion interventions. No matter where care begins, it ultimately leads to health promotion of the community.

INTERPROFESSIONAL APPLICATION TO NURSING AND PUBLIC HEALTH

The integrative community health promotion model reflects the basic beliefs and values of holistic nursing and health care practice and is consistent with the current emphasis on building a culture of health for all (RWJF, 2013) and the ecological perspective on multiple determinants of health (IOM, 2014; WHO, 2014a). The model depicts continuity and expansiveness of the client systems and foci of care. Health promotion is the central axis, or core, of the model. At its narrowest focus, individuals receive illness care. According to the model, at the broadest level of care, nurses work with community leaders, other community residents, and health professionals to plan programs to promote optimal health for the community and its people. The goals of nursing and health care actions in the integrative model, at any client level from the individual to the community, are to identify health potential and achieve maximal health. To achieve these goals across multiple populations, it is essential to have an active partnership between the nurse, health care providers, and the client system. By facilitating an active partnership with the client system, whether the focus of care is health promotion, illness prevention, or illness care, nurses involve clients in each step of the process of managing care from the assessment of their health needs and resources to implementation and evaluation of outcomes.

APPLICATION OF THE INTEGRATIVE MODEL FOR HEALTH EQUITY PROMOTION WITHIN COMMUNITIES

In the previous sections the importance of multiple levels of nursing and health care aimed at health promotion and illness prevention of individuals, families, aggregates, and the total community were described. In the remainder of this chapter an example using the integrative model to apply these concepts is presented.

Obesity and the Built Environment

Prevention Strategies Related to a Behaviorally Related Health Problem. In this case example (Table 18.1), a young woman recently learned that she was considered obese, and she was referred by the school health nurse to the PHN clinic. The nurse's immediate goal is to assist this client in reducing the risk of developing health problems that are related to obesity. Obesity rates have doubled over 20 years, with 16.9 percent of children ages 2 to 19 years and 34.9 percent of U.S. adults considered obese (Ogden et al., 2014). These rates are the result of a built environment that promotes increased unhealthy food consumption and decreased physical activity. The built environment includes all of the places were people live, work, learn, worship, and play and that are created or modified by people. According to the Centers for Disease Control and Prevention (CDC), in order for people to make healthy choices to combat obesity, both policy and environmental changes are needed to ensure affordable healthy food and safe places for activities (CDC, 2014b). Therefore teaching the client about the effects and side effects of her medications and how to monitor her weight, nutrition, and physical activity at home are important interventions. Since predisposing genetic, lifestyle, and environmental factors related to obesity exist, it is important to give family members information about this health problem, including early recognition of signs and symptoms for themselves.

TABLE 18.1 Community Health Levels of Care: Obesity and the Built Environment

	CLIENT SYSTEM			
Focus of Care	**Individual**	**Family**	**Aggregate**	**Community**
Illness care	Administer medications Monitor weight as well as adherence to nutrition and physical activity recommendations for individual client in the home setting	Teach family members about nutrition and physical activity practices to lose weight and prevent the onset of obesity-related diseases	Assess prevalence of obesity in the community Teach obesity classes community-wide in settings that high-risk groups frequent	Assess community for accessibility and adequacy of healthy food and safe physical activity venues in the local environment
Illness/disease prevention	Teach nutrition, progressive exercise, and lifestyle techniques to prevent additional weight gain	Teach nutrition and importance of regular exercise to all family members to prevent additional cases of obesity	Develop classes about obesity risk reduction for targeted high-risk groups and their community	Participate in community-wide multimedia education for obesity risk reduction
Health promotion	Empower individual to adopt a less sedentary and more active health promotion lifestyle	Plan with family to incorporate health promotion activities into lifestyle	Provide group education (classes) regarding benefits of regular exercise and healthy eating	Work with community leaders and citizens to establish safe physical activity space and healthy food options

QSEN FOCUS ON QUALITY AND SAFETY EDUCATION FOR NURSES

Targeted Competency: Teamwork and Collaboration

Function effectively within nursing and interprofessional teams, fostering open communication, mutual respect, and shared decision making to achieve quality client interventions and outcomes. Important aspects of teamwork and collaboration include:

- **Knowledge:** Know the scopes of practice of teammates and support them in practicing to their fullest level.
- **Skills:** Clarify roles when necessary to avoid duplication of efforts and to gain the most comprehensive approach to client care.
- **Attitudes:** Respect the unique perspectives and contributions of team members.

Teamwork and Collaboration Question

Consider the role of partnerships with the community to reduce childhood and adult obesity in the community in collaboration with school health, public health, occupational health, and home health. Are other team members needed to launch a community program to focus on obesity? If so, who would you include and what is your rationale?

Other important aspects to be addressed include assessing the prevalence of obesity among high-risk aggregates in the community and teaching obesity prevention and treatment classes in community-wide settings that high-risk, vulnerable groups frequent. An example is providing cooking classes in churches to at-risk women in the community. At the community level it is important to assess whether there are adequate and available providers and resources for healthy food and safe physical activity in the community.

Illness/Disease Prevention. Prevention care is also addressed at the individual level by teaching measures such as healthy nutrition, progressive exercise, and lifestyle techniques to prevent additional weight gain. Healthy nutrition and regular moderate to vigorous exercise are important preventive measures for all family members. Aggregate-level preventive interventions include providing showers at workplaces to encourage exercise before or during the workday. Community intervention examples include year-long multimedia campaigns to provide intensive education to the community about prevention of obesity or investment in public transit to promote active transportation and less sedentary time.

Health Promotion. Health promotion can motivate a person to adopt a less sedentary and more active lifestyle. Health promotion includes encouraging individuals to adopt a health-promoting lifestyle and helping them to become aware of their own power and self-efficacy to do so. Nurses can encourage families to make health-promoting activities a part of their daily lives. This might include taking walks, swimming together, or joining an intergenerational kickball or bowling team in which families compete with other families. Aggregates can also benefit from heart-healthy classes or activities that are culturally specific to particular subgroups, such as older Hispanic women or African American teenage girls. These activities can include stress management, well-balanced nutrition, exercise, dance classes, sports, or any other topic that can promote heart health. When looking at the total community, an example of a health promotion intervention is participating in a coalition to plan for supermarkets and community gardens, as well as parks or recreation areas, in specific locations in the community where they are absent and can be safe and accessible to the population with the greatest need.

LINKING CONTENT TO PRACTICE

This chapter explained the importance of public health nurses' roles in contributing to health equity, with emphasis on health promotion models, population health, and the challenges of building a culture of health (RWJF, 2013). The central focus of public health nursing (PHN) practice is health promotion, recognizing health disparities across populations and cultures. Public health nurses strive to improve the health status of communities and populations. Whether the client system is the family or a vulnerable population, and the focus of care is illness prevention or illness care, health promotion and disease prevention remain the central goals. No matter where PHN care begins, it ultimately leads to contributing to community and population health. Many PHN leaders, past and present, have conducted evidenced-based practice projects, developed and applied models of practice, and engaged in community-based participatory research. This work has provided the foundation for PHN practice.

In summary, the concepts of health, health promotion, community, and health equity are inextricably linked; it is difficult to discuss one without including the others. It is also important that nurses examine their definitions and beliefs about each concept as the basis for their practice. The essence of public health is the ability to see the totality of community while addressing its component parts and, at the same time, to see the total needs for health promotion, health protection, and illness and disease prevention. The relationship among these components distinguishes PHN from nursing in more circumscribed settings, such as hospitals and clinics.

PRACTICE APPLICATION

A rural health outreach program serves migrant workers, their families, and other vulnerable populations in the local community. The program's goals include increased knowledge about risk factors, services, and self-care; improved community health; increased access and affordability of individual- and community-level health promotion services; and reduced barriers to health services. The program offers health promotion and disease prevention educational materials and classes in English and Spanish throughout the region in churches, schools, community centers, fire departments, and migrant camps. In addition, clinics in eight local sites across the county provide services. Clinic services include health risk assessments, disease screening, immunizations, health education, counseling, and referral. The program staff trained community health workers (CHWs) from the migrant community to deliver basic health education and resource information. Funding from a variety of public and private sources supports the program. It is essential that the program show effective outcomes if it is to sustain funding.

Mary Ann Jones, a nurse with a bachelor of science in nursing degree, works for the outreach program. She is a member of a group asked to evaluate whether the outreach program (including the eight clinics) is effective in meeting the stated objectives.

A. Using community health promotion as a guide, how might you organize a comprehensive approach to assessment and data collection?

B. What are sources of data you might use for assessing individual, aggregate, and community health indicators?

C. What is the value of interviewing rural residents, migrant workers, and clinic participants about their perceptions of health and the value of health services?

D. Who else can you interview to elicit important information about the usefulness of the outreach program?

E. How can you best use CHWs to increase participation and partnership among concerned health professionals, community residents, and migrant families and to sustain the program?

Be creative and comprehensive in your approach, and consider how you might build a culture of health using the ecological perspective, the SDOH, and cultural factors associated with rural and migrant populations in the United States. Current spending limits on federal and state programs for health promotion and disease prevention require that nurses deal effectively with issues of outreach, sustainability, and success of community health programs.

Answers can be found on the Evolve site.

KEY POINTS

- The goals of a culture of health for America are for good health across geographic, demographic, and social sectors; for being healthy and staying healthy as a social value; and for everyone to have access to affordable, quality health care.
- The idea of health shapes the process of population-focused nursing practice, from assessment of health-related needs of individuals, families, aggregates, and communities to evaluation of health outcomes.
- The National Prevention Strategy foresees a prevention-oriented society where public and private sectors value health for individuals, families, and society and work together to achieve better health for Americans.
- The greatest benefits in public health are likely to come from efforts to improve individual and family lifestyles through community and population interventions that address the social determinants of health, including social conditions and the built environment.
- Public health nurses have a history of commitment to primary health care and to enhancing levels of wellness in communities and populations.
- When nurses examine their own definition of health, they recognize how this health definition directs the nursing care they provide.
- When nurses examine the client's definition of health, they are more likely to tailor care to the client's culture, needs, lifestyle, and social and physical environment.
- The Framingham Heart Study has provided more than 50 years of research about risk factors and lifestyle habits; Framingham researchers are currently studying how genes contribute to common disorders such as obesity, hypertension, and diabetes.
- The Stanford Heart Disease Prevention program, the North Karelia Project, the Pawtucket Heart Health program, and the Minnesota Heart Health program contributed to the scientific knowledge base for the design, implementation, and evaluation of community- and population-level risk-appraisal and risk-reduction programs.
- Public health nurses function beyond resolving a specific illness to preventing the illness and promoting optimal health for the individual, the family, the aggregate, and the total community. All of these levels are important to promote the health of the community and populations.
- Public health nurses can contribute to health equity using ecological perspectives with multilevel approaches and building a culture of health.

CLINICAL DECISION-MAKING ACTIVITIES

1. What are the first steps to build culture a of health to promote health equity within the community?
2. Write your own definition of health, and interview a nurse, client, and physician about their definitions of health. How are these definitions similar or different? How do they "fit" with your understanding of what nurses and health care providers need to do to build a culture of health?
3. What are some challenges encountered when you consider different definitions of health and health promotion from a disease-oriented versus an environmental or social-ecologically oriented perspective? Illustrate these challenges and opportunities with examples of strategies that are health promoting and will contribute to building a culture of health.
4. Discuss the importance of the built environment in community health promotion, and provide examples of environmental health promotion indicators for a specified community.

5. Develop a nursing care plan for addressing childhood obesity using the propositions of Milio (1976) as a frame of reference.
6. Use a model for community health promotion and social determinants of health to identify the most important strategies in a community-wide plan for childhood obesity.
7. Illustrate community health levels of care, including the client system and the focus of care:
   A. For teenage pregnancy: begin with community-level health promotion
   B. For childhood obesity: start with community-level illness prevention

ADDITIONAL RESOURCES

EVOLVE WEBSITE

http://evolve.elsevier.com/Stanhope/community/

- Answers to Practice Application
- Case Study
- Glossary
- Review Questions

REFERENCES

Adler N, Bachrach C, Daley D, et al.: *Building the Science for a Population Health Movement.* Discussion Paper. Washington, DC, 2013, Institute of Medicine. Retrieved from http://www.iom.edu.

American Academy of Pediatrics Committee on Community Health Services: The pediatrician's role in community pediatrics, *Pediatrics* 115:1092–1094, 2005.

American Nurses Association: *Public Health Nursing: Scope and Standards of Practice,* Washington, DC, 2013, ANA.

Anderson ET, McFarlane J: *Community-As-Partner: Theory and Practice in Nursing,* New York , 1998, Lippincott Williams & Wilkins.

Anderson ET, McFarlane J: *Community-As-Partner: Theory and Practice in Nursing,* ed 6, New York, 2011, Lippincott Williams & Wilkins.

Bekemeier B, Jones M: Relationships between local public health agency functions and agency leadership and staffing: a look at nurses, *J Public Health Manag Pract* 16:E8–E16, 2010.

Berkman LF, Breslow L: *Health and Ways of Living, the Alameda County Study,* New York, 1983, Oxford University Press.

Bigbee JL, Issel LM. Conceptual models for population-focused public health nursing interventions and outcomes: the state of the art, *Public Health Nurs* 29(4):370–379, 2012.

Botchwey ND: The religious sector's presence in local community development, *J Plan Educ Res* 27(1):36–48, 2007.

Bronfenbrenner U: Toward an experimental ecology of human development, *Am Psychol* 32:513–531, 1977.

Bronfenbrenner U: *The Ecology of Human Development,* Cambridge, MA, 1979, Harvard University Press.

Centers for Disease Control and Prevention: *CDC's Built Environment and Health Initiative,* 2013. Retrieved from http://www.cdc.gov.

Centers for Disease Control and Prevention: *Social determinants of health,* 2014a. Retrieved from http://www.cdc.gov.

Centers for Disease Control and Prevention: *Overweight and obesity,* 2014b. Retrieved from http://www.cdc.gov.

CDC National Health Report: *Leading Causes of Morbidity and Mortality and Associated Behavioral Risk and Protective Factors—United States, 2005–2013,* October 2014. Retrieved from www.cdc.gov.

Chopoorian TL: Reconceptualizing the environment. In Moccia P, editor: *New Approaches to Theory Development,* Pub. No. 15-1992, New York, 1986, National League for Nursing.

CDC: *Smoking and Tobacco Use,* 2018. Retrieved from https://www.cdc.gov.

Cunningham T, Botchwey N, Dillingham R, et al.: Understanding water perceptions in Limpopo Province: a Photovoice community assessment, *Environ Poll Public Health IEEE* 2009.

Edberg M: *Essentials of Health Behavior: Social and Behavioral Theory in Public Health,* ed 6, 2013, Jones & Bartlett.

Farley T, Cohen W: *Prescription for a Healthy Nation: A New Approach to Improving Our Lives by Fixing Our Everyday World,* Boston, 2005, Beacon Press, Chapter 4.

Farquhar JW, Maccoby N, Wood PD, et al.: Effects of community-wide education on cardiovascular disease risk factors: the Stanford Five-city Project, *JAMA* 264:359, 1990.

Fee, E. & Gonzalez, AR: The history of health equity: concept and vision, May 22, 2017. Diversity & Equality in Health and Care, Insight Medical Publishing. Retrieved from iMedPub.com.

Fuchs V: *Who Shall Live?* New York, 1974, Basic Books.

Gordon-Larsen P, Nelson MC, Page P, Popkin BM: Inequality in the built environment underlies key health disparities in physical activity and obesity, *Pediatrics* 1;117(2):417–424, 2006.

Gorin SS, Badr H, Krebs P, Das IP: Multilevel interventions and racial/ethnic health disparities, *J Natl Cancer Inst Monogr* 2012(44):100–111, 2012.

Institute of Medicine: *The Future of the Public's Health in the 21st Century,* Washington, DC, 2003, The National Academies Press. Retrieved from http://www.nap.edu.

Institute of Medicine: *The Impact of Social and Cultural Environment on Health. Defining the Social and Cultural Environment. Genes, Behavior, and the Social Environment: Moving Beyond the Nature/Nurture Debate,* Washington, DC, 2006, The National Academies Press.

Institute of Medicine: *Working definition of population health, Roundtable on population health,* 2014. Retrieved from http://www.iom.edu.

Keller LO, Strohschein S, Lia-Hoagberg G, et al.: Population-based public health nursing interventions: a model for practice, *Public Health Nurs* 15:207, 1998.

Keller LO, Strohschein S, Lia-Hoagberg B, Schaffer MA: Population-based public health nursing interventions: practice-based and evidence-supported. Part 1, *Public Health Nurs* 21:453–468, 2004.

Kindig D, Stoddart G: What is population health? *Am J Pub Health* 93(3):380–383, 2003.

Kulbok PA, Baldwin JH, Cox CL, Duffy R: Advancing discourse on health promotion: beyond mainstream thinking, *Ans Adv Nurs Sci* 20:12, 1997.

Kuehnert, PL: The interactive and organizational model of community as client: A model for public health nursing practice, *Public Health Nurs* 12(1):9–17, 1995.

Kulbok PA, Glick DF: "Something must be done!": The history of public health nursing education 1900-1950, *Fam Community Health* 37(3):170–178, 2014.

Kulbok P, Rhee H, Hinton I, et al.: Factors influencing adolescents' decisions not to smoke, *Public Health Nurs* 25:505–515, 2008a.

Kulbok P, Meszaros P, Hinton I, et al.: *Tobacco-Free Boys and Parents Use Photovoice to Tell Their Stories: Issues and Solutions [Abstract]*, San Diego, CA, October 25–29, 2008b, Proceedings of the 136th American Public Health Association, Annual Meeting.

Kulbok PA, Thatcher E, Park E, Meszaros P: Evolving public health nursing roles: focus on community participatory health promotion and prevention, *Online J Issues Nurs* 17(2):1, 2012.

Kumar S, Quinn SC, Kim KH, Musa D, Hilyard KM, Freimuth VS: The social ecological model as a framework for determinants of 2009 H1N1 influenza vaccine uptake in the United States, *Health Educ Behav* 39:229–243, 2013.

Lacson RS: *tb. Tuberculosis. pv. Photovoice*, 2007. Retrieved from http://tbphotovoice.org.

Laffrey SC, Kulbok PA: The integrative model for community health nursing: a conceptual guide to education, practice, and research, *J Holist Nurs* 17:88–103, 1999.

Laffrey SC, Loveland-Cherry CJ, Winkler SJ: Health behavior: evolution of two paradigms, *Public Health Nurs* 3:92–97, 1986.

LaLonde M: *A New Perspective on the Health of Canadians*, Ottawa, 1974, Government of Canada.

Lasater T, Abrams T, Artz L, et al.: Lay volunteer delivery of a community-based cardiovascular risk factor change program: the Pawtucket experiment. In Matarazzo JD, editor: *Behavioral Health: A Handbook of Health Enhancement and Disease Prevention*, Silver Spring, MD, 1984, Wiley.

Leavell HR, Clark EG: *Preventive Medicine for the Doctor in His Community: An Epidemiological Approach*, ed 3, New York, 1965, McGraw-Hill.

Li K, Seo DC, Torabi MR, Peng CY, Kay NS, Kolbe LJ: Social-ecological factors of leisure-time physical activity in black adults, *Am J Health Behav* 36:797–810, 2012.

Lieb W, Pencina MJ, Lanier KJ, et al.: Association of parental obesity with concentrations of select systemic biomarkers in nonobese offspring: The Framingham Heart Study, *Diabetes* 58(1):134–137, 2009.

Luepker RV, Murray DM, Jacobs DR Jr, et al.: Community education for cardiovascular disease prevention: risk factor changes in the Minnesota Heart Health Program, *Am J Public Health* 84:1383, 1994.

May KM, Phillips LR, Ferketich SL, Verran JA: Public Health Nursing: The Generalist in a Specialized Environment, *Public Health Nurs* 20(4):252-259. 2003.

McLeroy KR, Bibeau D, Steckler A, Glanz K: An ecological perspective on health promotion programs, *Health Educ Q* 15(4):351–377, 1988.

McQueen DV: Three challenges for the social determinants of health pursuit, *Int J Public Health* 54:1–2, 2009.

Milio N: A framework for prevention: changing health-damaging to health-generating life patterns, *Am J Public Health* 66:435, 1976.

Minkler M, Wallerstein N, editors: *Community-Based Participatory Research for Health*, ed 2, San Francisco, 2008, John Wiley & Sons.

National Prevention Council: *National Prevention Strategy*, Washington, DC, 2011, U.S. Department of Health and Human Services, Office of the Surgeon General.

National Research Council: *The Future of Public Health*, Washington, DC, 1988, The National Academies Press.

Navarro AM, Voetsch KP, Liburd LC, Giles HW, Collins JL: *Charting the future of community health promotion: recommendations from the National Expert Panel on Community Health Promotion, Prev Chronic Dis* 2007, [serial online]. Retrieved from http://www.cdc.gov.

Ogden CL, Carroll MD, Kit BK, Flegal KM: Prevalence of childhood and adult obesity in the United States, 2011-2012, *JAMA* 311: 806–814, 2014.

Owen N, Humpel N, Leslie E, Bauman A, Sallis JF: Understanding environmental influences on walking: review and research agenda, *Am J Prev Med* 27:67–76, 2004.

Paskett E, Thompson B, Ammerman AS, Ortega AN, Marsteller J, Richardson D. Multilevel interventions to address health disparities show promise in improving population health, *Health Aff* 35(8):1429–1434, 2016.

Pate RR, Colabianchi N, Porter D, Almeida MJ, Lobelo F, Dowda M: Physical activity and neighborhood resources in high school girls, *Am J Prev Med* 34:413–419, 2008.

Prentice AM, Jebb SA: Obesity in Britain; gluttony or sloth? *BMJ* 311:437–439, 1995.

Puska P, Salonen JT, Nissinen JT, et al.: Change in risk factors for coronary heart disease during 10 years of a community intervention programme (North Karelia Project), *Br Med J* 287:1840, 1983.

Riley RG, Manias E: The uses of photography in clinical nursing practice and research: a literature review, *J Adv Nurs* 48:397–405, 2004.

Robert Wood Johnson Foundation: *About the Culture of Health Blog*, 2013. Retrieved from http://www.rwjf.org.

Ronda G, Van Assema P, Ruland E, Steenbakkers M, Van Ree J, Brug J: The Dutch heart health community intervention 'Hartslag Limburg': results of an effect study at organizational level, *Public Health* 119:353–360, 2005.

Rose G: *The Strategy of Preventive Medicine*, New York, 1992, Oxford University Press.

Rosenbaum S: *Principles to Consider for the Implementation of a Community Health Needs Assessment Process*, 2013, The George Washington University School of Public Health and Health Services, Department of Health Policy. Retrieved from http://nnphi.org.

Rosenstock IM: Historical origins of the health belief model, *Health Educ Monog* 2(4):328–335, 1974.

Salmon M: Editorial: Public health nursing: the opportunity of a century, *Am J Public Health* 83:1674–1675, 1993.

Salmon M: An open letter to public health nursing, *Public Health Nurs* 26:483–485, 2009.

Sanders LM, Robinson TN, Forster LQ, Plax K, Brosco JP, Brito A: Evidence-based community pediatrics: building a bridge from bedside to neighborhood, *Pediatrics* 115:1142–1147, 2005.

Schulz AJ, Zenk S, Odoms-Young A, et al.: Healthy eating and exercising to reduce diabetes: exploring the potential of social determinants of health frameworks within the context of community-based participatory diabetes prevention, *Am J Public Health* 95:645–651, 2005.

Shuster G, Goeppinger J: Community as client: assessment and analysis. In Stanhope M, Lancaster J, editors: *Public Health Nursing: Population-Centered Health Care in the Community*, ed 8, St Louis, 2012, Mosby.

Simons-Morton B: Health behavior in ecological context, *Health Educ Behav* 40:6, 2013.

Skinner BF: *Why I am Not a Cognitive Psychologist in Reflections on Behaviorism and Society*, Englewood Cliffs, NJ, 1978, Prentice-Hall.

Smith JA: The idea of health: a philosophical inquiry, *Adv Nurs Sci* 3:43, 1981.

Strecher VJ: *Photovoice for tobacco, drug, and alcohol prevention among adolescents in South Africa [Abstract]*, 2004. Retrieved from http://apha.confex.com.

Task Force on Community Preventive Services: *The Guide to Community Preventive Services-What Works to Promote Health*, New York, 2005, Oxford University Press.

Terris M: Approaches to an epidemiology of health, *Am J Public Health* 65:1037–1045, 1975.

Thompson NC, Hunter EE, Murray L, Ninci L, Rolfs EM, Pallikkathayil L: The Experience of living with chronic mental illness: a Photovoice study [Abstract], *Perspect Psychiatr Care* 44(1):14–24, 2008. Retrieved from http://findarticles.com.

U.S. Department of Health, Education, and Welfare: *Forward Plan for Health*, FY 1978-82. DHEW Pub. No. (OS) 76-50046. Washington, DC, 1976, U.S. Government Printing Office.

U.S. Department of Health, Education, and Welfare: *Healthy People: The Surgeon General's Report on Health Promotion and Disease Prevention*, DHEW Pub. No. 79-55071, Washington, DC, 1979, U.S. Government Printing Office.

U.S. Department of Health and Human Services: *Healthy People in Healthy Communities: A Community Planning Guide Using Healthy People 2010*, Washington DC, 2001, U.S. Government Printing Office.

U.S. Department of Health and Human Services: *Healthy People 2030*. 2018a Retrieved from https://www.healthypeople.gov.

U.S. Department of Health and Human Services: *Healthy People 2020 topics and objectives*, 2018b. Retrieved from https://www.healthypeople.gov.

U.S. Department of Health and Human Services: *Implementing* Healthy People 2020. *MAP-IT: a guide to using* Healthy People 2020 *in your community*. 2018c. Retrieved from http://healthypeople.gov.

U.S. Department of Health and Human Services: *Social Determinants of Health*. 2018d Retrieved from https://www.healthypeople.gov.

U.S. Department of Health and Human Services: *Theory at a Glance: A Guide For Health Promotion Practice*, ed 2, NIH Pub. No. 05-3896. Washington, DC, 2005, National Cancer Institute, National Institutes of Health, (revised). Retrieved from http://www.cancer.gov.

U.S. Preventive Services Task Force: *Guide to Clinical Preventive Services: Report of the U.S. Preventive Services Task Force*, Baltimore, 1989, Lippincott, Williams & Wilkins.

U.S. Preventive Services Task Force: *Guide to Clinical Preventive Services, 2012: Recommendations of the U.S. Preventive Services Task Force*, Rockville, MD, 2011, Agency for Healthcare Research and Quality. Retrieved from http://www.ahrq.gov.

Wang C, Burris MA: Photovoice: concept, methodology, and use for participatory needs assessment, *Health Educ Behav* 24:369–387, 1997.

Wang C, Burris MA: Empowerment through photo novella: portraits of participation, *Health Educ Q* 21:171–186, 1994.

Watson M, Dannenberg AL: Investment in Safe Routes to School projects: public health benefits for the larger community, *Prev Chronic Dis* 5:1–7, 2008. Retrieved from http://www.ncbi.nlm.nih.gov.

Wight RG, Aneshensel CS, Botticello AL, Sepúlveda JE: A multilevel analysis of ethnic variation in depressive symptoms among adolescents in the United States, *Soc Sci Med* 60:2073–2084, 2005.

World Health Organization: *World conference on social determinants of health*, 2014a. Retrieved from http://www.who.int.

World Health Organization: *Health promotion: The Ottawa Charter for Health Promotion*, 2014b. Retrieved from http://www.who.int.

World Health Organization: *Preamble to the Constitution of the World Health Organization as adopted by the International Health Conference*, 1948. Retrieved from http://www.who.int\.

World Health Organization: *Social Determinants of Health*, Geneva, 2010. Retrieved from http://www.who.int.

Xu X, Bishop EE, Kennedy SM, Simpson SA, Pechacek TF: Annual Healthcare Spending Attributable to Cigarette Smoking: An Update, *Am J Prev Med* 48(3):326-333. 2015.

19

Health Education Principles Applied in Communities, Groups, Families, and Individuals for Healthy Change

Victoria P. Niederhauser, DrPH, RN, PPCNP-BC, FAAN

OBJECTIVES

After reading this chapter, the student should be able to do the following:

1. Describe the ways in which people learn.
2. Identify the steps and principles that guide community health education.
3. Discuss the importance of understanding the needs of learners, including their cultural background, educational and health literacy level, and their motivation to learn and change behavior.
4. Describe how nurses can work with groups to promote the health of individuals and communities.
5. Examine types of health education, including written, spoken, and the growing area of social media.
6. Explore ethical issues that arise in the practice of health education.

CHAPTER OUTLINE

Healthy People 2020 Objectives for Health Education
Education, Learning, and Change
How People Learn
The Educational Process
Educational Issues
Health Education for Community Groups

KEY TERMS

affective domain, p. 417
andragogy, p. 422
change, p. 416
cognitive domain, p. 416
cohesion, p. 427
democratic leadership, p. 430
education, p. 416
established groups, p. 430
ethics, p. 415
evaluation, p. 425
formal groups, p. 427
goals, p. 418
group, p. 427
health belief model, p. 425
health education, p. 416
health literacy, p. 424
informal groups, p. 427
learning, p. 416
long-term evaluation, p. 426
maintenance functions, p. 428
maintenance norms, p. 429
motivational interviewing, p. 420
norms, p. 428
objectives, p. 418
patriarchal leadership, p. 430
pedagogy, p. 422
process evaluation, p. 426
psychomotor domain, p. 417
reality norms, p. 429
short-term evaluation, p. 426
social media, p. 418
task function, p. 428
task norm, p. 428
transtheoretical model, p. 425

One of the best ways to manage health care costs is for people to stay healthy. Nurses are in an ideal role to help individuals, families, and groups learn about health education and health promotion in order to change their behavior. Nurses can help clients by (1) educating across all three levels of prevention: primary, secondary, and tertiary; and (2) working with individuals, families, groups, and communities. The goal is to assist clients with attaining optimal health, prevent health problems, identify and treat health problems early, and minimize disability. Education allows individuals to make knowledgeable health-related decisions, assume personal responsibility for their health, change behavior if needed, and cope effectively with alterations in their health and lifestyles. The Levels of Prevention box provides an example of how to use these three prevention levels in health education.

LEVELS OF PREVENTION

Related to Community Health Education

Primary Prevention

Provide education at health fairs about health promotion and/or disease prevention topics such as diet, exercise, or environmental hazards.

Secondary Prevention

Provide both education and health screenings at health fairs for such health issues as early diagnosis and treatment of diabetes and hypercholesterolemia in order to shorten the duration and severity of the disease.

Tertiary Prevention

Provide education in rehabilitation centers to teach ways to increase function to individuals who have been in an accident that left them with either an amputation or some paralysis.

This chapter discusses ways to develop community health promotion programs, group, and individual programs. Specific content in the chapter includes information about how people learn; the sequence of actions that a nurse follows when developing an educational program; the process of making change; literacy, especially health literacy; and the ethics related to health education. The role of groups in health promotion is also presented. Many of the objectives of *Healthy People 2020* address the importance of health promotion, and selected objectives are cited in this chapter.

HEALTHY PEOPLE 2020 OBJECTIVES FOR HEALTH EDUCATION

As mentioned in other chapters, *Healthy People 2020* lists national health needs and outlines goals and objectives designed to improve health. The *Healthy People 2020* educational objectives emphasize the importance of educating various populations (based on age and ethnicity) about health promotion activities in the priority areas of unintentional injury; violence; suicide; tobacco use and addiction; alcohol or other drug use; unintended pregnancy, human immunodeficiency virus/acquired immunodeficiency syndrome (HIV/AIDS), and sexually transmitted disease (STD); unhealthy dietary patterns; and inadequate physical activity (U.S. Department of Health and Human Services [USDHHS], 2010).

HEALTHY PEOPLE 2020

Selected examples of *Healthy People 2020* are provided here.

- **ECBP-2:** Increase the proportion of elementary, middle, and senior high schools that provide comprehensive school health education to prevent health problems in the following areas: unintentional injury; violence; suicide; tobacco use and addiction; alcohol or other drug use; unintended pregnancy, immunodeficiency virus/acquired immunodeficiency syndrome (HIV/AIDS), and sexually transmitted infection (STI); unhealthy dietary patterns; and inadequate physical activity.
- **ECBP-3:** Increase the proportion of college and university students who receive information from their institution on each of the priority health-risk behavior areas listed previously.
- **ECBP-8:** Increase the proportion of worksites that offer a comprehensive employee health promotion program to their employees.
- **ECBP-11:** Increase the proportion of local health departments that have established culturally appropriate and linguistically competent community health promotion and disease prevention programs.

ECBP, Educational and community-based programs.
From U.S. Department of Health and Human Services, Office of Health Promotion and Disease Prevention: *Healthy People 2020, Educational and community-based programs.* Available at https://www.healthypeople.gov. Accessed May 2018.

In designing, implementing, and evaluating health education activities, it is useful to understand the primary health problems in the community as well as education principles related to both learning and teaching. Also, effective educational programs are built on the premise that the best approach is to teach what people think they want to learn and in ways that facilitate their learning. For this reason, a core public health principle relates to asking the learners to participate in identifying their learning needs. Then health education programs are designed to meet the health need or problem in that population. In general, these programs involve educating individual members of the population about health promotion, illness prevention, and treatment. For example, in a community where childhood and adolescent asthma is a problem, a community-based asthma education and training program can be developed. If childhood obesity is a major health concern, a program to educate children in their schools and parents and other caregivers in an after-school program about healthy eating, cooking, and exercise may be useful.

To develop a community-based education program, nurses need to follow a set of steps. Typical steps that are discussed in detail throughout the chapter include the following: (1) *identify* a population-specific learning need for the community health client; (2) *select* one or more learning theories to use in the education program; (3) *consider* which educational principles are most likely to increase learning and choose those that are most appropriate and feasible; (4) *examine* educational issues, such as population-specific or cultural concerns, identify barriers to learning, such as limited literacy or limited or lack of health literacy, and choose the most appropriate teaching and learning strategies based on the age, gender, education, and learning needs of the learners; (5) *design and implement* the educational program, using carefully chosen strategies; and (6) *evaluate* the effects of the educational program. The steps used in designing educational programs parallel those of the nursing process.

EDUCATION, LEARNING, AND CHANGE

When helping people change their behavior, remember that people can most easily change knowledge. The next step is to help people change their attitudes, and the most difficult area to change is behavior. For this reason, nurses provide people with health information so they can improve their decision-making abilities and thereby decide if they will change their behavior. There is a difference between education and learning and between knowing and doing. **Education** is an activity "undertaken or initiated by one or more agents that is designed to effect changes in the knowledge, skill, and attitudes of communities, groups and individuals" (Knowles et al., 2005, p. 10). Education emphasizes the provider of knowledge and skills. In contrast, **learning** emphasizes the recipient of knowledge and skills and the person(s) in whom a change is expected to occur. Remember that learning involves change.

Change is not easy for most people. To **change** means to move away from one way of thinking, believing, and acting and move toward a new way. Thompson (2010) describes understanding and managing organizational change. Although much of the change regarding health education is directed toward clients, not organizations, the steps he uses also apply to health education. They are as follows: (1) identify the need for change—and this means that the client or clients being served need to believe that they need to make a change; (2) plan how to implement the change—and this step includes explaining the basis for the change, the benefits of the change, and seeking ideas from those being served about the best way to make an identified change; (3) implement the change; and (4) evaluate whether the change made a difference in health. Fielding (2013) offers a similar approach toward health education, consisting of the following five steps: (1) understanding the problem, (2) understanding what works, (3) agreeing on the approach or action, (4) implementing the plan, and (5) evaluating the effect. As nurses work with clients to make health changes, it is important to watch for resistance or reverting back to past behaviors.

HOW PEOPLE LEARN

People learn in a variety of ways. Some people learn better by hearing a message; others learn by observing and/or participating in what is being taught. Learners accept information on the basis of many factors, including what they already know, what they believe, and the culture in which they have been raised; as well as how well they can understand and relate to the information that they receive. What a person hears is filtered through his or her past experiences, the social groups to which he or she belongs, assumptions, values, level of attention and knowledge, and the respect he or she has for the person communicating the information. In some cultures, elders are considered to be valued sources of information. In other cultures, people value individuals with more education than they have. Also, because social groups play a critical role in the development of understanding or learning, concepts related to groups are discussed later in this chapter. Effective **health education** is a competency that is included in many documents that describe the role of public health professionals, including nurses. The Linking Content to Practice box illustrates the relationship between health education and selected standards, expectations, and competencies in public health.

LINKING CONTENT TO PRACTICE

Just as objectives in *Healthy People 2020* recommend that health education and promotion be used to provide public health care, so do other key documents such as the American Nurses Association's *Scope & Standards of Practice: Public Health Nursing,* second edition. Standard 5b, labeled "Health Teaching and Promotion," says that the "public health nurse employs multiple strategies to promote health, prevent disease, and ensure a safe environment for populations" (American Nurses Association, 2013, p. 23). Similarly, the *Core Competencies for Public Health Professionals* of the Council on Linkages between Academia and Public Health Practice (2014) lists eight competencies related to communication skills; seven of them relate directly to this chapter. These competencies, listed below, are discussed and illustrated throughout this chapter:

1. Assessing the health literacy of populations served
2. Communicating in writing and orally, in person, with linguistic and cultural proficiency
3. Soliciting input from individuals and organizations
4. Using a variety of approaches to disseminate public health information
5. Conveys data to professionals and the public using a variety of approaches
6. Communicates information to influence behavior and improve health
7. Facilitates communication among individuals, groups and organizations
8. Describes the roles of governmental public health, health care, and other partners in improving the health of a community

A variety of educational principles can be used to guide the selection of health information for communities and populations, including groups, and individuals. Three of the most useful categories of educational principles include those associated with the nature of learning, the educational process, and the skills of effective educators.

The Nature of Learning

One way to think about the nature of learning is to examine the cognitive (thinking), affective (feeling), and psychomotor (acting) domains of learning. Each domain has specific behavioral components that form a hierarchy of steps, or levels. Each level builds on the previous one. Understanding these three learning domains is crucial in providing effective health education (Bloom et al., 1956). First, consider assumptions about how adults learn. Specifically, adults are motivated to learn when (1) they think they need to know something, (2) the new information is compatible with their prior life experiences, (3) they value the person(s) providing the information, and (4) they believe they can make any necessary changes that are implied by the new information (Knowles et al., 2005).

Cognitive Domain. The **cognitive domain** includes memory, recognition, understanding, reasoning, application, and problem solving and is divided into a hierarchical classification of behaviors. Learners master each level of cognition in order of difficulty (Bloom et al., 1956). Start by assessing the cognitive abilities of the learners. This is especially important when learners have a limited level of literacy either of the language used in the instruction or of the content that is presented. A later section discusses both literacy in general and health literacy in particular. Teaching above or below a person's level of understanding can lead to frustration and discouragement. It is therefore important to be sensitive to the value of the cognitive domain in learning. The cognitive domain consists of the following components (Bloom et al., 1956):

1. *Knowledge:* Requires recall of information
2. *Comprehension:* Combines recall with understanding
3. *Application:* In which new information is taken in and used in a different way
4. *Analysis:* Breaks communication down into parts in order to understand both the parts and their relationships to one another
5. *Synthesis:* Builds on the first four levels by assembling them into a new whole
6. *Evaluation:* In which learners judge the value of what has been learned

Affective Domain. The affective domain includes changes in attitudes and the development of values. For affective learning to take place, nurses consider and attempt to influence what learners feel, think, and value. Because the attitudes and values of nurses may differ from those of their clients, it is important to listen carefully to detect clues to feelings or misperceptions that learners have that may influence learning. It is difficult to change deeply rooted attitudes, beliefs, interests, and values. To make such changes, people need support and encouragement from those around them. Affective learning, like cognitive learning, consists of a series of steps that the learner takes:

1. *Knowledge:* Receives the information
2. *Comprehension:* Responds to the information received
3. *Application:* Values the information
4. *Analysis:* Makes sense of the information
5. *Synthesis:* Organizes the information
6. *Evaluation:* Adopts behaviors consistent with new values

Psychomotor Domain. The psychomotor domain includes the performance of skills that require some degree of neuromuscular coordination and emphasizes motor skills (Bloom et al., 1956). Clients are taught a variety of psychomotor skills, including bathing infants, changing dressings, giving injections, measuring blood glucose levels, taking blood pressures, walking with crutches, as well as many skills related to health promotion exercises.

In teaching a skill, first show clients how to do a task requiring the skill being taught. You can use pictures, a model, or a device, or via a live demonstration, video, CD, or the Internet. Next, have clients practice through a repeat demonstration to validate that what is being taught was actually learned. Also, if the teaching is being done in a class, participants may learn by observing one another master a task. Psychomotor learning is dependent on learners meeting three conditions (Bloom et al., 1956). The learner must have the following:

- The *necessary ability:* This will include both cognitive and psychomotor ability. For example, you may find that a person with Alzheimer's disease can follow only one-step instructions. Thus, you need to tailor your education plan to that person.
- A *sensory image* of how to carry out the skill: For example, when teaching a group of women how to cook heart-healthy foods, ask the women to describe their kitchen and how they would actually go about the cooking process.
- *Opportunities to practice* the new skills: Provide practice sessions during the program to help the client adapt the skill to the home or work environment where the skill will be performed.

The following Quality and Safety Education for Nurses box describes the importance of clear and appropriate communication.

QSEN FOCUS ON QUALITY AND SAFETY EDUCATION FOR NURSES

Targeted Competency: Client-Centered Care

Important aspects of client-centered care include the following:

- **Knowledge:** Integrate understanding of multiple dimensions of client-centered care: information, communication, and education
- **Skills:** Communicate client values, preferences, and expressed needs to other members of the health care team
- **Attitudes:** Respect and encourage individual expression of client values, preferences, and expressed needs

Client-Centered Care Question

Providing health information in a way that is not understandable or useful to the recipient is a poor form of client-centered communication. If you were teaching a group of four women about wound care after surgery, what steps would you take to assure that the message the women received was the message that you intended to send?

Answer

In general, you would begin by providing the needed information by describing each step; you might include an easy-to-understand handout in the language that the four women understand, or if they have easy access to the Internet, provide them with valid and reliable websites with pertinent information. Next you would demonstrate how to clean the wound. Then you would ask each woman to repeat the cleaning process that you just demonstrated. Finally, you would ask each woman if she had the facilities and supplies to clean the wound at home; and then you would ask if they each had any questions or concerns that you might answer. What else would you do?

Source: Cronenwett L, Sherwood G, Barnsteiner J, et al.: Quality and safety education for nurses. *Nurs Outlook* 55:122–131, 2007.

In assessing a client's ability to learn a skill, be sure to evaluate intellectual, emotional, and physical ability, and then teach at the level of the learner's ability. Some clients do not have the intellectual ability to learn the steps that make up a complex procedure. Others may have cultural beliefs that conflict with healthy behaviors. Another client may be tremulous or have poor eyesight, making the client incapable of learning insulin self-injection.

THE EDUCATIONAL PROCESS

The educational process builds on an understanding of education, learning, and how people learn. The five steps of the educational process (identify educational needs, establish educational goals and objectives, select appropriate educational methods, implement the educational plan, and evaluate the educational process) are discussed next.

Identify Educational Needs and Develop Goals and Objectives

Begin with a needs assessment to learn about health education needs. The steps of such an assessment are listed in Box 19.1. Once you identify the needs, prioritize them to meet the most important needs first. Consider the many factors that influence a person's learning needs and the ability to learn, including demographic, physical, geographic, economic, psychological, social, and spiritual factors. Consider also the learner's knowledge, skills, and his or her motivation to learn, as well as what resources are available to support or prevent learning. Resources include printed, audio or visual materials, equipment, agencies, and other individuals. Barriers for the presenter include lack of time, skill and/or confidence, money, space, energy, and organizational support.

When you have identified the learning needs, develop the goals and objectives for the educational program. **Goals** are broad, long-term expected outcomes such as, "Each child in the third-grade class will participate in 30 minutes of daily physical exercise, 4 days per week for 2 months." Program goals should deal directly with the clients' overall learning needs. Regarding the third graders, their learning need is to know how important exercise is to their health and level of fitness.

Objectives are specific, short-term criteria that need to be met as steps toward achieving the long-term goal such as, "Within 2 weeks, each of the children will be able to demonstrate at least two exercises that they have learned." Objectives are written statements of an intended outcome or expected change in behavior and should define the minimal degree of knowledge or ability needed by a client. Objectives must be stated clearly and defined in measurable terms, and they typically imply an action (Knowles et al., 2005).

Select Appropriate Educational Methods

Educational methods should be chosen to facilitate the efficient and successful accomplishment of program goals and objectives. The methods should also be appropriately matched to the client's strengths and needs as well as those of the presenter. Choose the simplest, clearest, and most succinct manner of presentation and avoid complex program designs. Try to vary the methods in order to hold the attention of the learners and to meet the needs of different learners. Educators also need to be able to deliver presentations, lead group discussions, organize role plays, provide feedback to learners, share case studies, use media and materials, and, where indicated, administer examinations. You will want to think about what content to include, how to organize and sequence the information, what your rate of delivery will be, whether or not you need to include repetition, how much practice time should be included, how you will evaluate the effectiveness of the teaching, and ways that you can provide reinforcement and rewards. The Internet and use of **social media** have created an entirely new way of providing health information. According to the Pew Internet & American Life Project (Pew Charitable Trusts, 2013), 72 percent of Internet users sought health information online. Data from the Pew Charitable Trust (2018) demonstrates the popularity of social media in our society. Facebook and YouTube are the most popular social media platforms in the United States; in fact about two thirds of adults have active Facebook accounts. In the early adult population, 78 percent of 18- to 24-year-olds use Snapchat, 71 percent have Instagram accounts, and 45 percent use Twitter. These venues of access to—and sharing of—information affect the way in which health education is developed and delivered.

It is important to consider the ethical issues involved in using various forms of teaching tools, especially when using social media. Remember, not all websites are developed by health care professionals, nor have they all been peer reviewed. Also, when nurses use patient cases or data to illustrate a health education point, it is important to clearly understand the guidelines of the Health Insurance Portability and Accountability Act (HIPAA) and avoid privacy ethical violations of the ethics code. When nurses use social media to provide health education, they should consult the *ANA's Principles for Social Networking and the Nurse* (American Nurses Association, 2011) and the National Council of State Boards of Nursing's *White Paper: A Nurse's Guide to the Use of Social Media* (National Council of State Boards of Nursing, 2011). It is essential to protect the privacy of patients and their health data when making presentations in person or via social media or any other medium (Alder et al., 2017).

When choosing educational methods, consider age, gender, culture, hearing, sight or developmental disabilities or special learning needs, educational level, knowledge of the subject, and size of the group. For example, clients with a visual impairment need more verbal description than those with no impairment in sight. Persons who have hearing impairments or language deficits need more visual material and speakers or translators who can use sign language or speak their native language. Also, when the learners have limitations in attention and concentration, the educator will need to use creative methods and tools to keep them focused. For example, you might include frequent breaks; simple surroundings with few or no distractions; use of small group interactions to keep learners involved and interested; and

BOX 19.1 Steps of a Needs Assessment

1. Identify what the client wants to know. (Consider *Healthy People 2020* educational objectives.)
2. Collect data systematically about learning needs, readiness to learn, and barriers to learning.
3. Analyze assessment data that have been collected and identify cognitive, affective, and psychomotor learning needs.
4. Think about what will increase the client's ability and motivation to learn.
5. Assist the client to with prioritize prioritizing learning needs.

the use of hands-on equipment such as mannequins, models, interactive games, and other materials and devices that the learner can physically manipulate. Try to involve the learner appropriately, actively, and creatively in learning. Interactive educational programs may be more effective than non-interactive ones. Interactive strategies include discussion, small group work, games, and role-playing, whereas non-interactive strategies include lectures, videos, or demonstrations. The mnemonic TEACH is a useful way to teach clients. The steps are as follows:

Tune in: Listen before you start teaching. The client's needs should direct the content.

Edit information: Teach necessary information first. Be specific.

Act on each teaching moment: Teach whenever possible. Develop a good relationship.

Clarify often: Make sure your assumptions are correct. Seek feedback.

Honor the client: Respect the client as a partner, share responsibility, and build on the client's experience.

CHECK YOUR PRACTICE

You have been asked to serve on a community committee to develop and participate in the implementation of a health fair. What suggestions would you make to the committee? What would you do to prepare for your participation?

The goal of nurses who use *Healthy People 2020* as a guide in educating clients is to foster healthy communities mainly through primary and secondary prevention. Health fairs are a popular way to provide primary and secondary health education. The objectives of holding health fairs are to increase awareness by providing health screenings, activities, information and educational materials, and demonstrations. A health fair can target a specific population or focus on a specific health issue, as well as target a range of groups and cover a variety of health education and health promotion topics. The fair can be held in many locations and can be either inside or outside. The How To box lists guidelines to assist nurses who chair, co-chair, or serve on a planning committee for a health fair.

HOW TO Plan, Implement, and Evaluate a Health Fair

- Form a planning committee (2-12 people who represent the groups that will be part of the health fair) and select chair or co-chairs. Possibilities include health professionals, representatives from health agencies, schools, churches, employers, the media, and the target audience.
- Develop a budget and secure funding.
- Identify the target group; develop a theme.
- Establish goals, expected outcomes, and screening activities consistent with the needs and wishes of the target group. Your primary goal might be to improve the health of a specific population such as workers at one organization or children in one school. You might have secondary goals such as reduced health care costs for the workers and reduced absenteeism for the children.
- Develop a timeline and schedule.
- Choose a site and consider the site logistics: Do this about one year ahead. Think about the size of the site you will need and the traffic flow from one booth or demonstration to another, whether parking is available and free or low cost, and whether there are toilets and places to get food and drinks. If the site is inside, consider adequate exits; the possible risks to children, the elderly, or handicapped people; and other safety and security issues. You may need to create maps: one for how to get to the fair and another one to help attendees get from one table, exhibit, or screening station to another. Be sure to include on the map the location of amenities such as toilets and food vendors.
- Plan for supplies that you will need: Tables, chairs, electronic equipment, and accessories such as extension cords, office supplies, sign-in sheets (and what information should be included), release forms for screenings, name tags, bags for attendees to gather the educational information, and evaluation forms. Obtain these supplies in advance.
- Recruit and manage exhibitors: Do this about 6-12 months ahead. Develop a list of possible exhibitors and sponsors, and contact them via letter, fax, email, telephone, or in person. Follow-up with a confirmation letter (or fax) that outlines the details of the health fair.
- Recruit volunteers to assist with the health fair.
- Publicize the health fair: The planning committee will have many good ideas about how to publicize in the specific community. Examples might include fliers/posters, memos, brochures, social media, email blasts, local print, or radio/television.
- On the day of the fair: Arrive early. Greet volunteers, health care professionals, agency representatives, sponsors, and members of the population being served.
- Evaluate the health fair: By exhibitors, participants and volunteers. You will need a specific form for each of these groups. Schedule a meeting with the planning committee to review evaluations and discuss lessons learned.
- After the fair: Send thank-you letters to health care professionals, sponsors, and agencies, and pay bills associated with the fair.

Modified from Centers for Disease Control and Prevention: How to Plan a Health Fair, 2013. Available at https://www.cdc.gov; and UnitedHealthcare: Health Fair Planning Guide, 2010. Available at https://www.uhctools.com.

Skills of the Effective Educator

The educator needs to understand the basic sequence of instruction. The following steps are useful in planning an educational program. Begin by (1) gaining the attention of the learners and helping them understand that the information being presented is important and helpful to them; (2) tell the learners the objectives of the instruction; (3) ask the learners to recall previous knowledge related to this topic of interest so that they link new knowledge with previous knowledge; (4) present the essential material in a clear, organized, and simple manner and in a way consistent with the learners' strengths, needs, and limitations; (5) help learners apply the information to their lives and situations; (6) encourage learners to demonstrate what they have learned, which will help you correct any errors and improve skills; and (7) provide feedback to help learners improve their knowledge and skills. When you use each of these steps you can help clients increase their learning experiences.

Motivational Interviewing

Sometimes clients do not provide all of the information needed to help promote their health. It is important before developing an implementation plan to carefully assess the need. The goal in health education is to engage the clients in wanting to learn ways in which they can change their behavior. Pay attention to the words you use and avoid medical jargon. Instead, use conversational language. One tool to use in health education is **motivational interviewing** (MI), which is a tool designed to help clients state their motivations to change (Rosengran, 2017). It is a collaborative partnership between the teacher and the learner designed to help people make their own choices. It seeks to help clients resolve their ambivalence about change and uses the techniques of elaboration, affirmation, reflection, and summary to engage people in talking about change. MI often is used in conjunction with other communication techniques. MI has four essential steps: engaging, which includes person-centered, empathic listening; focusing, which includes a particular identified target for change; evoking of the client's own motivations for change; and planning (Rosengran, 2017).

MI was initially designed to treat problem drinkers and is used often with individuals rather than groups. However, the principles can be applied to health education. For example, if a public health nurse determines that she has four women in a community group she leads who are overweight, eat high-calorie foods, and indicate they exercise little if any on a regular basis, how could the nurse use MI? First, the nurse needs to form a partnership with each of the women, in which she and the clients can communicate easily and in which each woman trusts the nurse. The nurse draws each woman out and learns what, if anything, each wishes to change. The nurse also learns about each one's motivation to change and ability to do so. Consider the client, Anna, and examine her motivation to change her eating and activity patterns. Anna says that her family will eat only fried foods, so to get her husband and children to eat a meal she fries their meats and vegetables. The family does eat fresh fruit and drink milk. Anna says that she gets exercise by walking to the bus stop en route to work and cleaning her home. She has not considered other forms of regular exercise. If you want to use MI with Anna and incorporate these principles in designing your nursing plan, you could begin as follows:

1. Expressing empathy by trying to see the world through Anna's eyes
2. Building on Anna's strengths and helping her believe that she has the ability to make a change (self-efficacy)
3. Rolling with resistance when Anna is ambivalent about her ability to change
4. Developing discrepancy by helping Anna recognize that her current actions conflict with her expressed goals of eating healthy foods and exercising regularly

You could incorporate into your strategy the counseling skills that are part of MI: open-ended questions, affirmations, reflections, and summaries (OARS). These communication skills are useful in any nurse-client interaction. Open-ended questions refer to those that are not easily answered with yes or no or a short answer. These questions invite elaboration and more thinking about what is being asked. In helping Anna prepare healthier meals, ask her to describe the dinner she cooked the previous night. Affirmations are designed to recognize client strengths; they must be genuine and correct. Once Anna begins to explore the idea of preparing more nutritious food, you would affirm her progress and encourage her to continue working toward that goal. Reflections or reflective listening is possibly the most critical skill in that it conveys empathy because you are listening carefully. You can then guide Anna toward dealing with her ambivalence about change by examining the positive and negative aspects of the present situation. Using reflective listening, if Anna expresses concern or difficulty in her goal of preparing different meals, you can focus on her concern and possible ambivalence about sticking to the plan for change.

MI uses the term *change talk* to refer to statements by clients that they are motivated and willing to make change. An easy-to-use mnemonic is "DARN-CAT," which refers to the following:

Preparatory Change Talk	Implementing Change Talk
Desire (I want to change)	**C**ommitment (I will make changes)
Ability (I can change)	**A**ctivation (I am ready, prepared, willing to change)
Reason (It's important to change)	**T**aking steps (I am taking actions to change)
Need (I should change)	

Apply the DARN-CAT mnemonic to the goal you and Anna have for her to learn ways to prepare more nutritious meals. Although MI is a set of skills that requires training to use completely, nurses can incorporate some of the MI techniques into their communication with clients. See the website www.motivationalinterviewing.org for more information on motivational interviewing.

Develop Effective Health Education Programs

All programs, including sessions using MI skills, should include a clear message conveyed in a format appropriate to the learners and in an environment that is free from distractions and consistent with the message. Emotions such as anxiety, stress, anger, or fear can interfere with the listener actually hearing the message being sent. Also, provide information that is understandable to the listener. Use plain language and avoid jargon, multisyllable words, slang, and complex medical terms. Use words that the listener will know and recognize. For example, some people are more familiar with terms like *high blood pressure* and *high blood sugar levels* rather than *hypertension* and *increased glucose levels*. On the other hand, be careful not to oversimplify your terms if your audience is knowledgeable about health care. You want to avoid "talking down" or "over the head" of your listeners.

The type of learning format that you select will depend on the learners. If they are young, you will want an interactive format and many of your options will include the use of technology. You could use a game such as developing a bingo game with food groups to teach about healthy eating. The old adage "a picture is worth a thousand words" still holds true. People tend to remember what they see or hear; a lively format rather than a passive one encourages learning. Most people have a short attention span, so you need to make your point quickly and directly. It may help to provide take-home written materials or a CD for further reminders and follow-up of what is taught. Because people often learn better when they are actively

BOX 19.2 Examples of Learning Formats

Presentation: This method can be used when the group is large and you want to be consistent in the message that is delivered to all participants. Remember, people tend to have a short attention span, so what can you do to keep them engaged? You might ask them to spend some time talking with one another in small groups and then have the group respond to questions, or ask attendees to write answers to questions and invite several to share their answers. The presentation can also be a webinar or similar electronic tool, including Skype.

Demonstration: Use the demonstration technique to show attendees how to perform a task. You could demonstrate insulin injection, heart-healthy food preparation, and exercise.

Small Informal Group: Because learners often learn as much from one another as from the instructor, small groups can be valuable. For example, in working with women in a shelter for abused women, participants may share actions they took to remove themselves safely from the violent environment. They might also be able to jointly plan how each might move to the stage of independent living outside the shelter.

Health Fair: See the How To box on ways to plan, implement, and evaluate a health fair. For example, you might offer a health fair in a senior center and have displays such as posters; videos; live demonstrations; handouts on such topics as reducing fat in selected recipes (including samples) and age-appropriate exercises for flexibility; as well as screenings for elevated blood pressure, glucose, or cholesterol or for osteoporosis and vision.

Non native Language Sessions: You could adapt the health fair approach for a Hispanic group by holding the session in Spanish and providing all of the materials in Spanish. Then ask Spanish-speaking nurses to staff each of the stations for health learning.

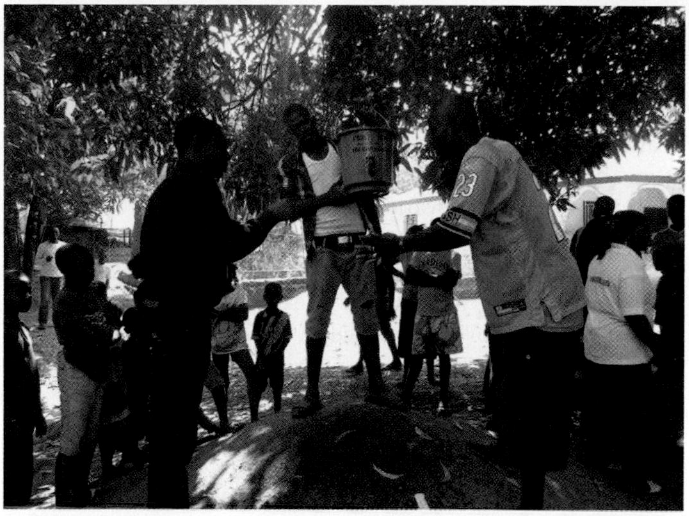

Fig. 19.1 Educating a community group about environmental health issues and gathering their concerns. (From Centers for Disease Control and Prevention, 2009. Courtesy Dawn Arlotta.)

BOX 19.3 Ways to Design Clear Educational Programs

1. Develop the content for your message.
2. Identify the most appropriate format and location for the program, taking into account your budget, location, and other available resources and constraints. See Box 19.2 for examples of formats.
3. Organize the learning experience to fit the audience; consider how to engage the learners in the process.
4. Plan how you will deliver the material, using the following points:
   - Limit the number of points that you wish to cover to the most important ones.
   - Begin with a strong opening and close with a strong ending; people remember most what is said first and last.
   - Fit your use of language to the learners; use an active voice and emphasize the positive. For example, "Many people are able to lose weight by reducing their intake by 500 calories a day and exercising 45 minutes at least four times a week."
   - Use examples, stories, and other vivid messages. Limit statistics and complex terminology.
   - Refer to trustworthy sources. In general, government, educational, or professional association sources are peer reviewed by professionals and dependable. The Centers for Disease Control and Prevention, National Cancer Institute, American Public Health Association, and the American Academy of Pediatrics are four examples of sites that offer useful information.
   - Use aids to highlight your message. For example, you might have posters, handouts, or CDs to give to attendees. You might also incorporate a clip from a website such as www.YouTube.com to emphasize your point. Be sure to verify that the content on the site is accurate; not all information is provided by professionals.
5. Don't forget to plan the evaluation when you are initially planning the program.

engaged in the learning, small group discussion, role-playing, and question-and-answer sessions may reinforce learning. See Box 19.2 for examples of types of learning formats.

Pontius (2013) offers many useful suggestions for developing both verbal and written messages. Her audience is composed of school nurses; however, her messages fit many areas of health education. For written material, first limit the content and make it relevant; use an active voice and conversational tone so that you engage the learner in the process; make the material easy to read and write the way you talk. You do not want to use a thesaurus to find terms to use, so say what you mean in understandable words. As has been mentioned, make the content relevant to the age, gender, and culture of the learner. For online and social media messages, send out one message at a time. Use 12-point print size for most people and 14 point for older people. Use bullets or numbers to easily catch the attention of the reader, and put your most important points early in the list. Leave some white space on the page, and choose ink that contrasts clearly with the background of the paper. Use examples to show the desired behavior. Fig. 19.1 shows a community group being educated, and Box 19.3 lists ways to design clear educational programs.

EDUCATIONAL ISSUES

There are three important educational issues to consider when you are planning educational programs. First, different populations of learners require different teaching strategies. Second, be prepared to overcome barriers to learning. And third, consider the appropriateness of using technology in the programs.

Population Considerations Based on Age and on Cultural and Ethnic Backgrounds

Nurses are an important source of health education in the community. The increase in populations of varying cultural and ethnic backgrounds and the aging of baby boomers require that community health education cross age and cultural boundaries. In terms of age, children, adults, and older adults have different learning needs and respond to different educational strategies. In each age group, learners vary also in their cognitive ability, personality, and prior knowledge. Some people learn better with more direct instruction, supervision, and encouragement than do other people.

Learning strategies for children and individuals with little knowledge about a health-related topic are characterized as **pedagogy**. In the pedagogical model of learning, the teacher assumes full responsibility for making decisions about what will be learned, and how and when it will be learned. This form of learning is teacher directed. Learning strategies for adults, older adults, and individuals with some health-related knowledge about a topic are called **andragogy**. In andragogy, learners play an important role in deciding what they need and want to learn. Andragogy is a more transactional way of learning than is the pedagogical model. Each model has useful elements (Knowles et al., 2005). For example, when learners are dependent and entering a totally new content area, they may require more pedagogical experiences. In addition to considering the age of the population to be educated, think about the learning needs of the population and use the pedagogical and andragogical principles that will best meet these needs. In educational programs for children, provide information that matches the developmental abilities of the group. The following age-specific strategies may help the nurse tailor educational programs for children.

- *With younger children use more concrete examples and word choices.* You might tell a group of three-year-old children that it is good to brush their teeth two times a day. With 10-year-olds, you can explain to them the benefits of brushing their teeth and the risks of not brushing and talk about issues such as the care of their teeth with braces.
- *Use objects or devices, rather than just discuss ideas, to increase attention.* When teaching a group of children with asthma how to use inhalers, it is better to hand out inhalers to each participant and have them practice proper technique with the inhalers rather than just giving them a handout with instructions or demonstrating how to use an inhaler while they watch you.
- *Incorporate repetitive health behaviors into games to help children retain knowledge and acquire skills.* Singing songs while acting out healthy activities such as washing hands before eating helps children get in the habit of washing their hands and makes this health promotion behavior fun. For example, the time a child should wash his or her hands is about the same amount of time it takes to sing "Twinkle, Twinkle Little Star."

In thinking about culture, it is important to know that by 2050 about 50 percent of the U.S. population will consist of ethnic minorities such as Asians, African Americans, Hispanic Americans, American Indians, and Pacific Islanders (Vespa, 2018). Culture influences family structure and interactions as well as views about health and illness. These demographic changes present new challenges to nurse educators. Nurses need to understand the health belief systems of the ethnic populations being served and be familiar with populations who are prone to develop certain health problems. When presenting seminars or providing written, audio, or visual information, provide information in a culturally competent manner.

For example, in a rural farming area, there might be a large population of Mexican migrant crop workers. Knowing that this Spanish-speaking group is more likely to have tuberculosis than other segments of the community, nurses may visit the migrant worker camp to present information on tuberculosis such as prevention, symptom identification, early diagnosis, and treatment. An interpreter may accompany the nurses and provide oral content in Spanish. Written handouts can be in Spanish and designed to be read and understood on a second- or third-grade reading level.

Think also about the generation of the learner. The generation born between 1980 and the present time have always had digital media and access to the Internet and may have very different learning styles and approaches to health compared to those born earlier. Baby boomers, born between 1943 and 1960, were raised without technology and are now reaching retirement age. They are accustomed to being dependent on the teacher, want to be in charge of their own learning, respond positively to feedback, and have a tendency to work many hours. They like to be engaged and connected to other people. Generation X, born between 1961 and 1979, are the children of the boomers and learned independence and self-sufficiency at an early age. Many Gen X children differ in work ethic of their parents (boomers); they want to do a good job, but may seek more work-life balance in their lives. Millennials, born after 1980, are digital savvy, raised using technology for daily communication, interaction, and entertainment (Smith & Nichols, 2015). They like working in teams and seek flexibility in their work life. Based on the understanding of generational difference, the nurse might have different approaches to educational program design (Smith & Nichols, 2015). For example, for the Gen X learners, one might have more independent learning activities build into the health educational program. And for the Millennials, the nurse could plan an asynchronous online educational offering that would allow for flexibility and self-directed, technology-enhanced education.

Use of Technology in Learning

Many kinds of technologies such as computer games and programs, videos, CDs, and Internet resources can increase learning. These technologies may enable the learner to control the pace of instruction, offer flexibility in the time and location of learning, present an appealing form of education, and provide immediate feedback. You may want to use a variety of technological applications in your teaching. It is also important to be aware that people increasingly are using the Internet as a source of health information. Why do people use the Internet? A major benefit is its convenience: It is available 24 hours a day, 7 days a week, and there is no need to drive there, take public transportation, or find a parking place.

Clients may ask nurses to provide them with information about ways to evaluate the quality and reliability of this information. According to the National Network of Libraries of Medicine (NNLM), there are several things that should be considered when evaluating health information on the Internet (NNLM, 2018). Heath information should be evaluated for:

- *Accuracy:* Is the information accurate? Does it come for a reputable source (for example, Centers for Disease Control and Prevention)? Is there an editorial review of the information? Are there spelling or grammatical errors?
- *Authority:* Are there references or citations? Are the authors, their credentials, and affiliations listed, and are they credible?
- *Bias/Objectivity:* Does the information come from a source that is biased (for example, anti-vaccination websites that provide only negative information about childhood immunizations)? Does the site clarify whether its function is to provide information or to market products?
- *Currency/Timeliness:* Are there dates when the information was updated on the website? Do the links on the page work?
- *Coverage:* Is the information complete? Are there links to additional information? Is an appropriate disclaimer provided?

The Evidence-Based Practice box below describes the effective use of a smartphone app for health promotion.

EVIDENCE-BASED PRACTICE

The authors describe the development and formative evaluation of a smartphone app that deals with physical activity promotion. They say that physical inactivity is the fourth leading risk factor for global mortality and that self-monitoring of physical activities levels can support a healthier life. Because the Internet is easily accessed by many people, the authors used "10,000 Steps," which is an online physical activity health program to encourage the use of step-counting pedometers to track daily exercise. Their goal was to evaluate the design and usability of this smartphone app. They used both qualitative (video-taping and having participants "think aloud") and quantitative (a four-item usability questionnaire that used a five-point Likert-type scale followed by a semistructured interview) measures. During the project they made modifications to the app. The results showed that the design changes significantly reduced the time it took for participants to complete their tasks. The study demonstrates the relevance of testing the design and then modifying a smartphone app designed for health promotion.

Nurse Use

Smartphones and their apps are an innovative medium for the delivery of health messages and health care interventions. It is a good idea to test the app before launching it to work out any areas that could be improved in terms of ease of use.

Kirwan M, Duncan MJ, Vandelanotte C, et al.: Design, development, and formative evaluation of a smartphone application for recording and monitoring physical activity levels: the 10,000 Steps "iStepLog." *Health Educ Behav* 40:140–151, 2013.

Barriers to Learning

Barriers to learning fall into two broad categories: one concerning the educator and the other concerning the learner.

Educator-Related Barriers. Some common educator-related barriers to learning, together with strategies to minimize them, follow (Knowles et al., 2005):

- *Fear of public speaking:* Be well prepared, use icebreakers, recognize and acknowledge the fear, and practice in front of a mirror or video camera or with a friend.
- *Lack of credibility with respect to a certain topic:* Increase your confidence by carefully preparing for the talk so that you have included useful information and you understand the information; avoid apologizing for lack of expertise, and instead convey the attitude of an expert by briefly sharing your personal and professional background.
- *Limited professional experiences related to a health topic:* You may want to describe personal experiences (brief ones), share experiences of others, or use analogies, illustrations, or examples from movies, current news, or famous people.
- *Inability to deal with difficult people who need to learn health-related information:* One strategy that may help with handling difficult learners is to confront the problem learner directly. Other strategies include using humor, using small groups to foster participation of timid people, asking disruptive people to give others a chance to speak, or, if this does not work, asking them to leave.
- *Lack of knowledge about how to gain participation:* You can foster participation by asking open-ended questions, inviting participation, and planning small group activities whereby a person responds based on the group rather than presenting his own information.
- *Lack of experience in timing a presentation so that it is neither too long nor too short:* Plan ahead and practice the presentation by speaking during the practice at the same pace that you will speak to the group.
- *Uncertainty about how to adjust instruction:* You can more easily adjust instruction when you know the participants' needs, request feedback, and redesign the presentation during breaks, based on what you have learned about the participants.
- *A sense of discomfort when learners ask questions:* Try to anticipate questions, concisely paraphrasing questions to be sure that you correctly understood the question, and recognizing that it is appropriate to admit that you do not know the answer to a question.
- *Lack of feedback from learners:* Solicit informal feedback during the program and at the end with program evaluation.
- *Concern about whether media, materials, and facilities will function properly:* Test the equipment before the program to make sure it runs and also that you know how to use it. Also, have back-up plans for how to get help if you have a problem.
- *Difficulty with openings and closings:* Strategies to foster successful openings and closings include developing several examples of openings and closings, memorizing the opening and closing, concisely summarizing information, and thanking participants for attending.

- *Overdependence on notes:* You may wish to use note cards or visual aids as prompts; also, practicing in advance is a proven way to increase skill at presenting.

Learner-Related Barriers. Two of the most important learner-related barriers are low literacy and lack of motivation to learn information and make needed behavioral changes.

Low Literacy Levels. Nurses often deal with individuals and populations who are illiterate or who have low literacy levels. These individuals may be embarrassed to admit this deficit to health care providers and educators and may try to appear to understand when they really do not. Specifically, they may not ask questions to clarify information even when they do not understand it. As society becomes more multicultural, the problem of low literacy can increase due to limited use of the primary language as well as limited education. One of the Core Competencies for Community/Public Health Nursing listed in the 2018 revisions by the Quad Council Coalition is to "assess the health literacy of individuals and families" (Quad Council Coalition Competency Review Task Force, 2018). The next paragraphs describe the significance of this problem and the need for nurses to address health literacy.

The National Assessment of Adult Literacy (NAAL) is the largest literacy assessment study done in the United States. This assessment was first conducted in 1992. At that time, out of five levels in the assessment, 50 percent of American adults were in the top two levels and 50 percent were in the bottom three levels of literacy. The minimal standard needed to function in the workplace is that of level 3 proficiency. In 2003, the tool measured literacy in four levels: *Below Basic, Basic, Intermediate,* and *Proficient.* The literacy scales used in 2003 were as follows: prose literacy, document literacy, and quantitative literacy. Prose examples include searching, comprehending, and using information from editorials, news stories, brochures, and instructional materials. Document literacy refers to searching, comprehending, and using information from documents such as job applications, payroll forms, transportation schedules, maps, tables, and drug and food labels. Quantitative literacy is the ability to identify and perform computations such as balancing a checkbook, completing an order form, or determining the interest on a loan from an advertisement. The 2003 test is more than just a survey and actually asks the test takers to perform tasks to demonstrate their literacy (Kutner et al., 2006). The 2003 NAAL included information about health literacy, which is an important topic for nurses.

Health literacy is gaining considerable attention for many reasons, including the costs of health illiteracy when people are unable to follow directions about health care. *Healthy People 2020* defines **health literacy** as "[t]he degree to which individuals have the capacity to obtain, process, and understand basic information and services needed to make appropriate health decisions" (USDHHS, 2010). Health literacy includes a range of abilities, including being able to "read, comprehend, and analyze information; decode instructions, symbols, charts and diagrams; weigh risks and benefits; and, ultimately, make decisions and take action" (National Institutes of Health [NIH], 2017). A person with limited literacy may be unable to understand instructions on prescription bottles, interpret health appointment cards, fill out health insurance forms, and read and understand self-care or hospital discharge instructions. What happens when someone has health illiteracy? A person with limited literacy may:

- Have a limited vocabulary and general knowledge and does not ask for clarification
- Focus on details and deal in literal or concrete concepts versus abstract concepts
- Select responses on a survey or questionnaire without necessarily understanding them
- Be unable to understand math (which is important in calculating medications)

In the past few years a great deal of federal and local attention has been paid to health literacy. Box 19.4 summarizes a sample of websites available to guide people in learning more about how to provide information in a way that learners who have varying levels of literacy can understand.

The *Plain Writing Act of 2010* requires the federal government to write all new publications, forms, and publicly distributed documents in a "clear, concise, well-organized" manner and according to plain writing guides (see Public Law 111-274 at http://www.gpo.gov). Similarly, the National Institutes of Health has developed materials on health literacy and clear communication and calls attention to the enormous costs associated with health illiteracy and how clear, understandable communication is needed for health care professionals (NIH, 2017). An especially helpful health literacy toolkit can be found on the Agency for Healthcare Research and Quality (AHRQ) website, http://www.ahrq.gov. This kit is filled with information on how to create a literacy plan and materials that will increase knowledge or change beliefs, attitudes, and behaviors by sending messages that are clear, relevant, and appropriate for the intended audience (AHRQ, 2017). Box 19.5 summarizes key sections in the toolkit.

Nurses may use pictures, including comic books, slides, and videos, including YouTube presentations, and models in educating clients with low literacy. Some people learn better in a series of educational sessions. For example, at the first session, identify learning capacity and provide a small amount of foundational information. During subsequent sessions, new information that builds on existing knowledge and skills is provided and evaluated. Give additional information when you believe that the information has been understood and can be

BOX 19.4 Examples of Useful Websites for Health Education

- Agency for Healthcare Research and Quality: *Health Literacy Universal Precautions Toolkit,* second edition (https://www.ahrq.gov)
- Centers for Disease Control and Prevention: *Plan and Act: What Is the National Action Plan to Improve Health Literacy?* (http://www.cdc.gov)
- Centers for Disease Control and Prevention: *Simply Put: A Guide for Creating Easy-to-Understand Materials* (http://www.cdc.gov)
- National Institutes of Health: *Health Literacy* (https://www.nih.gov)
- Motivational interviewing network of trainers (MINT): *Motivational Interviewing* (http://www.motivationalinterviewing.org)

BOX 19.5 An Approach to Implementing the AHRQ Health Literacy Universal Precautions Toolkit

Introduction
Quick Start Guide
Form a Team: Tool #1
Create a Health Literacy Improvement Plan: Tool #2
Raise Awareness: Tool #3
Communicate Clearly: Tool #4
Use the Teach-Back Method: Tool #5
Follow Up With Patients: Tool #6
Improve Telephone Access: Tool #7
Conduct Brown Bag Medicine Reviews: Tool #8
Address Language Differences: Tool #9
Consider Culture, Customs, and Beliefs: Tool #10
Assess, Select, and Create Easy-to-Understand Materials: Tool #11
Use Health Education Material Effectively: Tool #12
Welcome Patients: Tool #13
Encourage Questions: Tool #14
Make Action Plans: Tool #15
Help Patients Remember How and When to Take Their Medicine: Tool #16
Get Patient Feedback: Tool #17
Link Patients to Non-Medical Support: Tool #18
Direct Patients to Medicine Resources: Tool #19
Connect Patients With Literacy and Math Resources: Tool #20
Make Referrals Easy: Tool #21
Appendix Items
List of Internet Resources

AHRQ, Agency for Healthcare Research and Quality.
AHRQ Health Literacy Universal Precautions Toolkit. Content last reviewed August 2018. Agency for Healthcare Research and Quality, Rockville, MD. Available at http://www.ahrq.gov/professionals.

incorporated into learners' lives. To evaluate whether a person has limited health literacy, listen for the following clues: "I forgot my reading glasses," "I can read this when I get home," or "I will talk about this with my family—may I take the instructions home?" These comments may be quite straightforward or be a clue that the person actually cannot read the material.

Some people do not engage in learning because they have low levels of motivation to do so. Although adults respond to some external motivators, the most powerful motivators are internal. People are motivated to learn if they value the information and feel that they will benefit from the outcome, if they think they can follow through on what is being taught, and if it will improve their situation in life or increase their self-esteem (Wlodkowski & Ginsberg, 2017).

Models can be used to structure health education and health promotion plans. One model, the **health belief model** (HBM), is an individual-level model. This model can be useful in planning programs in which the motivation of learners might be a concern. Specifically, the HBM was one of the first theories of health behavior. It began in an interesting way when people failed to use free chest x-rays in the 1950s. A group of social psychologists were asked to try to explain the failure to use this screening. Specifically, what would motivate people to seek health care?

The HBM includes six components that attempt to answer the question of what motivates an individual to do something. These components are as follows: (1) perceived susceptibility ("Will something happen to me?"), (2) perceived severity ("If something does happen to me, will it be a big problem?"), (3) perceived benefits ("If I do what is suggested, will it really help me?"), (4) perceived barriers ("Assuming I do what is suggested, will there be barriers that will be unpleasant, costly, and so forth?"), (5) cues to action ("What might motivate me to actually do something?"), and (6) self-efficacy ("Can I really do this?"). This model has been applauded and criticized. It does offer guidance in planning health education programs in that it reminds nurses to think carefully about what motivates people to change. To understand motivation, it is important to learn (1) how the people involved feel about the health problem, (2) whether they think it is serious, (3) whether they believe that action on their part will make a difference, and (4) whether they think that they can both manage the barriers and actually perform the action (2018).

Consider the following example of how the HBM might be applied to a person in the community who has recently been diagnosed with diabetes. The person, June, is 25 years old and was diagnosed two months ago with diabetes mellitus. She has found it difficult to follow the recommendations of the public health nurse who has seen her in the community clinic. When the nurse asked June what seemed to be getting in the way of her complying, June said that she had asked herself these questions:

1. If I do not follow the nurse's advice about diet, exercise, and taking my insulin, will something really happen to me?
2. If I do not follow the advice and something does happen, will it really be a problem?
3. On the other hand, if I take my medicine, eat a diet that will keep my diabetes under control, exercise as recommended by the nurse, and take my insulin according to the nurse's directions, will I really reduce the seriousness of my disease?
4. How much will it cost me to purchase the foods in order to follow the diet? How much time will it take each week to exercise as recommended? Will it hurt me to give myself insulin injections?
5. I did see that my friend, Sue, who was diagnosed about two years ago with diabetes was careful about what she ate at the party, and she did talk about her exercise program where she walks 50 minutes five days a week. Sue did look better than she did when I saw her last year.
6. Is it possible for me to take care of myself like Sue does?

One additional model that is especially useful in health promotion discussed in Chapter 18 is the **transtheoretical model** (TTM). This model deals with change that occurs in stages and over time.

Evaluation

Evaluation is as important in the educational process as it is in the nursing process. Evaluation provides a systematic and logical method for making decisions to improve the educational program. You will need to evaluate the educator, the process, and the outcome.

Evaluating the Educator. Feedback to the *educator* provides the person an opportunity to modify the teaching process and enables the educator to better meet the learner's needs. The learner's evaluation of the educator occurs continuously throughout the educational program. The educator may receive written or verbal feedback from learners. Educators can get feedback by using return demonstrations to see what learners have mastered.

The educator should assume that inadequate learner responses reflect an inadequate program, not an inadequate learner. If the evaluation reveals that the learning objectives are not being met, the nurse must determine why the instruction is not effective. At this point, the educator will want to present the material creatively and meaningfully in new ways that will increase learner retention and the learner's ability to apply the new knowledge. Ultimately, the educator must assume responsibility for the success or failure of the educational process and the development of learner knowledge, skills, and abilities.

Evaluating the Educational Process. **Process evaluation** examines the dynamic, ongoing components of the educational program. It follows and assesses the movements and management of information transfer and attempts to make sure that the objectives are being met. Use process evaluation throughout the educational program to determine whether goals and objectives are being met and the time required for their accomplishment. Ongoing evaluation also allows the teacher to correct misinformation, misinterpretation, or confusion.

Periodically review program goals and objectives, and ask whether the desired health behavior change is really necessary. Such a question inevitably leads back to the original learning objectives and enables the nurse to rethink the practicality and merit of each of the objectives. If teaching seems not to be working, re-examine the factors that influence learner readiness and motivation. Process evaluation uses information gathered from the educator as well as from learner evaluations and assesses the dynamics of their interactions.

Evaluating the Educational Outcome. The educational outcome can be measured both qualitatively and quantitatively. For example, a qualitative assessment should answer the question, "How well does the learner appear to understand the content?" A quantitative assessment should answer the question, "How much of the content does the learner retain?" Thus, the quality of the product is measured by improvement and increase, or the lack thereof, in the learner's knowledge, skills, and abilities related to the content of the educational program. Selected outcomes for the population of interest need to be identified when the educational program is conceived. Measurement of changes in these outcomes determines the effectiveness of the program. In nursing, the educational outcome is assessed as a measurable change in the health or behavior of the client.

Evaluating Health and Behavioral Change. Many approaches, methods, and tools are used to evaluate health and behavioral changes. Examples include questionnaires, rating scales, surveys, checklists, skills demonstrations, testing, subjective client feedback, and client repeat demonstration. Whether you use qualitative or quantitative strategies depends on the expected educational outcome. Evaluation of outcomes measured includes changes in knowledge, skills, abilities, attitudes, behavior, health status, and quality of life. Approaches to evaluating health education effects will vary, depending on the situation. For example, when considering a client's ability to perform a psychomotor skill such as changing a dressing, observing the client doing the skill is the most appropriate means of evaluation.

If evaluation of the educational product shows positive changes in health status and health-related behaviors, the educator can expect good results in similar health educational programs. If evaluation shows no changes or negative changes in health status and health-related behaviors, then re-examine and modify the program to attain better results in the future.

It is important to evaluate short-term health and behavioral effects of health education programs and to determine whether they are really caused by the educational program. Short-term objectives are often easy to evaluate (see Chapter 23). For example, a **short-term evaluation** of whether a client can perform a return demonstration of a process being taught requires minimal energy, expense, or time; skill mastery can be determined within a matter of minutes. If the short-term objective is not met, the nurse determines why and identifies possible solutions so that successful learning can occur. If the short-term objective is met, the nurse can then focus on long-term evaluation designed to assess the lasting effects of the education program.

The goal of health education is to help clients make lasting behavioral changes that will improve their overall health status. Long-term follow-up with clients is a challenging task. **Long-term evaluation** is geared toward following and assessing the status of an individual, family, community, or population over time. The tools of evaluation are designed to assess whether specific goals and objectives were met. Also, monitor the extent and direction of client changes in health status and health behaviors (RHI, 2018). Often, for nurse educators, the goal of long-term evaluation is an analysis of the effectiveness of the education program for the entire community, not the health status of a specific client. Nurses track the achievement of community objectives over time, but not that of the individual community members. Thus, in a changing population, long-term evaluation of the results of an education program is still possible. The percent of objectives and goals met by sampling the target population gives valid statistics for program assessment, even though the population of individuals may have experienced a complete turnover.

For example, a nurse notes that according to annual health department data, 60 percent of all pregnant women in the nurse's catchment area received some prenatal care. Wanting to increase this percent to 100 percent, the nurse tries an educational intervention in which radio and television stations make public service announcements (PSAs) about the importance and availability of prenatal services.

After one year, the nurse discovers that 80 percent of all pregnant women now receive prenatal care. The nurse continues to use PSAs the next year because good results are evident. However, the long-term goal of the education program to influence the behavior of 100 percent of the pregnant women in the community has not yet been met. The nurse enlists volunteers to put informational posters in shopping malls, grocery stores, public transportation stops, laundries, and public transportation vehicles. In the second year after implementing the revised educational program, again using the statistics from the health department, the nurse finds that 95 percent of all pregnant women in the target area now receive prenatal care. The nurse can now evaluate and modify a community educational program over time to increase the rate, range, and consistency of progress made toward meeting the long-term goals of the project. It will be important and often difficult to keep track of clients; email, telephone calls, and text messages may be useful.

Because health education is often conducted in the community in groups rather than provided to one person at a time, the use of groups in health education is discussed.

HEALTH EDUCATION FOR COMMUNITY GROUPS

People are part of a variety of groups, and each can influence health behavior and support useful or poor health practices. Groups are an effective and powerful medium by which to initiate and implement changes for individuals, families, organizations, and the community. People naturally form groups in the home, and groups in the community dramatically influence the community's health. They may form for a clearly stated purpose or goal, or they may form naturally as shared values, interests, activities, or personal characteristics attract individuals to each other.

Community groups represent the collective interests, needs, and values of individuals; they provide a link between the individual and the larger social system. Throughout life, group membership influences thoughts, choices, behaviors, and values as people socialize and interact. Through groups, people may express personal views and relate them to the views of others. Groups serve as communication networks and can help organize various aspects of communities.

Community groups may be informal or formal. **Formal groups** have a defined membership and a specific purpose. They may or may not have an official place in the community's organization. In **informal groups**, the ties between members are multiple, and the purposes are unwritten yet understood by members. These groups often form spontaneously when participants have a common interest or need. You can find out about what formal and informal groups exist in a community by reading the local newspaper, listening to public service information on the radio or television, reading items on the Internet, and asking residents about the groups to which they belong. Nurses often serve as a catalyst for forming new groups or by creating linkages among groups that currently exist.

Group support often helps people make needed health changes. Skillful use of group methods can help a person analyze the problem, sustain motivation for change, experience support during vulnerable periods, and receive quick interpersonal feedback. The discomfort associated with change can be reduced through the relationships with others in beneficial groups. Many of the *Healthy People 2020* priorities can be addressed in health promotion and disease prevention groups, where individuals learn healthier behaviors and gain support from others in changing from risky to healthy lifestyle choices. For example, groups may support physical activity and fitness, sound nutrition, and safe sexual practices. Through group support, individuals may conquer smoking, drug abuse, or abusive relationships. They may identify and reduce exposure to environmental hazards and promote safer physical settings for all. Also, one of the core competencies for public health professionals is to "use group processes to advance community involvement" (Council on Linkages, 2014, p. 9).

Group: Definitions and Concepts

An understanding of several group concepts facilitates group work in the community. Some of the core concepts answer the following questions: (1) What is a group? (2) What is the purpose of the group? (3) How do groups develop and function? (4) What are their stages? and (5) What roles do members typically play in the group?

Definitions. A **group** is a collection of interacting individuals who have common purposes and are influenced by one another. Groups form for a variety of reasons. Families are an example of a community group. Families share kinship bonds, living space, and economic resources. They have many purposes such as teaching their members as well as providing psychological support and socialization. Groups also form in response to community needs, problems, or opportunities. For example, community residents may form a neighborhood association to protect their health and welfare. Community groups occur spontaneously because of mutual attraction between individuals and obvious and keenly felt personal needs such as those for socialization and recreation. Health-promoting groups may form when people meet to work together to support one another in achieving health goals such as weight loss, exercise, dealing with loss, and giving up smoking, gambling, or drinking.

Concepts. Groups need to identify a clear purpose. Having a clear purpose helps in establishing criteria for member selection and determining the action plan. For example, a clear statement of purpose proved valuable in forming a new group in one city's housing development. The local department of social services had received numerous reports of child abuse and neglect. Routine home visits for well-child care documented high stress between parents and their offspring, and some parents requested teaching and guidance from the nurse in child discipline. The nurse proposed that a parent group address this community need, and she chose this purpose for the group: dealing with kids for child and parent satisfaction. The purpose indicated both the process (to help parents deal with children) and the desired outcome (satisfaction for parents and children). As potential members were approached, this statement of group purpose helped them decide if they wanted to join.

Cohesion is the attraction between individual members and between each member and the group. Individuals in a highly cohesive group identify themselves as a unit, work toward common goals, endure frustration for the sake of the group, and defend the group against outside criticism. Attraction increases when members feel accepted and liked by others, see similar qualities in one another, and share similar attitudes and values. Group effectiveness also improves as members work together toward group goals while still satisfying the needs of individual members.

Members' traits that increase group cohesion and productivity include the following: (1) compatible personal and group goals, (2) attraction to group goals, (3) attraction to some members of the group, (4) a mix of leading and following skills, and (5) good problem-solving skills.

Groups have both task and maintenance functions. A **task function** is anything a member does that deliberately contributes to the group's purpose. Members with task-directed abilities become more attractive to the group. These traits include strong problem-solving skills, access to material resources, and skills in directing. Of equal importance are abilities to affirm and support individuals in the group. These functions are called **maintenance functions** because they help other members stay with the group and feel accepted. Other maintenance functions are the ability to help people resolve conflicts and create social and environmental comfort. Both task and maintenance functions are necessary for group progress. Naturally, those members who provide these functions are attractive, and an abundance of such traits within the membership tends to increase group cohesion.

The following group members' traits may decrease cohesion and productivity: (1) a sense of conflict between personal and group goals, (2) lack of interest in group goals and activities, (3) poor problem-solving and communication abilities, (4) lack of both leadership and supporter skills, (5) disagreement about types of leadership, (6) aversion to other members, and (7) behaviors and attributes that others do not understand.

Usually, the more alike group members are, the stronger a group's attraction, whereas differences tend to decrease attractiveness. Members' perceptions of differences can create marked competition and jealousy. At the same time, personal differences can increase group cohesion if they support complementary functioning or provide contrasting viewpoints necessary for decision making. Cohesive factors are complex, and many factors influence member attraction to each other and to the group's goal. High group cohesion positively affects productivity and member satisfaction. The following example illustrates factors that influence group cohesion. A nurse initiated a group for clients who had been treated for burns. Ten residents, all from one town, had been discharged after a month in the local burn unit. The stated purpose for the group was to teach coping skills to assist members in the difficult transition from hospital to home. Each person had been treated for extensive burns in an intensive care treatment center; each had relied heavily on health care workers for physical, social, and emotional rehabilitation; and each had faced the challenge of resuming work and family roles. Individuals shared some similar experiences and hopes for the future but varied in the amount of trauma and stress experienced. They also differed widely in psychological readiness for return to ordinary daily routines. One woman in the group was able to return quickly to her job as a cashier in a large supermarket. The strength of her determination to overcome public reaction to her scars, coupled with an ability to "use the right words" and an empathy for others, distinguished her from others in the group. These differences proved attractive to other members, inspiring them to work toward a return to their own roles in life. These members saw her differences as attainable.

This group's cohesion was provided by the members' attraction to the common purpose of returning to successful life patterns and managing relationships with others. Members also believed that interaction with others with similar burn experiences could help them reach that goal. This example shows that certain member experiences such as crises or traumas may help individuals identify with each other and may increase member attraction.

Being different from the general population and similar to the other group members can be positive for some members and negative for others. Some members may not want to be identified by an aversive characteristic such as disfigurement. Empathy for another's pain, learned only through mutual experience, may provide a person with a required perspective for problem solving or affirming another's view. This group was effective, and the nurse helped members use common experiences and learn from their differences.

Members' attraction to the group is influenced by factors such as the group programs, size, type of organization, and position in the community. Attraction to the group is increased when members view goals clearly and see group activities as effective.

The concept of cohesion helps to explain group productivity. Some cohesion is necessary for people to remain with a group and accomplish the set goals. Attractiveness positively influences members' motivation and commitment to work on the group task. Group cohesion may be increased as members better understand the experiences of others and identify common ideas and reactions to various issues. Nurses facilitate this process by pointing out similarities, contrasting supportive differences, or helping members redefine differences in ways that make those dissimilarities compatible.

Norms are standards that guide, control, and regulate individuals and communities. Group norms set the standards for group members' behaviors, attitudes, and perceptions. Norms suggest what a group believes is important, what it finds acceptable or objectionable, or what it perceives as of no consequence. This commonly held view of what ought to be motivates members to use the group for their mutual benefit (Northen & Kurland, 2001). All groups have norms and mechanisms to accomplish conformity. Group norms serve three functions: (1) to ensure movement toward the group's purpose or tasks; (2) to maintain the group through various supports to members; and (3) to influence members' perceptions and interpretations of reality.

Although certain norms keep the group focused on its task, some diversion can be present if members respect goals and feel committed to return to them. The **task norm** is the commitment to return to the central goals of the group, and its strength determines the group's ability to adhere to its work.

Maintenance norms create group pressures to affirm members and maintain their comfort. Individuals in groups seem most productive and at ease when their psychological and social well-being is nurtured. Maintenance behaviors include identifying the social and psychological tensions of members and taking steps to support those members at high-stress times. For example, maintenance norms often refer to things such as scheduling meetings at convenient times and in an accessible and comfortable space with parking as well as seating, refreshments, and toilets.

Groups also have **reality norms**, where members reinforce or challenge and correct their ideas of what is real. Groups can examine the life situations confronting individuals and help to make sense of them. As individuals gather information, attempt to understand that information, make decisions, and consider the facts and their implications, they can take responsible action, not only in relation to themselves and their group, but also for the community. Group (task, maintenance, and reality) norms combine to form a group culture. Although working with a group does not mean dictating its norms, the nurse can support helpful rules, attitudes, and behaviors. Norms form when these rules, attitudes, and behaviors become part of the life of the group, independent of the nurse. Reality norms influence each member to see relevant situations in the same way the other members see them. For example, suppose a group of individuals with diabetes defines an uncontrolled diet as harmful; members may try to influence one another to maintain diet control. The nurse's role in this group is to provide accurate information about diet and the disease process while continually displaying a belief that health through diet control is attainable and desirable.

Group members with similar backgrounds may have a limited scope of knowledge. For example, women in a spouse abuse group may believe that men are exploitive and harmful on the basis of common childhood and marriage experiences. Such a stereotypical view of men could be reinforced by similar perceptions in other members; this might lead to continuing anger or fear of interactions with men, and a hostile or helpless approach to family affairs. Nurses or group members who have known men in loving, helpful, and collaborative ways can describe their different and positive perceptions of men, thereby adding information and challenging beliefs. The health and condition of members improve as their perceptions of reality are based on a more complete range of data. Nurses bring an important perspective to groups in which similar backgrounds limit the understanding and interpretation of personal concerns.

The role structure of a group refers to the expected ways in which members behave toward one another. The role that each person assumes serves a purpose in the group. Examples of roles are leader, follower, task specialist, maintenance specialist, evaluator, peacemaker, and gatekeeper. Box 19.6 includes descriptions of each of these group roles.

BOX 19.6 Examples of Group Role Behavior

(There are many examples; this is a representative list of the types of roles members assume.)

- **Follower:** Seeks and accepts the authority or direction of others
- **Gatekeeper:** Controls outsiders' access to the group
- **Leader:** Guides and directs group activity
- **Maintenance specialist:** Provides physical and psychological support for group members, thereby holding the group together
- **Peacemaker:** Attempts to reconcile conflict between members or takes action in response to influences that disrupt the group process and threaten its existence
- **Task specialist:** Focuses or directs movement toward the main work of the group

Stages of Group Development

Tuckman (1965) developed a model of the stages of group development that has remained useful over time. He contended that any group, regardless of its type or setting, went through four stages: forming, storming, norming, and performing. In 1977 Tuckman and Jensen determined that there was actually a fifth stage: adjourning. This model can be used for health-related groups to identify in what stage the group is and what may be the next stage. Specifically, in the "forming" stage, members become acquainted with one another and the leader, become oriented to the group, and try to determine what their behaviors should be in relation to one another and to the goal of the group. In the "storming" stage, members begin to express their own individuality, which may run counter to that of others, and they may express hostility to one another and polarize because of interpersonal issues. In the third, or "norming," stage, members start to accept one another; develop some cohesion, norms, and roles; and become comfortable in expressing their opinions and offering ideas. Members begin to trust one another and their interaction takes on more depth. In the fourth stage, "performing," the group uses its interpersonal structure to accomplish its goals, and group energy is directed toward the tasks. In the fifth stage, "adjourning," the group engages in separating from one another.

Leadership is a complex concept. It consists of behaviors that guide or direct members and determine and influence group action. Positive leadership defines or negotiates the group's purpose, selects and helps implement tasks that accomplish the purpose, maintains an environment that affirms and supports members, and balances efforts between task and maintenance. An effective leader pays attention to communications and interactions among the members. Attention is paid to both spoken words and body language, and this information provides continuous feedback about the members and the group process. By paying close attention to communications and interactions, members detect changing group needs, and they can take responsibility and pride in their own involvement. One or more members may lead the group or many may share leadership. Shared leadership may increase productivity, cohesion, and satisfying interactions among members.

After initiating or establishing a group, nurses may facilitate leadership within and among members, frequently relinquishing central control and encouraging members to determine the ultimate leadership pattern for their group. In some settings

BOX 19.7 Examples of Leadership Behaviors

- **Advising:** Introducing direction on the basis of knowledgeable opinion
- **Analyzing:** Reviewing what has occurred as encouragement to examine behavior and its meaning
- **Clarifying:** Verifying the meanings of interaction and communication through questions and restatement
- **Confronting:** Presenting behavior and its effects to the individual and group to challenge existing perceptions
- **Evaluating:** Analyzing the effect or outcome of action or the worth of an idea according to some standard
- **Initiating:** Introducing topics, beginning work, or changing the focus of a group
- **Questioning:** Generating analysis of a view or views by questions that support examination
- **Reflecting behavior:** Providing feedback on how behavior appears to others
- **Reflecting feelings:** Naming the feelings that may be behind what is said or done
- **Suggesting:** Proposing or presenting an idea to a group
- **Summarizing:** Restating discussion or group action in brief form, highlighting important points
- **Supporting:** Giving the kind of emotionally comforting feedback that helps a person or group continue ongoing actions

and circumstances, a single authority seems necessary (e.g., when members have limited skills or limited time, or when groups claim discomfort with shared responsibility for leading). A leadership style that shares leading functions with other group members is effective when there are many alternatives and when issues of values and ethics are involved in the group's action. Examples of leadership behaviors are shown in Box 19.7. Leadership can be described as patriarchal (paternal) or democratic. Each of these styles has a particular effect on members' interaction, satisfaction, and productivity. Groups may reflect one or a combination of styles.

A patriarchal or paternal style is seen when one person has the final authority for group direction and movement. A person using **patriarchal leadership** may control members through rewards and threats, often keeping them in the dark about the goals and rationale behind prescribed actions. Paternal leaders win the respect and dependence of their followers by parent-like devotion to members' needs. The leader controls group movement and progress through interpersonal power. Patriarchal and paternal styles of leadership are authoritarian. These styles are effective for groups such as a disaster team in which immediate task accomplishment or high productivity is the goal. Group morale and cohesiveness are typically low under sustained authoritarian styles of leadership, and members may not learn how to function independently. Also, issues of authority and control may disrupt productivity if the group members challenge the power of the leader.

Democratic leadership is cooperative in nature and promotes and supports members' involvement in all aspects of decision making and planning. Members influence each other as they explore goals, plan steps toward the goals, implement those steps, and evaluate progress.

Choosing Groups for Health Change

Nurses choose the type of group that will be used after studying the overall needs of the community and its people. Such a study is based on client contacts, expressed concerns from various community spokespersons, health statistics for the area, available health resources, and the community's general well-being. These data point to the community's strengths and critical needs.

The nurse can identify goals for the community and for various groups through media reports, from community informants, and from colleagues. Goals may include visions for change as perceived by the people living and working in the local community. Data may be organized according to the opinions and behaviors of the identified groups. Such information about community groups and assessment data are used with community representatives to plan desired interventions. Alliances or coalitions unite diverse interest groups who share a common interest in perceived threats to community health, and nurses may work with groups both for community analysis and vehicles for change.

Deciding whether to work in **established groups** or to begin new ones is based on the clients' needs, the purpose of existing groups, and the membership ties in existing groups. There are advantages to using established groups for individual health change. Membership ties already exist, and the existing structure can be used. It is not necessary to find new members because compatible individuals already form a working group. Established groups usually have operating methods that have proved successful; an approach for a new goal is built on this history. Members are aware of each other's strengths, limitations, and preferred styles of interaction and may be comfortable working with and may be able to influence one another. If you choose to work with an established group, be sure to determine whether the new focus is compatible with the existing group purposes. Fig. 19.2 shows a breakout session during a community forum.

Groups can be used during a community assessment for information. Groups such as health-planning groups, better

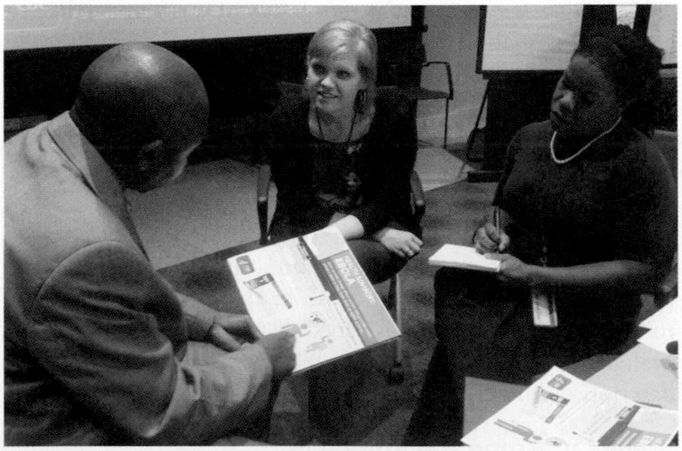

Fig. 19.2 Breakout session in a community forum on environmental health concerns. (From Centers for Disease Control and Prevention, 2009. Courtesy Dawn Arlotta.)

business clubs, women's action groups, school boards, and neighborhood councils are excellent information resources because part of their purpose is to determine and respond to community needs. In addition, they are already established as part of the community structure. When a group representing one community sector is selected for community health intervention, the total community structure is studied. Groups reflect existing community values, strengths, and norms.

How might nurses help established groups to work toward community goals? The same interventions recommended for groups formed for individual health change can be used for groups focused on community health. Such interventions include the following:

- Building cohesion through clarifying goals and individual attraction to groups
- Building member commitment and participation
- Keeping the group focused on the goal
- Maintaining members through recognition and encouragement
- Maintaining member self-esteem during conflict and confrontation
- Analyzing forces affecting movement toward the goal
- Evaluating progress

When nurses enter established groups, they need to assess the leadership, communications, and normative structures. This facilitates group planning, problem solving, intervention, and evaluation. The following example illustrates working with a community group. A nurse was asked to meet with a neighborhood council to help them study and "do something about" the number of homeless living on the streets. Residents knew this nurse from a local clinic and from his consulting work at a shelter for the homeless in an adjacent community. In their invitation to the nurse, council members said, "our intent is to be part of the solution rather than part of the problem." The nurse accepted the invitation to visit. He learned that this council had addressed neighborhood concerns for 20 years—protecting zoning guidelines, setting up a recreational program for teens, organizing an after school program for latchkey children, and generally representing the homeowners of the area. The neighborhood was made up of low-income families who took great pride in their homes. After meeting with the council and listening to their description of the situation, the nurse agreed to help and joined the council.

As the first step in addressing the problem, the council conducted a comprehensive problem analysis on the homeless situation. All known causes and outcomes of homeless persons on the street were identified, and the relationships between each factor and the problem were documented from literature and from the local history. The nurse brought expertise in health planning and knowledge of the homeless and their health risks. He suggested negotiation between the council and the local coalition for the homeless, recognizing that planning would be most relevant if homeless individuals participated. The council was cohesive and committed to the purpose, had developed working operations, and did not need help with group process. They made adjustments in their usual group operation to use the knowledge and health-planning skills of the nurse. Interventions for the homeless included establishing temporary shelters at homes on a rotating basis, providing daily meals through the city council or churches, and joining the area coalition for the homeless.

This example shows how an established, competent group addressed a new goal successfully by building on existing strengths in partnership with the nurse. Community groups, because of their interactive roles, are logical and natural ways for people who work together for community health change. As the decision-making and problem-solving capabilities of community groups are strengthened, the groups become more able representatives for the whole community. Nurses improve the community's health by working with groups toward that goal.

How can the nurse enter existing groups and direct their attention to individual health needs? One nurse employed by an industrial firm noted the harmful effect of managerial stress on several individuals. They had elevated blood pressure, stomach pain, and emotional tension. The nurse learned that the employees with stress were all members of a jogging team that met weekly for conversation in addition to regular workouts. High-level health had been a value shared by all team members, but although jogging was seen as an enjoyable and health-promoting activity, they had never talked about a shared purpose for improved health. The nurse saw a need for stress reduction, thought that the individuals at risk could achieve stress reduction if supported through a group process from valued friends, and proposed that a new purpose be added to the jogging team's activities. All in the group readily accepted and began to focus more on their stress levels as they jogged.

When it is neither desirable nor possible to use existing groups, the nurse can initiate a selected membership group. Choose members who have common health needs or concerns. For instance, individuals with diabetes can meet to discuss diet management and physical care and to share problem-solving remedies; community residents can meet for social support and rehabilitation after treatment for mental illness; or isolated older adults can meet to socialize, eat nutritious meals, and exercise.

Consider members' attributes when composing a new group. Members are attracted to others from similar backgrounds, with similar experiences, and with common interests and abilities. Members' behavior is influenced by the membership, purpose, attraction, norms, leadership, and group structure, and by memories of prior groups. Select members so that common ties or interests balance out dissimilar traits. Try to have members with expressive and problem-solving skills and others who serve in supportive roles; try to have a mix of people with both task and maintenance functions, and others who can develop these skills.

The size of the group influences effectiveness; generally, 8 to 12 is a good number for group work focused on individual health changes. Groups of up to 25 members may be effective when their focus is on community needs. Large groups often divide and assign tasks to subgroups, with the original large groups meeting less frequently for reporting and evaluation. Setting member criteria can facilitate recruitment and selection of the most appropriate members for any group. The criteria usually suggest a mixture of member traits, allowing for balance for the processes of decision making and growth.

Managing the Community Group

As soon as the group forms, begin to work on the stated purpose. Help members interact by paying attention to maintenance tasks of attending, eliciting information, clarifying, and recognizing contributions of members. Begin by talking about what brought each person to the group. Encourage each one to participate; recognize and support them as they take on leadership functions. The new group begins to take shape in the early sessions as members try out familiar roles and test their individual abilities. The core competency skills for communication recommended by the Public Health Foundation (Council on Linkages, 2014) are useful to nurses working with community groups. Box 19.8 lists these competencies. Subsequent steps are then planned not only according to the nurse's skill and preference, but also according to the group composition and the skills brought by members.

Conflict is normal in human relations. People may see conflict as the opposite of harmony and try to guard against it. This is an unfortunate view because the tensions of difference and potential conflict actually help groups work toward their purposes. "Conflict is defined as an interactive process manifested in incompatibility, disagreement, or dissonance within or between social entities (i.e., individual, group, organization, etc.)" (Rahim, 2017, p.16). Conflict signals that antagonistic points of view must be considered and that one must reexamine beliefs and assumptions underlying relationships. Some people are concerned about security, control of self and others, respect between parties, and access to limited resources. In groups, members may express frustrations about trust, closeness and separation, and dependence and independence. These themes of interpersonal conflict operate to some extent in all interactions and are not unique to groups.

People tend to repeat the same patterns of behavior in conflicts. Sometimes the pattern works; other times it does not. The best approach is to match the response style to the situation (Sportsman & Hamilton, 2007), which requires personal awareness and awareness of others. Specifically, when you respond with avoidance, forcing with power, capitulation, and exclusion of a member, the behaviors fail to satisfy the concerns of participants. Assertiveness (attempting to satisfy one's own concerns) and cooperativeness (attempting to satisfy the concerns of others) can be positive responses to conflict. Behaviors that reflect either assertiveness or cooperativeness and that may satisfy the frustrated parties include confrontation, competition, compromise, reconciliation, and collaboration. Resolving conflict within groups depends on open communication among all parties, diffusion of negative feelings and perceptions, concentration on the issues, and use of fair procedures and a structured approach to the process.

Conflict can be overwhelming, especially when members view the expression of controversy as unacceptable or unremitting. Conflict suppressed over time tends to build up and finally explode out of proportion to the current frustration. A group that repeatedly avoids expressing conflict becomes fragile, is unable to adapt and helpless to face challenges. Conflict may be destructive if contentious parties fail to respect the rights and beliefs of others.

Approaches for acknowledging conflict and solving problems that respect others and represent self-concerns are first learned in families and other small groups. These lessons teach people to embrace conflict as a natural occurrence that supports growth and change. Other people learn to avoid conflict or to disregard others in the promotion of self. Teams that try to be harmonious and avoid conflict may hinder collaboration and personal growth (Fogler et al., 2018).

It is important to evaluate individual and group progress toward health goals. Early in the planning, specify the action steps that should be taken to meet the goals. These small steps may be responses to learning objectives (listed as action steps designed to support facilitative forces and deal with resistive forces), or they may reflect the group's problem-solving plan. The action steps and the indicators of achievement are discussed and written in a group record. Recognition of accomplishments in the group and of the group is built into the group's evaluation system. Recognition may include concrete rewards such as special foods and drinks, or it may be the personal expression of joy and member-to-member approval. Celebration for group accomplishments marks progress, rewards members, and motivates each person to continue.

BOX 19.8 Core Competencies for Communication Skills of Educators

Communication Skills

- Communicates effectively both in writing and orally, including via email
- Solicits input from individuals and organizations
- Advocates for public health programs and resources
- Leads and participates in groups to address specific issues
- Uses the media, varied technologies, and community networks to convey information
- Effectively presents accurate demographic, statistical, programmatic, and scientific information for professional and lay audiences

Attitudes

- Listens to others in an unbiased manner
- Respects points of view of others
- Promotes the expression of diverse opinions and perspectives

Implementing the Educational Plan

Once educational methods have been selected, they should be implemented through management of the educational process. Implementation entails the following: (1) control over starting, sustaining, and stopping each method and strategy in the most effective and appropriate time and manner; (2) coordination and control of environmental factors, the flow of the presentation, and other contributory parts of the program; and (3) keeping the materials logically related to the core theme and overall program goals (Knowles, 1990). Administrative and political support is essential to successful program implementation.

Educators must be flexible and modify educational methods and strategies to meet unexpected challenges that confront both the educator and the learner. External influences (such as time limitations, expense, and administrative and political factors) and learner needs require an ongoing evaluation of their impact on the educational program. Implementation is a dynamic element in the educational process.

PRACTICE APPLICATION

During Kristi's BSN student public health practicum at a local health department, the health department got many calls from people wanting information about the newest flu virus. For Kristi's community health intervention project, she decided to do an educational piece on this topic. What is her best course of action?

A. Develop a poster presentation to have on display at the health department.
B. Make an educative pamphlet to mail to anyone calling with questions.
C. Work with the health department staff to develop a community forum presentation and information brochures on influenza.
D. Develop an in-service program for health department staff on potential spread of the virus and ways to prevent its spread.

Answers can be found on the Evolve site.

KEY POINTS

- Health education is a vital part of nursing because the promotion, maintenance, and restoration of health rely on clients' understanding of health care topics.
- Nurse educators identify learning needs, consider how people learn, examine educational issues, design and implement educational programs, and evaluate the effects of the educational program on learning and behavior.
- Nurses often use the *Healthy People 2020* educational objectives as a guide to identifying community-based learning needs.
- Education and learning are different. Education is the establishment and arrangement of events to facilitate learning. Learning is the process of gaining knowledge and expertise and results in behavioral changes.
- Three domains of learning are cognitive, affective, and psychomotor. Depending on the needs of the learner, one or more of these domains may be important for the nurse educator to consider as learning programs are developed.
- Nine principles associated with community health education are gaining attention, informing the learner of the objectives of instruction, stimulating recall of prior learning, presenting the stimulus, providing learning guidance, eliciting performance, providing feedback, assessing performance, and enhancing retention and transfer of knowledge.
- Often theory can guide the development of health education programs. Two useful ones are the health belief model (HBM) and the transtheoretical model (TTM).
- Principles that guide the effective educator include message, format, environment, experience, participation, and evaluation.
- Educational issues include population considerations, barriers to learning, and technological issues.
- Two important learner-related barriers are low literacy, especially health literacy, and lack of motivation to learn information and make the needed changes.
- The five phases of the educational process are identifying educational needs, establishing educational goals and objectives, selecting appropriate educational methods, implementing the educational plan, and evaluating the educational process and product.
- Evaluation of the product includes the measurement of short- and long-term goals and objectives related to improving health and promoting behavioral changes.
- Working with groups is an important skill for nurses. Groups are an effective and powerful vehicle for initiating and implementing healthful changes.
- A group is a collection of interacting individuals with a common purpose. Each member influences and is influenced by other group members to varying degrees.
- Group cohesion is enhanced by commonly shared characteristics among members and diminished by differences among members.
- Cohesion is the measure of attraction between members and the group. Cohesion or the lack of it affects the group's function.
- Norms are standards that guide and regulate individuals and communities. These norms are unwritten and often unspoken and serve to ensure group movement to a goal, to maintain the group, and to influence group members' perceptions and interpretations of reality.
- Some diversity of member backgrounds is usually a positive influence on a group.
- Groups also go through a set of stages in order to form, operate, and adjourn.
- Leadership is an important and complex group concept. Leadership is described as patriarchal (or paternal) or democratic.
- Group structure emerges from various member influences, including members' understanding and support of the group purpose.
- Conflicts in groups may develop from competition for roles or member disagreement about the roles ascribed to them.
- Health behavior is greatly influenced by the groups to which people belong and for which they value membership.
- An understanding of group concepts provides a basis for identifying community groups and their goals, characteristics, and norms. Nurses use their understanding of group principles to work with community groups toward needed health changes.

CLINICAL DECISION-MAKING ACTIVITIES

1. Think about an educational interaction that you had with each type of client (individual, family, community, and population) that did not seem to go well. For each type of client and on the basis of how people learn, identify what might have been the problem. Develop a plan for ways in which the interaction could have been improved, based on how people learn.
2. Recall a learning experience in which the message, format, environment, experience, participation, or evaluation was unsatisfactory. Then develop a plan for how the problem could have been overcome and turned from a negative or neutral learning situation into a positive one.
3. Review the phases of the educational process. Apply this process to a population of individuals with hypertension, a community in which tuberculosis is on the rise, and families with a child who has attention deficit disorder.
4. Select one of the *Healthy People 2020* educational objectives and design a population-specific education program to meet that objective. Consider how people learn, educational issues, educational process including teaching strategies, and evaluation procedures that you would use.
5. Consider three groups of which you are a member. What is the stated purpose of each group? Are you aware of unstated but clearly understood purposes? What is the nature of member interaction in each group? How do purpose and interaction differ in the three groups?
6. Observe two working groups in session, from the community, a health care agency, or a school. Notice the attractiveness of each group through the eyes of its members.
7. List actions that nurses may take to assist groups in various aspects of their work, such as member selection, purpose clarification, arrangements for comfort in participation, and group problem solving.
8. Observe a nurse working with a health promotion group. Does the nurse function in the way you anticipated? What nursing behavior facilitates the group process? List the areas of skill and knowledge that groups consisting of community residents would most likely expect of the nurse.

ADDITIONAL RESOURCES

EVOLVE WEBSITE

http://evolve.elsevier.com/Stanhope/community/

- Answers to Practice Application
- Case Study
- Glossary
- Review Questions

REFERENCES

Agency for Healthcare Research and Quality (AHRQ): *AHRQ Health Literacy Universal Precautions Toolkit*, ed 2, Rockville, MD, Content last reviewed May 2017, AHRQ. Retrieved from http://www.ahrq.gov.

Alder S, Kelleher A, Greene S: *HIPPA Compliance Guide*, 2017. Retrieved from https://www.hipaajournal.com.

American Nurses Association (ANA): *ANA's Principles for Social Networking and the Nurse*, Silver Spring, MD, 2011, ANA.

American Nurses Association (ANA): *Scope & Standards of Practice: Public Health Nursing*, ed 2, Silver Spring, MD, 2013, ANA.

Bloom BS, Englehart MO, Furst EJ, et al.: *Taxonomy of Educational Objectives: The Classification of Educational Goals—Handbook 1: Cognitive Domain,* White Plains, NY, 1956, Longman.

Centers for Disease Control and Prevention (CDC): *How to Plan a Health Fair*, 2013. Retrieved from https://www.cdc.gov.

Council on Linkages between Academia and Public Health Practice: *Core Competencies for Public Health Professionals*, Washington, DC, 2014, Public Health Foundation. Retrieved from http://www.phf.org.

Cronenwett L, Sherwood G, Barnsteiner J, et al.: Quality and safety education for nurses, *Nurs Outlook* 55:122–131, 2007.

Fielding JE: Heath education 2.0; the next generation of health education practice, *Health Educ Behav* 40:513–519, 2013.

Fogler J, Poole MS, Stutman RK: Communication & conflict. In *Working through Conflict: Strategies for Relationships, Groups and organizations*, New York, NY, 2018, Routladge/Taylor & Francis.

Kirwan M, Duncan MJ, Vandelanotte C, et al.: Design, development and formative evaluation of a smartphone application for recording and monitoring physical activity levels: the 10,000 steps "iStepLog." *Health Educ Behav* 40:140–151, 2013.

Knowles M: *The Adult Learner: A Neglected Species*, ed 4, Houston, 1990, Gulf.

Knowles MS, Holton EF III, Swanson RA: *The Adult Learner: The Definitive Classic in Adult Education and Human Resource Development*, ed 6, London, 2005, Elsevier/Butterworth Heinemann.

Kutner M, Greenberg E, Jin Y, et al.: *The Health Literacy of America's Adults: Results from the 2003 National Assessment of Adult Literacy,* Washington, DC, 2006, U.S. Department of Education, National Center for Education Statistics (NCES 2006-483). Retrieved from http://nces.ed.gov.

National Council of State Boards of Nursing (NCSBN): *A Nurse's Guide to the Use of Social Media*, Chicago, 2011, NCSBN. Retrieved from https://www.ncsbn.org.

National Institutes of Health (NIH): *Health Literacy*, 2017. Retrieved from https://www.nih.gov.

National Network of Libraries of Medicine (NNLM): *Evaluating Health Websites*, 2018. Retrieved from https://nnlm.gov/initiatives/topics/health-websites.

Northen H, Kurland R: *Social Work with Groups*, ed 3, New York, NY, 2001, Columbia University Press.

Pew Charitable Trust: *Health Online 2013*, 2013. Retrieved from http://www.pewinternet.org.

Pew Charitable Trusts: *Social Media Use in 2018*, 2018. Retrieved from http://www.pewinternet.org.

Pontius BJ: Health literacy: Part 2, *NASN School Nurse* 28:246–252, 2013.

Quad Council Coalition Competency Review Task Force: *Community/Public Health Nurse Competencies*, 2018. Retrieved from http://www.quadcouncilphn.org.

Rahim MA: Nature of Conflict. In *Managing Conflict in Organizations*, ed 4, Routledge, NY, 2017, pp 17–62.
Rosengran DB: *Building Motivational Interviewing Skills: A Practitioner Workbook*, ed 2, New York, 2017, Guilford Publication.
Rural Health Initiative: *A bridge to improve and sustain health and safety of farm families*, 2018. Thedacare, Appleton, Wisconsin. Retrieved from www.thedacare.org.
Smith TJ, Nichols T: Understanding the millennial generation, *J Bus Diversity* 15(1):39–47, 2015. Retrieved from https://login.proxy.lib.utk.edu.
Sportsman S, Hamilton P: Conflict management styles in the health professions, *J Prof Nurs* 23:157–166, 2007.
Thompson JM: Understanding and managing organizational change: implications for public health management, *J Public Health Manage Pract* 16:167–173, 2010.
Tuckman BW: Developmental sequence in small groups, *Psychol Bull* 63:384–399, 1965.
Tuckman BW, Jensen MAC: Stages of small-group development revisited, *Group Organ Manag* 2:419–427, 1977.
UnitedHealthcare: *Health Fair Planning Guide: Wellness Toolkit*, 2010. Retrieved from https://www.uhctools.com.
U.S. Department of Health and Human Services (USDHHS), Office of Health Promotion and Disease Prevention: *Healthy People 2020*, 2010. Retrieved from https://www.healthypeople.gov.
Vespa J, Armstrong D, Medina L: *Demographic Turning Points for the United States: Population Projections for 2020 to 2060*, Washington, DC, March 2018, US Census Bureau.
Wlodkowski RJ, Ginsberg MB: What Motivates Adults to Learn? *Enhancing Adult Motivation to Learn: A Comprehensive Gide for Teaching All Adults*, San Francisco, 2017, Jossey Bass, pp 81–106.

20

The Nurse-Led Health Center: A Model for Community Nursing Practice

Michele H. Talley, PhD, ACNP-BC, Connie White-Williams, PhD, RN, NE-BC, FAHA, FAAN, Maria R. Shirey, PhD, MBA, RN, NEA-BC, ANEF, FACHE, FNAP, FAAN, and Cynthia Selleck, PhD, RN, FAAN

OBJECTIVES

After reading this chapter, the student should be able to do the following:

1. Describe key characteristics of nurse-led center models.
2. Explain the concept of community collaboration.
3. Identify interventions that address *Healthy People 2020* goals.
4. Determine the feasibility of establishing and sustaining a nurse-led center.
5. Describe the roles and responsibilities of the advanced practice nurse in a nurse-led center.
6. Discuss the future of population-centered nursing practice, education, and research.

CHAPTER OUTLINE

Overview and Definitions
Nurse-Led Models of Care
The Team of a Nurse-Led Center
Other Key Roles in Addition to the Collaborative Team
Starting a Nurse-Led Clinic
Education and Research
Evaluating and Sustaining a Nurse-Led Clinic

KEY TERMS

behavioral health, p. 440
business plan, p. 445
community collaboration, p. 438
community health workers, p. 440
comprehensive primary health care, p. 440
cost-effectiveness, p. 449
enabling services, p. 442
health outcomes, p. 438
multilevel interventions, p. 438
nurse-led health center (NLHC), p. 438
nurse practitioners, p. 440
nursing models of care, p. 438
population health, p. 438
primary health care, p. 440
program evaluation, p. 449
public health nurses, p. 440
Quadruple Aim, p. 440
reimbursement systems, p. 440
safety net providers, p. 438
social determinants of health, p. 438
special care centers, p. 441
strategic planning, p. 439
wellness centers, p. 442

The authors offer a special acknowledgment to the previous contributors to this chapter, Katherine K. Kinsey, PhD, RN, FAAN, and Mary Ellen T. Miller, PhD, RN.

Considerable data document that nurse-led health centers (NLHCs) expand access to health care and improve **health outcomes**. The **nurse-led health center (NLHC)** model provides a comprehensive approach to health and illness; reduces disparities in health and health care; and has been shown to decrease the overall costs of health care (Talley et al., 2018). It is estimated that more than 250 NLHCs exist throughout the United States, providing care to primarily medically underserved, low-income populations that have traditionally lacked access to quality care (Holt et al., 2014). As **safety net providers**, NLHCs reach out to and engage underserved, vulnerable populations in public health and primary health care initiatives.

This chapter introduces the student to NLHCs, describes models of nurse-led care, the role of the collaborative team, the expanding role of the bachelor's prepared nurse in primary care, the business and clinical aspects of starting and managing a nurse-led clinic, as well as the importance of evaluating and sustaining the model. Emphasis is placed on the *Healthy People 2020* framework and the importance of **community collaboration**, community assessment, and **multilevel interventions** as necessary components to establishing and sustaining NLHCs.

BOX 20.1 American Nurses Association Nursing Centers Task Force: Nurse-Led Center Definition

Nurse-led centers—sometimes referred to as nursing centers, community nursing organizations, nurse-managed centers, nursing clinics, and community nursing centers—are organizations that give the client direct access to professional nursing services. Using nursing models of care, professional nurses in these centers diagnose and treat human responses to actual and potential health problems, and promote health and optimal functioning among target populations and communities. The services provided in these centers are holistic and client centered and are reimbursed at the reasonable fee level. Accountability and responsibility for client care and professional practice remain with the professional nurse. Overall accountability and responsibility remain with the nurse executive. Nurse-led centers are not limited to any particular organizational configuration. Nurse-led centers can be free-standing businesses or may be affiliated with universities or other service institutions such as home-health agencies and hospitals. The primary characteristic of the organization is responsiveness to the health needs of the population.

From Aydelotte MK, Barger S, Branstetter E, et al.: *The nursing center: concept and design*, Kansas City, MO, 1987, American Nurses Association, p. 1.

OVERVIEW AND DEFINITIONS

The terms *nurse-led health center, nursing center, nurse-managed health center,* and *nurse-managed health clinic* are interchangeable in this chapter and are used to describe a model developed by nurses to provide accessible, affordable, high-quality, patient-centered care. Nurse-led models of care originated with public health nursing and have existed in the United States for more than a century, with early examples such as Lillian Wald and the Henry Street Settlement in New York City. However, growth of NLHCs has occurred more rapidly within the past 30 years, paralleling not only the growth in the nation's uninsured population but also the growth in the preparation of nurse practitioners (NPs). The citations in this 10th edition of *Public Health Nursing: Population-Centered Health Care in the Community* include historical references that help frame the decades-long NLHC movement, as well as more current references regarding the evolution of NLHCs.

In the past, the most frequently cited and referenced definition of nurse-led health centers was the one developed by the American Nurses Association (ANA) Nursing Centers Task Force in the mid-1980s and shown in Box 20.1. However, the Patient Protection and Affordable Care Act (ACA) of 2010 provides a more current and functional definition of nurse-managed health clinics as seen in Box 20.2. The ACA envisioned NLHCs as having an expanded role in caring for many Americans newly covered by the expansion of Medicaid and other health insurance programs (Ely, 2015).

All NLHCs possess characteristics that reflect the values, beliefs, and scientific knowledge and skills inherent in **nursing models of care** and public health nursing, specifically. Furthermore, each NLHC is managed and staffed by registered nurses (RNs) and NPs, ensuring that decision making and ultimate accountability for the model of care rest with professional nurses.

BOX 20.2 Nurse-Managed Health Center Definition in Patient Protection and Affordable Care Act, 2010

A nurse-managed health center (NMHC) is defined as a community-based nurse practice led by advanced practice nurses, that provide primary care or wellness education, health promotion, and disease prevention primarily to underserved or vulnerable populations. These centers are usually affiliated with a school, university, college or nursing department, independent non-profit health agency or social service agency, or federally qualified health center.

Modified from Title 42-The Public Health and Welfare, Chapter 6A-Public Health Service, 2017, Section 254c-1a (42.U.S.C. § 254c-1a).

Nurse-led center models combine human caring, scientific knowledge about health and illness, and understanding of family and community characteristics, interests, assets, needs, and goals for health promotion, disease prevention, and disease management. NLHC models recognize and address the impact of the **social determinants of health** and subscribe to a holistic perspective on improving personal and **population health** and well-being.

Today's NLHCs are positioned to be responsive to the unique needs of the communities they serve (Hansen-Turton et al., 2015). Most centers focus on wellness promotion, disease prevention, primary care, and management of chronic conditions for vulnerable populations in the community (Ely, 2015). Personal respect, equity, and social justice perspectives serve as the foundation from which health is viewed as essential for everyday life. Efforts of the center focus on enhancing people's capacity to meet their personal, family, and community responsibilities and interests, and typically include the following:

- *Community-based, culturally competent care* that is accessible, acceptable, and responsive to the populations being served
- A *holistic approach* to care based on complex and interrelated bio-psychosocial factors
- *Interorganizational and interprofessional collaboration* that crosses health and human service systems and increases opportunities for comprehensive and seamless services among care providers, agencies, and payers
- *Multilevel interventions* that acknowledge organizational, environmental, health, economic, and social policy contributions to health, health problems, and issues of access to care
- *Community partnerships* that help establish and support the center's health efforts
- *Relationship-based practice* with individuals, families, organizations, and communities that fosters understanding of context, interests, and needs for health care

A nurse-led center's *health* and *community* orientation builds strong connections to the population served. These strong relationships with community leaders, residents, and clients foster a deep awareness of local factors as well as the social determinants (conditions in which people are born, grow, live, work, and age) that influence daily life (World Health Organization [WHO], 2010). This orientation builds on Lillian Wald's community work more than a century ago. Wald established The Henry Street Visiting Nurse Service and a cadre of public health nurses who treated social and economic problems—not just infections, diseases, and providing care to the chronically ill—is part of the nursing center legacy (Hansen-Turton et al., 2015).

The *Healthy People* initiative has framed the nation's health promotion and disease prevention agenda since 1980. Its framework, vision, mission, goals, and objectives are developed to achieve better health for all by 2020. *Healthy People* represents a collaborative federal, public, and stakeholder process and accounts for global and national environmental, social, demographic changes, and trends such as an increasing aging population. *Healthy People* accommodates the escalating technological influences on personal and population health and incorporates the ongoing transformation of the U.S. health care system, thus aligning well with the NLHC focus on integrating primary care and public health in community settings. Chapter 2 describes the history of *Healthy People,* and chapters throughout the text apply the objectives of *Healthy People 2020* to their content. The concept of *Healthy People 2020* builds on shared responsibility to improve the nation's health. Communities, individuals, and systems have the potential for change, yet no one person or organization can do this alone. Powerful, productive partnerships among diverse people and groups and long-term commitments to community collaboration are needed to achieve *Healthy People 2020* goals.

HEALTHY PEOPLE 2020

Nurse-led health centers (NLHCs) can help achieve the goals and objectives of *Healthy People 2020* and should emphasize those goals and objectives that fit their target populations' needs. For example, an NLHC providing care to patients with diabetes would review the 16 *Healthy People 2020* objectives related to diabetes and select ones to target such as:

D 5.1: Reduce the proportion of persons with diabetes with an A1c value greater than nine percent

D-7: Increase the proportion of persons with diagnosed diabetes whose blood pressure is under control

D-13: Increase the proportion of adults with diabetes who perform self-blood glucose-monitoring at least once daily.

The NLHC would also implement communication and education strategies that address the need for diabetes self-management.

Community Collaboration

Nurse-led centers and NPs are well positioned to guide and facilitate community collaboration and engagement surrounding the needs of the community. Building healthy communities is the work of public health nurses; however, it cannot be accomplished alone. It requires building coalitions and linking together others with the same goals, whether it is reducing violence in the community, improving the preterm birth rate, or addressing the local opioid epidemic. NLHCs should have a place at the table and can often lead these efforts because of their interest in improving community health.

Community collaboration involves gathering key stakeholders individuals, families, groups, organizations, policy makers, and staff—each with a unique perspective. Their individual knowledge and skills enhance the community's efforts to address critical needs, solve problems, and recognize unique strengths and resources. Long-term success of the NLHC is dependent on community collaboration and fully understanding the issues and concerns of the community (Sutter-Barrett et al., 2015).

Collaboration takes time, effort, and resources. It requires nurturing and support to make it work. Relationships among people and organizations serve as the foundation for the collaborative process and for community change. Relationships begin with introductions and open discussion to listen to and learn from one another. From this foundation, relationships grow toward a collective willingness to work together toward a common purpose, sharing *risks, responsibilities, resources,* and *rewards* along the way. The seminal definition of collaboration developed by Mattessich and Monsey (1992) describes the work involved; they view collaboration as a relationship entered into by two or more groups to achieve common goals that are well defined and beneficial to all. There must be a respectful commitment to these goals with mutual accountability and authority that allows for shared responsibilities, resources, and successes.

Each nurse-led center develops its philosophy, goals, and activities through a process of community collaboration, community assessment, and strategic planning. **Strategic planning** recognizes multiple levels of intervention required for bringing about and sustaining change. Often, community collaboration and assessment are concurrent activities.

Community Assessment

Nurse-managed centers should conduct an initial feasibility study and periodic community assessments. Data from an analysis of community needs and assets is important in determining the type of nursing center to establish or expand. Through the assessment process, nurses learn both the community's formal and informal infrastructure and the important communication networks. Systematic observations made through neighborhood walks, bus rides, or windshield surveys during car trips through the community as well as discussions with elected officials, health care administrators, public health department staff, and community members provide insight into the community's health and the many other influencing determinants.

Assessment activities identify community assets as well as challenges. For example, there may be a network of neighborhood presidents who serve as leaders and communication liaisons with the community. There may be a local community college that can provide space and support for meetings. If high rates of childhood asthma are discovered, there may be human service organizations that can help in disease prevention and management efforts.

As nurses conduct individual interviews and focus groups, develop surveys, review health care data, and examine social determinants of health (social, educational, employment, economic, housing, and others), they gather detailed information about the overall health and well-being of the community. These sources of information build an understanding of the community and its traditions, strengths, interests, concerns, problems, needs, and preferences. The assessment process also involves reporting back to the community about the information collected and encouraging involvement in collaborative decisions regarding the center's overall direction, services, and programs.

Multilevel Interventions

As the community and the center work together for comprehensive community health, a multilevel approach is needed. Some behavioral decisions or changes occur at the individual and family level. For comprehensive community health improvement, however, strategies are needed at organizational, community, population, and sociopolitical levels. NLHC staff may focus their efforts on system issues, community capacity, and family and individual health care access concurrently. Alternatively, the staff may concentrate programmatic efforts solely at the population level and address system and community issues. There is no one approach. In the twenty-first century, as the health care system is transforming and the focus has shifted to accomplishing the **Quadruple Aim** (better health outcomes, lower costs, improved patient satisfaction, and improved clinician experience) (Feeley, 2018), NPs involved in public health and nurse-led centers are well positioned to lead and influence change.

NURSE-LED MODELS OF CARE

NLHCs typically fit into one of three service models: comprehensive primary care centers, special care centers, or wellness

BOX 20.3 Nurse-Led Center Typologies

Service Model
- *Comprehensive primary care centers:* Provide health-oriented primary care and public health programs
- *Special care centers:* Provide programs targeting specific health conditions (such as diabetes) or population groups (such as the frail elderly)
- *Wellness centers:* Provide health promotion and disease prevention programs

Organizational Structure
- *Academic nurse-led center:* Affiliated with a school of nursing or academic health center
- *Freestanding center:* Independent center with its own governing board
- *Subsidiary:* Part of larger health care systems, home-health agencies, community centers, senior centers, schools, and others
- *Affiliated center:* Legal partnership association with health, human services, or other organization

Internal Revenue Service Designation
- *501(c)3:* Nonprofit business
- *Proprietary:* Incorporated as a for-profit business

Reimbursement Mechanism
- *Fee-for-service:* Payment at time of service; may include sliding-fee scale
- *Federally Qualified Health Center (FQHC):* Federal designation that allows cost-based reimbursement per encounter
- *Third-party reimbursement:* Client billing to public program or commercial/private insurance
- *Grant funded:* Federal, state, local or foundation awards that support personnel or services
- *Contributions:* Individual donations, philanthropic gifts, fund-raising activities to support a program

centers. Many are affiliated with an academic setting such as a school or college of nursing or academic health center; others may be freestanding and governed by a board. Still others may be subsidiaries of larger health care systems, community centers, schools, or other agencies. A smaller number of NLHCs are designated as Federally Qualified Health Centers (FQHCs) and receive federal funds to care for the local community's medically underserved population (Auerbach et al., 2013; Hansen-Turton et al., 2015). Organizational structure (academic, non-academic), federal tax status (profit or nonprofit), and **reimbursement systems** (fee-for-service, sliding scale fee rates, or no charge) also define centers. To date, most nurse-led centers fit into the types described in Box 20.3.

Comprehensive Primary Health Care Centers

In many communities, nurse-led centers offer **comprehensive primary health care** and serve as the primary care medical home for families in the communities where they are located. In these centers, **nurse practitioners** (NPs) and other health professionals provide primary care for individuals and families across the life span and are increasingly integrating **behavioral health** care services as well. **Public health nurses** and **community health workers** may provide outreach, social support, and an array of public health programs, including such things as health education, screening, immunizations, lead poisoning prevention, home visits, environmental health initiatives, and other preventive community-based health services.

A small number of NLHCs have received designation as FQHCs from the Bureau of Primary Health Care (BPHC) of the U.S. Department of Health and Human Services (USDHHS). Their purposes are to (1) provide population-based comprehensive care in medically underserved areas, and (2) maintain the appropriate mission, organizational, and governance structure according to the FQHC designation. These designations include community health center, migrant health center, public housing center, homeless center, or school-based center.

The FQHC designation is important from several perspectives. Most importantly, it supports a primary care center's efforts to serve low-income and uninsured populations and remain fiscally solvent. FQHCs receive federal grant funds from the Health Resources and Services Administration (HRSA) to support operational expenses. They also receive cost-based payment for services provided to Medicare and Medicaid patients, Federal Tort Claim coverage, reduced pharmaceutical costs through 340b drug pricing, and they have the option to recruit clinicians through the National Health Service Corps scholarship and loan repayment programs.

NLHCs that are affiliated with schools of nursing or academic health centers actively integrate service, education, and research in their model. They build on public health and primary care NP educational programs, draw on the knowledge and skills of faculty, and provide rich learning experiences for nursing students at all levels. Furthermore, these clinics often use the knowledge, skills, and resources of other academic programs such as social work, physical therapy, dentistry, optometry, medicine, as well as business, communications, and law to expand the center's service capacity.

Increasingly, interprofessional collaborative practice (IPCP) models of nurse-led care are gaining popularity. IPCP is defined as "multiple health workers from different professional backgrounds working together with patients, families, and communities to deliver the highest quality of care" (WHO, 2010, p. 13). In IPCP, members of the team are trained in the Interprofessional Education Collaborative's (IPEC) competencies, which require integration of four competency domains: values/ethics; roles/responsibilities; interprofessional communication; and teamwork (IPEC, 2016). Members within an IPCP model are health professionals from different disciplines who value the contributions of each team member and know enough about each discipline to understand their potential contributions to patient care quality and safety. Members within an IPCP model communicate with each other in a respectful manner, emphasizing teamwork rather than hierarchy.

The ultimate benefit of IPCP in nurse-led care is that the full interprofessional team approaches care from a more comprehensive fashion to enhance desirable care outcomes. Tapping into each member's full scope of knowledge, skills, and abilities to provide safe, timely, efficient, effective, and equitable care benefits patients, organizations, and communities. In emphasizing teamwork, care in an IPCP model facilitates care coordination and ensures smooth transitions across levels of care.

IPCP is often confused with multidisciplinary care; however, these two concepts are different (Table 20.1). In IPCP, multiple professionals, including community health workers, generally provide care under one roof and in close proximity to each other, thus facilitating just-in-time communication and consultation. Unlike the parallel work that might occur with multidisciplinary teams who are usually not co-located, in the IPCP model there is integrated work that is team-based, assuming full responsibility for a patient's plan of care. The emphasis in the IPCP model is to achieve desired patient outcomes, and all team members work as a unit to impact these outcomes. Similarly, in the IPCP model, the developmental investment is in building the team to produce an exceptional patient experience, improve patient health outcomes, and decrease the cost of care while simultaneously maintaining quality and safety goals.

Special Care Centers

Some nurse-led centers focus on a particular demographic group or on those with special health care needs. **Special care centers** provide services and specialized health knowledge and skills to a particular group; they may also provide comprehensive primary care services to those groups. Examples of special care centers are those that focus on the needs of people with

TABLE 20.1 Comparison of Multidisciplinary Practice With Interprofessional Collaborative Practice

Multidisciplinary Practice	Interprofessional Collaborative Practice
Multiple professionals working together not usually in close contact or proximity	Multiple professional working together usually in close proximity
Only professionals generally contribute to care delivery model	Multiple levels of personnel contribute to care delivery model (i.e., from licensed health professionals to lay community health workers)
Fragmented parallel work; not necessarily team based	Integrated work with team-based identity
Various professionals assume responsibility for parts of the patient plan of care; each discipline accomplishes its own goals	Full team assumes responsibility for the patient's full plan of care; team relies on each other and collaborates to accomplish care goals
Plan of care may be episodic and not necessarily focused along transitions	Plan of care is integrative and follows patients and families across transitions
Communication among multidisciplinary caregivers is episodic with check-ins only when deemed necessary	Communication among members of the IPCP team is ongoing with huddles and routine team checks
Care coordination may be an organizational function; staffed by organizational member outside multidisciplinary caregivers	Care coordination is team and population based; usually staffed by dedicated team member within the IPCP
Developmental resources may be invested in building individuals	Developmental resources may be invested in building the team

IPCP, Interprofessional collaborative practice.

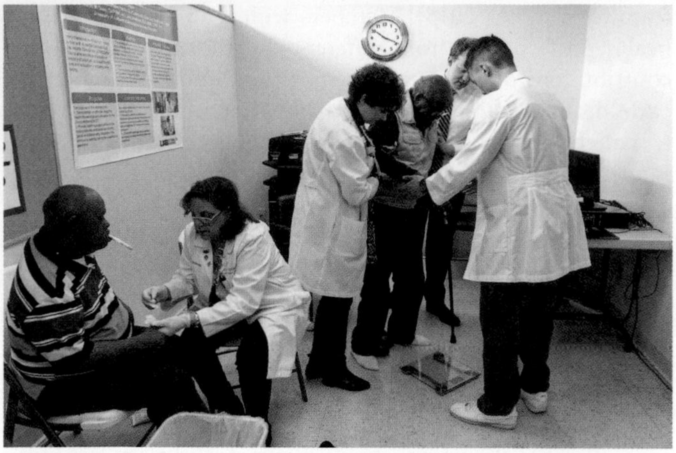

Fig. 20.1 Advanced practice nurses and undergraduate nursing students providing care for adults with developmental disabilities. (Courtesy The University of Alabama at Birmingham School of Nursing.)

diabetes or heart failure, human immunodeficiency virus (HIV)/acquired immunodeficiency syndrome (AIDS), women who have been victims of human trafficking, the frail elderly, or support services for people with mental or developmental disabilities. Other centers are the hub for public health nursing practice in home and community settings. Examples include house calls programs, transitional care home visits, and Nurse-Family Partnership models across the nation as well as other early childhood home visiting models, including Parents As Teachers and Early Head Start (Fig. 20.1).

House Calls Programs

House calls programs provide home-based primary or end-of-life care for vulnerable patients. These patients receive care at home because they cannot travel to their provider's office for appointments. The program goals can include improving (1) the outcomes of prenatal women during pregnancy, (2) mother and baby outcome after birth, and (3) care for frail elderly that are homebound. The house calls team may be led by an NP or physician who work closely together. A social worker, medical assistant, or RN could also be part of the team. Team members are chosen because of their skills, expertise, and needs of the patient. The house calls visit may include a review of medical history, a physical exam, medication review, social services assessment, education, and discussion about any health concerns.

Transitional Care Home Visits

The home visit may differ from a house calls program. As part of a transitional care model, a social worker and a nurse who functions as a transitional care coordinator make a home visit within the first seven days of hospital discharge and before the first clinic appointment. The home visit serves to meet any immediate needs since discharge and provides an opportunity to review the medication regimen and complete the social services assessment. The home visit team reports back to the NP or physician before the first clinic appointment, which assists in continuity of care and reduces re-hospitalization especially for vulnerable, high-risk clients.

Nurse-Family Partnership

Nurse-Family Partnership (NFP) is an evidence-based community health program that serves first-time low-income parents and their children through an intensive public health nurse home visit model. This model, originally developed by Dr. David Olds more than 40 years ago, is based on the most rigorously tested program of its kind (Nurse-Family Partnership, 2018). Eligible low-income women are enrolled during pregnancy, and each woman receives intensive home visit services by a bachelor's prepared RN until the child reaches age two (a total of 64 home visits through program graduation). NFP goals are to improve pregnancy outcomes, improve child health and development, and improve families' economic self-sufficiency over time. Nurse Home Visitors receive extensive education in NFP protocols, maternal-infant-toddler assessment measures, and motivational interviewing strategies (Fig. 20.2). Currently, there are more than 260 agencies implementing the NFP model across the United States.

Wellness Centers

Wellness centers focus on health promotion and disease prevention and management programs. Public health nurses, NPs, and others provide outreach and public awareness services, health education, immunizations, family assessment and screening services, home visiting, and social support services. Health education and support programs may include things such as smoking cessation and management of chronic conditions such as diabetes, asthma, and hypertension. Some centers also provide dental, behavioral health, environmental health risk reduction, and parenting education. Enabling services help people access language translation, registration for entitlement programs, transportation vouchers, and specialty services. *Healthy People 2020* goals and objectives provide direction to services planned, implemented, and evaluated through the wellness center model.

These centers complement existing primary care services. The staff maintains strong relationships with local health care providers in community health centers, clinics, private practices, long-term care facilities, and other organizations.

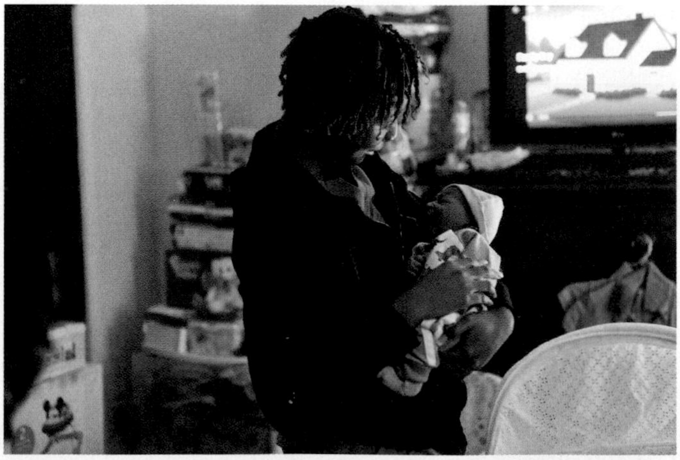

Fig. 20.2 Investing in the future: public health nurses and programs like Nurse-Family Partnership, Early Head Start, Parents As Teachers, and others improve the lives of vulnerable families. (Courtesy The University of Alabama at Birmingham School of Nursing.)

Financial support for wellness center programs typically comes from public health departments and other service contracts, foundation grants, fee-for-service, voluntary contributions, or shared resources from affiliated organizations. Wellness centers often serve as sites for community service learning activities for graduate and undergraduate students from multiple disciplines.

LINKING CONTENT TO PRACTICE

This chapter discusses the ways in which nurses provide care and public health services within the context of a nurse-led setting. Whether functioning in a clinic, community venue, or making a home visit, the skills of assessment, planning, implementation, evaluation, and policy development are integral to this role. The Core Competences for Public Health Professionals (Council on Linkages Between Academia and Public Health Practice, 2014) and the Community/Public Health Nursing (C/PHN) Competencies (Quad Council Coalition, Public Health Foundation, 2018), as well as Core Competencies of Public Health Nurses (2011) and the American Association of Colleges of Nursing (AACN) supplement to the 2010 *Essentials of Baccalaureate Nursing Education for Professional Nursing Practice* titled *Recommended Baccalaureate Competencies and Curricular Guidelines for Public Health Nursing* (AACN, 2013) provide nurses with the expected skills and resources to practice in a nurse-led setting.

THE TEAM OF A NURSE-LED CENTER

Roles of the Collaborative Team

The collaborative teams may include nurse practitioners, clinical nurse leaders, social workers, RNs, medical assistants, collaborating and specialty physicians, behavioral health specialists, dietitians, pharmacists, and support personnel. The clinic type and its services determine staff patterns and roles, responsibilities, and reporting lines. Every center must have an organizational chart that clearly shows staffing positions and reporting responsibilities. The organizational framework must be dynamic in nature and adaptive to new community-focused initiatives. A clinic's success also relates to how well the team works together to ensure the delivery of high-quality health care to target populations (Holt et al., 2014; Pilon & Hansen-Turton, 2015). Positive collegial and professional relationships set the tone for the work. The demand for services will be driven by the needs of the population served. Critical clinical and management positions are briefly highlighted in the following section.

Nurse Practitioners

Nurse practitioners have additional education and training beyond their basic nursing program and are certified or licensed in a specialty area. They provide an expanded level of health services to individuals and families. In nurse-led clinics, nurse practitioners provide on-site services. As NPs, nurse practitioners can be generalists (i.e., adult or family nurse practitioners who provide services to people of all ages) or specialists. The specialist nurse practitioner has skills with particular age groups (e.g., pediatric, adolescent, adult, or geriatric) or skills developed to meet the interests and needs of particular population. NPs are responsible for the daily operations and workflow of the clinic. These nurses use nursing and public health principles to promote and sustain the health of populations in various settings. Usually, NPs are responsible for the oversight of clinical staff accountable for program services and outcome measures.

Clinical Nurse Leader

The clinical nurse leader (CNL) is a master's educated nurse who is prepared to practice as a generalist across the health care continuum. The CNL role was developed to address the critical need to improve the quality of patient care outcomes. In a nurse-led clinic setting, the CNL may function as a transitional care coordinator, quality coordinator, and education specialist. These nurses work collaboratively with NPs to implement group health education classes and screenings and provide individual case management in community and home settings.

Social Workers

Social workers are an integral part of the collaborative team. Working directly with nurses, the social workers focus on the social assessment and address needs, which are often a consequence of social determinants of health. Areas of focus include food insecurity, access to medication, transportation, home and shelter, environmental safety, behavioral health counseling, employment, applying for insurance, and social support.

Other Collaborative Team Staff

Registered nurses or medical assistants help to triage patients and assist in workflow management. Community health workers may be part of the nurse-led clinic staff. Typically, they are neighborhood residents who have completed high school or two-year associate degree programs and who want to work with others in their community. The workers are trained in community outreach, family case management, or on-site services. Clinic receptionists or patient encounter specialists play an important role in the team. They schedule appointments and check in and check out patients from their appointments. In addition, they assist staff in obtaining needed supplies for patient care.

CHECK YOUR PRACTICE

In your care coordination role at the NLHC, you have called a 46-year-old uninsured client with diabetes scheduled for an appointment at your clinic next week. You ask if he has enough insulin to make it to his appointment, and he tells you he ran out of insulin two days ago.

- What follow-up questions do you ask this client?
- Do you confer with any of the other health care professionals at the clinic? Which ones?
- What do you instruct the client to do?

OTHER KEY ROLES IN ADDITION TO THE COLLABORATIVE TEAM

Director: Nurse Executive

The roles and responsibilities of the nurse executive are dynamic and diverse. Directors are visionary leaders and planners. The director has a current knowledge of the target community, the ability and willingness to work with many community organizations and groups, and a background in organizational planning, administration, and fiscal management. The nurse executive is responsible for oversight of contracts and grants, annual reports, and development of the advisory board or board of directors. Nurse executives constantly use data, collaborative feedback, existing resources, and partnerships to modify and adjust the overall direction of the clinic. Other responsibilities include hiring and retention of highly qualified staff. Nurse executives work closely with the leadership of the nurse-led clinics.

Operations Manager/Data Manager Program Coordinator/Technology Specialist

The operations of any nurse-led clinic require support staff. Staff members are dependent on the personnel budget. The operations manager handles contracts and grant budgets, advertising for staff, personnel hires, ordering supplies, and billing. Personnel management, staffing patterns, and site management, including data collection, are also responsibilities of an operations manager. A data manager or program coordinator is essential for clinic sustainability. Client-based and population-based outcomes are necessary for program evaluation, proposal development, and funding purposes. Rapid changes in technology related to billing and reporting requirements, and federal regulations regarding protection of information about an individual's health care status, require data operations personnel on site or as consultants. In today's litigious society, the operation of any nurse-led clinic involves ensuring privacy of client records and securing access to computerized data. At present and into the future, information systems (IS) and technology support (TS) personnel must be in place to meet the escalating expectation to institute and effectively use a computerized client-centered database. Computerized systems require upgrades and maintenance. Also, as hardware and software programs become obsolete and new programs are introduced, staff will need training and support to adapt to new data systems.

Educators, Researchers, Students

The education and research roles held by faculty, staff, and consultants are essential if the nurse-led clinic model is to advance in today's health care system (AACN, 2018; Holtman et al., 2011). The opportunity for faculty involvement through clinical training of students as well as community-focused research programs is evident and promising for community collaboration and well-being (McGraw, 2013; Nosek et al., 2017). Nursing students can learn about the intersection of health care economics, service, education, and research (Maru et al., 2018). Students also have opportunities to promote social justice while engaging in community service learning activities with underserved, vulnerable populations (ANA, 2016). If the clinic is part of a school of nursing, faculty roles include clinical oversight of graduate and undergraduate students assigned to the center or involved in related community projects, such as adult influenza inoculation campaigns.

Other members include community advocates, board of directors/advisory board members, and organizational partners. Community advocates are frequently known as key stakeholders. Community voices are often the most influential and listened to by elected officials and their staff.

Every nurse-led clinic should have a board of directors or advisory board. The organizational structure of a center as part of a larger institution or a freestanding entity dictates the type of board members that govern or advise staff on the direction of the center. A board of directors has oversight responsibilities, including fiscal management. An advisory board guides the work of the clinic but holds no fiduciary or voting responsibilities. The board should represent diverse professions and occupations and be knowledgeable about the target community and its residents.

In addition, organizational partners are valued members. Clinics that develop and maintain organizational relationships will benefit through service agreements and contracts with one or more of the partners.

Emphasizing the Role of the Bachelor's Prepared Nurse in Primary Care

Chronic diseases are responsible for 7 of 10 deaths each year, and treating people with chronic diseases accounts for most of our nation's health care costs (Centers for Disease Control and Prevention [CDC], 2018a). Given these overwhelming statistics, a need exists to address the full spectrum of community-based prevention interventions at the primary, secondary, and tertiary prevention levels. Similarly, to address challenges of rising health care costs, a need exists to maximize the talents of all appropriate health care professionals.

LEVELS OF PREVENTION

Nursing Center Application

Primary Prevention
Assess home for lead dust; educate family on lead poisoning prevention strategies.

Secondary Prevention
Conduct blood lead level screenings on a regular basis for children younger than age six.

Tertiary Prevention
Treat child who has an elevated blood lead level with appropriate therapies and eliminate environmental lead toxicity exposures.

According to the Josiah Macy Foundation (2016), primary care in the United States, which occurs mostly at the community level, is in urgent need of transformation. Much of that transformation requires maximizing scope of practice to better align health care professionals where the need for primary care exists. Although the NP provides a significant portion of the chronic disease management in the United States, a need exists to expand primary care services to address all levels of disease control and prevention. A relatively untapped resource for this purpose is the baccalaureate prepared RN workforce, which has been historically underutilized in addressing the nation's exponentially growing primary care service shortages (National Advisory Council on Nurse Education and Practice [NACNEP], 2010).

The role of the RN as integral to care coordination and management of transitions from hospital to home is well documented (Haas & Swan, 2014). However, over the past decades, the role of the RN has disappeared from most community-based primary care settings, often replaced by less trained medical assistants. When present in primary care settings, the role of the RN has often been limited to triaging phone calls and walk-ins (Anderson et al., 2012; Ladden et al., 2013). Consequently, RNs in primary care often do not practice to the full extent of their education and training. RNs in primary care are capable of assuming greater responsibility for care management of panels of patients with chronic conditions across all levels of prevention, following up on patients who are discharged from the hospital, and coordinating complex specialty care (NACNEP, 2010).

To address existing voids in primary care, a national paradigm shift is emerging in academic nursing to prepare baccalaureate nursing graduates for their full scope of practice as primary care RNs. The Health Resources and Services Administration is supporting this shift with significant grant funding dollars (HRSA, 2018). Growth in the integration of RNs in primary care will take some time to materialize as few RNs in primary care are currently available to precept students in these roles. As nurse-led clinics envision the future of care to maximize scope of practice and address the full spectrum of prevention not just chronic disease management, baccalaureate prepared primary care nurses should be considered valuable members of the health care team.

STARTING A NURSE-LED CLINIC

Overview of Business Aspects

Nurses who work in nursing centers are committed to working with diverse people in noninstitutional settings. In response to the needs of individuals, communities, population health indexes, and epidemiological findings, the role and scope of nursing practice has shifted to include a change in the model of the care provided (Randall et al., 2017). The model requires careful planning and structure to be a successful education, service, and business enterprise. During the planning and implementation phases, interrelated elements must be considered. These elements serve as an annual checklist to measure growth of a nursing center and guide sound decisions regarding sustainability and future planning. It is important to remember that this work is a business enterprise in which the art and science of nursing is practiced. Hence, the planning stages of the clinic require consultation with financial advisors and other experts. Final decisions about establishing a nursing center are made after exploration of the following essential areas:

1. Organizational goals, commitments, and resources
2. Community interests, assets, and needs
3. Feasibility study, internal and external to the parent organization
4. Strategic plan
5. Business plan
6. Information management plan and resources
7. Existing social policy and health care financing
8. Legal and regulatory considerations
9. Mission, vision, and commitment of the lead organization

The initial work of assessing the interests, resources, and capacity of an organization to undertake the nursing center model is interrelated yet separate. For example, conduct a feasibility study before developing a business plan and incorporate elements of the feasibility study into the business plan. A strategic plan builds on feasibility data as well as economic principles and practices. Planners must also consider workforce needs, personnel management, public information and outreach campaigns, community capacity, and the health care environment relative to funding streams. Feasibility studies must also analyze the national health care reform legislation dollars committed and funded programs. As a cautionary note, there will be widespread competition for program support.

The overall processes of community collaborations, assessment, and feasibility studies support the development of business plans, strategic plans, and timelines. A sound business plan considers all aspects of establishing a nursing center and describes the development and direction of the nursing center and how goals will be met (Box 20.4). A **business plan** is built on the known or more predictable sources of funding at the

BOX 20.4 Components of a Business Plan

1. *Cover page,* includes date, name, address, and phone number(s) of the person(s) responsible for the nursing center and any consultants to the business plan.
2. *Executive summary.* This is a one- or two-page overview of the center and the plan.
3. *Table of contents.*
4. *Description of the business plan* that details what the center is and what services it will provide.
5. *Survey of the industry.* This summarizes the past, present, and future of the local and regional health care market.
6. *Market research and analysis.* This description outlines existing competition and the potential market share and identifies target groups.
7. *Marketing plan.* This details how the center will reach its targeted clients.
8. *Organizational chart,* with a description of the management team.
9. *List of supporting professional staff (e.g., accountants).*
10. *Operations plan.* This describes how and where services will be provided.
11. *Research and development.* This projects program improvement and opportunities for new initiatives.
12. *Overall schedule.* The timeline establishes the start date and development phase of the nursing center.
13. *Critical risks and problems.* This examines the internal and external threats to the center and how these will be addressed.
14. *Financial plan.* The fiscal projections for the first three to five years are presented. A budget, cash flow forecast, and break-even point are included.
15. *Proposed funding.* Specific sources are listed that can provide funding.
16. *Legal structure of the center.* This describes the status of the center, such as freestanding, a corporation, or part of a larger organization.
17. *Appendixes and supporting documents.*

time the plan is developed. Modifications to the business plan may be needed, and anticipation of such modifications will support sustainability in the future. Legislative changes and reimbursement regulations can significantly alter the business plan. In addition, no grant allocation should ever be included in the business plan until the grant is awarded.

The strategic plan complements the business plan. A strategic plan anticipates future needs and guides the work of the nursing center in that direction. Strategic plans have a regular timeline and may change as indicated by local, national, and global events. Strategic planning meetings are periodically scheduled to review and refine the plan. The plan includes goals, objectives, and target timelines for implementation and evaluation of projected and ongoing services. The strategic plan should answer these questions: (1) What resources will the center need after start-up? (2) What economic and legislative factors may influence center productivity and sustainability? (3) What will be the center's core functions in five, seven, and nine years? (4) How can the staff move the center in the appropriate direction? (5) How will staff process and handle change?

Feasibility studies, business plans, and strategic plans lay the foundation for strong nursing centers. These components are crucial to the day-to-day functioning of a newly opened nursing center and reflect the abilities of the management team to build community coalitions and collaboratives. In addition, the management team must be knowledgeable about federal regulations, acts, and funding changes, especially Medicaid and Medicare reimbursement, and grant opportunities. One resource tool that should be on site for reference is the National Nursing Center Consortium (NNCC) guide: *Nurse-Managed Wellness Centers: Developing and Maintaining Your Center, a National Nursing Center Consortium Guide and Toolkit* (Hansen-Turton et al., 2009).

The organization cannot drive the desire for the nursing center. The center must be person- and community-centric, not provider-centric. If the establishment of a nursing center is solely done from the organization's vantage point, the possibility of long-term sustainability may be jeopardized.

The establishment of a nursing center is warranted if the model reflects the needs, interests, and strengths of the target population and is economically feasible. There should be long-term commitments by all involved in the planning process, including any parent organization. The parent organization's mission, vision, and commitment influence the viability of the nursing center model. Planners must determine the support of the parent organization before investing the time, effort, and collaborative work necessary to develop the model. If there is uncertainty at the administrative level, it is foolhardy to move forward until there is strong and documented commitment from the organization that matches the community commitment.

It is challenging for those involved in the planning process to forecast programs, determine service patterns, integrate outcome measures, and project costs. The planning process over time can be difficult. Planners need to devote sufficient time to ensure the optimization of financial outcomes (Polancich et al., 2017). If money matters are not thoroughly considered, sustaining a nursing center may not be possible.

The business plan provides information that forecasts the minimum funding necessary to begin a nursing center and project income one, three, and five years from inception. At a minimum, the nursing center must break even. However, a revenue generating, cost savings, and/or cost avoidance financial model is best. A business plan must be modified when any changes in reimbursement occur (e.g., Medicare and Medicaid reimbursements or commercial reimbursement) along with consideration of the provider's specialty in generating revenue for the nursing centers.

Potential income sources include fee-for-service, commercial reimbursement, and self-pay. Fee-for-service may be the most viable of economic strategies. Commercial reimbursement includes private health care insurers with established fee schedules. Clients without a source of health insurance are characterized as self-pay.

All costs and charges for services must be established in the planning stages. Nursing centers located in medically underserved areas or working with medically underserved populations may receive federal or local funding to provide care and may offer care at no charge to the patients. Other nursing centers may provide care while utilizing sliding-fee schedules based on published federal poverty guidelines. Managed care contracts with insurance companies, particularly Medicaid contractors, are other sources of income.

Financial support for nursing centers may also come from academic medical centers affiliated with schools of nursing, foundations, charitable contributions, private giving, and fund-raising. Fund-raising can take the form of direct mailings, pledges, and events that raise money. Grants are a source of initial and ongoing funding. The funding organization generally releases guidelines of what the organization will fund. The guidelines are frequently released as a request for proposals (RFP). A proposal developed in response to the RFP specifies how the nursing center would meet the goals of the granting organization in the given timeline. The description of services and client outcomes must be presented in relation to the RFP guidelines.

Nursing centers have agreements and contracts in place for specific services. Agreements and contracts may have different language as well as reporting and fiscal management requirements; however, the basic premise is similar. The nursing center enters into a written agreement to provide services to a select population group or develop a program that targets a specific area. For example, a center may have an agreement with an academic medical center to develop a diabetes clinic for adults who are uninsured. A memorandum of understanding is developed, and the agreement is for a defined time period, has target goals and objectives, outlines staff assignments and expectations, and includes a budget. A contract is a legal document that lists the purchase of services, reporting requirements, invoicing, and expected client outcomes. An example would be a city health department that issues a contract to a nursing center to immunize 100 adults against influenza for a specified sum per vaccine. Each nursing center may have one or many contracts and agreements; however, a nursing center should enter into each arrangement with clear understanding of the business side of the model. Any contract or agreement should be fiscally sound and not deplete center resources.

Overview of Clinical Aspects

Quality health indicators and related performance measures are priorities in any type of nursing center (Burston et al., 2013). These data are presented to the nursing center's board, funders, and the community at large and document the center's contributions to the health and welfare of the community. The concept of the "triple aim" used to measure clinical outcomes was first introduced by the Institute for Healthcare Improvement in 2007. This framework focused on three goals: (1) improved patient outcomes, (2) improved patient experience, and (3) reduced cost of care (Institute for Healthcare Improvement, 2018). Most recently, the framework was renamed the Quadruple Aim as an additional goal focused on attaining joy at work was added (Feeley, 2018). Improved patient clinical and cost-related outcomes are crucial concerns as providers deal with the instability of reimbursement rates and the variable number of underinsured people. Likewise, improving the satisfaction of patients and providers are key strategies to financial success.

Outcomes related to nursing centers assess growth and development and areas that need improvement. The outcomes may also include quality indicators (Table 20.2), population groups, performance targets, and measures. The indicators are grouped into the areas of prevention, utilization, client satisfaction, functional status, symptom severity, and others.

Utilization of the outcomes and select indicators and associated processes enable a nursing center to document evidence-based practice. The National Committee for Quality Assurance (NCQA) has developed health care performance measures known as the Healthcare Effectiveness Data and Information Set (HEDIS) (NCQA, 2018). HEDIS contains widely used evidence-based standards to ensure quality health care for a variety of disease processes.

The evidence-based practice application exemplifies what nurses can do to measure outcomes, strive to improve those outcomes given particular standards, and make meaningful contributions to the public's health (Box 20.5). Accurate data collection, measurement methods, summary statistics, and preparation of evidence-based practice reports are fundamental standards in any NLHC.

Cost-effective, quality care requires the incorporation of evidence-based practice. Evidence-based practice represents the clinical application of particular nursing (health care) interventions and documented client and population outcome data over time (Schaffer et al., 2013). Trends in health care services, client responses, and changes in community characteristics must be a good fit for the nursing center, be documented, and summarized periodically.

The cost of collecting and documenting outcome measures must be included in the NLHC budget (Harris et al., 2017). Measurement instruments require technological support, staff expertise, and ongoing monitoring and analyses. Defined outcome measures (evidence) will enable NLHC staff to determine program effectiveness and cost savings associated with clinical outcomes (Harris et al., 2017). The challenge is how to define the criteria, develop measurements and collection methods, compare the evidence with broader community findings, interpret the data to funders, and disseminate findings to the wider health care community. Nursing center staff can use a variety of forums to disseminate findings (e.g., professional conferences and publications, popular press, multimedia venues, and testimonies at public hearings).

TABLE 20.2 Examples of Quality Health Indicators for Nursing Centers

Indicator	Population	Performance Targets	Measure
Prevention			
Annual influenza vaccine	High-risk groups: Age 65, or those with heart or lung disease and other chronic conditions	*Healthy People 2020* = 90 percent age 65+ *Healthy People 2020* = 60 percent high-risk ages 18-64 years	Client self-report and/or clinical records/audit
Utilization			
Mammogram within past two years	HEDIS: Women age 52-69 years *Healthy People 2020:* Women 40 years and older	HEDIS 2001 = 81 percent *Healthy People 2020* = 70 percent	Client self-report and/or clinical records/audit
Client Satisfaction			
Client satisfaction, annual	100 consecutive clients per quarter	Performance targets to be determined by individual nursing center and/or health care plan	Surveys
Functional Status			
Quality-of-life indicator	Adults age 18 years and older	Determined by individual nursing center and related to baseline indicators and improvement goals	Screen using short form 12 or 36

HEDIS, Healthcare Effectiveness Data and Information Set.

BOX 20.5 Evidence-Based Practice

The steps of the EBP process:

1. Ask the burning question.
2. Collect the most relevant and best evidence.
3. Critically appraise the evidence.
4. Integrate the information to make a practice change or decision.
5. Evaluate the practice decision or change.

Title and author of article	Riegel B, Dickson V, Garcia L, et al.: Mechanisms of change in self-care in adults with heart failure receiving a tailored motivational interviewing intervention. *Patient Educ Couns* 100:283–288, 2017.
What clinical issue was discussed in the article?	The authors sought to evaluate which motivational interviewing techniques were most effective in changing patients' self-care behaviors.
What was "the *burning question*"?	In heart failure patients, does motivational interviewing vs. usual care methods improve self-care behaviors in this complex population?
What did the authors find in their literature review?	The literature search found that motivational interviewing was effective in heart failure patients in the areas of exercise, self-care, quality of life, and hospital readmissions.
What was the practice change? How did they *integrate* the information to make a practice decision or change?	Using motivational interviewing techniques, it was reported that reflection and reframing facilitated positive talk, genuine communication including empathy, affirmation, and humor assisted in overcoming barriers, and personalized problem solving stimulated openness to setting goals.
Did the practice change work? How did they *evaluate* their practice decision or change?	Using motivational interviewing in discussing self-care behaviors can help heart failure patients to engage in their own care. By looking at both quantitative and qualitative data, the researchers were able to report that motivational interviewing is effective and worth implementing into clinical practice.

EBP, Evidence-based practice.

Health Insurance Portability and Accountability Act

Staff committed to evidence-based practice, outcome measures, electronic health records (EHRs), data collection, and analyses must be knowledgeable about the Health Insurance Portability and Accountability Act (HIPAA). HIPAA, which is Public Law 104-191 passed by the 104th Congress to protect the privacy of individually identified health data referred to as protected health information (PHI). The regulations took into consideration the shift to paperless EHRs. Electronic records increase the potential for individuals to access, use, and disclose sensitive personal health data. The act enables consumers to have more control over their health information, establishes boundaries about the use and release of health records, sets safeguards about provider protection of private health information and penalizes violations of same, and enables consumers to obtain and/or make informed decisions about how their health information is used and disclosed. According to current regulations, all staff must monitor and keep secure client records, have mechanisms to transfer client information securely and appropriately, and strictly adhere to client confidentiality (Cohen & Mello, 2018).

Nurses in NLHCs who receive payment from the Centers for Medicare and Medicaid Services and or third-party payers are required to comply with HIPAA regulations, as well as be responsive to and report public health threats such as tuberculosis, disease outbreaks related to food contaminations, and influenza. Reference resources for individuals and professionals include the U.S. Department of Health and Human Services' website (http://www.hhs.gov) (USDHHS, 2018) and the CDC website on Privacy Rule guidelines (https://www.cdc.gov) (CDC, 2018b). Other chapters further detail public health responsiveness and HIPAA documentation challenges.

QSEN FOCUS ON QUALITY AND SAFETY EDUCATION FOR NURSES

Targeted Competency: Quality Improvement

Health care organizations focus on providing the best quality care to achieve excellent patient outcomes. The overall goal of QSEN is to prepare future nurses with the knowledge, skills, and attitudes they need to achieve excellence for their patients. There are several components to QSEN education: patient centered care, quality improvement, safety, evidence-based practice, informatics, and teamwork/collaboration.

Important aspects of quality improvement include:

- **Knowledge:** Be able to recognize that nursing and other health professions students are parts of systems of care and care processes that affect outcomes for patients and families
- **Skills:** These are the tools and information gathered to understand the care outcomes and opportunities for improvement.
- **Attitude:** Appreciate that continuous quality improvement is needed to improve the outcomes of care in local care settings

Quality Improvement Exemplar

QSEN defines quality improvement as using data to monitor the outcomes of processes along with designing and testing changes to continuously improve the care of patients in the health care system.

Influenza Vaccinations in a Nurse-Led Clinic for Underserved Patients With Heart Failure

You are a student doing a clinical rotation in a nurse-led clinic. During morning huddle, in addition to the patient's plan of care discussion, the recent clinic

QSEN Focus on Quality and Safety Education for Nurses—cont'd

quality metrics were reported. Metrics included hand hygiene, documentation of body mass index, documentation of endorsed results, proper patient identification, and documentation of pneumonia and influenza vaccines.

The clinic met all metrics except influenza vaccines. The expected metric was to achieve a 70 percent vaccination rate and the clinic was 25 percent. Using quality improvement tools such as the Plan-Do-Study-Act, what quality improvement process could be improved to increase the percent of influenza vaccinations given? What data do you need? What are the barriers to this patient population receiving the flu vaccine? What barriers does the clinic have to administering the vaccine?

Plan (Knowledge): Evidence states that persons with heart failure are at greater risk for becoming more seriously ill from the flu. Patients in this clinic have increased barriers to receiving the influenza vaccine such as cost, no previous medical home for care, and insufficient education regarding the importance of the vaccine. The clinic was currently under construction and did not have a refrigerator to keep the vaccines. **(Skill):** The clinic dashboard clearly displays a red dot for not meeting the metric. **(Attitude):** What change can be made to increase the number of influenza vaccinations given to this patient population?

Do: The clinic staff began to education their patients about the importance of a flu vaccination.

Clinic social workers partnered with a local pharmacy to supply 25 free influenza vaccinations. Then the clinic worked with Ambulatory Leadership, who provided 100 vaccinations. The clinic also purchased a medication refrigerator.

Study: The clinic was able to double the number of influenza vaccinations given from 25 percent to 50 percent.

Act: While the metric of 70 percent was not achieved, the medication refrigerator and donated flu vaccines came at the end of the flu season. The clinic will follow the same process next flu season and start earlier administering vaccinations to achieve the expected results.

This is an example of how nurses use evidence-based practice and quality improvement to improve the quality and safety outcomes of their patients.

EDUCATION AND RESEARCH

Nursing centers provide many education and research opportunities fostering an environment to develop clinical inquiry (Young et al., 2017). Clinical assignments through the nursing center model enable students at all levels to work with skilled clinicians, develop positive community collaboratives, and build their skills to become professionals. These students often develop an interest in working with underserved populations in medically underserved areas of the nation. The faculty brings skills that enable nursing center staff to develop and implement programs that integrate faculty-student contributions and enable the programs to engage more of the target population.

Research in nursing centers provides the opportunity to gain answers to questions and to share the findings with students, colleagues, and the community (Young et al., 2017). Nursing centers offer many opportunities for educational research by providing opportunities to answer questions about individual and population health status, client outcomes over time, roles and capacities to address health promotion with the existing health system, and the value and affordability of care (Young et al., 2017). Each center needs a research or program evaluation agenda. The research focus includes identification and clarification of client needs, particularly those not engaged in an existing health system; description of nursing interventions and linkages with consumer needs and resources; demonstration of effective interventions that produce appropriate outcomes; and cost analysis and documented cost-effectiveness of services (Young et al., 2017).

EVALUATING AND SUSTAINING A NURSE-LED CLINIC

Program Evaluation

Program evaluation is an essential organizational practice in NLHCs, and research questions emerge from program evaluation. The evaluation process is a systematic approach to improve and account for public health and primary care actions. Evaluation is thoroughly integrated in routine program operations. The process drives community-focused strategies, allows for program improvements, and identifies the need for additional services.

Program evaluation separates what is working from what is not and enables clinicians, faculty, and students to ask difficult questions and handle pressing challenges (CDC, 2018c). Resources are available to nursing center staff to enhance their understanding and application of program evaluation in their particular setting. Resources include the CDC's *Working Together: A Training Framework for Public Health and Planning Professionals* (2015) and other resources updated by the CDC Program Performance and Evaluation Office (2018c) (https://www.cdc.gov). These resources enable nursing center staff to implement the six essential program evaluation steps in the context of their model and in their particular community.

Logic Model As Framework

A logic model is a tool used to "design, implement, and evaluate new programs and projects" (Drayton-Brooks et al., 2016, p. 235). The logic model generally appears as a one-page visual depiction of the key elements of the proposed program or project. The appearance of a logic model may vary; however, it usually includes categories of inputs, activities, outputs, and outcomes. In designing a logic model, planning for a program or project incorporates addressing all categories of inputs, activities, outputs, and outcomes (Fig. 20.3).

Identifying the *inputs* entails determining the human, material, financial, and infrastructure resources needed to initiate and support an ongoing program or project. The *activities* required to make the program or project successful should be specified and include those processes (events or actions) that must be monitored to achieve results. The *outputs* refer to direct products of programs and may include number of people served or tangible items derived from the effort. The *outcomes* may be short, midterm, and long-term and represent desirable results at certain time targets. Outcomes must be specific and measurable.

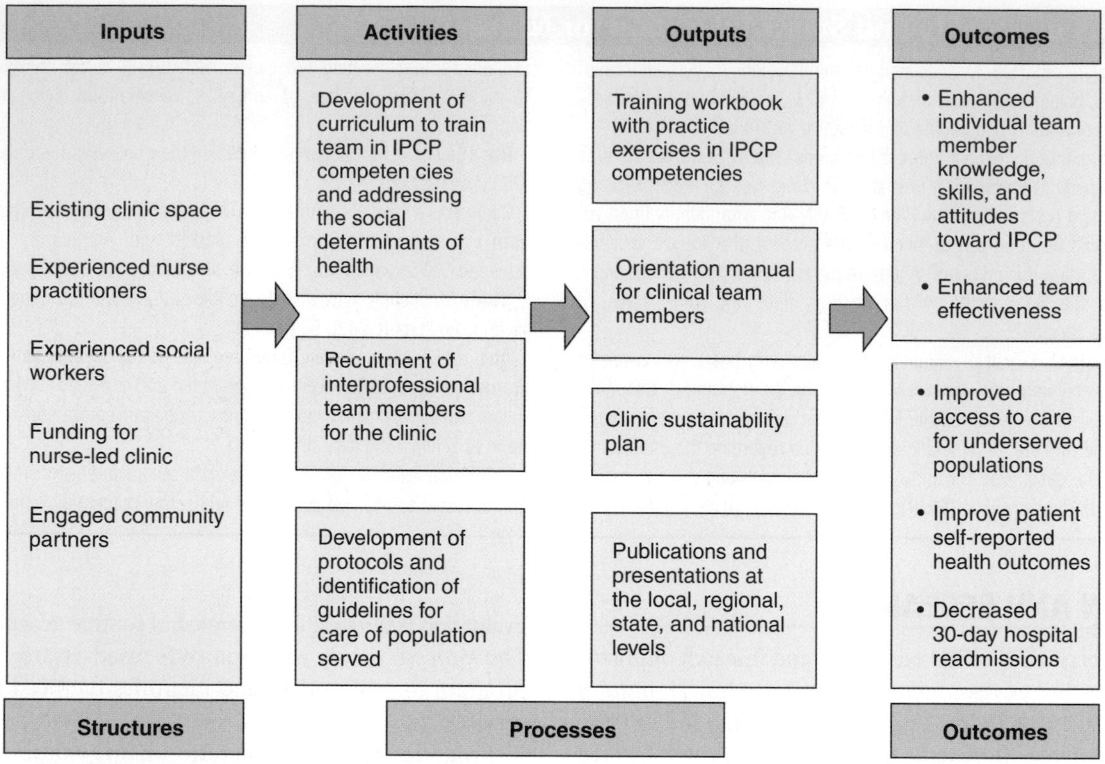

Fig. 20.3 Theory-based logic model for nurse-led IPCP clinic caring for primary care underserved population. *IPCP,* Interprofessional collaborative practice.

A logic model serves an important evaluation function. In specifying expected outcomes associated with program or project implementation, nurse leaders can monitor performance in a timely way and initiate just-in-time changes to ensure required goals are achieved.

Theory may be used to guide the development of logic models. Theory-driven logic models may incorporate systems theory, change theory, or health care quality theory, among other theories (Drayton-Brooks et al., 2016). In 1966, Donabedian developed a theory-based logic model pertinent to a nurse-led clinic and informed by classic health care quality theory.

In the case of nurse-led care, a logic model provides a road map of the program or project goals and aligns these with needed inputs, activities, outputs, and outcomes. The logic model can be used to engage members of the team around program or project goals and expectations. Although logic models may appear as simple, linear, or stagnant depictions, they actually may represent complex, dynamic, and changing elements of a program or project.

Sustaining the Program

Sustaining a nurse-led clinic financially can be challenging. In recent systematic reviews, nurse-led clinics were shown to have positive results in patient outcomes, patient satisfaction, and access to care while cost-effectiveness of the clinics had mixed results (Baker & Fatoye, 2017; Randall et al., 2017). The sustainability of nurse-led clinics depends on being able to achieve positive outcomes in addition to positive cost-effectiveness. There are three ways to finance nurse-led clinics: fee-for-service, contracts, and grants. Many nurse-led clinics emerge from academic-practice partnership grants between schools of nursing and hospital health systems (Pilon et al., 2015). Nurse-led clinics must be prepared to meet the daily needs of people they serve as well as the organizational needs of the partnering institution. These clinics often serve underserved or vulnerable populations. Unfortunately, many clinics close after grant funding has ended due inability to sustain funding (Pilon et al., 2015).

Sustaining a nurse-led clinic must begin early. Gathering clinic outcomes and cost-effectiveness data is essential. Clinic outcomes may include patient satisfaction, physical and mental health functioning, and access to care. Cost-effectiveness can include total cost savings and decreases in readmission or emergency department visits. Critical to the sustainability is a documented cost savings to the organization. Depending on the type of clinic funded, cash flow exceeding expenditures may be a requirement. Also, selecting the audience for your presentation of the outcome data is critically important. This audience typically includes key executive leadership personnel such as the chief nursing officer, chief financial officer, health system chief operating officer, and others in the organization's governing body. When presenting to the governing body, it is important to have a budget developed along with the resources needed such as space, equipment, and personnel. The fee-for-service model is based on payments for all clinical encounters. In this setting, it is important to know payer mix and have an annual budget. Lastly, in a contract model, the NP as provider has a contractual agreement with a partnering agency. Most commonly, these agreements are with universities or employee health (Pilon & Hansen-Turton, 2015).

PRACTICE APPLICATION

Annual summaries of client use patterns and program outcome data document erratic patterns of client access and ongoing use of one nursing center's services. The center, located in a public housing site, offers comprehensive primary health care to clients of all ages, a sliding-fee schedule so no one is turned away, managed care contracts, and a variety of public health and social services provided in home or community settings. The office is open six days a week with appointments available during day and early evening hours. The site is readily accessible by public or private transit, and it is less than a five-minute walk for any public housing resident. A large, attractive sign is in the front of the site for advertising purposes. Monthly outreach is conducted to local businesses, schools, social service agencies, and tertiary care centers. Outreach includes information such as the center's services, hours, and location. Personal contacts, flyers, and posters advertising unique programs such as flu clinics are strategically placed within the housing complex and proximal neighborhoods.

Despite these efforts, data indicate that other strategies are needed. A focus group held with staff, public housing residents, and users of the health center services began. Client users candidly shared their need to have more flexibility in the appointment schedule. Appointments made months in advance were often not kept because of conflicting schedules (such as work or school), despite the client's best intent. Staff said that too many clients were "no-shows" and their work schedules were "too light." Public housing residents were concerned about keeping their "business private."

Consensus was reached to establish an "open access" appointment model. Clients can schedule appointments or call the day before or day of a needed visit. Nurses would reinforce the open access model and the center's confidentiality standards with clients. All staff would reinforce the option during client visits as well as prepare press releases and community presentations. Staff would review client access and use patterns quarterly. By the next quarter, client access and adherence to appointments increased by 50 percent and primary care staff reported greater satisfaction in their work responsibilities. Nurses noted that clients in public housing expressed positive comments on how the nursing center had helped them manage their appointment schedules better. Overall, the increased access and use of appropriate primary health care services support the center's goal to promote community well-being.

KEY POINTS

- NLHCs provide unique opportunities to improve the health status of individuals, families, and communities through direct access to nursing care.
- Nurse-led center models combine people, place, approach, and strategy in everyday life to develop appropriate health care interventions.
- A nurse-led center's health and community orientation builds strong connections to the population served.
- A nurse-led center is defined by its particular array of services and programs, such as comprehensive primary health care centers and special care centers.
- The foundations for the nurse-led model include the perspective of the World Health Organization and the *Healthy People 2020* systematic approach to improving individual and community health.
- Each center develops its philosophy, goals, and activities through a process of community collaboration, assessment, and strategic planning.
- As the community and the center work together for health, a multilevel approach is used that includes individuals and key stakeholders.
- Nurse-led center development is rooted in public health nursing history and the evolution of the nursing profession.
- Most current nurse-led center models emerged from academic nursing centers and have expanded as a result of the Patient Protection and Affordable Care Act of 2010.
- Nurse-led models support the skill development and contributions of the interprofessional team, including advanced practice nurses such as NPs, baccalaureate prepared primary care nurses, and multiple colleagues such as physician colleagues, social workers, dietitians, and pharmacists.
- Any nurse-led center should have a board of directors or an advisory board to guide program development, fundraising, community networking, and other work.
- The nurse-led center requires careful planning and structure to be a successful education, service, and business enterprise.
- Start-up and sustainability are based on a community-focused feasibility study, a sound business and financial plan, operational support, and resource management.
- Evidence-based practice in nursing centers is essential and represents the clinical application of particular nursing interventions and documented client outcomes.
- The Health Insurance Portability and Accountability Act necessitates a center's investment in administrative and oversight services.
- Available technology and systems management must be used to collect, collate, and analyze center data.
- Education, community service, and research opportunities abound in the nurse-led center model, which fosters a culture of clinical inquiry.
- Program evaluation is an essential organizational practice in nurse-led centers, and research questions emerge from program evaluation.
- Threats to the viability of nursing centers include erratic funding resources, community decline, disenfranchised high-risk populations, and lack of outcomes to document sustainability.

- Nurses attracted to the nurse-led model discover professional fulfillment in advocating for people in need and becoming involved in public policy change.
- Nursing centers represent an innovative approach to the delivery of primary health care services.
- Nurses involved in the nurse-led model are front-line advocates for social justice and equality for all.

CLINICAL DECISION-MAKING ACTIVITIES

1. Discuss why a nurse-led center should be started or not started in your hometown.
2. What is your state's position on credentialing NPs who work in an NLHC model?
3. What existing public policy might adversely affect the viability of nurse-led centers?
4. Why would NPs and baccalaureate prepared nurses be attracted to this model of primary health care?
5. How many elected officials at the local level are familiar with the nurse-led center model, and, if the majority is uninformed, what could you do to educate the officials?
6. Where do you envision yourself professionally in 2030?

ADDITIONAL RESOURCES

EVOLVE WEBSITE

http://evolve.elsevier.com/Stanhope/community/
- Answers to Practice Application
- Case Study
- Glossary
- Review Questions

REFERENCES

American Association of Colleges of Nursing (AACN): *Essentials of Baccalaureate Nursing Education for Professional Nursing Practice: Recommended Baccalaureate Competencies and Curricular Guidelines for Public Health Nursing*, 2013, AACN. Retrieved from http://www.aacn.nche.edu.

American Association of Colleges of Nursing (AACN): *Curriculum Guidelines*, 2018, AACN. Retrieved from http://www.aacnnursing.org.

American Nurses Association (ANA): *The nurse's role in ethics and human rights: Protecting and promoting individual worth, dignity, and human rights in practice settings*, Silver Spring, 2016. Retrieved from Nursebooks.org

Anderson DR, St. Hilaire D, Flinter M: Primary care nursing role and care coordination: An observational study of nursing work in a community care setting, *Online J Issues Nurs* 17(2):3, 2012.

Auerbach DI, Chen PG, Friedberg MW, et al.: Nurse-managed health centers and patient-centered medical homes could mitigate expected primary care physician shortage, *Health Aff* 32(11): 1933–1941, 2013.

Baker E, Fatoye F: Clinical and cost effectiveness of nurse-led self-management interventions for patients with COPD in primary care: A systematic review, *Int J Nurs Stud* 71:125–138, 2017.

Burston S, Chaboyer W, Gillespie B: Nurse-sensitive indicators suitable to reflect nursing care quality: A review and discussion of issues, *J Clin Nurs* 23(13–14):1785–1795, 2013.

Centers for Disease Control and Prevention (CDC): *Chronic disease prevention and health promotion*, 2018a, CDC. Retrieved from https://www.cdc.gov.

Centers for Disease Control and Prevention (CDC): *HIPAA privacy rules guidelines*, 2018b, CDC. Retrieved from http://www.cdc.gov.

Centers for Disease Control and Prevention (CDC): *Program Performance and Evaluation Office*, 2018c, CDC. Retrieved from https://www.cdc.gov.

Centers for Disease Control and Prevention (CDC): *Working Together: A Training Framework for Public Health and Planning Professionals*, 2015, CDC. Retrieved from https://www.cdc.gov.

Cohen IG, Mello MM: HIPAA and Protecting Health Information in the 21st Century, *JAMA* 320(3):231–232, 2018.

Donabedian A: Evaluating the quality of medical care, *Milbank Mem Fund Q* 44(3):166–203, 1966.

Drayton-Brooks SM, Gray P, Desimone ME: In Bloch JR, Courtney MR, Clark ML, editors: *Practice-based clinical inquiry in nursing for DNP and PhD research: Looking beyond traditional methods*, New York, 2016, Springer, pp 235–255.

Ely LT: Nurse-managed clinics: Barriers and benefits toward financial sustainability when integrating primary care and mental health, *Nurs Econ* 33(4):193–202, 2015.

Feeley D: *The Triple Aim or the Quadruple Aim? Four Points to Help Set Your Strategy*, 2018, Institute for Healthcare Improvement. Retrieved from http://www.ihi.org.

Haas SA, Swan BA: Developing the value proposition for the role of the registered nurse in care coordination and transition management in ambulatory care settings, *Nurs Econ* 32(2):70–79, 2014.

Hansen-Turton T, Miller ME, Greiner P: *Nurse-Managed Wellness Centers: Developing and Maintaining Your Center, A National Nursing Center Consortium Guide and Toolkit*, Philadelphia, 2009, Saunders.

Hansen-Turton T, Valdez B, Ware JM, King ES: Anatomy of a nurse-led clinic: An Introduction to the Model of Care. In Hansen-Turton T, Sherman S, King ES, editors: *Nurse-led health clinics: Operations, policy and opportunity*, New York, 2015, Springer, pp 3–10.

Harris C, Allen K, Waller C, et al: Sustainability in Health care by Allocating Resources Effectively (SHARE) 7: Supporting staff in evidence-based decision-making, implementation and evaluation in a local healthcare setting, *BMC Health Serv Res* 17(1):430, 2017.

Health Resources & Services Administration (HRSA): *Nurse education, practice, quality, and retention (NEPQR)—Registered nurses in primary care (RNPC) training program*, 2018, HRSA. Retrieved from https://bhw.hrsa.gov.

Holt J, Zabler B, Baisch MJ: Evidence-based characteristics of nurse-managed health centers for quality and outcomes, *Nurs Outlook* 62:428–439, 2014.

Holtman MC, Frost JS, Hammer DP, McGuinn K, Nunez LM: Interprofessional professionalism: Linking professionalism and interprofessional care, *J Interprof Care* 25(5):383–385, 2011.
Institute for Healthcare Improvement (IHI): *Overview*, 2018, IHI. Retrieved from http://www.ihi.org.
Interprofessional Education Collaborative Expert Panel (IPEC): *Core competencies for interprofessional collaborative practice, 2016 update, IPEC.* Retrieved from https://s3.amazonaws.com.
Josiah Macy Foundation: *Registered nurses: Partners in transforming primary care*, 2016. Retrieved from http://macyfoundation.org.
Ladden JD, Bodenheimer T, Fishman NW, et al. The emerging primary care workforce: Preliminary observations from the primary care team learning from effective ambulatory practice project, *Acad Med* 88(2):1830–1834, 2013.
Maru S, Byrnes J, Carrington MJ, Chan YK, Stewart S, Scuffman PA; NIL-CHF Trial Investigators: Economic evaluation of a nurse-led home and clinic based secondary prevention programme to prevent progressive cardiac dysfunction in high-risk individuals: The Nurse-led Intervention for Less Chronic Heart Failure (NIL-CHF) randomized controlled study, *Eur J Cardiovasc Nurs* 17(5):439–445, 2018.
Mattessich P, Monsey B: *Collaboration: What Makes It Work?* St. Paul, MN, 1992, Amherst H. Wilder Foundation.
McGraw C: Preparing Nursing Students to Be Community Health Practitioners. (Research Focus), *Prim Health Care* 23(6):14, 2013.
National Advisory Council on Nurse Education and Practice (NACNEP): *The role of nurses in primary care*, 2010, NACNEP. Retrieved from http://www.hrsa.gov.
National Committee for Quality Assurance (NCQA): *Healthcare Effectiveness Data and Information Set*, 2018, NCQA. Retrieved from https://www.ncqa.org.
Nosek CM, Scheckel MM, Waterbury T, MacDonald A, Wozney N: The collaborative improvement model: An interpretive study of revising a curriculum, *J Prof Nurs* 33(1):38–50, 2017.
Nurse-Family Partnership: *First-time moms*, 2018. Retrieved from http://www.nursefamilypartnership.org.
Pilon BA, Ketel C, Davidson HA, et al.: Evidence-guided integration of interprofessional collaborative practice into nurse managed health centers, *J Prof Nurs* 31(4):340–350, 2015.
Pilon B, Hansen-Turton T: Nurse-managed health centers and sustainability. In Hansen-Turton T, Sherman S, King ES, editors: *Nurse-led health clinics: Operations, policy and opportunity*, New York, 2015, Springer, pp 67–82.
Polancich S, Williamson J, Selleck CS, et al.: Using Data Analytics as Evidentiary Support for Financial Outcome Success in Nurse-Led Population-Based Clinics, *J Healthc Qual* 39(6):391–396, 2017.
Public Health Foundation (PHF): *Council on Linkages Between Academia and Public Health Practice*, Washington DC, 2014, PHF. Retrieved from http://www.phf.org.
Quad Council Coalition, Public Health Foundation (PHF): *Quad Council Coalition for Public Health Nursing Competencies*, 2018, PHF. Retrieved from http://www.phf.org.
Randall S, Crawford T, Currie J, River J, Betihavas V: Impact of community based nurse-led clinics on patient outcomes, patient satisfaction, patient access and cost effectiveness: A systematic review, *Int J Nurs Stud* 73:24–33, 2017.
Schaffer MA, Sandau KE, Diedrick L: Evidence-based practice models for organizational change: Overview and practical applications, *J Adv Nurs* 69(5):1197–1209, 2013.
Sutter-Barrett RE, Sutter-Dalrymple CJ, Dickman K: Bridge care nurse-managed clinics fill the gap in health care, *J Nurse Pract* 11(2):262–265, 2015.
Talley MH, Polancich S, Williamson JB, et al.: Improving population health among uninsured patients with diabetes, *Popul Health Manag* 21(5):373–377, 2018.
U.S. Department of Health and Human Services: *Health Information Privacy*, 2018, USDHHS. Retrieved from http://www.hhs.gov.
World Health Organization: *Framework for action on interprofessional education and collaborative practice*, 2010, WHO. Retrieved from http://apps.who.int.
Young HM, Bakewell-Sachs S, Sarna L: Nursing practice, research and education in the west: the best is yet to come, *Nurs Res* 66(3):262–270, 2017.

21

Public Health Nursing Practice and the Disaster Management Cycle

Sherry L. Farra, PhD, RN, CNE, CHSE, NDHP-BC,
Sherrill J. Smith, RN, PhD, CNE, CNL, and Roberta Proffitt Lavin, PhD, FNP-BC, FAAN

"Wherever disaster calls there I shall go. I ask not for whom, but only where I am needed."

From Creed of the Red Cross Nurse, by Lona L. Trott, RN, 1953

OBJECTIVES

After reading this chapter, the student should be able to do the following:

1. Discuss how disasters, both human-made and natural, affect people and their communities.
2. Differentiate disaster management cycle phases to include prevention (mitigation and protection), preparedness, response, and recovery.
3. Examine the nurse's role in the disaster management cycle.
4. Describe competencies for public health nursing practice in disasters.
5. Explain how the community works together to prevent, prepare for, respond to, and recover from disasters.
6. Identify organizations where nurses can volunteer to work in disasters.

CHAPTER OUTLINE

Defining Disasters
Disaster Facts
National Disaster Planning and Response: A Health-Focused Overview
***Healthy People 2020* Objectives**
The Disaster Management Cycle and Nursing Role
Future of Disaster Management

KEY TERMS

alternate care centers, p. 474
American Red Cross, p. 455
bioterrorism, p. 455
CBRNE threats (chemical, biological, radiological, nuclear, and explosive), p. 458
Community Emergency Response Team, p. 461
community resilience, p. 457
crisis standards of care, p. 465
Disaster Medical Assistance Team, p. 461
Emergency Operations Center, p. 465
Emergency Support Function 8: Public Health and Medical, p. 457
Functional Needs Support Services, p. 473
general population shelter, p. 473
Homeland Security Act of 2002, p. 457
Homeland Security Exercise and Evaluation Program, p. 464
Homeland Security Presidential Directive 21: Public Health and Medical Preparedness, p. 457
human-made incident, p. 455
interprofessional, p. 458
Medical Reserve Corps, p. 461
mutual aid agreement, p. 465
National Disaster Medical System, p. 461
National Disaster Recovery Framework p. 475
National Health Security Strategy, p. 457
National Incident Management System, p. 457
National Preparedness Guidelines, p. 457
National Prevention Framework, p. 457
National Response Framework, p. 457
One Health, p. 467
pandemic, p. 455
Pandemic and All-Hazards Preparedness Reauthorization Act, p. 457
personal protective equipment, p. 460
points of dispensing, p. 459
Presidential Policy Directive 8: National Preparedness, p. 457
psychological first aid, p. 458
public health surge, p. 455

The authors wish to acknowledge the manuscript review and consultation of a review committee and to the many contributions of Susan Hassmiller, PhD, RN, FAAN and Sharon Stanley, PhD, RN, FAAN to prior editions of the chapter.

KEY TERMS—cont'd

public health triage, p. 458
rapid needs assessment, p. 458
risk communication, p. 471
Robert T. Stafford Disaster Relief and Emergency Assistance Act, p. 465
Strategic National Stockpile, p. 459
triage, p. 470
utilitarian framework, p. 473

Around the world, people are experiencing unprecedented disasters from natural causes ranging from hurricanes and earthquakes to human-made disasters such as oil spills, mass shootings, and terrorism. Disasters, whether human-made or natural, are inevitable, but there are ways to help communities prepare for, respond to, and recover from disaster. This chapter describes the disaster management cycle phases of prevention, preparedness, response, and recovery and the role of the public health nurse.

DEFINING DISASTERS

A disaster is any natural or **human-made incident** that causes disruption, destruction, and/or devastation requiring external assistance. Although natural incidents such as earthquakes or hurricanes trigger many disasters, predictable and preventable human-made factors can further affect the disaster. On March 11, 2011, northeastern Japan was rocked by a 9.0 magnitude earthquake that was quickly followed by a tsunami (Fig. 21.1). These dual natural disasters caused an estimated death toll of 20,000, but there was a third, human-made component to complete the incident triad: a nuclear reactor crisis. An independent parliamentary investigation later found the Fukushima nuclear disaster to be the result of a mix of several human-made factors (Inajima et al., 2012). Box 21.1 lists examples of natural and human-made disasters.

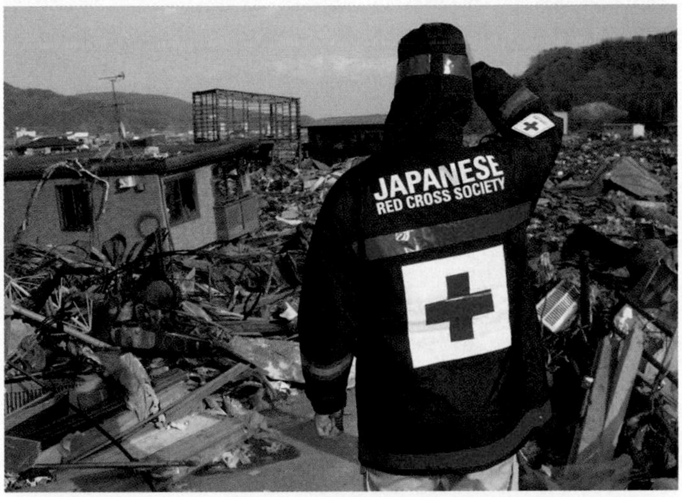

Fig. 21.1 A week after the earthquake struck and tsunami surged through northeast Japan, a Japanese Red Cross volunteer surveys the damage to Ōtsuchi in Iwate Prefecture. (Courtesy the American Red Cross Disaster Online Newsroom, Washington, DC. From http://newsroom.redcross.org.)

BOX 21.1 Types of Disasters

Natural	Human-Made
Hurricanes	Conventional warfare
Tornadoes	Unconventional warfare (e.g., nuclear, chemical)
Hailstorms	Transportation accidents
Cyclones	Structural collapse
Blizzards	Explosions/bombing
Drought	Fires
Floods	Hazardous materials incident
Mudslides	Pollution
Avalanches	Civil unrest (e.g., riots)
Earthquakes	Terrorism (chemical, biological, radiological, nuclear, explosives)
Volcanic eruptions	Cyber attacks
Pandemics and epidemics	Airplane crash
Lightning-induced forest fires	Radiological incident
Tsunamis	Nuclear power plant incident
Thunderstorms and lightning	Critical infrastructure failure
Extreme heat and cold	Water supply contamination

From U.S. Department of Health and Human Services: *Healthy People 2020*. Washington, DC, 2018, USDHHS.

In the disaster response phase, the incident type and timing predict subsequent injuries and illnesses. If there is prior warning (e.g., in hurricanes or slow-rising floods), the impact brings fewer injuries and deaths. Disasters resulting with little or no advance notice such as earthquakes or **bioterrorism** often have more casualties because those affected have little time to make evacuation preparations or to obtain adequate treatment. Individuals can also be injured attempting to prepare for the disaster or while evacuating. Public health disasters can create needs across a widespread region. In a **pandemic**, pressing and competing health needs occur within a close time frame, producing a **public health surge**. In the disaster recovery phase, the immediate threat shifts to adjusting to a new normal in the affected community or region.

DISASTER FACTS

Disasters can affect one family at a time, as in a house fire, or they can kill thousands and result in economic losses in the millions, as with floods, earthquakes, tornadoes, hurricanes, tsunamis, and bioterrorism. The **American Red Cross** reports that it responds to a disaster in the United States every eight minutes, resulting in response to more than 64,000 incidents each year (American Red Cross, 2018).

The number of reported natural and human-made disasters continues to rise worldwide, yet the number of lives lost has declined over the past two decades. Better forecasting and early warning systems have reduced the number of lives lost in a disaster (International Federation of Red Cross and Red Crescent Societies [IFRC], 2016).

Around the globe in 2015, the reported number of people (108 million) affected by natural disasters was low compared to previous peaks in 2010 and 2011. Droughts, floods, and storms contributed to the most common natural disasters. Almost 100,000 more were affected by disasters related to technological hazards, with fires accounting for the highest number of occurrences (IFRC, 2016).

In 2017, there were 137 disaster declarations in the United States, which included 59 major disasters, with another 15 emergency declarations and more than 60 fire management assistance declarations, up from 25 fire management emergencies in 2013 (Federal Emergency Management Agency [FEMA], 2018a). An additional explanation on how a disaster declaration is made is presented later in this chapter, but the point is that disaster incidents are a regular occurrence. Hurricane names such as Katrina (2005), Sandy (2012), and Irma (2017), and tornado pathways in Joplin, Missouri (2011), and Norman, Oklahoma (2013), are familiar to all. Irma, one of the most costly hurricanes recorded in the Atlantic, provided widespread devastation across Florida and the Caribbean Islands in 2017 (Cangialosi et al., 2018). Yet, the latest report card for our nation's emergency care environment in disaster preparedness grades our overall system with a C− for 2014, dropping from a C+ in 2009 (American College of Emergency Physicians [ACEP], 2014). The report states that this is due, in large part, to state variation. For example, although the average number of health professionals registering in the volunteer system (the Emergency System for Advance Registration of Volunteer Health Professionals [ESAR-VHP]) is 279.6 nurses per 1 million people overall, that number is 0 per 1 million in Mississippi and 1069 per 1 million in the District of Columbia (ACEP, 2014).

Disaster disproportionately strikes at-risk individuals, whether their day-to-day risk is physical, emotional, or economic. Disasters in less developed communities can also destroy decades of progress in a matter of hours, in a manner that rarely happens in more developed countries. The poor, elderly, ethnic minorities, people with disabilities, and women and children in developing communities are excessively affected and least able to rebound (World Health Organization, 2017). Unfortunately, by 2050, the percent of population areas more vulnerable to disasters will increase. Eighty percent of the world's population will live in developing countries, with 40 percent living in tornado and earthquake zones, near rivers, and on coastlines. The monetary cost of disasters is also increasing sharply with the average annual economic loss globally expected to rise from $250-300 billion to $415 billion in 2030 in urban areas alone (United Nations Development Programme, 2016). The cost in more developed countries is higher because of the extent of material possessions and complex infrastructures, including technology. In the United States, increases in population and development in areas vulnerable to natural disasters, especially coastal areas, have led to sharply increased insurance payouts. In 2017, the number of weather and climate-related disasters led to a record of $300 billion in losses (NOAA National Centers for Environmental Information [NCEI], 2018) (Table 21.1).

TABLE 21.1 Total Amount of Disaster Estimated Damage by Continent, Level of Human Development, and Year (2006-2015), in Millions of U.S. Dollars (2015 Prices)

	2006	2007	2008	2009	2010	2011	2012	2013	2014	2015	Total
Africa	277	885	982	197	66	1,103	988	246	688	2,662	8,094
Americas	8,643	18,630	73,540	16,878	86,948	73,720	109,417	35,485	24,999	25,550	473,811
Asia	28,472	40,692	134,255	20,126	42,693	297,840	28,848	59,468	64,459	33,853	750,705
Europe	2,942	25,949	5,340	13,774	21,393	3,188	25,734	22,817	8,383	4,697	134,217
Oceania	1,558	1,693	2,886	1,934	10,501	30,485	909	3,316	1,181	3,521	57,987
Very high human development	*14,055*	*53,878*	*73,868*	*30,914*	*94,277*	*330,450*	*1312,852*	*53,033*	*29,946*	*33,113*	*845,386*
High human development	*17,401*	*23,427*	*134,404*	*11,719*	*42,040*	67,759	*28,127*	*45,935*	*41,189*	*21,094*	*433,096*
Medium human development	*10,432*	*7,061*	*3,513*	*10,005*	*5,485*	*5,248*	*2,169*	*20,566*	*26,477*	*10,115*	*101,071*
Low human development	*4*	*3,484*	*5,217*	*271*	*19,801*	*2,878*	*3,748*	*1,799*	*2,097*	*5,962*	*45,261*
Total:	41,892	87,850	217,003	52,909	181,603	406,336	165,895	121,333	99,710	70,285	1,424,814

Notes: Some totals in Table 21.1 may not correspond, due to rounding.

Damage assessment is frequently unreliable. Even for existing data, methodologies are not standardized and the financial coverage can vary significantly. Depending on where the disaster occurred and who reported it, estimations may vary from zero to billions of U.S. dollars.

The total amount of damage reported in 2015 was the third lowest of the decade. Based on continent, damage was third lowest in Europe, fourth lowest in Asia, and fifth lowest in the Americas. In Africa, however, it was the highest, and the third highest in Oceania.

In terms of human development level, the amount of damage was third lowest in high human development countries and fourth in very high human development countries, however, in low human development countries it was second highest and in medium human development countries it was fourth highest.

From International Federation of Red Cross and Red Crescent Societies (IFRC): *World disasters report 2016: resilience: saving lives today, investing for tomorrow.* Geneva, Switzerland, 2017, IFRC, p. 239. Available at http://www.ifrc.org.

NATIONAL DISASTER PLANNING AND RESPONSE: A HEALTH-FOCUSED OVERVIEW

There is a concerted national effort to provide guidance to state and local planning regions to assist with the coordinated and successful responses and recovery efforts in all-hazard disasters and catastrophes. Many documents have been written at the national level, some of which are reviewed in this chapter. You may ask: "Isn't this all beyond what an individual nurse should have to know?"

As the single largest profession within the health care network, nurses must understand the national disaster management cycle. Without nursing integration at every phase, communities and clients lose a critical part of the prevention network, and the multidisciplinary response team loses a first-rate partner. Actually, it matters greatly how the nation dials 911, and it matters to individuals as well as communities, regions, and the country as a whole. It also matters globally, beyond our own borders. Our national response is not just about the United States, but our international ability to assist other nations in their times of need.

The U.S. Department of Homeland Security (DHS) was created through the **Homeland Security Act of 2002** (DHS, 2002), consolidating more than 20 separate agencies.

Presidential Policy Directive 8: National Preparedness (PPD-8) was signed and released by President Barack Obama on March 30, 2011. PPD-8 replaced Homeland Security Presidential Directive 8 from the Bush era and guides how the nation, from the federal level to private citizens, can "prevent, protect against, mitigate the effects of, respond to, and recover from those threats that pose the greatest risk to the security of the Nation" (DHS, 2011). The **National Preparedness Guidelines** (NPG) (DHS, 2007a) and the National Response Plan (NRP), which provide a national doctrine for preparedness that includes the **National Prevention Framework** and aids in securing the nation by preparing and preventing terrorist attacks (DHS, 2016a). The **National Response Framework** (NRF), was promulgated in January 2008. The third edition of the National Response Framework, updated in 2016, provides context for how the whole community works together and how response efforts relate to other parts of national preparedness (DHS, 2016c). Each of the five frameworks covers one mission area: Prevention, Protection, Mitigation, Response, or Recovery. In that framework there are also 15 emergency support functions. **Emergency Support Function 8: Public Health and Medical** provides coordinated federal assistance to supplement state, local, and tribal resources in response to public health and medical care needs (FEMA, 2016c).

Homeland Security Presidential Directive 5 (HSPD-5) created the **National Incident Management System** (NIMS), a unified, all-discipline, and all-hazards approach to domestic incident management (FEMA, 2018d; Naval Postgraduate School [NPS], 2018). The NIMS was established to provide a common language and structure enabling all those involved in disaster response to communicate with each other more effectively and efficiently.

Two national preparedness documents specifically guide disaster health preparedness, response, and recovery: **Homeland Security Presidential Directive (HSPD) 21: Public Health and Medical Preparedness** and the **National Health Security Strategy** (NHSS). HSPD-21 established a national strategy that enables a level of public health and medical preparedness sufficient to address a range of possible disasters. It did so through four critical components of public health and medical preparedness: (1) biosurveillance, (2) countermeasure distribution, (3) mass casualty care, and (4) **community resilience** (NPS, 2018). The NHSS is updated every four years and focuses on the national goals for protecting people's health in the case of disaster in any setting. National health security is achieved when "the nation and its people are prepared for, protected from, and resilient in the face of incidents with health consequences" (U.S. Department of Health and Human Services [USDHHS], 2015, para. 2). The NHSS was directed by the 2006 Pandemic and All-Hazards Preparedness Act (PAHPA), an act to improve the nation's ability to detect, prepare for, and respond to a variety of public health emergencies. The PAHPA was re-enacted in 2013 and is now called the **Pandemic and All-Hazards Preparedness Reauthorization Act** (PAHPRA). The PAHPRA funds public health and hospital preparedness programs, medical countermeasures under the BioShield Project, and enhances the authority of the Food and Drug Administration (FDA) (USDHHS, 2014).

In discussing community resiliency and impact of health care reform on public health preparedness, concerns have still been noted regarding the effects of the Affordable Care Act and how it has changed the role of public health in communities along with the increase in availability of primary care for more individuals (Institute of Medicine [IOM], 2014).

Our national system of homeland security includes public health preparedness and response as a core part of its national strategies. Some of the strategy documents introduced in this section are covered in greater detail throughout the chapter. Every aspect of disaster management involves the practice of public health nursing.

HEALTHY PEOPLE 2020 OBJECTIVES

Because disaster affects the health of people in many ways, disaster incidents have an effect on almost every *Healthy People 2020* objective. While there are specific objectives related to disaster preparedness, Access to Health Services and Public Health Infrastructure are two important *Healthy People 2020* topic areas with subsequent objectives that become even more significant when individual and community needs escalate in disaster (USDHHS, 2018). Disasters also play a direct role in the objectives related to environmental health, food safety, immunization and infectious disease, and mental health and mental disorders. Public health professionals, such as those who work at the Centers for Disease Control and Prevention (CDC), study the effect that disasters have on population health and continuously develop new prevention strategies. Other organizations, such as the American Psychological Association and the American Red Cross, work with communities in the preparedness, response, and recovery phases of a disaster and to revise and align the *Healthy People 2020* objectives related to mental health.

HEALTHY PEOPLE 2020

Objectives Related to Preparedness

- **PREP-1:** Reduce the time necessary to issue official information to the public about a public health emergency.
- **PREP-2:** Reduce the time necessary to activate designated personnel in response to a public health emergency.
- **PREP-3:** Increase the proportion of Laboratory Response Network (LRN) laboratories that meet proficiency standards.
- **PREP-4:** Reduce the time for state public health agencies to establish after-action reports and improvement plans following responses to public health emergencies and exercises.
- **PREP-5:** Increase the percentage of school districts that require schools to include specific topics in their crisis preparedness, response, and recovery plans

From U.S. Department of Health and Human Services (USDHHS): *Healthy People 2020,* Washington, DC, 2018, USDHHS. Available at https://www.healthypeople.gov.

THE DISASTER MANAGEMENT CYCLE AND NURSING ROLE

Disaster management includes four stages: prevention (including mitigation and protection), preparedness, response, and recovery. Fig. 21.2 shows the disaster emergency management cycle. Nurses have unique skills for all aspects of disaster, including assessment, priority setting, collaboration, and addressing both preventive and acute care needs. In addition,

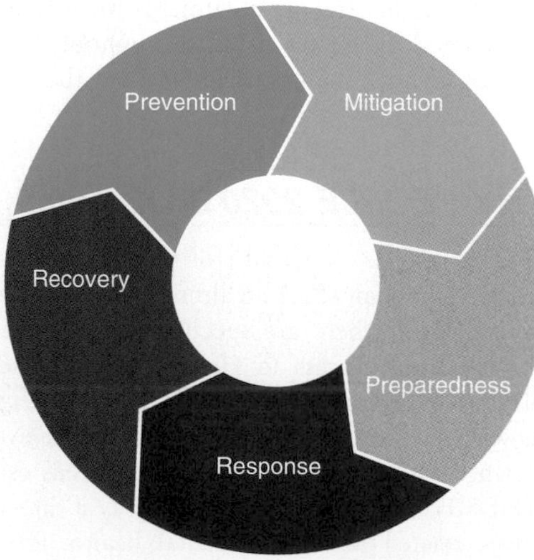

Fig. 21.2 Disaster management cycle. The original work for the disaster management cycle comes from National Governors' Association Center for Policy Research: *Comprehensive emergency management: a governor's guide,* Washington, DC, 1979, National Governors' Association. (Image from Ontario Agency for Health Protection and Promotion [Public Health Ontario]: Public health emergency preparedness: an IMS-based workshop. Base scenario. Toronto, ON, July 2015, Queen's Printer for Ontario, p. 7.)

public health nurses have a skill set that serves their community well in disaster, including health education and disease screening, mass clinic expertise, an ability to provide essential public health services, community resource referral and liaison work, population advocacy, **psychological first aid**, **public health triage**, and **rapid needs assessment**. Nurses have served globally in disaster care for over a century. They continue to provide a significant resource to both the employee and the volunteer disaster management workforce, and their numbers are unmatched by any other profession. In addition, nurses work closely with the **interprofessional** health team, community leaders, and organizations, engaging with and advocating for clients as needed across the disaster management cycle.

The World Association for Disaster and Emergency Medicine (WADEM) includes a nursing section. The Nursing Section of WADEM represents nurses from all countries to strengthen and improve the practice and knowledge of disaster nursing. The Nursing Section purposes are as follows (WADEM, 2018):

- Define nursing issues for public health care and disaster health care.
- Exchange scientific and professional information relevant to the practice of disaster nursing
- Encourage collaborative efforts enhancing and expanding the field of nursing disaster research.
- Encourage collaboration with other nursing organizations.
- Inform and advise WADEM of matters related to disaster nursing.

The International Council of Nurses (ICN) also hosts a disaster-focused response network to allow nurses to have access to resources for disaster response (ICN, 2016).

Prevention (Mitigation and Protection)

All-hazards mitigation (prevention, protection) is an emergency management term for reducing risks to people and property from natural hazards before they occur. The ability to provide primary prevention through national missions of prevention, mitigation, or protection can include structural measures, such as protecting buildings and infrastructure from the forces of wind and water, and nonstructural measures, such as land development restrictions. These primary prevention measures implemented at the local government level achieve effectiveness in an all-hazards approach to threats. Of course, prevention also includes human-made hazards and the ability to deter potential terrorists, detect terrorists before they strike, and take decisive action to eliminate the threat (DHS, 2016a). Prevention activities for terrorism may include heightened inspections; improved surveillance and security operations; public health and agricultural surveillance; and testing, immunizations, isolation, or neutralizing **CBRNE threats (chemical, biological, radiological, nuclear, and explosive)**.

The nurse may be involved in many roles in the primary prevention of a disaster. As community advocates, nurses promote environmental health by identifying environmental hazards and serving on the public health team for mitigation purposes. Public health nurses in particular are involved with organizing and participating in mass prophylaxis and

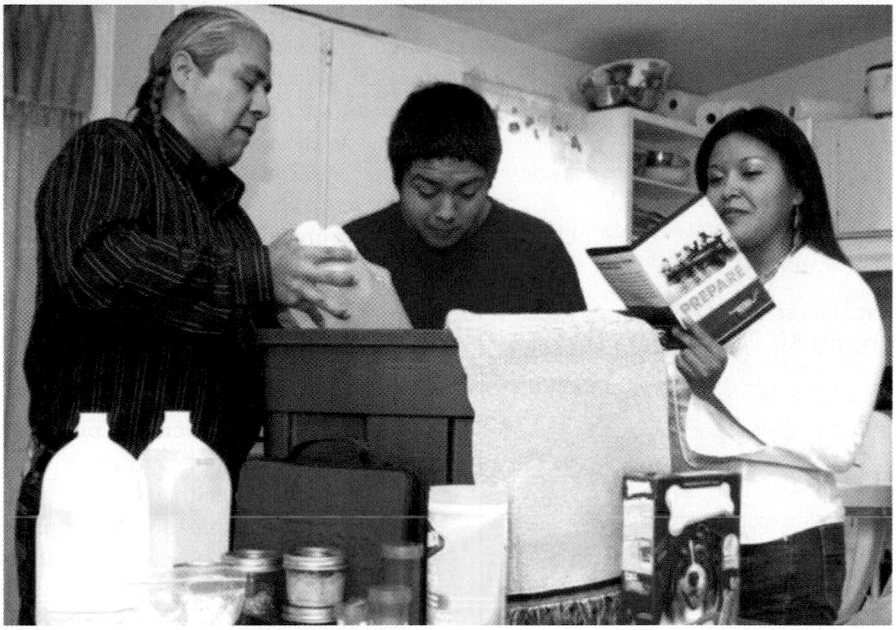

Fig. 21.3 Personal preparedness. Participants in National Preparedness Month, 2015, building a disaster kit. (Available at https://www.fema.gov.)

vaccination campaigns to prevent, treat, or contain a disease. The nurse should be familiar with the region's local cache of pharmaceuticals and how the **Strategic National Stockpile** (SNS) (described later in this chapter) will be distributed. Once federal and local authorities agree that the SNS is needed, medicine delivery to any state in the United States occurs within 12 hours (CDC, 2018c). State and local emergency planners then ensure **points of dispensing** (POD), to provide prophylaxis to the entire population within 48 hours.

In terms of human-made disaster prevention, the nurse should be aware of high-risk targets and current vulnerabilities and what can be done to eliminate or mitigate the vulnerability. Targets may include military and civilian government facilities, health care facilities, international airports and other transportation systems, large cities, and high-profile landmarks. Terrorists might also target large public gatherings, water and food supplies, banking and finance, information technology, postal and shipping services, utilities, and corporate centers.

Preparedness

Role of the Public Health Nurse in Personal and Professional Preparedness. Public health nurses play a key role in community preparedness, but they must accomplish the critical elements of personal and professional preparedness first.

Personal Preparedness. Disasters by their nature require nurses to respond quickly. Public health nurses without plans in place to address their own needs, to include family and pets, will be unable to fully participate in their disaster obligations at work or in volunteer efforts (Fig. 21.3). In addition, the nurse assisting in disaster relief efforts must be as healthy as possible, both physically and mentally. Disaster workers who do not practice self-health are of little service to their family, clients, and community (see the How To box entitled Be Red Cross Ready). Disaster kits should be made for the home, workplace, and car. There are emergency supplies specific to nursing that should be prepared and stored in a sturdy, easy-to-carry container (see the accompanying How To box). Important documents should always be in waterproof containers. Nurses should consider several contingencies for children and older adults with a plan to seek help from neighbors in the event of being called to a disaster. Many public shelters do not allow pets inside and other arrangements must be made. At present, local emergency management agencies include pet management in the local disaster plans and so should the pet owner (FEMA, 2018e).

HOW TO Be Red Cross Ready

1. Get a Kit
   Consider the following when assembling or restocking your kit to ensure that you and your family are prepared for any disaster:
   - Store at least three days of food, water, and supplies in your family's easy-to-carry preparedness kit. Keep extra supplies on hand at home in case you cannot leave the affected area.
   - Keep your kit where it is easily accessible.
   - Remember to check your kit every six months and replace expired or outdated items.
2. Make a Plan
   When preparing for a disaster, always:
   - Talk with your family.
   - Make a plan for your family that reflects the needs of the family and potential hazards in the area.
   - Learn how and when to turn off utilities and how to use lifesaving tools such as fire extinguishers.
   - Tell everyone where emergency information and supplies are stored. Provide copies of the family's preparedness plan to each member of the family. Always ensure that information is up to date and practice

evacuations, following the routes outlined in your plan. Don't forget to identify alternative routes.
- Include pets in your evacuation plans.

3. Get Informed

There are three key parts to becoming informed:
- Get Info: Learn the ways you would get information during a disaster or an emergency.
- Know Your Region: Learn about the disasters that may occur in your area.
- Action Steps: Learn first aid from your local Red Cross chapter.

Emergency Supplies That Nurses Should Have Ready in Addition to Personal Kit
- Identification badge and driver's license
- Proof of licensure and certification (e.g., RN, CPR/AED, First Aid)
- Pocket-size reference books (e.g., nursing protocols and intervention standards)
- Blood pressure cuff (adult and child) and stethoscope
- Gloves, mask, other personal protective equipment (PPE) for general care
- First aid kit with mouth-to-mouth cardiopulmonary resuscitation (CPR) barrier and tourniquet
- Crank radio and cell phone charger
- Cash, credit card
- Important papers and contact information in hard copy
- Sun protection and insect repellant
- Sturdy shoes with socks
- Medical identification of allergies, blood type
- Medications for self
- Weather-appropriate clothing to include rain gear
- Toiletries
- Watch, cell phone with pre-entered emergency numbers
- Flashlight, extra batteries
- Record-keeping materials, including pencil/pen
- Map of area

Courtesy the American Red Cross. Available at http://www.redcross.org.

One way a nurse can feel assured about family member protection is by working with them to develop the skills and knowledge necessary for coping in disaster. For example, long- term benefits occur by involving children and adolescents in activities such as writing preparedness plans, exercising the plan, becoming familiar with their school emergency procedures and family reunification sites, and learning about the range of potential hazards in their vicinity to include evacuation routes. This strategy also offers children and adolescents an opportunity to express their feelings.

Professional Preparedness. Every state needs a qualified workforce of public health nurses for solutions for today's public health problems that include natural disasters and the threat of terrorism. Public health nurses are leaders in coordinating interprofessional teams to promote community health (Robert Wood Johnson Foundation, 2017). Public health nurses are also lead by chief public health nurse officers at the state level who develop and maintain a strong public health nursing workforce and practice, especially when those nurses are scattered throughout state and local systems.

Disaster management in the community is about population health: The core public health functions of *assessment, policy development, and assurance* hold as true in disaster as in day-to-day operations. Operating in the chaos of disaster surge, however, demands a flexible and proficient practice base in each of public health's 3 core functions and 10 essential services (see http://www.cdc.gov).

Just as the mission of public health and its core functions and essential services do not change in disaster, neither does the practice of public health nursing. The public health nurse must be prepared to advocate for the community in terms of focus on population-based practice. The number of public health nurses available to get the job done is small when compared with those with generic or other specialty nurse preparation. Also, disaster produces conditions that demand an aggregate-care approach, increasing the need for public health nursing involvement in community service during disaster and catastrophe.

The Public Health Nursing Intervention Wheel (see Chapter 11) is a population-based practice model that encompasses 3 levels of practice (community, systems, and individual/family) and 16 public health interventions. Each intervention and practice level contributes to improving population health, providing a practice foundation. This Wheel holds true to public health nursing interventions whether the nurse is working in day-to-day or in disaster operations.

Interprofessional disaster care teams need nurses with disaster and emergency management training and experience. Although the majority of disaster work is not high tech, the knowledge one needs for CBRNE disasters must be developed to include access to a ready cache of information related to nursing care. The following sites provide useful information:
- CDC: *Emergency Preparedness and Response* (https://emergency.cdc.gov)
- National Library of Medicine: *Disaster Information Management Research Center* (http://disaster.nlm.nih.gov)
- Unbound Medicine: *Relief Central* (http://relief.unboundmedicine.com)
- National Library of Medicine: *WISER—Wireless Information System for Emergency Responders* (http://wiser.nlm.nih.gov) (see Box 21.2 for further information)

Depending on the assigned task and possible volunteer assignments, it is expected that nurses know how to use **personal protective equipment** (PPE), operate specialized equipment needed to perform specific activities, and safely perform duties in disaster environments.

Professional preparedness also requires that nurses become aware of and understand emergency and disaster plans at their workplace and in their community. Nurses should review the disaster history of the community, understanding how past disasters have affected the community's health care delivery system. It is important for nurses to understand and gain the competencies needed to respond in times of disasters *before* disaster strikes.

Disaster competencies for public health nursing practice have been proposed in a set of 25 competencies categorized into preparedness, response, and recovery (Polivka et al., 2008). However, it is recognized that disaster response needs to be interprofessional in nature to meet the needs of those in need. Box 21.3 displays core disaster competencies for those

BOX 21.2 Nurses and Technology Hazardous Material Information Delivered via Wireless

WISER (Wireless Information System for Emergency Responders) is a system designed to assist emergency responders in hazardous material incidents. Developed by the National Library of Medicine, WISER provides a wide range of information on hazardous substances, including substance identification support, physical characteristics, human health information, and containment and suppression guidance. By inputting a substance's physical properties and entering an individual's symptoms, WISER can help narrow the range of substances that may be involved. It provides detailed information about hazardous substances, health effects, treatment, personal protective equipment, toxicity, the emergency resources available, and the surrounding environmental conditions. In January 2018, WISER version 5.1 was released. This latest update includes up to date information from the EPA as well as the Hazardous Substances Data Bank (HSDB WISER is available as a standalone application on Microsoft Windows PCs, Apple's iOS devices (iPhone, iPad, and iPod touch), Google Android devices, and BlackBerry devices (Internet connectivity required).

From National Library of Medicine: *About WISER,* Bethesda, MD, 2018, National Library of Medicine. Available at http://wiser.nlm.nih.gov/about.html.

BOX 21.3 Core Competencies for Disaster Medicine and Public Health

1.0: Demonstrate personal and family preparedness for disasters and public health emergencies.
2.0: Demonstrate knowledge of one's expected role(s) in organizational and community response plans activated during a disaster or public health emergency.
3.0: Demonstrate situational awareness of actual/potential health hazards before, during, and after a disaster or public health emergency.
4.0: Communicate effectively with others in a disaster or public health emergency.
5.0: Demonstrate knowledge of personal safety measures that can be implemented in a disaster or public health emergency.
6.0: Demonstrate knowledge of surge capacity assets, consistent with one's role in organizational, agency, and/or community response plans.
7.0: Demonstrate knowledge of principles and practices for the clinical management of all ages and populations affected by disasters and public health emergencies, in accordance with professional scope of practice.
8.0: Demonstrate knowledge of public health principles and practices for the management of all ages and populations affected by disasters and public health emergencies.
9.0: Demonstrate knowledge of ethical principles to protect the health and safety of all ages, populations, and communities affected by a disaster or public health emergency.
10.0: Demonstrate knowledge of legal principles to protect the health and safety of all ages, populations, and communities affected by a disaster or public health emergency.
11.0: Demonstrate knowledge of short- and long-term considerations for recovery of all ages, populations, and communities affected by a disaster or public health emergency.

From National Center for Disaster Medicine and Public Health (NCDMPH): *Core competencies project,* 2014. Available at https://www.usuhs.edu.

working in public health that are applicable to public health professionals responding to a disaster. The preparedness competencies focus on personal preparedness and on comprehending disaster preparedness terms, concepts, and roles. The competencies also define the role of the public health nurse in a surge event. Response phase competencies include the ability to provide a rapid needs assessment, outbreak investigation and surveillance, public health triage, risk communication, and technical skills such as mass dispensing. Recovery competencies include after-action participation, disaster plan modifications, and coordinating efforts to address the psychosocial and public health impact. See Box 21.4 for education and training opportunities.

Nurses who seek increased participation or who seek a better understanding of disaster management can become involved in any number of community organizations. The National Disaster Medical System (NDMS) provides nurses the opportunity to work on specialized teams such as the Disaster Medical Assistance Team (DMAT). The Medical Reserve Corps (MRC) and the Community Emergency Response Team (CERT) provide opportunities for nurses to support emergency preparedness and response in their local jurisdictions. The American Red Cross offers training in disaster health services and disaster mental health for both local response and national deployment opportunities. In the Red Cross, nurses and nursing students can join a local disaster action team (DAT); act as a liaison with local hospitals; plan health services support for shelter sites; participate on an interprofessional team for optimal service

BOX 21.4 Websites Providing Education and Training Opportunities

Public Health Workforce Development Centers
- Centers for Disease Control and Prevention: https://emergency.cdc.gov
- Heartland Centers for Public Health and Community Capacity Development: http://www.heartlandcenters.slu.edu
- Public Health Learning Network: https://nnphi.org/phln
- Northwest Center for Public Health Practice: http://www.nwcphp.org

Government and Other Nurse-Specific Courses
- American Red Cross Disaster Health and Sheltering Course for Nursing Students: https://www.training-source.org
- Center for Domestic Preparedness: https://cdp.dhs.gov
- Emergency Management Institute: https://training.fema.gov
- Federal Emergency Management Agency (FEMA) Training: https://training.fema.gov
- Nurses on the Frontline: Preparing for Emergencies and Disasters: https://asprtracie.hhs.gov

Public Health Organizations
- American Public Health Association (APHA): http://www.apha.org
- Association of Public Health Nurses (APHN): http://www.phnurse.org
- Association of Schools and Programs of Public Health (ASPH): https://www.aspph.org
- National Association of County and City Health Offices (NACCHO): http://www.naccho.org
- Public Health Foundation (PHF): http://www.phf.org

BOX 21.5 Volunteer Opportunities in Disaster Work

- American Red Cross (ARC): http://www.redcross.org
- Buddhist Compassion Relief (Tzu Chi): http://www.tzuchi.org
- Certified Emergency Response Team (CERT): https://www.ready.gov
- Citizen Corps: https://www.ready.gov
- Disaster Medical Assistance Team (DMAT): https://www.phe.gov
- Medical Reserve Corps (MRC): https://mrc.hhs.gov
- National Voluntary Organizations Active in Disaster (NVOAD): http://www.nvoad.org
- One Nurse at a Time: http://onenurseatatime.org
- The Salvation Army: http://www.salvationarmyusa.org

delivery; address the logistics of health and medical supplies; and teach disaster nursing in the community. A list of opportunities is shown in Box 21.5.

The importance of being adequately trained and properly associated with an official response organization to serve in a disaster cannot be overstated. In a disaster, many untrained and ill-equipped individuals rush in to help. Spontaneous volunteer overload, leading to role conflict, anger, frustration, and helplessness, adds to the burden in an already tense situation. The World Trade Center attacks of September 11, 2001, brought many qualified but unassociated responders to the site. "Many well-intentioned local physicians in shirt sleeves and light footwear proceeded to the area and attempted to find victims, risking further injuries to themselves and getting in the way of structured rescue protocols. … [They were] prohibited from participating in rescue operations within any area designated as a disaster by the Fire Department of New York" (Crippen, 2002). After the bombing of the Alfred P. Murrah building in Oklahoma City in 1995, a nurse who rushed into the building to rescue people became the only fatality who was not killed or injured in the initial blast and collapse (Oklahoma City National Memorial & Museum, 2018). See Box 21.6 for more on the importance of national preparedness.

BOX 21.6 Trust for America's Health (TFAH): Bioterrorism and Public Health Preparedness

Health emergencies pose some of the greatest threats to our nation, because they can be difficult to prepare for, detect, and contain. Important progress has been made to improve emergency preparedness since September 11, 2001. However, while there has been significant progress toward improving public health preparedness over the past 10 years, particularly in core capabilities, there continue to be persistent gaps in the country's ability to respond to health emergencies, ranging from bioterrorist threats to serious disease outbreaks to extreme weather events.

In the 2017 annual *Ready or Not? Protecting the Public From Diseases, Disasters, and Bioterrorism* report, 25 states scored a 5 or lower on 10 key indicators of public health preparedness. Alaska scored lowest at 2 out of 10, and Massachusetts and Rhode Island scored the highest at 9 out of 10. Along with its annual report on public health preparedness, TFAH also offers a series of recommendations to further strengthen America's emergency preparedness.

What do you think about the recommendations through a public health nursing lens?

From Trust for America's Health: *TFAH initiatives—bioterrorism and public health preparedness,* 2017. Available at http://healthyamericans.org.

Community Preparedness. Presidential Policy Directive (PPD)-8 emphasizes that true preparedness is a *whole* community event. PPD-8 urges the strengthening of our nation's security and resilience through an integrated set of guidance, programs, and processes to implement the national preparedness goal, described earlier in this chapter (DHS, 2011). However, little evidence actually exists about community level capability gaps and such understanding is necessary to model the role of the health care system in preparedness planning (Zukowski, 2014).

This planning and implementation require a coordinated response that involves many stakeholders and must begin with consensus building efforts and development of a common agenda at the local level (Zukowski, 2014). Community preparedness also involves all levels of government, public health agencies, hospitals, first responders, emergency management, health care providers within the community, schools and universities, the private sector, and business and nongovernmental organizations (NGOs) such as the Red Cross. Mutual aid agreements and prior planning help to bridge perceived and actual barriers; good communication plans keep the public informed and prepared; establish relationships before the incident at the local, regional, state, and national levels; and ensure seamless service. Sometimes barriers involve regulatory authority and jurisdictional boundaries; sometimes the barriers involve organizational control versus the common good.

Emergency management is responsible for developing and coordinating emergency response plans within their defined area, whether local, state, federal, or tribal. The Federal Emergency Management Agency (FEMA) coordinates comprehensive, all-hazard planning at the national level, ensuring a menu of exercises and plan templates to address plausible incidents in any given community. Emergency management personnel at the state and local levels work closely with their communities and response partners, providing opportunities to train, exercise, evaluate, and update disaster plans. Stronger pre-disaster partnerships, which include all stakeholders, produce a more coordinated response. Fig. 21.4 shows FEMA regions across the nation.

Disaster planning involves simplicity and realism with backup contingencies because (1) the disaster will never be an "exact fit" for the plan, and (2) all plans must be implementation ready, no matter who is present to start them (DHS, 2018). The following Quality and Safety Education for Nurses box describes safety guidelines for the nurse's family.

Finally, the community must have an adequate warning system and an evacuation plan that includes measures to remove those individuals who hesitate to leave areas of danger. Some people refuse to leave their homes over fear that their possessions will be lost, destroyed, or looted. They also do not

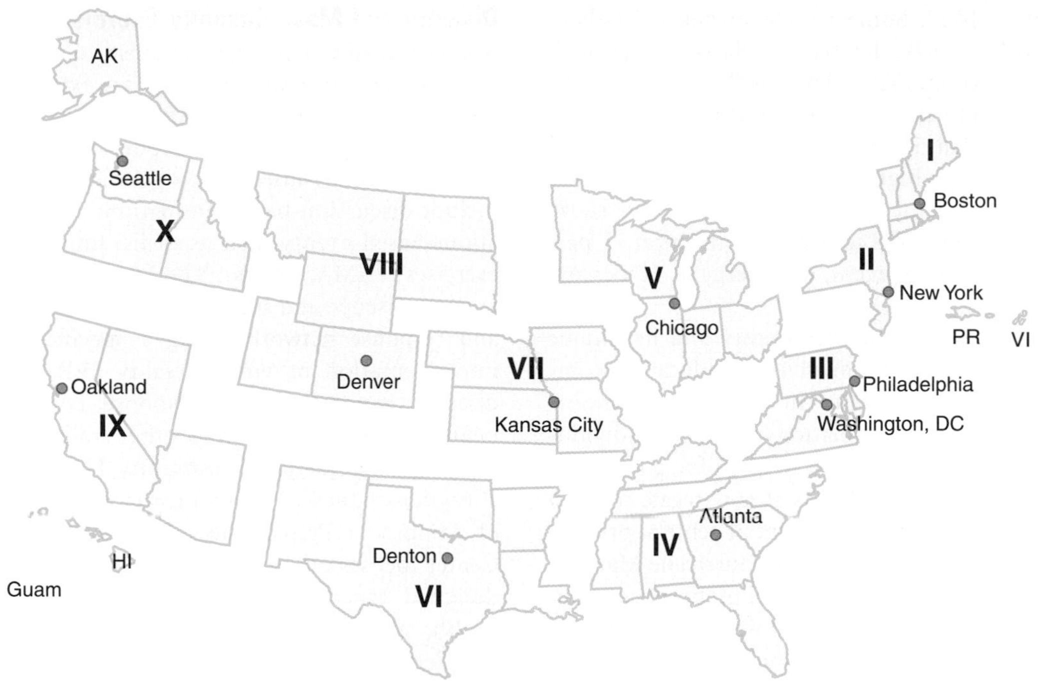

Fig. 21.4 FEMA regional contacts. (Courtesy Federal Emergency Management Agency [FEMA]: *Regional contacts,* Washington, DC, 2014, FEMA. Available at https://www.fema.gov.)

QSEN FOCUS ON QUALITY AND SAFETY EDUCATION FOR NURSES

Targeted Competency: Safety

Minimize risk of harm to clients and providers through both system effectiveness and individual performance. Selected knowledge, skills, and attitudes are cited below in order to develop a disaster safety plan:

Knowledge

Examine human factors and other basic safety design principles as well as commonly used unsafe practices (such as workarounds and dangerous abbreviations). Specific steps might be:

1. Learn how you can get information during the disaster or emergency.
   a. Determine what types of disasters are most likely to happen.
   b. Learn about warning signals in your community.
   c. Ask about post-disaster pet care (shelters usually will not accept pets).
   d. Review the disaster plans at your workplace, school, and other places where your family spends time.
   e. Determine how to help older adult or disabled family members or neighbors.
   f. What should you do?

Skills

Demonstrate effective use of strategies to reduce risk of harm to self or others.

1. Create a disaster plan:
   a. Talk with your family and create two places to meet, including outside your home and outside your neighborhood. Give each member of the family a copy of the plan.
   b. Discuss the types of disasters that are most likely to happen, and review what to do in each case and make a plan.
   c. Choose an out-of-state friend to be your family contact; this person will verify the location of each family member. After a disaster, it may be easier to call long distance than to make local calls.
   d. Review evacuation plans, including care of pets. Have alternative routes for evacuation.
2. Complete this checklist:
   a. Post emergency phone numbers next to telephones.
   b. Teach everyone how and when to call 911.
   c. Determine when and how to turn off water, gas, and electricity at the main switches.
   d. Check adequacy of insurance coverage for yourself and your home.
   e. Locate and review the use of fire extinguishers.
   f. Install and maintain smoke and carbon monoxide detectors.
   g. Conduct a home hazard hunt and fix potential hazards.
   h. Stock emergency supplies and assemble a disaster supplies kit.
   i. Acquire first aid and cardiopulmonary resuscitation (CPR) and tourniquet certification.
   j. Locate all escape routes from your home. Find two ways out of each room.
   k. Find safe spots in your home for each type of disaster.
3. Practice and maintain your plan:
   a. Review the plan every six months.
   b. Conduct fire and emergency evacuation drills.
   c. Replace stored water every three months and stored food every six months.
   d. Test and recharge fire extinguishers according to manufacturer's instructions.
   e. Test your smoke detectors monthly and change the batteries at least once a year.
   f. What more should you do?

Attitudes

Appreciate the cognitive and physical limits of human performance.

1. Monitor your personal reactions to the disaster and seek assistance if the stress of the losses and the potential work to re-establish a new normal seem overwhelming. Monitor also the reactions of your colleagues and the clients you serve and provide or refer to others anyone who needs stress management intervention.

Safety Question

To prepare more effectively for the event of a future disaster, what steps would you take to ensure the safety of your family, including any pets you may have?

want to leave pets behind. Some people mistakenly believe that experience with a particular type of disaster is enough preparation for the next one. The nurse's visibility in the community can help develop the trust and credibility needed to help in contingency planning for evacuation. In December 2017 nurses were rated the highest on honesty and ethics in a ranking of professions for the 16th straight year. Their ranking of 82 percent was compared to military officers at 71 percent, medical doctors at 65 percent, and clergy at 42 percent (Brenan, 2017).

Given their knowledge of the community and its unique characteristics, nurses should be involved in educating communities about their vulnerabilities in a disaster. Planning should include helping at-risk populations to address individualized preparedness needs. In addition to identifying high-risk individuals in neighborhoods, locations of congregate concern include schools, college campuses, residential centers, prisons, hospitals, and high-rise buildings. During Hurricane Maria in 2017 the impact was so severe that almost all of the 69 hospitals were left damaged and without power. Hospitals were in survival mode. There are times when no amount of planning is adequate for the situation or prepares providers for what they will face (Zorrilla, 2017).

The National Health Security Strategy and Community Resilience. The NHSS, mentioned earlier in this chapter, as part of the nation's national planning has been instrumental in bringing the concept of community resilience into all preparedness operations. The NHSS is designed to achieve two goals: (1) build community resilience and (2) strengthen and sustain health and emergency response systems (USDHHS, 2015). Some maintain, though, that the concept of community resilience is not fully defined at our national level and accountability measures to examine resilience pre-disaster and post-disaster are lacking (Uscher-Pines et al., 2013). Community resilience is a policy issue in all levels of planning (federal, state, and local) because limited resources post-disaster demand whole community resilience in order to move back into normalcy. Healthier communities, by default, will have better bounce-back ability.

Community resilience is defined as the sustained ability of a community to withstand and recover from adversity (Links et al., 2018). Healthy individuals, families, and communities with access to health care and protective, preventive knowledge that can be used to launch timely action become some of our nation's strongest assets in disaster incidents. Pre-incident capacity has a direct impact on resilience. Links et al. (2018) describe the pre-functioning domains as communication, economy, education, food and water, government, housing, health care and public health, nurturing care, transportation, and well-being. Strengths or deficits in these domains either increase or decrease resilience. Population factors that decrease resilience include vulnerability, inequity, and deprivation. Prevention/Mitigation factors include natural systems, engineered systems, and countermeasures. The nurse works to build on the strengths and mitigate areas of weakness as building resiliency in communities.

Disaster and Mass Casualty Exercises. Although practice will not ensure a perfect response to disaster, disaster and mass casualty drills and exercises are extremely valuable components of preparedness. After each exercise, the lessons learned through after-action reports are used to update disaster plans and subsequent operations. Exercise categories include discussion-based simulations or "tabletops" and operations-based events such as drills, functional, and full-scale exercises (FEMA, 2018b). The latter operation types involve escalating scope and scale testing of the disaster preparedness and response network, using a specific plan. In addition, implementation of virtual reality (VR)-based training for disaster preparedness and response, conducted either independently or combined with other training formats, is growing within the exercise community. For example, a virtual reality preparedness research project led through the University of Minnesota Preparedness Emergency Response Research Center focuses on an immersive simulation workshop that is designed especially for health science students in public health, medicine, nursing, pharmacy, veterinary medicine, and dentistry at the university. The researchers propose that engaging interprofessional health students in realistic simulated disaster response scenarios will improve system performance and quality disaster response through the acquisition of knowledge and team-based skills (University of Minnesota School of Public Health, 2018).

The National Exercise Program (NEP) serves to test and validate core capabilities. Participation in exercises, simulations or other activities, including real world incidents, helps organizations validate their capabilities and identify shortfalls, pulling in their partners and stakeholders including citizen participation (FEMA, 2018c). An annual Capstone Exercise, formerly titled the National Level Exercise (NLE), is conducted every two years as the final component of each NEP progressive exercise cycle. The Capstone Exercise for 2014 examined the nation's collective ability to coordinate and conduct risk assessments and implement National Frameworks and associated plans to deliver core capabilities (FEMA, 2015).

Most exercises conducted in hospitals, communities, colleges, counties, or regions are much smaller in scope and scale than the Capstone Exercises. The **Homeland Security Exercise and Evaluation Program** (HSEEP) was developed to help states and local jurisdictions improve overall preparedness with all natural and human-made disasters. It provides a standardized methodology and terminology for exercise design, development, conduct, evaluation, and improvement planning and assists communities to create exercises that will make a positive difference before a real incident (FEMA, 2018c). HSEEP is the national standard for all exercise development and implementation. Whether conducted as drills, tabletops, functional, or full-scale scenarios, and whether the scope is local or national in nature, nurses and other health care providers must be included as a part of the exercise's planning, response, and after-action activities. Nurses, as client and community advocates, are essential players in the exercise and preparedness arena.

HOW TO Conduct a Disaster Exercise

Formidable Footprint: A National Community/ Neighborhood Exercise Series

A team of national, regional, state, and local agencies and organizations has undertaken an effort to develop, conduct, and evaluate a recurring series of disaster exercises entitled "Formidable Footprint." This series of exercises serves as an opportunity for community and faith-based organizations along with governmental agencies to assess their capability to prepare for, respond to, and recover from a variety of natural disasters that affect communities and neighborhoods across the United States. There is no charge to participate in one or several of the neighborhood exercises, provided by the Disaster Resistant Communities (DRC) Group.

In addition, DRC provides the Disaster Health and Sheltering Course through nursing faculty and to their nursing students through the American Red Cross National Student Nurse Program.

Wherever and whenever you get to practice nursing in disaster response and recovery, you become a better-prepared health team member.

From Disaster Resistant Communities Group: *Formidable Footprint—a national community/neighborhood exercise series,* 2018. Available at http://www.drc-group.com.

Response

The first level of response to any event occurs at the local level with the mobilization of a team of responders such as the fire department, law enforcement, public health, and emergency services. If a disaster occurs and needs exceed local resources, the county or city emergency management agency (EMA) will coordinate activities through an **Emergency Operations Center** (EOC). The EOC provides central functions at a strategic level to oversee the emergency situation. In general, local responders within a county sign a regional or statewide **mutual aid agreement** to allow the sharing of needed personnel, equipment, services, and supplies.

The initial scope of disaster assessment is usually measured by injury, lost lives, health risks, and/or costs. The greater the destruction and lives at risk, the greater the degree of attention and resources provided at the local, regional, and state levels. When state resources and capabilities are overwhelmed, governors may, through provisions provided in the **Robert T. Stafford Disaster Relief and Emergency Assistance Act** (FEMA, 2016d), request federal assistance under a presidential disaster or emergency declaration. If the event is considered an incident of national significance (a potential or high-impact disaster), appropriate response personnel and resources are provided.

In a mass casualty incident, the goal is to maximize the number of lives saved and to do the greatest good for the greatest number of individuals. These circumstances could lead to changes in the usual standards of health and medical care in the affected locality or region. Rather than doing everything possible to save every life, **crisis standards of care** enable the health care operations necessary to allocate scarce resources in a different manner to save as many lives as possible (IOM, 2012). Crisis standards need to be explored and discussed with all community stakeholders in the preparedness phase. Community engagement is key to this process.

National Response Framework. As previously discussed, the NRF was written to provide an approach to domestic incidents in a unified, well-coordinated manner, enabling all responding entities the ability to work together more effectively and efficiently. The online component of the NRF Resource Center (https://training.fema.gov/nrfres.aspx) contains supplemental materials including annexes, partner guides, and other supporting documents and learning resources. The framework involves the entire community (individual families, community leaders, nongovernmental agencies, and the private sector) and is scalable, flexible, and adaptable to the given situation. It is a living document and is always in effect (DHS, 2016c).

The NRF includes the 15 emergency support functions (ESFs) (FEMA, 2016a):

ESF #1: Transportation
ESF #2: Communications
ESF #3: Public Works and Engineering
ESF #4: Firefighting
ESF #5: Information and Planning
ESF #6: Mass Care, Emergency Assistance, Temporary Housing and Human Services
ESF #7: Logistics
ESF #8: Public Health and Medical Services
ESF #9: Search and Rescue
ESF #10: Oil and Hazardous Materials
ESF #11: Agriculture and Natural Resources
ESF #12: Energy
ESF #13: Public Safety and Security
ESF #14: Long-Term Community Recovery
ESF #15: External Affairs/Standard Operating Procedures

Each ESF includes a coordinator function and the primary and support agencies that work together to coordinate and deliver federal capabilities. Specifically, the ESFs provide the structure for coordinating federal interagency support to align with state, regional, and local capabilities. The NRFs also include support annexes, incident specific annexes, and partner guides.

ESF-8, Public Health and Medical Services, provides guidance for medical and mental health personnel, medical equipment and supplies, assessment of the status of the public health infrastructure, and monitoring for potential disease outbreaks (FEMA, 2016c). The ESF-8 primary coordinating agency is the U.S. Department of Health and Human Services; supporting agencies include the DHS, the American Red Cross, the Department of Defense, and the Department of Veterans Affairs. The National Disaster Medical System (NDMS) is part of ESF-8.

National Incident Management System. The National Incident Management System (NIMS) is a comprehensive approach to incident management. The NIMS consists of concepts and principles that provide guidance in the management of all types of incidents. Topics cover the spectrum from preparedness to recovery regardless of incident cause, size, location, or complexity. NIMS provides an all hazard framework for government, nongovernment organizations and those in the private sector to work together using shared vocabulary, systems, and processes to prepare and respond to disasters (FEMA, 2018d).

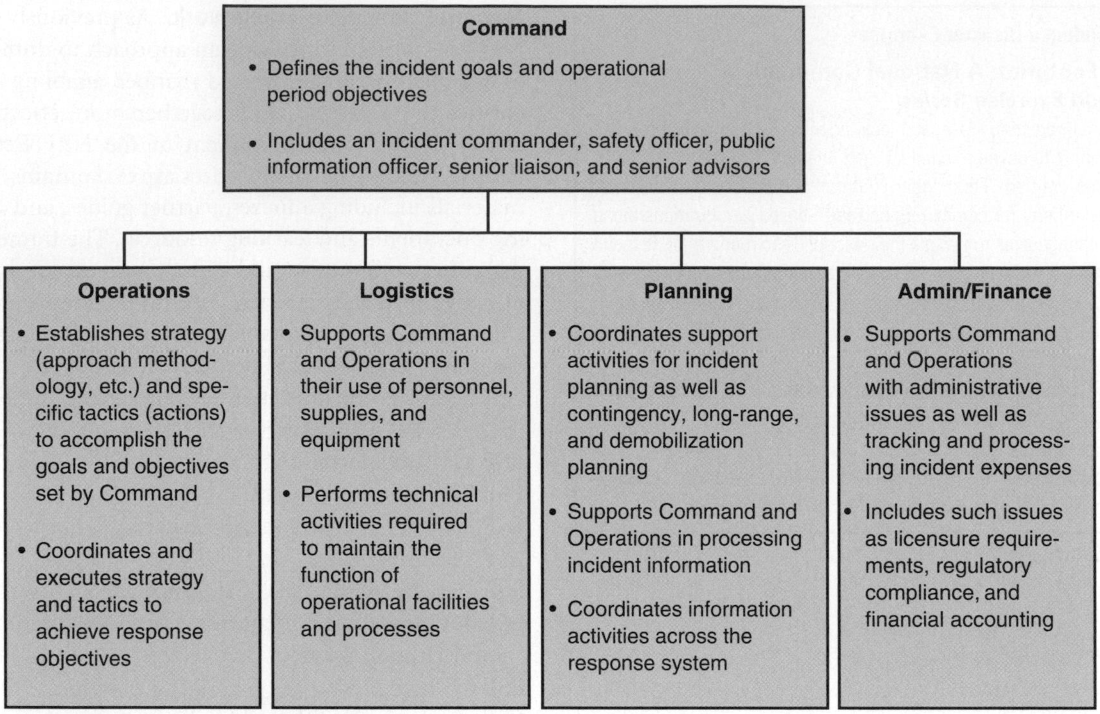

Fig. 21.5 Incident Command System (ICS). (Courtesy U.S. Department of Health and Human Services, Washington, DC. Available at http://www.phe.gov.)

No matter what type of nursing practice or which agency nurses choose, they will come into direct contact with NIMS, including the Incident Command System (ICS) (FEMA, 2018d). The ICS is a standardized approach to the command, control, and coordination of incident response. Fig. 21.5 displays basic ICS operations. FEMA provides varying levels of NIMS education and training, with many organizations requiring a base level of familiarization to comply with federal funding requirements (FEMA, 2018b).

A well-developed training program promotes nationwide NIMS implementation, producing an adequate number of trained and qualified emergency management/response personnel. The Emergency Management Institute (EMI) is the premier emergency management training institution. The mission of EMI is to improve the competence of government officials and emergency managers in preparing, responding, and recovering from all types of disasters (FEMA, 2018b). EMI is located at the National Emergency Training Center in Emmitsburg, Maryland, and offers a broad range of both onsite and online courses related to all phases of the disaster cycle. Some of the NIMS-related training offered includes the following online courses (FEMA, 2018b):

- IS-100.HCb: Introduction to the Incident Command System for Healthcare/Hospitals
- IS-200.HCa: Applying ICS to Healthcare Organizations
- IS-700.a: National Incident Management System (NIMS), an Introduction
- IS-701.a: NIMS Multiagency Coordination System
- IS-800.b: National Response Framework, an Introduction

Response to Biological Incidents. Biological agents pose a high risk to public health because only small amounts of the agents are needed to affect thousands of people and some of the agents are easy to conceal, transport, and disseminate. The CDC is an excellent source of biological agent information, including the latest agent fact sheets for health (CDC, 2018a). Important information provided includes the methods of transmission and communicability period. Through the Pandemic and All-Hazards Preparedness Reauthorization Act (PAHPRA), several biodefense programs exist to help public health professionals mount a proactive response to these events (USDHHS, 2014):

- *BioWatch* is an early warning system for biothreats that uses an environmental sensor system to test the air for biological agents in several major metropolitan areas.
- *BioSense* is a data-sharing program to facilitate surveillance of unusual patterns or clusters of diseases in the United States. It shares data with local and state health departments and is a part of the BioWatch system.
- *Project BioShield* is a program to develop and produce new drugs and vaccines as countermeasures against potential bioweapons and deadly pathogens.
- *Cities Readiness Initiative* is a program to aid cities in increasing their capacity to deliver medicines and medical supplies during a large-scale public health emergency such as a bioterrorism attack or a nuclear accident.
- *Strategic National Stockpile (SNS)* is a CDC-managed program with the capacity to provide large quantities of medicine and medical supplies to protect the public in a public health emergency to include bioterrorism. The SNS is deployed through a combination of a state-level request and the public health system (CDC, 2018c).

Some of the most important lessons from live biological incidents and exercises involve communication. In an effort to keep the public health community informed, the CDC developed the Public Health Information Network (PHIN). The PHIN provides for the electronic exchange of information among governmental agencies. It focuses on six components that help ensure information access and sharing—early event detection, outbreak management, connecting laboratory systems, countermeasure and response administration, partner communications and alerting, and cross-functional components—and is critical to information exchange (CDC, 2017b).

How Disasters Affect Communities. One Health recognizes that the health of humans is connected to the health of animals and the environment, and the One Health concept integration in disaster preparedness and response requires interprofessional efforts at global, national, and local levels (CDC, 2017a). The spread of infectious diseases and the relationships among humans, animals, and the environment are at the core of One Health. For example, animals serve as early warning signs of potential human illness; an example is that birds often die of West Nile virus before humans get sick with West Nile virus fever.

The first goal of any disaster response is to re-establish sanitary barriers as quickly as possible (Aronsson-Storrier, 2017). Water, food, waste removal, vector control, shelter, and safety are basic needs. Difficult weather conditions such as extreme heat or cold can hamper efforts, especially if electricity is affected. Continuous monitoring of the environment proactively addresses potential hazards. Disease prevention is an ongoing goal, especially if there is an interruption in the public health infrastructure. Infectious disease outbreaks can also occur in the recovery phase of disasters, and occasionally disaster workers introduce new organisms into the area.

People in a community will be affected physically and emotionally, depending on the type, cause, and location of the disaster; its magnitude and extent of damage; the duration; and the amount of pre-warning provided. Immediate effects may include loss of life and morbidity, but other health effects such as those during and after disaster disease outbreaks may be delayed.

Although the immediate emotional response to a disaster by civilians may be unpredictable, the response is not always a negative one. For example, the terrorist attacks of September 11, 2001, created extreme anger and grief but also led to a marked increase in compassion and patriotism. Thousands of people helped, from donating blood and money to rescuing individuals from the buildings. Four days after the attack, buying an American flag was nearly impossible, as most stores had sold out (Associated Press, 2001). Within one month of the attack, an estimated $757 million in cash contributions and hundreds of truckloads of goods had been donated to help the families of victims and rescue workers (Yates, 2001). This was the worst human-made disaster in American history, killing more than 2500 civilians and 460 emergency responders. Yet, the terrorist attacks of September 11 will also be remembered for how they unified the country (Rand Corporation, 2004). The psychological effects of September 11 were different from those of more contained, single-event disasters. The attack was unexpected and of great magnitude, with much uncertainty and fear about what might happen next. Not knowing when or if a subsequent attack will occur may sustain fear and anger.

To explore the community and individual resilience following the events of Hurricane Katrina, The Resilience in Survivors of Katrina (RISK) Project is a longitudinal study of Katrina survivors. Enrolled in the study are 1019 low-income parents from New Orleans, with the goal of increasing educational outcomes. The study measured participants' economic status, social ties, and mental and physical health prior to the hurricane. The investigators have performed surveys and two rounds of in-depth qualitative interviews. The interaction between health outcomes, genetic differences, and environmental factors is also being investigated. To explore the findings of the RISK project see findings and publications at the RISK project website, https://www.riskproject.org.

Stress Reactions in Individuals. A traumatic event can cause moderate to severe stress reactions. Individuals react to the same disaster in different ways depending on their age, cultural background, health status, social support structure, and general ability to adapt to crisis. Symptoms that will require the individual to seek assistance are listed in Box 21.7.

People who are affected by a disaster often have an exacerbation of an existing chronic illness. For example, the emotional stress of the disaster may make it difficult for people with diabetes to control their blood glucose levels. It is important that survivors take care of their bodies by getting appropriate nutrition and rest, stay informed, but avoid overexposure to news, and seek help as needed (CDC, 2018b).

Older adults' reactions to disaster depend a great deal on their physical health, strength, mobility, independence, and income (Miller & Farra, 2017) (Fig. 21.6). They can react deeply to the loss of personal possessions because of the high sentimental value attached to the items and their irreplaceable value. Their need for relocation depends on the extent of damage to their home or their compromised health. They may try and conceal the seriousness of their health conditions or losses if they fear loss of independence. It is important that the nurse aids vulnerable community members in preparing for disasters (Box 21.8).

BOX 21.7 Know When to Seek Help

Depending on the situation, some people may develop depression, experience grief and anger, turn to alcohol or drugs, and even think about hurting themselves or others. The signs of serious problems include:

- Excessive worry
- Crying frequently
- An increase in irritability, anger, and frequent arguing
- Wanting to be alone most of the time
- Feeling anxious or fearful, overwhelmed by sadness, confused
- Having trouble thinking clearly and concentrating, and difficulty making decisions
- Increased alcohol and/or substance use
- Increased physical (aches, pains) complaints such as headaches
- Trouble with your "nerves"

From Substance Abuse and Mental Health Services Administration (SAMHSA): *Coping with a traumatic event: know when to seek help*, 2011. Available at https://archive.samhsa.gov.

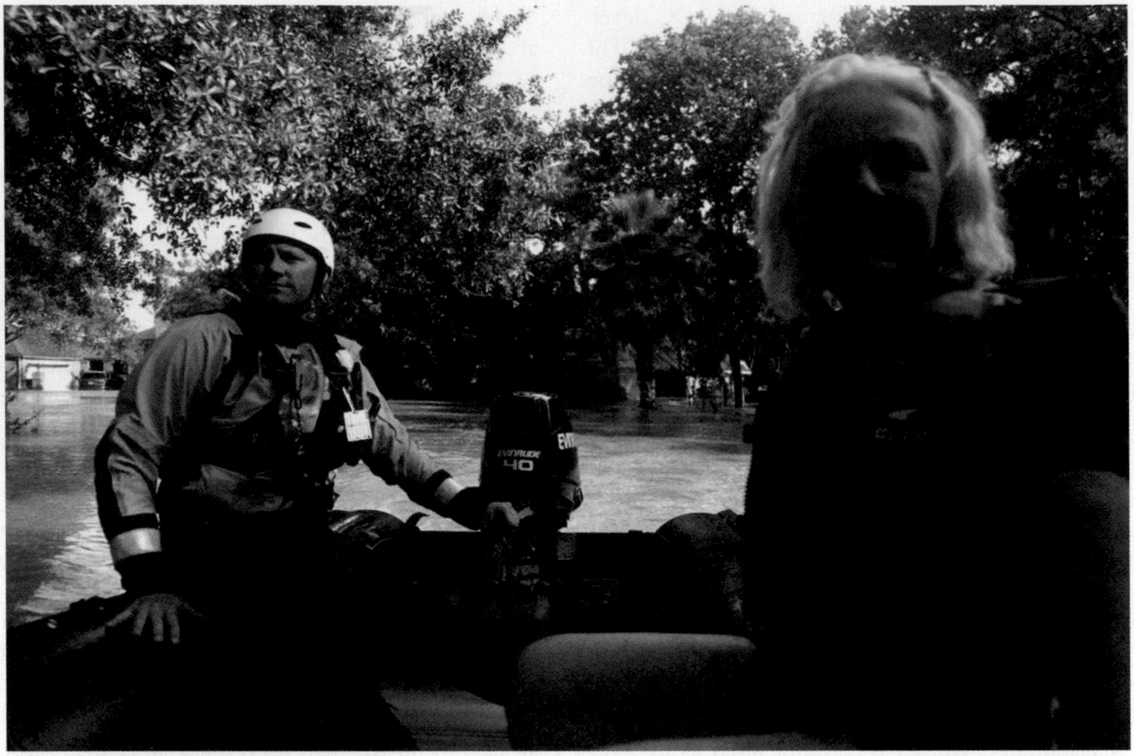

Fig. 21.6 A senior survivor is removed from her flooded neighborhood impacted by flooding from Hurricane Harvey by a member of FEMA's Urban Search and Rescue Nebraska Task Force One (NE-TF1). *FEMA,* Federal Emergency Management Agency. (Photo by FEMA News Photo, Aug. 30, 2017. Available at https://www.fema.gov.)

BOX 21.8 Populations at Greatest Risk for Disruption After Disaster

- Older adults
- Women
- Pregnant women
- Children
- Persons with disabilities
- Hearing impaired
- Visually impaired
- Individuals with chronic disease
- Individuals with chronic mental illness
- Low income
- Homeless
- Non–English-speaking
- Rural populations
- Tourists; persons new to an area
- Single-parent families
- Substance abusers
- Undocumented residents

Based on U.S. Department of Health and Human Services Outreach Activities and Resources: *Special populations: emergency and disaster preparedness,* 2017. Available at http://sis.nlm.nih.gov.

CHECK YOUR PRACTICE

Vulnerable Populations

You are a community home health nurse making a home visit to an elderly couple who recently retired to Florida. The 70-year-old wife was recently discharged from the hospital after a total hip replacement and is recovering at home. She uses a walker now, and both wear glasses and are on multiple medications for chronic health problems.

It is now hurricane season and the couple is new to the area. They ask you about preparing a disaster preparation plan specific to their unique needs as an elderly couple new to this community.

What do you tell them about how to prepare?

The effect of disasters on young children (Fig. 21.7) can be especially disruptive (National Institute of Mental Health [NIMH], 2013). Young children may respond with regressive behaviors such as thumb-sucking, bedwetting, crying, and clinging to parents. Older children tend to re-experience images of the traumatic event or have recurring thoughts or sensations, or they may intentionally avoid reminders, thoughts, and feelings related to disaster events. Children may have heightened sensitivity to sights, sounds, or smells and may experience exaggerated responses or difficulty with usual activities. Children not immediately impacted by a disaster can also be affected by it. The constant bombardment of disaster stories on television can cause fear in children. Parental reaction to a disaster will greatly influence children (NIMH, 2013). Professional assistance should be sought for children displaying behaviors beyond mild behavior changes.

Public health nurses should help those in the affected community talk about their feelings, including anger, sorrow, guilt, and perceived blame for the disaster or the outcomes of the disaster. Referrals should be made with for those who have persistent symptoms beyond mild disruptions. Community members should be encouraged to engage in healthy eating, exercise, rest, daily routine maintenance, limited demanding responsibilities, and time with family and friends.

Stress Reactions in the Community. Communities reflect the individuals and families living in them, both during and after a disaster incident. Four community phases as seen in Fig. 21.8 are commonly recognized: (1) heroic, (2) honeymoon,

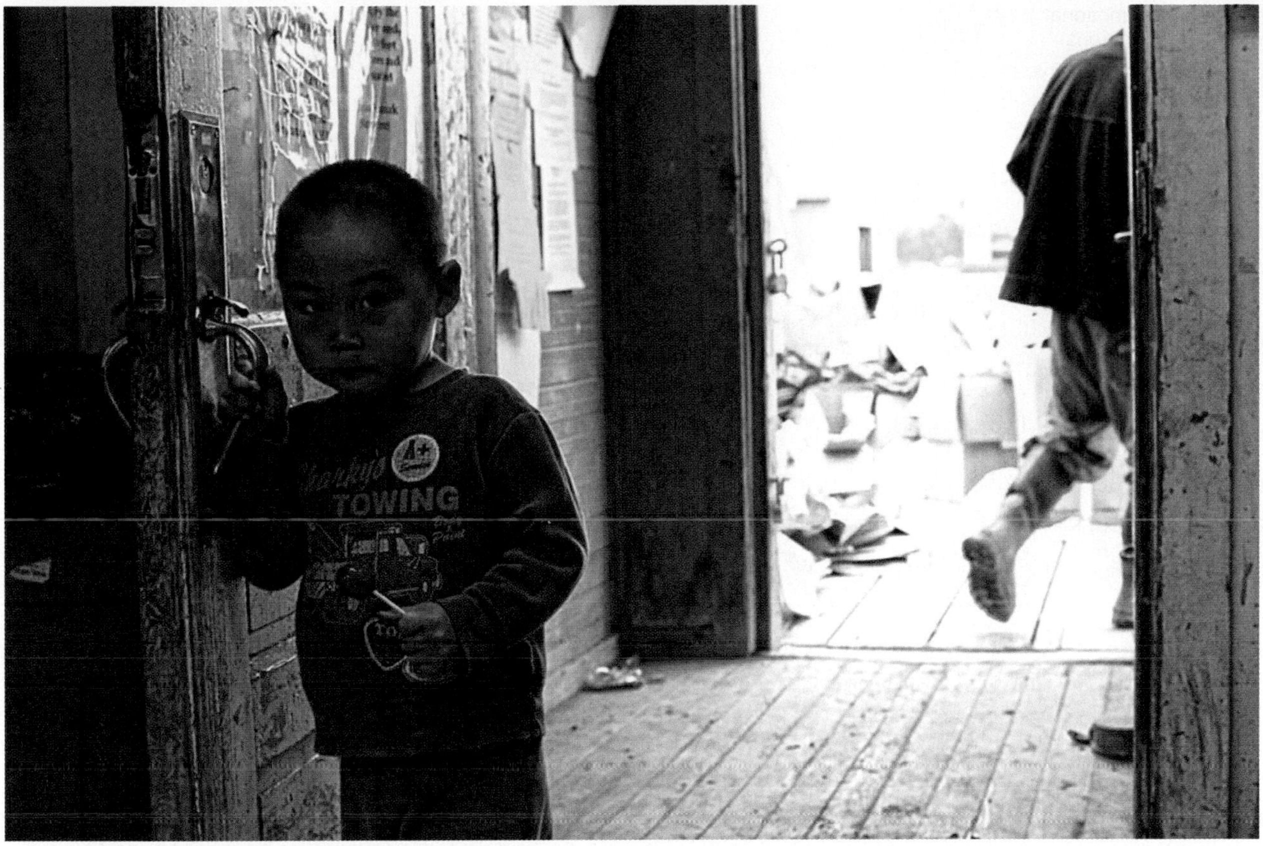

Fig. 21.7 Children in local general store following flooding in June 2013. Little Jameson Ayunerak of Alakanuk, Alaska, plays in the store while debris is removed after a severe flood devastated this community. A FEMA response team was in place working with the State of Alaska and the designated Alaska Native tribes to help business owners and individuals recover from the effects of the disaster. (Photo by Adam DuBrowa/FEMA. July 15, 2013, Alakanuk, AK. Available at https://www.fema.gov.)

(3) disillusionment, and (4) reconstruction (Department of Veterans Affairs, n.d.). The first two phases, the heroic and honeymoon phases, are most often associated with response efforts. The latter two phases, disillusionment and reconstruction, are most often linked with recovery.

During the heroic phase, there is an overwhelming need for people to do whatever they can to help others survive the disaster. First responders, including health and medical personal, will work long hours with no thought of their own personal or health needs. They may fight needed sleep and refuse rest breaks in their drive to save others. Moreover, deployed responders from outside the disaster area may be unfamiliar with the terrain and inherent dangers, exposing themselves in heroic attempts to aid survivors. Within the incident command structure it is the safety officer's responsibility to ensure worker safety (FEMA, n.d.). Exhausted, overworked responders present a danger to themselves and the community served.

In the honeymoon phase, survivors may be rejoicing that their lives and the lives of loved ones have been spared. Survivors will gather to share experiences and stories. The repeated telling to others creates bonds among the survivors. A sense of thankfulness over having survived the disaster is inherent in their stories.

The disillusionment phase occurs as time elapses and people notice that additional help and reinforcement are not coming as quickly as in the initial response. Fatigue and gloom can result and exhaustion starts to take its toll on volunteers, rescuers, and medical personnel. The community begins to realize that a return to the previous normal is unlikely and that they must make major changes and adjustments. Nurses in response must consider the psychosocial impact and the resulting emotional, cognitive, and spiritual implications. Public health nurses should identify groups/population segments particularly at risk for burnout and exhaustion, to include volunteers involved in response efforts. They may need breaks and reminders for nourishment. In addition, those in shock and those consumed by grief related to loss of loved ones will need compassionate care, with possible referrals to mental health counseling resources.

The last phase, reconstruction, is the longest. Recovery as a disaster cycle phase is addressed later in this chapter. Homes, schools, churches, and other community elements need to be rebuilt and reestablished. The goal is to return to a new state of normalcy. Community needs may still be extensive; the nurse continues to function as a member of the interprofessional team to provide and assure provision of the best possible coordinated care to the population.

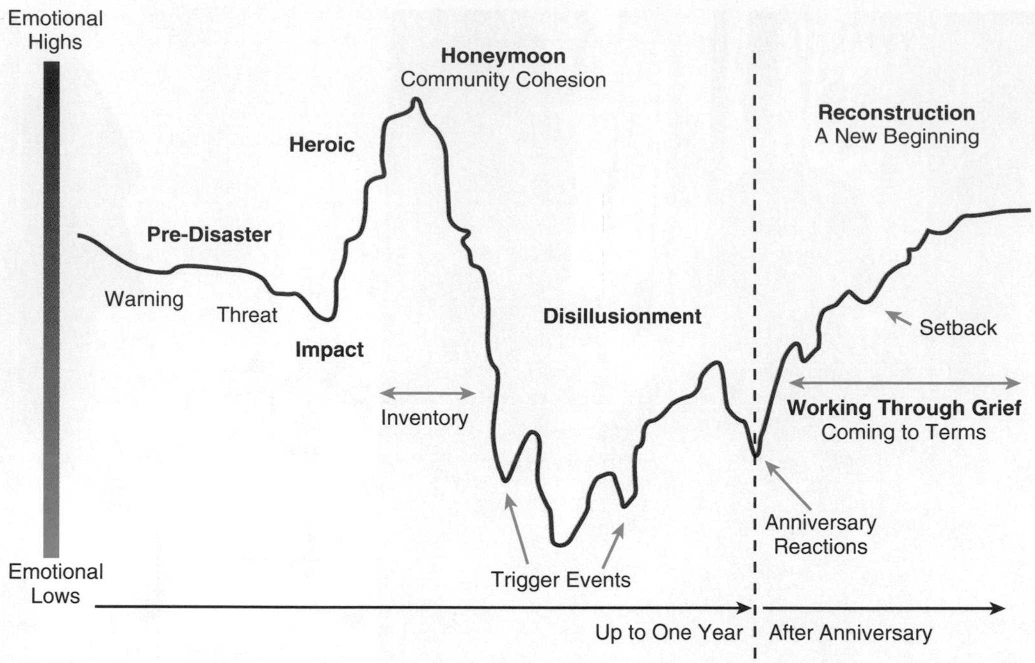

Fig. 21.8 Phases of disaster: collective reactions. (Courtesy U.S. Department of Health and Human Services, Substance Abuse and Mental Health Services Administration [SAMHSA]: *Training manual for mental health and human services workers in major disasters,* ed. 2, Washington, DC, 2000, SAMHSA. Available at ftp://ftp.snoco.org.)

Role of the Public Health Nurse in Disaster Response. The role of the public health nurse during a disaster depends a great deal on the nurse's experience, professional role in a community disaster plan, and prior disaster knowledge to include personal readiness. Public health nurses bring leadership, policy, planning, and practice expertise to disaster preparedness and response (Association of Public Health Nurses [APHN], 2014). One thing is certain about disasters: continuing change. Public health nursing roles in disaster are generally consistent with the scope of public health nursing practice, but that practice is often provided in chaotic surges. See Table 21.2 to visualize the role of the public health nurses in response, using the nursing process.

Nursing Role in First Response. Although valued for their expertise in community assessment, case finding and referring, prevention, health education, and surveillance, there may be times when the nurse is the first to arrive on the scene. In this situation, it is important to remember that life-threatening problems take priority. Triage should begin immediately. Triage at the individual level is the process of separating casualties and allocating treatment on the basis of the individuals' potentials for survival. Highest priority is given to those who have life-threatening injuries but, also, who have a high probability of survival once stabilized (AMA, 2011). There are many triage systems in use throughout the United States, yet there is little scientific evidence regarding their validity. Sort-Assess-Lifesaving Interventions-Treatment/Triage (SALT) triage is a method of triage developed by the Federal Interagency Committee on Emergency Medical Services. SALT is a free and non-proprietary system (Lerner et al., 2011). The following is an overview of the SALT triage process:

Sort: Casualties are sorted by their ability to move and respond to commands. Sorting is initiated by the call for survivors to move to a designated area. Individuals who can understand and relocate to the area are assessed last. The second step of sorting is to ask survivors to wave an extremity. Triage begins with the third group, those who did not respond to either call.

Assess:

1. Respiratory system
2. Cognition
3. Perfusion

Based upon findings in these three areas the victim is categorized into one of four triage categories.

1. Minimal (minor injury)
2. Delayed (severe injury such that delay in care will not adversely affect mortality
3. Immediate (severe injury; chances of survival are good if person receives immediate medical care)
4. Expectant (chances of survival are not good with current resources available)

Lifesaving Interventions: Lifesaving interventions (LSI) are provided as needed. The LSI that are included in the SALT triage algorithm include (1) Opening the airway, (two quick breaths for pediatric patients), (2) controlling hemorrhage, (3) needle decompression of the chest, and (4) the administration of auto injector antidotes.

Transport: Following assessment, casualties are moved to a collection point for transport. Those people in the Immediate category are transported first.

Fig. 21.9 depicts an overview of the SALT triage method.

Another type of triage called public health triage also exists, using a population-based approach for use in an incident undefined by a geographical location. Public health triage involves the sorting or identification of populations for priority

TABLE 21.2 The Disaster Cycle Linked to the Nursing Process

Disaster Cycle Phase: RESPONSE	Assessment	Planning	Implementation	Evaluation
Response activities address the short-term effects of the disaster. Including saving lives and meeting basic human needs.	Use public health, population-based triage to assess communicable disease outbreak impact and needed response (e.g., influenza) Use population-based triage involving surveillance to divide the affected population into susceptible, exposed, infected, removed, and vaccinated for expedient and life-saving treatment	Collaborate with response partners to develop plans for triage algorithms that determine appropriate care and sustenance logistics for populations, based on their symptoms and comorbid conditions (e.g., chronic disease)	Identify and place public health nurses and other support personnel to provide care according to the developed algorithms Assure that logistics are in place to support community care during the crisis period Conduct ongoing rapid needs assessments during the response phase in order to meet population needs	Maintain ongoing response planning during the incident (e.g., the Incident Management System and its Planning "P") Participate in service planning and provide real-time adjustment on the basis of real-time public health response evaluation Assure needed and necessary public health nursing care

From Association of Public Health Nurses (APHN): *The role of the public health nurse in disaster preparedness response, and recovery: a position paper,* 2014. Available at http://www.achne.org.

interventions (Burkle, 2006). In a public health emergency such as a bioevent the population may be triaged into categories of susceptible, exposed, infectious, deceased, and vaccinated. Those susceptible and/or exposed may need vaccination. Additional triage and prioritization may occur within this group if access to vaccine is limited. Those who require hospitalization will also need to be triaged to the appropriate level of care based upon condition and available resources. See Fig. 21.10 for an example of public health triage for a biological agent.

Nursing Role in Epidemiology and Ongoing Surveillance. Public health remains the first line of defense in disease outbreak. Epidemiology investigation components do not vary from normal operations in disaster; they simply become "field expedient" (Polivka et al., 2008). The need to collect surveillance data is heightened during a disaster. To detect adverse effects on the community, data are collected related to deaths, injuries, and illnesses. This information allows public health to determine impacts of disaster and assess for potential problems related to response and recovery. Surveillance includes disease tracking, injury trends, and vigilance for the potential for disease outbreaks. These data allow decision makers to plan and allocate resources. Ongoing assessments or surveillance reports are just as important as initial assessments. Surveillance reports indicate the continuing status of the affected population and the effectiveness of ongoing relief efforts. Surveillance continues into and through the recovery phase of a disaster, a vital part of establishing the new normal.

Nursing Role in Rapid Needs Assessment. The traditional model of community assessment presents the foundation for the rapid community assessment process. The acute needs of populations in disaster turn the community assessment into rapid appraisal of a sector or region's population, social systems, and geophysical features. Elements of a rapid needs assessment include the following: determining the magnitude of the incident, defining the specific health needs of the affected population, establishing priorities and objectives for action, identifying existing and potential public health problems, evaluating the capacity of the local response including resources and logistics, and determining the external resource needs for priority actions (Stanley et al., 2008). The Community Assessment for Public Health Emergency Response (CASPER) is a toolkit developed to assist public health practitioners and emergency management officials with determining the health status and basic needs of the affected community. The CASPER guides in the collection of health and basic need information (CDC, 2012).

Nursing Role in Disaster Communication. Nurses working as members of an assessment team need to report accurate information to facilitate situational awareness. This communication is critical to the rapid and ongoing needs assessment just described. A lack of or inaccurate information regarding the scope of the disaster and its initial effects can contribute to mismatched resources and increased morbidity. Times of crisis or great uncertainty call for great skills in communication. The community needs accurate information transmitted in a timely manner. Health care personnel are the best sources for essential health information that is technical in nature. The NIMS approach uses public affairs spokespersons for formal communication. The Public Information Officer (PIO) is an individual with the authority and responsibility to communicate information to the public at large (FEMA, n.d.). Still, nurses are considered trustworthy sources of information and may be approached for an interview. The nurse should refer the media to the PIO representing the agency. If the public approaches the nurse for health information, however, it should be conveyed. Nurses provide health education and information to assist in disaster response and recovery.

Although there are official spokespersons in all major disasters, there may be an occasion for the nurse to serve as a health consultant on the risk communication team. **Risk communication** includes providing critical information to the public. The information should be presented in a calm, brief, and concise manner. As a spokesperson in disaster, it is important to prepare key points in writing before speaking, verify all information is accurate, and never speculate or embellish.

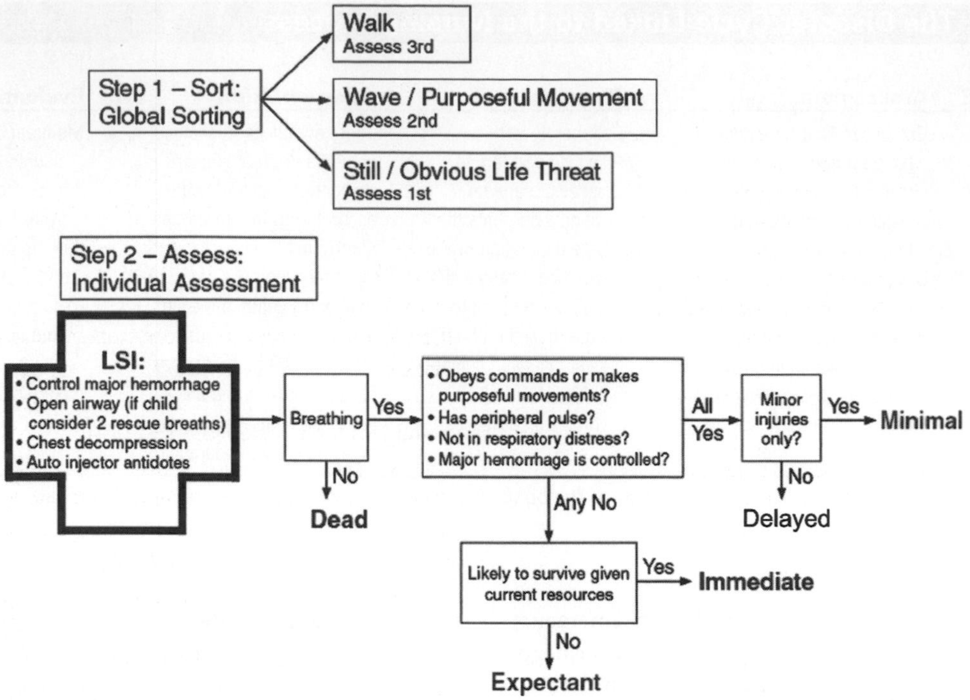

Fig. 21.9 SALT triage algorithm. *LSI,* Lifesaving interventions; *SALT,* sort-assess-lifesaving interventions-treatment/triage. (Available at https://www.ems.gov/pdf/2013/ficems_meet/07-FICEMS_MUCC_Implementation_Plan.pdf.)

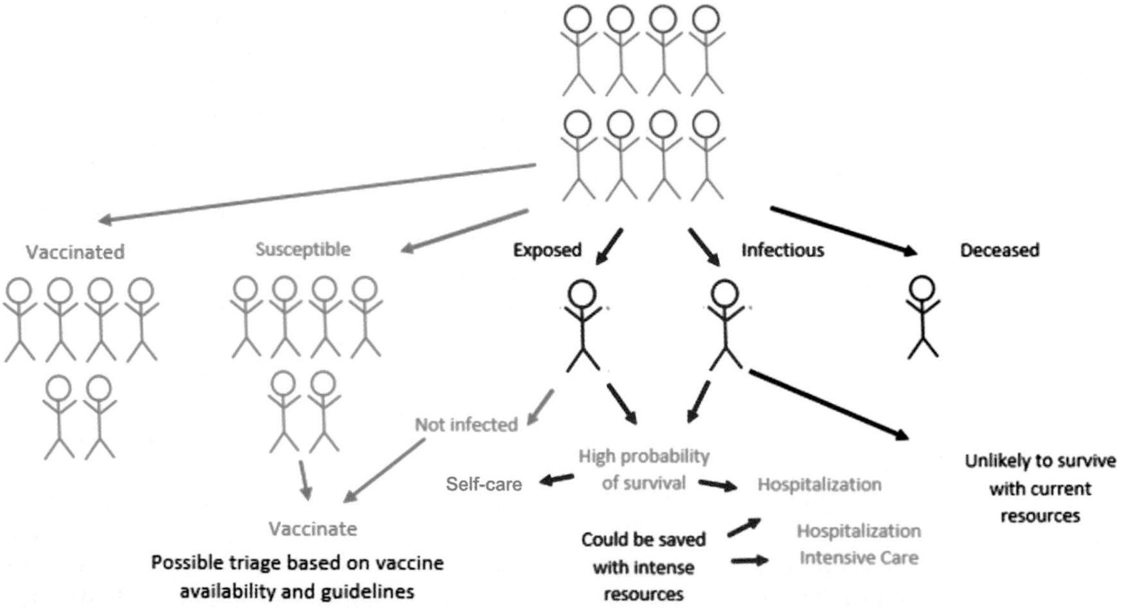

Fig. 21.10 Example of public health triage for a biological agent. (Modified from Burkle FM: Population-based triage management in response to surge-capacity requirements during a large-scale bioevent disaster. *Acad Emerg Med* 13:1118–1129, 2006.)

Social media, mobile technology, and their combined use in disaster are quickly changing disaster communication for the community as well as responders (see the example of using social media in Box 21.9). The Federal Emergency Management Agency (2013) National Preparedness Report states that during and immediately after Hurricane Sandy users sent more than 20 million Sandy-related Twitter posts despite the loss of cell phone service during the storm's peak. This trend is expected to rapidly increase, and relief organizations such as the American Red Cross are devoting separate response cells for the analysis of social media data in real time (American Red Cross, 2018). The Evidence-Based Practice box provides an example of communications in public health preparedness.

BOX 21.9 The Resilient Social Network: @OccupySandy #SuperstormSandy

A few hours after Superstorm Sandy made landfall in New Jersey, members of the Occupy Wall Street movement used social media to tap their established network for resources to combat the effects of the massive storm. Overnight, a corps of young, educated, tech-savvy individuals deployed to the region's hardest-hit neighborhoods. The network that came to be known as "Occupy Sandy" emerged as one of the leading humanitarian collectives providing relief to survivors across New York City and New Jersey. At its peak, it mobilized an estimated 60,000 volunteers, most having no prior disaster relief experience. Yet unlike traditional disaster relief organizations, there were no appointed leaders, no regulations to follow, no predefined mission.

Learn more about how social networks are changing the world of disaster response.

From Homeland Security Studies & Analysis Institute: *The resilient social network,* 2014. Available at http://us.resiliencesystem.org.

EVIDENCE-BASED PRACTICE

Labrague et al. (2018) performed a systematic review of the literature exploring nurses' preparedness for response to disasters (17 articles). A major finding from the literature review was the low level of preparedness reported by nurses. However, it was found that prior disaster experience and participation in disaster-related training enhanced disaster preparedness. The findings highlight the need for opportunities for both nursing students and practicing nurses to take part in disaster-related training experiences. An example of a training program that promotes training for both nursing students and health care practitioners in an interprofessional environment is the National Disaster Health Consortium (NDHC) training course (see https://nursing.wright.edu). These types of training programs promote nurses' readiness to work in interprofessional teams to promote positive outcomes. Training opportunities, like NDHC, can also help prepare nurses for the unique interprofessional disaster certification from the American Nurses Credentialing Center, documenting their expertise in disaster. (https://www.nursingworld.org).

From Labrague LJ, Hammad K, Gloe DS, et al.: Disaster preparedness among nurses: a systematic review of the literature. *Int Nurs Rev* 65:41–53, 2018.

Nursing Role in Disaster Response Ethics. Hurricane Katrina's impact was one of the largest catastrophic natural disasters in the United States. Thousands of health care personnel were stranded in New Orleans hospitals. These workers were faced with limited resources and rapidly deteriorating conditions as they awaited evacuations (Powell-Young et al., 2013). In disasters, nurses may work with limited resources. In disaster surge the nurse may no longer be focused on the care of individual clients, but on the entire community. In extreme conditions, traditional ethics of doing the best for every patient may shift to a **utilitarian framework** where nursing's goal becomes to do the "greatest good for the greatest number of individuals" (American Nurses Association [ANA], 2008, p. 10). In these circumstances, each patient may not receive all the care that would occur under normal conditions. Instead, the focus is on providing care that maximizes the benefit to the greatest number of people.

In addition to limited resources, nurses may be faced with situations that personally put them in harm's way. The ANA Code of Ethics (2010) states, "the nurse owes the same duties to self as to others" (p. 19). Yet, abandonment of patients may be grounds for disciplinary action in many states. Extreme conditions may cause the nurse to make many difficult decisions, and using an ethical framework will make these decisions easier. As part of disaster preparedness, nurses need to consider their role in their agency's disaster plan. Will they be needed in times of disasters? What plans have been made for their families if such a response is needed? Written policy should assure protections and make clear the expectations of the registered nurse, the employer, and the government response systems before the disaster occurs (ANA, 2017).

Nursing Role in Sheltering. **General population shelter** management is often the responsibility of the local Red Cross chapter within their ESF-6 colead function. In catastrophic disaster, however, governmental authority may establish "mega shelters" housing thousands. ESF-6 provides for both short- and long-term care (FEMA, 2016b). This responsibility includes the plan for structure, operations, management, and staffing of mass care sites.

Nurses, because of their comfort with delivering aggregate health promotion, disease prevention, and emotional support, make ideal shelter managers and team members. Nurses in shelter functions are involved in providing assessment and referral, health care needs (e.g., prescription glasses, medications), first aid, and appropriate dietary adjustment; keeping client records; ensuring emergency communications; and providing a safe environment (American Red Cross, 2013). The Red Cross provides training for shelter support and use of appropriate protocols and partners with other agencies such as the Medical Reserve Corps (MRC) and local public health agencies to accomplish this mission.

Common-sense approaches work best when dealing with the shelter community. Basic measures that can be taken by the shelter nurse include the following: listen to shelter residents tell and retell their disaster story and current situation; encourage residents to share their feelings with one another if it seems appropriate to do so, especially those suffering from similar circumstances; help residents make decisions; delegate tasks (e.g., reading, crafts, and playing games with children) to teenagers and others to help combat boredom; provide the basic necessities (e.g., food, clothing, rest); attempt to recover or gain needed items (e.g., prescription glasses or medication); provide basic compassion and dignity (e.g., privacy when appropriate and if possible); and refer to a mental health counselor or other sources of help as the situation warrants.

Emergency managers and shelter planners have the responsibility of planning to ensure that sheltering services and facilities are accessible to everyone. Children and adults with disabilities as well as those who have access and/or are functional should be integrated into general population shelters. According to FEMA (2010/2015), the needs of the whole community should be considered in every aspect of emergency shelter planning and response. To help assist these individuals, **Functional Needs Support Services** (FNSS) are implemented to help individuals maintain their independence with the general population shelter. Required FNSS include reasonable modification to policies, practices, and procedures to accommodate individuals with functional needs as well as access to durable medical equipment within the shelter environment (e.g., walkers, beds, ventilators), consumable medical supplies (e.g., ostomy supplies, dressings). All shelter residents should have access to personal assistance services and other goods and services as needed (FEMA, 2010/2015), and arrangements to make this so must be made in advance.

Alternate care centers may be used to shelter patients with medical needs designated as "Non-ambulatory care/Hospital overflow," for example, care of non-ambulatory patients with less intense medical needs. In addition, Federal Medical Stations (FMSs) are another alternate care area for clients. These units also provide basic care for non-ambulatory, hospital overflow, patients with minimal medical needs or to shelter patients with more advanced outpatient needs. Requested by state health or emergency management agencies, FMSs are designed to plug and play in "structures of opportunity" in the community, such as schools or convention centers (CDC, 2016). See the Linking Content to Practice box for ways to deal with a disaster.

LINKING CONTENT TO PRACTICE

About Federal Medical Stations

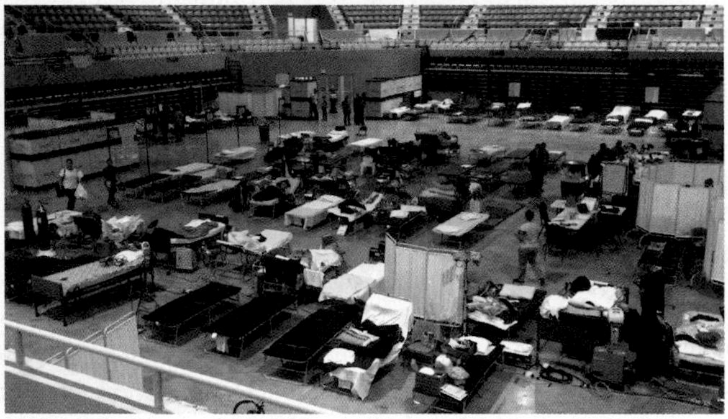

Following the impact of Hurricane Maria in Puerto Rico, the federal government set up medical facilities to serve people with needs due to Hurricane Maria. These facilities provided inpatient and outpatient care to the impacted population. The facility was located in Acropolis park in the town of Manati, Puerto Rico.

Courtesy FEMA Photo by Richard Cardona, Nov. 7, 2017. Federal Emergency Management Agency: Federal Medical Stations. Available at https://www.fema.gov.

Psychological Stress of Disaster Workers. Disaster relief work can be rewarding because it provides an opportunity to have a profound and positive impact on the lives of those who may be experiencing their greatest time of need. However, the work can also be challenging and stressful. During an assignment, responders may be exposed to chaotic environments, long hours, rapidly changing information and directives, long wait times before getting to work, noisy environments, and living quarters that are less than ideal. According to the National Institute for Occupational Safety and Health (NIOSH, 2013), responders may not recognize the need for self-care, and to monitor their own emotional and physical health. As recovery efforts span time frames of weeks to months, there is increasing risk of adverse effects to responders.

No one who experiences a disaster either personally or in a professional capacity is untouched by it. Nurses who work with survivors of disasters may be at risk for stress reactions. Self-care is as important as the care that is provided to community members. Symptoms that may signal a need for stress management assistance include the following: being reluctant or refusing to leave the scene until the work is finished; denying needed rest and recovery time; feelings of overriding stress and fatigue; engaging in unnecessary risk-taking activities; difficulty communicating thoughts, remembering instructions, making decisions, or concentrating; engaging in unnecessary arguments; having a limited attention span; and refusing to follow orders (USDHHS: SAMHSA, 2011).

The nurse should understand that everyone reacts differently after a disaster assignment. Most reactions are considered normal and are temporary, resolving in days to a few weeks. For some workers, disasters bring forth strong thoughts and emotions, both positive and negative. Other workers may experience mild reactions or hardly any reaction at all. According to the Department of Veterans Affairs (n.d.) some self-care measures that can be used by to reduce stress following deployment include having recovery time, keep the focus on what went well and accomplishments, try relaxation techniques, engage in hobbies, eat well, drink only in moderation, and ensure that you have appropriate sleep and exercise.

Recovery

Disaster recovery starts much sooner than most nurses may think. There is no clear defined change between response and recovery periods. Rather, the process is a transition. In recovery, the immediate response actions to address initial consequences subside, which could be within hours. Recovery is about returning to the new normal, a community balance of infrastructure and social welfare that is near the level that it would have had if the event had not occurred (DHS, 2016b).

The Department of Health and Human Services is responsible for the core recovery of health and social services, including educating the community and response workers about the long-term effects of a post-disaster environment. Their mission is to not only restore but improve the health and social services system while promoting "resilience, health (including behavioral health), independence, and well-being of the whole community" (USDHHS, 2017).

The recovery phase is often the hardest part of a disaster. It involves ongoing work beyond preparedness and the response rush. Recovery is where prior community resilience has the ability to make a real difference. Although the initial disaster response phase provides an onslaught of relief aid and resources, the reality of loss and enormity of the task involved in getting back to normalcy is soon felt (see Fig. 21.8). During the recovery phase for a large-scale incident, the federal government provides assistance with rebuilding property, restoring lifelines, and restoring economic institutions with the assistance of individuals, the private sector, and nongovernmental entities.

An incident that creates a need for a public health surge response is not a transitory event. Recovery involves a shift from short-term aid to long-term support for communities: sustainment of effort. Long-term support should include the disaster-affected population representation in the recovery effort, using local knowledge and skills to prioritize use of resources, personnel, and surviving systems and infrastructure. Assisting relief organizations will integrate and build on the existing community resilience.

Role of the Public Health Nurse in Disaster Recovery. The National Disaster Recovery Framework is a guide that enables effective recovery support to disaster-impacted states, tribes, territorial and local jurisdictions. It provides a flexible structure that enables disaster recovery managers to operate in a unified and collaborative manner. It also focuses on how best to restore, redevelop and revitalize the health, social, economic, natural and environmental fabric of the community and build a more resilient nation (www.fema.gov, 2018). This framework focuses on the restoration and redevelopment/revitalization of all aspects of the community, including health, social, economic, natural and environmental factors in order to build a more resilient Nation (DHS, 2016b).

The role of the public health nurse in the recovery phase of a disaster is as varied as in the preparedness and response phases, but the nurse's connection to the community puts the nurse in an incredible position of knowledge and awareness on the interprofessional recovery team. Flexibility is key to a successful recovery operation. Nurses need awareness of the potential public health challenges specific to the disaster area and should monitor the physical and psychosocial environment. Disruption of the public health infrastructure—water and food supply, sanitation system, vector control programs, and access to primary and mental health care—can lead to increased disease and community dysfunction for weeks and months after the incident.

Nurses can play a critical role in the success of the Health and Social Services Recovery Support Function (USDHHS, 2017) through their:

- Knowledge of ongoing and emerging post-disaster community needs and the availability of essential health services to meet those needs (Community Assessment)
- Holistic approach to well-being that includes promoting self-sufficiency and continuity of the health of all individuals and especially those with special needs such as children, seniors, people living with disabilities, people from diverse origins, people with limited English proficiency, and underserved populations (Resilience)
- Awareness of behavioral health needs of affected individuals, response and recovery workers, and the community and the resources available (Psychological Support)

Nursing Role in Ongoing Community Assessment. The reality of the recovery effort is that the rapid needs assessment continues into an ongoing community needs assessment. To determine effective interventions to ensure the best possible outcomes, it is essential to have ongoing accurate data about the population. Some conditions manifest only after time elapses. A major advantage of the recovery community assessment efforts is that they can be more in-depth, with greater confidence in the results. Some examples of community data points in the recovery phase include the following: ongoing illness and injuries related to the disaster; diseases related to disruption of environmental or health services; health facility infrastructure in terms of adequate personnel, beds, medical and pharmaceutical supplies; and environmental health assessment to include water quantity and quality, sanitation, shelter, solid waste disposal, and vector populations.

A realistic perspective is most useful to the community recovery effort. It will take months or perhaps years to achieve the new sense of normalcy, which may be significantly different from the normal pre-disaster state. The health care system and its related resources will continue to be taxed, perhaps beyond its abilities for adequate response.

Nurses should be aware that post-disaster cleanup creates opportunities for unintentional injury and hazards, including those occurring from falls, contact with live wires, accidents with cutting devices, heart attacks from overexertion and stress, and auto accidents resulting from road conditions and missing traffic controls (e.g., stoplights). In addition, risks from hazardous building materials such as asbestos and lead may exist. Nurses should educate the public about the hazards related to carbon monoxide poisoning stemming from using lanterns, gas ranges, or generators or from burning charcoal for a heat source in enclosed areas.

The Nursing Role in Community Resilience. The public health nurse understands that a resilient community is inter connected; it has strong horizontal and vertical relationships among its residents. There is evidence that both the sense of community created by these relationships and the individual connections of those relationships help improve disaster preparedness and, by default, disaster recovery (Chandra et al., 2011). The recovery period demands that these relationships be reactivated as soon as possible. The public health nurse will have knowledge of the previously existing relationships, and must work with the population to find creative ways to reinstitute those ties.

After disaster, for example, it may be easier for individuals to get to know their neighbors through the promotion of horizontal social relationships, and local NGOs can host social events that allow residents to interact (Chandra et al., 2011). Block associations and other local citizen-led efforts provide opportunities to develop social relationships in places that residents will frequent post disaster (e.g., schools or emergency distribution centers). Residents can connect with decision makers (i.e., vertical relationship) or join a local volunteer group focused on disaster response and recovery (e.g., the Community Emergency Response Team). A key to timely community recovery is in repairing or rebuilding social and community organizations, and this effort should be specifically referenced in response and recovery plans.

The Nursing Role in Psychosocial Support. Acute and chronic illnesses can become worse by the prolonged effects of disaster, including loss of family, sense of community, and personal identity. The psychological stress of cleanup and/or moving can cause feelings of severe hopelessness, depression, and grief in the disillusionment phase (see Fig. 21.8). Recent research, though, underscores the need for a tiered community approach where psychological disruption is viewed as normal in the immediate aftermath of the disaster, with a concurrent belief that community mental health wellness will return in time for most. In fact, leveraging primary prevention (i.e., community resilience education) and secondary prevention (e.g., use of early population-based mental health triage tools) can actually engage existing community resilience to promote population recovery (Stanley et al., 2012). Although the majority of individuals will eventually recover from disasters, especially at risk are the members of high-needs populations who continue to live in chronic adversity.

The needs of children differ from adults. Social support and problem-focused interventions are more appropriate with children, and therapeutic interventions should be reserved for those that appear to be in acute distress (Pfefferbaum et al., 2017). Interventions with children should involve both the family systems and the school system. A three-tiered approach is recommended: (1) communication strategy, (2) parent effectiveness and teacher training, and (3) Cognitive Behavioral Therapy (CBT screening) (Pfefferbaum et al., 2017). As with adults, all children bring with them their cultural perceptions on psychological services, which are further influenced by the perceptions of their parents or caregivers. It is important to remember that each person has a culture, and each provider responding to a disaster must be knowledgeable of cultural differences to provide the best care.

Schwartz et al. (2015) assessed the long-term psychological effects of Hurricane Sandy on New Yorkers. The prospective, cross-sectional study surveyed 669 adults from the New York region, including demographics, exposures to the hurricane impact, behavioral and psychological health (the main outcome measures were depression, anxiety, and post-traumatic stress disorder [PTSD]). The researchers found that study participants' exposures to Hurricane Sandy were predominately related to property damage/loss. Participants had an average number of 3.9 exposures. Slightly over 33 percent of participants reported probable depression, 46 percent experienced probably anxiety, and 21.1 percent experienced symptoms of probable PTSD. The higher the number of exposures, the greater the risk of depression, anxiety, or PTSD while controlling for previous mental health history. The impacts of Hurricane Sandy on mental health are similar to those reported in other studies. It is critical that response and recovery efforts are directed toward psychological first aid and ongoing mental health support through recovery.

Referrals to mental health professionals should continue throughout the recovery phase and as long as the need exists. The role of the nurse in case finding and referral remains critical during this phase. In the end, it is the leveraging of its resiliency that will help the community progress into its new normal. The public health nurse is the community and client advocate who ensures resilience is fostered in partnership with the population. The Levels of Prevention box provides examples of how nurses respond to preparation for and dealing with a disaster.

LEVELS OF PREVENTION

Primary Prevention

Participate in community disaster exercises; assist in development of the disaster management plan for the agency/community; pre-identify vulnerable populations.

Secondary Prevention

Assess disaster survivors; conduct rapid needs assessment; use individual and population-based triage for care; provide psychological first aid.

Tertiary Prevention

Ensure that community service linkages are available to individuals and families; conduct community outreach; participate in planning efforts for the community's "new normal."

FUTURE OF DISASTER MANAGEMENT

Mega disasters such as the terrorist events of September 11, 2001, Hurricane Katrina in 2005, the 2010 H1N1 pandemic and Haiti earthquake, and Japan's 2011 earthquake, tsunami, and nuclear reactor meltdown underscore the need for nursing involvement at every step of the disaster management cycle. To fully participate as a part of the interprofessional team across the disaster cycle, all nurses must continue to plan and train in an all-hazards environment, regardless of their specialty practice. With the largest numbers in terms of health care providers, nurses will remain leaders in disaster care.

Public health nurses are particularly critical members of the multidisciplinary disaster health team given their population-based nursing focus and specialty knowledge in epidemiology and community assessment skills. Although sophisticated technology and surveillance will continue to advance in response to both human-made and natural disasters, the nature of disasters will retain the element of unpredictability. That unpredictability and the disaster medicine and public health surge requirements make prevention and preparedness activities on the part of individuals and communities even more important. Disaster information changes rapidly because of the learning that occurs during and after each incident, producing progressive best practices. Staying current in disaster training requires the public health nurse's commitment in continuing to develop expertise related to community planning activities for disaster and everyday resilience.

Throughout this chapter, how nurses practice and provide care across the disaster cycle is aligned and applied using standards of public health nursing, various sets of disaster competencies for health professionals, and the Public Health Nursing Intervention Wheel. Other practice applications include discussion about the continuous processes of assessment, planning, implementation, evaluation, collaboration, and cooperation in disaster. The role of the nurse in disaster practice and care aligns with standards of nursing practice as well as public health practice. Specifically, in the disaster cycle the nurse must rapidly and continuously assess and then plan, implement, and evaluate nursing practice while simultaneously providing interprofessional, population-based care.

PRACTICE APPLICATION

You are a nurse working in your middle school when a level 7.4 earthquake strikes with the epicenter 40 miles away. As a single parent, you have two children in grade school at a neighboring school complex, and older parents who live 10 miles out of town, toward the epicenter. The high school building is also connected to your complex.

You are not hurt and the middle school does not appear extensively damaged, but there is structural glass breakage and some visible cracks and damage. Neither cell nor landline phones are working. Emergency auxiliary electricity is activated, but the computer system is down. A rapid damage assessment and visual survey within the immediate neighborhood reveals some structural damage, and 12 individuals with injuries have already approached your office for assistance. Two of the clients' injuries are serious but not life-threatening, with the remainder of the clients experiencing minor injuries and varying stress levels.

An hour passes and there is no word about damage outside of the immediate school area. School workers are very worried and concerned about their homes and family. Two staff members have already left on foot to check on their homes, which are within three miles of the school.

What are your priorities in this situation? List them in order and think through your position with another. Discuss the concepts of prevention and preparedness and how they relate to this disaster situation to include home, community, and workplace.

Answers can be found on the Evolve site.

KEY POINTS

- The number of disasters, both human-made and natural, continues to increase, as do the number of people affected by them.
- Professional preparedness involves personal planning as well as an understanding of the disaster plan at work and in the community.
- *Healthy People 2020* objectives are linked in many ways to the disaster management cycle, because a disaster incident affects the health of a community in many areas.
- For effectiveness in disaster prevention, preparedness, response, and recovery, nurses must get involved in their community's disaster plan: as a community member, through their workplace, or with a partnering community organization.
- Nurses must be adequately trained and properly associated with an official response organization to best serve those affected by a disaster.
- Becoming knowledgeable about available community resources before a disaster incident will ensure a better coordinated response and recovery.
- Flexibility is a key attribute in providing nursing care during disaster.
- The Public Health Nursing Intervention Wheel is appropriate for daily operations as well as during disaster chaos.
- With any disaster it is always best to use the resources, personnel, and infrastructure of the community itself to promote self-reliance and resilience.
- Our nation's planning efforts for disaster continue to develop, test, and evaluate the goal of a unified, well-coordinated public and private national response.
- The public health nursing role in the disaster management cycle includes helping clients maintain a safe environment and advocating for environmental safety measures in the community; risk communication and client education; community assessment to include rapid needs assessment; public health triage; and surveillance and field epidemiology.
- Triage in a disaster setting involves both individual and population-based approaches, and everything possible for one individual is provided while determining how to promote the greatest good for the greatest number of those affected.
- People in a community react differently to a disaster depending on the type, cause, and location of the disaster; its magnitude and extent of damage; its duration; and the amount of warning that was provided.
- Individual variables that cause people to react differently include their age, cultural background, health status, social support structure, and general adaptability to crisis.
- The affected community experiences four stages of stress during disaster: heroic, honeymoon, disillusionment, and reconstruction.
- The recovery phase begins almost immediately after a disaster occurs.
- Community organizations and social networks can foster community resilience across the disaster cycle.
- The nurse assisting in disaster relief efforts must maintain self-health, both physically and mentally, to be of service to his or her family and clients.
- Ongoing community assessment is just as important as initial rapid needs assessment. Surveillance reports indicate the continuing status of the affected population and the effectiveness of ongoing relief efforts.

CLINICAL DECISION-MAKING ACTIVITIES

1. Select a vulnerable population within your community and determine what needs the group would have in time of disaster. *What community resources are currently available to help this group? Where is the gap in services?*
2. Describe the role of the public health nurse across the disaster management cycle: prevention (mitigation and protection), preparedness, response, and recovery. *How do you practice nursing across these stages? How do you work with other members of the team?*

3. Interview a nurse who has responded to a disaster. *What role did the nurse play? Were his or her interventions provided at the individual, population level or both? Can you describe two specific examples?*
4. Conduct an interview with a leader from the Emergency Management Agency, American Red Cross, Medical Reserve Corps, or other agency involved with disaster management. *What is your community's plan for response to a disaster? What agencies are involved?*
5. Discuss the advantages and disadvantages of serving on a disaster team in your own community. *Are you a good candidate to serve on a disaster team? What about your personal preparedness? Is there a work conflict? How (or does) this differ from day-to-day nursing practice?*
6. Contact your local public health department to determine its role in a local disaster. Describe a specific nurse's role in disaster management. *How does that nurse navigate interprofessional practice?*
7. Determine what the disaster plan is where you work. Get specific details and share them with others who are important to you.

ADDITIONAL RESOURCES

EVOLVE WEBSITE

http://evolve.elsevier.com/Stanhope/community/

- Answers to Practice Application
- Case Study
- Glossary
- Review Questions

REFERENCES

American College of Emergency Physicians (ACEP): *America's emergency care environment: A state-by-state report card—2014*, 2014. Retrieved from https://www.annemergmed.com.

American Medical Association (AMA): Model uniform core criteria for mass casualty triage, *Disaster Med Public Health Prep* 5(2):125–128, 2011.

American Nurses Association (ANA): *Adapting standards of care under extreme conditions: Guidance for professionals during disasters, pandemics, and other extreme emergencies*, 2008. Retrieved from https://www.aft.org.

American Nurses Association (ANA): *Code of ethics for nurses*, Silver Spring, MD, 2010, ANA.

American Nurses Association (ANA): *Who will be there? Ethics, the law, and a nurse's duty to respond in a disaster*, 2017. Retrieved from https://www.nursingworld.org.

American Red Cross: *Disaster relief*, 2018. Retrieved from http://www.redcross.org.

Aronsson-Storrier M: Sanitation, human rights and disaster management, *Disaster Prev Mgmt* 25:514–525, 2017.

Associated Press: As patriotism soars, flags are hard to come by, *USA Today*, 2001. Retrieved from http://usatoday30.usatoday.com.

Association of Public Health Nurses (APHN): *The role of the public health nurse in disaster preparedness response, and recovery: A position paper*, 2014. Retrieved from http://www.achne.org.

Brenan M: Nurses keep healthy as most honest, ethical profession, *Gallup* 2017. Retrieved from https://news.gallup.com.

Burkle FM: Population-based triage management in response to surge-capacity requirements during a large-scale bioevent disaster, *Acad Emerg Med* 13:1118–1129, 2006.

Cangialosi JP, Latto AS, Berg R: National Hurricane Center Tropical Report: Hurricane Irma, *National Hurricane Center* 2018. Retrieved from https://www.nhc.noaa.gov.

Centers for Disease Control and Prevention (CDC): *Preparedness and response for public health disasters: Community Assessment for Public Health Emergency Response (CASPER)*, 2012. Retrieved from http://www.cdc.gov.

Centers for Disease Control and Prevention (CDC): *Strategic stockpile: Federal medical station*, 2016. Retrieved from https://www.cdc.gov.

Centers for Disease Control and Prevention (CDC): *Emergency preparedness and response: bioterrorism agents and diseases*, 2018a. Retrieved from http://www.bt.cdc.gov.

Centers for Disease Control and Prevention (CDC): *Emergency preparedness and response: Coping with a disaster or traumatic event*, 2018b. Retrieved from https://emergency.cdc.gov.

Centers for Disease Control and Prevention (CDC): *Strategic National Stockpile (SNS)*, 2018c. Retrieved from https://www.cdc.gov.

Centers for Disease Control and Prevention (CDC): *One health*, 2017a. Retrieved from https://www.cdc.gov.

Centers for Disease Control and Prevention (CDC): *Public Health Information Network (PHIN)*, 2017b. Retrieved from https://www.cdc.gov.

Chandra A, Acosta J, Sterns S, et al.: *Building community resilience to disasters: a way forward to enhance national health security*, Santa Monica, 2011, Rand Corporation. Retrieved from http://www.rand.org.

Crippen DW: *Disaster management: Lessons from September 11, 2001*, Sydney, Australia, 2002. Presented at the 8th World Congress of Intensive and Critical Care Medicine.

Department of Homeland Security (DHS): *Homeland Security Act of 2002: Title 1—Department of Homeland Security*, 2002. Retrieved from http://www.dhs.gov.

Department of Homeland Security (DHS): *National preparedness guidelines*, 2007a. Retrieved from https://www.fema.gov.

Department of Homeland Security (DHS): *Presidential Policy Directive/PPD-8: National Preparedness*, 2011. Retrieved from http://www.dhs.gov.

Department of Homeland Security (DHS): *National disaster prevention framework*, ed 2, 2016a. Retrieved from https://www.fema.gov.

Department of Homeland Security (DHS): *National disaster recovery framework*, ed 2, 2016b. Retrieved from https://www.fema.gov.

Department of Homeland Security (DHS): *National Response Framework (NRF)*, 2016c. Retrieved from https://www.fema.gov.

Department of Homeland Security (DHS): *FEMA regional contacts*, 2018. Retrieved from https://www.fema.gov.

Department of Health and Human Services (USDHHS): *Health and social services recovery support function*, 2017. Retrieved from https://www.phe.gov.

Department of Veterans Affairs: *Disaster mental health services: a guidebook for clinicians and administrators*, n.d. Retrieved from https://www.hsdl.org.

Federal Emergency Management Agency (FEMA): *2013 National Preparedness Report*, 2013. Retrieved from: http://www.fema.gov.

Federal Emergency Management Agency (FEMA): *Basic guidance for public information officers,* n.d. Retrieved from https://www.fema.gov.

Federal Emergency Management Agency (FEMA): *Disaster declarations for 2017,* 2018a. Retrieved from https://www.fema.gov.

Federal Emergency Management Agency (FEMA): *Emergency Management Institute (EMI),* 2018b. Retrieved from https://training.fema.gov.

Federal Emergency Management Agency (FEMA): *Homeland Security Exercise and Evaluation Program (HSEEP),* updated 2018c. Retrieved from https://www.fema.gov.

Federal Emergency Management Agency (FEMA): *National Incident Management System (NIMS),* 2018d. Retrieved from http://www.fema.gov.

Federal Emergency Management Agency (FEMA): *Ready: pets and animals,* 2018e. Retrieved from https://www.ready.gov.

Federal Emergency Management Agency (FEMA): *Emergency support function annexes,* 2016a. Retrieved from https://www.fema.gov.

Federal Emergency Management Agency (FEMA): *Emergency Support Function #6—Mass care, emergency assistance, temporary housing and human services annex,* 2016b. Retrieved from https://www.fema.gov.

Federal Emergency Management Agency (FEMA): *Emergency Support Function #8—Public health and medical services annex,* 2016c. Retrieved from https://www.fema.gov.

Federal Emergency Management Agency (FEMA): *Robert T. Stafford Disaster Relief and Emergency Assistance Act (Public Law 93-288) as amended,* 2016d. Retrieved from https://www.fema.gov.

Federal Emergency Management Agency (FEMA): *Guidance on planning for integration of functional needs support service in general population shelters,* 2010, updated 2015. Retrieved from https://www.fema.gov.

Inajima T, Adelman J, Okada Y: *Fukushima disaster was man-made, investigation finds. Bloomberg Businessweek,* July 2012. Retrieved from http://www.bloomberg.com.

Institute of Medicine (IOM): *Crisis standards of care: A systems framework for catastrophic disaster response.* [serial online], 2012. Retrieved from https://www.nap.edu.

Institute of Medicine (IOM): *Forum on medical and public health preparedness for catastrophic events,* Washington, DC, 2014, *National Academies Press.* Retrieved from https://www.ncbi.nlm.nih.gov.

International Council of Nurses (ICN): *Disaster response network,* 2016. Retrieved from http://www.icn.ch.

International Federation of Red Cross and Red Crescent Societies (IFRC): *World disasters report 2016: Resilience: saving lives today, investing for tomorrow,* Geneva, Switzerland, 2016, Imprimerie Chirat. Retrieved from http://www.ifrc.org.

Labrague LJ, Hammad K, Gloe DS, et al.: Disaster preparedness among nurses: a systematic review of literature, *Int Nurs Rev* 65:41–53, 2018.

Lerner EB, Cone DC, Weinstein ES, et al.: Mass casualty triage: an evaluation of the science and refinement of a national guideline, *Disaster Med Public Health Prep* 5(2):129–137, 2011.

Links JM, Schwart BS, Lin S, et al.: COPEWELL: a conceptual framework and system dynamics model for predicting community functioning and resilience after disasters, *Disaster Med Public Health Prep* 12(1):127–137, 2018.

Miller E, Farra S: Disaster preparedness, response and recovery. In Mauk K, editor: *Gerontological nursing: Competencies for care,* Burlington, ed 4, 2017, Jones & Bartlett Learning, pp 829–844.

National Institute of Mental Health (NIMH): *Helping children and adolescents cope with violence and disasters: what parents can do,* 2013. Retrieved from http://www.nimh.nih.gov.

National Institute of Occupational Health and Safety (NIOSH): *Traumatic incident stress,* 2013. Retrieved from http://www.cdc.gov.

Naval Postgraduate School (NPS): *Directives, instructions, specifications, and standards,* Monterey, 2018, Dudley Knox Library. Retrieved from http://libguides.nps.edu.

NOAA National Centers for Environmental Information (NCEI): *U.S. billion-dollar weather and climate disasters,* 2018. Retrieved from https://www.ncdc.noaa.gov.

Oklahoma City National Memorial & Museum: *Those who were killed,* 2018. Retrieved from https://oklahomacitynationalmemorial.org.

Pfefferbaum B, Jacobs AK, Jones RT, Reyes G, Wyche KF: A skill set for supporting displaced children in psychological recovery after disaster, *Curr Psychiatry Rep* 19:60, 2017.

Polivka BJ, Stanley SA, Gordon D, Taulbee K, Kieffer G, McCorkle SM: Public health nursing competencies for public health surge events, *Public Health Nurs* 25:159–165, 2008.

Powell-Young YM, Baker JR, Hogan JG: Disaster ethics and healthcare personnel: a model case study to facilitate the decision-making process, *Online J Health Ethics* 3, 2013. Retrieved from http://aquila.usm.edu.

Rand Corporation: *Compensating the victims of 9/11,* Santa Monica, 2004, RAND. Retrieved from https://www.rand.org.

Robert Wood Johnson Foundation: *Ten ways public health nurses (PHNs) improve health,* 2017. Retrieved from http://www.phnurse.org.

Schwartz RM, Sison C, Kerath SM, et al.: The impact of Hurricane Sandy on the mental health of New York area residents, *Am J Disaster Med* 10(4):339–346, 2015.

Stanley S, Bulecza S, Gopalani S: Psychological impact of disasters on communities. In Couig MP, Kelley PW, editors: *Annual review of nursing research: disasters and humanitarian assistance,* New York, 2012, Springer Publishing.

Stanley SA, Polivka BJ, Gordon D, et al.: The explore surge trail guide and hiking workshop: discipline-specific education for public health nurses, *Public Health Nurs* 25:166–175, 2008.

United Nations Development Programme: *Disaster recovery: challenges and lessons,* 2016. New York, NY, Author. Retrieved from http://www.undp.org.

University of Minnesota School of Public Health: *Grants and initiatives: emergency preparedness and response,* 2018. Retrieved from http://www.sph.umn.edu.

Uscher-Pines L, Chandra A, Acosta J: The promise and pitfalls of community resilience, *Disaster Med Public Health Prep* 7:603–606, 2013.

U.S. Department of Health and Human Services (USDHHS): *Healthy People 2020: A roadmap to improve all Americans' health,* June 2018. Retrieved from http://www.healthypeople.gov.

U.S. Department of Health and Human Services (USDHHS): *National health security strategy of the United States of America,* 2015. Retrieved from https://www.phe.gov.

U.S. Department of Health and Human Services (USDHHS): *Public Health Emergency. Pandemic and All-Hazards Preparedness Reauthorization Act (PAHPRA),* 2014. Retrieved from https://www.phe.gov.

U.S. Department of Health And Human Services: Substance Abuse and Mental Health Services Administration (SAMHSA): *Psychological first aid for first responders* [PDF], 2011. Retrieved from https://store.samhsa.gov.

World Association for Disaster and Emergency Medicine (WADEM): *Nursing section overview*, 2018. Retrieved from https://wadem.org.
World Health Organization (WHO): *Emergency response framework*, 2017. Retrieved from http://www.who.int.
Yates J: Gifts, letters piling up at N.Y. relief centers, *Chicago Tribune*, 2001. Retrieved from http://articles.chicagotribune.com.
Zorrilla CD: The view from Puerto Rico—Hurricane Maria and its aftermath, *N Engl J Med* 377:1801–1803, 2017.
Zukowski RS: The impact of adaptive capacity on disaster response and recovery: evidence supporting core community capabilities, *Prehosp Disaster Med* 29(4):380–387, 2014.

22

Public Health Surveillance and Outbreak Investigation*

Laura H. Clayton, PhD, RN, CNE

OBJECTIVES

After reading this chapter, the student should be able to do the following:

1. Define public health surveillance.
2. Analyze types of surveillance systems.
3. Identify steps in planning, analyzing, interviewing, and evaluating surveillance.
4. Recognize sources of data used when investigating a disease or condition outbreak.
5. Describe the role of the nurse in surveillance and outbreak investigation.
6. Relate the nurse's role in investigation to the national core competencies for public health nurses.

CHAPTER OUTLINE

Disease Surveillance
Notifiable Diseases
Case Definitions
Types of Surveillance Systems
The Investigation
Displaying of Data

KEY TERMS

algorithms, p. 484
BioSense Platform, p. 489
bioterrorism, p. 482
case definition, p. 485
chemical terrorism, p. 482
clusters of illness, p. 482
common source, p. 490
disease surveillance, p. 482
endemic, p. 490
epidemic, p. 490
event, p. 482
holoendemic, p. 490
hyperendemic, p. 490
infectivity, p. 490
intermittent or continuous source, p. 490
mixed outbreak, p. 490
National Electronic Disease Surveillance System, p. 488
National Notifiable Disease Surveillance System, p. 486
National Syndromic Surveillance Program, p. 489
outbreak, p. 481
outbreak detection, p. 490
outcome data, p. 482
pandemic, p. 490
pathogenicity, p. 490
point source, p. 490
process data, p. 482
propagated outbreak, p. 490
public health protection, p. 481
PulseNet, p. 489
sentinel, p. 485
sporadic, p. 490
syndromic surveillance systems, p. 489
virulence, p. 490

Disease surveillance has been a part of **public health protection** since the 1200s, during the investigations of the bubonic plague in Europe. During the 1600s John Graunt developed the fundamental principles of public health including surveillance and **outbreak** investigation, and in the 1700s Rhode Island passed the first public health laws to provide for the protection of health and care of the population of the state. In the eighteenth century, William Farr introduced the modern version of surveillance and, along with the United States, Italy, and Great Britain, began required reporting systems for infectious diseases. In 1901, the United States began the requirement for reporting cases of cholera, smallpox, and tuberculosis. By 1925 the United States began national reporting of morbidity causes. By 1935 the first national health survey had been conducted, and in 1949 the National Office of Vital Statistics published weekly mortality and morbidity statistics in the journal *Public*

---

*Special thank you to Dr. Lisa Turner who offered valuable guidance for the revision of this chapter.

Health Reports. This activity was later transferred to the Centers for Disease Control and Prevention (CDC), which began publishing the *Morbidity and Mortality Weekly Report* in 1961. Laws, regulations, reporting mechanisms, and data collections are all essential to surveillance and disease outbreak investigations (Richards et al., 2017).

The Constitution of the United States provides for "police powers" necessary to preserve safety of health as well as in other events (see Chapter 9). These powers include public health surveillance. State and local "police powers" also provide for surveillance activities. Health departments usually have legal authority to investigate unusual **clusters of illness** as well (Gostin & Wiley, 2018).

Florence Nightingale first demonstrated the nurse's role in responding to disasters. Public health nurses bring specific skills to events that require emergency responses. They are prepared for conducting and evaluating disaster response drills, exercises, and trainings. Public health nurses are first responders in emergency situations in the community, they can lead and manage in the field and in the incident command center, and they are able to collaborate with others to sustain the emergency infrastructure (Association of Public Health Nurses [APHN], 2014). It is important for nurses to be prepared to lead and be a team member if an unusual occurrence or event strikes a community, like the Ebola outbreak in 2014 (Michaud & Kates, 2018).

DISEASE SURVEILLANCE

Definitions and Importance

Disease surveillance is the ongoing systematic collection, analysis, interpretation, and dissemination of specific health data for use in public health (Blazes & Lewis, 2016; World Health Organization, 2018a). Surveillance provides a means for nurses to monitor disease trends in order to reduce morbidity and mortality and to improve health (McNabb et al., 2016; Veenema, 2018). The CDC indicates that public health surveillance is the foundation of public health practice (CDC, 2015a).

Surveillance is a critical role function for nurses practicing in the community. A comprehensive understanding and knowledge of the surveillance systems and how they work will help nurses improve the quality and the usefulness of the data collected for making decisions about needed community services, community actions, and public health programming (Chapter 21 provides additional information). The surveillance features indicate it:

- Is organized and planned
- Is the principal means by which a population's health status is assessed
- Involves ongoing collection of specific data
- Involves analyzing data on a regular basis
- Requires sharing the results with others
- Requires broad and repeated contact with the public about personal health issues
- Motivates public health action as a result of data analyses to:
  - Reduce morbidity
  - Reduce mortality
  - Improve health

Surveillance is important because it generates knowledge of a disease or **event** outbreak patterns (including timing, geographic distribution, and susceptible populations). The knowledge can be used to intervene to reduce risk or prevent an occurrence at the most appropriate point in time and in the most effective ways. Surveillance is built on understanding of epidemiologic principles of agent, host, and environmental relationships and on the natural history of disease or conditions (see Chapter 13). Surveillance systems make it possible to engage in effective continuous quality improvement activities within organizations and to improve quality of care (Kimble et al., 2017; Veenema, 2018).

Surveillance focuses on the collection of process and outcome data. **Process data** focus on what is done (i.e., services provided or protocols for health care delivery). **Outcome data** focus on changes in health status. The activities generated by analyses of these data aim to improve public health response systems. An example of process data is collection of data about the proportion of the eligible population vaccinated against influenza in any one year. Outcome data in this case are the incidence rates (new cases) of influenza among the same population in the same year.

Although surveillance was initially devoted to monitoring and reducing the spread of infectious diseases, it is now used to monitor and reduce chronic diseases and injuries, as well as environmental and occupational exposures (Latshaw et al., 2017; Perlman et al., 2017; Veenema, 2018), as well as personal health behaviors. Surveillance systems help nurses and other professionals monitor emerging infections and bioterrorist outbreaks (Veenema, 2018). Bioterrorism is one example of an event creating a critical public health concern that involves environmental exposures that must be monitored. This event also requires serious planning in order to be able to respond quickly and effectively. **Bioterrorism** is defined as "the intentional use of microorganisms or toxins derived from living organisms to cause death or disease in humans or the animals and plants on which we depend" (Ryan, 2016, p. 26). The CDC's bioterrorism website provides emergency preparedness and response information for the general public and health care professionals, as well as information on specific bioterrorism agents (http://emergency.cdc.gov) (CDC, 2017c). An example of a case of bioterrorism could occur when a religious cult located outside of town has applied to start its own school. The town voted the charter down initially and it is now on the ballot again. On election day, the majority of the town's residents become ill and are unable to vote. The police were called to the cult, and when searching the compound they uncovered a vial of *Salmonella typhimurium*. After questioning, one of the cult members reveals that the salmonella was used to contaminate the salad bar at a local restaurant, thus limiting the number of people who would vote against the cult starting a charter school (CDC, 2017b).

Chemical terrorism is the intentional release of hazardous chemicals into the environment for the purpose of harming or killing (CDC, 2016a; Ryan, 2016). An example of chemical terrorism occurred in 2016 when Islamic State militants near Mousl, Iraq, set fire to a sulfa mine producing widespread clouds of sulfur dioxide, resulting in two deaths and 1500 people injured (Johnston, 2017). The CDC (2016c) provides chemical emergency preparedness and response information to health care professionals and the public, along with information about specific chemical agents (https://emergency.cdc.gov). In the event of a bioterrorist attack, imagine how difficult it would be to control the spread of biological agents such as botulism or anthrax or chemical agents such as sarin or ricin if no data were available about these agents, their resulting diseases or symptoms, and their usual incidence patterns (new cases) in the community. The United States spent $612 million in annual public health preparedness and response funds in 2017 (CDC, 2018k). About $8 million was awarded to fund public health preparedness and increase the ability of the CDC to respond to public health emergencies and disasters (CDC, 2018k).

Uses of Public Health Surveillance

Public health surveillance can be used to facilitate the following (Brownson et al., 2018; McNabb et al., 2016):

- Estimate the magnitude of a problem (disease or event)
- Determine geographic distribution of an illness or symptoms
- Portray the natural history of a disease
- Detect epidemics; define a problem
- Generate hypotheses; stimulate research
- Evaluate control measures
- Monitor changes in infectious agents
- Detect changes in health practices and health behaviors
- Facilitate planning
- Guide public health policy and programs

Purposes of Surveillance

The overall purposes of surveillance are as follows:

- Assess public health status
- Define public health priorities
- Plan public health programs
- Evaluate programs
- Stimulate research
- Improve health

Surveillance helps public health departments identify trends and unusual disease patterns, set priorities for using scarce resources, and develop and evaluate programs for commonly occurring and universally occurring diseases or events. Surveillance activities can be related to the core functions of public health: assessment, policy development, and assurance. Disease surveillance helps establish baseline (endemic) rates of disease occurrence and patterns of spread. Surveillance makes it possible to initiate a rapid response to an outbreak of a disease or event that can cause a health problem. In the past two years the CDC has responded to 750 health threats (CDC, 2018c). For example, surveillance made it possible to respond quickly to outbreaks of Ebola (2014-2018), Zika (2016-2017), water contamination (2016), hepatitis A (2017), the opioid epidemic in the United States, and numerous foodborne outbreaks predominately related to salmonella and *Escherichia coli* (*E. coli*) in recent years (CDC, 2018c; CDC, 2018f). The CDC (2018b) maintains an active list of disease outbreak investigations and provides guidance for health care professionals regarding symptoms and treatment options.

Surveillance data are analyzed, and interpretations of these data analyses are used to develop policies that better protect the public from problems such as emerging infections; bioterrorist, biological, and chemical threats; and injuries from problems such as motor vehicle accidents. In 2006 a great deal of emphasis was placed on developing disaster management policies in health care organizations, industries, and homes so that the U.S. population could be prepared in the event of an emergency. Surveillance within individual organizations, such as infection control systems in hospitals, can be used to establish policies related to clinical practice that are designed to improve quality of care processes and outcomes. An example is documented by Sorour et al. (2016), where the standard of care of patients with Foley catheters was expanded to include the use of cranberry containing products and antimicrobial metal care for patients with Foley catheters, resulting in a reduced incidence of catheter-associated urinary tract infections.

Surveillance makes it possible to have ongoing monitoring in place to ensure that disease and event patterns improve rather than deteriorate. They can also make it possible to study whether the clinical protocols and public health policies that are in place can be enhanced, based on current science, so that disease rates actually decline (WHO, 2018a). For example, the ongoing monitoring of obesity in children in a community may show that new clinical and effective protocols need to be developed to be used in school-based clinics to reduce the prevalence of obesity among the school populations.

Surveillance data are very helpful in determining whether a program is effective. Such data make it possible to determine whether public health interventions are effective in reducing the spread of disease or the incidence of injuries. By determining the change in the number of cases at the beginning of a program (baseline) with the number of cases after program implementation, it is possible to estimate the effectiveness of a program. One could then compare the effectiveness of different approaches to reducing the problem or to improving health. Goldthwaite et al. (2015) investigated the impact of an initiative to prevent unintended pregnancy in the low-income population in Colorado through use of long-acting reversible contraceptive products (LARC). Funding was provided to 28 agencies specifically for providing of intrauterine devices (IUDs) and contraceptive implants to clients seeking care at one of the agencies; in addition to training for health care providers and staff. Their findings indicated that improved access to family planning services and increased use of LARC resulted in a significant reduction in preterm births.

Collaboration Among Partners

A quality surveillance system requires collaboration among a number of agencies and individuals: federal agencies, state and local public health agencies, hospitals, health care providers, medical examiners, veterinarians, agriculture, pharmaceutical agencies, emergency management, and law enforcement agencies, as well as 911 systems, ambulance services, urgent care and emergency departments, poison control centers, nurse hotlines, schools, and industry. Such collaboration promotes the development of a comprehensive plan and a directory of emergency responses and contacts for effective communication and information sharing. It is sometimes essential to include collaboration with international agencies as well. The type of information to be shared includes the following:

- How to use **algorithms** to identify which events should be investigated (i.e., this means using a precise step-by-step plan outlining a procedure that in a finite number of steps helps to identify the appropriate event)
- How to investigate
- Whom to contact
- How and to whom information is to be disseminated
- Who is responsible for appropriate action

Nurses are often in the forefront of responses to be made in the surveillance process whether working in a small rural agency or a large urban agency; within the health department, school, or urgent care center; or on the telephone performing triage services during a disaster. It is the nurse who sees the event first (Association of Public Health Nurses, 2014).

EVIDENCE-BASED PRACTICE

A systematic qualitative review was conducted by Klinger et al. (2017) to identify ethical issues in public health surveillance. The researchers noted that ethical issues sometimes arise in public health surveillance, particularly around informed consent and study design, yet there is a lack of clear ethics guidance and training for public health surveillance programs. In this systematic review, ethical issues were defined based on principlism, searching PubMed and Google Books for relevant publications. The search identified 525 references, of which 83 met the inclusion criteria and were reviewed. Most of the publications reviewed were journal articles (78 percent); the rest were books or book chapters (22 percent). The researchers identified 86 distinct ethical issues that come up over the surveillance life cycle. The researchers also identified 20 conditions in which foregoing informed consent procedures was more or less justifiable. From the systematic review, a comprehensive ethics matrix was developed which may be used to inform guidelines, reports, strategy papers, and educational material, and raise awareness among practitioners.

Nurse Use

In this example of using evidence to promote quality practice, the nurse can use this systematic review to change practice if necessary to adhere to the ethics matrix. Quality and ethical practices are essential components of surveillance.

Klingler, C, Silva, D, Schuermann, C, Reis, A. Saxena, A, Strech: Ethical issues in public health surveillance: a systematic qualitative review, *BMC Public Health* (2017) 17:295. Available at www.biomedcentral.com.

Cluster Detection

Cluster detection is a surveillance tool that public health nurses can use to determine geographic priority areas for health promotion and disease prevention interventions. Being able to focus on a specific area would enable the nurse to use public health resources in an efficient manner and provide outreach to the populations at highest risk for disease. For example, Maravi et al. (2017) used geospatial analysis to identify census tract areas in Denver, Colorado, that had high rates of *Bordetella pertussis* along with low immunization rates. Identification of these areas allowed public health officials to implement interventions resulting in increased immunization rates for pertussis in the identified areas.

Nurse Competencies

The national core competencies for public health nurses were developed from the Core Competencies for Public Health Professionals (Council on Linkages between Academia and Public Health Practice, 2014) and by the Quad Council of Public Health Nursing Organizations (beginning in 2011 and revised in 2018). These competencies are divided into eight practice domains: assessment and analytical skills; policy development/program planning; communication; cultural competence; community dimensions of practice; public health sciences; financial planning, evaluation, and management; and leadership and system thinking (Quad Council Coalition Competency Review Taskforce, 2018).

To be a participant in surveillance and investigation activities, the staff nurse must have the following knowledge related to the core competencies (Quad Council Coalition Competency Review Taskforce, 2018):

1. Assessment and analytical skills
   - Defining a problem
   - Determining a cause
   - Identifying and understanding relevant data
   - Using data to address community health problems
   - Developing community health assessments
   - Incorporating evidence in decision making
   - Identifying risks
2. Policy development/program planning skills
   - Planning, implementing, and evaluating policies and programs aimed at improving community health and strategic plans
3. Communication
   - Assessing and addressing population literacy levels
   - Providing effective oral and written reports
   - Soliciting input from others and effectively presenting accurate demographic, statistical, and scientific information to other professionals and the community at large
4. Community dimensions of practice
   - Establishing and maintaining links during the investigation
   - Collaborating with partners
   - Developing, implementing, and evaluating an assessment to define the problem
5. Basic public health science skills
   - Identifying individual and organizational responsibilities
   - Identifying and retrieving current relevant evidence-based practice
6. Leadership and systems thinking
   - Identifying internal and external issues that have an effect on the investigation
   - Promoting team and organizational efforts
   - Contributing to developing, implementing, and monitoring of the investigation

While the staff nurse participates in these activities, the advanced practice public health nurse should be proficient in applying these competencies. In addition, the nurse

TABLE 22.1 Phases of Nursing Process Linked to Preparedness

	DEFINITION OF:			
Preparedness	**Assessment**	**Planning**	**Implementation**	**Evaluation**
Assure capacity to respond effectively to disasters and emergencies	Assess the populations at risk for special needs during a disaster	Develop plans to care for special needs populations during a disaster	Conduct training, drills, and exercises related to care of special needs persons	Evaluate plans for serving populations with special needs

Excerpted from Association of Public Health Nurses: *The role of public health nurses in emergency preparedness and response: position paper* [Table 1: The Phases of Disaster Linked to the Nursing Process], 2013. Retrieved from https://www.phnurse.org.

applies the nursing process in preparedness as illustrated in Table 22.1.

The Minnesota model of *Public Health Interventions: Applications for Public Health Nursing Practice* (Minnesota Department of Health, 2001, pp. 15-16; also see Chapters 11 and 21) suggests that surveillance is one of the interventions related to public health nursing practice. The model gives seven basic steps of surveillance for nurses to follow:

1. Consider whether surveillance as an intervention is appropriate for the situation.
2. Organize the knowledge of the problem, its natural course of history, and its aftermath.
3. Establish clear criteria for what constitutes a case.
4. Collect sufficient data from multiple valid sources.
5. Analyze data.
6. Interpret data and disseminate to decision makers.
7. Evaluate the impact of the surveillance system.

Data Sources for Surveillance

Clinicians, health care agencies, and laboratories report cases to state health departments. Data also come from death certificates and administrative data such as discharge reports and billing records (McNabb et al., 2016; Veenema, 2018). The following are select sources of mortality and morbidity data:

1. Mortality data are often the only source of health-related data available for small geographic areas. Examples include the following:
   - Vital statistics reports (e.g., death certificates, medical examiner reports, birth certificates)
   - Mortality data can be obtained from the National Vital Statistics System. These data are available and one of the few sources of health-related data that are available for a long time period for small geographic areas (CDC, 2018g).
2. Morbidity data include the following:
   - Notifiable disease reports
   - Laboratory reports
   - Hospital discharge reports
   - Billing data
   - Outpatient health care data
   - Specialized disease registries
   - Injury surveillance systems
   - Environmental surveys
   - Sentinel surveillance systems

An example of a process in place to collect morbidity data is the National Program of Cancer Registries (NPCR) (CDC, 2018b). This program provides for monitoring of the types of cancers found in a state and the locations of the cancer risks and health problems in the state. Information about the health of a state or community can also be found at County Health Rankings and Roadmaps, a Robert Wood Johnson Foundation program (http://www.countyhealthrankings.org).

Each of the data sources has the potential for underreporting or incomplete reporting. However, if there is consistency in the use of surveillance methods, the data collected will show trends in events or disease patterns that may indicate a change needed in a program or a needed prevention intervention to reduce morbidity or mortality. Underreporting or incomplete reporting may occur for the following reasons: social stigma attached to a disease (such as human immunodeficiency virus [HIV]/acquired immunodeficiency syndrome [AIDS]); ignorance of required reporting system; lack of knowledge about the **case definition**, procedural changes in reporting, or changes in a database; limited diagnostic abilities; or low priority given to reporting (CDC, 2010; McNabb et al., 2016; Ryan, 2016).

Mortality data assist in identifying differences in health status among groups, populations, occupations, and communities; monitoring preventable deaths; and examining cause-and-effect factors in diseases (CDC, 2018c). Vital statistics can be used to plan programs and to monitor programs to meet *Healthy People 2020* goals (see the *Healthy People 2020* box for objectives related to surveillance).

The National Notifiable Diseases Surveillance System (NNDSS) as well as local public health laboratories, hospital discharge data, and billing data provide mechanisms for classifying diseases and events and calculating rates of diseases within and across groups, populations, and communities (CDC, 2018i).

The **sentinel** surveillance system provides for the monitoring of key health events when information is not otherwise available or for calculating or estimating disease morbidity in vulnerable populations (McNabb et al., 2016). Registries monitor chronic disease in a systematic manner, linking information from a variety of sources (health department, clinics, hospitals) to identify disease control and prevention strategies. Surveys then provide data from individuals about prevalence of health conditions and health risks. Such surveys allow for monitoring changes over time and assessing the individual's knowledge, attitudes, and beliefs (see QSEN box). This information can be used to assist health care professionals in providing education and planned interventions (Gostin & Riley, 2018).

QSEN FOCUS ON QUALITY AND SAFETY EDUCATION FOR NURSES

Targeted Competency: Safety

Minimizes risk of harm to patients and providers through both system effectiveness and individual performance.

- **Knowledge:** Discuss potential and actual impact of national patient safety resources, initiatives, and regulations.
- **Skill:** Use national patient safety resources for own development and to focus attention on safety in the community and health care settings.
- **Attitude:** Value relationship between national safety campaigns and implementation in practices and practice settings.

Safety Question

The Quad Council competency for communication skills indicates that the public health nurse uses a variety of methods to disseminate public health information to individuals, families, and groups within a population within a community and provides a presentation of targeted health information to multiple audiences at a local level: groups, professionals, peers, and agency peers (2018).

How would the nurse use the national sentinel surveillance system to identify health conditions and risks in the community? What types of data sources in this system would the nurse collect? After careful analysis of the data sources, what would the nurse include in a presentation to multiple audiences?

HEALTHY PEOPLE 2020

Surveillance Objectives

- **EH-5:** Reduce waterborne disease outbreaks arising from water intended for drinking among persons served by community water systems.
- **FS-1:** Reduce outbreaks of infections caused by key foodborne bacteria.
- **FS-2:** Reduce infections caused by key pathogens transmitted commonly through food.
- **GH-1:** Reduce the number of cases of malaria reported in the United States.
- **IID-26:** Reduce new hepatitis C cases.
- **PHI-2:** Increase the proportion of tribal, state, and local public health agencies that incorporate Core Competencies for Public Health Professionals into description and performance evaluation.
- **PHI-7:** Increase the proportion of population-based *Healthy People 2020* objectives for which national data are available for all major population groups.

From U.S. Department of Health and Human Services: *Healthy People 2020: a roadmap to improve all Americans' health*, Washington, DC, 2010, U.S. Government Printing Office.

NOTIFIABLE DISEASES

Before 1990, state and local health departments used many different criteria for identifying cases of reportable diseases. Using different criteria made the data less useful than it could have been because it could not be compared across health departments or states. For this reason some diseases may have been underreported and others may have been overreported. In 1990 the CDC and the Council of State and Territorial Epidemiologists assembled the first list of standard case definitions. This list was revised in 1997, and more information may be found at the CDC Division of Public Health Informatics and Surveillance website (CDC, 2018d). This site contains information about the National Notifiable Disease Surveillance System (NNDSS), and the standard case definitions which are updated on a case-by-case basis or otherwise remain the same. For example, the definition of carbapenemase producing carbapenem-resistant Enterobacteriaceae (CP-CRE) was updated in 2018. Additionally, beginning in January 2018, cases of salmonellosis were classified into two conditions: (1) salmonellosis (excluding paratyphoid fever and typhoid fever), and (2) paratyphoid fever (caused by *Salmonella* serotypes Paratyphi A, Paratyphi B [tartrate negative] and Paratyphi C) (CDC, 2017b). New case definitions are added as new diseases are identified.

National Notifiable Diseases

Box 22.1 shows the national notifiable infectious diseases. Reporting of disease data by health care providers, laboratories, and public health workers to state and local health departments is essential if trends are to be accurately monitored. "The data provide the basis for detecting disease outbreaks, for identifying person characteristics, and for calculating incidence, geographic distribution, and temporal trends. They are used to initiate prevention programs, evaluate established prevention and control practices, suggest new intervention strategies, identify areas for research, document the need for disease control funds, and help answer questions from the community" (CDC, 2018d). The CDC and the Council of State and Territorial Epidemiologists have a policy that requires state health departments to report selected diseases to the CDC National Notifiable Disease Surveillance System (NNDSS). The data for nationally notifiable diseases from 50 states, the U.S. territories, New York City, and the District of Columbia are published weekly in the *Morbidity and Mortality Weekly Report (MMWR)*. Data collection about these diseases and revision of statistics is ongoing. Annual updated final reports are published in CDC WONDER (CDC, 2018e).

State Notifiable Diseases

Requirements for reporting diseases are mandated by law or regulation. Although each state and Washington, DC, differ in the list of reportable diseases, the usefulness of the data depends on "uniformity, simplicity, and timeliness." Because state requirements differ, not all nationally notifiable diseases are legally mandated for reporting in a state. For legally reportable diseases, states compile disease incidence data (new cases) and transmit the data electronically (weekly) through the National Electronic Disease Surveillance System (CDC, 2018h).

Ongoing analysis of this extensive database has led to better diagnosis and treatment methods, national vaccine schedule recommendations, changes in vaccine formulation, and the recognition of new or resurgent diseases (CDC, 2017c). Selected data are reported in the CDC MMWR report (https://www.cdc.gov). Adverse health data for the calendar year are documented on the reportable disease form, entitled EPID, to the local health department or the state department for public health. Local health department surveillance personnel investigate case reports and proceed with recommended public health measures, requesting assistance from the state's department

BOX 22.1 Infectious Diseases Designated as Notifiable at the National Level During 2018

- Anthrax
- Arboviral diseases, neuroinvasive and non-neuroinvasive
- California serogroup virus diseases
- Chikungunya virus disease
- Eastern equine encephalitis virus disease
- Powassan virus disease
- St. Louis encephalitis virus disease
- West Nile virus disease
- Western equine encephalitis virus disease
- Babesiosis
- Botulism
- Botulism, foodborne
- Botulism, infant
- Botulism, wound
- Botulism, other
- Brucellosis
- Campylobacteriosis
- Carbapenemase producing carbapenem-resistant Enterobacteriaceae (CP-CRE)
- CP-CRE, *Enterobacter* spp.
- CP-CRE, *Escherichia coli (E. coli)*
- CP-CRE, *Klebsiella* spp.
- Chancroid
- *Chlamydia trachomatis* infection
- Cholera
- Coccidioidomycosis
- Congenital syphilis
- Syphilitic stillbirth
- Cryptosporidiosis
- Cyclosporiasis
- Dengue virus infections
- Dengue
- Dengue-like illness
- Severe dengue
- Diphtheria
- Ehrlichiosis and anaplasmosis
- *Anaplasma phagocytophilum* infection
- *Ehrlichia chaffeensis* infection
- *Ehrlichia ewingii* infection
- Undetermined human ehrlichiosis/anaplasmosis
- Giardiasis
- Gonorrhea
- *Haemophilus influenzae*, invasive disease
- Hansen's disease
- Hantavirus infection, non-Hantavirus pulmonary syndrome
- Hantavirus pulmonary syndrome
- Hemolytic uremic syndrome, post-diarrheal
- Hepatitis A, acute
- Hepatitis B, acute
- Hepatitis B, chronic
- Hepatitis B, perinatal virus infection
- Hepatitis C, acute
- Hepatitis C, chronic
- Hepatitis C, perinatal infection
- HIV infection (AIDS has been reclassified as HIV stage III)
- Influenza-associated pediatric mortality
- Invasive pneumococcal disease
- Latent TB infection (TB infection)
- Legionellosis
- Leptospirosis
- Listeriosis
- Lyme disease
- Malaria
- Measles
- Meningococcal disease
- Mumps
- Novel influenza A virus infections
- Pertussis
- Plague
- Poliomyelitis, paralytic
- Poliovirus infection, nonparalytic
- Psittacosis
- Q fever
- Q fever, acute
- Q fever, chronic
- Rabies, animal
- Rabies, human
- Rubella
- Rubella, congenital syndrome
- Salmonellosis
- Severe acute respiratory syndrome-associated coronavirus disease
- Shiga toxin-producing *Escherichia coli*
- Shigellosis
- Smallpox
- Spotted fever rickettsiosis
- Streptococcal toxic shock syndrome
- Syphilis
- Syphilis, primary
- Syphilis, secondary
- Syphilis, early non-primary non-secondary
- Syphilis, unknown duration or late
- Tetanus
- Toxic shock syndrome (other than streptococcal)
- Trichinellosis
- Tuberculosis
- Tularemia
- Typhoid fever
- Vancomycin-intermediate *Staphylococcus aureus* and vancomycin-resistant *Staphylococcus aureus*
- Varicella
- Varicella deaths
- Vibriosis
- Viral hemorrhagic fever
- Crimean-Congo hemorrhagic fever virus
- Ebola virus
- Lassa virus
- Lujo virus
- Marburg virus
- New World arenavirus—Guanarito virus
- New World arenavirus—Junin virus
- New World arenavirus—Machupo virus
- New World arenavirus—Sabia virus
- Yellow fever
- Zika virus disease and Zika virus infection
- Zika virus disease, congenital
- Zika virus disease, non-congenital
- Zika virus infection, congenital
- Zika virus infection, non-congenital

AIDS, Acquired immunodeficiency syndrome; *HIV,* human immunodeficiency virus; *TB,* tuberculosis.
From Centers for Disease Control and Prevention: *National notifiable infectious diseases,* 2018. Retrieved from https://www.cdc.gov.

assigned to monitor the reports when needed. Reports are forwarded by mail or fax or, in urgent circumstances, by telephone 24 hours a day, 7 days a week. When reports are received, they are scrutinized carefully and, when appropriate, additional steps are initiated to assist local health departments in planning interventions.

To determine which of the national notifiable diseases are reportable in your state, go to your state health department website.

CASE DEFINITIONS

Criteria

Criteria for defining cases of different diseases are essential for having a uniform, standardized method of reporting and monitoring diseases. A case definition provides understanding of the data that are being collected and reduces the likelihood that different criteria will be used for reporting similar cases of a disease. Case definitions may include clinical symptoms, laboratory values, and epidemiologic criteria (e.g., exposure to a known or suspected case). Each disease has its own unique set of criteria based on what is known scientifically about that particular disease. Cases may be classified as *suspected, probable,* or *confirmed,* depending on the strength of the evidence supporting the case criteria.

Although some diseases require laboratory confirmation, even though clinical symptoms may be present, other diseases do not have laboratory tests to confirm the diagnosis. Other cases are diagnosed on the basis of epidemiologic data alone, such as exposure to contaminated food. If a case definition has been established by the CDC or another official source, it should be used for reporting purposes. The case definition should not be used as the only criterion for clinical diagnosis, quality assurance, standards for reimbursement, or taking public health action. Action to control a disease should be taken as soon as a problem is identified, although there may not be enough information to meet the case definition.

Case Definition Examples

For example, from September 1, 2017, through January 23, 2018, there were 590 cases of Hepatitis A in San Diego County, California, resulting in 68 percent of the individuals being hospitalized and 3.4 percent deaths. The majority of those affected by Hepatitis A were homeless and/or illicit drug uses (San Diego County, 2018). The CDC (2018m) identified the clinical case definition for Hepatitis A as a "discrete onset of symptoms consistent with Hepatitis (e.g., fever, headache, malaise, anorexia, nausea, vomiting, diarrhea, and abdominal pain) and either jaundice or elevated serum aminotransferase levels." The clinical symptoms of patients with all types of acute viral Hepatitis are the same; therefore a person with acute Hepatitis A must (1) have a positive immunoglobulin M (IgM) antibody for Hepatitis A or (2) meet the clinical symptoms and "occur in a person who has an epidemiologic link with a person who has laboratory-confirmed Hepatitis A (i.e., household or sexual contact with an infected person during the 15-50 days before the onset of symptoms)" (https://www.cdc.gov).

The World Health Organization (WHO) used the following cases definitions in response to the Ebola outbreak in 2014 (2014a). A suspected case was defined as "Any person, alive or dead, who has (or had) sudden onset of high fever and had contact with a suspected, probable or confirmed Ebola case, or a dead or sick animal OR any person with sudden onset of high fever and at least three of the following symptoms: headache, vomiting, anorexia/loss of appetite, diarrhea, lethargy, stomach pain, aching muscles or joints, difficulty swallowing, breathing difficulties, or hiccup; or any person with unexplained bleeding OR any sudden, unexplained death." Probable cases were defined as "Any suspected case evaluated by a clinician OR any person who died from 'suspected' Ebola and had an epidemiologic link to a confirmed case but was not tested and did not have laboratory confirmation of the disease." The definition of a confirmed case was "A probable or suspected case is classified as confirmed when a sample from that person tests positive for Ebola virus in the laboratory" (http://apps.who.int).

TYPES OF SURVEILLANCE SYSTEMS

Informatics is essential to the mission of protecting the public's health. Surveillance systems are designed to assist public health professionals in the early detection of disease and event outbreaks in order to intervene and reduce the potential for morbidity or mortality, or to improve the public's health status (Blazes & Lewis, 2016; CDC, 2018j). Surveillance systems in use today are defined as *passive, active, sentinel,* and *special.*

Passive System

In the passive system, case reports are sent to local health departments by health care providers (e.g., physicians, public health nurses), or laboratory reports of disease occurrence are sent to the local health department. The case reports are summarized and forwarded to the state health department, national government, or organizations responsible for monitoring the problem, such as the CDC or an international organization such as the WHO.

The **National Electronic Disease Surveillance System** (NEDSS) is a voluntary system monitored by the CDC and includes a total of 682 infectious diseases or conditions with case definitions that are considered important to the public's health (CDC, 2018d). Each state determines for itself which of the diseases and conditions are of importance to the state's health and legally requires the reporting of those diseases to the state health department by health care providers, health care agencies, and laboratories. The passive system may not provide an accurate picture of the problem because of delayed reporting by providers and laboratories and incomplete reporting across providers and laboratories. This system, however, has the ability to provide disease-specific demographic, geographic, and seasonal trends over time for reported events. An example is a cancer registry system in which cases of cancer are required to be reported to the state on the basis of the type of cancer, the demographics of the client, and the geographic location. Because the system has limits, a disease outbreak may be occurring before all reports are received by the state health department (CDC, 2018d; Veenema, 2013).

Active System

In the active system, the nurse, as an employee of the health department, may begin a search for cases through contacts with local health care providers and health care agencies. In this system, the nurse names the disease or an event and gathers data about existing cases to try to determine the magnitude of the problem (how widespread it is).

For example, the CDC defines a foodborne disease outbreak as occurring when two or more people get the same illness after ingesting the same contaminated food or drink. Numerous examples of multistate foodborne illness occur annually in the United States. For example, in 2018, foodborne outbreaks were linked to ingestion of contaminated coconut, raw sprouts, lettuce, fast-food chain salads, and precut melon (CDC, 2018c). Bacteria most commonly associated with the outbreaks included various strains of *E. coli* and Salmonella.

Other examples of active systems include ongoing tracking systems within an occupational setting that are designed to monitor work-related injuries or illnesses and symptoms . Many organizations share results of surveillance studies with The National Institute for Occupational Safety and Health (NIOSH) (CDC, 2018l). The active surveillance system is often used to detect a need for an investigation but is of limited use during an actual investigation.

Sentinel System

In the sentinel system, trends in commonly occurring diseases or key health indicators are monitored (*Healthy People 2020*). A disease or event may be the sentinel, or a population may be the sentinel. In this system a sample of health care providers or agencies is asked to report the problem. The system is useful because it helps to monitor trends in community occurring diseases and events. Some of the questions that may be asked include the following: What really happened? What are the consequences? What was different in this event? What was the outcome? Could the occurrence have been prevented? Did providers follow procedures? Did providers know what to do? Has this happened before? If so, how was it fixed? Who reported the event? What might prevent it from happening again?

For example, certain providers and/or agencies in a community may be asked to report the number of cases of Influenza seen during a given time period in order to make projections about the severity of the "flu season." Another example would be monitoring the population of children in the local elementary school to determine the rate of obesity among school-age children. Although much may be learned about diseases and conditions using the sentinel system, because the system data are based on a sample of a problem or a specific population, they cannot be used to monitor specific clients or to initiate prevention and control interventions for individuals. The system is useful because it helps monitor trends in commonly occurring diseases or events.

Special Systems

Special systems are developed for collecting particular types of data and may be a combination of active, passive, and/or sentinel systems. As a result of bioterrorism, newer systems called syndromic surveillance systems are being developed to monitor illness syndromes or events. This approach requires the use of automated data systems to report continued (real time) or daily (near real time) disease outbreaks (CDC, 2016e) (Box 22.2).

The CDC's Syndromic Surveillance website discusses the impact of increasing electronic health record systems: "Public health syndromic surveillance using inpatient and ambulatory clinical care electronic health record (EHR) data is a relatively new practice. As eligible health professionals and hospitals adopt, implement, and upgrade their EHR systems through the Centers for Medicare and Medicaid Services EHR Incentive programs (Meaningful Use programs), there is an opportunity for public health agencies (PHAs) to routinely receive health data from settings other than emergency departments and urgent care centers. Given the number of factors and complex relationships that affect EHR data quality, a collaborative approach that includes public health, health care, and EHR technology developers is the best way to determine how EHR data can be meaningfully used for surveillance." (http://www.cdc.gov).

An example of a special system is the PulseNet system developed by the CDC, the Association of Public Health Laboratories, and federal food regulatory agencies to "fingerprint" foodborne bacteria. This system is designed to provide data for early recognition and investigation of foodborne outbreaks in all 50 states. Similarly, the BioSense Platform provides for analysis and exchange of data across regional boundaries regarding potential community health threats and expanded situational awareness for all-hazards preparedness and response. (CDC, 2018k). The National Syndromic Surveillance Program (NSSP) promotes timely exchange and monitoring of syndromic data, including patient encounter data from emergency departments, urgent care, ambulatory care, and inpatient health care settings, as well as pharmacy and laboratory data. The real-time data are used as potential indicators of an event, disease, or outbreak concern (CDC, 2018j). For example, syndromic surveillance data were useful in tracking Influenza trends in New York City through monitoring emergency department visits, detecting clusters of carbon monoxide poisoning due to power outages after a windstorm, identifying an outbreak of ciguatera fish poisoning, and correlating opioid-related emergency department visits with sales of prescription opioids (Gould et al., 2017).

Although all of the systems are important, the public health nurse is most likely to use the active or passive systems. An

BOX 22.2 Bioterrorism and Response Networks

Integrating of training and response preparedness can be supported by the following networks:

- Health Alert Network (http://emergency.cdc.gov)
- The Emerging Infections Program (http://www.cdc.gov)
- Epidemiology and Laboratory Capacity for Prevention and Control of Emerging Infectious Diseases (ELC) (http://cdc.gov)
- Hazardous Substances Data Bank (toxnet.nim.nih.gov)
- Influenza surveillance in the United States
- Community emergency response systems (check local health department)

example of when one might use a passive system is the use of the state reportable disease system to complete a community assessment or MAPP (Mobilizing for Action through Planning and Partnerships; see Chapters 17 and 23). The active system is used when several schoolchildren become ill after eating lunch in the cafeteria or at the local hot dog stand, to investigate the possibility of food poisoning, or following up on contacts of a newly diagnosed tuberculosis or sexually transmitted disease (STD) client at the local homeless shelter (CDC, 2013). An example of a use of the active system occurred in 2012, when a Liberian citizen in Dallas, Texas, was found to be infected with Ebola virus (CDC, 2014e).

THE INVESTIGATION

Investigation Objectives

Any unusual increase in disease incidence (new cases) or an unusual event in the community should be investigated. The system used for investigation depends on the intensity of the event, the severity of the disease, the number of people or communities affected, the potential for harm to the community or the spread of disease, and the effectiveness of available interventions (CDC, 2016d). The objectives of an investigation are as follows:

- To control and prevent disease or death
- To identify factors that contribute to the outbreak of the disease and the occurrence of the event
- To implement measures to prevent occurrences

Defining the Magnitude of a Problem/Event. The following definitions provide a way to describe the level of occurrence of a disease or event for purposes of communicating the magnitude of the problem. A disease or an event that is found to be present (occurring) in a population is defined as **endemic** if there is a persistent (usual) presence with low to moderate number of cases of the disease or event. The endemic levels of a disease or an event in a population provide the baseline for establishing a public health problem. For example, foodborne botulism is endemic to Alaska. The baseline must be known to determine the existence of a change or increase in the number of cases from baseline. If a problem is considered **hyperendemic**, there is a persistently (usually) high number of cases. An example is the high cholera incidence rate among Asian and Pacific Islanders. **Sporadic** problems are those with an irregular pattern, with occasional cases found at irregular intervals.

Epidemic means that the occurrence of a disease within an area is clearly in excess of expected levels (endemic) for a given time period. This is often called the outbreak. **Pandemic** refers to the epidemic spread of the problem over several countries or continents (e.g., severe acute respiratory syndrome [SARS] outbreak). **Holoendemic** in a population implies a highly prevalent problem that is commonly acquired early in life. The prevalence of this problem decreases as age increases (Nmadu et al., 2015). **Outbreak detection**, or identifying an increase in the frequency of disease above the usual occurrence of the disease, is the function of the investigator (CDC, 2015b).

Patterns of Occurrence

Patterns of occurrence can be identified when investigating a disease or event. These patterns are used to define the boundaries of a problem to help investigate possible causes or sources of the problem. A **common source** outbreak refers to a group exposed to a common noxious influence such as the release of noxious gases (e.g., ricin in the Japanese subway system several years ago and in a water system in the United States [Merrill, 2017]). In a **point source** outbreak, all persons exposed become ill at the same time, during one incubation period. A **mixed outbreak** is "when a victim of a common source epidemic has person-to-person contact with others and spreads the disease, further propagating the health problem" (Merrill, 2017, p. 316), as in the spreading of influenza. **Intermittent or continuous source** cases may be exposed over a period of days or weeks, as in the recent food poisonings at a restaurant chain throughout the United States as a result of the restaurant's purchase of contaminated green onions. A **propagated outbreak** does not have a common source and spreads gradually from person to person over more than one incubation period, such as the spread of tuberculosis from one person to another.

Causal Factors From the Epidemiologic Triangle. Factors that must be considered as causes of an outbreak are categorized as agents, hosts, and environmental factors (see Chapter 13). The belief is that these factors may interact to cause the outbreak and therefore the potential interactions must be examined. The following presents definitions used to classify agents in an attack:

- **Infectivity**: Refers to the capacity of an agent to enter a susceptible host and produce infection or disease
- **Pathogenicity**: Measures the proportion of infected people who develop the disease
- **Virulence**: Refers to the proportion of people with clinical disease who become severely ill or die

Box 22.3 lists the types of agent factors that may be present. The host factors associated with cases may be age, sex, race,

BOX 22.3 Types of Agent Factors

1. Biological
   - Bacteria (e.g., tuberculosis, salmonellosis, streptococcal infections)
   - Viruses (e.g., hepatitis A, herpes)
   - Fungi (e.g., tinea capitis, blastomycosis)
   - Parasites (protozoa causing malaria, giardiasis; helminths [roundworms, pinworms]; arthropods [mosquitoes, ticks, flies, mites])
2. Physical
   - Heat
   - Trauma
3. Chemicals
   - Pollutants
   - Medications/drugs
4. Nutrients
   - Absence
   - Excess
5. Psychological
   - Stress
   - Isolation
   - Social support

socioeconomic status, genetics, and lifestyle choices (e.g., cigarette smoking, sexual practices, contraception, eating habits). The environmental factors that may be related to a case are physical (e.g., weather, temperature, humidity, physical surroundings) or biological (e.g., insects that transmit the agent). Some of the socioeconomic factors that might affect development of a disease or an event are behavior (e.g., terrorist behaviors), personality, cultural characteristics of group, crowding, sanitation, and the availability of health services.

When to Investigate

An unusual increase in disease incidence should be investigated. The amount of effort that goes into an investigation depends on the severity or magnitude of the problem, the numbers in the population who are affected, the potential for spreading the disease, and the availability and effectiveness of intervention measures to resolve the problems. Most of the outbreaks of diseases (or increased incidence rates) occur naturally and/or are predictable when compared with the consistent patterns of previous outbreaks of a disease, such as influenza, tuberculosis, or common infectious diseases. When a disease or an event outbreak occurs as a result of purposeful introduction of an agent into the population, then predictable patterns may not exist. Sobel and Watson (2009) provide clues to be used when trying to determine the existence of bioterrorism. These clues are simplified and appear in the How To box entitled "Recognize the Epidemiologic Clues That May Signal a Covert Bioterrorism Attack."

HOW TO Recognize the Epidemiologic Clues That May Signal a Covert Bioterrorism Attack

- Large number of ill persons with similar disease or syndrome
- Large number of unexplained disease, syndrome, or deaths
- Unusual illness in a population
- Higher morbidity and mortality than expected with a common disease or syndrome
- Failure of a common disease to respond to usual therapy
- Single case of disease caused by an uncommon agent
- Multiple unusual or unexplained disease entities coexisting in the same person without other explanation
- Disease with an unusual geographic or seasonal distribution
- Multiple atypical presentations of disease agents
- Similar genetic type among agents isolated from temporally or spatially distinct sources
- Unusual, atypical, genetically engineered, or antiquated strain of agent
- Endemic disease with unexplained increase in incidence
- Simultaneous clusters of similar illness in noncontiguous areas, domestic or foreign
- Atypical aerosol, food, or water transmission
- Ill people presenting at about the same time
- Death or illness among animals that precedes or accompanies illness or death in humans
- No illness in people not exposed to common ventilation systems, but illness among those people in proximity to the systems

Steps in an Investigation

First confirm whether a real disease or condition outbreak exists or if there has been a false alarm. Review the information available about the situation. Determine the nature, location, and severity of the problem. Verify the diagnosis and develop a case definition to estimate the magnitude of the problem; this may change as new information is made available. Compare current incidence (number of new cases) with the usual or baseline incidence. Use local data if available and compare them with the literature, or call the state health department. Assess the need for outside consultation. Report the situation to state public health authorities if required. Check the state reportable disease list. Early and continually changing control measures should be used on the basis of the magnitude and nature of the condition (infectious disease, chronic disease, injuries, personal behaviors, environmental exposure). Control measures may include eliminating a contaminated product, modifying procedures, treating carriers, or immunizing those who might contract the infectious disease. A request should be made that laboratory specimens be saved until the investigation is completed (if applicable to the case definition).

CHECK YOUR PRACTICE

You are working at the health department and the hospital emergency department has reported to you that they have seen 16 patients, of various ages, who have been admitted in the last two hours with complaints of nausea, vomiting, severe abdominal cramping, and diarrhea. When questioned, all of the patients report eating at a local fast-food restaurant within the last 24 hours. As you are on a team at the health department to investigate this, what should you do?

HOW TO Conduct an Investigation

- Confirm the existence of an outbreak.
- Verify the diagnosis and/or define a case.
- Estimate the number of cases.
- Orient the data collected to person, place, and time.
- Develop and evaluate a hypothesis.
- Institute control measures and communicate findings.

Centers for Disease Control and Prevention: *Steps to investigation*, 2014. Retrieved July 2018 from http://www.cdc.gov.

As the investigation continues, seek additional cases and collect critical data and specimens. Encourage immediate reporting of new cases from laboratory reports (e.g., radiology in cases of pneumonia) and physicians and other health care providers, including public health nurses, health care agencies, and others in the community as appropriate. In addition, search for other cases that may have occurred in the past or are now occurring by reviewing laboratory reports, medical records, and patient charts and questioning physicians, other health care providers and agencies, and others in the community. Use a specific data collection form such as a questionnaire or a data abstract summary form. Characterize the cases by person, place, and time. Evaluate the client characteristics (i.e., age, sex, underlying disease, geographic location) and possible exposure sites. The place where the outbreak occurs provides clues to the population at risk. Did the problem occur in a community, school, or homes? Drawing tables or spot maps helps to

TABLE 22.2 Potential Epidemiologic Factors That Call for Increased Investigation or Monitoring

Factors	Reason
Disease located in one geographic area	Might indicate a point source of a disease agent that can be discovered and controlled
Severe symptoms/diagnoses such as encephalitis or death	Indicates disease process that needs rapid investigation because of severity
Rapid rise to very high numbers of illness two to three times normal baseline with steep epidemic curve	Potential for continuing rapid rise in numbers; requires immediate investigation to institute control measures
Outbreak detected and confirmed by multiple data sources	Unlikely to be attributable to error; possibly widespread
Outbreak occurring at an unusual time or place (e.g., respiratory/influenza-like symptoms in summer)	Might indicate targeted population or early signs in a susceptible population (e.g., very young or very old)
Outbreak confined to one age or gender group	Might indicate targeted population or early signs
Number of cases continuing to rise over time	Indicates sustained outbreak that might continue to grow

From Andersson T, Bjelkmar P, Hulth A, et al.: Syndromic surveillance for outbreak detection and investigation. *Online J Public Health Inform* 5:e78, 2013.

visualize the clusters of the disease condition in specific areas of the community. The exact time period of the outbreak or an occurrence is important (be sure to go back to the first case or first indication of outbreak or an occurrence activity). Given the diagnosis, describe what appears to be the period of exposure. Record the date of onset of morbidity/mortality cases and draw an epidemic curve. Determine whether the outbreak/condition originates from a common source or is propagated. Table 22.2 suggests factors to monitor and explains the reasons for their use. It provides clues to the use of time, place, and person.

As the investigation continues, develop a tentative hypothesis (the best guess about what is happening). Do a quick evaluation of the outbreak by assessing previous findings. Record, tabulate, and review data collected from the previously described activities to summarize common agent, environment, host factors, and exposures. On the basis of this analysis (and literature review if necessary), develop a hypothesis (best guess) on (1) the likely cause, (2) the source(s), and (3) the mode of transmission of the disease. The hypothesis should explain the majority of cases. Frequently, there will be concurrent cases not explained by the hypothesis that may be related to endemic or sporadic cases, a different disease or condition (similar symptomatology), or a different source or mode of transmission.

Test your hypothesis with other public health team members (e.g., epidemiologists). Many investigations do not reach this stage because of lack of available personnel, lack of severity of the problem, and lack of resources available. Situations that should be studied include disease or events associated with a commercial product, disease or events associated with considerable morbidity and/or mortality, and disease or events associated with environmental exposures (e.g., terrorist attack). Analyze data collected to determine sources of transmission and risk factors associated with disease/condition. Determine how this problem differs in incidence or exposure for other population groups. Refine the hypothesis (best guess) and carry out additional studies if necessary.

Evaluate the effects of control measures. Cases may cease to occur or return to endemic (normal) level. If the control interventions do not produce change, return to the beginning and start the investigation over or reevaluate cases. Use the opportunity of an outbreak to review and correct practices related to the current situation that may contribute to an outbreak in the future.

Communicate findings to those who should be notified. Communication of findings may take two forms: an oral briefing for local authorities or a written report. Describe the problem, the data collected, the case definition with verification of the diagnosis, data sources, the hypothesis, and testing of the hypothesis. Present only the facts of the situation, the data analysis, and the conclusions.

DISPLAYING OF DATA

Reporting of data in an investigation needs to be valid: Does the event reported reflect the true event as it occurs? It must also be reliable: Is the same event reported consistently by different observers? A number of tools can be used to display data according to time, place, or person. The spatial map shows where the event is occurring and allows prevention resources to be targeted. Fig. 22.1 provides a map of the location of reported cases of hepatitis A in the United States. From looking at this map, priority prevention target areas appear to be Georgia, the District of Columbia, California, New Mexico, Kansas, and Florida. Table 22.3 shows the number of cases of an infectious disease compared by month and year over four years. In this table, cases have increased by year with a serious outbreak in

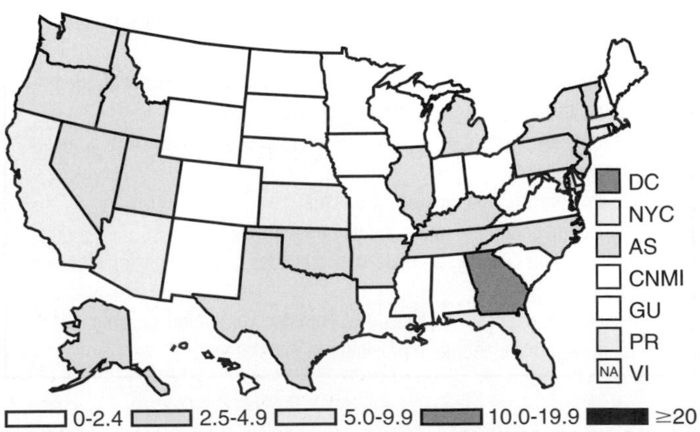

Fig. 22.1 Hepatitis A cases reported in the United States and U.S. territories in one year.

TABLE 22.3 Example of Ways to Display Data[a] or Number of Clients With Hepatitis A, by Month, for Four Years

	Year 1	Year 2	Year 3	Year 4
January	12	20	21	16
February	14	19	26	19
March	7	21	8	27
April	12	10	11	13
May	5	0	11	0
June	4	11	1	6
July	5	5	9	8
August	5	9	12	7
September	6	7	13	8
October	15	8	10	70
November	?	8	11	0
December	0	11	20	0
Total	85	129	153	174

[a]This table shows the number of persons who match a case definition of a select infectious disease over a four-year period. Note that for Year 4, there were overall more cases, especially in March and October, with a serious outbreak in October. This is a simple display of the raw data which can help show changes over time.

Modified from Centers for Disease Control and Prevention: Notifiable diseases and mortality tables. *MMWR* 63(28):ND-382-ND-395, July 18, 2014. Retrieved from http://www.cdc.gov.

October of Year 4. When cases are reported by person, they are usually reported by a person's characteristics. Data displays are a step in analysis that shows graphically what is happening. It reduces the assumptions made about the event and provides a means for describing the event using quantitative data. Data help in stating your hypothesis or your best guess about what is happening (refer to the CDC website for additional information on outbreak investigations). Fig. 22.2 shows another way to display data. This histogram depicts suspected meningitis cases over a seven month period.

LEVELS OF PREVENTION

Surveillance Activities

Primary Prevention

Develop an approach for mass immunizations of citizens to prevent the occurrence of H1N1 (H1N2 or H3N3) in the community.

Secondary Prevention

Investigate an outbreak of flulike illness in a local school.

Tertiary Prevention

Provide health care and treatment for those infected by H1N1 or the new strains of the virus.

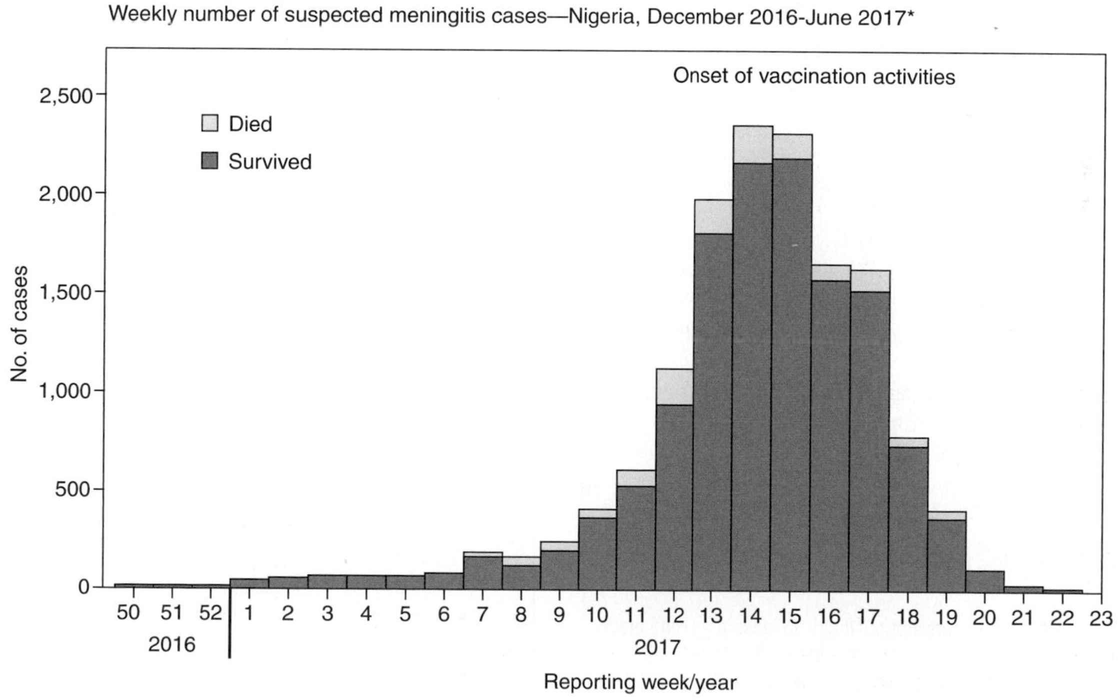

*Reporting week 15 corresponds to April 16-22, 2017; week 21 corresponds to June 4-10, 2017.

Fig. 22.2 Weekly number of suspected meningitis cases—Nigeria, December 2016-June 2017. This is an example of displaying data in a histogram. It shows the number of cases on the vertical axis, and the horizontal axis shows the cases per week of about 22 weeks, and the numbers of survivors for each week and the numbers of the deceased per week. (From Centers for Disease Control and Prevention: Large outbreak of *Neisseria meningitides* serogroup C—Nigeria, December 2016-June 2017. *MMWR* 66(49):1352–1356. Retrieved from https://www.cdc.gov.)

LINKING CONTENT TO PRACTICE

Remember that disease and event surveillance systems exist to help improve the health of the public through the systematic and ongoing collection, distribution, and use of health-related data. A nurse can contribute to such systems and best use the data collected through such systems to help manage endemic health problems and those that are emerging, such as evolving infectious diseases and bioterrorist (human-made) health problems. Functions of surveillance and investigation include detecting cases, estimating the impact of disease or injury, showing the national history of a health condition, determining the distribution and spread of illness, generating hypotheses, evaluating prevention and control measures, and facilitating planning (CDC, 2018g; McNabb et al., 2016). Response to bioterrorism or large-scale infectious disease outbreak may require the use of emergency public health measures such as quarantine, isolation, closing public places, seizing property, mandatory vaccination, travel restrictions, and disposal of the deceased. In 2008 in preparation for a projected H1N1 flu epidemic, information was distributed about the use of several of these interventions, including isolation and closure of public places (see Appendix XX).

Suggestions for protecting health care providers from exposure include use of standard precautions when coming into contact with broken skin or body fluids, the use of disposable nonsterile gowns and gloves followed by adequate hand washing after removal, and the use of a face shield (CDC, 2018g).

The Robert Wood Johnson Foundation (RWJF) funded a project initiative focusing on the development of competencies and resources to enhance the ability of nursing professionals to deliver high-quality and safe nursing care. The Quality and Safety Education for Nurses (QSEN) collaboration identified and defined six quality and safety competencies for nursing. In addition, the project allowed for the development of proposed targets for the knowledge, skills, and attitudes of students for each of the six competencies that were identified by the Institute of Medicine as client-centered care, teamwork and collaboration, evidence-based practice, quality improvement, safety, and informatics. The overall goal for the QSEN project is to meet the challenge of preparing future nurses who will have the knowledge, skills, and attitudes (KSAs) necessary to continuously improve the quality and safety of the health care systems within which they work. This chapter focuses on the importance of using informatics to identify, monitor, and intervene in unusual occurrences and events to protect the public and to keep communities safe (see Chapter 24 for further discussion of quality management).

Informatics in the QSEN project is defined as the use of information and technology to communicate, manage knowledge, mitigate error, and support decision making. The knowledge requirement for the public health nurse and student is to explain why information and technology skills are essential for safety. The skill to be developed is the seeking of education about how information is managed in the setting before providing an intervention. This chapter applies this by looking at trends of occurrences and events before investigating the situation and deciding on an intervention. It is also important to be able to use the databases and the tools of investigation to ensure safe processes of care. The attitude of engaging in continuous learning and the development of new technology skills is essential. In the case of influenza pandemic and to assist community residents in being safe during such an outbreak, the How To box entitled "Plan for Pandemic Flu, Using a Planning Checklist for Individuals and Families" provides steps for assisting individuals and families in preparation for such an occurrence.

HOW TO Plan for Pandemic Flu, Using a Planning Checklist for Individuals and Families

Nurses are responsible for assisting clients by providing them the means for safety. One of the roles of the nurse, to assure safety, is to assist clients in being prepared for an occurrence or an event in an emergency and urgent situations that could compromise their health status or health outcomes. Following is a checklist to assist individual and family clients in preparing for a pandemic. Although this presents a process in preparation for pandemic flu this process may be used in other communicable disease outbreaks that may reach pandemic proportions.

Use this as a guide to educate clients if an epidemic or pandemic is forecast.

Prepare for an influenza pandemic as soon as it is forecast. Prepare clients with the knowledge of both the magnitude of what can happen during a pandemic outbreak and what actions can be taken to help lessen the impact of an influenza pandemic on the client(s). This checklist helps to gather the information and resources needed in case of a flu pandemic.

1. To plan for a pandemic; the client(s) will want to:
   - Store a two-week supply of water and food.
   - During a pandemic, if client(s) cannot get to a store, or if stores are out of supplies, it will be important to have extra supplies on hand.
   - This can be useful in other types of emergencies, such as power outages and disasters.
   - Periodically check regular prescription drugs to ensure a continuous supply at home.
   - Have nonprescription drugs and other health supplies on hand, including pain relievers, stomach remedies, cough and cold medicines, fluids with electrolytes and vitamins.
2. To limit the spread of germs and prevention infection:
   - Teach children to wash hands frequently with soap and water, and suggest that family members model the current behavior.
   - Teach children to cover coughs and sneezes with tissues, and be sure to model that behavior in families.
   - Teach children to stay away from others as much as possible if they are sick.
   - Encourage family members to stay home from work and school if sick.
3. Items to have on hand for an extended stay at home:
   - Examples of food and nonperishables
     - Ready-to-eat canned meats, fish, fruits, vegetables, beans, soups
     - Protein or fruit bars
     - Dry cereal or granola
     - Peanut butter or nuts
     - Dried fruit
     - Crackers
     - Canned juices
     - Bottled water
     - Canned or jarred baby food and formula
     - Pet food
   - Examples of medical, health, and emergency supplies
     - Prescribed medical supplies such as glucose and blood pressure–monitoring equipment
     - Soap and water, or alcohol-based (60-95 percent) hand wash
     - Medicines for fever, such as acetaminophen or ibuprofen
     - Thermometer
     - Anti-diarrheal medication
     - Vitamins
     - Fluids with electrolytes
     - Cleansing agent/soap
     - Flashlight
     - Batteries
     - Portable radio
     - Manual can opener
     - Garbage bags
     - Tissues, toilet paper, disposable diapers

Excerpted and adapted from the Centers for Disease Control and Prevention: *Get your household ready for pandemic flu*, 2017. Available at https://www.cdc.gov.

PRACTICE APPLICATION

As a clinical project, the health department asked the public health nursing class at the university to develop a community service message to air on local radio about the potential of a pandemic flu outbreak. What does the message need to contain to help the community prepare?

Answers can be found on the Evolve site.

KEY POINTS

- Disease surveillance has been a part of public health protection since the 1200s during the investigations of the bubonic plague in Europe.
- Surveillance provides a means for nurses to monitor disease trends to reduce morbidity and mortality and to improve health.
- Surveillance is a critical role function for nurses practicing in the community.
- Surveillance is important because it generates knowledge of a disease or event outbreak patterns.
- Surveillance focuses on the collection of process and outcome data.
- Although surveillance was initially devoted to monitoring and reducing the spread of infectious diseases, it is now used to monitor and reduce chronic diseases and injuries, as well as environmental and occupational exposures.
- Surveillance activities can be related to the core functions of public health assessment, policy development, and assurance.
- A quality surveillance system requires collaboration among agencies and individuals.
- The Minnesota model of *Public Health Interventions: Applications for Public Health Nursing Practice* (Minnesota Department of Health, 2001) suggests that surveillance is one of the interventions related to public health nursing practice.
- Clinicians, health care agencies, and laboratories report cases to state health departments.
- Data also come from death certificates and administrative data such as discharge reports and billing records.
- Each of the data sources has the potential for underreporting or incomplete reporting. However, if there is consistency in the use of surveillance methods, the data collected will show trends in events or disease patterns that may indicate a change needed in a program or a needed prevention intervention to reduce morbidity or mortality.
- The sentinel surveillance system provides for the monitoring of key health events when information is not otherwise available or for calculating or estimating disease morbidity in vulnerable populations.
- Reporting of disease data by health care providers, laboratories, and public health workers to state and local health departments is essential if trends are to be accurately monitored.
- Requirements for reporting diseases are mandated by law or regulation.
- Surveillance systems in use today are defined as passive, active, sentinel, and special.
- Any unusual increase in disease incidence (i.e., new cases) or an unusual event in the community should be investigated.
- Patterns of occurrence can be identified when investigating a disease or event. These patterns are used to define the boundaries of a problem to help investigate possible causes or sources of the problem.
- Factors that must be considered as causes of outbreak are categorized as agents, hosts, and environmental factors.
- An unusual increase in disease incidence should be investigated.
- Functions of surveillance and investigation include detecting cases, estimating the impact of disease or injury, showing the natural history of a health condition, determining the distribution and spread of illness, generating hypotheses, evaluating prevention and control measures, and facilitating planning.

CLINICAL DECISION-MAKING ACTIVITIES

1. Call the local health department and attend an emergency response team planning meeting. How many agencies are involved? Determine the roles of each agency. Does the nurse have a role on the team? Explain.
2. Go to the Health Hazard Evaluation program website. What is the purpose of this program? How would information from the website be used in a disease investigation?
3. Explain the purpose of applying the sentinel system to improve population health outcomes.

ADDITIONAL RESOURCES

EVOLVE WEBSITE

http://evolve.elsevier.com/Stanhope/community/

- Answers to Practice Application
- Case Study
- Glossary
- Review Questions

REFERENCES

Association of Public Health Nurses (APHN): *The role of the public health nurse in disaster preparedness, response, and recovery: a position paper,* APHN Public Health Preparedness Committee, 2014. Retrieved from http://www.achne.org.

Blazes DL, Lewis SH: *Disease surveillance—technology contributions to global health security,* Boca Raton, FL, 2016, CRC Press.

Brownson RC, Baker EA, Deshpande AD, Gillespie KN: *Evidence-based Public Health,* ed 3, New York, 2018, Oxford University Press.

Centers for Disease Control and Prevention (CDC): *Public health preparedness and response core competency model,* 2010. Retrieved from https://www.cdc.gov.

Centers for Disease Control and Prevention (CDC): *Bioterrorism overview,* 2012a. Retrieved from http://emergency.cdc.gov.

Centers for Disease Control and Prevention (CDC): CDC's vision for public health surveillance in the 21st century, *MMWR Morb Mortal Wkly Rep* 61(Suppl), 2012b. Retrieved from http://www.cdc.gov.

Centers for Disease Control and Prevention (CDC): *Emergency and Terrorism Preparedness for Environmental Health Practitioners,* 2013. Retrieved from http://www.cdc.gov.

Centers for Disease Control and Prevention (CDC): *2014 National Notifiable Infectious Diseases,* 2014a. Retrieved from http://www.cdc.gov.

Centers for Disease Control and Prevention (CDC): *Introduction to public health Surveillance 101 Series,* Atlanta, GA, 2014b. U.S. Department of Health and Human Services, CDC. Retrieved from http://www.cdc.gov.

Centers for Disease Control and Prevention (CDC): *Public health 101 series: Introduction to public health surveillance,* 2014c. Retrieved from https://www.cdc.gov.

Centers for Disease Control and Prevention (CDC): *Steps to investigation,* 2014d. Retrieved from http://www.cdc.gov.

Centers for Disease Control and Prevention (CDC): *Cases of Ebola diagnosed in the United States,* 2014e. Retrieved from http://www.cdc.gov.

Centers for Disease Control and Prevention (CDC): *National Notifiable Disease Surveillance System (NNDSS),* 2015a. Retrieved from https://www.cdc.gov.

Centers for Disease Control and Prevention (CDC): *Outbreak response and prevention branch, Division of Foodborne, Waterborne, and Environmental Diseases (DFWED),* 2015b. Retrieved from http://www.cdc.gov.

Centers for Disease Control and Prevention (CDC): *Surveillance Resource Centers,* 2015c. Retrieved from https://www.cdc.gov.

Centers for Disease Control and Prevention (CDC): *Chemical emergencies,* 2016a. Retrieved from https://emergency.cdc.gov.

Centers for Disease Control and Prevention (CDC): *Lesson 6: investigating an outbreak,* 2016b. Retrieved from https://www.cdc.gov.

Centers for Disease Control and Prevention (CDC): *Nationally notifiable infectious diseases: United States,* 2016c, CDC. Retrieved from https://www.cdc.gov.

Centers for Disease Control and Prevention (CDC): *Preparation & planning. Emergency Preparedness and Response,* 2016d. Retrieved from https://emergency.cdc.gov.

Centers for Disease Control and Prevention (CDC): *Syndromic surveillance (SS),* 2016e. Retrieved from http://www.cdc.gov.

Centers for Disease Control and Prevention (CDC): *Bioterrorism,* 2017a. Retrieved from https://emergency.cdc.gov.

Centers for Disease Control and Prevention (CDC): *Emergency Preparedness and Response: Bioterrorism,* 2017b. Retrieved from https://emergency.cdc.gov.

Centers for Disease Control and Prevention (CDC): *National Biomonitoring Program: Chemical threat agents,* 2017c. Retrieved from https://www.cdc.gov.

Centers for Disease Control and Prevention (CDC): *National Electronic Disease Surveillance System (NEDSS) Base System (NBS),* 2017d. Retrieved from https://www.cdc.gov.

Centers for Disease Control and Prevention (CDC): *NETSS,* 2017e. Retrieved from https://www.cdc.gov.

Centers for Disease Control and Prevention (CDC): *National Notifiable Disease Surveillance System (NNDSS): Surveillance case definitions for current and historical conditions,* 2017f. Retrieved from https://www.cdc.gov.

Centers for Disease Control and Prevention (CDC): *CDC current outbreak list,* 2018a. Retrieved from https://www.cdc.gov.

Centers for Disease Control and Prevention (CDC): *CDC WONDER,* 2018b. Retrieved from https://wonder.cdc.gov.

Centers for Disease Control and Prevention (CDC): *Division of Health Informatics and Surveillance,* 2018c. Retrieved from https://www.cdc.gov.

Centers for Disease Control and Prevention (CDC): *Foodborne outbreaks: List of selected multistate foodborne outbreak investigation,* 2018d. Retrieved from https://www.cdc.gov.

Centers for Disease Control and Prevention (CDC): *Improving public health surveillance data,* 2018e. Retrieved from https://www.cdc.gov.

Centers for Disease Control and Prevention (CDC): *National Center for Health Statistics. National Vital Statistics Reports,* 2018f. Retrieved from https://www.cdc.gov.

Centers for Disease Control and Prevention (CDC): *National Notifiable Diseases Surveillance System (NNDSS),* 2018g. Retrieved from https://www.cdc.gov.

Centers for Disease Control and Prevention (CDC): *National Notifiable Diseases Surveillance System (NNDSS): Data collection and reporting,* 2018h. Retrieved from https://www.cdc.gov.

Centers for Disease Control and Prevention (CDC): *National Notifiable Disease Surveillance System (NNDSS): Why we do notifiable disease surveillance,* 2018i. Retrieved from https://www.cdc.gov.

Centers for Disease Control and Prevention (CDC): *National Syndromic Surveillance Program (NSSP): NSSP Overview,* 2018j. Retrieved from https://www.cdc.gov.

Centers for Disease Control and Prevention (CDC): *NNDSS—2018 National Notifiable Conditions,* 2018k. Retrieved from https://www.cdc.gov.

Centers for Disease Control and Prevention (CDC): *Public health preparedness and response 2018 national snapshot,* 2018l. Retrieved from https://www.cdc.gov.

Centers for Disease Control and Prevention (CDC): *The National Institute for Occupational Safety and Health (NIOSH),* 2018m. Retrieved from https://www.cdc.gov.

Center for Disease Control and Prevention (CDC): *Viral hepatitis: 2017—Outbreaks of hepatitis A in multiple states among people who use drugs and/or people experiencing homelessness,* 2018n. Retrieved from https://www.cdc.gov.

Centers for Disease Control and Prevention (CDC): *National Program of Cancer Registries (NPCR),* 2018o. Retrieved from https://www.cdc.gov.

Council on Linkages between Academia and Public Health Practice: *Core competencies for public health professionals,* Washington, DC, 2014, The Council. Retrieved from http://www.phf.org.

Goldthwaite LM, Duca L, Johnson RK, et al.: Adverse birth outcomes in Colorado: assessing the impact of a statewide initiative to prevent unintended pregnancy, *Am J Public Health* 105:e60–e66, 2015.

Gostin LO, Wiley LF: *Public Health Law and Ethics: A Reader,* ed 3, Oakland, CA, 2018, University of California Press.

Gould DW, Walker D, Yoon PW: The evolution of BioSense: lessons learned and future directions, *Public Health Rep* 132(Suppl 1): 7S–11S, 2017.

Kimble, LE, Massoud MR, Heiby J: *Using quality improvement to address hospital-acquired infections and antimicrobial resistance*, AMR Control, 2017. Retrieved from http://resistancecontrol.info.

Latshaw MW, Degeberg R, Patel SS, et al.: Advancing environmental health surveillance in the U.S. through a national human biomonitoring network, *Int J Hyg Environ Health*, 220(2, PT A):98–102, 2017.

McNabb S, Conde JM, Ferland L, et al.: *Transforming public health surveillance—proactive measures for prevention, detection, and response*, Jordan, 2016, Elsevier.

Maravi, ME, Snyder LE, McEwen LD, DeYoung K, Davidson AJ: Using spatial analysis to inform community intervention strategies, *Biomed Inform Insights* 9:1178222617700626. 2017.

McNabb SJN, Conde JM, Ferland L, et al., editors: *Transforming public health surveillance: proactive measures for prevention, detection, and response*, Amman, Jordan, 2016, Elsevier.

Merrill RM: *Introduction to epidemiology*, ed 7, Burlington, Mass, 2017, Jones & Bartlett.

Minnesota Department of Health: *Division of Community Health Services, Public Health Nursing Section: Public Health Interventions -Applications for Public Health Nursing Practice*, 2001. Retrieved from http://www.health.state.mn.us.

Michaud J, Kates J: *The Latest Ebola Outbreaks: What Has Changed in the International and U.S. Response Since 2014?* Kaiser Family Foundation, 2018. Retrieved from www.kff.org.

Nmadu PM, Peter E, Alexander P, et al.: The prevalence of malaria in children between the ages 2–15 visiting Gwarinpa General Hospital Life-Camp, Abuja, Nigeria, *J Health Sci* 5:47–51, 2015.

Perlman SE, McVeigh KH, Thorpe LE, Jacobson L, Greene CM, Gwynn RC: Innovations in population health surveillance: using electronic health records for chronic disease surveillance, *Am J Public Health* 107(6):853–857, 2017.

Public Health Nursing Section: *Public health interventions: applications for public health nursing practice*, St Paul, Minnesota, 2001, Public Health Nursing Section.

Quad Council Coalition Competency Review Task Force: *Community/Public Health Competencies*, 2018. Retrieved from http://www.quadcouncilphn.org.

Richards CL, Iademarco MF, Atkinson D, et al.: Advances in public health surveillance and information dissemination at the Centers for Disease Control and Prevention, *Public Health Rep* 132(4):403–410, 2017.

Ryan J: *Biosecurity and bioterrorism*, ed 2, Cambridge MA, 2016, Elsevier.

San Diego County: *Health and Human Services: San Diego Hepatitis A Outbreak*, 2018. Retrieved from https://www.sandiegocounty.gov.

Shannon K: *Suspicious biological outbreaks: benefits of conducting joint law enforcement and public health investigations*, October 15, 2015, National Association of County & City Health Officials, Preparedness Brief. Retrieved from http://nacchopreparedness.org.

Sobel J, Watson JC: Intentional Terrorist contamination of food and water. In Lutwick SM, Lutwick LI, editors: *Beyond Anthrax: The Weaponization of Infectious Diseases*, ed 2, New York, 2009, Springer.

Sorour K, Nuzzo E, Tuttle M, et al.: Addition of bacitracin and cranberry to standard Foley care reduces catheter-associated urinary tract infections, *Can J Infect Control* 3:166–168, 2016.

U.S. Department of Health and Human Services: *Healthy People 2020: a roadmap for health*, Washington, DC, 2010, U.S. Government Printing Office.

U.S. Department of Homeland Security: *Chemical Threats*, n.d. Retrieved from https://www.ready.gov.

Veenema TG: *Disaster nursing and emergency preparedness for chemical, biological, and radiological terrorism and other hazards*, ed 3, New York, 2013, Springer.

World Health Organization (WHO): *Integrated disease surveillance and response*, 2018a. Retrieved from http://www.who.int.

World Health Organization (WHO): *EBOLA Response Roadmap Situation Report Update*, 2014a: Retrieved from http://apps.who.int.

23

Program Management

Catherine Carroca, MSN, RN, Lisa M. Turner, PhD, RN, PHCNS-BC, and Marcia Stanhope, PhD, RN, FAAN

OBJECTIVES

After reading this chapter, the student should be able to do the following:

1. Compare and contrast the program management process and the nursing process.
2. Analyze the application of the program planning process to nursing.
3. Critique a program planning method to use in nursing practice.
4. Analyze the components of program evaluation methods, techniques, and sources.
5. Compare different types of cost studies applied to program management.

CHAPTER OUTLINE

Definitions and Goals
Historical Overview of Health Care Planning and Evaluation
Benefits of Program Planning
Assessment of Need
Planning Process
Program Evaluation
Advanced Planning Methods and Evaluation Models
Program Funding

KEY TERMS

case registers, p. 517
community assessment, p. 502
community health planning, p. 499
cost studies, p. 509
evaluation, p. 499
evidence-based practice, p. 505
formative evaluation, p. 498
grant writing, p. 518
health program planning, p. 503
outcome, p. 517
planning, p. 499
planning process, p. 509
population needs assessment, p. 502
process, p. 517
program, p. 499
program effectiveness, p. 499
program evaluation, p. 499
program management, p. 498
projects, p. 499
quality assurance, p. 509
strategic planning, p. 501
structure, p. 517
summative evaluation, p. 498
tracers, p. 517

Program management consists of assessing, planning, implementing, and evaluating a program. This chapter focuses primarily on planning and evaluation. Although presented in separate discussions, these factors are related and interdependent processes that work together to bring about a successful program. This chapter does not address implementing programs because other chapters in this text focus on implementation.

The program management process is parallel to the nursing process. One process is applied to a program that addresses the needs of a specific population, whereas the other process is applied to individuals or families. The process of program management, like the nursing process, consists of a rational decision-making system designed to help nurses know when to make a decision to develop a program (through the needs assessment and defining the problem), where they want to be at the end of the program (goal setting), how to decide what encompasses a successful program (planning), how to develop a plan to go forward so they will know where they want to be (implementing), how to know that they are getting there (**formative evaluation**), and what to measure to know that the program has successful outcomes (**summative evaluation**).

Today there is a greater need for the nurse to be accountable for nursing actions and client outcomes. Prospective payment systems, pay for performance, health care reform, and integrated care delivery models have changed the focus of nursing. Planning for nursing services is necessary today if the nurse is to survive in the health care delivery field. Nurses are expected to demonstrate leadership in addressing community-based health problems.

This chapter examines how nurses can act, instead of react, by planning programs that can be evaluated for their effectiveness. The discussion focuses on the historical development of health planning and evaluation, a general program planning and evaluation method, the benefits of planning and evaluation, the elements of planning and evaluation, how cost studies are applied to program evaluation, and how programs may be funded. Some sections of this chapter can be used by undergraduate students, whereas other sections are more appropriately used by graduate students.

DEFINITIONS AND GOALS

Community health planning is population focused, and it positions the well-being of the public to promote health equity, community empowerment, and social justice above private interests (American Planning Association, 2018; American Public Health Association, 2018). A **program** is an organized approach to meet the assessed needs of individuals, families, groups, populations, or communities by reducing the effect of or eliminating one or more health problems. Community health programs are planned to meet the needs of designated populations or subpopulations in a community. Many programs exist as specific efforts within the umbrella of large, complex organizations such as state health departments, universities, health systems, and private organizations such as insurance companies. Unlike these complex organizations, smaller programs are endeavors that focus on more specific services and communities or groups. Specific examples in population-focused nursing are home health, immunization and infectious disease programs, health-risk screening for industrial workers, and family planning programs. These are usually conducted under the direction of the total plan of a local health department, a managed care agency, or, in some instances, an insurance company. Examples of more complex broadly based group and community programs are the community school health, occupational health and safety, environmental health, and community programs directed at preventing specific illnesses through special-interest groups (e.g., American Heart Association, American Cancer Society, March of Dimes). Disaster preparedness is a type of program that may be conducted through collaborative efforts of several community organizations or agencies.

Programs are ongoing organized activities that become part of the continuing health services of a community or organization, whereas **projects** are smaller, organized activities with a limited time frame. A health fair and a blood pressure screening day at the mall are examples of projects that nurses may implement.

Planning is defined as the selecting and carrying out of a series of activities designed to achieve desired improvements (Issel & Wells, 2018). The *goal* of planning is to ensure that health care services are acceptable, equal, efficient, and effective. Planning provides a blueprint for coordination of resources to achieve these goals.

Evaluation is determining whether a service is needed and can be used, whether it is conducted as planned, and whether the service actually helps people in need (Royse, 2016). Evaluation is a process of accountability. Evaluation for the purpose of assessing whether objectives are met or planned activities are completed is referred to as *formative* or *process evaluation.* This type of evaluation begins with an assessment of the need for a program and involves ongoing monitoring of the activities conducted by the program. Evaluation to assess program outcomes or as a follow-up of the results of the program activities is called *summative* or *impact evaluation.*

Program evaluation is an ongoing, systematic process that begins during the planning phase and continues until the program ends. It is used to make evidenced-based judgments about improving, managing, and continuing programs. The major goals of program evaluation are to determine the relevance, adequacy, progress, efficiency, effectiveness, impact, and sustainability of program activities (Issel & Wells, 2018; USDHHS, 2011).

HISTORICAL OVERVIEW OF HEALTH CARE PLANNING AND EVALUATION

As the health care delivery system has grown during the last century, emphasis on health planning and evaluation has increased. Factors that have intensified interest in planning and evaluation are advances in health care technology and consumer education, escalating health care costs, increased consumer expectations, third party payers, focus on health care as a business, personnel shortages, unionizing of health care workers, professional conflicts, focus on preventive care, recognition of increasing health disparities, and the threats from terrorism, natural disasters, and emerging infectious diseases. From the 1920s to the 1940s, specific actions were initiated that related to health planning. Table 23.1 outlines the development of health planning.

The post–World War II era brought an interest in evaluating **program effectiveness**. As government and third-party payers began to finance health care services and money became more plentiful, public demand for health services grew. As a result, numbers and kinds of health care agencies increased; laws were passed to increase the scope of and control over health care, and the health care delivery system began to be held accountable for its actions. During this time, legislation was passed to require health care providers and consumers to work together in groups to address issues in health care.

Through the 1970s, laws were passed to provide more comprehensive structure and more power over federal program funds. In 1974 Congress enacted the National Health Planning and Resources Development Act. This legislation had the goal of reducing the growth of health care costs by ensuring that only needed services and facilities would be added to the health care system. Under this legislation, health care providers were required to obtain a certificate of need (CON) in order to add services or facilities. However, very little authority existed to carry out some of the more critical tasks of improving the health of clients, increasing access and quality of services,

TABLE 23.1 Historical Development of Health Planning and Evaluation

Year	Initiator	Action-Purpose
Late 1800s	Lumber, railroad, mining, and other industry	Contract with providers for health care to maintain health of workers.
1920	Committees on administrative practice and evaluation of American Public Health Association	Called for public health officers to engage in better program planning. Reduced haphazard methods used to develop public health programs.
1920s	Committee on costs of medical care	Studied social and economic aspects of health services. Cited the need for comprehensive health care planning because of rising costs and unequal health care services to target populations.
1921	Congress	Sheppard-Towner Act on Maternity and Infancy provided first continuing program of federal grants-in-aid for state health departments to provide direct care. States established maternal-child divisions with the funding.
1930s	Federal government, Congress	Blue Cross Insurance founded for provision of prepayment for hospital services in response to Great Depression and increased cost of health care.
1935	Federal government, Congress	Social Security Act passed. This was an early movement to provide resources for the elderly and impoverished.
1944	American Hospital Association	Established committee on postwar planning.
1946	Federal government, Congress	Passed the Hospital Survey and Construction Act (Hill-Burton Act) to legislate health planning, which resulted in increase in number of hospitals.
1963	Federal government, Congress	Community Mental Health Centers Act (PL 88-464) passed to provide mental health programs in the states; defined the role of consumers in making decisions and of professionals as advisors in the planning process.
1965	U.S. Department of Health and Human Services	Office of Health Planning opened; no direct authority for health planning given.
1965	Federal government, Congress	Passed regional medical program legislation (PL 89-239); upgraded quality of tertiary health care services for the leading causes of death. Coined the term *Partnership for Health.*
1966	Federal government, Congress	Passed the Comprehensive Health Planning (CHP) and Public Health Services amendments (Public Law 89-749). Developed a national health planning system.
Late 1960s to early 1970s	Individual state legislation	Certificate of Need established as a check against duplication of services. Limited new construction, plant modernization, and major technology.
1973	President Nixon	Government encouragement for health maintenance organizations (HMOs) for prepaid health insurance with emphasis on preventive health efforts.
1974	Federal government, Congress	Passed National Health Planning and Resources Development Act (Public Law 93-641), which provided specific directions for developing the structure, process, and functions of a national health planning system.
1980	U.S. Department of Health and Human Services	Began *Healthy People* initiative. Support for national level assessment, data collection, analysis, goal setting, and evaluation for the U.S. population.
1982	Congress	Tax Equity and Fiscal Responsibility Act (TEFRA) imposed financial cuts to Medicare and Medicaid and directed the Department of Health and Human Services (DHHS) to instill a prospective payment system for hospitals. Capitation through prospective payment was created with diagnosis-related groups (DRGs).
1993	President Clinton	Introduced Health Security Act to provide for health care reform and planning based on population needs (not passed).
2000	Congress	Home Health Prospective Payment System placed capitation on Medicare home health expenses based on clinical assessment of recipients using the Outcome and Assessment Information Set (OASIS).
2001	Congress	Creation of Department of Homeland Security following the terrorist attacks of September 11, 2001. Consolidated selected government departments into one entity for providing national security.
2004	CDC	Development of guidelines for distribution of flu vaccine to the U.S. population following flu vaccine recall.
2005	Hurricane Katrina	This natural disaster on the Gulf Coast and New Orleans shed light on deficiencies of government for emergency planning at local, state, and national levels.
2010	President Obama	Passage into law of the Patient Protection and Affordable Care Act (Public Law 111-148).

CDC, Centers for Disease Control and Prevention.

restraining costs, and preventing the duplication of unnecessary services. Power over the private health care sector continued to be absent.

As "the new federalism" became the catch phrase of the 1980s and emphasis was placed on shifting costs, reducing costs, and providing more competition within the health care system, President Ronald Reagan proposed eliminating the federal government's role in health planning. In 1981, with cutbacks in federal spending, states began the takeover or dismantling of their own health planning systems. The national health planning system came to a halt. The federal, state, and consumer partnership for health care was ended.

In an attempt to provide equitable health care, in 1993, President Bill Clinton sent the Health Security Act to congress. The Act was opposed by both the health care industry and the health insurance industry and was declared dead by the end of 1993 (Griffin, 2017). The government, however, would use its power to set limits on health insurance costs and limit overall health care spending. In this way, it would influence health planning decisions made by the private health care agencies and providers (Sparer & Thompson, 2015). Although national health care reform did not occur, many states engaged in reforming their systems. President Clinton was successful in signing the Health Insurance Portability and Accountability Act (HIPAA) and the Children's Health Insurance Program (CHIP) into law (Griffin, 2017).

Today, in the early years of the twenty-first century, the process of health planning is not coordinated but is for the most part in the control of different interests in the health care industry. The health care system has been mainly shaped by decisions of hospitals, physicians, pharmaceutical companies, equipment companies, insurance companies, and managed care organizations, which determine where, how, and for whom health care will be delivered. Although the federal health planning legislation is no longer in effect, some states continue to have health system agencies (HSAs), even though these organizations have much less authority than when they were established in the 1970s. In some states, the HSA must approve the planned expanding of agencies or services, and a CON must be issued by the state before these plans may proceed. The primary purpose of such health planning is to improve the health of local communities by increasing available and accessible services, preventing the duplication of services, and controlling health care costs.

The political party in power often influences the outcome of the national and state health planning efforts. An example of this was the passage of the Affordable Care Act, led by President Obama and the Democratic party in March 2010, which addresses planning at national, state, and local levels (PL 111-148). The American Nurses Association (2018) reports numerous activities nurses participated in related to the health care reform effort (see https://www.nursingworld.org).

To impact the direction of health care reform now and in the future, nurses must always be involved in all aspects of health planning for the community in which they live.

In addition to health planning in the external environment, internal health care agency planning is necessary to meet the goals and objectives of providing efficient, effective health care services to clients at a reasonable cost. Health care planning within the community and national health care planning affect health planning within an agency. For example, following the attack on the World Trade Center in 2001, there was much emphasis on developing national and community health plans for emergency preparedness and to prevent terrorism. In a comprehensive reorganization of the federal government, President George W. Bush created the Department of Homeland Security. This reorganization consolidated 22 federal agencies into a single department with the goal of protecting America from terrorism. In addition, states and communities have been given federal monies to develop their own plans. Agencies within communities were charged to develop emergency preparedness plans and to be a part of community plans.

Public health personnel have a responsibility to participate in internal planning and evaluation to solve the problems of a client population and to ensure the delivery of health services that are accessible, acceptable, and affordable. Emphasizing population health means focusing on the health outcomes of a group of persons, including the health outcome distribution in that group (Robert Wood Johnson Foundation [RWJF], 2017).

BENEFITS OF PROGRAM PLANNING

Systematic planning for meeting the health needs of populations in a community has benefits for clients, nurses, employing agencies, and the community. It ensures that available resources are used to address the actual needs of people in the community, and it focuses attention on what the organization and health provider are attempting to do for clients. Planning assists in identifying the resources and activities that are needed to meet the objectives of client services. It also reduces role ambiguity (uncertainty) by giving responsibility to specific providers to meet program objectives (Issel & Wells, 2018).

Furthermore, planning reduces uncertainty within the program environment and increases the abilities of the provider and the agency to cope with the external environment. Everyone involved with the program can anticipate what will be needed to implement the program, what will occur during the implementation process, and what the program outcomes will be. Planning helps the provider and the agency anticipate events. Also, planning allows for quality decision making and better control over the actual program results by setting specific goals, examining those goals regularly to determine whether the agency continues with the existing programs or makes changes based on the needs of the population they serve. Today, this type of planning is referred to as **strategic planning**, and it involves the successful matching of client needs with specific provider strengths and competencies and agency resources.

Managers of programs engage in *management planning*. This type of planning assists managers to determine whether the resources of the agency are used properly to actually implement the agency programs. The type of planning emphasized in this chapter is the program planning process (Kettner et al., 2017). This planning process shifts from a focus on the agency as a unit to one aspect of the agency. Program planning reflects the desire to implement a reality-based program that can be readily evaluated and can reduce the number of unexpected events that occur in a defined population. There can be numerous programs within an agency, and each needs to engage in program planning and evaluation. A major national program to assist communities to plan, organize, and develop programs specific to their needs is the Centers for Disease Control and Prevention's program planning model (CDC, 2014).

ASSESSMENT OF NEED

Planning for effective and efficient programs must be based on identifying the needs of populations within a community. Identification of at-risk groups and documentation of the health needs of the targeted population provide the basic justification and rationale for the proposed program plan. Such documentation of need is essential if funding will be required to implement the plan. Unless the program is totally voluntary, funding is most often required either from the agency that requires the program plan or the community at large. An assessment of health needs may be approached as either a community assessment or a population needs assessment.

QSEN FOCUS ON QUALITY AND SAFETY EDUCATION FOR NURSES

Targeted Competency: Quality Improvement

Uses data to monitor outcomes of care processes and uses improvement methods to design and test changes to continually improve quality and safety of health care systems.

- **Knowledge:** Describe approaches for changing processes of care
- **Skill:** Identify gaps between local and best practice
- **Attitude:** Value measurement and its role in good client care

QI Question

The Quad Council Coalition of Public Health Nursing Organizations has identified a beginning public health nurse (PHN) competency as policy development and program planning skills. The beginning PHN participates in developing organizational plans to implement programs and policies and participates as a team member. (2018). How could the new PHN best contribute to program management? What type of activity might the PHN participate in to determine gaps in existing programs?

Community Assessment

A thorough assessment of a community is necessary to provide a clear understanding of the overall health status of a community, to identify populations at risk, and to document health needs. Public health agencies, health planners, nurses, and agencies wishing to address the true needs of a community benefit from accurate and thorough community assessment data (The Community Toolbox, 2018; NACCHO, 2018).

A **community assessment** is comprehensive. It is a population-focused approach that views the entire community as the client. Community assessment considers all of the people in a community for the purpose of identifying the most vulnerable populations and determining unmet health needs. All of the services of a community are examined to assess their effect on the health of the population, and the environment is assessed for its impact on the health of the people. For example, some vulnerable groups may lack access to existing services because of lack of transportation, or there may be a high prevalence of asthma because of air pollution from a particular industrial source (see Chapter 17).

CHECK YOUR PRACTICE

As a student assigned to the local mayor's office, you have been asked to participate in completing an assessment of the community to identify the characteristics of the population of the community. What would you do? How would you approach this assignment?

Community assessment begins with the collection of existing data (secondary data). Variables related to the characteristics of the population in the community include demographic data such as age, sex, ethnic group/race, income, occupation, education, and health status. Such data, which for most communities are readily available on the Internet, are derived from census data and morbidity and mortality statistics. Much can be learned about a community through use of secondary data found on the Internet (UNC, 2017). In addition, data about communities may be found in local libraries, courthouse records, service agencies, newspapers, the phone book, and other local resources. Public health departments are also good sources of secondary data.

New data about the community may be collected through surveys or interviews with community members and key informants. When community members have a voice in clarifying norms and values of their community, in identifying needs, and in planning programs, community acceptance and use of that program are likely to be increased (The Community Toolbox, 2018).

Variables related to people, resources, and the environment of a community may be determined by using existing models that provide an organizing framework for the collection and analysis of data. (For more information about community assessment and the community-as-partner model, see Chapter 17.)

Population Needs Assessment

Agencies or health care providers are frequently interested in providing a specific service in a community and want to assess the need for that service in a target population. In this case, an assessment may be focused on determining the needs of a specific population in a community. Population health is the basis for doing the *assessment of need,* which is defined as a systematic appraisal of type, depth, and scope of problems as perceived by clients or health providers, or both (The Community Toolbox, 2018; NACCHO, 2018).

A **population needs assessment** focuses on the characteristics of a specific population, its health needs, and the resources available to address those needs. For example, a nurse may want to initiate a health education program for older adults with diabetes, to establish an immunization program for children of a certain age, or to provide health services for migrant workers. In each case, assessment would focus on the characteristics and health status of the target population and the resources

TABLE 23.2 Summary of Needs Assessment Tools

Name	Definition	Advantages	Disadvantages
Community forum	Community, group, organization, open meeting	Low cost Learn perspectives of large number of persons	Limited data Limited expression of views Discourages less powerful Becomes arena to discuss political issues
Focus groups	Open discussion with small representative groups	Low cost Clients participate in identification of need Initiates community support for the program	Time consuming Allows focus on irrelevant or political issues
Key informant	Identify, select, and question knowledgeable leaders	Provides picture of services needed	Bias of leaders Community characteristics may be incorrectly perceived by informants
Indicators approach	Existing data used to determine problem	Excellent data on problems and characteristics of client groups	Growth and change in population may make data outdated
Survey of existing agencies	Estimates of client populations via services used at similar community agencies	Easy method to estimate size of client group Know extent of services offered in existing programs	Records and data may be unreliable All cases of need may not be reported Exaggeration of services may occur
Surveys	Measurement of total or sample client population by interview or questionnaire	Direct and accurate data on client population and their problems	Expensive Technically demanding Need many interviews or observations Interviews may be biased

available to address the identified need for that group. When assessing a population, the same types of data collected for community assessment are collected and entered for the population, such as demographic data.

It is important to avoid planning services that do not focus on the health needs of the target population and services already provided by other agencies. A needs assessment determines gaps in or duplication of needed services (i.e., their availability), examines the quality of existing resources to meet the identified needs (i.e., their adequacy), and identifies barriers to the use of existing resources (i.e., their acceptability).

A number of needs assessment tools exist to assist the nurse in the needs assessment process. The major sources of information used for needs assessment, summarized in Table 23.2, are census data, key informants, community forums, surveys of existing community agencies with similar programs, surveys of residents of the community to be served (client population), and statistical indicators (Kettner et al., 2017).

Nurses working in community agencies who identify unmet needs among vulnerable populations can initiate program development and find funding to provide needed services and modify health disparities. For example, staff public health nurses in one community identified a need for schools to have more school health nurses, especially to meet the needs of unserved children in poverty. The nurses held a series of meetings with key informants, surveyed health departments of surrounding counties, and found an unknown source of funds through the state Medicaid program that would reimburse public health nurses for providing school health services. The result was the development of a program to increase the numbers of school health nurses in the community.

PLANNING PROCESS

Health program planning is affected by government control over licensure and funding by political forces, and by the culture and belief system of the population in which the program must function. Program planning is required by federal, state, and local governments; by philanthropic organizations; and by the employing agency. Planning programs and planning for the evaluation of programs are two very important activities, whether the program being planned is a national health insurance program such as Medicare, a state health care program such as an early childhood development screening program, or a local program such as vision screening for elementary school children. Regardless of the type of program, the planning process is the same.

Nutt (1984) described a basic planning process that is reflected in the steps of most planning methods and remains a great influence on strategic planning for population health and health programs today (Issel & Wells, 2018). The process includes five planning stages: formulating, conceptualizing, detailing, evaluating, and implementing (Table 23.3).

Basic Program Planning Model Using a Population-Level Example

Formulating. The initial and most critical step in planning a health program is defining the problem and assessing client need. This stage in the planning process can be *preactive,* projecting a future need; *reactive,* defining the problem based on past needs; *inactive,* defining the problem on the basis of the existing health state of the population to be served; or *interactive,* describing the problem using past and present data to project future population needs.

TABLE 23.3 Basic Planning Process

Basic Planning	Elements
1. Formulating	Client identifies problems.
2. Conceptualizing	Provider group identifies solutions.
3. Detailing	Client and provider analyze available solutions.
4. Evaluating (the plan)	Client, providers, and administrators select best plan.
5. Implementing	Best plan is presented to administrators for funding.

Needs assessment is a key component of the planning process in the formulating stage. The target population or client to be served by any program must be identified and involved in every stage of designing the program. To avoid duplication or gaps in services, program planners must verify that a current health problem exists and is being either ignored or unsuccessfully treated in a client group. Data provide the rationale to establish a new program or revise existing programs to meet the needs of the client group. The client population should be defined specifically by its demographic and psychosocial characteristics, by geographic location, and by problems to be addressed (Fig. 23.1).

For example, in a community with a large number of preschool children who require immunizations to enter school, the client population may be described as all children between 4 and 6 years of age residing in Central County who have not had up-to-date immunizations. A health education program may be necessary to alert the population to the existing need. In the example of the need for immunizing preschool children, public service announcements on television and radio and in newspapers may be used to alert parents to laws requiring immunizations, to the continuing problems with communicable diseases, and to the outcomes of successful immunizing programs, such as vaccination programs that have been successful in eliminating smallpox worldwide. A good example of the use of media can be found in a press release by the Centers for Disease Control and Prevention highlighting the threat of measles to health security locally and globally (CDC, 2013).

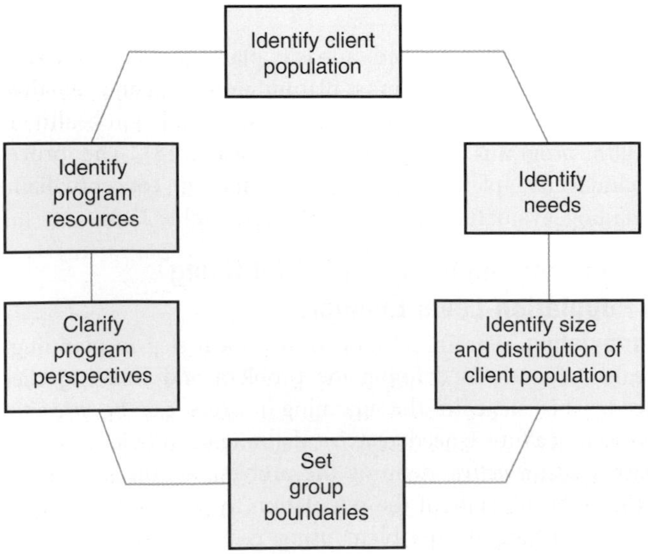

Fig. 23.1 Steps in the needs assessment process.

Specifying the size and distribution of a client population for a program involves more than counting the number of persons in the community who may be eligible for the program. It involves determining the number of persons with the problem who are not being served by existing programs and the numbers of eligible persons who have and have not taken advantage of existing services. For example, consider again the community need for a preschool immunization program. In planning the program, the size of the population of preschool children in the county may be obtained from census data or state vital statistics. The nurse then must determine the number of children unserved and the number of children who have not used services for which they are eligible. Today there are many opportunities to locate the unserved children through early start programs for preschool children.

Boundaries for the client population are primarily established by defining the size and distribution of the client population. The boundaries will stipulate who is included in and who is excluded from the health program. If the fictional immunization program were designed to serve only preschool children of low-income families, all other preschool children would be excluded.

Perspectives on the program, or what people think about the need for a program, might differ between health providers, agency administrators, policy makers, and potential clients. These groups are considered the stakeholders in the program. Collecting data on the opinions and attitudes of all persons, whether directly or indirectly involved with the program, is necessary to determine if the program is feasible, if there is a need to redefine the problems, or if a new program should be developed or an existing program should be expanded or modified. If a new or changed program is to be successful, it must not only be *available,* but also be *accessible* and *acceptable* to the people who will use it. For example, policy makers in the 1970s decided that neighborhood health clinics were the answer to providing services for low-income residents. They discovered that their perspective was not the same as those of most health providers and clients, who did not support development of neighborhood clinics.

The neighborhood health clinics have evolved over time to better reflect clients' perspectives. It is important for policy makers to explore the perspectives of the clients when planning the program. Clients might choose another type of service to offer rather than the one the policy maker or provider thinks best for them. The needs to be met for the client population must be identified by both the client and the health provider if the program is to be accepted by the client population. If the client population does not recognize the need, the program will usually be unsuccessful. Today community health centers have replaced the concept of the neighborhood health centers, and these centers are being supported and increased in number by health care reform (Rosenbaum et al., 2018).

Before implementing a health program, the nurse must also identify available resources. *Program resources* include financing, personnel, facilities, and equipment and supplies.

The source and amount of funds must be adequate to support the program. The number and kinds of personnel required and available must be determined. There must be a place for the program to operate, and up-to-date equipment and supplies are essential. If any one of the four categories of resources is unavailable, the program is likely to be inadequate to meet the needs of the client population. If planners consider the problem to be a critical one, funding may be sought by seeking donations or by writing a proposal for grant funds to support the program. A well-done assessment provides direction and suggests strategies for appropriate interventions (see the Evidence-Based Practice box).

EVIDENCE-BASED PRACTICE

Thorland et al. (2017) evaluated the impact of the Nurse-Family Partnership (NFP) program on status of breastfeeding and child immunization outcomes of the program participants. This home-visiting program serves first-time, low-income mothers, who are regularly visited by a specially trained registered nurse from the program. The nurse helps the mother receive the care and support needed for a healthy pregnancy, teaches responsible, competent child care (up to 2 years old), and supports the mother in becoming economically self-sufficient. The program participant data were compared to National Survey of Children's Health data and National Immunization Survey data. The researchers found that NFP clients were significantly more likely to have ever breastfed and maintain breastfeeding at 6 and 12 months, but less likely exclusively breastfeed at 6 months, compared to the national data. NFP clients were also significantly more likely to be up-to-date on immunizations at 6, 18, and 24 months (no significant difference at 12 months). The researchers concluded that NFP clients had more beneficial breastfeeding and immunization outcomes than children of mothers with similar demographic profiles; however, further improvement with exclusive breastfeeding at 6 months could be sought after.

Nurse Use

Nurse home-visiting programs for new, low-income mothers can positively impact breastfeeding and immunization outcomes of clients. Evaluating a program's impact on health outcomes provides evidence for continuing or discontinuing/changing the program in question. Nurses can teach leaders in the community how to identify and evaluate evidence-based prevention programs. By educating key stakeholders, community mobilization on priority health needs is strengthened.

From Thorland W, Currie D, Wiegand ER, et al.: Status of breastfeeding and child immunization outcomes in clients of the Nurse-Family Partnership. *Matern Child Health J* 21:439–445, 2017.

Conceptualizing. The need and demand for a program are determined through the formulating process. The conceptualizing stage of planning creates options for solving the problem and considers several solutions. Each option for program solution is examined for its uncertainties (risks) and consequences, leading to a set of outcomes. The outcomes sought are improvements in the health status of the population served by the program.

A first step in the conceptualizing process is a review of the literature to determine what approaches have been used in other places with similar problems, and with what success. Such review can assist nurses to improve the quality, effectiveness, and appropriate outcomes of health programs by combining the evidence and translating it into practice (**evidence-based practice**). Review of the literature should be guided by the following question: What can be learned from the experience of others in similar circumstances?

Some alternative solutions to the problem will have more risks or uncertainties than others. The nurse must decide between a solution that involves more risk and a solution that is free of risk. A "do nothing" decision is always the decision with the least risk to the provider. When choosing a solution, the nurse looks at whether the desired outcome can be achieved. After careful thought about each possible solution to the problem, the nurse rethinks the solutions. The assessment data compiled during the formulation stage should be used to develop alternative solutions.

Decision trees are useful graphic aids that give a picture of the solutions and the risks of each solution. Such a picture graph of the process of identifying a solution helps clients and administrators rank the consequences of a decision (Issel & Wells, 2018). Fig. 23.2 shows an example of a decision tree.

As shown in Fig. 23.2, the best consequence would be for each low-income child to be given flu immunization by their private physician. One must consider the value of this action to the person, the odds that immunizations will be obtained, the cost to families as opposed to the taxpayer, and the cost to the community. Costs to the community include the possibility of increased incidence of communicable disease or mortality and increased need for more expensive services to treat the diseases if vulnerable people are not immunized. Conversely, if families self-pay for the immunizations, costs to the taxpayer and to the community are low.

Detailing. In this phase, the provider, with client input, considers the possibilities of solving a problem using one of the solutions identified. The provider details (or is specific about) the costs, resources, and program activities needed to choose one of the solutions from the conceptualizing phase. For each of the three proposed alternatives shown in the immunization scenario in Fig. 23.2, the program planner lists the activities that would need to be implemented. Using the proposed solution of encouraging families to see their private physicians for the vaccine (the best consequence), examples of activities include developing a script for a health education program and implementing a television program to encourage parents to see a physician. If an alternative that produced the second, third, fourth, or fifth best consequence was chosen, offering a clinic at the health department or providing a mobile clinic to each daycare center to provide the immunizations would be possible activities.

For each alternative, the nurse lists the resources needed to implement each activity. The resources to be considered include all costs of personnel, supplies, equipment, and facilities, and the potential acceptance by the clients and the administrators of the program. In the example, personnel could include nurses, volunteers, and clerks; supplies might include handouts, Band-Aids, vaccines, records, and consent forms; equipment might include syringes, needles, stethoscopes, and blood pressure cuffs; and facilities might include a television studio for a media

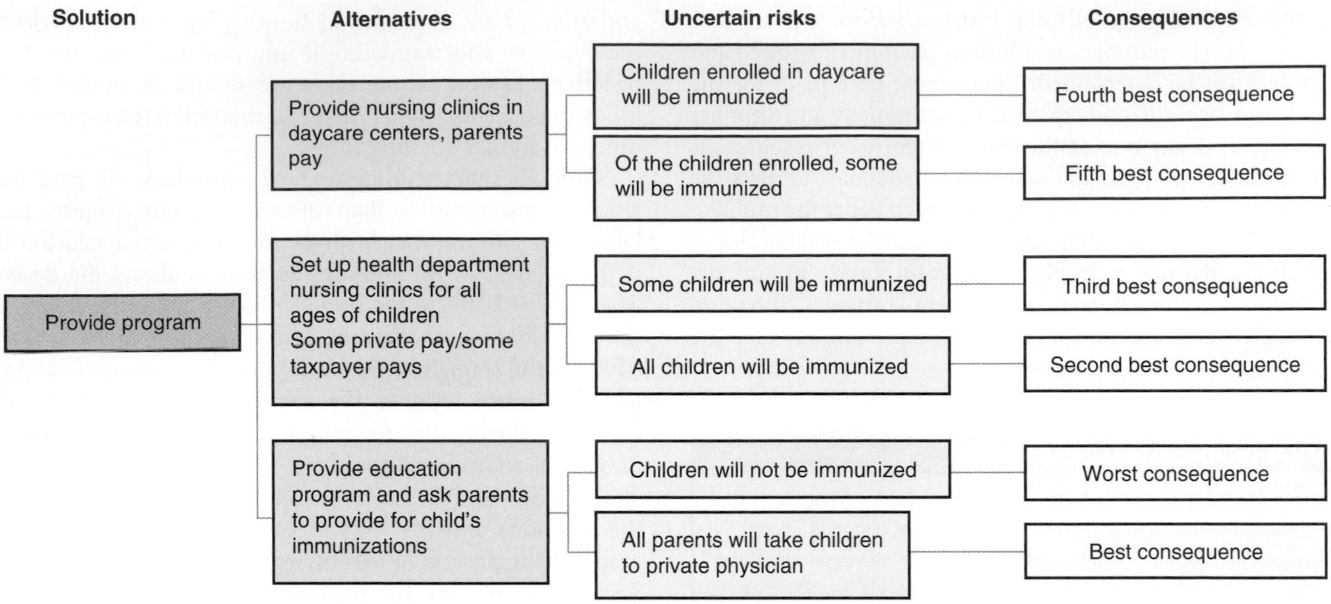

Fig. 23.2 Ranking of solutions to a problem: providing a preschool immunization program to low-income children using a decision tree.

blitz on the education program and a room with examination tables, chairs, and emergency carts. The total costs of each solution must be considered. As indicated, clients should review each solution for acceptance.

Evaluating. In the evaluation phase of the plan, each alternative is weighed to judge the costs, benefits, and acceptance of the idea to the client population, community, and providers. The information outlined in the detailing phase would be used to rank the solutions for choice by the client population and provider on the basis of cost, benefit, and acceptance. Consideration must be given to the solution that will provide the desired outcomes. Review of the literature or interviews might disclose whether someone else had previously tried each of the options in another place, and what costs and outcomes occurred. The experience of others in similar circumstances is helpful in deciding whether a chosen solution would be useful.

Implementing. In the planning process, the clients, providers, and administrators selected the best plan to solve the original problem. Providing reasons why a particular solution was chosen will help the provider get the approval of the agency administration for the plan. Once approved, the plan is implemented.

Implementation requires obtaining and managing the resources required to operationalize the program in a way that is consistent with the plan. Program implementation requires accountability and responsibility (Issel & Wells, 2018). Change theory can be useful to help create an environment in which the program is supported.

Community members may participate in implementing the program either as volunteers or as paid staff. Program success will be increased if community residents are included in the work of the program and if they are on advisory boards and participate in program evaluation. The greater the participation of community members in developing a program, the greater the sense of ownership of that program by members of the target population, and therefore the greater the probability that the program will achieve its objectives and result in positive changes in health (Issel & Wells, 2018).

Program management may be compared with the nursing process (Table 23.4). The nursing process is a standardized and systematic process utilized by nurses to ensure quality client care. The first and second steps of the nursing process involve accurate assessment and nursing diagnosis of the client. The client is then involved in the next step of planning and outcome identification with the nurse to ensure that realistic and appropriate goals are formulated. Nurses must then choose suitable interventions and implement them to achieve the goals that were set. The last step involves evaluation of the plan and carefully evaluates if the measurable goals were achieved.

Program management utilizes similar steps as the nursing process. Creating a successful program relies on careful assessment of the population or community to identify needs. All stakeholders should then be involved in the formulation of goals and outcomes. Appropriate interventions should be implemented to achieve the set goals and outcomes after careful consideration of the benefits, risks, and consequences. Lastly, evaluation must occur, in a formative and summative nature to ensure the intended goals and objectives for the program were met.

Objectives Development for Program Planning and Evaluation

The most important step in the planning and evaluation process is the writing of program objectives. The objectives provide direction for conducting the program, and they provide the mechanism for evaluating specific activities and the total program. The following discussion addresses the

TABLE 23.4 Comparison of the Nursing Process and Program Planning

Nursing Process	Basic Planning Process
Assessment Subjective and objective data are systematically collected.	**Formulation** Assess the client's need and define the problem.
Nursing Diagnosis Client's problem is defined by using the assessment data to guide the nurse in looking for similar patterns in the systematically collected subjective and objective data.	**Conceptualization** Provider group identifies solutions; each solution is examined for its risks, consequences, and expected outcomes.
Nursing Intervention Any direct care treatment or nursing action based on the nursing diagnosis is performed by a nurse and includes rationale that justifies the treatment or nursing action. Treatment or action is evaluated by the nurse for its appropriateness and acceptability to the client before implementation.	
Implementation Direct care treatment or nursing action established in the intervention is implemented.	**Detailing** Client and provider analyze solutions proposed in the conceptualizing phase for costs, resources, and program activities.
Evaluation Implementation of the nursing intervention is evaluated.	**Evaluation of the Plan** Client, providers, and administrators select best plan based on costs, benefits, and acceptability of the plan to the client and provider.
	Implementation Best plan (solution) based on input from the client and provider is presented to administration and implemented.
	Program Evaluation Implemented best plan (solution) is evaluated.

development of well-written objectives. Development of program objectives begins with the initial phases of program planning.

Specifying Goals and Objectives. A program may begin with a mission statement. This is a broad general statement of the overall conceptual framework or philosophy of the program. The mission statement clarifies the values and overall purpose of the program and provides a framework for the goals and objectives that follow.

A goal is a statement that describes the general direction of logical response to a demonstrated need. One or two goals are often sufficient for a program to state how it will resolve or lessen the problem defined in the need statement. The goals should be consistent with the values and overall intent set forth in the mission statement. Their purpose is to focus on the major reason for the program, to support the mission. The goals are also the basis for writing the objectives for the program and the action steps that reflect the overall goal accomplishment.

- Mission—statement of values
- Goal—overall aim
- Objectives—specific measurable outcomes
- Action steps—explicit actions to accomplish objectives

Objectives are concise statements describing in measurable and time-bound terms precisely what specific outcome is to be accomplished. *Measurable* means that the objective contains the specific outcome anticipated that could be documented with collectable data. *Time-bound* means that the objective contains the target date when the specific outcome will be accomplished. Objectives should be realistic and attainable means to meet the program goal (The Community Toolbox, 2018; UNC, 2017).

Clear, concise, and measurable objectives help with evaluating the program. If the objectives are too general, program evaluation becomes impossible. The objectives must be specific and stated so that anyone reading them could conduct the program without further instruction. The document *Healthy People 2020* (USDHHS, 2010) may be used as a template to guide the development of more specific objectives that are tailored to address the needs of a given community.

Useful program objectives include a statement of the specific behaviors that the program will accomplish, and success criteria, or expected results, for the program. Each program objective requires a *strong, action-oriented verb* to specify the behavior; *a statement of a single purpose; a statement of a single result;* and *a time frame for achieving the expected result.*

For example, a general program goal may be to reduce the incidence of low-birth-weight babies in Center County by 2020 by improving access to prenatal care. Several specific objectives are required to meet a general program goal. A specific objective for this program may be to open (action verb) a prenatal clinic in each health department within the county by January 2025 (time frame) to serve the population within each census tract of the county (purpose) to improve pregnancy outcomes (result).

As objectives are developed, an *operational indicator* for each objective should be considered so the evaluator knows when and if the objective has been met. For instance, an operational indicator for the previous objective would be a 10 to 25 percent increase in the use of prenatal care by women in Center County. Such indicators provide a target for persons involved with implementing programs. A review of *Healthy People 2020* health objectives will give the reader examples of objectives that include all the elements just listed.

Action steps are written for each program objective. An action step is defined as a concise statement describing precisely how (by what method), when, and by whom each activity will be accomplished to achieve the objective for which it was written. These activities address resources, such as number of nurses, equipment, supplies, and location. A time frame is planned for each activity. It is assumed that as each specific objective is met, progress is made toward achieving the general program objective (or goal) (Box 23.1).

BOX 23.1 Planning Programs for Elders in the Community

The Jefferson Area Board for Aging (JABA) has created a vision for the one-city, five-county planning district. In concert with 85 public and private organizations and more than 500 individuals, they developed a comprehensive community plan, known as the "2020 Community Plan on Aging." The plan started with a comprehensive community assessment that addressed the livability for elders in the community. The "2020 Community Plan on Aging" has been an asset for the community in providing guidance for specific programs at JABA and throughout the community. In September 2005 the city of Charlottesville and the surrounding counties were honored when presented with the U.S. Department of Health and Human Services, Administration on Aging (AOA), "Livable Communities for All Ages" award. Seven communities received the award for their model efforts to make their communities more supportive places to live and grow for seniors and all populations. The competition was administered by the Center for Home Care and Policy Research, Visiting Nurse Service of New York, with the participation of the American Planning Association and the International City/County Management Association.

Excerpted from Jefferson Area Board of Aging: *About JABA*, 2018. Available at http://www.jabacares.org. Accessed August 14, 2018.

HOW TO Develop a Program Plan

A. Define the problem
B. Formulate the plan
  1. Assess population need
    a. Who is the program population?
    b. What is the need to be met?
    c. How large is the client population to be served?
    d. Where are they located?
    e. How does the target population define the need?
    f. Are there other programs addressing the same need? (Describe.)
    g. Why is the need not being met?
  2. Establish program boundaries
    a. Who will be included in the program?
    b. Who will not be included? Why?
    c. What is the program goal?
  3. Program feasibility
    a. Who agrees that the program is needed (stakeholders: administrators, providers, clients, funders)?
    b. Who does not agree?
  4. Resources (general)
    a. What personnel are needed? What personnel are available?
    b. What facilities are needed? What facilities are available?
    c. What equipment is needed? What equipment is available?
    d. Is funding available to support the project? Is additional funding needed?
    e. Are resources being donated (space, printing, paper, medical supplies)?
      • *Type*
      • *Amount*
  5. Tools used to assess need
    a. Census data
    b. Key informants
    c. Focus groups
    d. Community forums
    e. Existing program surveys
    f. Surveys of client population
    g. Statistical indicators (e.g., demographic and morbidity/mortality data)
C. Conceptualize the problem
  1. List the potential solutions to the problem.
  2. What are the risks of each solution?
  3. What are the consequences?
  4. What are the outcomes to be gained from the solutions?
  5. Draw a decision tree to show the problem-solving process used.
D. Detail the plan
  1. What are the objectives for each solution to meet the program goal?
  2. What activities will be done to conduct each of the alternative solutions listed under C1 and based on objectives?
  3. What are the differences in the resources needed for each of the alternative solutions?
  4. Which of the alternative solutions would be chosen if the resources described under B4 were the only resources available?
  5. Who would be responsible or accountable for implementing the plan?
E. Evaluate the plan
  1. Which of the alternative solutions is most acceptable to the following:
    a. The client population
    b. The agency administrator
    c. You
    d. The community
  2. Which of the alternative solutions appears to have the most benefits to the following:
    a. The client population
    b. The agency administrator
    c. You
    d. The community
  3. On the basis of cost, which alternative solution would be chosen by the following:
    a. The client population
    b. The agency administrator
    c. You
    d. The community
F. Implement the program plan
  1. On the basis of data collected, which of the solutions has been chosen?
  2. Why should the agency administrator approve your request? Give a rationale.
  3. Will additional funding be sought?
  4. When can the program begin? Give date.

Developed by M. Stanhope and based on the Basic Program Planning Model (Issel & Wells, 2018; Nutt, 1984).

HEALTHY PEOPLE 2020

Example of* Healthy People 2020 *Goals for Program Planning

Focus Area	Overall Goal	Objective	Measuring the Objective
IID-23: Immunization and infectious diseases	Attain high-quality, longer lives free of preventable disease, disability, injury, and premature death.	IID-11: Increase routine vaccination coverage levels for adolescents.	IID: 11-1: Increase (action verb) to one dose of tetanus-diphtheria-acellular pertussis (Tdap) booster vaccine by 13 to 15 years (purpose) for 80 percent of this age group (operational indicator) by 2020 (time frame).

From U.S. Department of Health and Human Services: *Healthy People 2020: a roadmap for health,* Washington, DC, 2010, U.S. Government Printing Office.

PROGRAM EVALUATION

Benefits of Program Evaluation

Program evaluation is a method of ensuring that a program has met its goals (CDC, 1999; Issel & Wells, 2018). It is a means of documenting accountability by the program managers to the clients and the funding sources. The major benefit of program evaluation is that it shows whether the program is fulfilling its purpose and whether the program addresses merit or quality, worth or value (such as cost-effectiveness), and significance or importance (CDC, 1999; Issel & Wells, 2018). It should answer the following questions:

1. Are the needs for which the program was designed being met?
2. Are the problems it was designed to solve being solved?

This is critical information for program managers, funding agencies, top-level decision makers, program accreditation reviewers, health providers, and the community. Evaluation data are used to make judgments about a program and may be used to justify sustaining the program, making adjustments in the program, expanding or reducing the program, or even discontinuing it.

Process evaluation, also referred to as formative evaluation or the evaluation of implementation, occurs while the program is being implemented. This type of evaluation makes it possible to do mid-program corrections to ensure achievement of program goals. Designing the evaluation during the planning phase of the program allows the evaluation to be guided by the program goals (Issel & Wells, 2018). Brownson et al. (2018) describe process evaluation as an ongoing function of examining, documenting, and analyzing the progress of a program. Changes are required when there is an unacceptable difference between what was observed and what was anticipated from the implementation of program activities. Corrective action may then be taken to get the program back on track. This description of process evaluation is consistent with what the USDHHS (2011) referred to as implementation evaluation. Four critical questions are addressed when monitoring the implementation of a program (USDHHS, 2011): (1) Are the activities taking place, (2) who is conducting the activities, (3) who is reached through the activities, and (4) have sufficient inputs been allocated or mobilized (CDC, 1999; Issel & Wells, 2018)?

Quality assurance programs are prime examples of program evaluation in health care delivery. Evaluation data are used to justify continuing programs in public health. Program evaluation focuses on whether goals were met and the efficiency and effectiveness of program activities. Many methods of program evaluation are described in the literature. One of the primary methods of evaluation used in health care today is Donabedian's (1982; updated in 2003) classic evaluative framework, which examines the structure, process, and outcomes of a program. Other models and frameworks have been developed using this approach, such as the Structure-Process-Outcome (SPO) Framework for Quality Assessment in Nursing (Jones, 2016). The tracer method and case register are examples of other methods applied to program evaluation. (See Chapter 24 for further discussion.)

Program records and a community index serve as the major source of information for program evaluation. Surveys, interviews, observations, and diagnostic tests are ways to assess client and community responses to health programs. **Cost studies** help identify program benefits and objectiveness (refer to Chapter 5) (Issel & Wells, 2018).

As financial resources become scarce, nursing and the health care system must be able to justify their existence, prove that their services are responsive to client needs, and show their concern for being accountable. Planning and evaluation will assist in meeting these objectives.

Planning for the Evaluation Process

Planning for the evaluation process is an important part of program planning. When the **planning process** begins, the plan for evaluating the program should also be developed. All persons to be involved in implementing a program should be a part of the plan for program evaluation. Assessment of need is one component of evaluation. The basic questions to be answered, after carefully considering the data collected from a census, key informants, community forums, surveys, or health statistics indicators, are as follows:

1. Will the objectives and resources of this program meet the identified needs of the client population?
2. Is the program relevant?

Once need has been established and the program is designed, the nurse must continue plans for program evaluation. As a part of the planning process, Linfield and Posavac (2018) described six steps to use for continuing program evaluation (Fig. 23.3):

1. Identify the key people for evaluation. Program personnel, program funders, and the clients of the program should be included in planning for evaluation.

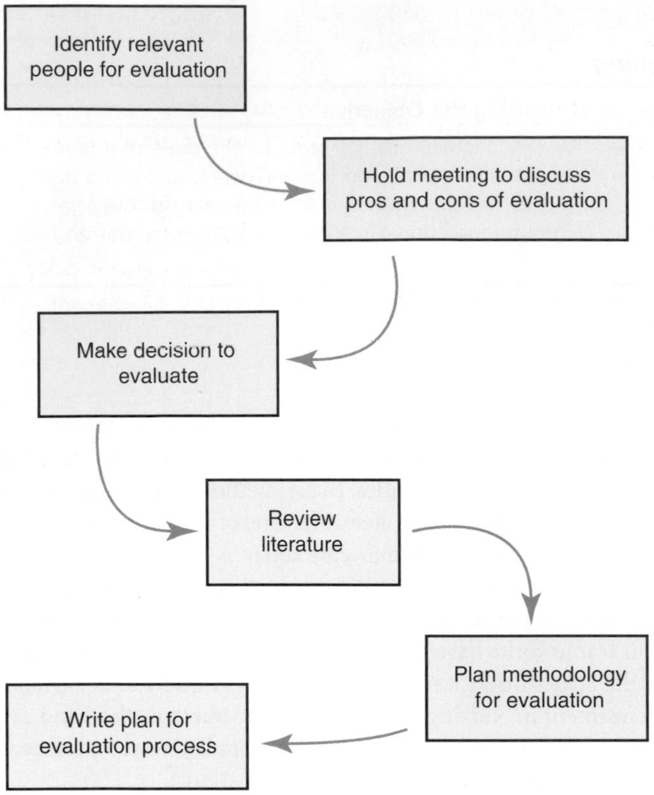

Fig. 23.3 Six steps in planning for program evaluation.

2. Arrange preliminary meetings to discuss the question of how the group wants to evaluate the program and where to start. If the program planners and others agree on an evaluation, the resources needed to do the evaluation must be identified. Evaluation is necessary even though some may not be interested in it. Nurses can help others see that without evaluation, money to support programs will not be available, or the need for a new nurse to help with the work cannot be justified. In health care today, there is great emphasis on outcomes of care. The only way to see outcomes is through evaluation.
3. After the key people have met and considered the questions in the previous steps, they are ready to begin the evaluation process. Even though evaluation may be desired, the decision to conduct the evaluation may be an administrative one, based on available resources and existing circumstances. For example, if a program evaluation were attempted in a situation in which program personnel wanted it but clients chose to be uncooperative, evaluation efforts would be unsuccessful.
4. Examine the literature for suggestions about the appropriate methods and techniques for evaluation and their usefulness in program evaluation. If an agency has chosen to use an external evaluator, this person may make suggestions about the questions to be answered in the evaluation process. These questions are based on the program goals. Nurses who have reviewed the literature and communicated with others affected by the evaluation can determine whether the evaluation suggestions are appropriate for the situation.
5. Plan the method to be used, including decisions about what goals and objectives will be measured, how they will be measured, and for what population.
6. Write a plan that outlines the mission and goals of the overall program, the type of evaluation to be done, the operational measures to be used to evaluate the program goals, the choice of who will do the evaluation (i.e., internal or external personnel), the available resources for conducting the evaluation, and the readiness of the organization, personnel, and clients for program evaluation. Nurses at all levels of education and preparation can participate in program planning and evaluation.

Evaluation Process

A framework for evaluation in public health has been developed by the Centers for Disease Control and Prevention (CDC) to guide understanding about program evaluation and to facilitate integration of evaluation in the public health system. This framework defines program evaluation as a systematic way to improve and to account for public health actions by using methods that are useful, feasible, ethical, and accurate. The purpose of utilizing this framework in program evaluation is to systematically summarize the essential elements, clarify steps, provide standards, and address misconceptions regarding the purposes and methods of program evaluation. Further, public health professionals can utilize the framework as they go through the steps of program evaluation in a systematic and organized way (Longest, 2015). Six interdependent steps are identified in Fig. 23.4 that must be part of an evaluation process (CDC, 1999; Issel & Wells, 2018):

1. *Engage stakeholders*—This includes those who are involved in planning, funding, and implementing the program, those who are affected by the program, and the intended users of its services.
2. *Describe the program*—The program description should address the need for the program and should include the

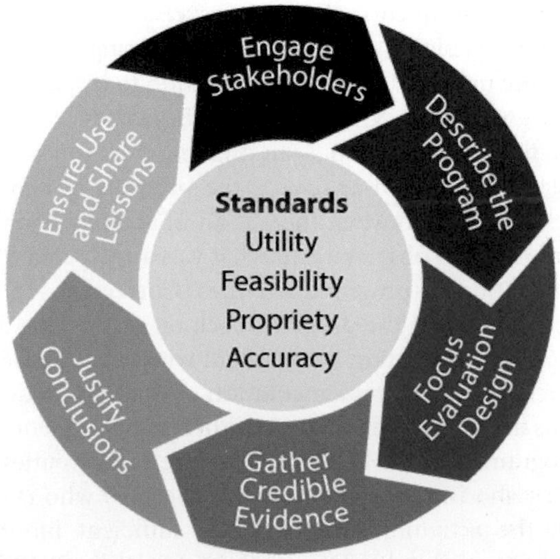
Engage Stakeholders
Describe the Program
Focus Evaluation Design
Gather Credible Evidence
Justify Conclusions
Ensure Use and Share Lessons
Standards
Utility
Feasibility
Propriety
Accuracy

Fig. 23.4 Visual picture of steps of program evaluation. (From Centers for Disease Control and Prevention: Framework for program evaluation in public health. *MMWR* 1999;48[No. RR-11], https://www.cdc.gov.)

mission and goals. This sets the standard for judging the results of the evaluation.

3. *Focus the evaluation design*—Describe the purpose for the evaluation, the users who will receive the report, how it will be used, the questions and methods to be used, and any necessary agreements.
4. *Gather credible evidence*—Specify the indicators that will be used, sources of data, quality of the data, quantity of information to be gathered, and the logistics of the data gathering phase. Data gathered should provide credible evidence and should convey a well-rounded view of the program.
5. *Justify conclusions*—The conclusions of the evaluation should be validated by linking them to the evidence gathered and then appraising them against the values or standards set by the stakeholders. Approaches for analyzing, synthesizing, and interpreting the evidence should be agreed on before data collection begins to ensure that all needed information will be available.
6. *Ensure use and share lessons learned*—Use and dissemination of findings require deliberate effort so that the lessons learned can be used in making decisions about the program

Sources of Program Evaluation

Both quantitative and qualitative methods may be used to conduct an evaluation; however, the strongest evaluation designs combine both qualitative and quantitative methods. Major sources of information for program evaluation are the program clients, program records, and community indexes.

Qualitative methods such as site visits, structured observations of interventions, or open-ended interviews may be used (Newcomer et al., 2015). The program participants, or clients of the service, have a unique and valuable role in program evaluation. Whether the clients, for whom the program was designed, accept the services will determine to a large extent whether the program achieves its goal. Thus, their reactions, feelings, and judgments about the program are very important to the evaluation. For example, to garner feedback from participants in a program, an evaluator may use a written survey in the form of a questionnaire or an attitude scale. Interviews and observations are other ways of obtaining feedback about a program. Attitude scales are probably used most often, and they are usually phrased in terms of whether the program met its objectives. The client satisfaction survey is an example of an attitude scale often used in the health care delivery system to evaluate the program objectives (Kelly et al., 2018). Client input into the development of evaluation tools ensures that the questions and approaches are more acceptable to the clients and that the tools effectively elicit the information needed.

The second major source of information for program evaluation is program records, especially clinical records. Clinical records provide the evaluator with information about the care given to the client and the results of that care. To determine whether a program goal has been met, one might summarize the data from a group of records. For example, if one overall goal were to reduce the incidence of low-birth-weight babies through prenatal care, records would be reviewed to obtain the number of mothers who received prenatal care and the number of low-birth-weight babies born to them. Records would be reviewed from the beginning of the program and at the end of a specific time frame, such as at the end of each year. Care must be taken to ensure that any review and use of clinical records complies with HIPAA regulations. (For details about HIPAA compliance, see https://aspe.hhs.gov.)

The third major source of evaluation is epidemiologic data. Mortality and morbidity data measuring health and illness are probably cited more frequently than any other single index for program evaluation. These health and illness indicators are useful in evaluating the effects of health care programs on the total community. Incidence and prevalence data are valuable indexes for measuring program effectiveness and impact, and these data are readily available on the Internet. Useful sites for such data include vital statistics available at state department of health sites, the CDC, and the U.S. Census site. Most counties and communities have their own sites, and many of these contain very useful demographic and health data.

An example of a national program based on a needs assessment of the U.S. population is the national health objectives program *Healthy People 2020* (USDHHS, 2010). *Healthy People* documents have been published every 10 years since 1980. The data gathered from each 10-year period have been used to evaluate the population needs met and the assessment of needs for the next *Healthy People* document.

The example shown in the *Healthy People 2020* box on p. 504 highlights injury and violence prevention. This box shows that objectives include an action verb, a result, an operational indicator, and a time frame for implementing the objective (10 years, begun in 2010).

The Levels of Prevention box provides examples of applying levels of prevention to program planning and evaluation.

Aspects of Evaluation

The aspects of program evaluation include the following (CDC, 1999; Issel & Wells, 2018):

1. *Relevance*——Need for the program
2. *Adequacy*—Program addresses the extent of the need
3. *Progress*—Tracking of program activities to meet program objectives
4. *Efficiency*—Relationship between program outcomes and the resources spent
5. *Effectiveness*—Ability to meet program objectives and the results of program efforts
6. *Impact*—Long-term changes in the client population
7. *Sustainability*—Enough resources to continue the program

The How To box suggests questions that may be asked about program evaluation using this process.

The following paragraphs provide an explanation of each step in program evaluation.

Relevance. Evaluation of relevance is an important component of the initial planning phase. As money, providers, facilities, and supplies for delivering health care services are more closely monitored, the needs assessment done by the nurse will determine whether the program is needed.

Adequacy. Evaluation of adequacy looks at the extent to which the program addresses the entire problem defined in the

HEALTHY PEOPLE 2020

Objectives Focus Areas

1. Access to Health Services
2. Adolescent Health
3. Arthritis, Osteoporosis, and Chronic Back Conditions
4. Blood Disorders and Blood Safety
5. Cancer
6. Chronic Kidney Diseases
7. Dementias, including Alzheimer's
8. Diabetes
9. Disability and Health
10. Early and Middle Childhood
11. Educational and Community-Based Programs
12. Environmental Health
13. Family Planning
14. Food Safety
15. Genomics
16. Global Health
17. Healthcare-Associated Infections
18. Health Communication and Health IT
20. Hearing and Other Sensory or Communication Disorders (Ear, Nose, Throat—Voice, Speech, and Language)
21. Heart Disease and Stroke
22. HIV
23. Immunization and Infectious Diseases
24. Injury and Violence Prevention
26. Maternal, Infant, and Child Health
27. Medical Product Safety
28. Mental Health and Mental Disorders
29. Nutrition and Weight Status
30. Occupational Safety and Health
31. Older Adults
32. Oral Health
33. Physical Activity and Fitness
34. Preparedness
35. Public Health Infrastructure
36. Respiratory Diseases
37. Sexually Transmitted Diseases
38. Sleep Health
40. Substance Abuse
41. Tobacco Use
42. Vision

Three other objectives are under development: numbers 19, 25, 39.

HIV, Human immunodeficiency virus; *IT,* information technology.
U.S. Department of Health and Human Services: *Healthy People 2020: a roadmap for health,* Washington, DC, 2010, U.S. Government Printing Office.

HEALTHY PEOPLE 2020

Example of a Measurable National Health Objective

In the *Healthy People* focus area of injury and violence prevention, one objective is:

- **IPV-5:** Increase (action verb) the number of states and the District of Columbia where 90 percent of deaths of children aged 17 years and under (operational indicator) due to external causes are reviewed by a child fatality review team (purpose), by 2020 (time frame).

U.S. Department of Health and Human Services: *Healthy People 2020: a roadmap for health,* Washington, DC, 2010, U.S. Government Printing Office.

LEVELS OF PREVENTION

Program Planning and Evaluation

Primary Prevention

Plan a community-wide program with the local school system and health department to serve healthy meals and snacks in all schools to promote good childhood nutrition.

Secondary Prevention

Develop screening programs for all school children to determine the incidence/prevalence of childhood obesity before implementing the program.

Tertiary Prevention

Evaluate the incidence/prevalence of obesity among school children after the implementation of the program and provide programs to reduce complications from the condition.

needs assessment. The magnitude of the problem is determined by vital statistics, incidence, prevalence, and expert opinion.

Progress. The monitoring of program activities, such as hours of services, number of providers used, number of referrals made, and amount of money spent to meet program objectives, provides an evaluation of the progress of the program. This type of evaluation is an example of formative or process evaluation, which occurs on an ongoing basis while the program exists. This provides an opportunity to make effective day-to-day management decisions about the operations of the program. Progress evaluation occurs primarily while implementing the program. The nurse who completes a daily or weekly log of clinical activities (e.g., number of clients seen in clinic or visited at home, number of phone contacts, number of referrals made, number of community health promotion activities) is contributing to progress evaluation of the nursing service.

Efficiency. If the reason for evaluation is to examine the efficiency of a program, it may occur on an ongoing basis as formative evaluation or at the end of the program as a summative evaluation. The evaluator may be able to determine whether the program provides better benefits at a lower cost than a similar program, or whether the benefits to the clients, or number of clients served, justify the costs of the program.

Effectiveness and impact. An evaluation of program effectiveness may help the nurse evaluator determine both client and provider satisfaction with the program activities, as well as whether the program met its stated objectives. However, if evaluation of impact is the goal, long-term effects such as changes in morbidity and mortality must be investigated. Both effectiveness and impact evaluations are usually summative evaluation functions primarily performed as end-of-program activities.

Sustainability. A program can be continued only if there are resources for the program. Ongoing evaluation of sustainability is important!

HOW TO Do a Program Evaluation

To do a program evaluation, first choose the type of evaluation you wish to conduct. Second, identify the goal and objectives for the evaluation. Third, decide who will be involved in the evaluation. Fourth, answer the questions related to the type of evaluation as follows:

A. Program relevance: needs assessment (formative)
   1. Use answers to all questions listed in section B of How To Develop a Program Plan.
   2. On the basis of the needs assessment, was the program necessary?

B. Adequacy
   1. Is the program large enough to make a positive difference in the problem/need?
   2. Are the boundaries of the services defined so that the problem/need can be addressed for the target population?

C. Program progress (formative)
   1. Monitor activities (circle which this reflects: daily, weekly, monthly, annually).
      a. Name the activities provided.
      b. How many hours of service were provided?
      c. How many clients have been served?
      d. How many providers are there?
      e. What types of clients have been served?
      f. What types of providers were needed?
      g. Where have services been offered (e.g., home, clinic, organization)?
      h. How many referrals have been made to community sources?
      i. Which sources have been used to provide support services?
   2. Budget
      a. How much money has been spent to carry out activities?
      b. Will more/less money be needed to conduct activities as outlined?
      c. Will changes to objectives and activities be needed to sustain the program?
      d. What changes do you recommend and why?

D. Program efficiency (formative and summative)
   1. Costs
      a. How do costs of the program compare with those of a similar program to meet the same goal?
      b. Do the activities outlined in C1 compare with the activities in a similar program?
      c. Although this program costs more/less than expected, is it needed? Why?
   2. Productivity (may use national or state averages for comparison)
      a. How many clients does each type of staff see per day (e.g., registered nurses, clinical nurse specialists, nurse practitioners)?
      b. How does this compare with similar programs?
      c. Although the productivity level of this program is low/high, is the program needed? Why?
   3. Benefits
      a. What are the benefits of the program to the clients served?
      b. What are the benefits to the community?
      c. Are the benefits important enough to continue the program? Why? (Look at cost, productivity, and outcomes of care.)

E. Program effectiveness (summative)
   1. Satisfaction
      a. Is the client satisfied with the program as designed?
      b. Are the providers satisfied with the program outcomes?
      c. Is the community satisfied with the program outcomes?
   2. Goals
      a. Did the program meet its stated goal?
      b. Are the client needs being met?
      c. Was the problem solved for which the program was designed?

F. Impact (summative)
   1. Long-term changes in health status (1 year or more)
      a. Have there been changes in the community's health?
      b. What are the changes seen (e.g., in morbidity or mortality rates, teen pregnancy rates, pregnancy outcomes)?
      c. Have there been changes in individuals' health status?
      d. What are the changes seen?
      e. Has the initial problem been solved or has it returned?
      f. Is new or revised programming needed? Why?
      g. Should the program be discontinued? Why?

G. Sustainability
   1. Was the program funded as a demonstration or by an external agency?
   2. Can money and resources be found to continue the program after the initial funding is gone?

Depending on the answers to the questions, the program can be found to be successful or unsuccessful.

Developed by Marcia Stanhope.

ADVANCED PLANNING METHODS AND EVALUATION MODELS

After a need and a client demand for a program have been determined through the needs assessment process, the next step in the development of the program is to choose a procedural method that will assist the nurse in planning the program to be offered. The following is offered for students who are more advanced in their career and need to consider several methods of program planning plus more extensive evaluation models for program management.

Five planning methods are discussed in this section:

1. Program planning method (PPM)
2. Multi-attribute utility technique (MAUT)
3. Planned Approach to Community Health (PATCH)
4. Assessment Protocol for Excellence in Public Health (APEXPH)
5. Mobilizing for Action through Planning and Partnerships (MAPP)

PPM is a more general approach to program planning, whereas MAUT offers guidelines for identifying and tracking specific program activities essential to program success. PATCH, APEXPH, and MAPP are PPMs that were designed by the CDC and the National Association of County Health Officials with input from local and state health departments. All of these approaches establish the basis for program evaluation.

Program Planning Method

PPM is a technique using the nominal group technique described by Delbecq and Van de Ven in 1971. The nurse can use this method to involve clients more directly in the planning process. PPM is a five-stage process to identify program needs. It focuses on three levels of planning groups composed of clients, providers, and administrators. The client or consumer group relays a list of problems to the provider group, who in turn aids the client group by presenting the solutions to the problems to the administrative group (Issel & Wells, 2018).

TABLE 23.5 Planning Methods Compared With Basic Planning Process

Basic Planning	PPM	PATCH	APEXPH	MAUT	MAPP
Formulating	Problems identified by client.	Community members identify health priorities.	Assess community capacity to address health problems.	Identify target populations and program objectives.	Assess community themes and strengths, health status, and strategic issues.
Conceptualizing	Provider group identifies solution.	Stakeholders use data to develop program activities.	Assess with community the strengths and health problems.	Identify alternative problem solutions.	Formulate goals and strategies.
Detailing	Analyze available solutions.	Design comprehensive program to meet identified health priorities.	Choose plan based on community capacity resources.	Identify criteria for choice; rank and weight; calculate value.	Develop plan for action; engage in visioning.
Evaluating	Clients, providers, and administrators select best plan.	Use process evaluation to improve program.	Support recommendations for program change.	Choose best alternatives.	Evaluate the plan.
Implementing	Best plan presented to administrators for funding.		Partners implement the plan.		Assess community ability to change and implement the plan.

APEXPH, Assessment Protocol for Excellence in Public Health; *MAPP,* Mobilizing for Action through Planning and Partnership; *MAUT,* multi-attribute utility technique; *PATCH,* Planning Approach to Community Health; *PPM,* program planning method.

The stages of PPM are compared with MAUT's planning process in Table 23.5. The five stages are as follows:

1. *Problem diagnosis.* Each client in the group works with all other members of the group to develop a written problem list, one problem at a time. After all problems have been shared and recorded, they are discussed by the total client group. After the discussion, clients select the problems with the highest priority by voting on the ranking of each problem.
2. *Expert provider group identifies solutions for each of the problems identified by the clients.*
3. *Client and provider groups present their problems and suggested solutions* to the administrative group to determine the possibilities of developing a program to resolve one or more of the problems using one or more of the solutions. In this phase, clients and providers are seeking acceptance from the administrators who control the program resources.
4. *Alternative solutions to the problem are identified,* and the pros and cons of each are analyzed.
5. *Clients, providers, and administrators select the best plan* for program implementation. In this phase, the link between the planned solutions and the problem is evaluated, pointing out strengths and limitations of the proposed program plan.

A nurse might use this technique for developing school health services within the total community or in one school. A nurse working with a senior citizens group might use this method to identify the priority needs for nursing clinic services at the health department. It is important to note that this method is used to obtain consensus among all persons involved in the program: clients, providers, and administrators. Consensus is most helpful in having a successful program. The process may also be used in a community decision-making activity in which community representatives come together to decide health care service needs for the entire community.

Multi-Attribute Utility Technique

MAUT is a planning method based on decision theory (Kabak & Ervural, 2017). This method can be adapted for making decisions about the care of a single client or about national health care programs (Claudio et al., 2014). The purpose of MAUT is to separate all elements of a decision and to evaluate each element separately for its effects on the overall decision, considering available options.

If money is no object, then the option with the highest use value is the best decision. However, if this option exceeds the budget, the next best option may be the alternative to choose. The steps of MAUT listed in Box 23.2 relate closely to the basic planning process described by Nutt (1984) as shown in Table 23.5.

Steps 1 and 2 of MAUT relate to problem formulating. Step 3 involves conceptualizing the program alternatives, and steps 4 through 9 focus on detailing and the implications of each option. Step 10 involves the evaluating phase of planning or the choice of the best solution as identified in steps 4 through 9. Placing quantitative values on solutions to meet program needs is most helpful in the implementing phase of planning (e.g., convincing administrators of the need for such a program). However, caution must be taken in using all planning methods, because the best solution reflects the bias of the planner.

Planning Approach to Community Health

The PATCH model, which has not been emphasized as much in recent years, was developed in the 1980s by the CDC with input from state and local health departments. The PATCH model was developed using as a framework the PRECEDE model developed by Laurence Green in the 1970s. The PRECEDE model was used for planning health education programs (Green & Kreuter, 1992; Glanz & Bishop, 2010).

Although this model was originally developed to strengthen health promotion activities, the PATCH model is used by communities and agencies to plan, develop, implement, and evaluate both health promotion and disease prevention programs. Application of PATCH emphasizes community participation

BOX 23.2 Ten Basic Steps of the Multi-Attribute Utility Technique (MAUT) Method

1. Identify the person or aggregate for whom a problem is to be solved. Who is the client for whom the program is being planned?
2. Identify the issue(s) or decision(s) that is (are) relevant. This step involves the identification of the program objectives.
3. Identify the options to be evaluated. The program planner identifies the available options or action alternatives to accomplish the program goals.
4. Identify the relevant criteria related to the value of each option. The program planner places a value on competing options or alternatives or identifies criteria to be considered in making a choice between them.
5. Rank the criteria in order of importance. The program planner decides which of the criteria are most important and which are least important for meeting program goals.
6. Rate criteria in importance. In this step the program planner assigns an arbitrary rating of 10 to the least important criterion. In considering the next least important criterion, the planner decides how many times more important it is than the least important criterion. If it is considered twice as important, the dimension will be assigned a 20. If it is only considered half as important, it will be assigned a 15. If it is considered four times as important, it will be assigned a 40. The process is continued until all criteria have been rated.
7. Add the importance rate, divide each by the sum, and multiply by 100. This process is called *normalizing* the weights. It is recommended that the number of criteria be kept between 6 and 15. Therefore, in this initial process, the planner can be concerned with only general criteria for choosing action alternatives.
8. Measure the location of the option being evaluated by each criterion. The planner may ask a colleague or expert to estimate on a scale of 0 to 100 the probability that a given option from step 3 will maximize the value of the criterion from step 4.
9. Calculate the use of options. The program planner will obtain the usefulness of each identified action alternative by multiplying the weight for each criterion (step 7) by the rating of an option for each criterion (step 8) and adding the products. The sum of the products for each action is termed the *aggregate utility*.
10. Decide on the best alternative to meet the program objective. The action alternative with the highest aggregate use is considered the best decision for meeting the program objectives.

Data from Kabassi K, Vroom M: MAUT and adaptive techniques for web based educational software. *Instruct Sci* 34(2):313–358, 2006.

and ownership by all who are involved. The PATCH process includes the following:

- Mobilizing the community
- Collecting and analyzing data to support local health issues
- Choosing health priorities
- Setting objectives and standards to denote progress and success
- Developing and implementing multiple intervention strategies to meet objectives
- Evaluating the process to detect the need for change
- Securing support of the public health infrastructure within the target community

These elements are essential to the success of any community-based program:

- Participation in the planning process by community members (stakeholders)
- Use of data to help stakeholders select health priorities and develop and evaluate program activities
- Development by stakeholders of a comprehensive approach to design the program to meet the identified health needs
- Use of process (formative) evaluation to improve the program and provide feedback to the stakeholders
- Increase in the capacity of the community to address a variety of health priorities by improving the health program planning skills of the stakeholders

The PATCH model has been useful in developing programs to address *Healthy People 2020* goals (www.healthypeople.gov). The PATCH framework and other commonly used models for decision making are available online at the CDC (https://www.cdc.gov).

Assessment Protocol for Excellence in Public Health

Following the development of the PATCH model in 1987, the CDC, partnering with the National Association of County and City Health Officials (NACCHO) and other organizations, developed its APEXPH model. The model was introduced for use in 1999.

The APEXPH model incorporates the three core functions of public health in assessment, assurance, and policy development. Although the model was developed for use by local health departments, it can be adapted to fit other situations and resources. The model framework includes the following:

- Process for assessing agency organization and management
- Process for working with communities to assess the health of a community as well as a community's strengths and health problems
- Process for integrating plans for resolving health problems based on the capacity, resources, and community members partnering to implement the plan

This model uses the strategic planning process of Nutt (1984) and has three elements:

1. Assessing internal organization capacity to address the community's health problems
2. Assessing and priority setting for the community's health problems
3. Implementing the plan to address these problems

Application of the APEXPH process is useful for the following:

- Supporting recommendations for change in programs/services
- Highlighting the need for improvements in program functions

If APEXPH is applied along with the project budget process, key stakeholders may unite to discuss health and program priorities and options for providing services as well as to make plans for the year (https://www.cdc.gov). Workbooks and other resources are available through NACCHO at their website (http://www.naccho.org).

Mobilizing for Action Through Planning and Partnership

MAPP is a strategic planning model that can be applied at the community level to improve the community's health. Application of this model helps to identify public health issues and priorities and to identify resources to address the priorities. As

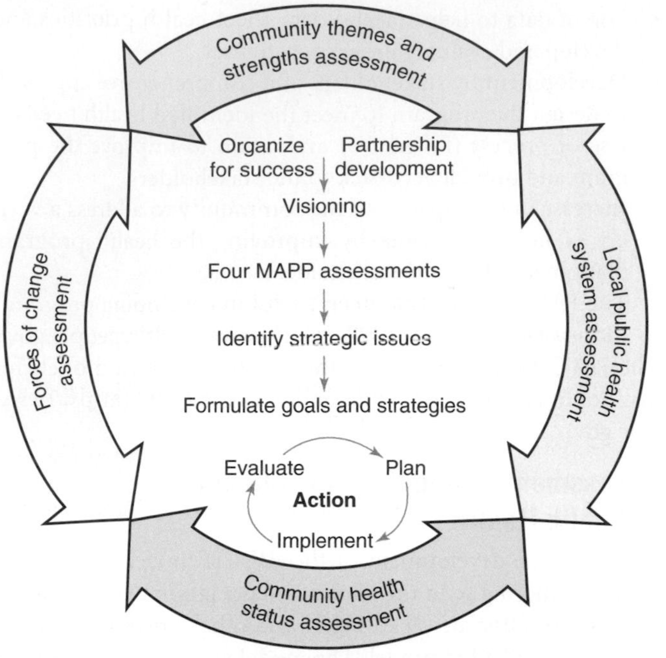

Fig. 23.5 MAPP process. *MAPP*, Mobilizing for Action through Planning and Partnership.

with PATCH and APEXPH, it is important that the community feels ownership of the process. The community's strengths, needs, and wishes are integral to the process.

Two figures (Figs. 23.5 and 23.6) show the MAPP process and the community roadmap to a healthier community. The phases of the MAPP process are as follows:

A. Organize for success/partnership development.
   1. Organize agencies.
   2. Recruit partners.
   3. Prepare to implement MAPP.

B. Visioning.
   1. Work toward long-range goals through a shared vision and common values.

C. Engage in four assessment processes.
   1. Assess community themes and strengths.
      a. Identify issues.
      b. Identify interest to community.
      c. Explore quality of life perceptions.
      d. Identify community assets.
   2. Assess local public health system.
      a. Identify all agencies and other partners who contribute to the public's health.
      b. Measure each partner's capacity to participate; what can each partner contribute?
      c. Measure the performance of each partner; how have they addressed issues in the past?
   3. Assess the health status of the community.
      a. Assess available data.
      b. Assess quality of life.
      c. Assess community risk factors.
   4. Assess ability of community to change.
      a. Identify forces for change.
      b. Identify forces against change.

D. Identify strategic issues.
   1. What are the health issues that need to be addressed?
   2. Which are the most important?
   3. Where should the community begin?

E. Formulate goals and strategies.
   1. Which goals will be met?
   2. Which strategies will be used to meet the goals?

F. Act.
   1. Participants develop plan for action.
   2. Implement the plan.
   3. Evaluate the implementation.

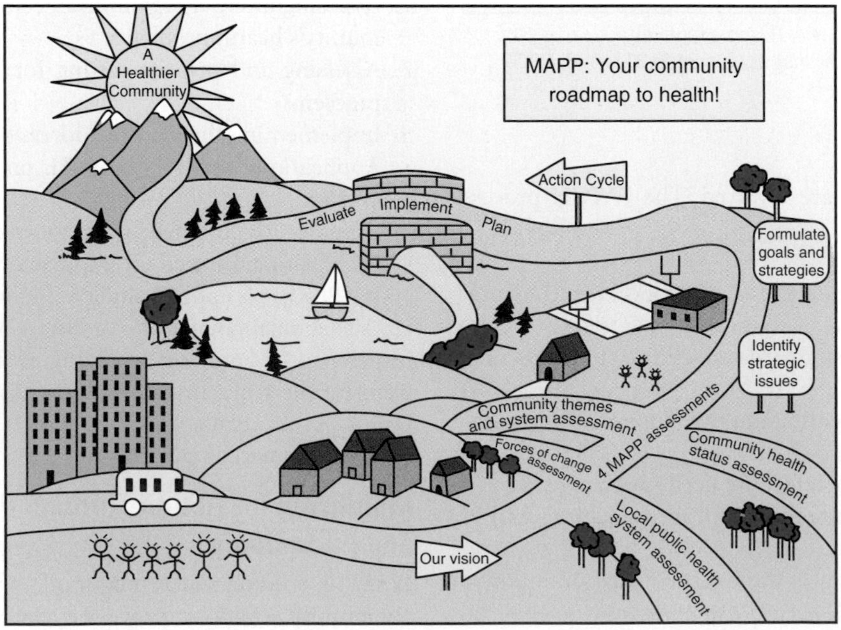

Fig. 23.6 MAPP roadmap to community's health. *MAPP,* Mobilizing for Action through Planning and Partnership.

Two products are available to assist in implementing the MAPP process (see Fig. 23.5): the NACCHO website and the MAPP toolbox (http://www.naccho.org).

The five models of program planning presented here may be adapted to use with a single program or with a community.

Evaluation Models and Techniques

Structure-Process-Outcome Evaluation. The method for evaluation of programs by Donabedian (1982) was initially directed primarily toward medical care but is applicable to the broader area of health care. He describes three approaches to assessment of health care: structure, process, and outcome.

- Structure refers to settings in which care occurs. It includes materials, equipment, qualification of the staff, and organizational structure (Donabedian, 1982). This approach to evaluation is based on the assumption that, given a proper setting with good equipment, good care will follow. However, this assumption is not strongly supported.
- Process refers to whether the care that was given was "good" (Donabedian, 1982), competent, or preferred. Use of process in program evaluation may consist of observing practice but more likely consists of reviewing records. The review could focus on whether documentation of preventive teaching was on the clinical record. Audits using specific criteria are examples of the use of process.
- Outcome refers to results of client care and restoration of function and survival (Donabedian, 1982) but is also used in the sense of changes in health status or changes in health-related knowledge, attitude, and behavior. Thus program outcomes may be expressed in terms of mortality, morbidity, and disability for given populations, such as infants, but they could be expressed in a broader sense through health promotion behaviors such as weight control, exercise, and abstinence from tobacco and alcohol.

Donabedian's model of evaluating program quality is widely used for evaluation in the health care field and is useful in evaluating program effectiveness. The Centers for Medicare and Medicaid Services and other third-party payers are currently placing more emphasis on outcome evaluation. It is essential that nurses begin to develop outcome criteria for client interventions.

Tracer Method. The Institute of Medicine (1973) of the National Academy of Sciences developed a program to evaluate health service delivery called the tracer method. The tracer method of evaluation of programs is based on the premise that health status and care can be evaluated by viewing specific health problems called tracers. Just as radioactive tracers are used to study the thyroid gland, specific health problems are selected to evaluate the delivery of health and nursing services. Examples of conditions selected as tracers are cardiovascular disease, diabetes, obesity, smoking patterns, and breast and cervical cancer. This approach can be used to compare the following:

- Health status among different population groups and in different geographic locations
- Health status in relation to social status, economic level, medical care, nursing care, and behavioral variables
- Various arrangements for health care delivery

The tracer method is a useful technique for looking at the efficiency, effectiveness, and effect of a program.

BOX 23.3 Examples of Questions Asked About Cases for Case Register

1. What is the incidence of disease? What is the prevalence? What differences in incidence and prevalence are there between one community and another?
2. What percent of clients recover? What percent die?
3. Where does death occur?
4. How long do clients wait before contacting a health care provider?
5. How long is it before they are seen by a health care provider?
6. How many cases are associated with other major risk factors?
7. How many cases are associated with environmental factors such as water hardness or air pollution?
8. What happens after clients leave the hospital and when they return to work? Are there rehabilitation programs?
9. How many clients had been seen by a health care provider shortly before the problem occurred?
10. What prevention measures are taken for persons considered susceptible?

Case Register

Systematic registration of a contagious disease has been a practice for many years. Denmark began a national register of tuberculosis in 1921 (Friis & Sellers, 2019). Its contribution to the reduction in the incidence of contagious diseases has been widely recognized. Case registers (Issel & Wells, 2018) are also used for acute and chronic diseases (e.g., cancer and myocardial infarction).

Registers collect information from defined groups, and the information may be used for evaluating and planning services, preventing disease, providing care, and monitoring changes in patterns and care. The method is described here because of its use in evaluation of services. The answers to the questions listed in Box 23.3, asked before and after implementing a program, give information about the effects of the program. A tuberculosis register indicates the degree to which infection is being controlled. Cancer registers make state, regional, national, and international comparisons possible, and they provide clues to causes of disease. They are also used to direct the development of programs specific to population needs.

PROGRAM FUNDING

Providing adequate funding for programs to meet the needs of populations can be a challenge to nurse managers in communities. When money is not available to support endeavors that serve the public good, nonprofit organizations may seek funding from outside the organization. Such funding may be in the form of gifts, contracts, or grants.

Gifts are philanthropic contributions from individuals, foundations, businesses, religious or civic organizations, or voluntary associations. Many organizations engage in extensive development efforts to solicit monetary gifts that support the agency's goals. Contracts are awarded for the performance of a specific task or service, usually to meet guidelines specified by the organization making the award. Contracts are frequently used by the government to purchase services of others to perform certain services. Grants are awards to nonprofit organizations to allow recipients to implement activities of their own design that address the interests of the funding agency. Grants are given by the government, foundations, and corporations.

Nurse leaders working in nonprofit agencies may write grants to fund community programs that meet the needs of at-risk populations. Development of a proposal is guided by concepts and principles of program planning and evaluation that have been discussed in this chapter. Successful **grant writing** meshes the plan for the envisioned program of the applying organization with the criteria set forth by the funding agency. A grant proposal is a means of recording plans for establishing, managing, and evaluating a program into a written document. Funding agencies provide guidelines for grant applications, and it is essential to follow those specific guidelines if grant funding is to be acquired. In general, however, most grant proposals include certain essential components.

First, it is important to identify the target population and define the problem(s) that the project intends to address. Specific data, conditions, or circumstances that illustrate the problem and that document the need (e.g., environmental characteristics, economic conditions, population characteristics, and health status indicators) should be included and discussed. Health services should be discussed in relationship to availability, accessibility, and acceptability to the target population within both the public and private sectors. Identification of duplication or gaps in services that result in unmet needs should be addressed.

The second component is the description of the program that is being proposed. The program description should provide details about what is planned, how it will be done, where it will be done, and by whom. This section should present the reviewer with a clear understanding of the details of the program structure and function. It should be apparent that the program is realistic and can be accomplished. This section includes goals, objectives, action steps, and anticipated outcomes that describe how, when, and by whom each activity will be accomplished to achieve the outcome of the objective for which it was written.

Plans for evaluation address the method that will be used to ensure ongoing and timely review of the specific action steps and objectives involved in achieving the stated goal (formative) and to assess program outcomes (summative).

Applicants for grant funds should develop a realistic operating budget that is appropriate to the requirements of the project. The budget represents the plan for how the program will be implemented and reflects the project's proposed spending plan.

LINKING CONTENT TO PRACTICE

Program planning skills and knowledge are essential for public health nurses. In *Public Health Nursing: Scope and Standards of Practice* (ANA, 2013), the first standard is that of assessment. This addresses the issue of conducting needs assessments and having the ability to collect multiple sources of data, analyze population characteristics, problem solve, and set priorities based on the data collected. Standard 2 speaks to using the assessment data to diagnose health problems with input from the client population. Standards 3 through 5 address the nurses' roles in identifying health status outcomes, planning and implementing processes to address the health problem, and directing strategies to meet the outcomes. Standard 6 discusses the nurses' role in evaluation, including participating in process and outcome evaluation by monitoring activities in programs.

The four professional organizations dedicated to public health nursing—the Association of State and Territorial Directors of Nursing (now APHN), the Association of Community Health Nursing Educators, the Public Health Nursing Section of the APHA, and the Alliance of Nurses for Healthy Environments— form an organization called the Quad Council Coalition. This coalition recently updated a document identifying the domains of practice for public health nurses. One of the domains is Policy Development and Program Planning Skills. The skills the nurse needs for this domain of practice related to program management are:

- A focus on determining needed policies and programs
- The ability to advocate for policies and programs
- Knowledge of how to plan, implement, and evaluate policies and programs
- The ability to develop and implement strategies for program continuous quality improvement
- Skills to develop and implement community health improvement plans and strategic plans

New baccalaureate nurses will want to be knowledgeable and be able to participate in program management; graduate nurses will want to be able to direct programs. Appendix B describes a Program Planning and Design process to use for practicing the content from this chapter. Try out this process on the development of a small program of interest to you and the client population you want to serve and the community level health problem of interest to you.

From Quad Council Coalition of Public Health Nursing Organizations, 2018.

PRACTICE APPLICATION

The following is a real-life example of the application of the program management process by an undergraduate nursing student. This activity resulted in the development and implementation of a nurse-managed clinic for the homeless. This example shows how students as well as providers can make a difference in health care delivery. It also illustrates that no mystery surrounds the program management process.

Eva was listening to the radio one Sunday afternoon and heard an announcement about the opening of a soup kitchen within the community for the growing homeless population. She was beginning her public health nursing course and wanted to find a creative clinical experience that would benefit herself as well as others. The announcement gave her an idea. Although it mentioned food, clothing, shelter, and social services, nothing was said about health care.

Eva was interested in finding a way to provide nursing and health care services at the soup kitchen. Which of the following should she do?

A. Talk with key leaders to determine their interest in her idea.

B. Review the literature to find out the magnitude of the problem.
C. Survey the community to determine if others are providing services.
D. Discuss the idea with members of the homeless population.
E. Consider potential solutions to the health care problems.
F. Consider where she would get the resources to open a clinic.
G. Talk with church leaders and nursing faculty members to seek acceptance for her idea.

Answers can be found on the Evolve site.

KEY POINTS

- Planning and evaluation are essential elements of program management and vital to the survival of the nursing discipline in health care delivery.
- The program management process is population focused and is parallel to the nursing process. Both are rational decision-making processes.
- The health care delivery system has grown in the past century, making health planning and evaluation very important.
- Comprehensive health planning grew out of a need to control costs.
- A program is an organized approach to meet the assessed needs of individuals, families, groups, populations, or communities by reducing or eliminating one or more health problems and addressing health disparities.
- Planning is defined as selecting and carrying out a series of actions to achieve a stated goal.
- Evaluation is defined as the methods used to determine if a service is needed and will be used, whether a program to meet that need is carried out as planned, and whether the service actually helps the people it intended to help.
- To develop quality programs, planning should include four essential elements: assessment of need and problem diagnosis, identification of problem solutions, analysis and comparison of alternative methods, and selection of the best plan and planning methods.
- The initial and most critical step in planning a health program is assessment of need. Assessment focuses on the needs of the population who will use the services planned.
- Some of the major tools used in needs assessment are census data, community forums, surveys of existing community agencies, surveys of community residents, and statistical indicators about demographics, morbidity, and mortality of the population.
- The major benefit of program evaluation is to determine whether a program is fulfilling its stated goals. Quality assurance programs are prime examples of program evaluation.
- Plans for implementing and evaluating programs should be developed at the same time.
- Program records and community indexes and health data serve as major sources of information for program evaluation.
- Planning programs and planning for their evaluation are two of the most important ways in which nurses can ensure successful program implementation.
- Cost studies help identify program benefits, effectiveness, and efficiency.
- Program planning helps nurses and agencies focus attention on services that clients need.
- Planning helps everyone involved understand their role in providing services to clients.
- The assessment of need process provides an evaluation of the relevance that a new service may have to clients.
- A decision tree is a useful tool to choose the best alternative for solving a problem.
- Setting goals and writing objectives to meet the goals are necessary to evaluate program outcomes.
- *Healthy People 2020* is an example of a national program based on needs assessment that has stated goals and objectives on which the program can be evaluated.
- Program planning models include PPM, MAUT, PATCH, APEXPH, and MAPP.
- Program evaluation includes assessing structure, process, and outcomes of care.
- Grant writing is a tool used by nurse managers to provide resources for needed services.
- Grant proposals are documents that incorporate principles of program planning and evaluation.

CLINICAL DECISION-MAKING ACTIVITIES

1. Choose the definitions that best describe your concepts of a program, planning, and evaluation. Explain how each of these definitions can help you in accomplishing planning and evaluation.
2. Apply the program planning process to an identified clinical problem for a client group with whom you are working in the community. Give specific examples.
   A. Assess the client needs and existing resources.
   B. Choose tools appropriate to the assessment of unmet needs.
   C. Analyze the overall planning process of arriving at decisions about implementing a program.
   D. Summarize the benefits for program planning that apply to your situation.
3. Given the situation just described, choose three or four of your classmates to work with you on the following projects:
   A. Plan for evaluation of the program in activity 2.
   B. Apply the evaluation process to the situation.
   C. Identify the measures you will use to gather data for evaluating your program.
   D. Identify the sources you will tap to gain information for program evaluation.
   E. Analyze the benefits of program evaluation that apply to your situation.

F. Talk with a nurse or an administrator working in the community about the application of program planning and evaluation processes at the local agency. Compare their answers to your research. What are some of the difficulties that your group and the agency had in evaluating a program?

ADDITIONAL RESOURCES

EVOLVE WEBSITE

http://evolve.elsevier.com/Stanhope/community/

- Answers to Practice Application
- Case Study
- Glossary
- Review Questions

REFERENCES

American Nurses Association (ANA): *Health System Reform*, July 2018. Retrieved from https://www.nursingworld.org.

American Nurses Association (ANA): *Public Health Nursing: Scope and Standards of Practice*, ed 2, Silver Springs, MD, 2013, American Nurses Association.

American Planning Association (APA): *What is planning?* 2018. Retrieved from https://www.planning.org.

Brownson RC, Baker EA, Deshpande AD, Gillespie KN: *Evidence-Based Public Health*, ed 3, New York, 2018, Oxford University Press.

Centers for Disease Control and Prevention (CDC): Framework for program evaluation in public health, *MMWR Recomm Rep* 48(RR-11):1–40, 1999.

Centers for Disease Control and Prevention (CDC): *Measles still threatens health security, press release*, 2013. Retrieved from https://www.cdc.gov.

Centers for Disease Control and Prevention (CDC): *Conducting a community needs assessment, field guidelines*, 2014. Retrieved from https://www.cdc.gov.

Delbecq A, Van de Ven A: A group process model for problem identification and program planning, *J Appl Behav Sci* 7:466–492, 1971.

Donabedian A: *Explorations in Quality Assessment and Monitoring*, vol 2, Ann Arbor, MI, 1982, Health Administration Press.

Donabedian A: *An Introduction to Quality Assurance in Health Care*, New York, 2003, Oxford University Press.

Friis RH, Sellers TA: *Epidemiology for Public Health Practice*, ed 5, Burlington MA, 2019, Jones and Bartlett Learning.

Glanz K, Bishop DB: The role of behavioral science theory in development and implementation of public health interventions, *Annu Rev Public Health* 31:399–418, 2010.

Green LW, Kreuter MW: CDC's Planned Approach to Community Health as an application of PRECEED and an inspiration for PROCEED, *J Health Educ* 23:140–147, 1992.

Griffin J: *The history of healthcare in America*, 2017. Retrieved from https://www.griffinbenefits.com.

Institute of Medicine (IOM): *A strategy for evaluating health services.* In Kessner DM, Kalk CE, editors. Washington DC, 1973, National Academy of Sciences.

Issel LM, Wells R: *Health Program Planning and Evaluation: A Practical, Systematic Approach for Community Health*, ed 4, Burlington MA, 2018, Jones and Bartlett Learning, LLC.

Jefferson Area Board of Aging: *About JABA*, 2018. Retrieved from http://www.jabacares.org.

Jones TL: Outcome measurement in nursing: imperatives, ideals, history, and challenges, *Online J Issues Nurs* 21(2):1, 2016.

Kabak O, Ervural B: Multiple attribute group decision making—a generic conceptual framework and a classification scheme, *Knowl Based Syst* 123(1):13–30, 2017.

Kabassi K, Vroom M: MAUT and adaptive techniques for web based educational software, *Instruct Sci* 34(2):313–358, 2006.

Kelly PJ, Kyngdon F, Ingram I, Deane FP, Baker AL, Osborne BA: The client satisfaction questionnaire-8—psychometric properties in a cross-sectional survey of people attending residential substance abuse treatment, *Drug Alcohol Rev* 37(1):79–86, 2018.

Kettner PM, Moroney RM, Martin LL: *Designing and Managing Programs: An Effectiveness-Based Approach*, ed 5, Washington DC, 2017, Sage Publications, Inc.

Linfield KJ, Posavac EJ: *Program Evaluation: Methods and Case Studies*, ed 9, New York NY, 2018, Routledge.

Longest Beaufort B Jr: *Health Program Management: From Development Though Evaluation*, ed 2, San Francisco, CA, 2015, Jossey-Bass & Pfieiffer.

National Association of City and County Health Officers (NACCHO): *Community health assessment and improvement planning*, 2018. Retrieved from https://www.naccho.org.

Newcomer KE, Hatry HP, Wholey JS: *Handbook of Practical Program Evaluation*, ed 4, Hoboken NJ, 2015, Jossey-Bass.

Nutt P: *Planning Methods for Health and Related Organizations*, New York, 1984, Wiley.

Quad Council of Public Health Nursing Organizations: *Community/Public Health Nursing Competencies*, 2018, Quad Council Coalition Competency Review Task Force. Retrieved from http://www.quadcouncilphn.org.

Robert Wood Johnson Foundation (RWJF): *Catalysts for change – harnessing the power of nurses to build population health in the 21st* century, *executive summary*, 2017. Retrieved from https://www.rwjf.org.

Royse D, Thyer BA, Padgett DK: *Program Evaluation: An Introduction to an Evidence-Based Approach*, ed 6, Boston MA, 2016, Cengage Learning.

Sparer MS, Thompson FJ: Government and health insurance – the policy process. In Kovner AR, Knickman JR, editors: *Jonas and Kovner's Health Care Delivery in the United States*, ed 11, New York NY, 2015, Springer Publishing Company, LLC.

The Community Toolbox. 2018. The Center for Community Health and Development, University of Kansas, Lawrence, Kansas.

Thorland W, Currie D, Wiegand ER, Walsh J, Mader N: Status of breastfeeding and child immunization outcomes in clients of the Nurse-Family Partnership, *Matern Child Health J* 21:439–445, 2017.

University of North Carolina Health Services Library: *Finding information for a community health assessment*, 2017. Retrieved from https://guides.lib.unc.edu.

U.S. Department of Health and Human Services: *Healthy People 2020: A Roadmap for Health.* Washington, DC, 2010, U.S. Government Printing Office.

U.S. Department of Health and Human Services: *Introduction to Program Evaluation for Public Health Programs: A Self-Study Guide*, Atlanta, GA, 2011, Centers for Disease Control and Prevention.

24

Quality Management

Marcia Stanhope, PhD, RN, FAAN

OBJECTIVES

After reading this chapter, the student should be able to do the following:

1. Explain differences in total quality management/continuous quality improvement (TQM/CQI).
2. Evaluate the role of QA/QI in CQI.
3. Analyze the historical development of the quality process in nursing and describe the changes developing under managed care.
4. Evaluate approaches and techniques for implementing CQI and the method of documentation.
5. Plan a model QA/QI program.
6. Identify the purposes for the types of records kept in community and public health agencies.

CHAPTER OUTLINE

Definitions and Goals
Historical Development
Approaches to Quality Improvement
TQM/CQI in Community and Public Health Settings
Client Satisfaction
Model CQI Program
Records

KEY TERMS

accountability, p. 525
accountable care organizations (ACOs), p. 523
accreditation, p. 527
audit process, p. 533
certification, p. 528
charter, p. 528
client-centered care, p. 530
concurrent audit, p. 533
continuous quality improvement, p. 522
credentialing, p. 527
evaluative studies, p. 535
evidence-based practice, p. 530
licensure, p. 527
malpractice litigation, p. 537
managed care, p. 524
managed care organizations (MCOs), p. 523
Nurse Licensure Compact Administrators (NLCAs), p. 527
outcome, p. 535
partnerships, p. 524
practice guidelines, p. 532
peer review organization (PRO), p. 526
process, p. 535
professional review organizations (PROs), p. 534
Professional Standards Review Organization (PSRO), p. 534
quality assurance/quality improvement (QA/QI), p. 525
quality improvement, p. 523
quality improvement organization (QIO), p. 526
recognition, p. 528
records, p. 540
report cards, p. 523
retrospective audit, p. 533
risk management, p. 534
safety, p. 530
sentinel, p. 535
staff review committees, p. 533
structure, p. 535
teamwork and collaboration, p. 530
total quality management, p. 522
tracer, p. 535
utilization review, p. 533

Although the concept of quality assurance has been a part of the health care arena for a number of years, it is only in the last few years that major movement to improve health care quality has begun in the United States. The Institute of Medicine (IOM, 2001), not confident of the health care systems' ability to deliver the quality of care expected, set forth a series of recommendations to transform systems to meet Americans' expectations. Very little is known about quality of care in this country for two reasons: (1) a variety of definitions of *quality* are used, and (2) it is difficult to obtain comparable data from all providers and health care agencies.

However, in the Healthcare Research and Quality Act of 1999 (PL 106-129), Congress mandated that the Agency for Healthcare Research and Quality (AHRQ) produce an annual report on health care quality in the United States beginning in fiscal year 2003. This National Healthcare Quality Report (NHQR) is a collaborative effort among the agencies of the U.S. Department of Health and Human Services (USDHHS) and includes a broad set of performance measures that will be used to monitor the nation's progress toward improved health care quality. The NHQR represented the broadest examination of quality of health care, in terms of number of measures and number of dimensions of care, ever undertaken in the United States. The report represents progress toward improving quality as well as recommendations for how to improve quality outcomes (USDHHS, 2017). Starting in 2014, the AHRQ (2015) integrated the NHQR with their annual disparities report to become the National Healthcare Quality and Disparities Report (NHQDR).

The NHQDR is intended to serve a number of purposes, such as demonstrating the validity (or lack) of concerns about quality; documenting whether health care quality is stable, improving, or declining over time; and providing national benchmarks against which specific states, health plans, and providers can compare their performance (AHRQ, 2017; NCQA, 2018).

In a changing health care market, the demand for quality has become a rallying point for health care consumers. All consumers, including private citizens, insurance companies, industry, and the federal government, are concerned with the highest quality outcomes at the lowest cost (Clancy & Fraser, 2015). In addition to the demand for higher quality and lower cost, the public wants health care delivered with greater access, and health care that is accountable, efficient, and effective. Moreover, consumers want information about quality. Information is empowering to the consumer. With the expanded use of the Internet, access to information about quality in health care is readily available, ranging from talking to consumers about quality health care (https://www.ahrq.gov) to clinical practice guidelines that promise to improve care for all (http://www.guideline.gov). **Total quality management** (TQM) is a management philosophy that includes a focus on client, **continuous quality improvement** (CQI), and teamwork (Spath & Kelly, 2017). Although relatively new in public health care, the concepts of TQM/CQI have been tried and proven in industry at large. The terms *total quality management, continuous quality improvement, total quality,* and *organization-wide quality improvement* are often used interchangeably. However, they have different meanings. As indicated, TQM refers to a management philosophy that focuses on the statistical processes by which to assess work done with the goal of organization-wide quality effectiveness. TQM is often referred to as TQ, and both acronyms have the same meaning. CQI, while different from the other three terms, can be implemented not only to address system problems but also to maintain and enhance good performance through the use of differing techniques. Everyone in the public health or community-based organization is involved in CQI—the leaders, the staff, and the client. By obtaining facts about work processes (e.g., all the steps in certifying a child for the women, infants, and children nutritional program [WIC]), it is possible to discover which steps are unnecessary (i.e., non–value adding) and to eliminate those steps to produce better health outcomes for individuals and communities (Oakland, 2014). Table 24.1 presents several abbreviations that are commonly used in health care and quality management.

Both consumers and providers have a vested interest in the quality of the health care system to do the following:

1. Improve safety of care to save lives
2. Reduce costs by using effective interventions
3. Increase client confidence in health care delivery regardless of setting (National Quality Forum [NQF], 2010, 2017)

Kovner and Jonas state that in health care there is a direct link between doing a good job and individual and professional survival. Health care providers pride themselves on individual achievement and responsibility for good client outcomes (Knickman & Kovner, 2015). Health care organizations are natural extensions of health care providers and thus can demonstrate their responsibility for optimal outcomes through a

TABLE 24.1 Commonly Used Abbreviations

AACN	American Association of Colleges of Nursing
ACHNE	Association of Community Health Nursing Educators
AHRQ	Agency for Healthcare Research and Quality (formerly AHCPR)
ANA	American Nurses Association
APHA	American Public Health Association
CCNE	Commission on Collegiate Nursing Education
CHAP	Community Health Accreditation Partner
CMS	Centers for Medicare and Medicaid Services (formerly HCFA)
CQI	Continuous Quality Improvement
HEDIS	Health Plan Employer Data and Information Set
IOM	Institute of Medicine
JCAHO	Joint Commission on Accreditation of Healthcare Organizations
MCO	Managed Care Organization
NCQA	National Committee for Quality Assurance
NHQDR	National Healthcare Quality and Disparities Report
NLN	National League for Nursing
NPHPSP	National Public Health Performance Standards Program
OBQI	Outcomes-Based Quality Improvement
QA	Quality Assurance
QI	Quality Improvement
QIO	Quality Improvement Organization
TQI	Total Quality Improvement
TQM	Total Quality Management

rigorous **quality improvement** process. The application of quality improvement strategies through the following six areas of performance could affect both process and outcomes of health care:

1. Consistently providing appropriate and effective care
2. Reducing unjustified geographic variation in care
3. Eliminating avoidable mistakes
4. Lowering access barriers
5. Improving responsiveness to clients
6. Eliminating racial/ethnic, gender, socioeconomic, and other disparities and inequalities in access and treatment (USDHHS, 2016)

In the 1990s the United States entered a new era of population-centered, community-controlled delivery of care in which **managed care organizations (MCOs)** played an integral role. MCOs are agencies such as health maintenance organizations (HMOs) and preferred provider organizations (PPOs) designed to monitor and deliver health care services within a specific budget. Currently providers, clients, payers, and policy makers all have input into the quality measurement process. The Health Plan Employer Data and Information Set (HEDIS), a data collection arm of the National Committee for Quality Assurance (NCQA), provides performance information, or report cards, for 90 percent of America's health plans. Since the release of HEDIS 2.0, nearly 90 percent of all health insurance plans, including HMOs and PPOs, reported audited HEDIS data to show the level of quality performance (NCQA, 2017). In the Affordable Care Act (ACA) **accountable care organizations (ACOs)** are being promoted (Kaiser Health News [KHN], 2015). The ACO may involve a network of physicians.

Although introduced in the 1990s, **report cards** for public health agencies are currently being developed and promoted to measure quality health care in communities. The term *community health report card* refers to different types of reports, community health profiles, needs assessments, scorecards, quality-of-life indicators, health status reports, and progress reports. All of these reports are critical components of community-based approaches to improving the health and quality of life of communities (Community Tool Box, 2018).

An example at the national level was the Community Health Status Indicator (CHSI) Project, which was a collaborative effort between the Health Resources and Services Administration (HRSA), the Association of State and Territorial Health Officials (ASTHO), the National Association of County and City Health Officials (NACCHO), and the Public Health Foundation (http://www.countyhealthrankings.org). In 2000, the project published and disseminated community health status reports for all U.S. counties. These reports provided county-level data, including peer county and national comparisons, for every county in the country. The goal of CHSI was to provide an overview of key health indicators for local communities and to encourage dialogue about actions that can be taken to improve a community's health. The CHSI report was designed not only for public health professionals but also for members of the community who are interested in the health of their community. They were designed to support health planning by local health departments, local health planners, community residents, and others interested in community health improvement. The CHSI report contained over 200 measures for each of the 3141 U.S. counties. Although CHSI presented indicators like deaths resulting from heart disease and cancer, it is imperative to understand that behavioral factors such as tobacco use, diet, physical activity, alcohol and drug use, and sexual behavior substantially contribute to these deaths (NICHSR, 2012).

These community health improvement initiatives grew out of three major trends: (1) an increasing recognition of the importance of local community action to solve local problems, (2) an increasing emphasis on outcomes and accountability, and (3) the Healthy Communities movement (see Chapter 16). The Healthy Communities movement views community health and its determinants broadly, and they use a set of indicators (to track their progress) that reflects this broad definition. These indicators might include the following:

- Demographics
- Functional health status or health-related quality of life
- Public health systems
- Socioeconomics
- Culture
- Political and historical context
- Environment
- Behavior (Pennel et al., 2017)

Beginning in 2017, the CHSI was replaced by the County Health Rankings and Roadmaps program. This program is a collaboration between Robert Wood Johnson Foundation and the University of Wisconsin Population Health Institute. Data about any county in the United States can be found at http://www.countyhealthrankings.org (Remington et al., 2015).

Community health report cards can be a useful tool in efforts to help identify areas where change is needed, to set priorities for action, and to track changes in population health over time (Egen et al., 2017; Hood et al., 2016). The report card may be used to track leading causes of morbidity and mortality in a community, looking at trends over time to see if public health interventions have improved health care outcomes. The card may also be used to assess a specific chronic disease, like diabetes, to determine the health status of the community for this particular disease (Record et al., 2015). The report card may be used as an internal measure of public health program outcomes and CQI measures within the agency (Yeager et al., 2013). HEDIS measures of care include several that address public health issues, including body mass index (BMI) reduction and maintenance, smoking or tobacco use quit rates, and physical activity levels (NCQA, 2018).

As a part of a movement to provide quality health care in communities, health departments are increasingly examining their place in promoting quality (CDC, 2017). Sollecito and Johnson (2013) state that public health and CQI are connected because of the use of systems approaches that public health takes in identifying problems and developing interventions. Aspects of planning, implementing, and evaluating by TQM fall under each of the core public health functions of assessment, assurance, and policy development. However, it is with the assurance core function, related to ensuring available access to the health care services essential to sustain and improve the health of the population, that TQM programs must be undertaken. Public health cannot ensure services that improve health if those services lack quality. Public health will want to maintain quality in its workforce and continually evaluate the effectiveness of its services whether service is delivered to the individual, the community, or the population.

At least four documents provide report cards on how well the United States is performing on improving safety of health care delivery, quality of and access to care across population groups, progress and opportunities for improving health care quality, and the state of health care quality. These reports are published regularly by the Agency for Health Care Research and Quality, the National Quality Forum, and the National Committee for Quality Assurance.

Nurses are in a perfect position to implement strategies to improve population-centered health care. Community assessments, identification of high-risk individuals, use of targeted interventions, case management, and management of illnesses across a continuum of care are strategies suggested as part of the focus in improving the health of communities (Quad Council Coalition of Public Health Nursing Organizations, 2018). These strategies have long been used by nurses.

The growth of the **managed care** industry has changed the face of health care in the United States, both in how health care is delivered and in how it is received by consumers. Consumers are forming **partnerships** in communities to counteract the power of MCOs by holding them accountable for health outcomes in relation to costs. The ACA's (KHN, 2015) emphasis on ACOs is promoting the managed care approach to health care delivery with quality indicators. Partnerships are using data-based community assessments to improve health and to ensure that communities receive quality services. Projects are being funded to meet this goal (Kresge Foundation, 2017).

Because of managed care agencies and consumer demands for quality nursing, objective and systematic evaluation of nursing care is a priority for the nursing profession. Since organized nursing is committed to direct individual accountability, is evolving as a scientific discipline, and is concerned about how costs of health services limit access, it demands delivery and evaluation of quality service aimed at superior client outcomes (ANA, 2013). In the public health arena, the Quad Council Coalition of Public Health Nursing Organizations (2017, 2018), which includes four nursing organizations—the Association of Community Health Nursing Educators (ACHNE), the Public Health Nursing Section of the American Public Health Association (PHN Section), the Alliance of Nurses for Healthy Environments (ANHE), and the Association of Public Health Nurses (APHN)—has identified competencies for public health nursing based on the Council on Linkages Between Academia and Public Health Practice's *Core Competencies for Public Health Professionals* (2001, updated 2014). Other states have developed models to document outcomes attributable to nursing interventions and are adding methods for evaluating total quality (Fawcett & Ellenbecker, 2015; Keller et al., 2004a, 2004b; Minnesota Department of Health, 2001; Sakamoto & Avila, 2004; Smith & Bazini-Barakat, 2004; University of Wisconsin-Madison, 2009). Table 24.2 is a list of the areas of nursing interventions that nurses will want to be able to use. (See Chapter 11 for the most recent updates on the Keller et al. model of the Intervention Wheel.)

TABLE 24.2 The Public Health Nursing Interventions for Quality Population-Centered Health Care by Chapter

Interventions	Chapter
Advocacy	5-7, 19, 25, 29, 31, 34, 36, 37, 46
Case finding	15, 31, 33, 42
Case management	25, 29, 31-33, 42, 46
Coalition building	9, 16, 17
Collaborating	20, 24, 25, 31, 39, 41, 45
Community organizing	11
Consulting	40, 42
Counseling	11, 15, 29, 31, 36, 39, 42, 45, 46
Delegated functions	11, 40
Disease and health event investigation	13-15, 21, 22
Health teaching	11, 14-16, 18, 19, 36, 38-40, 42-45
Outreach	33, 35, 46
Policy development and enforcement	1, 6, 9, 17, 26, 29, 33
Referral and follow-up	6, 25-27, 31, 46
Social marketing	14, 17, 34, 38
Survey	16

Interventions based on Minnesota Department of Health, Division of Community Health Services: *Public health interventions: applications for public health nursing practice,* St. Paul, MN, March 2001, p. 1, Public Health Nursing Section, updated 2009.

The competencies for public health leadership developed by the Council on Linkages (2001, updated 2014) are crucial to ensure the quality and performance of the public health workforce. The Council on Linkages Between Academia and Public Health Practice (the Council) is a coalition of representatives from 23 national public health organizations. Since 1992, the Council has worked to further academic/practice collaboration to ensure a well-trained, competent workforce and a strong, evidence-based public health infrastructure. The Council is funded by the CDC and staffed by the Public Health Foundation. These competencies are used in quality assurance/quality improvement (QA/QI) as performance measurements of providers, including nurses, to ensure quality of services. See Resource Tool 46.A on the Evolve website for a list of the competencies.

Records are maintained on all health care system clients to provide complete information about the client and to show the quality of care being given to the client within the system. Records are a necessary part of a CQI process, as are the tools and methods for evaluating quality. Electronic health records are becoming more common and are aiding in decreasing errors, increasing quality, and monitoring interventions (Birnbaum et al., 2018; Vogel et al., 2014).

DEFINITIONS AND GOALS

The IOM definition of quality is "the degree to which health services for individuals and populations increase the likelihood of desired health outcomes and are consistent with current professional knowledge" (2001, p. 1000). The AHRQ (2017) defines quality health care as doing the right thing, for the right client, and having the best possible results. Quality in public health is defined as "the degree to which policies, programs, services, and research for the population increase desired health outcomes and conditions in which the population can be healthy" (IOM, 2013, p. 3).

However, a definition of quality rests largely on the perception of the client, the provider, the care manager, the purchaser, the payer, or the public health official. Whereas the physician views quality in a more technical sense, the client may look at the personal outcome; the manager, purchaser, or payer may consider the cost-effectiveness; and the public health official will look at the appropriate use of health care resources to improve population health (AHRQ, 2017).

According to the AHRQ (2018), problems with quality of care were divided into five groups: variation of service, underuse of service, overuse of service, misuse of service, and disparities in quality. Variation of service refers to the lack of standards of practice continuity. This variation is often seen between regional, state, and local health care services and stems from lack of evolutionary health care practice and not keeping abreast of the constant changes taking place in health care (evidence-based practice) (AHRQ, 2018; IOM, 2001, 2013). Variation of service refers to coordination of care. As an example, avoidable hospital admissions for certain health care problems like hypertension continue to occur (AHRQ, 2017). Underuse of service refers to conservative treatment practices. Overuse of service refers to the over-ordering of unnecessary tests, surgeries, and treatments. This overuse drives up the cost of already expensive health care. Misuse of service refers to client safety issues and how disability and mortality can be reduced. With diligent care by health care providers, client injury and death can be avoided (IOM, 2001, 2013). Disparities in quality refer to racial, ethnic, and socioeconomic disparities in accessibility and affordability of health care (AHRQ, 2017).

The term *health services* applies to a wide range of health delivery institutions. Of particular interest to public health is the question of access to appropriate and needed services, a well-prepared workforce, and improvement in the status of the population's health. Client satisfaction and well-being and the processes of client–provider interaction should be considered as well.

TQM is a process-driven, customer-oriented management philosophy that includes leadership, teamwork, employee empowerment, individual responsibility, and continuous improvement of system processes to yield improved outcomes (Oakland, 2014). Under TQM, quality is defined as customer satisfaction. **Quality assurance/quality improvement (QA/QI)** is the promise or guarantee that certain standards of excellence are being met in the delivery of care. The *Juran Trilogy* consists of quality planning, quality control, and quality improvement (Juran, 1986). This trilogy combines components of QA as well as CQI to improve client outcomes in health care delivery.

QI is defined as "systematic and continuous actions that lead to measurable improvement in health care services and the health status of targeted patient groups" (USDHHS, 2011). QI in public health is the use of a deliberate and defined improvement process, such as plan-do-study-act (PDSA), which is focused on activities that are responsive to community needs and improving population health. It refers to a continuous and ongoing effort to achieve measurable improvements in the efficiency, effectiveness, performance, accountability, outcomes, and other indicators of quality in services or processes that achieve equity and improve the health of the community (Riley et al., 2010).

QA is concerned with the accountability of the provider and is only one tool in achieving the best client outcomes. **Accountability** means being responsible for care and answerable to the client (Sollecito & Johnson, 2013). Under QA/QI, quality may have a variety of definitions. According to Edwards (2013), QA should consist of peer review leading to QI to improve health care delivery. Client standards of care and safety issues are the core of QA.

Quality traditionally has been an important issue in the delivery of health care. QA programs historically have ensured this accountability. The goals of QA and QI are on a continuum of quality, and in public health they are (1) to continuously improve the timeliness, effectiveness, safety, and responsiveness of programs, and (2) to optimize internal resources to improve the health of the community (Riley et al., 2010).

Under a CQI philosophy, QA and QI are but two of the many approaches used to ensure that the health care agency fulfills what the client thinks are the requirements for the service. QA focuses on finding what providers have done wrong in the past (e.g., deviations from a standard of care found through a chart audit). CQI operates at a higher level on the quality continuum but requires the commitment of more organization resources to move in a positive direction. CQI focuses on the sources of differences in the ongoing process of health care delivery and seeks to improve the process (Spath & Kelly, 2017; Sullivan, 2013).

The process of health care includes two major components: technical interventions (e.g., how well procedures are accomplished, accurate assessments, and effective interventions) and interpersonal relationships between public health practitioner and client. Both contribute to quality care, and both can be evaluated. Several approaches and techniques are used in quality programs. *Approaches* are methods used to ensure quality, and *techniques* are tools for measuring differences in quality (Knickman & Kovner, 2015).

Traditional approaches to quality focus on assessing or measuring performance, ensuring that performance conforms to standards, and providing remedial work to providers if those standards are not met. Such a definition of quality is too narrow in health care systems that try to meet the needs of many clients, both internal and external to the agency. CQI requires constant attention and should involve surveillance of all records while there is still the opportunity to intervene in both the client's care and the practitioner's actions. Comprehensive data analysis is necessary to detect process failure. Many agencies use some of the TQM/CQI concepts, such as client satisfaction questionnaires, but have not adopted the entire management philosophy. However, because QA/QI methods have traditionally been used and are still in use in many agencies, the QA/QI concepts will be covered.

HEALTHY PEOPLE 2020

Goal: Improving access to comprehensive, high-quality health care

Examples of objectives to eliminate health disparities:

- **AHS-1:** Increase the proportion of persons with health insurance.
- **AHS-5:** Increase the proportion of persons who have a specific source of ongoing care.
- **AHS-7:** Increase the proportion of persons who receive evidence-based clinical preventive services.

From U.S. Department of Health and Human Services: *Healthy People 2020,* Washington, DC, 2010, U.S. Government Printing Office.

HISTORICAL DEVELOPMENT

Improving the quality of care has been a part of nursing since the days of Florence Nightingale. In 1860 Nightingale called for the development of a uniform method to collect and present hospital statistics to improve hospital treatment. Nightingale was a pioneer in setting standards for nursing care. The movement to establish nursing schools in the United States came in the late 1800s from a desire to set standards that would upgrade nursing care. In the early 1900s, efforts were begun to set similar standards for all nursing schools. From 1912 to 1930, interest in quality nursing education led to the development of nursing organizations involved in accrediting nursing programs. Licensure has been a major issue in nursing since 1892. By 1923 all states had permissive or mandatory laws directing nursing practice.

After World War II, the attention of the emerging nursing profession focused on establishing a scientific method of practice. The nursing process was the chosen method and included evaluation of how nursing activities helped clients (Maibusch, 1984). QA/QI was the evaluative step in the nursing process.

The 1950s brought the development of QA measurement tools. One of the first tools was Phaneuf's nursing audit method (1965), which has been used extensively in population-centered nursing practice.

In 1966, the American Nurses Association (ANA) created the Divisions on Practice. As a result, in 1972, the Congress for Nursing Practice was charged with developing standards to institute QA programs. The Standards for Community Health Nursing Practice were distributed to ANA Community Health Nursing Division members in 1973. In 1986, 1999, and in 2005, with updates in 2007, in 2013, the scope and standards were again revised with a change in focus from community health nursing to public health nursing (ANA, 2013).

In 1972, the Joint Commission on Accreditation of Hospitals (JCAH) clearly stated the responsibilities of nursing in its description of standards for nursing services. The JCAH called on the nursing industry to clearly plan, document, and evaluate nursing care provided. In the mid-1980s, the JCAH became the Joint Commission on Accreditation of Healthcare Organizations (JCAHO) and began developing quality control standards for hospital and home health nursing. JCAHO is now known as The Joint Commission (TJC) and presently incorporates CQI principles in its standards.

Also in 1972, the Social Security Act (PL 92-603) was amended to establish the Professional Standards Review Organization (PSRO) and to mandate the process review of the delivery of health care to clients of Medicare, Medicaid, and maternal and child health programs. The PSRO program later became the **Peer Review Organization (PRO)** under the 1983 Social Security amendments. The purpose of the PROs was to monitor the implementation of the prospective reimbursement system for Medicare clients (the diagnosis-related groups [DRGs]). Although PSROs were intended for physicians, PROs made QI a primary issue for all health care professionals. The PRO was renamed the QIO, or the **quality improvement organization (QIO)**, and is mandated to improve the quality and efficiency of Medicare funded services (CMS, 2018).

In response to increasing charges of malpractice, the government passed the National Health Quality Improvement Act of 1986. Although it was not funded until 1989, its two major goals were to encourage consumers to become informed about their practitioner's practice record and to create a national clearinghouse of information on the malpractice records of providers. The emphasis of this act continued to be on the structure of care rather than the process or outcomes of care (NAHQ, 1993). (See Chapter 23 for discussion of structure, process, and outcome.)

Efforts to strengthen nursing practice in the community have been carried out by several nursing organizations, including the ANA, the Public Health Nursing Section of the American Public Health Association (APHA), the Association of State and Territorial Directors of Nursing (now APHN), and the Association of Community Health Nursing Educators (ACHNE). The quality of nursing education is a major concern of the ACHNE, which was established in 1978. In 1993, 2000, 2003, and 2007, five reports published by this organization identified the curriculum content required to prepare nursing students for practice in the community (ACHNE, 1993, 2000a/2009, 2000b, 2003, 2007). In 2005, and again in 2007, the Quad Council reviewed scopes and standards of population-focused (public health) and community-based nursing practice and worked with the American Nurses Association to develop new standards to guide the profession in obtaining the best health outcomes for the populations they serve. These standards were updated again in 2013. QA/QI programs remain the enforcers of standards of care for many agencies that have not elected to engage in a program of CQI. These activities are called *assurance activities* because they make certain that those policies and procedures are followed so that appropriate quality services are delivered.

APPROACHES TO QUALITY IMPROVEMENT

Two basic approaches exist in QI: *general* and *specific.* The general approach involves a large governing or official body's evaluation of a person's or agency's ability to meet criteria or standards. Specific approaches to QI are methods used to manage a specific health care delivery system in an attempt to deliver care with outcomes that are acceptable to the consumer. QA/QI programs that evaluate provider and client interaction through compliance with standards historically have been used alone to monitor quality care. In a TQM approach, CQI with QA/QI methods are an integral, but not the only, tool for ensuring quality or customer satisfaction.

General Approaches

General approaches to protect the public by ensuring a level of competency among health care professionals are *credentialing, licensure, accreditation, certification, charter, recognition,* and *academic degrees.* Although there has been a long history of public oversight of quality in the United States, this public oversight increasingly involves the private sector. Public oversight for quality emerged when the private market failed to focus on health care quality. Previously mentioned reports about quality are indicators of public sector involvement in public oversight of quality.

Credentialing is generally defined as the formal recognition of a person as a professional with technical competence, or of an agency that has met minimum standards of performance. These mechanisms are used to evaluate the agency structure through which care is provided and the outcomes of care given by the provider. Credentialing can be mandatory or voluntary. Mandatory credentialing requires laws. State nurse practice acts are examples of mandatory credentialing. Voluntary credentialing is performed by an agency or an institution. The certification examinations offered by the ANA through the American Nurses Credentialing Center are examples of voluntary credentialing. Licensing, certification, and accreditation are all examples of credentialing (ANCC, 2018a).

Licensure is one of the oldest general QA approaches in the United States and Canada. Individual licensure is a contract between the profession and the state. Under this contract, the profession is granted control over entry into, and exit from, the profession and over quality of professional practice (NCSBN, 2018a).

The licensing process requires that written regulations define the scope and limits of the professional's practice. Job descriptions based on these regulations set minimum and maximum limits on the functions and responsibilities of the practitioner. Licensure of nurses has been mandated by law since 1903. Today all 50 states have mandatory nurse licensure, which requires all individuals who practice nursing, whether it be for money or as a volunteer, to be licensed. A new approach to interstate practice requires a pact between states so that nurses can practice across state borders (NCSBN, 2018b). Although reciprocity (which means nurses can have their license accepted through an application process if there is agreement between the states requiring application) exists among states for nursing licensure, interstate practice without approval is an issue for state boards of nursing. The states' compact agreements were to reduce the barriers for interstate practice. The mutual recognition model of nurse licensure allows a nurse to have one license (in his or her state of residency) and to practice in other states (both physically and electronically when giving advice through programs like "ask a nurse"), subject to each state's practice law and regulation. Under mutual recognition, a nurse may practice across state lines unless otherwise restricted. This is referred to as a multistate nurse licensure model, specifically referred to as the Enhanced Nurse Licensure Compact (eNLC). All states that currently belong to the eNLC also operate the single-state licensure model for those nurses who do not reside legally in an NLC state or do not qualify for multistate licensure. To achieve mutual recognition, each state must enact legislation or regulation authorizing the NLC. States entering the compact also adopt administrative rules and regulations for implementation of the compact.

Once the compact is enacted, each compact state designates a Nurse Licensure Compact Administrator to facilitate the exchange of information between the states relating to compact nurse licensure and regulation. On January 10, 2000, the **Nurse Licensure Compact Administrators (NLCAs)** were organized to protect the public's health and safety by promoting compliance with the laws governing the practice of nursing in each party state through the mutual recognition of party state licenses (NCSBN, 2018b).

Accreditation, a voluntary approach to QI, is used for institutions. Since 1954 the National League for Nursing (NLN), a voluntary organization, has had established standards for inspecting nursing education programs. In 1997 the NLN board established an accrediting body as an independent organization: the NLN Accrediting Commission (NLNAC). The name of this organization is now the Nursing Commission for Nursing Education Accreditation (CNEA) (NLN, 2018). In 1997 the American Association of Colleges of Nursing (AACN), also a voluntary organization supporting baccalaureate and higher degree programs, established an affiliate—the Commission on Collegiate Nursing Education (CCNE)—to accredit baccalaureate and higher degree nursing programs (CCNE, 2018). In 1966 community health/home health program standards were established by the NLN for the purpose of accrediting these programs through their Community Health Accreditation Partner (CHAP), now an independent organization (CHAP, 2018). In addition, state boards of nursing accredit basic nursing programs so that their graduates are eligible for the licensing examination. In some states, state boards of nursing accredit graduate programs.

The accreditation function is quasi-voluntary. Although accreditation appears to be a voluntary program, it is often linked to government regulation that encourages programs to participate in the accrediting process. Examples include the federal Medicare regulations restricting payments only to accredited public health and home health care agencies (CMS, 2016).

Accreditation, whether voluntary or required, provides a means for effective peer review and an opportunity for in-depth review of program strengths and limitations. Accreditation applies external pressure and places demands on institutions to improve quality of care. In the past, the accreditation process primarily evaluated an agency's physical structure, organizational structure, and personnel qualifications. However, beginning in 1990, more emphasis was placed on evaluation of the outcomes of care and on the educational qualifications of the person providing the care.

In the past there has not been a mechanism for accrediting public health agencies. In 2007 the Public Health Accreditation Board (PHAB) was incorporated, after public health leaders explored the feasibility of a national accreditation program. The field saw the need for, and value of, public health accreditation and advocated for the implementation of a national voluntary program. The PHAB was developed in accordance with the recommendations generated by the Exploring Accreditation Steering Committee. The Steering Committee was composed primarily of state and local public health officials, including boards of health. The committee called on the expertise from other specialty areas engaged in accreditation. The PHAB is a nonprofit organization and is developing and testing national standards and processes that will be used to assess the strengths and areas for improvement in public health (PHAB, 2018).

The PHAB mission is to promote and protect the health of the public by advancing the quality and performance of *all* public health departments in the United States. The PHAB works toward creating a high-performing public health system that will make the United States the healthiest nation. The CDC and the Robert Wood Johnson Foundation are funders, and partners, of PHAB. The goal is for the accreditation program and the accrediting process, which began in 2011, to be self-sustaining. As of March 29, 2019, 218 local, 36 state, and 3 tribal public health departments have been accredited, with many more in the process of accreditation (PHAB, 2019).

Certification, another general approach to quality, combines features of licensure and accreditation. Certification is usually a voluntary process within professions. Educational achievements, experience, and performance on an examination determine a person's qualifications for functioning in an identified specialty area. The American Nurses Credentialing Center provides certification in several areas of nursing (ANCC, 2018a). Many other professional nursing specialty credentialing organizations also provide for individual certification.

Although usually a voluntary process, certification can also be a quasi-voluntary process. For example, to function as a nurse practitioner in all but three states, one must show proof of educational credentials and take an examination to be certified to practice within the boundaries of the state (Fitzgerald, 2013; NursingLicensure.org, 2018).

Major concerns exist about certification as a QA mechanism. Data are lacking about the clinical competence of the practitioner at the time of certification because clinical competency is usually not measured by a written test. Although better data exist about the quality of the practitioner's work after the certification process, the American Nurses Credentialing Center conducted a research program to look at how certification is related to the work of the certified nurse (Blegen, 2012; Boltz et al., 2013; Kendall-Gallagher et al., 2011; Martinez, 2011). Except for occupational health nurses and nurse anesthetists, certification was not universally recognized by employers as an achievement beyond basic preparation, so financial rewards were few (Keefe, 2010). But with the introduction of the Magnet program for health care organizations by the American Nurses Credentialing Center, the emphasis on certification and rewards improved.

Although the nursing profession has accepted the certification process as a mechanism for recognizing competence and excellence, certifying bodies must help nurses communicate the importance of certified nurses to the public.

Charter, recognition, and academic degrees are other general approaches to QA. **Charter** is the mechanism by which a state government agency, under state laws, grants corporate status to institutions with or without rights to award degrees (e.g., university-based nursing programs).

Recognition is a process whereby one agency accepts the credentialing status of and the credentials conferred by another. For example, most state boards of nursing accept nurse practitioner credentials that are awarded by the American Nurses Credentialing Center or by one of the specialty credentialing agencies. Academic degrees are titles awarded to individuals recognized by degree-granting institutions as having completed a predetermined plan of study in a branch of learning. There are four academic degrees awarded in nursing, with some variety at each degree level: Associate of Arts/Sciences; Bachelor of Science in Nursing; master's degrees, such as Master of Science in Nursing and Master of Nursing; and doctoral degrees, such as Doctor of Philosophy and Doctor of Nursing Practice.

Although these general quality management methods are important and should continue, newer and better approaches must be devised. If performance in the area of quality health care is to advance, better diagnosis of performance problems and corrective strategies that are effective will be necessary. The National Network of Public Health Institutes (2014) designed a modular guide to assist emerging and public health institutes interested in continued growth and success. The guide with the support of the Robert Wood Johnson Foundation was developed first in 2005.

An approach to recognition is the Magnet nursing services recognition status given by the American Nurses Credentialing Center to agency nursing services that, after an extensive review, are considered excellent. This program began with recognition of excellent hospital nursing services. The Magnet program has expanded to include nursing home and home health agencies. Reapplication for Magnet status must occur every four years to ensure that Magnet organizations stay at the top of their games. Achieving Magnet status depends on the quality and standards of the nursing service of the organizations. Thus certification by the individual nurse now has increasing importance to meeting the standards for Magnet status (ANCC, 2018b).

Specific Approaches

Historically, QA programs conducted by health care agencies have measured or assessed the performance of individuals and how they conformed to standards set forth by accrediting agencies. TQM as a management philosophy uses CQI methods that incorporate many tools, including QA, to increase customer satisfaction with quality care. According to the AHRQ, quality health care means doing the right thing, at the right time, in the right way, for the right people—and having the best possible results (AHRQ, 2017). To the Institute of Medicine (IOM, 2001, p. 3), quality health care is care that is as follows:

- *Effective*—Providing services based on scientific knowledge to all who could benefit and refraining from providing services to those not likely to benefit

- *Safe*—Avoiding injuries to clients from the care that is intended to help them
- *Timely*—Reducing waits and sometimes harmful delays for both those who receive and those who give care
- *Client-centered*—Providing care that is respectful of and responsive to individual client preferences, needs, and values and ensuring that client values guide all clinical decisions
- *Equitable*—Providing care that does not vary in quality because of personal characteristics such as gender, ethnicity, geographic location, and socioeconomic status
- *Efficient*—Avoiding waste, including waste of equipment, supplies, ideas, and energy

QA seeks to eliminate errors before negative outcomes can occur rather than waiting until after the fact to correct individual performance.

Health care agencies have only recently paid heed to the tenets of TQM. This management philosophy has been used in Japanese industry since the post–World War II era when W. Edwards Deming was invited to Japan to help rebuild its broken economy. In addition to Deming, people associated with the total quality concept are Walter Stewart (who first published on the subject), Joseph M. Juran, Armand F. Feigenbaum, Phillip B. Crosby, Genichi Taguchi, and Kaoru Ishikawa. Unlike traditional QA programs, the focus of CQI is the *process* of delivering health care. This focus on process avoids placing personal blame for less-than-perfect outcomes. Applying TQM in health care allows management to look at the contribution of all systems to outcomes of the organization.

Deming's (1986, p. 23) guidelines are summarized by his 15-point program:

1. Create, publish, and give to all employees a statement of the aims and purposes of the company or other organization. The management must demonstrate constantly their commitment to this statement.
2. Learn the new philosophy, top management and everybody.
3. Understand the purpose of inspection, for improvement of processes and reduction of costs.
4. End the practice of awarding business on the basis of price tag alone.
5. Improve constantly and forever the system of production and service.
6. Institute training.
7. Teach and institute leadership.
8. Drive out fear. Create trust. Create a climate for innovation.
9. Optimize toward the aims and purposes of the company the efforts of teams, groups, and staff areas.
10. Eliminate exhortations for the workforce.
11. Eliminate numerical quotas for production. Instead, learn and institute methods for improvement.
12. Eliminate management by objective. Instead, learn the capabilities of processes and how to improve them.
13. Remove barriers that rob people of pride of workmanship.
14. Encourage education and self-improvement for everyone.
15. Take action to accomplish the transformation.

Deming's first point emphasizes that an organization must have purpose and values. Health care providers have a clear idea of their values and have been committed to quality in the past, as demonstrated by codes of ethics and standards of care. However, successful TQM and CQI processes rely on a cultural change within an organization and the full support of management. With respect to providing quality health care, a paradigm shift from individual provider responsibility to team responsibility must occur (Sollecito & Johnson, 2013). A guiding principle is a customer orientation focused on positive health outcomes and perceived satisfaction. Customer (client) satisfaction surveys must be done for both internal and external users of services.

Personnel policies that are motivating as well as continuous training/learning opportunities are crucial to any CQI program. Deming's eighth point addresses driving out fear. Fear in this context means the fear of being fired for being innovative or taking risks. In the CQI process, individuals are not blamed for failures in the system and therefore are motivated through the group to continually look for problems and improve system performance.

TQM works best in a flat organizational structure. This means there are very few supervisors between the staff and the director. This organization operates with an interprofessional team approach and a separate but parallel management quality council that monitors strategy and implementation. Teams are empowered to solve problems and locate opportunities for system improvement. Shewhart's plan-do-check-act cycle serves as a guideline for the team approach to problem solving. This approach was modified by Deming to the plan-do-study-act model of TQM and is known as the Deming wheel. Steps include the following (Deming, 1986, p. 88; Deming Institute, 2018):

1. PLAN: Ask questions, such as: What could be the most important accomplishments of this team? What changes might be desirable? What data are available? Are new observations needed? If yes, plan a change or implement a test. Decide how to use the observations.
2. DO: Carry out the change or test decided upon.
3. STUDY: Observe the effects of the change. Study the results. What did we learn? What can we predict?
4. ACT: Repeat the cycle, if the changes worked, or implement a different strategy if the first plan was flawed, or revise the initial strategy based on the changes needed.

A suggested way to start the problem-solving process with a team in step 1 is brainstorming (Harel et al., 2016). Brainstorming is getting everyone's input about a possible process situation with no team member criticizing the suggestion. Because TQI organizations are data driven, moving to step 2 requires that ongoing statistics be collected. Differences from the mean (average) or norm are detected through consistent use of tools, such as the flow chart, the Pareto chart (used to compare the importance of differences between groups of data), cause-and-effect diagrams, check sheets, histograms, control charts, regression, and other statistical analyses (e.g., QA data and techniques, risk management data, risk-adjusted outcome measures, and cost-effectiveness analysis) (Sollecito & Johnson, 2013). Steps 3 and 4 are self-explanatory.

Joseph Juran built on Deming's initial quality work and became a supporter of building quality into all processes. The

Juran trilogy provides an effective way to compare the tasks of quality planning, QA, and QI (Juran, 1986). Quality planning involves determining who the clients are, the needs of those clients, the service that fulfills the needs, and the process to produce that service. QA evaluates the performance of that service, compares it with the service goals, and then makes corrections if necessary. QI makes sure the infrastructure exists to enable individuals to identify improvement projects. Management of QI establishes project teams and provides those teams with the resources needed to carry out improvement projects (Beitsch et al., 2015; Van den Heuvel et al., 2013).

QSEN FOCUS ON QUALITY AND SAFETY EDUCATION FOR NURSES

Targeted Competency: Quality Improvement

Use data to monitor the outcomes of intervention processes, and use improvement methods to design and test changes to continuously improve the quality and safety of health care systems.

Important aspects of quality improvement include:

- **Knowledge:** Recognize that nursing and other health professions students are parts of systems and intervention processes that affect outcomes for clients and families
- **Skills:** Identify gaps between local practices and best practice
- **Attitudes:** Value own and others' contributions to outcomes in local community settings

Quality Improvement Question

You are working as a home care nurse and are discovering a trend of frequent readmissions to the hospital of many of your clients with heart failure. Using the quality assurance approach, consider the following questions:

- What is being done now?
- Why is it being done?
- Is it being done well?
- Can it be done better?
- Should it be done at all?
- Are there improved ways to deliver service?
- How much is it costing?
- Should certain activities be abandoned or replaced?

To which aspects of your clients' quality of life and care transitions will you apply these questions?

Answer

It would be helpful to look at a group of clients discharged from the hospital. Are they receiving adequate education and preparation to return home? You could also gather data about how clients are being managed by the community. How often are they following up with their primary care clinician? Are clients adequately educated to monitor their own fluid status, weight, and dietary restrictions? Are there community-based cardiovascular care programs that can help clients maintain optimum health and avoid exacerbations?

Prepared by Gail Armstrong, PhD(c), DNP, ACNS-BC, CNE, Associate Professor, University of Colorado Denver College of Nursing.

QUALITY AND SAFETY EDUCATION FOR NURSES

The Robert Wood Johnson Foundation (RWJF) funded a project initiative focusing on the development of competencies and resources to enhance the ability of nursing professionals to deliver high-quality and safe nursing care. The Quality Safety Education for Nurses collaboration identified and defined six quality and safety competencies for nursing. In addition, the project allowed for the development of proposed targets for the knowledge, skills, and attitudes of students for each of the six competencies identified by the Institute of Medicine as: client-centered care, teamwork and collaboration, evidence-based practice, quality improvement, safety, and informatics.

QSEN FOCUS ON QUALITY AND SAFETY EDUCATION FOR NURSES

QSEN Project

The overall goal for the Quality and Safety Education for Nurses (QSEN) project is to meet the challenge of preparing future nurses who will have the knowledge, skills, and attitudes (KSAs) necessary to continuously improve the quality and safety of the health care systems within which they work. The following are the definitions for each of the six competencies and examples of the chapters in the text where content can be found and related to the competency.

Client-Centered Care

Recognize the client or designee as the source of control and full partner in providing compassionate and coordinated care based on respect for client's preferences, values, and needs. (Chapters 4, 7, 8, 10, 11, 13, 15, 32)

Teamwork and Collaboration

Function effectively within nursing and interprofessional teams, fostering open communication, mutual respect, and shared decision making to achieve quality client care. (Chapters 5-7, 9, 16, 17, 19, 20, 24-27, 29, 31, 33-35, 37, 39, 41, 45, 46)

Evidence-Based Practice (EBP)

Integrate best current evidence with clinical expertise and client/family preferences and values for delivery of optimal health care. (All chapters, with emphasis in Chapters 10 and 24)

Quality Improvement (QI)

Use data to monitor the outcomes of care processes and use improvement methods to design and test changes to continuously improve the quality and safety of health care systems. (Chapters 3, 6, 9, 13, 15-17, 22-24)

Safety

Minimizes risk of harm to clients and providers through both system effectiveness and individual performance. (Chapters 13-15, 21, 22, 27, 39-46)

Informatics

Use information and technology to communicate, manage knowledge, mitigate error, and support decision making. (Chapters 21-24)

All of these competencies are addressed in this text as the competencies relate to public health nursing practice. The knowledge, skills, and attitudes related to QI are addressed in this chapter and one area of the QI competency appears in the following table.

Knowledge	Skills	Attitudes
Describe approaches for changing processes of care	Design a small test of change in daily work (using an experiential learning method such as PDSA)	Value local change (in individual practice or team practice on a unit) and its role in creating joy in work
	Practice aligning the aims, measures, and changes involved in improving care	Appreciate the value of what individuals and teams can to do to improve care
	Use measures to evaluate the effect of change	

TQM/CQI IN COMMUNITY AND PUBLIC HEALTH SETTINGS

Guidelines provided by the 1991 APHA *Model Standards* linked standards to meeting the health goals for the nation in the year 2000 (Sollecito & Johnson, 2013). *Healthy People 2000* and APHA *Model Standards* (APHA, 1991) provided not only lists of priority health objectives for the nation and a way for public health to implement TQM/CQI but also the most current statistics and scientific knowledge about health promotion and disease prevention. *Healthy People in Healthy Communities* (USDHHS, 2001) provided the objectives with their stated targets, measurement tools, and reflected intended performance expectations.

Healthy People 2010 built on *Healthy People 2000* and contained modified and additional objectives for promoting health and preventing disease (USDHHS, 2000). An important part of the framework of *Healthy People 2010* was eliminating health disparities and ensuring access to quality health care for all. After extensive review of the *Healthy People 2010* objectives, new goals and objectives were developed for *Healthy People 2020* (USDHHS, 2010). The goals for *Healthy People 2020* are as follows:

- Attain high-quality, longer lives free of preventable disease, disability, injury, and premature death.
- Achieve health equity, eliminate disparities, and improve the health of all groups.
- Create social and physical environments that promote good health for all.
- Promote quality of life, healthy development, and healthy behaviors across all life stages.

Although all of the goals speak to quality of life and health, the second goal specifically addresses issues related to quality of health care delivery.

In addition, the *Planned Approach to Community Health* (PATCH) (CDC, 1995, with update in 2010); the Assessment Protocol for Excellence in Public Health (APEXPH), *APEXPH in Practice* (NACCHO, 1995, 2014); and most recently the *Mobilizing for Action through Planning and Partnerships* (MAPP) process (NACCHO, 2014) provide methods of assessing community needs to see how well health departments are operating to meet existing standards (see Chapter 23).

As health care reform continues, especially with the implementation of the Affordable Care Act, public health agencies face competition and are trying to reform themselves. A promising outcome of reform is how private health care and public health can come together in a community-level effort to monitor performance and improve health (see Chapter 3).

Recognizing the many factors that cause health problems and the fragmenting that continues to exist in the health care system, the public–private collaborative framework supported by the *Healthy People* documents involves many stakeholders, including public health, in monitoring the health of entire communities. Performance monitoring is defined as "a continuing community-based process of selecting indicators that can be used to measure the process and outcomes of an intervention strategy for health improvement (making the results available to the community as a whole) to inform assessments of an effective intervention and the contributions of accountable agencies to this" (USDHHS, 2014). These indicators would measure processes or states that contribute to health, and thus the processes are potentially alterable. As previously noted, there are three documents highlighted here that monitor the quality and safety of health care, including the contributions of public health. Table 24.3 provides highlights from each of these reports.

Home health care agencies have increasingly adopted QI programs because of the competition that exists. Congruent with the TQM philosophy, meeting customer expectations is essential for home health care agencies. Models for QA/QI in home health care have been developed to improve the quality of

TABLE 24.3 National Quality and Safety Reports

Name of Report	Most Recent Results
The National Healthcare Quality and Disparities Report, Agency for Healthcare Research and Quality, began publication in 2003 and has published for 16 years	The *National Healthcare Quality and Disparities Report* assesses the performance of our health care system and identifies areas of strengths and weaknesses, as well as disparities, for access to health care and quality of health care. Quality is described in terms of six priorities: patient safety, person-centered care, care coordination, effective treatment, healthy living, and care affordability. The report is based on more than 250 measures of quality and disparities covering a broad array of health care services and settings. The outcomes for these measures are presented by state and can be found on the website https://nhqrnet.ahrq.gov.
The State of Health Care Quality, 2017; The National Committee for Quality Assurance	The National Committee for Quality Assurance is an independent 501 nonprofit organization in the United States that works to improve health care quality through the administration of evidence-based standards, measures, programs, and accreditation The organization assesses HEDIS to determine quality improvement across third-party payers. Reports after more than a decade of progress in quality of care related to access and availability of care, use of services, risk adjusted use, and collects data related to health care interventions, like depression screening and pneumonia vaccinations.
The National Quality Forum Reports	National Quality Forum (NQF) is a not-for-profit, nonpartisan, membership-based organization that works to catalyze improvements in health care. Beginning in 1999, NQF has focused on an array of cross-cutting issues and builds upon 15 years of evidence-based measure endorsement that is the gold standard for health care quality measurement.

HEDIS, Health Plan Employer Data and Information Set.

care in TQM frameworks emphasizing processes, empowerment, collaboration, consumers, data and measurement, and standards and outcomes (Oakland, 2014). Datasets of clinical information, such as those developed through the Omaha System (see Chapter 41) and the OASIS toolkit from the National Association of Home Care and Hospice (NAHC, 2014), are useful in measuring quality of care. In 2003 the Home Health Care Quality Initiative (HHQI) was developed by the USDHHS to provide consumers with data on the quality of home health services. *Home Health Compare,* posted on the Medicare website, is a home health agency report card available to consumers nationwide (USDHHS, 2018).

Finally, in the area of standards and guidelines, Honoré and Scott (2010) address six priority areas of performance that need improvement. One of these areas is consistently providing appropriate and effective care. This area is applicable to all health care practitioners, including nurses. Evidence-based **practice guidelines** are one way to deliver consistent, up-to-date care and to improve outcomes for individuals, communities, and populations. Every year the American Cancer Society (ACS) provides a summary of current cancer screening guidelines for health care professionals and updates the guidelines at least every five years, or sooner if new evidence warrants an update (Smith et al., 2018). The use of guidelines helps in gathering data on the effectiveness and outcomes of nurse interventions (Jones, 2016; Matthew-Maich et al., 2013). The AHRQ, formerly the Agency for Healthcare Policy and Research (AHCPR), has played a major role in developing clinical practice guidelines.

Guidelines are protocols or statements of recommended practice developed by governmental and health care agencies and by professional organizations; they are based on the distilling of scientific evidence and expert opinion that guide a clinician in decision making. Guidelines provide research-based evidence for interventions and promote improved health outcomes. Using research findings as guidelines or frames of reference can improve nurses' awareness of new or better ways to practice, allow for documentation of nurse interventions, and improve outcomes at all levels of public health nursing practice (Jones, 2016; Matthew-Maich et al., 2013) (see Chapter 11). Keystones of evidence-based practice guidelines arise from client concerns, clinical experience, best practices, and clinical data and research (Melnyk & Fineout-Overholt, 2015). Clinical practice guidelines are systematically developed statements to assist practitioner and client decisions about appropriate health care for specific clinical circumstances (as discussed in Chapter 10).

One of the quality reports published by AHRQ each year is the *National Healthcare Quality and Disparities Report*, the most recent being 2018. Primary care practice guidelines are available in the *Guide to Clinical Preventive Services* (U.S. Preventive Services Task Force [USPSTF], 2014) and the population-based *Guide to Community Preventive Services* available on the CDC website. This guide is an ongoing process of the Taskforce on Community Preventive Services that offers information on changing risk behaviors; reducing specific diseases, injuries and impairments, and environmental concerns; and state-of-the-art public health activities. Nurses need guidelines to reduce differences in care practices, to improve outcomes on the basis of the best research available, and to deliver effective care to individuals, communities, and populations.

Using QA/QI in CQI

QA/QI methods and tools help agencies conform to standards required by external accrediting agencies. QA/QI provides a way to identify examples of substandard care and to improve that care when standards are not met. QA is focused on problem detection, whereas CQI is focused on problem prevention and continuous improvement. In QA, little attention is paid to preventing errors or problems and finding out who owns the quality issues. Furthermore, the QA process may stop unless another problem is found. Sollecito and Johnson (2013) point out differences in traditional management models that use performance standards versus those that use TQM (Table 24.4). The most important difference is in the emphasis on QA, or simply identifying the problem in the traditional management model versus the emphasis on CQI in the total quality management model. In TQM the problem is identified and measures are implemented to correct the problem. The TQM model is required in health care delivery because of the standards set by the national accrediting agencies such as TJC. Public health, through the public health accrediting process begun in 2011, is required to emphasize TQM.

Positive steps of a known QA program can be integrated into a CQI approach. Strengths of QA include a history of expertise in developing evaluation of structure, identifying high-priority problems, and developing knowledge in QA and information systems (Burstin et al., 2016). These strengths can be used advantageously in a CQI effort.

Traditional Quality Assurance

Traditional QA programs can fit well with the CQI process. The overall goal of specific QA approaches is to monitor the process and outcomes of client care. The goals of CQI are as follows:

1. To identify problems between provider and client through QA methods
2. To intervene in problem cases
3. To provide feedback regarding interactions between client and provider
4. To provide documentation of interactions between client and provider

TABLE 24.4 Traditional Management Model Compared With Total Quality Management (TQM) Model

Traditional Model	TQM Model
Legal or professional authority	Collective or managerial responsibility
Specialized accountability	Process accountability
Administrative authority	Participation
Meeting standards	Meeting process and performance expectations
Longer planning horizon	Shorter planning horizon
Quality assurance	Continuous improvement

Specific approaches are often implemented voluntarily by agencies and provider groups interested in the quality of interactions in their setting. However, state and federal governments require mandatory programs within public health agencies. For example, periodic utilization review, peer reviews (audits), and other QA measures are required in public health agencies that receive funds from state taxes, Medicaid, Medicare, and other public funding sources. Examples of specific approaches to QA are agency staff review committees for peer review (Edwards, 2013), utilization review committees for Medicare and Medicaid, research studies, quality improvement organization (QIO) monitoring, client satisfaction surveys, risk management, and malpractice lawsuits.

Staff Review Committee. Staff review committees are the most common specific approach to QA in the United States. Staff review committees are designed to monitor client-specific aspects of certain levels of care. The audit is the major tool used to evaluate quality of care.

The audit process (Fig. 24.1) consists of six steps:

1. Select a topic for study.
2. Select explicit criteria for quality care.
3. Review records to determine whether criteria are met.
4. Do a peer review for all cases that do not meet criteria.
5. Make specific recommendations to correct problems.
6. Follow up to determine whether problems have been eliminated.

Two types of audits are used in nursing peer review: concurrent and retrospective. The concurrent audit is a process audit that evaluates the quality of ongoing care by looking at the nursing process. Concurrent audit is used by Medicare and Medicaid to evaluate care being received by public health/home health clients. The audit data look at the group, population, or community served. The advantages of this method are as follows:

- Identification of problems at the time care is given
- Provision of a mechanism for identifying and meeting client needs during the intervention
- Implementation of measures to fulfill professional responsibilities
- Provision of a mechanism for communicating on behalf of the client

The disadvantages of the concurrent audit are as follows:

- It is time consuming.
- It is more costly to implement than the retrospective audit.
- Because the intervention is ongoing, it does not present the total picture of the outcomes of the intervention that the client ultimately will receive.

The retrospective audit, or outcome audit, evaluates quality of care through evaluation of the nursing process at the end of a program or as an audit of the long-term impact of a program within the health care system. The advantages of the retrospective audit are that it provides the following:

- Comparison of actual practice to standards of care
- Analysis of actual practice findings
- A total picture of care given to a population or group of clients
- More accurate data for planning corrective action

Disadvantages of the retrospective audit method are as follows:

- The focus of evaluation is directed away from ongoing care.
- Client problems (group or population or community) are identified after care is offered through the program; thus corrective action can be used only to improve the care of future clients.

Currently in public health, program record audits are done to determine the processes and outcomes of care, such as family planning audits, WIC audits, breast and cervical cancer screening audits, billing coding (to audit costs), and registration audits. Programs regarding physical activity, nutrition, obesity, arthritis, smoking cessation, and others are all designed to address the major causes of morbidity and mortality locally, statewide, and nationwide. The audits assist in determining the progress being made in reducing morbidity and mortality.

Utilization Review. The purpose of utilization review is to ensure that care is needed and that the cost is appropriate. Utilization review is more likely used in HMOs, other MCOs, and ACOs including Medicaid or Medicare state-level managed care programs. There are three types of utilization review:

1. *Prospective:* An assessment of the necessity of care before giving service
2. *Concurrent:* A review of the necessity of services while care is being given
3. *Retrospective:* An analysis of the necessity of the services received by the client after the care has been given

Each of these reviews assesses the appropriate cost of care. Prospectively, care can be denied and money saved. Concurrently, services can be cut if they are not found to be essential.

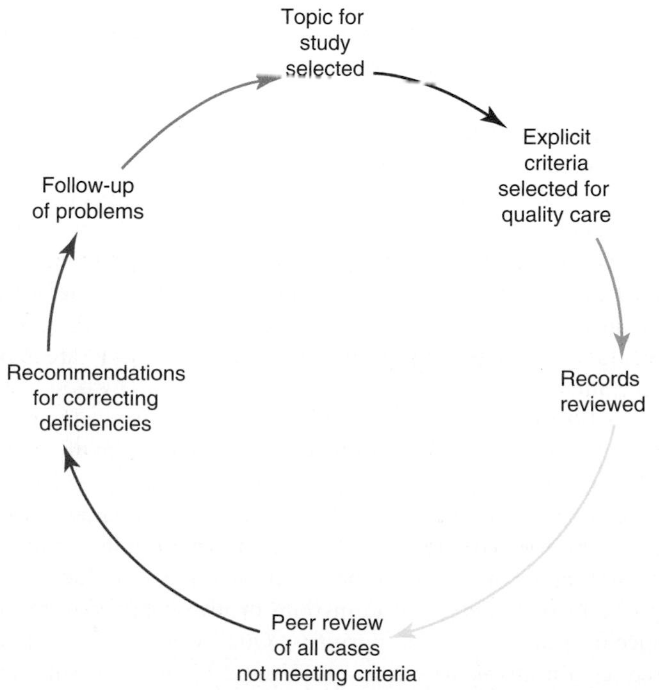

Fig. 24.1 The audit process.

Retrospectively, payment can be denied to the provider if the care was not necessary.

Utilization review began in the middle part of the twentieth century out of concern for increasing health care costs. The first committees were developed by insurance companies and professional groups. Utilization review committees became mandatory under the 1965 Medicare law as a way to control hospital costs.

The utilization review process includes development of explicit criteria regarding the need for services and the length of service. Utilization review has been used primarily in hospitals to establish the need for client admission and to determine the length of hospital stay. In community and public health, especially home health care, utilization review establishes criteria for admission to agency service, the number of visits a client may receive, the eligibility for client services (e.g., a nursing aide or physical therapist), and discharge.

Utilization review has several advantages:

- It helps clients avoid unnecessary care.
- It may encourage clients to consider alternative care options, such as home health care rather than hospital care.
- It can provide guidelines for staff and program development.
- It provides for agency accountability to the consumer.

The major disadvantage of utilization review is that not all clients fit the classic picture presented by the explicit criteria used to determine approval or denial of care. For example, an older adult client was admitted to a home health care agency for management after hospital discharge. The client was paraplegic as a result of a cerebrovascular accident. After several weeks of physical and speech therapy, the client showed little sign of progress. The utilization review committee considered the client's condition to be stable and did not recognize the continued need for management to prevent future complications; therefore, Medicare payment was denied.

Appeal mechanisms have been built into the utilization review process used by Medicare and Medicaid. The appeal allows providers and clients to present additional data that may help reverse the original decision to deny payment.

EVIDENCE-BASED PRACTICE

The Public Health Accreditation Board (PHAB) contracted with a social science research organization, NORC at the University of Chicago, to evaluate the accreditation process to identify opportunities for improvement and to assess the impact of accreditation (Kronstadt et al., 2016). The researchers surveyed health departments one year after accreditation, asking a series of Likert-style accreditation-related statements and conducted focus group and one-on-one interviews. Data collection was completed on a quarterly basis from October 2013 through January 2016. Surveys were sent to 60 health departments, of which 52 (87 percent) responded. Three focus groups and 18 interviews were conducted with health department personnel and stakeholders. A vast majority of survey respondents agreed or strongly agreed that accreditation stimulated quality and performance improvement opportunities within the health department (98 percent), allowed the department to better identify strengths and weaknesses (96 percent), and helped the department document capacity to deliver the core functions of public health and the Essential Public Health Services (95 percent), and improved the management process used by department leadership (92 percent). Respondents also reported increased accountability and improved transparency for the health department. The researchers noted that their study findings were consistent with previous similar studies, which reported accreditation activities improved quality improvement and collaboration. The researchers noted that the foremost reported benefit of accreditation reported was the increased use of quality improvement information in decision making and in supporting a culture of quality improvement.

Nurse Use

Accreditation has the potential to strengthen health departments' capacities and infrastructure by fostering quality improvement, strengthening management processes, and improving accountability. Community/public health nurses are in a prime position to be leaders in their organizations in leading accreditation activities and developing a quality improvement environment.

From Kronstadt J, Meit M, Siegfried A, et al.: Evaluating the impact of national public health department *accreditation*—United States, 2016. *MMWR Morb Mortal Wkly Rep* 65(31):803-806, 2016.

Risk Management. Risk management committees are often a part of the CQI program of a community agency. Risk management seeks to reduce the agency's liability because of grievances brought against them. The risk management committee reviews all risks to which an agency is exposed. It reviews client and personnel safety policies and procedures and determines whether personnel are following the rules. Examples of problems reviewed by a risk management committee in public health clinics include administering incorrect vaccination dosage, pediatric client injury caused by a fall from an examination table, or injury to the nurse from a needlestick in the sexually transmitted diseases clinic at the health department or as a result of an accident while making a home visit. Incident reports are reviewed by the risk management committee for appropriate, accurate, and thorough documentation of any problem that occurs relating to clients or personnel. In addition, patterns are identified from looking at program data that may require changes in policy or staff development to correct the problem. As a part of risk management, grievance procedures are established for both clients and personnel (Institute for Health Care Improvement, 2018).

Professional Review Organizations/Quality Improvement Organizations. The Professional Standards Review Organization (PSRO) was established in 1972 in an amendment to the Social Security Act (PL 92-603) as a publicly mandated utilization and peer review program. This law provided that medical, hospital, and nursing home care under Medicare, Medicaid, and Title V Maternal and Child Health Programs would be reviewed for appropriateness and necessary care to be reimbursed.

In 1983 Congress passed the Peer Review Improvement Act (PL 97-248), creating professional review organizations (PROs). PROs replaced PSROs and are directed by the federal government to reduce hospital admissions for procedures that can be performed safely and effectively in an ambulatory surgical setting on an outpatient basis. The goal was to reduce inappropriate or unnecessary admissions or invasive procedures by specific practitioners or hospitals. Quality measures include reducing unnecessary admissions caused by previous substandard care, avoidable complications and deaths, and unnecessary surgery or invasive procedures (CMS, 2018). The PRO is now known as the Quality Improvement Organization (QIO).

Institutions contracting with QIOs for quality reviews are usually state organizations that establish criteria for care on the basis of local patterns of practice, and they are private contractors to CMS and mostly not-for-profit organizations. They may have on their board health care providers who are independent from the QIO, and the board must have at least one consumer. QIOs must define their operational objectives; monitor access to care, cost of care, and quality concerns; and protect the Medicare Trust. Professionals working under the regulation of QIOs should develop accurate and complete documenting procedures to ensure compliance with the criteria of the QIO (CMS, 2018).

Debate has occurred over the limits and benefits of the federally mandated quality review process. Limits include jeopardizing professional autonomy because decision making regarding care includes professionals, consumers, and government representatives. Another limitation of this process is the development of a costly control mechanism whereby client care activities may be determined by cost rather than by professional criteria. The benefit of the QIO system has been the development of standards and the peer review mechanisms to increase accountability for care provided.

TQM provides direction for managing a system of care, whereas CQI using QA/QI focuses on the care a client receives within the system.

Evaluative Studies. Evaluative studies for quality health care increased during the twentieth century. Studies demonstrate the effect of nursing and health care interventions on client populations. Three key models have been used to evaluate quality: Donabedian's structure-process-outcome model, the tracer method, and the sentinel method.

Donabedian's model (1981, 1985, 2003) introduced three major methods for evaluating quality care:

1. Structure: Evaluating the setting and instruments used to provide care; examples of structure are facilities, equipment, characteristics of the administrative organization, client mix, and the qualifications of health providers
2. Process: Evaluating activities as they relate to standards and expectations of health providers in the management of client care
3. Outcome: The net change or result that occurs as a result of health care

The three methods may be used separately to evaluate a part of care. However, to get an overall picture of quality of care, they should be used together.

The tracer method described by Kessner and Kalk (1973) is a measure of both process and outcome of care and is used today. This method is more effective in evaluating health care of groups than of individual clients. It is also more effective in evaluating care delivered by an institution than care delivered by an individual provider. The following are essential characteristics for implementing the tracer method (Kessner & Kalk, 1973; Papanicolas & Smith, 2013; Spath & Kelly, 2017):

1. A tracer, or a problem, that has a definite impact on the client's level of functioning
2. Well-defined and easily diagnosed characteristics
3. Population prevalence high enough to permit adequate data collection
4. A known variation resulting from use of effective health care
5. Well-defined management techniques in prevention, diagnosis, treatment, or rehabilitation
6. Understood (documented) effects of nonmedical factors on the tracer

Client groups selected for tracer outcome studies in nursing would have the following:

1. A shared health problem
2. Receiving a similar intervention
3. Sharing similar needs
4. Located in the same community
5. Having a similar lifestyle
6. Being at the same illness stage

The tracer method provides nurses with data to show the differences in outcomes as a result of nursing care standards.

The sentinel method of quality evaluation is based on epidemiologic principles. This method is an outcome measure for examining specific instances of client care (Spath & Kelly, 2017). Changes in the sentinel indicate potential problems for others. For example, increases in encephalitis in certain communities may result from increases in mosquito populations. Data may be collected at the health department through a state or local required disease reporting system. The health department would be notified and an immediate mosquito control strategy would be put into place. Such an intervention would include, for example, nurses notifying the population to remove standing water around the outside of homes, such as animal water bowls, rain barrels, and gutter downspout water collection pools. Flyers may be sent home with school children or given to clients visiting the public health clinics, and media announcements may be used. In addition, the environmental office at the health department may inspect local swimming pools and may also implement a nighttime mosquito spraying program throughout the community.

HOW TO Conduct a Sentinel Evaluation

- Identify cases of unnecessary disease, disability, and complications (for example, tuberculosis).
- Count the deaths from these causes.
- Examine the circumstances surrounding the unnecessary event (or sentinel), in detail.
- Review morbidity and mortality rates as an index for comparison; determine the critical increase in the untimely event, which may reflect changes in quality of care. Example: Compare the incidence and prevalence of TB cases before the increased population occurred.
- Explore health status indicators, such as changes in social, economic, political, and environmental factors that may have an effect on health outcomes. Example: Overcrowding in the shelter where migrant workers stay (environmental) and the inability to follow-up on testing because of the transient nature of the population (social).

CLIENT SATISFACTION

Client satisfaction is another approach to measuring quality of care. Client satisfaction can be assessed using in-person or telephone interviews and mailed questionnaires. Satisfaction surveys are used to assess care received during an admission to a specific agency, to assess a client's personal nursing care, or to assess the total care that the client received from all services.

Satisfaction surveys may measure the interventions used for client care, attitudes about the care received and the providers of care, and perceptions of the situation (environment) in which the care was received. Clients are often more critical of interpersonal and situational components of care than of the interventions of care.

Satisfaction surveys are an essential aspect of QA. Survey data provide clues to reasons for client compliance or noncompliance with plans of care. Although consumers may not view quality in the same light as the health professional, surveys provide data about health-seeking behaviors, the probability of malpractice litigation, and the likelihood of continuing client-provider–agency relationships—always an important measure for community-based and public health agencies (Oakland, 2014) (Fig. 24.2).

Please mark the following questions using the scale.

Domain	Example	Strongly Agree	Somewhat Agree	Agree	Somewhat Disagree	Strongly Disagree
Affective support	1. The visiting nurse was understanding of my health concerns.					
	2. The nurse gave me encouragement in regard to my health problems.					
Health information	3. I got my questions answered in an individual way.					
	4. The information I received from the nurse helped me to take care of myself at home.					
Decision control	5. I was included in decision making.					
	6. I was included in the planning of my care.					
Technical competencies	7. The care I received was of high quality.					
	8. Decisions regarding my health care were of high quality.					
Accessibility	9. The nurse was available when I needed help.					
	10. The nurse was on time.					
Overall satisfaction	11. Overall, I was satisfied with my health care.					
	12. The care I received was of high quality.					

Fig. 24.2 Client satisfaction tool domains and examples.

Malpractice Litigation

Malpractice litigation (i.e., a lawsuit) is a specific approach to QA imposed on the health care delivery system by the legal system. Malpractice litigation typically results from client dissatisfaction with the provider and with the content of the care received. Nursing is not immune from malpractice litigation. Nursing must continue to have a sound QA program that ensures quality care. This will reduce the risk of quality control measures being imposed by an external source, such as the legal system. As a true example, a public health nurse was individually sued by a new family to the community because the nurse repeated an immunization the child had already received prior to moving to the community. The result was Guillain-Barré syndrome. The nurse was found at fault even though the parents did not provide the physician's record of immunizations to the nurse. It was the nurse's responsibility to follow standard guidelines and to obtain the essential records prior to proving the immunization. The public health department was dismissed from the lawsuit because of immunity granted to state agencies.

MODEL CQI PROGRAM

The primary purpose of a QA/QI program is to ensure that the results of an organized activity are consistent with the expectations. All personnel affected by a QI program should be involved in its development and implementation. Although administration and management are responsible for the quality of services, the key to that quality is in the personnel who deliver the service: their knowledge, skills, and attitudes.

Fig. 24.3 shows a model that identifies the basic components of a QI program. QI programs answer the following questions about health care services and nursing care:

1. What is being done now?
2. Why is it being done?
3. Is it being done well?
4. Can it be done better?
5. Should it be done at all?
6. Are there improved ways to deliver the service?
7. How much does it cost?
8. Should certain activities be abandoned or replaced?

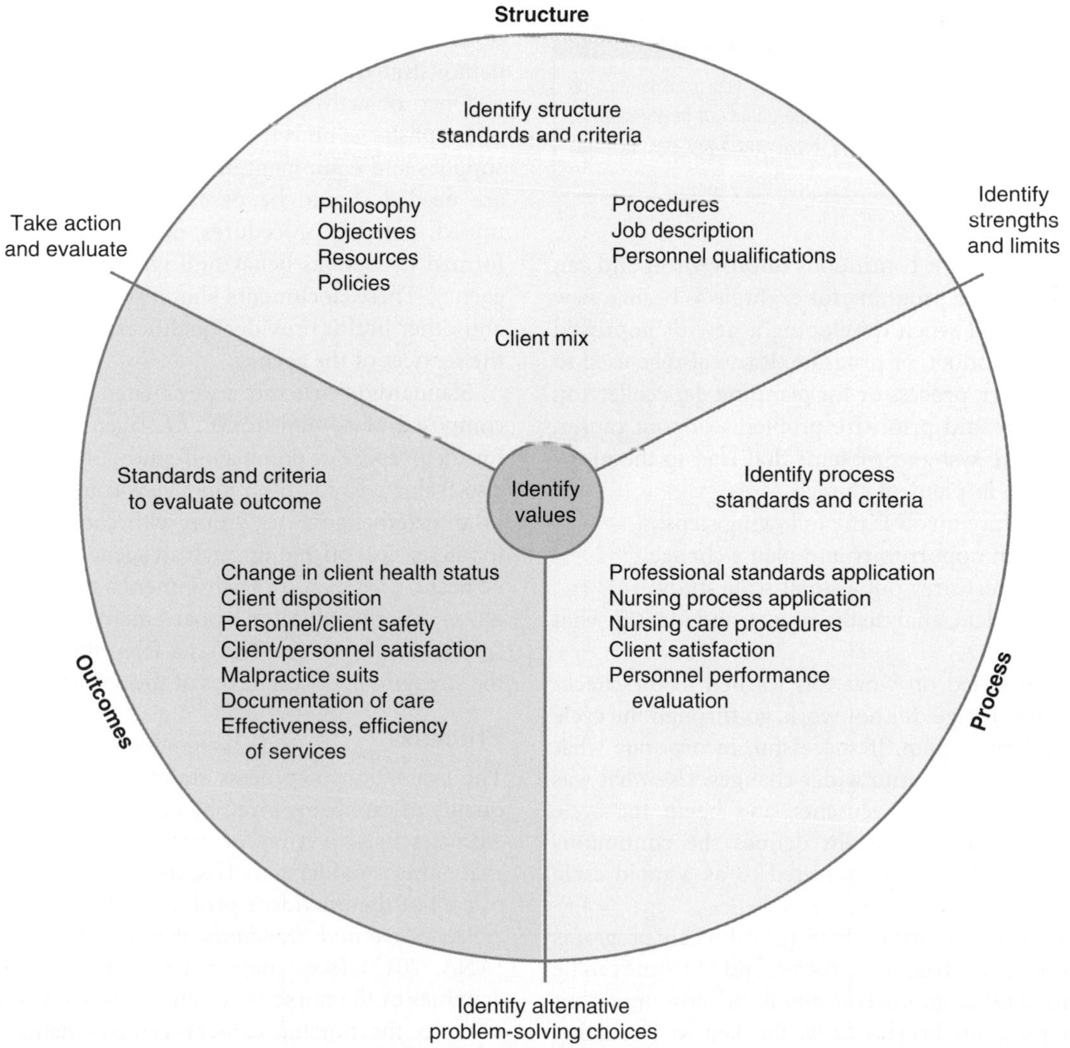

Fig. 24.3 Model quality improvement programs.

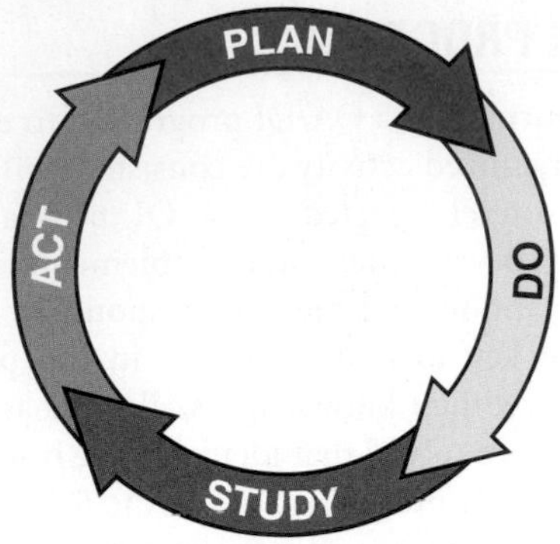

Fig. 24.4 The plan-do-study-act (PDSA) model of continuous quality improvement. The concept of the PDSA cycle was originally developed by Walter Shewhart, the pioneering statistician who developed statistical process control in the Bell Laboratories in the United States during the 1930s. It is often referred to as the "Shewhart Cycle." It was adopted in the 1950s by W. Edwards Deming and is often referred to as the "Deming Wheel."

As a part of answering the questions and determining changes that can improve services, public health can use the PDSA model. The steps of the model are shown in Fig. 24.4.

> **CHECK YOUR PRACTICE**
>
> As a member of a committee in the school system of your community, you have been asked to determine how to improve the quality of health care for the population of children in your community. How would you approach this project? What would you do?

The PDSA is a model for continuous improvement and can be used after an audit of a program, for example to begin a new improvement project or when developing a new or improved design of a process, product, or program. It can also be used to define a repetitive work process or for planning data collection and analysis to verify and prioritize problems or root causes, which are actually the system problems that lead to the problem. It is also used to implement change.

The PDSA procedure involves the following steps:

1. **Plan.** Recognize an opportunity and plan a change.
2. **Do.** Test the change. Carry out a small-scale study.
3. **Study.** Review the data, analyze the results, and identify what has been learned.
4. **Act.** Take action based on what was learned in the check/study step: If the change did not work, go through the cycle again with a different plan. If successful, incorporate what you learned from the test into wider changes. Use what was learned to plan new improvements, and begin the cycle again. Beginning the cycle again defines the continuous program of CQI. This is also referred to as a rapid cycle improvement process in health care.

Donabedian's framework for evaluating health care programs using the components of structure, process, and outcome can be used in developing a QI program. *Outcome* is the most important ingredient of a program because it is the key to evaluating providers and agencies by accrediting bodies, by insurance companies, and by Medicare and Medicaid through QIOs, report cards, and other accrediting agencies.

Structure

The vision, values, philosophy, and objectives of an agency serve to define the structural standards of the agency. Evaluation of structure is a specific approach to looking at quality. In evaluating the structure of an organization, the evaluator determines whether the agency is adhering to the stated philosophy and objectives and to its vision and stated values. Is the agency providing services to populations across the life span? Are primary, secondary, and/or tertiary preventive services offered? Standards of structure are defined by the licensing or accrediting agency (e.g., the Community Health Accreditation Partner [CHAP's] standards for accrediting home health agencies).

Identifying values, the first step in a QA program, serves to define the beliefs of the agency about humanity, nursing, the community, and health. The beliefs of the community, the population to be served, and the providers of care are equally important to the agency, and all need to be considered to provide quality service.

Identifying standards and criteria for QA begins with writing the philosophy and objectives of the organization. Program objectives define the intended results of nursing care, descriptions of client behaviors, and/or change in health status to be demonstrated on discharge.

Once objectives are formulated, the resources needed to accomplish the objectives should be identified. The personnel, supplies and equipment, facilities, and financial resources that are needed should be described. Once resources are determined, policies, procedures, and job descriptions should be formed to serve as behavioral guides to the employees of the agency. These documents should reflect the essential nursing and other health provider qualifications needed to implement the services of the agency.

Standards of structure are evaluated internally by a committee composed of administrative, management, and staff members for the purpose of doing a self-study. Standards of structure are also evaluated by a utilization review committee, often composed of an external advisory group with community representatives for all services offered through an agency, such as a nurse, a public health physician, an environmental engineer, a sanitation engineer, a health educator, a board member, and an administrator from a similar agency. The data from these committees identify the strengths and weaknesses of the agency structure.

Process

The evaluation of process standards is a specific look at the quality of care being given by agency providers, such as nurses. Agencies use a variety of methods to determine criteria for evaluating provider activities: conceptual models; the standards of care of the provider's professional organization, such as the ANA's *Scope and Standards of Public Health Nursing Practice* (ANA, 2013) (see Chapter 1); or the nursing process. The activities of the nurse are evaluated to see whether they are the same as the nursing care procedures defined by the public health agency.

The primary approaches used for process evaluation include the peer review committee and the client (often community) satisfaction survey. The techniques used for process evaluation are direct observation, focus groups, questionnaire, interview, written audit, and video or digital recordings of client and provider encounters.

Once data are collected to evaluate nursing process standards, the peer review committee reviews the data to identify strengths and weaknesses in the quality of care delivered. The peer review committee is usually an internal committee composed of representatives of the nursing staff who are trained to administer audit instruments and conduct client interviews.

Outcome

The evaluation of outcome standards, or the result of nursing care, is one of the more difficult tasks facing nursing today. Identifying changes in the client's health status that result from nursing care provides nursing data that demonstrate the contribution of nursing to the health care delivery system. Research studies using the tracer or sentinel method to identify client outcomes and client satisfaction surveys can be used to measure outcome standards. Measures of outcome standards include client data about the changes in the community in low-birth weight babies as a result of improved prenatal care and client compliance with care through the WIC program.

From these data, strengths and weaknesses in nursing care delivery can be determined. The most common measurement methods are direct physical observations and interviews. Instruments have also been developed to measure general health status indicators in home health. The Omaha Visiting Nurse Association problem classification system includes nursing diagnosis, protocols of care, and a problem rating scale to measure nursing care outcomes. Nursing has been involved primarily in evaluating program outcomes to justify program expenses rather than in evaluating client outcomes.

Outcome evaluation assumes that health care has a positive effect on client status. The major problem with outcome evaluation is determining which nursing care activities are primarily responsible for causing changes in client status. Recently, studies have been conducted on nurse-sensitive indicators, such as failure to rescue, that show the importance of nurse staffing in adverse client outcomes (McHugh et al., 2016; Sherwood & Barnsteiner, 2017). In nursing, many uncontrolled factors in the field, such as environment, community services, and family relationships, have an effect on client status. Often it is difficult to determine whether these factors are the cause of changes in client status or whether nursing interventions have the most effect.

Types of problems studied in a QA program include reasons for the following:

- Client death (population mortality)
- Client injury (population morbidity)
- Personnel and client safety
- Agency liability
- Increased costs
- Denied reimbursement by third-party payers (decreased program funding by government)

TABLE 24.5 Quality Assurance Measures

Structure	Process	Outcome
Internal agency	Peer review committees	Internal agency committees
Self-study	Prospective audit	Evaluative studies
Review agency documents	Concurrent audit	Survey health status
	Retrospective audit	
External agency	Client	Client
Regulatory audit	Satisfaction survey	Malpractice suits
	Utilization review	Satisfaction survey

- Client complaints
- Inefficient service
- Staff noncompliance with standards of structure
- Lack of resources
- Unnecessary staff work and overtime
- Documenting of care
- Client health status (population health status)

Table 24.5 summarizes QA measures.

Evaluation, Interpretation, and Action

Interpreting the findings of a quality care evaluation is an important part of the process. It allows differences between the quality care standards of the agency and the actual practice of the nurse or other health providers to be identified. These patterns reflect the total agency's functioning over time and generate information for decisions to be made about the strengths and limits of the agency. Regular intervals for evaluation should be established within the agency, and periodic reports should be written so that the combined results of structure, process, and outcome efforts can be analyzed and health care delivery patterns and problems can be identified. These reports should be used to establish an ongoing picture of changes that occur within an agency to justify nursing services.

Identifying choices of possible courses of action to correct the weaknesses within the agency should involve both the administration and the staff. The courses of action chosen should be based on their importance, cost, and timeliness. For example, if there is a nursing problem in the recording of client health education, the agency administration and staff may analyze the problem to see why it is occurring. Reasons for lack of record-keeping given by the nurses include a lack of time to do paperwork properly, workloads that reduce the amount of time spent with clients, and lack of available resources for health education. If such reasons are given, it would not be appropriate for management to deal with the problem by providing a staff development program on the importance of doing and recording health education; it would be more important to assess how to provide the time and resources necessary for the nurses to offer health education to the clients. Economically, it may be more beneficial to provide personal data assistants or laptop computers and clerical assistance so that nurses can make notes at the point of implementation, thereby providing more client contact time, or it may be more beneficial economically to employ an additional nurse and reduce workloads.

Taking action is the final step in the QA/QI model. Once the alternative courses of action are chosen to correct problems, actions must be implemented for change to occur in the overall operation of the agency. Follow-up and evaluation of actions taken must occur to improve quality of care. Although health provider evaluation will continue to be included in a QI effort, the focus of a CQI effort emphasizes the process and not the person. The assumption here is that health care professionals and other employees customarily want to do the best job possible for the client, and problems or differences in a process should not be automatically attributed to their behavior. Although frequent feedback should be given to all employees, the hallmark of QI is continuous learning. Staff development must be ongoing for all employees. (The Levels of Prevention box shows prevention levels related to quality management.)

LEVELS OF PREVENTION

Quality Management

Primary Prevention

The nurse participates in a parent education program to improve the immunization level of children in the local elementary school and develops a strategy for follow-up.

Secondary Prevention

Agency evaluation, using a retrospective audit of records of the immunization program, determines that the vaccine-preventable infectious disease rates have declined in the elementary school after the implementation of the parent education program.

Tertiary Prevention

A review of the public health report card indicated that community incidence of complications from vaccine-preventable diseases have declined over a two-year period after the implementation of the parent education program.

Documentation is essential to evaluating quality care in any organization. The following section focuses on the kinds of documentation that normally occur in a community agency.

RECORDS

Records are an important part of the communication structure of the health care organization. Accurate and complete records are required by law and must be kept by all government and nongovernment agencies. In most states, the state departments of health stipulate the kinds of records to be kept and their content requirements for community agencies.

Records provide complete information about the client (whether a family, group, population or community), indicate the extent and quality of services being given, resolve legal issues in malpractice suits, and provide information for education and research.

Community and Public Health Agency Records

Within the community or public health agency, many types of records are kept and used to predict population trends in a community, to identify health needs and problems, to prepare and justify budgets, and to make administrative decisions. The kinds of records kept by the agency may include reports of accidents, births, census, chronic disease, communicable disease, mortality rates, life expectancy, morbidity rates, child and spouse abuse, occupational illness and injury, and environmental health.

Other types of records kept within the agency are those used to maintain administrative contact and control of the organization. Three types of records make up this category: clinical, provider service, and financial. The *clinical record* is the client health record. The *provider service records* include information about the number of clinic clients seen daily, the immunizations given, home visits made daily, transportation and mileage, the provider's time spent with the client, and the amount and kinds of supplies used. The service record is completed on a daily basis by each provider and is summarized monthly and annually to indicate trends in health care activities and costs related to personnel time, transportation, maintenance, and supplies. The provider service records are used to compare with the agency's *financial records* of salaries, overhead, and transportation costs, and they serve as the basis for the cost accounting system. These records are basic to peer review and audit.

Three additional kinds of service records seen in the community agency are the central index system, the annual implementation plan, and the annual summary of agency activities. The *central index system* is a data-filing system that indicates the services requested, services offered, active and inactive clients of the agency, and a profile of the agency's clients.

The *annual implementation plan* (often referred to as the strategic plan or tactical plan) is developed at the beginning of each fiscal year to define the short- and long-term goals of the agency. The annual implementation plan serves as the basis for the agency's annual summary. The *annual summary* reflects the success of the agency in meeting the annual objectives, the changes in population trends and health status during the year, the actual versus the projected budget requirements, the number of services offered, the number of clients served, and the plans and changes recommended for the future. This plan serves as the basis for the evaluation of agency structure.

As an outgrowth of QA efforts in the health care system, comprehensive methods are being designed to document and measure client progress and client outcome from agency admission through discharge. An example of such a method is the client classification system developed at the Visiting Nurses Association of Omaha, Nebraska (Martin, 2005; Omaha System, 2018). This comprehensive method for evaluating client care has several components: a classification system for assessing and categorizing client problems, a database, a nursing problem list, and anticipated outcome criteria for the classified problem. Such schemes are viewed as having the potential to improve the delivery of nursing care, documentation of care, and the descriptions of client care. Briefly, implementing a comprehensive documentation method improves nursing assessment, planning, implementation, and evaluation of client care; it also allows the organization of important client information for more effective and efficient nurse productivity and communication (see Fig. 24.2).

LINKING CONTENT TO PRACTICE

How To Apply the PDSA Model With a Population

The PDSA model is being used in public health to promote CQI. A brief example of how to apply this model is given below.

This approach was designed to improve population health outcomes by improving nurse/school management and teacher communication processes.

1. The goal of the project is to improve health outcomes for the elementary school population in the community by offering an assessment of the most common health problems among the children in the community elementary school children.
2. The performance measures include:
   A. An assessment of the numbers of school personnel, including the school health nurse, who could successfully answer the questions about the illnesses of the children in each school.
   B. DEVELOPMENT OF a summary report of the most common health problems shared by the children in the school system.
3. APPLICATION OF THE PDSA PROCESS

Plan: Plan with the school health nurses and school personnel to implement a process for reducing the risk of the most common health problems throughout the community.

Do: Prioritize the health problems to be addressed and develop interventions for the most common to the least common problems

Study: Assess the abilities of each of the nurses to respond to the health problems in their school.

Assess how efficient the nurse is in implementing a plan to reduce the health risk and the ability to independently answer the questions of families and school personnel about what is needed to make this happen to improve the health of the children in the population

Act: If the school nurses were able to efficiently implement an approach to address the most common health problems of the children, after the school year, conduct a survey to see if the numbers of children in the community with the problem has been reduced. Use the PDSA process until the nurses are able to efficiently address other common health problems on the priority list.

The PDSA cycle is continuously repeated until the school administration, the nurses, and the families and children are satisfied that the process is working.

Data from PDSA will provide realistic estimates of the percent of the nurses who can successfully improve and reduce the health risk of their school population. The purpose of the initial assessment and implementation plan is to provide healthier child populations so children's ability to learn will improve. The process may enlist the support of all community families with children and the school system and create a change in the school environment As students develop questions, they also develop a PDSA approach to answering those questions.

PRACTICE APPLICATION

Oscar, a nursing student, has been working in the migrant farmworker clinic and has noted that each practitioner uses a different educational method for teaching good nutrition practices to newly diagnosed diabetic clients. The clinic has seen a substantial increase in the number of new diabetic clients in the Hispanic farmworker population. Oscar knows that practice guidelines for teaching nutrition practices exist in his clinical facility and that charts have an area to note nutrition education information. He also knows that for nurses to be most effective and ensure quality client outcomes, research-based practice guidelines should be used by all nurses in the health department.

As part of his course, Oscar must prepare a teaching plan and conduct a class on a health care problem. He obtains permission from his instructor and the director of the clinic to conduct an in-service program. The purpose of Oscar's in-service program is to instruct the nursing staff in how to teach newly diagnosed diabetic clients good nutrition practices. He obtains and studies the literature about teaching good nutrition practices for Diabetes type 1 and 2 evidence-based nutrition practice. Oscar's native language is Spanish, so this will help him in determining whether brochures for newly diagnosed diabetic clients regarding good nutrition convey the appropriate message.

As part of his in-service program, Oscar keeps demographic records on attendees and conducts before-and-after tests of knowledge, adding questions about the present use of the guidelines. He plans to follow up with the nurses in 6 months with a further test and questions about use of the guidelines. The director will help him determine an outcome measure that can be used with the client population to show effective use of the guidelines.

A. What outcome measure would be useful in this project?

B. How will this help in the overall assessment of quality in the nursing service?

Answers can be found on the Evolve site.

KEY POINTS

- The health care delivery system is the largest employing industry in the United States; society is demanding increased efficiency and effectiveness from the system.
- The actual quality and safety of care in the United States is being assessed regularly and reported in four reports.
- Because of varying definitions, logistics, and data collection methods, quality is difficult to assess accurately.
- Responding to the quality of care question, the federal government has instituted several quality improvement programs. Among these are the National Healthcare Quality and Disparities Report (NHQDR) that is used to monitor the nation's progress toward improved health care quality; the Center for Medicare and Medicaid Services (CMS) Outcomes Based Quality Improvement (OBQI) for home health; and the National Committee for Quality Assurance (NCQA), which provides performance information, or report cards, for health care agencies.
- Quality improvement is the tool used to ensure effective and efficient care.
- The managed care industry is changing the face of the American health care delivery system and how quality is defined and measured.

- Objective and systematic evaluation of nursing care has become a priority within the profession for several reasons, including the effects of cost on health care access, consumer demands for better-quality care, and increasing involvement of nurses in formulating public and health agency policy.
- Total quality management is a management philosophy new to the public health care arena. It is prevention oriented and process focused. Its primary focus is to deliver quality health care. One measure of quality is customer satisfaction.
- Public and private sectors are forming partnerships to monitor the performance of all players in health care delivery to improve the health of communities. The different players in the health care system have different perceptions of quality.
- Quality assurance/quality improvement (QA/QI) is the monitoring of client care activities to determine the degree of excellence attained in implementing activities.
- Quality assurance has been a concern of the profession since the 1860s, when Florence Nightingale called for a uniform format to gather and disseminate hospital statistics.
- Licensure has been a major issue in nursing since 1892.
- Two major categories of approaches exist in QA/QI today: general and specific.
- Accreditation is an approach to quality control used for institutions, whereas licensure is used primarily for individuals.
- Certification combines features of both licensing and accreditation.
- Three major models have been used to evaluate quality: Donabedian's structure-process-outcome model, the sentinel model, and the tracer model.
- A fourth model to evaluate quality—the PDSA model—has been adopted by the public health system.
- Seven basic components of a quality improvement program are (1) identifying values, (2) identifying structure, process, and outcome standards and criteria, (3) selecting measurement techniques, (4) interpreting the strengths and weaknesses of the care given, (5) identifying alternative courses of action, (6) choosing specific courses of action, and (7) taking action.
- Records are an integral part of the communication structure of a health care organization. Accurate and complete records are by law required of all agencies, whether governmental or nongovernmental.
- QA/QI mechanisms in health care delivery are the mechanisms for controlling the system and requesting accountability from individual providers within the system. Records help establish a total picture of the contribution of the agency to the client community.
- Delivering quality care to individuals, communities, and populations falls under the 10 essential services of public health.
- Evidence-based practice guidelines can help population-centered nurses document the outcomes and effectiveness of their interventions.

CLINICAL DECISION-MAKING ACTIVITIES

1. Write your own definition of TQM; compare your definition with the one given in the text. Are they the same or different? Give justification for your answer.
2. How does traditional QA/QI fit with the CQI effort? Explain the relative importance of a continuing QA/QI effort.
3. Interview a nurse who is a coordinator of or is responsible for QA/QI in a local health agency. Ask the following questions and add your own. Do the answers to the questions relate to what you have learned about QA/QI? Explain.
   - **A.** Does the agency subscribe to the TQM approach to management?
   - **B.** If not, is the agency incorporating elements of the TQM process as outlined by Deming (1986) in his 15 points?
   - **C.** Is a traditional method of management used to ensure quality?
   - **D.** Describe the components of the QA/QI program.
   - **E.** How are records used in your QA/QI effort?
   - **F.** Discuss the approaches and techniques that are used to implement the QA/QI program.
   - **G.** How has the QA/QI program changed in the health agency over the past 20 years?
   - **H.** What influence has the QA/QI program had on decreasing problems attributable to process? To provider accountability?
   - **I.** List and describe the types of records usually kept in a community health agency. Explain the purpose of each type of record.
4. Identify partnerships necessary to ensure quality health outcomes for your community from data gathered in a community assessment. Explain why these partners are necessary.
5. Find the *Guide to Community Preventive Services* on the CDC website, and look for the segments on smoking cessation or tuberculosis control. How could you use this information in your practice in health?
6. Explain the nurse's responsibilities and role in the CQI program.

ADDITIONAL RESOURCES

EVOLVE WEBSITE

http://evolve.elsevier.com/Stanhope/community/

- Answers to Practice Application
- Case Study
- Glossary
- Review Questions

REFERENCES

Agency for Healthcare Research and Quality: *2013 National Healthcare Quality Report*, Rockville, MD, 2014, USDHHS. AHRQ Pub. No. 14-0005.

Agency for Healthcare Research and Quality (AHRQ): *2014 National Healthcare Quality and Disparities Report*, Rockville MD, 2015, USDHHS. AHRQ Pub. No. 15-0007.

Agency for Healthcare Research and Quality (AHRQ): *2016 National Healthcare Quality and Disparities Report*, Rockville MD, 2017, USDHHS. AHRQ Pub. No. 17-0001.

Agency for Healthcare Research and Quality (AHRQ): *The Challenge and Potential for Assuring Quality Health Care for the 21st Century*, Content last reviewed June 2018, Agency for Healthcare Research and Quality, Rockville, MD. Retrieved from http://www.ahrq.gov.

American Nurses Association (ANA): *Public Health Nursing: Scope and Standards of Practice*, ed 2, Silver Springs, MD, 2013, American Nurses Association.

American Nurses Credentialing Center (ANCC): *About ANCC*, 2018a. Retrieved from https://www.nursingworld.org.

American Nurses Credentialing Center (ANCC): *Magnet recognition program*. 2018b. Retrieved from https://www.nursingworld.org.

American Public Health Association (APHA): *Healthy Communities 2000: Model Standards, Guidelines for Community Attainment of the Year 2000 National Health Objectives*, ed 3, Washington, DC, 1991, APHA.

Association of Community Health Nursing Educators (ACHNE): *Perspectives on Doctoral Education in Community Health Nursing*, Lexington, KY, 1993, ACHNE.

Association of Community Health Nursing Educators (ACHNE): *Essentials of Baccalaureate Nursing Education for Entry Level Community Health Nursing Practice*, Chapel Hill, NC, 2000a, updated 2009, ACHNE.

Association of Community Health Nursing Educators (ACHNE): *Graduate Education for Advanced Practice Education in Community/Public Health Nursing*, Chapel Hill, NC, 2000b, ACHNE.

Association of Community Health Nursing Educators (ACHNE): *Graduate Education for Advanced Practice in Community Public Health Nursing*, New York, 2003, ACHNE.

Association of Community Health Nursing Educators (ACHNE): *Graduate Education for Advanced Practice Public Health Nursing: at the Crossroads*, Chapel Hill, NC, 2007, ACHNE.

Beitsch LM, Yeager VA, Moran J: Deciphering the imperative: translating public health quality improvement into organizational performance management gains, *Annu Rev Public Health* 36: 273–287, 2015.

Birnbaum G, Gretsinger K, Antonio MG, Loewen E, Lacroix P: Revisiting public health informatics – patient privacy concerns, *Int J Health Gov* 23(2):149–159, 2018.

Blegen MA: Does certification of staff nurses improve patient outcomes? *Evid Based Nurs* 15:54–55, 2012.

Boltz M, Capezuti E, Wagner L, Rosenberg MC, Secic M: Patient safety in medical-surgical units: can nurse certification make a difference? *Medsurg Nurs* 22(1):26–37, 2013.

Burstin H, Leatherman S, Goldmann D: The evolution of healthcare quality measurement in the United States, *J Intern Med* 279: 154–159, 2016.

Centers for Disease Control and Prevention (CDC): *Planned Approach to Community Health: Guide for Local Coordinators*, Atlanta, 1995, CDC, National Center for Chronic Disease Prevention and Health Promotion, and updated 2010.

Centers for Disease Control and Prevention (CDC): *National Public Health Performance Standards*, 2017. Retrieved from https://www.cdc.gov.

Centers for Medicare and Medicaid (CMS): *Accreditation*, 2016. Retrieved from https://www.cms.gov.

Centers for Medicare and Medicaid (CMS): *Quality improvement organizations*, 2018. Retrieved from https://www.cms.gov.

Clancy C, Fraser I: High quality health care. In Knickman JR, Kovner AR, editors: *Jonas and Kovner's Health Care Delivery in the United States*, ed 11, New York, NY, 2015, Springer Publishing Company, LLC.

Commission on Collegiate Nursing Education (CCNE). *CCNE homepage*, 2018. Retrieved from http://www.aacnnursing.org.

Community Health Accreditation Partner (CHAP): *Why CHAP*, 2018. Retrieved from http://www.chapinc.org.

Community Tool Box: *Creating and using community report cards*, 2018, Center for Community Health and Development, University of Kansas. Retrieved from https://ctb.ku.edu.

Council on Linkages Between Academia and Public Health Practice: *The Core Competencies for Public Health Professionals*, Washington, DC, originally published 2001, updated 2014, The Public Health Foundation. Retrieved from http://www.phf.org.

Deming Institute: *PDSA cycle*, 2018, Retrieved from https://deming.org.

Deming WE: *Out of the Crisis*. Cambridge, MA, 1986, Massachusetts Institute of Technology, Center for Advanced Engineering Study.

Donabedian A: *Explorations in Quality Assessment and Monitoring*, vol 2, Ann Arbor, MI, 1981, Health Administration Press.

Donabedian A: *Explorations in Quality Assessment and Monitoring*, vol 3, Ann Arbor, MI, 1985, Health Administration Press.

Donabedian A: *An Introduction to Quality Assurance in Health Care*, New York, 2003, Oxford University Press.

Edwards MT: A longitudinal study of clinical peer review's impact on quality and safety in U.S. hospitals, *J Healthc Manag* 58(5):369–384, 2013.

Egen O, Beatty K, Blackley DJ, Brown K, Wykoff R: Health and social conditions of the poorest versus wealthiest counties in the united states, *Am J Public Health* 107(1):130–135, 2017.

Fawcett J, Ellenbecker CH: A proposed conceptual model of nursing and population health, *Nursing Outlook* 63(3):288–298, 2015.

Fitzgerald M: *State Licensure and Certification: Myths and Realities*, 2013, Fitzgerald Health Education Association. Retrieved from https://www.fhea.com.

Harel Z, Silver SA, McQuillan RF, et al: How to diagnose solutions to a quality of care problem, *Clin J Am Soc Nephrol* 11(5):901–907, 2016.

Hood CM, Gennuso KP, Swain GR, Catlin BB: County health rankings—relationship between determinant factors and health outcomes, *Am J Prev Med* 50(1):129–135, 2016.

Honoré PA, Scott W: *Priority Areas for Improvement of Quality in Public Health*, Washington, DC, November 2010, USDHHS.

Institute for Health Care Improvement: *Quality Improvement Essentials Toolkit*, 2018. Retrieved from www.ihi.org. Accessed Nov 11, 2018

Institute of Medicine (IOM): *Crossing the Quality Chasm*, Washington, DC, 2001, National Academy Press.

Institute of Medicine (IOM): *Health Professions Education: A Bridge to Quality*, Washington, DC, 2003, National Academies Press.

Institute of Medicine (IOM): *Toward Quality Measures for Population Health and the Leading Health Indicators*, Washington, DC, 2013, The National Academies Press.

Jones TL: Outcome measurement in nursing: imperatives, ideals, history, and challenges, *Online J Issues Nurs* 21(2):1, 2016.

Juran JM: *The quality trilogy—a universal approach to managing for quality*, paper presented at the ASQC 40th annual Quality Congress, Anaheim California, May 20, 1986. Retrieved from http://andrewgelman.com.

Kaiser Health News (KHN): *Accountable Care Organizations Explained*, 2015, Gold J, Kaiser Family Foundation. Retrieved from https://khn.org.

Keefe S: *Advance: nurses salary survey: results in! Many hospitals don't need to increase salaries to be competitive—for now,* March 1, 2010. Retrieved from www.advanceweb.com.

Keller LO, Strohschein S, Lia-Hoagberg B, Schaffer MA: Population-based public health interventions: practice-based and evidence-supported. Part I, *Public Health Nurs* 21:453–468, 2004a.

Keller LO, Strohschein S, Schaffer MA, Lia-Hoagberg B: Population-based public health interventions: innovations in practice, teaching and management. Part II, *Public Health Nurs* 21:469–487, 2004b.

Kendall-Gallagher D, Aiken LH, Sloane DM, Cimiotti JP: Nurse specialty certification, inpatient mortality, and failure to rescue, *J Nurs Scholarsh* 43(2):188–194, 2011.

Kessner DM, Kalk CE, Singer J: Assessing health quality—the case for tracers, *N Engl J Med* 288:189–194, 1973.

Knickman JR, Kovner AR, editors: *Jonas and Kovner's Health Care Delivery in the United States*, ed 11, New York, NY, 2015, Springer Publishing Company, LLC.

Kresge Foundation: *Community health partnerships*, 2017. Retrieved from https://kresge.org.

Kronstadt J, Meit M, Siegfried A, Nicolaus T, Bender K, Corso L: Evaluating the impact of national public health department accreditation–United States, 2016, *Morb Mortal Wkly Rep* 65(31):803–806, 2016.

Maibusch RM: Evolution of quality assurance for nursing in hospitals. In Schroder PS, Maibusch RM, editors: *Nursing Quality Assurance*, Rockville, MD, 1984, Aspen.

Matthew-Maich N, Ploeg J, Dobbins M, Jack S: Supporting the uptake of nursing guidelines: what you really need to know to move nursing guidelines into practice, *Worldviews Evid Based Nurs* 10(2):104–115, 2013.

Martin S: *The Omaha System: A Key to Practice, Documentation, and Information Management*, ed 2, St. Louis, 2005, Mosby.

Martinez JM: Hospice and palliative nursing certification: the journey to defining a new nursing specialty, *J Hosp Palliat Nurs* 13(6): S29–S34, 2011.

McHugh MD, Rochman MF, Sloane DM, et al: Better nurse staffing and nurse work environments associated with increased survival of in-hospital cardiac arrest patients, *Med Care* 54(1):74–80, 2016.

Melnyk BM, Fineout-Overholt E: *Evidence-based practice in nursing & healthcare,* ed 3, New York, 2015, Wolters Kluwer Health.

Minnesota Department of Health, Division of Community Health Services: *Public Health Interventions: Applications for Public Health Nursing Practice*, St Paul, MN, March 2001, Public Health Nursing Section.

National Association of City and County Health Officials: *APEXPH in Practice*, Washington, DC, 1995, NACCHO.

National Association of City and County Health Officials: *Mobilizing for Action Through Planning and Partnerships: Web-Based Tool*, Washington, DC, 2014, NACCHO. Retrieved from http://mapp.naccho.org.

National Association of Home Care and Hospice: *Uniform data set for home care and hospice,* 2014. Retrieved from http://www.nahc.org.

National Committee for Quality Assurance (NCQA): *HEDIS Compliance Audit Certification,* 2017. Retrieved from http://www.ncqa.org.

National Committee for Quality Assurance (NCQA): *HEDIS: Health Plan for Employee and Data Information set*, Washington, DC, 2018, NCQA. Retrieved from http://www.ncqa.org.

National Council of State Boards of Nursing (NCSBN): *NCLEX and other exams,* 2018a. Retrieved from https://www.ncsbn.org.

National Council of State Boards of Nursing (NCSBN): *Licensure compacts,* 2018b. Retrieved from https://www.ncsbn.org.

National Information Center on Health Services Research and Health Care Technology (NICHSR): *Community Health Status Indicators (CHSI): Questions and Answers*, Bethesda, MD, 2012, National Institute of Health, U.S. National Library of Medicine. Retrieved from http://www.nlm.nih.gov.

National League for Nursing: *National League for Nursing Commission for Nursing Education Accreditation (CNEA),* 2018. Retrieved from http://www.nln.org.

National Network of Public Health Institutes: *Modular Guide for Developing and Thriving as a Public Health Institute,* 2014. Retrieved from www.nnphi.org.

National Quality Forum: *Safe practices for better healthcare*, 2017. Retrieved from https://www.qualityforum.org.

National Quality Forum: *Patient Safety 2016*, 2017. Retrieved from https://www.qualityforum.org.

NursingLicensure.org: *Nurse Practitioner license requirements – change is in the air*, 2018. Retrieved from https://www.nursinglicensure.org.

Oakland JS: *Total Quality Management and Operational Excellence: Text with Cases*, ed 4, New York, NY, 2014, Routledge.

Omaha System: *Omaha system overview*, 2018. Retrieved from http://www.omahasystem.org.

Papanicolas I, Smith PC: *Health System Performance Comparison: An Agenda for Policy, Information and Research*, New York, NY, 2013, Open University Press.

Pennel CL, Burdine JN, Prochaska JD, McLeroy KR: Common and critical components among community health assessment and community health improvement planning models, *J Public Health Manag Pract* 23:S14–S21, 2017.

Phaneuf M: A nursing audit method, *Nurs Outlook* 5:42–45, 1965.

Public Health Accreditation Board: *About PHAB*, 2018a. Retrieved from http://www.phaboard.org.

Public Health Accreditation Board: *Accreditation Activity Map,* 2019. Retrieved from http://www.phaboard.org.

Quad Council of Public Health Nursing Organizations: *Operating guidelines*, 2017. Retrieved from http://www.quadcouncilphn.org.

Quad Council Coalition of Public Health Nursing Organizations: *Community/Public Health Nursing Competencies*, 2018: Quad Council Coalition Competency Review Task Force. Retrieved from http://www.quadcouncilphn.org.

Remington PL, Catlin BB, Gennuso KP: The county health rankings – rationale and methods, *Popul Health Metr* 13:11, 2015.

Record BN, Onion DK, Prior RE, et al: Community-wide cardiovascular disease prevention programs and health outcomes in a rural county, 1970-2010, *JAMA,* 313(2):147–155, 2015.

Riley WJ, Moran JW, Corso LC, Beitsch LM, Bialek R, Cofsky A: Defining quality improvement in public health, *J Public Health Manag Pract* 16(1):5–7, 2010.

Sakamoto SD, Avila M: The public health nursing practice manual: a tool for public health nurses, *Public Health Nurs* 21:179–182, 2004.

Sherwood G, Barnsteiner J: *Quality and safety in nursing – a competency approach to improving outcomes,* Hoboken NJ, 2017, John Wiley & Sons, Inc.

Smith K, Bazini-Barakat N: A public health nursing practice model: melding public health principles with the nursing process, *Public Health Nurs* 20:42–48, 2004.

Smith RA, Andrews KS, Brooks D, et al: Cancer screening in the United States, 2018 – a review of current American Cancer Society guidelines and current issues in cancer screening, *CA Cancer J Clin* 68(4):297–316, 2018.

Sollecito WA, Johnson JK: *McLaughlin and Kaluzny's Continuous Quality Improvement in Health Care*, ed 4, Burlington, MA, 2013, Jones & Bartlett.

Spath PL, Kelly D: *Applying Quality Management in Health Care: A Systems Approach*, ed 4, Washington, DC, 2017, Health Administration Press.

Sullivan DT: Healthcare quality. In DeNisco SM, Barker AM, editors: *Advance Practice Nursing: Evolving Roles for the Transformation of the Profession*, ed 2, Burlington, MA, 2013, Jones & Barlett.

University of Wisconsin-Madison, School of Nursing: *Wisconsin Public Health Nursing Practice Model*, 2009. Retrieved from http://academic.son.wisc.edu.

U.S. Department of Health and Human Services (USDHHS): *Healthy People 2010: Understanding and Improving Health*, ed 2, Washington, DC, 2000, U.S. Government Printing Office.

U.S. Department of Health and Human Services (USDHHS): *Healthy People in Healthy Communities*, Washington, DC, February 2001, U.S. Government Printing Office.

U.S. Department of Health and Human Services (USDHHS): *Healthy People 2020*, Washington, DC, 2010, U.S. Government Printing Office.

U.S. Department of Health and Human Services (USDHHS): *Quality Improvement*, Rockville, MD, 2011, Health Resources and Services Administration.

U.S. Department of Health and Human Services (USDHHS): *Program Planning - MAP-IT: A guide to using Healthy People 2020 in your community*, 2014. Retrieved from https://www.healthypeople.gov.

U.S. Department of Health and Human Services (USDHHS): *Home health compare*, 2018. Retrieved from https://www.medicare.gov.

U.S. Department of Health and Human Services (USDHHS): *HHS Action Plan to Reduce Racial and Ethnic Health Disparities*, Washington, DC, April 2016, USDHHS, Retrieved from https://minorityhealth.hhs.gov.

U. S. Preventive Services Task Force (USPSTF): *US clinical preventive services*, 2014. Retrieved from https://www.uspreventiveservicestaskforce.org.

Van den Heuvel J, Niemeijer GC, Does RJ: Measuring healthcare quality: the challenges, *Int J Health Care Qual Assur* 26(3):269–278, 2013.

Vogel J, Brown JS, Land T, Platt R, Klompas M: MDPHnet: secure, distributed sharing of electronic health record data for public health surveillance, evaluation, and planning, *Am J Public Health* 104(12):2265–2270, 2014.

Yeager VA, Menachemi N, Ginter PM, Sen BP, Savage GT, Beitsch LM: Environmental factors and quality improvement in county and local health departments, *J Public Health Manag Pract* 19(3):240–249, 2013.

25

Case Management

Ann H. Cary, PhD, MPH, RN, FNAP, FAAN

OBJECTIVES

After reading this chapter, the student should be able to do the following:

1. Define continuity of care, care management, case management, care coordination, population health management, transitional care, integrated care, social determinants of health, and advocacy.
2. Describe the scope of practice, roles, and functions of a case manager.
3. Compare and contrast the nursing process with processes of case management and advocacy.
4. Identify methods to manage conflict, as well as the process of achieving collaboration.
5. Define and explain the legal and ethical issues confronting case managers.

CHAPTER OUTLINE

Definitions
Concepts of Case Management
Evidence-Based Examples of Case Management
Essential Skills for Case Managers
Issues in Case Management

KEY TERMS

accountable care organizations, p. 547
advocacy, p. 560
affirming, p. 562
allocation, p. 564
amplifying, p. 561
assertiveness, p. 565
autonomy, p. 568
beneficence, p. 568
brainstorming, p. 563
care coordination, p. 551
care management, p. 548
care maps, p. 556
case management plans, p. 555
case manager, p. 556
clarifying, p. 561
collaboration, p. 557
cooperation, p. 565
coordinate, p. 551
critical pathways, p. 549
dashboard indicators, p. 547
demand management, p. 549
disease management, p. 549
distributive outcomes, p. 564
fidelity, p. 568
information exchange process, p. 561
informing, p. 561
integrative outcomes, p. 564
justice, p. 568
life care planning, p. 557
Medical/Health Home or Patient/Client-Centered Medical Home model, p. 551
negotiating, p. 564
nonmaleficence, p. 568
patient engagement, p. 555
population management, p. 547
problem-purpose-expansion method, p. 563
problem solving, p. 563
social mandate, p. 548
supporting, p. 562
transitions of care, p. 551
utilization management, p. 548
value-based health care, p. 547
veracity, p. 568
verifying, p. 562

Since the Patient Protection and Affordable Care Act (ACA) was initiated in 2010 and has evolved throughout implementation, the health care industry continues to re-evaluate systems and processes that attempt to integrate financing, management, quality, and service delivery models that will ultimately improve population health. Challenges abound for clients and providers as they attempt to coordinate care, transition clients among providers and systems, access and share information and documentation about clients and communities, and navigate the complexity of integrated care to optimize quality and access while managing costs and achieving value-based health care. The new models of health care financing provide incentives to value care outcomes over the volume of care provided. **Value-based health care** is a term that can describe this aspirational approach to health care outcomes where care is reimbursed based on quality care and outcomes for patients as opposed to fee-for-service, which is reimbursed on volume of care regardless of outcomes. Delivery of care is now organized through a network of providers, such as negotiated contracts with hospitals and other levels of care, physicians, nurse practitioners, pharmacies, ancillary health services, outpatient centers, and home health care. Providers can be selected based on the outcomes of care they provide for their population of patients—a new approach to health care quality.

Managing the health of populations served by any integrated system is essential whether the definition includes a geographic area or shared characteristics of the population such as age, race, gender, occupation, education, or health status, as examples (NACNEP, 2016). Organizations managing population health include current **accountable care organizations** (ACOs) and health care systems. While there are historical and varied definitions of population health, the Institute of Medicine (2014) definition is simple: "an approach that treats the population as a whole (including the environment and community contexts) as the patient." Nurse case managers and nurse care managers play a pivotal role in population health delivery, building on the foundation created by Florence Nightingale, who studied the population of sick and wounded soldiers and reduced the mortality rate from infection in this population. **Population management** includes wellness and health promotion, illness prevention, acute and subacute care, chronic disease, rehabilitation, end-of-life care, care coordination, and community engagement. Case managers and care coordination are at the core of population health strategies to improve the community outcomes (Kimmel, 2016). Population health management can maintain and improve the physical and psychosocial status of clients through cost-effective and customized solutions, such as coordinating and transitioning care to reduce gaps and costs; supporting evidence-based practices; selecting quality care that is culturally competent; and providing disease management and self-management educational programming (Case Management Society of America [CMSA], 2016). Examples include planning and delivery strategies for adolescents in a school-based clinic system or the chronic disease management of elderly in a rural community to avoid nursing home placement (Sebelius, 2011). The care coordination process strengthens the nurses' care coordination management of population health.

The ACA endorses the use of integrated systems to realize the following important consequences on the focus of care:

- Emphasis is on population health management across the continuum, rather than on episodes of illness for an individual.
- Management has shifted from inpatient care as the point of management to primary care providers as points of entry.
- Care management services and programs provide access and accountability for the continuum of health.
- Successful outcomes are measured by systems performance and pay for performance for providers to meet the needs of populations.

The contemporary focus of integrated health systems defines the nature of the client as a population in addition to that as an individual. In these systems, population management involves the following activities:

- Assessing the needs of the client population through health histories (and, in the future, genograms), claims, use-of-service patterns, and risk factors, and communicating through interoperable information systems to ascertain patterns, trends, and responses to health programming in a population
- Creating benefits and network designs to address these needs
- Selecting **dashboard indicators** to measure performance
- Prioritizing actions to produce a desired outcome with available resources
- Selecting evidence-based programs related to wellness, prevention, health promotion, and demand management; patient/client engagement; and educating the population about them
- Instituting evidence-based care management processes that ensure transitional and coordinated care across the health continuum for a population aggregate
- Deploying case managers within a variety of delivery and insurance systems to clients and providers
- Evaluating provider patterns of performance and client dashboard indicators for impact

In 2018 Pifer reported that Medicare ACOs with a higher emphasis on primary care and care management strategies were more likely to have lower costs and higher quality scores.

Nurses will be called upon to work with and lead teams while functioning as transition and care coordinators in order to achieve health outcomes at the population level. The nursing discipline with unique preparation in care management and coordination plays a key role in care and case management across delivery sites and within populations (AACN, 2016). Nurses are in the unique position, based on baccalaureate education, to identify and incorporate in planning the social determinants affecting health and well-being, analyze patterns across patient populations, link patients with value-based resources, and secure interventions at the individual, institutional and health policy level (Bachrach & Thomas, 2016; Fink-Samnick, 2018; Van Dijk, 2016). In fact, social determinants of health (SDOH) drive the effectiveness of a case manager's outcomes.

Major federal advisory committees to the secretary of health and human services and the U.S. Congress have placed in the public domain documents acknowledging and recommending that the education and practice of nurses include the competencies necessary to execute population health management and the respective essential value-based components (National Advisory Council for Nurse Education and Practice, 2016). As illustrated in the Macy Foundation Report (2016) and in Barton (2017), nurses interested in working in community-based primary care will need to have both primary care knowledge and competencies in areas that include chronic disease management, care coordination, care transitions, prevention and wellness, interprofessional teamwork, and triaging.

The *Healthy People 2020* goals are to attain both quality of life and increase years of healthy life, achieve health equity and eliminate health disparities, and create social and physical environments as a **social mandate** for health care. In the coming decade of the twenty-first century case management, care coordination, and planned transitional care will be an essential intervention provided by nurses who incorporate the SDOH dimensions of their clients into effective care planning to achieve the Healthy People goals and population management outcomes. Many of the interventions nurses use with clients and health care systems will further the *Healthy People 2020* objectives. These include case management and care coordination interventions to minimize fragmented care and promote quality transitions of care; incorporate standardized practice tools and adherence guidelines; improve safety of care; and use interprofessional teams to deliver services.

Establishing evidence-based strategies for all functions is critical to the success of case management and care coordination for individuals and populations. Using the current best evidence blended with clinical expertise is a critical skill of the case manager (American Nurses Association [ANA], 2013b; CMSA, 2016; Lamb & Newhouse, 2018). In their practice, nurse case managers and community/public health nurses have the following core values: increasing the span of healthy life, reducing disparities in health among Americans, and promoting access to care and to preventive services.

The Quad Council Coalition (2018) edition of the *Community/Public Health Nursing Competencies* clearly illustrates the importance of evidence-based practice and ongoing research to retain competencies in this discipline. The ANA (2015b) *Standards of Practice 5A: Care Coordination* specify the complexities of this practice. The American Academy of Ambulatory Care Nursing specifies nine dimensions of care coordination and transition management practice (2014). In addition, the Commission for Care Manager Certification and the American Nurses Credentialing Center specify areas of competency evaluated through their certification programs.

In the Intervention Wheel model for public health nursing practice, the nursing actions of case management, collaboration, and advocacy are 3 of 17 evidence-based interventions for individuals, families, and populations served by public health nurses (Keller et al., 2004; and see Chapter 11). Case management incorporates many of the Quad Council Coalition of *Community/Public Health Nursing Competencies* (Quad Council, 2018) because it involves individual and family care as well as community resources, population health, interprofessional teams, and policy implementation.

HEALTHY PEOPLE 2020

Case management strategies offer opportunities for nurses to help meet the following *Healthy People 2020* objectives for target populations:

Access to Care

- **AHS-2:** Increase the proportion of insured persons with coverage for clinical preventive services.
- **AHS-3:** Increase the proportion of persons with a usual primary care provider.
- **AHS-6:** Reduce the proportion of individuals who experience difficulties or delays in obtaining necessary medical care, dental care, or prescription medications.
- **ECBP-14 and -14.1:** Increase the inclusion of clinical prevention and population content in undergraduate nursing, including counseling training for health promotion and disease prevention.
- **SA-9:** Increase the portion of persons who are referred for follow-up for substance abuse problems.

From USDHHS: *Healthy People 2020: A roadmap for health*, Washington, DC, 2010, U.S. Government Printing Office.

DEFINITIONS

Care management is a health care delivery process that helps achieve better health outcomes by anticipating and linking populations with the services they need more quickly (CMSA, 2016). It is an enduring process in which a population manager establishes systems and processes to monitor the health status, resources, and outcomes for a targeted aggregate of the population. The population manager is the tactical architect for a population's health in the delivery system. According to a report by McKesson Corporation (2014) and affirmed by URAC (2018), nurse care managers are predicted to hold the primary responsibility for the care management process in health systems. Building blocks that are used by the manager include risk analysis; data mapping; predictive modeling; dashboard indicators; monitoring for health processes, indicators, and unexpected illnesses; epidemiologic investigation of unexpected illnesses; development of multidisciplinary action plans and programs for the population; and identifying case management triggers or events (e.g., when dramatic results are obtained by prevention or early intervention) that indicate the need for early referrals of high-risk clients (ANA, 2013; Stricker, 2014).

Care management strategies were initially developed by health maintenance organizations (HMOs) in the late 1970s to manage the care of different populations. The purpose then and now is to promote quality and ensure appropriate use and costs of services. Care management strategies include utilization management, critical pathways, case management, disease management, and demand management.

Utilization management attempts to promote optimal use of services to redirect care and monitor the appropriate use of provider care/treatment services for both acute and community/ambulatory services. Providers are offered multiple options for care with different economic implications. Through the use of utilization management, clients who have repetitive readmissions (i.e., they fail to respond to care) are often referred to care management programs.

Critical pathways and maps, which were initiated in the early 2000s, are tools that specify activities providers may use in a timely sequence to achieve desired outcomes for care. The outcomes are measurable, and the pathway tools strive to reduce variation in client care. Today, agencies are more likely to call these clinical paths, evidence-based practice protocols, clinical decision supports or guidelines, or case management plans of care.

Care management services are used for clients with specific diagnoses who may have high-use patterns, noncompliance issues, cost caps (e.g., no more than $10,000 to $20,000 can be spent on their case), or threshold expenses, which means highest amount of medical expenses that can be deducted against income taxes.

Disease management constitutes systematic activities to coordinate health care interventions and communications for populations with disease conditions in which client self-care efforts are significant (CMSA, 2016). For example, chronic conditions like diabetes, asthma, and depression and catastrophic conditions like trauma are typically targeted by providers and insurers. With 71 percent of the U.S. health care dollar going to treating patients with more than one chronic condition, the possibilities for cost-effectiveness are great (URAC, 2018). Disease management programs work with providers and consumers to educate on self-care, shared decision making, and knowledgeable use of medicines. These programs are eligible for accreditation by URAC.

Demand management seeks to control use by providing clients with correct information and education strategies to make healthy choices, to use healthy and health-seeking behaviors to improve their health status, and to make fewer demands on the health care system (Tufts Managed Care Institute, 2011).

In contrast to care management—which was developed as a population approach to manage care—*case management* is composed of the activities implemented with individual clients/families in the system. In the 2016 *Standards of Practice for Case Management,* case management is defined as "a collaborative process of assessment, planning, facilitation, care coordination, evaluation and advocacy for options and services to meet an individual's and family's comprehensive health needs through communication and available resources to promote patient safety, quality of care, and cost effective outcomes" (p. 12). "Case management interventions focus on improving care coordination and reducing the fragmentation of the services the recipients of care often experience especially when multiple health care providers and different care settings are involved. Taken collectively, case management interventions are intended to enhance client safety, well-being, and quality of life. These interventions carefully consider health care costs through the professional case manager's recommendations of cost-effective and efficient alternatives for care. Thus, effective case management directly and positively impacts the health care delivery system especially in realizing the goals of the 'Triple Aim' which include improving the health outcomes of individuals and populations, enhancing the experience of health care, and reducing the cost of care" (p. 13).

The case manager builds on the basic functions of the traditional nurse's role and adapts new competencies for managing transitions among health care facilities, such as wellness and prevention, workflow, informatics, and interprofessional teams. Tahan and Treiger (2017) illustrate the core curriculum areas for case managers who chose this practice by professional development or in their educational programs. Although Medicare reimburses advanced practice registered nurses (APRNs) for case management services, a registered nurse provision of this service is not directly reimbursed as payment is bundled in ordinary hospital services (Lamb & Newhouse, 2018).

Case management is provided by the disciplines of nursing, social work, and rehabilitation counseling, to name a few. Research by Park and colleagues (2009) found that common knowledge exists for case management providers from the disciplines of nursing, social work, and rehabilitation counseling: case recording and documentation, conflict resolution strategies, negotiation, ethics, relevant legislation, interpersonal communication, and roles and functions required in various settings. These areas were further described by Fabbri et al. (2017) noting that the case manager is a central figure in ensuring quality in the patient-centered experience. Fig. 25.1 illustrates the unified knowledge domains for professionals in case management and emphasizes the fluidity of common knowledge used by case managers regardless of discipline.

Treiger (2013) indicates that the challenges of academic preparation for future case managers will be to prepare them in interprofessional case management programs rather than through the lens of a particular clinical practice. In addition, case managers in case management programs are expanding their clinical expertise to embrace the process of disease management, a successful strategy for population outcomes. Specialty case management in advanced nursing practice is a critical role in this field (Treiger, 2013). In implementing case management, advanced practice nurses work with clients or community aggregates as well as systems managing disease and outcomes, whereas nurses with bachelor's degrees more often focus on care at the individual level. Treiger (2013) also observes that there are many individuals working under the title of case manager who fail to perform the full scope of roles and functions, leading to the question of title protection for case managers.

This chapter describes the nature and process of case management for individual and family clients. Case management has a rich tradition in public health nursing as practiced by Lillian Wald and now is frequently found in hospitals, transitional and long-term care, home and hospice care, and health insurance companies. Case management is at the top of the care management pyramid, reserved for a subset of the population. In Fig. 25.2, Coggeshall Press (2008) illustrates a classic case management model pyramid that recognizes the tenets of risk stratification and case finding, coordination, and ultimately case management of a smaller proportion of clients in the population. This model recognizes the interchange of public health and populations at risk for service intensity resulting from economic needs or the need to integrate care.

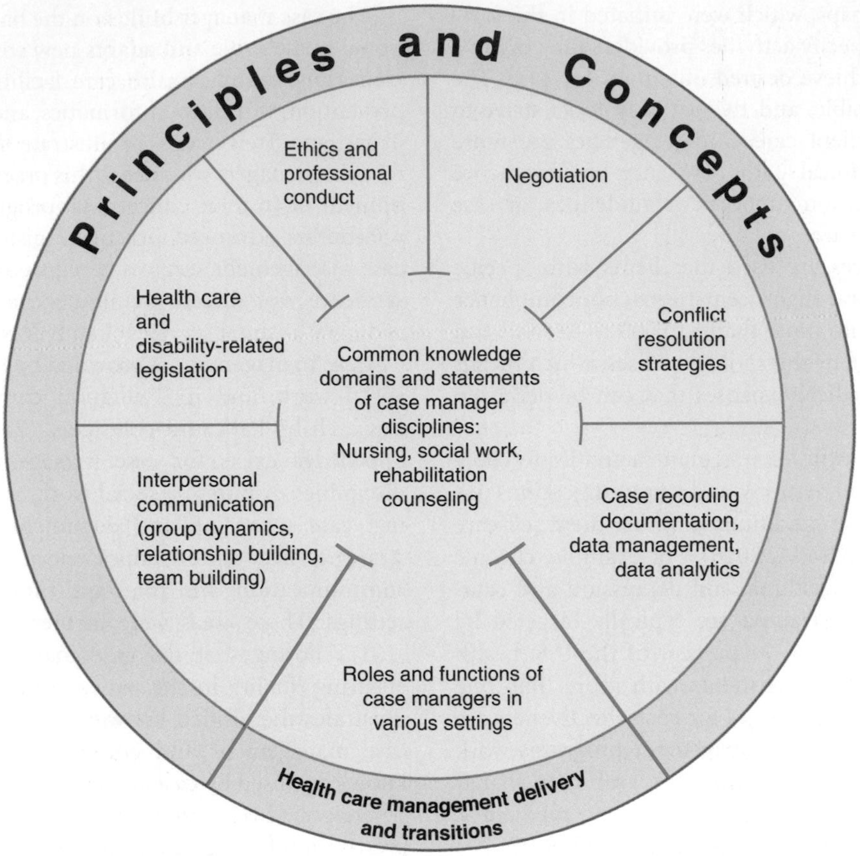

Fig. 25.1 Evidence-based knowledge of case managers from disciplines of nursing, social work, and rehabilitation counseling. (Courtesy Ann H. Cary.)

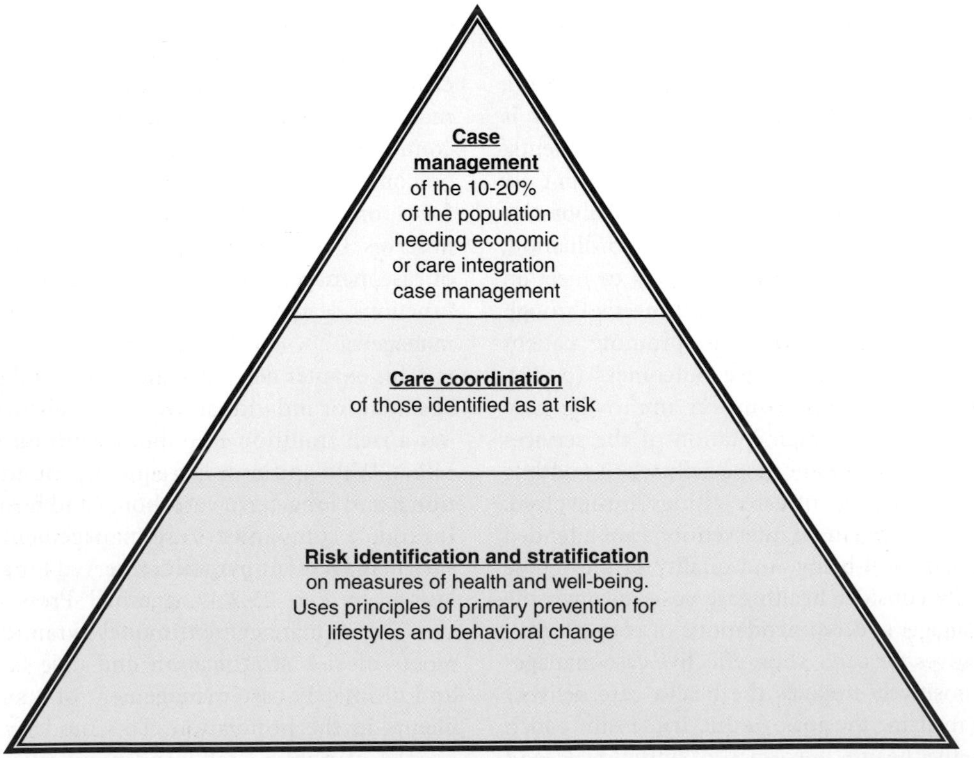

Fig. 25.2 Case management model. (From Coggeshall Press: *Case management model,* Coralville, IA, 2008, Coggeshall Press; as cited in Huber DL: *Leadership and nursing care management,* ed. 4, St. Louis, 2010, Elsevier.)

CONCEPTS OF CASE MANAGEMENT

Reviewing multiple or historical definitions of case management helps to demonstrate the complex process and the concept of case management over time. Weil and Karls, in 1985, described case management as a "set of logical steps and process of interacting within a service network, which ensures that a client receives needed services in a supportive, effective, efficient and cost-effective manner" (p. 4). Case management was defined by the American Hospital Association (1986) as the process of planning, organizing, coordinating, and monitoring services and resources needed by clients, while supporting the effective use of health and social services. Secord (1987) defined case management as a systematic process of assessing, planning, and coordinating the service, referrals, and monitoring that meets the multiple needs of clients. Bower (1992) described the continuity, quality, and cost containment aspects of case management as a health care delivery process, the goals of which are to provide quality health care, decrease fragmentation, enhance the client's quality of life, and contain costs.

A focus on collaboration is important in the National Case Management Task Force definition. The definition emphasizes a collaborative process between the case manager, the client, and representatives of other agencies and provider groups. The process includes assessments, plans, implementation, coordination, monitoring, and the evaluation of options and services to meet an individual's health needs. Effective communication is essential to identify available resources to promote quality, cost-effective outcomes (CMSA, 2016; Mullahy, 2010; Stricker, 2013).

As a competency, case management was classically defined in the public health nursing literature as the "ability to establish an appropriate plan of care based on assessing the client/family and coordinating the necessary resources and services for the client's benefit" (Muller & Flarey, 2003, p. 230). In 2018 the Quad Council Coalition updated the *Community/Public Health Nursing Competencies,* and case management for populations can be assumed in Domain 5 (Community Dimensions of Practice Skills) and Domain 8 (Leadership and Systems Thinking Skills). Case management has been a term prevalent in the social work literature as well as in public health nursing beginning in the mid-1900s. Knowledge and skills required to achieve this competency include the following:

- Knowledge of community resources and financing mechanisms
- Written and oral communication and technology-enhanced documentation
- Proficient negotiating and conflict-resolving practices
- Critical-thinking processes to identify and prioritize problems from the provider and client viewpoints
- Application of evidence-based practices and outcomes measures
- Advocacy for patients, populations, and policy (Tahan, 2016a)

Case management practice is complex as evidenced by the need to **coordinate** activities of multiple providers, payers, and settings throughout a client's continuum of care. **Care coordination**, one function of case management, is "the deliberate synchronization of activities and information to improve health outcomes by ensuring that care recipients and families' needs and preferences for health care and community services are met over time" (NQF, 2014, p. 2). For example, in a contemporary model of primary care practice, the **Medical/Health Home or Patient/Client-Centered Medical Home model** provides accessible, continuous, coordinated, comprehensive care and is managed centrally by a physician/nurse practitioner with the active involvement of nonphysician practice staff. Care provided must be assessed, planned, implemented, adjusted, and evaluated on the basis of goals designed by many disciplines as well as goals of the client, the family, significant others, and community organizations. Although likely employed and located in one setting, the nurse as case manager will be influencing the selection, monitoring, and evaluation of care provided in other settings by formal and informal care providers.

With the increased use of electronic care delivery through telehealth activities and robotics, case management activities are now handled via tablets like iPads, phones, email, and fax, and through telehealth transmission visits with the electronic monitoring of physiological status at a client's residence from a case manager who is located elsewhere. Case managers may also deliver care to a global network of clients located in different countries. A challenging problem is the fragmentation of services and miscommunication handoffs, which can result in overuse, underuse, gaps in care, and miscommunication. These can result in costly client outcomes and quality issues in handoffs and transitions from provider to provider. Health information technology interoperability and electronic health records are benefiting collaborative care team communication, real-time data, and timely adjustments in care (AAACN/AMSN, 2017).

Case management, including the care coordination function, is part of a wider concept of **transitions of care** illuminated by the National Transitions of Care Coalition (NTOCC, 2011). The Transitional Care Model was developed and led by APRN providers for care coordination for chronic diseases or patients with complex needs at risk for poor outcomes at discharge to the home (Naylor & Sochalsik, 2010). This work resulted in Medicare payment for transitional care within the first 30 days of discharge (CMS, 2016). Another model of care coordination that has produced positive outcomes, cost-effectiveness, and lower costs is the Aging in Place model by Rantz et al. (2014) (http://www.agingmo.com). Transitional care services bridge the gaps among diverse services, providers, and settings through the systematic application of evidence-based interventions that improve communication and transfer of information within and across services, enhance post–acute care follow-up, and decrease gaps in care by the use of a single consistent provider (cited in ANA, 2013, p. 19). To advance knowledge on the outcomes of transitions of care, NTOCC has developed a number of tools and resources for case managers to ensure effective communication between clients, caregivers, and providers, and published a compendium of transition models in practice that provides evidence of cost savings and lower 30-day hospital readmission rates and emergency department visits. The Transitional Care Bundle includes seven essential interventions: medication management, transition planning, client/family engagement and education, information transfer, follow-up care, provider engagement, and shared accountability across providers (Lattimer, 2013). Research indicates that the models employing the "Transitions" concept are currently ensuring higher quality and health care savings (http://www.ntocc.org).

Case management differs between urban and rural settings. In the rural setting, where the distance between populations is more expansive, there are fewer organized community-based systems, and communication and distance are often a greater challenge. Furthermore, the economics, pace and style of life, values, and social organization all differ. In a study referenced in Stanton and Dunkin (2009), rural residents identified four barriers to access to care that confront case managers in rural areas: lack of proximity to providers, limited services, scarcity of providers, and reduced availability of emergency and acute care services. Transportation, both for nurses and for clients, and lack of health insurance and benefits were documented challenges to rural clients of case managers. However, in federal study findings on the creation of Programs of All-Inclusive Care for the Elderly (PACE) sites in rural areas, which included the services of case management, researchers discovered that the rural PACE model restored health, well-being and independence, and reduced family caregiving burden. It also provided employment opportunities in rural communities to stimulate local economies (Sebelius, 2011).

In a study of rural Veterans Affairs (VA) mental health patients who received case management services, Mohamed, with Neale and Rosenheck (2009) and Mohamed, with colleagues Rosenheck and Cuerdon (2010) found that intensive case management services were characterized as slightly less frequent, less intensive, and less recovery oriented than services delivered to the urban VA population. Travel distances and times were longer for rural case managers. Case management service intensity was related to premature termination of services for the veteran populations. Because case management is part of a transitional care model and coordination of care can reduce readmissions and promote safety, appropriate delivery of case management is essential to support The Joint Commission's National Safety Goals (2009) as well as the National Quality Strategy (AHRQ, 2016). In the 2016 publication of the National Quality Strategy Report it has been emphasized that more research and the use of standardized protocols are needed to understand and solve disparities in care coordination interventions. For example evidence has detected that lower quality of care is experienced by more people with low incomes who are non-white (AHRQ, 2016).

CHECK YOUR PRACTICE

As an employee of the school system, you have been asked to become the case manager for the population of asthmatic children in the school system. What will this involve? What will you be responsible for doing?

Case Management and the Nursing Process

Case management activities with individual clients and families will reveal the broader picture of health services and health status of the community. *Community assessment, policy development,* and *assurance activities* that frame core functions of public health actions are often the logical next step for a nurse's practice. The nurse views the process of case management through the broader health status of the community. Clients and families receiving service represent the microcosm of health needs within the larger community. Through a nurse's case management activities, general community deficiencies in quality and quantity of health services are often discovered. When observing lack of care or services at the individual and family intervention levels, the nurse can, through case management, intervene at the community level to make changes. For example, the management of a severely disabled child by a nurse case manager may uncover the absence of respite services or parenting support and education resources in a community. While managing the disability and injury claims within a corporation, the nurse may discover that alternative care referrals for home-health visits and physical therapy are generally underused by the acute care providers in the community. Through a nurse's case management of brain-injured young adults, the absence of community standards and legislative policy for helmet use by bicyclists and motorcyclists may be revealed, stimulating advocacy efforts for changing community policy. Clearly, the core components of case management and the nursing process are complementary (Table 25.1).

While Secord's classic illustration of case management (1987) remains an appropriate picture of the process, the CMSA model (2016) is a contemporary illustration of the case manager's process in the continuum of care (Fig. 25.3), and Table 25.1 also compares the case management process and nursing process.

Characteristics and Roles

Case management can be labor intensive, time consuming, and costly. Because of the rapid growth in complexity in clients' problems managed by the case manager, the intensity and duration of activities required to support the case management function may soon exceed the demands of direct caregiving. Managers and clinicians in community health are exploring methods to make case management more efficient, including the use of providers who can perform to the limit of their licenses, auxiliary case management providers/services, and evidence-based practices. These provider characteristics include:

1. The technical/intellectual qualifications to understand and evaluate specific diagnoses, generally requiring clinical credentials (and experience), social determinants of health, financial resources, health information technology knowledge and analyses, risk arrangements
2. Capability in language and terminology (able to understand and then to explain to others in simple terms)
3. Cultural and linguistic knowledge of patients and communities for effective practice
4. Assertiveness, diplomacy, and negotiation skills with people at all levels
5. The ability to *assess* situations objectively and to *plan* appropriate case management services
6. Knowledge of available clinical evidence and resources as well as their strengths and weaknesses
7. The ability to act as *advocate* for the client and payer in models relying on third-party payment
8. The ability to act as a counselor or *facilitator* to clients to provide support, information curation and education, understanding, and intervention
9. An interprofessional team player

TABLE 25.1 The Nursing Process and Case Management

Nursing Process	Case Management Process	Activities
Assessment	• Case finding • Identification of incentives and barriers for target population • Screening, selection, and intake • Determination of eligibility • Assessment of challenges, opportunities, and problems	• Develop networks with target population • Disseminate written materials • Seek referrals • Apply screening tools according to program goals and objectives • Use written and on-site screens • Apply comprehensive assessment methods (physical, social, emotional, cognitive, economic, and self-care capacity) • Obtain consent for services if appropriate
Diagnosis	• Identification of problem/opportunity and challenges	• Hold interprofessional, team, family, and client conferences • Determine conclusion on basis of assessment • Use interprofessional team
Planning for Outcomes	• Problem prioritizing • Planning to address care needs • Identification of resource match	• Validate and prioritize problems with all participants • Select evidence-based interventions • Develop goals, activities, time frames, and options • Create case management plan • Gain client's consent to implement • Have client choose options
Implementation	• Advocating for client interests • Frequent monitoring to assess alignment with goals and changing nature of client needs • Facilitation for executing right services, right time, right patient, right place	• Contact providers • Coordinate care activities • Negotiate services and price • Adjust as needed during implementation • Document processes and monitor progress
Evaluation	• Measuring attainment of activities and goals of service delivery plan • Continued monitoring and follow-up of client status during service • Reassessment • Bringing closure to care when client needs are achieved or change • Appropriate discharge to ensure effective transitional care and termination of case management processes	• Ensure quality of transitional communication and coordination of service delivery • Monitor for changes in client or service status • Follow up as needed • Examine outcomes and metrics against goals • Examine needs against service • Examine costs • Examine satisfaction of client, providers, and case manager • Examine best practices and outcomes for this client • Examine readmissions, ED visits

ED, Emergency department.

In 1998, Cary described the roles of case managers in the practice setting. These roles are clearly affirmed today by the CMSA (2016) (Box 25.1) (assessor, planner, facilitator, coordinator, monitor, evaluator, and advocate.) The roles demanded of the nurse as case manager are greatly influenced by the forces that support or detract from the role. Fig. 25.4 presents factors that demand the attention of both the nurse and the system during the case management process.

Knowledge and Skill Requisites

Nurses, like those in other disciplines, are not automatically experts in the role of case manager. First, they develop and refine the knowledge and skills that are essential to implementing the role successfully. Knowledge domains useful for nurses in systems desiring to implement quality case management roles are found in Box 25.2 (Cary, 1998; Stanton & Dunkin, 2009; Treiger, 2013).

When a nurse seeks a case manager position, some of the skills and knowledge will need to be acquired through academic and continuing education programs, literature reviews, onboarding, orientation, and mentoring experiences. Broad nursing knowledge may need to be updated, and practical experiences in case management may be required (CMSA, 2016). Treiger (2013) recommended that case managers pursue advanced education in case management. In fact, professional development activities for case managers in public health have been demonstrated to contribute to job satisfaction (Schutt et al., 2010). Finally, title protection for case managers is an issue under discussion in the literature in order to ensure credibility of services provided by professional, skilled case managers.

Tools of Case Managers

The six "rights" of case management are right care, right time, right provider, right setting, right price/value, and right outcomes. How does the nurse judge the effectiveness of case management? Three tools are useful for case management practice: case management plans, disease management, and life care planning tools. An underlying principle for the use of each of these tools is to use robust evidence as the basis for the selection of activities; technology, health information systems (HIS) and electronic health records (EHRs), and analytics are now the drivers of these tools.

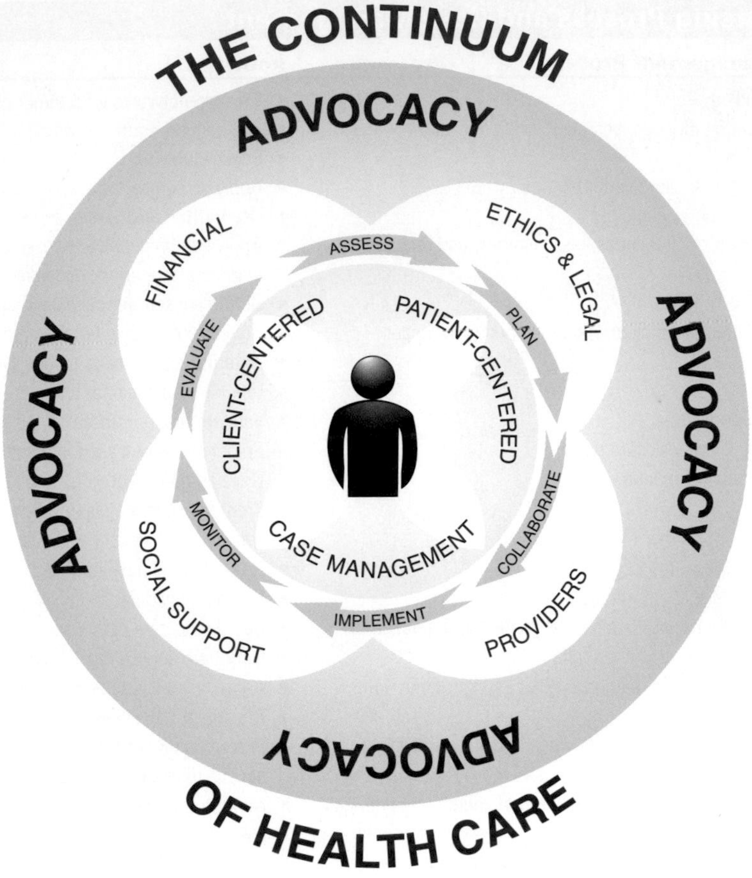

Fig. 25.3 The continuum of care case management model. (Reprinted with permission, the Case Management Society of America, 6301 Ranch Drive, Little Rock, AR 72223, www.cmsa.org.)

BOX 25.1 Case Manager Roles

- **Broker:** Acts as an agent for provider services that are needed by clients to stay within coverage according to budget and cost limits of health care plan
- **Client advocate:** Acts as advocate, provides information, and supports benefit changes that assist member, family, primary care provider, and capitated systems
- **Consultant:** Works with providers, suppliers, the community, and other case managers to provide case management expertise in programmatic and individual applications
- **Coordinator:** Arranges, regulates, and coordinates needed health care services for clients at all necessary points of services. Effectively participates and leads interprofessional teams
- **Educator:** Educates client, family, and providers about case management process, delivery system, community health resources, and benefit coverage so that informed decisions can be made by all parties
- **Facilitator:** Supports all parties in work toward mutual goals
- **Liaison:** Provides a formal communication link among all parties concerning the plan of care management
- **Mentor:** Counsels and guides the development of the practice of new case managers
- **Monitor/reporter:** Provides information to parties on status of member and situations affecting client safety, care quality, and client outcome, and on factors that alter costs and liability
- **Negotiator:** Negotiates the plan of care, services, and payment arrangements with providers; uses effective collaboration and team strategies
- **Researcher:** Accesses and applies evidence-based practices for programmatic and individual interventions with clients and communities; participates in protection of clients in research studies; initiates/collaborates in research programs and studies; accesses real-time evidence for practice
- **Standardization monitor:** Formulates and monitors specific, time-sequenced critical path and care map plans (see page XXX) as well as disease management protocols that guide the type and timing of care to comply with predicted treatment outcomes for the specific client and conditions; attempts to reduce variation in resource use; targets deviations from standards so adjustments can occur in a timely manner; uses dashboards and predictive modeling to anticipate outcomes
- **Systems allocator:** Distributes limited health care resources according to a plan or rationale

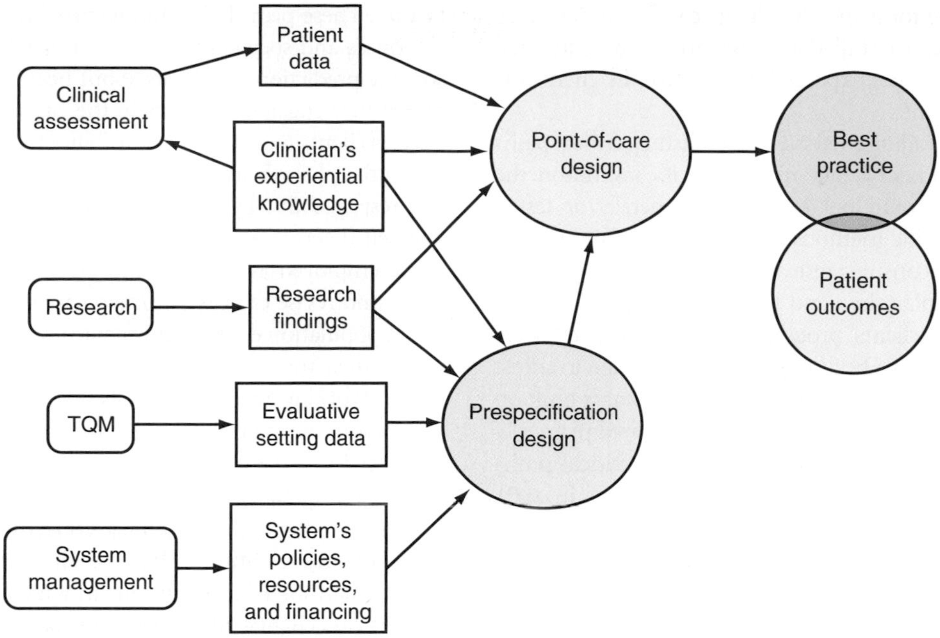

Fig. 25.4 Factors that require the attention of the nurse and the system in the case management process. *TQM,* Total quality management.

BOX 25.2 Knowledge Domains for Case Management

- Standards of practice for case management
- Evidence-based practice guidelines for specific health and disease conditions and communities
- Knowledge of health care financial environment and the financial dimension of client populations managed by nurses
- Clinical knowledge, skill, and maturity to direct quality timing and sequencing of care activities
- Care resources for clients within institutions and communities: facilitating the development of new resources and systems to meet clients' needs
- Transition planning for ideal timing, sequencing, and levels of care
- Management skills: communication, delegation, persuasion, use of power, consultation, problem solving, conflict management, confrontation, negotiation, management of change, marketing, group development, accountability, authority, advocacy, ethical decision making, and profit management
- Teaching, counseling, and education skills
- Program evaluation and research
- Performance improvement techniques
- Peer and team consultation, collaboration, and evaluation
- Requirements of eligibility and benefit parameters by third-party payers
- Legal and ethical issues
- Information management systems: clinical and administrative
- Health care legislation/policy
- Technical information skills, interoperable information systems, dashboard monitoring, data management and analysis, predictive modeling software, facile use of EHRs
- Outcomes management and applied research

EHR, Electronic health record.

Technology and technology enabled information and decision support such as artificial intelligence—still in early development—can optimize the delivery of processes used by the case manager. The technology sector is refining software in the areas of documentation, decision support, dashboard tools, predictive modeling, workflow automation, reporting capabilities, electronic health records, **patient engagement** strategies and social media, and remote monitoring (Carneal & Pock, 2014; Lamb & Newhouse, 2018; Stricker, 2014; Treiger, 2013). For example, health information technology (HIT) allows the case manager to access real-time data to improve timeliness of decisions or program changes for any number of adjustments in care protocols to ensure optimal outcomes. Data analytic software and dashboards allow for rapid decisions for clinical, administrative, and financial outcomes. Dashboard functions typically include (1) manipulation of report data, (2) access to information, (3) observing individual/population trends, and (4) observing trends in large datasets (Stricker, 2014). These data-reporting tools can vary from off-the-shelf, to customized, to simple Excel spreadsheets—each with their own advantages and gaps.

Historically, **case management plans** have evolved through various titles and methods (e.g., critical paths, critical pathways, care maps, multidisciplinary action plans, nursing care plans). Regardless of the title given, standards of client care, standards of nursing practice, and clinical guidelines using evidence-based practices for case management serve as core foundations of case management plans. Likewise, in interprofessional action plans, core professional standards of each discipline guide the development of the standard process.

As early as 1985, the New England Medical Center (Boston, Massachusetts) instituted a system of critical path development to guide the case management process in the acute care setting. This method of designing structures and processes of care laid the groundwork for the critical paths, care maps, and clinical decision tools now used in the industry. A *critical path* was described as a case management tool composed of abbreviated versions of discipline-specific processes; it was used to achieve a measurable outcome for a specific client "case" (Zander et al., 1987). The critical path detailed the essential and sequential activities in care, so that the expected progress of the client was known at a point in time.

At that time the prevailing method of establishing critical paths was by internal, "expert knowledge" from a specific institution, the result being that they could not be applied generally or tested under systematic, scientific methods. In the New England model, key incidents included consults, tests, activities, treatments, medication, diet, discharge planning, and teaching. The paths showed the differences between clients' progress. However, the paths were generally not revised unless a body of evidence was found to adjust the expected actions. Contemporary case management is built on clinical knowledge, predictive analysis, and personalized plans.

Care maps became the second generation of critical pathways of care. Rather than give definitions, as early as in 2001 Brown discussed the "various types of evidence that must be accessed, interpreted, and integrated into care design" (p. 3). Brown proposed the best practice health care map (BPHM) as a model for providing quality clinical care within an interprofessional practice. This model discussed all the components of knowledge development and care planning activities that must occur to have positive client outcomes. The author noted that care designed in advance takes the form of "clinical guidelines, care maps, decision algorithms, and clinical protocols for specified populations of clients" (Brown, 2001, p. 3). Furthermore, the author emphasized that at the point of care, these prespecified plans must be adapted to the individual client or population. The Brown BPHM was (1) client centered, (2) scientifically based, (3) population-outcomes based, (4) refined through quality assessment and compared with other maps, (5) individualized to each client, and (6) compatible with the larger system of health care in the United States.

Such activities today are more likely referred to as case management plans, care maps, integrated clinical pathways, and decision support tools and are the foundation for the methods to establish standardized, evidence-based case management plans. Clinical paths today are defined as structures of care based on interventions translated from evidence for use with clients; include detailed steps in a course of care; are based on pilot applications; and are modified (Kinsman et al., 2010). However, as Lamb and Newhouse (2018) articulate, much of the work of care coordination and case management has not been translated into the HIT infrastructure. More translation of the nature of the work, connection with patient status and needs and system interoperability to talk from one to another need to be developed to optimize the promise of HIT. Care guidance formats (critical paths, care maps) once optimized must be integrated into the EHR to be used by the case manager for clinical decision support. They may appear as prompts, checklists, references, for example, that will auto-populate a documented service and remind providers as to the array of procedures to be implemented. Case managers need to ensure that any "guidance care plans" embrace the unique needs of the client and care in order to optimize outcomes of care for clients.

Adaptation of any standardized case management plan to each client's characteristics is a crucial skill for the process and outcome of care. These plans link multiple provider interventions to client responses and social determinant of health factors and offer reasonable predictions to clients about health outcomes. Institutions report that engaging patients in the case management plans empowers clients to assume responsibility for monitoring and adhering to the plan of care and ensures the plan is culturally sensitive. Self-responsibility by clients incorporates the values of autonomy and self-determination as the core of case management. For the nurse employed as a **case manager**, ample opportunity exists to apply and revise critical path/map care guidance prototypes for a target population experiencing acute and chronic health problems within their unique cultural, social determinants, and population needs. Working with the architects and designers of these next generation information systems can assist in optimizing for greater accuracy for patient engagement and outcomes.

Disease management is an organized program of coordinated health care interventions that use consensus-driven performance measures and scientifically based evaluations in clinical outcomes for populations with conditions in which client self-care efforts are critical (URAC, 2018). This approach focuses on the natural progression of diseases in high-risk populations. Due to comorbidities, a whole person model is the basis for a disease management program (Population Health Alliance, 2016).

HOW TO Apply Telehealth Interventions for Clients

To utilize telehealth interventions for clients, case managers:

- Understand the patient, synthesize relevant information.
- Formulate conclusions about patient needs and what will be effective care strategies.
- Adopt the goal of a patient-centered approach in a virtual environment.
- Demand skills in clinical judgment and safe clinical relationships.
- Enter the relationship and connect with the patient.
- Share and review information.
- Recognize patterns and trends, documenting and reflecting on patient information.
- Synthesize information over time.
- Exit the relationship with transitional planning in mind (American Academy of Ambulatory Care Nursing, 2018).
- Make it a point to learn how telehealth works in your community and in the industry.
- Examine the evidence base for telehealth as an option for the types of clients you are servicing when considering available resources.
- Seek continuing education to prepare you on the art and science of telehealth application and client receptivity. Read the literature on e-communication and monitoring impact effectiveness.
- Be aware of the strengths and weaknesses of this delivery and plan to adjust the delivery model to optimize effectiveness for your clients.
- Seek networking opportunities with professional organizations and other case managers about the uses of telehealth.
- Examine the clinical guidelines and practice algorithms for telehealth adoption, application, and use.
- Sharpen your personal interaction and program evaluation skills to better assist in decision making about the use of telehealth services.

From Hagan L, Morin D, Lépine R: Evaluation of telenursing outcomes: satisfaction, self-care practices, and cost savings. *Public Health Nurs* 17:305–313, 2000; American Association of Ambulatory Care Nurses: *Scope and standards of practice for professional telehealth nursing,* ed. 6, Pitman, NJ, 2018.

Disease management can give clients the tools needed to better manage their lives (CMSA, 2016; Newman et al., 2014). Clients with chronic diseases may benefit from a disease management approach. The goals are to interrupt the continued development of a disease and prevent future disease and complications through secondary and tertiary prevention interventions. Promotion of wellness is necessary for success. For specific client populations that consume a disproportionate share of resources, disease management programs allocate the correct resources in an efficacious manner. Disease management programs may reduce emergency department visits, result in fewer inpatient days and rehospitalizations, greater client satisfaction, and reduced school absences (NTOCC, 2011; Sidorov, 2010; URAC, 2018). As the science of disease management evolves to predict direct relationships between outcomes and protocols of care, case managers will need to demonstrate cost-effective, optimal clinical care across the continuum—a goal of care management for populations. In fact, disease management is viewed as a top strategy by employers. The Joint Commission (TJC) certifies and URAC accredits disease management organizations and programs on the basis of their respective standards (see websites www.jointcommission.org and www.urac.org). This may influence the choice of programs a case manager selects to use with clients.

Life care planning is another tool used in case management. A life care plan assesses the current and future needs of a client for catastrophic or chronic disease over a life span. The life care plan is a customized, medically based organized plan to estimate reasonable and necessary current and future medical and nonmedical needs of clients with associated costs and frequencies of goods and services. Typically these needs incorporate medical, financial (income), psychological, vocational, built environment, and social costs during the remaining life of the client (Sambucini, 2013). Life care plans are typically used for clients experiencing catastrophic illness or adverse events resulting from professional malpractice or accidents/injuries or those who have sustained an injury when younger and subsequently have changes in resource requirements as they age. For example, conditions may include spinal cord injury, traumatic brain injury, chronic pain, amputation, cerebral palsy, and burns. Life care plans are also used to set financial awards, which can be used to secure resources for care in the future and create a lifetime care plan. A systematic process like the nursing process is used and interprofessional input is required.

The American Association of Nurse Life Care Planners (AANLCP) has published a *Code of Professional Ethics and Conduct for Nurse Life Care Planners with Interpretive Statements* (2012a) as well as the *Nurse Life Care Planners Standards of Practice with Interpretive Statements* (2012b). Nurse life care planners have access to academic course work, continuing education activities, and *A Core Curriculum for Nurse Life Care Planning* (Apuna-Grummer & Howland, 2013). There is also a certification examination for nurse life care planners that awards the designation of Certified Nurse Life Care Planner (CNLCP) as a specialty designation (www.cnlcp.org).

The first phase of the plan includes a thorough assessment of the client, financial/billing agreements, an information release signed by the client, and a targeted date for report completion. Development of the plan is the second phase. Plans are based on a number of factors: social and cultural situation, leisure activities, educational and employment status, medical history, physical and psychological abilities, current status, assistance required for completing activities of daily living, and regulatory requirements.

HOW TO Ensure High-Quality Care

The following actions can ensure high-quality care for clients and have implications for case managers in their practice:

- Provide access to easily understood information for each client based on his or her needs and health literacy level.
- Remember that the client is the source of control and that patient/family engagement is critical.
- Provide access to appropriate specialists with coordination and communication transparency.
- Ensure continuity of care for those with chronic and disabling conditions (transition care).
- Provide access to emergency services when and where needed.
- Disclose financial incentives that could influence medical decisions and outcomes.
- Prohibit "gag clauses" (which mean that providers cannot inform clients of all possible treatment options).
- Provide antidiscrimination protections.
- Provide internal and external appeal processes to solve grievances of clients.
- Make decisions on the basis of evidence.

From McClinton DH: Protecting patients, *Contin Care* 17:6, 1998; Institute of Medicine (IOM): *Crossing the quality chasm: a new health system for the 21st century,* Washington, DC, 2001, National Academies Press.

The execution of a life care plan is typically managed by a case manager who will work with the life care planner, especially when re-evaluation of the plan is necessary (AANLCP, 2013).

All of these tools/programs, in coordination, constitute individual and population health management strategies to educate clients, promote self-management and wellness, provide nurse coaching support, promote safe care transitions, improve care management and coordination, and enhance quality.

EVIDENCE-BASED EXAMPLES OF CASE MANAGEMENT

Historical Evidence

Carondelet Health at St. Mary's Hospital in Tucson, Arizona, developed a community nursing network in which enrollees are distributed among a number of community health centers. Professional nurse case managers assisted older clients to attain healthier lifestyles and maintain themselves in the community. Nurses were successful in delivering economical services per month for Medicare enrollees. Through nurse case management services, this nursing HMO was reported to have reduced the number of inpatient days per 1000 enrollees by one third, at an average cost of $900 per day, for a savings of $300,000 for every 1000 enrollees (ANA, 1993; American Nurses Foundation

[ANF], 1993). These strengths have been critical to allow the model to evolve to provide group and telephonic case management, telehealth, and automated standardized care instruments. Future endeavors will capitalize on the advances in information technology to capture clinical and cost data so that the case manager relies on data and analytics for decision and outcome reporting in a timely manner (Phillips-Jones, 2018).

Community-based statewide programs in New Jersey used case management methods to promote early identification, selection, evaluation, diagnosis, and treatment of children who are potentially physically compromised. Local case management units provided coordinated and comprehensive care. Collaboration with existing local and regional agencies serving children supported this process. The nurse case manager (1) provided counseling and education to parents and children about identifying problems and increasing their knowledge, (2) developed individual plans incorporating multidisciplinary services (education, social issues, medical development, rehabilitation), (3) obtained appropriate community services, (4) acted as a family resource in crises and service concerns, (5) facilitated communication between child and family, and (6) monitored services for outcomes. Interprofessional teams include nurses and social workers (with master's degrees) for larger caseloads. A recommended caseload was 300 to 350 children per case manager (Bower, 1992).

A national study of 2437 people who tested positive for human immunodeficiency virus (HIV) and who had case managers demonstrated that, regardless of the model, these clients were more likely to use life-prolonging HIV medications and meet the needs for income, health insurance, home care, and supportive emotional counseling than those without case management. Having contact with a case manager was not significantly related to use of outpatient care, hospital admission, or emergency department visits. Case managers in this study included social workers, nurses, and acquired immunodeficiency syndrome (AIDS) service organization staff (Katz et al., 2001).

Liberty Mutual Insurance Company had used case management principles for more than 30 years in workers' compensation cases and expanded services for employees whose conditions were noted as chronic or catastrophic. Case managers coordinated all clients, providers, and services to reduce expenses caused by lack of coordination; failure to use beneficial alternatives; and duplication and fragmentation of services (Bower, 1992).

Reducing the rate of readmission within 30 days of hospital discharge is a quality goal in health care. For psychiatric clients, the risk of rehospitalization is greatest and most costly during this time. Kolbasovsky (2009) replicated a model of intensive case management (ICM) in the United States that had been successful in Europe in reducing 30-day readmission rates (Burns et al., 2001, 2007) and found that ICM significantly reduced readmissions and the associated costs of 305 clients at a cost of $41.39 per member during the 30-day period. Had these persons been rehospitalized, the hospital psychiatric costs would have been $1528.14 per member.

In a randomized controlled trial of 450 clients post–cardiac bypass surgery, case management intervention by nurses using telephone-based collaborative care improved the mental and physical health of persons experiencing depression after cardiac bypass in an 8-month case management intervention. Outcomes included increased mental health scores, improved physical and functional status, and fewer readmissions among males with subsequent cost savings (AHRQ, 2010a).

Within the states, the types of agencies designated to conduct case management are often district offices of state government, area agencies on aging, county social services departments, and private contractors. States maintain the oversight responsibilities for case management agencies to (1) ensure they are complying with program standards, contracts, reporting, and fiscal controls, (2) identify emerging problems and issues to be resolved by additional state policies, and (3) provide on-site technical assistance and consulting to improve performance. States' payment methods for case management include daily/monthly rates, hourly/quarterly rates, capped rates for services, and capped aggregate rates to cover both case management and provider costs (Health Resources and Services Administration [HRSA], 2004; U.S. Department of Health and Human Services [USDHHS], 2008).

The models of case management vary today as they did in the recent past. In 1999, Taylor described three models by their focus: client, system, and social service. *Client-focused models* are concerned with the relationship between case manager and client to support continuity of care and to access providers of care. *System-focused models,* in contrast, address the structure and processes of using the population-based tools of disease management and case management plans to offer care for client populations. The *social service models* provide services to clients to assist them in living independently in the community and in maintaining their health by eliminating or reducing the need for hospital admissions or long-term care.

These models offer a solution to unnecessary health care expenses by reducing costs and accessing appropriate health care services. Imagine the impact on health status if these saved expenses were shifted to primary prevention and health promotion activities.

Contemporary Evidence

Evidence is mounting today in our evolving systems of care to reduce rehospitalizations, promote wellness, and understand the impact of transitional, coordinated, case management. Most of the new data directing the new models of care transitions are being constructed by leveraging technology and data to improve quality, integrate care, coordinate next services, and promote smooth handoffs to the next level and provider. These applications apply for those patients in the community who are managing their wellness and chronic conditions as well as to those in home care, hospitals, and nursing homes.

For example, Geisinger Health System sought to reduce the communication gap among providers by embedding advanced practitioners into their skilled nursing facilities (SNFs). By getting a patient ready for discharge when they are admitted through identification of home care needs, they have reduced the 30-day readmission to the hospital from 30 percent to 15 percent—beating the national average of 25 percent (URAC, 2018).

Another risk factor for readmission to the hospital that can be influenced by quality case management is the lack of medication adherence and adverse reactions. The Geisinger *ProvenHealthNavigator* program connects a nurse with patients 24-48 hours after discharge to review medications, and the community home worker ensures that patients have food, transportation, and social support. In this program about 70 nurse case managers work in primary care systems with patients with complex needs. The suite of transition and case management services in aggregate implemented by Geisinger Health System has now pushed the average readmission rates to those who participate to 10-12 percent with the aspiration to get that number even lower (URAC, 2018).

About 35 percent of hospitals now provide a "Meds to Bed" program to improve compliance by providing one on one pharmacy support prior to discharge for patients with multiple meds. The case manager matches patients with financial assistance programs such as copay reductions, free trial cards, and price matching. In fact, Tallahassee Memorial Transitions Center works with underinsured and uninsured patients to ensure they obtain their outpatient medications. During a patient's stay, postdischarge clinic appointments are made within a few days of discharge and a multidisciplinary team meets with the patient to craft a personalized health care plan to connect them with needed resources. Evidence from this approach shows emergency department and hospital visits are reduced by 68 percent—saving more than $1 million annually in unnecessary acute care use (URAC, 2018).

Le (2016) reviewed studies on transitional handoffs that used research approaches of phenomenology, qualitative, survey, and systematic reviews. Transitional findings showed that the best practice for communication included the review of the health provider information, reason for transfer, medical diagnosis, cognitive/functional abilities, medical orders, allergies, vital sign problems, and safety considerations.

Camicia and Lutz (2016) in a systematic review of descriptive and qualitative studies noted that 60 percent of stroke patients require post–acute care services after inpatient discharge to include rehabilitation services, SNFs, community-based services such as outpatient and home care. Safe timely and efficient transitions are created through effective transfer of information, patient and caregiver engagement as advocates for health care, and community support, documenting transition issues early, implementing strategies to intervene, and communicating transition plans to the next provider.

The evidence shows that strong transitional care services delivered in a timely manner by multidisciplinary teams of which nurses and nurse case managers are an essential provider result in fewer unnecessary acute care services, stronger community-based care outcomes in wellness and disease management, higher-quality patient care, and cost savings, which can be reinvested in expanded appropriate care. Employers who fund employee health insurance (nearly half of all insured Americans) are looking for new ways to bend the cost curve of rising health care costs by seeking high-value health care, providers and options for employees that are demonstrated centers of excellence and that can manage employees' chronic diseases in a cost-effective manner (Olson et al., 2018). Nurse case management is a centerpiece of these innovations by insurers and provider systems and can guide the use of evidence-based practices by nurses and systems.

EVIDENCE-BASED PRACTICE

A Classic Example of Research in Case Management

A successful pilot program led to the execution of a randomized controlled trial—After Discharge Care Management of Low Income Frail Elderly (AD-LIFE)—for community-based elderly. The care management model uses the integration of medical and social care to improve the outcomes of low-income and chronically and functionally impaired elderly after hospital discharge. AD-LIFE uses an interprofessional team, comprehensive geriatric assessment, and care management by a team nurse. Throughout the first year after hospital discharge, the nurse works with the area Agency on Aging social services program, performs a hospital and home assessment, uses a client goal-setting approach, creates a plan for development of self-care skills, and provides care planning for chronic illnesses and geriatric syndromes (e.g., incontinence, depression, nutrition, skin problems, and memory impairment). The interprofessional team can access specialists, and the primary care provider performs frequent evaluations and revises care plans as needed.

Ninety-two percent of the 118 clients had the need for at least one medical or social intervention. Half were taking 5 to 10 prescription drugs, 40 percent were living alone, 28 percent had congestive heart failure, 28 percent had diabetes, and many were unable to perform some activities of daily living (ADLs) or experienced geriatric syndrome. About 70 percent of clients said the care management program improved their health, allowed them to more easily access health care services, and provided them with a greater understanding of their disease(s). Hospital admissions decreased, and the care cost savings were $1000 per client per month.

- As a nurse working in public health, aspects of this program could be built on to design an interprofessional program for community-based clients with Alzheimer's disease, people living with acquired immunodeficiency syndrome (AIDS), chronically ill or disabled children, or clients with unstable psychiatric conditions.
- Contemporary evidence cited below from health systems affirms the use of transitional care and case management to provide appropriate services to keep patients in their communities and avoid unnecessary readmission for costly care.

Nurse Use

Postdischarge care management that integrates medical, nursing, and socially and culturally proficient care can improve outcomes of the low-income elderly as well as other groups named above. It is important to identify the interprofessional team members who could be assembled to conduct the program with each client group, to identify measures of success for each of the programs, and to relate the case management process to *Healthy People 2020* objectives that could be addressed for each of these client groups.

From Wright K, Hazelett S, Jarjoura D, et al.: The AD-LIFE trial. *Home Healthc Nurse* 25(5):308–314, 2007.

The impact of using a nurse case manager (NCM) and community health worker (CHW) team on diabetic control, emergency department (ED) visits, and hospitalizations among urban African Americans with type 2 diabetes in a randomized controlled clinical trial comparing intensive case management with minimal case management revealed the positive effects of the intensity of case management services on outcomes. Intensive services included mailings and telephone calls about preventive screenings, culturally tailored care provided by the NCM and CHW team, and evidence-based clinical algorithms with feedback to the primary care providers. Those clients receiving intensive case management were 23 percent less likely to have ED visits, and this effect was strongest for clients who received the most nurse and community health worker visits for their care (Gary et al., 2009). Culturally tailored interventions are essential to approaching health equity outcomes. Social determinants of health (SDOH) must be clearly addressed by the case manager in allocation of resources where communities experience disproportionate shares of SDOH impact.

In fact, studies show race-related disparities in the availability and need for education by diabetic African American patients (Hooks-Anderson et al., 2015). In a study of 19 ACOs, gross resource inadequacies were reported by 68 percent of providers for their communities where social determinants of health impacted their clients to include inadequate funding, services, data interoperability, and reimbursement issues (Anctil, 2017). A case manager involved in community-based programming focused on public health initiatives can be an asset to creating programs to address SDOH (Jackson, 2015). As an example, in a 2012 study with 83 clients in an urban setting, most of whom were uninsured, a community-based case management program with clients experiencing one or more chronic diseases yielded impressive results: acute outpatient encounters decreased by 62 percent and inpatient admissions by 53 percent. Primary care visits increased by 162 percent with an overall reduction in aggregate costs of 41 percent—from $16,208 pre-intervention to $9541 post-intervention (Glendenning-Napoli et al., 2012).

ESSENTIAL SKILLS FOR CASE MANAGERS

Three skills are essential to the role performance of the case manager: advocacy, conflict management, and collaboration.

Advocacy

Case managers report that they are first and foremost client advocates (CMSA, 2016; Tahan, 2016a). The definition of nursing includes advocacy: "Nursing is the protection, promotion and optimization of health and abilities, prevention of illness and injury, alleviation of suffering through the diagnosis and treatment of human response, and advocacy in the care of individuals, families, communities and populations" (ANA, 2010, p. 6). For nurses, advocacy involves a number of activities, ranging from exploring self-awareness to lobbying for health policy. Advocacy is essential for practice with clients and their families, communities, organizations, and colleagues on an interprofessional team. The functions of advocacy require scientific knowledge, expert communication, facilitating skills, and problem-solving and affirming techniques.

As the *Guide to the Code of Ethics for Nurses* (ANA, 2015a) states, "The nurse, in all professional relationships, practices with compassion and respect…" (p. 4). This means the nurse has the obligation to move beyond his or her own personal feelings of agreement or disagreement to respond compassionately. However, this goal is a contemporary one; the perspective regarding the advocacy function has shifted through history. The nurse advocate has been described in earlier writings as one who acted on behalf of or interceded for the client. An example of the nurse interacting on behalf of the client is the nurse who calls for a well-child appointment for a mother visiting the family planning clinic when the mother is capable of making an appointment on her own.

The advocate role evolved to that of mediator and is described as a response to the complex configuration of social change, reimbursement, and providers in the health care system (Tahan, 2016b). Mediating is an activity in which a third party attempts to provide assistance to those who may be experiencing a conflict in obtaining what they desire. The goal of the nurse advocate as mediator is to assist parties to understand each other on many levels so that agreement on an action is possible. In the example of a nurse as case manager for an HMO, mediating activities between an older adult client and the payer (the HMO) could accomplish the following results: the client may understand the options for community-based skilled nursing care, and the payer may understand the client's desires for a less restrictive environment for care, such as the home. The case manager as mediator does not decide the plan of action but facilitates the decision-making processes between the client and the payer so that the desired care can be reimbursed within the options available or new options created.

In contemporary practice, nurse advocates place the client's rights as the highest priority. The goal of promoter for the client's autonomy and self-determination may result in an optimal degree of patient engagement and empowerment and independence in decision making. For example, when a group of young pregnant women is the collective "client" (the aggregate), the nurse advocate's role may be to inform the group of the benefits and consequences of breastfeeding their infants. However, if the new mothers decide on formula feeding, the nurse advocate should support the group and continue to provide parenting, infant, and well-child services. This example shows a different perspective of the nurse as advocate. It notes that the nurse's role as advocate may demand a variety of functions that are influenced by the client's physical, psychological, social, and environmental abilities. Advocacy can result in clients becoming their own "client expert" in problem solving, decision making, maximization of resources, partnership development with providers, and ultimately using appropriate interventions (Burton et al., 2010; Tahan, 2016a).

The advocacy role aims to achieve engagement—a process in which clients are invested in their health and care through programs that provide information and tools to empower them to take control and evaluate their care (ANA, 2013; Tahan, 2016a). The nurse adapts the advocacy function to the client's dynamic capabilities as the client moves from one health state to another. Even clients who desire access to more substantial health promotion activities can benefit from a partnership with the nurse advocate. Case managers are called to mediate between client needs and payer requirements/economic constraints without becoming a barrier to quality care. Examples of advocacy in such cases might include promoting a client's (as an aggregate) access to on-site physical fitness programs in the occupational setting, or supporting parents' and students' concerns about the high fat and high sugar content of cafeteria and vending machine food in the school system. With the cost of health care exceeding $3 trillion annually and consumers assuming a larger financial portion of the care they choose, the promoter role of advocacy for those clients capable of autonomy is expected to increase.

Advocacy: Link to Public Health Nursing

The clinical practice skill of advocacy is an inherent concept in the practice of case management. Advocacy is a function of public health nurses described in the Intervention Wheel model (see Chapter 11), and in the ANA and CMSA Standards of Practice for Case Management. Advocacy can be applied at the policy, community, systems, individual, and/or family levels. For example, case managers can demonstrate advocacy when they establish new services and when they promote patient-centered changes in organizational and government policy (CMSA, 2016). In fact, when a public health nurse advocates for clients at any of these levels, the source of conflict and collaboration will likely come from competing values, that is, those of the client and any of these other levels of population or system values. For example:

- A client may want access to unlimited treatment; financial values may pose a source of conflict as the system attempts to justify the comparative effectiveness or costs.
- Family members may pose conflicting values for the nature of care they wish a family member to receive, even as the client refuses care.
- Communities can divert budget allotments to needs that are in competition for other population services such as community policing, health care access, and environmental services.

The nurse as advocate must listen carefully to his or her client in order to truly represent the interest of the client and encourage "win-win" processes and outcomes for the client. Advocacy occurs in all three of the core functions of public health: assessment, policy development, and assurance.

Process of Advocacy. The goal of advocacy is to promote self-determination and patient empowerment in a client (Tahan, 2016). The client may be an individual, family, peer, group, or community. The classic process of advocacy has been historically defined by Kohnke (1982), Mallik and Rafferty (2000), and Smith (2004) to include informing, supporting, and affirming. All three activities are more complex than they may initially seem, and they require self-reflection by the nurse as well as skill development. It is often easier for the nurse to inform, support, and affirm another person's decision when it is consistent with the nurse's values. When clients make decisions within their value systems that are different from the nurse's values, the advocate may feel conflict about contributing to the process of informing, supporting, and affirming those decisions. Promoting self-determination in others demands that the nurse have a philosophy of free choice once the information necessary for decision making has been discussed.

Informing. Knowledge is essential, but it is not sufficient to make decisions that affect outcomes. Interpreting knowledge is affected by the client's values and the meanings assigned to the knowledge. Interpreting facts is the result of both objective and subjective processing of information. Subjective processes greatly influence client decisions as prior experiences, myths, and fears can influence patients' decisions.

Informing clients about the nature of their choices, the content of those choices, and the consequences to the client is not a one-way activity. The **information exchange process** is composed of interactions that reflect three subprocesses: amplifying, clarifying, and verifying. **Amplifying** occurs between the nurse and the client to assess the needs and demands that will eventually frame the client's decision. Information is exchanged from both viewpoints. Although the exchange may be initiated at the objective, factual level, it is likely to proceed to incorporate the subjective perspectives of both parties.

The tone of the amplifying process can direct the remainder of the information exchange. It is important to relate with clients in a manner that reflects the advocate's endorsement of the client's self-determination. Setting aside the time necessary to listen to clients is critical. Clients will sense they are part of a mutual process if the nurse can engage them during the information exchange with a message that says, "I respect your needs and desires as I share my knowledge with you." Nonverbal behaviors, including using direct eye contact, sitting at the client's level, arriving and concluding at a prescribed time, and using verbal patterns that foster exchange (e.g., open-ended statements, questions, probes, reflections of feelings, paraphrasing), convey the nurse's desire to promote the client's ability to self-determine. Recent research indicates that clients' race and ethnicity may influence how providers and clients communicate with one another, thus contributing to disparities in health. Active communication among clients and providers has been linked to better treatment compliance and health outcomes (Schraeder & Shelton, 2011; URAC, 2018).

A client may not desire to exchange information because of lack of self-esteem, fear of the information, fear of disclosure, or inability to comprehend the content of the communication. In such a case, the focus is to understand the client's desire to be given no information and to express to the client the consequences of such inaction. The nurse may invite the client to ask for the information exchange at a later time, when the client is ready, and can periodically check with the client whether information exchange and amplifying are desired. In these cases, the nurse should document the implemented nursing actions to reflect the guidelines just discussed. This can reduce the basis for lawsuits and misunderstanding by other parties.

Clarifying is a process in which the nurse and client strive to understand meanings in a common way. Clarifying builds on the breadth and depth of the exchange developed during amplifying to determine whether the nurse and client understand each other. During this process, misunderstandings and confusions are examined. The goal of clarifying is to avoid confusion between the nurse and the client. To foster clarifying, nurses can use certain verbal prompts such as the following:

- "What do you understand about…?"
- "Please tell me more about how you…"
- "I don't think I am clear. Let me explain the situation in another way."
- "As an example, …"
- "What other information would be helpful so that we both understand?"

Verifying is the process used by the nurse advocate to establish accuracy and reality in the informing process. Low health literacy is a challenge for 90 million Americans who have difficulty understanding and acting on health information. Peterson and colleagues (2011) report that only 40 percent of whites and 41 percent of those from Asia and the Pacific Islands living in the United States are proficient in reading English. Low health literacy has been related to increased rates of chronic disease and hospitalizations (Fink-Samnick, 2018). In 2014, a *Public Broadcasting Newshour* publication cited the Department of Education findings that only about 1 in 10 people in the United States has a proficient level of health literacy (Gorman, 2014).

If the nurse discovers that a client is misinformed, the nurse may return to the clarifying or amplifying stage and begin the process again. Verifying produces the chance for the advocate and client to examine "truth" from their points of view, which may include knowledge, intuition, previous experiences, and anticipated consequences.

Promoting a client's self-determination may take the advocate and client through the information exchange process several times, as new dimensions, or obstacles, to an issue develop. Information exchange is a critical process for advocacy and is applicable to all advocacy clients: individuals, families, groups, and communities (see the How To box).

HOW TO Provide for Information Exchange Between Nurse and Client

1. Assess the client's present understanding of the situation. Have you considered your client's literacy level? Health literacy level? Cultural and ethnic values? Age and any disabilities that would interfere with learning? Do they convene myths, legends, and/or previous experiences that would influence their understanding?
2. Provide correct information.
3. Communicate on the client's literacy level, making the information as understandable as possible. Use interpreters and translators where needed.
4. Use a variety of media sources and teach-back methods to increase the client's comprehension.
5. Discuss other factors that affect the decision, such as financial, legal, and ethical issues.
6. Discuss the possible consequences of a decision.

Supporting. The second major process, **supporting**, involves upholding a client's right to make a choice and to act on it. People who are aware of clients' decisions fall into three general groups: supporters, dissenters, and obstructers. Supporters approve and support clients' actions. Dissenters do not approve and do not support clients. Obstructers cause difficulties when clients try to implement their decisions.

In 1998, Cary noted that the nurse advocate needs to implement several actions to fulfill the supporting role. Important interventions are assuring clients that they have the right and responsibility to make decisions, and reassuring them that they do not have to change their decisions because of others' objections.

Affirming. The third process in the advocacy role is **affirming**. It is based on an advocate's belief that a client's decision is consistent with the client's values and goals. The advocate validates that the client's behavior is purposeful and consistent with the choice that was made. The advocate expresses a dedication to the client's mission, and a purposeful exchange of new information may occur so that the client's choice remains possible. Recognizing that a client's needs may fluctuate with changing resources, the affirming activity must encourage a process of re-evaluation and rededication to promote client self-determination.

The importance of affirming activities cannot be emphasized strongly enough. Many advocacy activities stop with assuring and reassuring, but affirming is often critical in promoting a client's self-determination. Table 25.2 compares the nursing process with the advocacy process.

The advocate's role in the decision-making process is *not* to tell the client that an option is correct or right. The advocate's role is to provide the opportunity for information exchange, and to arm clients with tools that can empower them in making the best decision from their point of view. Enabling clients to make an informed decision is a powerful tool for building self-confidence. It gives clients the responsibility for selecting the options and experiencing the success and consequences of their decisions. Clients are empowered in their decision making when they recognize that although some events are beyond

TABLE 25.2 Comparison of Nursing Process and Advocacy Process

Nursing Process	Advocacy Process
Assessment/diagnosis	• Exchange information • Gather data • Illuminate values
Planning/outcome	• Generate alternatives and consequences • Prioritize actions • Engage the client
Implementation	• Empower the client to make decisions as possible • Support the client • Assure • Reassure
Evaluation	• Affirm • Evaluate • Reformulate • Close client case

their control, other events are predictable and can be affected by decisions they can make. Ultimately patient engagement brings improvements in patients' lives (Tahan, 2016a).

Nurses can promote client decision making by using the information exchange process, promoting the use of the nursing process, incorporating written techniques (e.g., contracts, lists), using reflecting and prioritizing techniques, and using role playing and sculpturing to "try on" and determine the "fit" of different options and consequences for the client. By engaging clients in the information-sharing process and assisting them to recognize the progression of activities they experience as they build their informed decision-making base, the nurse advocate is providing clients the opportunity to empower themselves with skills that can strengthen their autonomy and confidence in the future.

Advocacy is a complex process that maintains a delicate balance between doing for the client and promoting autonomy. The process is influenced by the client's physical, emotional, and social capabilities. The goal of advocacy is to promote the maximal degree of client self-determination, given the client's current and potential status; for most clients, this goal can be realized. When clients are comatose, unborn, or legally incompetent, nurse advocates have unique functions. The advocate's role is usually determined by the legal system; however, in some cases, nurses must decide what roles they will play. These are areas requiring intensive self-exploration, research, and collaboration with professionals, family members, and significant others. We are reminded that every encounter with a client is an opportunity to serve in the advocacy role that constitutes a necessary competency of a case manager to deliver quality and safe care (Cesta & Tahan, 2016; CMSA, 2016; Treiger & Fink-Samnick, 2016).

Skill Development. Skills needed by the nurse advocate are not unique to their profession. Nursing demands scientific, technical, relationship, and problem-solving knowledge and skills. Advocacy applies nursing skills of communication and competency to promote client self-determination.

Knowledge of nursing and other disciplines as well as of human behavior is essential for the advocacy role in establishing authority, promoting authenticity, and developing skills. The capacity to be assertive for personal rights and the rights of others is essential.

Systematic Problem Solving. The nursing process—assessment, diagnosis, planning, implementing, and evaluating—is an example of a method of **problem solving** that can be used in the advocacy role. Advocates can be particularly helpful with clients in identifying values and generating alternatives.

Illuminating Values. People's values affect their behavior, feelings, and goals. In the process of amplifying, clarifying, and validating, the advocate understands a client's values. Through the process of self-revelation, an emerging value (such as environment, people, cost, or quality) may become more apparent to a client. This can have an effect in two ways. The client may be able to focus on actions on the basis of the value, or the value may confuse the decision process. The nurse can assist the client in prioritizing action and clarifying the value. Values can also change as new or relevant data are processed. The advocate's role is to assist clients in discovering their values. This process can be particularly demanding in the information exchange and affirming process.

Generating Alternatives. Clients and advocates may feel limited in their options if they generate solutions before completely analyzing the problems, needs, desires, and consequences. Several techniques can be used to generate alternatives, including brainstorming and a technique known as the problem-purpose-expansion method. In **brainstorming**, the nurse, client, professionals, or significant others generate as many alternatives as possible, without placing a value on them. Brainstorming creates a list that can then be examined for the critical elements the client seeks to preserve (e.g., environmental preferences, degree of control). The list can be analyzed according to the consequences and the effect of the alternatives on self and others.

The classic **problem-purpose-expansion method**, as described by Volkema (1983), and later expanded on by Heslin and Moldoveanu (2002) and Winston and Albright (2012), is a way to broaden limited thinking. It involves restating the problem and expanding the problem statement so that different solutions can be generated. If problem formulation yields to solution generation too early, important dimensions of the problem may go undetected and opportunities are missed. For example, if the problem statement is to convince the insurance company to approve a longer length of service, the nurse and client have narrowed their options. However, if the problem statement is to improve the client's convalescence and safety, several solutions and options are available, such as the following:

- Obtaining skilled nursing facility placement
- Obtaining home-health skilled services
- Arranging physician home visits
- Paying for custodial care
- Paying for private skilled care
- Obtaining informal caregiving

Impact of Advocacy. Advocacy empowers clients to participate in problem-solving processes and decisions about health care. Clients try to understand changing opportunities in the health care system for access, use, and achieving continuity of care. Nurse advocates promote client engagement and self-determination and management of behavior as it relates to health and the adherence to therapeutic regimens. Clients are part of larger systems: the family, the work environment, and the community. Each system interacts with the client to shape the available options through resources, needs, and desires. Each system also exhibits both confirming and conflicting goals and processes that need to be understood for client self-determination to be successful. For example, the practice of advocacy among minority groups may involve the ability to focus attention on the magnitude of problems caused by diseases affecting minority clients. Whether the client is an individual, family, group, or community, the advocacy function can promote the interest of self-determination, which influences the progress of societies.

Advocacy is not without opposition. Clients and advocates may find barriers to services, vendors, providers, and resources. A community may experience a shortage in nursing home beds or providers, a childcare facility may experience staffing shortages, a family may not have the money to keep a child at home, and a client may find that the school system cannot fund a full-time nurse for its clinic. The reality of scarce resources creates a difficult barrier for advocates. However, events such as these often stimulate a community's self-determination and lead to innovative actions to correct gaps in service (see the Levels of Prevention box).

LEVELS OF PREVENTION

Case Management

Primary Prevention

Use information exchange process to increase health literacy as a requisite to impact wellness and to use the health care system, adopt health promotion strategies that will maintain health, and engage in health education to create and maintain healthy lifestyles.

Secondary Prevention

Use case finding and dashboard data to identify existing health problems in your caseload and the population served by your agency. Timely, holistic assessments and interventions can slow disease trajectories and promote healing and health.

Tertiary Prevention

Monitor and adjust the use of prescription medications and adherence to treatment to reduce the risk of complications. Institutionalize this approach in your agency.

Allocation and Advocacy: Complement or Conundrum?

Whereas advocacy holds a traditional role in the nursing profession, **allocation** is a staple of market competition. Nurses perform allocation roles when they triage clients or perform the gatekeeping and rationing functions. Nurses often reflect that clinical judgments are influenced by their values and ethics as well as organizational demands (ANA, 2015a). When working in organizations, nurses experience allocation demands at the systems level through budgetary decisions and staffing assignments. At the clinical level, demands relate to implementing treatment protocols. When nurses act as client advocates by clarifying a client's desires or needs, they can conflict with systems procedures for allocation of limited resources within these systems. Case managers need to balance efficient use of resources.

Nurses who shoulder both advocacy and allocation responsibilities may benefit from a clear understanding of their personal and professional values. A systematic procedure for mediating conflict between the two competing responsibilities is also helpful (Cary, 1998; Fink-Samnick & Muller, 2010; Tahan, 2016b). The role of patient advocate is now germane to health care as evidenced by the new certification and training programs in Professional Patient Advocacy by the Patient Advocate Certification Board, which can be accessed at www.pacboard.org.

Conflict Management

Case managers help clients manage conflicting needs and scarce resources. Techniques for managing conflict include a range of active communication skills. These skills are directed toward learning all parties' needs and desires, detecting their areas of agreement and disagreement, determining their abilities to collaborate, and assisting in discovering alternatives and activities for reaching a goal. Mutual benefit with limited loss is a goal of conflict management.

Conflict and its management vary in intensity and energy in a number of ways. The effort needed to manage a conflict depends on various factors: the existing evidence to support facts and the objective and subjective perceptions of the parties involved.

Negotiating is a strategic process used to move conflicting parties toward an outcome. A major focus is to reach agreement where parties feel results are fair, equitable, free of bias, and satisfactory (Tahan, 2016b). The outcome can vary from one in which one party gains benefit at the other's expense (**distributive outcomes**) or in which mutual advantages override individual gains (**integrative outcomes**) (Thompson et al., 2010).

The process of negotiating can be characterized in three stages: prenegotiating (preparing and discussing), negotiating (discussing, proposing, bargaining), and aftermath (closing, renegotiating, willingness to negotiate again). Prenegotiating activities are designed to have parties agree to collaborate. Parties must see the possibility of agreeing and the costs of not agreeing (Lee & Lawrence, 2013). Preparations must be made as to time, place, and ground rules concerning participants, procedures, and confidentiality.

The negotiation stage consists of phases in which parties must develop trust, credibility, distance from the issue (to limit the feeling of "one best way"), and the ability to retain personal dignity. Bazarman (2005) and Lee and Lawrence (2013) agree that stages occur in negotiation:

Phase 1: Establishing the issues and agenda. This is accomplished by identifying, clarifying, presenting, and prioritizing the issues.

Phase 2: Advancing demands and uncovering interests. Negotiations center on presenting parties' interests and differentiating parties' demands and positions on the conflict.

Phase 3: Bargaining and discovering new options. Debates include gathering facts, based on reasoning, that will generate understanding and promote relearning. Bargaining reduces differences on issues by giving or removing rewards or desired objects. Creating new solutions or options through brainstorming, reflective thinking, and problem-purpose-expansion techniques is important in achieving options that provide mutual benefits.

BOX 25.3 Categories of Behaviors Used in Conflict Management

Accommodating: Individual neglects personal concerns to satisfy the concerns of another.
Avoiding: Individual pursues neither his or her concerns nor another's concerns.
Collaborating: Individual attempts to work with others toward solutions that satisfy the goals of both parties.
Competing: Individual pursues personal concerns at another's expense.
Compromising: Individual attempts to find a mutually acceptable solution that partially satisfies both parties.

Modified from Volkema RJ, Bergmann TJ: Conflict styles as indicators of behavioral patterns in interpersonal conflicts. *J Social Psychol* 135:5–15, 2001; CPP: *History and Validity of the Thomas-Kilmann Conflict Mode Instrument (TKI)*. Mountainview, CA, CPP, Inc. Available at asia.themyersbriggs.com

Phase 4: Working out an agreement. This may involve settling on some but not all points. Parties can agree to re-examine the issues later, and steps for implementing and follow-up must be clarified.

The aftermath of negotiation is the period following an agreement in which parties are experiencing the consequences of their decisions and will discern the degree to which they are willing to work together in the future (Thompson et al., 2010). The reality of their decisions may lead to re-evaluating their values. In a conflict situation, parties engage in behaviors that reflect the dimensions of assertiveness and cooperation. **Assertiveness** is the ability to present one's own needs. **Cooperation** is the ability to understand and meet the needs of others. Each person uses a primary and secondary orientation to engage in conflict (Box 25.3).

Clearly, flexibility in conflict management behavior can facilitate an outcome that meets the client's goals. Helping parties navigate the process of attaining a goal requires effective personal relations, knowledge of the situation and alternatives, and a commitment to the process.

Collaboration

In case management, the activities of many disciplines (social workers, nurses, physicians, insurers, physical therapists, etc.) are needed for success. Clients, the family, significant others, payers, and community organizations contribute to achieving the goal. Collaboration can include working with communities; local, state, and federal resources; providers; team members; payers; and family, to name a few. It can include the techniques of motivational interviewing, mediation, and negotiation to facilitate communication and relationships (CMSA, 2016). **Collaboration** is achieved through a developmental process. Collaboration is a dynamic, highly interactive, and interdependent process in which people work together, sharing resources and even a vision for a goal (Morales Arroyo, 2003). Androwich and Cary (1989) found that collaboration occurs in a sequence and is reciprocal and can be characterized by seven stages and activities (Fig. 25.5).

The goal of communication in the collaborative development process is to amplify, clarify, and verify all team members' points of view. Although communication is essential in collaboration, it is not sufficient to result in or maintain collaboration. While the collaboration model recognizes the contributions of joint decision making, one member of the team should be accountable to the system and to the client. This team member should be responsible for monitoring the entire process (see the following QSEN box).

QSEN FOCUS ON QUALITY AND SAFETY EDUCATION FOR NURSES

Targeted Competency: Teamwork and Collaboration

Function effectively within nursing and interprofessional teams, fostering open communication, mutual respect, and shared decision making to achieve quality client interventions and outcomes.

Important aspects of teamwork and collaboration include:

- **Knowledge:** Describe scopes of practice and roles of health care team members
- **Skills:** Clarify roles and accountabilities under conditions of potential overlap in team member functioning. Use negotiation when disputes exist.
- **Attitudes:** Value the perspectives and expertise of all health team members

Teamwork and Collaboration Question

Observe a typical workday of a nurse case manager in an acute care, community health or public health setting, noting the types of activities that are done in coordination and handoffs, the team members involved, and the amount of time spent in these areas. Interview several staff members to determine whether they perceive that the amount of their time spent in case management is changing. To what degree are the staff members involved in care management activities? Ask about colleagues with whom case managers collaborate. Besides primary care physicians, which health care team members are often involved in managing clients' care across time and across settings? Reflect and state the skills that are needed by the case management nurse to best facilitate these interdisciplinary teams.

Prepared by Gail Armstrong, PhD(c), DNP, ACNS-BC, CNE, Associate Professor, University of Colorado Denver College of Nursing, and adapted by Ann Cary, 2018.

Case managers encounter conflict on a daily basis. Competing needs, resources, organizational demands, and professional role boundaries present opportunities and pitfalls for conflict management and collaboration (Box 25.4). Providers report that in the collaborative role of serving as advocates for clients, they encounter competing expectations by other providers in the system—even other case managers (Sands, 2013; Tahan, 2016b).

Teamwork and collaboration clearly demand knowledge and skills about clients, health status, resources, treatments, and community providers. The ability to assess clients' and families' complex needs involves knowledge of intrapersonal, interpersonal, medical, nursing, and social dimensions. Demonstrating team member and leadership skills in facilitating a

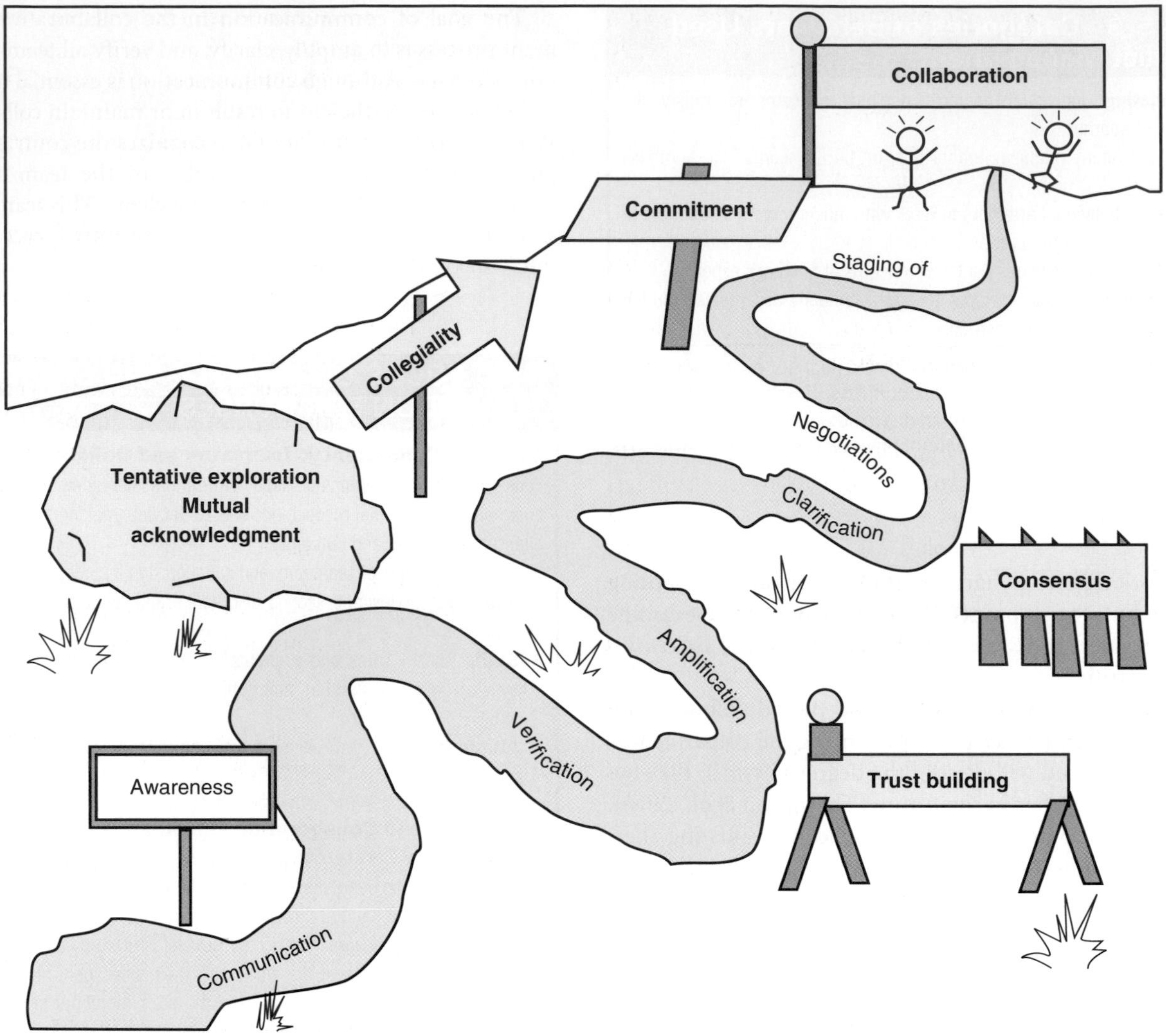

Fig. 25.5 Collaboration is a sequential yet reciprocal process. (From Androwich I, Cary AH: *A collaboration model: a synthesis of literature and a research survey.* Paper presented at the Association of Community Health Nurse Educators Spring Institute, Seattle, June 1989.)

BOX 25.4 Stages of Collaboration

1. Awareness
   - Make a conscious entry into a group process; focus on goals of convening together; generate a definition of collaborative process and what it means to team members.
2. Tentative exploration and mutual acknowledgment
   - Exploration: Disclose professional skills for the desired process; disclose areas where contributions cannot be made; disclose values reflecting priorities; identify roles and disclose personal values, including time, energy, interest, and resources.
   - Mutual acknowledgment: Clarify each member's potential contributions; verify the group's strengths and areas needing consultation; clarify members' work style, organizational supports, and barriers to collaborative efforts.
3. Trust building
   - Determine the degree to which reliance on others can be achieved; examine congruence between words and behaviors; set interdependent goals; develop tolerance for ambiguity.
4. Collegiality
   - Define the relationships of members with each other; define the responsibilities and tasks of each; define entrance and exit conditions.
5. Consensus
   - Determine the issues for which consensus is required; determine the processes used for clarifying and making decisions to reach consensus; determine the process for re-evaluating consensus outcomes.
6. Commitment
   - Realize the physical, emotional, and material actions directed toward the goal; clarify procedures for re-evaluating commitments in light of goal demands and group standards for deviance.
7. Collaboration
   - Initiate a process of joint decision making reflecting the synergy that results from combining knowledge and skills.

Modified from Cary A, Androwich I: *A collaboration model: a synthesis of literature and a research survey.* Paper presented at the Association of Community Health Nurse Educators Spring Institute, Seattle, June 1989; Mueller WJ, Kell B: *Coping with conflict,* Englewood Cliffs, NJ, 1972, Prentice Hall.

goal-directed group process is essential. It is unlikely that any single professional possesses the expertise required in all dimensions. It is likely, however, that the synergy produced by all can result in successful outcomes.

ISSUES IN CASE MANAGEMENT

Legal Issues

Case managers today face pressure to control costs, to use evidence-based guidelines for practice, and to reduce risks for legal liability. They are vulnerable to legal risks because of inadequate preparation, changing legislation and policy, health systems changes, the advent of new workers and the absence of title protection, insufficient support, and role expectations. CMSA (2016) notes in their legal standard (J) that confidentiality, client privacy, and consent for professional case management services are essential in addition to those that follow. Liability concerns of case managers exist when the following three conditions are met: (1) the provider had a duty to provide reasonable care, (2) a breach of contract occurred through an act or an omission to act, and (3) the act or omission caused injury or damage to the client. Case managers must strive to reduce risks, practice wisely within acceptable practice standards, and limit legal defense costs through professional insurance coverage. Areas of risk are adapted from Hendricks and Cesar (2003), Cunningham (2007), Llewellyn and Leonard (2009), and Sambucini (2013):

1. Liability for managing care
   a. Inappropriate design or implementation of the case management system
   b. Failure to obtain all pertinent records on which case management actions are based
   c. Failure to have cases evaluated by appropriately experienced and credentialed clinicians
   d. Failure to confer directly with the treating provider (physician or nurse practitioner) at the onset and throughout the client's care
   e. Substituting a case manager's clinical judgment for that of the medical provider
   f. Requiring the client or his or her provider to accept case management recommendation instead of any other treatment
   g. Harassment of clinicians, clients, and family in seeking information, and setting unreasonable deadlines for decisions or information
   h. Claiming orally or in writing that the case management treatment plan is better than the provider's plan
   i. Restricting access to otherwise necessary or appropriate care because of cost
   j. Referring clients to treatment furnished by providers related to the case management agency without proper disclosure
   k. Connecting case managers' compensation to reduced use and access of services
   l. Inappropriate delegation of care
   m. Inappropriate use of clinical practice guidelines
2. Negligent referrals
   a. Referral to a practitioner known to be incompetent
   b. Substituting inadequate treatment for an adequate but more costly option
   c. Curtailing treatment inappropriately when treatment was actually needed
   d. Referral to a facility or practitioner inappropriate for the client's needs
   e. Transfer to another facility that lacks care requirements
   f. Communication and transition handoff failures
3. Experimental treatment and technology
   a. Failure to apply the contractual definition of "experimental" treatment found in the client's insurance policy
   b. Failure to review sources of information referenced in the applicable insurance policy (e.g., Food and Drug Administration, or published medical literature)
   c. Failure to review the client's complete medical record
   d. Failure to make a timely determination of benefits in light of timeliness of treatment
   e. Failure to communicate coverage determined to be needed, to the insured client or participant
   f. Improper economic considerations determining the coverage
   g. Failure to understand and retrieve information from HIT sources.
4. Confidentiality/security
   a. Failure to deny access to sensitive information that is awarded special protection by federal or state law
   b. Failure to protect access to computerized medical records
   c. Failure to adhere to regulatory provisions (e.g., Health Insurance Portability and Accountability Act provisions [http://hipaa.cms.gov]; Americans with Disabilities Act)
5. Fraud and abuse
   a. Making false statements of claims or causing incorrect claims to be filed
   b. Falsifying the adherence to conditions of participation of Medicare and Medicaid
   c. Submitting claims for excessive, unnecessary, or poor-quality services
   d. Engaging in remuneration, bribes, kickbacks, or rebates in exchange for referral
   e. Upcoding intensity of care or intervention requirements

Legal citations relevant to case management and managed care include negligent referrals, provider liability, payer liability, breach of contract, denial of care, and bad faith. As in any scope of nursing practice and with the potential growth in tort reform, it behooves the nurse to seek preventive education on contemporary practice and legal trends to lower exposure to legal liability.

Sambucini (2013) notes that court cases and federal and state tort reforms influence the legal considerations of case managers generally. When courts find that cost considerations affect medical care decisions, all parties to the decision will be liable for resulting damages. Guidelines to reduce risk exposure include the following:

1. Clear documentation of the extent of client participation in decision making and reasons for decisions
2. Records demonstrating accurate, timely, and complete information on interactions and outcomes
3. Use of reasonable care in selecting referral sources, which may include verifying of licensure of providers

4. Written agreements when arrangements are made to modify benefits other than those in the contract
5. Good communication with clients
6. Informing clients of their rights of appeal
7. Applying the ethical guidelines of case management (CMSA, 2016; Valiant & Jensen, 2012)

Ethical Issues

Case managers as nursing professionals are guided in ethical practice by the *Code of Ethics for Nursing* (ANA, 2015a) and *Code of Professional Conduct for Case Managers* (Commission for Case Management Certification [CCMC], 2015), by performance indicators for ethics in the *Standards of Practice for Case Management* (CMSA, 2016), and by the contract expressed in *Nursing's Social Policy Statement* (ANA, 2015a).

By integrating these guidelines and philosophies, nursing practice is ideally suited to preserve the ethical principles of autonomy, beneficence, fidelity, justice, nonmaleficence, and veracity in case management processes. Numerous authors, notably Hendricks and Cesar (2003), McCollom (2004), Llewellyn and Leonard (2009), Fink-Samnick and Muller (2010), Apuna-Grummer and Howland (2013), and Tahan (2016a) describe how case managers may confront dilemmas in these areas:

- Case management may hamper a client's **autonomy**, or the individual's right to choose a provider, if a particular provider is not approved by the case management system. If a new provider must be found who can be approved for coverage, continuity of care may be disrupted.
- **Beneficence**, or doing good, can be impaired when excessive attention to containing costs supersedes the nurse's duty to improve health or relieve suffering.
- **Fidelity** is defined as faithfulness to the obligation of duty (www.merriam-webster.com), in this case to the client by keeping promises and remaining loyal within the nurse-client relationship. Duty to clients to secure benefits on their behalf and to limit unnecessary expenditures can create dilemmas when the goals are not uniform.
- **Justice** as an ethical principle for case managers considers equal distribution of health care with reasonable quality. Tiers of quality and expertise among provider groups can be created when quality providers refuse to accept reimbursement allowances from the managed system, leaving less experienced or lower quality providers as the caregiver of choice for clients being managed.
- **Nonmaleficence** is defined as doing no harm. When case managers incorporate outcomes measures, evidence-based practice, and monitoring processes in their plans of care, this principle is addressed.
- **Veracity**, or truth telling, is absolutely necessary to the practice of advocacy and building a trusting relationship with clients. Clients particularly complain that in the changing health care system, payers do not seem to be able to provide comprehensive yet inexpensive options for care.

Three of the most common legal dilemmas have been historically classified as conflicts in advocacy, priorities, and duties (Hendricks & Cesar, 2003; Mahlin, 2010). For example, a case manager may advocate for many perspectives—clients, organizations, and society—that are not harmonious. When considering priorities in values, the case manager will ultimately be considering personal, professional, organizational, and client values. Selecting which values to honor can result in violating the values of the other, and asking the question "Whose best interests can be served?" may create a dilemma. Finally, conflicts in duties can result when placing the best interest of a client first adversely affects the other party.

Standards of practice and care, codes of ethics, licensure laws, credentialing through certification, and organizational policies and procedures (e.g., ethics committees, risk management units) offer the case manager information and support in managing ethical conflicts and dilemmas in the case management system. Maintaining familiarity with ethical issues published in the case management literature can offer specific assistance for practicing case managers (Tables 25.3 and 25.4).

TABLE 25.3 Credentialing Resources for Case Managers (Individual Certification Options)

Organization	Website	Credentials
American Nurses Credentialing Center	http://www.nursecredentialing.org	Nurses: RN-BC, for Registered Nurse-Board Certified for Case Management
American Case Management Association	https://www.acmaweb.org	ACM-RN accredited case manager
Certification of Disability Management Specialists Commission	http://www.cdms.org	Interprofessionals: CDMS, for Certified Disability Management Specialist
Commission for Case Manager Certification	http://www.ccmcertification.org	CCM, for Interprofessionals as a Certified Case Manager
Certification Board for Certified Nurse Life Care Planners	http://cnlcp.org	CNLCP, for Certified Nurse Life Care Planner (specialty certification for nurses who are life care planners)
National Academy of Certified Care Managers	http://www.naccm.net	Interprofessionals: CLM, for Certified Long-term Care Manager
Rehabilitation Nursing Certification Board	http://www.rehabnurse.org	CRRN, for Certified Rehabilitation Registered Nurse
Patient Advocate Certificate	http://www.patientadvocatetraining.com	BCPA—credential in patient advocacy

TABLE 25.4 **Websites for Case Management Resources**

Resource	Website	Details
URAC	www.urac.org	Accredits disease management, case management, and health plan programs and other services. Supports efforts for clinical benchmarking, quality of care, chronic care evidence-based models
America's Health Insurance Plans	http://www.ahip.org	Trade association representing health insurance industry
American Nurses Credentialing Center	http://www.nursecredentialing.org	Offers review course materials for nurse case managers
American Medical Association	http://www.ama-assn.org	Includes continuing medical education unit (CEU) programs
Case Management Society of America	http://www.cmsa.org	Specialty organization for case managers
Centers for Medicare and Medicaid Services	http://www.cms.gov	Oversees execution of rules and regulations for clients of state and federally funded services
CenterWatch Clinical Trial Listing Service	http://www.centerwatch.com	Global source for clinical trials information
Centers for Disease Control and Prevention	http://www.cdc.gov	Provides education, training, and research for disease, emergency preparedness, environmental health, traveler health, workplace safety and health, population health, and healthy living
The Joint Commission (TJC)	http://www.jointcommission.org	Accredits health care–related delivery organizations and disease-specific care programs
Medscape	http://www.medscape.org	Features clinical updates and education for professionals
National PACE Association On Lok	http://www.npaonline.org Http://OnLOK.org	Provides information on models and locations of PACE services for the elderly as well as On Lok services
National Transitions of Care Coalition (NTOCC)	http://www.ntocc.org	Provides information on transitions of care models and outcomes
National Committee for Quality Assurance	http://www.ncqa.org	Publishes HEDIS performance indicators for provider systems and accredits managed care organizations. Provides certification of disease management, utilization management, and credentialing verification organizations. Also ACOs, case management, and patient-centered medical homes (among other organizations)
National Library of Medicine	http://www.nlm.nih.gov	Global medical library
NurseWeek	http://www.nurse.com	Provides information links to other sites and nursing professional education course work
Oncology	http://www.oncolink.upenn.edu	Oncology links
Online Journal of Issues in Nursing	http://www.nursingworld.org	Publication on issues in nursing
Commission on Accreditation of Rehabilitation Facilities	http://www.carf.org	Accredits services globally that may be used by case management clients such as adult day care, assisted living, behavioral health, disability rehabilitation, addiction and substance abuse rehabilitation, employment and community services, and medical rehabilitation

ACO, Accountable care organization; *HEDIS*, Healthcare Effectiveness Data and Information Set.

LINKING CONTENT TO PRACTICE

Important guidance in developing a community-based case management program can be found in the United States. Case management is a key component of federally financed and many state-financed health delivery options. The experiences of states over the past two decades provide testimony to the importance of case management for populations at risk. For older clients, state-derived case management provides objective advice and assistance with care needs. It also provides access to interprofessional providers and services. For payers (federal, state, clients), case management serves as a way to ensure that funds are allocated appropriately to those in greatest need. Case management serves a policy assurance and accountability function for communities. The PACE (Program of All-Inclusive Care for the Elderly) program addresses the needs of chronically ill seniors who wish to remain in their homes rather than be admitted to nursing homes. PACE participants are enrolled in a managed care model of medical, nursing and support services, case management, medications, respite, hospital, and nursing home care when necessary. These services are financed by Medicare and Medicaid and some seniors will pay a monthly premium. The PACE model uses interdisciplinary care teams to provide services. PACE prevents institutionalization in nursing homes, uses a strong social model of health care delivery, and case manages transitions of clients between delivery systems and providers. Studies (Fretwell & Old, 2011; On Lok, 2017; Sebelius, 2011; Wieland et al., 2013) have demonstrated cost savings with PACE programs in both urban and rural areas compared with nursing home costs. The PACE model has been permanently recognized as a provider type under both Medicare and Medicaid and operates in the majority of the states (On Lok, 2017).

PRACTICE APPLICATION

During her regularly scheduled visit to a blood pressure clinic in a local apartment cluster, a Hispanic resident, Mrs. B., 45 years old, complained of feeling dizzy and forgetful. She could not remember which of her six medications she had taken during the last few days. Her blood pressure readings on reclining, sitting, and standing revealed gross elevation. The nurse and Mrs. B. discussed the danger of her present status and the need to seek medical attention. Mrs. B. called her physician from her apartment and agreed to be transported to the emergency department.

In the emergency department, Mrs. B. manifested the progressive signs and symptoms of a cerebrovascular accident (a CVA, or stroke). During hospitalization, she lost her capacity for expressive language and demonstrated hemiparesis and loss of bladder control. Her cognitive function became intermittently confused, and she was slow to recognize her physician and neighbors who came to visit. The utilization review/discharge planning nurse at the hospital contacted the case manager from the home health agency to screen and assess for the continuum of care needs as early as possible, because Mrs. B. lived alone and family members resided out of town.

It became apparent that family caregiving in the community could only be intermittent because family members lived too far away. Mrs. B. had residual functional and cognitive deficits that would demand longer-term care.

As the case manager contracted by the plan, place the following actions in the correct sequence to construct a case management plan:

A. Discuss with the family their schedule of availability to offer care in the client's home.
B. Discuss their cultural values in caring for family members.
C. Call the client and introduce yourself, as a prelude to working with her.
D. Obtain information on the scope of services covered by the benefit plan for your client.
E. Arrange a skilled nursing facility site visit for the client and family.

Answers can be found on the Evolve site.

KEY POINTS

- An important role of the nurse is that of client advocate.
- The goal of advocacy is to promote the client's engagement in the plan and self-determination.
- When performing in the advocacy role, conflicts may emerge about the full disclosure of information, territoriality, accountability to multiple parties, legal challenges to clients' decisions, and competition for scarce resources.
- The functions of advocacy and allocation can pose dilemmas in practice.
- Amplification, clarification, and verification are three communication skills necessary in the advocacy process.
- Information systems and interoperability are critical to communication and successful handoffs from provider to provider and patients during the case management process
- Additional skills important to fulfilling the role of client advocate include the helping relationship, assertiveness, and problem solving.
- Problem solving is a systematic approach that includes understanding the values of each party and generating alternative solutions.
- Brainstorming and the problem-purpose-expansion method are two techniques to enhance the effectiveness of problem-solving skills.
- During conflict, negotiations can move conflicting parties toward an outcome.
- Prenegotiation, negotiation, and aftermath are three phases of managing a conflict.
- Each individual has a predominant orientation when engaging in conflict: competing, accommodating, avoiding, collaborating, or compromising.
- Collaboration may result by moving through seven stages: awareness, tentative exploration and mutual acknowledgment, trust building, collegiality, consensus, commitment, and collaboration.
- Care management is a strategic program to maintain the health of a population enrolled in a delivery system.
- Continuity of care is a goal of nursing practice. It requires making linkages with services and information systems to improve the client's health status.
- As the structure of the health care system moves toward delivering more services in the community, the achievement of continuity of care will present a greater challenge.
- Case management is typically an interprofessional process in which the client is the focus of the plan.
- Documentation and use of dashboards for case management activities and outcomes are essential to nursing practice.
- Case management is a systematic process of assessment, planning, service coordination, referral, monitoring, and evaluation that meets the multiple service needs of clients.
- A nurse's scope of practice includes advocacy, allocation, and case management functions.
- Nurses functioning as advocates and case managers need to be aware of the ethical and legal issues confronting these components of their practice.
- Standardization of care for predictable outcomes can be achieved through critical paths, disease management protocols, dashboards, data analytics, clinical guidelines, interprofessional action plans, and a caring-based practice in which processes of diagnosis and treatment are applied to the human experiences of health and illness.
- Nurses are guided by a philosophy of caring and advocacy.
- Nurses have a high regard for client self-determination, independence, and informed choice in decision making.

- Recognizing that responses to illness and disability may limit independence and self-determination, nurses focus on the rights of individuals, families, and communities to define their own health and evidence-based guidelines for practice.
- Telehealth application provides expansive alternatives within resource delivery options but must be customized for clients.

CLINICAL DECISION-MAKING ACTIVITIES

1. Observe a typical workday of a nurse working with a population, noting the types of activities that are done in coordination, transition care, case management, and documentation as well as the amount of time spent in these areas. Interview several staff members to determine whether they perceive that their time spent in case management is changing. To what degree are the staff members involved in care management activities? What are the top three legal and ethical issues they encounter in their practice? What are the sources of conflict and negotiation they experience in their practice? What do the nurses report as their greatest sources of satisfaction and dissatisfaction in their jobs?
2. Initiating, monitoring, and evaluating resources are essential components of nursing practice. Describe a client situation and the case management process that might occur in the following practices:
   A. A school nurse in an elementary school and one in a high school working with brain-injured students
   B. An occupational health nurse in a hospital and one in a manufacturing plant
   C. A nurse working in a primary care well-child clinic
   D. A case manager employed by a managed care organization
   E. A care manager employed in a health benefits corporation; an insurer; an ACO
3. Explain how the case management processes affected client outcome in each of these situations.
4. The values and beliefs held by a nurse influence the nurse's ability to be an advocate for clients. Analyze your values and beliefs about rationing health care and describe how they may affect your ability to be a client advocate. How did you develop your values and beliefs?
5. Read the following and respond to the respective questions: Fink-Samnick E: Managing social determinants of health: part I Fundamental knowledge for professional case management. *Prof Case Manag* 23(3):107-129, 2018. Discuss your reactions to the statement: for case managers, the social determinants of health (SDOH) pose major challenges to providing effective patient resources, health and behavioral health treatment plans, patient adherence, and overall coordination of care.
   A. What are the major types of SDOH in patients we care for?
   B. What are the social, psychological, and ecosocial factors that influence patients' health and recovery from illness?
   C. For persons with disabilities behavioral risk factors add to the SDOH influence. What are some of these factors that have been identified in the article and how would you assess for these as part of your case management plan to strengthen successful outcomes?
   D. Given that the article describes various factors related to SDOH, identify the food deserts and household locations for food insecurity in your community by location, zip code, or census tract. Is this gap in food supply assessed in any of the case management assessments or assessment tools you have examined? Is it addressed in the plan?

   Or read: Phillips-Jones C: Accountable care organizations and the impact on care management. *CMSA Today,* April 6, 2018. Retrieved from https://www.cmsatoday.com.
   A. Describe the interventions used by ACOs as they relate to the skills of case and care managers.
   B. Based on the needs of organizations today, what are the two differences between the traditional and contemporary care managers' skills in the process of validating their outcomes?
   C. What can organizations do to ensure the care manager and case manager is an integral part of the patient-centered team? Give two examples.

ADDITIONAL RESOURCES

EVOLVE WEBSITE

http://evolve.elsevier.com/Stanhope/community/

- Answers to Practice Application
- Case Study
- Glossary
- Review Questions

REFERENCES

Agency for Healthcare Research and Quality (AHRQ): Nurse-Led, Telephone-Based Collaborative Care Improves Mental and Physical Health of Depressed Clients after Cardiac Bypass Surgery [Health Care Innovations Exchange], 2010a. Retrieved from https://innovations.ahrq.gov.

Agency for Healthcare Research and Quality (AHRQ): Care coordination, 2016a. Retrieved from https://www.ahrq.gov.

Agency for Healthcare Research and Quality (AHRQ): Effective communication and Care Coordination-Priorities in Focus, 2016b. Retrieved from https://www.ahrq.gov.

Agency for Healthcare Research and Quality (AHRQ): National Healthcare quality and Disparities Report and 5th Anniversary update on the National Quality Strategy, 2015 AHRQ Pub. No 16-0015 Rockville, MD: AHRQ.

American Association of Ambulatory Care Nurses and Academy of Medical Surgical Nurses: Care Transition Hand off Tool Task Force Evidence Table, 2017, AAACN.org. Retrieved from https://www.aaacn.org.

American Association of Ambulatory Care Nurses (AAACN): Scope and Standards of Practice for Professional Telehealth Nursing, ed 6, Pitman, NJ, 2018, AAACN.

American Association of Colleges of Nursing (AACN): Advancing healthcare transformation: a new era for academic nursing, Washington, DC, 2016, Author.

American Association of Nurse Life Care Planners (AANLCP): Code of Professional Ethics and Conduct for Nurse Life Care Planners with Interpretive Statements. AANLCP membership guide, 2012a. Retrieved from www.AANLCP.org.

American Association of Nurse Life Care Planners (AANLCP): Nurse Life Care Planners: Standards of Practice with Interpretive Statements. AANLCP membership guide, 2012b. Retrieved from www.AANLCP.org.

American Association of Nurse Life Care Planners (AANLCP): A core curriculum for nurse life care planners, Bloomington Indiana, October 2013, Universe LLC.

American Hospital Association (AHA): Glossary of Terms and Phrases for Health Care Coalitions, Chicago, 1986, AHA Office of Health Coalitions and Private Sector Initiatives.

American Nurses Association (ANA): Managed Care: Cornerstone for Health Care Reform—A Fact Sheet, Washington, DC, 1993, ANA.

American Nurses Association (ANA): A guide to Nursing's Social Policy Statement: From *Social contract to social covenant*, ed 1, Silver Spring, MD, 2013a. Retrieved from Nursesbooks.org.

American Nurses Association (ANA): Framework for Measuring Nurses' Contributions to Care Coordination, Silver Spring, MD, 2013b, ANA.

American Nurses Association (ANA): Guide to the Code of Ethics for Nurses with Interpretative Statements, Silver Spring, MD, 2015a. Retrieved from Nursesbooks.org.

American Nurses Association (ANA). *Nursing scope and standards of practice,* ed 3, Silver Spring, MD: 2015b, ANA.

American Nurses Foundation (ANF): America's Nurses: An Untapped Natural Resource, Washington, DC, 1993, ANF.

Anctil B: Social determinants in a new era of healthcare. Premier Blogs, 2017. Retrieved from http://learn.premier.com.

Androwich I, Cary AH: A Collaboration Model: A Synthesis of Literature and a Research Survey. Paper presented at the Association of Community Health Nurse Educators Spring Institute. Seattle, June 1989.

Apuna-Grummer D, Howland WA, editors: *A Core Curriculum for Nurse Life Care Planning,* Bloomington, IN, 2013, iUniverse.

Bachrach C, Thomas Y: Training nurses in population health science: what, why, how? Presentation at the 133rd meeting of the National Advisory Council for Nurse Education and Practice, Rockville, MD, June 2016.

Barton AJ: Role of the RN in Primary Care: Implications for Nursing Education, *J Nurs Educ* 56(3):127–128, 2017.

Bazarman MH, editor: *Negotiating, Decision Making and Conflict Management,* Cheltenham, UK, 2005, Edward Elgar Publishing United.

Bower KA: Case Management by Nurses, Washington, DC, 1992, American Nurses Association.

Brown SJ: Managing the complexity of best practice health care, *J Nurs Care Qual* 15:1–8, 2001.

Burns T, Catty J, Dash M, Roberts C, Lockwood A, Marshall M: Use of intensive case management to reduce time in hospital in people with severe mental illness: systematic review and meta-regression, *BMJ* 335:336, 2007.

Burns T, Fioritti A, Holloway F, Malm U, Rössler W: Case management and assertive community treatment in Europe, *Psychiatr Serv* 52:631–636, 2001.

Burton J, Murphy E, Riley P: Primary immunodeficiency disease: a model for case management of chronic disease, *Prof Case Manag* 15:5–14, 2010.

Camicia M, Lutz BJ: Nursing's role in successful transitions across settings, *Stroke* 47, e246–e249, 2016.

Carneal G, Pock R: Six year of study reveals the impact of IT on the practice of case management, *CMSA Today* 2:16–17, 2014.

Cary AH: Advocacy or allocation, *Nurs Connect* 11:1–7, 1998.

Case Management Society of America (CMSA): Standards of Practice for Case Management, Little Rock, AR, 2016, CMSA. Retrieved from http://www.cmsa.org.

Centers for Medicare and Medicaid Services (CMS). Transitional care management services, 2016. Retrieved from https://www.cms.gov.

Cesta TG, Tahan HM: *The Case manager survival guide: Winning strategies for the new healthcare environment*, ed 3, Lancaster, 2016, DEStech Publications Inc.

Coggeshall Press: Case Management Model, Coralville, IA, 2008, Coggeshall Press. As cited in Huber, 2010.

Commission for Case Management Certification (CCMC): Code of Professional Conduct for Case Managers with standards, rules, procedures, and penalties, Mt. Laurel, 2015, Author.

CPP: History and Validity of the Thomas-Kilmann Conflict Mode Instrument (TKI), Mountain View, CA, CPP, Inc. Retrieved from https://www.cpp.com.

Cunningham B, Powell SK, Tahan HA, editors: *CMSA Core Curriculum for Case Management,* Philadelphia, 2007, Lippincott, Williams & Wilkins.

Fabbri E, De Maria M, Bertolaccini L: Case Management: An up-to-date review of literature and a proposal of a county utilization, *Ann Transl Med* 5(20):396, 2017.

Fidelity [Def. 2]: Merriam-Webster Online. In *Merriam-Webster,* n.d. Retrieved from http://www.merriam-webster.com.

Fink-Samnick E, Muller LS: Case management across the life continuum: ethical obligations versus best practice, *Prof Case Manag* 15:153–156, 2010.

Fink-Samnick E: Managing social determinants of health: Part I Fundamental knowledge for case managers, *Prof Case Manag* 23(3):107–129, 2018.

Fretwell MD, Old JS: The PACE program: home-based care for nursing home-eligible individuals, *N C Med J* 72:209–211, 2011.

Gary TL, Batts-Turner M, Yeh HC, et al.: The effects of a nurse case manager and a community health worker team on diabetic control, emergency department visits, and hospitalizations among urban African Americans with type 2 diabetes mellitus: a randomized controlled trial, *Arch Intern Med* 169:1788–1794, 2009.

Glendenning-Napoli A, Dowling B, Pulvino J, Baillargeon G, Raimer BG: Community-based case management for uninsured patients with chronic diseases: effects on acute care utilization and costs, *Prof Case Manag* 17:267–275, 2012.

Gorman A: Many new patients overwhelmed by health care jargon, Kaiser Health News 2014. Retrieved from http://www.pbs.org.

Hagan L, Morin D, Lépine R: Evaluation of telenursing outcomes: satisfaction, self-care practices, and cost savings, *Public Health Nurs* 17:305–313, 2000.

Health Resources and Services Administration (HRSA): Health Systems and Financing Group: Medicaid Case Management Services by State, archived Webcast, 2004. Retrieved from http://www.hrsa.gov.

Hendricks AG, Cesar WJ: How prepared are you? Ethical and legal challenges facing case managers today (CEU), *Case Manager* 14:56–62, 2003.
Heslin PA, Moldoveanu M: What's the "real" problem here? A model of problem formulation. Presented at Managing the Complex IV: Conference on Complex Systems and the Management of Organizations, Fort Myers, FL, December 2002.
Hooks-Anderson, DR, Crannage EF, Salas J, Scherrer JF: Race and referral to diabetes education in primary care patients with prediabetes and diabetes, *Diabetes Educ* 41(3):281–289, 2015.
Institute of Medicine (IOM): Crossing the Quality Chasm: A New Health System for the 21st Century, Washington, DC, 2001, National Academies Press.
Institute of Medicine (IOM): Population health implications for the Affordable Care Act: workshop summary, Washington, DC, 2014, The National Academies Press.
Jackson K: Public health social work: Now more than ever, *Social Work Today* 15(6):12, 2015.
Josiah Macy Jr, Foundation: Registered nurses: Partners in transforming primary care. Recommendations from the Macy Foundation Conference on preparing registered nurses for enhanced roles in primary care, New York, 2016, Author.
Katz MH, Cunningham WE, Fleishman JA, et al.: Effect of case management on unmet needs and utilization of medical care and medications among HIV-infected persons, *Ann Intern Med* 135:557–565, 2001.
Keller LO, Strohschein S, Schaffer MA, Lia-Hoagberg B, et al.: Population-based public health interventions: innovations in practice, teaching and management, Part II, *Public Health Nurs* 21:469–487, 2004.
Kimmel KC: Current Health IT Challenges and opportunities in population health. Presentation at the 133rd meeting of the National Advisory Council for Nurse Education and Practice, Rockville, MD, January 2016.
Kinsman L, Rotter T, James E, Snow P, Willis J: What is a clinical pathway? Development of a definition to inform the debate, *BMC Med* 8:31, 2010.
Kohnke MF: Advocacy: Risk and Reality, St. Louis, 1982, Mosby.
Kolbasovsky A: Reducing 30-day inpatient psychiatric recidivism and associated costs through intensive case management, *Prof Case Manag* 14:96–105, 2009.
Lamb G, Newhouse R: Care Coordination—A blueprint for Action for RNs, Silver Spring, MD, 2018, ANA.
Lattimer C: Working to improve transitions of care, *CMSA Today* 5:12–14, 2013.
Lee R, Lawrence P: *Organizational Behavior: Politics at Work,* New York, NY, 2013, Routledge.
Le L: Patient: Transfer (intrahospital) [Monograph] Evidence Summaries. Retrieved from the Joanna Briggs Institute Library Database, 2016, AAACN/AMSN Care Transition Hand-Off Tool Table.
Llewellyn A, Leonard M: *Case Management Review and Resource Manual,* ed 3, Silver Spring, MD, 2009, Nursesbooks.org.
Mahlin M: Individual patient advocacy, collective responsibility and activism within professional nursing associations, *Nurs Ethics* 17:247–254, 2010.
Mallik M, Rafferty AM: Diffusion of the concept of patient advocacy, *J Nurs Scholarsh* 32:399–404, 2000.
McClinton DH: Protecting patients, *Contin Care* 17:6, 1998.
McCollom P: Advocate versus abdicate, *Case Manager* 15:43–45, 2004.
Improvement Strategies, 2007. Technical Review 9 (prepared by Stanford-UCSF Evidence-Based Practice Center under Contract No. 290-02-0017). Retrieved from http://www.ahqr.gov.
McKesson Corporation: How Care Management Evolves with Population Management—A White Paper, 2014. Retrieved from http://www.healthleadersmedia.com.
Mohamed S, Neale M, Rosenheck RA: VA intensive mental health case management in urban and rural areas: veteran characteristics and service delivery, *Psychiatr Serv* 60:914–921, 2009.
Mohamed S, Rosenheck R, Cuerdon T: Who terminates from ACT and why? Data from the National VA Mental Health Intensive Case Management Program, *Psychiatr Serv* 61:675–683, 2010.
Morales Arroyo MA: *The physiology of collaboration: an investigation of library-museum-university partnerships.* Dissertation, August 2003. Retrieved from http://digital.library.unt.edu.
Mullahy C: *The Case Manager's Handbook,* ed 4, Sudbury, MA, 2010, Jones & Bartlett.
Muller LS, Flarey DL: Defining advanced practice nursing, *Lippincotts Case Manag* 8:230–231, 2003.
National Advisory Council on Nurse Education and Practice (NACNEP): Preparing Nurses for New Roles in Population Health Management, Rockville, 2016, HRSA.
National Quality Forum (NQF): Priority setting for healthcare performance measurement: Addressing performance measure gaps in care coordination, Washington, DC, 2014, National Quality Forum.
National Transitions of Care Coalition (NTOCC): Improved Transitions of Patient Care Yield Tangible Savings, 2011. Retrieved from http://www.ntocc.org.
Naylor MD, Sochalski JA: Scaling up: Bringing the transitional care model into the mainstream, Issue Brief (Commonw Fund) 103: 1–12, 2010.
Newman MB, Kowlsen T, Beckworth V: An integrated approach: the impact of health care reform from a managed care perspective, *CMSA Today* 1:20–23, 2014.
Olson A, Japinga M, Crook H, Saunders R, Taylor Jr, DH: Value innovations by employers: Examples beyond cost sharing, Raleigh, 2018, Duke/Margolis Center for Health Policy. Retrieved from https://healthcarediv.com.
On Lok: Annual Report, San Francisco, On Lok Inc. 2017.
Park EJ, Huber DL, Tahan HA: The evidence base for case management practice, *West J Nurs Res* 31:693–714, 2009.
Peterson PE, Woessmann L, Hanushek EA, et al.: Globally Challenged: Are U.S. Students Ready to Compete? PEPG report #11-03, 2011. Harvard Kennedy School. Retrieved from http://www.hks.harvard.edu.
Pifer R: ACOs using medical home physicians save money, yield higher quality report finds, Health Care Dive Brief 2018. Retrieved from https://www.healthcaredive.com.
Population Health Alliance PHM Glossary: Disease Management, Washington DC, 2016, Population Health Alliance. Retrieved from http://www.populationhealthalliance.org.
Quad Council Coalition Competency Review Task Force: Community/Public Health Nursing Competencies, 2018. Retrieved from http://www.quadcouncilphn.org.
Rantz M, Popejoy LL, Galambos C, et al.: The continued success of registered nurse care coordination in a state evaluation of aging in place in senior housing, *Nurs Outlook* 62:237–246, 2014.
Sambucini A: History and evolution of the nurse life care planning specialty. In Apuna-Grummer D, Howland WA, editors: *A Core Curriculum for Nurse Life Care Planners,* Bloomington, IN, 2013, iUniverse.

Sands JR: Where was care coordination? *CMSA Today* 8:14–17, 2013.
Schraeder C, Shelton PS: *Comprehensive Care Coordination for Chronically Ill Adults,* West Sussex, UK, 2011, John Wiley & Sons.
Schutt RK, Fawcett J, Gall GB, Harrow B, Woodford ML: Case manager satisfaction in public health, *Prof Case Manag* 15:124–134, 2010.
Sebelius K: Report to Congress-Evaluation of the rural PACE provider grant program, 2011. Retrieved from https://www.cms.gov.
Secord LJ: *Private Case Management for Older Persons and Their Families,* Excelsior, MN, 1987, Interstudy.
Sidorov J: TRICARE saves taxpayers millions on chronic illness disease management [Disease Management Care Blog], 2010. Retrieved from http://diseasemanagementcareblog.blogspot.com.
Smith AP: Patient advocacy: roles for nurses and leaders, *Nurs Econ* 22:88–90, 2004.
Stanton MP, Dunkin J: A review of case management functions related to transitions of care at a rural nurse managed clinic, *Prof Case Manag* 14:321–327, 2009.
Stricker P: Collaborative care teams and the benefits of communicating across disciplines, *CMSA Today* 4:20–23, 2013.
Stricker P: Data analytics: a critical tool, *CMSA Today* 4:20–23, 2014.
Tahan HA: Essentials of advocacy in case management: Part 1: Ethical underpinnings of advocacy-theories, principles, and concepts, *Prof Case Manag* 21:163–179, 2016a.
Tahan HA: Essentials of advocacy in case management: Part 2: Client advocacy model and case manager's advocacy strategies and competencies, *Prof Case Manag* 21:217–232, 2016b.
Tahan HM, Treiger TM: *Case Management Society of America (CMSA) Core Curriculum for Case Management,* ed 3, Philadelphia, PA, 2017, Wolters Kluwer.
Taylor P: Comprehensive nursing case management. An advanced practice model, *Nurs Case Manag* 4:2–10, 1999.
The Joint Commission (TJC): 2009 National Patient Safety Goals for Ambulatory Care, Oakbrook Terrace, IL, 2009, TJC.
Thompson LL, Wang J, Gunia BC: Negotiation, *Annu Rev Psychol* 61:491–515, 2010.
Treiger TM: Case management today and its evolution into the future, *CSMA Today* 7:16–20, 2013.
Treiger T, Fink-Samnick E: Collaborate for professional case management: A universal competency based paradigm, Philadelphia, PA, 2016, Wolters Kluwer.
Tufts Managed Care Institute: Demand Management: Introduction and References, 2011. Retrieved from http://jobfunctions.bnet.com.
URAC: Disease Management. Retrieved from https://www.urac.org.
URAC: Transitions of Care-Proven strategies to close care gaps, 2018. Retrieved from http://URAC.org.
U.S. Department of Health and Human Services (USDHHS): Redefining Case Management, Rockville, MD, 2008, USDHHS, HRSA, HIV/AIDS Bureau.
U.S. Department of Health and Human Services (USDHHS): *Healthy People 2020: A Roadmap for Health,* Washington, DC, 2010, U.S. Government Printing Office.
Valiant C, Jensen S: Ethical and legal issues: ten guidelines the professional case manager cannot afford to ignore, *CCMC Issue Brief* 3(4):2012. Retrieved from http://ccmcertification.org.
Van Dijk J: Population health: a foundation for nursing action. 2016 Presentation at the 132nd meeting of the National Advisory Council for Nurse Education and Practice. Rockville, 2016.
Volkema RJ: Problem-Purpose-Expansion: A Technique for Reformulating Problems [unpublished manuscript], Madison, WI, 1983, University of Wisconsin.
Weil M, Karls JM: Historical origins and recent developments. In Weils M, Karls JM, et al., editors: *Case management in Human Service Practice,* San Francisco, 1985, Jossey-Bass.
Wieland D, Kinosian B, Stallard E, Boland R: Does Medicaid pay more to a program of all-inclusive care for the elderly (PACE) than for fee-for-service long term care? *J Gerontol A Biol Sci Med Sci* 68:47–55, 2013.
Winston W, Albright S: *Practical Management Science,* ed 4, Mason, OH, 2012, South-Western.
Wright K, Hazelett S, Jarjoura D, Allen K: The AD-LIFE trial: working to integrate medical and psychosocial care management models, *Home Healthc Nurse* 25:308–314, 2007.
Zander K, Etheredge ML, Bower KA: Nursing Case Management: Blueprints for Transformation, Waban, MA, 1987, Winslow Printing Systems.

26

Working With Families in the Community for Healthy Outcomes

Jacqueline Webb, DNP, FNP-BC, RN

OBJECTIVES

After reading this chapter, the student should be able to do the following:

1. Explain the multiple ways public health nurses work with families and communities.
2. Identify challenges to working with families in the community.
3. Describe family function and structure.
4. Describe family demographic trends and demographic changes that affect the health of families.
5. Compare and contrast three social science theoretical frameworks nurses use when working with the family in the community.
6. Work with families using a strength-based approach to assess, develop, and evaluate family action plans.

CHAPTER OUTLINE

Challenges for Nurses Working With Families in the Community
Family Functions and Structures
Family Demographics
Family Health
Four Approaches to Family Nursing
Theories for Working With Families in the Community
Working With Families for Healthy Outcomes
Social and Family Policy Challenges

KEY TERMS

balanced families, p. 585
bioecological systems theory, p. 587
blended family households, p. 583
capacity building model, p. 590
chronosystems, p. 590
cohabitation, p. 581
dysfunctional families, p. 585
ecomap, p. 593
exosystems, p. 590
family, p. 577
family as a component of society, p. 587
family as a system, p. 587
family as client, p. 587
family as context, p. 585
family cohesion, p. 585
family demographics, p. 580
family developmental and life cycle theory, p. 587
family flexibility, p. 585
family functions, p. 579
family health, p. 585
family health literacy, p. 595
family nursing, p. 576
family nursing theory, p. 587
family policy, p. 598
family structure, p. 579
family systems theory, p. 587
functional health literacy, p. 595
genogram, p. 593
limited services, p. 578
macrosystems, p. 590
mesosystems, p. 590
microsystems, p. 590
social and family policies, p. 598
transitions of care, p. 577
under-insured, p. 577
underserved, p. 578
uninsured, p. 578

Appreciation is given to Dr. Joanna Rowe Kaakinen, who contributed greatly to previous editions of this chapter.

Advances in health care, changes in our health care system and health economics impacting length of hospital stays, distribution of resources, and access to health care are some of the factors contributing to the shift from tertiary health care systems to community and family home care (Kaakinen, 2018a; Salmond & Echevarria, 2017). Factors driving health care transformation into community settings mean many more individuals and their families are now relying on nurses who have knowledge of family structure, function, and process (Kaakinen, 2018a). The health of communities is directly related to the health of its families (American Nurses Association [ANA], 2013; American Public Health Association [APHA], 2013; Eddy et al., 2018). Nurses working in community settings are ideally positioned for this role, as nursing has consistently embraced an approach to care that is holistic, inclusive of patients, families, and communities, and oriented toward empowering patients in their care to assume responsibility for self-care and disease management (ANA, 2013; George & Shocksnider, 2014; Salmond & Echevarria, 2017).

The importance of establishing collaborative relationships with families for providing care has been well documented in public health nursing literature (Jonsdottir et al., 2003; Paavilainen & Astedt-Kurki, 1997; Porr et al., 2012; Wald, 1915; Wu et al., 2017). Public health nurses must have skills to move competently between working with individual families, bridge relationships between families and the community, advocate for family and community legislation, and influence policies that promote and protect the health of populations. Therefore, public health nurses must integrate knowledge and practice of family nursing and community health nursing (APHA, 2013) in meeting the needs of families.

Family nursing is a philosophy and a science that is based on the following assumptions: health and illness are family events; what affects one family member affects the whole family; and health care practices, decisions, and behaviors are made within the context of the family (Kaakinen, 2018a). Currently there is no universal agreement as to how to define a family. For example, the U.S. Census Bureau since 1930 defines *family* as two or more people living together who are related by birth, marriage, or adoption (Pemberton, 2015; U.S. Census Bureau, 2015). Often definitions of family differ by disciplines and definition of what constitutes a family.

Public health nursing practice has a secondary focus: the "synthesis of nursing theory and public health theory applied to promoting, preserving and maintaining the health of populations through the delivery of personal health care services to individuals, families, and groups. The focus of practice is the health of individuals, families and groups and the effect of their health status on the health of the community as a whole" (p. XXX).

Nurses practicing in the community use the core competencies for public health professionals (Public Health Foundation [PHF], 2014) and the core public health functions of assessment, assurance, and policy development to promote the interconnectedness of individual health with the health of families and communities (Eddy et al., 2018). The Linking Content to Practice box shows the applications of public health nursing practice from a family perspective. The *Healthy People 2020* box highlights four new objectives that have been identified as leading health issues that address ways to improve the health of families and the nation. Nurses who practice with a family nursing philosophy and theory base will improve the health of families, their members, and the community. *Note:* U.S. Department of Health and Human Services (USDHHS) planning is now under way for *Healthy People 2030.* Check out the development and objectives of *Healthy People 2030* at https://www.healthypeople.gov.

LINKING CONTENT TO PRACTICE

In this chapter the public health core functions with the essential services below are applied to family nursing.

Assessment
- Monitor health status of families to identify community health problems.
- Diagnose and investigate health problems and health hazards in the community that affect families.
- Evaluate effectiveness, accessibility, and quality of personal and population-based health services.

Policy Development
- Develop policies and plans that support family and community health efforts.
- Enforce laws and regulations that protect health and ensure safety of families in the community.
- Research for new insights and innovative solutions to health problems.

Assurance
- Link people to needed personal health services and assure the provision of health care when otherwise unavailable.
- Assure a competent public health and personal health care workforce.
- Inform, educate, and empower family members about health issues
- Mobilize community partnerships to identify and solve health problems.

HEALTHY PEOPLE 2020

Objectives specific to families and family nursing that relate to a leading health issue:
- **AHS 1:** Increase the proportion of persons with health insurance.
- **AH-5-1:** Increase the proportion of students who graduate with a regular diploma four years after starting the ninth grade.
- **DIA-1:** Increase the proportion of adults aged 65 years and older with diagnosed Alzheimer's disease and other dementias, or their caregiver, who are aware of the diagnosis.
- **D-5:** Improve glycemic control among persons with diabetes, especially those with A1C greater than nine percent.
- **NWS-9 & 10:** Reduce the proportion of adults and children who are obese.
- **PREP-5.1:** Increase the percent of school districts that required schools to include family reunification plans.

From: U.S. Department of Health and Human Services, Office of Disease Prevention and Health Promotion: *2020 Topics and objectives,* 2010. Available at https://www.healthypeople.gov. Accessed on July 11, 2018.

CHALLENGES FOR NURSES WORKING WITH FAMILIES IN THE COMMUNITY

Numerous challenges exist that affect the practice of family nursing in a community setting. Many of the following challenges have been recognized in the family nursing literature for a long time, yet they persist in the current health care system. One role for the nurse would be to advocate that the following challenges be addressed in federal and state health care policies and programs.

Definition of Family

As more health care organizations move toward patient-centered care, family involvement becomes an essential component for providing compassionate and inclusive care (Barnsteiner & Disch, 2018). Traditional definitions of family are being challenged with social changes such as the increase in the number of families headed by single mothers, an increase in cohabitation, and the legalization of same-sex marriages (Cohen, 2018; U.S. Census Bureau, 2017a) There is still no universally agreed on definition of family (Kaakinen, 2018a).

Public health nurses and family nurses struggle on a daily basis with the conflict between the narrow traditional legal definition of family used in the health care system and by social policy makers and the broader term used by the family. Family, as defined and implemented in the health care system, continues to be based on the legal notions of relationships such as biological/genetic blood ties and contractual relationships such as adoption, guardianship, or marriage. However, the family system and family nurses use the following broader definition of family: "Family refers to two or more individuals who depend on one another for emotional, physical, and/or financial support. The members of the family are self-defined" (Hanson, 2005, p. 8).

Many policies related to families assume legal marriage and that children will be raised by married-couple families. For example, Social Security benefits are based on earnings of a spouse to determine retirement security for the living survivor. According to the U.S. Census Bureau, 4 million out of about 12 million single-parent families have children under the age of 18, and more than 80 percent are headed by single mothers (Cohen, 2018). Given the current social and political climate, nurses need to adopt the open definition described earlier because the families they work with have a wide variety of family structures. Nurses who work with the people in the individual's everyday world have a higher likelihood of helping them to achieve better health outcomes.

Transitions of Care

Nurses have a pivotal role relative to communication of information in transitions of care between agencies that frequently result in hospital admission or readmission. Hospital readmission rates have been declining among Medicare patients from home health settings (Agency for Healthcare Research and Quality [AHRQ], 2016). Specifically home health rehospitalization rates for Medicare patients decreased from 19.17 percent in 2011 to 17.39 percent in 2012 and to 16.92 percent by 2013. The increased emphasis on better coordination of care and home health care are viewed as being a part of the solution to readmissions (AHRQ, 2016; Liepelt, 2015). However, overall hospital readmission rates are still high, and it is estimated that about 20 percent of individuals discharged from a hospital in the United States are readmitted within 30 days (Kripalani et al., 2014). Of the estimated $26 billion in Medicare spending on readmissions, about $17 billion is potentially preventable (Center for Health Information and Analysis, 2015). Individuals most at risk for readmissions are males over 75 years of age, African American, hospitalized with a medical diagnosis, and without insurance other than Medicare (Felix et al., 2015). Studies also suggest that primary drivers of variability in 30-day readmission rates are related to the available resources in the community and the composition of a hospital's patient population (Joynt & Jha, 2012).

There are communication issues between health care providers within the community agencies, such as incomplete or missing documentation, that result from rushed assessments. Rushed procedures and failure to follow the plan of action and standards of care are known causes of hospital readmissions (Kripalani et al., 2014). Studies analyzing claims data found that the highest 30-day readmission rates were observed among patients with diagnoses such as congestive heart failure, schizophrenia/psychoses, and recent vascular surgery (U.S. Department of Health and Human Services [USDHHS], 2010; Kripalani et al., 2014). Persons at high risk for readmission rates parallel those of the population with low health literacy rates (Bailey et al., 2015; Cloonan et al., 2013).

About 35 percent of adults in the United States have limited literacy skills. In the United States literacy rates have not changed much in the past 10 years, even with an additional 30 million adults who have below basic literacy skills (Berkman et al., 2011). A systematic review of the literature indicated that low health literacy was associated with increased health care use, inappropriate drug use, low use of preventive services, and overall poorer health (Berkman et al., 2011). It is crucial that home health care staff have current updates on evidence-based practice, standards of care, and interventions to ensure quality health outcomes. Nurses practicing in the community have a significant role in working with multiple health care systems to improve communication and evidence-based design protocols as well as becoming familiar with community resources to improve the quality of care and the health of the home health population (Joynt & Jha, 2012). When health literacy concerns are added to the primary drivers of hospital readmission rates such as mental health, poor social support, and poverty the value of community nursing becomes apparent (Joynt & Jha, 2012). Nurses can assess the many variables affecting individuals and their families and develop patient-centered management plans that contribute to a better patient outcome.

Nurses must develop and refine excellent negotiation skills because they spend a significant amount of time arranging for limited services for their under-insured and uninsured clients and families. In working with families, communication and teaching will be more effective if hours of service match the times of day when family members, specifically the family care provider, can attend appointments. Bringing a companion to office visits benefits communication (Wolff et al., 2009; Wolff et al., 2018), especially for those with low health literacy and cognition difficulties (Rosland et al., 2011); enhances shared decision making (Zwijnenberg et al., 2012); and improves the sharing of information (Eggly et al., 2006). Involving the family in the care of the client improves self-management of health care, results in fewer medication errors (Kinnersley et al., 2007; Wolff et al., 2009), and improves health outcomes (Grady & Gough, 2014). Based on this information about companion participation, it is crucial that nurses involve the family as much as possible in their interactions and decisions with clients.

Uninsured, Underinsured, and Limited Services

Nursing practice in the community presents various challenges such as knowing how to access health care resources for clients and understanding how recent health care reforms are transforming the landscape of our current health care system. **Uninsured** clients are those who do not have health insurance for any family member. **Underserved** are individuals who have minimal insurance coverage and usually have a high deductible. Individuals with **limited services** are people who may have trouble accessing health care and/or experience barriers to health care. For example, a family with insurance coverage may live in a rural area that does not have a primary health care provider or services near them. The main goals of the Affordable Care Act (ACA) of 2010 were to provide U.S. citizens with patient protection and affordable health care, and decrease the overall cost of health care (see Chapter 3 for more discussion of health care systems). The ACA is designed to offer premium subsidies to help eligible individuals and their families purchase insurance coverage when affordable employer-sponsored insurance is not available. Questions remain about how this affordability protection will be applied in situations where self-only coverage offered by an employer is affordable but family coverage is not.

The U.S. Supreme Court ruled that the ACA Medicaid expansion is a voluntary program for states. As a result, not all states have expanded Medicaid coverage. What this means for persons living in states that have expanded Medicaid coverage is that they qualify for either Medicaid or reduced costs on a private insurance plan if they earn up to $16,753 a year for one person or $28,676 for a family of three (CMS, 2018). According to a review of CMS policies by the Kaiser Family Foundation since January 2018, 49 states cover children with family incomes up to at least 200 percent of the federal poverty level (Brooks et al., 2018). However, only 34 states cover pregnant women with incomes at or above 200 percent of the federal poverty level, and only 16 states extend partial and/or full coverage for pregnant women regardless of immigration status. According to the U.S. Department of Health and Human Services, since the ACA was enacted in 2010 an estimated 20 million people have become newly insured and 24 million people have gained access to subsidized or free care through tax credits and Medicaid expansion (Eibner & Nowak, 2016). Most uninsured people are low-income families and have at least one worker in the family (Kaiser Family Foundation [KFF], 2018). Undocumented immigrants, who are prohibited from enrolling in Medicaid and purchasing coverage through the new health insurance exchanges, are projected to constitute 25 percent of the uninsured after the major provisions of the ACA are fully implemented (USDHHS, 2012). A Kaiser Family Foundation review of health coverage found that in 2016, 25 percent of uninsured nonelderly lawfully present immigrants were eligible for Medicaid, and 43 percent were eligible for various state-sponsored tax credit subsidies. Many uninsured lawfully present immigrants are eligible but not enrolled in coverage because they may face a range of enrollment barriers, including fear, confusion about eligibility policies, difficulty navigating the enrollment process, and language and literacy challenges (Brooks et al., 2018). Community nursing requires understanding the challenges of the population nurses are serving. Nurses must be adept at working among health care systems to find resources and services for the large population of uninsured clients and families. Over 27 million people in the United States remained uninsured in 2016 and of these 45 percent of the adults said that they remained uninsured because the cost of coverage was too high. Hispanic and African Americans have higher uninsured rates (16.9 percent and 11.7 percent, respectively) than whites (7.6 percent) (Kaiser Family Foundation, 2018). The uninsured rate among children under the age of 18 was 5 percent, which is a significant decrease from 9.8 percent in 2010 (Kaiser Family Foundation, 2018). Since the enactment of the 2010 Affordable Care Act, children can now remain on their parents' insurance plans until the age of 26.

Employer-sponsored insurance continues to be the largest source of health insurance coverage, with 66 percent of nonelderly workers of the U.S. population covered (Long et al., 2016). The demand for primary care will be driven over the next decade and a half not only by the ACA mandates, but also by an aging population and an overall growth in the size of the U.S. population. This growth in demand also accompanies a shift from acute care services to more chronic care management as the nation's disease patterns change as the population ages (Ariosto et al., 2018). Various studies projecting current or imminent shortages in primary care providers are shifting attention away from the traditional physician model of care to nurse practitioners, who now account for about 19 percent of the U.S. primary care workforce, and physician assistants, who account for 7 percent of the U.S. workforce (Green et al., 2013; Spetz & Muench, 2018). Nurse practitioners and physician assistants not only provide effective care but they can also meet the growing demands for primary care providers (Spetz & Muench, 2018).

The lack of insurance makes finding adequate services for clients and families difficult. In some areas federal and state funding for care in health clinics is free or available for a minimal fee. However, because the number of primary health care clinics is limited, care is often provided based on the number of volunteer health care providers working that day in the clinic. Many clinics are program based, such as family planning clinics, sexually transmitted disease (STD) clinics, and immunizations clinics. Thus, it is difficult to meet the needs of the uninsured or underinsured populations.

Nurses need to understand the effects of the ACA reforms and how they are being implemented in their states. Nurses help clients and families negotiate and maneuver through the health care system. They must work closely with the family to remove barriers and provide services and resources that enhance the families' abilities to provide quality care to family members. To successfully address these challenges, community health nurses must integrate principles of family nursing with those of community/public health (see Evidence-Based Practice and Levels of Prevention boxes).

EVIDENCE-BASED PRACTICE

A systematic review of various programs targeting parents to manage childhood obesity found including the family is an important strategy, which demonstrates improvement in child body mass index (BMI) (Jang et al., 2015). Reducing obesity in the United States is a *Healthy People 2020* objective. A study by the Centers for Disease Control and Prevention (2013) found a 43 percent drop in obesity rates among children two to five years of age over a 10-year period. Part of this decline is directly related to the change in the social policy of improvements in the food packages available to these parents through the Women, Infants, and Children (WIC) Program. The improvements include adding healthy items like fruits and vegetables and whole grain foods while reducing the amount of fruit juice and whole milk. This change, coupled with nutrition education for families with infants and young children led to parents selecting healthier food choices and improved access to healthy foods for at risk families. Physical activity plays an important role in helping children maintain a healthy weight yet nearly half (47 percent) of children in the United States are not exercising regularly (Annie B. Casey Foundation, 2018).

Nurse Use

Nurses have a significant role in advocating for social policies that improve the health of families and educating parents of young children to make healthy food choices. Public health nurses should be actively involved in helping to decrease childhood obesity. Refer to the Levels of Prevention box for reducing childhood obesity.

Data from Centers for Disease Control and Prevention: *Vital signs: obesity among low income, preschool aged children—United States, 2008–2011*, 2013. Available at https://www.cdc.gov. Accessed September 2, 2018.

LEVELS OF PREVENTION

Reduce the proportion of children and adolescents aged 2-19 years who are considered obese (*Healthy People 2020* objective NWS 10.4).

Primary Prevention

- Educate parents about healthy nutritional choices for young children and the risks associated with obesity.
- Provide counseling and weight management for overweight children and teens.
- Help mothers who qualify for the Women, Infants, and Children Program complete the extensive paperwork.

Secondary Prevention

- Screen teens for obesity with body mass index (BMI) greater than or equal to 30.
- Analyze children's height and weight growth as part of annual health assessments.

Tertiary Prevention

- Work with schools to improve quality of food offered in school lunch.
- Help communities establish local farm to school networks, create school gardens, and ensure that more local foods are used in the school setting.

FAMILY FUNCTIONS AND STRUCTURES

Knowledge of **family functions** and structures is essential for understanding how families influence health, illness, and well-being. Nurses who understand family functions and structures can use this knowledge to empower families through evidence-based interventions.

Family functions are the ways in which families meet the needs of (1) each family member, (2) the family as a whole, and (3) their relationship to society. Throughout history, the following functions have been performed by families (Kaakinen, 2018a):

1. *Economic function:* Family income is a substantial part of family economics, but it is also related to family consumerism, money management, housing decisions, insurance choices, retirement, and savings. Family economics affect and reflect the nation's economy.
2. *Reproductive function:* The survival of a society is linked to patterns and rates of reproduction. The family has been the traditional structure in which reproduction was organized. Today, the reproductive function of family has become more separated from traditional family structure as more children are born outside of marriage and into nontraditional family structures.
3. *Socialization function:* A major expectation of families is that they are responsible for raising their children to fit into society and take their place in the adult world. In addition, families disseminate their culture, including religious faith and spirituality.
4. *Affective function:* Families provide boundaries and structure that provide a sense of belonging and identity of who the family members are individually and to their family. The purpose of the affective function is to learn about intimate reciprocal caring relationships, to learn about dependency and how to nurture future generations.
5. *Health care function:* It is in the family that one learns the concepts of health, health promotion, health maintenance, disease prevention, and illness management. Family members provide informal caregiving to ill family members and are primary sources of support.

Family structure refers to the characteristics and demographics (e.g., sex, age, number) of individual members who make up family units. More specifically, the structure of a family defines the roles and the positions of family members (Box 26.1).

Family structures have changed over time to meet the needs of the family and society. The great speed at which changes in family structure, values, and relationships are occurring makes working with families at the beginning of the twenty-first century exciting and challenging. According to Kaakinen (2018a), the following aspects need to be addressed when determining the family structure:

1. The individuals that compose the family
2. The relationships between them
3. The interactions between the family members
4. The interactions with other social systems

As social norms have become more tolerant of a range of choices in relation to managing one's life, there is no longer a

BOX 26.1 Family and Household Structures

Married Family
- Traditional nuclear family
- Dual-career family
- Spouses reside in same household
- Commuter marriage
- Husband/father away from family
- Stepfamily
- Stepmother family
- Stepfather family
- Adoptive family
- Foster family
- Voluntary childlessness

Single-Parent Family
- Never married
- Voluntary singlehood (with children, biological or adopted)
- Involuntary singlehood (with children)
- Formerly married
- Widowed (with children)
- Divorced (with children)
- Custodial parent
- Joint custody of children
- Binuclear family

Multi-Adult Household (With or Without Children)
- Cohabitating couple
- Communes
- Affiliated family
- Extended family
- Newly extended family
- Home-sharing individuals
- Same-sex partners

general consensus that the traditional nuclear family model, consisting of father, mother, and children, is the "best" model. There is no "typical" family model or family structure. For example, the single-mother household may be represented by the unmarried teenage mother with an infant (unplanned pregnancy), the divorced mother with one or more children, or the career-oriented woman in her late 30s who elects to have a baby and remain single.

The family structure changes and modifies over time. An individual may participate in a number of family life experiences over a lifetime (Fig. 26.1). For example, a child may spend the early, formative years in the family of origin (mother, father, siblings); experience some years in a single-parent family because of divorce; and participate in a stepfamily relationship when the single parent who has custody remarries.

This same child as an adult may experience several additional family types: cohabitation while completing a desired education, and then a commuter marriage while developing a career. As an adult, the individual may divorce and become a custodial parent. The adult may eventually cohabitate with another partner and finally marry a different partner who also has children. As couples age, they have to address issues of the aging family, and subsequently the woman may become an older single widow. Thus, nurses work with various families representing different structures and living arrangements.

Prospects for families in the twenty-first century are numerous. New family structures that are currently experimental will emerge as everyday "natural" families (e.g., families in which the members are not related by blood or marriage, but who provide the services, caring, love, intimacy, and interaction needed by all persons to experience a quality life).

At times it is helpful to understand families through a narrow framework of family function and structure. However, a family is a system within itself as well as the basic unit of a society. Some would argue that the traditional concept of family is disintegrating based on how the structure and functions of the family have changed over time. On the other side of that debate, families change in response to the societal changes and are ever evolving and thriving as they seek different ways of interconnectedness (Kaakinen, 2018a).

FAMILY DEMOGRAPHICS

Historically, **family demographics** can be analyzed by looking at data about the families and household structures and

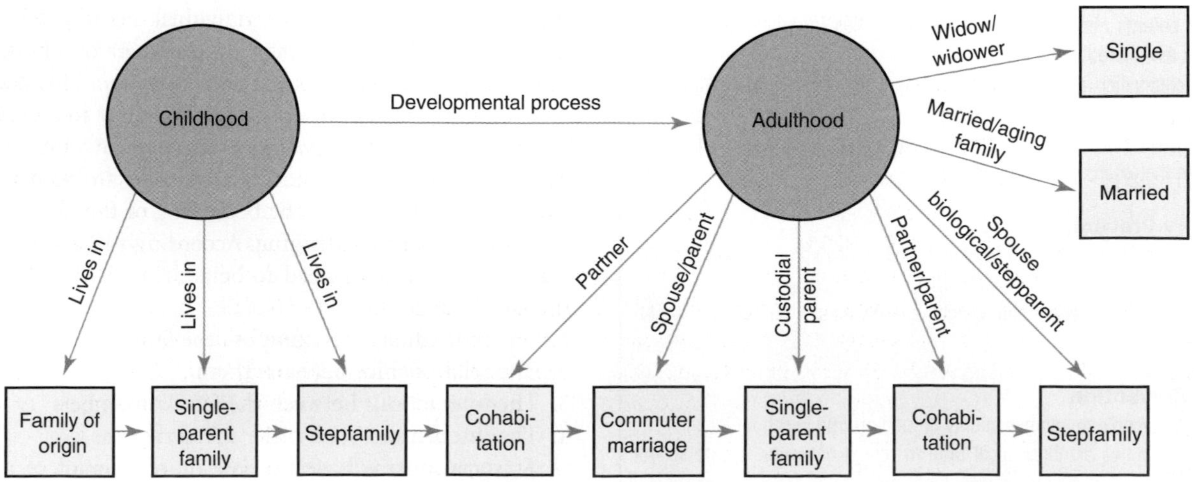

Fig. 26.1 An individual's family life structure over time.

the events that alter these structures. Recent trends in family demographics show that there has been a quieting of the rapid changes that were found in family structure and living arrangements in the twenty-first century. Nurses draw on family demographic data to forecast and predict family community needs, such as family developmental changes, stresses, and ethnic issues affecting family health, as they formulate possible solutions to identified family community problems. In this chapter, major family demographic trends valuable to nurses practicing in the community are presented. The development of ancestry DNA testing has also brought changes in how we perceive our racial identity and our family structure. Although our ancestral differences reflect only about a 0.1 percent difference, DNA studies demonstrate we often cling to those differences (Foeman et al., 2014).

Living Arrangements

The number of households in the United States has more than tripled from 35 million households in 1940 to 126 million households in 2017 (U.S. Census Bureau, 2017b). Of these 126 million households, 65 percent were considered family households and the remaining 35 percent being nonfamily households (U.S. Census Bureau, 2017a). Family households include a householder and at least one other member related by birth, marriage, or adoption, whereas a nonfamily household is either a person living alone or a householder who shares the house only with nonrelatives, such as boarders or roommates (U.S. Census Bureau, 2015).

The fastest growth was among persons living alone, with much of this growth occurring during the 1960s and 1970s. The proportion of households with just one person more than doubled from 13 percent to 27 percent between 1960 and 2017 (U.S. Census Bureau, 2017b).

Family demographic trends have continued in the direction of fewer married couples with children households. Two-parent households are on the decline in the United States as divorce, remarriage, and cohabitation rise. Families are smaller now, both due to the growth of single parent households and the drop in fertility. From 2009 to 2017 no change was noted in the number of married couples with children. This number has remained steady at about 23 million compared to 30 million in 1980 (Pew Research Center, 2015; U.S. Census Bureau, 2017b).

Americans are living longer. According to the Centers for Disease Control and Prevention (CDC) between 1975 and 2015, life expectancy at birth increased from 72.6 to 78.8 years for the total U.S. population. For males, life expectancy increased from 68.8 years in 1975 to 76.3 years in 2015, and for females, life expectancy increased from 76.6 years in 1975 to 81.2 years in 2015 (CDC, 2016a). From 1975 to 2015 the number of Americans 65 years of age and older doubled from 22.6 million to 47.8 million. Women have experienced the most rapid growth in the 85 and over age group. It is projected that by 2030 one in five Americans will be 65 years or older (CDC, 2016b). Among adults ages 18-64 and 65 and over, women have a higher percent living below 200 percent of poverty level compared to men. See also National Center for Health Statistics (2017) for demographics of the population in the United States.

The likelihood of living alone has grown since 1990 for older men and for women ages 85 and older. Women continue to make up the majority of adults living alone but their rates have fallen significantly (Stepler, 2016). In 1990 women made up nearly 79 percent of older adults living alone and by 2014 this number had dropped to 32 percent. Women are more likely to live with their spouse or their children. The percent of men living alone has increased from15 percent in 1990 to 18 percent in 2014 (Stepler, 2016). Older men ages 65 to 84 are less likely to live with a spouse. A Pew Research Center survey found that adults living alone have more financial difficulties and have less frequent contact with their children and grandchildren than adults who live with others (Stepler, 2016). Living alone can mean delays in getting attention for illness or injury and can complicate arrangements for informal care or transportation to formal care when needed. What this means is that elderly individuals are more likely to access and need community-based services. In addition, with the geographic mobility of American society, many of these elderly do not live close to family; therefore they do not have as many family members to care for them. Despite the trend toward independent living among older Americans, many of them are not able to live alone without assistance.

Marriage, Divorce, and Cohabitation

Marriage, although still a popular American ideal, has assumed a forerunner: cohabitation. **Cohabitation** is a couple living together who are having a sexual relationship without being married. This delay in marriage has implications for the delay in child birthing. The number of divorces has leveled off and remained constant.

Rates for divorce have decreased since 2001, when there were 4.0 divorces per 1000 total population, to the 2016 rate of 3.2 divorces per 1000 total population (CDC, 2016c). However, the divorce rates among married people 50 years or older doubled between 1990 and 2010 with one in four divorces in 2010 being people over 50 years of age (Stepler, 2016). As cohabitation has become more acceptable, fewer divorced people are getting remarried, and the remarriage rate has dropped especially for those younger than 35 years (Livingston, 2018a). However, in the 55-64 adult category the trend is increasing with about 67 percent remarrying, up from 55 percent in 1960 (Livingston, 2018a). According to the U.S. Census Bureau about 18 million U.S. adults were cohabitating in 2016. This is about a 29 percent increase since 2007 (U.S. Census Bureau, 2017b). It is estimated that there are about 1.2 million adults living in a same-sex domestic partnership and about 390,000 married same-sex couples in the country (Schwarz, 2015).

Attitudes related to marriage, cohabitation, and divorce have changed in the last four decades. The 2011-2013 National Survey of Family Growth (NSFG) found 60 percent of women and 67 percent of men agreed that living together before marriage may help prevent divorce. In the 2011-2013 NSFG survey 78.3 percent of women and 69.2 percent of men agreed it was okay for an unmarried female to have and raise a child outside of marriage compared to the 2002 survey when 69.5 percent of women and 58.8 percent of men agreed. The same survey found that since 2002 there has been an increase in both men and women agreeing gay or lesbian adults have the right to adopt children (CDC, 2016d).

Casper and Coritz (2018) suggest the increased uncertainty and stability of marriage, increased social acceptance of people living together, and economic changes all contribute to the increase in cohabitation. More than 67 percent of couples that married in 2012 had lived together in cohabitation prior to their marriage (Daugherty & Copen, 2016). Different factors were associated with duration of marriage and cohabitation. Duration of marriage was associated with two factors: age of first marriage and timing of first child. Marriage at a younger age had a lower probability of the marriage lasting 10 years. Women who gave birth 8 months or more after the marriage began compared with women who had no first birth during the marriage had a 79 percent chance versus a 34 percent chance of the marriage lasting 10 years. Education was a factor in both men's and women's duration of cohabitation, with lower education being associated with longer cohabitation (Goodwin et al., 2010).

As cohabitation increases, ensuring STD reduction and family planning services becomes essential. The most frequently reported infectious disease in the United States is chlamydia (CDC, 2017). In 2016 more than 1.59 million cases of chlamydia were reported. Women between the ages of 15 and 19 years of age and minority women are at the highest risk (CDC, 2017). Untreated chlamydia can cause severe and costly reproductive health problems. A model collaborative program is Get Yourself Tested (GYT) launched in 2009 to reduce stigma and promote STD communication and testing. GYT is a partnership program between MTV, the Kaiser Family Foundation, and Planned Parenthood Federation of America. Evaluation of the program that used social media and outreach events demonstrated an increase in STD testing especially among youth aged 15-24 years of age (Friedman et al., 2014).

Effects of Cohabitation on Children. Cohabitating couples in the United States live together for shorter periods of time than cohabiting couples in other countries (Cherlin, 2010). Parental separation is five times greater for children born to cohabiting parents than to married parents (Brown, 2010). The unstable living arrangements for children born outside of marriage remains an important question relative to the well-being of these children. The number of transitions is associated with negative child well-being (Osborne & McLanahan, 2007). Many of these children experience about three transition relationships from birth to three years of age (Osborne & McLanahan, 2007). The research shows that children in cohabitating relationships have more behavioral and cognitive problems (Ray, 2013).

Fully one fourth (26 percent) of children younger than age 18 are now living with a single parent, up from just 9 percent in 1960 and 22 percent in 2000. Some 15 percent are living with parents in a remarriage and 7 percent are living with parents who are cohabiting. About 5 percent of children are living without either parent, and most of these children are being raised by grandparents (Pew Research Center, 2015). The majority of white, Hispanic, and Asian children are living in two-parent households, while less than half of African American children are living in this type of arrangement (Pew Research Center, 2015).

Mothers living in the United States today are also far better educated than they were in the past. While in 1960 just 18 percent of mothers with infants at home had any college experience, today that number is at 67 percent. Research by the Pew Research Center has found that this increase in college experience is partly due to more women graduating from high school and having greater opportunities to continue their education. While about half (49 percent) of women ages 15 to 44 in 1960 lacked a high school diploma, today the largest share of women (61 percent) has at least some college experience, and just 19 percent lack a high school diploma. However the majority of mothers (55 percent) ages 40-44 who lack a high school diploma have had three or more children compared to 38 percent of mothers of similar age who have completed high school (Pew Research Center, 2015).

The poverty rate for single-mother families in 2016 was 35.6 percent, nearly five times more than the rate (6.6 percent) for married-couple families. One third (31.6 percent) of single-mother families were "food insecure" while one seventh (13 percent) used food pantries; one third spent more than half their income on housing, which is generally considered the threshold for "severe housing cost burden" (Lee, 2018; U.S. Census Bureau, 2017a).

Nurses working with various family structures must be familiar with the challenges of growing up in single-parent homes and become familiar with community resources available to assist and enrich the lives of all family members.

Births

Replacement-level fertility refers to the required number of children each woman in the population would have to bear on average to replace herself and her partner, and it is conventionally set at 2.1 children per woman for countries with low mortality rates (Casper & Coritz, 2018). The fertility rate in the United States has been in continual decline over the last century, with occasional boosts, such as the baby boom after World War II in the late 1940s and early 1950s. In 2017 the USDHHS division of vital statistics reported births in the United States were down two percent from 2016 rates, and the lowest in nearly 30 years (Hamilton et al., 2018). When looking at the various age groups the report found, although birth rates had declined for nearly all age groups, women over the age of 40 had increased by two percent since 2016. Almost 30 percent of foreign-born women giving birth are ages 35 or older. Researchers found women from Vietnam, the Philippines, China, and India have some of the highest rates of women giving births ages 35 or older. Researchers also found that low birth weight among African American and Hispanic births have increased and have remained unchanged for white women (Hamilton et al., 2018).

Community nurses working with vulnerable populations must become familiar with prenatal resources in their communities. There are greater health risks for older women becoming pregnant after the age of 40 and having low-birth-weight babies.

Low-birth-weight babies may have serious health problems that may impact the entire family. Health risks such as gestational diabetes, preterm births, emergency cesarean delivery as well as risk of maternal mortality increases with maternal age, impacting family members.

Compared with U.S.-born women, birth rates for foreign-born women are higher. Fertility rates differ by race and ethnicity. Hispanic women have the highest fertility rates at 2.3, followed by African American women at 2.0, and Asian women have the lowest fertility rate at 1.84 (Belluz, 2018; Casper & Coritz, 2018). Not all cultures value limiting the number of children in a family, and nurses may be challenged to understand these values and provide services where the woman assumes the value of limiting the number of children while the husband and or partner does not. For example, a Hispanic woman comes to the public health clinic for family planning services. It is not uncommon for the husband to come in at the end of the week to pay for those services. If the wife is on birth control, such as Depo, but does not want her husband to know, itemizing services on the receipt would present a problem. The nurse needs to understand these changing values and facilitate the family planning services requested by the woman without violating her confidentiality.

Since 2008 the number of births outside of marriage has remained constant for U.S.-born women but has been decreasing for foreign-born women. The overall number of births outside of marriage in the United States is about 40 percent (Livingston, 2018a). Births outside of marriage for U.S.-born women have remained constant at about 42 percent compared to 33 percent for foreign-born women. Women from Latin America have the highest rate of births outside of marriage. As women are delaying marriage, so too are they older at the birth of their first child. In 2014, the average age at first birth was 26.3 (Hamilton et al., 2018). This means that nurses will likely have older mothers who are at risk of having more complications with pregnancy and birth. The birth rate for teenagers has decreased substantially, but the United States still has one of the highest rates of teenage pregnancies in the industrialized world. The birth rate for teenagers aged 15-19 in 2017 was 18.8 births per 1000, which has declined by 55 percent since 2007, when the rate was 41.5 per 1000 births for this age group (Hamilton et al., 2018).

Parenting

Even with divorce and cohabitation, postponement of marriage, and decline in childbearing, most North American adults have children, and most children live with two parents. The majority of Americans do marry with close to 50 percent of adults marrying in 2016. Although this number has remained relatively stable in recent years, it is down nine percentage points over the past quarter century (U.S. Census Bureau, 2017a). Factors driving this change are that Americans—particularly men—are staying single longer, cohabitation rates have increased, and a delay in the age of first marriage (Daugherty & Copen, 2016). According to the U.S. Census Bureau, in 2017, the median age at first marriage had reached its highest point on record: 29.5 years for men and 27.4 years for women (Geiger & Livingston, 2018).

Blended family households are when two people marry and at least one of these individuals brings a child with them into the marriage (American Psychological Association [APA], 2018). Today more than half of all marriages are remarriages. About 62 percent of children are living with two married parents, and about 15 percent are living with parents in a remarriage and an additional 7 percent are living with parents in a cohabitating relationship (Pew Research Center, 2016). Research suggests members who may have the most difficult time adjusting to a blended family are adolescents 10 to 14 years of age (APA, 2018). Because the blended family makes up a significant proportion of families with children, nurses are likely to interact with parents and children whose roles and responsibilities are not well defined. Obtaining legal authorization can be challenging when legal obligations are unclear; therefore it is important that nurses identify which parent(s) have legal responsibility for medical decision making. It is also important for nurses to be aware that they may also need to notify nonresidential parents when their children require medical attention because these parents may share the legal right to make medical decisions.

Single mothers, never married, are particularly disadvantaged; they are younger, less well educated, and less often employed than are divorced single mothers and married mothers (Casper & Coritz, 2018). Mothers who never married (26 percent) are much less likely to get child support from the father than are mothers who are divorced or separated (46 percent) (Casper & Coritz, 2018). Divorced mothers are substantially better educated and more often employed than are mothers who are separated or who never married. However, the average income of families headed by divorced mothers is less than half that of two-parent families (Casper & Coritz, 2018). Increases in cohabitating parents are changing the profile of unmarried parents. Most recently a Pew Research Center analysis of Census Bureau data reports 35 percent of unmarried parents are living with a partner. Single parents are also more likely to live with one of their own parents. It is estimated that about 23 percent of single parents share a household with one of their own parents (Livingston, 2018b).

The National Center for Children in Poverty (NCCP) estimates that about 15 million children in the United States or 21 percent of all children are living in poverty with family incomes below the federal poverty threshold (NCCP, 2017). Most of these children are living with parents who work but have jobs with low-paying wages and unstable employment. Poverty not only contributes to poor health and mental health outcomes but also to lower educational opportunities. Families need an income equal to about two times the federal poverty threshold to meet their basic needs. A family of two with one child earning $33,086 annually is living at poverty-level income according to 2016 federal poverty thresholds (NCCP, 2017). Nurses working with various populations need to be able to identify high-risk families living at poverty thresholds. Children living with immigrant parents have the highest risk of living in poverty. African American, American Indian, and Hispanic children have the highest risk of living in low- to poverty-income families.

The slow but steady increase in the number of single-father households is one changing aspect of family life in America. The number of unmarried parents who are single fathers has more than doubled over the past 50 years. Rates of single fathers who reside with their children have increased to 29 percent from 12 percent in 1968 (Livingston, 2018b). Fathers who are divorced are more likely to share child custody than in the past; however, that does not mean that there are fewer obstacles in such complicated family arrangements (Carlson & McLanahan, 2010). In general, fathers are spending more time with their children and are more involved with housework than in the past (Casper & Coritz, 2018).

Many children are raised by or receive regular care from their grandparents. These grandparents may or may not have legal responsibility for their grandchildren, but may seek medical care for them. In 2011, about 7.7 million children lived in a home with a grandparent (Desilver, 2013). Of these children 80 percent had at least one parent also living in the same household. However, three million of these children had their grandparent as their primary caregiver and provider (Desilver, 2013). Although there are many rewards for both the grandparent and grandchild, taking care of children at such an "off family" time creates stress and can be very difficult.

Immigration

It is estimated that in 2015 there were about 43.2 million residents born outside of the country (López & Radford, 2017). Because immigrants tend to arrive in the United States early in their working careers, they are younger, on average, than the overall U.S. population and account for a larger share of young families (Casper & Coritz, 2018). It has been estimated that in 2014 about 32 percent of all births in the United States were to mothers born outside of the country (Livingston, 2018a). Over half of these women had lived in the United States an average of 11 years, with only nine percent having recently immigrated to the United States within the preceding two years (Livingston, 2018a). Most likely to be recent immigrants were new mothers from the Middle East and North Africa. While births to Mexican-born mothers have declined, they still account for about 32 percent of all U.S. births to foreign-born mothers. These statistics help nurses understand the importance of having a solid understanding of culture and health beliefs because they are essential components of practice with families. Nurses need to become familiar with some of the differences between foreign-born and U.S.-born mothers. For example foreign-born new mothers tend to be older and have lower levels of education and many have little experience in the workforce. These factors contribute to having lower annual family incomes and higher rates of poverty (Livingston, 2018a). Understanding demographic differences may also help nurses evaluate age appropriate resources. Mothers born in Latin America tend to be younger, also less educated; however, they also tend to have lived in the United States longer and may be more familiar with American culture and beliefs.

Family Caregivers

A national survey conducted in 2015 by the National Alliance for Caregiving and AARP found an estimated 43.5 million adults in the United States have provided unpaid care to an adult or child (National Alliance for Caregiving, 2015). Sixty percent of caregivers are women (40 percent are male) with an average being 49 years of age and 7 percent being 75 years of age or older. A majority (85 percent) provided care for a relative, with 49 percent caring for a parent or parent-in-law, and 12 percent or 1 in 10 providing care for a spouse. With roughly 24 percent providing care for five years or more, caretaking fatigue needs to be an important variable to assess for when working with families who have members requiring caretaking. The typical person being cared for is female, and over half of care recipients are 75 years or older with long-term physical conditions and memory problems. Prevalent reasons for providing care include an aging family member who needs assistance with activities of daily living (ADLs) and some type of dementia, mobility, and mental/emotional health issues (National Alliance for Caregiving, 2015).

Many of these caretakers are increasingly performing tasks that nurses have typically performed, such as giving injections, managing tube feedings, providing catheter care, and providing colostomy care (Reinhard et al., 2012). In addition to the stress of performing these types of skills, many report their own health has suffered and report financial, physical, and emotional stress. Employed caregivers need to negotiate flexible working hours or paid sick days with their employers. Only about 23 percent of working caretakers have been offered employee assistance programs or the ability to work from home (National Alliance for Caregiving, 2015). Being involved within the health care system does not guarantee that health care providers such as physicians, nurses, or social workers are meeting the information needs or caregiving support of caregivers. Less than a third of caregivers report being asked by their health care providers about what was needed to care for their family member. Only 16 percent of caregivers who entered the health care system had been asked about their own self-care needs (National Alliance for Caregiving, 2015). Nurses working with caregivers need to provide information and caregiving support. Information about making end-of-life decisions and supportive services were important topics for many caregivers surveyed.

An invisible trend that needs attention is the number of children under 19 years of age who are providing care for a family member. In the United States there are 1.3 to 1.4 million children, ranging in age from 10 to 20 years who provide care for sick or disabled relatives, with about a third caring for a grandparent (National Alliance for Caregiving, 2005). Three in ten child caregivers are ages 8 to 11 (31 percent), 38 percent are ages 12 to 15, and the remaining 31 percent are ages 16 to 18. Child caregivers are evenly balanced by gender (male 49 percent, female 51 percent). Caregivers tend to live in households with lower incomes than do noncaregivers, and they are less likely than noncaregivers to have two-parent households (76 percent versus 85 percent) (National Alliance for Caregiving, 2005, p. 5). In a large study conducted by Siskowski (2006) of 12,681 public school children in Palm Beach County, Florida, more than 1 in 2 middle and high school children (6210) were providing care for a family member. Of these young caregivers 67 percent missed school or after school activities, did not complete their homework, or were interrupted in their studying to provide care for a family member. About 22 percent of high school dropouts leave school to provide care for a family member (Bridgeland et al., 2006).

As family caregivers are the primary care providers, it is crucial that they be supported in all ways possible. Nurses can work with families who are providing care to their family member in the following ways (National Alliance for Caregiving, 2015):

1. Identify and help caregivers who are most at risk for deteriorating health, financial security, and quality of life.
2. Identify and advocate for programs that could make a real difference in caregivers' well-being and in their ability to continue providing care, including helping them balance paid employment and unpaid care.
3. Give caregivers resources to cope with the sometimes unexpected and sudden entry into providing care.
4. Extend training to caregivers who perform ADLs, medical/nursing tasks, and other activities, including communicating and interacting with the formal care system.
5. Encourage families to proactively plan for and discuss aging and health/disability, including plans for future care and scenarios where the current unpaid caregiver may no longer be able to provide care.

FAMILY HEALTH

The meaning of family health is not precise and lacks consensus, despite the increased focus on family health within the nursing profession. The term **family health** is often used interchangeably with the concepts of family functioning, healthy families, and familial health. Hanson (2005, p. 7) defines family health as "a dynamic changing relative state of well-being, which includes the biological, psychological, spiritual, sociological, and cultural factors of the family system." This holistic approach refers to individual members as well as the family unit as a whole entity and in turn the family within the community context. An individual's health (the wellness and illness continuum) affects the functioning of the entire family, and in turn, the family's functioning affects the health of individuals. Thus assessment of family health involves simultaneous assessment of individual family members, the family system as a whole, and the community in which the family is embedded.

Health professionals have tended to classify clients and their families into two groups: healthy families and nonhealthy families, or those in need of psychosocial evaluation and intervention. The term *family health* implies mental health rather than physical health. A popular term for *nonhealthy families* is **dysfunctional families**, also called noncompliant, resistant, or unmotivated—phrases that label families who are not functioning well with each other or in their communities.

Families are neither all good nor all bad; rather, all families have both strengths and difficulties. All families have seeds of resilience and strengths upon which the nurse should work with the family to build interventions and design plans of action.

Families with strengths, functional families, and **balanced families** are terms often used to refer to *healthy families* that are doing well. Studies have identified traits of healthy families as well as family stressors that are useful for nurses to include in their assessment (Kaakinen, 2018a; Olson & Gorall, 2003). Box 26.2 shows characteristics of families who are healthy and functioning well in society.

BOX 26.2 Characteristics of Healthy Families

1. The family tends to communicate well and listen to all members.
2. The family affirms and supports all of its members.
3. Teaching respect for others is valued by the family.
4. The family members have a sense of trust.
5. The family plays together, and humor is present.
6. All members interact with each other, and a balance in the interactions is noted among the members.
7. The family shares leisure time together.
8. The family has a shared sense of responsibility.
9. The family has traditions and rituals.
10. The family shares a religious core.
11. Privacy of members is honored by the family.
12. The family opens its boundaries to admit and seek help with problems.

Adapted from Kim-Godwin, Y, Robinson, M: Family health promotion. In Kaakinen JR, Coehlo DP, Steele R, & Robinson M, editors: *Family health care nursing; theory, practice and research,* ed. 6, Philadelphia, 2018, FA Davis.

The most recent concept described in the family literature pertains to ways families function across the family life cycle. Balanced families are those that have the ability to adapt to situations; therefore, they demonstrate **family flexibility** in leadership, relationships, rules, control, discipline, negotiation, and role sharing (Kaakinen, 2018a; Olson & Gorall, 2003). Balanced families have the ability to allow family members to be independent from the family yet remain connected to the family as a whole, which is termed **family cohesion** (Olson & Gorall, 2003).

FOUR APPROACHES TO FAMILY NURSING

Central to the practice of family nursing is conceptualizing and approaching the family from four perspectives. All have legitimate implications for family nursing assessment and intervention (Figs. 26.2 and 26.3). The approaches that nurses use are determined by many factors, including the issues for which the individuals or families as a whole are seeking help, the environment in which they coexist with other family members and the community, the interaction among all of these factors, and of course the nursing resources available to deal with all of these factors (Hanson, 2005).

Family As Context

The family has a traditional focus that places the individual first and the family second. The **family as context** serves as either a strength or a stressor to individual health and illness issues. The nurse is most interested in the individual and realizes that the family influences the health of the individual. A nurse using this focus might ask an individual client the following questions: "Is your family available to help you get to your doctor appointments?"

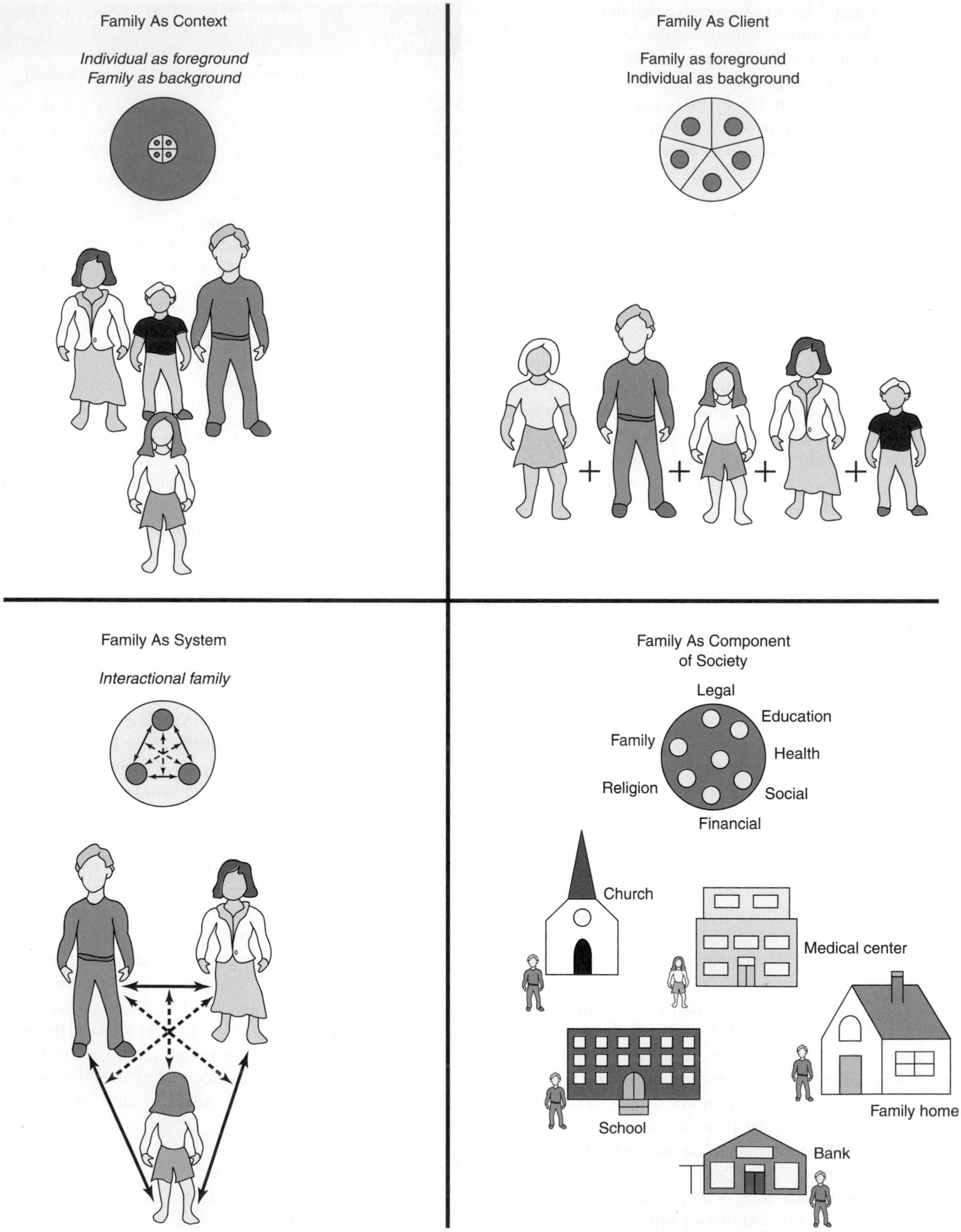

Fig. 26.2 Approaches to family nursing. (From Hanson SMH, Gedaly-Duff V, Kaakinen JR, editors: *Family health care nursing: theory, practice and research*, ed. 3, Philadelphia, 2005, FA Davis.)

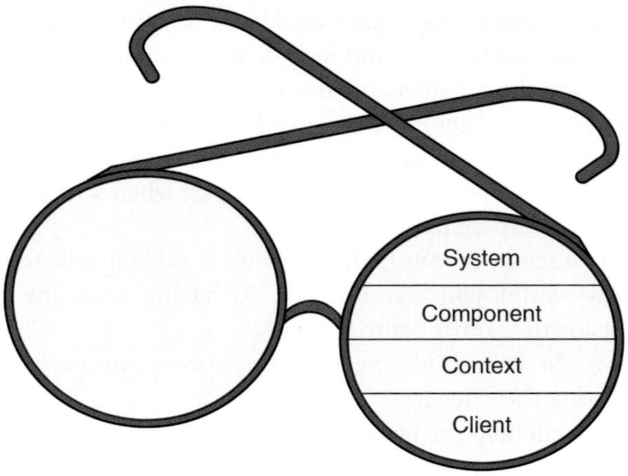

Fig. 26.3 Four views of the family.

"Can your wife help you with your insulin injections?" or "Perhaps your son could help you go up and down the stairs since your mother is so much smaller than you and your dad."

Family As Client

When the nurse views the family as client the family is the primary focus and individual family members are secondary. The family is seen as the sum of individual family members. The focus is concentrated on how the family as a whole is reacting to the event when a family member experiences a health issue. In addition, the nurse looks to see how each family member is affected by the health event. From this perspective, a nurse might say the following to a family member who has recently become ill: "How is the family reacting to your mother's recent diagnosis of liver cancer?" "How have you experienced your mother's recent diagnosis of liver cancer?" "How has your diagnosis of insulin-dependent diabetes affected your family?" "Will your need for medication at night be a problem for your family?"

Family As a System

The focus is on the family as client, and the family is viewed as an interactional system in which the whole is more than the sum of its parts. This approach focuses on individual members and the family as a whole at the same time. The interactions among family members become the target for nursing interventions (e.g., the interactions among both parents and children, and between the parental dyad). The systems approach to families always implies that when something happens to one family member, the other members of the family system also are affected, and vice versa. Questions nurses ask when approaching the family as a system are the following: "What has changed between you and your spouse since your child's head injury?" "How do you feel about the fact that your son's long-term rehabilitation will affect the ways members of your family are functioning and interact with one another?"

Family As a Component of Society

The family as a component of society is seen as one of many institutions in society, along with health, education, and religious and financial institutions. The family is a basic or primary unit of society, as are all the other units, and they are all a part of the larger system of society. The family as a whole interacts with other institutions to receive, exchange, or give services. Nurses who work with families have derived many of their tenets of practice from this component of society, because they focus on the interface between families and community agencies. Nurses using this approach see families as a population. Questions the nurse might ask using this lens are, "How do we meet the needs of adolescent pregnant women?" or "What plan should we develop to increase the H1N1 immunization rates in the families living in the lower-income housing developments?" This is the approach used by public health nurses as they implement population-centered strategies to improve the health of the overall community.

THEORIES FOR WORKING WITH FAMILIES IN THE COMMUNITY

There is no single theory or conceptual framework that fully describes the relationships and dynamics and can be used to understand and intervene with families. Thus, an integrated theoretical approach is necessary because one theoretical perspective does not provide nurses with enough knowledge to work effectively with families. Public health nurses must also blend family nursing theories with public health theories and frameworks to work both with individual families and populations of families.

Family nursing theory is an evolving synthesis of the scholarship from three different traditions: family social science, family therapy, and nursing (Fig. 26.4). Of the three categories of theory, the family social science theories are the most well-developed and informative with respect to how families function, the environment-family interchange, interactions within the family, how the family changes over time, and the family's reaction to health and illness. Therefore, in this chapter, three family social science theories that blend well with public health nursing are reviewed. These social science theories are the family systems theory, family developmental and life cycle theory, and the bioecological systems theory.

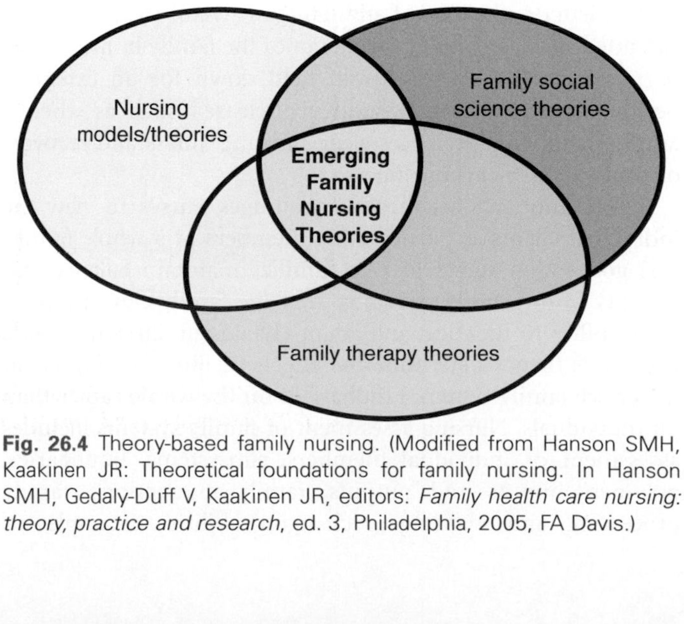

Fig. 26.4 Theory-based family nursing. (Modified from Hanson SMH, Kaakinen JR: Theoretical foundations for family nursing. In Hanson SMH, Gedaly-Duff V, Kaakinen JR, editors: *Family health care nursing: theory, practice and research*, ed. 3, Philadelphia, 2005, FA Davis.)

Family Systems Theory

Families are social systems and much can be learned from the systems approach. A system is composed of a set of organized, complex, interacting elements. Nurses use family systems theory to understand how a family is an organized whole as well as composed of individuals (Kaakinen, 2018b). The purpose of the family system is to maintain stability through adaptation to internal and external stresses that are created by change (Kaakinen, 2018b; White & Klein, 2008). Assumptions of family systems theory include the following:

- Family systems are greater than and different from the sum of their parts.
- There are many hierarchies within family systems and logical relationships between subsystems (e.g., mother-child, family-community).
- Boundaries in the family system can be open, closed, or random.
- Family systems increase in complexity over time, evolving to allow greater adaptability, tolerance to change, and growth by differentiation.
- Family systems change constantly in response to stresses and strains from within and from outside environments.
- Change in one part of a family system affects the total system.
- Family systems are an organized whole; therefore, individuals within the family are interdependent.
- Family systems have homeostatic features to maintain stable patterns that can be adaptive or maladaptive.

An excellent way to understand family systems theory is to visualize a mobile that consists of different members of a family suspended from each arm of the mobile; this represents the family as a whole. The parts of the mobile move about in response to changes in the balance. The amount of movement and length of time it takes to achieve a calm, balanced state depends on the severity of the imbalance. The family is a system similar to that of the mobile. When one member is affected by a health event, the whole family and each member of the family is affected differently by this change in balance. Imagine what would happen to the mobile if one of the parts was cut off as in the death of a family member, an additional part was added as in the birth or adoption of an infant, an arm of the mobile was extended such as a child moving out of the family home, or one part is yanked really hard and held down for an extended period of time and then suddenly released such as when a family member experiences a life-limiting illness and recovers or proceeds to a chronic illness.

The family systems theory encourages nurses to view the individual clients as participating members of a whole family. The goal is for nurses to help families maintain balance and stability in the family system so that the family can maximize their ability to function and adapt (Kaakinen, 2018b). Nurses using this theory determine the effects of illness or injury on the entire family system. Emphasis is on the whole rather than on individuals. Nursing assessment of family systems includes assessment of individual members, subsystems, boundaries, openness, inputs and outputs, family interactions, family processing, and adapting or changing abilities. Examples of assessment questions nurses could ask a family based on a family systems theory would include the following:

- Who are the members of your family?
- How has one member's illness affected the family?
- Who in the family is or will be affected the most?
- What has helped your family in the past when you have had a similar experience?
- Who outside of your family do you see as being able to help?
- How would your family react to having someone from outside the family come to help?
- How do you think the children, spouse, or parents are meeting their needs?
- What will help the family cope with the changes?

Interventions need to build on the strengths of the family to improve or support the functioning of the individual members and the whole family. Some nursing strategies based on a family systems theory include establishing a mechanism for providing families with information about their family members on a regular basis, helping the family maintain routines and rituals, and discussing ways to provide for everyday functioning when a family member becomes ill.

The major strength of the systems framework is that it views families from both a subsystem and a suprasystem approach. That is, it views the interactions within and between family subsystems as well as the interaction between families and the larger supersystems, such as the community and the world. The major weakness of the systems framework is that the focus is on the interaction of the family with other systems rather than on the individual, which is sometimes more important.

Family Developmental and Life Cycle Theory

Family developmental and life cycle theory provides a framework for understanding normal predicted stresses that families experience as they change and transition over time. In the original theory of family development by Duvall and Miller (1985) they applied the principles of individual development to the family as a unit. The stages of family development are based on the age of the eldest child. Overall family tasks are identified that need to be accomplished for each stage of family development. Table 26.1 shows the stages of the family life cycle and some of the family developmental tasks. One developmental concept of this theory is that families as a system move to a different level of functioning, thus implying progress in a single direction. Family disequilibrium and conflicts occur during these expected transition periods from one stage of family development to another. The family begins as a married couple. Then the family becomes more complex with the addition of each new child until it becomes simpler and less complex as the younger generation begins to leave the home. Finally, the family comes full circle to the original husband-wife pair. Recognizing that families of today are different in structure, function, and processes, Carter and McGoldrick (2005) expanded the work of Duvall and Miller (1985) to have the family developmental and life cycle theory include different family structures such as divorced families and blended families.

TABLE 26.1 Traditional Family Life Cycle Stages and Family Developmental Tasks

Stages of Family Life Cycle	Family Developmental Tasks
Married couple	Establish relationship as a family unit, role development Determine family routines and rituals
Childbearing families with infants	Adjust to pregnancy and then birth of infant Learn new roles as mother and father Maintain couple time, intimacy, and relationship as a unit
Families with preschool children	Understand growth and development, including discipline Cope with energy depletion Arrange for individual time, family time, and couple time
Families with school-aged children	Learn to open family boundaries as child increases amount of time spent with others outside of the family Manage time demands in supporting child's interest and needs outside of the home Establish rules, new disciplinary actions Maintain couple time
Families with adolescents	Adapt to changes in family communication, power structure, and decision making as teen increases autonomy Help teen develop as individual and as a family member
Families launching young adults	As young adult moves in and out of the home allocate space, power, communication, roles Maintain couple time, intimacy, and relationship
Middle-aged parents	Refocus on couple time, intimacy, and relationship Maintain kinship ties Focus on retirement and the future
Aging parents	Adjust to retirement, death of spouse, and living alone Adjust to new roles (i.e., widow, single, grandparent) Adjust to new living situations, changes in health

Traditional Family Life Cycle Stages and Family Developmental Tasks. Family developmental and life cycle theory explains and predicts the changes that occur to families and its members over time. Achievement of family developmental tasks helps individual family members to accomplish their tasks. Two of the major assumptions of this theory are as follows:

- Families change and develop over time based on the age of the family members and the social norms of the society. Families have predictable stressors and changes based on changes in the family development and family structure. For example, when a family has their first child, there are predictable stresses and goals to accomplish. Also, families who experience a divorce have some predictable stresses based on when in the life cycle of the family the divorce occurs.
- Families experience disequilibrium when they transition from one stage to another stage. These transitions are considered "on time" or "off time." For example, a couple in their late 20s having their first child would be considered "on time," whereas a teenager having a child or a 30-year-old wife and mother dying from breast cancer would be considered "off-time" transitions.

This theory assists nurses in anticipating stresses families may experience based on the stage of the family life cycle and if the family is experiencing these changes "on time" or "off time." Nurses can also use these predictable stresses to identify family strengths in adaptation to the changes. In conducting an assessment of families, the following are examples of the types of questions nurses can ask based on the family developmental and life cycle theory.

- How has time that the family spends together been affected?
- How has communication among and between the family members been altered?
- Has physical space in the home been changed to meet the needs of the evolving family?
- In what ways have the informal roles of the family been changed?
- What changes are being experienced in family meals, recreation, spirituality, or sleep habits?
- How are the family finances affected as the family members age?
- Who should be included in the family decision making?

Nursing intervention strategies that derive from the family developmental and life cycle theory help individuals and families understand the growth and development stages and manage the normal transition periods between developmental periods (e.g., tasks of the school-age family member versus tasks of the adolescent family member) with the least amount of stress possible. Family nurses must recognize that in every family there are both individual and family developmental tasks that need to be accomplished for every stage of the individual or family life cycle that are unique to that particular family.

The major strength of this approach is that it provides a basis for forecasting normative stresses and issues that families will experience at any stage in the family life cycle. The major weakness of the model is that it was developed at a time when the traditional nuclear family was emphasized and that some theory development has been conducted on how family life cycles or stages are affected in divorced families, stepparent families, and domestic-partner relationships (Carter & McGoldrick, 2005).

Bioecological Systems Theory

The bioecological systems theory was developed by Urie Bronfenbrenner (1972, 1979, 1997) to describe how environments and systems outside of the family influence the development of a child over time. Even though this theory was designed around how both nature and nurture shape the development of a child, the same underlying principles can be applied when the client is the family. This theory is very useful for public health nurses since it helps identify the stresses and potential resources that can affect family adaptation. Fig. 26.5 depicts the five systems in this theory at different levels of engagement that can affect family development and adaptation. The family as the client is at the center of the concentric circles. Each of the levels contains roles, norms, and rules that influence the current situation of the family.

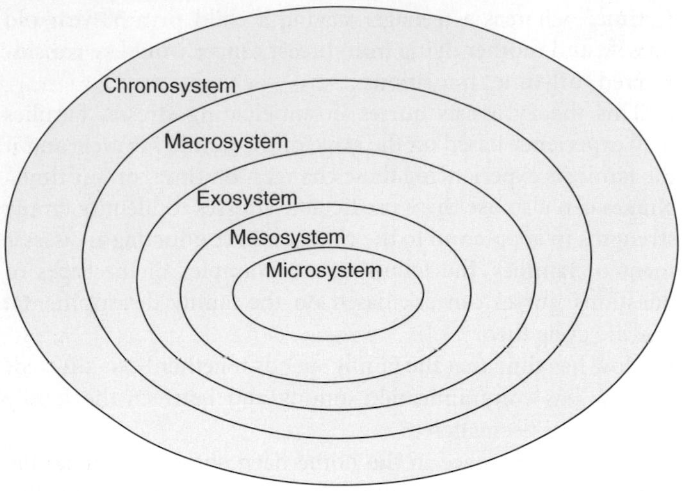

Fig. 26.5 Bioecological family systems model: levels of systems.

Microsystems are composed of the systems and individuals that the family directly interacts with on a daily basis. These systems vary for each family, but could include their home, neighborhood, place of work, school systems, extended family, health care system, community/public health system, or close friends.

Mesosystems are the systems that the family interacts with frequently but not on a daily basis. These systems vary based on the situation in which the public health nurse is working with a family. Some ideas for systems at this level could be a home health aide who comes to the home twice a week, a hospice nurse who comes to the home once a week, a social worker, church members who come to deliver food to the family, the transportation system, the school system, specialty physicians, pharmacy, or extended family.

Exosystems are external environments that have an indirect influence on the family. For example, some of these systems could be the economic system, local and state political systems, religious system, the school board, community/health and welfare services, the Social Security office, or protective services.

Macrosystems are broad overarching social ideological and cultural values, attitudes, and beliefs that indirectly influence the family. Examples include a Jewish religious ethic, a cultural value of autonomy in decision making, or ethnicity.

Chronosystems refer to time-related contexts in which changes that have occurred over time may influence any or all of the other levels/systems. Examples include the death of a young parent, a divorce and remarriage, war, or natural disasters.

One assumption of this model is that what happens outside of the family is equally as important as what happens inside the family. The interaction between the family and the systems in which it interacts is bidirectional in that the family is affected by the outside systems and the family affects these systems. The strength of this model is that it provides a holistic view of interactions between the family and society. In working with the family, a critical intervention strategy is drawing a family ecomap that shows the systems with which the family interacts, including the flow of energy from that system into the family or out of the family. The family ecomap is explained in more detail later in the chapter. The weakness of this model is that it does not address how families cope or adapt to the interaction with these systems.

WORKING WITH FAMILIES FOR HEALTHY OUTCOMES

Family nurses should transcend the traditional nursing approach as a service model and change their practice to a **capacity building model** (Bomar, 2004; Kim-Godwin & Bomar, 2015). In a capacity building model nurses assume the family has the most knowledge about how their health issues affect the family, supports family decision making, empowers the family to act, and facilitates actions for and with the family. The goal of family nursing is to focus care, interventions, and services to optimize the self-care capabilities of families and to achieve the best possible outcomes.

Nurses work with all types of family structures in a variety of settings. Each family is unique in how it responds to the stresses that evolve when a family member experiences a health event. Public health nurses are in a unique position to help families by providing direct care, removing barriers to needed services, and improving the capacity of the family to take care of its members (Kaakinen, 2018c).

Pre-encounter Data Collection

Using excellent communication skills, nurses help families determine the priority of issues they are confronting, identify their needs, and develop a plan of action. Family members are experts in their own health. They know the family health history, their health status, and their health-related concerns (Smith, 2009).

Nurses gather information about the family from many sources as well as directly from the family. Data collection begins when an actual or potential problem is identified by a source, which may be the family, the health care provider, a school nurse, or a caseworker. Several examples follow:

1. A family is referred to the home health agency because of the birth of the newest family member. In that district, all births are automatically followed up with a home visit.
2. A family calls hospice to request assistance in providing care to a family member with a terminal illness.
3. A school nurse is asked to conduct a family assessment by a teacher who noticed that the student has frequent absences and has demonstrated significant behavior changes in the classroom.
4. A nurse practitioner requests a family assessment for a child who has failure to thrive.
5. An individual seeks health care in a primary care county clinic or a program-specific clinic such as family planning or an STD clinic.

The assessment process and data collection begin as soon as the referral occurs or the appointment is made. Sources of pre-encounter data the nurse gathers include the following:

- *Referral source.* The information collected from the referral source includes data that led to the identification of a problem for this family. Demographic information and subjective and objective information may be obtained from the referral source.

- *Family.* A family may identify a health care concern and seek help. During the initial intake or screening procedure, valuable information can be collected from the family. Information is collected during phone interaction with the family member, even when calling to set up the initial appointment. This information might include family members' views of the problem, surprise that the referral was made, reluctance to set up the meeting, avoidance in setting up the interview, or recognition that a referral was made or that a probable health care concern exists.
- *Previous records.* Previous records may be available for review before the first meeting between the nurse and the family. Often, a record release for information is necessary to obtain family or individual records. However, one challenge may be that many of the electronic health records are premade templates that ignore family information.

Determine Where to Meet the Family

Before contacting the family to arrange for the initial appointment, the nurse decides the best place to meet with the family, which might be in the home, clinic, or office. The How To Plan for Family Assessment box identifies reflection questions nurses need to address before meeting the family. The type of agency in which the nurse works may determine where the family meeting is held (e.g., home health is conducted in the home, and mental health agencies meet the family in the clinic).

> **HOW TO Plan for Family Assessment**
>
> Assessment of families requires an organized plan before you see the family. This plan is developed through the following questions:
>
> 1. Why are you seeing the family?
> 2. Are there any specific family concerns that have been identified by other sources?
> 3. Is there a need for an interpreter?
> 4. Who will be present during the interview?
> 5. Where will you see the family and how will the space be arranged?
> 6. What are you going to be assessing?
> 7. How are you going to collect the data?
> 8. What services do you anticipate the family will need?
> 9. What are the insurance sources for the family?
> 10. What cultural factors need to be considered in working with this family?

One major advantage to meeting in the family home is seeing the everyday family environment. Family members are likely to feel more relaxed in their home, thereby demonstrating typical family interactions. Meeting with a family in their home emphasizes that the whole family and not one family member is the client. This approach allows the whole family to participate in the identification and resolution of the health problem. Conducting the interview in the home may increase the probability of having more family members present. There are two important disadvantages of meeting in the family home: (1) the family home may be the only sanctuary or safe place for the family or its members to be away from the scrutiny of others, and (2) meeting with a family on their ground requires the nurse to be highly skilled in communication by setting limits and guiding the interaction.

Conducting the family appointment in the office or clinic allows easier access to other health care providers for consultation. An advantage of using the clinic may be that the family situation is so intense that a more formal, less personal setting may be necessary for the family to begin discussion of emotionally charged issues. A disadvantage of not seeing the everyday family environment is that it may reinforce a possible culture gap between the family and the nurse.

Making an Appointment With the Family

After the decision is made regarding where to meet the family, the nurse contacts the family. It is important to remember that the family gathers information about the nurse from this initial phone call to arrange a meeting, so the nurse should be confident and organized. After the introduction, the nurse concisely states the reason for requesting the family visit and encourages all family members to attend the meeting. The How To Make an Appointment With the Family box reviews steps for making an appointment with the family. Determine if you need an interpreter with you or if you need to arrange to have one available by phone during the visit. Several possible times for the appointment can be offered, including late afternoon or evening, which allows the family to select the most convenient time for all members to be present. It is important to remember that families ultimately retain control of the situation and they do not have to let the nurse enter their home (Smith, 2009).

> **HOW TO Make an Appointment With the Family**
>
> Data collection starts immediately upon referral to the nurse. The following are suggestions that will make the process of arranging a meeting with the family easier:
>
> 1. Remember that the assessment is reciprocal and the family will be making judgments about you when you call to make the appointment.
> 2. Introduce yourself and the purpose for the contact.
> 3. Do not apologize for contacting the family. Be clear, direct, and specific about the need for an appointment.
> 4. Arrange a time that is convenient for all parties and allows the most family members to be present.
> 5. If appropriate, ask if an interpreter will be needed during the meeting.
> 6. Confirm place, time, date, and directions.

Planning for Your Own Safety

It is critical to plan for your own safety when you make a home visit. Learn about the neighborhood you will be visiting, anticipate needs you may have, and determine if it is safe for you to make the home visit alone or if you need to arrange to have a security person with you during the visit. Always have your cell phone fully charged and readily available. In addition, the following strategies will help to ensure your own safety when you visit families in their homes (Smith, 2009, p. 316):

1. Leave a schedule at your office.
2. Plan the visit during safe times of day.

3. Dress appropriately, bringing little jewelry or money.
4. Avoid secluded places if you are by yourself.
5. Obtain an escort; take a coworker or neighborhood volunteer.
6. Sit between the client and the exit.
7. If you feel unsafe, do not visit or leave immediately.
8. Check in with your work at the end of the day.

Interviewing the Family: Defining the Problem

One of the underlying central tenets of family nursing is to build a trusting family-nurse relationship. Working with families requires nurses to use therapeutic communication efficiently and skillfully by moving between informal conversation and skilled interviewing strategies. Prepare your family questions before your interview based on the best family theory given what is known about the family situation.

Although it seems commonplace, it is important for nurses to introduce themselves to the family and to initiate conversation with each member present. Spending some initial time on informal conversation helps put the family at ease, allows them time to assess the person/nurse, and disperses some of the tension surrounding the visit (Tabacco, 2010). Involving each family member in the conversation, including children, elderly, or any disabled family member, demonstrates respect and caring and sends the message that the purpose of the visit is to help the whole family and not just the individual family member. Too much disclosure during the early contacts between the family and nurse may scare the family away. Slow down the process and take time to build trust.

Shifting the conversation into a more formal interview can be accomplished by asking the family to share their story about the current situation. If the nurse focuses only on the medical aspect or illness story, much valuable information and the priority issue confronting the family may be missed in the data collection. The purpose of the interview is to gather information and help the family focus on their problem and determine solutions. The following specific therapeutic questions have been found to provide important family information (Leahey & Svavarsdottir, 2009, p. 449):

- What is the greatest challenge facing your family now?
- Who in the family do you think the illness has the most impact on?
- Who is suffering the most?
- What has been most and least helpful to you in similar situations?
- If there is one question you could have answered now, what would that be?
- How can we best help you and your family?
- What are your needs/wishes for assistance now?

Box 26.3 lists a variety of additional interview questions that will help uncover the family story. Encourage several members of the family to provide input into the discussion. One strategy is to ask the same question of several different family members. It is critical for the nurse to not take sides in the family discussion and to focus on guiding them in their decision making. In addition to the family story, the nurse will likely need to ask specific assessment questions about the family member who is in need of services.

BOX 26.3 Family Interview Questions

- What do you believe is the most important or pressing issue right now?
- What have you done to improve the situation?
- Share with me your primary goal in the immediate situation.
- What are the main problems you are having related to ____?
- What is causing you the most stress?
- How has this stress affected you and the members of your family?
- How are the everyday needs of the family getting done (e.g., cooking, shopping, cleaning, laundry, transportation, sleeping)?
- How well is your family managing this stress?
- What results or outcomes do you hope for?
- What do you feel you need to help solve this situation?
- What can your family do for you?
- Who do we need to involve in this situation?
- What information do you need to know?
- Walk me through a typical 24-hour day in your home.
- During times of need, where can you go for support and resources?
- What do you think would help me better understand what you are experiencing?
- How does your family anticipate caring for ___?
- How does this situation affect you financially?
- Where, how, and from whom do you receive your support, inspiration, and energy to maintain the responsibilities required of you?
- What has been the biggest surprise to you about all of this?
- How do you think your family roles and routines are going to change in this situation?
- How have you and your family prepared to provide care for ____?
- What are your family plans for when you have to return to work?
- What does your family do to feel relief or take a break?
- What are some specific changes that you and your family members have had to make?
- What do you fear the most about ____?

Family Assessment Instruments

One quick way for nurses to gather information from a family is to use reliable and valid short assessment instruments that are specifically focused on the relevant family situation. Well over 1000 different family assessment instruments exist (Touliatos et al., 2001); therefore, it is critical that the following criteria be used to help determine the most appropriate assessment instrument (Kaakinen, 2018c):

- Written in uncomplicated language at a fifth-grade level
- Only takes 10 to 15 minutes to complete
- Relatively easy and quick to score
- Offers valid data on which to base decisions
- Sensitive to gender, race, social class, and ethnic background

Families should always be asked their permission to use an assessment instrument and be informed of how the information will be used by the nurse in helping to plan their care. Nurses should review the results or interpretation of the information with the family.

Genograms and ecomaps are both assessment instruments that actively engage the family in their care. In addition, they both provide visual diagrams of the current family story and offer ideas about the plan of action, solutions, and resources (Harrison & Neufeld, 2009; Kaakinen, 2018c). The genogram and ecomap are essential components of any family assessment, and they should be used concurrently with any other specific assessment instruments used in the interview.

Genogram. The genogram displays pertinent family information in a family tree format that shows family members and their relationships over at least three generations (McGoldrick et al., 2008). The genogram shows family history and patterns of health-related information, which is a rich source of information for planning interventions. The identified client and his or her family are highlighted on the genogram. Genograms enhance nurses' abilities to make clinical judgments and connect them to family structure and history.

Nurses have various resources available to them to assist families with the collection of family history. In 2002, the Office of Public Health Genomics (OPHG) through the CDC started the Family History Public Health Initiative to increase awareness of family history as an important risk factor for common chronic diseases such as cancer, heart disease, and diabetes, and to promote its use in programs aimed at reducing the burden of these diseases in the U.S. population (CDC, 2013). The initiative has four main activities (for more information, check out their website: http://www.cdc.gov):

- Conducting research to define, measure, and assess family history in populations and individuals
- Developing and evaluating tools for collecting family history
- Evaluating whether family history-based strategies work
- Promoting evidence-based applications of family history to health professionals and the public

The diagramming of the genogram must adhere to a specific format to ensure that all parties understand the information. A form that can be used for developing genograms is depicted in Fig. 26.6, and the symbols most often used in a genogram are shown in Fig. 26.7.

An outline for gathering information during the genogram interview is presented in Box 26.4, and genogram interpretive categories are found in Box 26.5. The health history for all family members (morbidity, mortality, onset of illness) is important information for family nurses and can be the focus of analysis of the family genogram. The more information that can be added to the family genogram, the more the family and nurse understand the family situation. Most families are cooperative and interested in completing the genogram, which does not have to be completed in one sitting. The genogram becomes a part of the ongoing health care record.

Ecomap. The ecomap is a visual diagram of the family unit in relation to other units or subsystems in the community. The ecomap serves as a tool to organize and present factual information and thus allows the nurse to have a more holistic and integrated perception of the family situation. The ecomap shows the nature of the relationships among family members, and between family members and the community; it is an overview of the family, picturing both the important nurturing and the important stress-producing connections between the family and its environment. The nurse starts with a blank ecomap, which consists of a large circle with smaller circles around it (Fig. 26.8). The identified client and his or her family are placed in the center of the large circle. The outer smaller circles around the family unit represent significant people, agencies, or organizations in the family's environment that interact with the family members (Kaakinen, 2018b, 2018c). The nature and quality of the relationships and the direction of energy flow between the family members and the subsystems are shown by different connecting lines.

The ecomap serves as a tool to organize and present information, allowing the nurse and family to have a more holistic and integrated perception of the current situation. Not only

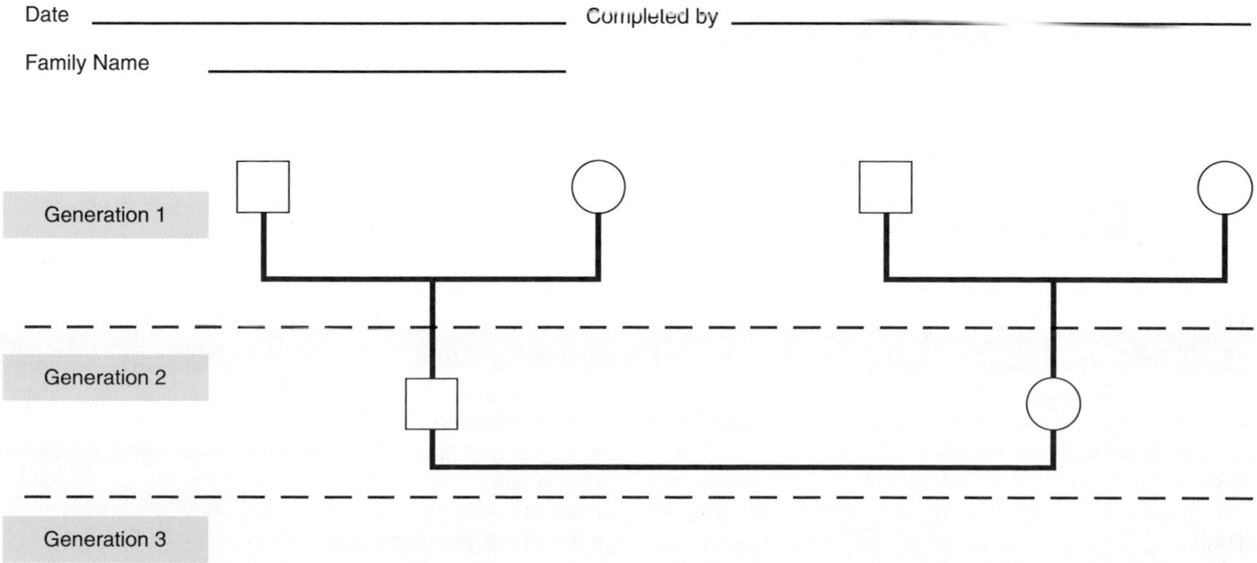

Fig. 26.6 Genogram form. (Modified from McGoldrick M, Gerson R, Shellenberger S: *Genograms: assessment and intervention*, ed. 2, New York, 1999, Norton.)

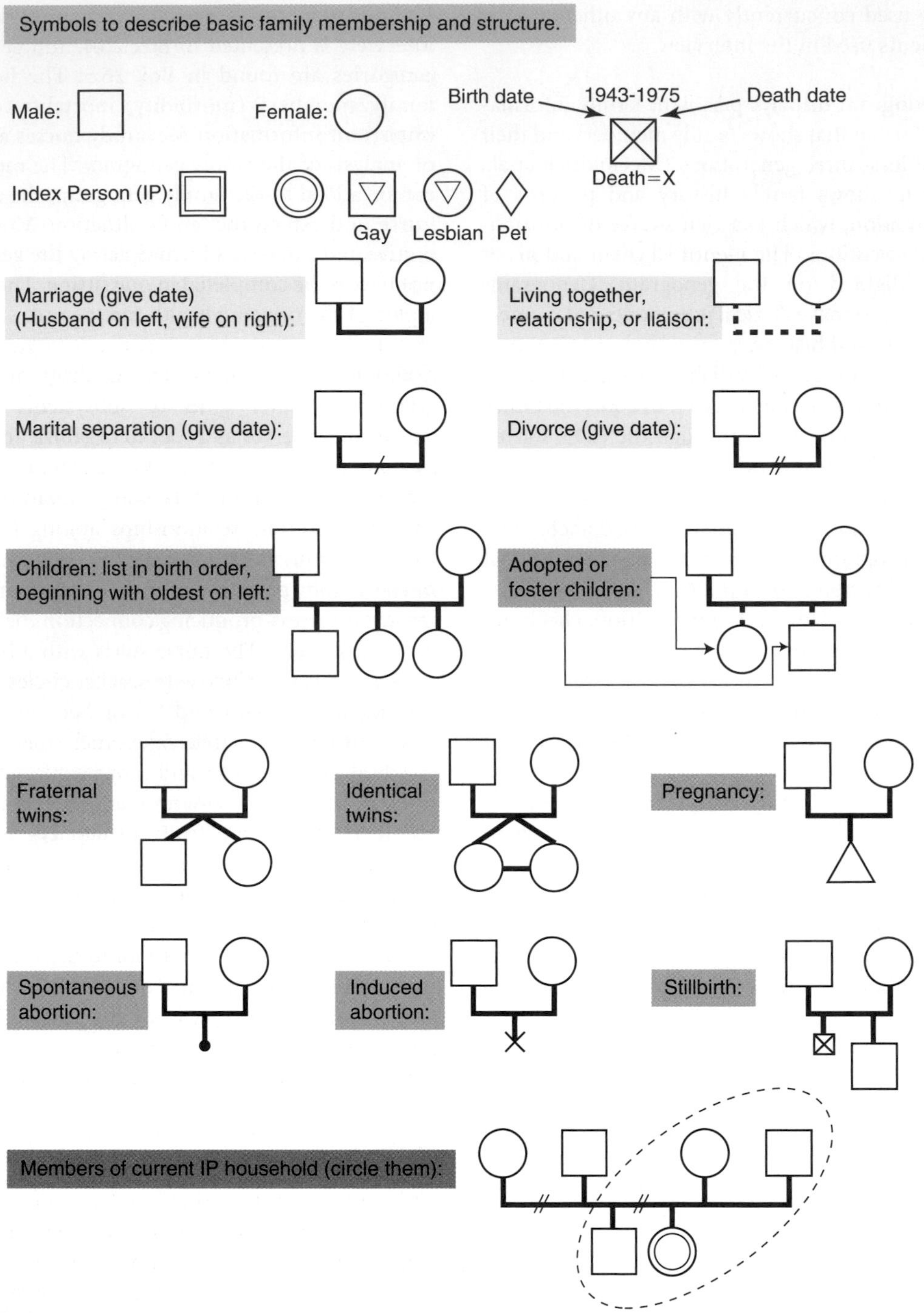

Fig. 26.7 Genogram symbols. (Modified from Gerson, R, McGoldrick M, Petry, S: *Genograms: assessment and intervention*, ed. 3, New York, 2008, Norton.)

BOX 26.4 Outline for a Genogram Interview

For each person on the genogram, the nurse should determine which of the following pieces of information to include on the genogram. The information should be relevant to the issues the family is facing.

- First name
- Age
- Date of birth
- Occupation
- Health problems
- Cause of death
- Dates of marriages, divorces, separations, commitments, cohabitations, and remarriages
- Education level
- Ethnic or religious background

Modified from McGoldrick M, Gerson R, Petry SS: *Genograms: assessment and interventions*, ed. 3, New York, 2008, W.W. Norton.

BOX 26.5 Genogram Interpretive Categories

The following areas are important to note in the family genogram:

- Family structure: nuclear, blended, single-parent household, gay/lesbian relationship, cohabitation, divorces, and separations
- Sibling subsystem group: birth order, sex, distance between ages of children
- Patterns of repetition: patterns across the generations related to family structure, behaviors, health problems, relationships, violence, abuse, poverty
- Life events: repeated similar events across generations, such as transitions, traumas

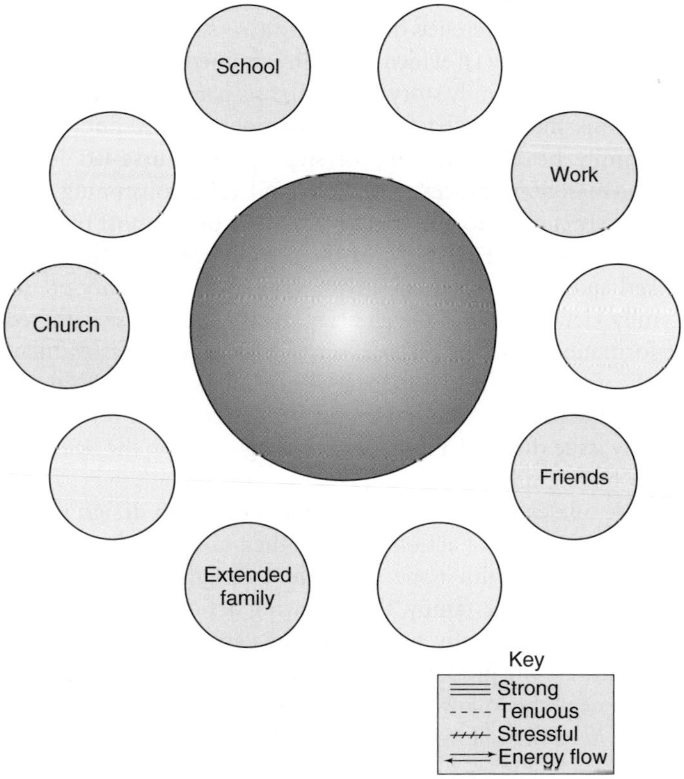

Fig. 26.8 Ecomap form. (Modified from Kaakinen JR, Hanson SMH: Family nursing assessment and intervention. In Hanson SMH, Gedaly-Duff V, Kaakinen JR, editors: *Family health care nursing: theory, practice and research*, ed. 3, Philadelphia, 2005, FA Davis.)

does it portray the present situation, but it can also be used to set goals for the future by encouraging connection and exchange with individuals and agencies in the community. A more detailed discussion of ecomapping can be found in Kaakinen (2018b, 2018c) and McGoldrick et al. (2008).

Family Health Literacy

Family health literacy is necessary for the family or its members to be actively involved in their care. Family health literacy includes the ability to understand information in order to make appropriate health care decisions, accurately carry out plans of action, and successfully advocate for the family in the complex health care systems in which they receive care (Kaakinen, 2018c). Health care providers and researchers have recognized the importance of assessing health literacy as a means of mitigating health disparities (Mantwill et al., 2015). Those with poor health literacy skills have been strongly associated with lower health outcomes (Mantwill et al., 2015).

Functional health literacy includes the ability to read and understand numbers in order to use this health information to make informed decisions (DeWalt et al., 2007) and to understand the consequences when instructions or plans of action are not followed. Health literacy affects medical decision-making preferences especially in vulnerable populations such as those that are underserved (Seo et al., 2016). Nurses can assess for health literacy in conversations and when completing genograms and ecomaps. Rather than spend time determining the extent of the health literacy in a family, it is most important that nurses use the following techniques when writing out plans of care, listing directions, discussing medication management, or writing telephone numbers (Kaakinen, 2018b, 2018c). As more emphasis is placed on clients taking a more active role in their health care, nurses will need to assist their clients with managing the amount of information they receive about their care (Zwijnenberg et al., 2012).

- Use black ink on white paper
- Use short sentences
- Use bullets no longer than seven items
- Information should be written at the fifth-grade level
- Remove all extra words
- Print in upper- and lower-case letters
- If using a computer, use 14 point font with high contrasting Arial or sans serif print
- Have plenty of white space

Families retain more information when nurses use a variety of communication methods, including both visual materials and visual language (Zwijnenberg et al., 2012). Families need direct, clear information to assist in their decision making and carrying out the plans of action (Salmond, 2008).

Designing Family Interventions

Nurses will be challenged to help families identify the primary problem confronting them and to step aside and accept the family priority as they work in partnership with the family to keep their interventions simple, specific, timely, and realistic. It is essential that the family participate in determining the primary need and in designing interventions.

It is important to view the family with an open approach, since the central issue identified by the referral source may not be the actual problem the family is experiencing. See the following case study:

The Raggs family is referred to the home health clinic by a physician for medication management. Sam, the 73-year-old husband, has been a type 2 diabetic for 13 years and now requires insulin to manage his condition. He is being discharged from the hospital. The potential area of concern that prompted the referral was the administration of insulin. After the initial meeting with the family, the primary problem the family uncovers is really not the administration of the medication, but managing his nutrition. The inference of the referral source was that the family knew how to manage the dietary aspects of diabetes because Sam had type 2 diabetes for 13 years.

CHECK YOUR PRACTICE

Based on this case study with the Raggs family, what would your immediate and then long-term nursing approaches be?

If the primary family issue is not accurately identified, the family and the nurse will collect data, design interventions, and implement plans of care that do not meet the most pressing family needs. The importance of identifying the family issue of concern and accurately making the family nursing diagnosis is demonstrated by comparing the following two scenarios:

Scenario #1: The hypothesized central issue for the Raggs family was identified by the referral source: Is insulin being administered correctly? Based on this question from the referral source, the nurse asked only for information pertaining to this specific problem. The nurse asked questions that elicited information about (1) concerns of giving injections, (2) difficulty drawing up the accurate amount of insulin, and (3) the storage of insulin. The nurse focused the interventions on (1) the psychomotor skills of family members necessary to give the insulin injection, (2) the correct amount of insulin to give according to blood glucose level, and (3) the correct storage and handling of the medication and the equipment. By not looking at the whole family, the care was based on the nurse's perception of the problem confronting the family.

Scenario #2: The central question asked by a nurse who knows how to integrate family theory into practice was, "What is the best way to ensure that the Raggs family understands how to manage his type 2 diabetes?" By asking the family to share their story of the situation together, they determined that the primary issue was not medication administration but rather a lack of family knowledge related to health care management of a family member who now requires the addition of insulin to his management plan.

The immediate approach for the nurse incorporating family systems theory is to ask open-ended and broader-based questions that can provide information about what the family perceives to be the biggest or more complex challenges. The immediate focus is how the family is responding to Sam's condition and health care needs.

Asking broader-based questions uncovers the whole picture of the family dealing with this specific health concern and directs a more comprehensive holistic data-collection process. More evidence was collected in this case scenario because more options for possible interventions were considered concurrently. Areas of data collection based on the whole family story were (1) administration of medication, (2) nutritional management, (3) blood glucose monitoring, (4) activity/exercise, (5) coping with a changed management plan, and (6) knowledge of pathophysiology of diabetes. Out of all these issues, the nurse worked with the family to help them identify that their major concern centered on nutritional management of hyperglycemia and hypoglycemia, both of which ultimately affect the administration of medication. The long-term nursing approaches would include discussions, for example, of who else in the family may be at risk for type II diabetes. For example, discussing how the children and grandchildren of this family are also at risk and dietary and lifestyle changes incorporated now may have lasting effects for the next generation. Helping families understand how conditions such as diabetes can be managed by having members participate in the care, decision making, and supportive lifestyle changes can have intergenerational effects.

The major difference between the two scenarios presented here was the way in which the nurse framed questions while listening to the family story. In the first scenario the nurse asked questions that allowed for consideration of only one aspect of family health. This type of step-by-step nurse-led linear problem-solving process is tedious and time consuming, and will likely cause errors in the identification of the most pressing family concern (Fig. 26.9). In the second scenario, the nurse asked questions that allowed for critical thinking about the family view of their challenges (Fig. 26.10). The nurse gathered information from the referral source, conducted an assessment of the impact of the new management plan on the whole family, and collaboratively the nurse and family identified the critical family issue that had a more far-reaching effect on the health of the whole family.

The nurse works with the family to help them design realistic steps or a plan of action based on their ability to successfully adapt to the health issue given the strengths of the family. Working with the family, the following action plan approach helps focus the family on things they can immediately do to help address the problem:

1. We need the following type of help.
2. We need the following information.

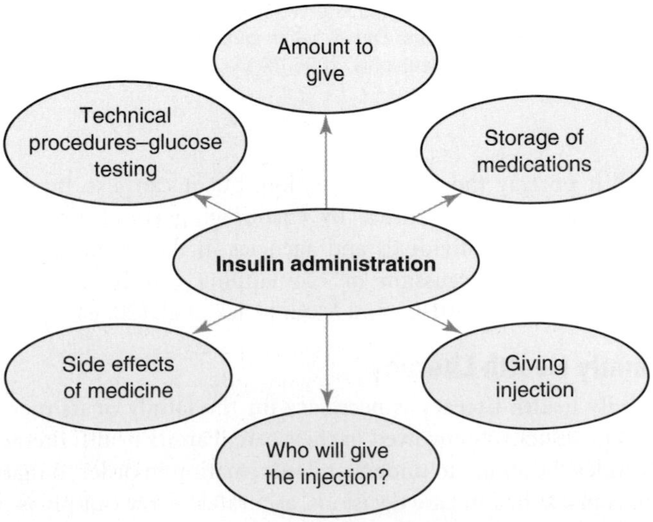

Fig. 26.9 Scenario 1: Nurse-led linear problem-solving identification process.

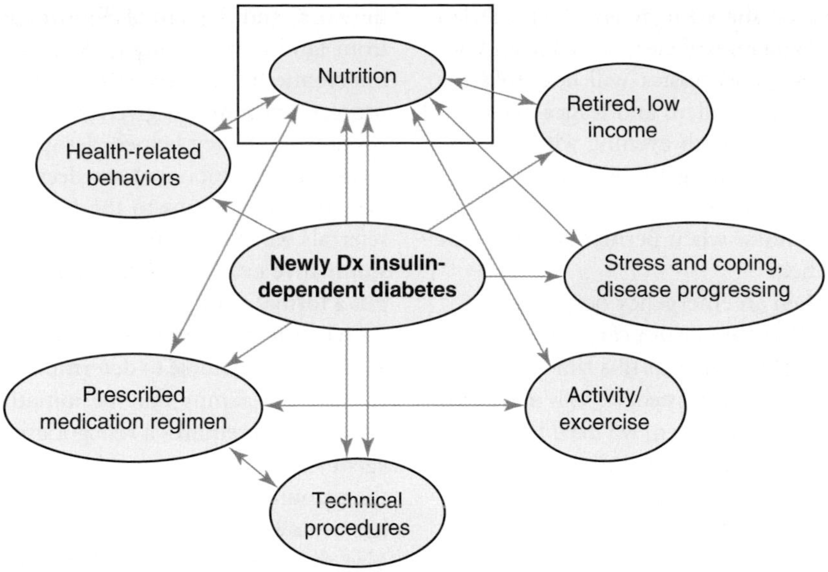

Fig. 26.10 Scenario 2: An example of complex relationships between issues affecting the whole family because of the new diagnosis.

3. We need the following supplies.
4. We need to involve or tell the following people.
5. To make our family action plan happen, we need to . . . (list five things in the order they need to have happen).

Using knowledge and evidence-based practice, the nurse guides the family in outlining ways to prevent a potential problem, minimize the problem, stabilize the problem, or help the family recognize it as a deteriorating problem. The following scenario shows how nurses work with families to determine their strengths, identify the problem, and design interventions.

Scenario #3: The home hospice nurse has been working with the Brush family for three weeks. The Brush family consists of the members outlined in Fig. 26.11.

Family story: Beatrice was diagnosed with terminal liver cancer four weeks ago. The Brush family—Bernice, Dylan, Myra, William and Jessica—agreed that Bernice should live with them and be cared for until her death in their home. Bernice has other children who live in the same city. The hospice nurse in collaboration with the Brush family identified that the primary problem is that Myra is experiencing role stress, strain, and overload in her new role as the family caregiver. Myra showed her role conflict by stating, "Sometimes I do not know who I am—daughter, nurse, mother, or wife." As Myra took a family leave from her job to stay home to care for her mother, some members of the family were surprised by her statement as they did not realize she was so overwhelmed. The family worked with the nurse to find ways to minimize her role strain by spreading the caregiver role among the extended family members.

By understanding the family systems theory, the nurse knows that what affects one member of the family affects all members of the family. One of the strengths this family has is the shared belief that caring for the dying grandmother in their home is the "right" ethical choice for them. The nurse brings knowledge

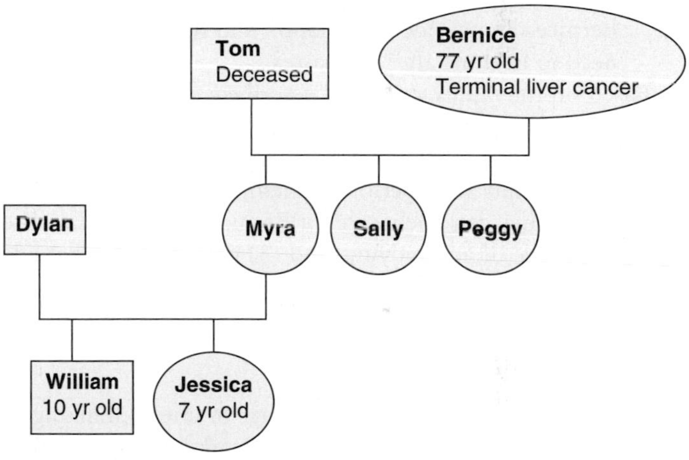

Fig. 26.11 The Brush family genogram.

and evidence into this situation because he or she knows that the disruption to the family and their expected roles will be short term because the grandmother will probably not live for more than four months. However, experience with families also supports this nurse's knowledge that Myra's role conflict may likely increase as her caregiver role becomes more intense as her mother's health declines. By conducting a family genogram, another strength of this family is uncovered: it has a strong internal and external support system. The family determines that the extended family is willing to be involved in the care of Bernice. The intervention is aimed at mobilizing resources to minimize Myra's role conflict. Using the simple action plan outlined previously, the family determined the following:

1. We need the following type of help:
   - Other family members to come every day to relieve Myra
   - Every other weekend, one of Bernice's other daughters will provide care through the night to relieve Myra

- Jobs in the family will be shared to relieve Myra. Dylan will do the shopping, William will clear the table and put dishes in the dishwasher, and Jessica will help fold the clothes and put them away. William and Jessica agreed to help by spending some time each evening with Bernice, such as reading to her or watching TV with her.

2. We need the following information:
   - How to call the hospice nurse when Bernice gets worse or they need immediate help
   - A list of who to call when an emergency occurs
   - A list and numbers of Bernice's health care team
3. We need the following supplies: None at this time
4. We need to involve or tell the following people: Sally and Peggy
5. To make our family action plan happen, we need to . . . (list five things in the order they need to happen):
   - Invite Sally and Peggy over for a family meeting, and include the home hospice nurse
   - Make a list of what weekends Sally and Peggy will help with Bernice
   - Make a calendar with whose turn it is to spend time with Bernice every evening, which will relieve Myra of the care
   - Know what arrangements need to be made now when Bernice can provide information and what arrangements need to be done after she passes

Based on the family story just described, as viewed through the frame of family systems theory, the following interventions were implemented: (1) assisting the family in the role negotiation of tasks and who performs them, (2) educating family members so they can safely care for Bernice now and when she enters the stage of active dying, and (3) determining what additional resources the family needs. After a plan is put into place, it needs to be evaluated periodically.

Evaluation of the Plan

In evaluating the outcome, nurses engage in critical thinking to determine if the plan is working, if it is working fast enough to address the problem, if it is addressing only part of the problem, or if the plan needs to be revised based on changes. When the plan is not working, the nurse and the family work together to determine the barriers interfering with the plan or figure out if something changed in the family story. Family apathy and indecision are known to be barriers in family nursing (Friedman et al., 2003). Friedman et al. (2003) also identified the following nurse-related barriers that can affect achievement of the outcome: (1) nurse-imposed ideas, (2) negative labeling, (3) overlooking family strengths, and (4) neglecting cultural or gender implications. Family apathy may occur because of value differences between the nurse and the family, because the family is overcome with a sense of hopelessness, because the family views the problems as too overwhelming, or because family members have a fear of failure. Additional factors to be considered are that the family may be indecisive because they cannot determine which course of action is better (because they have an unexpressed fear or concern) or because they have a pattern of making decisions only when faced with a crisis.

An important part of the evaluation step in working with families is the decision to terminate the relationship between the nurse and the family. Termination is phasing out the nurse from family involvement. When termination is built into the interventions the family benefits from a smooth transition process. The family is given credit for the outcomes of the interventions that they helped design. Strategies often used in the termination component are decreasing contact with the nurse, extending invitations to the family for follow-up, and making referrals when appropriate. The termination should include a summative evaluation meeting, in which the nurse and family put a formal closure to their relationship.

When termination with a family occurs suddenly, it is important for the nurse to determine the forces bringing about the closure. The family may be initiating the termination prematurely, which requires a renegotiating process. The insurance or agency requirements may be placing a financial constraint on the amount of time the nurse can work with a family. Regardless of how termination comes about, it is important to recognize the transition from depending on the family nurse on some level to having no dependence. Strategies that help with the termination are to (1) increase time between the nurse's visits, (2) develop a plan for the transition, (3) assess the family support systems, (4) make referrals to other resources, and (5) provide a written summary to the family.

SOCIAL AND FAMILY POLICY CHALLENGES

National, state, and local **social and family policies** provide various challenges to nurses' practices. As professionals, public health nurses are accountable for participating in the three core public health functions: assessment, policy development, and assurance.

National **family policy** is government actions that have a direct or indirect effect on families. The range of social policy decisions that affect families is vast, such as health care access and coverage, low-income housing, Social Security, welfare, food stamps, pension plans, affirmative action, and education. Although all government polices affect families in both negative and positive ways, the United States has little overall explicit family policy (Coehlo et al., 2018). Most government policy indirectly affects families. The Administration for Children and Families was created in 1991 as part of the USDHHS to promote the economic and social well-being of families, children, individuals, and communities. However, because of how the government defines family individuals who are members within a family but do not meet the legal definition of "family" as two or more people related by birth, marriage, or adoption are not eligible for many of the services provided by USDHHS (Coehlo et al., 2018). Some of the programs offered by USDHHS include Temporary Assistance to Needy Families (TANF), Head Start, and the Healthy Marriage Initiative. The Family Medical Leave legislation passed in 1993 by the U.S. Congress is an example of a type of family policy that has been positive for families. A family member may take a defined amount of leave for family events (e.g., births, deaths) without fear of losing his or her job. The ACA of 2010 is an example of a national policy that has effects on family policy.

Nurses must become familiar with programs developed by USDHHS and some of the key features of the ACA reforms affecting individuals and their families, which include the following (check out www.HHS.gov/healthcare): DO you want this to be www.USDHHS?

- Health plans can no longer limit or deny benefits to children under the age of 19 due to a pre-existing condition.
- Young adults under the age of 26 may be eligible to be covered under their parent's health plan.
- Insurance companies can no longer arbitrarily cancel a person's health insurance coverage.
- An individual's right to appeal is guaranteed.
- Health plans are prohibited from putting a lifetime dollar limit on most benefits individuals receive.
- Insurance companies must now publicly justify any unreasonable rate hikes.
- Insurance companies are required to spend premium dollars primarily on health care. It does this by enforcing a policy called the "80/20 rule" to hold insurance companies accountable.
- Insurance companies are required to cover certain preventive services at no cost to the individual. There are specific covered preventive services for adults, women, and children.
- The ACA reforms ensure that individuals can seek emergency care at a hospital outside their plan's network without prior approval from their health plan.

State assistance for families varies by state.

The challenges of social policy for families are numerous. Given the ongoing debate as to what constitutes a family, social policies may specify a definition that is not consistent with the family's own definition. Examples include same-sex partnerships and/or marriage, legal definition of parents, reproductive and fertility issues (e.g., a surrogate mother decides she wants to keep the baby), or issues involving care of older adults (e.g., a niece wants to institutionalize an older aunt with dementia because her children are not available). Besides how families define themselves, governments define health care services that affect families.

Teen pregnancy prevention is a monitored health status throughout the United States and a good example of the challenges of family health policy. In some states, any child who is sexually active may have access to reproductive health services. This is a family policy to which some families object, yet the sexually active teenager is protected by a number of laws, both state and federal. The teenager who requests confidential services is protected by Title X and Health Insurance Portability and Accountability Act of 1996 (HIPAA) federal regulations given the state law allowing access to services. Providers can encourage the teen to talk with his or her parents, but ultimately it is the teen's decision. Nurses need to be knowledgeable about these policies since they participate in carrying out family policy and have a responsibility to inform the state regarding the services they provide.

Nurses participate in enforcing laws and regulations that affect the family such as state immunization laws. Most states have some school immunization laws that exclude children from school who are not vaccinated. If the child does not have that state's particular set of immunizations and the parents do not want the child vaccinated, two sets of laws are in conflict: the immunization laws and the school attendance laws. The state could provide a mechanism for a waiver, or the child could be excluded from school, thus making home schooling the only option.

Health care insurance is a social and family policy issue. Medicare and Medicaid, enacted in 1965, provide some health care for the elderly and low-income families. Today Medicare covers nearly 44 million beneficiaries with enrollments expected to rise to 79 million by 2030 (CMS, 2018). Insuring the elderly has proven to be beneficial, yet is fraught with numerous problems. Both living wills and durable power of attorney for health care, legal contracts that designate a person to make health care decisions when the individual is incapacitated, are more commonplace today than in the past. However, without these legal instruments, families are faced with making end-of-life decisions for their loved ones. Although Medicare and Medicaid provide health care to many, a significant population is still uninsured. Emergency departments continue to be the only access to health care for the uninsured and a convenient and accessible source of health care for many without access to a health care provider (Marco et al., 2012).

The H1N1 pandemic was an excellent example of mobilizing community partnerships to solve health problems. In one county health department, space for storing vaccines was insufficient in the county health clinics, so arrangements were made with the law enforcement departments to store vaccines in their secure evidence refrigerators. Other examples of partnering included collaboration with Health and Human Services departments and homeless programs to get at-risk populations and the homeless vaccinated. County health departments and pediatricians worked together to get members of families who had infants under six months of age vaccinated, since these infants were too young to receive the H1N1 vaccine.

These are only a few examples of social and family policy in which nurses are involved. Population-focused nurses need to be involved in making policy at the local, state, and national level that affects families. Using the core public health functions as a framework allows the population-focused nurse to view the broad spectrum of activities that improve the lives of communities, families, and the individuals within those families.

QSEN FOCUS ON QUALITY AND SAFETY EDUCATION FOR NURSES

Targeted Competency: Client-Centered Care

Recognize the client or designee as the source of control and full partner in providing compassionate and coordinated care based on respect for client's preferences, values, and needs.

Important aspects of client-centered care include:

- **Knowledge:** Describe strategies to empower clients or families in all aspects of the health care process.
- **Skills:** Assess level of client's decisional conflict and provide access to resources.
- **Attitudes:** Value active partnership with clients or designated surrogates in planning, implementation, and evaluation of care.

Client-Centered Care Question

Describe how a family assessment is different from an individual client assessment. Beyond immediate family members, who might be included in a client's "family"? Think about the difference between being an advocate for an individual (the client) and an advocate for a family. What different skills are needed?

Prepared by Gail Armstrong, PhD, DNP, ACNS-BC, CNE, Associate Professor, University of Colorado Denver College of Nursing.

PRACTICE APPLICATION

One of the most notable changes in the twenty-first century is women and mothers working outside of the home. In 2017 about 65 percent of women with children under the age of six worked outside the home. In the same year the Bureau of Labor found 71.1 percent of women and 92.5 percent of fathers with children under the age of 18 worked outside the home (Bureau of Labor Statistics, 2018).

A. In what ways does this influence family socialization and affective functions?
B. In what ways does this situation affect the family health care function?
C. How does this impact family nursing?

Answers can be found on the Evolve site.

KEY POINTS

- Families are the context within which health care decisions are made.
- Nurses are responsible for assisting families in meeting health care needs.
- Family nursing is practiced in all settings.
- Family nursing is a specialty area that has a strong theoretical base and is more than just common sense.
- Community health nurses must integrate both family theory and public health theory in their practice.
- There are a variety of family definitions, such as a group of two or more, a unique social group, and two or more persons joined together by emotional bonds.
- The five functions performed by families are economic, reproduction, socialization, affective, and health care.
- Family structure refers to the characteristics, sex, age, and number of the individual members who make up the family unit.
- Family demographics is the study of structures of families and households as well as events that alter the family, such as marriage, divorce, births, and cohabitation. Demographic trends affect the family.
- Family health is difficult to define, but it includes the biological, psychological, sociological, cultural, and spiritual factors of the family system.
- There are four approaches to viewing families: family as context, family as client, family as a system, and family as a component of society.
- Systems theory describes families as a unit of the whole composed of members whose interactional patterns are the focus of attention, in that what affects one member affects all members.
- Family developmental and life cycle theory emphasizes how families change over time and focuses on interactions and relationships among family members.
- Bioecological family theory helps community/public health nurses identify the stressors and potential resources that can affect family adaptation.
- One of the underlying central tenets of family nursing is to build a trusting family-nurse relationship.
- Working with families requires nurses to use therapeutic communication efficiently and skillfully by moving between informal conversation and skilled interviewing strategies.
- Nurses should ask clients whom they consider to be their family and then include those members in the health care plan. Genograms and ecomaps are essential components of any family assessment.
- Families want to be involved in identifying their major problem and designing solutions that are family focused.
- It is important for the nurse to recognize that the family has the right to make its own health decisions.
- The goal of family nursing is to focus care, interventions, and services to optimize the self-care capabilities of families and to achieve the best possible outcomes.
- Nurses working with families must understand the effects of health care reforms at the local, state, and federal levels as all government actions affect the family.

CLINICAL DECISION-MAKING ACTIVITIES

1. Select six or more health professionals and ask them to define family. Analyze the responses for common points and differences. Write your own definition of family.
2. Characterize the different family structures and household arrangements represented in your community. This information may be available from various sources, such as the health department, schools, other social and welfare agencies, and census data. Be specific.
3. Draw your own family genogram and ecomap. Discuss how they are used in family nursing.
4. Discuss the role of nursing related to family policy. Be specific about issues related to family culture.
5. Break into small groups and have students discuss the Brush family presented in the chapter in terms of the three family social science theories. What questions would they ask the family from the different theoretical perspectives? Examine different situations when one theory might be more appropriate to use than another.
6. How might you go about obtaining services for a Hispanic woman who tests positive for diabetes who is uninsured or underinsured?
7. Break into small groups to discuss how you have found judging or reacting to family structure situations that are different from those you personally bring to practice. What helps you try to reframe this situation in order to practice family nursing?
8. You are working with a lesbian family with three children. What barriers or problems do you anticipate with social policies while trying to access resources?

ADDITIONAL RESOURCES

EVOLVE WEBSITE

http://evolve.elsevier.com/Stanhope/community/

- Answers to Practice Application
- Case Study
- Glossary
- Review Questions

REFERENCES

Agency for Healthcare Research and Quality: *National healthcare quality and disparities report*, 2016, USDHHS. Retrieved from http://www.ahrq.gov.

American Nurses Association: *Public Health Nursing: Scope and Standards of Practice*, Silver Spring, MD, 2013, ANA.

American Psychological Association (APA): *Making stepfamilies work*, 2018. Retrieved from http://www.apa.org.

American Public Health Association: *The definition and practice of public health nursing*, 2013. Retrieved from http://www.apha.org.

Annie E. Casey Foundation: *Three in 10 U.S. kids are overweight or obese*, January 30, 2018. Retrieved from https://www.aecf.org.

Ariosto DA, Harper EM, Wilson ML, Hull SC, Nahm ES, Sylvia ML: Population health: a nursing action plan, *J Am Med Inform Assoc* 1:7–10, 2018.

Bailey SC, Fang G, Annis IE, O'Conor R, Paasche-Orlow MK, Wolf MS: Health literacy and 30-day hospital readmission after acute myocardial infarction, *BMJ Open* 5(6):e006975, 2015.

Barnsteiner J, Disch J: Role of the chief nurse officer in ensuring person- and family-centered care, *Nurs Adm Q* 42(3):284–290, 2018.

Belluz J: *The historically low birthrate, explained in 3 charts: Vox*, 2018. Retrieved from https://www.vox.com.

Berkman ND, Sheridan SL, Donahue KE, Halpern DJ, Crotty K: Low health literacy and health outcomes: an updated systematic review, *Ann Inter Med* 155:97–107, 2011.

Bomar PJ: *Nurses and family health promotion: concepts, assessment, and interventions*, ed 3. Philadelphia, PA, 2004, Saunders.

Bridgeland JM, DiIulio JJ, Morison KB: *The silent epidemic: perspectives of high school dropouts*, 2006. Retrieved from https://docs.gatesfoundation.org.

Bronfenbrenner U: *Influences on human development*, Hinsdale, IL, 1972, Dryden Press.

Bronfenbrenner U: *The ecology of human development*, Cambridge, MA, 1979, Harvard University Press.

Bronfrenbrenner U: Ecology of the family as a context for human development: research perspectives. In Paul JL, Churton M, Rosselli-Kostoryz H, et al., editors: *Foundations of special education*, Pacific Grove, CA, 1997, Brooks/Cole.

Brooks T, Wagnerman K, Artiga S, Cornachione E: *Medicaid and CHIP eligibility, enrollment, renewal, and cost sharing policies as of January 2018: findings from a 50-state survey*, Washington, DC, 2018, Kaiser Family Foundation. Retrieved from https://www.kff.org.

Brown SL: Marriage and child well-being: research and policy perspectives, *J Marriage Fam* 72:1059–1077, 2010.

Bureau of Labor Statistics: *Employment characteristics of families summary 2017*, 2018. Retrieved from https://www.bls.gov.

Carlson MJ, McLanahan SS: Fathers in fragile families. In Lamb ME, editor: *The role of the father in child development*, ed 5, Hoboken, NJ, 2010, John Wiley & Sons, pp 241–269.

Carter B, McGoldrick M, editors: *The expanded family life cycle: individual, family, and social perspectives*, ed 3. New York, NY, 2005, Allyn & Bacon.

Casper LM, Coritz A: Family demography. In Kaakinen JR, Gedaly-Duff V, Coehlo DP, et al., editors: *Family health care nursing: theory, practice, and research*, ed 6. Philadelphia, PA, 2018, F.A. Davis, pp 53–81.

Center for Health Information and Analysis: *Performance of the Massachusetts health care system series: a focus on provider quality*, 2015. Retrieved from http://www.chiamass.gov.

Centers for Medicare & Medicaid Services (CMS): *CMS fast facts*, July 2018. Retrieved from https://www.cms.gov.

Centers for Disease Control and Prevention: *Vital signs: obesity among low-income, preschool-aged children-United States, 2008–2011*, 2013. Retrieved from https://www.cdc.gov.

Centers for Disease Control and Prevention: *National Vital Statistics Reports, Volume 66 Number 4: United States Life Tables, 2013*, 2016a. Retrieved from https://www.cdc.gov.

Centers for Disease Control and Prevention: *National Center for Health Statistics. Health, United States, 2016 Report;* DHHS Publication No. 2017-1231, 2016b.

Centers for Disease Control and Prevention: *Provisional number of marriages and marriage rate: United States, 2000-2016; CDC/NCHS National Vital Statistics System*, 2016c. Retrieved from https://www.cdc.gov.

Centers for Disease Control and Prevention: *National Survey of Family Growth*, 2016d. Retrieved from https://www.cdc.gov..

Centers for Disease Control and Prevention: *Reported STDs in the United States*, 2017. Retrieved from https://www.cdc.gov.

Cherlin AJ: *The marriage-go-round: the state of marriage and the family in America today*, Evansville, IN, 2010, Vintage.

Cloonan P, Wood J, Riley JB: Reducing 30-day readmissions: health literacy strategies, *J Nurs Adm* 43:382–387, 2013.

Coehlo DP, Henderson TL, Lester C: Family policy: the intersection of family policies, health disparities, and health care policies. In Kaakinen JR, Coehlo DP, Steele R, Robinson M, editors: *Family health care nursing: theory, practice, and research*, ed 6, Philadelphia, PA, 2018, F.A. Davis, pp 83–112.

Cohen PN: *The family: diversity, inequality, and social change*, New York, NY, 2018. W.W. Norton.

Daugherty J, Copen C: Trends in attitudes about marriage, childbearing, and sexual behavior: United States, 2002, 2006–2010, and 2011–2013, *Natl Health Stat Report* (92):1–10, 2016.

Department of Health & Human Services: *Health care cost and utilization project (HCUP)*, 2010. Retrieved from https://hcup-us.ahrq.gov.

Desilver D: *After recession, more children living with Grandma or Grandpa*, 2013. Retrieved from http://www.pewresearch.org.

DeWalt DA, Boone RS, Pignone M: Literacy and its relationship with self-efficacy, trust and participation in medical decision making, *Am J Health Behav* 31(Suppl3): S27–S35, 2007.

Duvall EM, Miller BC: *Marriage and family development*, ed 6, New York, NY, 1985, Harper & Row.

Eddy L, Bailey A, Doutrich D: Families and community and public health nursing. In Kaakinen JR, Coehlo DP, Steele R, Robinson M, editors: *Family health care nursing: theory, practice, and research*, ed 6, Philadelphia, PA, 2018, F.A. Davis.

Eggly S, Penner LA, Greene M, Harper FW, Ruckdeschel JC, Albrecht TL: Information seeking during "bad news" oncology interactions: question asking by patients and their companions, *Soc Sci Med* 63(11):2974–2985, 2006.

Eibner C, Nowak SA: *Evaluating the CARE Act: implications of a proposal to repeal and replace the Affordable Care Act*, The Commonwealth Fund; May 2016. Retrieved from https://www.rand.org.

Felix HC, Seaberg B, Bursac Z, Thostenson J, Stewart MK: Why do patients keep coming back? Results of a readmitted patient survey, *Soc Work Health Care* 54(1):1–15, 2015.

Foeman A, Lawton BL, Rieger RH: Questioning race: ancestry DNA and dialog on race; *Commun Monogr* 82(2):271–290, 2014.

Friedman AL, Brookmeyer KA, Kachur RE, et al.: An assessment of the GYT: Get yourself tested campaign: an integrated approach to sexually transmitted disease prevention communication, *Sex Transm Dis* 41(3):151–157, 2014.

Friedman MM, Bowden VR, Jones EG: *Family nursing: research, theory, and practice*, ed 5, Upper Saddle River, NJ, 2003, Prentice Hall.

Geiger A, Livingston G: *8 facts about love and marriage in America*, Pew Research Center: Fact-Tank News in the numbers (2), 2018. Retrieved from http://pewrsr.ch/2En5IoI.

George VM, Shocksnider J: Leaders: are you ready for change? The clinical nurse as care coordinator in the new health care system, *Nurs Adm Q* 38(1):78–85, 2014.

Goodwin PY, Mosher WD, Chandra A: Marriage and cohabitation in the United States: a statistical portrait based on cycle 6 (2002) of the National Survey of Family Growth, *Vital Health Stat 23* (28):1–45, 2010.

Grady PA, Gough LL: Self-management: a comprehensive approach to management of chronic conditions, *Am J Public Health* 104(8):e25–e31, 2014.

Green LV, Savin S, Lu Y: Primary care physician shortages could be eliminated through use of teams, nonphysicians, and electronic communication, *Health Aff (Millwood)* 32(1):11–19, 2013.

Hamilton BE, Martin JA, Osterman M, et al.: *Births: provisional data for* 2017, U.S. Department of Health and Human services, Centers for Disease Control and Prevention, National Vital Statistics Systems, Report No 884, May 2018. Retrieved from https://www.cdc.gov.

Hanson SMH: Family health care nursing: an overview. In Hanson SMH, Gedaly-Duff V, Kaakinen JR, editors: *Family health care nursing: theory, practice and research*, ed 3, Philadelphia, PA, 2005, F.A. Davis.

Harrison M, Neufeld A: *Nursing and family caregiving: social support and Nonsupport*, New York, NY, 2009, Springer.

Jang M, Chao A, Whittemore R: Evaluating intervention programs targeting parents to manage childhood overweight and obesity: a systematic review using the RE-AIM framework, *J Pediatr Nurs* 30:877–887, 2015.

Jonsdottir H, Litchfield M, Pharris MD: Partnership in practice, *Res Theory Nurs Pract* 17:51–62, 2003.

Joynt KE, Jha AK: Thirty-day readmissions—Truth and consequences. *N Engl J Med* 366:1366–1369, 2012.

Kaakinen JR: Family health care nursing: an introduction. In Kaakinen JR, Coehlo DP, Steele R, Robinson M, editors: *Family health care nursing: theory, practice, and research*, ed 6, Philadephia, PA, 2018a, F.A. Davis.

Kaakinen JR: Theoretical foundations for the nursing of families. In Kaakinen JR, Coehlo DP, Steele R, Robinson M, editors: *Family health care nursing: theory, practice, and research*, ed 6, Philadelphia, PA, 2018b, F.A. Davis.

Kaakinen JR: Family nursing assessment and intervention. In Kaakinen JR, Coehlo DP, Steele R, Robinson M, editors: *Family health care nursing: theory, practice, and research*, ed 6. Philadelphia, PA, 2018c, F.A. Davis.

Kaiser Family Foundation: *Key facts about the uninsured population*, 2018. Retrieved from https://www.kff.org.

Kim-Godwin YS, Bomar PJ: Family health promotion. In Kaakinen JR, Coehlo DP, Steele R, Robinson M, editors: *Family health care nursing: theory, practice, and research*, ed 5, Philadelphia, PA, 2015, F.A. Davis.

Kinnersley P, Edwards A, Hood K, et al.: Interventions before consultations for helping patients address their information needs, *Cochrane Database Syst Rev* (3):CD004565, 2007.

Kripalani S, Theobald CN, Anctil B, Vasilevskis EE: Reducing hospital readmission rates: current strategies and future directions, *Annu Rev Med* 65:471–485, 2014.

Leahey M, Svavarsdottir EK: Implementing family nursing: how do we translate knowledge into clinical practice? *J Fam Nurs* 15(4):445–460, 2009.

Lee D: *Single mother statistics*, 2018, Retrieved from https://singlemotherguide.com.

Liepelt K: *Home health readmission numbers keep getting better*, 2015, Home Health Care News. Retrieved from https://homehealthcarenews.com.

Livingston G: *Births outside of marriage decline for immigrant women*, October 2018a, Pew Research Center Social & Demographic Trends. Retrieved from http://www.pewsocialtrends.org.

Livingston G: *The changing profile of unmarried parents*, October 2018b, Pew Research Center Social & Demographic Trends. Retrieved from http://www.pewsocialtrends.org.

Long M, Rae M, Claxton G, Damico A: *Trends in employer-sponsored insurance offer and coverage rates, 1999–2014*, 2016, Kaiser Family Foundation Report. Retrieved from https://www.kff.org.

López G, Radford J: *2015, foreign-born population in the United States statistical portrait*, May 3, 2017, Pew Research Center. Retrieved from http://www.pewresearch.org.

Mantwill S, Monestel-Umaña S, Schulz PJ: The relationship between health literacy and health disparities: a systematic review, *PLoS One* 10(12):e0145455, 2015. Retrieved from https://www.ncbi.nlm.nih.gov.

Marco CA, Moskop JC, Schears RM, et al.: The ethics of health care reform: impact on emergency medicine, *Acad Emerg Med* 19(4):461–468, 2012.

McGoldrick M, Gerson R, Petry S: *Genograms: assessment and intervention*, ed 3, New York, NY, 2008, W.W. Norton.

National Alliance for Caregiving: *Young caregivers in the United States*, 2005. Retrieved from https://www.caregiving.org.

National Alliance for Caregiving: *2015 report caregiving in the U.S.*, 2015. Retrieved from https://www.caregiving.org.

National Center for Children in Poverty (NCCP): *Child Poverty*, 2017. Retrieved from http://www.nccp.org.

National Center for Health Statistics: *Health, United States, 2016: with chartbook on long-term trends in health.* Hyattsville, MD, 2017, National Center for Health Statistics.

Office of Disease Prevention and Health Promotion: *2020 Topics and Objectives*, 2010. Retrieved from https://www.healthypeople.gov.

Olson DH, Gorall DM: Circumplex model of marital and family systems. In Walsh F, editor: *Normal family processes*, ed 3, New York, NY, 2003, Guilford, pp 514–517.

Osborne C, McLanahan S: Partnership instability and child well-being, *J Marriage Fam* 69:1065–1083, 2007.

Paavilainen E, Astedt-Kurki P: The client-nurse relationship as experienced by public health nurses: toward better collaboration, *Public Health Nurs* 14:135–188, 1997.

Pemberton D: *Statistical definition of 'family' unchanged since 1930*, 2015, U.S. Census Bogs. Retrieved from https://www.census.gov.

Pew Research Center (PEW): *Parenting in America: the American family today*, 2015. Retrieved from http://www.pewsocialtrends.org.

Porr C, Drummond J, Olson K: Establishing therapeutic relationships with vulnerable and potentially stigmatized clients, *Qual Health Res* 22:384–396, 2012.

Public Health Foundation: *Core competencies for public health professionals*, 2014. Retrieved from http://www.phf.org.

Ray B: Cohabitation's effect on kids, *Psychol Today* March 19, 2013. Retrieved from https://www.psychologytoday.com.

Reinhard SC, Levine C, Samis S: *Home alone: family caregivers providing complex chronic care*, 2012, AARP Public Policy Institute. Retrieved from https://www.aarp.org.

Rosland AM, Piette JD, Choi H, Heisler M: Family and friend participation in primary care visits of patients with diabetes or heart failure: patient and physician determinants and experiences, *Med Care* 49:37–45, 2011.

Salmond SW, Echevarria M: Healthcare transformation and changing roles for nursing, *Orthop Nurs* 36(1):12–25, 2017.

Salmond S: Who is family? Family and decision making. In Lewenson SB, Truglio-Londrigan M, editors: *Decision-making in nursing: thoughtful approaches for practice*, Sudbury, MA, 2008, Jones and Bartlett, pp. 89–104.

Seo J, Goodman MS, Politi M, Blanchard M, Kaphingst KA: *Effect of health literacy on decision-making preferences among medically underserved patients*, *Med Decis Making* 36(4):550–556, 2016.

Siskowski C: Young caregivers: effect of family health situations on school performance, *J Sch Nurs* 22:163–169, 2006.

Smith CM: Home visit: opening the doors for family health. In Maurer FA, Smith CM, editors: *Community public health nursing practice: health for families and populations*, ed 4, St. Louis, MO, 2009, Saunders, pp. 302–326.

Spetz J, Muench U: California nurse practitioners are positioned to fill the primary care gap, but they face barriers to practice, *Health Aff (Millwood)* 37(9):1466–1474, 2018. Retrieved from https://www.healthaffairs.org.

Stepler R: *Smaller share of women ages 65 and older are living alone: More are living with spouse or children*, 2016, Pew Research Center Social & Demographic Trends. Retrieved from http://www.pewsocialtrends.org.

Schwarz H: There are 390,000 gay marriages in the U.S. the Supreme Court could quickly make it half a million, *The Washington Post*, 2015.

Tabacco A: Nursing assessment of the family. In Votroubek W, Tabacco A, editors: *Pediatric home care for nurses: a family-centered approach*, ed 3. Boston, MA, 2010, Jones & Bartlett, pp. 59–80.

Touliatos J, Perlmutter B, Straus M: *Handbook of family measurement techniques*, Newbury Park, CA, 2001, Sage.

U.S. Census Bureau: *Current Population Survey (CPS): Subject Definitions*, 2015. Retrieved from https://www.census.gov.

U.S. Census Bureau: *Table A3. Parents with coresident children under 18, by living arrangement, sex, and selected characteristics*, 2017a. Retrieved from https://www.census.gov.

U.S. Census Bureau: *Table HH-1. Historical Households Tables*, 2017b. Retrieved from https://www.census.gov.

U.S. Department of Health and Human Services: *A comprehensive review of immigrant access to health and human services*, 2012. Retrieved from https://aspe.hhs.gov.

Wald L: *The house on henry street*, New York, NY, 1915, Holt.

White JM, Klein DN: *Family theories: an introduction*, ed 3, Thousand Oaks, CA, 2008, Sage.

Wolff JL, Roter DL, Given B, Gitlin LN: Optimizing patient and family involvement in geriatric home care, *J Healthc Qual* 31(2): 24–33, 2009.

Wolff JL, Roter DL, Boyd CM, et al.: Patient-family agenda setting for primary care patients with cognitive impairment: the SAME page trial, *J Gen Intern Med* 33(9):1478–1486, 2018.

Wu J, Dean KS, Rosen Z, Muennig PA: The cost-effectiveness analysis of nurse-family partnership in the United States, *J Health Care Poor Underserved* 28(4):1578-1597, 2017.

Zwijnenberg NC, Hendriks M, Damman OC, et al.: Understanding and using comparative healthcare information; the effect of the amount of information and consumer characteristics and skills, *BMC Med Inform Decis Mak* 12:101, 2012. Retrieved from https://bmcmedinformdecismak.biomedcentral.com.

27

Family Health Risks

Mollie E. Aleshire, DNP, MSN FNP-BC, PPCNP-BC, FNAP,
Kacy Allen-Bryant, PhD(c), MSN, MPH, RN, and
Debra Gay Anderson, PhD, PHCNS-BC

OBJECTIVES

After reading this chapter, the student should be able to do the following:

1. Evaluate the various approaches to defining and conceptualizing family health.
2. Analyze the major risks to family health.
3. Analyze the interrelationships among individual health, family health, and community health.
4. Explain the relevance of knowledge about family structures, roles, and functions for family-focused nursing in the community.
5. Discuss the implications of policy and policy decisions, at all governmental levels, on families.
6. Explain the application of the nursing process (assessment, planning, implementation, evaluation) to reducing family health risks and promoting family health.

CHAPTER OUTLINE

Early Approaches to Family Health Risks
Concepts in Family Health Risk
Major Family Health Risks and Nursing Interventions
Nursing Approaches to Family Health Risk Reduction
Community Resources

KEY TERMS

Affordable Care Act, p. 605
behavioral risk, p. 614
biological risk, p. 609
contracting, p. 618
economic risk, p. 612
empowerment, p. 619
family crisis, p. 608
family health, p. 605
health risk appraisal, p. 608
health risk reduction, p. 608
health risks, p. 608
home visits, p. 615
in-home phase, p. 617
initiation phase, p. 616
life-event risk, p. 610
policy, p. 605
post-visit phase, p. 618
pre-visit phase, p. 616
risk, p. 607
social risks, p. 612
telehomecare, p. 620
termination phase, p. 618
transitions, p. 610

What is a "family"? Is there one definition that fits all families? Is there a new normal? Was there ever a true "normal" family? Trying to identify only one definition of the family is like trying to cheat death: it doesn't work and you end up feeling foolish for trying. Rather than settling for a universal definition, it seems more appropriate to define families according to the particular issue involved (Purdue University, 2015).

Since the 1960s there has been an evolution of family structure, which includes "more unmarried couples raising children; more gay and lesbian couples raising children; more single women having children without a male partner to help raise them; more people living together without getting married; more mothers of young children working outside the home; more people of different races marrying each other; and more women not ever having children" (Livingston, 2018).

As noted by Pew, history demonstrates that the makeup of families is in constant flux, depending on the current socioeconomic pragmatism. We are reminded of Abraham

Lincoln's father leaving his two children following the death of their mother for the purpose of bringing back a new mother. Was that a "normal" family? Sarah Bush Johnston Lincoln, with three children, married Thomas Lincoln, following the deaths of both of their spouses and, in addition to their combined five children, raised a cousin of Nancy Hank Lincoln. Today, we might call that a "blended" family. We refer to Lincoln's family simply to demonstrate that the "traditional" family was never the "normal" family. As family makeup transitions, those families are often the ones that are the most vulnerable because they do not conform to traditional societal expectations.

Regardless of makeup, the family as a client unit is basic to the practice of population-centered nursing, and nurses are responsible for promoting healthy families in society. As such, families are described as a unique population in public health. The purpose of this chapter is to make the reader aware of influences, both individual and societal, that place families at risk for poor health outcomes, and to discuss how positive outcomes for diverse families can be accomplished through appropriate nursing interventions.

The expanding definition of the family unit presents today's nurse with an array of challenges and opportunities to address the health needs of families. First, it is essential to place the family in the context of the twenty-first century. Some Americans tend to idealize *family* and wish for a return to family values of the past and a golden time for families. However, historical demographic statistics reveal that this prevalence of the idealized family that has often been portrayed in the media never actually existed. Rather than arguing for a return to the "traditional family," serious discussions are needed about how to help today's diverse families succeed. A focus on all family structures is a moral and ethical imperative in the promotion of the health of individuals as well as the health of the community (Nightingale et al., 1978; WHO, 2018).

The varying family structures of today need to be recognized and examined to better understand both the strengths and weaknesses associated with each. Only by doing this will we be able to help all families live healthy and productive lives. Nurses can play an active role in leading and facilitating this learning process. This facilitation can enable better-informed health care policy decisions that have a positive effect on single-parent families, remarried and stepfamilies, gay and lesbian families, grandparent-headed families, and ethnically diverse families, as well as "traditional" families.

A nation's family health care **policy** is a primary determinant of **family health**. Family policy means anything that is done by the government that directly or indirectly affects families. Family health policy and its relative effectiveness demonstrates a government's understanding of families and its role in promoting their health, with an important desired outcome being that families derive a sense of empowerment and are able to take responsibility for their own health (KFF, 2018). The responsibility for family health programs is shared by the federal government with state and local governments. Each state, as well as regions within states, has programs and laws related to family services. The United States is one of the richest and most technologically advanced countries in the world today and yet, despite the profusion of technological advances and the continually growing proportion of the national budget spent on health care, the disparities in health status between different populations of families has continued to grow (Families USA, 2015). These disparities have resulted, at least in part, from previous attempts to develop and implement "family policies" that either directly or indirectly affect specific issues related to family health but which have failed to take a comprehensive system-wide approach.

Although many disparities and inequities continue in the United States, the health care disparities related to health insurance coverage have decreased as a result of the Patient Protection and **Affordable Care Act** (ACA) as more low-income families and families of color have gained health insurance coverage (Artiga et al., 2017). At the 2014 Health Action Conference, Families USA, Vice President Joe Biden spoke of the importance of the Affordable Care Act (discussed throughout this text) and the importance of the ACA for families in the United States. The specific benefits he highlighted were the coverage of pre-existing conditions, mental health coverage, the disparity in the cost of insurance for women and men, the more than three million young adults on their parents' insurance policies, and not receiving medical care simply because one does not have insurance (Biden, 2014). In 2017, federal legislation eliminated the Affordable Care Act's individual health insurance mandate, which is predicted to negatively affect the health insurance coverage and cost of insurance for families (Congressional Budget Office, 2017). Nursing has a rich history in social activism and social justice which should be continued, emphasizing advocacy and policy work to help families and communities become healthier for all populations.

Evidence to date suggests that the United States could benefit from a cohesive family policy designed to enhance the well-being of all families. Such a policy would go a long way toward preventing future crises in vulnerable family populations, such as those in or on the verge of poverty or families overwhelmed with abuse and neglect, by providing a structural safety net to help families to maintain their health in times of disaster, economic downturns, unemployment, health crises, and other situations. An effective family health policy may consider as its foundational element an infrastructure of programs designed to provide access to primary and preventive health care. The building of this foundation requires a multiprofessional process in which nurses can be actively involved. Nurses are educated in community assessment, planning, development, and evaluation activities that emphasize and address issues crucial to promoting and sustaining primary family health. Nurses looking to positively influence family health will want to be aware of and actively participate in the ongoing national debate and dialogue on family health policy that embraces their role as principal constituents in building healthy families.

In establishing health objectives for the nation, an emphasis has been placed on both health promotion and risk reduction. Reducing the risks to segments of the population is a direct way to improve the health of the general population. Specific objectives have been identified related to specific health risks for families. The family is an important environmental factor that affects the health of individuals as well as a social unit whose health is basic to that of the community and the larger population. It is within the family that health values, health habits, and health risk perceptions are developed, organized, and carried out. Individuals' health behaviors are affected by and acted out within the family environment, the larger community, and society.

Family health habits are developed in the same manner in the context of community norms and values, and on the basis of availability and accessibility. For example, in a television commercial for an over-the-counter stimulant, a man is featured who is able to coach his child's basketball team, work at a rehabilitation center, and work as a borough inspector for the city, all while pursuing a college degree at night. The commercial credits the drug for providing the man with the energy needed to be successful in all of these areas. The message is clear: you can, and must, do it all, and taking drugs to succeed is a viable option. The health risks to individual and family health are affected by the societal norms—in this example, the norm is increasing productivity through drugs.

To intervene effectively and appropriately with families to reduce their health risk and thereby promote their health, nurses need to understand not only family structure and functioning, but also family theory, nursing theory, and models of health risk (see Chapters 26 and 27. In addition, the effective nurse needs to look beyond the individual and the family in order to understand the complex environment in which the family exists. Increasing evidence of the effects of social, biological, economic, and life events on health requires a broader approach to addressing health risks for families. Nurses and the communities they serve have a vital interest in exploring new and appropriate options for structuring nursing interventions with families to decrease health risks and to promote health and well-being for all families. It is important for the nurse to focus on families who share similar health risks as a population. Working and planning interventions to reduce health risks in family populations provides a mechanism for shared communication and support among families as well as efficient and effective health care interventions that will not only make the families, but the community as a whole, healthier.

EARLY APPROACHES TO FAMILY HEALTH RISKS

Health of Families

Historically, the study of the family relative to health and illness focused on three major areas: (1) the effect of illness on families, (2) the role of the family in the cause of disease, and (3) the role of the family in its use of services. In his classic review of the family as an important unit, Litman (1974) pointed out the important role that the family (as a primary unit of health care) plays in health and illness and emphasized that the relationship between health, health behavior, and family "is a highly dynamic one in which each may have a dramatic effect on the other" (p. 495). At about this same time, Mauksch (1974) proposed the idea of distinguishing between family health and individual health. Pratt's (1976) examination of the role of the family in health and illness included the role of family health in the promotion of healthy or unhealthy behavior. Pratt proposed and described the *energized family* as being an ideal family type that was most effective in meeting health needs. The energized family is characterized as promoting freedom and change, active contact with a variety of other groups and organizations, flexible role relationships, equal power structure, and a high degree of autonomy in family members. Doherty and McCubbin (1985) proposed a family health and illness cycle consisting of six phases, beginning with family health promotion and risk reduction and continuing through the family's vulnerability to illness, their illness response, their interaction with the health care system, and finally their ways of adapting to illness. This framework continues to be relevant today in caring for families.

Health of the Nation

In recent years, increased attention has been given to improving the health of everyone in the United States. As a result of major public health and scientific advances, the leading causes of morbidity and mortality have shifted from infectious diseases to chronic diseases, accidents, and violence, all of which have strong lifestyle and environmental components. A classic population-focused study in Alameda County, California (Belloc & Breslow, 1971) demonstrated the relationships between seven lifestyle habits and decreased morbidity and mortality. These habits were (1) sleeping seven to eight hours daily, (2) eating breakfast almost every day, (3) never or rarely eating between meals, (4) being at or near recommended height-adjusted weight, (5) never smoking cigarettes, (6) moderate or no use of alcohol, and (7) regular physical activity. These same lifestyle health habits are still important for improved health in the twenty-first century.

The Alameda study has been supported by Dan Buettner's (2009) work with The National Geographic Society and their examination of communities around the world who have not only longevity, but quality of life. Public health nurses (PHNs) will want to read *The Blue Zones: 9 Lessons for Living Longer* for in-depth case studies. The nine lessons include the following:

1. Move naturally: Be active without thinking about it;
2. Hara Hachi Bu: Painlessly cut calories by 20 percent;
3. Plant slant: Avoid meat and processed foods;
4. Grapes of life: Drink red wine in moderation;
5. Purpose now: Take time to see the big picture;
6. Downshift: Take time to relieve stress;
7. Belong: Participate in a spiritual community;
8. Loved ones first: Make family a priority; and
9. Right tribe: Be surrounded by those who share Blue Zone values (Buettner, 2008-2018).

A growing body of literature supports the notion that lifestyle and the environment interact with heredity to cause disease. In response to these findings and to the limited effect of medical interventions on the growing incidence and prevalence of injuries and chronic disease, the government launched a major effort to address the health status of the population. Part of this effort was a report by the Division of Health Promotion and Disease Prevention of the Institute of Medicine that examined the critical components of the physical, socioeconomic, and family environments related to decreasing risk and promoting health (Nightingale et al., 1978). *The Surgeon General's Report on Health Promotion and Disease Prevention* (Califano, 1979) described the risks to good health in the United States at that time. As a result of these reports, health objectives for the nation were established and then evaluated and restated for the year 2000 and again for 2010 (USDHHS, 2000). The *Healthy People 2020* objectives extend the work of the three past documents. An innovative part of this latest *Healthy People* (USDHHS, 2010) update has been a move to become more creative and inclusive. The focus challenges health care providers with a national goal of improving health and will provide the necessary background for future policy initiatives to reduce risk in all populations. Of the four goals, three are particularly important to families:

- Achieve health equity, eliminate disparities, and improve the health of all groups.
- Create social and physical environments that promote good health for all.
- Promote quality of life, healthy development, and healthy behaviors across all life stages.

With the notion of **risk**, any factor resulting in a predisposition toward or an increased likelihood of ill health takes on increased importance. Specific attention is being paid to those environmental and behavioral factors that lead to ill health with or without the influence of heredity. Reducing health risks is a major step toward improving the health of the nation. Although the family is considered an important environment related to achieving important health objectives, limited attention and research have been directed at family health risks and the role of society in promoting healthy families.

HEALTHY PEOPLE 2020

Objectives Related to Family and Home Health

- **EH 18:** Decrease the number of U.S. homes that are found to have lead-based paint or related hazards.
- **MICH-11:** Increase abstinence from alcohol, cigarettes, and illicit drugs among pregnant women.
- **NWS-12:** Eliminate very low food security among children in U.S. households.
- **TU-14:** Increase the proportion of smoke-free homes.

From U.S. Department of Health and Human Services: *Healthy People 2020*, Washington, DC, 2010, U.S. Government Printing Office.

CONCEPTS IN FAMILY HEALTH RISK

The Health Promotion Model (2019) continues to be useful in research that is done with families. This health promotion model states there are two factors that motivate individuals to participate in positive health behaviors. One is a desire to promote one's own health, using behaviors that have been determined to increase the individual, family, community, and society's well-being, and in the process, actually moving toward not only individual self-actualization, but a society actualization as well. The second factor is a desire to protect health, using those same behaviors in an effort to decrease the probability of ill health and provide active protection against illness and dysfunction in families (Murdaugh et al., 2019). Understanding family health risk requires an examination of several related concepts: family health, family health risk, risk appraisal, risk reduction, life events, lifestyle, and family crisis. These concepts will be defined and discussed here. It is important to remember that *health* can be defined in a number of ways, and it is defined by individuals and families within their own culture and value system.

Family Health

Family theorists refer to healthy families but generally do not define family health (White et al., 2015). Based on the variety of perspectives on family (see Chapters 26 and 27), definitions of healthy families can be derived within the guidelines of the framework associated with that perspective. For example, within the perspective of the developmental framework, family health can be defined as possessing the abilities and resources to accomplish family developmental tasks. Thus, the accomplishment of stage-specific tasks is one indicator of family health.

CHECK YOUR PRACTICE

As a student in public health nursing you have been assigned to work with a group of families in a low-income community in your city. Your assessment indicates that these families are not accomplishing their stage specific tasks, which may affect their family health. What would you do to assist these families as a community work toward improved family health?

Because the family unit is a part of many societal systems, the systems perspective will be discussed in more detail. Using the Neuman Systems Model (Beckman & Fawcett, 2017), family health is defined in terms of system stability as characterized by five interacting sets of factors: physiological, psychological, sociocultural, developmental, and spiritual. The client family is seen as a whole system with the five interacting factors. The Neuman Systems Model is a wellness-oriented model in which the nurse uses the strengths and resources of the family to keep the system stable while adjusting to stress reactions that lead to health change and wellness. In other words, this model focuses on family wellness in the face of change. Because change is inevitable in every family, the Neuman Systems Model proposes that families have a flexible external line of defense, a normal line of defense, and an internal line of resistance. When a life event is big enough to contract the flexible line of defense (a protective mechanism) and breaks through the normal line of defense, the family feels stress. The degree of wellness is determined by the amount of energy it takes for the system to become and remain stable. When more energy is available than is being used, the system remains stable.

Examples of energy-building characteristics in this system are social support, resources, and prevention (or avoidance) of stressors. Nurses can use preventive health care both to reduce the possibility that a family encounters a stressor and to help strengthen the family's flexible line of defense. The following clinical example applies the Neuman Systems Model to one family's situation:

The Harris family consists of Ms. Harris (Gloria), 12-year-old Kevin, 8-year-old Leisha, and Ms. Harris's mother, 75-year-old Betty. Kevin was recently diagnosed with insulin-dependent diabetes mellitus, and the family was referred by the endocrinology clinic to the nursing service at the local health department to work with the family in adjusting to the diagnosis.

The focus of the Neuman Systems Model would be to assess the family's ability to adapt to this stressful change and then focus on their strengths in the stabilizing process. The *five interacting variables* would compose an important component of the assessment:

- *Physiological:* Is the Harris family physically able to deal with Kevin's illness? Is everyone else in the family currently healthy? Are there current health stressors?
- *Psychological:* How well will the family be able to deal with the illness psychologically? Are their relationships stable and healthy? Are there any memories of other family members with diabetes?
- *Sociocultural:* How will the sociocultural variable come into play in Kevin's illness? Does the family have social support? Are the treatment and diagnosis culturally sensitive? Can family members support each other?
- *Developmental:* How will Kevin's development as a preadolescent be affected by diabetes? How will the family's development change? How will Kevin's diagnosis affect Leisha?
- *Spiritual:* How will the family's spiritual beliefs be affected by the diagnosis? What effect will they have on his treatment and willingness to adhere to therapy?

Health Risk

Several factors contribute to the development of healthy or unhealthy outcomes. Clearly, not everyone exposed to the same event will have the same outcome. The factors that determine or influence whether disease or other unhealthy results occur are called **health risks**. Control of health risks is done through disease prevention and health promotion efforts. Health risks can be classified into three general categories: (1) inherited biological risks (including age-related risks), (2) environmental risks (composed of social factors, economic, and physical aspects), and (3) behavioral risks (USDHHS, 2010). These three categories of risk are discussed later in terms of family health risk, under Major Family Health Risks and Nursing Interventions (USDHHS, 2010).

Although single risk factors can influence outcomes, the combined effect of accumulated risks is often greater than the sum of the individual effects. For example, a family history of cardiovascular disease is a single biological risk factor that is exacerbated by smoking (a behavioral risk that is more likely to occur if other family members also smoke). This risk factor can also be affected either positively or negatively by diet and exercise. Diet and exercise are influenced both by family and society's norms. Although the demographics may be changing, residents of the Northwest and West have historically been more likely to eat heart-healthy diets and to exercise compared with people who live in the Midwest and South; thus, communities in the Northwest and West are often more supportive of exercise programs, bicycle paths, and diets lower in fat than communities in other parts of the United States. This illustrative example of how the combined effect of a family history, family behavioral risks, and society's influences is more than just the sum of the three individual behavioral risk factors (smoking, diet, and exercise) and demonstrates how a nurse working with populations of families and intervening within a community is more likely to reduce the effects of the health risks overall and produce a healthier community as well as a healthier family unit.

Health Risk Appraisal

Health risk appraisal refers to the process of assessing for the presence of specific factors in each of the categories that have been identified as being associated with an increased likelihood of an illness, such as cancer, or an unhealthy event, such as an automobile accident. Several techniques have been developed to accomplish health risk appraisal, including computer software programs and paper-and-pencil instruments. One technique is the Youth Risk Behavior Surveillance instruments of the Centers for Disease Control and Prevention (CDC, 2017). The general approach is to determine whether and to what degree a risk factor is present. On the basis of scientific evidence, each factor is weighted, and a total score is derived. This appraisal method provides an individual score that can be examined as a whole within the family being assessed, thus appraising the health risks that are likely to be experienced by other members of the family. Additional research is needed to determine if the individual appraisals can be used to determine family risk.

Health Risk Reduction

Health risk reduction is based on the assumption that decreasing the number of risks or the magnitude of risk will result in a lower probability of an undesired event occurring. For example, to decrease the likelihood of adolescent substance abuse, family behaviors such as parents not drinking, alcohol not available in the home, and family contracts related to alcohol and drug use may be useful. Health risks can be reduced through a variety of approaches, such as those just described. It is important to note the specific risk and the family's tolerance of it. Murdaugh et al. (2019) provide examples of different kinds of risks:

- Voluntarily assumed risks are better tolerated than those imposed by others.
- Risks over which scientists debate and as a result have some level of uncertainty as to their magnitude are more feared than risks on which scientists agree.
- Risks of natural origin are often considered less threatening than those created by humans.
- Thus, risk reduction is a complex process that requires knowledge of the specific risk and the family's perceptions of the nature of the risk.

Family Crisis

A **family crisis** occurs when the family is not able to cope with an event or multiple events and becomes disorganized or dysfunctional. When the demands of the situation exceed the resources of the family, a family crisis exists. When families experience a crisis or a crisis-producing event, they attempt to gather their resources to deal with the demands created by the situation. Price et al. (2017) differentiate between family resources and family coping strategies. The former are the resources, such as money and extended family, that a family has available to them. The latter are the family's efforts to manage, adapt, or deal with the stressful event in order to achieve balance in the family system (Price et al., 2017). Thus, if a family were to experience an unexpected illness of the primary wage earner, family resources might include financial assistance from relatives or emotional support. Family coping strategies, in contrast, would include whether the family was able to ask a relative to loan them emergency funds or was able to talk with relatives about the worries they were experiencing. On the basis of the existing literature, Friedman et al. (2003) developed a system of coping strategies (Table 27.1).

It is important to note that the amount of support available to families in times of crisis from government and nongovernment agencies varies in different regions, states, and locales. In addition, the rules and conditions of support often differ and may inhibit families from seeking support, particularly if the conditions are demeaning. Nurses must be aware and sensitive to these differences in assessing the accessibility of support resources to families.

TABLE 27.1 Framework of Coping Strategies

Internal Strategies (From Within Family)	Processes for Coping
1. Cognitive	1. Be accepting of the situation and others.
	2. Gain useful knowledge. Use of Internet helpful.
	3. Collaborate in problem solving (reframe the situation).
2. Relationships	4. Increase cohesion (togetherness).
	5. Increase flexibility.
	6. Share feelings and thoughts.
	7. Increase family structure.
3. Communication	8. Be open and honest.
	9. Listen to one another.
	10. Be sensitive to nonverbal communication.
	11. Use humor when appropriate.
External Strategies	**Processes for Coping**
4. Community links	12. Maintain links in organizations.
5. Spiritual	13. Be more involved in religious activities.
	14. Increase faith or seek help from God.
6. Social support	15. Seek help and support from others.

From Friedman M, Bowden V, Jones E: *Family nursing: research, theory and practice*, ed. 5, Upper Saddle River, NJ, 2003, Prentice Hall.

MAJOR FAMILY HEALTH RISKS AND NURSING INTERVENTIONS

As mentioned earlier, risks to a family's health arise in three major areas: biological, environmental, and behavioral. In most instances, a risk in one of these areas may not be enough to threaten family health, but a combination of risks from two or more categories could threaten health. For example, a family history of cardiovascular disease by itself may not indicate an increased risk, but the health risk is often increased by an unhealthy lifestyle. An understanding of each of these categories provides the basis for a comprehensive perspective on family health risk assessment and intervention.

Healthy People 2020 targets areas in health promotion, health protection, preventive services, and surveillance and data systems to describe age-related objectives (USDHHS, 2010). Included in the area of health promotion are physical activity and fitness, nutrition, tobacco use, use of alcohol and other drugs, family planning, mental health and mental disorders, and violent and abusive behavior. Health protection activities include issues related to unintentional injuries, occupational safety and health, environmental health, food and drug safety, and oral health. Preventive services, designed to reduce risks of illness, include maternal and infant health, heart disease and stroke, cancer, diabetes and other chronic disabling conditions, human immunodeficiency virus (HIV) infection, sexually transmitted diseases, immunization for infectious diseases, and clinical preventive services. The interrelationships among the various groups of risk are clear when the objectives for the nation are considered. Most of the national health objectives are based on risk factors of groups or populations in a variety of categories like age, gender, and health problems. However, it is important to recognize that some of these factors also relate to and have potential effects on the individuals' families, work, school, and communities.

Family Health Risk Appraisal

Assessment of family health risk requires many approaches. As in any assessment, the first and most important task is to get to know the family, their strengths, and their needs (see Chapter 26). The following discussion focuses on appraisal of family health risks in the areas of biological and age-related risk, social and physical environmental risk, and behavioral risk. Box 27.1 provides some definitions related to family health.

Biological and Age-Related Risk. The family plays an important role in both the development and the management of a disease or condition. Several illnesses have a family component that can be accounted for by either genetics or lifestyle patterns. These factors contribute to the **biological risk** for certain conditions. Patterns of cardiovascular disease, for example, can often be traced through several generations of a family. Such families are said to be at risk for cardiovascular disease. How or whether cardiovascular disease is found in a family is often influenced by the lifestyle of the family. Research evidence consistently supports the positive effects of diet, exercise, and stress management on preventing or delaying cardiovascular disease. The

BOX 27.1 Definitions Related to Family Health

Determinants of health: An individual's biological makeup influences health through interaction with social and physical environments as well as behavior.

Behaviors: These may be learned from other family members.

Social environment: This includes the family, and it is where culture, language, and personal and spiritual beliefs are learned.

Physical environment: Hazards in the home may affect health negatively, and a clean and safe home has a positive influence on health.

development of hypertension can be managed by following a low-sodium diet, maintaining a normal weight, exercising regularly, and using effective stress management techniques, such as meditation (Vooradi & Mateti, 2016). Diabetes mellitus is another disease with a strong genetic pattern, and the family plays a major role in the management of the condition. Family patterns of obesity increase the risk in individuals for a number of conditions, including heart disease, hypertension, diabetes, some types of cancer, and gallbladder disease (Bouchard, 2010; Choquet & Meyre, 2011; USDHHS, 2010). The role of genetics is becoming increasingly important in health care and is discussed in Chapter 12. It is often difficult to separate biological risks from individual lifestyle factors.

Transitions (movement from one stage or condition to another) are times of potential risk for families. Age-related or **life-event risks** often occur during transitions from one developmental stage to another. Transitions present new situations and demands for families. These experiences often require that families change behaviors, schedules, and patterns of communication; make new decisions; reallocate family roles; learn new skills; and identify and learn to use new resources. The demands that transitions place on families have implications for the health of the family unit and individual family members and can be considered as life-event risks. How well prepared families are to deal with a transition depends on the nature of the event. If the event is normative, or anticipated, then it is possible for families to identify needed resources, make plans, learn new skills, or otherwise prepare for the event and its consequences. This kind of anticipatory preparation can increase the family's coping ability and lessen stress and negative outcomes. If, on the other hand, the event is non-normative, or unexpected, families have little or no time to prepare and the outcome can be increased stress, crisis, or even dysfunction. Table 27.2 lists family stages and the developmental tasks associated with each stage (Friedman et al., 2003).

Several normative events have been identified for families. The developmental model organizes these events into stages and identifies important transition points. It provides a useful framework for identifying normative events and preparing families to cope successfully with related demands. The developmental tasks associated with each stage identify the types of skills families need. The kinds of normative events families

TABLE 27.2 Eight Major Stages and Eight Family Development Tasks in the Family Life Cycle

Stages of the Family Life Cycle	Positions in the Family	Family Developmental Tasks
Stage 1. The married couple	Wife/husband	Establishing a mutually satisfying marriage. Adjusting to pregnancy Fitting into the kin network
Stage 2. Childbearing	Wife/mother Husband/father Infant(s)	Having and adjusting to an infant Establishing a satisfying home for parents
Stage 3. Preschool-aged children	Wife/mother Husband/father Daughter/sister Son/brother	Adapting to the needs of preschool children Coping with energy depletion and lack of privacy as parents
Stage 4. School-aged children	Wife/mother Husband/father Daughter/sister Son/brother	Fitting into the community Encouraging children's educational achievements
Stage 5. Teenage children	Wife/mother Husband/father Daughter/sister Son/brother	Balancing freedom with responsibility Establishing post-parental interests
Stage 6. Launching the children	Wife/mother/grandmother Husband/father/grandfather	Launching youth into adulthood Maintaining a supportive home base
Stage 7. Middle-aged parents	Wife/mother/grandmother Husband/father/grandfather	Refocusing on the marriage relationship Maintaining kin ties with older and younger generations
Stage 8. Aging family members	Widow/widower Wife/mother/grandmother Husband/father/grandfather	Coping with death and living alone Selling the family home Adjusting to retirement

From DeFrain J: *Getting connected, staying connected: loving one another, day by day,* June 20, 2012, iUniverse, Board of Regents of the University of Nebraska, Lincoln, Nebraska, Table 2-1.

experience are usually related to the addition or loss of a family member, such as the birth or adoption of a child, the death of a grandparent, a child moving out of the home to go to school or take a job, or the marriage of a child. There are health-related responsibilities associated with each of these tasks. For example, the birth or adoption of a child requires that families learn about human growth and development, parenting, immunizations, management of childhood illnesses, normal childhood nutrition, and safety issues.

Non-normative events present different kinds of issues for families. Unexpected events can be either positive or negative. Getting a job promotion or inheriting a substantial sum of money may be unexpected but are usually positive events. More often, non-normative events are unpleasant, such as a major illness, divorce, death of a child, or loss of the main family income.

Both normative and non-normative life events pose potential risks to the health of families. Even events that are generally viewed as being positive require changes and can place stress on a family. The normative event of the birth of a child, for example, requires considerable changes in family structures and roles. Furthermore, family functions are expanded from previous levels, requiring families to add new skills and establish additional resources. These changes can in turn result in strain and, if adequate resources are not available, stress. Therefore, to adequately assess life risks, both normative and non-normative events occurring in the family need to be considered. Regardless of whether a life event is normative or non-normative, it is often a source of stress for families. Several theoretical frameworks have been developed to examine the processes of family stress and coping. Perhaps the most widely used is the ABC-X model. The model was originally developed by Hill (1949) and was based on work with families separated by war. In the model, crisis (X) was proposed to be a product of the nature of the event (A), the family's definition of the event (B), and the resources available to the family (C). Doherty and McCubbin (1985) extended the model to the Double ABC-X model to encompass the period after the initial crisis and introduced the idea of a pile-up of stressors. Adaptation or maladaptation by the family is proposed to be determined by the pile-up of stressors (Aa), the family's perception of the crisis (Bb), and new resources and coping strategies (Cc).

Conger et al. (2014) challenged this step-by-step view of families and stress and coping. They advocated a more systems-oriented concept of family stress. They pointed out that families develop a series of processes to manage or transform inputs to the system (e.g., energy, time) to outputs (e.g., cohesion, growth, love) known as *rules of transformation.* Over time, families develop these patterns in enough quantity and variety to handle most changes and challenges; this is referred to as *requisite variety of rules of transformation.* However, when families do not have an adequate variety of rules to allow them to respond to an event, the event becomes stressful. Rather than being able to deal with the situation, they fall into a pattern of trying to figure out what it is they need to do, and the usual tasks of the family are not adequately addressed. Rules that were implicit in the family are now reconsidered and redefined.

Furthermore, the family stress theory of Conger et al. (2014) proposed three levels of stress: level I is change "in the fairly specific patterns of behavior and transforming processes" (e.g., change in who does which household chores); level II is change "in processes that are at a higher level of abstraction" (e.g., change in what are defined as family chores); and level III is change in highly abstract processes (e.g., family values) (Conger et al., 2014). Coping strategies can be identified to address each level of stress that families go through in sequence, if necessary (see the Evidence-Based Practice box).

EVIDENCE-BASED PRACTICE

Building the evidence based case for the effectiveness of a nursing intervention program is not a goal that can be accomplished quickly. Rather, such a case requires many years of testing and refining interventions, as well as the ongoing and arduous task of obtaining funding from federal and state entities. It is also dependent on the intense advocacy involved in influencing legislators to achieve health and social policy reform necessary to enable lasting change. The Nurse-Family Partnership (NFP) is one such program that was begun in the late 1970s by a social and behavioral sciences major who focused on psychology, specifically with early infant attachment. Dr. David Olds would later complete his doctoral studies under the mentoring of Dr. Urie Bronfenbrenner, a professor at Cornell University, and continued his research with the goal of improving the lives of children. Using nurses only for the intervention study, Olds set out to study the impact that home visitation to new mothers by nurses would have on social and health outcomes of both mother and baby. The home visitation began during pregnancy. Olds conducted randomized controlled studies in diverse locations and diverse populations. He also completed a study that compared the use of nurses with the use of paraprofessionals and determined that the use of nurses had more positive outcomes than did the use of paraprofessionals.

Outcomes of these studies have demonstrated that new mothers receiving nurse home visits, beginning during pregnancy and continuing for two years, exhibit improvements to maternal health, decrease in childhood injuries, lower rates of child abuse, and greater spacing of subsequent pregnancies when compared with new mothers not receiving nurse home visits. The results have also shown that these mothers are more likely to enter the workforce, and longitudinal data have demonstrated that the nurse-visited families are more economically self-sufficient and that criminal behavior has been less in both mothers and children. The Olds model, developed in 2004, became the NFP, a nonprofit organization, in an effort to make it more accessible as well as to ensure quality control, educate nurses, and monitor existing programs. NFP is currently operating in 32 states. Criteria have been established to keep the program true to Olds' fundamental principles outlined here to ensure consistent quality and positive outcomes (Nurse-Family Partnership, 2018)

Of his model, Olds says, "It reduces injuries to children. It helps families plan future pregnancies and create better spacing between the birth of the first and second children. It helps women find employment. It helps improve prenatal health. It improves children's school readiness."

Nurse Use

The NFP developed by Dr. Olds and his team provides the ultimate example of the effects of nursing on the individual, family, and community. From care of the pregnant woman, to the care of her newborn and family, to the policy implications that provide for healthier families and healthier communities, the NFP makes a difference in outcomes. The NFP is nursing at its very best—it provides evidence-based early nursing interventions that result in the positive outcomes listed earlier rather than the poor societal outcomes often described with teen pregnancies and single parenting. The evidence-based NFP model should continue to be tested in other populations and environments, such as in foster and adoptive homes early in the foster or adoption process, thus allowing the benefits of the program to have an even broader reach.

References

The Nurse-Family Partnership: *The David Olds story*, Denver, CO, 2018, Nurse-Family Partnership.

The Nurse-Family Partnership: *From a healthy babies program to crime prevention, Nurse-Family Partnership is validated by research*, Denver, CO, 2018, Nurse-Family Partnership.

Eckenrode J, Campa M, Luckey DW, et al.: Long-term effects of prenatal and infancy nurse home visitation on the life course of youths: 19-year follow-up of a randomized trial, *Arch Pediatr Adolesc Med* 164(1):9–15, 2010.

Biological Health Risk Assessment. One of the most effective techniques for assessing the patterns of health and illness in families is the genogram (see Chapter 26 for further discussion and an example). Briefly, a genogram is a drawing that shows the family unit of immediate interest and includes several generations using a series of circles, squares, and connecting lines. Basic information about the family, relationships in the family, and patterns of health and illness can be obtained by completing the genogram with the family. Dates of birth, marriage, death, and other important events can be indicated where appropriate. Major illness or conditions can be listed for each family member. Patterns can be quickly assessed and provide a guide for the health interviewer about health areas that need further exploring.

A more intensive and quantitative assessment of a family's biological risk can be achieved through the use of a standard family risk assessment. Because such assessments involve other areas in addition to biological risk, one will be described later, after the description of assessment of other types of risk.

Community-level support groups (e.g., Families Anonymous, Bereaved Parents, Parents and Friends of Lesbian and Gay Persons, Single Parents) have been successful in assisting families in dealing with a variety of stressful situations and crises that arise from both life events and age-related events. Nurses have been instrumental in developing and moderating such groups. These are examples of intervening with families as a specific population.

Environmental Risk. The importance of **social risks** to family health is gaining increased recognition (see Chapters 8 and 26. Living in high-crime neighborhoods, in communities without adequate recreation or health resources, in communities that have major noise pollution or chemical pollution, or in other high-stress environments increases a family's health risk. One social stress is discrimination, whether racial, cultural, or other. The psychological burden resulting from discrimination is itself a stressor, and it adds to the effects of other stressors. The implication of these examples of risky social situations is that they contribute to the stressors experienced by the families. If adequate resources and coping processes are not available, breakdowns in health can occur (Artigia, 2018)

The poor are at greater risk for health problems (see Chapter 33. **Economic risk**, which is related to social risk, is determined by the relationship between family financial resources and the demands on those resources. Having adequate financial resources means that a family is able to purchase the necessary commodities related to health. These include adequate housing, clothing, food, education, and health or illness care. The amount of money that a family has available is relative to situational, cultural, and social factors. A family may have an income well above the poverty level, but because of a devastating illness in a family member, they may not be able to meet financial demands. Likewise, families from ethnic populations or families with same-sex parents frequently experience discrimination in finding housing. Even if they find housing, they may not be welcome and may be harassed, resulting in increased stress.

Unfortunately, not all families have access to health care insurance. For families at the poverty level, programs such as Medicaid are available to pay for health and illness care. Families in the upper-income brackets usually have health insurance through an employer, or they can afford to either purchase health insurance or pay for health care out of pocket. An increasing number of middle-income families have major wage earners in jobs that do not have health benefits. These people often do not have enough income to purchase health care but earn too much money to qualify for public assistance programs. Consequently, many families have financial resources that allow them to maintain a subsistence level but that limit the quality of their purchasing power. Illness care may be available, but preventive care may not; food high in fat and calories may be affordable, whereas fresh fruit and vegetables are not. Nutritious diets are important in preventing illness and promoting health. Along with providing children, pregnant women, and breastfeeding mothers with nutritious foods, the Women, Infants, and Children (WIC) program links low-income families to the health care system through referrals and collaboration with health care organizations. Children in WIC are more likely to receive both preventive and curative care, such as the receipt of immunizations, more often than children not participating in WIC (Thomas et al., 2014). WIC continues to be touted as one of the most effective federally funded nutrition programs in the United States (Carlson & Neuberger, 2017; USDA, 2018).

Environmental Risk Assessment. Assessment of environmental health risk is less well-defined and developed. While the genogram portrays the family relationships, details on the relationships that the family has with others (e.g., relatives and neighbors), their connections with other social units (e.g., church, school, work, clubs, and organizations), and the flow of energy (positive or negative) can be assessed through the use of an ecomap (Holtslander et al., 2014). The genogram (the Graham family in Fig. 27.1) represents the family structure, sibling subsystem, patterns of repetition, and life events. This

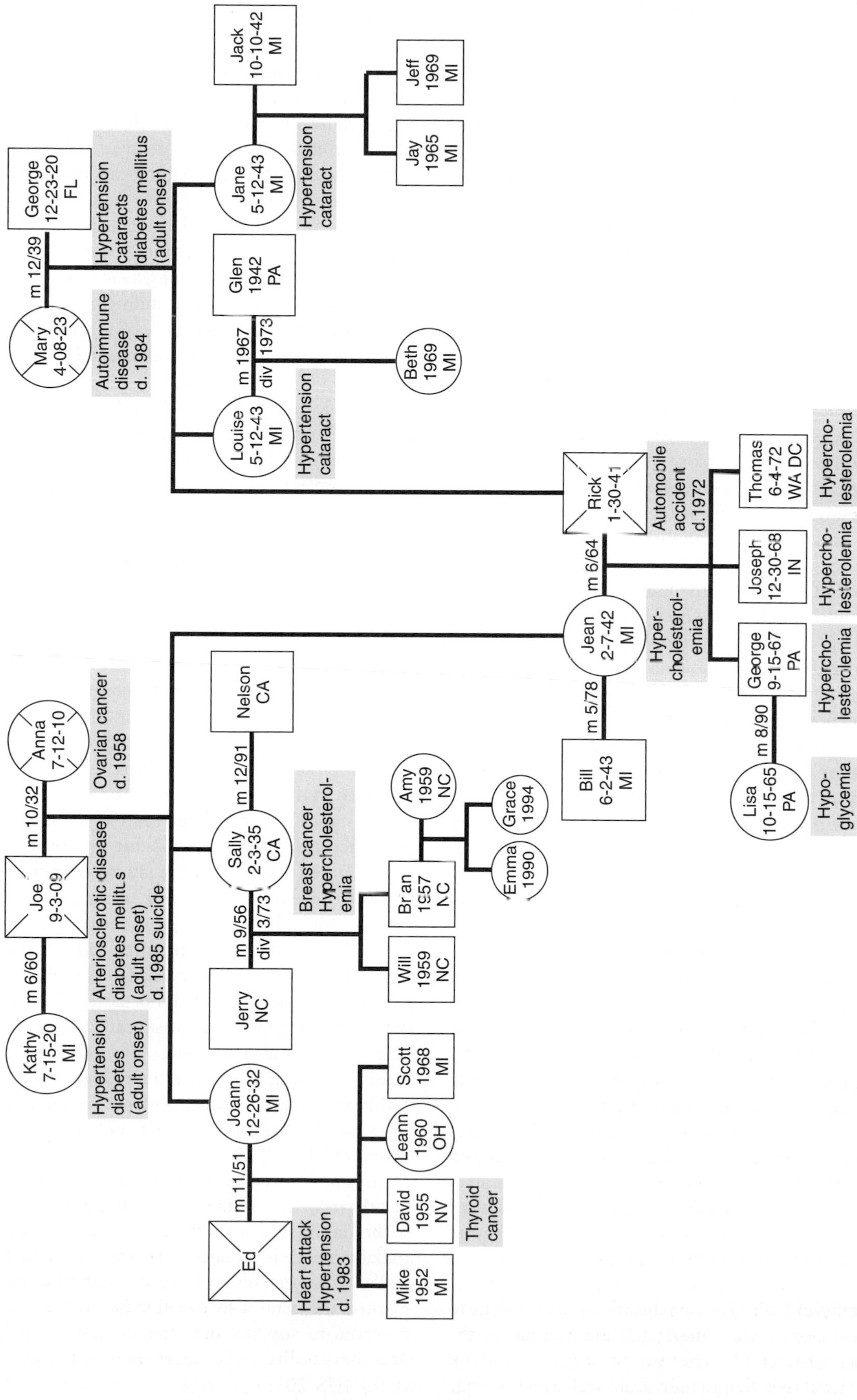

Fig. 27.1 Family genogram of the Graham family. (Developed by Carol Loveland-Cherry for the fifth edition of this book.)

family genogram can be used to develop an ecomap showing interactions with other groups and organizations, accomplished using a series of circles and lines (see Chapter 26). The family of interest is represented by a circle in the middle of the page; other groups and organizations are then indicated by other circles. Lines, representing the flow of energy, are drawn between the family circle and the circles representing other groups and organizations. An arrowhead at the end of each line indicates the direction of the flow of energy (into or out of the family), and the darkness of the line indicates the intensity of the energy. A Graham family ecomap would indicate that much of the family energy goes into work (also a source of stress for the parents). Major sources of energy for the Grahams would be their immediate and extended families and friends.

In addition to the support network shown by the ecomap, other aspects of social risk include characteristics of the neighborhood and community where the family lives. A nurse who has worked in the general geographic area may already have performed a community assessment (see Chapter 17) and have a working knowledge of the neighborhood and community. It is important, however, for the nurse to obtain information from the family to understand their perceptions of the community.

Information about the origins of the family is useful to understand other social resources and stressors. Information about how long the family has lived in their current location and the immigration patterns of the family and their ancestors provides insight into the pressures they experience.

Economic risk is one of the foremost predictors of health. Families often consider financial information private, and both the nurse and the family may be uncomfortable when discussing finances. It is not necessary to know actual family income except in certain instances when it is necessary to determine whether families are eligible for programs or benefits. It is useful to know whether the family's resources are adequate to meet their needs, and it is important to understand that the family may be quite comfortable with their finances and standard of living, which may be different from those of the health care provider. The provider should not try to push financial values onto the family. In terms of health risk, it is important to understand the resources that families have to obtain health/illness care; adequate shelter, clothing, and food; and access to recreation. Families with limited resources may qualify for programs such as Medicaid, WIC, or Maternal Support Systems/Infant Support Systems. Families with wage earners with medical benefits and those with enough income are usually able to afford adequate health care. Unfortunately, in a growing number of families, the main wage earner is employed but receives no medical benefits and the salary is not sufficient for health promotion or illness care. This is a policy issue for which nurses are very capable of drafting legislation and providing testimony related to the stories of families in their caseloads. (See Chapter 9 for a discussion of policy involvement by nurses.)

Behavioral (Lifestyle) Risk. Personal health habits continue to contribute to the major causes of morbidity and mortality in the United States (see Chapter 13). The pattern of personal health habits and **behavioral risk** defines individual and family lifestyle risk. The family is the basic unit within which health behavior—including health values, health habits, and health risk perceptions—is developed, organized, and performed. Families maintain major responsibility for determining what food is purchased and prepared, setting sleep patterns, planning family activities, setting and monitoring norms about health and health risk behaviors, determining when a family member is ill, determining when health care should be obtained, and carrying out treatment regimens. In 2016 more than half of all deaths in the United States were attributed to heart disease or cancer, both of which identify diet as a causative factor (NCHS, 2017). General guidelines from the U.S. Department of Health and Human Services and the U.S. Department of Agriculture include eating a variety of foods; maintaining healthy weight; choosing a diet low in fat and cholesterol, including plenty of vegetables, fruits, and grain products; limiting use of sugars, salt, and sodium; and consuming alcohol only in moderation (USDHHS, 2015; USDA, 2018).

Multiple health benefits of regular physical activity have been identified; regular physical exercise is effective in promoting and maintaining health and preventing disease. Physical activity can help to prevent obesity, diabetes, heart disease, cancer, osteoporosis, and depression (CDC, 2018).

Among the benefits of regular physical activity are increased muscle strength, endurance, and flexibility; management of weight; prevention of colon cancer, stroke, and back injury; and prevention and management of coronary heart disease, hypertension, diabetes, osteoporosis, and depression (USDHHS, 2010). Families can structure time and activities for family members. It is helpful when the community in which they live promotes exercise by having accessible parks and walking or biking paths that help families select activities that provide moderate, regular physical exercise, rather than sedentary activities in the home setting.

Substance use and abuse, such as the use of drugs, alcohol, or tobacco, is a major contributor to morbidity and mortality in the United States. Drug use is a major social and health problem. Drug use is associated with transmission of HIV, fetal alcohol syndrome, liver disease, unwanted pregnancy, delinquency, school failure, violence, and crime (NIDA, 2014). Drunk driving is also a public health hazard. It is well known that tobacco use increases morbidity and mortality. When caring for families with a smoking member, nurses can consider not only smoking cessation, but also education regarding secondhand smoke. Passive smoking has been associated with several types of cancer, heart disease, chronic obstructive pulmonary disease, low birth weight, premature births, and sudden infant death syndrome (USDHHS, 2010).

Although violence and abusive behavior are well-known health risks for individuals, the extent of their prevalence within families is not well understood. The amount of intrafamilial violence is thought to be underestimated. It is difficult to collect data and obtain accurate statistics on family violence because the issue is so sensitive for families. There is evidence, however, to support the intergenerational nature of violence and abuse—that is, abusers were often abused as children (USDHHS, 2018).

Behavioral (Lifestyle) Health Risk Assessment. Families are the major source of factors that can promote or inhibit positive lifestyles. They regulate time and energy and the boundaries of the system. A number of tools exist for assessing individuals' lifestyle risks, but few are available for assessing family lifestyle patterns. Although assessment of individual lifestyle contributes to determining the lifestyle risk of a family, it is important to look at risks for the family as a unit. One approach is to identify family patterns for each of the lifestyle components included in *Healthy People 2020.* In the areas of health promotion, health protection, and preventive services, lifestyle can be assessed in several dimensions. From the literature on health behavior research (USDHHS, 2010), the critical dimensions include the following: value placed on the behavior; knowledge of the behavior and its consequences; effect of the behavior on the family; effect of the behavior on the individual; barriers to performing the behavior; and benefits of the behavior.

It is important to assess the frequency, intensity, and regularity of specific behaviors. It also is important to evaluate the resources available to the family for implementing the behaviors. Thus, items for assessment of physical activity include the value that a family places on physical activity, the hours that a family spends in exercise, the kinds of exercise in which the family participates, and resources available for exercise.

NURSING APPROACHES TO FAMILY HEALTH RISK REDUCTION

Home Visits

Home visits have been effective and have been used since the early days of nursing. Most notable are the Visiting Nurse Services of New York (VNSNY, n.d.), founded by Lillian Wald in the late 1800s, and the Frontier Nursing Service (Allen & Birdwhistell, 1987) of Kentucky, founded by Mary Breckinridge in 1925. Both visiting nurse services were developed to work with extremely vulnerable populations, particularly pregnant women and young children. Today's home visitation programs often build on the values of the VNSNY and the FNS, working with young families to help the families learn principles of parenting as well as develop life skills, including resources for employment, education, and housing. Although nurses work with families in a variety of settings, including clinics, schools, support groups, and offices, the home setting remains an important aspect of the nurse's role in reducing health risks and promoting the health of populations.

Purpose. Home visits, as compared with clinical visits, give a more accurate assessment of the family structure, the natural or home environment, and behavior in that environment. Home visits also provide opportunities to identify both barriers and supports for reaching family health promotion goals. The nurse can work with the client directly to adapt interventions to match resources. Visiting the family in their home may also contribute to the family's sense of control and active participation in meeting their health needs. The majority of historical studies evaluating home visits have focused on the maternal–child population (Fraser et al., 2000; Hammond-Ratzlaff & Fulton, 2001; Wager et al., 2004). Studies of home visits are often conducted for maternal–child health (Nurse-Family Partnership, 2018). The Health Access Nurturing Development Services (HANDS) program is a voluntary home visitation program offered to new parents in the Commonwealth of Kentucky (Kentucky's HANDS, n.d.). The purpose of HANDS is to provide a positive beginning for families, building on the family's strengths, and improving the well-being of the family.

Home visiting programs have been receiving increased attention and provide a broad range of services to achieve a variety of health-related goals. Long-term effects of home visits are positive and are shown to be cost effective for society. As a result, several states have reinstituted home visits for high-risk families. If the home visit is to be a valuable and effective intervention, careful and systematic planning must occur (Klein & Daro, 2017).

Advantages and Disadvantages. The effectiveness of health promotion services in the home has been critically reexamined by agencies such as health departments and visiting nurses associations. Advantages include client convenience, client control of the setting, availability of an option for those clients unwilling or unable to travel, the ability to individualize services, and a natural, relaxed environment for the discussion of concerns and needs. Costs are a major disadvantage; the cost of pre-visit preparation, travel to and from the home, time spent with one client, and post-visit preparation is high. Many agencies have actively explored alternative modes of providing service to families, particularly group interventions. The important issue is determining which families would benefit the most and how home visits can most effectively be structured and scheduled. With increasing demands for home health care, the home visit is again becoming a prominent mode for delivery of nursing services. When looking at cost versus effectiveness, it is not always the least costly service that is the most effective (Sewell & Marczak, 2014); rather the social value produced may be more compelling. An example is that of home visits. Although more costly in the short term, some services are more effective in family health outcomes using home visitation rather than visits to the health department or clinic.

Process. The components of a home visit are summarized in Table 27.3. The phases include the initiation phase, the pre-visit phase, the in-home phase, the termination phase, and the post-visit phase. Building a trusting relationship with the family client is the cornerstone of successful home visits. Five skills are fundamental to effective home visits: observing, listening, questioning, probing, and prompting. The need for these skills is evident in all phases of the home visit process. Cultural competency cannot be over-stressed when discussing home visits. The PHN is a visitor in the client (or community) setting and every effort should be made to understand our clients' cultures in order to provide the best and most effective interventions for each one. Fadiman's (1997) book, *The Spirit Catches You and You Fall Down,* offers incredible insight into the negative impacts that occur when health care providers and systems do not make the

TABLE 27.3 Phases and Activities of a Home Visit

Phase	Activity
I. Initiation phase	Clarify source of referral for visit. Clarify purpose for home visit. Share information on reason and purpose of home visit with family.
II. Pre-visit phase	Initiate contact with family. Establish shared perceptions of purpose with family. Determine family's willingness for home visit. Schedule home visit. Review referral and/or family record.
III. In-home phase	Introduce self and professional identity. Interact socially to establish rapport. Establish nurse-client relationship. Implement nursing process.
IV. Termination phase	Review visit with family. Plan for future visits.
V. Post-visit phase	Record visit. Plan for next visit.

From Whitley DM, Kelley SJ, Sipe TA: Grandmothers raising grandchildren: are they at increased risk of health problems? *Health Soc Work* 26:105–114, 2001.

effort to understand a culture other than their own. It is recommended (required) that this book be read by all public health and research students to demonstrate the outcomes based on lack of communication and understanding by health care providers, even those with "good intentions."

Initiation Phase. Usually, a home visit is initiated as the result of a referral from a health or social agency. However, a family may request services, or the nurse may initiate the home visit as a result of case-finding activities. The **initiation phase** is the first contact between the nurse and the family. It provides the foundation for an effective therapeutic relationship. Subsequent home visits should be based on need and mutual agreement between the nurse and the family. Frequently, nurses are not sure of the reason for the visit. This carries with it the potential for the visit to be compromised and to progress aimlessly or abruptly come to a premature halt. Regardless of the reason for making a home visit, it is necessary that the nurse be clear about the purpose for the visit and that this purpose or understanding be shared with the family.

Pre-visit Phase. The **pre-visit phase** has several components. For the most part, these are best accomplished in order, as presented in the How To box.

HOW TO Prepare for the Home Visit: Pre-Visit Phase

- First, if at all possible, the nurse should contact the family by telephone before the home visit to introduce self, to identify the reason for the contact, and to schedule the home visit. A first telephone contact should be brief, a maximum of 15 minutes. The nurse should give name and professional identity. For example, the nurse might say, "This is Karen Smith. I'm a community health nurse from the Fayette County Health Department." If the client has a first language other than English, it is important to include an interpreter during this first contact, as well as with their continuing care, as this will set the tone for the phone call and the following phases of home visits. The National Standards for Culturally and Linguistically Appropriate Services in Health and Health Care (The National CLAS Standards) should be used to provide respectful and quality care to clients with limited English proficiency (USDHHS, n.d.). The purpose of the CLAS Standards is to improve health care quality and equity in increasingly diverse U.S. neighborhoods.
- The family should be informed of how they came to the attention of the nurse—for example, as the result of a referral, or a contact from observations, or records in the school setting. If a referral has been received, it is important and useful to ascertain whether the family is aware of the referral.
- A brief summary of the nurse's knowledge about the family's situation will allow the family to clarify their needs. For example, the nurse might say, "I understand that your baby was discharged from the hospital yesterday and that you requested some assistance with learning more about how to care for your baby at home."
- A visit should be scheduled as soon as possible. Letting the family know agency hours available for visits, the approximate length of the visit, and the purpose of the visit are helpful to the family in determining when to set the visit. Although the length of the visit may vary, depending on circumstances, about 30 to 60 minutes is usual.
- If possible, the visit should be arranged when as many family members as possible will be available for the entire visit. It is also important for the nurse to tell the client about any fee for the visit and subsequent visits and possible methods for payment.
- The telephone call can terminate with a review by the nurse of the time, place, and purpose for the visit and a means for the family to contact the nurse in case they need to verify or change the time for the visit or to ask questions. If the family does not have a telephone, another method for setting up the visit can be used. A note can be dropped off at the family home or sent by mail informing the family of when and why the home visit will occur and providing a way for the family to contact the nurse if necessary.

The possibility exists that the family may refuse a home visit. Less-experienced nurses or students may mistakenly interpret this as a personal rejection. Families make decisions about when and which outsiders are allowed entry into their homes. The nurse needs to explore the reasons for the refusal; there may be a misunderstanding about the reason for a visit, or there may be a lack of information about services. The contact may be terminated as requested if the nurse determines either that the situation has been resolved or that services have been obtained from another source, and if the family understands that services are available and how to contact the agency if desired. There are instances when the nurse will be mandated to persist in requesting a home visit because of legal obligations, such as follow-up of certain communicable diseases. This has become more obvious in this era of increasing contagious and infectious diseases in our highly mobile society.

Before visiting a family, the nurse should review the referral or, if this is not the first visit, the family record. If there is a time lapse between the contact and the visit, a brief telephone call to confirm the time often prevents the nurse from finding no one at home.

Personal safety is an issue that may arise either while approaching the family home or when the family has opened the door to the nurse. Nurses need to evaluate personal fears and objective threats to determine if safety is indeed an issue. Certain precautions can be taken in known high-risk situations. Agencies may provide escorts for nurses or have them visit in pairs; readily identifiable uniforms may be required; or a sign-out process indicating timing and location of home visits may be used routinely. Home visits are generally very safe; however, as with all worksites, the possibility of violence exists. Therefore, the nurse needs to use caution. If a reasonable question exists about the safety of making a visit, the visit should not be made..

The nurse should be aware that families may feel that they are being scrutinized, that they are seen as being inadequate or dysfunctional, or that their privacy is being intruded upon. Nursing services, especially those from health departments, have been perceived by the public as being "public services" for needy families or those with inadequate funds to pay for care. These potential areas of concern underlie the need for sensitivity on the part of the nurse, the need for clarity in information regarding the reason for visits, and the need to establish collaborative, trusting relationships with the family.

Another factor that may affect the nature of the home visit is whether the visit is viewed as voluntary or required. A *voluntary* home visit (visit requested by the client) is characterized by easier entry for the nurse, client-controlled interaction, an informal tone, and mutual discussion of frequency of future visits. An example of a voluntary visit is a new mother who has requested the nurse come to the home and assist her with learning how to care for the infant. In contrast, the client may feel little need for *required* home visits that often may be legally mandated. In these instances, entry may be difficult for the nurse; the interaction may be nurse controlled; there may be a more formal, investigatory tone to the visit with distorted nurse-client communication; and there may be no mutual discussion of scheduling or frequency of future visits. Two examples of a required home visit are (1) when a family member has been diagnosed with tuberculosis and the nurse needs to make certain that the client is taking medications regularly, and (2) when there is known child abuse and a new baby has arrived. The nurse may need to visit the home to observe the interaction between the parents and the child.

The changing nature of the American family can make it difficult to schedule visits during what have been traditional agency hours. The number of working single-parent or dual-income, two-parent families is increasing, which means that families have more demands on their time. Even if one parent is at home during the usual workday, the ideal is to work with the entire family unit. This often is not possible because of conflict between agency hours and school or work schedules. It may be possible to schedule a visit at the beginning or end of a day to meet with working or school-age members. In some parts of the country, agencies have reconsidered the traditional hours and Monday through Friday visits and include evening and weekend work hours. These issues are important to assess and address during the pre-visit phase so the nurse and the family will be better prepared for the visit.

Culture influences a person's interpretation of and response to health care (Shi & Singh, 2019). It is impossible, given the diversity of the United States and the diversity within cultural groups, to cover every group extensively. Instead, practitioners need to take the responsibility to learn about their client's culture as they prepare for visits with families or communities. Again, refer to the Office of Minority Health's website for additional information regarding culture and diversity.

In-Home Phase. The actual visit to the home constitutes the **in-home phase** and affords the nurse the opportunity to assess the family's neighborhood and community resources, as well as the home and family interactions. The actual home visit includes several components. Once at the family home, the nurse provides personal and professional identification and tells the client the location of the agency. Then, a brief social period allows the client to assess the nurse and establish rapport. The next step is a description by the nurse of his or her role, responsibilities, and limitations. Another important component of the home visit is to determine the client's expectations.

The major portion of the home visit is concerned with establishing the relationship and implementing the nursing process. Assessment, intervention, and evaluation are ongoing. What then occurs in the home visit is determined by the reason for the visit. It is recommended that the nurse use the Intervention Wheel to guide nursing practice during home visits. The Intervention Wheel provides appropriate guidelines for the purpose of the home visit. Some reasons for visits are listed in Box 27.2.

A nurse must be flexible and anticipate that families may or may not be able to control interruptions during the visit. Telephones ring, pets join in the visit, people come and go, and televisions may be left on. The nurse can ask that televisions be turned off for a limited time or that other disruptive activities be limited. Families may be so accustomed to the background

BOX 27.2 Reasons for the Home Visit

Nursing interventions may include some or all of the 17 resources identified by the Minnesota Department of Health, Section of Public Health Nursing:

- Advocacy
- Case management
- Coalition building
- Collaboration
- Community organizing
- Consultation
- Counseling
- Delegated medical treatment and observations
- Disease and other health investigation
- Health teaching
- Outreach
- Policy development and enforcement
- Case finding
- Referral and follow-up
- Screening
- Social marketing
- Surveillance

Keller LO, Strohschein S, Lia-Hoagberg B, et al.: Population-based public health interventions: practice-based and evidence-supported, Part I. *Public Health Nurs* 21:453–468, 2004. See Chapter 11 for updates.

noises and routine activities that they do not recognize them as being potentially disruptive.

It is important that the nurse be realistic about what can be accomplished in a home visit. In some situations, one visit may be all that is possible or appropriate. In this instance, needs and the resources available to meet them are explored with the family, and it is determined whether further services are desired or indicated. If further services are indicated and the nurse's agency is not appropriate, the nurse can assist the family in identifying other services available in the community and can help in initiating referrals. Although it is not unusual to have only one home visit with a family, multiple visits are often made. The frequency and intensity of home visits vary not only with the needs of the family, but also with the eligibility of the family for services as defined by agency policies and priorities. It is realistic to expect an initial assessment and at least the beginning of building a relationship to occur on a first visit.

Termination Phase. When the purpose of the visit has been accomplished, the nurse reviews with the family what has occurred and what has been accomplished. This is the major focus of the **termination phase**, and provides a basis for planning further home visits. Ideally, termination of the visit and, ultimately, termination of service begin at the first contact with the establishment of a goal or purpose. If communication has been clear to this point, the family and nurse can now plan for future visits, specifically the next visit. Planning for future visits is part of another issue: setting goals and planning service. Contracting is a constructive approach to working with clients to specify and achieve agreed-on goals and is receiving increasing attention by health professionals (Duiveman & Bonner, 2012). The purpose and components of contracting with clients are discussed in more detail later.

Post-visit Phase. Even after the nurse has concluded the home visit and left the client's home, responsibility for the visit is not complete until the interaction has been recorded. A major task of the **post-visit phase** is documenting the visit and services provided. Agencies may organize their records by families. That is, the basic record may be a "family" folder with all members included. However, this often does not occur, although it is useful for the family history and background. More often, each family member has a separate record, and other family members' records are cross-referenced. This is because the focus often shifts from the family to the individual. Consequently, nursing diagnoses, goals, and interventions are directed toward individual family members rather than the family unit. This approach has its shortcomings and it is important for the nurse to recognize these. Chapter 41 provides an approach for offering nursing diagnoses, stating goals, and identifying interventions for the individual. It is important for the nurse to focus on the continuing assessment of the individual behaviors, responses, or health status and the impact on the family. Interventions at the family level may become necessary, such as educating all family members on hygiene and cleanliness or on the appropriate disposal of supplies of the tuberculosis client in the home.

Record systems and formats vary from agency to agency. The nurse needs to become familiar with the particular system used in the agency. All systems should include a database; a nursing diagnosis and problem list; a plan, including specific goals; actual actions and interventions; and evaluation. These are the basic elements needed for legal and clinical purposes. The format may consist of narratives; flow sheets; problem-oriented medical records (POMRs); subjective, objective, assessment plans (SOAP); or a combination of formats. It is important that recording be current, dated, and signed.

The nurse should be sure to use theoretical frameworks that are appropriate to the family-centered nursing process. For example, a nursing diagnosis of *ineffective mothering skill,* related to lack of knowledge of normal growth and development, is an individual-focused nursing diagnosis. The *inability for family to accomplish stage-appropriate tasks of providing a safe environment for a preschooler* related to lack of knowledge and resources is a family-focused nursing diagnosis based on knowledge of the developmental approach to families. At times, it may be necessary to present information for a specific family member. However, the emphasis should be on the individual as a member of, and within the structure of, the family.

Contracting With Families

Increasingly, health professionals are looking at working with clients in an interactive, collaborative style. This approach is consistent with a more knowledgeable public and the recent self-care movement in the United States. However, it may not be consistent with other cultures that look to health care providers for more direct guidance; therefore, it is important to determine the family's value system before assuming that contracting will work.

Contracting is a strategy aimed at formally involving the family in the nursing process and jointly defining the roles of both the family members and the health professional. Contracting involves making an agreement between two or more parties and seeks to create a shift in responsibility and control toward a shared effort by client and professional as opposed to an effort by the professional alone. The motivational premise of contracting is family control. It is assumed that when the family has legitimate control, their ability to make healthful choices is increased.

Purposes. The nursing contract is a working agreement that is continuously renegotiable and may or may not be written. It may be either a contingency or a noncontingency contract. A *contingency contract* states a specific reward for the client after completion of the client's portion of the contract; a *noncontingency contract* does not specify rewards. The implied rewards are the positive consequences of reaching the goals specified in the contract.

For family health risk reduction, it is essential that the contract be made with all responsible and appropriate members of the family. Involving only one individual is not sufficient if the goal is family health risk reduction, which requires a total family system effort and change. Scheduling a visit with all family members present may require extra effort. If meeting with the entire family is not possible, each family member can review a contract, give input, and sign it. This allows active participation

TABLE 27.4 Phases and Activities in Contracting

Phase	Activity
I. Beginning phase	Mutual data collection and exploration of needs and problems
	Mutual establishment of goals
	Mutual development of a plan
II. Working phase	Mutual division of responsibilities
	Mutual setting of time limits
	Mutual implementation of plan
	Mutual evaluation and renegotiation
III. Termination phase	Mutual termination of contract

by all family members without the necessity of finding a time when everyone involved can be present.

Process of Contracting. Contracting is a learned skill on the part of both the nurse and the family (Duiveman & Bonner, 2012). All persons involved need to know the purpose and process of contracting. There are three general phases: beginning, working, and termination. The three phases can be further divided into eight sets of activities, as summarized in Table 27.4.

The first activity is collection and analysis of data, and it involves both the family and the nurse. An important aspect of this step is obtaining the family's view of the situation and its needs and problems. The nurse can present his or her observations, validate them with the family, and obtain the family's view.

It is important that goals be mutually set and be realistic. A pitfall for nurses and clients who are new to contracting is to set overly ambitious goals. The nurse should recognize that there may be discrepancies between their professional priorities and those of the client and determine whether negotiating is required. Because contracting is a process characterized by renegotiation, the goals are not static.

Throughout the process, the nurse and family continually learn and recognize what each can contribute to meeting health needs. The exploring of resources allows both parties to become aware of their own and one another's strengths and requires a review of the nurse's skills and knowledge, the family support systems, and community resources.

Developing a plan to meet the goals involves specifying activities, prioritizing goals, and selecting a starting point. Next, the nurse and the family need to decide who will be responsible for which activities. Setting time limits involves determining the frequency of contacts for evaluating progress toward accomplishing goals and deciding on a deadline for accomplishing the goal. At the agreed-on time or times, the nurse and family together to evaluate progress both in terms of process and outcome. The contract can be modified, renegotiated, or terminated on the basis of the evaluation.

Advantages and Disadvantages of Contracting. Contracting takes time and effort and may require the family and nurse to reorient their roles (Duiveman & Bonner, 2012). Increased control on the part of the family also means increased responsibility. Some nurses may have difficulty relinquishing the role of the controlling expert professional. Contracts are not always successful, and contracting is neither appropriate nor possible in some cases. Some clients do not want to have this kind of involvement; they prefer to defer to the "authority" of the professional. Included in this group are individuals with minimal cognitive skills, those who are involved in an emergency situation, those who are unwilling to be more active in their care, and those who do not see control or authority for health concerns as being within their domain. Some of these clients may learn to contract; others never will.

The nursing process does not necessarily provide an active role for the family as a client; the assumption that a need exists is based on professional judgment only, and it is also assumed that changes can and should be made within the family unit. Contracting is one alternative approach that depends on the value of input from both nurse and family, on the competency of the family, on the family's ability to be responsible, and on the dynamic nature of the process. This not only allows for but requires continual renegotiating. Although it may not be appropriate in all situations or with all families, contracting can give direction and structure to health risk reduction and health promotion in families.

Empowering Families

Approaches for helping individuals and families assume that an active role in promoting their health care should be characterized by **empowerment** rather than enabling or providing help (Chen et al., 2018). Interventions in which help is given do not always have positive outcomes for clients. If families do not perceive a situation as a problem or need, offers of help may cause resentment. Providing help also may have negative consequences if there is not a match between what is expected and what is offered. A nurse's failure to recognize a family's competencies and to define an active role for them can lead to the family's dependency and lack of growth. This can be frustrating for both the nurse and the family. For families to become active participants, they need to feel a sense of personal competence and a desire for and willingness to take action. Definitions of empowerment reflect three characteristics of the empowered family seeking help: access and control over needed resources; decision-making and problem-solving abilities; and the ability to communicate and to obtain needed resources

The last characteristic refers to the fact that families may need to learn how to identify sources of help, how to contact agencies, how to ask critical questions, and how to negotiate with agencies to meet family needs. These characteristics generally reflect a process by which people (individuals, families, organizations, or communities) take control of their own lives. The outcomes of empowerment are positive self-esteem, the ability to set and reach goals, a sense of control over life and change processes, and a sense of hope for the future (Chen et al., 2018). The Levels of Prevention box shows prevention strategies applied to families.

LEVELS OF PREVENTION

Strategies Applied to Families

Primary Prevention

Completing a family genogram and assessing health risks with the family to contract for family health activities to prevent diseases from developing.

Secondary Prevention

Using a behavioral health risk survey and identifying the factors leading to obesity in the family.

Tertiary Prevention

Developing a contract with the family to change nutritional patterns to reduce further complications from obesity.

Empowerment requires a viewpoint that often conflicts with the views of many helping professions, including nursing. Empowerment's underlying assumption is one of a partnership between the professional and the client as opposed to one in which the professional is dominant. Families are assumed to be either competent or capable of becoming competent. This implies that the professional is not an unchallenged authority who is in control. Empowerment promotes an environment that creates opportunities for competencies to be used. Finally, families need to identify that their actions result in behavior change. A nursing intervention that incorporates the principles of empowerment is directed toward the building of nurse-family partnerships that emphasize health risk reduction and health promotion. The nurse's approach to the family should be positive and focused on competencies rather than on problems or deficits. The interventions need to be consistent with family cultural norms and the family's perception of the problem. Rather than making decisions for the family, the nurse supports the family in primary decision making and bolsters their self-esteem by recognizing and using family strengths and support networks. Interventions that promote desired family behaviors increase family competency and decrease the need for outside help, resulting in families viewing themselves as being actively responsible for bringing about desired changes. The goal of an empowering approach is to create a partnership between the nurse and the family characterized by cooperation and shared responsibility.

COMMUNITY RESOURCES

Families have varied and complex needs and problems. The nurse is often involved in mobilizing several resources to effectively and appropriately meet family health promotion needs. Although the specific resources vary from community to community, general types can be identified. Government resources such as Medicare, Medicaid, Aid to Families with Dependent Children, Supplementary Security Income, Food Stamps, and WIC are available in most communities. These programs primarily provide support for basic needs (e.g., illness/health care, nutritional needs, funds for housing and clothing), and funds are based on meeting eligibility criteria (Families USA, 2012, 2013, 2018). As discussed earlier, the Affordable Care Act is important to assure access to insurance for people, particularly important for those with pre-existing conditions and older Americans. It is important to pay attention to those trying to sell "junk insurance" as ACA plans (Families USA, 2017).

In addition to government agencies providing health-related services to families, most communities have voluntary (nongovernmental) programs. Local chapters of such organizations as the American Cancer Society, the American Heart Association, the American Lung Association, and the Muscular Dystrophy Association provide education, support services, and some direct services to individuals and families. These agencies provide primary prevention and health promotion services, as well as screening programs and assistance after the disease or condition is diagnosed. Local social service agencies, such as Catholic Social Services, provide direct services such as counseling to families. Other voluntary organizations provide direct service (e.g., shelters for homeless or battered individuals, substance abuse counseling and treatment, Meals on Wheels, transportation, clothing, food, furniture).

Health resources in the community may be proprietary, voluntary, or public. In addition to private health care providers, nurses should be aware of voluntary and public clinics, screening programs, and health promotion programs.

Identifying resources in a community requires time and effort. Although the telephone book was once a valuable resource, it has been replaced, in many cases by Internet browsers and search engines. Google Chrome, Safari, and Firefox are just a few examples of internet browsers that provide a vast amount of resources within a matter of minutes. Often community service organizations, such as the local chamber of commerce, churches, and health departments, publish community resource listings. Coalitions composed of interfaith communities provide a wealth of information related to resources. These resources may be listed on the organizations' websites. Regardless of how the resource is identified, the nurse must be familiar with the types of services offered and any requirements or costs involved. If this information is not available, the nurse can contact the resource via their webpage or via phone.

Locating and using these systems often requires skills and patience that many families lack. Nurses work with families to identify community resources, and as client advocates they help families learn to use resources. This may involve sharing information with families, rehearsing with families what questions to ask, preparing required materials, making the initial contact, and arranging transportation. The appropriateness and effectiveness of resources should be evaluated with families afterward. Navigating the maze of resources is often difficult, even for the nurse. It is important to remember that if a family is in crisis or does not have a phone, computer, or a home base from which to call or receive return calls, this process is even more difficult, and their sense of helplessness may be increased. Therefore, the nurse's assistance, while promoting the family's sense of empowerment, is both necessary and often complex.

Telehomecare

Telehomecare (also referred to as telehealth or telemedicine) is a practice that continues to develop. It is vital in the provision of care to vulnerable populations, including the rural and place-bound urban, allowing clients to communicate with and transfer health information to providers from home. Researchers have found that telehomecare can improve certain health outcomes, such as reducing the duration of hospitalization, increasing access to care, improving patient satisfaction, and improving patient education and self-care (Bowles et al., 2011; Shea & Chamoff, 2012). Telehomecare monitoring requires less time per client interaction, so it allows nurses to feasibly care for more clients per day. Nurses may increasingly rely on this technology to assist with home visits to families. Patients with chronic diseases benefit from receiving the care they need in their own home setting, decreasing time spent receiving health care and education.

Telehomecare can also be a particularly useful option in situations where ongoing and frequent monitoring of a family member's condition is necessary; however, it should be recognized that it is not a substitute for the in-home trust and relationship building and assessment of both family and community resources that can only be accomplished by an attentive and engaged nurse spending time with the family in their home environment. Telehomecare is currently used in several areas, including Maine General Health in Augusta, Maine, and Ontario, Canada (Canada Health Infoway, 2017; Maine General Health, 2015). It is used to manage chronic conditions such as heart failure, diabetes, and respiratory illnesses, connecting patients to their home care nurse and/or doctor, while allowing the patient to stay at home, decreasing emergency department visits and hospital stays.

Family Policy

This chapter ends where it began, with a discussion of the nurse's role in policy development and implementation. Florence Nightingale, Lillian Wald, and Mary Breckenridge were all strongly committed and involved nurses who advocated for families and influenced policy to improve the health of families and consequently the health of communities. Building on the gains made possible by these influential women is essential. Families are affected by the rules and values of their surrounding society in general. If families—all families—are valued, the community will be strong and connected. If any family is neglected and not supported, the community will be weak and disconnected. The United States is one of the few countries without a family policy, including a lack of paid maternity leave. The United States currently has 12 weeks of protected leave, Family Medical Leave Act (FMLA); however paid leave is not part of that Act.

Family Medical Leave Act. The FMLA was signed into law on February 5, 1993, by then President Clinton (PL 103-3) (Waldfogel, 2001). This act allows covered employees to take up to 12 weeks of leave each year for certain family and medical reasons (National Partnership for Women and Families, 2016). Under the FMLA, employees may take a leave of absence for many reasons: for their own serious illness; for the illness of their child, parent, or spouse; and for the birth or adoption of a child (PL 103-3). While on leave, employees still receive their medical benefits and are guaranteed that their position or one similar to it will be available to them upon returning to work.

The FMLA was needed to help Americans meet the needs of their families while maintaining employment. Women in particular were experiencing hardship in keeping a job while having a family. The Affordable Care Act (although currently in a precarious position due to political ideologies) and family policies such as the FMLA reflect a growing recognition and valuing of the healthy family unit as a key factor and contributor to the health of not only individuals, but our communities and society at large. Nurses are positioned to improve the health of families, thus leading to healthier communities, as well as improving the health of communities, thus leading to healthier families.

Affordable Care Act. Many of the family health risks discussed in this chapter involve how family stressors can negatively affect health outcomes and suggest strategies and interventions to cope with rectifying these issues. Health policy can also be part of a solution to mitigate the financial and emotional effects of family stress by increasing access and affordability of health care. The Patient Protection and Affordable Care Act of 2010 (ACA) helps women, children, and families by increasing access to health care, improving health care quality, lowering health care costs, and instituting new consumer protections ("The Affordable Care Act," n.d.). However, as with all policies, health care providers must be diligent in the follow through and continued maintenance of policies that improve the health of our families, including advocating for vulnerable populations with our legislative bodies. Improving access and control over resources such as health care can lead to greater empowerment of families.

LINKING CONTENT TO PRACTICE

Vulnerable Populations: Teenage Parent Families at Risk

Although endless hours have been spent researching ways to help parents of teenagers, it is also important to remember the teenagers who *are* parents. This family structure faces multiple health-related and social challenges, the most prominent being affordable and accessible health care. A closely related challenge is the recruitment and development of mentors to help teen parents acquire this health care, as it is uncharted water for nearly all teenagers. The humiliation teens experience when visiting doctors and agencies is a pain analyzed and discussed incessantly, and yet little has been done for the teenage parents.

The most common issue raised by teenage parents is their uncertainty and low self-confidence in handling adult responsibilities *other* than actual parenting. There is a great need for more teenage-instructional literature on family health policy information and health care service accessibility written from the perspective of teenagers. Single teenage parents need to be able to understand welfare and how to apply, as well as how to find support communities. Teenage parents who decide not to be involved in a child's life must be able to understand child support, adoption, and legal visitation and involvement issues.

The rising numbers of teenagers giving birth must be met with stronger and more extensive plans for families led by teens. Education, vocational opportunity, and social acceptance are "luxuries" often missed by adolescent parents. While the last of these issues can only be solved by eventual cultural assimilation, schooling and careers should be made possible.

Although it is not advisable to simply hand out opportunities to teenagers with children, it is definitely necessary to offer assistance, not only so that they may have a second chance at a successful life, but for their children as well. It is recognized that the children of teenage parents often make the same mistakes as their parents, due to factors of poor living conditions, low socioeconomic status, and a rough childhood. Without adequate family care, there will be no end to the cycle of child parents. Today, many people are advocating for sex education and prevention, but it is also time *now* for postpregnancy programs, which accept that there is a child born to two teenagers; although they may have made a poor choice, these teenagers now have *no* choice but to accept parental responsibility and be shown the tools to do so.

Vulnerable Populations: LGBTQIA+ Families at Risk

Lesbian, gay, bisexual, transgendered, queer/questioning, intersex, ally/asexual, and a plus sign to designate those not included (LGBTQIA+) (Gold, 2018). This listing is just a beginning of terms for persons who do not identify as heterosexual. It is ever evolving, along with the scope of familial and other relationships and groupings to which these persons belong. Over the past decade, there has been an explosion of visibility for this population. Debates and legal battles centering on LGBTQIA+ rights have taken place nationally and in states across the country. Notable examples include same-sex marriage, which was established in a civil rights case in 2015 by the U.S. Supreme Court; adoptions by same-sex couples; opening of the military to gays, lesbians and transgendered individuals (although the debate continues in the administrative branch of government); and a plethora of antidiscrimination laws. However, antidiscrimination laws often are not clearly written or adhered to, as shown in the 2018 Supreme Court decision that ruled in favor of a Christian baker who refused to bake a wedding cake for a gay couple while at the same time, voicing support for gay rights (Savage, 2018).

As noted in the introduction to this section, nurses have an ethical obligation to provide culturally competent care to LGBTQIA+ families. To fulfill this obligation, nurses should first seek to provide a safe environment for clients to discuss their sexual orientation. Although some nurses may feel a degree of discomfort discussing sexual orientation with their clients, it is important to develop learning strategies to help overcome this barrier to care for LGBTQIA+ families.

Just as there is great variation among heterosexual families, all LGBTQIA+ families are not the same. Nurses are well prepared to learn to better assess and contribute to a growing understanding of the dynamics of LGBTQIA+ families and their associated health care needs as well as the obstacles to care which they may face. Same-sex couples have historically had special barriers within the health care system. Although the Supreme Court settled the issue of same-sex marriage, there continues to be a great variation in LGBTQIA+ adoption rights. The lack of legal recognition for LGBTQIA+ relationships in most areas of the country has resulted in barriers that often present challenges for LGBTQIA+ families seeking to access the health care system as well. Despite the Supreme Court's recognition of same-sex marriage nationwide, there continues to be discrimination (Wordon, 2014).

On April 15, 2010, President Obama signed a directive instructing hospitals that accept Medicaid and Medicare to allow adult clients the right to designate specific individuals who can visit them in the hospital or make medical decisions on their behalf. This helped to alleviate some issues that LGBTQIA+ partners face when interacting with the health care system. (See https://obamawhitehouse.archives.gov for more information.)

Nurses are in an optimal position to fulfill a vital role in helping LGBTQIA+ families achieve equitable access to health care. Nurses can assist with assessing the implementation of health care policy such as President Obama's directive. In addition, nurses can help to advocate for more policies designed to reduce barriers within the health care system for LGBTQIA+ families, such as the inclusion of culturally competent care and the education of all health care providers in providing culturally appropriate health care.

Another type of family at risk is the more "traditional" family with a non-heterosexual member. After a family member declares his or her sexual preferences, families may need initial support to process the information. Nurses may be in a position to provide support during this time. Nurses may also refer families to community resources, such as Parents and Friends of Lesbians and Gays (www.pflag.org). Check within your local community for other appropriate resources.

In addition to providing support for the family unit as a whole, nurses may also be in a position to assess LGBTQIA+ individuals. As in all family units, the health of individual members of a family affects the entire family unit. Sexual and gender minorities face a higher risk for depression, anxiety, substance abuse, thoughts of suicide, and suicide. Addressing mental health issues in these populations may help reduce the mental health disparities the LGBTQIA+ population faces.

QSEN FOCUS ON QUALITY AND SAFETY EDUCATION FOR NURSES

Targeted Competency

Evidence-based practice integrates the best current clinical evidence with client and family preferences and values to provide optimal care.

- **Knowledge:** Describe how the strength and relevance of available evidence influences the choice of interventions in providing client-centered care.
- **Skills:** Question rationale for routine approaches to care that result in less than desired outcomes or adverse events.
- **Attitudes:** Value the need for continuous improvement in clinical practice based on new knowledge.

EBP Question

The Quad Council of PHN Organizations initially identified the core competency of policy development and program planning and suggests the beginning public health nurse (PHN) will identify policy issues relevant to the health of individuals, families, groups, and within a community.

In this chapter several family policy issues are discussed. Choose one policy that has been passed legislatively to explore. Policy is one level of evidence used in practice. Before a policy becomes law, the strength and relevance of scientific and other data sources are explored to support the argument for developing the policy. Determine what evidence was used to support the policy. How strong and relevant was the evidence? What reasons were given for the policy becoming law or standard practice? Will the policy improve practice? Is it currently being implemented to improve family health care?

PRACTICE APPLICATION

The initial contact between a nursing service and a family provides limited information, and the situation that develops may be much more complex than originally anticipated. The following example, based on an actual case, illustrates the issues and approaches outlined in this chapter.

The Local County Health Department was notified that Amy C., age 16, had been referred by the school counselor at the local high school for prenatal supervision. Amy was four months pregnant, apparently in good health, and in the 10th grade. She lived at home with her mother, stepfather, and younger sister. The family lived in a rural area outside of a small farming community. The father of the baby also lived in the community and continued to see Amy on a regular basis. The referral information provided the nurse with a beginning, but limited, assessment of the family situation.

A. What would you do first as the nurse assigned to this family?

B. How would you help this family empower themselves to take responsibility for this situation?

C. After the initial contact, how would you extend the assessment to the entire family system?

D. Would you contract with this family? How? On what terms?

Answers can be found on the Evolve site.

KEY POINTS

- The importance of the family as a major client system for nurses in reducing health risks and promoting the health of individuals and populations is well documented.
- The family system is a basic unit within which health behavior, including health values, health habits, and health risk perceptions, is developed, organized, and performed.
- Knowledge of family structure and functioning, family theory, nursing theory, and models of health behavior is fundamental to implementing the nursing process with families in the community.
- Nurses need to go beyond the individual and family, and to understand the complex environment in which the family functions, to be effective in reducing family health risks. Categories of risk factors that are important to family health are biological risk, environmental risk (including economic factors), and behavioral risk.
- Several factors contribute to the experience of healthy/unhealthy outcomes. Not everyone exposed to the same event will have the same outcome. The factors that influence whether disease or other unhealthy results occur are called health risks. The accumulated risks are synergistic; their combined effect is more than the sum of the individual effects.
- An important aspect of nursing's role in reducing health risk and promoting the health of populations has been the tradition of providing services to individual families in their homes.
- Home visits afford the opportunity to gain a more accurate assessment of the family structure and behavior in the natural environment. Home visits also provide opportunities to make observations of the home environment and to identify both barriers and supports to reducing health risks and reaching family health goals.
- Health professionals increasingly have come to look toward working with clients in a more interactive, collaborative style.
- Contracting, which is making an agreement between two or more parties, involves a shift in responsibility and control, from the professional alone to a shared effort by client and professional.
- Families have varied and complex needs and problems. The nurse often mobilizes several resources to effectively and appropriately meet family health needs.
- Policy development and implementation is an important skill that the nurse uses to improve the health of families and thus improve the health and livability of communities.

CLINICAL DECISION-MAKING ACTIVITIES

1. Select one of the *Healthy People 2020* objectives and identify how biological risk (including age-related risk), environmental risk (including economic risk), and behavioral risk contribute to family health risks for that objective. Give examples.
2. Select three to four families (hypothetically or from actual situations) that represent different ethnic and socioeconomic backgrounds. Complete a family genogram and ecomap for each family, and identify and compare major health risks. Summarize your findings.
3. Select one or more agencies in which nurses work, and examine the agency and nursing philosophies and objectives with emphasis on individual care, family care, illness care, risk reduction, and health promotion. If you were to accept a position with this agency, what approach to family risk reduction would you be required to use? Is there a better way?
4. Identify three public health problems in your community, and discuss the implications of these problems for the health of families. How did you arrive at your conclusions?
5. Identify three health problems common to families in your community, and discuss the implications of the problems for the health and/or health care resources of the community. What strategies might you use to address the health problems?

ADDITIONAL RESOURCES

EVOLVE WEBSITE

http://evolve.elsevier.com/Stanhope/community/
- Answers to Practice Application
- Case Study
- Glossary
- Review Questions

REFERENCES

Allen SE, Birdwhistell TL: *The Frontier Nursing Service oral history project: An annotated guide*, 1987, University of Kentucky Library Occasional Papers Series 2. Retrieved from https://uknowledge.uky.edu.

Artiga S, Hinton E: *Beyond Health Care: The Role of Social Determinants in Promoting Health and Health Equity*. May 10, 2018. Retrieved from: www.kff.org.

Artiga S, Ubri P, Foutz J: What is at stake for health and health care disparities under ACA repeal? Henry J, Kaiser Family Foundation, 2017. Retrieved from https://www.kff.org.

Beckman S, Fawcett J, editors: *Neuman Systems Model: Celebrating Academic-Practice Partnerships*, Fort Wayne, IN, 2017, Neuman Systems Model Trustee Group, Inc.

Belloc NB, Breslow L, Hochstim JR: Measurement of physical health in a general population survey, *Am J Epidemiol* 93:328–336, 1971.

Biden J: *Speaker at 2014 Health Action Conference*, Washington, DC, 2014, Families USA.

Bouchard C: Defining the genetic architecture of the predisposition to obesity: A challenging but not insurmountable task, *Am J Clin Nutr* 91:5–6, 2010.

Bowles KH, Hanlon AL, Glick HA, et al.: Clinical effectiveness, access to, and satisfaction with care using a telehomecare substitution intervention: a randomized controlled trial, *Int J Telemed Appl* 12:540138, 2011.

Buettner D: *The Blue Zones, 9 Lessons for Living Longer*, ed 2, Washington, DC, 2009, National Geographic.

Buettner D: *Blue Zones, 2008–2018*: *Power 9®, Reverse Engineering Longevity*, 2008–2018, Washington, DC, National Geographic.

Califano JA Jr: *Healthy People: The Surgeon General's Report on Health Promotion and Disease Prevention*, Washington, DC, 1979, U.S. Government Printing Office.

Canada Health Infoway: *Telehomecare Centre*, 2017. Retrieved from http://telehomecare.otn.ca.

Centers for Disease Control and Prevention (CDC): *Adolescent and School Health*, 2017. Retrieved from https://www.cdc.gov.

Centers for Disease Control and Prevention (CDC): *Physical Activity and Health*, 2018. Retrieved from https://www.cdc.gov.

Chen L, Chen Y, Chen X, Shen X, Wang Q, Sun C: Longitudinal study of effectiveness of a patient-centered self-management empowerment intervention during predischarge planning on stroke survivors, *Worldviews Evid Based Nurs* 15(3):197–205, 2018.

Choquet H, Meyre D: Genetics of obesity: What have we learned? *Curr Genomics* 12(3):169–179, 2011.

Conger RD, Lorenz FO, Wickrama KAS, editors: *Continuity and Change in Family Relations: Theory, Methods, and Empirical Findings*, reprint, New York, NY, 2014, Taylor and Francis.

Congressional Budget Office: *Repealing the Individual Health Insurance Mandate: An Updated Estimate*, Washington, DC, 2017, Congressional Budget Office. Retrieved from http://www.cbo.gov.

DeFrain J: *Getting Connected, Staying Connected: Loving One Another, Day by Day*, June 20, 2012, iUniverse, Board of Regents of the University of Nebraska.

Doherty WJ, McCubbin HI: Family and health care: an emerging arena of theory, research and clinical intervention, *Family Relat* 34:5, 1985.

Duiveman T, Bonner A: Negotiating: experiences of community nurses when contracting with clients, *Advances Contemp Nurse* 41:120–125, 2012.

Eckenrode J, Campa M, Luckey DW, et al.: Long-term effects of prenatal and infancy nurse home visitation on the life course of youths: 19-year follow-up of a randomized trial, *Arch Pediatr Adolesc Med* 164(1):9–15, 2010.

Fadiman A: *The Spirit Catches You and You Fall Down*, New York, 1997, Farrar, Straus and Giroux.

Families USA: *A 50-state look at Medicaid expansion*, 2018. Retrieved from http://familiesusa.org.

Families USA: *Affordable Care Act*, 2017. Retrieved from http://familiesusa.org.

Families USA: *Help is at hand: new health insurance tax credits*, 2013. Retrieved from http://familiesusa.org.

Families USA: *Medicaid leads to better education*, 2012. Retrieved from http://familiesusa.org.

Families USA: *To tackle health disparities make care more affordable*, 2015. Retrieved from http://familiesusa.org.

Fraser JA, Armstrong KL, Morris JP, Dadds MR: Home visiting intervention for vulnerable families with newborns: follow-up results of a randomized controlled trial, *Child Abuse Negl* 24:1399–1429, 2000.

Friedman M, Bowden V, Jones E: *Family Nursing Theory and Practice*, ed 5, Upper Saddle River, NJ, 2003, Prentice Hall.

Gold M: *The ABCs of L.G.B.T.Q.I.A. The New York Times*, June 21, 2018. Retrieved from https://www.nytimes.com.

Hammond-Ratzlaff A, Fulton A: Knowledge gained by mothers enrolled in a home visitation program, *Adolescence* 36:435–442, 2001.

Hill R: *Families Under Stress*, New York, 1949, Harper.

Holtslander L, Solar J, Smith NR: The 15-minute family interview as a learning strategy for senior undergraduate nursing students, *J Fam Nurs* 19:230–248, 2014.

Kentucky's HANDS: *What is HANDS?* n.d. Retrieved from http://www.kyhands.com.

Kaiser Family Foundation: *Beyond Health Care*, 2018, Retrieved from http://www.kff.org.

Klein S, Daro D: *The Pew home visiting data for performance initiative: Phase II final report on feasibility study*, 2017. Retrieved from https://www.chapinhall.org.

Litman TJ: The family as a basic unit in health and medical care: a social-behavioral overview, *Soc Sci Med* 8:495–519, 1974.

Maine General Health: *Home Care Services*, 2015. Retrieved from https://www.mainegeneral.org.

Mauksch HO: A social science basis for conceptualizing family health, *Soc Sci Med* 8:521–528, 1974.

Livingston G. *Family life is changing in different ways in the US*, Washington, DC, 2018, PEW Foundation.

Murdaugh CL, Parsons MA, Pender NJ: *Health promotion in nursing practice*, ed 8, Upper Saddle River, NJ, 2019, Pearson.

National Center for Health Statistics (NCHS): *Health, United States, 2016: with chartbook on long-term trends in health*, Hyattsville, MD, 2017, NCHS.

National Institute on Drug Abuse (NIDA): *Addiction and health*. Washington, DC, 2014, USDHHS. Retrieved from http://www.drugabuse.gov.

Nightingale EO, Cureton M, Kalmar V, Trudeau MB: *Perspectives on health promotion and disease prevention in the United States.* Washington, DC, 1978, Institute of Medicine, National Academy of Sciences.

Nurse-Family Partnership: *About us.* 2018. Retrieved from https://www.nursefamilypartnership.org.

Pratt L: *Family structure and effective health behavior.* Boston, MA, 1976, Houghton Mifflin.

Price CA, Bush, KR, Price SJ: *Families and change: coping with stressful events and transitions,* ed 5, Thousand Oaks, CA, 2017, Sage.

Purdue University: *What is a family?* July, 2015. Retrieved from: https://www.purdue.edu.

Savage DG: Supreme Court rules for Christian cake baker but voices support for gay rights too. *Los Angeles Times,* June 4, 2018. Retrieved from http://www.latimes.com.

Sewell M, Marczak M: *Using cost analysis in evaluation,* 2014. Retrieved from http://ag.arizona.edu.

Shea K, Chamoff B: Telehomecare communication and self-care in chronic conditions: moving toward a shared understanding, *Worldviews Evid Based Nurs* 9(2):109–116, 2012.

Shi L, Singh D: *Delivering health care in America: a systems approach,* ed 7. Burlington, MA, 2019, Jones & Bartlett Learning.

The Affordable Care Act: *What it means for children, families, and early childhood programs,* n.d. Retrieved from http://www.acf.hhs.gov.

The National CLAS Standards, 2004 with updates 2018. USDHHS. Retrieved from https://www.minorityhealth.hhs.gov.

National Partnership for Women and Families: *Guide to Family Medical Leave Act,* ed 8, Washington, DC, 2016, National Partnership for Women and Families.

Thomas TN, Kolasa MS, Zhang F, Shefer AM: Assessing immunization interventions in the Women, Infants, and Children (WIC) program, *Am J Prev Med* 47(5):624–628, 2014.

U.S. Department of Agriculture, Food and Nutrition Service: *Women, Infants and Children. About WIC- how WIC helps,* 2018. Retrieved from http://www.fns.usda.gov.

U.S. Department of Health and Human Services, Administration for Children and Families: *Administration on Children, Youth and Families, Children's Bureau: Child maltreatment 2016,* 2018. Retrieved from https://www.acf.hhs.gov.

U.S. Department of Health and Human Services (USDHHS): *Healthy People 2010: understanding and improving health,* ed 2. Washington, DC, 2000, USDHHS, Public Health Service.

U.S. Department of Health and Human Services (USDHHS): *Healthy People 2020.* Washington, DC, 2010, U.S. Government Printing Office.

U.S. Department of Health and Human Services, Office of Minority Health (USDHHS): *The National CLAS standards,* n.d. Retrieved from https://minorityhealth.hhs.gov.

U.S. Department of Health and Human Services, U.S. Department of Agriculture (USDHHS): *Dietary guidelines for Americans 2015–2020,* ed 8, 2015. Retrieved from https://health.gov.

U.S. Department of Labor, Wage and Hour Division: *Fact sheet #28: the Family and Medical Leave Act.* 2012. Retrieved from http://www.dol.gov.

Visiting Nurse Services of New York: *History,* n.d. Retrieved from http://www.vnsny.org.

Vooradi S, Mateti UV: A systemic review on lifestyle interventions to reduce blood pressure, *J Health Res Rev* 3:1–5, 2016.

Wager KA, Lee FW, Bradford WD, Jones W, Kilpatrick AO: Qualitative evaluation of South Carolina's postpartum/infant home visit program, *Public Health Nurs* 21:541–546, 2004.

Waldfogel J: Family and medical leave: evidence from the 2000 surveys, *Monthly labor review,* 2001. Retrieved from https://stats.bls.gov.

Worden A, Couloumbis A: *Pennsylvania governor won't appeal gay marriage ruling,* 2014. Retrieved from http://www.governing.com.

White JM, Klein DM, Martin TF: *Family theories: an introduction,* ed 4. Thousand Oaks, CA, 2015, Sage Publications.

World Health Organization (WHO): *The determinants of health: health impact assessment,* Geneva, Switzerland, 2018, World Health Organization.

28

Child and Adolescent Health

Cynthia Rubenstein, PhD, RN, CPNP-PC

OBJECTIVES

After reading this chapter, the student should be able to do the following:

1. Describe significant physical and psychosocial developmental factors characteristic of the child and adolescent population.
2. Examine the role of the nurse and discuss appropriate nursing interventions that promote and maintain the health of children and adolescents as individuals, as members of their family, and as members of the community.
3. Discuss the built environment and how it relates to major health issues of children and adolescents.
4. Explain the current status of children and their physical, emotional, behavioral, and environmental health issues.
5. Differentiate between the models for delivery of health care to the pediatric populations in the community and other settings.

CHAPTER OUTLINE

Status of Children
Child Development
Immunizations
The Built Environment
Injuries and Accidents
Health Problems of Childhood
Models for Health Care Delivery to Children and Adolescents
Role of the Population-Focused Nurse in Child and Adolescent Health

KEY TERMS

abusive head trauma, p. 640
body mass index, p. 634
built environment, p. 632
bullying, p. 644
child feeding practices, p. 634
child maltreatment, p. 640
Children's Health Insurance Program, p. 628
cognitive development, p. 630
development, p. 629
developmental screening, p. 630
digital media, p. 635
electronic nicotine delivery system (ENDS), p. 646
environmental tobacco smoke (ETS), p. 646
family-centered medical home, p. 647
federal poverty level (FPL), p. 627
food deserts, p. 634
food insecurity, p. 627
food landscape, p. 634
growth, p. 629
human ecology theory, p. 630
immigrant children, p. 627
immunization, p. 631
Medicaid, p. 628
motivational interviewing, p. 647
obesity, p. 633
overweight, p. 632
psychosocial development, p. 630
social media, p. 635
sports specialization, p. 639
sudden infant death syndrome (SIDS), p. 643
sudden unexpected infant death (SUID), p. 642
sudden unexpected death in infancy (SUDI), p. 642
unintentional injuries, p. 637

Walt Disney identified the greatest natural resource of any nation as the minds of its children. The future of the world depends on how well it cares for its youth. If this population is to thrive, it must be nurtured in an appropriate environment. Focusing on the health needs and health promotion of children increases the chances that they will become adults who value and practice healthy lifestyles. Population-focused nurses have two major roles in the area of child and adolescent health:

1. Providing direct services to children and their families: assessing, managing care, educating, and counseling.
2. Assessment of the community and the establishment of programs to ensure a healthy environment for this population.

The population-focused nurse has the opportunity to teach healthy lifestyles to children and caregivers and to provide family-centered care in the community setting. This chapter provides information on the assessment of children and adolescents as well as activities to promote their health. The content includes basic principles of childhood growth and development and major health problems seen in this population. The concept of evaluating child health and implementing health education and models of health behavioral change will be explored within the context of the child's home and community. The pediatric medical home model and motivational interviewing are discussed in this chapter as strategies to promote improved health behaviors within families. *Healthy People 2020* objectives (USDHHS, 2010) are used as a framework for focusing on needs of children in the community.

STATUS OF CHILDREN

Poverty Status

It is well established that living in poverty is associated with poorer health outcomes regardless of age, and youth disproportionately represent those Americans living in poverty. There were 73.6 million children ages birth to 17 years in the United States in 2016, representing 22.9 percent of the population. About 20 percent of these children lived in poverty in 2015 (Federal Interagency Forum on Child and Family Statistics [Federal Interagency Forum], 2017). More children born to immigrant parents live at or below the federal poverty level compared to children of U.S. native-born parents (AAP, 2017). Just under a third of children live in households receiving supplemental security income (SSI), cash public assistance income, and/or Supplemental Nutrition Assistance Program (SNAP) benefits (National Center for Children in Poverty, 2016). The **federal poverty level (FPL)** for 2018 was defined as a family income of less than $25,100 for a family of four, whereas low income (the amount of income necessary to provide for the family's basic needs) is defined as a family income that does not exceed 150 percent of the poverty level ($37,650 for a family of four in 2018). The National Center for Children in Poverty (2018) notes that families need about twice the federal poverty defined income to meet their most basic needs, yet 44 percent of children live in low-income families.

Minority children, most notably African American and American Indian children, have higher proportions living at poverty and African American and Hispanic in families with the lowest-income levels (Fig. 28.1).

Characteristics that put children at risk for living in low-income families are parents without a high school degree, having a lack of parental employment, and living in a single-parent household. Children's ability to learn in school and reach their full cognitive ability is affected by low-income status with children living in poverty experiencing a higher incidence of behavioral, social, and emotional problems (Jiang et al., 2014).

In addition, U.S. children face other challenges. About 13.1 million U.S. children experienced **food insecurity** in 2015 (Federal Interagency Forum on Child and Family Statistics, 2017). Food insecurity, a lack of available food and access to food on a regular basis, negatively affects children's physical health, development, and school performance. Homelessness is increasing for American children and is highly correlated to poverty status and the lack of affordable housing. At an alarming increased prevalence, up to 2.5 million U.S. children experience homelessness each year (American Institutes for Research, 2018). The full impact of homelessness and poverty on families can be further explored in Chapter 33 (Poverty and Homelessness).

Immigrant Children

Children of immigrant families represent a large portion of the U.S. population. **Immigrant children** are defined as those children who are foreign-born or native-born children who live with a foreign-born parent(s). In 2016, 22 percent of all U.S. children were native-born children with at least one foreign-born parent (Federal Interagency Forum on Child and Family Statistics, 2017). When compared to nonimmigrant

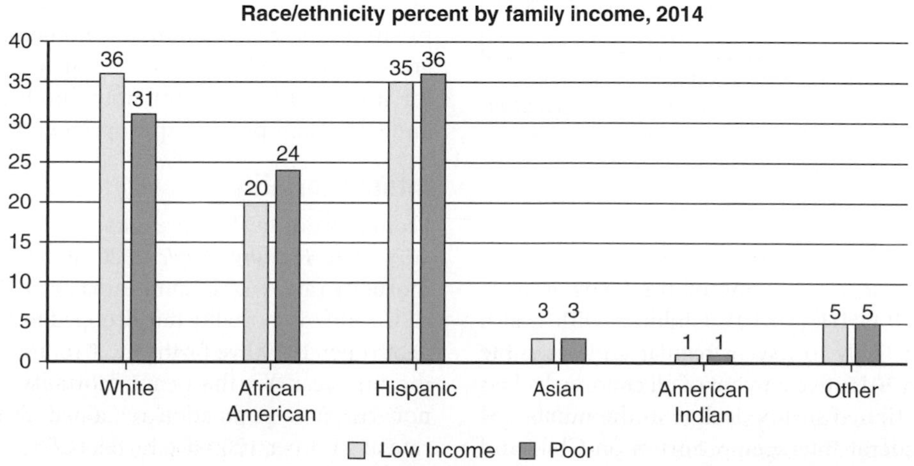

Fig. 28.1 Percent of children living in poverty and low income by ethnicity in 2014. (From National Center for Children in Poverty: Basic facts about low income children, 2016. Available at www.nccp.org.)

children, immigrant children are more likely to have poor to fair health.

Immigrant children face many barriers to good health, including a lack of health insurance, poverty, language barriers, and substandard housing. These families often experience fear of discrimination related to anti-immigration sentiment and this impacts access to health care and child health outcomes. Nurses should advocate for culturally and linguistically effective comprehensive health care, provide preventive screenings and referrals as appropriate, and encourage early education services for the support of optimal development in immigrant children (AAP, 2013a). (See Evidence-Based Practice box.)

EVIDENCE-BASED PRACTICE

With immigration enforcement, U.S. native children of undocumented immigrants are or may be separated from parents and/or siblings. It is assumed that the stress of actual or potential family destabilization negatively impacts the children's psychosocial health. The authors conducted a study to evaluate the psychological status of three groups of citizen-children (those living in Mexico with their deported parents; those living in the United States with parents affected by detention or deportation; and those living in the United States with undocumented parents not affected by detention or deportation. The study identified that all three groups of U.S. native children experienced elevated levels of distress with differences between the children who had experienced a parent's detention or deportation (Zayas et al., 2015).

Nurse Use

There is an assumption that U.S. native children with an undocumented parent do not have increased distress if they have not been affected by detention or deportation. This study demonstrates that all children, whether experiencing actual or potential family destabilization, have significant distress that impacts overall functioning. Children from all three groups experienced higher levels of attention deficits, depressive symptoms and emotional problems, and lower levels of freedom from anxiety and happiness. Cultural differences can be influential in making health care decisions. By identifying this specific population of concern, nurses can direct mental health assessment strategies and refer at-risk children for counseling and support. Public health nurses can collaborate with federal immigration officials and local social services to help prepare families and children for family destabilization to minimize the detrimental long-term distress impact on this population of children.

Based on Zayas LH, Aguilar-Gaxiola S, Yoon H, et al.: The distress of citizen-children with detained and deported parents. *J Child Fam Stud* 24(11):3213-3223, 2015. Available at https://www.ncbi.nlm.nih.gov.

Access to Care

Access to quality health services is one of the focus areas of *Healthy People 2020* (USDHHS, 2010). Children with health care coverage are more likely to have a regular and accessible source of health care. In 2015, five percent of all children had no health insurance, a continued steady decline in the number of uninsured children (Federal Interagency Forum on Child and Family Statistics, 2017).

The **Medicaid** program, established by the Social Security Act in 1965, is a state-administered health insurance program financed jointly by the federal and state governments. Children under 18 years of age living in a household with an income level up to 138 percent of the federal poverty level (FPL) or children meeting disability requirements qualify for this program. The program provides health services at no cost to participants and includes outpatient visits, hospitalization, laboratory testing, immunizations, well care/preventive services, and dental care (Children's Defense Fund, 2018).

The **Children's Health Insurance Program** (CHIP) is the result of federally mandated legislation passed in 1997 to expand health insurance to the nation's uninsured children. The Children's Health Insurance Program Reauthorization Act of 2009 has continued to provide insurance to 9.4 million American children as of 2017 (CMMS, 2017). CHIP is a federal and state partnership directed toward uninsured children and pregnant women in families with incomes too high to qualify for state Medicaid programs but usually too low to afford private coverage. Following federal guidelines, each state determines the model of its particular CHIP program, which includes the eligibility parameters, benefit package, payment levels for coverage, and administrative process. The program is jointly financed by the federal and state governments, and administered by the states (CMMS, 2017). CHIP enrollment eligibility requirements are:

- Family income too high for Medicaid qualification (varies by state with ranges of 200-300 percent above FPL)
- Uninsured children under 19 years of age in the home

CHIP coverage includes:

- Primary care provider/specialist visits
- Immunizations
- Hospitalizations and emergency department (ED) visits

With recent efforts to expand insurance coverage for children, more than 43 million children (57 percent of all children in the population) receive comprehensive and affordable health insurance through Medicaid and CHIP. With the expanded Affordable Care Act (ACA) legislation, 94 percent of children have had access to health coverage with the expansion of health insurance options (Children's Defense Fund, 2018). With the recent legislation removing individual mandates and premium increases, a number of eligible children continue to go uninsured. This remains an area of outreach opportunity for nurses to identify potential families eligible for Medicaid and CHIP and provide appropriate referrals to state agencies.

Infant Mortality

Promotion of healthy pregnancies is a focus of *Healthy People 2020*. The *Healthy People 2020* target goal for the U.S. infant mortality rate is 6.0 infant deaths per 1000 live births. The overall U.S. infant mortality rate dropped to a record low of 5.9 infant deaths per 1000 live births in 2016, meeting the target goal for the first year. Yet the infant mortality rate for the non-white, non-Hispanic population remained almost double the overall rate at 11.3 per 1000 live births (CDC, 2016a). Geographically, infant mortality rates are highest in Southern states with a total of 23 U.S. states meeting the *Healthy People 2020* target goal. Although infant death rates have decreased, the United States continues to have a higher infant mortality rate than 55 other nations (Central Intelligence Agency, 2017) and its position in a global ranking has consistently fallen over the past years.

Infant mortality rates are critical indicators of a country's overall health. Infant mortality rates are associated with a variety of factors such as maternal health, socioeconomic circumstances, quality and access to medical care, and community health practices. Nurses should promote proper prenatal care, educate on the benefits of breastfeeding and immunizations, and refer pregnant women, new mothers, and infants to appropriate health care and social services. These strategies alone, particularly in high-risk populations, can effectively reduce the infant mortality rate.

Risk-Taking Behaviors

Risk behaviors are any behaviors that place early and middle adolescents at risk for physical, emotional, or psychological harm. Much progress has been made through health promotion and education to decrease risk factors in adolescents. The Youth Risk Behavior Surveillance System (YRBSS) indicates that many teens engage in health-risk behaviors correlated with the leading causes of death in teens—unintentional injuries, suicide, and homicide. Within the previous 30 days, 39.2 percent of teens shared that they texted while driving with 5.9 percent of adolescents reporting never wearing a seat belt, and 16.5 percent of teens riding in cars with an intoxicated driver. While teens reported a decrease in drinking and driving (5.5 percent), a new survey item noted that 13 percent of teens had driven a vehicle while using marijuana. With 22 percent of teen deaths attributed to motor vehicle crashes in 2016, primary prevention is focused on education and strategies to reduce the overall risk-taking behaviors of teens in relation to vehicular associated deaths (Kann et al., 2018).

Although a large percent of teens (28.9 percent) report ever trying cigarette smoking, the number of teens smoking regularly has continued to decline annually (8.8 percent smoke at least once per month with 2.6 percent reporting smoking 20 or more times per month). Of great concern is the apparent acceptability for youth to try an electronic nicotine delivery system (ENDS) product (42.2 percent) and use on a monthly basis (13.2 percent). ENDS products include vape pipes, vaping pens, e-cigarettes, e-cigars, e-pipes, e-hookahs, and hookah pens. When you combine monthly use of smoking cigarettes, cigars, smokeless tobacco, and electronic vapor products, almost 20 percent of teens report monthly use. Also, on the increase in teens is the use of marijuana with 35.6 percent of teens reporting using marijuana at least once and 19.8 percent of youth reporting using marijuana on a regular basis (Kann et al., 2018). With the recent legalization of recreational marijuana in a number of states, teens' perception of the harmlessness of marijuana has increased significantly (Cerdá et al., 2017). While teen alcohol consumption has remained relatively stable, alcohol intake for youth remains high with 29.8 percent reporting that they drink alcohol monthly and 60.4 percent of all teens reporting they have ever tried alcohol (Kann et al., 2018).

Increasingly, drugs of abuse are prescription pain medications taken without a provider's prescription or taken differently than prescribed. Nationally, 14 percent of high school students have taken prescription pain medications in this manner (Kann et al., 2018). This prevalence was higher in Hispanic males and females. It is vital to promote community and family awareness of this problem and educate children and adolescents on the dangers of taking others' prescription medications in light of the current opioid epidemic our country is facing. Of significant concern is 20 percent of youth reported being offered, sold, or given illegal drugs on school property during the previous 12 months. The overall prevalence of all drugs of abuse (including nicotine) risk behaviors in teens indicates the continued emphasis on primary and secondary prevention and education with the adolescent population. This requires collaboration with health care professionals, school systems, community leaders, and parents to effectively implement programs and surveillance to reduce risk behaviors and improve associated outcomes in teens.

Despite extensive education campaigns, adolescents continue to engage in sexual activity (39.5 percent) with only 53.8 percent using condoms during intercourse and 9.7 percent of teens reporting that they had sexual intercourse with four or more partners (Kann et al., 2018). These risk behaviors increase the risk for unintended pregnancies and sexually transmitted infections. Concurrently, the birth rate for teenagers (15-19 years) has dropped to an all-time low of 20.3 births per 1000 teens in 2016 (USDHHS, 2016). This number remains a significant concern for public health nurses because teen pregnancy creates a significant socioeconomic burden on society and the family.

Nurses should be aware of the factors associated with increased adolescent risk-taking behaviors: poor academic performance, poor parental role models, low self-esteem, lack of a supportive social environment, and poverty. Individual assessment of an adolescent's risk-taking behavior can provide the direction to focus education and interventions. Providing after-school extracurricular activities, identifying a positive adult role model, and engaging teens in support systems to build self-esteem can reduce risk-taking behaviors in at-risk adolescents.

CHILD DEVELOPMENT

Growth and Development

Growth is the measurable aspect of the individual's size and follows a predictable pace that is evaluated at regular intervals to determine if a child is growing based on standard parameters. **Development** involves the observable changes in the individual and relates to physical, psychosocial, and cognitive achievements. Growth and development in children are ongoing, dynamic processes that result in physical, cognitive, and emotional changes (Fig. 28.2).

Health visits or well-child checkups are scheduled at key ages to monitor these processes and provide anticipatory guidance to families. Nursing assessments include growth and health

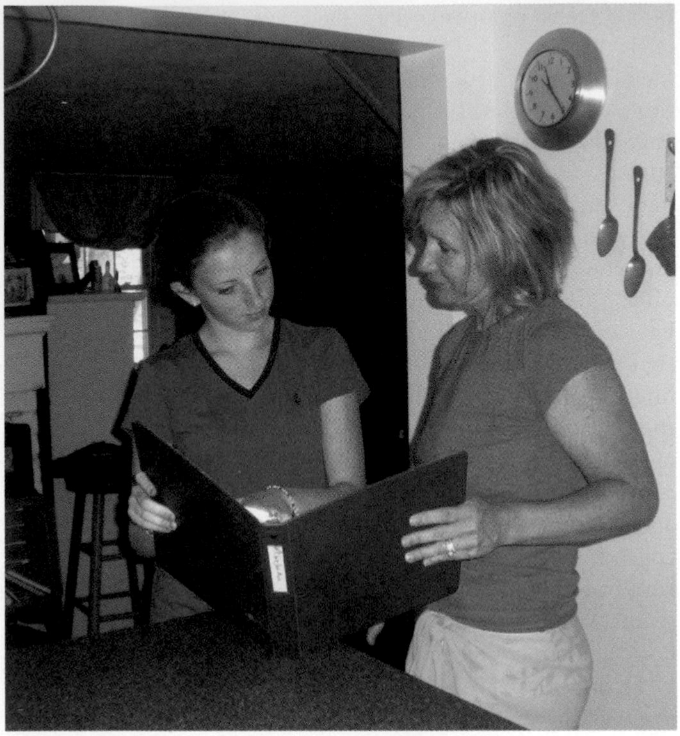

Fig. 28.2 Conflict between parents and teenagers is normal as teenagers experience physical and emotional growth processes.

status, developmental level, and the quality of the parent-child relationship. (See Tables 28.2, 28.3, 28.4, and 28.5 for considerations and issues to address at each stage.) The recommendations for preventive pediatric health care (see Resource Tool XX on the Evolve site) list components of well-child assessments. Other tools are included on the Evolve website.

Developmental Theories

Many developmental theories provide perspectives on children's growth and development. The work of Erik Erikson on **psychosocial development** emphasizes that personality development culminates in the achievement of ego identity, which involves accepting oneself and having the skills for healthy functioning in society. According to Erickson, development is a continual process that occurs in distinct stages with a developmental crisis needing resolution at each stage and some degree of mastery being achieved before proceeding successfully to the next stage. All new development is rooted in prior experiences, and difficulty resolving the crisis will cause problems progressing through the subsequent stages.

The work of Jean Piaget is widely used to understand the process of **cognitive development**. According to Piaget, learning results from actively manipulating objects and information followed by a mental processing of the event. As the child interacts with the environment, new objects and problems are discovered. The child creates mental schemes or thought patterns to understand the encounter. This permits the child to receive information from the world, make sense of it, and predict future events. Development occurs as the schemes increase in scope and complexity. Piaget identified four stages of cognitive development that represent increasing problem-solving ability. As one will remember from pediatric courses, these stages are sensorimotor, preoperational, concrete, and formal operations (Shaffer & Kipp, 2013).

Bronfenbrenner's **human ecology theory** emphasizes the complex relationship between the growing child and his or her immediate environment. Children are greatly influenced by the environments in which they spend time and one of the most important environments in affecting growth is the family environment. Educational programs, communities, and other environmental factors also influence the child's development. Children learn to accommodate to their environment and alter themselves based on environmental interactions. This theory explains that individuals do not develop in isolation but in relation to their home and family, school, community, and society (Shaffer & Kipp, 2013).

Developmental Screening

Developmental screening is a process designed to identify children who should receive more intensive assessment or diagnosis of potential developmental delays. These delays may be in any of the developmental domains—gross motor, fine motor, language, or social skills. Developmental screening promotes early detection of delays and improves child health and well-being for identified children. In the United States, 15 percent of children have a developmental disability such as autism, attention-deficit disorder, hearing loss or a language delay (Boyle et al., 2011; CDC, 2018a). Nurses are critical to early screening and identification of developmental delays in young children and appropriately initiating referrals to maximize school readiness and maximum achievement. Multiple screening tools are available and are selected based on the nurse's role in the community (Table 28.1).

Children with delayed skills or other disabilities may qualify for special services that provide individualized education programs in public schools that are free of charge to families. Nurses can be effective health advocates for these children within educational settings. The passage of the updated version of the Individuals with Disabilities Education Act 2004 (IDEA) promotes a collaborative focus on meeting the needs of children with disabilities (Department of Education, 2006). Parents, educators, administrators, nurses, and other team

TABLE 28.1 Developmental Screening Tools

Tool	Purpose
Denver II	Domain specific development (gross and fine motor, social, language)
Ages and Stages Questionnaire	Social and emotional development
Parents' Evaluation of Developmental Status (PEDS)	General developmental and behavioral screening
Modified Checklist for Autism in Toddlers (M-CHAT)	Autism spectrum disorder
Pediatric Symptom Checklist	Coping and mental health concerns

members collaboratively develop a plan—the individualized education plan (IEP)—to help children succeed in school. The IEP explains the goals the team sets for a child during the school year as well as any special support needed to help achieve these goals.

IMMUNIZATIONS

Increasing immunization coverage for children remains a significant focus of the *Healthy People 2020* objectives. Immunizations have contributed significantly over the past decades to the reduction in morbidity and mortality from many communicable diseases. Unfortunately, communicable disease outbreaks such as measles, mumps, and pertussis continue to rise in the United States.

In 2015, only 72 percent of the nation's 19- to 35-month-old children had received the recommended combined seven-vaccine series (Federal Interagency Forum, 2017). For adolescents, vaccination rates continue to rise steadily for this age group. For those aged 13 to 17 years, 86.4 percent received the recommended tetanus-diphtheria-acellular pertussis vaccine (Tdap) and 81.3 percent received the meningococcal conjugate vaccine (MCV4). Lowest immunization rates are noted for the human papillomavirus vaccine (HPV4) series, with 41.9 percent of girls receiving one dose and only 28.1 percent receiving the full three-dose series by 17 years of age (National Center for Health Statistics, 2018). Routine immunization of children is very successful in the prevention of selected diseases. The ultimate challenge is making sure that children receive immunizations within the recommended time frame.

Barriers

There are several barriers to successful immunizations. These include vaccine cost, vaccine delay or refusal by parents, vaccine shortages, and changes in vaccine scheduling and recommendations. Health disparities in vaccination rates continue to exist. Children living in poverty have lower immunization rates than their peers, and African American children have lower immunization rates compared with white children (Ventola, 2016). Socioeconomic factors such as lack of access to care and health insurance, lack of transportation, and inconvenient clinic hours contribute to lower rates of immunization. It is important to educate and counsel parents to obtain immunizations for their children and to focus on the issue at every encounter with families. Administering combination vaccines, referring at-risk families for social services to gain health insurance, and improving access to immunizations can improve vaccination rates.

Vaccines and vaccine administration costs are high, and those families without health insurance often find following the vaccination recommendations financially prohibitive. A federal program established in 1995, Vaccines for Children (VFC), provides free vaccines to eligible children, including those without health insurance coverage, children enrolled in Medicaid, American Indians and Alaska Natives, and children whose health insurance does not cover vaccines. Identifying children who qualify for VFC is a primary prevention strategy of population-focused nurses.

Parental fears about vaccines can prevent or delay some children from getting immunized. Although vaccination is compulsory for public school enrollment, exemptions for medical reasons are allowed in all 50 states with 48 states permitting religious exemption and 20 states allowing philosophical exemptions. Most communities only have an average of 1-3 percent of children exempted for vaccinations, but some communities have rates as high as 20 percent (Ventola, 2016). These communities are particularly at risk for communicable disease outbreaks due to the loss of herd immunity.

Parents report a number of reasons for delaying, refusing, or following an alternative immunization schedule. These include a fear of autism as well as concern for side effects and number of injections. Parents today have limited exposure or experience with communicable diseases and may fail to realize the danger these diseases posed to previous generations before vaccines were readily available. It is critical for nurses to educate families on the safety and efficacy of vaccinations. Scientific studies have not found a relationship between immunizations and autism, sudden infant death syndrome, diabetes, neurological disabilities, deafness, or cancer (CDC, 2016b). When a parent chooses not to vaccinate their child, this puts the child and others at risk.

Immunization Theory

The goal of immunization is to protect by using immunizing agents to stimulate antibody formation (see Chapter 14 for types of immunity). Immunizing agents for active immunity are in the form of toxoids and vaccines. A toxoid is a bacterial toxin (e.g., from the bacteria that cause tetanus and diphtheria) that has been heated or chemically treated to decrease virulence but not antibody-producing ability. Vaccines are suspensions of attenuated (live) or inactivated (killed) microorganisms. Examples include pertussis (inactivated bacteria); measles, mumps, and rubella (live attenuated viruses); and hepatitis B (inactivated virus) (see Chapter 15) (CDC, 2017a).

The neonate receives placental transfer of maternal antibodies. This natural passive immunity lasts for about two months. Protection is temporary and is only to diseases to which the mother has adequate antibodies. The immune system of both term and preterm infants is capable of adequate antibody response to immunizations by two months of age. Generally, this is the recommended age to start immunizations; the exception is the hepatitis B series which begins at birth (CDC, 2017b).

The interval between immunizations is important to the immune response. After the first injection, antibodies are produced slowly and in small concentrations (the primary response). When subsequent injections of the same antigen are given, the body recognizes the antigen and antibodies are produced much faster and in higher concentration (the secondary response). Because of this secondary response, once an initial immunization series has been started, it does not need to be restarted if interrupted, regardless of the length of time elapsed.

Once the initial series is completed, boosters are required at appropriate intervals to maintain an adequate concentration of antibodies. (Further information about immunizing agents is available on the Evolve website).

Recommendations

Immunization recommendations rapidly change as new information and products are available. The recommended immunization schedule guidelines for children from birth through 18 years and the catch-up immunization schedule have been approved by the U.S. Public Health Services Advisory Committee on Immunization Practices (ACIP), the American Academy of Pediatrics (AAP), the American Academy of Family Physicians (AAFP), and the American College of Obstetricians and Gynecologists (ACOG) (CDC, 2018b). Current recommendations for children and adolescents can be found on the Evolve website. The main goal of the guidelines is to provide flexibility to ensure that the largest number of children will be immunized. All health care providers are urged to assess immunization status at every encounter with children and to update immunizations whenever possible.

Contraindications

There are relatively few contraindications to giving immunizations. Minor acute illness is not a contraindication. Immunizations should be deferred with moderate or acute febrile illnesses because the reactions may mask the symptoms of the illness. The side effects of the immunization may be accentuated by the illness (CDC, 2018b).

People with the following conditions are not routinely immunized and require medical consultation: pregnancy, generalized malignancy, immunosuppressive therapy or immunodeficiency disease, sensitivity to components of the agent, or recent administration of immune serum globulin, plasma or blood (CDC, 2018b).

Legislation

The National Childhood Vaccine Injury Act became effective in 1988. It requires providers to counsel parents and clients about the risks and benefits of the immunizing agent as well as possible side effects. Informed consent is recommended. Vaccine information statements (VIS) are used for this purpose. The VIS is an information sheet produced by the CDC that explains both the benefits and risks of a vaccine. Federal law requires that a VIS be given to parents or legal guardians before each vaccine dose is given (CDC, 2017c).

The Vaccine Adverse Event Reporting System (VAERS) is a national safety surveillance program. It requires providers and vaccine manufacturers to report any adverse effects following the administration of routinely recommended vaccinations. The program has been effective in tracking and identifying adverse effects associated with vaccinations. In 1999, VAERS detected reports of intussusception above what would be expected to occur by chance alone after the administration of the RotaShield rotavirus vaccine. Subsequently, this vaccine was pulled from manufacturing and the vaccine formulation was redeveloped (CDC, 2017d).

QSEN FOCUS ON QUALITY AND SAFETY EDUCATION FOR NURSES

Targeted Competency: Teamwork and Collaboration:
Ability to function effectively with nursing and interprofessional teams and to foster open communication, mutual respect, and shared decision making to provide quality client care

- **Knowledge:** Recognize the contributions of other individuals and groups in helping clients achieve health goals.
- **Skills:** Integrate contributions of others who play a role in helping clients achieve health goals.
- **Attitudes:** Respect the unique attributes and contributions of others.

Teamwork and Collaboration Question

The Quad Council of Public Health Nursing Organizations defines one competency for public health nurses (PHNs) as analytic and assessment skills. The PHN uses available data and resources related to social determinants of health when planning care for clients. From this chapter you know that the built environment includes the physical environment where the child client lives, plays, goes to school, shops, and seeks safety. This environment assists the child in managing health risks. Many persons and groups assist the child in this endeavor. To determine the potential or real health risks of a child client, what information would you gather and from whom? How would you use the data from your assessment? Name a health risk and discuss the interventions you might plan and the health education you would offer to promote the child's health. What would you see as the role of other individuals and groups in the community to assist you or to take the lead in assisting the child and family? Be specific.

CHECK YOUR PRACTICE

The pediatric population is vulnerable to environmental hazards. You have been asked, as a part of your public health rotation, to determine the risk factors for the pediatric population at the local elementary school. What would you do? What would be your plan for identifying these risk factors?

THE BUILT ENVIRONMENT

A **built environment** is simply defined as the person's human-made or modified surroundings in which they live, work, and partake in recreation (Villanueva et al., 2013). This is the actual physical environment in which children live and includes neighborhood access to recreation opportunities, grocery stores, the home environment, and the consideration of general safety for children in their physical environments. A child's built environment influences the risk factors for obesity, amount and type of physical activity, risk for injuries, and exposure to environmental toxins. Therefore, as nurses, assessing a child's built environment provides a foundation for identifying interventions and education to promote health and prevent injuries and diseases.

Obesity

Obesity rates in American children have risen to epidemic levels over the past few decades. These increases are noted for all children aged 2 to 18 years regardless of gender or ethnicity. The CDC defines **overweight** as a body mass index (BMI) at or above the 85th percentile and lower than the 95th percentile,

TABLE 28.2 Centers for Disease Control and Prevention Classification of Body Mass Index (BMI) for Children Age 2 Years and Above

Plotted Percentile for Age and Gender	BMI Interpretation
<5th percentile	Underweight
5th-85th percentile	Normal
85th-95th percentile	Overweight
>95th percentile	Obese

From Centers for Disease Control and Prevention: Classification of body mass index, 2015. Available at www.CDC.gov.

and **obesity** is defined as a BMI at or above the 95th percentile for children of the same age and sex when plotted on the CDC growth charts (Table 28.2) (CDC, 2016c, 2018c).

Research has been conducted to analyze infants for obesity using both World Health Organization (WHO) growth standards for children younger than two years (weight for length) and BMI to determine if infant obesity measures are predictive of obesity in later childhood. Both weight for length and BMI for infants six months and older are consistent predictors of early childhood obesity with BMI noted as an accurate predictor as early as two months of age (Roy et al., 2016).

The 2015-2016 prevalence of obesity is 13.9 percent in children ages 2 to 5 years, 18.4 percent for children ages 6 to 11 years, and 20.6 percent for adolescents 12 to 19 years (Fig. 28.3). For ages 2-19 years combined, the prevalence of obesity is higher in non-Hispanic African American and Hispanic children and teens as compared to non-Hispanic white and non-Hispanic Asian children and teens (Hales et al., 2017). The current obesity prevalence rates have increased overall for youth to 18.5 percent from 17.2 percent in 2014. This continues to exceed the *Healthy People 2020* goal of an obesity prevalence rate at or below 14.5 percent for children and teens.

The physiological consequences of childhood obesity are extensive and significantly impact the health status of American children. Research has clearly identified strong relationships between being obese as a child and increased disease risk and disease burden in the cardiovascular, metabolic, musculoskeletal, respiratory, and renal systems (Chandrasekhar et al., 2017; Hruby & Hu, 2015). Another critical consequence for children is the negative psychological and social impact of obesity with decreased self-esteem; higher incidence of depression, sadness, and anxiety; problems with social relationships; and higher reports of being the victim of bullying (Gibson et al., 2017; Latzer & Stein, 2013; van Geel et al., 2014).

Multiple factors contribute to the likelihood that a child will become overweight or obese. Genetics and genetic susceptibility are certainly contributing components, although the genetic composition of the population has been stable over time, thereby failing to account for a sudden rise in obesity in the past two decades (Chandrasekhar et al., 2017; Garver et al., 2013). Within the literature, modifiable risk factors for the development of childhood obesity have been identified. These risk factors are sleep duration, digital media engagement (including television, computer/tablet, phone, and video games), physical activity engagement, and dietary intake/eating behaviors (Börnhorst et al., 2015; Domingues-Montanari, 2017; Felső et al., 2017; Hruby & Hu, 2015; Chassiakos et al. (2016).)

A rising comorbidity for childhood obesity is type 2 diabetes mellitus (T2DM). Currently, about 5300 U.S. children and adolescents have T2DM (CDC, 2017e). Children and adolescents diagnosed with T2DM are usually between 10 and 19 years old, are obese with a strong family history for T2DM, and have insulin resistance (Springer et al., 2013). Most children and adolescents with T2DM have poor glycemic control with hemoglobin A1C levels between 10 percent and 12 percent. T2DM affects all ethnic groups but occurs more frequently in non-white groups with the highest prevalence in American Indian youth (CDC, 2017e).

Screening for T2DM is recommended for children with a BMI of 85th to 95th percentile with two risk factors of family history of diabetes, belonging to a racial minority group, or with signs of insulin resistance; all children with a BMI above the 95th percentile; and at age 10 years or onset of puberty. In addition, these children should be screened for hypercholesterolemia and hypertension, which are also associated with childhood obesity (Springer et al., 2013). Nurses can be instrumental

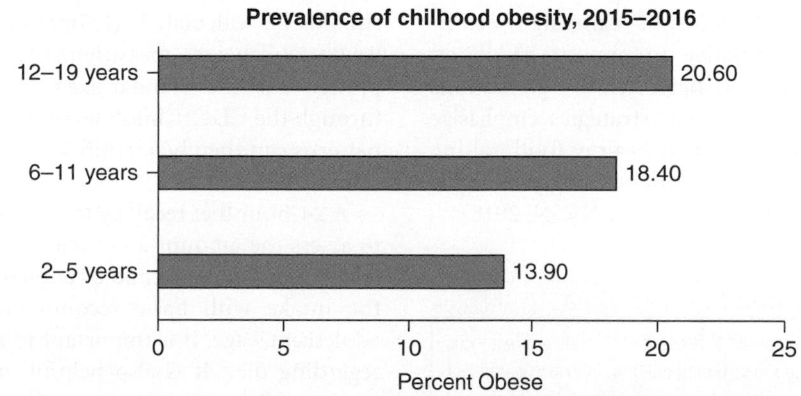

Fig. 28.3 Obesity prevalence for 2 to 19 years, 2015-2016. (Data from Hales C, Carroll, M Fryar C, et al.: Prevalence of obesity among adults and youth: United States, 2015-2016, NCHS Data Brief, no. 288, 2017. Available at www.cdc.gov.)

in the management of T2DM in children by educating and counseling.

Built Environments

A discussion on the risk factors for childhood obesity should be considered within the context of a child's built environment. The emerging research on the relationship of built environments and obesity evaluates the factors within an individual's environment that may contribute on a macro- or micro-level to the development of obesity. The current literature focuses on the role of the built environment in physical activity levels, nutrition, and health outcomes (Gose et al., 2013; Smith et al., 2017).

For children, the built environment as it relates to nutrition includes both macro- and micro-level considerations. On the community, or macro level, the factors of the built environment that influence nutrition and risk factors for obesity include a greater reliance on convenience foods and fast foods, increasing portion sizes, and the **food landscape**. The food landscape evaluates the accessibility and availability of healthy foods, and it is clear that low-income neighborhoods have limited access to stores offering fruits and vegetables (Dutko et al., 2012).

Close proximity to fast-food restaurants and convenience stores are negatively correlated with daily fruit and vegetable consumption for school-age children (Hager et al., 2017). Many urban and rural Americans live in areas termed as **food deserts**, which are defined as having limited access to affordable and nutritious foods. The inability to easily obtain nutritious foods has been identified as a contributing factor to the development of obesity and obesity-related diseases. More than 23.5 million American households live in low-income areas more than one mile from a supermarket (Dutko et al., 2012).

The factors on the macro level interact closely with those factors on the micro level. For children, the micro-level factors of the built environment that influence nutrition include the home food environment. The home food environment factors include home availability and accessibility of fruits and vegetables, parent role modeling, child feeding practices, and general parenting style (Couch et al., 2014).

Obesity Prevention

A united national movement is under way to reduce risk factors for developing obesity in children. Building upon the prior White House administration's "Let's Move!" campaign, a comprehensive and coordinated initiative to prevent childhood obesity, governmental agencies and health care organizations have continued the efforts. The current strategies emphasize healthy schools, access to affordable and healthy food, raising children's physical activity levels, and empowering families to make healthy choices (AAP, 2015; AAP, 2016a; NASN, 2018).

HEALTHY PEOPLE 2020

The *Healthy People 2020* priority focus areas of prevention include a direct focus on achieving the goals of reducing the proportion of children who are overweight or obese, increasing the proportion of daily servings of fruits for children, and increasing the proportion of daily servings of vegetables for children.

From U.S. Department of Health and Human Services: *Healthy People 2020*, Washington, DC, 2010, U.S. Government Printing Office.

Promoting good nutrition and dietary habits is a key to maintaining child health. The first six years are the most important for developing sound lifetime eating habits. Parents as primary caregivers are most influential in teaching children specific eating behaviors through their own child feeding practices. **Child feeding practices** are a primary factor in the development of eating behaviors for children and include the level of control the parent or caregiver exerts over the type and amount of food the child eats, the role modeling of eating behaviors, the feeding cues given to the child, and the actual mealtime environment and routine. The resulting learned eating behaviors then follow an individual through adolescence and into adulthood (Birch, 2006; Park et al., 2015).

Collaboration between agencies is critical to implementing community-based interventions to reduce childhood obesity. Shape NC is an innovative partnership that provides grant funding and training resources to improve obesity risk factors for young children. The resources extend to 100 North Carolina counties and improve policies, practices, and outdoor environments in childcare centers and communities so that more children are entering kindergarten at a healthy weight. Within three years of implementation in 2010, Shape NC has shown an increase from 34 percent to 80 percent of children consuming fruit two or more times a day. Currently, over 10,000 children birth to five years have benefited from Shape NC, and data have demonstrated a statistically significant decrease in BMI percentile for these children. The collaborative program is an exemplar of a successful team-based strategy to implement best practices and support young children and families in maintaining a healthy weight (The North Carolina Partnership for Children, Inc., 2018).

Nutrition Assessment

Physical growth serves as an excellent measure of adequacy of the diet. Measurements of height and weight, plotted on appropriate growth curves at regular intervals, allow assessment of growth patterns. Head circumference is followed until age three. For children less than two years, the weight for recumbent length is assessed at regular intervals. Those infants and toddlers who measure above the 97.7th percentile of WHO growth standards are considered high risk for obesity. For children two years and older, the **body mass index** (BMI) should be calculated (kilograms/[meters]^2) based on the weight and height measurements. BMI for age and gender is plotted on the standardized BMI-for-age charts available through the CDC. Children falling outside the expected growth patterns can then be identified and interventions implemented (CDC, 2015).

A 24-hour diet recall by the parent is a helpful screening tool to assess the amount and variety of food intake. If the recall is fairly typical for the child or adolescent, the nurse can compare the intake with basic recommendations for the child's or adolescent's age. It is important to ask about parent's concerns regarding diet. It is also helpful to look at the family's meal patterns. Other important parts of the nutrition assessment include amount of physical activity and any behavior problems that occur during meals. Table 28.3 offers guidelines to daily requirements for all ages.

TABLE 28.3 Daily Dietary Recommendations: Childhood and Adolescence

Food Group[a]	2-3 Years	4-8 Years	9-13 Years	14-18 Years
Milk: Try to select low-fat sources of milk, cheese, yogurt	2 cups	2-2½ cups	3 cups	3 cups
Meat and Beans: Lean meats, beans, eggs, seafood	2 oz	4 oz	5 oz	5-6½ oz
Vegetables: Fresh vegetables best choice	1 cup	1-1½ cups	2-2½ cups	2½-3 cups
Fruits: Limit fruit juices	1 cup	1-1½ cups	1½ cups	2 cups
Grains: Half of grains should be whole grains; cooked pasta or rice, bread, cereals	3 oz	5 oz	5-6 oz	6-8 oz

[a]Recommendations are per day for each group.
Modified from U.S. Department of Agriculture: Choose my plate, 2015. www.USDA.gov.

Physical Activity

Physical activity levels contribute significantly to the overall health of children, particularly related to their risk for obesity. Fewer children are meeting the recommended physical activities levels today compared with previous generations. There are several contributing factors, including the physical built environment, changes in school practices for physical education, and increased screen time.

Some children are at higher risk for not getting enough physical activity, particularly those children living in poverty in urban neighborhoods that are unsafe for outdoor playtime and with limited access to playgrounds and parks (AAP, 2013b). Even in suburban areas, parents are wary of allowing their children to play unsupervised outdoors. Few families live in locations where they can regularly walk or bike to school or for errands. As a society, Americans have become increasingly sedentary, which contributes greatly to obesity and the development of many chronic diseases.

The CDC recommends that every child and adolescent gets 60 minutes of physical activity daily. This should primarily consist of moderate-intensity aerobic activity and it is recommended that vigorous-intensity aerobic, muscle strengthening, and bone strengthening activities be incorporated at least three times a week (CDC, 2017f). This can be accumulated throughout the day with smaller increments of activity, those obtained during school, at home, and while engaged in leisure or sports activities. According to the most recent National Health and Nutrition Examination Survey (NHANES) data, all age groups are failing to meet recommended daily activity levels. For children 6 to 19 years of age, only 21.6 percent participate in 60 minutes of moderate activity at least 5 days a week (CDC, 2018d). It is important to encourage families to be active together since this promotes greater physical activity levels in children. It also provides family time for promoting family engagement, connection, and communication. Table 28.4 shows developmental guidelines for physical activity promotion.

Schools

Children and adolescents spend much of each weekday in school. Physical activity improves academic achievement with grades, cognitive performance, classroom behavior, and school attendance (CDC, 2018d). Currently, 51.7 percent of high school students attend physical education classes one or more days a week with only 29.9 percent attending physical education classes five days per week (Kann et al., 2018). In addition, 54.3 percent of adolescents in the United States play on at least one sports team, with more males participating in sports than females.

Schools have a vital ability to influence student health and academic achievement through federal and state school policies. Quality physical education requires adequate time (at least 150 minutes for elementary schools and 225 minutes for secondary schools per week), teacher preparation and professional support, and adequate facilities and class size. Recommendations to meet high levels of physical activity in schools include strategies that integrate physical activity into structured classroom activities, encouraging more unstructured play, expanding extracurricular activities promoting physical activity, and guiding adolescents in developing their own personal fitness goals and plans (CDC, 2013).

The *Healthy People 2020* objectives include a focus on increasing the proportion of adolescents and children who engage in moderate to vigorous activity on a daily basis, increasing the proportion of adolescents who spend at least 50 percent of school physical education class time being physically active, and increasing the proportion of adolescents who participate in daily school physical education. Nurses will want to be active in educating school administrators and school boards on the benefits of physical activity in improving children's and adolescents' physical health, cognitive performance, and behavior. Nurses should be engaged in policy revisions in the school systems to restore compulsory, quality, daily physical education classes; retain school recess; and expand extracurricular activities that promote physical activity before and after schools.

Digital Media

The concept of "media" has changed significantly over the past decades. In addition to television, **digital media** now includes social media, apps, videos, podcasts, ebooks, and blogs. These can be viewed on a multitude of devices, including televisions, computers, tablets, and smartphones. **Social media**, any technology platform that allows social interaction, is a primary avenue in which children and teens interact with peers, family, and friends. With the rapid shifts in technology platforms, the impact on children and adolescents is significant. Almost all adolescents (95 percent) have a smartphone or access to a smartphone with 45 percent of teens reporting that they are online on a near-constant basis (Anderson & Jiang, 2018). Teens identify social media primarily as a means to remain connected and in touch with others—family, friends, and new

TABLE 28.4 Physical Activity Recommendations by Age Group

Age Group	Recommendations
Infants and toddlers (0-2 years)	Safe, minimally structured play environment Promote outdoor activities and exploration under supervision of a responsible adult No use of screen media except video chats; at 18 months, may introduce high-quality digital media programming (watching with child) Organized exercise classes are not recommended
Preschoolers (2-6 years)	Encourage free play and exploration under proper supervision Provide unorganized play with opportunity for running, swimming, tumbling, throwing, catching with supervision Take short walks with family member; limit use of strollers for transportation Limit screen use to one hour per day of high-quality programs
Elementary school age (6-9 years)	Encourage free play with emphasis on basic skills acquisition Promote walking, dancing, jumping rope Organized sports (soccer, baseball) can be started but should be flexible with rules, allowing free time in practice Take walks, short bike rides together as a family Place consistent limits on time using media, types of media. Ensure media does not replace adequate sleep, physical activity and other health promoting behaviors
Middle school age (10-12 years)	Encourage physical activities enjoyed with families and friends Emphasize skills acquisition with increased focus on strategies Participation in diversity of complex sports (football, basketball) is appropriate Weight training can begin with good supervision and small weights Place consistent limits on time using media, types of media Ensure media does not replace adequate sleep, physical activity and other health promoting behaviors
Adolescents	Encourage physical activities that are enjoyed with friends and considered fun to the teen Diversity of team-based sport teams Promote personal fitness—running, yoga, dance, swimming Encourage active transportation—biking and walking Weight training is safe for this age Place consistent limits on time using media, types of media. Ensure media does not replace adequate sleep, physical activity and other health promoting behaviors

Data from Hagan JF, Shaw JS, Duncan PM, editors: *Bright futures: guidelines for health supervision of infants, children, and adolescents,* ed. 4, Elk Grove Village, IL, 2017, American Academy of Pediatrics.

people. Of concern is the 24 percent of teens describing social media as a negative impact, sharing that it allows teens to speak hurtfully without consequences and provides a platform that negatively influences teen behavior through distortion of reality (Anderson & Jiang, 2018). Gaming, the playing of video games via a technology platform, is almost universal with male teens (97 percent) and has increased in females to 83 percent. Videos games have evolved from solo play to multi-player, interactive team play.

Research has shown both positive and negative effects of social media on children and teens. Benefits for youth include the ability to stay connected and develop a deeper sense of self within the community through online civic engagement and opportunity for creative endeavors (blogs, podcasts, or video creations). Electronic bullying, discussed in the Mental Health section, can have a detrimental effect on youth. Additionally, 20 percent of teens report engaging in sexting which can have grave negative consequences for youth (AAP, 2016b). Sexting is defined as sending, receiving, or forwarding sexually explicit messages, photographs, or images via digital devices. There is strongly correlated increased use of digital media with an increased sedentary lifestyle, obesity, hypercholesterolemia, and hypertension. In addition to the negative physiological effects, exposure to such extensive digital media with aggressive, violent, or sexual overtones has been correlated to desensitization to violence and increased aggression, greater sexual content exposure, and increased sexual activity (AAP, 2016b).

Interventions need to be based on the goal of lifestyle changes for the entire family. The AAP recommends that all families identify media-free family times (i.e., dinner, driving), media-free locations at home (i.e., bedrooms), and communicate regularly about online citizenship and safety. Specific age recommendations include the following (AAP, 2016c):

- Birth–18 months: No use of screen media except video chats
- 18-24 months: Option of introducing high-quality digital media programming (watching it with the child)
- 2-5 years: Limit screen use to one hour per day of high-quality programs
- 6 years and older: Place consistent limits on time using media, types of media. Ensure media does not replace adequate sleep, physical activity, and other health promoting behaviors

Nurses are uniquely positioned within the community to effect change in the childhood obesity rates. With the knowledge and skills to identify children as at risk or obese, nurses can develop interventions for healthy change for these families and refer to providers appropriately. Education on healthy eating, child feeding practices, and physical activity levels are necessary for individuals, families, and groups within the community. Nurses have the abilities and knowledge to develop creative programs to provide families with the skills to grow their own gardens and cook healthy meals. Advocating for exercise trails and physical activity programs within the community will improve the health of families living in the vicinity. It is clear from obesity research that a community-based approach is most effective at reducing obesity rates and improving health. The following list highlights some guidelines on nutrition education for families:

- Breastfeeding is the recommended exclusive feeding choice for infants from birth to six months and should be continued until one year of age. Breastfeeding is associated with a lower risk for developing childhood obesity.
- Parents' responsibilities are to provide healthy meals and snacks for their children. It is their child's responsibility to decide how much to eat.
- Limit 100 percent fruit juices and avoid all other sugary beverages. These are empty calories and fill children up so they are not hungry at meals. Appropriate beverages are milk and water.
- For toddlers and preschoolers, it sometimes takes 10 to 15 tastes of a new food before they learn to like that food. Be persistent!
- Parents should role model good eating behaviors—lots of fruits and vegetables, no sugary beverages, and little to no "junk" food or "fast" food.
- Family meals are important for teaching manners, listening to hunger cues, and having quality family time together.
- Encourage children to help with food selection and preparation as appropriate to developmental skills. Allow them to select new foods to try in the produce section of the grocery store.
- Avoid using food as a punishment or reward. Do not expect your child to "clean their plate." These feeding techniques have been associated with increased risk for obesity.
- Turn off all digital media (including phones) during meals. Children do not listen to their cues of satiety when distracted.
- Cook meals at home. Broil, bake, stir-fry, or poach foods rather than frying.
- Modify family eating habits to include low-fat food choices. Serve calorically dense foods that incorporate the food guide pyramid: whole grains, fruits, vegetables, lean protein foods, and low-fat dairy products.
- Encourage family members to stop eating when they are satisfied. Encourage recognizing hunger and satiation cues.
- Schedule regular times for meals and snacks. Include breakfast and do not skip meals.
- Have low-calorie, nutritious snacks ready and available. Avoid having empty-calorie junk foods in the home. Plan for healthy snacks when eating "on the run," such as granola, fruits, and nuts.
- Decrease salt, sugar, and fat. Increase complex carbohydrates—whole grains.
- Maintain regular activity (e.g., exercise, sports) and limit digital media time.
- Select family activities and vacations that include or focus on physical activity (hiking, bicycling, swimming).

INJURIES AND ACCIDENTS

Unintentional Injuries

Unintentional injuries are the leading cause of morbidity and mortality in the United States for young people ages 1 to 19 years. Unintentional injuries are any injuries sustained by accident such as falls, drowning, or motor vehicle accidents. It is one of the most under-recognized public health problems facing the United States today, with more than 13,000 youth dying from a preventable injury in 2015. Reducing injuries from unintentional causes, as well as from violence and abuse, is a goal of *Healthy People 2020*. More than 22,200 children are seen in emergency departments daily for treatment from a nonfatal unintentional injury (Ballesteros et al., 2018).

Motor vehicle crashes (MVCs) remain the leading cause of death for unintentional injuries in children and teens. Studies have noted that more than 618,000 children 0-12 years have been unrestrained passengers in vehicles, and for children under the age of 12 years who died from a MVC in 2015, 35 percent were not restrained (CDC, 2017g). It is recommended by the National Highway Traffic Safety Administration for children to remain in booster seats until they are at least 8 years of age and he or she is big enough to fit in a seat belt properly (Fig. 28.4). Child safety seats are estimated to reduce fatal injury by 71 percent for infants and 54 percent for toddlers (NHTSA, 2017). National standards recommend that all children ages 12 years and younger ride in the back seat because they are at significant risk of injury from airbag deployment with the back seat known as the safest part of the vehicle if a crash occurs (CDC, 2017g).

Drowning, poisonings, and burns account for most of the other deaths. For infants, the leading cause of death is suffocation (Table 28.5). From 1999 to 2015, the rates of unintentional

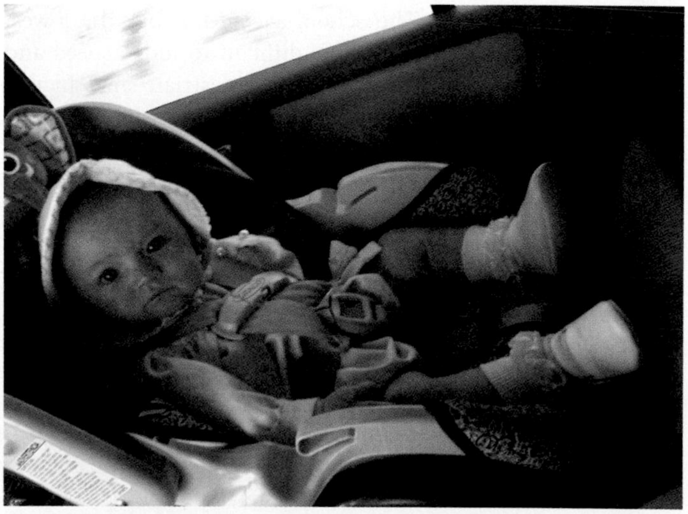

Fig. 28.4 Children should always be restrained while riding in a vehicle.

TABLE 28.5 Leading Causes of Unintentional Injury Death Among U.S. Children 0 to 19 Years, 2016

Rank	0-1 Years	1-4 Years	5-9 Years	10-14 Years	15-19 Years
1	Suffocation	Drowning	MVT-related[a]	MVT-related[a]	MVT-related[a]
2	Homicide	MVT- related[a]	Drowning	Suicide	Poisoning
3	MVT-related[a]	Suffocation	Burns/fire	Drowning	Homicide
4	Drowning	Homicide	Homicide	Homicide	Suicide
5	Adverse effects from injury	Fire/burns	Suffocation	Burns/fire	Drowning

[a]MVT-related: Motor vehicle traffic–related includes motor vehicle injuries, pedestrian injuries.
Data from National Center for Health Statistics (NCHS), National Vital Statistics System. 2018. Retrieved from www.CDC.gov

infant deaths increased by 46 percent with unintentional injury deaths in teens decreasing by 44 percent (NHTSA, 2017). To effectively implement prevention strategies, nurses need to understand the developmental factors that place this population at risk.

Developmental Considerations

Infants. Infants have the second highest injury rate of all groups of children; their small size contributes to some types of injury. The small airway may be easily occluded. The small body fits through places where the head may be entrapped. In motor vehicle crashes, small size is a great disadvantage and increases the risk for crushing or being propelled into surfaces.

The second half of infancy brings major accomplishments in gross motor activities. Rolling, sitting, pulling up, and walking bring safety concerns. Their developing motor skills remain immature, which limits their ability to escape from injury and places them at risk for drowning, suffocating, and burns (CDC, 2012).

Toddlers and Preschoolers. This population experiences a large number of nonfatal falls and being struck by or against an object. They are active and lack an understanding of cause and effect, and their increasing motor skills make supervision difficult (CDC, 2012). They are inquisitive and have relatively immature logic abilities.

School-Age Children. The school-age group has the lowest injury death rate. At this age, it is difficult to judge speed and distance, placing them at risk for pedestrian and bicycle accidents. Boys are twice as likely as girls to sustain a nonfatal bicycle injury, and the highest injury rate is at 10 to 14 years of age. Universal use of bicycle helmets would prevent most deaths. Peer pressure and lack of parental role modeling often inhibits the use of protective devices such as helmets and limb pads (CDC, 2012).

Adolescents. Motor vehicle–related injuries and violence are the leading causes of morbidity and mortality for adolescents. Risk-taking becomes more conscious at this time, especially among boys. The injury death rates for boys are twice as high as those for girls. Adolescents are at the highest risk of any age group for motor vehicle deaths and fatal poisonings. Use of weapons and drug and alcohol abuse play an important role in injuries in this age group. Suicides are the second leading cause of death for U.S. adolescents. Poor social adjustment, psychiatric problems, and family disorganization increase the risk for suicide (Ballesteros et al., 2018; CDC, 2012).

In a survey of adolescents, 23.6 percent reported being in a physical fight at least one time in the previous 12 months and 6.7 percent reported missing school at least one day in the previous month because they felt unsafe at school or on their way to school. Homicide is the third leading cause of death among youths between the ages of 10 and 19 years (Kann et al., 2018).

For all ages, families should be given anticipatory guidance in the high-risk areas for each age group to promote safety and injury prevention. Nurses can use community centers, schools, workplaces, and health centers to provide teaching to families on how to prevent injuries in their children.

Sports Injuries

Encouraging participation in team sports and individual sports and active leisure activities can increase the physical activity of children and adolescents. It has the added benefits of providing opportunity for developing teamwork and leadership skills, socializing with peers, and improving self-esteem. Children who are active in sports should have annual sports physicals, and guidelines for sports safety should be discussed as follows:

- Children should be grouped according to weight, size, maturation, and skill level.
- Qualified and competent persons should be available for supervision during games and practices.
- Adequate and appropriate-size equipment should be available.
- Goals should be developmentally and physically appropriate for the child.

About 3.2 million children 5-14 years of age are seen each year in the emergency department for sports and recreational injuries with injuries from organized and unorganized sports responsible for 775,000 of those emergency department visits (CDC, 2017h). To protect children and adolescents during sports, families require education on selecting age and physically appropriate activities, using the correct safety gear, maintaining the safety gear in good condition, and practicing good body mechanics (Fig. 28.5). Management of acute injuries sustained during sports should be monitored closely by coaches and primary care providers. The incidence of concussions, or

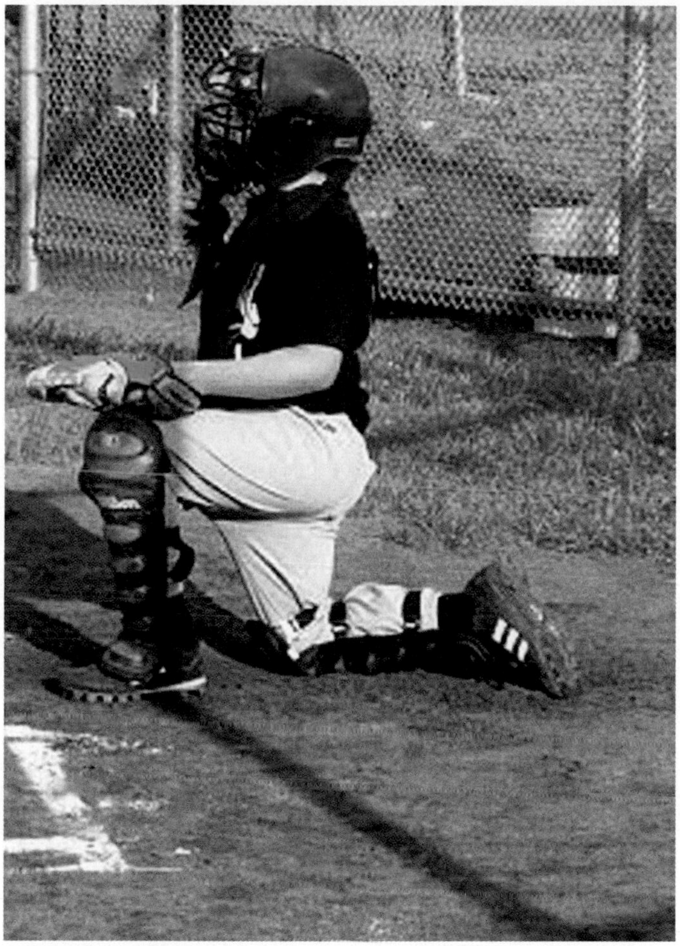

Fig. 28.5 Involvement in developmentally appropriate sports promotes physical activity and skills acquisition.

brain injuries, is 3.8 million per year in the United States (USDHHS, 2013) with sports-related concussions accounting for 4.5 percent of sports-related injuries (Sheu et al., 2016).

The state of Washington passed the first law on concussion in sports in 2009, the Zackery Lystedt Law. Between 2009 and 2012, 43 states (as well as the District of Columbia) passed laws on concussions in sports for youth and/or high school athletes. Many of these laws are known as "Return to Play" laws. The CDC's *Heads Up* program provides recommendations and educational materials to health professionals, coaches, and parents to increase knowledge related to sports-related concussions in youth.

Recognition of concussions and proper treatment is critical to prevent repeat concussions, which can cause long-term problems (USDHHS, 2013) (Table 28.6). While there is no device at present that protects against sports-related concussions and the only primary prevention mechanism is to avoid sports participation, there are recommendations to reduce the incidence of concussions. These include law and public policy, modification and enforcement of rules of the sport, educational programs, protective equipment, and changes to the youth sports culture (Patel et al., 2017). With recent media attention to the concussion-related chronic traumatic encephalopathy

TABLE 28.6 Recognizing a Concussion in an Athlete

Signs Observed by Coaches/Parents	Symptoms Reported by Athlete
Appears dazed, stunned, confused	Headache or "pressure" in head
Forgets sports plays	Nausea or vomiting
Moves clumsily	Balance problems, dizziness, double/blurred vision
Answers questions slowly	Sensitivity to light and/or noise
Loses consciousness (even briefly)	Feeling sluggish, foggy, or groggy
Shows behavior or personality changes	Concentration or memory problems
Cannot recall events prior to or after hit or fall	Confusion or does not "feel right"

From U.S. Department of Health and Human Services: Heads up, concussion in youth sports: a fact sheet for coaches, 2013b. Available at www.cdc.gov.

(CTE) in professional athletes, parents are driving changes in the youth sports culture out of concerns for long-term health consequences in their children and teens.

The trend of **sports specialization** where a youth athlete focuses on one sport to the exclusion of other sports and plays year-round has increased dramatically over the past decade as compared to the multisport athlete of previous decades. Sports specialization has contributed significantly to the increase in overuse injuries, overtraining, and youth athlete burnout. Pressure from coaches and parents leads to youth athletes participating on single sports travel and school teams with intensive training beginning as early as age 7 years. As many as 70 percent stop playing organized sports by age 13 due to burnout and/or injuries. With visions and goals of college and professional sport play, over 50 percent of youth athletes with single sport specialization experience overuse and training injuries. Yet, only 1 percent of high school athletes receive sports-related college scholarships and only 0.03-0.5 percent of high school athletes reach professional level sports (Brenner, 2016).

With a focus towards creating the elite athlete, sports specialization fails to accommodate the physiological developmental needs of youth. As children and teens grow and experience continual physical changes, sports specialization places undue stress to joints and connective tissue with growth cartilage particularly vulnerable in young athletes. An example of a common overuse injury is "Little League elbow" in baseball and softball youth players from repetitive throwing motions. Previously a rare occurrence, it now affects 45 percent of 13- to 14-year-old single sport athletes, and teens account for 57 percent of "Tommy John" surgeries (ulnar collateral ligament surgery) with a concerning number of teens electing to have surgery "proactively" to improve their pitching arm (Gregory et al., 2016; Zaremski et al., 2017).

Best practices in sports specialization to minimize risk of injury and lead to a higher likelihood of athletic success include delaying sports specialization until after puberty. Diversification in sports for young athletes provides an avenue to develop fundamental athletic skills while reducing the risk for injury and burnout. The following are recommendations that nurses can provide to youth athletes, parents, and coaches (Brenner, 2016):

- Participate in multiple sports until puberty.
- Monitor the training and coaching environment of "elite" sports programs to ensure best practices.
- Adhere to guidelines of pitch counts or other developmentally specific guidelines.
- Provide at least three months off throughout the year in increments of one month for single sports to allow for recovery.
- Provide one to two days off per week from the single sport to reduce risk of injury.
- Limit single sport teams to one team at a time (i.e., youth athletes should not play on school team and travel team concurrently).

Child Maltreatment

In 2015, 3.4 million children were reported abused or neglected with about 683,000 cases confirmed by Child Protective Services. Of these reports, 27.7 percent of victims of child maltreatment were less than three years of age and infants less than one year of age had the highest incidence of abuse. Of all victims, 75.3 percent were neglected, 17.2 percent physically abused, and 8.4 percent sexually abused. It is estimated that 1670 children died nationally in 2015 as a result of abuse with 80 percent of cases involving at least one parent (USDHHS, 2017).

Child maltreatment is defined by the Child Abuse Prevention and Treatment Act (CAPTA), as "any recent act or failure to act on the part of a parent or caretaker which results in death, serious physical or emotional harm, sexual abuse or exploitation; or an act or failure to act, which presents an imminent risk of serious harm" to a child or teen under the age of 18. Acts of commission (abuse) include physical abuse, sexual abuse, and psychological abuse; acts of omission (neglect) include failure to provide (physical neglect, emotional neglect, medical/dental neglect, educational neglect) and failure to supervise (inadequate supervision, exposure to violent environments) (Fig. 28.6) (CDC, 2014a).

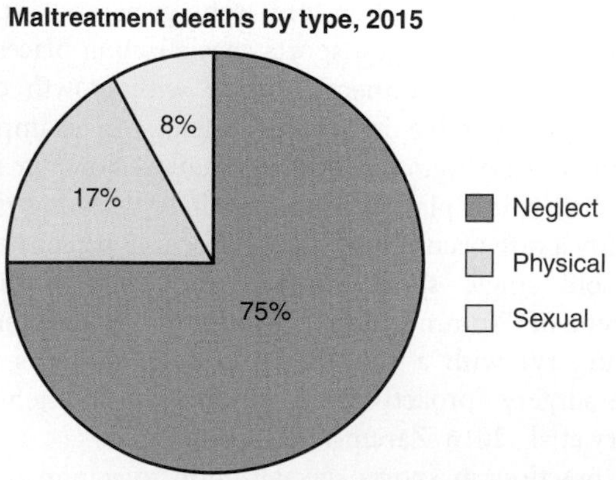

Fig. 28.6 U.S. child deaths from maltreatment, 2015. Estimated 1670 deaths in 2015. (U.S. Department of Health and Human Services, Administration for Children and Families, Administration on Children, Youth and Families, Children's Bureau: Child Maltreatment, 2017.)

Child maltreatment occurs in all socioeconomic, racial, and ethnic groups with African American and American Indian children experiencing higher rates of victimization. Children under the age of four years and those children with special needs are also at highest risk. Children are most likely to be maltreated by their parents, and common parental characteristics include a poor understanding of child development and children's needs, history of abuse in the family of origin, substance abuse in the household, and nonbiological transient caregivers in the home (e.g., mother's boyfriend). Nationally, domestic violence in the household was a risk factor for 25 percent of victims. Families at highest risk for maltreatment are those families experiencing social isolation, family violence, parenting stress, and poor parent-child relationships (CDC, 2014a; USDHHS, 2017).

The consequences of child maltreatment are often devastating. Children experience long-term physical consequences as well as negative psychological and behavioral consequences. **Abusive head trauma** (AHT), also known as shaken baby syndrome, results from violent shaking or shaking and impacting of the head of an infant or young child. Intracranial injury, subdural bleeding, retinal hemorrhages, and skull fractures can result, leading to death or survival with associated motor impairments, visual deficits, and cognitive deficits (CDC, 2018e).

Preventive strategies are necessary to reduce the incidence of child maltreatment. Parental education should be started prenatally to prevent AHT. Nurses can use home visiting programs, peer mentoring programs, preschool and Head Start programs, and public health centers to identify at-risk families and provide support and education to prevent child maltreatment. Nurses can provide education to those individuals in the community who work with children on recognizing signs of abuse and how to report suspected maltreatment. Increased awareness within the community and early intervention can prevent maltreatment from occurring and rescue children from violent and unsafe abuse situations.

Injury Prevention

Health care provider offices, schools, community centers, public health centers, and daycare/preschool facilities provide opportunities to teach children, adolescents, and their families about prevention of injuries. Safety and health promotion can be incorporated into required health education courses within the school systems. Community-sponsored car seat and seat belt safety checks and safety fairs are another way to educate families (CDC, 2012). Early home visitation programs to high-risk families are a strategy to reduce risk for child maltreatment, unintentional injuries, and improve health outcomes overall (Casillas et al., 2016; Rushton et al., 2015).

Reducing Gun Violence. Although total child firearm homicide rates have decreased by 36 percent since 2007, about 19 youth are killed or injured by guns each day in the United States (McBride, 2018). The YRBSS survey of adolescents found that 4.8 percent had carried a gun on at least one day during the previous month (Kann et al., 2018). Males (82 percent) are more likely to die from firearms and receive nonfatal injuries (84 percent) than females. Ethnic disparities in unintentional gun deaths are significant. African American children have the highest firearm homicide rate and are twice as likely to die from unintentional gun violence than white children. Suicide rates involving firearms are highest among American Indian and white youth (McBride, 2018).

For firearm-related mortality rates in urban and rural settings, there are no significant differences in the death rates between the settings but a difference in the firearm intent was evident. Urban victims died from high rates of firearm homicide while the rural victims experienced high rates of firearm suicide and unintentional firearm-related accidental deaths (Nance et al., 2010). Only about a third of gun owners with children follow firearm storage safety guidelines, and those parents with children with a mental health condition were no more likely to safely store firearms at home (Scott et al., 2018). These findings provide evidence that to reduce firearm mortality effectively, prevention strategies should be geared for the specific type of firearm injury issue within the community of interest.

Characteristics associated with gun violence include a history of aggressive behaviors, poverty, school problems, substance abuse, and cultural acceptance of violent behavior. Young children are inquisitive and often imitate in play what they see in the media and on television. A significant number of accidental firearm injuries and deaths in children occur in the homes of friends and family members (AAP, 2017). Interventions must begin early and address each of these factors. Nurses must advocate FOR sensible, effective solutions and use a culturally-sensitive, well-reasoned approach to prevent firearm deaths when educating families and communities about risks of gun violence to youth. Awareness and knowledge of the political landscape and strong industry influence on gun policy and surveillance is necessary to advocate for primary and secondary prevention to reduce firearm morbidity and mortality in America's youth.

The *Healthy People 2020* objectives seek to reduce the number of high school students who carry weapons. Nurses can actively participate in efforts to reduce gun violence among young people in the following ways (AAP, 2017; McBride, 2018):

- Urge legislators to support gun control legislation, assault weapons bans, and eliminate gun show loopholes.
- Collaborate with schools to develop programs to discourage violence among children.
- Encourage families to remove guns from their homes. If unable to do this, educate families to:
  - Store all firearms unloaded and uncocked in a securely locked container. Only the parents should know where the container is located.
  - Store the guns and ammunition in separate locked locations.
  - When handling or cleaning a gun, never leave it unattended, even for a moment; it should be in the parent's view at all times.
- Initiate community programs focusing on gun storage and safety at school.
- Educate parents on communicating with the homeowners of the homes their children visit regarding gun access and safety.
- Children and adolescents learning to hunt in rural areas should take gun safety courses.
- Identify populations at risk for violence and target aggression or anger management.
- Discourage mixing alcohol or drugs with guns.
- Encourage families to avoid gun violence in media sources at home.

Promoting Safe Playgrounds and Recreation Areas. Schools, daycare centers, families, and community groups often need guidance toward developing safe places for children to play. Each year, more than 200,000 children are treated in emergency departments for injuries sustained on playgrounds and play sets. About 56 percent of playground-related injuries are fractures and contusions/abrasions with a significant increase in traumatic brain injury in recent years. Between 2001 and 2008, 40 children died from playground-related injuries with an average age of six years. These deaths were attributable to strangulation (68 percent) and falls (15 percent) to the playground surface (CDC, 2016d).

The U.S. Consumer Product Safety Commission has published guidelines for public and home playground safety. Guidelines cover structure, materials, surfaces, and maintenance of equipment:

- Playgrounds should be surrounded by a barrier to protect children from traffic.
- Activity centers should be distributed to avoid crowding in one area.
- Surfaces should be finished with substances that meet Consumer Product Safety Commission (CPSC) regulations for lead.
- Durable materials should be used.
- Sand, gravel, wood chips, and wood mulch (not chromated copper arsenate [CCA] treated) are acceptable surfaces for limiting the shock of falls.
- Equipment should be inspected regularly for protrusions that could puncture skin or entangle clothes.
- Inspect equipment for openings/angles that allow for possible head entrapment.
- Multiple-occupancy swings, animal swings, rope swings, and trampolines are not recommended.

The developmental skills of specific ages are incorporated, as well as recommendations for physically challenged children. Nurses can use these guidelines to help the community establish standards for play areas (Fig. 28.7).

Nurses share responsibility in the prevention of intentional and unintentional injuries in the pediatric population. Assessment of the characteristics of the child, family, and environment identifies risk factors. Interventions include anticipatory guidance, modification of the environment, and safety education. Education focuses on age-appropriate interventions based on knowledge of leading causes of death and risk factors. Topics to consider are listed in Box 28.1.

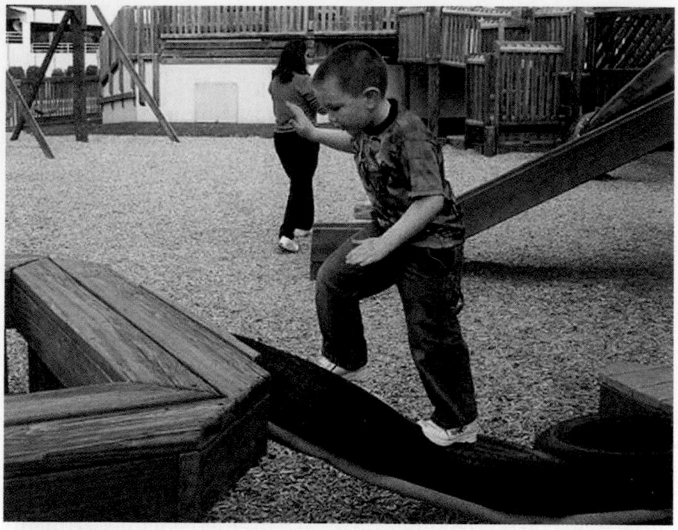

Fig. 28.7 Playground injuries are frequent among young children.

BOX 28.1 Injury Prevention Topics

- Car restraints, seat belts, airbag safety
- Preventing fires, burns
- Poison prevention
- Preventing falls
- Preventing drowning, water safety
- Bicycle safety
- Safe driving practices
- Sports safety
- Pedestrian safety
- Firearm safety
- Decreasing gang activities
- Substance abuse prevention

HEALTH PROBLEMS OF CHILDHOOD

Acute Illnesses

Acute illnesses are those illnesses with an abrupt onset and are usually of a short duration. For children, it is common for viruses to spread easily through daycares, preschools, and school systems. Nurses use developmental factors at each age to plan assessment and intervention strategies to prevent the spread of illnesses between children. Community-focused interventions, education, and programs can prevent many childhood illnesses.

Hand washing is a simple and reliable strategy to reduce the incidence of acute illnesses in children. The following How To box provides guidelines for the nurse to teach families about hand washing. Infants and young children are particularly at risk for contracting viral and bacterial illnesses spread by contact because their immune systems are not yet fully developed. Focusing community education on preschools, daycare centers, and other programs that serve the families of infants and young children can reduce the occurrence of acute illnesses (Aronson & Shope, 2016).

HOW TO Teach Families About Hand Washing

Use the guidelines below when counseling families about hand washing.

Always wash your hands *before:*

- Preparing foods
- Eating
- Touching someone who is sick
- Inserting or removing contact lenses

Always wash your hands *after:*

- Preparing foods, particularly raw meats or poultry
- Using the toilet
- Changing a diaper
- Touching animals, animal toys, leashes, or animal waste
- Blowing your nose, coughing, or sneezing into your hands
- Touching someone who is sick
- Or anytime you feel that your hands need washing!

How to wash your hands:

- Wet your hands with warm running water
- Apply soap (liquid, bar, or powder)
- Lather your hands well
- Rub your hands vigorously for at least 20 seconds (sing the "Happy Birthday" song)—scrub all surfaces including between your fingers, under your nails, backs of your hands, and your wrist
- Rinse your hands well
- Dry your hands with a clean towel, disposable towel, or air dryer
- Use your towel to turn off the faucet if possible

Several strategies can be used to reduce the occurrence of acute illnesses as follows: sanitizing objects such as toys that are handled by multiple children each day to prevent the spread of diseases; practicing good hand hygiene and diaper disposal techniques in daycares to prevent the spread of illnesses; and educating parents, daycares, and schools on when to keep children home to prevent putting others at risk for illness (Aronson & Shope, 2016).

Influenza is a common viral illness that affects children and adolescents primarily during the winter months. It is a highly contagious acute febrile illness of the nose, throat, and lungs that leads to missed school days and can result in complications including pneumonia and infrequently death. The best prevention strategy is vaccinations for all children ages six months and above. It is important to educate families about the need for vaccination and home management of symptoms (Aronson & Shope, 2016).

Nurses can focus on preventive measures and promote high vaccination rates, good hand washing hygiene and early identification to prevent the spread of illness. If a child or adolescent is diagnosed with influenza, parents can be instructed to keep children at home until symptoms have improved and fever has been gone for 24 hours. Nurses can be actively involved in developing community-based policies in the event of a pandemic, and this may include plans for mass immunizations, specific flu clinics, and protocols for school closures (Aronson & Shope, 2016).

SUIDS (SUDI)/ SIDS

Sudden unexpected infant death (SUID), also known as **sudden unexpected death in infancy (SUDI)**, is a term that describes any sudden and unexpected death that occurs in infancy; this includes both explained (i.e., suffocation, infection, trauma) and unexplained cases. Sudden infant death syndrome (SIDS) is a subcategory of SUID and is ascribed to infant deaths under one year of age that remain unexplained after a thorough case investigation, including performance of a complete autopsy, examination of the death scene, and review of the clinical history (AAP, 2016d). Although mortality rates declined dramatically in the 1990s with the "Back to Sleep" campaign, mortality rates have been stable for several years and SIDS remains the leading cause of mortality in young infants (Moon et al., 2016).

With over 3500 resulting deaths each year, the peak age for SUID deaths occurs between one and four months of age with 90 percent occurring before six months of age. SUID is rare after eight months of age. The rates of SUID in non-Hispanic African American and American Indian infants is more than twice that of white infants. There are both modifiable and nonmodifiable risk factors for SUID. Following are the sleep recommendations to reduce the risk of SUID, SIDS, and sleep-associated suffocation, asphyxia, and entrapment for infants (Moon et al., 2016):

- Supine (wholly on the back) position for every sleep
- Use a firm sleep surface; keep soft objects and loose bedding away from infant sleep area
- Room-sharing with the infant on a separate sleep surface
- Breastfeeding
- No smoking, alcohol, or illicit drug use during pregnancy or after birth
- Offer a pacifier at naptime and bedtime
- Regular prenatal care for pregnant women
- Immunize infants in accordance with AAP and CDC recommendations
- Do not use cardiopulmonary monitors as a strategy to reduce the risk of SUID

When an infant dies from SUID, the family requires tremendous support. The nurse provides empathetic support and assists the family as they progress through the grief process and provides guidance for siblings and other family members. Referral to support groups may be helpful.

Oral Health

Oral health is recognized as an integral component of overall health for children and adolescents. Dental caries in early childhood has been identified as one of the most prevalent infectious diseases with more than 40 percent of children diagnosed with caries by entrance to kindergarten. The incidence is more common in preschool children living in poverty or low socioeconomic status (42 percent) as compared to children (18 percent) in higher socioeconomic families. Disparities also exist for Hispanic and non-Hispanic African American children with twice the incidence of caries as compared to non-Hispanic white children. Access to pediatric dental care is a barrier to meeting the oral health care needs of children in the United States (AAPD, 2016).

Nurses are well positioned to provide oral health screenings and to educate families on preventive oral health topics. Children should be referred to a qualified dentist by one year of age. Families should receive anticipatory guidance on optimal use of fluorides, caries prevention, proper nutrition and dietary practices, age-appropriate dental injury prevention, and proper care of teeth and gingival tissue (AAPD, 2013).

Chronic Health Conditions

Improved medical technology has increased the number of children surviving with chronic health problems. In addition, environmental factors are leading to an increase in certain chronic health conditions. At present, it is estimated that about 26 percent of American children have a chronic health condition (Van Cleave et al., 2010). Some examples of common chronic conditions in children are Down syndrome, spina bifida, cerebral palsy, asthma, attention-deficit/hyperactivity disorder (ADHD), diabetes, congenital heart disease, cancer, hemophilia, bronchopulmonary dysplasia, and acquired immunodeficiency syndrome (AIDS). Prevalence of certain chronic diseases is higher in children receiving public insurance and in certain minority populations. For example, children in poverty have a 23 percent higher incidence of asthma, and non-Hispanic African American youth are twice as likely to be diagnosed with asthma as compared to non-Hispanic white youth (Miller et al., 2016).

Despite the differences in the specific diagnoses, all of these families have complex needs and face similar problems. Several variables exist to assess for each child and family:

- What is the actual health status? Is the condition stable or life threatening?
- What is the degree of impairment to the child's ability to develop?
- What types of treatments and therapy are required and with what frequency?
- How often are health care visits and hospitalizations required?
- To what degree are the family routines disrupted?

The common issues nurses will want to evaluate for these families include the following:

- All children and adolescents with chronic health problems need routine health care. The same issues of pediatric health promotion and acute health care need to be addressed with this group. The use of the medical home (discussed later in the chapter) is very important for this population.
- Ongoing medical care specific to the health problem needs to be provided. Examples include monitoring for complications of the health problem, medications management, dietary adjustments, and coordination of therapies. Evaluation of the effectiveness of the treatment plan is critical.
- Care is often provided by multiple specialists. There is a need for coordinating the scheduling of visits, tests or procedures and the treatment regimen.
- Skilled care procedures are often required and may include suctioning, positioning, medications, feeding techniques, breathing treatments, physical therapy, and use of appliances.
- Equipment needs are often complex and may include monitors, oxygen, ventilators, positioning or ambulation devices, infusion pumps, and suction machines.
- Educational needs are often complex. Communication between the family, the team of health care providers, school administrators, and teachers is essential to meet the child's health and educational needs.
- Safe transportation to health care services and school must be available. Several barriers may exist, including family resources, location, and the burden of supportive equipment.

- Financial resources may not be adequate to meet the needs.
- Behavioral issues include the effect of the condition on the child's behavior as well as on other family members.

The ultimate goal is for children with chronic health conditions to achieve optimal health and functioning. Identifying barriers for individual families and overall community barriers is a focus for nurses. Developing support groups, advocating for improved community access to resources, and educating those working with these children on their conditions and needs will promote the family's functioning. The following How To box details a community nursing approach to supporting a child with ADHD.

HOW TO Implement a Community Nursing Approach to a Chronic Illness: ADHD

The following describes the steps the nurse in the community will follow to support a child with ADHD:

- **Assessment:** Obtaining history, physical, parent/family assessment, environmental assessment, learning, and psycho-educational evaluations
- **Behavioral modifications:** (home and school) Teaching families techniques to support clear expectations, consistent routines, positive reinforcement for appropriate behavior, and consequences for negative behaviors
- **Classroom modifications:** Consulting with family and teachers to meet individual needs for remediation or alternative instruction methods if necessary; structuring activities to respond to the child's needs
- **Support:** Referring family to family therapy/counseling, support groups, or mental health services to assist development of positive coping behaviors
- **Medications:** Consulting with physician to monitor and evaluate therapeutic and adverse effects
- **Follow-up:** Assessing at three- to six-month intervals when stable; dynamic process affected by relationships with others; behaviors will change with age; problem may persist through adulthood

Mental Health

Psychosocial stressors have increased over the years for children and mental health issues are a priority health concern for children and adolescents. There are many underlying causes for mental health problems in children, ranging from lead poisoning to exposure to violence in the home. For U.S. children two to eight years, one out of every seven was reported to have a diagnosed mental, behavioral, or developmental disorder with a higher occurrence in boys, children who live in poverty, and non-Hispanic white children (Bitsko et al., 2016).

Nationally, 31.5 percent of high school students reported feeling so sad or hopeless almost every day for 2 or more weeks in a row that they stopped doing some usual activities. This risk factor for depression and suicide has continued to increase over time. The rate of teens reporting seriously considering a suicide attempt has remained stable (17.2 percent) for the past three years with 7.4 percent of teens reporting an actual suicide attempt. Suicide ideation and attempts are higher in females of all ethnicities as compared to males (Kann et al., 2018).

Some of the common mental health problems diagnosed in children and adolescents are anxiety disorders, autism spectrum disorders, depression, bipolar disorder, conduct disorder, oppositional defiant disorder, and substance abuse. Each of these mental health diagnoses has a specific set of criteria for diagnosis found in the *Diagnostic and Statistical Manual of Mental Disorders*, fifth edition (DSM-5). Early recognition and coordinated management of pediatric mental health issues is critical to a child's functioning in school, home, and the community.

More than two million U.S. children during the past 10 years have experienced the stress and emotions associated with being separated from a parent deployed for active duty. These children experience symptoms of depression (25 percent), excess worry (50 percent), and sleep problems (50 percent). By understanding the stressors of military deployment, nurses can identify and provide the support (and referrals) needed to help these children (Siegel & Davis, 2013).

Bullying, an ongoing issue for youth today, is defined as an individual or a group of youth with a perceived or actual power leverage who repeatedly and intentionally cause hurt or harm to another youth(s) who feels helpless to respond. With the extensive use of texting, emails, social networking, and other means of electronic communication among tweens and adolescents, electronic bullying has become a significant problem within communities. In the 2017 YRBSS, 14.9 percent of teens report being electronically bullied and 19 percent of teens reported being bullied on school property in the previous 12 months (Kann et al., 2018). Electronic bullying occurs through texts, Instagram, or other social media. Girls are more likely to be victims of both types of bullying, and victims report thinking about self-harm and/or suicide as a result of bullying. Many electronic bullies use avatars or other ways of disguising their true identity, which makes it difficult for the victim to know who the bully is. The victims often do not report cyber bullying for fear of retaliation from the bully and experience emotional and behavioral symptoms along with school-related problems (Suzuki et al., 2012).

Many families can be at a loss for the mental health behaviors or symptoms they observe in their child. A sense of embarrassment may prohibit parents from seeking help. Nurses can be instrumental in promoting community awareness about common mental health problems in children and identifying resources for families. The use of the medical home to coordinate management of mental health problems is important in the ability to provide oversight of subspecialties, medications, and therapies. A challenge for treating pediatric mental health disorders is an inadequate number of practitioners specializing in pediatric mental health, which may leave some families without adequate support and resources (AAP, 2018).

Environmental Health

The built environment that children and adolescents live in directly affects their health. Growth, size, and behaviors place the pediatric population at greater risk for damage from various toxins. Lead poisoning is one of the most common environmental health hazards. Pesticides, mercury exposure, plasticizers, and poor air quality also pose serious risks (National Institute of Environmental Health Science, 2014). Common toxins and sources of pediatric exposure are listed in Table 28.7.

Growing tissues absorb toxins readily. Developing organ systems are more susceptible to damage. Smaller size means increased concentration of toxins per pound of body weight.

TABLE 28.7 **Common Environmental Agents Hazardous to Children**

Toxins	Sources
Arsenic	Food, water
Asbestos	Building materials: insulation, ceilings, floor tiles
Carbon monoxide	Space heaters, woodstoves, fireplaces, engine exhaust, tobacco smoke
Dioxins	Contaminated foods, water, and soil
Lead	Paint, dust, soil, water, occupational exposure (e.g., battery plant), hobbies (e.g., stained glass)
Mercury	Water contamination, fish, thermometer/sphygmomanometer breakage
Molds	Food, ubiquitous to moist outdoor and indoor environment
Nitrites, nitrates	Water, food
Nicotine, benzene, tars	Environmental tobacco smoke
Particulate matter-nanomaterials	Outdoor air pollution, dust mites, animal dander, roach parts
Pesticides	Food, soil, plants, water, air, topical application for lice treatment, home and school insect management
Phthalates and bisphenol (BPA)	Linings of canned foods, children's toys, vinyl flooring, hard plastics made of polycarbonate (many sports water bottles and baby bottles)
Radon	Soil and rock, the air, ground water, surface water
Solvents/volatile organic compounds	Furniture, carpet, building materials, solvents and degreasers, cleaning products, acetone, formaldehyde
Styrene	Vapors from building materials, photocopiers, tobacco smoke
Ultraviolet light	Outdoor sun exposure, tanning beds

From National Institutes of Environmental Health: Your environment your health, 2015, Triangle Park, NC. Available at www.NIEHS.Nih.gov.

The fact that children are short exposes them to lower air spaces, where heavy chemicals tend to concentrate. Outdoor play, especially during summer months, increases the opportunity for exposure to air pollutants. Chewing and mouthing behaviors offer contact to toxins such as lead. Playing on the floor increases exposure to chemicals in rugs and flooring. Rolling and playing in grass can result in pesticide exposure, and playground materials that are treated with chemicals put children at risk. Exposure risks for adolescents are similar to those for adults and are primarily through work, school, and hobbies (NIEHS, 2015).

It is critical to assess for these environmental health hazards during health care visits. Referral for treatment may be necessary. Counseling families on risk reduction is important to children's health. Population-focused nurses identify environmental problems within the community and target at-risk populations with community interventions (see Table 28.8 for examples).

Bringing screening programs into neighborhoods at risk may facilitate early identification and prevent complications. Lobbying efforts and education can affect public policy to make the environment healthier. The following case presentation

TABLE 28.8 **Prevention Strategies Applied to Environmental Hazards**

Prevention Strategies	Examples
Primary	
Identification of at-risk populations	Substandard housing communities
	Pregnant women
	Children with asthma
Health education about environmental risks	Poison prevention
	Responses to poor air quality alerts
	Discontinue use of plasticizers
Formation of public health policies	Air/water quality standards
	Safety inspections: playgrounds, schools, daycare centers
	Standards for lead levels in imported products intended for children
Research to assess impact of environmental hazards on the pediatric population	Developing reference ranges/biological markers to assess toxic levels in children
	Identify long-term physiological and cognitive consequences of exposure to environmental toxins
Secondary	
Early detection, treatment, and referral for management of environmental toxins	Removal of at-risk persons when lead hazards are detected
	Assessment of lead levels of populations of at-risk children with treatment of individuals as indicated
Tertiary	
Restoration of environment and occupants to healthier state	Asbestos/lead abatement of buildings
	Radon remediation of homes
	Replacement of heating, ventilation, air conditioning, systems contaminated with mold
	Chelating agents for individuals with lead toxic levels

Modified from the Office of Disease Prevention and Health Promotion, Environmental Health, 2018. Retrieved from www.HealthyPeople.gov

gives an example of how a school environment can lead to health problems.

A child's built environment includes exposure to media and the resulting influence on behavior and choices. Food and beverage corporations spend over $1.6 billion each year on advertising that specifically targets children. Much of this advertising uses child-directed marketing strategies to promote food products, and the majority of those products are of poor nutritional value. The heart of the question is whether this advertising is effective in influencing children's food choices. A meta-analysis found that children exposed to unhealthy food marketing were more likely to eat more after seeing the advertisements and tended to select the advertised unhealthy food and beverages seen in the marketing ad (Sadeghirad et al., 2016). Nurses in the community can use this information to provide guidance to parents to limit exposure to television and media, make healthy food choices for their children, and avoid unhealthy foods promoted via media marketing to children. Nurses can also advocate for stricter advertising laws for those unhealthy foods targeted to children.

Lead Poisoning. Lead is a heavy metal that is absorbed into the body primarily through ingestion. Lead poisoning is defined as a serum lead level above 10 μg/dL and it causes significant neurological, cardiovascular, and renal disease. A *Healthy People 2020* goal is to eliminate elevated blood lead levels in all children. More than 88,000 children younger than five years have elevated lead levels in 2016, and the most common exposure is through lead-based paints and lead-contaminated soil and dust in houses built before 1987. Currently, more than four million housing units are home to young children. Children under the age of six years are at highest risk for lead poisoning due to rapid physiological growth and the developmental trait of putting their hands and other objects, which may be contaminated with lead dust, in their mouths (CDC, 2014b; CDC, 2016e).

Universal screening for lead poisoning of all children at ages one and two years is recommended. This screening is recommended when children receive well-child or early and periodic screening, diagnosis, and treatment (EPSDT) screening at regular intervals. In addition, families should be assessed for environmental risk factors to determine the need for screening at other ages. Specific guidelines for minimizing lead exposure through contaminated toys are included in Box 28.2.

BOX 28.2 Steps to Minimize Lead Exposure in Contaminated Toys and Products

- Read recall notices from the CPSC (www.cpsc.gov) and do not buy recalled toys.
- Check old toys at home to make sure they have not been recalled.
- Avoid purchasing toys secondhand from yard sales and flea markets.
- Check labels and recommended ages on all toy labels and follow recommendations.
- Do not purchase children's costume jewelry or allow children to play with adult costume jewelry.

CPSC, Consumer Product Safety Commission.

LEVELS OF PREVENTION

Lead Poisoning	Obesity
Primary Prevention Community education about lead exposure, lead sources in the community, and the adverse health consequences for children.	**Primary Prevention** Offer healthy cooking classes for families in the community.
Secondary Prevention Implement universal screening for all children ages one and two years that present to the community health centers and primary care practices.	**Secondary Prevention** Conduct child body mass index screenings in community daycares and preschools.
Tertiary Prevention Provide families with guidance and resources for lead abatement and to eliminate lead exposure for children with blood lead levels >5 μg/dL.	**Tertiary Prevention** Develop individualized weight loss plans and counsel children identified as obese on lifestyle changes.

Environmental Tobacco Smoke. Environmental tobacco smoke (ETS) is exhaled smoke, smoke from burning tobacco, or smoke from the mouthpiece or filter end of a cigarette, cigar, or pipe. Cigarettes have many known poisons, and both cigarettes and ETS were classified as Class A known human carcinogens in 1992 by the Environmental Protection Agency (EPA). Parents often do not understand or believe the effects of smoking on children. Children, particularly those under age five years and those living in poverty, have higher levels of exposure to ETS. The recent introduction of electronic nicotine delivery systems (ENDS) is also considered to be a risk for ETS. These products produce an aerosolized mixture containing flavored liquids that appeal to youth and nicotine inhaled by the user. As previously noted, ENDS are the most commonly used tobacco product among American youth (AAP, 2016e). An initial study found cancer-causing substances in all of the ENDS samples that were tested (Goniewicz et al., 2014).

Children exposed to ETS experience increased episodes of middle ear infections, asthma, upper respiratory tract infections, and more missed school days. Prenatal exposure to ETS is linked to preterm births, low birth weight, and increased risk for several childhood cancers. Prenatal exposure is also linked to the fetal brain becoming sensitized to nicotine, leading to greater addiction when exposed at an older age. Children living in smoking households with a parent role modeling smoking are more likely to start smoking (Tanski & Wilson, 2012).

Interventions to discourage smoking focus on the parent, the child or adolescent, and public policy. Nurses in public health should offer educational programs for parents dealing with the negative effects of smoking on children, specific interventions to stop smoking, and ways to create a smoke-free environment. Antismoking programs directed toward children and teenagers are more successful if the focus is on short-term effects rather than on long-term effects. Developmentally, children and teenagers cannot visualize the future to imagine the consequences of smoking. Teaching social skills to resist peer pressure is critical.

Nurses should become politically active in the area of smoking. Policies to ban tobacco advertising, enforce restrictions of sale to minors, increase funds for antismoking education, and restriction of public smoking may reduce the incidence of smoking. Community-based interventions to reduce smoking and ETS exposure are included here.

- Collaborate with schools to provide tobacco-free environments (for all school facilities, vehicles, and events).
- Work with schools to provide prevention curricula in elementary, middle, and high schools.
- Develop or identify smoking cessation programs and provide information to health care providers and workplaces in the community.
- Provide education to families on the dangers of ENDS and ETS exposure for children and adolescents.
- Partner with community merchants to enforce minors' access laws.
- Advocate for local policy change to limit smoking in public and private enterprises (CDC, 2016f).

MODELS FOR HEALTH CARE DELIVERY TO CHILDREN AND ADOLESCENTS

Nurses are in a position to work with specific populations through programs targeting the health care needs of children and particularly those at risk. In the following section, strategies for promoting the health care of children and adolescents are described.

Family-Centered Medical Home

A **family-centered medical home** is a partnership between a child or adolescent, the child or adolescent's family, and the pediatric team who oversees the child or adolescent's health and well-being within a community-based system that provides uninterrupted care to promote optimal health outcomes. The medical home incorporates preventive, acute, mental health, and chronic care from birth through transition to adulthood. The medical home emphasizes an integrated health system with collaboration of care from an interprofessional team of primary care physicians, specialists and subspecialists, nurses, other health professionals, hospitals and health care facilities, public health, and the community working with children and families (Malouin, 2013).

About 48.7 percent of all children have a medical home in the United States (KFF, 2016). It is imperative to increase the use of medical homes for all children, particularly children with special health care needs. A child with special health care needs will greatly benefit from collaborative care from the primary care provider, subspecialty physicians, school system, community therapists, family support groups, and other community resources to achieve optimal health and reduce the time burden on families (Miller et al., 2015). Research has demonstrated a significant reduction in emergency department visits (17 percent) and decrease in inpatient admissions (47 percent) for children with a medical home (Matiz et al., 2016).

A successful medical home relies on the multitude of supports that are brought to the service delivery system that surrounds the family and community. Families can trust that there is a place where their child or adolescent is provided holistic care that addresses all aspects of physical, mental, and emotional health. The medical home is not a specific building, but it is a system of care that is accessible, continuous, comprehensive, coordinated, compassionate, and culturally effective. Nurses in the community play an active role as a team member of the medical home by identifying resources for families, referring families to a medical home, and participating in the health care of children in medical homes.

Motivational Interviewing

Motivational interviewing is a focused communication strategy in which the parents are encouraged to set goals, identify personal barriers, and identify potential mechanisms to overcome the barriers to make safety and health promotion changes for their child. This can be an effective intervention to promote healthy changes within the family environment (Resnicow et al., 2015). It can be easily implemented by nurses in primary care settings and public health clinics under limited time constraints and is readily incorporated into the medical home model.

Motivational interviewing emphasizes a collaborative approach to behavior change instead of a prescriptive approach (Fig. 28.8). Nurses use open-ended questioning and reflection to encourage the parent or adolescent to share their identified barriers to change. When individuals demonstrate positive comments toward change, the nurse expands upon those comments and provides further support for that change. This strategy is very effective with positive health behavior changes such as smoking cessation, healthy eating, and safety behaviors.

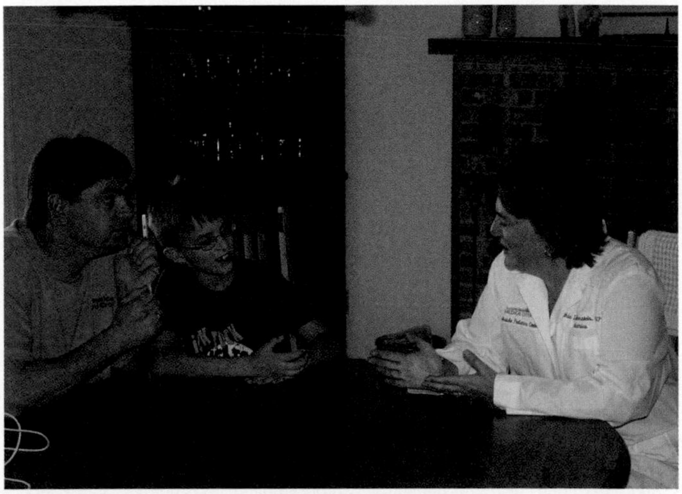

Fig. 28.8 Motivational interviewing is an effective way for nurses to intervene with families and promote positive behavioral change in the home.

ROLE OF THE POPULATION-FOCUSED NURSE IN CHILD AND ADOLESCENT HEALTH

Population-focused nurses have the opportunity to work with families to achieve growth toward many of the *Healthy People 2020* objectives. They practice in a variety of settings, including community health centers, school-based clinics, and home health programs. They provide care through well-child clinics, immunization programs, federally mandated programs (such as the nutrition program Women, Infants, and Children [WIC]) or specific state-funded programs, such as Head Start.

With passage of the ACA, strategies to implement improved access include expanding the role of nurses and the settings for practice. The nursing process and a knowledge base of the factors unique to the pediatric population provide a framework of care. Nursing, through developing and coordinating community services and through formation of public policies, promotes the well-being of children and families within the community. Assessments are made to identify the needs and target populations at risk. Programs based on the needs of specific at-risk populations are developed for the delivery of health care.

The nursing plan of care includes three major components. The first is the management of actual or potential health problems. The second involves both education and anticipatory guidance. This enables families to understand what to expect in the areas of growth and development as well as social, emotional, and cognitive changes. Nurses offer information to promote healthy lifestyles and to prevent acute and chronic health problems as well as unintentional injuries. A third role is case management or coordination of care. For example, the nurse coordinates referrals to community agencies, other health care services or providers or assistance programs. Box 28.3 lists community resources.

LINKING CONTENT TO PRACTICE

In this chapter, emphasis is placed on the community health needs of children and adolescents within the context of the family. The public health core functions of disease prevention, health promotion, and the three levels of health services are directly related to the pediatric population and their specific population needs. To meet the core public health competencies, nurses must learn how to assess children and adolescents using developmental principles to determine safety risks for injury and environmental health exposures. Policy and program development for the pediatric population is geared toward improving the built environment in which a child grows and providing parents with education on health promotion strategies like smoking cessation to improve their child's health. Nurses develop competencies in communication strategies with children of varying developmental levels and recognize the various locations in the community that need education on promoting the health of children (e.g., daycare centers, schools). Basic health services such as well-child care and immunizations are critical to the health of the pediatric population, and the nurse is poised as a leader within the medical home model of health care delivery for children and adolescents. This chapter prepares the community health nurse to provide comprehensive, developmentally appropriate education to families; deliver basic health care services in a holistic approach; and develop community programming to improve safety and environmental wellness for children and adolescents.

BOX 28.3 Community Resources for Pediatric Health Care

- Children's service clinics
- Well-child clinics
- Immunization clinics
- Infectious disease clinics
- Children's specialty services
- Family violence/child abuse centers
- Homeless shelters
- School health programs
- Head Start
- Parents Anonymous
- Crisis hotlines
- Community education classes
- Early intervention/developmental services
- Childbirth education classes
- Breastfeeding support groups
- Parent support groups
- Family planning clinics
- Women, Infants, and Children (WIC) programs
- Medicaid and CHIP
- Youth employment/training programs

HEALTHY PEOPLE 2020

Objectives Focused on Children and Adolescents

Education and Community-Based Programs

ECB-4: Increase the proportion of elementary, middle, and senior high schools that provide school health education to promote personal health and wellness.

ECB-7: Increase the proportion of middle, junior high, and senior high schools that provide comprehensive school health education to prevent health problems.

Environmental Health

EH-8: Eliminate elevated blood lead levels in children.

Immunizations and Infectious Disease

IID-7: Achieve and maintain effective vaccination coverage levels for universally recommended vaccines among young children.

Injury/Violence Prevention

IVP-16: Increase use of age appropriate child restraints in cars.

Nutrition and Weight Status

NWS-10: Reduce the proportion of children and adolescents who are overweight or obese.

Physical Activity and Fitness

PA-4: Increase the proportion of the nation's public and private schools that require daily physical education for all students.

Tobacco Use

TU-15: Tobacco-free environments in schools, including all school facilities, property, vehicles, and school events.

From U.S. Department of Health and Human Services: *Healthy People 2020,* Washington, DC, 2010, U.S. Government Printing Office.

PRACTICE APPLICATION

Sam is a 4-year-old boy brought to the clinic by his mother for his 4-year well-child check and immunizations. Sam will be attending the local Head Start program in the fall. He is the oldest of three children and his siblings are 9 months and 35 months. His mother is a single parent who works at a local restaurant as a waitress. Sam and his siblings are insured by Medicaid. Sam's mother is 24 years old and the family lives with the maternal grandparents. Sam's mother is in good health and does not smoke or abuse drugs. Sam has been watched by his grandmother since birth and is exposed to cigarette smoke in the home by both grandparents.

On the developmental exam, Sam is very cooperative, eager to please, and speaks clearly. His development is significant for failure to identify three colors, count to five, or recognize any letters. His gross motor skills are appropriate but he only scribbles when given a crayon. Sam reports watching television shows with his family for fun. On physical examination, Sam has a >95th percentile BMI for age/gender but no other abnormal exam findings are noted. Hearing and vision are within normal limits for age.

Based on the previous scenario, answer the following questions:

A. What additional history and assessment information should you collect based on the child's home environment?
B. What immunizations and lab tests are indicated based on his age and risk factors?
C. What education should you give this mother on changes in the home to promote development? To reduce ETS exposure? To ensure safety?
D. Based on the BMI percentile, what additional nutrition and dietary practices information should you obtain?
E. What interventions and education should you provide to this mother regarding Sam's obesity and associated risk factors?
F. In an analysis of the Medicaid child population in Sam's medical home, the population-focused nurse found that a number of children had similar risk factors. Is there a population-level intervention the nurse may want to use to reduce the risk in the future child population?

Answers can be found on the Evolve site.

KEY POINTS

- Physical growth and development are ongoing processes resulting in physical, cognitive, and emotional changes that affect health status.
- Good nutrition is essential for healthy growth and development, and it influences disease prevention in later life.
- Childhood obesity is increasing in prevalence. Modifiable risk factors include dietary intake, physical activity, sleep, and digital media time.
- Immunizations are successful in prevention of selected diseases. Barriers to immunizing children are parental concerns, cost, vaccine shortages, and changes in recommended vaccine scheduling.
- The built environment is influential on a child's physical, emotional, and psychosocial health. Nurses can design interventions for families and communities to improve a child's environment if improvement is indicated.
- The family is critical to the growth and development of the child. Social support has a powerful influence on successful parenting.
- Unintentional injuries are the major cause of morbidity and mortality in the child and adolescent population. Most are preventable. Nurses have a major role in anticipatory guidance and prevention.
- Population-focused nurses have a strong role in the prevention of, identification of, and education about child maltreatment.
- Child advocacy is critical to reduce the incidence of abuse and neglect in childhood.
- Minimizing complications of the major health risks to the pediatric and adolescent population follows the goals of *Healthy People 2020* initiatives.
- The pediatric population is vulnerable to environmental hazards. Decreasing exposure and identifying problems early are important areas for interventions by population-focused nurses.
- Nurses are involved in strategies to meet the needs of the pediatric population and their families in the community.
- The family-centered medical home is a successful system for coordinating health care for children and for facilitating continuous family support and health management.
- Children who are low income or live in poverty are at increased risk for violence, injuries, and environmental hazards.
- The use of motivational interviewing can facilitate positive health behavior changes for families with children.

CLINICAL DECISION-MAKING ACTIVITIES

1. Develop a plan of immunization for a 5½-year-old who has had one dose of diphtheria, tetanus, and acellular pertussis (DTaP), *Haemophilus influenzae* type b (Hib), and inactivated poliovirus (IPV). Be specific about due dates for immunizations.
2. Develop a screening program for children and adolescents who live in a low-income older neighborhood with a large percent of Hispanic residents. What risk factors would you consider in the process? Have you examined the thoughts of

others in the community that might affect the success of the screening program? Be specific.
3. Plan a survey of a school district to determine its "friendliness" to children with chronic health problems. How would you implement changes?
4. Develop a community program for smoking cessation. Identify how you will target parents and caregivers of children. Discuss how you will incorporate the concept of ETS (including ENDS) exposure in your program.
5. Develop nutrition education programs for (1) mothers who are breastfeeding their infants, (2) a group of five-year-olds in a kindergarten class, and (3) a group of high school sophomores. What factors do these programs have in common? How do they differ?
6. Administer a safety survey (e.g., the Injury Prevention Program [TIPP] from the American Academy of Pediatrics, or develop your own) to assess the home environment of a six-month-old and a five-year-old. Develop a plan of education and anticipatory guidance for the family. How would you apply this information to a larger population?

ADDITIONAL RESOURCES

EVOLVE WEBSITE

http://evolve.elsevier.com/Stanhope/community/

- Answers to Practice Application
- Case Study
- Glossary
- Review Questions

REFERENCES

American Academy of Pediatric Dentistry: *Guideline on periodicity of examination, preventive dental services, anticipatory guidance/counseling, and oral treatment for infants, children, and adolescents*, 2013. Retrieved from http://www.aapd.org.

American Academy of Pediatric Dentistry: *Policy on oral health care programs for infants, children, and adolescents*, 2016. Retrieved from http://www.aapd.org.

American Academy of Pediatrics: Policy statement: providing care for immigrant, migrant, and border children, *Pediatrics* 131(6): e2028–e2034, 2013a.

American Academy of Pediatrics: Policy reaffirmation: the built environment: designing communities to promote physical activity in children, *Pediatrics* 131(5):e1707, 2013b.

American Academy of Pediatrics: *AAP updates recommendations on obesity prevention: it's never too early to begin living a healthy lifestyle*, 2015. Retrieved from https://www.aap.org.

American Academy of Pediatrics: *Blueprint for children: how the next president can build a foundation for a healthy future*, 2016a. Retrieved from https://www.aap.org.

American Academy of Pediatrics: Media use in school-aged children and adolescents, *Pediatrics* 138(5), 2016b. Retrieved from https://www.aap.org.

American Academy of Pediatrics: *Recommendations for children's media use*, 2016c. Retrieved from https://www.aap.org.

American Academy of Pediatrics: SIDS and other sleep-related infant deaths: updated 2016 recommendations for a safe infant sleeping environment, *Pediatrics* 138(5), 2016d.

American Academy of Pediatrics: *Electronic nicotine delivery systems*, 2016e. Retrieved from https://www.aap.org.

American Academy of Pediatrics: Policy affirmation: firearm-related injuries affecting the pediatric population, *Pediatrics* 139(3), 2017.

American Academy of Pediatrics: *Promoting children's mental health*, 2018. Retrieved from https://www.aap.org.

American Institutes for Research: *National center on family homelessness*, 2018. Retrieved from https://www.air.org.

Anderson M, Jiang J: *Teens, social media & technology 2018*, 2018. Retrieved from http://www.pewinternet.org.

Aronson SS, Shope TR: *Managing infectious diseases in child care and schools*, ed 4, Elk Grove, CA, 2016, American Academy of Pediatrics.

Ballesteros MF, Williams DD, Mack KA, Simon TR, Sleet DA: The epidemiology of unintentional and violence-related injury morbidity and mortality among children and adolescents in the United States, *Int J Environ Res Public Health* 15(4):616, 2018.

Birch LL: Child feeding practices and the etiology of obesity, *Obesity* (Silver Spring) 14(3):343–344, 2006.

Bitsko RH, Holbrook JR, Robinson LR, et al.: Health care, family, and community factors associated with mental, behavioral, and developmental disorders in early childhood—United States, 2011–2012, *MMWR Morb Mortal Wkly Rep* 65:221–226, 2016.

Börnhorst C, Wijnhoven TM, Kunešová M, et al.: WHO European childhood obesity surveillance initiative: associations between sleep duration, screen time and food consumption frequencies, *BMC Public Health* 15:442, 2015.

Boyle CA, Boulet S, Schieve LA, et al.: Trends in the prevalence of developmental disabilities in US children, 1997–2008, *Pediatrics* 127(6):1034–1042, 2011.

Brenner JS: Sports specialization and intensive training in young athletes, *Pediatrics* 138(3):e20162148, 2016.

Casillas KL, Fauchier A, Derkash BT, Garrido EF: Implementation of evidence-based home visiting programs aimed at reducing child maltreatment: a meta-analytic review, *Child Abuse Negl* 53:64–80, 2016.

Centers for Disease Control and Prevention: *National action plan for child injury prevention*, 2012. Retrieved from http://www.cdc.gov.

Centers for Disease Control and Prevention: *High quality physical education*, 2013. Retrieved from http://www.cdc.gov.

Centers for Disease Control and Prevention: *Understanding child maltreatment*, 2014a. Retrieved from https://www.cdc.gov.

Centers for Disease Control and Prevention: *Lead: prevention tips*, 2014b. Retrieved from https://www.cdc.gov.

Centers for Disease Control and Prevention: *About child & teen BMI*, 2015. Retrieved from https://www.cdc.gov.

Center for Disease Control and Prevention: *Infant mortality*, 2016a. Retrieved from https://www.cdc.gov.

Centers for Disease Control and Prevention: *Common vaccine safety concerns*, 2016b. Retrieved from https://www.cdc.gov.

Centers for Disease Control and Prevention: *Defining childhood obesity*, 2016c. Retrieved from https://www.cdc.gov.

Centers for Disease Control and Prevention: *Playground safety*, 2016d. Retrieved from https://www.cdc.gov.

Centers for Disease Control and Prevention: *Childhood lead poisoning data, statistics, and surveillance*, 2016e. Retrieved from https://www.cdc.gov.

Centers for Disease Control and Prevention: *Smoking and tobacco use: guide to community preventative services*, 2016f. Retrieved from https://www.cdc.gov.

Centers for Disease Control and Prevention: *Immunity types*, 2017a. Retrieved from https://www.cdc.gov.

Centers for Disease Control and Prevention: *Making the vaccine decision*, 2017b. Retrieved from https://www.cdc.gov.

Centers for Disease Control and Prevention: *Facts about VISs*, 2017c. Retrieved from https://www.cdc.gov.

Centers for Disease Control and Prevention: *Chapter 21: surveillance for adverse events following immunization using the vaccine adverse event reporting system (VAERS)*, 2017d. Retrieved from https://www.cdc.gov.

Centers for Disease Control and Prevention: *National diabetes statistics report*, 2017e. Retrieved from https://www.cdc.gov.

Centers for Disease Control and Prevention: *Youth physical activity guidelines*, 2017f. Retrieved from https://www.cdc.gov.

Centers for Disease Control and Prevention: *Child passenger safety: get the facts*, 2017g. Retrieved from https://www.cdc.gov.

Centers for Disease Control and Prevention: *Sports and recreation-related injuries*, 2017h. Retrieved from https://www.cdc.gov.

Centers for Disease Control and Prevention: *Facts about developmental disabilities*, 2018a. Retrieved from https://www.cdc.gov.

Centers for Disease Control and Prevention: *Recommended child and adolescent immunization schedule for ages 18 years or younger, United States*, 2018b. Retrieved from https://www.cdc.gov.

Centers for Disease Control and Prevention: *Childhood obesity facts*, 2018c. Retrieved from https://www.cdc.gov.

Centers for Disease Control and Prevention: *Physical activity facts*, 2018d. Retrieved from https://www.cdc.gov.

Centers for Disease Control and Prevention: *Abusive head trauma*, 2018e. Retrieved from https://www.cdc.gov.

Centers for Medicare & Medicaid Services (CMMS): *Children's Health Insurance Program (CHIP)*, 2017. Retrieved from https://www.medicaid.gov.

Central Intelligence Agency: *The World Factbook: Infant Mortality Rate*, 2017. Retrieved from https://www.cia.gov.

Cerdá M, Wall M, Feng T, et al.: Association of state recreational marijuana laws with adolescent marijuana use, *JAMA Pediatr* 171(2):142–149, 2017.

Chandrasekhar R, et al.: Social determinants of influenza hospitalization in the United States, *Influenza Other Respir Viruses.* 11(6): 479–488 2017.

Chassiakos Y, Radesky J, Christakis D, Moreno M, Cross C: Children and adolescents and digital media, *Pediatrics* 138(5), 2016.

Children's Defense Fund: *The state of America's children 2017 report*, 2018. Retrieved from http://www.childrensdefense.org.

Couch SC, Glanz K, Zhou C, Sallis JF, Saelens BE: Home food environment in relation to children's diet quality and weight status, *J Acad Nutr Diet*, 114(10):1569–1579.e1, 2014.

Department of Education: Assistance to states for the education of children with disabilities and preschool grants for children with disabilities, *Fed Regist* 71(156):46541–46845, 2006. Retrieved from www.idea.ed.gov.

Domingues-Montanari S: Clinical and psychological effects of excessive screen time on children, *J Paediatr Child Health* 53(4): 333–338, 2017.

Dutko P, Ver Ploeg M, Farrigan T: *USDA characteristics and influential factors of food deserts*. Economic Research Service, Economic Research Report Number 140, August 2012.

Federal Interagency Forum on Child and Family Statistics: *America's children: key indicators for well-being*, 2017. Retrieved from https://www.childstats.gov.

Felső R, Lohner S, Hollódy K, Erhardt É, Molnár D: Relationship between sleep duration and childhood obesity: systematic review including the potential underlying mechanisms, *Nutr Metab Cardiovasc Dis* 27(9):751–761, 2017.

Garver WS, Newman SB, Gonzales-Pacheco DM, et al.: The genetics of childhood obesity and interaction with dietary macronutrients, *Genes Nutr* 8:271–287, 2013.

Gibson LY, Allen KL, Davis E, Blair E, Zubrick SR, Byrne SM: The psychosocial burden of childhood overweight and obesity: evidence for persisting difficulties in boys and girls, *Eur J Pediatr* 176(7):925–993, 2017.

Goniewicz ML, Knysak J, Gawron M, et al.: Levels of selected carcinogens and toxicants in vapour from electronic cigarettes, *Tob Control* 23(2):133–139, 2014.

Gose M, Plachta-Danielzik S, Willié B, Johannsen M, Landsberg B, Müller MJ: Longitudinal influences of neighbourhood built and social environment on children's weight status, *Int J Environ Res Public Health* 10:5083–5096, 2013.

Gregory B, Nyland J: Medial elbow injury in young throwing athletes, *Muscles Ligaments Tendons J* 3(2):91–100, 2016.

Hager ER, Cockerham A, O'Reilly N, et al.: Food swamps and food deserts in Baltimore City, MD, USA: associations with dietary behaviours among urban adolescent girls, *Public Health Nutr* 20(14):2598–2607, 2017.

Hales CM, Carroll MD, Fryar CD, Ogden CL: Prevalence of obesity among adults and youth: United States, 2015–2016, *NCHS Data Brief* (288):1–8, 2017. Retrieved from www.cdc.gov.

Hruby A, Hu FB: The epidemiology of obesity: a big picture, *PharmacoEconomics* 33(7):673–689, 2015.

Jiang Y, Ekono M, Skinner C: *Basic facts about low-income children, children under 18 years, 2012*, 2014, National Center for Children in Poverty. Retrieved from http://www.nccp.org.

Kaiser Family Foundation: *Percent of children with a medical home*, 2016. Retrieved from https://www.kff.org.

Kann L, McManus T, Harris WA, Shanklin SL, et al.: Youth risk behavior surveillance—United States, 2017, *MMWR Surveill Summ* 67(8):1–114, 2018.

Latzer Y, Stein D: A review of the psychological and familial perspectives of childhood obesity, *J Eat Disord* 1:7, 2013.

Malouin RA: *Positioning the family and patient at the center: a guide to family and patient partnership in the medical home*, Elk Grove Village, IL, 2013, American Academy of Pediatrics, National Center for Medical Home Implementation.

Matiz LA, Robbins-Milne L, Krause MC, Peretz PJ, Rausch JC: Evaluating the impact of information technology tools to support the asthma medical home, *Clin Pediatr (Phila)* 55(3):165–170, 2016.

McBride DL: Pediatric firearm deaths and injuries in the United States, *J Pediatr Nurs* 38:138–139, 2018.

Miller GF, Coffield E, Leroy Z, Wallin R: Prevalence and costs of five chronic conditions in children. *J Sch Nurs* 32(5):357–364, 2016.

Miller JE, Nugent CN, Russell LB: Which components of medical homes reduce the time burden on families of children with special health care needs? *Health Serv Res* 50(3):440–461, 2015.

Moon RY, Task Force On Sudden Infant Death Syndrome: SIDS and other sleep-related infant deaths: evidence base for 2016 updated recommendations for a safe infant sleeping environment, *Pediatrics* 138(5):e20162940, 2016.

Nance ML, Carr BG, Kallan MJ, Branas CC, Wiebe DJ: Variation in pediatric and adolescent firearm mortality rates in rural and urban US counties, *Pediatrics* 125(6):1112–1118, 2010.

National Association of School Nurses: *Position statement, overweight and obesity in children and adolescents in schools—the role of the school nurse*, 2018. Retrieved from https://www.nasn.org.

National Center for Children in Poverty: *Basic facts about low income children*, 2016. Retrieved from www.nccp.org.

National Center for Health Statistics (NCHS): *National Vital Statistics System*, 2018. Retrieved from www.cdc.gov.

National Highway Traffic Safety Administration: *Traffic safety facts, occupant protection in passenger vehicles*, 2017. Retrieved from https://crashstats.nhtsa.dot.gov.

National Institute of Environmental Health Sciences: *Your environment your health*, Triangle Park, North Carolina, 2015. Retrieved from www.NIEHS.Nih.gov.

North Carolina Partnership for Children: *Shape NC: healthy starts for young children*, 2018. Retrieved from http://www.smartstart.org.

Park S, Li R, Birch L: Mothers' child-feeding practices are associated with children's sugar-sweetened beverage intake, *J Nutr* 145(4):806–812, 2015.

Patel DR, Fidrocki D, Parachuri V: Sport-related concussions in adolescent athletes: a critical public health problem for which prevention remains an elusive goal, *Transl Pediatr* 6(3):114–120, 2017.

Resnicow K, McMaster F, Bocian A, et al.: Motivational interviewing and dietary counseling for obesity in primary care: an RCT, *Pediatrics* 135(4):649–657, 2015. Retrieved from http://pediatrics.aappublications.org.

Roy SM, Spivack JG, Faith MS, et al.: Infant BMI or weight-for-length and obesity risk in early childhood, *Pediatrics* 137(5):e20153492, 2016. Retrieved from http://pediatrics.aappublications.org.

Rushton FE, Byrne WW, Darden PM, McLeigh J: Enhancing child safety and well-being through pediatric group well-child care and home visitation: the Well Baby Plus Program, *Child Abuse Negl* 41:182–189, 2015.

Sadeghirad B, Duhaney T, Motaghipisheh S, Campbell NR, Johnston BC: Influence of unhealthy food and beverage marketing on children's dietary intake and preference: a systematic review and meta-analysis of randomized trials, *Obes Rev* 17(10):945–959, 2016.

Scott J, Azrael D, Miller M: Firearm storage in homes with children with self-harm risk factors, *Pediatrics* 141(3), 2018.

Shaffer DR, Kipp K: *Developmental psychology: childhood and adolescence*, ed 9, Independence, KY, 2013, Cengage Learning.

Sheu Y, Chen LH, Hedegaard H: Sports- and recreation-related injury episodes in the United States, 2011–2014, *Natl Health Stat Report* (99):1–12, 2016.

Siegel BS, Davis BE: Health and mental health needs of children in US military families, *Pediatrics* 131(6):e2002–e2015, 2013.

Smith M, Hosking J, Woodward A, et al.: Systematic literature review of built environment effects on physical activity and active transport—an update and new findings on health equity. *Int J Behav Nutr Phys Act*, 14:158, 2017.

Springer SC, Silverstein J, Copeland K, et al.: Management of type 2 diabetes mellitus in children and adolescents, *Pediatrics* 131:e648–e664, 2013.

Suzuki K, Asaga R, Sourander A, Hoven CW, Mandell D: Cyberbullying and adolescent mental health, *Int J Adolesc Med Health* 24(1):27–35, 2012.

Tanski SE, Wilson KM: Children and secondhand smoke: clear evidence for action, *Pediatrics* 129(1):170–171, 2012. Retrieved from http://pediatrics.aappublications.org.

U.S. Department of Agriculture: *Choose my plate*, 2015. Retrieved from www.USDA.gov.

U.S. Department of Health and Human Services: *Healthy People 2020*, Washington, DC, 2010, U.S. Government Printing Office. Retrieved from www.cdc.gov.

U.S. Department of Health and Human Services: *Heads up, concussion in youth sports*, 2013. Retrieved from http://www.cdc.gov.

U.S. Department of Health and Human Services: *Trends in teen pregnancy and childbearing*, 2016. Retrieved from https://www.hhs.gov.

U.S. Department of Health & Human Services, Administration for Children and Families, Administration on Children, Youth and Families, Children's Bureau: *Child maltreatment 2015*, 2017. Retrieved from http://www.acf.hhs.gov.

Van Cleave J, Gortmaker SL, Perrin JM: Dynamics of obesity and chronic health conditions among children and youth, *JAMA* 303(7):623–630, 2010.

Van Geel M, Vedder P, Tanilon J: Are overweight and obese youths more often bullied by their peers? A meta-analysis on the correlation between weight status and bullying, *Int J Obes* (Lond) 38(10):1263–1267, 2014.

Ventola CL: Immunization in the United States: recommendations, barriers, and measures to improve compliance: Part 1: childhood vaccinations, *P T* 41(7):426–436, 2016.

Villanueva K, Pereira G, Knuiman M, et al.: The impact of the built environment on health across the life course: design of a cross-sectional data linkage study, *BMJ Open* 3(1):e002482, 2013. Retrieved from https://bmjopen.bmj.com.

Zaremski JL, McClelland J, Vincent HK, Horodyski M: Trends in sports-related elbow ulnar collateral ligament injuries, *Orthop J Sports Med* 5(10):2325967117731296, 2017.

Zayas LH, Aguilar-Gaxiola S, Yoon H, Rey GN: The distress of citizen-children with detained and deported parents, *J Child Fam Stud* 2015. Retrieved from https://www.ncbi.nlm.nih.gov.

29

Major Health Issues and Chronic Disease Management of Adults Across the Life Span

Monty Gross, PhD, MSN, RN, CNE, CNL, Andrea Knopp, PhD, MPH, MSN, FNP-BC, and Hazel Brown, DNP, RN

OBJECTIVES

After reading this chapter, the student should be able to:

1. Define terms commonly used in the care of adults.
2. Describe historical and current perspectives of adult health and health policy.
3. Discuss sources of population-based public health data and health status indicators about adults to be used to align community resources to support adults with chronic illnesses.
4. Identify useful resources and development strategies to care for populations of adults across the life span.
5. Discuss the concepts of self-management and the implementation of the Chronic Care Model to support adults with chronic illness.
6. Explain the dynamic forces that contribute to shared and gender-specific diseases, health disparities, and cultural diversity.
7. Identify and validate social and behavioral factors that contribute to culturally competent care of adults in their communities.

CHAPTER OUTLINE

Historical Perspectives on Adult Men and Women's Health
Health Policy and Legislation
Health Status Indicators
Adult Health Concerns
Women's Health Concerns
Men's Health Concerns
Health Disparities Among Special Groups of Adults
Community-Based Models for Care of Adults

KEY TERMS

abuse, p. 656
adult day health, p. 672
advanced medical directives, p. 656
Americans with Disabilities Act (ADA), p. 655
anorexia, p. 664
assisted living, p. 673
bisexual, p. 670
body mass index, p. 663
bulimia, p. 664
cancer, p. 662
cardiovascular disease, p. 661
caregiver burden, p. 656
Chronic Care Model (CCM), p. 660
chronic disease, p. 654
community-based model, p. 672
diabetes, p. 661
do-not-resuscitate order, p. 656
durable medical power of attorney, p. 656
erectile dysfunction, p. 669
Family and Medical Leave Act (FMLA), p. 655
financial exploitation, p. 656
frail elderly, p. 671
gay, p. 670
gestational diabetes mellitus (GDM), p. 665
health screenings, p. 666
health status indicators, p. 657
heart disease, p. 660
home health, p. 672
hospice, p. 672
hypertension, p. 661
impoverished, p. 671
injury, p. 672
lesbian, p. 670
life expectancy, p. 658
living will, p. 656
long-term care, p. 673
menopause, p. 665
men's health, p. 664
mental health, p. 662
morbidity, p. 658
mortality, p 658
neglect, p. 656
obesity, p. 664
Office on Women's Health, p. 664
Older Americans Act (OAA), p. 655
osteoporosis, p. 666
palliative care, p. 672
patient-centered medical home, p. 672

Continued

KEY TERMS—cont'd

Patient Self-Determination Act, p. 656
Personal Responsibility and Work Opportunity Reconciliation Act, p. 656
preconceptual counseling, p. 664
prostate cancer, p. 668
rehabilitation, p. 673
reproductive health, p. 664
respite care, p. 672
self-management, p. 660
sexually transmitted disease, p. 663
sexually transmitted infection, p. 663
stroke, p. 663
Temporary Assistance for Needy Families (TANF), p. 656
testicular cancer, p. 668
unintended pregnancy, p. 664
veteran, p. 659
weight control, p. 664
women's health, p. 654

This chapter provides an overview of major health issues of adults that occur at various stages of life. Nurses struggle with these numerous and complex topics. Changes in population demographics signal challenges of limited resources and increased prevalence of persons living with multiple chronic conditions. Unhealthy lifestyles, environmental pollution, and politics are a sample of factors a nurse will need to consider in population-centered health care. Descriptive statistics are provided to help illustrate the significance of a disease or condition. Despite many pressing issues and political debates, there are many opportunities to improve the health of the population. The key is to focus on effective public health interventions and policies targeting chronic diseases, which will lead to a healthier population with lower health care spending, less school and workplace absenteeism, increased economic productivity, and an improved quality of life (American Public Health Association [APHA], n.d.). Significant changes are rapidly occurring in health care and in the communities through policy changes and research. Nurses will be better prepared to practice by having a better understanding of these major health issues.

HISTORICAL PERSPECTIVES ON ADULT MEN AND WOMEN'S HEALTH

Men and women have always faced a wide array of health issues that transition over time to impact their lives and the community. Gender is a major social determinant of health. Gender equity positively affects a variety of factors, such as decision making, income generation/allocation, and application and observance of norms, which affect health. Gender inequalities span throughout time and all societies, damaging the health of both genders, but in the majority of societies, particularly middle- and lower-income areas, women are secondary citizens to men. Social and political climates influence research and funding agendas that ultimately affect how health care is delivered in the community. A gender gap has existed where the emphasis on health issues and community focus has given priority to one gender over the other through research, policies, and funding. This has resulted in the focus of prevention and treatment being predominantly on males, depending on social and political time period.

Historically men have dominated the medical and research professions because of cultural and societal norms. At the beginning of the twentieth century, discussions of **women's health** focused primarily on reproduction and women's roles as mothers. In the 1920s, with the birth control movement in its initial stages, women's health expanded to address family planning and reproductive health. Women began to be empowered by the suffragette movement, winning the right to vote in 1920. As the women's rights movement gained momentum, women's health issues and the research of those issues displaced many issues of men. In the 1980s recommendations were made by the U.S. Public Health Services Task Force on Women's Health Issues to increase gender equity in biomedical research and the establishment of guidelines for including women in federally sponsored studies (Alexander et al., 2007). In 1990 the Society for Women's Research was founded. Through political action of the National Institutes of Health (NIH), legislation once again included women and other minorities in research studies (NIH, 1993).

During the nineteenth and twentieth centuries, illness and death rates from infectious diseases decreased and those of **chronic diseases** increased for men and women in Western countries. Due to refinement and understanding of germ theory and the use of medical and public health strategies such as immunizations, pasteurization, and antibiotics, primary infections declined (Egger, 2012). Health policies and programs were implemented to reduce the spread of infections and increase life span. These activities began the shift in focus to chronic illnesses, such as cardiovascular disease and cancers.

HEALTH POLICY AND LEGISLATION

Health policy is action taken by public and private agencies to promote health. It is a reflection of the values held in society and can greatly influence the health of the citizens overall. The development of health policy is driven in a cascade down through the hierarchy of national policy. At the apex of this hierarchy is the Constitution. Legislation in the form of acts, laws, and regulations, must be congruent with the Constitution as the overarching umbrella for national guidance. The hierarchy contains nested systems, or fractals, that represent the state and organizational components that drive practice at the point

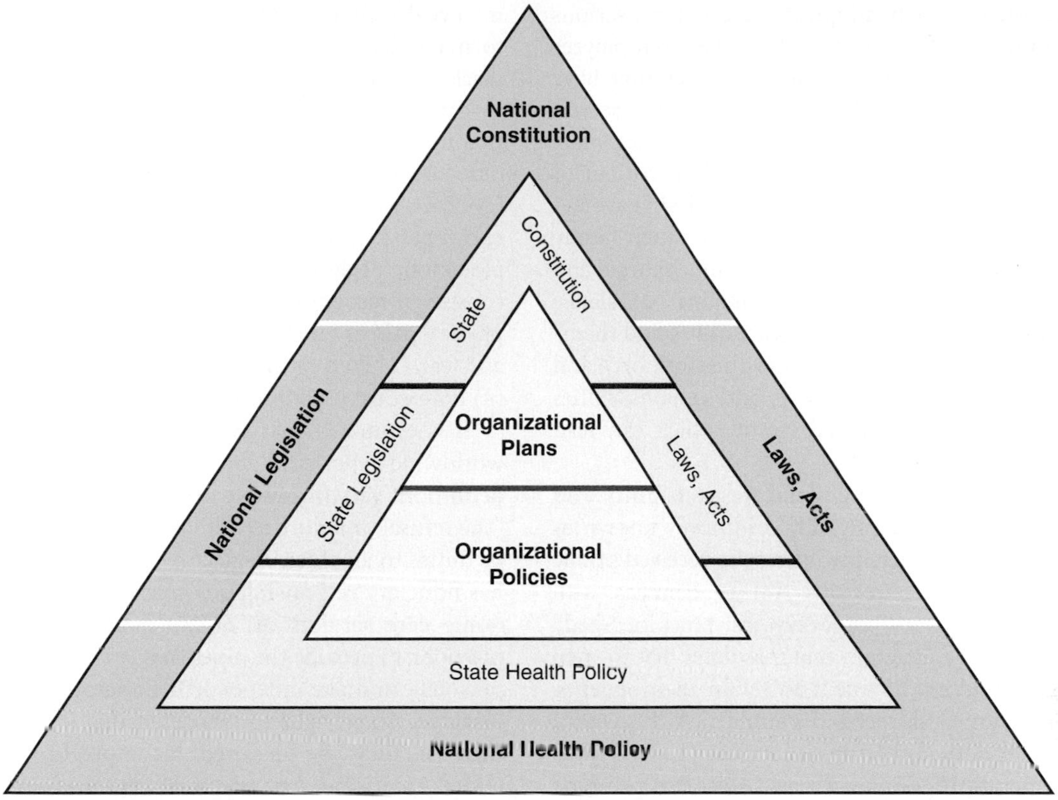

Fig. 29.1 Nest of cascading policy frameworks from national to organizational levels demonstrating the dependency of the latter on the former and the fractals that characterize complex adaptive systems. (Developed by Hazel Brown, RN, DNP, June 2018.)

of care delivery (Fig. 29.1). Because of their education, experience, and perspectives, registered nurses are uniquely qualified to be engaged in policy formation. When involved with influencing policies that affect decisions, nurses can make large contributions to improving health.

The following are five examples of important federal legislation that has influenced the health of adults and their lives in communities: The Older Americans Act of 1965, the Americans with Disabilities Act of 1990, the Family and Medical Leave Act of 1993, the Personal Responsibility and Work Opportunity Reconciliation Act of 1996, and the Patient Protection and Affordable Care Act of 2010.

The **Older Americans Act (OAA)**, originally passed in 1965, established the Administration on Aging (AOA) and state agencies to provide for the social service needs of older people. The mission of the AOA is to help older adults maintain dignity and live independently in their communities through a comprehensive and coordinated network across the United States (AOA, 2017). Title III of the OAA authorizes funding for nonprofit area agencies on aging to coordinate social services that provide supportive and nutritional services, family caregiver support, and disease prevention and health promotion activities. The services are available to all people age 60 or over, specifically targeted to those with the greatest economic or social need. The 2016 OAA Act Reauthorization Act (P.L. 114–144) reauthorized programs from FY 2017 through FY 2019 and includes provisions to protect vulnerable elders (AOA, 2016). In 2012, the U.S. Department of Health and Human Services (HHS) created the Administration for Community Living (ACL), which brought together the AOA, the Administration of Intellectual and Developmental Disabilities (AIDD), and the HHS Office on Disability to serve as the Federal agency responsible for increasing access to community supports that focus on the unique needs of older Americans and people with disabilities (ACL, 2018).

In 1990, the **Americans with Disabilities Act (ADA)** was passed, providing protection against discrimination to millions of Americans with disabilities. A disability is generally defined by the ADA as a physical or mental impairment that substantially limits one or more major life activities, having a record of such an impairment, or being regarded as having such an impairment (Americans with Disabilities Act of 1990, as amended with ADA Amendments Act of 2008, n.d.). The ADA legislation requires government and businesses to provide disabled individuals with equal opportunities for jobs, education, access to transportation and public buildings, and other accommodations for both physical and mental limitations.

The **Family and Medical Leave Act (FMLA)**, initially passed in 1993, provides job protection and continuous health benefits where applicable for eligible employees who need extended leave for their own illness or to care for a family member. Gender equality was expanded with FMLA to offer women the ability to better manage both a career and a family (Guy, 2013). However, FMLA is limited. It only permits eligible employees to take 12 weeks of unpaid leave during a 12-month period for limited situations such as birth, adoption, or care for a serious illness of self or family members. It also only applies to employees who worked for at least 12 months in companies that have 50 or more employees . The FMLA definition of spouse was revised in 2015 to allow eligible employees in same-sex marriages to take family and medical leave (U. S. Department of Labor Wage and Hour Division, Family and Medical Leave Act n.d.). Frequently caregivers provide unpaid care for their family members, including aging parents, children, grandchildren, and partners. Often adults find themselves struggling to balance work and caring for a family member. More families find themselves in this struggle as more women enter the workforce and work full time. Caregivers' multiple roles and responsibilities are frequently coupled with financial strain, which can lead them to experience **caregiver burden**.

In 1996 Congress passed the **Personal Responsibility and Work Opportunity Reconciliation Act**, commonly known as "welfare reform." This law targeted women who received public assistance and changed the previous Aid to Families with Dependent Children (AFDC) to **Temporary Assistance for Needy Families (TANF)**—a work program that mandates that women heads-of-household find employment to retain their benefits. The Administration for Children and Families (ACF), within the Department of Health and Human Services (USDHHS) is responsible for federal programs such as TANF that promote the economic and social well-being of families, children, individuals, and communities (ACF, n.d.).

The Patient Protection and Affordable Care Act (2010), also known as the Affordable Care Act (ACA), was passed by Congress and signed into law by President Obama in March 2010. The ACA has been considered the most significant reform law passed since Medicare and Medicaid were enacted in 1965. Some of the key features of the ACA include an end to health plans limiting or denying benefits to children under 19 years of age due to a pre-existing condition. Effective in 2010, children under the age of 26 can be covered under their parent's health plan, lifetime coverage limits were stopped, no copayment is needed for preventive care, and access to insurance is provided for uninsured individuals. The percent of adults aged 19–25 who were uninsured decreased from 33.8 percent in 2010 to 16 percent in 2015 (NCHS, 2017). The law is complex and expensive. As such, ACA is a continuing source of debate and will undoubtedly be modified over time.

The nurse serves in a unique position for advocacy and support of health legislation and policy that supports the physical, mental, and social well-being of adults. Advocacy can be accomplished in a variety of ways such as lobbying, public speaking, participating in grassroots activities, and staying abreast of proposed legislation that influences the health of men and women, their families, and communities.

Ethical and Legal Issues and Legislation for Older Adults

Ethical issues regarding the care and treatment of older adults arise regularly. As the population continues to age and technological advances continue to be developed, complex ethical and legal questions will increase. The most common of these issues involve decision making—assessment of the ability of the client to make decisions, the appropriate surrogate decision maker, disclosure of information to make informed decisions, level of care needed on the basis of function, and termination of treatment at the end of life. One often-overlooked concern of older persons is **abuse**. The National Center on Elder Abuse (NCEA), within the Administration on Aging, notes that abuse encompasses physical, emotional, and sexual abuse, as well as exploitation, neglect, and abandonment. Identification of abuse consists of recognizing the following: (1) The willful infliction of physical pain or injury, (2) infliction of debilitating mental anguish and fear, (3) theft or mismanagement of money or resources, and (4) unreasonable confinement or the depriving of services.

It is estimated that every year one out of six older adults worldwide experience abuse (Yon et al., 2017). Although legal definitions vary from state to state, the NCEA defines **neglect** as "the refusal or failure to fulfill any part of a person's obligations or duties to an elder. Neglect may also occur if the person who has fiduciary responsibilities fails to pay for items or necessary home care services or, on the part of the in-home service provider, to provide the necessary care (NCEA, n.d., p. 2). Older persons can make independent choices with which others may disagree. Their right to self-determination can be taken from them if they are declared incompetent. According to the Older Americans Act, **financial exploitation** is the "illegal or improper act or process of an individual, including a caregiver, using the resources of an older individual for monetary or personal benefit, profit or gain" (Administration on Aging, 2016).

During the assessment process, nurses need to be aware of contradictions between injuries and the explanation of their cause, codependency issues between client and caregiver, and substance abuse by the caregiver. To solicit valuable information, pose open-ended questions to patients presenting with signs of injuries or abuse, such as, "Can you tell me what happened? and "What do you remember about how this injury occurred?" The local social services agency or area agency on aging can help with information on reporting requirements. Nurses can play a key role in reducing elder abuse.

The **Patient Self-Determination Act** of 1991 requires those providers receiving Medicare and Medicaid funds to give clients written information regarding their legal options for treatment choices if they become incapacitated. A routine discussion of **advanced medical directives** can help ease the difficult discussions faced by health care professionals, families, and clients. The nurse can help an individual complete a values history instrument. These instruments ask questions about specific wishes regarding different medical situations. There are two parts to the advanced directives. The **living will** enables the client to express wishes regarding the use of medical treatments in the event of a terminal illness. A **durable medical power of attorney** is the legal way for the client to designate someone else to make health care decisions when he or she is unable to do so. A **do-not-resuscitate order** (DNR) is a specific order from a physician not to use cardiopulmonary resuscitation. Physician Orders for Life-Sustaining Treatment (POLST) are becoming common to specify end-of-life care or resuscitation orders for patients not in cardiopulmonary arrest. The POLST document is brightly colored and signed by the physician and the patient, depending on the state, and specifies medical orders to be carried out by health care workers when the patient is unable to speak. State laws vary widely regarding the implementation of these tools, so it is important to consult a knowledgeable source for information. By the end of 2016, 36 states had adopted some version of POLST (Thomas & Sabatino, 2017). The key to successful end of life care is involving the family, and especially the designated decision maker or agent, in these discussions so that everyone is clear about the client's choices.

Environmental Impact

The World Health Organization (WHO, 2016) defines environment, as it relates to health, as "all the physical, chemical, and biological factors external to a person, and all the related behaviors" (p. x). Globally, 23 percent of all deaths and 26 percent of deaths among children under the age of five are due to preventable environmental factors. Because humans are constantly interacting with the environment, the impact of an unhealthy environment adds significantly to the burden of disease. Environmental risks lead to a quantifiable disease burden. Knowing the modifiable environmental risks can lead to identifying prevention opportunities though policies and interventions (WHO, 2016).

Men and women are often exposed to different environmental factors because of upbringing, employment, cultural, or tradition variations. Although the environmental fraction of the global burden of disease is similar among men and women (22.8 percent and 20.6 percent respectively), it is important to understand that the hosts (men and women) may experience environmental health risks differently. For example, in some cultures, women and small children are exposed to higher levels of household air pollution than men because more women cook over cook stoves that give off pollutants (WHO, 2016). Globally, men are employed more often than women causing a higher exposure to occupational environment health risks.

Governmental programs are in place to improve environmental health. The Centers for Disease Control and Prevention (CDC) Environmental Hazards and Effects Program (EHEP) is designed to prevent and control disease or death and to promote health and quality of life that result from interactions between people and their environments. The program uses indicators to assess and monitor progress on goals to improve the environmental health (CDC, 2018c). It is incumbent on community health nurses to decrease the burden of disease resulting from an unhealthy environment. The effect of climate change on the environment has been discussed in recent years; nurses must be aware of the scientific evidence and maintain currency of knowledge on the phenomenon and its impact on health.

CHECK YOUR PRACTICE

You are serving on a state ad hoc committee as the Public Health Department nurse representative. The purpose of the task force is to determine the location for a proposed nursing home. The proposed location is next to a river and near a landfill. What are some potential health risks that could impact the future residences if the proposed location is chosen? What stakeholders and agencies could be consulted to help determine the best location for the new nursing home?

HEALTH STATUS INDICATORS

Health status indicators are the quantitative or qualitative measures used to describe the level of well-being or illness present in a defined population or to describe related attributes or risk factors. They can be represented in the form of rates, such as mortality and morbidity, or proportions, such as percent of a given population that receive immunizations. A variety of sources are available to obtain data on health indicators such as *Healthy People 2020* (USDHHS, 2010). HealthData.gov (2018) provides access to valuable health data to allow for entrepreneurs, researchers, and policy makers to make better health outcomes.

While health status indicators in the United States show persistent health disparities among ethnic and racial groups, the awareness of social determinants of health and health care disparities persists among health care providers and the general public (Holm et al., 2017). Persons with low socioeconomic status are more likely to be affected by chronic illness such as diabetes, hypertension, human immunodeficiency virus (HIV). They are less likely to be screened for colorectal cancer or vaccinated against influenza.

The prevalence of diabetes, serious heart conditions, and hypertension among adults 45 to 64 years of age is strongly associated with poverty status. In lower-income populations, modifiable risk factors for these diseases are more common. The number of poor adults 45 to 64 with hypertension was similar to the percent of higher-income persons who were 65 to 74 years of age (NCHS, 2017).

Efforts to reduce chronic disease and their risk factors in adults are ongoing. Programs like Healthy People regularly update objectives and monitor progress of meeting health indicators to encourage collaboration and provide data to inform health decisions and measure the impact of prevention activities. Only by ongoing measurement to identify health improvement priorities, engaging the multiple sectors of the public, and delivering effective interventions can higher levels of health be achieved.

EVIDENCE-BASED PRACTICE

Using data to inform decisions is essential for best practice. Critically thinking about how the data is analyzed can reveal new perspectives and potential new solutions. Looking at certain data at the county level is often used to understand health disparities. These counties are usually grouped by state or region. Egen et al. (2017) chose to look at the poorest counties in the nation, regardless of where they were geographically located, and compare them with the wealthiest counties. The researchers reclassified the 3141 counties in the United States into 50 new "states" by socioeconomic status indicators of 5-year median income. The 1st percentile (least number of years of life lost) to the 99th percentile (greatest number of years of potential life lost) on the X axis and years of potential life lost on the Y axis were plotted for the wealthiest "state" and the counties that constitute the poorest "state." The wealthiest "state" had a median household income of $89,723, whereas the poorest "state" had a median household income of $24,960. Looking at the data in a new way illustrated that women and men in the poorest "state" will live, on average, 7 to 10 fewer years than those in the wealthiest "state. It also illustrated that life expectancies in the poorest "state" falls below that of more than half of the countries in the world, hence "there are several developing countries hidden within the borders of the United States" (p. 135).

Nurse Use

Results of this study highlight the need to look at data in new ways to reveal hidden information. It serves as a reminder that poverty has a significant impact on health and is found throughout the country.

Data from Egen O, Beatty K, Blackley DJ, et al.: Health and social conditions of the poorest versus wealthiest counties in the United States. *Am J Public Health* 107(1):130–135, 2017.

Morbidity

Morbidity is a term used to describe the number of cases of a disease in a population. Measures of morbidity frequency reflect the number of persons in a defined population who become ill or new cases (incidence in a given time period or the total number of persons who are ill at a given time period (prevalence). Although not all people who get sick die, morbidity is the cause of mortality or deaths.

When healthy years of life are increased, longer life spans are generally considered desirable. However, increasing morbidity, especially associated with chronic diseases and other conditions associated with aging, can increase functional limitations and affect quality of life. Of particular concern is the high prevalence of adults with risk factors related to disability-adjusted life-years (DALYs) in the United States including dietary risks, tobacco smoking, high body mass index, hypertension, high fasting plasma glucose, physical inactivity, and alcohol use (U.S. Burden of Disease Collaborators, 2013).

Mortality

Mortality data is helpful to present characteristics of people dying, to determine life expectancy, and to compare mortality trends with other countries. The National Vital Statistics System (NVSS) is a valuable source of this type of data. Monitoring levels of premature mortality is critical to identifying the main sources of premature deaths and understanding how they can be resolved and also improving health equity so everyone, regardless of social group or status, has the opportunity to be as healthy as possible. **Life expectancy** and infant mortality are measures that are used to gauge the overall health of a population. Life expectancy at birth for the United States in 2016 decreased to 78.6 years from 78.7 years in 2015. Women live a full 5 years longer than men: 81.1 years versus 76.1 years. The top five leading causes of death in 2015 were heart disease, cancer, chronic lower respiratory diseases, unintentional injuries, and stroke (NCHS, 2017).

Infant mortality rate was 5.9 infant deaths per 1000 live births in 2015. This represents a 63 percent decrease in infant mortality since 1975, but the rate of decline has slowed to 1.8 percent per year during 2007–2015, compared with 4.7 percent per year during 1975–1982. Although the rate of infant mortality declined for all racial and ethnic groups, the rates are higher for infants of non-Hispanic African Americans and non-Hispanic American Indian or Alaska Natives (NCHS, 2017). Although the United States spends more money per capita on health than any other country, other developed countries have a longer life expectancy. The Organization for Economic Co-operation and development (OECD, 2017), using 2008 data, ranked the United States life expectancy 25th out of 37 countries and territories for men (75.2 years) and 23rd for women (80.4 years). Thakrar et al. (2018) report that from 2001 to 2010 the risk of death in the United States was 76 percent greater for infants and 57 percent greater for children ages 1–19. The lagging U.S. performance amounted to over 600,000 excess deaths over the 50-year study period. The outstanding conclusion of numerous morbidity and mortality reports is that the United States needs to make significant changes in policy and interventions to reverse the trends in health care outcomes for all ages, ethnic and socioeconomic groups (Figs. 29.2 and 29.3).

HEALTHY PEOPLE 2020

Selected Objectives Relevant to Major Health Issues and Chronic Disease of Adults

Arthritis, Osteoporosis, and Chronic Back Conditions
- **AOCBC-7:** Increase the proportion of adults with doctor-diagnosed arthritis who receive health care provider counseling.
- **AOCBC-10:** Reduce the proportion of adults with osteoporosis.

Cancer
- **C-1:** Reduce the overall cancer death rate.

Diabetes
- **D-3:** Reduce the diabetes death rate.

Educational and Community-Based Programs
- **ECBP-9:** (Developmental) Increase the proportion of employees who participate in employer-sponsored health promotion activities.

Environmental Health
- **EH-3:** Reduce air toxic emissions to decrease the risk of adverse health effects caused by airborne toxics.

Genomics
- **G-1:** Increase the proportion of women with a family history of breast and/or ovarian cancer who receive genetic counseling.
- **G-2:** (Developmental) Increase the proportion of persons with newly diagnosed colorectal cancer who receive genetic testing to identify Lynch syndrome (or familial colorectal cancer syndromes).

Heart Disease and Stroke
- **HDS-2:** Reduce coronary heart disease deaths.
- **HDS-3:** Reduce stroke deaths.

Older Adults
- **OA-1:** Increase the proportion of older adults who are up to date on a core set of clinical preventive services.

Physical Activity and Fitness
- **PA-2:** Increase the proportion of adults that meet current federal physical activity guidelines for aerobic physical activity and for muscle strength training.

U.S. Department of Health and Human Services: *Healthy People 2020*, 2010. Available at https://www.healthypeople.gov.

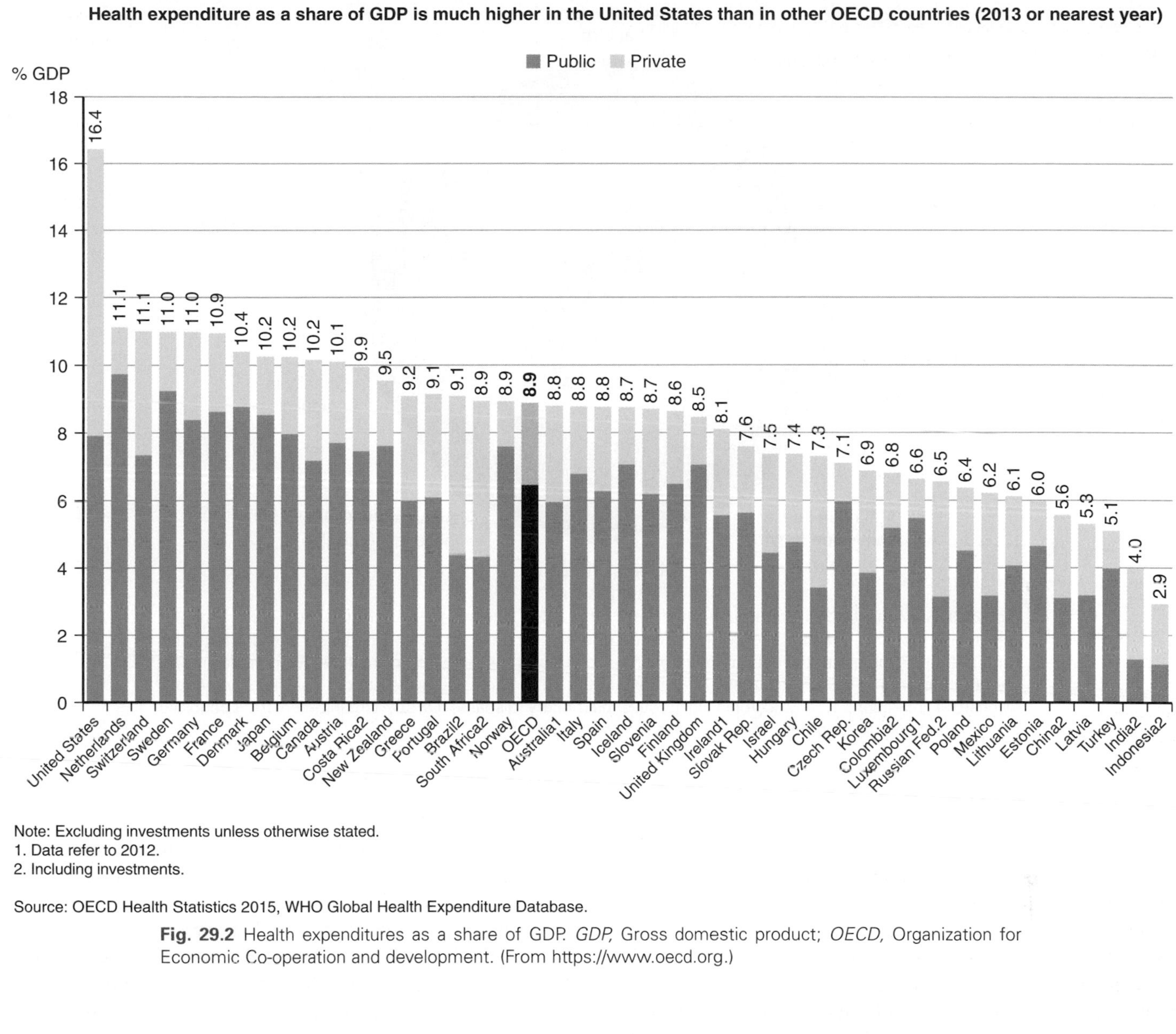

Note: Excluding investments unless otherwise stated.
1. Data refer to 2012.
2. Including investments.

Source: OECD Health Statistics 2015, WHO Global Health Expenditure Database.

Fig. 29.2 Health expenditures as a share of GDP. *GDP,* Gross domestic product; *OECD,* Organization for Economic Co-operation and development. (From https://www.oecd.org.)

Although women live about five years longer than men, they do not necessarily live those extra years in good physical and mental health. Women are more likely to use health services and report greater rates of disability. For instance, men have higher blood pressure levels than women through middle age. However, after menopause, women may be more affected by increased blood pressure. Women also present with different risk factors and symptoms for cardiac-related conditions. Women often report more jaw/neck pain, dyspnea, back pain, fatigue, paroxysmal nocturnal dyspnea, and palpitations. Men and women were equally likely to report midsternal chest pain or pressure.

ADULT HEALTH CONCERNS

A group that often has chronic diseases including those related to mental health are **veterans**. Since veterans are both men and women, each of the diseases discussed in this section could apply. In addition veterans often suffer from Post Traumatic Stress Disorder related to what they saw and had to do while in the war zone. Often veterans find it difficult or impossible to integrate back into their families, communities and society when they complete their military service. They can become a high risk group for the chronic diseases discussed in the following sections.

Chronic Disease

In 1988 the CDC created the National Center for Chronic Disease Prevention and Health Promotion (NCCDPHP). Chronic illness has become a major public health problem. The most common and costly chronic diseases are heart disease, diabetes, stroke, cancer, and arthritis. According to the RAND report *Multiple Chronic Conditions in the United States* (2017), in 2014 6 in 10 adults had a least one chronic condition and 4 in 10 had more than one. People with chronic and mental health conditions consume 86 percent of the nation's $2.7 trillion annual health care expenditures. Chronic disease is the leading cause of

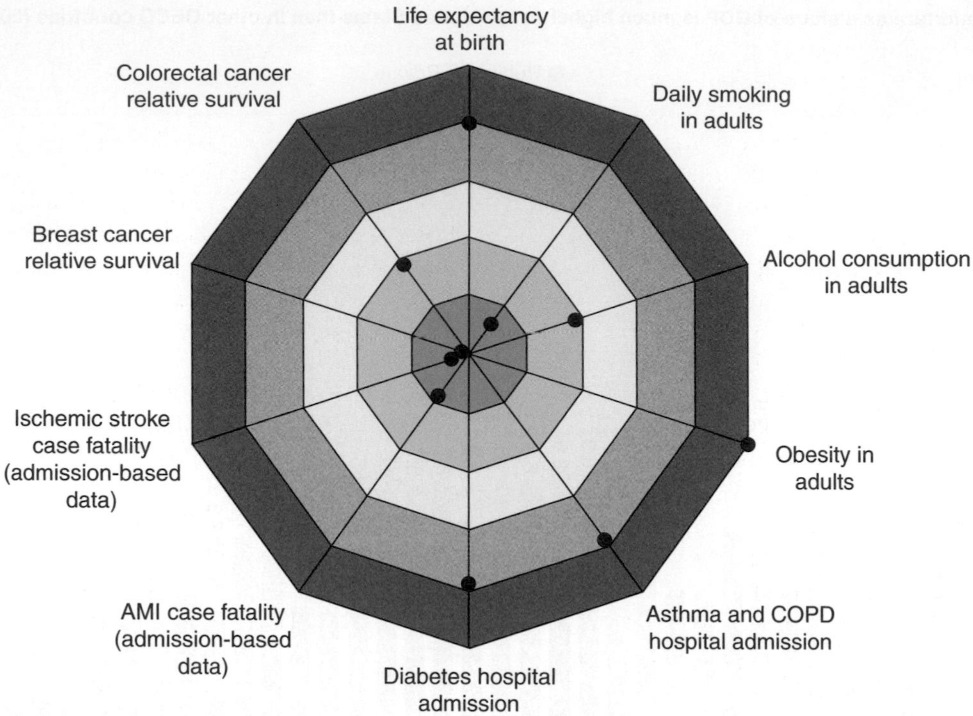

Fig. 29.3 How the United States compares with other OECD countries on selected indicators of health status, risk factors to health, and quality of care (2013 or nearest year). *Note:* The closer the dot is to the center "target," the better the country performs. The countries in the inner circle are in the top quintile among the best performing OECD countries, while those in the outer circle are in the bottom quintile. *AMI,* Acute myocardial infarction; *COPD,* chronic obstructive pulmonary disease; *OECD,* Organization for Economic Co-operation and development. (Source: https://www.oecd.org.)

preventable deaths, disability, and decreased quality of life. The CDC has identified four modifiable health risk behaviors for the prevention of chronic disease. These are lack of physical activity, poor nutrition, tobacco use, and excessive alcohol use (NCCDPHP, 2014). Many models have been developed to guide the delivery of care to people with chronic illness. A complex health care system and community model was developed with the funding of the Robert Wood Johnson Foundation. This model is Wagner's **Chronic Care Model (CCM)**.

The CCM identifies the essential elements of a health care system that encourages high-quality chronic disease care. These elements are the community, the health system, self-management support, delivery system design, decision support, and clinical information systems. Evidence-based change concepts under each element, in combination, foster productive interactions between informed clients who take an active part in their care and providers with resources and expertise (Model Elements, 2014). The CCM continues to be implemented and evaluated. In a structured literature review, authors found qualitative (patient and clinician satisfaction) and quantitative (health status, mortality) data showing positive outcomes even when some components of the CCM are implemented in a health system and "the potential to improve the seamless transition between hospital and ambulatory settings for those older than 65 years with two or more chronic conditions" (Sendall et al., 2016, p. 10).

Another model that focuses on reducing the burden of chronic disease through education and empowerment is the Chronic Disease **Self-Management** Program (CDSMP). The program offers interventions that have shown positive outcomes for people with chronic diseases. The U.S. Administration on Aging initiated CDSMP in 2009. Within two years 9305 workshops were offered to more than 100,000 middle-aged and older adults (Ory et al., 2013). Studies have shown improvement in health behaviors, health outcomes, and reduced health care utilization. A recent study showed significant reductions in emergency department visits and hospitalizations. Potential savings of $364 per participant and a national savings of $3.3 billion could result if only five percent of the U.S. population participated (Ahn et al., 2013). Opportunities exist for additional studies to identify effective models and strategies. Nurses should consider using models and strategies that have shown improvements in health behaviors or outcomes when planning community interventions.

Cardiovascular Disease

The leading cause of death for both men and women, African Americans, American Indians or Alaska Natives, Hispanics, and whites in the United States is **heart disease** (HD). Heart disease has been diagnosed in 11.5 percent, or 27.6 million, of American adults. More than 360,000 people died of coronary heart disease, the most common type of HD (Benjamin et al., 2018).

By 2030, the annual direct medical costs associated with cardiovascular disease (CVD) are projected to rise to more than $818 billion with productivity costs that could exceed $275 billion (CDC Foundation, 2015). In response to the high incidence and mortality rates of heart disease, the American Heart Association (AHA) has the following goal: "By 2020, to improve the cardiovascular health of all Americans by 20 percent while reducing deaths attributable to cardiovascular disease (CVD) and stroke by 20%" (Benjamin et al., 2018). Progress is being made. The mortality trends for males and females in the United States have declined from 1979 to 2015. With the increased rates of obesity and diabetes in children, future prevalence may increase.

About 23 of the *Healthy People 2020* objectives focus on cardiovascular disease. Reaching these objectives means intervening with all ethnicities and health promotion and disease prevention in the United States. Presently, there continue to be gaps in knowledge and awareness for heart disease. For example, one study revealed that CVD was not a top concern for women or physicians (Bairey Merz et al., 2017). Community health educational campaigns must emphasize the significance of CVD and behavioral changes to reduce risk factors.

Hypertension

In November of 2017, the American Heart Association announced changed guidelines classifying high blood pressure, or hypertension, as a reading of 130 mm Hg for systolic (instead of 140 mm Hg) and 80 mm Hg for diastolic. Blood pressure (BP) should now be categorized as normal, elevated, or stage 1 or 2 hypertension. Normal BP is defined as <120/<80 mm Hg. Elevated BP is 120–129/<80 mm Hg. Hypertension stage 1 is defined as a systolic BP of between 130 and 139 mm Hg or a diastolic between 80 and 89 mm Hg. Hypertension stage 2 is defined as a systolic blood pressure of equal to or greater than 140 mm Hg or a diastolic blood pressure equal to or greater than 90 mm Hg (Carey & Whelton, 2018).

The prevalence estimates are hypertension change significantly based on the cutoff points that categorize high blood pressure. The prevalence of hypertension based on the new guidelines among U.S. adults is 46 percent versus 32 percent using older cutoff points. In 2011 to 2012, 11.0 percent of children and adolescents 8 to 17 years of age had either high blood pressure or borderline high blood pressure (Benjamin et al., 2018). Uncontrolled hypertension leads to heart attack, stroke, kidney damage, and a host of other complications. Between 2011 and 2014, 84.1 percent of people with hypertension were aware that they had the disease (NCHS, 2017). There is no significant difference in prevalence between men and women, but there are racial and ethnic differences in hypertension rates among both men and women. African Americans in the United States have the highest prevalence of hypertension compared to other racial and ethnic groups (AHA, 2017).

Stroke

Strokes have decreased in the United States since the 1950s. An estimated 7.2 million Americans over 20 years self-reported having a stroke (Benjamin et al., 2018). About 795,000 people each year experience a new or recurrent stroke. Of all strokes 87 percent are ischemic, 10 percent are intracranial hemorrhages, and 3 percent are subarachnoid hemorrhages. The lifetime risk for stroke is higher in women (about one in five) than in men (about one in six), and since women live longer than men and strokes increase with age, more women than men are likely to die of stroke. African Americans have almost twice the risk of first-time strokes as whites. Mexican Americans also have an increased incidence of stroke over non-Hispanic whites (Benjamin et al., 2018).

One *Healthy People 2020* objective is to reduce stroke deaths to 48 in 100,000. Community-based programs and policies regarding stroke care from initial signs and symptoms to aftertreatment have been developed by the AHA and other organizations. The CDC's Division for Heart Disease and Stroke Prevention (DHDSP) is promoting the use of community health workers (CHWs) to support healthy living strategies that would reduce the prevalence of stroke as well as other chronic conditions (Brownstein et al., 2013). Collaboration between health care institutions, community leaders, emergency medical services, CHWs, and support groups within the community is needed for programs to be effective. Because there is a strong dose-response relationship between smoking and ischemic stroke, nurses can direct efforts toward smoking reduction (Markidan et al., 2018).

Diabetes

Diabetes is a serious public health challenge for the United States. The American Diabetes Association reports that diabetes is the seventh leading cause of death (ADA, 2018a). The prevalence of both diagnosed (23.1 million) and undiagnosed diabetes (7.2 million) people of all ages is 30.3 million, which is 9.4 percent of the population in 2015. Between 1988–1994 and 2011–2014, the overall prevalence increased from 8.8 percent to 11.9 percent. The ADA (2018b) estimates that the cost of diabetes to the nation is $327 billion. For every four people who have diabetes there is another who does not know he or she has it. The rates of diagnosed diabetes in adults by race/ethnic background are 7.4 percent of non-Hispanic whites, 8.0 percent of Asian Americans, 12.1 percent of Hispanics, 12.7 percent of non-Hispanic African Americans, and 15.1 percent of American Indians/Alaska Natives (ADA, 2018a).

More than 18 of the goals of *Healthy People 2020* are related to diabetes. The increasing prevalence of this complex condition, and the wide ranging impact on individual and community health demands a multilevel approach to prevention.

Primary prevention includes educating adults about nutrition and the risks of obesity, smoking, and physical inactivity. Community interventions addressing healthy eating, exercise, and weight reduction can also benefit adults at risk for diabetes. Secondary prevention includes screening for diabetes with finger-stick blood glucose tests or glucose tolerance tests. Screening is also accomplished by thorough history and physical examination. Tertiary prevention targets activities aimed at reducing the complications of the disease (see Levels of Prevention box).

LEVELS OF PREVENTION

Cardiovascular Disease in Women and Prevention of HIV in Men

Primary Prevention

Collaborating with a variety of organizations such as the American Heart Association to design and implement interventions aimed at reducing women's risk for cardiovascular disease.

The nurse advises men who have sex with other men to use a new latex condom during oral or anal sex. In group and individual counseling about HIV, the nurse indicates to clients that they should not share needles, syringes, razors, or toothbrushes.

Secondary Prevention

Establishing screening clinics in community settings for cholesterol and hypertension.

The nurse advises an infected man to swallow all of his highly active antiretroviral therapy (HAART) medication on schedule. The nurse advises a man who had unprotected sex to be tested with a standard enzyme-linked immunosorbent assay (EIA), followed by a confirmatory Western blot test.

Tertiary Prevention

Developing a community-based exercise program for a group of women who have cardiovascular disease.

The nurse teaches men newly diagnosed with HIV to exercise regularly, eat a balanced nutritious diet, sleep at least eight hours a day, and stop or limit alcohol. The nurse advises clients not to donate blood, plasma, or organs.

HIV, Human immunodeficiency virus.

Mental Health

Mental health is defined as a state of well-being in which every individual realizes his or her own potential, can cope with normal stresses of life, can work productively and fruitfully, and is able to make a contribution to her or his community (WHO, 2014). Mental health is more than the absence of mental disorders. It is an integral and essential component of health, including emotional, psychological, and social well-being at every stage of life. Mental health is complex. *Healthy People 2020* lists factors linked to mental health as race, ethnicity, gender, age, income level, education level, sexual orientation, and geographic location. Social conditions, as well, can positively and negatively influence mental health. These include interpersonal, family, and community dynamics, housing quality, social support, employment opportunities, and work and school conditions (USDHHS, 2010).

Mental health disorders are a common cause of disability. They disrupt a person's thinking, feelings, relationships, and ability to carry out activities of daily living. According to the National Institute of Mental Health (NIMH, 2017), there were an estimated 44.7 million (18.3 percent) adults in the United States with any mental illness in the prior year and 10.4 million (4.2 percent) of those were categorized as serious mental illness. Mental health treatment accounted for $186 billion of spending in 2014 (NCHS, 2017).

Mental illness is generally viewed by society in a negative manner and stigmas surrounding mental health are among the barriers that discourage people from treatment options. Public stigma and self-stigma are two dimensions of stigma surrounding mental health that create barriers that discourage people from utilizing mental health services in the United States (Wu et al., 2017). Public stigma refers to the negative societal prejudices that include cognitive, effective, and behavioral communication that is either overt or subtle about persons seeking help or struggling with mental health issues. Self-stigma is a negative view one holds toward oneself related to the mental health concern. Both stigma dimensions inhibit those wanting mental health services.

Because negative stigmas are tied to the decreased utilization of mental health services, public health nurses are advised to take steps to decrease negative stigmas surrounding mental health issues. Community education programs will want to focus messages that address audiences to educate them and dispel the stereotypes and fears often applied by society to individuals with mental illness. Local and mass media outlets can be incorporated to broadcast positive aspects of those living with mental disabilities and functioning as a productive part of society.

Cancer

Cancers of all types are a serious public health concern (Table 29.1). Cancer is the second leading cause of death in the United States, surpassed only by heart disease. As of January 1, 2016, about 15.5 million Americans with a history of cancer were alive, some of whom were cancer free. The American Cancer Society's (ACS, 2018a) *Cancer Facts and Figures 2018* reports an estimated 609,640 cancer deaths in 2018. In 2018, about 1.7 million new cancer cases were projected to be diagnosed. Cancer costs billions of dollars in direct medical costs and indirect costs or those resulting from lost productivity related to illness or premature death. These costs could be reduced by removing barriers to care such as lack of health insurance and improving the health literacy of Americans.

American Cancer Society epidemiologists estimate that 42 percent of newly diagnosed cancers, or 729,000 cases in 2018, are potentially avoidable (ACS, 2018a). Of these cases, 19 percent are attributed to smoking and 18 percent are caused by a combination of excess body weight, physical inactivity, excess alcohol consumption, and poor nutrition. Early screening and detection, promotion of healthy lifestyles, expansion of access to services, and improvement in cancer treatments will help reduce the burden of cancer and disparities. Declining death rates from colorectal cancer, the second leading cause of

TABLE 29.1 Deaths Caused by Cancers[a]

Population	Men	Women
White	218.7	153.4
African American	278.8	176.9
Hispanic	145.4	101.4
American Indian	137.0	108.9
Asian/Pacific Islander	128.2	93.3

[a]Rates are per 100,000.

From United States Cancer Statistics: *Leading cancer cases and deaths*, 2015. Available at https://gis.cdc.gov.

cancer-related deaths among men and women, are largely attributed to screening and risk factor reduction. An example of a systematic and replicable program that increased colorectal screening is when the Alabama Department of Public Health partnered with the University of Alabama in Huntsville and the University of South Alabama to provide colorectal cancer (CRC) screening to eligible university employees and dependents (O'Keefe et al., 2018). Finding cancer lesions in a precancerous state, such as those found in cervical, colorectal, and breast cancer, allows for treatment while in a highly treatable stage. Obesity, physical inactivity, smoking, heavy alcohol consumption, a diet high in red or processed meats, and insufficient intake of fruits and vegetables are risk factors for colorectal cancer. Reducing these risk factors will reduce the incidence of the disease.

Public health agencies, health care providers, and communities must work together to reduce the burden of cancer on society. The *Healthy People 2020* goal is to reduce the number of overall cancer cases as well as the illness, disability, and death caused by cancer. Education on the hazards of tobacco use and secondhand smoke, eating a healthy diet and limiting daily consumption of alcohol, and exposure to ultraviolet rays are examples of topics for education programs that will reduce the burden of cancer on society.

STDs/HIV/AIDS

Sexually transmitted diseases (STDs) refer to more than 25 infectious organisms, such as viruses, bacteria, or parasites, transmitted primarily through sexual activity. Some other means of transmission include lice, mother-to-child transmission during pregnancy or breastfeeding, or contaminated needles used in drug use or surgery. The term **sexually transmitted infections** (STIs) is also used synonymously, although there are distinctions. The broader term *STI* means that the body has had an invasion and multiplication of microorganisms, whereas *STD* signifies that pathology or damage has occurred with or without symptoms. STDs continue to be a major burden to society and have tremendous health and economic consequences in the United States despite their relatively preventable nature. The costs to the U.S. health care system related to STDs are as much as $16 billion in health care costs annually (CDC, 2017a).

The CDC (2017a) estimates there are about 20 million new STD infections each year, with almost half occurring in people from 15 to 24 years of age. Because many cases go undiagnosed and untreated, there is a high risk for severe lifelong health outcomes such as chronic pain, severe reproductive health complications, and HIV. The true burden is not fully known. In 2016, more than 1.6 million cases of chlamydia and gonorrhea occurred, making them the two most reported infectious diseases. Females are at greater risk for STDs as a result of biological differences and other factors. Syphilis, once close to elimination, has reemerged, with rates of primary and secondary syphilis increasing 18 percent from 2015 to 2016. People with an STD are more susceptible to and two to five times more likely to acquire an HIV infection (CDC, 2017a).

In the United States about 1.1 million people were living with HIV at the end of 2015 (CDC, 2017a). In 2016, 39,782 people received a diagnosis of HIV. Seventy percent of new HIV infections were gay and bisexual men. Heterosexual contact accounted for 23 percent of new cases. Other cases involved intravenous (IV) drug use. African Americans accounted for 44 percent of the HIV/acquired immunodeficiency syndrome (AIDS) cases, whereas Hispanics/Latinos accounted for 25 percent of new cases in 2016.

The *Healthy People 2020* goal is to promote responsible sexual behaviors, strengthen community capacity, and increase access to quality services to prevent STDs and their complications (USDHHS, 2010). Nurses have a role in this goal and can serve as advocates by focusing on the high-risk behaviors of men and women, as well as on the factors in their communities that lead to STDs. High-risk populations should be considered when assessing for clients' risk for STDs, including pregnant women, adolescents, men who have sex with men (MSM), women who have sex with women (WSW), and older clients. Interventions to improve education, employment opportunities, and adequate housing—as well as those to decrease drug use, isolation, and poverty—can have a critical impact on this epidemic (see How To box).

HOW TO Estimate the Impact of Budget Changes on Disease Burden and Direct Medical Costs

SPACE Monkey (STD Prevention Allocation Consequences Estimator) is a tool created for state and local sexually transmitted disease (STD) programs to make evidence-based calculations that show how budget changes impact disease burden and direct medical costs. SPACE Monkey also illustrates how budget changes can affect intermediate outcomes such as partner services.

Based on Centers for Disease Control and Prevention: *STD prevention allocation consequences estimator,* 2018. Available at https://www.cdc.gov.

Weight Control

In the United States, the prevalence of obesity among adults was 39.8 percent; prevalence among youth 2–19 years of age was 18.5 percent with an estimated annual cost of obesity at $147 billion (CDC, 2018a). In 1998 the NIH began using the calculation of **body mass index** (BMI) to define overweight and obesity in individuals (Table 29.2). BMI is the relationship of body

TABLE 29.2 BMI Determination and Interpretation

BMI[a]	Category
≤18.5–24.9	Normal weight
25.0–29.9	Overweight
30.0–39.9	Obesity
≥40	Extreme obesity

[a]Body mass index is a method used to determine optimal weight for height and is an indicator for obesity or malnutrition.
BMI, Body mass index.
From National Institutes of Health: Do you know the health risks of being overweight? National Heart, Lung, and Blood Institute (NHLBI). *Calculate your body mass index,* 2018. Available at https://www.nhlbi.nih.gov.

weight and height. A BMI of 25 to 29.9 is defined as overweight, whereas a BMI of 30 and above is considered obese (NHLBI, 2018). Childhood BMIs in the highest quartile were associated with premature death as an adult in a cohort of 4857 American Indian children (Benjamin et al., 2018).

Because obesity affects so many people of all ages, races, and the overall health of the United States, the issue is a recurring theme in *Healthy People 2020* objectives. For example, *Healthy People 2020* objective NWS-9 focuses on obesity in adults and NWS-10.4 focuses on obesity in children and adolescents. Other objectives like PA-2.4 focus on physical activity levels and NWS-15.1 on total vegetable intake.

Obesity has many effects on health and is linked to a number of major health problems, including type 2 diabetes, hypertension, dyslipidemia, sleep disordered breathing, subclinical atherosclerosis, coronary heart disease, stroke, and dementia (Benjamin et al., 2018). Nurses can provide education regarding obesity's risks to health. The educational offerings can be fashioned after a community health model using the levels of prevention (see Levels of Prevention box) to establish effective interventions for adults at risk for **weight control** issues. A community prevention project aimed at increasing activity levels would help in prevention of obesity and subsequent illnesses of diabetes and heart disease.

In addition to obesity, other eating disorders have increased among U.S. women. Common eating disorders seen in women include anorexia nervosa and bulimia. **Anorexia** is defined as a fear of gaining weight coupled with disturbances in perceptions of the body. Excessive weight loss is the most noticeable clue to this disorder. Individuals with anorexia rarely complain of weight loss because they view themselves as normal or overweight. Many of these women also struggle with psychological problems, including depression, obsessive symptoms, and social phobias. **Bulimia** is characterized by a persistent concern with the shape of the body along with body weight, recurrent episodes of binge eating, a loss of control during these binges, and use of extreme methods to prevent weight gain, such as purging, strict dieting, fasting, use of laxatives or diuretics, or vigorous exercise (NIMH, 2014).

Through comprehensive physical and psychosocial assessments, as well as histories of dietary practice, nurses identify women with eating disorders and provide appropriate referrals. Weight control strategies include promoting healthy eating habits and regular physical activity. At a population level, nurses advocate against advertising that promotes exceptionally thin bodies for women. They also promote community-wide exercise and healthy eating programs.

WOMEN'S HEALTH CONCERNS

It is preferable to emphasize prevention in adult health care. Screening, immunizations, and a healthy lifestyle are important for women of all ages. The **Office on Women's Health** (USDHHS, 2014) works through policy, education, and model programs to improve the health of women and girls. This agency has guidelines that include screening tests and disease-specific information for women. The Agency for Healthcare Research and Quality (AHRQ) was mandated by Congress to provide annual reports on health care quality and disparities. Women are one of the populations addressed in this report.

Reproductive Health

Women often use health care services for **reproductive health** concerns. A number of *Healthy People 2020* objectives address areas related to women's reproductive health (see the Maternal Infant and Child Health section of the *Healthy People 2020*).

Nurses are in a unique position to advocate for policies that increase women's access to services for reproductive health. In addition, many nurses discuss contraception with women of childbearing age. Contraceptive counseling requires accurate knowledge of current contraceptive choices and an open nonjudgmental approach. The goal of contraceptive counseling is to ensure that women have appropriate instruction to make informed choices about reproduction. The choice of contraceptive method depends on many factors, including the woman's health, frequency of sexual activity, number and types of partners, and plans to have future children. Except for abstinence, no method provides a 100 percent guarantee against **unintended pregnancy** or disease (USDHHS, 2014).

Preconceptual counseling addresses risks before conception and includes education, assessment, diagnosis, and intervention. The purpose is to reduce and/or eliminate health risks for women and infants. One major health problem that could be significantly impacted by preconceptual counseling is the problem of neural tube defects. More than 300,000 babies annually are born with neural tube defects (anencephaly and spina bifida). In the United States, it is estimated that the annual health care costs for people with spina bifida exceed $200 million. The United States is part of a global initiative to reduce these numbers. Research has shown that intake of folic acid can significantly reduce the occurrence of these very serious and often fatal neural tube defects by 50 to 70 percent. The goal of one *Healthy People 2020* objective is to increase the proportion of women who plan to become pregnant who have the recommended folic acid level intake. The current recommendation is for healthy women capable of or planning a pregnancy to take 400–800 mcg of folic acid daily (CDC, 2018b). Supplementation with enriched foods such as pastas, breads, and cereals, surveillance, and detection of levels are part of the initiatives currently being conducted with worldwide partners (CDC, 2017b).

Another concern critical to preconception awareness is substance abuse, including alcohol, opioids, marijuana, and other illegal drugs. A major preventable cause of birth defects, mental retardation, and neurodevelopmental disorders is fetal exposure to alcohol during pregnancy. Although fetal alcohol spectrum disorders (FASDs) are declining in the United States, they remain a preventable public health problem. Older data suggested the prevalence of FASD in the United States was 10 per 1000 children, but May et al. (2018) estimated FASD in first-graders in four U.S. communities range from 1.1 percent to 5.0 percent. The CDC and the American Academy of Pediatrics recommend no alcohol during pregnancy. Cannon et al. (2012) sought to prevent FASD by studying the characteristics of birth mothers. They discovered that predictors were older age, American Indian/Alaska Native or African American ethnicity, unmarried, unemployed, and without prenatal care. In addition, they were more likely to be smokers, Medicaid recipients, have a history of treatment for alcohol abuse or confirmed alcoholism, and to have used marijuana or cocaine during their pregnancy. Community interventions have been shown to help decrease the consumption of alcohol during pregnancy. Studies are needed with interventions that target this risk group for children with FASD.

Marijuana use in all pregnant women has increased since 2009 (Young-Wolff et al., 2017). In adolescent mothers-to-be the marijuana use rates rose to 14.6 percent during pregnancy. This has become a pertinent issue as use of marijuana is legalized for recreational use in states and the District of Columbia area. Even though the long-term effects of marijuana use on a fetus are still being studied, the data show tetrahydrocannabinol (THC) could contribute to low birth weight and developmental issues (Volkow et al., 2017). Teen mothers who are already at higher risk for alcohol use create a double effect with the additional consideration that THC stays in the system for 30 days after use when mothers may not even be aware of a pregnancy.

Nurses will want to be involved in community-based interventions for women. They can conduct educational classes and participate in campaigns that print and broadcast advertisements informing women of childbearing age that drinking during pregnancy can cause birth defects. Nurses can serve as advocates not only to encourage their clients to use prenatal care services, but also to work toward the establishment of services that are accessible, affordable, and available to all pregnant women.

Gestational Diabetes

Gestational diabetes mellitus (GDM) is a condition characterized by carbohydrate intolerance that is first identified or develops during pregnancy. According to the CDC (2017c), between 2 percent to 10 percent of pregnancies in the United States are affected by GDM. Women with gestational diabetes have up to a 50 percent chance to develop diabetes in the future. Secondary complications from gestational diabetes for mother and child are large for gestational age (LGA) baby, higher rates of Cesarean section, pre-eclampsia or elevated blood pressure in the mother, and rebound hypoglycemia where the medications used drop the blood glucose level of the mother too low and cause hypoglycemia for the baby at delivery (CDC, 2017c).

Clearly, interventions are needed to prevent gestational diabetes and its consequences for both mother and baby. A meta-analysis of studies regarding physical activity and gestational diabetes was conducted by Aune et al. (2016). Higher levels of physical activity prior to or in early pregnancy were significantly associated with a lower risk of developing gestational diabetes mellitus. Nursing interventions related to activity levels are imperative in reproductive women and their unborn children.

Menopause

During **menopause** the levels of the hormones estrogen and progesterone decrease in a woman's body causing a cessation of menstruation usually occurring around the age of 51. Decline in these hormone levels can affect the vaginal and urinary tract, cardiovascular system, bone density, libido, sleep patterns, memory, and emotions as estrogen receptors are prevalent in many organ systems (Santoro et al., 2015). Recent research shows additional impact on body composition and obesity due to women's waning hormone levels. The impacts are noticeable even in the peri-menopausal time prior to actual cessation that is an absence of menstruation for a full 12 months (Cheng et al., 2018).

Women's attitudes toward menopause vary greatly and are influenced by culture, age, support, and the recounted experiences of other women. For decades, however, the prevailing medical view of menopause was a state of deficiency that required hormone replacement to reduce heart disease and osteoporosis. A more positive outlook on menopause encourages women to view it as a transitional and natural stage in the life of a woman.

For decades, many U.S. women used hormone replacement therapy (HRT) or menopausal hormone therapy (MHT), although MHT remained untested by rigorous scientific study. A clinical trial launched in 1991, the Women's Health Initiative, set out to test specific effects HRT had on women's health, especially its effects on heart disease and osteoporosis. In the past, MHT was recommended for prevention of osteoporosis and coronary heart disease; however, long-term studies showed adverse effects such as increased risk of stroke, coronary heart disease, and thromboembolism with use of MHT (USPSTF, 2018). MHT is still considered useful for management of vasomotor symptoms or "hot flashes" but only for a limited amount of time to avoid the adverse side effects (Martin & Barbieri, 2018).

Use of Complementary and Alternative Therapies in Menopause. The changes in the recommendations regarding MHT led many women to seek alternative approaches for the management of menopausal symptoms. Women experiencing menopause frequently report symptoms including hot flashes, vaginal dryness, and irregular menses. Examples of alternative therapies are those actions that are taken by women instead of MHT/HRT. Complementary therapies are those taken to augment (or as a complement to) MHT/HRT. The listing of alternative/complementary therapies for menopausal symptoms can be an endless task, but Box 29.1 provides common examples. The National Center for Complementary and Integrative Health (2016) notes that alternative therapies may or may not be helpful in reducing menopausal symptoms and that more research should be done to determine the scientific benefits and risks of these therapies. Befus et al. (2018) performed a systemic review indicating acupuncture is effective as an adjunctive or as a sole treatment for vasomotor symptoms of menopause. The National Center for Complementary and Integrative Health (NCCIH) found insufficient evidence to determine effectiveness for managing symptoms of menopause with alternative methods such as using black cohosh, red clover, or mind and body practices, such as yoga or hypnotherapy (NCCIH, 2016).

BOX 29.1 Examples of Alternative/Complementary Therapies for Menopausal Symptoms

- Acupuncture
- Acupressure
- Massage therapy
- Healing touch
- Aromatherapy
- Guided imagery
- Chiropractic healing
- Yoga
- Tai chi
- Qi gong
- St. John's wort
- Black cohosh
- Soy and isoflavones
- Ginseng
- Kava
- Red clover
- Dong quai

Breast Cancer

Breast cancer is the most common cancer, except for skin cancers, for American women. The American Cancer Society (2018a) estimated that there would be 266,120 new cases of breast cancer in 2018 for U.S. women. An estimated 40,920 women would die in 2018 even though the breast cancer death rate in the United States peaked in 1989 at 33.2 per 100,00 and declined to 20.3 in 2015 (ACS, 2018a). Although the incidence of breast cancer is higher in white women than in African American women, the death rate for African American women is higher due to low screening activity, social determinants such as low income, and poor health access (DeSantis et al., 2017). The researchers also concluded higher rates of other diseases such as obesity contributed to the disparity between races with non-Hispanic white and non-Hispanic African Americans having higher breast cancer incidences and death rates. Secondary prevention that includes screening activities, such as mammography every two years after the age of 50, makes a difference in death rates. Family history of breast cancer stratifies a woman into screening between ages 40 and 49. Early detection can promote a cure, whereas late detection typically ensures more aggressive therapy and a poorer prognosis (National Cancer Institute, 2018).

Osteoporosis

Osteoporosis, or *porous bone,* is a disease marked by reduced bone strength leading to an increased risk of fractures, or broken bones. This is the most common bone disease, affecting 44 million people in the United States, and is most common in white and Asian women. Among women over 50 years of age, about one out of every two will have an osteoporosis-related fracture—that is, more than two million fractures annually are attributed to osteoporosis. Hip fractures have the most impact on quality of life, and one in five people who suffer hip fractures over the age of 50 will die in the year following their fracture (National Osteoporosis Foundation [NOF], 2014).

Prevention includes diets rich in calcium and vitamin D and avoiding medications that cause bone loss. Exercise also improves bone density, especially weight-bearing activities such as walking, running, stair climbing, and weight lifting. Limiting alcohol consumption and avoiding smoking are also important. Home assessment and correction of risk factors for falls, bone density testing, and annual height measurements help with fracture prevention. Finally, several medications are approved for the prevention of osteoporosis in the United States (NOF, 2014).

A systemic review of research by Qaseem et al. (2017) resulted in six main recommendations for treatment of osteoporosis/low bone density based on strength of evidence. Treatment guidelines include treatment for five years with bisphosphonates in women with known osteoporosis to reduce risk of hip and vertebral fracture. Conversely, the evidence leans toward not recommending MHT for the treatment of osteoporosis in post-menopausal women (Qaseem et al., 2017).

MEN'S HEALTH CONCERNS

The health status of one gender impacts the health status of the other gender, the children, and ultimately society. For example, in dual income families, when either spouse is ill and cannot work, the family and society are affected economically and work productivity is reduced. The family can suffer from lack of income. If one spouse dies, the other spouse generally experiences the loss of companionship and assumes the responsibilities of the lost spouse. Resources to promote and sustain health outcomes of both genders must be balanced for the overall health of the community. However, although a vital aspect of community health, **men's health** is often overlooked and factors exist that prevent men from reaching their full health potential. Factors such as "socioeconomic status, access to health care, male acculturation to health issues, harmful perceptions about masculinity, and lack of understanding of male health behaviors contribute to poor health outcomes for men" (Giorgianni et al., 2013, p. 343). There are a wide range of poorer overall health status and health outcomes for men in the United States that result in an about five-year shorter life span for men than women. Giorgianni et al. (2013) provide examples of these different outcomes; for example, more men than women smoke (21.5 percent versus 17.3 percent), more men are overweight (72.3 percent versus 64.1 percent), and men are less likely to receive routine care or seek out care early in the disease process than women. Changing these health behaviors could significantly improve the health outcomes of men.

Although health policies, campaigns, and community health organizations offer services for men, there are disparities that emphasize women's health and other barriers that negatively impact men's health. Several barriers to men reaching their full health potential have been identified. In 2015, women aged 18 or older were more likely than men to have seen or talked to a doctor or health professional (CDC, 2017). Men are socialized to ignore pain, be self-reliant, and be achievement oriented. Large numbers of men do not receive the **health screenings** intended to prevent and identify disease. Not only do these behaviors limit the opportunity to prevent disease through screening, health education, and counseling, but also once they are diagnosed, management and treatment is more difficult. Another barrier impacting to a greater degree is the work environment. Even though more women have the opportunity and are choosing careers that place them in dangerous work environments, men are more often employed in dangerous jobs and incur more work-related injuries than women, especially those in the military (Box 29.2).

BOX 29.2 Highlighting Military and Veteran Health Issues and Supporting Health System Resources

Military members and veterans naturally would have all the risks for diseases that the average person would in the United States; however, their exposure to health risk is more severe. They are exposed to environments and situations not experienced by the nonmilitary citizen. To make caring for this population more complicated is the fact that these exposures and the sequelae vary based on the time and war zone in which they served. The U.S. Department of Veterans Affairs (VA) provides a valuable resource that identifies major issues based on the time frame and location where the service member served: https://www.va.gov.

There are about 1.4 million active duty and 331,000 reserve-component personnel and 21.8 million veterans, according to the Census Bureau, between 9 and 10 percent of whom are women. Military members and veterans can obtain health care services from federal agencies and/or private and public hospitals, so nurses should be familiar with the potential ways health care can be accessed and provided. The Military Health System (MHS) is operated within the U.S. Department of Defense and provides health care to activity duty and retired U.S. military personnel and their dependents as well as retirees and their dependents aged 65 and over. The VA operates the nation's largest integrated health care system, clinics, community living centers, and other facilities. The VA has over 1200 sites of care and serves 8.76 million enrolled veterans each year. Due to access to care difficulties, the Veterans Choice Program (VCP), or "Choice Program," was initiated in 2014 through which veterans can receive care from community providers paid for by the VA. The VCP has gone through many updates since it was initiated in 2014, causing confusion for both the veterans and the providers. The VA is also a leader in veterans' health issues. For example, the Million Veteran Program (MVP) is collecting data from veteran volunteers to learn more about how genes affect health. As of April 2017, more than 560,000 participants enrolled in the program to create the largest database of its kind to help screen, diagnose, and treat a wide range of illnesses.

Environmental exposures in a war zone can include dust and smoke, extreme heat and cold temperatures, and biochemical weapons use, or a combination of all elements may result in significant health problems. Weaponry used in battle is designed to kill and maim combatants. Often, people have serious wounds and amputations. The violence and stress in war places a heavy burden on military and veteran personnel's mental capacity to manage in a healthy manner. Post-traumatic stress disorder (PTSD) is a common sequela of being in such life-threatening and traumatic situations. About 10 percent of women and 4 percent of men are estimated to develop PTSD after a trauma. It is normal to have disturbing memories by reliving it and to have feelings of anxiousness and trouble sleeping. Although difficult at first, most people are able to return to work, go to school, or return to normal activities and spend time with family and friends. But if these symptoms continue or occur sometime after the traumatic event, PTSD should be suspected.

Although the battle and training environment is dangerous, it is not the only threat to military personnel resulting in PTSD. Military sexual trauma has been a recurrent issue that has plagued the military services. In May of 2018, the U.S. Department of Defense released a report on sexual assault in the military (U.S. Department of Defense, 2018). The report stated that there were 6769 reports of sexual assault involving service members as either victims or subjects of criminal investigation in fiscal year 2017, which was a 9.7 percent increase from reports made in fiscal 2016. This increase, in part, is attributed to more sexual assaults being reported.

Homelessness in the veteran population has been a major concern in the nation. The U.S. Department of Housing and Urban Development's (HUD's) 2017 Annual Homeless Assessment Report to Congress found that on a single night in January 2017, 40,056 veterans were homeless (HUD, 2017). Veterans Affairs, veteran organizations, and numerous community organizations have partnered to decrease the homelessness among veterans. For example, according to the Los Angeles Homeless Services Authority 2018 Point-In-Time (PIT) count, Los Angeles County had an 18 percent decline in veteran homelessness. Veterans Affairs and community partners collaborated to help more veterans maintain their housing and help vulnerable veterans into permanent supportive housing (U.S. Department of Veterans Affairs, 2018).

Besides governmental agencies supporting current military personnel and veterans, numerous nongovernmental organizations support veterans. The United Service Organizations (USO), although chartered by Congress, is not part of the federal government. Since 1941, it has provided care packages and entertainment worldwide. The Fisher House Foundation, started in 1990, provides comfort homes where military and veterans' families can stay at no cost, while a loved one is receiving treatment. The Disabled American Veterans (DAV) Charitable Service Trust supports physical and psychological rehabilitation programs that provide direct support to ill or wounded veterans. DAV also funds programs that provide food, shelter, and other necessary items to homeless or at-risk veterans and their families. The Wounded Warrior Project, founded in 2003, supports programs for wounded veterans, their families, and caregivers.

References

U.S. Department of Defense: DoD releases annual report on sexual assault in military. Available at https://www.defense.gov.

U.S. Department of Veteran Affairs: National Center for Veterans Analysis and Statistics, n.d. Available at https://www.va.gov.

U.S. Census Bureau: Veterans, 2018. Available at https://www.census.gov.

U.S. Department of Housing and Urban Development: HUD 17–109, 2017. Available at https://www.hud.gov.

U.S. Department of Veteran Affairs: Veterans homelessness decreases 18% in Los Angles, 2018. Available at https://www.losangeles.va.gov.

U.S. Department of Veteran Affairs: Taking a personal health history, n.d. Available at https//www.va.gov.

Common health issues in the Military and Veteran Population: Olenick M, Flowers M, Diaz VJ: US veterans and their unique issues: enhancing health care professional awareness, Ad Med Educ Pract, 2015; 6:635–639.

Disparities and barriers such as these provide opportunities and challenges for nurses. By being aware of disparities and barriers in the health care system and recognizing that something should be done, nurses can help reduce the bias and remove barriers to health for both genders. Nurses can develop strategies to get men involved in lifestyle changes that prevent illness. Health care providers can reach out to men and offer the guidance and knowledge to improve men's health. Nurses can take an active role in public policy development and implementation. Nurses also can encourage men to identify primary care providers and obtain a physical examination and the appropriate recommended screening tests.

Men who can establish a working relationship with their health care provider and participate in the recommended screening tests may live healthier, happier, and longer lives. Refer to Box 29.3 for a variety of screening tests with suggested frequencies. Health screenings as well as other prevention strategies for adults are regularly updated by AHRQ. Some health screenings are clearly beneficial while health care providers and researchers debate the benefit of other screening procedures. As

BOX 29.3 Prevention Strategies for Adults

Dental Health
- Regular dental examinations
- Floss; brush with fluoride toothpaste

Health Screening
- Blood pressure
- Height and weight
- Nutritional screening (obesity)
- Lipid disorders (men 35 and older; women 45 and older)
- Papanicolaou (Pap) test (all women sexually active with a cervix)
- Colorectal cancer (adults 50 and older)
- Mammogram (women 40 and older)
- Osteoporosis (postmenopausal women 60 and older)
- Problem drinking
- Depression screening
- Tobacco use/tobacco-causing diseases
- Rubella serology or vaccination (women of childbearing age)
- Chlamydia (sexually active women age 25 and younger; women older than 25 with new/multiple sexual partners)
- Testicular cancer (symptomatic males)
- Coronary heart disease screening (EEG; exercise treadmill)
- Syphilis screening (for at-risk population only)
- Diabetes mellitus (adults with hypertension or hyperlipidemia)

Chemoprophylaxis
- Multivitamin/folic acid (women planning or capable of pregnancy)
- Aspirin prevention (CAD at-risk adults)

Immunizations
- Tetanus-diphtheria (TD) boosters
- Rubella (women of childbearing age)
- Pneumococcal vaccine (adults 65 and older)
- Influenza vaccine (adults 65 and older/at risk/annually)

CAD, Coronary artery disease; *EEG,* electroencephalogram.
From Agency for Health Care Research and Quality (AHRQ), U.S. Preventive Services Task Force: *The guide to clinical preventive services,* 2014, Rockville, MD, AHRQ.

a health care professional, it is important to be knowledgeable about current research and literature to identify appropriate screenings for specific populations.

Nurses can make significant contributions to improve men's health by learning more about men's health and how to work with men effectively. Nurses can assume many roles to fulfill responsibilities to improve the health of men in the community. As an educator, the nurse provides the knowledge and skill for replacing unhealthy behaviors with a healthy lifestyle. As a client advocate, the nurse supports and interacts with agencies to obtain the needed resources. The nurse acts as a change agent to assess needs and system influences, identify and set priorities, plan and implement programs for men, and evaluate results. Working within groups and communities, nurses can identify needs and priorities and develop interventions to reduce health risks and improve the health status not only of men, but also of their wives, mothers, daughters, and sisters and the communities in which they live.

Cancers Unique to Men

Prostate Cancer. The CDC identified prostate cancer as the most common non-skin cancer among American men. It also is one of the leading causes of cancer death among men of all races and Hispanic origin populations. In 2018, 164,690 new cases of prostate cancer were expected to be diagnosed and 29,430 died of the disease in the United States (ACS, 2018c). Having one or more close relatives with prostate cancer increases the risk for having prostate cancer for men. However, African American men have higher lifetime rates of prostate cancer compared to other races (4.2 percent for African American men, 2.9 percent for Hispanic men, 2.3 percent for white men, and 2.1 percent for Asian and Pacific Islanders).

The American Cancer Society (ACS) recommends men be informed about risks and possible benefits of prostate cancer screening and talking about the pros and cons of screening and treatment. The information should be provided at age 50 for men of average risk for prostate cancer and age 45 for men at high risk, such as African American men and men who have had a father, brother, or son diagnosed with prostate cancer before age 65. Men who have had family members diagnosed with prostate cancer at an early age should be informed about prostate screening at age 45. The 10-year survival for all stages of prostate cancer is 98 percent (ACS, 2018b).

After the discussion with the health care provider, two screening tests include the prostate-specific antigen (PSA) and the digital rectal examination (DRE). The PSA test is not accurate in terms of sensitivity or specificity. This blood test produces many false-positive results because many factors can elevate the PSA, such as infections, ejaculation, exercise such as bike riding, and benign prostatic hyperplasia (BPH). The DRE is a procedure where the physician inserts a well-lubricated, gloved index finger into the rectum to palpate the prostate gland and examine the rectum for masses (ACS, 2016). The examiner is unable to palpate the anterior aspects of the prostate, reducing the accuracy of this examination. Men find this examination unpleasant and another reason for avoiding health care.

Testicular Cancer. Testicular cancer is not common with about 1 of every 250 males developing it at an average age of 33 (ACS, 2018a). The risk of dying of testicular cancer is only about 1 in 5000. The ACS predicted 9310 new cases of testicular cancer and 400 deaths in 2018 (ACS, 2018b). Unfortunately, the cause of testicular cancer is unknown. Risk factors for testicular cancer include an undescended testicle, personally having or family history of testicular cancer, or HIV infection. White men are four to five times more likely than are African American and Asian American men to have testicular cancer. The only established relationship to testicular cancer is cryptorchidism. The good news is that testicular cancer is rare, and the five-year survival rate by race was reported as 95.7 percent for white men and 88.4 percent for African American men.

The ACS recommends a testicular exam by a doctor as part of a routine cancer-related checkup (ACS, 2018b). Because painless testicular enlargement is commonly the first sign of testicular cancer, the testicular self-examination has traditionally been recommended for men. The ACS recommends that men be aware of testicular cancer and see a doctor if a lump is found in a testicle. However, testicular self-exams are not to be known to be effective in reducing the death rate and some testicular cancers might not cause symptoms until they have grown and/or metastasized. In 2004 the U.S. Preventive Services Task Force (USPSTF) updated previously published guidelines that significantly altered that tradition for asymptomatic adolescent and adult males (USPSTF, 2004). The new guidelines state:

> *The USPSTF found no new evidence that screening with clinical examination or testicular self-examination was effective in reducing mortality from testicular cancer. Even in the absence of screening, the current treatment interventions provided very favorable health outcomes. Given the low prevalence of testicular cancer, limited accuracy of screening tests, and no evidence for the incremental benefits of screening, the USPSTF concluded that the harms of screening exceeded any potential benefits.*

Depression

Although more women than men are classified as having depression (8.5 percent and 4.8 percent, respectively), it is frequently unrecognized, undiagnosed, and untreated among men (Roche et al., 2016). Of particular concern for men is that higher rates of depression can be found in the unemployed, socially disadvantaged, those who abuse substances, and those with more than one medical condition. There are reasons to believe that men with depression often go unrecognized and underreported. Men do not express feelings of depression because it does not fit with the masculine role (Salk et al., 2017). Men tend to be stoic and do not verbalize how they feel and are reluctant to talk about health issues, and men often do not have positive relationships with their health care provider. For example, the death of a spouse, divorce, or job loss are risk factors for both genders for suicide, but males and females usually respond differently. Women tend to maintain their social network of family and friends for support. Men are less likely to seek support but attempt to maintain their gender role that includes strength and independence.

The suicide rate is four times greater for men, although women are diagnosed twice as often with major depression. Serious suicide attempts (SSAs) occur significantly more frequently in males than female (Freeman et al., 2017). This may be due to the gender bias in the criteria used to diagnose depression and suggests that men may have more difficulty recognizing or acknowledging depression related to the socially reinforced masculinity norms, including self-reliance, restrictions of emotions, and wanting to appear more masculine. Much of how gender is manifested in individuals is learned through socialization. How men manifest signs and symptoms of depression may result in low numbers of men diagnosed with depression because men are socialized to hide their feelings. Ultimately, men are seen with more incidences of avoidance behavior, anger, violence, and finally suicide. Nurses should recognize how men can manifest depression and be aware of the importance of developing a therapeutic relationship. Through the therapeutic relationship the experience of depression can be normalized, the biological and social factors in depression can be explained, and the positive outcome of depression treatment can be communicated.

Erectile Dysfunction

Erectile dysfunction (ED), also known as impotence, is the consistent inability to achieve or maintain an erection sufficient for satisfactory sexual performance. Up to 52 percent of men between the ages of 40 and 70 are affected by ED, and it is associated with decreased quality of life. ED can lead to withdrawal from intimacy, emotional stress, lower self-esteem, and avoidance of physical contact. Although the incidence of ED significantly increases with age, 55 percent to 70 percent of men aged 77 to 79 years are sexually active (McMahon, 2014). Psychogenic or organic factors or a combination of the two can cause ED. Psychogenic factors include stress, performance anxiety, or psychological disorders such as depression or schizophrenia. Organic factors include cardiovascular disease, diabetes, hypertension, hypercholesterolemia, smoking, spinal cord injury, prostate cancer, and genitourinary surgery. Alcohol and drug use, including medications used to treat a variety of both organic and psychological illness, are associated with ED (Muneer et al., 2014).

It is now known that ED is an independent marker for increased cardiovascular disease with vascular disease of the penile arteries (Jackson & Kirby, 2014). Men with ED and no cardiac symptoms should have a thorough health assessment. Lifestyle changes to reduce weight, manage hypertension and diabetes, stop smoking, reduce alcohol consumption and stress, and start exercising regularly will reduce risk.

Although ED may be discussed more openly with health care providers since the increased publicity generated from the marketing of the medications for ED, many men will still be embarrassed and reluctant to discuss the subject. A variety of treatments are available and can be discussed with the health care provider. Men who respond positively to treatment for ED report significantly better quality of life. With this evidence of positive response, health care providers should be proactive in discussing ED with men.

In summary, regardless of the prevalence differences in the health problems described in this section between men and women, appropriate health care services must be provided. Men and women need to be encouraged equally to take advantage of these services.

HEALTH DISPARITIES AMONG SPECIAL GROUPS OF ADULTS

Health disparities present political implications and influence government actions, including the commitment of resources to address them. In the United States, the government describes health disparities as differences that exist among specific population groups in the attainment of full health potential that can be measured by differences in incidence, prevalence, mortality, burden of disease, and other adverse health conditions (National Academies of Sciences, Engineering, and Medicine,

2017). There are two clusters of root causes of health inequity. The first is the intrapersonal, institutional, and systematic mechanisms that organize the distribution of power and resources differently across lines of race, gender, class, sexual orientation, gender expression, and other dimensions of individual and group identity. The second is the unequal allocation of power and resources (i.e., goods, services, and environmental conditions), which manifest in unequal social, economic, and environmental conditions also known as the social determinants of health. It is important to understand the complex and diverse factors that compose the root causes of health inequities to inform public health nurses to develop effective interventions to promote health equity.

Certain groups have been recognized as experiencing health disparities and have become a priority for policy efforts in reaching *Healthy People 2020* goals. Many factors contribute to disparities in health and health care for special groups of adult men and women, including education, insurance status, segregation, immigration status, health behaviors and lifestyle choices, health care provider behavior, employment, and the nature and operation of the health system in communities. While some outcomes measures have improved such as uninsurance rates, care coordination, and healthy living, great demarcations are still seen in care affordability, income, and poorer care for the uninsured (National Healthcare Quality and Disparities Report [NHQDR], 2018). As noted, poverty is a strong underlying current throughout all of the special groups.

Adults of Color

In 2000, about 44 percent of the U.S. population identified themselves as members of racial or ethnic minority groups. By 2050, these groups are projected to account for almost half of the U.S. population (NHQDR, 2018). Improvements in preventive care, chronic care, and access to care have led to improvements to the health of some populations in areas such as mammograms and smoking cessation counseling. However, the complete picture of disparities is different for each population. For instance, non-Asian racial/ethnic minorities continue to experience higher rates of HIV diagnoses than whites. When compared with whites, a lower percent of African Americans diagnosed with HIV were prescribed antiretroviral therapy and a lower percent of both African Americans and Hispanics had suppressed viral loads (McCree et al., 2017). Diabetes prevalence is highest among non-Hispanic African Americans, Hispanics, American Indians, and those of mixed races (ADA, 2018a). Although addressing these disparities appears daunting, the intent is to close the gap with regard to health disparities while at the same time preserving and respecting the richness and unique influences of various cultures. Population-focused nurses are positioned to advocate for culturally sensitive and gender-sensitive programs necessary in communities where adults of color may reside.

Incarcerated Adults

From 2007 to 2016 the U.S. prison population decreased to a nine-year low (U.S. Department of Justice, 2016). However, there are more than 10 million prisoners worldwide, and the prevalence of mental disorders is higher than in the general population (Fazel et al., 2016). Caring for the incarcerated or recently incarcerated population poses challenges to nurses who will be caring for this special population in other community settings.

African American males were incarcerated at a rate six and one-half times higher than white males. The proportion of prisoners under state or federal jurisdiction was 93 percent men and 7 percent women (Carson, 2015). Women are more likely to be serving time for property and drug offenses rather than violent crimes.

Inmates have been shown to have higher rates of chronic diseases such as hypertension, diabetes, asthma, chronic liver disease, and HIV than the general population (Maruschak & Berzofsky, 2016). Upon release from correctional institutions, ex-offenders face interruptions in their medical care stemming from limited resources, limited ability to access health care, and a lack of adequate discharge planning.

Incarcerated populations with major psychiatric disorders (major depressive disorder, bipolar disorders, schizophrenia, and non-schizophrenic psychotic disorders) have a substantially increased risk of multiple incarcerations. The greatest increase may be among inmates with severe mental disorders such as bipolar disorders. Nurses can support and deliver beneficial continuity of care reentry programs to help those who have been incarcerated to connect with community-based health programs at the time of release from prison to decrease recidivism rates.

Lesbian/Gay/Bisexual/Transgender/Queer/ Intersexual Adults

Lesbian/gay/bisexual/transgender/queer/intersex (LGBTQI) adults represent a sometimes hidden special population, in part because of the social stigma associated with alternate approaches to sexuality coupled with the fear of discrimination. Several studies have documented health disparities by sexual orientation in population-based data and have revealed differences in health between LGBTQI adults and their heterosexual counterparts, including higher risks of mental health issues, suicide and substance abuse (Fredriksen-Goldsen et al., 2013; McLaughlin et al., 2010) To improve the health of LGBTQI adults, services that address their unique needs are warranted. Safe places where this special population can voice their concerns and receive effective health promotion, disease prevention, and treatment are critical. Clarification of ways in which sexual orientation is associated with health outcomes will be critical to developing appropriate health interventions (Fredriksen-Goldsen et al., 2014).

Adults With Physical and Mental Disabilities

Many issues confront adults with disabilities. Concerns associated with health, aging, civil rights, abuse, and independent living are but a few examples of the types of problems facing this population. In 2015, 77 million adults 18 years of age and over had either basic actions difficulty (including movement or emotional difficulty or trouble seeing or hearing) or complex activity limitation (such as work or self-care limitations). This was an increase of over 8 million over the past 10 years. One third of adults 18 to 64 years of age had at least one basic actions difficulty or complex activity limitation in 2015, compared with 62 percent of adults 65 years of age and over (NCHS, 2017).

Adults with lifelong disabilities are more likely to have chronic conditions and multiple comorbidities than adults with no limitations (Dixon-Ibarra & Horner-Johnson, 2014). For instance, adults with developmental disabilities may be at a high risk for obesity and its sequelae (CDC, 2017b). This may be due to individual and community factors, including physical challenges, cognitive limitations, medications, lack of accessible adaptive fitness facilities, and segregation from the community in general.

Nurses can develop an awareness of the many health-related issues facing adults with disabilities. In particular, care should be taken to recognize the physical barriers that prevent disabled adults from accessing health care, such as structures that are not accessible despite the ADA recommendations. Developing health promotion programs targeted at this vulnerable, high-risk group can assist in overall well-being.

Impoverished and Uninsured Adults

The official poverty rate was 12.7 percent in 2016 with an estimated 40.6 million people in poverty. The child poverty rate was 18 percent, or 13.3 million children, in that same time period indicating a slight decline since 2015 (U.S. Census Bureau, 2017). Poverty affects acute and chronic conditions, accumulates over the life course, and is transmitted across generations. It limits education and employment opportunities, leaving individuals susceptible to weaker social integration, low control, depressive symptoms, and often a fatalistic outlook. For children, poverty has even greater effects on neurological development, behavior, and educational attainment. The stress of poverty may lead to poor dietary habits, tobacco use, and inconsistent personal hygiene. Health disparities, including chronic illness and health care services, are consistently associated with socioeconomic differences. The vulnerable homeless, **impoverished** rural, migrant, and public housing communities suffer from an increased burden of disease and greater morbidity and mortality than the general population. Veterans may fall in to this category due not being able to find or retain adequate employment upon military discharge.

Insured adults access health care services more often, including obtaining recommended screening and care for chronic conditions, thus reducing the overall costs of potential catastrophic illness. Although President Obama signed the Patient Protection and Affordable Care Act along with the Health Care and Education Reconciliation Act in March 2010 (United States Congress, 2010), many changes will occur as the law evolves and administrations change.

Under the ACA, states can extend Medicaid eligibility to nearly all adults with income no more than 138 percent of the federal poverty level. However, compared with adults who were already enrolled in Medicaid prior to the ACA, a substantial proportion of uninsured adults with chronic conditions do not have good disease control and may require intensive medical care following Medicare enrollment (Decker et al., 2013). The Kaiser Family Foundation (Artigaet al., 2017) reports the expansion in Medicaid and Marketplace improved coverage for low-income individuals leading to better health outcomes.

Nurses can be uniquely involved in community assessments to document pockets of poverty within their communities. For example, housing is a fundamental determinant of health and provides shelter and privacy. Exposure to cracks in ceilings and walls, inadequate heat, mold, poor ventilation, pesticide residue, excessive moisture, leaky pipes, and lead paint are all health hazards that can be addressed by nurses. Recent research has also found that health resilience to poverty was supported by protective factors in built and social environments. When poverty itself cannot be eliminated, improving access to care and identification of health risks improve individual and population outcomes.

Frail Elderly

In the past decade, the United States experienced a 30 percent increase in the population 65 years of age and older with a coinciding reduction in birth rates. Frailty is a geriatric syndrome that places older adults at risk for adverse health outcomes, including falls, worsening disability, institutionalization, and death. It is a complex state of impairment that signifies loss in areas of physical functioning, physiological resiliency, metabolism, and immune response.

By 2060, this group is expected to double and by 2040 the older elderly, 85 years and frail elderly will triple to 14.6 million (Administration on Aging, 2016). Most older persons have at least one chronic condition and many have multiple conditions, putting them at risk of experiencing frailty while living in a community setting. The number of elderly living in poverty is at 9.3 percent, increasing their health disparities and health status. Another major risk factor for health is elder abuse (U.S. Census Bureau, 2017).

The prevalence of **frail elderly** in the population poses a major public health dilemma since the majority of this group resides in a community setting, placing new demands on health care systems, family caregivers, and community resources. To improve the health of frail elderly, community-based nursing programs need to address racial/ethnic and socioeconomic disparities.

The elder-friendly community model identifies four domains needed by the elderly, including having basic needs met, social and civic engagement, physical and mental health and well-being, and independence for the frail and disabled (Greenfield et al., 2015). Age friendly community models identify independence for the frail elderly as the ability to "age in place" with specific indicators that focus on activities of daily living, transportation, and caregivers' ability to complement formal services. Community-level characteristics, including security issues, accessible shopping, and adequate transportation services are important community resources (Greenfield et al., 2015). Nurses can use this model to incorporate both individual and community factors that are necessary for elderly to live and thrive in community settings.

COMMUNITY-BASED MODELS FOR CARE OF ADULTS

Nursing Roles

Communities are where people live, work, and socialize. Community health settings include public health departments, nurse-managed health centers, ambulatory care clinics, and home health agencies. Nurses are involved in direct care, providing self-care information, contributing to the supervision of paraprofessionals, or collaborating with other disciplines to provide the most appropriate, high-quality, cost-effective care at the most appropriate level and location.

Knowledge of community resources is a fundamental part of caring for the adult with special needs in any community. The nurse assesses the need for and helps develop the resources. Every community has an area agency on aging that coordinates planning and delivery of needed services, and it can be a good resource for the nurse. Most communities have information and referral systems as well as a public directory of services available.

The complex nature of chronic illness with care focused primarily on maximizing functional status and well-being is particularly suited to nursing's holistic focus. The Doctor of Nursing Practice (DNP)-prepared advanced practice nurse role brings specific competencies and nursing backgrounds to the role of primary care provider. A recent community-based model to provide care for frail elders highlights three areas of expertise that advanced practice nurses in the DNP role can provide: management of complex chronic illness, illness and injury prevention, and promotion of quality of life.

Community Care Settings

Patient-Centered Medical Homes. A traditional part of community care for adults with chronic illness is the use of primary care practices. Health care systems with a primary care focus have better outcomes, including better quality, lower costs, less inequality in health care and health, and better population health when compared with systems based on other approaches to health care. The patient-centered medical home (PCMH) moves beyond primary care to include new approaches to organizing practice to enhance its responsiveness to individual patient needs. PCMH has been associated with a lower probability of inpatient hospitalization and may be associated with a reduction in health care utilization (Adaji et al., 2018). The following are basic tenets for the concept of PCMH:

1. A relationship between the patient and medical provider
2. A provider who takes charge of total patient care, including arrangements for specialty care
3. Open access to health care
4. Ongoing care managed by the same provider to assure coordination and collaboration
5. Quality and safety as key aspects of the system
6. Transparent and fair payment

For patients with chronic illnesses, one approach to PCMH is to include physician assistants (PAs) and nurse practitioners (NPs) on primary care teams. This approach has demonstrated positive outcomes in the measure of quality of diabetes care and use of health care services (Everett et al., 2013).

Senior Centers. Senior centers were developed in the early 1940s to provide social and recreational activities. Now many centers are multipurpose, offering recreation, education, counseling, therapies, hot meals, and case management, as well as health screening and education. Some even offer primary care services. Nurses have a unique opportunity to provide services to a group of older persons who wish to remain independent in the community.

Adult Day Health. Adult day health is for individuals whose mental or physical function requires them to obtain more health care and supervision. It serves as more of a medical model than the senior center, and often individuals return home to their caregivers at night. Some settings offer respite care for short-term overnight relief for caregivers. This provides caregivers the opportunity to work or have personal time during the day. Nurses may provide support groups for caregivers.

Home Health, Palliative Care, and Hospice. Home health can be provided by multidisciplinary teams. Nurses provide individual and environmental assessments, direct skilled care and treatment, and provide short-term guidance and instruction. Nurses often function independently in the home and must rely on their own resources and knowledge to improvise and adapt care to meet the client's unique physical and social circumstances. They work closely with the family and other caregivers to provide necessary communication and continuity of care. (See Chapter 41 for more details.)

Palliative care is the broad term used to describe the care provided by an interdisciplinary team consisting of physicians, nurses, social workers, chaplains, and other health care professionals. Coyle (2010) describes the distinctive features of palliative care nursing as "a whole person" philosophy of care. This care is provided across a continuum of different settings, including the life span, the illness trajectory, the patient's death, and the family's bereavement. Often, the terms *hospice* and *palliative care* are used interchangeably. Palliative care is a broader concept and includes the entire continuum of care. Hospice care is always palliative care, but not all palliative care is hospice care (Coyle, 2010).

Hospice represents a philosophy of caring for and supporting life to its fullest until death occurs. The hospice team encourages the client and family to jointly make decisions to meet physical, emotional, spiritual, and comfort needs (see palliative care in the Content Resources section of the Evolve website).

QSEN FOCUS ON QUALITY AND SAFETY EDUCATION FOR NURSES

Targeted Competency: Client-Centered Care

Recognize the client or designee as the source of control and full partner in providing compassionate and coordinated care based on respect for the client's preferences, values, and needs.

Important aspects of client-centered care include the following:

- **Knowledge:** Describe strategies to assist clients and their families in all aspects of the health care process.
- **Skills:** Communicate client values, preferences, and expressed needs to other members of the health care team.
- **Attitudes:** Willingly support client-centered care for individuals and groups whose values differ from your values.

Client-Centered Care Question

You are making a home visit to the Jones family—Mr. and Mrs. Jones and their children, John (10 years), Sally (6 years), and Tommy (3 years). Mr. and

Mrs. Jones are considered obese using the body weight index measures of the American Heart Association. John is considered overweight by this same measure, and you note that both Sally and Tommy are at the upper range for weight for their age. You observe during the visit that the family appears to eat a lot of processed food, including lunch meats, chips, and carbonated drinks with sugar. What steps would you take to help this family (1) understand the importance of maintaining an average weight, (2) learn about the different ways in which foods can be prepared, and (3) learn about the relationship among calorie consumption, physical activity, and weight?

Answer

First, you would need to assess their knowledge about weight management. Next, you would need to determine if they have the skill to purchase and prepare lower calorie, nutritious food and if they are capable of engaging in physical activities. You would also need to evaluate their attitude toward body size and image. Their willingness to change their behavior will be influenced by whether they view themselves as needing to change. If there is a willingness to make weight management behavior change, you can refer them to a nutrition expert for a consultation or to attend a class(es). You can find out how they spend their leisure time and what options they can identify that would include the entire family in a physical activity such as a walk, a game, or a trip to the park

Assisted Living. Assisted living covers a wide variety of choices, from a single shared room to opulent independent living accommodations in a full-service, life-care community. The differences are related to the type and extent of the amenities provided and the contract signed for them. The role of the nurse varies depending on the philosophy and leadership of the management of the facility. The nurse generally provides assessment and interventions, medication review, education, and advocacy.

Long-Term Care and Rehabilitation. Nursing homes, or long-term care facilities, house only about 5 percent of the older population at a given time; however, 25 percent of those adults older than 65 will spend some time in a nursing home. Nursing homes provide a safe environment, special diets and activities, routine personal care, and the treatment and management of health care needs for those needing rehabilitation, as well as for those needing a permanent supportive residence. Rehabilitation is a combination of physical, occupational, psychological, and speech therapy to help debilitated persons maintain or recover their physical capacities. Rehabilitation is typically needed for older adults after a hip fracture, stroke, or prolonged illness that results in serious deconditioning.

LINKING CONTENT TO PRACTICE

There are many health issues burdening the public's health. The steps of the nursing process (assessment, diagnosis, planning, intervention, and evaluation) are foundational to all services rendered by the public health nurse to address these issues. However, nurses must clearly understand that neither the process nor the services occur in isolation. Nurses must learn to apply systems thinking skills and be able to communicate and work collaboratively in an interprofessional and multicultural environment to improve community health. Public health nursing is a complex calling requiring a commitment to continued learning and professional development.

PRACTICE APPLICATION

The nurse in a local public health department talks with the director of the department, who needs to determine what major public health issues exist in the community and prioritize them to better allocate resources. The director formed a committee to assist in this process. The director asks the nurse to participate on the committee because of the nurse's interest in men's health. The director asks the nurse to identify up to 10 major health issues in the community, prioritize them, and recommend strategies to improve men's health in the community. The director wants a report supporting conclusions and strategies that the department could implement.

Based on the previous scenario, answer the following questions:

A. What information do you want to collect?

B. How would you identify priorities in your area?

C. What positive and negative factors may be influencing these issues?

D. How would you select strategies to improve health issues?

1. What interventions, if any, are currently being used, and are they effective?
2. Who are the key participants that would need to be involved in improving the issues?
3. Have these issues been addressed effectively in other communities? If they have, what have they done?

Answers can be found on the Evolve site.

KEY POINTS

- The health of adults is embedded in their communities.
- Societal factors influence the distribution of health and disease.
- Women's health advocates have widened the framework of women's health by focusing on social, psychological, cultural, political, and economic as well as biological factors.
- The complexities of women's lives—their educational levels, income, culture, ethnicity/race, and a host of other identities and experiences—shape their health.
- The Office on Women's Health (OWH) works to address inequities in research, health services, and education that have traditionally placed women at risk for health problems.
- The problem of unintended pregnancy exists among adolescents as well as adult women.
- Women's attitudes toward menopause vary greatly and are influenced by culture, age, support, and the shared experiences of other women.

- Cardiovascular disease (CVD) is the leading cause of death among U.S. adults.
- Diabetes has increased dramatically in the United States during the last decade.
- Women in the United States experience depression at higher rates than do men.
- Overall, white women have a higher incidence rate for all cancers while African American women have higher mortality rates.
- Research shows that older women, especially women of color from lower socioeconomic groups, experience higher rates of chronic illness and disability than their white and more affluent counterparts.
- One out of every two American women more than 50 years of age will experience an osteoporosis-related fracture in her lifetime.
- Men are reluctant to seek health care and are not well connected to the health care system.
- Large numbers of men do not receive the health screenings intended to prevent and identify disease.
- To improve health outcomes for men, chronic disease prevention and control programs should combine individual and population-based strategies developed in collaboration with community members and developing infrastructure to address environmental and policy change.
- Although adverse working conditions and numerous pathological conditions clearly are detrimental to men's health, there is a great need to focus on the mental health of men.
- The nurse acts as a change agent to assess needs and system influences, identify and set priorities, plan and implement programs, and evaluate results.

CLINICAL DECISION-MAKING ACTIVITIES

1. Interview three women, each from a different culture, about their experiences accessing health care. Are there differences in their stories about how they meet their health care needs? Do variances in ethnicity and culture present barriers to accessing health care?
2. Review current legislation that deals with women's health. Note patterns or trends in the issues that are being considered by the Senate or the House of Representatives. Are there obvious gaps in legislation that adversely affect women's health?
3. Considering breast cancer, apply the levels of prevention to women in underserved areas. Describe approaches to meeting their health care, social needs, and psychological needs. What barriers might prevent an effective program addressing breast cancer?
4. Contact your local public health office to determine what services are available for women. Identify community resources and agencies targeted for women. How do these organizations communicate their services to women in the community?
5. Propose a community-based intervention for women with HIV. Describe various program components such as goals and objectives, evaluation methods, and program outcomes.
6. Identify a men's health issue in your community. Contact local health agencies in your area to determine what strategies are currently in place to address the issue.
7. Based on the issue identified in question 6, search the Internet for evidence-based practices related to the issue.
8. Think about television, movie, or magazine portrayals of men and identify both positive and negative influences the media may have on men's health.
9. Locate several websites focusing on men's health topics. Using criteria for credible websites from Health on the Net Foundation (https://www.hon.ch/en/), evaluate those sites for credible health information.

ADDITIONAL RESOURCES

EVOLVE WEBSITE

http://evolve.elsevier.com/Stanhope/community/

- Answers to Practice Application
- Case Study
- Glossary
- Review Questions

REFERENCES

Adaji A, Melin GJ, Campbell R, Lohse CM, Westphal JJ, Katzelnick DJ: Patient-centered medical home membership is associated with decreased hospital admissions for emergency department behavioral health patients, *Popul Health Manag* 21(3), 2018.

Administration for Children and Families: *About ACF*, n.d. Retrieved from https://www.acf.hhs.gov.

Administration for Community Living: *About ACL*, 2018. Retrieved from https://www.acl.gov.

Administration on Aging (AOA). *A profile of older Americans: administration on aging*, 2016, USDHHS. Retrieved from https://www.acl.gov.

Administration on Aging: *Older Americans Act*, 2017. Retrieved from https://www.acl.gov.

Agency for Healthcare Research and Quality: *Guide to clinical preventive services*, 2014. Retrieved from https://www.ahrq.gov.

Ahn S, Basu R, Smith ML, et al.: The impact of chronic disease self-management programs: healthcare savings through a community-based intervention, *BMC Public Health* 13:1141, 2013.

Alexander LL, LaRosa JH, Bader H, et al.: *New dimensions in women's health*, ed 4, Boston, MA, 2007, Jones & Bartlett.

American Cancer Society (ACS): *American Cancer Society Recommendations for prostate cancer early detection*, Atlanta, GA, 2016, ACS. Retrieved from https://www.cancer.org.

American Cancer Society (ACS): *Cancer facts & figures 2018*, Atlanta, GA, 2018a, American Cancer Society. Retrieved from https://www.cancer.org.

American Cancer Society (ACS): *Cancer facts for men*, Atlanta, GA, 2018b, ACS. Retrieved from https://www.cancer.org.

American Cancer Society: *Prostate Cancer Overview*, 2018c. Retrieved from http://www.cancer.org.

American Diabetes Association (ADA): *Statistics about diabetes: overall numbers, diabetes and prediabetes*, 2018a. Retrieved from http://www.diabetes.org.

American Diabetes Association: Economic costs of diabetes in the U.S. in 2017, *Diabetes Care* 41(5):917–928, 2018b. Retrieved from http://care.diabetesjournals.org.

American Heart Association (AHA): *What about African Americans and high blood pressure?* 2017. Retrieved from http://www.heart.org.

American Public Health Association (APHA): *Public health and chronic disease: cost savings and return on investment*, n.d. Retrieved from https://www.apha.org.

Americans with Disabilities Act of 1990, as amended with ADA Amendments Act of 2008, n.d. Retrieved from http://www.ada.gov.

Artiga S, Ubri P, Foutz J: What is at stake for health and health care disparities under ACA repeal? *Kaiser Family Fund* 2017. Retrieved from kff.org.

Aune D, Sen A, Henriksen T, Saugstad OD, Tonstad S: Physical activity and the risk of gestational diabetes mellitus: a systematic review and dose–response meta-analysis of epidemiological studies, *Eur J Epidemiol* 31(10):967–997, 2016.

Bairey Merz CN, Andersen H, Sprague E, et al.: Knowledge, attitudes, and beliefs regarding cardiovascular disease in women: the women's heart alliance, *J Am Coll Cardiol* 70:123–132, 2017.

Befus D, Coeytaux RR, Goldstein KM, et al.: Management of menopause symptoms with acupuncture: an umbrella systematic review and meta-analysis, *J Altern Complement Med* 24:314–323, 2018.

Benjamin EJ, Virani S, Clifton W, et al.: 2018: Heart disease and stroke statistics—2018 Update: a report from the American Heart Association, *Circulation* 135.e1–e45. Retrieved from http://circ.ahajournals.org.

Brownstein JN, Mirambeau AM, Roland KB: News from the CDC: using web-based training to translate evidence on the value of community health workers into public health action, *Transl Behav Med* 3(3):229–230, 2013.

Cannon MJ, Dominique Y, O'Leary L, Sniezek JE, Floyd RL: Characteristics and behaviors of mothers who have a child with fetal alcohol syndrome, *Neurotoxicol Teratol* 34(1):90–95, 2012.

Carey RM, Whelton PK, for the 2017 ACC/AHA Hypertension guideline writing committee: Prevention, detection, evaluation, and management of high blood pressure in adults: synopsis of the 2017 American College of Cardiology/American Heart Association Hypertension Guideline, *Ann Intern Med* 168: 351–358, 2018. Retrieved from http://annals.org.

Carson E: *Prisoners in 2014*, 2015, Bureau of Justice Statistics. Retrieved from https://www.bjs.gov.

CDC Foundation: *Heart disease and stroke cost America nearly $1 billion a day in medical costs, lost productivity*, 2015. Retrieved from https://www.cdcfoundation.org.

Centers for Disease Control and Prevention (CDC): QuickStats: percentage of adults aged ≥18 years who have seen or talked to a doctor or other health care professional about their own health in the past 12 months, by sex and age group, National Health Interview Survey, United States, 2015, *MMWR Morb Mortal Wkly Rep* 66:65, 2017. Retrieved from https://www.cdc.gov.

Centers for Disease Control and Prevention: *CDC Fact Sheet: Reported STDs in the United States, 2017*, 2017a. Retrieved from https://www.cdc.gov.

Centers for Disease Control and Prevention: *Disability and Obesity*, 2017b. Retrieved from https://www.cdc.gov.

Centers for Disease Control and Prevention: *CDC Fact sheet: adult obesity facts*, 2018a. Retrieved from https://www.cdc.gov.

Centers for Disease Control and Prevention: *Folic acid basics*, 2018b. Retrieved from https://www.cdc.gov.

Centers for Disease Control and Prevention: *National center for environmental health*, 2018c. Retrieved from http://www.cdc.gov.

Centers for Disease Control and Prevention: *STD prevention allocation consequences estimator*, 2018d. Retrieved from https://www.cdc.gov.

Centers for Disease Control and Prevention: *Gestational diabetes and pregnancy*, 2017, Atlanta, GA, 2017c, CDC. Retrieved from http://www.cdc.gov.

Centers for Disease Control and Prevention: *National Center on Birth Defects and Developmental Disabilities (NCBDDD) annual report*, 2017b, USDHHS, CDC. Retrieved from https://www.cdc.gov.

Centers for Disease Control and Prevention: *Sexually Transmitted Disease Surveillance 2016*, Atlanta, GA, 2017c, U.S. Department of Health and Human Services. Retrieved from https://www.cdc.gov.

Cheng CC, Hsu CY, Liu JF: Effects of dietary and exercise intervention on weight loss and body composition in obese postmenopausal women: a systematic review and meta-analysis, *Menopause* 25(7):772–782, 2018.

Coyle N: Introduction to palliative nursing care. In Ferrell BR, Coyle N, editors: *Textbook of Palliative Nursing*, ed 3, Oxford, UK, 2010, Oxford University Press, pp 3–11.

Decker SL, Kostova D, Kenney GM, Long SK: Health status, risk factors, and medical conditions among persons enrolled in Medicaid vs uninsured low-income adults potentially eligible for Medicaid under the Affordable Care Act, *JAMA* 309(24): 2579–2586, 2013.

DeSantis CE, Ma J, Goding Sauer A, Newman LA, Jemal A: Breast cancer statistics, 2017, racial disparity in mortality by state, *CA Cancer J Clin* 67:439–448, 2017.

Dixon-Ibarra A, Horner-Johnson W: Disability status as an antecedent to chronic conditions: National Health Interview Survey, 2006–2012, *Prev Chronic Dis* 11:130251, 2014.

Egen O, Beatty K, Blackley DJ, Brown K, Wykoff R: Health and social conditions of the poorest versus wealthiest counties in the United States, *Am J Public Health* 107(1):130–135, 2017.

Egger G: In search of a germ theory equivalent for chronic disease, *Prev Chronic Dis* 9:110301, 2012.

Everett C, Thorpe C, Palta M, Carayon P, Bartels C, Smith MA: Physician assistants and nurse practitioners perform effective roles on teams caring for Medicare patients with diabetes, *Health Aff (Millwood)* 32(11):1942–1948, 2013.

Fazel S, Hayes A, Bartellas K, Clerici M, Trestman R: Mental health of prisoners: prevalence, adverse outcomes, and interventions, *Lancet Psychiatry* 3:871–881, 2016.

Fredriksen-Goldsen KI, Kim HJ, Barkan SE, Muraco A, Hoy-Ellis CP: Health disparities among lesbian, gay, and bisexual older adults: results from a population-based study, *Am J Public Health* 103(10):1802–1809, 2013.

Fredriksen-Goldsen KI, Simoni JM, Kim HJ, et al.: The health equity promotion model: reconceptualization of lesbian, gay, bisexual, and transgender (LGBT) health disparities, *Am J Orthopsychiatry* 84(6):653–663, 2014.

Freeman A, Mergl R, Kohls E, et al.: A cross-national study on gender differences in suicide intent, *BMC Psychiatry* 17:234, 2017.

Giorgianni SJ, Porche DJ, Williams ST, Matope JH, Leonard BL: Developing the discipline and practice of comprehensive men's health, *Am J Mens Health 7*(4):342–349, 2013.

Greenfield EA, Oberlink M, Scharlach AE, Neal MB, Stafford PB: Age-friendly community initiatives: conceptual issues and key questions, *Gerontologist* 55(2):191–198, 2015.

Guy ME: *American Political Science Association 2013 annual meeting*, 2013. Retrieved from http://ssrn.com.

HealthData.gov: 2018. Retrieved from www.healthdata.gov.

Holm AL, Rowe Gorosh M, Brady M, White-Perkins D: Recognizing privilege and bias: an interactive exercise to expand health care providers' personal awareness, *Acad Med* 92:360–364, 2017.

Jackson G, Kirby M: Erectile dysfunction increases cardiovascular risk: time to reduce it, *Trends Urol Men's Health* 5(1):28–30, 2014.

Markidan J, Cole JW, Cronin CA, et al.: Smoking and risk of ischemic stroke in young men, *Stroke* 49:1276–1278, 2018.

Martin KA, Barbieri RL: *Treatment of menopausal symptoms with hormone therapy*, 2018. Retrieved from https://www.uptodate.com.

Maruschak LM, Berzofsky M: *Medical problems of state and federal prisoners and jail inmates, 2011–12*, 2016. Retrieved from https://www.bjs.gov.

May PA, Chambers CD, Kalberg WO, et al. Prevalence of fetal alcohol spectrum disorders in 4 U.S. communities, *JAMA* 319:474–482, 2018.

McCree DH, Sutton M, Bradley E, Harris N: Changes in the disparity of HIV diagnosis rates among black women—United States, 2010–2014, *MMWR Morb Mortal Wkly Rep* 66:104–106, 2017.

McLaughlin KA, Hatzenbuehler ML, Keyes KM: Responses to discrimination and psychiatric disorders among Black, Hispanic, female, and lesbian, gay, and bisexual individuals, *Am J Public Health* 100(8):1477–1484, 2010.

McMahon CG: Erectile dysfunction, *Intern Med J* 44(1):18–26, 2014.

Model Elements: *Improving chronic illness care*, 2014. Retrieved from http://www.improvingchroniccare.org.

Muneer A, Kalsi J, Nazareth I, Ary M: Erectile dysfunction, *BMJ* 348:g129, 2014.

National Academies of Sciences, Engineering, and Medicine: *Communities in action: pathways to health equity*, Washington, DC, 2017, National Academies Press. Retrieved from https://www.ncbi.nlm.nih.gov.

National Cancer Institute (NCI): *Breast cancer screening*, 2018. Retrieved from https://www.cancer.gov.

National Center for Chronic Disease Prevention and Health Promotion (NCCDPHP): *Health risk factors that cause chronic disease*, 2014. Retrieved from http://www.cdc.gov.

National Center for Complementary and Integrative Health (NCCIH): *Menopausal symptoms and complementary health practices: what the science says*, 2016. Retrieved from https://nccih.nih.gov.

National Center for Elder Abuse (NCEA): *Why should I care about elder abuse?* n.d. Retrieved from https://ncea.acl.gov.

National Center for Health Statistics (NCHS): *Health, United States, 2016: with chartbook on long-term trends in health*, 2017. Retrieved from https://www.cdc.gov.

National Healthcare Quality and Disparities Report (NHQDR): *2016 National healthcare quality and disparities report*, Rockville, MD, 2018, Agency for Healthcare Research and Quality. Retrieved from https://www.ahrq.gov.

National Heart, Lung, and Blood Institute (NHLBI): *Calculate your body mass index*, 2018. Retrieved from https://www.nhlbi.nih.gov.

National Institute of Mental Health: *Mental illness*, 2017. Retrieved from https://www.nimh.nih.gov.

National Institutes of Health: Revitalization Act of 1993. Retrieved from https://www.govtrack.us.

National Institutes of Mental Health (NIMH): *What are eating disorders?* Rockville, MD, 2014, USDHHS, National Institutes of Health.

National Osteoporosis Foundation (NOF): *Clinician's guide to prevention and treatment of osteoporosis*, Washington, DC, 2014, National Osteoporosis Foundation. Retrieved from https://www.ncbi.nlm.nih.gov.

O'Keefe LC, Sullivan MM, McPhail A, Van Buren K, Dewberry N: Screening for colorectal cancer at the worksite, *Workplace Health Saf* 66:183–190, 2018.

Organization for Economic Co-operation and Development (OECD): *Health at a glance: how does the United States compare?* 2017. Retrieved from https://www.oecd.org.

Ory MG, Smith ML, Patton K, Lorig K, Zenker W, Whitelaw N: Self-management at the tipping point: reaching 100,000 Americans with evidence-based programs, *J Am Geriatr Soc* 61(5):821–823, 2013.

Qaseem A, Forciea MA, McLean RM, Denberg TD, for the Clinical Guidelines Committee of the American College of Physicians: Treatment of low bone density or osteoporosis to prevent fractures in men and women: a clinical practice guideline update from the American College of Physicians, *Ann Intern Med* 166:818–839, 2017.

Research and Development (RAND). *Multiple chronic conditions in the United States*, Santa Monica, CA, 2017, RAND Corporation. Retrieved from https://www.rand.org.

Roche AM, Pidd K, Fischer JA, Lee N, Scarfe A, Kostadinov V: Men, work, and mental health: a systematic review of depression in male-dominated industries and occupations, *Saf Health Work* 7:268–283, 2016. Retrieved from https://www.ncbi.nlm.nih.gov.

Salk RH, Hyde JS, Abramson LY: Gender differences in depression in representative national samples: meta-analyses of diagnoses and symptoms, *Psychol Bull* 143(8):783–822, 2017.

Santoro N, Epperson CN, Mathews SB: Menopausal symptoms and their management, *Endocrinol Metab Clin North Am* 44(3):497–515, 2015.

Sendall M, McCosker L, Crossley K, Bonner A: A structured review of chronic care model components supporting transition between healthcare service delivery types for older people with multiple chronic disease, *Health Inf Manag* 46(2):58–68, 2016.

Thakrar AP, Forrest AD, Maltenfort MG, Forrest CB: Child mortality in the U.S. and 19 OECD comparator nations: a 50-year time-trend analysis, *Health Aff (Millwood)* 37:140–149, 2018.

Thomas J, Sabatino C: Patient preferences, policy, and POLST: how innovations and legislation are transforming advanced illness in a digital age, *J Am Soc Aging* 41:102–109, 2017.

United States Cancer Statistics: *Leading cancer cases and deaths, male and female*, 2015. Retrieved from https://gis.cdc.gov.

United States Congress: *Public Law 111–148*, Washington, DC, 2010, United States Government Printing Office. Retrieved from https://democrats.senate.gov.

U.S. Burden of Disease Collaborators: The state of U.S. health, 1990–2010: burden of diseases, injuries, and risk factors, *JAMA* 310(6):591–608, 2013.

U.S. Census Bureau: *Income, poverty and health insurance coverage in the United States: 2016*, September 12, 2017. Release Number: CB17–156. Retrieved from www.census.gov

U.S. Department of Defense (DOD): *DoD releases annual report on sexual assault in military*, 2018. https://www.defense.gov.

U.S. Department of Health and Human Services (USDHHS): *Healthy People 2020*, 2010. Retrieved from https://www.healthypeople.gov.
U.S. Department of Health and Human Services (USDHHS): *Office of Women's Health*, 2014. Retrieved from https://www.hrsa.gov.
U.S. Department of Housing and Urban Development. *HUD.17–109*, 2017. Retrieved from https://www.hud.gov.
U.S. Department of Justice, Bureau of Justice Statistics: *Correctional populations in the United States*, 2016. Retrieved from www.bjs.gov.
U.S. Department of Labor Wage and Hour Division (WHD): *The Family and Medical Leave Act of 1993*, n.d. Retrieved from http://www.dol.gov.
U.S. Department of Veterans Affairs: *VA Greater Los Angeles Healthcare System: veteran homelessness decreases 18% in Los Angeles*, 2018. Retrieved from https://www.losangeles.va.gov.
U.S. Preventive Services Task Force (USPSTF): Hormone therapy for the primary prevention of chronic conditions in postmenopausal women: recommendation statement, *Am Fam Physician* 97(8), 2018. Retrieved from https://www.aafp.org.
U.S. Preventive Services Task Force (USPSTF): Screening for testicular cancer: U.S. Preventive Services Task Force reaffirmation recommendation statement, 2004, *Ann Intern Med* 154: 483–486, 2004.
Volkow ND, Compton WM, Wargo EM: The risks of marijuana use during pregnancy, *JAMA* 317(2):129–130, 2017.
World Health Organization (WHO): *Mental health: a state of well-being*, 2014. Retrieved from http://www.who.int.
World Health Organization (WHO): *Preventing disease through healthy environments: a global assessment of the burden of disease from environmental risks*, Geneva, Switzerland, 2016, WHO. Retrieved from http://www.who.int.
Wu IHC, Bathje GJ, Kalibatseva Z, Sung D, Leong FTL, Collins-Eaglin J: Stigma, mental health, and counseling service use: a person-centered approach to mental health stigma profiles, *Psychol Serv* 14:490–501, 2017.
Yon Y, Mikton CR, Gassoumis ZD, Wilber KH: Elder abuse prevalence in community settings: a systematic review and meta-analysis, *Lancet Glob Health* 5:e147–e156, 2017.
Young-Wolff KC, Tucker LY, Alexeeff S, et al.: Trends in self-reported and biochemically tested marijuana use among pregnant females in California from 2009–2016, *JAMA* 318(24):2490–2491, 2017.

30

Disability Health Care Across the Life Span

Lynn Wasserbauer, RN, FNP, PhD

OBJECTIVES

After reading this chapter the student should be able to do the following:

1. Define terms related to disability.
2. Discuss implications of developmental disability, physical disability, or chronic illness.
3. Discuss the effects of being disabled on the individual, the family, and the community.
4. Discuss the objectives of *Healthy People 2020* as they relate to disability.
5. Examine the nurse's role in caring for people who are disabled.
6. Identify key disability rights legislation.

CHAPTER OUTLINE

Understanding Disabilities
Scope of the Problem
The Effects of Disabilities
Selected Issues
Role of the Nurse
Disability Rights Legislation

KEY TERMS

Americans with Disabilities Act, p. 678
bullying, p. 688
burden of chronic disease, p. 681
children with special health care needs (CSHCN), p. 680
chronic disease, p. 680
developmental disability, p. 680
disability, p. 679
disability rights legislation, p. 691
dual diagnosis, p. 683
front line staff/entry level, p. 681
functional limitations, p. 680
health promotion, p. 688
medical model of disability, p. 679
program management/supervisory level, p. 681
senior management/executive level, p. 681
social model of disability, p. 679

Foundational to the American system of government is the belief that all citizens are entitled to protection of individual civil rights. Unfortunately, individuals with disabilities were among the last groups in the United States to receive civil rights protection. Until the late twentieth century, widespread discrimination against the disabled made it difficult for them to feel fully integrated into society. As a result of this discrimination, the disabled often were literally shut in and shut out of much of American society. The **Americans with Disabilities Act** (ADA) of 1990 was the first comprehensive civil rights legislation for individuals with disabilities. One effect of this legislation is a greater emphasis on community care for the disabled, rather than institutionalization, and there is a growing emphasis on providing that care in as "home-like" an environment as possible.

One of the many challenges for the disabled is access to appropriate health care. Although not all care can be delivered at home, public health nurses are uniquely positioned to serve as care providers and managers for community-dwelling disabled individuals. Having an understanding of disabilities, disability rights, and the legislation specifically enacted to decrease discrimination will assist nurses in intervening and advocating for the disabled.

This chapter provides an overview of disabilities, defines key terms, and reviews the effects of disabilities on individuals, families, and communities. The relationships between disabling conditions and *Healthy People 2020* are discussed. Also reviewed is the nurse's role in planning and providing or securing appropriate interventions for individuals, families, and communities to manage or prevent these health problems.

UNDERSTANDING DISABILITIES

Models of Disability

There is no single accepted definition for disability. The definition of disability varies depending on common use of the word or the specific agency defining the term. With regard to health care, the **medical model of disability** is generally used to conceptualize disability. In this model, disability is considered to be a function of physical characteristics or conditions that place an individual at a disadvantage compared with those who do not have the characteristic or condition. This model places emphasis on the disabled person and the need to modify the course of illness, or as much as possible to give the disabled person a "normal" life. The Social Security Administration uses this model for determination of disability. In the **social model of disability**, emphasis is placed on systemic barriers as well as societal attitudes and stigmas that contribute to the perception that those with limitations or physical illnesses are disabled. In this model the focus is on the need to change society and not the individual with a disability. This model has led to a focus on civil rights for the disabled and the need for legislation addressing discrimination (Goering, 2015).

Disability Defined

Disability is defined by Webster's as "a physical, mental, cognitive, or developmental condition that impairs, interferes with, or limits a person's ability to engage in certain tasks or actions or participate in typical daily activities and interactions; impaired function or ability; an impairment (such as a chronic medical condition or injury) that prevents someone from engaging in gainful employment; an impairment (such as spina bifida) that results in serious functional limitations for a minor; a program providing financial support to a person affected by a disability; the financial support provided by such a program; a disqualification, restriction, or *disadvantage*; lack of legal qualification to do something" (Merriam-Webster, 2018).

Census Determination of Disability

The way the Census determines disability has changed over time. Data used to be collected with the standard long-form and additional disability data were obtained from a cross section of the United States. These test questions were part of the American Community Survey (ACS), an early supplement to the decennial census, and the Survey of Income and Program Participation (SIPP), a continuous survey of a national panel of households with each panel lasting about four years. In 2000 the population was assessed to determine and define disability based on functional limitations. The Census Bureau collected data on the number of individuals with disabilities. Six specific subpopulations of disability were identified and included sensory disability, mental disability, physical disability, self-care disability, go-outside-the-home disability, and employment disability (ACS, 2017).

After the 2000 Census there was concern that the definition of disability was too limiting and not inclusive of the effects of disabilities on overall functioning. In 2008 the ACS disability questions were changed. In addition to focusing more on the effects of a disability, the revised questions were also an attempt to improve the response rate and gather more reliable information. For the ACS, the current definition of disability includes the following: hearing difficulty, vision difficulty, cognitive difficulty, ambulatory difficulty, self-care difficulty, and independent living difficulty data (ACS, 2017).

The SIPP disability questions are expanded in an effort to obtain more detailed disability data. The questions include the following:

- "Limitations in functional activities—seeing, hearing, speaking, walking, using stairs, grasping, lifting and carrying
- Activities of daily living (ADLs)—difficulty getting around inside the home, getting in/out of a bed/chair, bathing, dressing, eating, and toileting
- Instrumental activities of daily living (IADLs)—difficulty going out, managing money, preparing meals, doing housework, taking prescriptions, and using the phone
- Use of assistive aids such as wheelchairs, crutches, canes, or walkers
- Presence of conditions related to mental functioning
- Difficulty working at a job or business
- Disability status of children including developmental disabilities, learning disabilities, and difficulty with schoolwork" (ACS, 2017).

According to the Centers for Disease Control and Prevention (CDC) about 22 percent of adults in the United States have a disability. Box 30.1 provides details on percent of several types of disabilities.

Social Security Disability

The Social Security Administration (SSA), who ultimately determines the individual's status for disability benefits, defines disability as the inability "to engage in any substantial gainful activity (SGA) because of a medically-determinable physical or mental impairment(s): That is expected to result in death, or That has lasted or is expected to last for a continuous period of at least 12 months" (SSA, 2017, p. 5). An individual's inability to perform any SGA is the criteria used by the Social Security Administration to determine disability. A gainful work activity is "Work performed for pay or profit; or Work of a nature generally performed for pay or profit; or Work intended for profit, whether or not a profit is realized" (SSA, 2017, p. 5).

BOX 30.1 Percent of Adults in the United States With Select Functional Disability Types

1. Mobility, 13.0
2. Cognition, 10.6
3. Independent Living, 6.5
4. Vision, 4.6
5. Self-care, 3.6

Modified from Centers for Disease Control and Prevention: *A snapshot of disability in the United States*, 2017a, Author. Available at www.cdc.gov.

The Social Security Administration and Worker's Compensation Programs determine the patient's disability based on clinical evidence. Health care providers should consult the office of Disability Determination Services in the Social Security Administration or the Worker's Compensation Programs for guidelines from individual states because requirements may vary.

Americans with Disabilities Act

According to the ADA, the term *disability* means, with respect to an individual, (1) a physical or mental impairment that substantially limits one or more of the major life activities of such an individual, (2) a record of such an impairment, or (3) being regarded as having such an impairment (ADA, 1990, Section 3 [2]).

Thus, individuals who are clearly diagnosed with an illness that limits functioning in one or more major life activities are covered. According to ADA guidelines disability status is based on a person's ability to complete major life activities independently. Major life activities refer to self-care, receptive and expressive language, learning, mobility, self-direction, capacity for independent living, and financial sufficiency.

Also covered by the ADA are individuals who have a history of an illness, those who have been considered (possibly erroneously) to have had an illness, or those who have been treated as if they had a disabling illness. The intent of the ADA is to reduce "discrimination based not only on simple prejudice, but also on stereotypical attitudes and ignorance about individuals with disabilities" (Jones, 1991, p. 34). This means that individuals may have been misdiagnosed or inappropriately treated as if they had an illness or disability. Because of this, these individuals may not have had the same opportunities as do nondisabled individuals. An example of this is intelligence testing or assessment of cognitive ability. If there was an underestimate of intelligence or functioning, an individual may not have been allowed full access in education. This then may have limited his or her ability to be prepared for higher education

Functional Disability

In 2001 the World Health Organization (WHO) redefined The International Classification of Impairments, Disabilities, and Handicaps from 1980. This new classification, called the International Classification of Functioning, Disability, and Health (ICF), provides standardized language for measuring, classifying, and defining disability. The new definition of disability considers not only medical problems, but also physical, social, attitudinal, and personal factors (WHO, 2002). In the new classification, functioning and disability are determined by the complex interaction between the health condition of the individual and environmental and personal factors. It recognizes that external factors beyond body structures and functions contribute to the disability. The emphasis is on function rather than the condition or the disease. It is relevant across cultures, age groups, and genders and is a useful way to measure health outcomes (WHO, 2002).

Functional limitations occur when individuals experience difficulty performing basic activities of daily living because of their disability. Examples of functional limitations include difficulty standing, walking, climbing, grasping, and reading. Emphasis is placed on the level of function rather than on the purpose of the activity, so that functional limitation can be associated with the disability. For example, impairment in the strength or range of motion of the arm could lead to functional limitations in grasping or reaching. Affected individuals may have difficulty performing basic self-care activities such as bathing and dressing.

Additional Definitions

The term **children with special health care needs (CSHCN)** is defined by the Maternal and Child Health Bureau (MCHB) of the U.S. Department of Health and Human Services as "those who have or are at increased risk for a chronic, physical, developmental, behavioral or emotional condition and who also require health and related service of a type or amount beyond that required by children generally" (MCHB, 2013, p. 1). This definition is broad and includes children with many conditions and risk factors. The prevalence of special health care needs increases with age and varies with race and ethnicity. The children with the highest prevalence of special health care needs are American Indian/Alaska Native children, multiracial children, and non-Hispanic white children. The lowest rates are in Hispanic children and non-Hispanic Asian children (MCHB, 2013).

The term **developmental disability**, as defined by the National Center on Birth Defects and Developmental Disabilities of the Centers for Disease Control and Prevention (CDC), is a chronic impairment that occurs during development and up to age 22 and lasts throughout the person's lifetime. The disability limits the functioning of an individual in at least three of the following areas: self-help, language, learning, mobility, self-direction, independent living, and economic self-sufficiency (CDC, 2015).

Chronic disease, or illness, refers to any long-lasting condition or illness. Disease processes (e.g., diabetes mellitus, cancer, heart disease) and congenital or acquired conditions (e.g., Down syndrome, severe burns, amputation of a limb) are examples of chronic diseases. Therefore, concepts related to disabilities and functional limitations may apply to individuals with a chronic disease or other conditions. For nurses working with these clients, the onset, course, outcome, and degree of limitation are important factors to consider when determining the meaning of the disease to individuals and the families.

Persons with disabilities have often been defined by their illness or disability. Defining someone by their disease or disability is devaluing and disrespectful. It can also place artificial limitations on an individual's potential and value. Language is powerful. The word *handicapped* symbolized the person with a disability begging with a "cap in his hand." The term *disabled* is often used to describe cars that are disabled, indicating they are broken, not functioning, or defective. Whereas we may refer to *things* that are broken or defective, people with disabilities are not broken. Rather than saying a baby has a birth defect, a better term would be to say a child has a congenital disability. The Person First Movement was initiated in an effort to promote acceptable language for people with disabilities. The Person First Movement advocates for sensitivity in defining persons with disabilities. In other words, refer to a "woman who is blind" rather than a "blind woman" or a "person with diabetes" rather than a "diabetic" (Disability Is Natural, 2018).

Definitions of disability need to take into account the degree of disability, the limitations it imposes, and the degree of dependence that occurs as a result of the disability. These definitions can range from minor to severe. Situational factors also affect the disability experience and influence the individual's ability to cope and function in society. Nurses and the interdisciplinary team need to be included, informed, and involved in the science of disability and rehabilitation to be influential in the decision making related to practice, policy, training, research, and funding.

LINKING CONTENT TO PRACTICE

Within public health nursing, there has been a commitment to caring for people in their communities and working to build the health of communities. The Council on Linkages (2014) has identified several core competencies for public health professionals, including public health nurses.

Tier 1—Front Line Staff/Entry Level: applies to public health professionals, including nurses, who are involved in day to day activities, and who are not in management. Responsibilities of these public health professionals may include basic data collection and analysis, fieldwork, program planning, outreach activities, programmatic support, and other organizational tasks.

Tier 2—Program Management/Supervisory Level: applies to individuals with program management and/or supervisory responsibilities. Responsibilities may include program development, program implementation, program evaluation, establishing and maintaining community relations, managing timelines and work plans, presenting arguments and recommendations on policy issues.

Tier 3—Senior Management/Executive Level: applies to individuals at a senior/management level and leaders of public health organizations. In general, an individual who is responsible for the major programs or functions of an organization, setting a strategy and vision for the organization, and/or building the organization's culture can be considered to be a Tier 3 public health professional.

Public health nurses working in any tier are needed to ensure that disabled individuals are properly cared for in the community. This may involve providing or directing care, or understanding disability legislation and programs for which individual/families are eligible. Public health nurses may also be involved in developing and implementing programs for the disabled or being the chief executive officer of an agency that advocates for the disabled.

SCOPE OF THE PROBLEM

Number of Disabled Americans

According to the most recent data from the American Community Survey completed in 2016, about 12.8 percent, or 40.8 million civilian, noninstitutionalized men, women, and children of all races and educational levels in the United States reported a disability. Prevalence rates by type of disability are as follows: vision 2.4 percent; hearing 3.6 percent; ambulatory 3.6 percent; cognitive 5.2 percent; self-care 2.7 percent; and independent living 5.2 percent (Cornell University, 2018).

Number of Disabled Worldwide

According to the World Health Organization, an estimated one billion people, or 15 percent of the global population has some type of disability. Moreover, the number of people who are over the age of 15 who have significant difficulty with functioning is estimated at 110 million (2.2 percent) to 190 million (3.8 percent) people. This number is increasing annually in part because of the increase in chronic diseases, injuries, automobile crashes, violence, an aging population, and improvements in the methodologies used to measure disability. Minorities, including women, and the poor are disproportionately affected by being disabled. Worldwide, most of the people with disabilities have limited access to basic public health services and rehabilitation (WHO, 2018a).

Burden of Chronic Disease

Another way to consider disability data is to look at the burden of chronic disease. According to 2016 worldwide data obtained from The Global Burden of Disease Study, the five leading causes of years lived with disability (YLD) are low back pain, migraine, hearing loss, iron deficiency anemia, and major depressive disorder. The YLD for these types of noncommunicable chronic diseases is growing faster than malnutrition and infectious disease, which used to be considered typical public health concerns. There is growing emphasis on global prevention strategies to decrease the burden of chronic disease (Vos et al., 2017).

Although not all individuals with chronic diseases are disabled, the following data from the CDC provide convincing evidence that chronic diseases contribute significantly to the development of disability. Chronic diseases such as heart disease, stroke, cancer, diabetes, arthritis, and obesity are some of the most common, costly, and preventable of all health problems in the United States. In 2014 about 7 out of 10 deaths among Americans were from chronic diseases. Heart disease and cancer accounted for 46 percent of all deaths. In 2012 nearly 50 percent of the adult population, or almost 117 million Americans, had at least one chronic illness and 1 in 4 had two chronic health concerns (CDC, 2017b).

Additional Causes of Disability

Disabilities among the chronically ill are common, and the CDC reports that about one fourth of people with chronic conditions have one or more daily activity limitations. For example, arthritis is the most common cause of disability, with nearly 23 million Americans reporting activity limitations due to their arthritis. Diabetes continues to be the leading cause of kidney failure, non-traumatic lower-extremity amputations, and blindness among adults (CDC, 2017b).

There is an obesity epidemic in the United States, and according to the CDC (2017c) more than one third of adults (36 percent), or 72 million Americans, are obese. Moreover, about one in six children and youth (17 percent) aged 2 to 19 years old obese. People who are obese are more likely to develop chronic medical problems and have higher medical costs than people of normal weight. Moreover, older adults who are obese are more likely to have disabilities related to functional impairment.

Several other conditions and inherited problems can cause disability as seen in Fig. 30.1. These include genetic disorders, acute and chronic illnesses, violence, tobacco use, lack of access to health care, as well as failure to eat correctly, exercise regularly, or manage stress effectively. In addition, substance abuse, environmental problems, and unsanitary living conditions can cause disability. The people reporting these causes identified difficulty with functional limitations, difficulty with activities of daily living (ADLs)/instrumental activities of daily living (IADLs), or inability to do housework, or to work at a job or business (CDC, 2017c).

Falls among the elderly, especially the frail elderly, are common and about one quarter of adults over the age of 65 fall every year. Of these falls about 20 to 30 percent result in moderate to severe injury and can cause temporary or permanent disability. This places the elderly at greater risk for loss of independence and decreased physical mobility that can in turn cause additional medical problems. This loss of independence places additional burdens on family members and caregivers to provide assistance with ADLs and IADLs (CDC, 2017d). A thorough nursing assessment can identify factors placing a community-dwelling elder at risk for falls. The assessment should include functional impairments, medications, and environmental factors that increase fall risk. Early assessment and intervention can prevent a fall and decrease development of additional medical problems and disability

Childhood Disability

An estimated 15.1 percent of children in the United States have special needs, which may be developmental, behavioral, or emotional in nature. Moreover, 23.0 percent of households with children have at least one child with a special health need. Children with special health care needs require such things as prescription medication (86 percent), specialty medical care (48 percent), vision care (35 percent), mental health care (28 percent), specialized therapies (27 percent), and medical equipment (11 percent). Many families with children with special needs have difficulty obtaining services due to waiting lists and difficulty getting to appointments (17.8 percent), child not eligible for the service (10.8 percent), trouble getting the needed information (9.0 percent), the cost of the service (14.9 percent), and the service not being available in the area (11.2 percent) (MCHB, 2013).

Of the children with special health care needs, 20.8 percent are under the age of 5; 38.7 percent are between the ages of 6 and 11; and 40.5 percent are age 12 through 17. Moreover, children with special health care needs are more likely to be boys (59.3 percent) than girls (40.7 percent) (MCHB, 2013).

Childhood disability may be developmental or acquired and may be a result of prenatal damage, perinatal factors, acquired neonatal factors, or early childhood factors. These may include genetic factors, prematurity, infections, traumatic or toxic exposure, or nutritional factors. Although the etiology of many

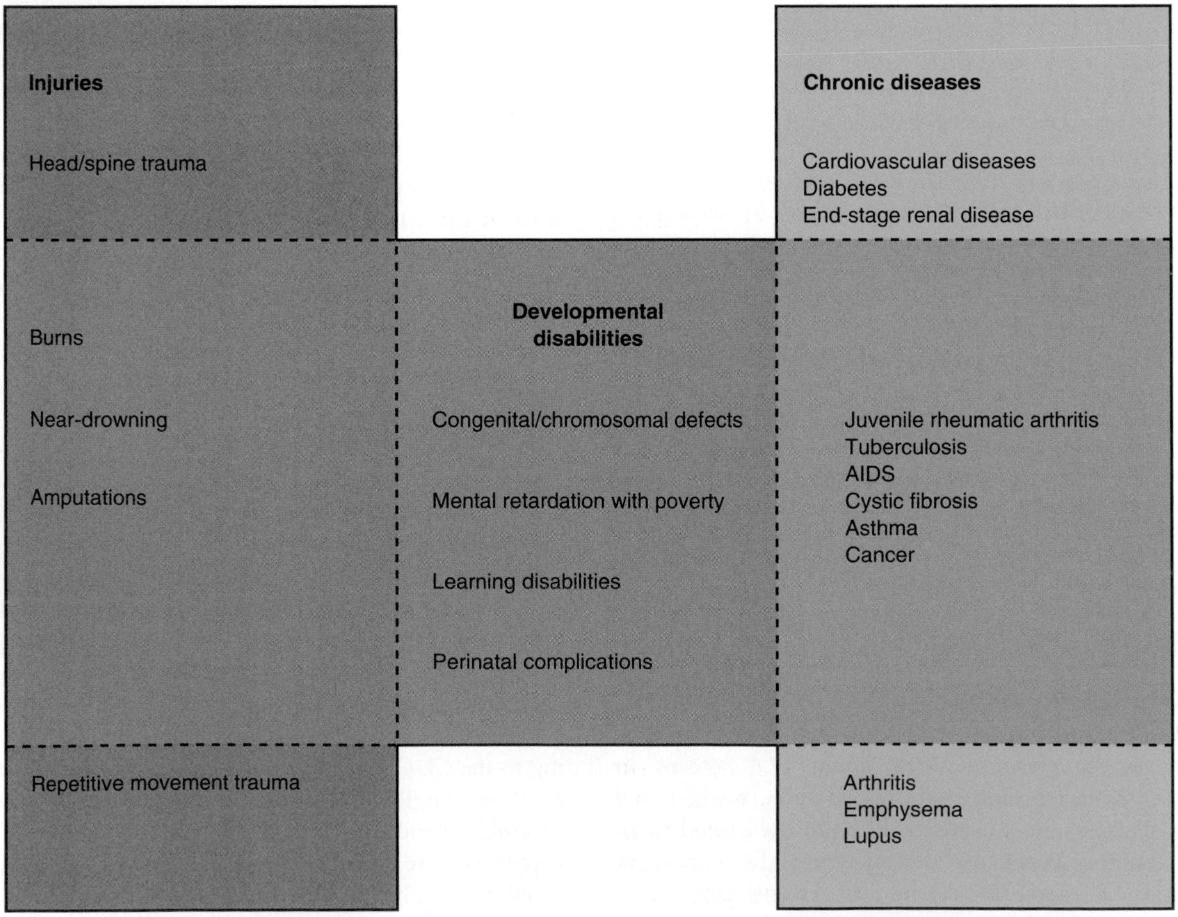

Fig. 30.1 Examples of conditions related to being physically compromised. *AIDS,* Acquired immunodeficiency syndrome.

BOX 30.2 Children With Special Health Care Needs

- Nearly 20 percent of U.S. children under 18 years of age have a special health care need.
- One in five U.S. families has a child with a special health care need.
- Children and youth with special health care needs and their families often need services from multiple systems—health care, public health, education, mental health, and social services.

Modified from Maternal and Child Health Bureau: *Children with special health care needs,* 2018, Author. Available at www.mchb.hrsa.gov.

childhood disabilities remains unknown, preventive screening for genetic disorders including developmental disabilities is critical for early detection and medical intervention. Newborn screening, immunization programs, and genetic counseling prevent disabilities. Neonatal screening for phenylketonuria (PKU), hypothyroidism, thalassemias, and other disorders has greatly reduced childhood disabilities. Box 30.2 lists information regarding children with special health care needs.

Mental Illness

An often overlooked source of disability is that related to mental disorders. Depression is the leading cause of disability worldwide. More than 300 million people have depression, yet less than half that number receive appropriate treatment The prevalence of depression, as well as the lack of treatment, contributes significantly to the global burden of disease (WHO, 2018b).

In the United States, the National Institute of Mental Health (2017) estimates that about one in six Americans over the age of 18 have a diagnosable mental disorder. One of the leading causes of mental health disability among both adults and adolescents is major depression. In 2016 data were collected on both adult and adolescent depression. About 16.2 million (6.7 percent) of adults in the United States reported at least one major depressive episode. For adolescents aged 12 to 17 years old, about 2.2 million (9.0 percent) experienced at least one major depressive episode with severe impairment. For individuals with one diagnosable mental illness, almost 45 percent meet criteria for a second or third mental illness. Multiple diagnoses, including individuals with a **dual diagnosis** of mental illness and substance use, increase the severity of disability and functional impairment.

THE EFFECTS OF DISABILITIES

The costs of chronic disability to the disabled, as well as to their families, their employers, and society are significant. The unemployment rate for many minority groups in the United States improved between the years 1980 and 2015. However, the unemployment rate for individuals with a disability increased. In 2015, of the adults between the ages of 18 and 64 who had a disability, about 35 percent were employed as compared to an employment rate of 76 percent for the nondisabled. These data represent adults across all education levels (Donnelly, 2017).

Disability status also affects annual income as can be seen in a 2016 survey of the median annual income among individuals over the age of 16 with or without a disability. The median annual income for individuals with a disability was $21,572, which is about two thirds of the median annual income of $31,874 for individuals without a disability. Perhaps of more significance is the number of individuals with disabilities who live in poverty. An estimated 26.6 percent of non-institutionalized persons aged 21 to 64 years with a disability in the United States were living below the poverty line (Donnelly, 2017; Kraus, 2017).

Nurses provide care for persons who are disabled, for their families, for the populations and subpopulations they make up, and for the communities in which they live. It is important to remember that some clients prefer to be regarded as being physically or mentally challenged or compromised, whereas others may think such terms minimize the importance of the needs and problems of people who are disabled. The extent to which the disabled person may need extra support, care, and services from the family unit and the community is shown in Box 30.3. These relationships are best understood by looking at the stress placed on the individual.

Effects on the Individual

According to the U.S. Department of Health and Human Services, disabilities are characteristics of the body, mind, or senses that affect a person's ability to engage independently in some or all aspects of day-to-day life. Many types of disabilities exist, and they affect people in various ways. People may be born with a disability, develop a disability from being sick or injured, or acquire a disability with the aging process. Most men, women, and children of all ages, races, and ethnicities will experience disability at some time during their lives (Kraus, 2017).

The number of disabled varies by age group, and as one expects, the number of individuals with a disability increases

BOX 30.3 Potential Effects of Being Physically Compromised

Individuals, Families, and Communities

Individuals

- Related health problems (e.g., nutrition, oral health, hygiene, limited activity/stamina)
- Self-concept/self-esteem
- Life expectancy and risk for infection and secondary injury
- Developmental tasks; change in role expectations

Families

- Stress on family unit
- Need for use of external resources to help family meet role expectations
- Options limited in use of any discretionary income
- Social stigma

Communities

- Need/demand to reallocate resources
- Discomfort or fear from lack of knowledge of disability
- Need to comply with legislation
- Services provided by health department, health care providers
- Need for other services beyond medical diagnosis (e.g., transportation)

with age. According to 2015 data, the percent of individuals with disabilities by age group was as follows: 0–5 (0.4 percent), 5–17 (7.2 percent), 18–64 (51.1 percent), and 65 and over (41.2 percent). Disability is not a sickness, and most people with disabilities are healthy and without a documented chronic illness. However, persons with disabilities may be at greater risk for developing illnesses as a result of their condition. For example, someone with decreased mobility can suffer from the problems of immobility such as obesity, skin breakdown, osteoporosis, pneumonia, malnutrition, or loneliness. Most persons with disabilities can and do work, play, learn, and enjoy healthy lives (Kraus, 2017).

Many disabled people try to discourage the image that they are helpless and pitiful. For example, the United States Quad Rugby Association is an organization formed for individuals in wheelchairs to play competitive rugby. Their motto is "Smashing stereotypes one hit at a time!" These individuals promote the idea of living and working independently (U.S. Quad Rugby Association, 2018).

Children: Infancy Through Adolescence. Children who live with a disability are affected in many ways. According to the Children and Young People With Disabilities Fact Sheet, disability can be conceptualized as a human rights issue. Children and adolescents with disabilities are considered to be one of the most marginalized groups in the world. They are more likely to live in poverty, and as a result of this poverty, they are at higher risk for developing a disability through illness or accidents. Moreover, children with disabilities are less likely than their nondisabled peers to engage in physical activity. This is often due to inaccessible play equipment or play places with limited or no handicapped accessibility. As a result, they are more likely to have increased health problems associated with inactivity. These problems include being overweight or obese, general deconditioning, and poor exercise tolerance (Perkins & Agrawal, 2018; UNICEF, 2013).

Children and adolescents with special health care needs are also at higher risk to experience psychological maladjustment compared with their healthy peers. The risk of psychological problems such as depression and anxiety is correlated with the degree of physical impairment, not with the level of disease activity. For some, the inability to participate in certain physical activities affects their feelings of belonging and self-worth. Children and adolescents with disabilities are more likely to live in institutions. This leads to more depression, anxiety, social isolation, and marginalization (Perkins & Agrawal, 2018; WHO, 2018b).

Providing access to schools, play places, stores, and other community spaces is primarily focused on those with physical disabilities. However, children and adolescents with intellectual or developmental disabilities also have access needs in order for them to participate fully in their social environment. They often misinterpret social cues and often have difficulty when interactions are not usual and predictable. There is evidence that rehabilitation can help these children and adolescents. Appropriate interventions can be designed with regard to population health and health equity for all children (Umeda et al., 2017)

For other children, managing the effects of their disability may cause embarrassment and they may choose to isolate themselves from others. For example, students who have spina bifida or renal disease might need to leave classrooms or other school settings quickly to use the bathroom. Having to explain this need to their classmates could call unwanted attention to these children and their diseases. However, disabled children can overcome some of these obstacles if they have families who are able to provide the support necessary for the development of more positive self-images and a feeling of inclusiveness. The use of assistive technology such as computers can enhance learning and decrease obstacles related to inadequate education (WHO 2011; WHO, 2015).

The unique issues and challenges experienced by adolescents with disabilities has not been studied as well as those that affect younger children and adults. This population is often overlooked by advocacy groups for the disabled and by most of the new initiatives developed for disabled persons. However, the years between 10 and 18 are difficult ones for most adolescents, and the needs of those who are disabled are similar to those of their healthy peers (i.e., education, peer relationships, recreation, and planning for the future). In addition to the expected challenges experienced by adolescents, those who are disabled must also deal with prejudice, discrimination, and social isolation because of their disability (UNICEF, 2013; WHO, 2015).

Disabled adolescents are often viewed as asexual by their healthy peers. However, they are as sexually active as healthy adolescents. They view themselves as "normal" even though they realize that others perceive them differently. Moreover, disabled adolescents are just as likely as their nondisabled peers to engage in risky sexual activity. This places them at risk for unplanned pregnancy and sexually transmitted diseases. Therefore, they should receive the same amount of sexual education as their unaffected peers (WHO, 2015).

EVIDENCE-BASED PRACTICE

Researchers conducted a secondary analysis of the 2011–2015 National Survey of Family Growth to determine the population-based use of family planning services for women 15–44 years, and if there were differences in use of family planning services based on the woman's disability status. The study included 11,300 women who completed interviews conducted in their homes. The researchers found that 17.8 percent of women reported having at least one disability. The results showed a statistically significant difference between disabled and nondisabled women. Women who were disabled were less likely to receive family planning services. Moreover, the study concluded that disabled women with low education, low income or who were not working were especially at risk.

Nurse Use

This study provides additional evidence that individuals with disabilities, in this case women, can be at higher risk for not receiving essential health information, specifically information related to family planning. Family planning services are important for all women of childbearing age and should be available to all without regard for disability status. The reasons for this disparity need additional study. However, nurses working with the disabled should be prepared to provide information on sexuality and family planning

Data from Mosher J, Bloom T, Hughes R, et al.: Disparities in receipt of family planning services by disability status: new estimates from the national survey of family growth. *Disabil Health J* 10(3):394–399, 2017.

Adults. According to the Center for an Accessible Society (CAS) (2014), more than three million people in the United States require help from another person to live independently. Many adults receive some, but not enough, help to meet their needs. With inadequate community support, an individual may experience hunger, injuries, falls, or other problems that contribute to the development of secondary health problems, disabilities, and possibly early death. Becoming disabled increases the risk of placement in a nursing home or other long-term care facility, contributing to both decreased community participation and limited social integration for individuals with disabilities.

It is estimated that those persons who live by themselves receive only 56 percent of the help they need, while those living with family members or friends receive 80 percent of what they need. Informal supports such as family members and friends frequently have multiple work, family, and community responsibilities. This makes it difficult for them to consistently meet the needs of the disabled. Those without informal supports must rely on formal supports, which are increasingly limited in difficult financial times (CAS, 2014).

In addition, millions of Americans depend on Medicaid to finance their long-term services. For example, 80 percent of all Medicaid long-term care funds go to nursing homes or other institutional service providers, even though many of these people could receive services in their own homes. A personal assistant could make it possible for a disabled person to live at home instead of in an institution. Many Americans think that nursing homes are the only alternative for long-term care. However, the elderly often prefer the freedom and control of living at home. Many states offer community-based services such as home health care services and senior services. In home supportive services (IHSS) provide home health services to the aged, blind, or disabled. In addition, adult protective services exist to receive reports of abuse of elders or dependent adults (CAS, 2014).

Computer technology and use of the Internet can increase the independence of people with disabilities. Homebound persons can access a computer and order groceries, shop for needed items, research issues, participate in online discussions, and communicate with friends and family. With newer technologies, blind persons can access the computer as well as sighted persons. Even persons who cannot hold a pen or who lack fine-motor skills can use speech recognition and other technologies to write letters, pay bills, and perform other tasks using the computer and Internet (CAS, 2014). However, only one fourth of persons with disabilities own computers, and only one tenth use the Internet. The elderly and African Americans with disabilities, especially low-income or low-education-level elders, rarely take advantage of these new technologies. Fortunately, computers and associated equipment for the disabled has become less expensive. Moreover, there are organizations that provide low-cost or free computer equipment for qualified disabled individuals (CAS, 2014).

Effects on the Family

Most people who are physically disabled are cared for at home by one or more family members. Fig. 30.2 lists some of the issues and concerns that occur when a family member is disabled and shows the effect of the disability on the family unit. As this figure shows, the entire family system is affected when one member is disabled.

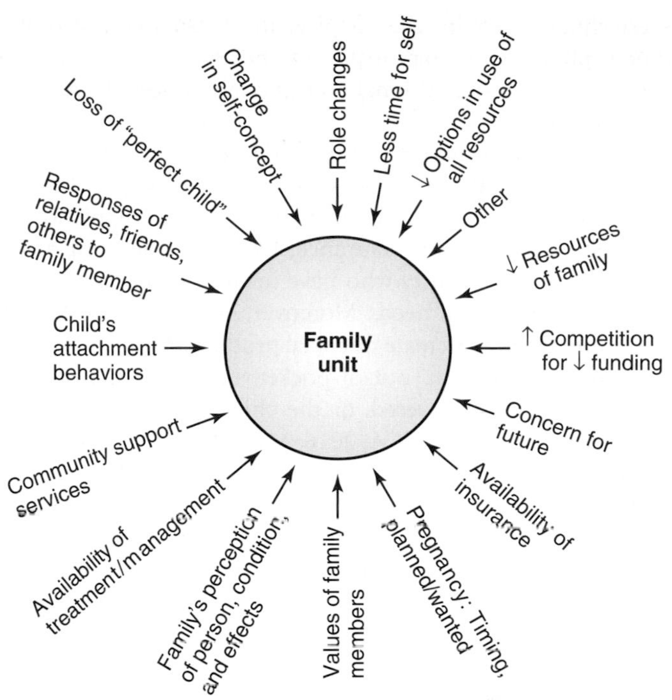

Fig. 30.2 Factors influencing a family unit when a member is physically compromised.

The number of individuals providing care to family members is increasing and the care provided is more complex. Family members provide a wide range of services, including coordinating care, transportation to medical care, providing direct medical care, and using medical equipment. This caregiver burden can result in stress, depression, and financial problems, as well as physical and social isolation. Moreover, adults caring for family members frequently have to juggle work and caregiver responsibilities. Fortunately for some families, it is now possible to get paid to provide care to their own family members. Organizations like the Family Caregiver Alliance (FCA) and the National Home Sharing and Short Breaks Network (NHSN) provide information on many issues of importance to family members caring for a family member with a disability (Carl, 2017; FCA, 2016; NHSN, 2016).

Children: Infancy Through Adolescence. A child's disability may have long-term effects on the family, primary caregiver, and the marital relationship. Providing care for these children places additional demands on the family, particularly the mother. Mothers of children with special health care needs report higher levels of stress, anxiety, depression, and feelings of isolation compared with mothers of unaffected children. In addition, employment is difficult and sometimes impossible to secure for the parents of children who require extensive care. This is especially true for mothers, single parents, and low-income families who may be unable to afford child care for their disabled children. In addition to the day-to-day physical care these children require, the caregiver must also access and coordinate physical, occupational, and speech therapy, as well as specialty care and additional educational services (FCA, 2016; NHSN, 2016)

The cost of caring for a child with a disability often affects the family's financial well-being. Children with special health care needs are more likely than the general population of children to have health insurance. However, one third of the children with disabilities who have insurance have inadequate coverage to meet their needs. Moreover, 21.6 percent of CSHCN have conditions that create financial problems for their families. This is due to high out-of-pocket expenses; the services required not being covered, or the child not having access to appropriate providers (FCA, 2016; MCHB, 2013).

Some children with special health care needs are more likely to have health insurance through Medicaid. However, children from low-income families who lack medical insurance are at a particular disadvantage because their families may be unable to afford the care they need. Siblings of children with special health care needs are at higher risk for developing emotional and psychological problems compared with their unaffected peers. For example, they tend to express more psychosomatic illnesses, anxiety disorders, and aggressive behaviors compared with siblings of nondisabled children (CDC, 2017b; MCHB, 2013).

Conversely, these siblings are often found to be more mature, altruistic, responsible, and independent when compared with siblings of nondisabled children. Whether a child suffers or benefits from having a disabled brother or sister depends on the attitude of the parents toward the disability and their coping methods, the economic circumstances of the family, the communication among family members, and the degree of parental affection and attention received by the nondisabled child (MCHB, 2013).

Adults. Having a physically disabled adult in a family causes enormous stress on the rest of the members. There may be a significant loss of income when a parent is unable to work because of a disability, and the disability prevents people from earning a living. Another effect on multigenerational families is caregiver burden. Well children in the family may have unmet needs due to the disability of a parent. Moreover, the children may have to assume the role of caregiver if other supports are not available. Adults who are responsible for caring for their own children as well as one or both of their parents have been termed the "sandwich generation." These adults often struggle with burnout as well as increased marital stress when faced with caring for an elderly parent with a disability (Council for Disability Awareness, 2013; FCA, 2016).

Effects on the Community

The presence of physically disabled people and their families in the community has far-reaching effects on all aspects of community life. The prevention of disability and providing community support for caretakers need to be priorities. The community may be called on to respond in new ways to these citizens as a result of federal laws affecting those who are disabled. Moreover, the initiative on providing population health needs to include care for those with disabilities.

Children: Infancy Through Adolescence. Families of children with disabilities need the support of their communities as they care for their disabled children at home. Children with disabilities have rights, including the right to remain at home rather than become institutionalized. The concept of providing mainstream inclusive health care is essential. Moreover, family services should also include education regarding available services and how to access them (WHO, 2015).

Children who are chronically ill or disabled and who enter school for mainstream education require educational support from the public school system as mandated in the Individuals with Disabilities Education Act (IDEA). IDEA is outlined in Box 30.4. In addition, IDEA requires states to provide appropriate services to infants and children from birth to age five who have or are at risk for disability. Examples of such services include speech therapy, occupational therapy, physical therapy, play therapy, and behavioral therapy (U.S. Department of Education [USDE], 2018). Although the provision of appropriate services for disabled infants and children is mandated by IDEA, states vary in the nature and quantity of services they provide for eligible children. In addition, public schools must evaluate their effectiveness with students who are disabled. This can add to the cost of educating children. Increased education for pediatricians and nurses can increase supportive and knowledgeable collaboration for the development of early intervention programs in schools (USDE, 2018).

Adults. Former Surgeon General Richard H. Carmona sought to improve the health and wellness of persons with disabilities. To achieve this goal, in 2005 he published a call to action that encouraged (1) health care providers to see and treat the whole person, not just the disability, (2) educators to teach about disability, (3) the public to focus on a person's abilities, not just the disability, and (4) the community to ensure accessible health care and wellness services to persons with disabilities (Carmona, 2005).

BOX 30.4 Individuals with Disabilities Education Act

The Individuals with Disabilities Education Act (IDEA) federal law was developed:

- To ensure that all children with disabilities have available to them a free, appropriate public education that emphasizes special education and related services designed to meet their unique needs and prepare them for employment and independent living
- To ensure that the rights of children with disabilities and their parents are protected
- To assist states, localities, educational service agencies, and federal agencies to provide for the education of all children with disabilities
- To assess and ensure the effectiveness of efforts to educate children with disabilities

Modified from U.S. Department of Education: *IDEA website*, 2018, Author. Available at www.ed.gov.

These goals have been only partially achieved as evidenced by the data from multiple agencies. Countries with developed health systems and economic resources are more likely to have increased accessibility for individuals with disabilities. However, in areas of the world where there is significant poverty, as well as political conflicts and war, providing access or services to the disabled are not priorities. Global agencies such as the World Health Organization (2015) and UNICEF (2013) have recommendations for removing barriers and improving the quality of life for adults with disabilities. The recommendations include making frequently used community areas accessible to those with any type of disability. There is also acknowledgment that the changes needed for the disabled require an investment of resources. Little will be done without adequate planning, an investment in adequate staffing, and financial support. Moreover, the recommendations include involving individuals with disabilities in the process. Many agencies continue to work to raise public awareness of the problems, to improve disability data collection, and to strengthen and support research on disabilities.

Persons with disabilities that affect mobility are at risk for health problems of the multiple body systems related to mobility/immobility. Persons with mobility-associated problems can suffer damage to any system. Some of the problems that develop with the musculoskeletal system include foot drop, muscular atrophy, contractures, or fractures. Respiratory and circulatory function can be compromised by pneumonia or deep vein thrombosis. Renal problems such as infection, incontinence, or renal calculi are common problems related to immobility. Decubiti and skin breakdown and rashes can develop from immobility and/or incontinence of bowel and bladder. Malnutrition or obesity could also be related to effects of immobility. All of these complications of being disabled place additional burdens on communities and health care systems.

Low-Income Populations

Physically compromised individuals often experience poverty, as do other special population groups, including single parents and their children, the aged, the unemployed, and members of racial and ethnic minorities. Persons with low income have less access to health care throughout their lives and are less likely to participate in all levels of prevention. Therefore, they are at greater risk for the onset of disabling conditions and for more rapid progression of disease processes. Those in poverty may also be at greater risk for disabling conditions related to accidental injuries and poor nutrition.

People who are disabled and live in poverty are less likely to have the resources to provide for their own special needs. Those who are disabled are often unemployed, even though they may be able to work and are seeking jobs. Employers may be reluctant to hire people whose conditions may increase employer-provided health insurance costs. This can create another barrier to adequate insurance and access to health care for the disabled. Inadequate transportation, lack of coordination of care, and limited locally available services for those who cannot pay for them are other factors that affect this population and the ability to access needed services. Fig. 30.3 illustrates the relationship between poverty and disabilities.

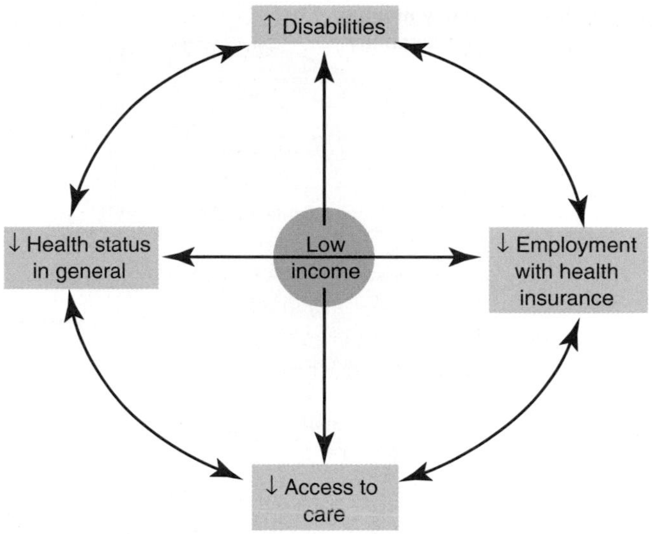

Fig. 30.3 Relationships of poverty and disability.

SELECTED ISSUES

Abuse and Neglect

Individuals with disabilities are more likely to experience some form of abuse or neglect during their lifetime compared with individuals without disabilities. Examples of abuse and neglect include physical harm, inappropriate sexual contact, emotional or verbal threats, withholding care, not providing adequate supervision, and not providing needed medical care. Abuse and neglect also include withholding medical information, denying the opportunity to participate in decision making, including decisions about medical care and the right to refuse care, and financial exploitation (Missouri Department of Health & Senior Services [MDHSS], 2018; WHO, 2018a). Fig. 30.4 illustrates the relationships among the family member with a disability, the caregiver, the environment and the intersection with abuse.

While all individuals with disabilities are at risk for abuse and neglect, children, the elderly, and women are at particular risk. Children are dependent on adults and require care, supervision, guidance, and financial support to achieve normal growth and development. The responsibility for and care of healthy, nondisabled children poses many challenges for parents. When a child is born with or develops a disability, the developmental, physical, and financial needs can become overwhelming. According to the U.S. Department of Health and Human Services (USDHHS) (2018) risk factors for the abuse/neglect of disabled children can be stratified to societal factors, such as believing disabled children are asexual or do not feel pain; family or parental factors, which include the child being viewed as different, parents who are embarrassed by their disabled child, or families with inadequate social support or resources; and child-related factors, which include being male,

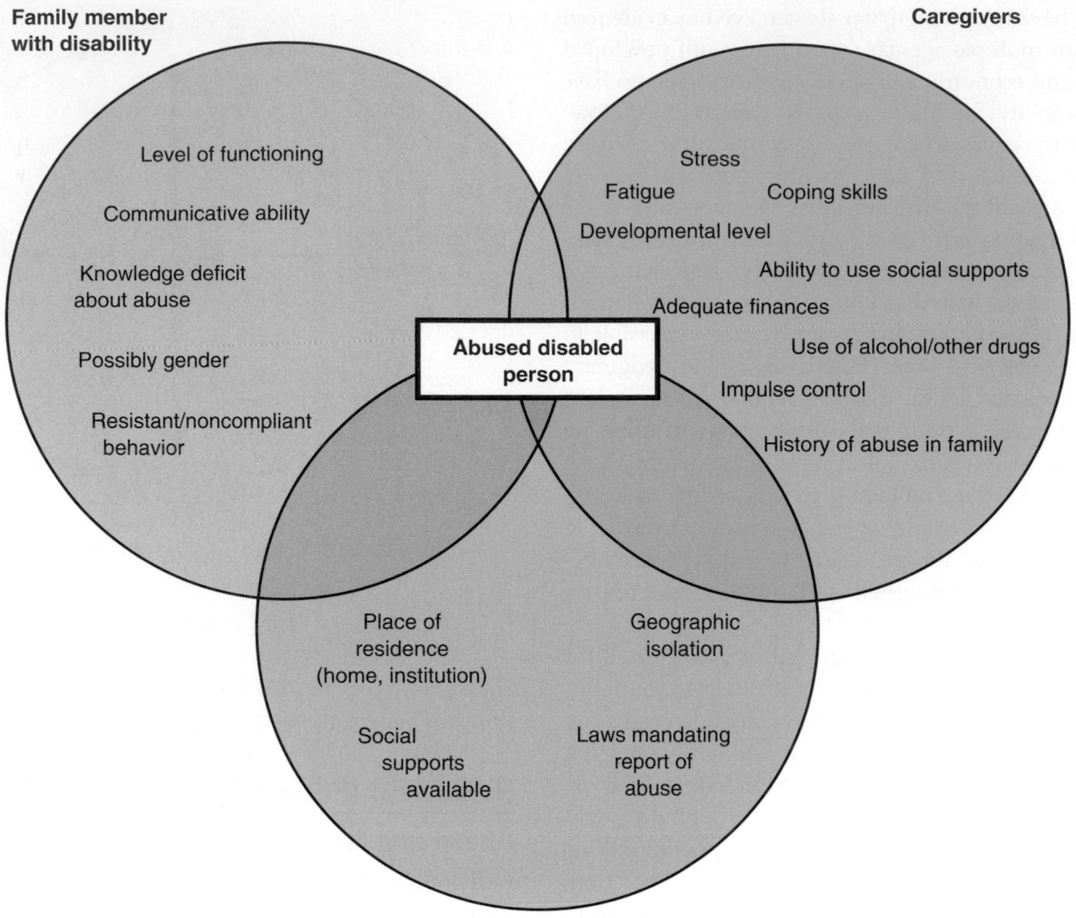

Fig. 30.4 Factors influencing the abuse of those who are physically compromised.

having challenging/difficult behaviors, or requiring extensive physical care.

Individuals with autism spectrum disorders (ASDs) can be especially vulnerable to abuse in the form of **bullying** and social exclusion. This is due to their impaired communication and impaired social interactions. Moreover, they can exhibit repetitive behaviors that are often difficult for others to understand. Types of bullying include physical, verbal, social, and cyber. Social bullying includes things like mimicking behaviors of a person, playing practical jokes designed to embarrass or shame someone, or socially excluding someone (National Center Against Bullying, 2018).

CHECK YOUR PRACTICE

You are working in a high school based health clinic, and a 15-year-old boy with autism comes to the office. He is in special education classes and eats in the general cafeteria. He reports that he is being bullied at lunch by several nondisabled students You ask who is bullying him, but he prefers not to give you any specific names.

- What would you say to him?
- What types of intervention could you design to decrease bullying in the school?

In general, the elderly are at increased risk for abuse and neglect. Elderly individuals with a disability are at additional risk due to their increased dependency needs. The most common type of abuse reported by disabled individuals is care related. Because many disabled individuals are dependent on others for basic care, they are at risk for experiencing neglect and at times cruel physical care from providers. Financial abuse is another common way elderly disabled persons are mistreated. Community-dwelling elderly living with family may be threatened with institutionalization in a nursing home if they report the abuse or complain (MDHSS, 2018; WHO, 2018a).

Women and girls with disabilities face many challenges and often have to face "double discrimination." There is worldwide gender discrimination in such areas as access to housing, education, training, employment, and salary equity. Being female also places one at risk for sexual exploitation, abuse, neglect, and violence. Women with disabilities are at increased risk of this type of abuse because of the powerlessness of women in many parts of the world, the lack of resources, and women being undervalued (United Nations, 2015; WHO, 2018a).

Health Promotion

Health promotion usually focuses on the primary prevention of conditions that may lead to disability (e.g., smoking cessation to prevent lung cancer). Actually all three levels of prevention apply to physically compromised clients (see the Levels of Prevention box). They need information and counseling for health-promoting behaviors and for prevention of the progression of a condition or pathology.

LEVELS OF PREVENTION

Physically Compromised Clients

Primary Prevention

- Educate community residents about behaviors during pregnancy that will reduce the risk of having a baby with a disability.
- Push for a congressional mandate for addition of folic acid to cereals in the United States to reduce neural tube defect in infants.
- Promote exercise and physical fitness programs in schools to lessen obesity in that population and decrease incidence of metabolic syndrome.

Secondary Prevention

- Initiate early detection actions to identify any chronic or disabling condition.
- Initiate blood pressure screening programs to identify those at risk for strokes or heart damage as soon as possible.
- Push programs for early detection of cancer (e.g., mammography, malignant melanoma), since co-occurring morbidities are more common with later detection of cancer.

Tertiary Prevention

- Take action to maintain or increase functional abilities for persons who have a physically compromising condition.
- Encourage exercise programs for sedentary clients with osteoporosis to reduce the likelihood of fractures.
- Initiate a diabetes type 1 education program for children and parents, with a focus on disease management and prevention of disease complications.

Health promotion is a multidimensional concept that applies to all individuals regardless of disability. Strategies are needed to expand the knowledge base of health promotion for those who are disabled. Persons with chronic disabilities have frequently defined themselves in terms of their physical problems and sick role. However, they need all the prevention activities available to the nondisabled. This includes immunizations, exercise, weight control, use of safety precautions, safe sex practices, stress reduction, as well as screening and treatment of disease not related to their disability.

In addition, health promotion and prevention programs for persons with disabilities should focus on preventing complications from the effects of immobility and the disease process. The complications of immobility and the disease process need to be prevented to ensure optimal independent and healthy living, thus allowing the individual with disabilities the opportunity to have a productive and happy life.

Many health promotion and disease prevention needs are similar across the life span (e.g., exercise, diet, avoidance of excess substance use, and injury prevention). However, specific problems and interventions to deal with these needs vary according to age, specific disabling condition, and developmental status. For example, nutritional needs of premature infants are related to obtaining adequate energy, protein, fat, vitamins, and minerals. An older adult with type 2 diabetes mellitus may be concerned primarily with reducing the risk of experiencing a myocardial infarction.

Persons with disabilities need appropriate nutrition. Therefore, nurses may consult with or refer appropriate individuals to dietitians for nutrition teaching. Speech therapists may also be needed for those with chewing or swallowing difficulties. Occupational health professionals focus on the activities of daily living and often use adaptive equipment to promote success and independence with ADLs. Families and professionals can work together to meet the nutritional needs of persons with disabilities and chronic health care problems.

Health promotion and disease prevention for those who are physically compromised have not been emphasized in primary care or in rehabilitation. It is especially important to establish lifelong health-promoting behaviors in children who are disabled. Unfortunately, parents may be so overwhelmed by caring for such children that this aspect of care is not considered.

Healthy People 2020 Objectives

Selected objectives from *Healthy People 2020* for persons with disabilities are highlighted in the *Healthy People 2020* box. Many of the objectives address concerns discussed in this chapter regarding increasing health promotion and wellness activities for individuals with disabilities. In addition, there is greater emphasis on increasing access to services, which can increase independence and foster community living.

HEALTHY PEOPLE 2020

Selected objectives are listed here that pertain to persons with disabilities.

Systems and DH-1 Policies

- **DH-1:** Increase the number of population-based data systems used to monitor *Healthy People 2020* objectives that include in their core a standardized set of questions that identify people with disabilities.
- **DH-2:** Increase the number of tribes, states, and the District of Columbia that have public health surveillance and health promotion programs for people with disabilities and caregivers.

Barriers to Health Care

- **DH-5:** Increase the proportion of youth with special health care needs whose health care provider has discussed transition planning from pediatric to adult health care.
- **DH-7:** Reduce the proportion of older adults with disabilities who use inappropriate medications.

Environment

- **DH-8:** Reduce the proportion of adults with disabilities aged 18 and older who experience physical or program barriers that limit or prevent them from using available local health and wellness programs.
- **DH-9:** Reduce the proportion of people with disabilities who encounter barriers to participating in home, school, work or community activities.

Activities and Participation

- **DH-13:** Increase the proportion of adults with disabilities aged 18 years and older who participate in leisure, social, religious or community activities.
- **DSC-14:** Increase the proportion of children and youth with disabilities who spend at least 80 percent of their time in regular education programs.

Data from U.S. Department of Health and Human Services: *Healthy People 2020: disability and health*, 2015, Author. Available at www.healthypeople.gov.

The *Healthy People 2020* objectives are a useful tool available to nurses to evaluate if individuals with disabilities are receiving adequate services. Moreover, these objectives can serve as national benchmarks for individuals with disabilities with regard to their health, use of community services, leisure activities, and overall quality of life. Nurses can use the *Healthy People 2020* objectives to advocate for increased physical activity and wellness programs for the disabled. This can be done by working with community and disability organizations to ensure compliance with the ADA and by educating others about the *Healthy People 2020* objectives (USDHHS, 2015).

ROLE OF THE NURSE

Many factors influence the role of nurses who work with individuals with disabilities. These factors include the community's awareness of these persons and the commitment to their health needs. Also, the missions of the agencies where nurses work influence the type of services they provide to special groups. For example, the structure and priorities of a community-based agency determine whether a nurse will care for the general population or focus on service to a specific population. If funding sources are dedicated to particular programs (e.g., tuberculosis control, maternal–child health services), care for those who are disabled may be dispersed throughout several program areas and may be difficult to identify.

In dealing with those who are disabled, a nurse's role may also change as the focus varies among the levels of individuals, families, groups, or entire communities. For example, at the level of the individual, nurses may provide nursing care for ventilated patients at home. Nurses also serve as educators who provide clients at any level with sufficient knowledge to enable them to care for their own needs. At the community level, nurses may provide information about certain causes of disability and aim to reduce the behaviors that precede the development of disability, such as spinal cord injury. The closely related counseling role is of value because clients learn to improve their problem-solving skills with guidance from the nurse. The How To box that follows discusses ways to promote the appropriate use of asthma medications by children.

HOW TO Promote Appropriate Use of Asthma Medications by Children

A. Collaborate/coordinate efforts with health care provider managing child's asthma.
   1. Personnel in all areas in which a child uses drugs need to be informed of regimen.
   2. Be aware of factors that could affect adherence to regimen:
      - Prolonged therapy
      - Medications used prophylactically
      - Delayed consequences of nonadherence
      - Drugs expensive, hard to use
      - Family concerns about side effects
      - Adherence less likely with mild or severe asthma; most likely with moderate asthma
      - Child with cognitive or emotional problems
      - Poorly functioning family
      - Strong alternative health beliefs
      - Multiple caregivers

B. Assess child's adherence to regimen.
   1. Count pills; use float test for remaining amount in inhalers (gross estimate).
   2. Ask child, "In an average week, how many puffs of your inhaler do you actually get?"
   3. Obtain refill history from pharmacist (information can be obtained from child's health care provider).

C. Interventions
   1. Educate child, parents, and other caregivers.
   2. Encourage adaptation of regimen to family's needs.
      - Health care provider may need additional information about family situation.
      - Signed, dated, written permission to exchange information with such a provider is needed.
   3. Encourage consideration of acceptability of medication to child, family.
   4. Be encouraging, caring, supportive, and willing to work with family.
   5. Follow-up and monitor progress closely, including school attendance, when appropriate.
   6. Consider home visits (e.g., to assess/manage environmental triggers).
   7. Identify an "asthma partner" (i.e., another adult besides parents when they do not reliably monitor child).
   8. Use a contract for adherence.
   9. In extreme cases, especially with young and/or ill children, consider reporting family to child protective services for medical neglect.

Nurses serve as advocates for individuals and families or groups. An advocate is a person who speaks on behalf of those who are unable to speak for themselves. One of the potential problems with this role is that nurses may unintentionally foster excessive dependence by individuals, families, or other groups. Nurses should focus on using advocacy to support those who need this service. Moreover, having an opportunity to observe nurses using their advocacy skills may assist others to feel more comfortable in being advocates for themselves or for family members. For example, nurses might advocate for a school environment that is adapted to the specific needs of children who require wheelchairs but who do not necessarily have to be limited to their chairs, without explicitly telling the children when they should use their wheelchairs. In addition, nurses may help family caregivers of individuals with disabilities by validating that the caregiver may have unmet needs and by helping them to identify ways their needs can be met.

As referral agents, nurses maintain current information about agencies with services that are of potential use to those who are disabled. Referral, a common practice for nurses, is the process of directing clients to the resources that can meet their needs. For self-directed individuals and families, information about an agency's services, phone number, and address may be adequate. For families with little understanding of how systems work, more specific guidance and case conferences may be necessary to coordinate clients' health-related and educational needs.

As health care providers with a goal of making basic care universally accessible, nurses are positioned well to ensure that the full range of prevention and information about health promotion is made available to individuals with disabilities. On a more individualized basis, the nurse in a case manager role works to meet the needs of people by developing a plan of care for them to help them reach individual goals. Although nurses may direct others to carry out the plan, they are responsible for evaluating the plan's effectiveness. For example, clients who have been disabled because of complications from diabetes mellitus may have several immediate problems. They may need to adjust to the amputation of one or more limbs, as well as learn new skills to improve management of their diabetes in an effort to prevent additional complications. Nurses (as case managers) will develop plans with clients and families to meet these needs and establish time frames to evaluate specific outcomes.

In the coordinator role, nurses are not responsible for developing overall plans of care. Instead, responsibilities include assisting individuals and families by organizing and integrating the resources of other agencies or care providers to meet needs most efficiently. For example, with the family's agreement, a nurse may arrange for the family to see a social worker on the same day they bring their children to an appointment in a pediatric cardiology clinic.

Nurses are collaborators when they take part in joint decision making with individuals, families, groups, and communities. Collaboration with other care providers is of particular importance in coordinating care and assisting a person with a disability to understand the full range of services available. For example, nurses may work with agencies or groups who make decisions about community housing for those who are physically disabled.

In the nursing as case finder role, nurses identify individuals with disabilities who have unmet service needs. For example, nurses may arrange developmental, vision, and hearing screenings for young children. Although a nurse's efforts are for particular individuals, the focus of case finding is on monitoring the health status of entire groups or communities. Nurses may also identify those who are members of vulnerable populations and who, although not presently affected by an illness, are at high risk for acquiring the disease. Such people may have limited or no access to health promotion or disease prevention services, or they may be unaware of those for which they are eligible.

Nurses may function as change agents at all levels, including the health care delivery system. A change agent is one who originates and creates change. This process includes identifying a need for change, enlightening and motivating others as to this need, as well as starting and directing the proposed change. Nurses may function in the role by helping to obtain more appropriate health care services for those who are disabled. The most up-to-date information on national and local resources for individuals with disabilities can be found on the Internet. Two excellent resources are Connecting the Disability Community to Information and Opportunities (www.disability.gov) and Disability Resource (www.disability-benefits-help.org). The following Focus on Quality and Safety Education for Nurses box provides useful information regarding teamwork and collaboration in caring for a person who is part of a special needs population.

QSEN FOCUS ON QUALITY AND SAFETY EDUCATION FOR NURSES QUALITY AND SAFETY FOCUS

Targeted Competency: Teamwork and Collaboration

Function effectively within nursing and interprofessional teams, fostering open communication, mutual respect, and shared decision making to achieve quality patient care.

Important aspects of teamwork and collaboration include:

- **Knowledge:** Recognize contributions of other individuals and groups in helping patient/family achieve health goals
- **Skills:** Integrate the contributions of others who play a role in helping patient/family achieve health goals
- **Attitudes:** Respect the unique attributes that members bring to a team, including variations in professional orientations and accountabilities

Teamwork and Collaboration Question

You are a U.S. Department of Veterans Affairs (VA) home care nurse who has extensive experience in caring for returned veterans who are recovering from spinal cord injuries. You have been approached by the VA Hospital to help develop a program to reduce recurring admissions to the acute care setting for this population. Specifically, there are models from leading rehabilitation hospitals that a Spinal Cord Injury Nurse Advice Line can effectively help clients and families address commonly recurring complications like neurogenic bladder and skin breakdown. Employing an "Ask-A-Nurse" model, a Spinal Cord Injury Nurse Advice Line is a call-in resource. The development team is asking your input on which team members should be involved in development of this local initiative. If successful, the model may be implemented nationally across the VA Medical System.

What contributions will the following team members make to a Spinal Cord Injury Nurse Advice Line?

- Patients with spinal cord injuries
- Families of patients with spinal cord injuries
- Primary care providers
- Neurologists
- Urologists
- Wound care nurses
- Emergency department physicians
- Case managers

Prepared by Gail Armstrong, PhD, DNP, ACNS-BC, CNE, Associate Professor, University of Colorado Denver College of Nursing.

DISABILITY RIGHTS LEGISLATION

A nurse who works with the physically disabled may have a caseload of all ages, while another nurse, such as a school nurse, may see clients in a specific age group. Nurses need to be knowledgeable about the legislation that relates to populations for whom they provide nursing care. Box 30.5 summarizes key **disability rights legislation**. The U.S. Department of Justice (USDOJ, 2017b) website provides an overview of federal civil rights laws designed to ensure equal opportunity for people with disabilities. This website is an excellent reference about legislation and disability rights information.

Rehabilitation services were originally developed through legislation for veterans of World War I. In time, others who were physically disabled were regarded less as sources of embarrassment to their families and more as citizens who should participate as fully as possible in all aspects of society. This

BOX 30.5 Summary of Legislation

- Communications Act of 1934 and Telecommunications Act of 1996
- Elementary and Secondary Education Act of 1965
- Architectural Barriers Act of 1968
- Rehabilitation Act of 1973
- Individuals with Disabilities Education Act (IDEA) of 1975
- Civil Rights of Institutionalized Persons Act of 1980
- Voting Accessibility for the Elderly and the Handicapped Act of 1984
- The Air Carrier Access Act of 1986
- The Fair Housing Act of 1988
- Americans with Disabilities Act (ADA) of 1990
- National Voter Registration Act of 1993
- The Developmental Disabilities Act and Bill of Rights Act of 2000
- No Child Left Behind Act of 2001
- The Individuals with Disabilities Education Improvement Act of 2004

From U.S. Department of Justice: *Disability rights section*, 2017a, Author. Available at www.ada.gov.

change in attitude was reflected in changing laws affecting the disabled.

Rehabilitation Act of 1973

The Rehabilitation Act of 1973 was the first legislation designed specifically to eliminate discrimination against the disabled. This act required all federal agencies and programs receiving federal funds to hire disabled workers. The Rehabilitation Act was an important piece of legislation that defined disability clearly and increased opportunities for some disabled Americans. However, additional legislation was needed to provide more inclusive protection for individuals with disabilities and to extend the benefits of the Rehabilitation Act to encompass more than federal programs. The ADA of 1990 was designed to decrease discrimination and increase opportunities for all disabled Americans by providing more comprehensive protection for them (Allarie, 2005; Lair & Kale, 2005).

Americans with Disabilities Act

The ADA was signed into law July 26, 1990. The act makes it illegal for state and local governments, private employers, employment agencies, labor organizations, and labor-management committees to discriminate against the disabled in employment, public accommodations, transportation, state and local government operations, and telecommunications (ADA, 1990). Cutting across the specific policy provisions of the ADA are four global goals that clarify the intent of the legislation. For persons with a disability, the ADA is designed to promote (1) equality of opportunity, (2) full participation in society and social integration, (3) independent living, and (4) economic self-sufficiency (ADA, 1990). "The ADA provides comprehensive civil rights protection for qualified individuals with disabilities" (Walk et al., 1993, p. 92). The ADA addresses four areas as shown in Box 30.6.

According to the ADA (1990), a qualified employee or applicant with a disability is a person who, with or without reasonable accommodation, can perform the essential functions

BOX 30.6 Components of the Americans with Disabilities Act

Title 1 (Employment): Employers, including religious organizations that employ 15 or more employees, cannot exclude individuals with disabilities from being hired solely on the basis of disability with or without accommodations, unless they can prove that provision of such accommodations may cause undue burden on the business.

Title 2 (Access to state and local governments, and public transportation): All state and local government agencies, programs, services, and activities must be accessible to individuals with disabilities. In addition all public transportation systems, including city buses and public rail transit systems must be accessible, unless they can prove that provision of such accommodations will cause an undue burden. In such cases, an alternative paratransit system must be made available to individuals with disabilities who are unable to use the regular transportation system.

Title 3 (Public accommodations): All business and nonprofit organizations that offer public accommodations, private entities that offer services, privately operated transportation and commercial facilities, must not exclude, separate, or discriminate against individuals with disabilities who are trying to access their programs and services otherwise available to the public. They must remove any architectural barriers that prevent individuals with disabilities from using their facilities.

Title 4 (Telecommunications relay services): Covers access to communication and media for people with hearing and speech disabilities. It requires common carriers (telephone companies) to establish interstate and intrastate telecommunications relay services (TRS) 24 hours a day, 7 days a week. It also requires closed captioning of federally funded public service announcements.

From U.S. Equal Employment Opportunity Commission: *Facts about the Americans with disabilities act*, 2015, Author. Available at www.eeoc.gov.

of the job in question. Reasonable accommodations may include but are not limited to the following:

- Making existing facilities that are used by employees readily accessible to and usable by persons with disabilities
- Job restructuring, modifying work schedules, reassignment to a vacant position
- Acquiring or modifying equipment or devices; adjusting or modifying examinations, training materials, or policies; and providing qualified readers or interpreters

Employers may not ask qualified job applicants questions about the existence, nature, or severity of a disability. Qualified applicants may be asked about their ability to perform job functions. A job offer may be made conditional based on the results of a medical examination, but only if that examination is required for all applicants for the same job. In addition, the examination must be job related and consistent with the employer's business needs. Individuals who use illegal drugs or who are intoxicated at work are not covered under the ADA. Tests for illegal drugs are not subject to the ADA's restrictions on examinations. Employers may hold illegal drug users and alcoholics to the same performance standards as other employees.

Service animals are defined and protected under the ADA. Service animals are working animals that are individually trained to perform tasks for persons with disabilities. These tasks may include guiding someone who is blind, alerting persons who are deaf, pulling wheelchairs, and other special tasks. Under the ADA, businesses and other organizations who serve the public, including restaurants, hotels, taxis, stores, medical offices and hospitals, theaters, and parks, are required to allow service animals to accompany a disabled person into all areas open to the general public.

Individuals with Disabilities Education Act

IDEA of 1975 is federal legislation that guarantees all children with disabilities ages 3 through 21 years the right to a free and appropriate public school education that will meet their individual needs. This law protects the rights of parents, guardians, and surrogate parents to fully participate in educational decisions. Special education including physical education is defined in this law, and special instruction is to be provided at no cost to parents. Special education was created to meet the special needs of children with disabilities.

According to IDEA, children with disabilities are those who have one or a combination of the following conditions and therefore would benefit from special education: autism, blindness, deafness, hearing impairment, mental retardation, multiple disabilities, orthopedic impairment, serious emotional disturbance, specific learning disabilities, traumatic brain injury, visual impairment, and other health impairments (USDE, 2018).

Basic Rights Under IDEA

Free and appropriate public education (FAPE)—The child's education must be designed to meet the child's special needs.

Appropriate evaluation/assessment—Each child with a disability must receive a complete educational assessment before being placed in a special education program.

Individualized education plan (IEP)—This plan must be focused and modified on a set of goals and objectives to meet the child's individual needs.

Education in the least restrictive environment (LRE)—Children with disabilities should be educated as much as possible with their peers who do not have disabilities.

Parent and student participation in decision making—Parent and student participation and communication are encouraged. Parents are members of the IEP team and are included in evaluation, eligibility, and placement.

Early intervention services for children and their families—Funds are allocated to infants who have disabling conditions and/or developmental delays. An individualized family service plan (IFSP) is developed that details the early intervention services to enhance the child's development and strengthen the family (USDE, 2018).

No Child Left Behind

The No Child Left Behind Act of 2001 expands parental roles in their child's education. This law reauthorized the Elementary and Secondary Education Act of 1965, the principal federal law governing elementary and secondary education. According to the USDE, it is built on four concepts: accountability, doing what works according to the scientific research, expanding parental options, and expanding local control and flexibility. This bill does the following:

- Supports learning in the early years, hopefully preventing learning disabilities
- Provides more information for parents about their child's programs
- Alerts parents to important information about their child's performance
- Gives more resources to schools
- Gives children and parents a lifeline
- Improves teaching and learning by providing better information to teachers
- Ensures that teacher quality is a high priority
- Allows more flexibility

Administration of Developmental Disabilities

The Developmental Disabilities Act and Bill of Rights Act of 2000 requires the Administration on Developmental Disabilities (ADD) under the USDHHS to ensure that people with developmental disabilities and their families receive the services and support they need. The disabled and their families must also be given the opportunity to participate in the planning and implementation of these services. The ADD is a federal agency within the USDHHS and is responsible for implementation and administration of The Developmental Disabilities Act and Bill of Rights Act of 2000 and the disability provisions of the Help Americans Vote Act. There are eight areas of emphasis for ADD: employment, education, child care, health, housing, transportation, recreation, and quality assurance. The ADD meets these requirements through four programs:

1. *State Councils on Developmental Disabilities (SCDD)*: Each state has a council whose function is to increase the independence, productivity, inclusion, and community integration of persons with developmental disabilities.
2. *Protection and Advocacy Agencies (P&As)*: Every state has a system to empower, protect, and advocate on the behalf of persons with developmental disabilities. The system investigates incidents of abuse, neglect, or discrimination based on disability.
3. *University Centers for Excellence in Developmental Disabilities—Education, Research, and Services (UCEDD):* This program provides support to a national network of university centers to carry out interdisciplinary training, services, technical assistance, and information dissemination activities. Its purpose is to increase independence, productivity, and integration into communities.
4. *Projects of National Significance:* The purpose of this program is to focus on emerging issues, provide technical assistance, conduct research regarding disability issues, and develop state and federal policy. Additional information is available at the following website: www.acf.hhs.gov. In addition, most states and many large cities and counties have their own laws prohibiting discrimination on the basis of disability. Such laws offer greater protection to employees by extending coverage to smaller employers, by using more expansive definitions of disability than those used under the ADA, and by expanding the duty of employers to assist

BOX 30.7 Federal Agencies With Developmental Disability Activities

- Administration on Developmental Disabilities (ADD)
- Center for Medicaid and Medicare Services—Medicaid and the State Children's Health Insurance Program can help children and adults obtain health care coverage
- DisabilityInfo.gov—provides information about disability resources in the federal government
- Maternal and Child Health Bureau (MCHB)—promotes the health of mothers and children; provides newborn hearing screening, information on child health and safety, and information on genetics
- MedlinePlus Health Information, National Library of Medicine—online resource for information
- National Council on Disability (NCD)—ensures that persons with disabilities have the same opportunities as others; promotes policies and programs that assist people with disabilities
- National Institutes of Health (NIH)—conducts and funds research on developmental disabilities
- National Institute on Disability and Rehabilitation Research (NIDRR)—promotes the participation of persons with disabilities in their communities
- Office of Disability Employment—focus is to increase job opportunities for people with disabilities; this office is within the U.S. Department of Labor
- Office of Special Education Programs (OSEP)—improves the lives of children and youth with disabilities from birth to adulthood through education and support services; this office is within the U.S. Department of Education
- Office on Disability—oversees the implementation of federal disability policies and programs; fosters interactions between the U.S. Department of Health and Human Services, other federal and state agencies, and private-sector groups
- Rehabilitative Services Administration (RSA)—helps persons with disabilities get jobs and live more independently; RSA is part of the U.S. Department of Education

employees with disabilities to move to new positions for which they are qualified. Box 30.7 lists federal agencies with developmental disability activities.

Additional Legislation

The Fair Housing Act of 1988 prohibits housing discrimination based on race, color, religion, sex, disability, familial status, and national origin. This includes private as well as public housing. The Act also requires new multifamily housing with four or more units to be accessible for persons with disabilities.

The Civil Rights of Institutionalized Persons Act of 1997 authorizes the attorney general to investigate conditions of confinement in state and local institutions such as prisons, detention centers, jails, nursing homes, and institutions for persons with psychiatric or developmental disabilities. Civil lawsuits may be initiated on the behalf of the person if harmful or neglectful conditions are found (USDOJ, 2015).

According to the Department of Justice, the Voting Accessibility for the Elderly and the Handicapped Act of 1984 requires polling places across the United States to be accessible for persons with disabilities during federal elections. In addition, states are responsible for ensuring available registration and voting aids for disabled and elderly voters, including telecommunication devices for the deaf (USDOJ, 2017b).

The Individuals with Disabilities Education Improvement Act of 2004 is the nation's special education law and serves millions of children and youth with disabilities (USDE, 2018).

The National Voter Registration Act of 1993, also known as the Motor Voter Act, makes it easier for all Americans to vote. Because of the low registration turnout of minorities and persons with disabilities, this act requires all offices of state-funded programs to provide program applicants with voter registration forms, to assist them in completing the forms, and to transmit the forms to the appropriate office (USDOJ, 2017b).

The Air Carrier Access Act of 1986 prohibits discrimination by airlines. Persons with disabilities do not have to give advance notice before they fly. Moreover, unless there is a safety concern, they cannot be discriminated against with regard to seat assignment. Facilities in airports and on board planes need to be fully accessible for the disabled. Moreover, passengers with disabilities are entitled to bring needed adaptive equipment and service animals (U.S. Department of Transportation [USDOT], 2015).

PRACTICE APPLICATION

A referral was made to a public health department from a nearby regional level III neonatal intensive care unit (NICU) regarding discharge plans for a developmentally delayed infant. The infant, Joel, was born at 27 weeks' gestation and had remained in intensive care for 7 months. His hospital course was complicated by respiratory distress syndrome, bronchopulmonary dysplasia, and intraventricular hemorrhage. At the time of discharge, Joel was receiving neither supplemental oxygen nor medications and was taking all of his feedings orally. There were strong indications of spastic diplegia and he was diagnosed as having severe retinopathy of prematurity with the expectation of eventual blindness.

Family financial resources were extremely limited. Although Medicaid coverage was available for subsequent needs, the family owed more than $100,000 to the hospital. Joel's grandmother agreed to care for him while his 17-year-old mother Mary finished high school. Joel's father, who is also 17 years old and unemployed, had not been active with Mary and her mother in the hospital discharge-planning program. His involvement with Mary and Joel was expected to be minimal. The hospital was seeking a home evaluation before discharge.

What would you consider to be the first step in completing the home evaluation?

Answers can be found on the Evolve site.

KEY POINTS

- Nurses have many opportunities to influence the care of individuals with disabilities through health promotion activities. Health education is important for parents who might be at high risk for having a disabled child, for children at risk for accidents and injuries, and for adults with chronic illnesses who might prevent disability through careful health practices.
- Many of the *Healthy People 2020* objectives apply to physically compromised individuals, their families, and communities.
- Physically compromised individuals need to participate in health promotion to prevent the onset of a new health disruption, to strengthen their well-functioning aspects, and to prevent further deterioration of their health.
- Nursing interventions for physically compromised clients require attention to their health as well as to the environment in which they live.
- Nurses influence policy decisions that affect the health and well-being of compromised individuals.
- Nurses must know both federal and state laws pertaining to disabilities to most effectively assist clients and their families.

CLINICAL DECISION-MAKING ACTIVITIES

1. Divide the class or the clinical group into two teams and debate the following: Children with developmental disabilities should or should not be mainstreamed into classrooms with nondisabled children.
2. During a home visit first to an adult and then to a child who have a chronic illness that leaves them physically compromised, answer the following questions:
   A. Could this disability have been prevented? If so, what steps could a nurse have taken to provide health promotion activities that would have prevented the occurrence of the disabling condition?
   B. What role, if any, does the environment play in the onset of this compromising health condition?
   C. What preventive activities are currently needed to ensure the highest possible quality of life for this person?
3. For the next week, look at each building you enter and consider the following:
   A. What accommodations have been made to allow physically compromised people to enter this building?
   B. What accommodations should still be made?
   C. Who should pay for these architectural accommodations?
4. Spend one day following your usual schedule using either crutches or a wheelchair, so that you can understand better what it means to be physically compromised and have special needs.
5. Using a telephone book, community resource directories, or the web pages for your town, identify all agencies whose scope of work is devoted to assisting special needs individuals and their families.

ADDITIONAL RESOURCES

EVOLVE WEBSITE

http://evolve.elsevier.com/Stanhope/community/

- Answers to Practice Application
- Case Study
- Glossary
- Review Questions

REFERENCES

Allarie SH: Employment and satisfaction outcomes from a job retention intervention delivered to persons with chronic diseases, *Rehabil Couns Bull* 48:100–109, 2005.

American Community Survey: *Disability*, 2017, Author. Retrieved from www.census.gov.

Americans with Disabilities Act of 1990, PL 101–336, 1990.

Carl C: *Can I get paid to be a family caregiver?* 2017, The Caregiver Space. Retrieved from https://thecaregiverspace.org.

Carmona R: *The surgeon general's call to action to improve the health and wellness of persons with disabilities*, 2005: author. Retrieved from www.surgeongeneral.gov.

Center for an Accessible Society: *Independent living for a million adults jeopardized by a shortfall of a few hours of help*, 2014, Author. Retrieved from www.accessiblesociety.org.

Centers for Disease Control and Prevention (CDC): *Classifications of diseases functioning, and disability*, 2015, Author. Retrieved from www.cdc.gov.

Centers for Disease Control and Prevention (CDC): *A snapshot of disability in the United States*, 2017a, Author. Retrieved from www.cdc.gov.

Centers for Disease Control and Prevention (CDC): *Chronic diseases overview*, 2017b, Author. Retrieved from www.cdc.gov.

Centers for Disease Control and Prevention (CDC): *Disability and health*, 2017c, Author. Retrieved from www.cdc.gov.

Centers for Disease Control and Prevention (CDC): *Important facts about falls*, 2017d, Author. Retrieved from www.cdc.gov.

Cornell University: *Disability statistics*, 2018, American community survey. Retrieved from www.disabilitystatistics.org.

Council for Disability Awareness: *Disability statistics*, 2013, Author. Retrieved from www.disabilitycanhappen.org.

Council on Linkages Between Academia and Public Health Practice: *Core competencies for public health professionals: Tiers*, 2014, Author. Retrieved from www.phf.org.

Disability Is Natural: *People first language*, 2018, Author. Retrieved from www.disabilityisnatural.com.

Donnelly G: *Employment rate for workers with disabilities, Fortune* [serial online], February, 2017. Retrieved from http://fortune.com.

Family CareGiver Alliance: *Caregiver statistics: Work and caregiving*, 2016, Author. Retrieved from www.caregiver.org.

Goering S: Rethinking disability: The social model of disability and chronic disease, *Curr Rev Musculoskelet Med* 8(2):134–138, 2015.

Jones NL: Essential requirements of the act: A short history and overview, *Milbank Q* 69(Suppl 1–2):25–54, 1991.

Kraus L: *2016 disability statistics annual report*, 2017: Durham, NH: University of New Hampshire. Retrieved from disabilitycompendium.org.

Lair PL, Kale KD: Post-offer medical exam was premature, *HR Magazine* 50:163, 2005.

Maternal and Child Health Bureau: *The national survey of children with special health care needs chartbook 2009–2010*, 2013, Author. Retrieved from www.mchb.hrsa.gov.

Maternal and Child Health Bureau: *Children with special health care needs*, 2018, Author. Retrieved from www.mchb.hrsa.gov.

Merriam-Webster On-Line Dictionary: *Disability*, 2018, Author. Retrieved from www.merriam-webster.com.

Missouri Department of Health & Senior Services: *Stop abuse & neglect*, 2018, Author. Retrieved from www.health.mo.gov.

Mosher J, Bloom T, Hughes R, Horton L, Mojtabai R, Alhusen JL: Disparities in receipt of family planning services by disability status: New estimates from the national survey of family growth, *Disabil Health J* 10(3):394–399, 2017.

National Center Against Bullying: *Autism spectrum disorder and bullying*, 2018, Author. Retrieved from www.ncab.org.au.

National Home Sharing and Short Breaks Network: *The impact of disability on a family*, 2016, Author. Retrieved from nhsn.ie.

National Institute of Mental Health: *Mental health information*, 2017, Author. Retrieved from www.nimh.nih.gov.

Perkins J, Agrawal R: Protecting rights of children with medical complexity in an era of spending reduction, *Pediatrics* 141 (Suppl 3):S242–S249, 2018.

Social Security Administration: *Red book*, 2017, Author. Retrieved from www.ssa.gov.

Umeda CJ, Fogelberg DJ, Jirikowic T, Pitonyak JS, Mroz TM, Ideishi RI: Expanding the implementation of the Americans with Disabilities Act for populations with intellectual and developmental disabilities: the role of organization-level occupational therapy consultation, *Am J Occup Ther* 71(4): 7104090010p1–7104090010p6, 2017.

Unicef: *Children and young people with disabilities fact sheet*, 2013: author. Retrieved from www.unicef.org.

United Nations: *The world's women 2015: trends and statistics*, 2015, Author. Retrieved from www.un.org.

USQRA: *United States Quad Rugby Association*, 2018, Author. Retrieved from www.usqra.org.

U.S. Department of Education: *IDEA website*, 2018, Author. Retrieved from www.ed.gov.

U.S. Department of Health and Human Services: *Healthy People 2020: disability and health*, 2015, Author. Retrieved from www.healthypeople.gov.

U.S. Department of Health and Human Services, Children's Bureau: *The risk and prevention of maltreatment of children with disabilities*, 2018, Author. Retrieved from www.childwelfare.gov.

U.S. Department of Justice: *Civil rights of institutionalized persons*, 2015, Author. Retrieved from www.justice.gov.

U.S. Department of Justice: *Disability rights section*, 2017a, Author. Retrieved from www.ada.gov.

U.S. Department of Justice: *Law and regulations*, 2017b, Author. Retrieved from www.ada.gov.

U.S. Department of Transportation: *Passengers with disabilities*, 2015, Author. Retrieved from www.transportation.gov.

U.S. Equal Employment Opportunity Commission: *Facts about the Americans with Disabilities Act*, 2015, Author. Retrieved from www.eeoc.gov.

Vos T, Abajobir AA, Abate KH, et al.: Global, regional, and national incidence, prevalence, and years lived with disability for 328 diseases and injuries for 195 countries, 1990–2016: a systematic analysis for the Global Burden of Disease Study 2016. *The Lancet [serial online]*, September 2017. Retrieved from www.thelancet.com.

Walk EE, Ahn HC, Lampkin PM, Nabizadeh SA, Edlich RF: Americans with Disabilities Act, *J Burn Care Rehabil* 14:92–98, 1993.

World Health Organization (WHO): *Towards a common language for functioning, disability and health*, 2002, author. Retrieved from www.who.int.

World Health Organization (WHO): *World report on disability*, 2011, Author. Retrieved from www.who.int.

World Health Organization (WHO): *WHO global disability action plan 2014–2021: Better health for all people with disability*, 2015, Author. Retrieved from www.who.int.

World Health Organization (WHO): *Disability and health*, 2018a, Author. Retrieved from www.who.int.

World Health Organization (WHO): *Depression*, 2018b, Author. Retrieved from www.who.int.

31

Health Equity and Care of Vulnerable Populations

Carole R. Myers, PhD, MSN, BS

OBJECTIVES

After studying and reflecting on this chapter, the student should be able to do the following:

1. Discuss health equity and its importance to nurses.
2. Describe population health and its application to nursing practice.
3. Discuss health determinants.
4. Describe population groups who might be considered vulnerable.
5. Identify the ways in which these populations often have health disparities compared with the general population.
6. Analyze trends that have influenced both the development of vulnerability among certain population groups and social attitudes toward vulnerability.
7. Analyze the effects of public policies on vulnerable populations and on reducing health disparities experienced by these populations.
8. Examine the multiple individual and social factors that contribute to vulnerability.
9. Evaluate strategies that nurses can use to improve the health status and eliminate health disparities of vulnerable populations including governmental, community, and private programs.

CHAPTER OUTLINE

Health Equity
Health Determinants
Vulnerability
Reducing Disparities and Improving Population Health Outcomes
Assessment Issues

KEY TERMS

advocacy, p. 704
case management, p. 709
comprehensive services, p. 707
cross-sectoral approach, p. 698
determinants of health, p. 698
disadvantaged, p. 703
disenfranchisement, p. 703
equality, p. 698
federal poverty level, p. 703
health determinants, p. 698
health disparities, p. 700
health equity, p. 698
health/wealth gradient, p. 700
human capital, p. 701
income inequality, p. 703
inequities, p. 698
linguistically appropriate health care, p. 707
marginalization, p. 701
population health, p. 698
poverty, p. 698
resilience, p. 701
risk, p. 698
safety net providers, p. 707
social determinants of health, p. 699
social justice, p. 701
vulnerability, p. 701
wrap-around services, p. 706

Appreciation goes to Jeanette Lancaster, who authored earlier versions of this chapter.

This chapter includes a discussion of the concept of health equity and how nurses can advance equity at multiple levels for significant and sustainable change and improved outcomes. To understand health equity we must first define **population health** and understand the multitude of **health determinants** that contribute to or distract from health, the differences or disparities in health and health determinants among different populations, and distinguish equity from equality. The relationships among health and health determinants and vulnerability, health disparities, and equity are explored. The concept *vulnerability* is discussed and a description of selected population groups that are at a greater **risk** than others for poor health outcomes is included. This foundational information is then used as a basis for discussing how nurses can implement strategies to reduce disparities and foster improvement in health equity and population outcomes.

HEALTH EQUITY

The Robert Wood Johnson Foundation uses the following definition of **health equity**: "Health equity means that everyone has a fair and just opportunity to be healthier. This requires removing obstacles to health such as **poverty**, discrimination, and their consequences, including powerlessness and lack of access to good jobs with fair pay, quality education and housing, safe environments, and health care" (Braveman et al., 2017). The American Public Health Association (APHA) describes health equity as meaning "everyone has the opportunity to attain their highest level of health" (n.d.).

Health **inequities** are barriers that prevent individuals and populations from attaining maximal health. Addressing health equity starts with recognizing the inherent value of all people and populations regardless of their circumstances and is achieved by "[optimizing] the conditions in which people are born, grow, live, work, and age" (APHA, n.d.).

An equity mindset leads to actions aimed at ameliorating health inequities for the purpose of maximizing health for all people. Achieving health equity requires a **cross-sectoral approach**. This means that nurses and other health professionals must partner with stakeholders outside of traditional public health and health care delivery systems to design multilevel solutions for improving health. Effective cross-sectoral work is collaborative. When diverse people and organizations collaborate, they work together in inter-connected ways to achieve a common goal. Collaboration is synchronized and coordinated.

Equality is a quintessential American value that permeates the American vision codified in the country's Declaration of Independence, Constitution, Bill of Rights, and many laws. Equality is often likened to equity, but they are not the same. Health equity is a means to achieve health equality. An equity approach to health equality means that those individuals and populations who have the least actually need more opportunities and resources, not equal opportunities and resources, to achieve equal health. More simply put: *those people and groups who have the least need the most.*

Population Health

The focus of public health nursing is population health. Population health is "an approach to health that aims to improve the health of an entire population and reduce inequities among population groups" (Kindig, 2007; Kindig & Stoddart, 2003). Population health is largely a product of individual, collective behaviors. The importance of personal health practices and individual knowledge, skills, and ability must be acknowledged, along with social, economic, and physical environments that make health more likely. The goal of population health is to provide evidence-based care to targeted groups of people with similar needs in order to improve outcomes and reduce disparities.

Population health strategies work to create conditions in which individuals and families can be healthy. Population health encompasses wellness, prevention, and health promotion; a focus on upstream causes of health problems; addressing health determinants; and partnerships among a broad complement of health and other stakeholders. Improving health requires actions directed at a broad range of conditions that influence health. Characteristics of population health and population health practice are shown in Table 31.1.

Populations. A population is a collection of individuals who have one or more personal or environmental characteristics in common. Populations can be defined by (1) *geography*, (2) *enrollment* in a system (e.g., health plan, accountable care organization [ACO]), or (3) common *characteristic* (e.g., older adults with multiple chronic conditions or pregnant teenagers).

Several terms are associated with populations. *Aggregates* are subpopulations that may be based on ethnicity, geographic location, age, occupation, or shared diagnosis or risk factor. A *community* is composed of multiple aggregates, most commonly high-risk aggregates. Likewise we frequently focus on *populations at risk.*

Health. Population health is based on a broad perspective of what health is and what constitutes health. The World Health

TABLE 31.1 Population Health and Population Health Practice

Population Health Characteristics	Population Health Practice
• Beyond the patient population; beyond medical care • Looks upstream at multiple **determinants of health** • Prioritizes measurement/distribution of outcomes, health disparities, and health equity • Outcomes-focused; oriented to reducing disparities and inequities • Shared accountability • Supports authority of the individual (Minnesota Department of Health, 2003)	• Focused on entire population • Grounded in an assessment of the population's health status • Considers broad determinants of health • Emphasizes all level of prevention • Intervenes with communities, systems, individuals, and families (Stevens & Aly, 2014)

Organization (WHO) definition of health is aspirational, holistic, and consistent with a nursing and population perspective. The WHO definition of health is "a state of complete physical, mental, and social well-being, and not merely the absence of disease or infirmity" (1946).

HEALTH DETERMINANTS

Health determinants include a range of individual characteristics and behaviors, social and economic circumstances, and physical environmental factors that influence health status or outcomes (USDHHS-ODPHP, n.d.a; WHO, n.d.). Health outcomes include mortality, morbidity, life expectancy, health care expenditures, health status, and functional limitations (Artiga & Hinton, 2018).

The *County Health Rankings model* (UWPHI, 2018) shown in Fig. 31.1 is a useful depiction of the many factors that impact population health and should be addressed to improve health. The model focuses on modifiable determinants and highlights the key points that health outcomes are more influenced by contextual factors than individual choices or access to and use of health care. The majority of health outcomes result from behaviors and actions; only 10-20 percent is a result of medical care (Hacker & Walker, 2013). This is important since a significant portion of the $2.8 trillion we spend on health care is allocated to direct medical care services, although the availability and quality of medical care services account for just 10 to 15 percent of health outcomes.

Social Determinants of Health

Social determinants of health include a range of social, political and economic factors that include socioeconomic status, living conditions, geographic location, social class, education, environmental factors, nutrition, stress, and prejudice that lead to resource constraints, poor health, and health risk (Lathrop, 2013). From an international perspective, the World Health Organization (WHO, 2015) states that many factors in combination affect the health of individuals and communities. Specifically, "whether people are healthy or not is determined by their circumstances and environment." The WHO, consistent with *Healthy People 2020,* describes three overall determinants of health to be (1) the social and economic environment, (2) the physical environment, and (3) the person's individual characteristics and behaviors. The WHO also notes that individuals are unlikely to be able to directly control many of the determinants of health, and this is directly related to vulnerability. That is, when people experience adverse determinants of health that they cannot control, they are predisposed to becoming vulnerable. The WHO (2015) cites seven examples of factors that affect health. There are many more factors that affect health, as noted later in the *Healthy People 2020* document. The seven WHO factors are as follows (WHO, 2015, pp. 1-2).

1. Income and social status: Higher income and social status are associated with better health.
2. Education: Low education is linked with poor health, more stress, and lower self-confidence.

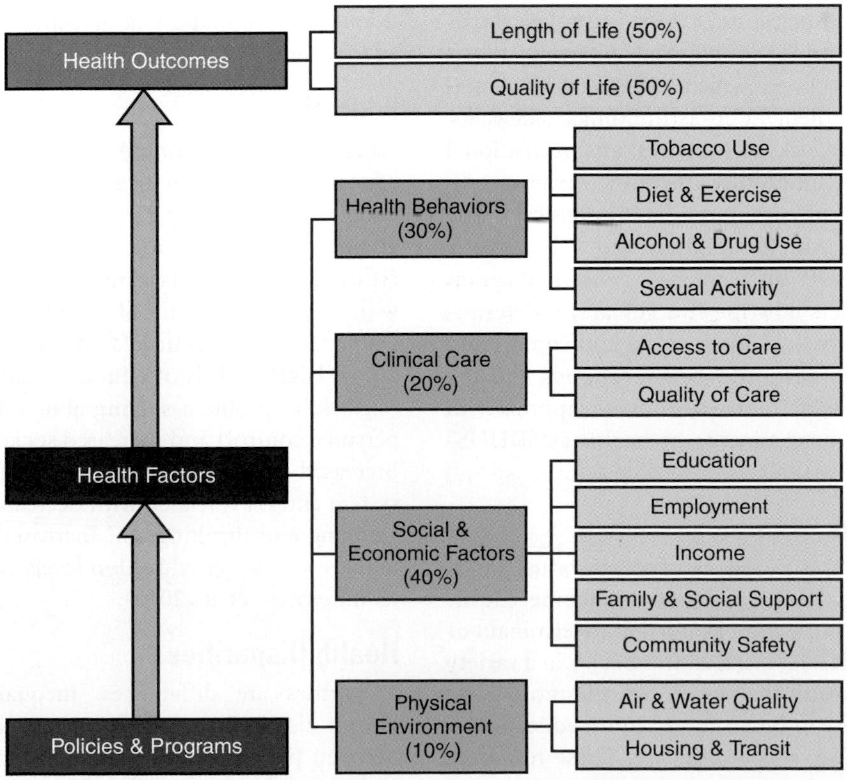

Fig. 31.1 County Health Rankings model. (University of Wisconsin Population Health Institute. County Health Rankings & Roadmaps 2019. www.countyhealthrankings.org.)

3. Physical environment: Safe water and clean air; healthy workplaces; safer homes, communities, and roads; and good employment and working conditions, especially when the person has more control, all contribute to good health.
4. Social support networks: Family, friends, and community as well as culture, customs, traditions, and beliefs affect health.
5. Genetics, as well as personal behavior and coping skills, affects health.
6. Health services: Access and use of services affect health.
7. Gender: Men and women suffer from different types of diseases at different ages.

Healthy People 2020 (USDHHS-OHPDP, 2010) discusses the importance of social determinants of health by including "Create social and physical environments that promote good health for all" as one of the four overarching goals. This document explains that it is important to understand the relationship between how population groups experience "place" and the effect that "place" has on the social determinants of health. This concept is consistent with an ecological framework that examines the effect that people have on the environment and vice versa. *Healthy People 2020* lists 15 examples of social determinants of health: (1) availability of resources to meet daily needs; (2) access to educational, economic, and job opportunities; (3) access to health services; (4) quality of education and job training; (5) availability of community-based resources in support of community living and opportunities for recreation; (6) transportation options; (7) public safety; (8) social support; (9) social norms and attitudes; (10) exposure to crime, violence, and social disorder; (11) socioeconomic conditions; (12) residential segregation; (13) language/literacy; (14) access to mass media and emerging technologies; and (15) culture. This document also lists seven examples of physical determinants of health: (1) natural environment, such as green space and weather; (2) built environment, such as buildings, sidewalks, bike lanes, and roads; (3) worksites, schools, and recreational settings; (4) housing and community design; (5) exposure to toxic substances and other physical hazards; (6) physical barriers, especially for people with disabilities; and (7) aesthetic elements (USDHHS-OHPDP, 2010, pp. 3-4). A useful diagram is also provided that depicts how the five key areas (determinants) of economic stability, education, social and community context, health and health care, and neighborhoods and the built environment serve as a framework for an approach to understanding the social determinants of health (USDHHS-OHPDP, 2010, p. 4).

Socioeconomic Status

Socioeconomic status (SES) is a measure of social status, standing, or class of an individual or group based on income, education, and occupation. SES is the most important determinant of health. As mentioned, social status influences health in a variety of ways. First, the more wealth the person has, the more likely the person is to have access to better foods, more education, a safer community, recreation, and health care. These resources serve as protective barriers against chronic disease, injury, and premature mortality (Lathrop, 2013). Nursing interventions are designed to help vulnerable populations gain the resources needed for better health and reduction of risk factors.

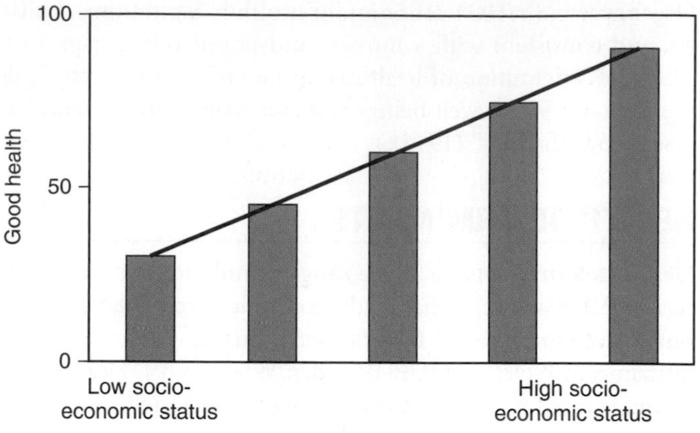

Fig. 31.2 Health/wealth gradient. (Reprinted from The Sycamore Institute: How socioeconomic factors affect health in Tennessee, 2018. Available at https://www.sycamoreinstitutetn.org.)

The **health/wealth gradient** (Fig. 31.2) shows that lower income is linked to poorer health. The reverse is true. In addition, the greater the gap or inequality between the wealthiest members of a group and the poorest members, the greater the differences in health. Addressing social determinants of health is important for improving overall health and reducing disparities. Health care is essential for health, but it is a relatively weak determinant when compared to health behaviors and socioeconomic factors. It is important to note that socioeconomic factors shape health behaviors, therefore exerting an additive effect (Artiga & Hinton, 2018).

Education

Education plays an important role in health status. Although education is related to income, educational level seems to influence health separately. Health disparities related to educational attainment are alarming. In aggregate, life expectancy is increasing among Americans. However life expectancy among white Americans without a high school diploma, especially women, has actually decreased since 1990 (Montez & Berkman, 2014). Higher levels of education contribute to human capital (e.g., skills, problem-solving ability, learned effectiveness, and personal control) and increased social and economic resources. Increased education enhances navigation of the health care system and is associated with decreased risky behaviors such as smoking and drinking and increased healthy behaviors. Individuals with lower education levels are at greater risk for stress (Zimmerman et al., 2015).

Health Disparities

Disparities are differences, inequalities, or incongruences. **Health disparities** are differences in health status or outcomes between people and populations (APHA, n.d.) closely linked with social or economic disadvantages (USDHHS-CDC, n.d.a). Health disparities result in a disproportionate burden of poor health, premature mortality, and morbidity among individuals and populations.

Health disparities viewed through a **social justice** lens are considered unjust if the differences are unnecessary and avoidable (Whitehead, 1991, 2000) as they reflect deeply rooted structural factors such as discrimination and/or **marginalization** of people or populations. Social justice is a concept that has been broadly interpreted and consequently means different things to different people. For the purposes of this discussion, social justice entails recognizing the dignity of every human being and group irrespective of ethnicity, gender, sexual orientation, economic status, educational level, possessions, race, religion, or other characteristics and treating every person or group without prejudice. Marginalization results when people or populations are relegated to a position on the periphery of society where they have diminished importance, influence, or power. Health disparities and inequities differ in that inequities are barriers that prevent people and populations from achieving maximal health status. In contrast disparities are the resultant differences in health status or outcomes.

For more than two decades, *Healthy People* has had an overarching goal that focused on intervening in disparities. The goal in *Healthy People 2000* was to reduce health disparities, and the goal moved to remove health disparities in *Healthy People 2010*. *Healthy People 2020* has expanded the goal to aim to achieve health equity, eliminate disparities, and improve the health of all groups. *Healthy People 2020* describes health equity as attaining the highest possible level of health for all people and includes eliminating health disparities (USDHHS-OHPDP, 2010). Thirty-eight topic areas in *Healthy People 2020* emphasize access, chronic health problems, injury and violence prevention, environmental health, food safety, education and community-based programs, health communication, health information technologies, immunization and infectious diseases, and public health infrastructure, among others. These topic areas are discussed in chapters throughout the text.

The *Healthy People 2030* goals have been expanded as seen in the following box, but the emphasis on elimination of health disparities and promotion of health equity and the highest possible level of health for all populations is unchanged (USDHHS-OHPDP, n.d.b).

HEALTHY PEOPLE 2030

Overarching Goals

- Attain healthy, thriving lives and well-being, free of preventable disease, disability, injury, and premature death.
- Eliminate health disparities, achieve health equity, and attain health literacy to improve the health and well-being of all.
- Create social, physical, and economic environments that promote attaining full potential for health and well-being for all.
- Promote healthy development, healthy behaviors and well-being across all life stages.
- Engage leadership, key constituents, and the public across multiple sectors to take action and design policies that improve the health and well-being of all.

From U.S. Department of Health & Human Services, 2019. Available at www.healthypeople.gov.

VULNERABILITY

Vulnerability is defined as susceptibility to actual or potential stressors that may lead to an adverse effect. According to the WHO (n.d.), vulnerability is the degree to which an individual is "unable to anticipate, cope with, resist, or recover from potential or actual stressors." Vulnerable populations are typically considered to be those that are at greater risk for poor health status and that have poor access to health care. The definition applies to populations too.

Limitations in physical resources, environmental resources, personal resources (or human capital), and biopsychosocial resources (e.g., the presence of illness, genetic predispositions) combine to cause vulnerability (Aday, 2001; Leight, 2003). Poverty, limited social support, and working in a hazardous environment are examples of limitations in physical and environmental resources. People with pre-existing illnesses, such as those with communicable or infectious diseases or chronic illnesses such as cancer, heart disease, or chronic airway disease, have less physical ability to cope with stress than those without such physical problems. **Human capital** refers to all of the strengths, knowledge, and skills that enable a person to live a productive, happy life. People with little education have less human capital because their choices are more limited than those of people with higher levels of education.

The interaction among many variables causes a more powerful impact that predisposes vulnerable individuals to illness and injury. Risks come from environmental hazards (e.g., lead exposure from lead water pipes, lead-based paint from peeling walls, or paint used in toy manufacturing and melamine added to milk supplies), social hazards (e.g., crime, violence), personal behavior (e.g., diet, exercise habits, smoking), or biological or genetic makeup (e.g., congenital addiction, compromised immune status). Members of vulnerable populations often have multiple illnesses, with each affecting the other. Some members of vulnerable populations do not succumb to the health risks that impinge on them. It is important to learn what factors help these people to resist, or have **resilience** to, the effects of vulnerability. Vulnerability is a global concern, with different populations being more vulnerable in different countries.

Vulnerable people are at greater risk for poor health status. Risk is an epidemiologic term indicating that some people have a higher probability of illness than others. In the *epidemiologic triangle* as shown in Chapter 13) the agent, host, and environment interact to produce illness or poor health. This multifactor perspective aligns well with models that depict health as a result of complex personal and other environmental factors. *The natural history of disease model* explains how certain aspects of physiology and the environment, including personal habits, social environment, and physical environment, make it more likely that a person will develop particular health problems (USDHHS-CDC, n.d.b). See Chapter 13 for more information on the natural history of disease model. *The web of causation model* (USDHHS-CDC, n.d.c) can be used to depict vulnerability and risk. Chapter 12 discusses the web of causation. Many factors increase a person's vulnerability such as the individual's living conditions, poor nutrition, and likely other factors. Vulnerability refers to general conditions such as being poor or afflicted with a stigmatizing disease such as human immunodeficiency virus (HIV)/acquired immunodeficiency syndrome (AIDs) or mental illness. In contrast risk refers to exposure to a specific stressor.

Age imposes vulnerabilities. People at both ends of the life continuum are less able to physiologically adapt to stressors. For example, children who survive disasters may experience difficulties in later life if they do not receive adequate counseling. Examples of protective social factors include social support, self-esteem, and self-efficacy (thinking you can handle situations and cope) (Braveman & Gottlieb, 2014). Specifically, higher levels of confidence in one's ability or internal locus of control appear to protect children (particularly adolescents) from the negative effects of disaster and trauma. Persons with an internal locus of control believe that they control their behavior and do not depend entirely on external people, events, or forces to control behavior. It is the person's perception of his or her level of personal control that influences the person's decisions. Persons with a high level of internal locus of control are more likely to participate in health screenings and take responsibility for their health. That is, they believe they can control to some extent their health outcomes. For example, a woman with a high internal locus of control would participate regularly in yoga and exercise classes to increase flexibility and build strength to preserve her bone and muscle tone. Vulnerable population groups often develop an external locus of control. They may believe that events are outside their control and result from bad luck or fate. People with an external locus of control have more difficulty taking action or seeking care for health problems. They may minimize the value of health promotion or illness prevention because they do not think they have control over their health destinies. Also, people who have been abused or have experienced chronic stress may have used up a lot of the reserves that others would normally have for coping with new forms of stress.

Elderly individuals are more likely to develop active infections from communicable diseases such as the flu or pneumonia and generally have more difficulty recovering from infectious processes than younger people because of their less effective immune systems. Older people also may be more vulnerable to safety threats and loss of independence because of their age, multiple chronic illnesses, and impaired mobility.

There is often a cycle to vulnerability. Predisposing factors that lead to poor health and other outcomes can exacerbate predisposing factors, creating an additive effect. Vulnerability is associated with a heavy stress load, which creates yet another barrier to the attainment of good health. Fig. 31.3 is an illustration of a cycle of vulnerability related to homelessness.

Differences in mortality among homeless individuals illustrate how additive effects worsen outcomes and provide insight into the value of interventions designed to break the cycle, such as the Housing First initiative. Mortality rates among unsheltered homeless people are 3 times higher than people who were sheltered and 10 times higher than the general population (Roncarati et al., 2018).

Vulnerability should be considered at two levels, the individual and aggregate levels. Nurses, including public health nurses, care for both individuals and groups or populations. Group are aggregates of individuals. It is important that we not stereotype individuals based on group affiliation or characteristics. Being a member of a vulnerable group does not necessarily make an individual vulnerable. Conversely, individuals can be vulnerable even if they are not members of a vulnerable group (deChesnay, 2016).

Chronic stress can also contribute to vulnerability. Chronic stress associated with marginalization, adverse childhood experiences (ACEs), poverty, unemployment, poor education, and many other factors can lead to maladaptive physical responses and diseases (Lathrop, 2013).

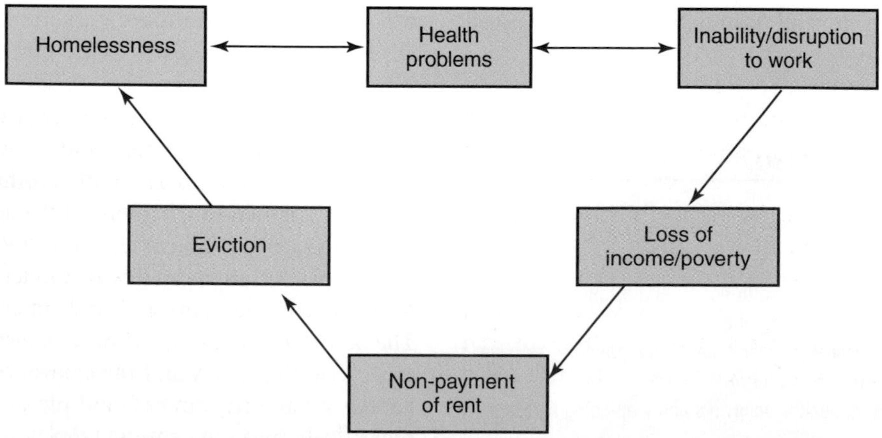

Fig. 31.3 A vicious cycle of vulnerability. (Source: Coumarelos C, Pleasence P, Wei Z: *Law and disorders: illness/disability and the experience of everyday problems involving the law*, Justice issues, no. 17, Law and Justice Foundation of NSW, Sydney. http://www.lawfoundation.net.au/ljf/site/articleIDs/187BFC9DE888BE81CA257BEA0019ECDF/$file/JI17_LawAndDisorders_FINAL_web.pdf.)

Marginalization

Vulnerable people and populations are in a marginalized, disadvantaged, or disenfranchised position. Marginalization results when people or populations are relegated to a position on the periphery of society where they have diminished importance, influence, or power. Marginalization is both a cause and outcome of vulnerability. The likelihood of developing health problems and having worse outcomes among vulnerable people and groups is higher because of general societal and environmental factors and increased exposure to risks.

Marginalized people are disconnected from mainstream society, lacking emotional ties to any group or with the larger society. Some groups such as the poor, the homeless, and migrant workers are "invisible" to society as a whole and tend to be forgotten in health and social planning. Vulnerable populations are at risk for disenfranchisement because their social supports are often weak, as are their linkages to formal community organizations such as churches, schools, and other types of social organizations. They also may have few informal sources of support, such as family, friends, and neighbors. In many ways, vulnerable groups have limited control over potential and actual health needs. In many communities, these groups are in the minority and disadvantaged because typical health planning focuses on the majority. Disadvantage also results from lack of resources that others may take for granted. Vulnerable population groups have limited social and economic resources with which to manage their health care. For example, women may endure domestic violence rather than risk losing a place for them and their children to live. Women who are among the working poor are more likely to become homeless when they leave an abusive partner. They may not be able to pay for a place to live when they lose their partner's income.

ACEs

ACEs include emotional, physical, and sexual abuse; emotional and physical neglect; mother treated violently; household substance abuse and mental illness; parental separation or divorce; and an incarcerated household member (AAP, 2014). ACEs exert negative impacts via a number of mechanisms, including disrupted neurodevelopment; social, emotional, and cognitive impairment; adoption of risky behaviors; disease; disability; social problems; and premature death (USDHHS-CDC, n.d.d).

Researchers studying ACEs conceptualized stress arrayed on a continuum. There are three major types of stress: (1) positive stress, which comes from short-lived adverse events and which children can manage with the help of supportive adults; (2) tolerable stress, which is more intense but still short-lived, such as stress arising from a natural disaster or frightening accident; or (3) toxic stress, which results from intense adverse experiences sustained over time. Stress conferred by ACEs can become toxic. Toxic stress can be profoundly destructive and last a lifetime (AAP, 2014).

Poverty

Poverty is one of the most deeply rooted and significant contributors to poor health and disparities. Adequate income facilitates (buys) access to resources that support a healthier life, including safe housing and neighborhoods, clean air and water, and nutritious food to eat. Low income is associated with low life expectancy. Someone born in 1960 in the lowest income quintile can expect to live until age 76. In contrast, the life expectancy of those in the highest quintile is 89 years (Stein & Galea, 2018a).

People who are poor are more likely to live in hazardous environments that are overcrowded and have inadequate sanitation, work in high-risk jobs, have less nutritious diets, and have multiple stressors, because they do not have the extra resources to manage unexpected crises and may not even have adequate resources to manage daily life. Poverty often reduces an individual's access to health care. In the developed countries of the world, this is more likely to be a problem for those just above the poverty line, who are not eligible for public support, whereas in developing countries poverty is correlated with decreased access to health care. The chronic stress of factors such as poverty, unemployment, and poor education can lead to maladaptive physical responses and disease (Lathrop, 2013).

The U.S. Census Bureau (Semega et al., 2017) reported that in 2016, 40.6 million Americans, or 12.7 percent, lived in poverty. The South has the highest rate of poverty (14.1 percent). Poverty rates are highest in rural areas. A review of poverty trends reveals other troubling disparities. Metrics that illustrate this point include the following: (1) pre-tax income for the poorest Americans has held steady for the past 40 years, but after tax income has dropped due to increasing taxes, which disproportionately burden poor people (Stein & Galea, 2018b); (2) income inequality has grown (Stein & Sandro, 2018)—the disparity between the wealthiest Americans and everyone else multiplied by 27 percent between 1970 and 2016 (Kochar & Cilluffo, 2018); (3) the national minimum wage is stuck at $7.25 per hour, an amount that traps many full-time workers, depending on family size, below the wage needed to be above the federal poverty level (Koucher & Cilluffo, 2018); and (5) the real value of the current minimum wage has declined (Center for Poverty Research, 2018). The major Organisation for Economic Co-Operation and Development (OECD) countries spend on average of $1.70 for social services for every $1.00 on health services. The United States spends 56 cents per health care dollar (Butler, 2016), and there are calls from some federal policy makers to decrease social safety net spending.

Poverty among children is a particular concern. Poverty grew among children from 14 percent in 1969 to 21 percent in 2014 (AEI/Brookings, 2015). A May 2018 Save the Children report demonstrates how hard poverty hits children, particularly those who live in rural areas and the South. In the United States, 19.5 percent of children live in poverty. In rural America, 23.5 percent of children live in poverty (compared to 18.8 percent of urban children). Five states in the United States, all but one in the Southeast, have rural child poverty rates at or above 33 percent.

Children are particularly susceptible to the effects of poverty. Healthy development and learning are negatively impacted by poverty, and poverty increases a child's exposure to risk. The effects of childhood poverty can persist across the life span and be conferred to the next generation (Save the Children, 2018).

Poverty is both a cause and an outcome of poor health. Poor health often results in lost labor income that can result in poverty, and poverty is linked with poorer health outcomes. This is another example the cyclic nature of vulnerability.

Addressing poverty will require broad-based and sustained initiatives addressing family composition (more households headed by single women are in poverty than two-parent households), work and wages, and education (AEI/Brookings, 2015). The need for this type of approach that addresses deep-rooted social problems to reduce disparities and improve health is the impetus for the *Health in All Policies* initiative (Rudolph et al., 2013).

Vulnerable Populations

A population is deemed vulnerable based on status that is unfavorable compared to other groups (deChesnay, 2016). Select examples of vulnerable populations of concern to nurses are persons who are poor, homeless, displaced, victims of abuse or neglect, rural residents, incarcerated, or have special needs or are suffering from stigmatizing diseases such as mental illness, addiction disorders, and HIV/AIDS. Other vulnerable populations include certain groups of children, pregnant teens, migrant workers, immigrants, refugees, and people at risk for infectious or communicable diseases, including persons who are HIV positive or have hepatitis B virus (HBV) or sexually transmitted diseases (STDs).

Resiliency and Hope

Objections have been raised about the use of the term *social determinants of health.* The objections stem from the connotation of the term *determinant.* The word implies that individual and population resiliency and recovery are not possible. Adopting a deterministic rather than probabilistic view of social and other influences allows us to understand important interactions that can explain to whom a factor matters most or least and the environmental conditions that interact to impact outcomes and to what degree (Simon, 2017). Useful nursing interventions to increase resilience include case finding, health education, care coordination, and policy making related to improving health for vulnerable populations.

REDUCING DISPARITIES AND IMPROVING POPULATION HEALTH OUTCOMES

Working with vulnerable populations to reduce disparities and improve population health outcomes requires informed strategies and practices. These strategies must rely on the latest evidence and be patient- and population-centric and sensitive. It is important that nurses honor the individuals and populations they work with and advocate for changes that reduce inequities, disparities, marginalization, and stigmata and improve health. Nurses have long been leaders in efforts to enhance equity.

Social-Ecological Model

The social-ecological model (SEM) is a theory-based framework that promotes understanding of the interaction of personal, social, and environmental factors that shape behavior and ultimately health (Unicef, 2009; Wendell et al., 2017). The SEM is derived from a social ecology perspective that seeks explanations for "how individuals and their environments mutually affect each other" (Wendell et al., 2017). The SEM is a tool for promoting the overarching goals which have been developed for *Healthy People 2030.* The SEM facilitates understanding of the upstream cause of health disparities. Multilevel interventions are more effective and sustainable.

The SEM includes five levels: individual, interpersonal, community, organization, and policy environment (Fig. 31.4.). Each of these levels is discussed in Table 31.2.

Advocacy and Policy Making As Caring

Advocating on behalf of individuals and populations and being engaged in policy making are essential nursing roles. Advocacy refers to actions taken on behalf of another.

Advocacy and policy involvement extend the caring ethos of nursing. A profession that establishes a relationship with people or groups, based on a social contract, like nursing, is morally obligated to uphold justice within its domain (Ballou, 2000; Fawcett & Russell, 2001). Nurses may function as advocates for vulnerable populations by working for the passage and implementation of policies that lead to improved public health services for these populations. For example, a nurse may serve on a local coalition for uninsured people, and another may work to develop a plan for sharing the provision of free or low-cost health care by local health care organizations and providers.

Social justice includes the concepts of *egalitarianism* and *equality.* Braveman (2014) says that at the heart of social justice is "justice with respect to the treatment of more advantaged versus less advantaged socioeconomic groups when it comes to health and health care" (p. 129). A society that subscribes to the concept of social justice would be one that values equality and recognizes the worth of all members of that society. Such a society would provide humane care and social supports for all people. Nurses who function in advocacy roles and facilitate change in public policy are intervening to promote social justice.

Nurses can be advocates for policy changes to improve social, economic, and environmental factors that predispose vulnerable populations to poor health. The legacy of the nursing profession is replete with exemplary nursing leaders who fulfilled the moral obligation to advocate on behalf of individuals and groups and understand and be involved in policy making to advance health equity.

Public Policies Advancing Health

Health in All Policies is a strategy designed to influence health and equity by addressing social determinants of health in policy.

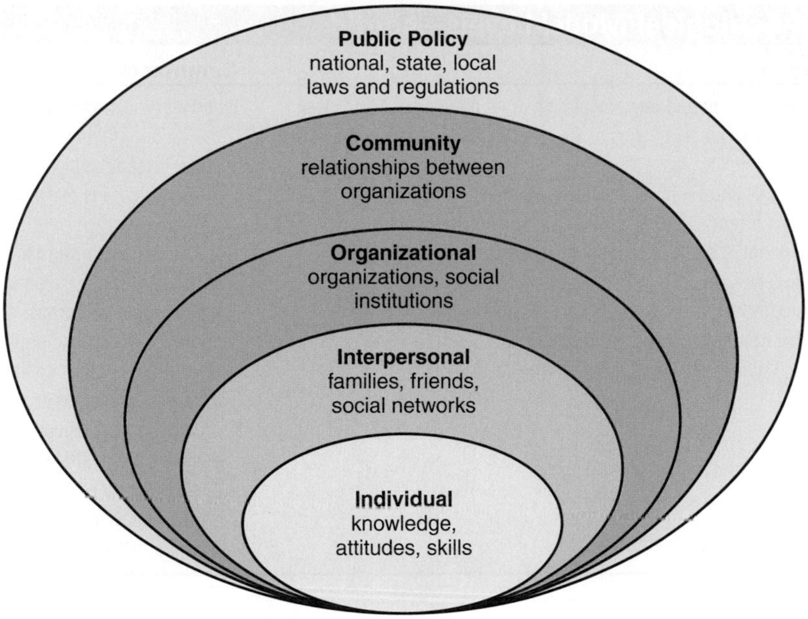

Fig. 31.4 Social-ecological model. (Modified from Centers for Disease Control and Prevention [CDC]: The social ecological model: a framework for prevention. Available at http://www.cdc.gov.)

TABLE 31.2 Social-Ecological Model Levels

Level	Description	Comments
Individual	Includes individual characteristics, traits, and identities and knowledge, attitudes, and behaviors that influence behavior change; examples: • Age • Developmental history • Education levels • Financial resources • History of abuse or trauma • Literacy • Racial and ethnic identity • Religious identity • Sexual orientation • Social status	Socioeconomic status is the most influential determinant of health. Poverty often is associated with lower educational attainment.
Interpersonal	Includes personal relationships and social networks and support systems that influence behavior and create circumstances that encourage or impede health attainment; examples: • Family • Friends • Partners • Peers • Formal and informal social networks • Co-workers • Religious networks • Customs, traditions	An individual's personal relationships and social networks have profound direct and indirect effects on health. There is mounting evidence of the adverse impact of social isolation on affected individuals and groups. The health impact of social isolation has been equated with smoking 15 cigarettes/day (Flowers et al., 2018).
Community	Includes relationships among organizations, institutions, and informational networks within a defined boundary that influence behavior of a population and their values, cultures, and customs; examples: • Built environment • Community leaders • Local businesses • Neighborhoods • Schools • Stigma • Transportation • Workplaces	The rate of mental illness among young people of color is similar to that of white, young adults, but they are less likely to be diagnosed or seek help (Primm, 2018).

Continued

TABLE 31.2 Social-Ecological Model Levels—cont'd

Level	Description	Comments
Organization	Includes development and implementation of regulations and rules that enable or thwart certain behaviors, as well as enforcement of regulation and rules; examples: • Organizations and social institutions with policies, rules, and regulations affecting the availability of support and services	National discussions about how to address gun violence in the United States is increasingly centered on the organizational level as arming school teachers is debated and large retail businesses make decisions about whether or not to sell guns.
Policy	Includes national, state, and local governmental laws, policies, and regulations; includes: • Access to prevention and health care resources • Allocation of resources and policy priorities • Social and other policies that promote or inhibit equity	Rural Americans often face challenges in accessing health care. Increasingly telehealth services are seen as one way to improve access, address health care needs, and improve patient and population health outcomes. However, the requisite broadband availability and access is frequently deficient in rural areas, which impedes the provisions of telehealth services. Policy can be used to increase the availability of broadband access in rural areas. Improved broadband access will have direct impact on telehealth services and indirect positive employment benefits.

There are numerous governmental policies that have improved conditions of vulnerable people and populations. The Seattle/King County Health Department is facilitating cross-sectoral partnerships with planning, transportation, and housing officials to integrate efforts and create synergies to enhance equity and health. Examples of recent initiatives include (1) inclusion of health-based metrics and objectives in city and county land use and transportation plans, (2) educational initiatives to improve outcomes in low-income and migrant populations and reduce the number of students expelled from school, and (3) better opportunities for physical activity in low-income neighborhoods by building trails (Wernham & Teutsch, 2014).

There are numerous governmental policies that have improved conditions and outcomes for vulnerable populations. The Social Security Act of 1935, a federal law, was designed to ensure a minimal level of support for people at risk for problems from inadequate financial resources. The Social Security Amendments of 1965 created Medicare and Medicaid to address the health care needs of older adults, people living in poverty, and disabled people. Poverty among elderly Americans declined from 35 percent in 1959 to 10 percent in 2014, in large part because of Medicare (AEI/Brookings, 2015).

Since the enactment of the Affordable Care Act in 2010, there have been states that have expanded existing Medicaid programs and other states that have not pursued expansion. This scenario has created natural experiments that allow us to look at whether Medicaid improves health outcomes. The evidence is mounting in states that have expanded Medicaid that Medicaid coverage does improve outcomes. Improvements seen in Medicaid expansion states include (1) significant increases in rates of cancer diagnoses, especially early-stage diagnosis rates, (2) increased probability of early, uncomplicated patient presentations for five common surgical procedures, (3) improvements in access to medications and other treatments for people with behavioral and mental health conditions, (4) declines in hospital lengths-of-stay, and (5) improved hypertension control (Antonisse et al., 2018).

Nursing Approaches to Advance Health Equity

Nurses have a rich legacy of promoting health equity. Florence Nightingale understood that the physical and social environments influenced the health of patients and worked hard to introduce improvements in both domains with good results. Lillian Wald, the founder of the Henry Street Settlement and mother of modern public health nursing, provided nursing care and education to the community through health promotion, including education, modification of the environment, and disease control. Dorthea Dix was a staunch advocate for indigent, mentally ill individuals whose lobbying was instrumental in policies that established mental asylums. Mary Breckenridge established the Frontier Nursing Service that was successful in improving the health of poor women and children in rural Kentucky.

There is a trend toward providing more comprehensive, family-centered services when treating vulnerable population groups. It is important to provide comprehensive, family-centered, "one-stop" services. Providing multiple services during a single clinic visit is an example of one-stop services. If social assistance and economic assistance are provided and included in interdisciplinary treatment plans, services can be more responsive to the combined effects of social and economic stressors on the health of special population groups. This situation is sometimes referred to as providing **wrap-around services**, in which comprehensive health services are available and social and economic services are "wrapped around" these services. Although this is an excellent approach to care, it is not available in all or even most areas in the United States.

It is helpful to provide comprehensive services in locations where people live and work, including schools, churches, neighborhoods, and workplaces. *Comprehensive services* are health services that focus on more than one health problem or concern. For example, some nurses use stationary or mobile outreach clinics to provide a wide array of health promotion, illness prevention, and illness management services in migrant camps, schools, and local communities. A single client visit may focus on an acute health problem such as influenza, but it also may include health education about diet and exercise, counseling for smoking cessation, and a follow-up appointment for immunizations once the influenza is over. The shift away from hospital-based care includes a renewed commitment to the public health services that vulnerable populations need to prevent illness and promote health, such as reductions of environmental hazards and violence and assurance of safe food and water.

Referring clients to community agencies involves much more than simply making a phone call or completing a form. Nurses should make certain that the agency to which they refer a client is the right one to meet that client's needs. Nurses can do more harm than good by referring a stressed, discouraged client to an agency from which the client is not really eligible to receive services. Nurses should help the client learn how to get the most from the referral. Nurses are critical to vulnerable populations.

Nurses are critical safety net providers. Safety net health providers deliver essential primary care to marginalized populations such as poor people, minority groups, homeless and uninsured people, and groups with stigmatizing illnesses and conditions such as HIV/AIDS and behavioral, mental health, and addiction disorders. Safety net facilities and providers have been referred to as *providers of last resort.*

One successful model that is associated with bridging gaps in health and health care is nurse-managed health centers (NMHCs). NMHCs are community-based primary care clinics and centers led by advanced practice registered nurses (APRNs). The hallmarks of NMHCs are the emphasis on health education and promotion, disease prevention, and the focus on underserved populations, including populations that have low incomes, may be members of minority groups, may be homeless, or may lack adequate insurance coverage, as well as other groups of vulnerable people. NMHCs are generally non-profit and usually employ a sliding scale fee schedule (Campaign for Action, 2010). NMHCs provide comprehensive care that includes referrals, follow-up, and advocacy.

There is growing recognition of the importance of the role of the registered nurse (RN) in community-based and primary care. Roles for RNs include (1) protocol-based management of chronic disease, (2) leading complex care teams, (3) care coordination, (4) management of common episodic conditions using protocols, and (5) prevention, health education/promotion, and family support (Bodenheimer & Mason, 2017).

QSEN FOCUS ON QUALITY AND SAFETY EDUCATION FOR NURSES

Targeted Competency: Quality Improvement

Use data to monitor the outcomes of care processes and use improvement methods to design and test changes to continuously improve the quality and safety of health care systems.

Important aspects of quality improvement include:

- **Knowledge:** Explain the importance of variation and measurement in assessing quality of care.
- **Skills:** Use quality measures to understand performance.
- **Attitudes:** Value measurement and its role in good client care.

Quality Improvement Question

Examine health statistics and demographic data in your geographic area to determine which vulnerable groups are predominant. Look on the web for examples of agencies you think provide services to these vulnerable groups. If the agency has a web page, read about the target population they serve, the types of services they provide, and how they are reimbursed for services. Learn about different agencies and share results during class. On the basis of your findings, identify gaps or overlaps in services provided to vulnerable groups in your community. Which data do these agencies collect to demonstrate the efficacy of their services? How could you deal with these gaps and overlaps to help clients receive needed services?

Prepared by Gail Armstrong, PhD, DNP, ACNS-BC, CNE, Associate Professor, University of Colorado Denver College of Nursing.

It is important for nurses to provide culturally and linguistically appropriate health care. *Linguistically appropriate health care* means communicating health-related information in the recipient's primary language when possible and always in a language the recipient can understand. It also means using words that the recipient can understand. The factors that predispose people to vulnerability and the outcomes of vulnerability create a cycle in which the outcomes reinforce the predisposing factors, leading to more negative outcomes. Unless the cycle is broken, it is difficult for vulnerable populations to improve their health. Nurses can identify areas in which they can work with vulnerable populations to break the cycle. The nursing process guides nurses in assessing vulnerable individuals, families, groups, and communities; developing nursing diagnoses of their strengths and needs; planning and implementing appropriate therapeutic nursing interventions in partnership with vulnerable clients; and evaluating the effectiveness of interventions.

It is also important to consider that there can be ethical dilemmas associated with working with vulnerable populations. Ethical dilemmas that arose in an academic-community partnership designed to learn about the experiences of undocumented immigrants who sought health care in Toronto, Canada, are described in the Evidence-Based Practice box.

In some situations, the nurse works with individual clients. The nurse also develops programs and policies for populations of vulnerable persons. In both examples, planning and

EVIDENCE-BASED PRACTICE

Using an academic-community partnership, a study was conducted to understand the experiences of undocumented immigrants seeking health care in Toronto, Canada. A team composed of the principal investigator, three researchers, and a group of nine undocumented immigrants used a community-based participatory research process to examine the experiences of the immigrants. Representatives from the community-based organization (CBO) had a pre-existing, strong, and trusting relationship with the study participants. Two ethical dilemmas arose. Two of the participants thought that the researcher who was asking them questions was a spy for the Canadian Border Services Agency (CBSA). These two participants had not attended the orientation session. They were concerned when asked about their immigration status during the informed consent process. To solve this dilemma, the team decided that the CBO worker should ask for the informed consent because trust was present in that relationship. A second ethical dilemma arose when one participant told the principal investigator (PI) that she was suicidal. The PI was unprepared to deal with this information, and the team decided that in future interviews the PI would tell the participants that she was not a mental health professional. They also determined that the team needed to have access to a mental health professional in the event they learned information that needed follow-up.

Nurse Use

When ethical dilemmas arise in either research or client care, it is essential to identify them and immediately try to seek a solution. This study is a good example of how the team learned a great deal from their project. They put the project on hold in order to reflect, analyze, synthesize, and evaluate the facts.

Data from Campbell-Page RM, Shaw-Ridley MS: Managing ethical dilemmas in community-based participatory research with vulnerable populations. *Health Promot Pract* 17:485-490, 2013.

implementing care for members of vulnerable populations involve partnerships between the nurse and client and build on careful assessment. Nurses need to avoid directing and controlling clients' care because this might interfere with their being able to establish a trusting relationship and may inadvertently foster a cycle of dependency and lack of personal health control. The most important initial step is for nurses to demonstrate they are trustworthy and dependable. For example, nurses who work in a community clinic for substance abusers must overcome any suspicion that clients may have of them and eliminate any fears clients may have of being manipulated.

Nurses working with vulnerable populations may fill numerous roles, including those listed in Box 31.1. They identify vulnerable individuals and families through outreach and case finding. They encourage vulnerable groups to obtain health services, and they develop programs that respond to their needs. Nurses teach vulnerable individuals, families, and groups strategies to prevent illness and promote health. They counsel clients about ways to increase their sense of personal power and help them identify strengths and resources. They provide direct care to clients and families in a variety of settings, including storefront clinics, mobile clinics, shelters, homes, neighborhoods, worksites, churches, and schools.

BOX 31.1 Nursing Roles When Working With Vulnerable Population Groups

Case manager
Health educator
Counselor
Direct care provider
Population health advocate
Community assessor and developer
Monitor and evaluate care
Advocate
Health program planner and implementer
Participant in developing policies

CHECK YOUR PRACTICE

If you were a nurse working with families who are picking peaches in a southern state and one of the adults steps on a rusty nail, what actions would you take? What would your first action be? What additional actions might you take to assure this client of the best outcome?

The following are some examples of care to clients, families, and groups: (1) a nurse in a mobile migrant clinic might administer a tetanus booster to a client who has been injured by a piece of farm machinery and may also check that client's blood pressure and cholesterol level during the same visit; (2) a home health nurse seeing a family referred by the courts for child abuse may weigh the child, conduct a nutritional assessment, and help the family learn how to manage anger and disciplinary problems; (3) a nurse working in a school-based clinic may lead a support group for pregnant adolescents and conduct a birthing class; and (4) a nurse may work with people being treated for TB to monitor drug treatment compliance and ensure that they complete their full course of therapy.

LINKING CONTENT TO PRACTICE

Generalist and staff public health nurses should have competencies in eight domains as defined by the Quad Council Coalition of Public Health Nursing Organizations (2018). Each of the eight competencies is important in working with vulnerable populations. Public health nurses working with vulnerable populations should be able to analyze data and determine when a problem exists with an individual and within a vulnerable population group. They should be able to identify options for programs or policies that could be helpful to these populations and communicate their ideas and recommendations clearly. Public health nurses should be able to provide culturally competent interventions for individuals or for vulnerable populations. As an example, a public health nurse should be able to collect and analyze data related to the prevalence of violence among women in the community; identify key stakeholders; evaluate the cultural preferences of the population; work with others to develop a program to meet a defined need within this population, including preparation of a basic budget for the program; and ensure that the program is culturally appropriate for the population. The Council on Linkages Between Academia and Public Health Practice (2014) published a similar list for public health professionals, including but not limited to public health nurses. This list includes an emphasis on evaluation and ongoing improvement of programs. In this example, the nurse would evaluate the program developed for women who are victims of violence and work with others to develop and implement quality improvements on a regular basis.

Public health nurses also serve as population health advocates and work with local, state, or national groups to develop and implement policies that promote health. They also collaborate with community members and serve as community assessors and developers, and they monitor and evaluate care and health programs. Nurses often function as case managers for vulnerable clients, making referrals and linking them to community services. **Case management** services are especially important for vulnerable persons because they often do not have the ability or resources to make their own arrangements. They may not be able to speak the language, or they may be unable to navigate the complex telephone systems that many agencies establish. Nurses also serve as advocates when they refer clients to other agencies, work with others to develop health programs, and influence legislation and health policies that affect vulnerable populations.

The nature of nurses' roles varies depending on whether the client is a single person, a family, or a group. For example, a nurse might teach an HIV-positive client about the need for prevention of opportunistic infections, may help a family with an HIV-positive member understand myths about transmission of HIV, or may work with a community group concerned about HIV transmission among students. In each case, the nurse teaches individuals how to prevent infectious and communicable diseases. The size of the group and the teaching method for each group differ.

Health education is often used in working with vulnerable populations. The nurse should teach members of populations with low educational levels what they need to do to promote health and prevent illness rather than directing health education to groups that the nurse thinks might be at high risk even though there is no evidence to support the perception.

Levels of Prevention

Healthy People 2020 (USDHHS, 2010) objectives emphasize improving health by modifying the individual, social, and environmental determinants of health. One way to do this is for vulnerable individuals to have a primary care provider who both coordinates health services for them and provides their preventive services. This primary care provider may be an advanced practice nurse or a primary care physician. Another approach is for a nurse to serve as a case manager for vulnerable clients and, again, coordinate services and provide illness prevention and health promotion services. See the Levels of Prevention box for an example that relates to different vulnerable populations.

One example of primary prevention is to give influenza vaccinations to vulnerable populations that are immunocompromised (unless contraindicated). Secondary prevention is seen in conducting screening clinics for vulnerable populations. For example, nurses who work in homeless shelters, prisons, migrant camps, and substance abuse treatment facilities should know that these groups are at high risk for acquiring communicable diseases. Both clients and staff need routine screening for TB. Screening homeless adults and providing isoniazid to those who test positive for TB are examples of secondary prevention. An example of tertiary prevention is conducting a therapy group with the residents of a group home for severely mentally ill adults. Nurses who work with abused women to help them enhance their levels of self-esteem are also providing tertiary preventive activities.

LEVELS OF PREVENTION

Levels of Prevention Related to Vulnerable Populations

Primary	Secondary	Tertiary
• Provide culturally and economically sensitive health teaching about balanced diet and exercise. • Develop a portable immunization chart, such as a wallet card, that mobile population groups such as the homeless and migrant workers can carry with them.	• Conduct screening clinics to assess for things such as obesity, diabetes, heart disease, or tuberculosis (TB). • Develop a way for homeless individuals to read their TB skin test, if necessary, and to transfer the results back to the facility at which the skin test was administered.	• Develop community-based exercise programs for people identified as obese or who have increased blood pressure or increased blood glucose. • Provide directly observed medication therapy for people with active TB.

ASSESSMENT ISSUES

Nurses who work with vulnerable populations need good assessment skills, current knowledge of available resources, and the ability to plan care based on client needs and receptivity to help. They also need to be able to show respect for the client. The How To box entitled "Assess Members of Vulnerable Population Groups" lists guidelines for assessing members of vulnerable population groups.

HOW TO Assess Members of Vulnerable Population Groups

Setting the Stage

- Create a comfortable, nonthreatening environment.
- Learn as much as you can about the culture of the clients you work with so that you will understand cultural practices and values that may influence their health care practices.
- Provide a culturally competent assessment by understanding the meaning of language and nonverbal behavior in the client's culture.
- Be sensitive to the fact that the individual or family you are assessing may have other priorities that are more important to them. These might include financial or legal problems. You may need to give them some tangible help with their most pressing priority before you will be able to address issues that are more traditionally thought of as health concerns.
- Collaborate with others as appropriate; you should not provide financial or legal advice. However, you should make sure to connect your client with someone who can and will help them.

Nursing History of an Individual or Family

- You may have only one opportunity to work with a vulnerable person or family. Try to complete a history that will provide all the essential information you need to help the individual or family on that day. This means that you will have to organize in your mind exactly what you need to ask. You should also understand why you need any information that you gather.

- It will help to use a comprehensive assessment form that has been modified to focus on the special needs of the vulnerable population group with whom you work. However, be flexible. With some clients, it will be both impractical and unethical to cover all questions on a comprehensive form. If you know that you are likely to see the client again, ask the less pressing questions at the next visit.
- Be sure to include questions about social support, economic status, resources for health care, developmental issues, current health problems, medications, and how the person or family manages their health status. Your goal is to obtain information that will enable you to provide family-centered care.
- Determine whether the individual has any condition that compromises his or her immune status, such as AIDS, or if the individual is undergoing therapy that would result in immunodeficiency, such as cancer chemotherapy.

Physical Examination or Home Assessment

- Again, complete as thorough a physical examination (on an individual) or home assessment as you can. Keep in mind that you should collect only data for which you have a use.
- Be alert for indications of physical abuse, substance use (e.g., needle marks, nasal abnormalities), or neglect (e.g., underweight, inadequate clothing).
- You can assess a family's living environment using good observational skills. Does the family live in an insect- or rat-infested environment? Do they have running water, functioning plumbing, electricity, and a telephone?
- Is perishable food left sitting out on tables and countertops? Are bed linens reasonably clean? Is paint peeling on the walls and ceilings? Is ventilation adequate? Is the temperature of the home adequate? Is the family exposed to raw sewage or animal waste? Is the home adjacent to a busy highway, possibly exposing the family to high noise levels and automobile exhaust?

Because members of vulnerable populations often experience multiple stressors, assessment must balance the need to be comprehensive while focusing only on information that the nurse needs and the client is willing to provide. Remember to ask questions about the client's perceptions of his or her socioeconomic resources, including identifying people who can provide support and financial resources. Support from other people may include information, caregiving, emotional support, and help with instrumental activities of daily living, such as transportation, shopping, and babysitting. Financial resources may include the extent to which the client can pay for health services and medications, as well as questions about eligibility for third-party payment. The nurse should ask the client about the perceived adequacy of both formal and informal support networks.

When possible, assessment should include an evaluation of clients' preventive health needs, including age-appropriate screening tests such as immunization status, blood pressure, weight, serum cholesterol, Papanicolaou (Pap) smears, breast examinations, mammograms, prostate examinations, glaucoma screening, and dental evaluations. It may be necessary to make referrals for some of these tests. Assessment should also include preventive screening for physical health problems, for which certain vulnerable groups are at particularly high risk. For example, people who are HIV positive should be evaluated regularly for CD4 cell counts and common opportunistic infections, including TB and pneumonia. Intravenous drug users should be evaluated for HBV, including liver palpation and serum antigen tests as necessary. Alcoholic clients should also be asked about symptoms of liver disease and should be evaluated for jaundice and liver enlargement. Severely mentally ill clients should be assessed for the presence of tardive dyskinesia, indicating possible toxicity from their antipsychotic medications.

Vulnerable populations should be assessed for congenital and genetic predisposition to illness and either receive education and counseling as appropriate or be referred to other health professionals as necessary. For example, pregnant adolescents who are substance abusers should be referred to programs to help them quit using addictive substances during their pregnancies and, ideally, after delivery of their infants. Pregnant women older than 35 years should receive amniocentesis testing to determine whether genetic abnormalities exist in the fetus.

The nurse should also assess the amount of stress the person or family is having. Does the family have healthy coping skills and healthy family interaction? Are some family members able and willing to care for others? What is the level of mental health in each member? Also, are diet, exercise, and rest and sleep patterns conducive to good health?

The nurse should assess the living environment and neighborhood surroundings of vulnerable families and groups for environmental hazards such as lead-based paint, asbestos, water and air quality, industrial wastes, and the incidence of crime.

Planning and Implementing Care for Vulnerable Populations

Nurses who work in community settings may have considerable involvement with vulnerable populations. The relationship with the client will depend on the nature of the contact. Some will be seen in clinics and others in homes, schools, and at work. Regardless of the setting, the following key nursing actions should be used:

- **Create a trusting environment:** Trust is essential, because many of these individuals have previously been disappointed in their interactions with health care and social systems. It is important to follow through and do what you say you are going to do. If you do not know the answer to a question, the best reply is "I do not know, but I will try to find out."
- **Show respect, compassion, and concern:** Vulnerable people have been defeated again and again by life's circumstances. They may have reached a point at which they question whether they even deserve to get care. Listen carefully, because listening is a form of respect, as well as a way to gather information to plan care.
- **Do not make assumptions:** Assess each person and family. No two people or groups are alike.
- **Coordinate services and providers:** Getting health and social services is not always easy. Often people feel like they

are traveling through a maze. In most communities a large number of useful services exist. People who need them simply may not know how to find them. For example, people may need help finding a food bank or a free clinic or obtaining low-cost or free clothing through churches or in secondhand stores. Clients often need help in determining whether they meet the eligibility requirements. If gaps in service are found, nurses can work with others to try to get the needed services established. Care for vulnerable populations requires interprofessional collaboration to meet their multiple needs. For example, nurses can work with business and public health leaders to reduce hazardous exposures, develop accessible services, and improve working conditions for low-income employees (Lathrop, 2013). Nurses may need to work with lawmakers, union leaders, urban developers, business leaders, and a range of public health and other health care workers. The case study in Box 31.2 describes a situation in which a mother faced many obstacles in getting care for her three children.

- **Advocate for accessible health care services:** Vulnerable people have trouble getting access to services. Neighborhood clinics, mobile vans, and home visits can be valuable for them. Also, coordinating services at a central location is helpful. These multiservice centers can provide health care, social services, daycare, drug and alcohol recovery programs, and case management. When working with vulnerable populations, it is a good idea to arrange to have as many services as possible available in a single location and at convenient times. This "one-stop shopping" approach to care delivery is very helpful for populations experiencing multiple social, economic, and health-related stresses. Although it may seem difficult and costly to provide comprehensive services in one location, it may save money in the long run by preventing illness.

BOX 31.2 Case Study

Felicia is a 22-year-old single mother of three children whose primary source of income is Temporary Assistance for Needy Families (TANF). She is worried about the future because she will no longer be eligible for welfare by the end of the year. She has been unable to find a job that will pay enough for her to afford childcare. Her friend Maria said that Felicia and her children can stay in Maria's trailer for a short time, but Felicia is afraid that her only choice after that will be a shelter.

Felicia recently took all three children with her to the health department because 15-month-old Hector needed immunizations. Felicia was also concerned about 5-year-old Martina, who had had a fever of 100°F to 101°F on and off for the past month. Felicia and her friends in the trailer park think that some type of hazardous waste from the chemical plant next door to the park is making their children sick. Now that Martina was not feeling well, Felicia was particularly concerned. However, the health department nurse told her that no appointments were available that day and that she would need to bring Martina back to the clinic on the next day. Felicia left discouraged because it was so difficult for her to get all three children ready and on the bus to go to the health department, not to mention the expense. She thought maybe Martina just had a cold and she would wait a little longer before bringing her back. However, she wanted to take care of Martina's problem before losing her medical card. Felicia is desperate to find a way to manage her money problems and take care of her children.

- **Focus on prevention:** Use every opportunity to teach about preventive health care. Primary prevention may include child and adult immunizations and education about nutrition, foot care, safe sex, contraception, and the prevention of injuries or chronic illness. It also includes providing prophylactic anti-tuberculosis drug therapy for HIV-positive people who live in homeless shelters or giving flu vaccine to people who are immune-compromised or older than 65 years of age. Secondary prevention would include screening for health problems such as TB, diabetes, hypertension, foot problems, anemia, or drug use or abuse. People who spend time in homeless shelters, substance abuse treatment facilities, and prisons often get communicable diseases such as influenza, TB, and methicillin-resistant *Staphylococcus aureus* (MRSA). Nurses who work in these facilities should plan regular influenza vaccination clinics and TB screening clinics. When planning these clinics, nurses should work with local physicians to develop signed protocols and should plan ahead for problems related to the transient nature of the population. For example, nurses should develop a way for homeless individuals to read their TB skin test if necessary and transfer the results back to the facility where the skin test was administered. It is helpful to develop a portable immunization chart, such as a wallet card, that mobile population groups such as the homeless and migrant workers can carry with them.
- **Know when to "walk beside" the client and when to encourage the client to "walk ahead":** At times it is difficult to know when to do something for people and when to teach or encourage them to do for themselves. Nursing actions range from providing encouragement and support to providing information and active intervention. It is important to assess for the presence of strength and the ability to problem solve, cope, and access services. For example, a local hospital might provide free mammograms for women who cannot pay. The nurse would need to decide whether to schedule the appointments for clients or to give them the information and encourage them to do the scheduling.
- **Know what resources are available:** Be familiar with community agencies that offer health and social services to vulnerable populations. Also follow up after you make a referral to make sure the client was able to obtain the needed help. Examples of agencies found in most communities are health departments, community mental health centers, voluntary organizations such as the American Red Cross, missions, shelters, soup kitchens, food banks, nurse-managed or free clinics, social service agencies such as the Salvation Army or Travelers Aid, and church-sponsored health and social services.
- **Develop your own support network:** Working with vulnerable populations can be challenging, rewarding, and at times exhausting. Nurses need to find sources of support and strength. This can come from friends, colleagues, hobbies, exercise, poetry, music, and other sources.
- In addition to the nursing actions described, the How To box entitled "Intervene With Vulnerable Populations" summarizes goals and interventions and evaluates outcomes with vulnerable populations.

HOW TO Intervene With Vulnerable Populations

Goals

- Set reasonable goals based on the baseline data you collected. Focus on reducing disparities in health status among vulnerable populations.
- Work toward setting manageable goals with the client. Goals that seem unattainable may be discouraging.
- Set goals collaboratively with the client as a first step toward client empowerment.
- Set family-centered, culturally sensitive goals.

Interventions

- Set up outreach and case-finding programs to help increase access to health services by vulnerable populations.
- Do everything you can to minimize the "hassle factor" connected with the interventions you plan. Vulnerable groups do not have the extra energy, money, or time to cope with unnecessary waits, complicated treatment plans, or confusion. As your client's advocate, you should identify possible hassles and develop ways to avoid them. For example, this may include providing comprehensive services during a single encounter, rather than asking the client to return for multiple visits. Multiple visits for more specialized aspects of the client's needs, whether individual or family group, reinforce a perception that health care is fragmented and organized for the professional's convenience rather than that of the client.
- Work with clients to ensure that interventions are culturally sensitive and competent.
- Focus on teaching skills in health promotion and disease prevention. Also, teach clients how to be effective health care consumers. For example, role-play asking questions in a physician's office with a client.
- Help clients learn what to do if they cannot keep an appointment with a health care or social service professional.

Evaluating Outcomes

- It is often difficult for vulnerable clients to return for follow-up care. Help your client develop self-care strategies for evaluating outcomes. For example, teach homeless individuals how to read their own tuberculosis (TB) skin test, and give them a self-addressed, stamped card they can return by mail with the results.
- Remember to evaluate outcomes in terms of the goals you have mutually agreed on with the client. For example, one outcome for a homeless person receiving isoniazid therapy for TB might be that the person returns to the clinic daily for direct observation of compliance with the drug therapy.

In general, more agencies are needed that provide comprehensive services with nonrestrictive eligibility requirements. Communities often have many agencies that restrict eligibility to make it possible for more people to receive services. For example, shelters may prohibit people who have been drinking alcohol from staying overnight and limit the number of sequential nights a person can stay. Food banks usually limit the number of times a person can receive free food. Agencies are often very specialized as well. For vulnerable individuals and families, this means that they must go to several agencies to obtain services for which they qualify and that meet their health needs. This is tiring and discouraging, and people may forgo help because of these difficulties.

Nurses need to know about community agencies that offer various health and social services. It is important to follow-up with the client after a referral to ensure that the desired outcomes were achieved. Sometimes excellent community resources may be available but impractical because of transportation or reimbursement issues. Nurses can identify these potential problems by following through with referrals, and they can also work with other team members to make referrals as convenient and realistic as possible. Although clients with social problems such as financial needs should be referred to social workers, it is useful for nurses to understand the close connections between health and social problems and know how to work effectively with other professionals. A list of community resources can often be found in the telephone directory or online. The following are examples of agency resources found in most communities:

- Health departments
- Community mental health centers
- American Red Cross and other voluntary organizations
- Food and clothing banks
- Missions and shelters
- Nurse-managed clinics
- Social service agencies such as Travelers Aid and the Salvation Army
- Church-sponsored health and service assistance
- Free clinics and other community services

Nurses who work with vulnerable populations often need to coordinate services across multiple agencies for members of these groups. It is helpful to have a strong professional network of people who work in other agencies. Effective professional networks make it easier to coordinate care smoothly and in ways that do not add to clients' stress. Nurses can develop strong networks by participating in community coalitions and attending professional meetings. When making referrals to other agencies, a phone call can be a helpful way to obtain information that the client will need for the visit. When possible, having an interdisciplinary, interagency team plan care for clients at high risk for health problems is effective. Obtain the clients' written and informed consent before engaging in this kind of planning because of confidentiality issues. The following list of tips can be helpful:

- Involve clients in making decisions about the kinds of services they are willing and able to use.
- Work with community coalitions to coordinate services for targeted vulnerable populations.
- Collaborate with legal counsel from the agencies involved in the coalitions to ensure that legal and ethical issues related to care coordination have been properly addressed. Examples of issues to address include privacy and security of clinical data and ensuring compliance with the Health Insurance Portability and Accountability Act of 1996 (HIPAA), contractual provisions for coordinating care across agencies, and consent to treatment from multiple agencies.
- Develop policies and protocols for making referrals, following up on referrals, and ensuring that clients receiving care from multiple agencies experience the process as smooth and seamless. The following discussion and box provide information about how to use case management with vulnerable groups.

HOW TO Use Case Management in Working With Vulnerable Populations

- Know available services and resources.
- Find out what is missing; look for creative solutions.
- Use your clinical skills.
- Develop long-term relationships with the families you serve.
- Strengthen the family's coping and survival skills and resourcefulness.
- Be the roadmap that guides the family to services, and help them get the services.
- Communicate with the family and the agencies that can help them.
- Work to change the environment and the policies that affect your clients.

Two other important categories of resources for vulnerable people are their own personal coping skills and social supports (Aday, 2001). These groups often are resourceful and creative in managing multiple stressors. Nurses can work with clients to help them identify their strengths and draw on those strengths when managing their health needs. Also, clients may be able to depend on informal support networks. Even though social isolation is a problem for many vulnerable clients, nurses should not assume they have no one who can or will help them. *Case management* involves linking clients with services and providing direct nursing services to them, including teaching, counseling, screening, and immunizing. Lillian Wald was the first case manager. She linked vulnerable families with various services to help them stay healthy (Buhler-Wilkerson, 1985). Nurses are often the link between personal health services and population-based health care. Linking, or brokering, health services is accomplished by making appropriate referrals and following up with clients to ensure that the desired outcomes from the referral were achieved. Nurses are effective case managers in community nursing clinics, health departments, hospitals, and various other health care agencies. Nurse case managers emphasize health promotion and illness prevention with vulnerable clients and focus on helping them avoid unnecessary hospitalization.

As can be seen, many of these nursing actions are in the realm of case management, in which the nurse makes referrals and links clients with other community services. In the case manager role, the nurse often is an advocate for the client or family. The nurse serves as an advocate when referring clients to other agencies, when working with others to develop health programs, and when trying to influence legislation and health policies that affect vulnerable population groups.

PRACTICE APPLICATION

Ms. Green, a 46-year-old farm worker pregnant with her fifth child, has come to the clinic requesting treatment for swollen ankles. During your assessment, you learned that she had seen the nurse practitioner at the local health department two months ago. The nurse practitioner gave her some sample vitamins, but Ms. Green lost them. She has not received regular prenatal care and has no plans to do so. Her previous pregnancies were essentially normal, although she said she was "toxic" with her last child. She also said that her middle child was "not quite right." He is in the seventh grade at age 15. Ms. Green is 5 feet 2 inches tall, weighs 180 pounds, and has a blood pressure of 160/90 mm Hg. She has pitting edema of the ankles and a mild headache.

Ms. Green says that she usually takes chlorpromazine hydrochloride (Thorazine) but has run out of it and cannot afford to have her prescription refilled. She says that she has been in several mental hospitals in the past and that she has been more agitated lately, and now has problems managing her daily activities. As her agitation grows, she says that she usually hears voices and this really makes her aggressive.

None of her children lives with her, and she has no plans for taking care of the infant. She thinks she will ask the child's father, a race track worker, to help her, because she usually travels around the country with him.

A. What additional information do you need to help you adequately assess Ms. Green's health status and current needs?

B. What nursing activities are suggested by her history, physical, and psychological descriptions?

Answers can be found on the Evolve website.

KEY POINTS

- All countries have population subgroups that are more vulnerable to health threats than the general population.
- Vulnerable populations are more likely to develop health problems as a result of exposure to risk or to have worse outcomes from those health problems than the population as a whole.
- Vulnerable populations are more sensitive to risk factors than those who are more resilient, because they are often exposed to cumulative risk factors. These populations include poor or homeless persons, pregnant adolescents, migrant workers, severely mentally ill individuals, substance abusers, abused individuals, people with communicable diseases, and people with sexually transmitted diseases.
- Factors leading to the growing number of poor people in the United States include reduced earnings, decreased availability of low-cost housing, more households headed by women, inadequate education, lack of marketable skills, welfare reform, and reduced Social Security payments to children.
- Poverty has a direct effect on health and well-being across the life span. Poor people have higher rates of chronic illness and infant morbidity and mortality, shorter life expectancy, and more complex health problems.
- Child poverty rates are twice as high as those for adults. Children who live in single-parent homes are twice as likely to be poor than those who live with both parents.
- The complex health problems of homeless people include the inability to obtain adequate rest, sleep, exercise, nutrition,

and medication; exposure; infectious diseases; acute and chronic illness; infestations; and trauma and mental health problems.
- Health care is increasingly moving into the community. This began with deinstitutionalization of the severely mentally ill population and is continuing today as hospitals reduce inpatient stays. Vulnerable populations need a wide variety of services, and because these are often provided by multiple community agencies, nurses coordinate and manage the service needs of vulnerable groups.
- Socioeconomic problems, including poverty and social isolation, physiological and developmental aspects of age, poor health status, and highly stressful life experiences, predispose people to vulnerability. Vulnerability can become a cycle, with the predisposing factors leading to poor health outcomes, chronic stress, and hopelessness. These outcomes increase vulnerability.
- Nurses assess vulnerable individuals, families, and groups to determine which socioeconomic, physical, biological, psychological, and environmental factors are problematic for clients. They work as partners with vulnerable clients to identify client strengths and needs and develop intervention strategies designed to break the cycle of vulnerability.

CLINICAL DECISION-MAKING ACTIVITIES

1. Identify nurses in your community who work with vulnerable groups. Invite these nurses to come to class and talk about their experiences. What is their typical day? What are the rewards? What are the challenges? How do they deal with frustration, competing demands, and stress?
2. Discuss welfare reform with your classmates. How does the U.S. welfare system work? Who gets welfare? What should be done to improve the system? Is your state a leader in welfare reform?
3. Suppose you are making a home visit to a person whose home is not clean. Food is everywhere, and roaches are crawling around the house. What do you do if the person asks you to sit down? What if you are offered food?

ADDITIONAL RESOURCES

EVOLVE WEBSITE

http://evolve.elsevier.com/Stanhope/community/
- Answers to Practice Application
- Case Study
- Glossary
- Review Questions

REFERENCES

Aday LA: At risk in America: the health & health care needs of vulnerable populations in the United States, San Francisco, 2001, Jossey-Bass.

AEI/Brookings Working Group on Poverty & Opportunity (AEI/Brookings): Opportunity, responsibility, & security: a consensus plan for reducing poverty & restoring the American dream, 2015. Retrieved from https://www.brookings.edu.

American Academy of Pediatrics (AAP): Adverse childhood experiences & the lifelong consequences of trauma, 2014. Retrieved from https://www.aap.org.

American Public Health Association (APHA): Health equity, n.d. Retrieved from https://www.apha.org.

Antonisse L, Garfield R, Rudowitz R, Artiga S: The effects of Medicaid expansion under the ACA: updated findings from a literature review, March 28, 2018, Kaiser Family Foundation. Retrieved from https://www.kff.org.

Artiga S, Hinton E: Beyond health care: the role of social determinants in promoting health & health equity, May 10, 2018, Kaiser Family Foundation Disparities Policy. Retrieved from https://www.kff.org.

Ballou KA: A historical-philosophical analysis of professional nurse obligation to participate in sociopolitical activities, *Policy, Politics, & Nurs Pract* 1:172–184, 2000.

Bodenheimer T, Mason D: Registered Nurses: partners in transforming primary care, Proceedings of a conference sponsored by the Josiah Macy Jr. Foundation in June 2016; New York, 2017, Josiah Macy Jr. Foundation.

Braveman P: What are health disparities and health equity? We need to be clear, *Public Health Rep* 129(Suppl 2):5–8, 2014.

Braveman P, Arkin E, Orleans T, Proctor D, Plough A: What is health equity? May 01, 2017, Robert Wood Johnson Brief. Retrieved from https://www.rwjf.org.

Braveman P, Gottlieb L: The social determinants of health: It's time to consider the causes of the causes, *Public Health Rep* 129(Suppl 2): 19–31, 2014.

Buhler-Wilkerson K: Public health nursing: in sickness or in health, *Am J Public Health* 75(10):1155–1161, November 1985.

Butler SM: Social spending, not medical spending, is key to health, July 13, 2016. Brookings. Retrieved from https://www.brookings.edu.

Campaign for Action: Nurse Managed Health Centers (NMHCs), 2010, Center to Champion Nursing in America. Retrieved from https://campaignforaction.org.

Campbell-Page RM, Shaw-Ridley MS: Managing ethical dilemmas in community-based participatory research with vulnerable populations, *Health Promot Pract* 17:485–490, 2013.

Center for Poverty Research: What are the annual earnings for a full-time minimum wage worker? January 12, 2018, University of California Davis. Retrieved from https://poverty.ucdavis.edu.

Coumarelos C, Pascoe P, Wei Z: Law & disorders: illness/disability & experience of everyday problems involving the law. *Justice Issues*, Paper 17, 2013. Retrieved from https://www.researchgate.net.

Council on Linkages between Academia and Public Health Practice: *Core competences for public health professionals,* 2014, Author. Retrieved from www.phf.org.

deChesnay M: Vulnerable populations: vulnerable people. In DeChesnay M, Anderson BA, editors: Caring for the vulnerable: perspectives in nursing theory, practice, and research, ed 4, Burlington, MA, 2106, Jones & Bartlett, pp 3–18.

Fawcett J, Russell G: A conceptual model of nursing & health policy, *Policy, Politics, & Nurs Pract* 2:1527–1544, 2001.

Flowers L, House A, Noel-Miller C, et al. Medicare spends more on socially isolated older adults, 2018. Retrieved from https://www.aarp.org.

Hacker K, Walker DK: Achieving population health in Accountable Care Organizations, *Am J Public Health* 103:1163–1167, 2013.

Kindig DA: Understanding population health terminology, *Milbank Q* 85(1):139–161, 2007.

Kindig D, Stoddart G: What is population health? *Am J Public Health* 93(3):380–383, 2003.

Kochar R, Cilluffo A: Income inequality is rising most rapidly among Asians, July 12, 2018, Pew Research Center. Retrieved from http://www.pewsocialtrends.org.

Lathrop B: Nursing leadership in addressing the social determinants of health, *Policy, Politics, & Nurs Pract* 14:41–47, 2013.

Leight SB: The application of the Vulnerable Populations conceptual model to rural health, *Public Health Nurs* 20:440–448, 2003.

Minnesota Department of Health. Definition of population-based practice, 2003. Retrieved from http://www.health.state.mn.us.

Montez JK, Berkman LF: Trends in the educational gradient of mortality among U.S. adults aged 45 to 84 years: bringing regional context into the explanation, *Am J Public Health* 104(1): e82–e90, 2014.

Primm AB: College students of color: overcoming mental health challenges, July 16, 2018, National Alliance of Mental Illness. Retrieved from https://www.nami.org.

Quad Council Coalition of Public Health Nursing Organizations: *Community/public health nursing competencies*, 2018. Retrieved from: www.quadcouncil/phn.org.

Roncarati JS, Baggett TP, O'Connell JJ, et al. Mortality among unsheltered homeless adults in Boston, Massachusetts, 2000–2009, *JAMA Intern Med* 178:1242–1248, 2018. Retrieved from https://jamanetwork.com.

Rudolph L, Caplan J, Ben-Moshe K, Dillon L: Health in all policies: a guide for state and local governments, Washington, DC and Oakland, CA, 2013 American Public Health Association and Public Health Institute. Retrieved from http://www.phi.org.

Save the Children: The many faces of exclusion: end of childhood report 2018, 2018. Retrieved from https://reliefweb.int.

Semega JL, Fontenot KR, Kollar MA: Income and Poverty in the United States: 2016, 2017, U.S. Census Bureau, Current Population Reports, P60-259. Retrieved from https://www.census.gov.

Simon G: What's wrong with the term 'social determinants of health'? July 27, 2017, KP Washington Health Research. Retrieved from https://medium.com.

Stein M, Galea S: The health of the poorest 50 percent, Public Health Post July 18, 2018a. Retrieved from https://www.publichealthpost.org.

Stein M, Galea S: Income inequality & our health, Public Health Post April 11, 2018b. Retrieved from https://www.publichealthpost.org.

Stevens AB, Aly R: Health policy brief: What is "population health"? 2014. Retrieved from http://www.healthpolicyohio.org.

Unicef: Communication for development (C4D) Capability Development Framework, 2009. Retrieved from http://intranet.unicef.org.

University of Wisconsin Population Health Initiative (UWPHI): 2018 County Health Rankings key findings report, March 2018. Retrieved from http://www.countyhealthrankings.org.

U.S. Department of Health & Human Services-Centers for Disease Control & Prevention (USDHHS-CDC): Definitions, n.d.a. Retrieved from https://www.cdc.gov.

U.S. Department of Health & Human Services-Centers for Disease Control & Prevention (USDHHS-CDC): Lesson 1: Introduction to epidemiology-Section 8: Concepts of disease occurrence, n.d.b. Retrieved from https://www.cdc.gov.

U.S. Department of Health & Human Services-Centers for Disease Control & Prevention (USDHHS-CDC): Lesson 1: Introduction to epidemiology-Section 9: Natural history & spectrum of disease, n.d.c. Retrieved from https://www.cdc.gov.

U.S. Department of Health & Human Services-Centers for Disease Control & Prevention (USDHHS-CDC): Adverse childhood experiences (ACEs), n.d.d. Retrieved from https://www.cdc.gov.

U.S. Department of Health and Human Services-Office of Disease Prevention & Health Promotion (USDHHS-ODPHP): Healthy People 2020, 2010. Retrieved from www.healthypeople.gov.

U.S. Department of Health & Human Services-Office of Disease Prevention & Health Promotion (USDHHS-ODPHP): Determinants of health, n.d.a. Retrieved from https://www.healthypeople.gov.

U.S. Department of Health & Human Services-Office of Disease Prevention & Health Promotion (USDHHS-ODPHP): Healthy People 2030 framework, n.d.b. Retrieved from https://www.healthypeople.gov.

Wendell ML, Garney WR, McLeroy KR: Ecological approaches, 2017. Retrieved from https://www.researchgate.net.

Wernham A, Teutsh SM: Health in All Policies for big cities, *J Public Health Manag Pract* 21(Suppl 1):S56–S65, 2014. Retrieved from https://www.ncbi.nlm.nih.gov.

Whitehead M: The concepts and principles of equity and health, *Health Promot* 6(3):217–228, 1992, and updated in 2000 for the World Health Organization. Retrieved from http://www.who.int.

World Health Organization (WHO): Health Impact Assessment (HIA): The determinants of death, 2015. Retrieved from http://www.who.int.

World Health Organization (WHO): Constitution of WHO: principles, 1946. Retrieved from http://www.who.int.

World Health Organization (WHO): *The determinants of health*, n.d. Retrieved from http://www.who.int.

Zimmerman EB, Woolf SH, Haley A: *Population health: behavioral & social science insights*, 2015, Agency for Healthcare Quality & Research. Retrieved from https://www.ahrq.gov.

32

Population-Centered Nursing in Rural and Urban Environments

Angeline Bushy, PhD, RN, FAAN

OBJECTIVES

After reading this chapter, the student should be able to do the following:

1. Compare and contrast definitions of *rural* and *urban*.
2. Describe residency as a continuum, ranging from farm residency to core inner city.
3. Compare and contrast the health status of rural and urban populations on select health measures.
4. Analyze barriers to care in health professional shortage areas and for underserved populations.
5. Evaluate issues related to the delivery of public health services for rural underserved populations.
6. Describe characteristics of rural and small-town residency.
7. Examine the role and scope of public health nursing practice in rural and underserved areas.
8. Evaluate two professional-client-community partnership models that can effectively provide a continuum of health care to residents living in an environment with sparse resources.

CHAPTER OUTLINE

Historic Overview
Definition of Terms
Rural-Urban Continuum
Current Perspectives
Rural Health Care Delivery Issues and Barriers to Care
Nursing Care in Rural Environments
Future Perspectives
Building Professional-Community-Client Partnerships in Rural Settings

KEY TERMS

farm residency, p. 717
frontier, p. 722
health professional shortage area (HPSA), p. 721
medically underserved, p. 731
metropolitan area, p. 718
micropolitan area, p. 718
non-core areas, p. 718
non-farm residency, p. 717
rural, p. 717
rural-urban continuum, p. 717
suburbs, p. 718
urban, p. 717

Access to health care is a national priority, especially in regions with an insufficient number of health care providers. Recruiting and retaining qualified health professionals is often difficult in underserved communities, particularly inner cities and rural areas of the United States. Until recently, however, only limited research has been undertaken on the special challenges, problems, and opportunities of nursing practice—especially public health in rural settings. This chapter presents major issues surrounding health care delivery in rural environments, which sometimes differs from that in urban or more populated settings. Common definitions for the term *rural* are discussed, as are its associated lifestyle, the health status of rural populations, barriers to obtaining a continuum of health care services, and public health nursing practice issues. Strategies are discussed to help nurses deliver more effective population-focused nursing services to clients who live in more isolated environments with sparser resources. This chapter describes rural public health nursing practice and could be used by students, nurses who practice in rural public health departments, and those who work in agencies located in urban areas that offer outreach services to rural populations in their catchment area.

HISTORIC OVERVIEW

Formal rural nursing originated with the Red Cross Rural Nursing Service (RCRNS), which was organized in November 1912. The Committee on Rural Nursing was directed by Mabel Boardman (Chair), Jane Delano (Vice-Chair), and Annie Goodrich, along with other Red Cross leaders and philanthropists (Bigbee & Crowder, 1985). Prior to the formation of the

Red Cross Rural Nursing Service, care of the sick in a small community was provided by informal social support systems. When self-care and family care were not effective in bringing about healing, this task was assigned to traditional or cultural healers, who often were women who lived in the local community. Historically, rural Americans have had many health care needs, and they may differ in some ways from those of urban populations. Problems of maldistribution of health professionals, poverty, limited access to services, lack of education, and social isolation have plagued many rural communities for generations.

The history of the RCRNS consistently moved away from its initial rural focus, as seen in its frequent name changes. Unfortunately, concern about rural health is often temporary and replaced by other areas of greater need. Hopefully, health care reform initiatives will ensure equitable access to care for rural and urban residents alike (NACRHHS, 2017a).

DEFINITION OF TERMS

Rurality: A Subjective Concept

Everyone has an idea as to what constitutes rural as opposed to urban residence. However, the two cannot be viewed as opposing entities. With the increased degree of urban influence on rural communities, the differences may not be as distinct as they may have been even a decade ago (Bureau of the Census, 2016). In general, **rural** may be defined by geographic location and population density, or it may be described in terms of the distance from (e.g., 20 miles) or the time (e.g., 30 minutes) needed to commute to an urban center. See Box 32.1 for selected terms and definitions.

Both urban and rural communities are highly diverse and vary in their demographic, environmental, economic, and social characteristics. In turn, these characteristics influence the magnitude and types of health problems that communities face. Urban counties, however, tend to have more health care providers in relation to population, and residents of more rural counties often live farther from health care resources (RHI-Hub, 2018).

Some equate the idea of rural with **farm residency**, and **urban** with **non-farm residency**, whereas others consider *rural* to be a "state of mind." For the more affluent, rural may bring to mind a recreational, retirement, or resort community located in the mountains or in lake country where one can relax and participate in outdoor activities, such as skiing, fishing, hiking, or hunting. For the less affluent, the term can impose rather grim scenes. For example, some people may think of an impoverished Indian reservation as comparable to an underdeveloped country, while others think of a migrant labor camp with several families living in a one-room shanty with no access to safe drinking water or adequate sanitation.

Just as each city has its own unique features, also it is difficult to describe a "typical rural town" because of the wide population and geographic diversity. For example, rural towns in Florida, Oregon, Alaska, Hawaii, and Idaho are different from one another, and quite different from those in Vermont, Texas, Alabama, or California. Also, there can be vast differences between rural areas within one state. Still, descriptions and definitions for *rural* tend to be more subjective and relative in nature than those for *urban*.

For example, "small" communities with populations of more than 20,000 have some features that one may expect to find in a city. Then again, residents who live in a community with a population of less than 2000 may consider a community with a population of 5000 or 10,000 to be a city. Although some communities may seem geographically remote on a map, the residents who live there may not feel isolated. Those residents believe they are within easy reach of services through telecommunication and dependable transportation, although extensive shopping facilities may be 50 to 100 miles from the family home, obstetric care may be 150 miles away, or nursing services in the district health department in an adjacent county may be 75 or more miles away (Bolin & Bellamy, 2015).

BOX 32.1 Terms and Definitions

Farm residency: Residency outside area zoned as "city limits"; usually infers involvement in agriculture
Frontier: Regions having fewer than six persons per square mile
Large central: Counties in large (1 million or more population) metro areas that contain all or part of the largest central city
Large fringe: Remaining counties in large (1 million or more population) metro areas
Metropolitan county: Regions with a central city of at least 50,000 residents
Non-farm residency: Residence within area zoned as "city limits"
Micropolitan county: Counties that do not meet SMSA (see below) criteria
Rural: Communities having fewer than 20,000 residents or fewer than 99 persons per square mile
Small: Counties in metro areas with fewer than 1 million people
Standard metropolitan statistical area (SMSA): Regions with a central city of at least 50,000 residents
Suburban: Area adjacent to a highly populated city
Urban: Geographic areas described as non-rural and having a higher population density; more than 99 persons per square mile; cities with a population of at least 20,000 but less than 50,000

Modified from Rural Health Information Hub (RHI-Hub): *What is rural?* 2018. Available at https://www.ruralhealthinfo.org.

RURAL-URBAN CONTINUUM

Frequently used definitions to describe rural and urban and to differentiate between them are provided by several federal agencies (RHI-Hub, 2018; USDA, 2017) (see Box 32.1). These definitions, which in many cases are dichotomous in nature, fail to take into account the relative nature of ruralness. Rural and urban residencies are not opposing lifestyles. Rather, the two should be conserved as a **rural-urban continuum**, ranging from living on a remote farm, to a village or small town, to a larger town or city, to a large metropolitan area with a *core inner city*. See Fig. 32.1, which describes the continuum of rural-urban residency.

Several federal agencies classify U.S. counties and county equivalents (N = 3142) according to population density, specifically, metropolitan counties (84 percent of the total population) and non-metropolitan counties (16 percent of the

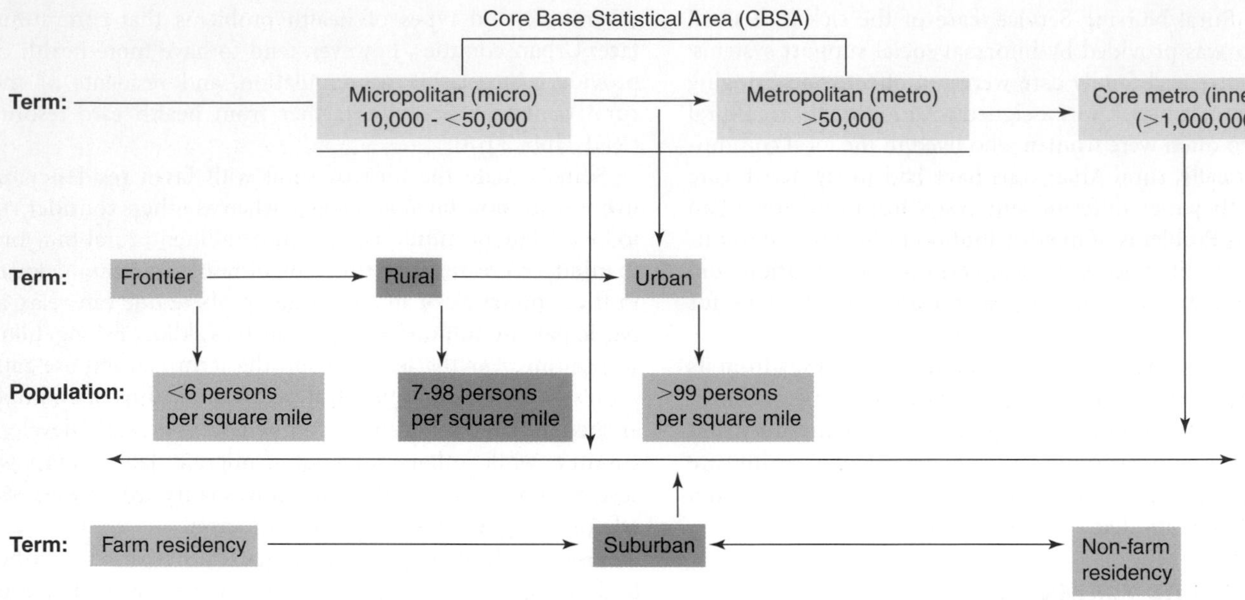

Fig. 32.1 The continuum of rural-urban residency.

total population) (RHI-Hub, 2018). The terms **metropolitan area** and **micropolitan area** (metro and micro areas) refer to geographic entities primarily used for collecting, tabulating, and publishing federal statistics. Core-based statistical area (CBSA) is a collective term for both metro and micro areas. A metro area contains a core urban area of 50,000 or more population. A micro area contains an urban core of at least 10,000 (but less than 50,000) population. Each metro or micro area consists of one or more counties containing the core urban area. Likewise, adjacent counties have a high degree of social and economic integration (as measured by commuting to work) with their urban core.

Demographically, micro areas contain about 60 percent of the total non-metro population, with an average of 43,000 people per county. In contrast, **non-core areas**, with no urban cluster of 10,000 or more residents, have on average about 14,000 residents. In general, lack of an urban core and low overall population density may place these counties at a disadvantage in efforts to expand and diversify their economic base. The designation of micro areas is an important step in recognizing non-metro diversity. The term also provides a framework to understand population growth and economic restructuring in small towns and cities that have received less attention than metro areas. Nationally and regionally, many measures of health, health care use, and health care resources among rural populations vary by the level of urban influence in a particular region.

Micro areas embody a widely shared residential preference for a small-town lifestyle—an ideal compromise between large highly populated urban cities and sparsely populated rural settings. As information about these places makes its way into government data and publications alongside metro areas in the coming years, hopefully the notion of "micropolitan" will draw increased attention from policy makers and the business community.

In recent years there has been a population shift from urban to less-populated regions of the United States. Demographers metaphorically refer to this demographic phenomenon as the "doughnut effect." That is to say, people are moving away from highly populated areas to outlying **suburbs** of urban centers. Most of the population growth has been in rural counties with a booming economy coupled with the geographic area to expand that is evident in some western and southern states (RHI-Hub, 2018).

Clearly, a notable population shift will also affect the health status and lifestyle preferences of communities in which this phenomenon occurs. As beliefs and values change over time, urban-rural differences narrow in some respects while others became more pronounced. Depending on the definition that is used, the actual rural population might vary slightly. According to Bureau of the Census estimates (2016), while about 97 percent of the land's area is rural, about 20 percent (or 60 million) of all U.S. residents live in rural settings. In this chapter, rural refers to areas having fewer than 99 persons per square mile and communities having 20,000 or fewer inhabitants.

CURRENT PERSPECTIVES

Population Characteristics

Adding to the confusion about what constitutes rural versus urban residency are the special needs of the numerous underrepresented groups (minorities, subgroups) who reside in the United States. In general, there are a higher proportion of whites in rural areas than in urban areas. There are, however, regional variations, and some rural counties have a significant number of minorities. Little is documented on the actual needs and health status of special rural populations (AHCPR, 2017; Bolin & Bellamy, 2015; USDHHS, 2013). Anthropologists note that, within a group, there often exists a wide range of lifestyles.

Consequently, even in the smallest or most remote town or village, a subgroup may behave differently and have different values about health, illness, and patterns of accessing health care. Also, a group's lifestyle may be associated with health problems that are different from those of the predominant cultural group in a given community. Background information on selected populations can be found in Chapters 8 and 31 that discuss cultural diversity and vulnerable populations.

Demographically, rural communities include a higher proportion of younger and older residents. Nurses often encounter more residents under the age of 18 and over 65 years of age in rural areas compared with an urban setting. Rural residents 18 years of age and older are more likely to be, or to have been, married than are their urban counterparts. As a group, rural adults are more likely to be widowed and have fewer years of formal education than urban adults (Bureau of the Census, 2016; CDC, 2018a; United States Census Bureau, 2010).

Although there are regional variations, rural families tend to be poorer than their urban counterparts. Comparing annual incomes with the standardized index established, more than one fourth of rural Americans live in or near poverty, and nearly 40 percent of all rural children are impoverished. Compared with those in metropolitan settings, a substantially smaller proportion of rural families are at the high end of the income scale. Accompanying the recent population shifts from urban to formerly rural areas, the average income level may change; however, no data are available at this time to substantiate this estimate. Regardless, level of income is a critical factor in whether a family has health insurance or qualifies for public insurance. Consequently, rural families are less likely to have private insurance and more likely to receive public assistance or to be uninsured (RHI-Hub, 2018).

The working poor in rural areas are particularly at risk for being underinsured or uninsured. In working poor families, one or more of the adults are employed but still cannot afford private health insurance. Furthermore, their annual income is such that it disqualifies the family from obtaining public insurance. Several factors help explain why this phenomenon occurs more often in rural settings (Bushy, 2013). For example, a high proportion of rural residents are self-employed in a family business, such as ranching or farming, or they work in small enterprises, such as a service station, restaurant, or grocery store. Also, an individual may be employed in part-time or in seasonal occupations, such as farm laborer and construction, in which health insurance often is not an employee benefit. In other situations, a family member may have a pre-existing health condition that makes the cost of insurance prohibitive, if it is even available to them. At present it remains to be seen if this situation will change with the recent health care reform. A few rural families fall through the cracks and are unable to access any type of public assistance because of other deterrents, such as language barriers, including a low level of English reading and writing even if they appear comfortable speaking the language, compromised physical status, the geographic location of an agency, lack of transportation, or undocumented worker status. Insurance, or the lack of it, has serious implications for the overall health status of rural residents and the nurses who provide services to them (AHCPR, 2017; NCHS, 2018).

Health Status of Rural Residents

Even though rural communities constitute about one fourth of the total population, the health problems and the health behaviors of the residents in them are not fully understood. This section summarizes what is known about the overall health status of rural adults and children. The health status measures that are addressed are perceived health status, diagnosed chronic conditions, physical limitations, frequency of seeking medical treatment, usual source of care, maternal–infant health, children's health, mental health, minorities' health, and environmental and occupational health risks (Bolin & Bellamy, 2015; OSHA, n.d.). Residents of rural areas suffer some of the same health problems as migrant farmworkers, as described in Chapter 34, including exposure to environmental factors and accidents.

Perceived Health Status. In general, people in rural areas have a poorer perception of their overall health and functional status than their urban counterparts. Rural residents over 18 years of age assess their health status less favorably than do urban residents. Studies show that rural adults are less likely to engage in preventive behavior, which ultimately increases exposure to risk. Specifically, they are more likely to use tobacco products and self-report higher rates of alcohol consumption and obesity; furthermore, they are less likely to engage in routine physical activity during leisure time, wear seat belts, have regular blood pressure checks, have Pap smears, complete breast self-examinations, and have colorectal screenings. Ultimately, failure to participate in health-promoting lifestyle behaviors impacts the overall health status of rural residents, their level of function, physical limitations, degree of mobility, and level of self-care activities (NCHS, 2018).

Chronic Illness. Rural adults are more likely than urban adults to have one or more of the following chronic conditions: heart disease, chronic obstructive pulmonary disease, hypertension, arthritis and rheumatism, diabetes, cardiovascular disease, and cancer. Nearly half of all rural adults have been diagnosed with at least one of these chronic conditions, compared with about one fourth of non-rural adults. Also, the prevalence of diagnosed diabetes in rural adults is about 7 out of 100, as opposed to 5 out of 100 in non-rural environments. Rural adults are more likely to have cancer (almost seven percent) compared with urban adults (about five percent). Although most cases of acquired immunodeficiency syndrome (AIDS) are still found in urban areas, the rate is increasing in some rural populations (NCHS, 2018).

Rural-urban health disparities have been documented in health status (Box 32.2) and for health behaviors (Box 32.3). For example, there are disparities in the proportion of rural adults who receive medical treatment for both life-threatening illness and degenerative or chronic conditions compared with urban adults. The proportion of rural residents who receive these treatments is high in rural versus urban areas.

BOX 32.2 Disparities Among U.S. Urban (Metropolitan) and Rural (Micropolitan) Residents' Health Status

Residents of fringe counties near large metro areas have the following:

- Lowest levels of premature mortality, partly reflecting lower death rates for unintentional injuries, homicide, and suicide
- Lowest levels of smoking, alcohol consumption, and childbearing among adolescents
- Lowest prevalence of physical inactivity during leisure time among women
- Lowest levels of obesity among adults
- Greatest number of physician specialists and dentists per capita
- Lowest percent of the population without health insurance
- Lowest percent of the population who had no dental visits

Residents in the most rural counties have the following:

- Highest death rates for children and young adults
- Highest death rates for unintentional and motor vehicle traffic–related injuries
- Highest death rates among adults for ischemic heart disease and suicide
- Highest levels of smoking among adolescents
- Highest levels of physical activity during leisure time among men
- Highest levels of obesity among adults
- Highest percent of adults with activity limitations caused by chronic health conditions
- Fewest physician specialists and dentists per capita
- Least likely to have seen a dentist
- Highest percentage of the population without health insurance

Modified from Centers for Disease Control and Prevention: *Strategies for reducing health disparities,* 2016. Available at https://www.cdc.gov; Bolin JN, Bellamy G: *Rural Healthy People: 2020,* 2015. Retrieved from https://srhrc.tamhsc.edu; Meit M, Knudson A, Gilbert T, et al.: *The 2014 update of the rural-urban chartbook,* 2014. Available at https://ruralhealth.und.edu.

Life-threatening conditions include malignant neoplasms, heart disease, cardiovascular problems, and liver disorders. Degenerative or chronic diseases include diabetes, kidney disease, arthritis, and chronic diseases of the circulatory, nervous, respiratory, and digestive systems. Chronic health conditions, coupled with their poor health status, limit the physical activities of a larger proportion of rural residents than of their urban counterparts (Bolin & Bellamy, 2015; NCHS, 2018).

Physical Limitations. Limitations in mobility and self-care are strong indicators of an individual's overall health status. Specific assessed measures on a national health survey included walking one block, walking uphill or climbing stairs, bending, lifting, stooping, feeding, dressing, bathing, and toileting. In fact, almost 10 percent of rural adults report at least three or more of these physical limitations, compared with about 6 percent of metropolitan adults. The increased prevalence of poor health status and impaired function is not necessarily attributable to the increased number of older adults found in rural areas. Similar patterns are evident in adults 18 to 64 years of age. Rural adults under 65 years of age are more likely than urban adults to assess their health status as fair to poor, and a greater percent have been diagnosed with a chronic health condition (NCHS, 2018; USDA, n.d.; USDHHS, 2013).

BOX 32.3 Rural-Urban Disparities: Lifestyle and Health Behaviors

- Residents in any rural areas are more likely to report fair to poor health status (19.5 percent) than were residents of urban counties (15.6 percent).
- Rural residents are more likely to report having diabetes (9.6 percent) versus urban adults (8.4 percent).
- Rates of diabetes are markedly higher among rural American Indians (15.2 percent) and African American adults (15.1 percent).
- Rural residents are more likely to be obese (27.4 percent) versus urban residents (23.9 percent).
- Rural black adults are particularly at risk for obesity; ranging from 38.9 percent in rural micropolitan counties to 40.7 percent in remote rural counties.
- Rural residents are less likely to meet CDC recommendations for moderate or vigorous physical activity (44 percent) versus urban residents (45.4 percent).
- Rural African American adults are less likely to meet recommendations for physical activity than other rural residents; this difference persists across all levels of rurality.

Access to Health Care Services

- Rural residents are more likely to be uninsured (17.8 percent) versus urban residents (15.3 percent).
- Hispanic adults are more likely to lack insurance, with uninsured rates ranging from 40.8 percent in rural micropolitan counties to 56.1 percent in small remote counties.
- Most rural residents (81 percent) and urban residents (79.4 percent) report having a personal health care provider. However, residents in remote rural counties were least likely to have a personal physician (78.7 percent).
- Rural white adults are more likely to have a personal health care provider than were other adults. Among Hispanic adults, the proportion with a personal provider ranged from 60.4 percent in rural micropolitan counties to 47.7 percent in remote rural counties.
- Rural adults are more likely than urban adults to defer seeking health care because of cost (15.1 percent versus 13.1 percent)
- Rural adult African Americans, Hispanics, and American Indians are more likely to report having deferred care due to cost compared with white rural residents.

Receipt of Preventive Services

- Rural women are less likely (70.7 percent) than urban women (77.9 percent) to be in compliance with mammogram screening guidelines.
- Rural women are less likely (86 percent) than urban women (91.4 percent) to have had a Pap smear within the past three years.
- Rural residents over age 50 years are less likely (57.7 percent) to have had a colorectal screening versus urban counterparts (61.4 percent).

Quality of Diabetes Care

- The proportion of adults with diabetes who reported receiving at least two hemoglobin A1c tests within the past year was low among both rural (33.1 percent) and urban residents (35 percent).
- White rural residents with diabetes were more likely than African American or Hispanic residents to receive at least two hemoglobin A1c tests in the past year.
- Only 64.2 percent of rural and 69.1 percent of urban residents with diabetes reported receiving an annual dilated eye examination.

Adapted from Centers for Disease Control and Prevention: *Strategies for reducing health disparities,* 2016. Available at https://www.cdc.gov; Bolin JN, Bellamy G: *Rural Healthy People: 2020,* 2015. Available at https://srhrc.tamhsc.edu; Meit M, Knudson A, Gilbert T, et al.: *The 2014 update of the rural-urban chartbook,* 2014. Available at https://ruralhealth.und.edu.

Based on data from national health surveys, the overall health status of rural adults leaves much to be desired. This is attributed to several factors, including impaired access to health care providers and services, coupled with other rural factors. Thus, nurses who practice in rural areas are essential in providing a continuum of care for clients. Specifically, nurses can help clients have healthier lives by teaching them how to prevent accidents, engage in more healthful lifestyle behaviors, and reduce the risk of chronic health problems. Once clients in rural environments have been diagnosed with a long-term problem, nurses can help them manage chronic conditions to achieve better health outcomes and functioning (Bolin & Bellamy, 2015; IOM, 2010).

Patterns of Health Service Use. When the use of health care services is measured, it is found that more than three fourths of adults in rural areas received medical care on at least one occasion during a year. Despite their overall poorer health status and higher incidence of chronic health conditions, rural adults seek medical care less often than urban adults. In part, this discrepancy can be attributed to scarce resources and the several other barriers cited earlier, including lack of providers in rural areas. Other reasons are discussed later under Rural Health Care Delivery Issues and Barriers to Care (AHCPR, 2017; CDC, 2017, 2018a). Nurses must be thorough in their health assessment of rural clients who may not receive regular care for chronic health conditions.

CHECK YOUR PRACTICE

When you conduct an the initial client assessment and discharge planning have you asked these questions:

- Context of residency (urban versus rural)? If rural ... then ...
- Occupation of the individual?
- Potential health risks associated with employment or place of residence?
- Access to health-related and support services available in the community?
- Veteran's status? If so ... any actual or potential impact on health? If so, then ...
- Does individual have access to veterans services?

Availability and Access to Health Care. The ability of a person to identify a usual source of care is considered a favorable indicator of access to health care and a person's overall health status. Essentially, a person who has a usual source of care is more likely to seek care when ill and adhere to prescribed regimens. Having the same provider of care can enhance continuity of care, as well as a client's perception of the quality of that care. Rural adults are more likely than urban adults to identify a particular medical provider as their usual source of care. Rural adults are more likely to receive care from general practitioners and advanced practice registered nurses (APRNs) compared to urban adults who are more likely to seek care from a medical specialist. However, this trend may be changing with health care reform, which emphasizes the importance of primary care (BHWF, 2017; Jakobs & Bigbee, 2016; IOM, 2010).

Another measure of access to care is traveling time and/or distance to ambulatory care services. Rural persons who seek ambulatory care are more likely to travel more than 30 minutes to reach their usual source of care. Extended commuting time may also be a factor for residents in highly populated urban areas and those who must rely on public transportation. Once the person arrives at the clinic or physician's office, no differences between rural and urban residents are found in the waiting time to see the provider. Also, many rural residents live on unpaved dirt roads that vehicles that transport clients to health care simply cannot reach.

In general, there is a maldistribution of health professionals among rural and urban counties. For instance, 1 out of 17 rural counties is reported to have no physician. Among rural respondents on national surveys, the ability to identify a usual site of care or a particular provider often stems from a community or county having only one, perhaps two, health care providers. The limited number of health care facilities is reinforced by the finding that nearly all rural residents who seek health care use ambulatory services that are provided in a physician's office as opposed to a clinic, community health center, hospital outpatient department, or emergency department (NACRHHS, 2017a; USDA, 2017, n.d.). One can speculate about the indicator of *usual place and usual provider*; that is to say, it suggests that rural residents are at least as well off as urban residents regarding access to care. However, this finding may be related to the fact that rural physicians tend to live and practice in a particular community for decades, thus providing care to multigenerational families who seek care from this particular provider.

Moreover, in a **health professional shortage area (HPSA)**, a physician or a nurse practitioner may provide services to residents who live in surrounding counties. One or two nurses in a public health department usually offer a full range of services for all residents in a rural catchment area of 100 or more miles from one end to the other end of a county or health district. Consequently, rural physicians and nurses frequently report, "I provide care to individuals and families with all kinds of conditions, in all stages of life, and across several generations." It should not come as a surprise that rural respondents who participate in national surveys are able to identify a usual source and a usual provider of health care (BHWF, 2018; Meit et al., 2014).

Maternal–Infant Health. Reports in the literature conflict regarding pregnancy outcomes in rural areas. Overall, rural populations have higher infant and maternal morbidity rates, especially counties designated as HPSAs, which often have a high proportion of racial minorities. Here one also finds fewer specialists, such as pediatricians, obstetricians, and gynecologists, to provide care to at-risk populations. There are extreme variations in pregnancy outcomes from one part of the country to another, and even within states. For example, in several counties located in the north-central and intermountain states, the pregnancy outcome is among the finest in the United States. However, in several other counties within those same states, the pregnancy outcome is among the worst. Particularly at risk are women who live on or near Indian reservations, are migrant workers, and are of African American descent residing in rural areas in southeastern states (Bolin & Bellamy, 2015; USDHHS, 2013).

Public health nurses recognize the interactive effects of socioeconomic factors, such as income level (poverty), education level, age, employment-unemployment patterns, and use of prenatal services, on pregnancy outcomes. There are other, less well-known health determinants, such as environmental hazards, occupational risks, and the cultural meaning placed on childbearing and child-rearing practices by a community. The interaction effects of these multifaceted factors vary and often are difficult to measure (Nelson, 2009).

Health of Children. Reports on the health status of rural children show regional variations and conflicting data. Comparing rural children with urban children under 6 years of age on the measures of access to providers and use of services reveals the following (AHCPR, 2017; Bolin & Bellamy, 2015; USDHHS, 2013):

- Urban children are less likely to have a usual provider but are more likely to see a pediatrician when they are ill.
- Like rural adults, rural children are more likely to be cared for by a general practitioner who is identified as their usual caregiver.

School nurses play an important role in the overall health status of children in the United States. The availability of school nurses in rural communities also varies from region to region. Specifically, in **frontier** and rural areas of the United States, school nurses usually are scarce. In part, this deficit can be attributed to limited resources associated with very low local tax revenues and shortages of health personnel in those counties. In other words, there are fewer taxpayers living in those large geographic areas. Some frontier areas have fewer than four persons per square mile and a few areas have fewer than two persons per square mile. Consequently, rural county commissioners, like their urban counterparts, must prioritize the allocation of scarce resources for essential public services such as maintaining the infrastructures of utilities, roads, bridges, and education; supporting a financially suffering county hospital; hiring a county health nurse; and offering school health services. In rural communities there are fewer resources overall, yet certain public services must be provided to local residents—albeit in many situations with aging and outdated infrastructures (RHI-Hub, 2017).

Clearly, creativity is required by both community residents and local public health care providers to resolve health care and school nursing needs. Partnership arrangements, for example, have been negotiated by two or more counties that agree to share the cost of a "district" public health nurse. Other county commissioners have forged partnerships with an agency in an urban setting and contracted for specific health care services. In both of these situations, it is not unusual for the nurse to provide services to *all* children attending *all* schools in the health district's participating counties. In some frontier states, schools may be situated more than 100 miles apart, and as many miles or more from the district health office. Because of the number of schools and distances between them, the county nurse may be able to visit each school only once or twice in a school term. Usually the nurse's visit is to update immunizations and perhaps teach maturation classes to students in the upper grades.

The health status of rural women, infants, and children is less than optimal. In part this can be attributed to inadequate preventive, primary, and emergency services to meet their particular health care needs. Scarce resources can pose a challenge to a nurse who provides care to rural residents, especially those in underserved areas. Resource deficits encourage creativity and innovation; both of these behaviors are characteristic of nursing in general and of rural nurses in particular (BHWF, 2017).

Mental Health. Like many other measures of health, the facts about the mental health status of rural people are also ambiguous and conflicting (CDC, 2018a; NACRHHS, 2017a; NCHS, 2018). Stress, stress-related conditions, and mental illness are prevalent among economically deprived populations. Increasing federal regulations imposed on agriculture, timber, and marine- and mining-related industries as well as trade agreements with other counties in the past two decades led to many job losses in rural communities. The term *farm stress* is associated with the economic downturn in the agriculture industry as it affects an individual, family, and the community. This same term or diagnosis could be applied to other communities experiencing economic recessions in their predominant enterprises, such as marine-, automobile-, and timber-related industries. Economic factors also contribute to a family's being underinsured or uninsured. Even if mental health services are available and accessible, rural residents delay seeking care when they have an emotional problem until there is an emergency or a crisis. This behavior is reflected in the lower number of annual visits for mental health services and chronic health conditions by rural residents (Bolin & Bellamy, 2015; NACRHHS, 2017b).

Mental health professionals who serve rural populations report a persistent, endemic level of depression among residents in economically stressed rural areas. They speculate this condition is exacerbated by elevated levels of poverty, geographic isolation, and an insufficient number of mental health services. Depression may also contribute to the escalating incidence of accidents and suicides, especially among rural male adolescents and young men. These incidents have increased dramatically over the last decade and continue to rise within this group, to the point of being epidemic in some small communities. Likewise, the stigma associated with mental illness remains, especially in communities having fewer health care providers to educate the public about mental and behavioral health conditions (RHI-Hub, 2018).

There are conflicting reports on the prevalence of interpersonal violence and alcohol and substance use among rural populations. These behaviors are less likely to be reported in areas where residents are related or personally acquainted. Over time, destructive coping behaviors in small, tight-knit communities may be accepted by local residents as "business as usual" for a particular family. Family problems may also be ignored if formal social services and public health services are sparse or nonexistent, or if residents do not trust the professionals who provide services at a local agency. In underserved rural areas, there are gaps in the continuum of mental health services, which, ideally, should include preventive education, anticipatory guidance, screenings, early intervention programs, crisis and acute care services, and follow-up care. As with other aspects of health care, nurses in rural areas play an important role in community education, case finding, advocacy, and case management of client systems experiencing acute and chronic emotional and behavioral health problems (Booth & Graves, 2018; Eisenhauer et al., 2016; Montgomery et al., 2017).

Health of Minorities. As mentioned previously, a considerable number of at-risk minority groups in rural America have some rather distinctive concerns (particularly children, older adults, American Indians, Alaska Natives, Native Hawaiians, migrant workers, African Americans, immigrants, and the homeless) (CDC, 2018a; MHN, 2017; USDHHS, 2013). The rural homeless, for example, may be migrant farmworkers or local families whose homes were foreclosed. Sometimes the family may be allowed by law to continue living in the house that once was theirs. The family no longer has a means of livelihood and often remains hidden in the community with insufficient income to purchase food or other necessary services. The particular health problems of these at-risk groups are discussed in several chapters in the book. Nurses should be aware, however, that at-risk and underrepresented groups may experience some unique challenges associated with rural social structures, lifestyle, and sparse resources.

Environmental and Occupational Health Risks. A community's primary industry or industries are a determinant in the local lifestyle, the health status of its residents, and the number and types of health care services it may need. For example, four high-risk industries identified by the Occupational Safety and Health Administration (OSHA) and found in predominantly rural environments are forestry, mining, marine-related fields, and agriculture. See Table 32.1 for a description of rural groups, their typical health care needs, and their health risks or conditions. Associated health risks of these industries are machinery and vehicular accidents, trauma, selected types of cancer related to environmental factors, and allergies and respiratory conditions associated with repeated exposure to toxins, pesticides, and herbicides (NCHS, 2018; OSHA, n.d.; USDA, 2017).

For example, agriculture production industries such as farming and ranching are often owned and operated by a family. Small enterprises with a small number of employees do not fall under OSHA guidelines. For that reason, safety standards are not enforceable on most farms and ranches, since these often are family enterprises. Moreover, small businesses, such as farms, are not covered under workers' compensation insurance. Additional concerns arise because family members participate in the farm or ranch work. This means that some adults and children may work with animals and operate

TABLE 32.1 Select Health Care Needs, Risks/Conditions of Select Rural Aggregates

Rural Aggregates	Health Care Needs	Health Risks/Conditions
Farmers/ranchers	Advanced life support/emergency services	Agricultural chemicals and environmental hazards
	Oral/dental care	Dermatitis
	Obstetric/perinatal/pediatric services	Stress/depression/anxiety disorders
	Mental/behavioral health services	Respiratory conditions (e.g., farmer's lung)
	Agricultural health nurses	Accidents (vehicular/machinery)
	Geriatric specialists	Trauma-related chronic conditions
	Health promotion/illness prevention education	Dental caries/loss
	Veterans services	Interpersonal/domestic violence
	Pain management education	Pain management/opioid misuse
	Independent/progressive care living facilities for aging population	Interpersonal/domestic violence
	Home health care services	
	Interpersonal/domestic violence services	
	Women's health services	
	LGBTQ sensitive services	
American Indians	Advanced life support/emergency services	Infectious diseases (e.g., hepatitis, TB)
	Oral/dental care	Sudden infant death syndrome (SIDS)
	Obstetric/perinatal/pediatric services	Interpersonal/domestic violence
	Mental/behavioral health services	Diabetes
	Culturally appropriate substance abuse treatment programs	Alcohol/substance abuse
	Epidemiologists	Cirrhosis of the liver
	Diabetes screening and educators	Vehicular accidents
	Community health workers/education	Hypothermic/environmental injuries
	Health promotion/illness prevention education	Trauma-related injuries/chronic conditions
	Veterans services	Dental caries/loss
	Interpersonal/domestic violence services	Chronic pain management
	Women's health services	Interpersonal/domestic violence
	LGBTQ sensitive services	
	Veterans services	
	Pain management education	
	Independent/progressive care living facilities for aging population	

Continued

TABLE 32.1 Select Health Care Needs, Risks/Conditions of Select Rural Aggregates—cont'd

Rural Aggregates	Health Care Needs	Health Risks/Conditions
African Americans	Community nursing health promotion and screening services Diabetes screening and educators Hypertension screening/education Prenatal and perinatal health care services Oncology services (education/screening/follow-up interventions) HIV/AIDS prevention education/screening/follow-up care Mental/behavioral health services Health promotion/illness prevention education Veterans services Pain management education Independent/progressive care living facilities for aging population Interpersonal/domestic violence services Women's health services LGBTQ sensitive services	Diabetes Hypertension Sickle cell anemia Infectious diseases (e.g., hepatitis, HIV/AIDS) Cancer (e.g., prostate, breast) Dental caries/loss Depression Interpersonal/domestic violence Pain management/opioid misuse
Migrant farmworkers	Environmental protection policies (safe drinking water/sanitation) Community nursing/migrant health services (primary, secondary, tertiary prevention) Diabetes screening and educators Hypertension screening/education Maternal/child services Oncology services (education/screening/follow-up interventions) Mental/behavioral health services Interpersonal/domestic violence services Women's health services LGBTQ sensitive services Immunizations	Infectious diseases (e.g., hepatitis, typhoid, TB, HIV/AIDS, STDs) Environmental exposure effects of pesticides/herbicides Otitis media (children) Substance abuse (alcohol, recreational drugs, imported medicinal/herbs) Dental caries/loss Interpersonal/domestic violence Substandard living conditions with inadequate safe water/waste disposal Inadequate immunizations across the life span
Alaska Natives	Advanced life support/emergency care services Medical transport services Oral/dental care Obstetric/perinatal/pediatric services Mental/behavioral health services Culturally appropriate substance abuse treatment programs Epidemiologists Diabetes screening and educators Health promotion/illness prevention education Veterans services Pain management education Independent/progressive care living facilities for aging population Interpersonal/domestic violence services Women's health services LGBTQ sensitive services Culturally sensitive grief counselors	Infectious diseases (e.g., hepatitis, TB) Dental caries/loss Depression Interpersonal/domestic violence Environmental health risks (e.g., exposure to toxic substances/contaminants, hypothermia) Diabetes Alcohol/substance abuse Cirrhosis of the liver Vehicular accidents/trauma/long-term chronic residual effects Interpersonal/domestic violence Suicide awareness/prevention
Coal miners	Occupational Safety and Health Administration policy/standards Mental/behavioral health services Emergency/advanced life support services Occupational health nurses Grief counselors Health promotion/illness prevention education Veterans services Pain management education Independent/progressive care living facilities for aging population	Depression/substance abuse Occupational-related accidents/trauma Respiratory conditions (e.g., black lung, chronic obstructive pulmonary disease) Interpersonal/domestic violence Chronic pain management/opioid misuse Alcohol/substance abuse Interpersonal/domestic violence

HIV/AIDS, Human immunodeficiency virus/acquired immunodeficiency syndrome; *LGBTQ,* lesbian/gay/bisexual/transgender/queer; *TB,* tuberculosis.

Data from Bolin JN, Bellamy G: *Rural healthy people: 2020,* 2015. Available at https://srhrc.tamhsc.edu; Centers for Disease Control and Prevention: *Strategies for reducing health disparities,* 2016. Available at https://www.cdc.gov; Meit M, Knudson A, Gilbert T, et al.: *The 2014 update of the rural-urban chartbook,* 2014. Available at https://ruralhealth.und.edu; Migrant Clinicians Network: *FHN key resources for migrant health,* 2017. Available at https://www.migrantclinician.org; National Center for Health Statistics (NCHS): *Data visualization* gallery, 2018. Available at https://www.cdc.gov.

dangerous machinery with minimal operating instructions on the hazards and on safety precautions. Also, many agriculture workers do not speak or read English. Consequently, agriculture-related accidents result in a sizeable number of deaths and long-term injuries, particularly among children and women. The morbidity and mortality rates associated with agriculture vary from state to state. The rising incidence of these injuries and deaths, however, has become a national concern. Nurses in rural settings can help address this problem by including farm safety content in school and community education programs (Prengaman et al., 2017).

In summary, it is risky to generalize about the health status of rural Americans because of their diversity coupled with conflicting definitions of what differentiates rural from urban residences. Many vulnerable individuals and families live in rural communities across the United States, but little is known about most of them. This information deficit is a rich area of research for nurses who practice in rural environments.

RURAL HEALTH CARE DELIVERY ISSUES AND BARRIERS TO CARE

Although each rural community is unique, the experience of living in a rural area has several common characteristics (Bushy & Winters, 2013; Montgomery et al., 2017). Barriers to health care may be associated with these characteristics (e.g., whether services and professionals are available, affordable, accessible, or acceptable to rural consumers). Box 32.4 lists characteristics of rural life.

Availability implies the existence of health services as well as the necessary personnel to provide essential services. Sparseness of population limits the number and array of health care services in a given geographic region. Lacking a critical mass, the cost of providing special services to a few people often is prohibitive, particularly in frontier states where there are an insufficient number of physicians, nurses, and other types of health care providers. Consequently, where services and personnel are scarce, these must be allocated wisely. Accessibility implies that a person has logistical access to, as well as the ability to purchase, needed services. Affordability is associated with both availability and accessibility of care. It infers that services are of reasonable cost and that a family has sufficient resources to purchase these when needed. Acceptability of care means that a particular service is appropriate and offered in a manner that is congruent with the values of a target population. This can be hampered by a client's cultural preference and the urban orientation of health professionals (AHCPR, 2017; Bushy & Winters, 2013). Box 32.5 lists barriers to health care in rural areas.

Providers' attitudes, insights, and knowledge about rural populations are also important. A patronizing or demeaning attitude, lack of accurate knowledge about rural populations, or insensitivity about the rural lifestyle on the part of a nurse can make it difficult to relate to those clients. Also, insensitivity fosters mistrust, resulting in rural clients' perceiving professionals as outsiders to the community. Some nurses in rural public health practice settings express feelings of professional isolation and community nonacceptance. To address disparate views, nursing faculty members should expose students to the rural environment and the people who live there. Clinical experiences must include opportunities to provide care to clients in their natural (e.g., rural) setting to gain accurate insight about a given community (Hawkins et al., 2018).

To design population-focused programs that are available, accessible, affordable, and appropriate, nurses must implement interventions that mesh with clients' beliefs. This implies that a family and a community are actively involved in planning and delivering care for those who receive it. Nurses must have an accurate perspective on rural clients. Although the importance of forming partnerships and ensuring mutual exchange seems obvious, most current research about rural communities has been for policy or reimbursement purposes. Empirical data about rural family systems are sparse in terms of their health beliefs, values, perceptions of illness, and health care–seeking behaviors as well as what is deemed to be appropriate nursing care. Therefore, nurse scholars must assume a more active role

BOX 32.4 Characteristics of Rural Life

- More space; greater distances between residents and services
- Cyclical/seasonal work and leisure activities
- Informal social and professional interactions
- Access to extended kinship systems
- Residents who are related or acquainted
- Lack of anonymity
- Challenges in maintaining confidentiality stemming from familiarity among residents
- Small (often family) enterprises; fewer large industries
- Economic orientation to land and nature with industries that are extractive in nature (e.g., agriculture, mining, lumbering, marine-related, outdoor recreational activities)
- More high-risk occupations
- Town as center of trade
- Churches and schools as socialization centers
- Preference for interacting with locals (insiders)
- Mistrust of newcomers to the community (outsiders)

BOX 32.5 Barriers to Health Care in Rural Areas

- Lack of health care providers and services
- Great distances to obtain services
- Lack of personal transportation
- Unavailable public transportation
- Lack of telephone services
- Unavailable outreach services
- Inequitable reimbursement policies for providers
- Unpredictable weather and/or travel conditions
- Inability to pay for care/lack of health insurance
- Lack of "know how" to procure publicly funded entitlements and services
- Inadequate provider attitudes and understanding about rural populations
- Language barriers (caregivers not linguistically competent)
- Care and services not culturally and linguistically appropriate

in implementing research on the needs of rural populations for nursing services to expand the profession's theoretical base and subsequently implement community-oriented, empirically based clinical interventions; they must understand the barriers to health care that many rural residents experience (Paré et al., 2017; Oosterbroek et al., 2017).

NURSING CARE IN RURAL ENVIRONMENTS

Theory, Research, and Practice

Information on nursing practice in small towns and rural environments is growing, and several themes have emerged as shown in Box 32.6. A nurse who practices in this setting can view each of these dimensions either as an opportunity or as a challenge.

Nationally and internationally, nurse researchers contend that existing theories do not fully explain rural nursing practice (Bell et al., 2018; Bushy & Winters, 2013; Williams et al., 2012). Their focus has been on the key concepts pertinent to nursing theory (health, person, environment, and nursing/caring) and proposed relational statements that are relevant to clients and nurses in rural environments (see the Evidence-Based Practice box). Because the focus of their research was primarily with non-Hispanic whites living in the Rocky Mountain area, care must be taken about generalizing those findings to other geographic regions and minorities. These researchers propose that rural residents often judge their health by their ability to work. They consider themselves healthy, even though they may suffer from several chronic illnesses, as long as they are able to continue working. For the rural person, being healthy is the ability to be productive. Chronically ill people emphasize emotional and spiritual well-being rather than physical wellness.

BOX 32.6 Characteristics of Nursing Practice in Rural Environments

- Variety/diversity in clinical experiences
- Broader/expanding scope of practice
- Generalist skills
- Flexibility/creativity in delivering care
- Sparse resources (e.g., materials, professionals, equipment, fiscal)
- Professional/personal isolation
- Greater independence/autonomy
- Role overlap with other disciplines
- Slower pace
- Lack of anonymity
- Increased opportunity for informal interactions with clients/coworkers
- Opportunity for client follow-up upon discharge in informal community settings
- Discharge planning allowing for integration of formal and informal resources
- Care for clients across the life span
- Exposure to clients with a full range of conditions/diagnoses
- Status in the community (viewed as prestigious)
- Viewed as a professional role model
- Opportunity for community involvement and informal health education

Adapted from Rural Health Information Hub (RHI-Hub): *What is rural?* 2018. Available at https://www.ruralhealthinfo.org. Winters C, Lee H: *Rural nursing: concepts, theory and practice*, ed. 3, New York, 2009, Springer Publishing.

EVIDENCE-BASED PRACTICE

Early on, nurse researchers at Montana State University related nursing theoretical concepts to rural practice (Long & Weinert, 1989; Winters, 2013; Winters & Lee, 2009). Since then, researchers have studied the relevance of the proposed rural nursing concepts to various populations and settings to expand the knowledge base of the profession.

- **Health:** Defined by rural residents as the ability to work. Work and health beliefs are closely related for rural Montana sample.
- **Environment:** Distance and isolation are particularly important for rural dwellers. Those who live long distances neither perceive themselves as isolated nor perceive health care services as inaccessible.
- **Nursing:** Lack of anonymity, outsider versus insider, old-timer versus newcomer. Lack of anonymity is a common theme among rural nurses who report knowing most people for whom they care, not only in the nurse-client relationship, but also in a variety of social roles, such as family member, friend, or neighbor. Acceptance as a health care provider in the community is closely linked to the outsider/insider and newcomer/old-timer phenomena. Gaining trust and acceptance of local people is identified as a unique challenge that must be successfully negotiated by nurses before they can begin to function as effective health care providers.
- **Person:** Self-reliance and independence in relationship to health care are strong characteristics of rural individuals. They prefer to have people they know care for them (informal services) as opposed to an outsider in a formal agency.

Nurse Use

In working with rural residents, it is important to know how they define their health and their environment, because their definitions may differ from yours. Understand that you may not find acceptance and trust immediately; rural residents often trust informal caregivers more than those in a formal organization.

From Bell J, Crawford R, Holloway K: Core components of the rural nurse specialist role in New Zealand. *Rural Remote Health* 18(2), 2018. Available at https://www.rrh.org.au; Rural Health Information Hub (RHI-Hub): *What is rural?* 2018. Available at https://www.ruralhealthinfo.org.

Distance, isolation, and sparse resources characterize rural life and are seen in residents' independent and innovative coping strategies. Self-reliance and independence are demonstrated through their self-care practices and preference for family and community support. Community networks provide support but still allow for each person's and family's independence. Ruralites prefer and usually seek help through their informal networks, such as neighbors, extended family, church, and civic clubs, rather than seeking a professional's care in the formal system of health care, including services such as those provided by a mental health clinic, social service agency, or health department.

Although nursing is generally similar across settings and populations, there are some unique features associated with practice in a geographically remote area or in small towns where most people know one another. The following paragraphs highlight a few of the variations that nurses in rural practice report.

A nurse's professional and personal boundaries often overlap and are diffuse. It is not unusual for a nurse to have more than one work-related role in the community. For example, a nurse may work at the local hospital or in a physician's office and may also be actively involved in managing the family farm, a local grocery store, or pharmacy. For nurses, this means that many, if not all, clients they encounter are known also as neighbors, as friends of an immediate family member, or as part of one's extended family. Associated with social informality is a corresponding lack of anonymity in a small town. Some rural nurses say, "I never really feel like I am off duty because everybody in the county knows me through my work." In part, this can be attributed to nurses being highly respected and viewed by local people as experts on health and illness. Often rural residents informally ask a nurse's advice before seeing a physician for a health problem. Rural residents may ask health-related questions when they see a local nurse (who may be a neighbor, friend, or relative) in a grocery store, at a service station, during a basketball game, or at church functions (Ortiz et al., 2018).

Nurses in rural public health practice must make decisions about the care of individuals of all ages with a variety of health conditions. They assume many roles because of the range of services they provide in a rural health care facility and because of the scarcity of nurses and other health professionals. Nurses who work in rural areas need to have skills that include technical and clinical competency, adaptability, flexibility, strong assessment skills, organizational abilities, independence, interest in continuing education, sound decision-making skills, leadership ability, self-confidence, and skills in handling emergencies, teaching, and public relations. The nurse administrator is also expected to be a jack-of-all-trades (i.e., a generalist) and to demonstrate competence in several clinical specialties in addition to managing and organizing staff within the facility for which he or she is responsible (Pavloff et al., 2017; Prengaman et al., 2017).

Rural nursing practice provides challenges, opportunities, and rewards. The way in which each factor is perceived depends on individual preferences and the situation in a given community. Challenges of rural practice sometimes include professional isolation, limited opportunities for continuing education, lack of other kinds of health personnel or professionals with whom one can interact, heavy workloads, an ability to function well in several clinical areas, lack of anonymity, and, for some, a restricted social life (Molinari & Bushy, 2012).

The most often cited opportunities and rewards in rural nursing practice are close relationships with clients and co-workers, diverse clinical experiences that evolve from caring for clients of all ages who have a variety of health problems, caring for clients for long periods of time (in some cases, across several generations), opportunities for professional development, and greater autonomy. Many nurses value the solitude and quality of life found in a rural community personally and for their own family. Others thrive on the outdoor recreational activities. Still others thoroughly enjoy the informal, face-to-face interactions coupled with the public recognition and status associated with living and working as a nurse in a small community. Disease prevention is also an important consideration in rural communities. The Levels of Prevention box shows the levels of prevention that a nurse in a rural locale might use.

LEVELS OF PREVENTION

Rural Health

Primary Prevention

- The public health nurse partners with a women's organization in a faith community located in a small Midwestern town to instruct members on meal planning as a strategy to offset the tendency to develop diabetes in family members.
- The public health nurse advocates for policy changes regarding sexual education content (to include information on contraception that goes beyond abstinence) in the schools with the district commissioners of education.

Secondary Prevention

- The public health nurse screens congregation members of the faith community in the Midwestern town for the presence of diabetes.
- The public health nurse partners with the local critical access hospital to offer free cholesterol, blood pressure, and blood glucose screening as well as the influenza vaccine to adults attending the annual county health fair.

Tertiary Prevention

- The public health nurse collaborates with the senior center in the small community town, which provides meals on a routine basis to the elderly, to reach individuals with a diagnosis of diabetes.
- The public health nurse provides consultation on diabetic nutrition, exercise habits, foot care, and, if needed, assists clients in obtaining medications through a mail-order pharmaceutical vendor.

Although most of the publications about rural health care and nursing focus on hospital practice, much of that information is applicable to both community agencies and community-focused nursing (Davis & Droes, 1993). An early study by Case (1991) focused on work-related stressors of nursing in rural communities in Oklahoma public health departments. Anecdotal reports reinforce these same stressors are present in rural practice, including: political/bureaucratic problems and intraprofessional and interpersonal conflicts associated with inadequate communication; unsatisfactory work environment and understaffing; difficult or unpleasant nurse-client encounters, such as with relatives who refuse to deliver needed care to clients, and with clients who are hostile, apathetic, dependent, or of low intelligence; fear for personal safety; difficulty locating clients; and clients falling through the cracks of the health care system. These same stressors continue to be cited by nurses who work in rural as well as urban public health agencies. Essentially, stressors for rural nurses in general, and specifically for those in community practice, are associated with geographic distance, isolation, sparse resources, and environmental factors that characterize rurality (Pare et al., 2017).

Nursing in rural areas is characterized by physical isolation that may lend itself to any one of the following: professional isolation; scarce financial, human, and health care resources; and a broad scope of practice. Associated with personal familiarity with local residents, nurses often possess in-depth

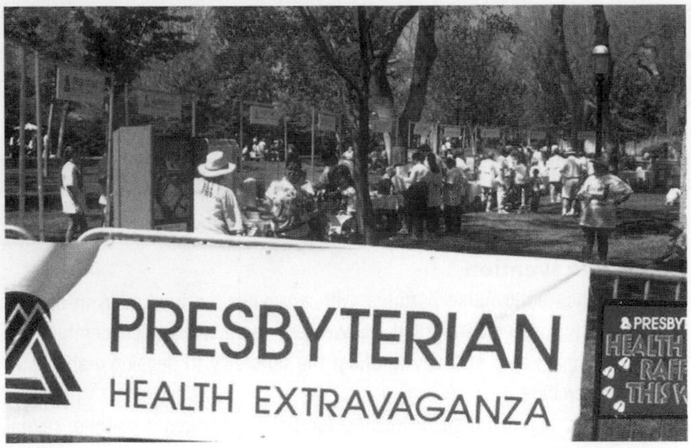

Fig. 32.2 A hospital-sponsored health fair is one example of a community event to provide health services to individuals in a rural area.

knowledge about clients and their families. Along with the acknowledged benefits, informal (face-to-face) interactions can significantly reduce a nurse's anonymity in the community and at times be a barrier to completing an objective assessment on a client. Like urban practice, rural community nursing as shown in Fig. 32.2 takes place in a variety of locations, including homes, clinics, schools, occupational settings, and correctional facilities, and at community events such as county fairs, rodeos, civic and church-sponsored functions, and school athletic events.

Research Needs

There is a paucity of empirical studies focusing on rural nursing practice, but anecdotal reports by nurses confirm earlier studies on practice in this setting (Bushy & Winters, 2013). Specific research topics of importance to nursing practice in rural environments include the following:

1. Most nurses indicate that they enjoy practicing in rural areas and are proud of what they do. They believe that their work deserves more recognition by professional nursing organizations. Also, the retention rate of nurses in some practice settings is poor. The perspective of nurses who are dissatisfied with rural nursing provides a more complete picture of the rural experience. This information can be useful to a variety of people: other nurses who are considering rural practice, nurse managers in need of better screening tools to assess the fit between the nurse and the environment when interviewing applicants, planners of continuing nursing education programs, and faculty members who teach public health to undergraduate and graduate students.
2. More information is needed about the stressors and rewards of rural practice, in particular public health nursing. These data could lead to the development of stress management techniques to be used by nurses and their supervisors to retain nurses and to improve the quality of their workplace environment.
3. With the increasing number of rural residents in all regions of the United States, empirical data are needed on the particular nursing needs of rural client systems, especially under-represented groups, minorities, and other at-risk populations that vary by region and state.
4. A need also exists for the international perspective on the health of rural populations, and on nursing practice within the rural community. Australian, New Zealand, and Canadian nurse scholars have provided some insights into rural practice in these nations. Information is needed from less-industrialized nations as well as from those that are highly industrialized.
5. Technology increasingly is used in health care and seems to hold great potential in improving access to health care in rural and underserved areas. However, research is needed to determine the most efficient and effective way to meet the needs and preferences of rural clients, and to ensure quality.
6. Communication technology increasingly is used by institutions of higher learning to deliver educational programs to nurses who live and work some distance from campus. Empirical studies are needed to measure the most effective modalities to achieve desired learning outcomes and the impact on recruitment and retention of nurses in rural settings.
7. Rural-urban disparities in health status and health behaviors need closer examination from the nursing perspective. Evidence-based practice nursing guidelines are needed that take into consideration the rural context and preferences of residents who obtain health care in these settings.

Preparing Nurses for Rural Practice Settings

Nurses in rural practice need broad knowledge about nursing, including health promotion, primary prevention, rehabilitation, obstetrics, medical-surgical specialties, pediatrics, planning and implementing community assessments, and understanding the public health risks and needs for emergency preparedness in a particular state. A community's demographic profile and its principal industry(ies) can provide a snapshot of local social determinants that can affect health. Using demographic information, a nurse can anticipate the particular nursing skills that will be needed to care for clients in a catchment area (BHWF, 2018; Booth & Graves, 2018; Jackman et al., 2016; Nelson, 2009; Oosterbroek et al., 2017; Pavloff et al., 2017). In rural areas nurses use their knowledge of resources and their ability to coordinate formal and informal services to coordinate a continuum of services for clients even when resources are sparse and fragmentation exists in the health care delivery system (Hawkins et al., 2018).

Technology has great potential for connecting rural public health providers and consumers with resources outside of their community. The concept of *telehealth* is an expansion of the term *telemedicine*. Essentially, telemedicine more narrowly focuses on the curative aspect of health care, whereas telehealth encompasses preventive, promotive, and curative aspects of health care and can include delivery of education/information to a more distant site. Telehealth uses a variety of technology solutions such as a health care provider communicating by email with clients, ordering medications from a pharmacy, consulting with other health care providers, or accessing advanced or continuing education offered by a university located some distance from the receiving site. More specifically, telecommunication technology could be as simple as nurses in two or more different public health settings consulting over the telephone or via computer video conferencing coordinating local health fairs, or as complex as nurse scholars collaborating with international peers on a community health–focused research project or a medical specialist located at a health science center using complex robotic surgical technology on a client who is located in another country. Regardless of the practice setting, the nurse must be computer literate and be proficient in using the communication technology that is available in that community. Increasingly, the Internet is linking nurses in rural public health practice with nursing colleagues, educators, and researchers in urban-based academic settings, thereby addressing often-cited concerns associated with professional isolation (ANCC, 2017).

FUTURE PERSPECTIVES

It is important for all people involved in providing health care in rural areas to understand the possible problems they might encounter when trying to provide the continuum of needed services in an area with a disproportionally high number of underserved persons. Those who should be involved include residents, their elected representatives, the administrators of public and private health care agencies, and members of the media. The media need to focus on public health as well as hospital care and the lack of primary care providers in rural areas. As discussed later, both case management and community-oriented primary health care (COPHC) are effective models for dealing with some of the care deficits and resolving rural health disparities.

Scarce Resources and a Comprehensive Health Care Continuum

The current fragmented health care system makes it difficult to provide a comprehensive continuum of care to populations living in areas having scarce resources, such as money, personnel, equipment, and ancillary services. In rural communities, the most critically needed services are usually preventive services, such as health screening clinics, nutrition counseling, tobacco cessation, and wellness education (Bolin & Bellamy, 2015; CDC, 2017a, 2018a, 2018b). Box 32.7 lists several health-related priorities for rural communities.

Although the nursing needs vary by community, there is generally a need in most rural areas for the following:

- School and parish nurses
- Family planning services
- Prenatal and postpartum services
- Resources for individuals diagnosed with human immunodeficiency virus (HIV)/AIDS and their families
- Emergency medical services
- Resources for families of children with special needs, including those who are physically and mentally challenged
- Mental health services
- Resources for older adults (especially the frail elderly and those with declining mental capacity) to include a continuum of residential and respite services, including adult day care, hospice, homemaker assistance, and provision of nutritional meals along with public transportation for those who remain at home

BOX 32.7 Health-Related Priorities for Many Rural Communities

- Access to care
- Cancer (screening, early intervention, oncology services)
- Diabetes (prevention, screening, tertiary care)
- Maternal–infant and children services
- Mental illness and behavioral health services
- Nutrition/obesity
- Drugs, alcohol, and substance abuse
- Use of tobacco products
- Education and an array of community-based programs
- Public health infrastructures
- Immunizations and infectious diseases
- Trauma-related injury and violence prevention
- Family planning
- Environmental and occupational health exposure education/prevention
- Emergency medical services infrastructures
- Long-term care/assistive living facilities
- Veterans services
- Safety education on outdoor recreational activities (all-terrain vehicles, water, weapons, etc.)
- Grief counseling
- High-risk occupation safety education
- Suicide awareness/prevention
- Prevention of motor vehicle accidents/injuries

Adapted from Meit M, Knudson A, Gilbert T, et al.: *The 2014 update of the rural-urban chartbook*. Available at https://ruralhealth.und.edu; Bolin JN, Bellamy G: *Rural Healthy People: 2020*, 2015. Available at https://srhrc.tamhsc.edu.

Providing a continuum of care has been further hindered by the closure of many small hospitals in the past two decades. Of those that remain, many report financial problems that could lead to closure (NACRHHS, 2017). A shortage or the absence of even one provider, most often a physician or nurse, could mean that a small hospital must close its doors. Closure of the hospital has a ripple effect on the health of local residents, other health care services, recruitment and retention of health professionals, as well as on economic development efforts in a small community (USDA, 2017a, n.d.; USDHHS, 2013).

The short supply and increasing demand for primary care providers in general, and nurses in particular, will continue for some time. To help solve this problem, elected officials and policy developers need nurses, especially those in advanced practice roles, to provide vital services in underserved areas. In an effort to effectively respond to this opportunity, nurses must be creative to ensure delivery of appropriate and acceptable services to at-risk and vulnerable populations who live in rural and underserved regions. Nurses must be sensitive to the health beliefs of clients, and then plan and provide nursing interventions that mesh with the community's cultural values and preferences.

Healthy People 2020 National Health Objectives Related to Rural Health

Because the demographic profile varies from community to community, each state has variations in the health status of its population. *Healthy People 2020,* along with *Rural Healthy People 2020* (vol. 1, vol. 2), has important implications for nurses in that a significant number of at-risk populations cited in that policy-guiding document live in rural areas across the United States (Bolin & Bellamy, 2015). Consequently, priority objectives vary, depending on population mix, health risks, and health status of residents in the state.

HEALTHY PEOPLE 2020

These selected objectives pertain to residents of both rural and urban areas:

- **AHS-3:** Increase the proportion of persons with a usual primary care provider.
- **IVP-13:** Reduce motor vehicle crash–related deaths.
- **MHMD-9:** Increase the proportion of adults with mental disorders who receive treatment.
- **HDS-2:** Reduce coronary heart disease deaths.
- **IVP-1:** Reduce fatal and nonfatal injuries.

From U.S. Department of Health and Human Services: *Healthy People 2020,* 2010. Available at https://www.healthypeople.gov.

At the local level, communities have been using *Healthy People* as a guide for action and to identify objectives and establish meaningful goals. The two-volume *Rural Healthy People 2020* focuses on particular concerns relative to vulnerable populations in rural environments (Bolin & Bellamy, 2015).

The Centers for Disease Control and Prevention's (CDC's) (2017a) *Healthy Places Initiative* addresses chronic disease prevention in both rural and urban communities. Individuals and groups at the local level collaborated with state health departments, the CDC, and other organizations to implement programs that promote and support good health in their community. This CDC initiative is a useful tool for state and local officials and health care planners to use to tailor *Healthy People* objectives to fit a community's specific needs, both rural and urban. Translating national objectives highlighted in *Healthy People 2020* (USDHHS, 2013) into achievable community health goals requires integration of the following components to ensure that services will be acceptable and appropriate for rural clients:

- Health statistics must be meaningful and understandable, and they must include appropriate process and outcome objectives that can be readily measured.
- Strategies must be designed that involve the public, private, and voluntary sectors of the community to achieve agreed-on local objectives.
- Coordinated efforts are needed to ensure that the community works together to achieve the goals.

Consider, for example, general objectives in developing a health plan for a rural county having a large population of young people. *Healthy People 2020* objectives for the county should target women of childbearing age, children, and adolescents. Priority objectives should include offering accessible prenatal care programs, improving immunization levels, providing preventive dental care instructions, implementing vehicular accident prevention and firearm safety programs, and educating teachers and health professionals for early identification of cases of interpersonal violence. On the other hand, consider a rural county that has a higher number of residents over the age of 65 years, compared with the national average. Priority objectives in the health plan should target health risks and problems of older adults in that community. Specific objectives might include developing health-promoting programs to prevent chronic health problems, or establishing community programs to meet the needs of those having chronic illness, specifically cardiovascular disease, diabetes, hypertension, and accident-related disabilities; or organizing a partnership to build progressive/assistive care residential facilities in the community. In general, the objectives in *Healthy People 2020* are pertinent to people living in all areas and not unique to rural residents. The *Healthy People 2020* box illustrates selected objectives that fit people in rural as well as more urban areas.

When implementing community-focused health plans that emerge from *Healthy People 2020,* consideration must always be given to the rural context, such as sparse population, geographic remoteness, scarce resources, personnel shortages, and physical, emotional, and social isolation. In addition to being actively involved in empowering the community and planning and delivering care, nurses play an important role in representing their community's perspective to local, state, regional, and national health planners and to their elected officials.

BUILDING PROFESSIONAL-COMMUNITY-CLIENT PARTNERSHIPS IN RURAL SETTINGS

Health care reform initiatives are focusing on cutting costs while improving access to care with equitable quality for all citizens, especially vulnerable and underserved populations. State and local grassroots organizations must be actively involved for health care reform to succeed in rural areas. Specifically, professional-client-community partnerships are essential to accomplish reform at the local level. As seen in the Linking Content to Practice box, nursing practice in rural areas is comprehensive and incorporates skills from nursing and public health. Two models have been found to be particularly useful for nurses in rural environments: case management and Community-Oriented Primary Health Care (COPHC).

Case Management

Case management is a client-professional partnership that can be used to arrange a continuum of care for rural clients, with the case manager tailoring and blending formal and informal resources. Collaborative efforts between a client and the case manager allow clients to participate in their plan of care in an acceptable and appropriate way, especially when local resources are few and far between. The Practice Application at the end of this chapter demonstrates how nursing case management can

LINKING CONTENT TO PRACTICE

As discussed, practice in rural areas relies on excellent nursing and public health skills in assessment, communication, cultural competency, problem solving, coalition building, coordination, and policy development, among others. Documents that guide the practice include the American Nurses Association Standards of Nursing Practice, the core competencies as identified by the Council on Linkages, and the Quad Council Coalition for Public Health Nursing Competencies. As one example of the congruence, consider assessment. The Council on Linkages' Core Competency of "Assess the health status of populations and their related determinants of health and illness" under their analytic assessment skills is then elaborated on by the Quad Council as a public health nursing skill of "Conducts thorough health assessments of individuals, families, communities and populations" and the public health nursing practice standard under assessment of "the public health nurse collects comprehensive data pertinent to the health status of populations" (p. XXX.) The relationship among these three sets of standards continues through all phases of the public health care provision process.

Data from American Nurses Association (ANA): *Public Health Nursing: Scope and Standards of Practice*, ed. 2, Silver Spring, MD, 2013. Available at https://www.nursingworld.org . Council on Linkages between Academia and Public Health Practice: *Core competencies for public health professionals*, 2014. Available at http://www.phf.org Quad Council: *Public health nursing competencies*, 2018. Available at http://www.quadcouncilphn.org.

allow an older adult resident to stay at home in a rural environment if adequate supports can be provided. Outcomes are often remarkably different when case management is used. Additional information on case management is found in Chapter 25.

Community-Oriented Primary Health Care

COPHC is an effective model for delivering available, accessible, and acceptable services to vulnerable populations living in **medically underserved** areas. This model emphasizes flexibility, grassroots involvement, and professional-community partnerships. It blends primary care, public health, and prevention services, which are offered in a familiar and accessible setting. As shown in Box 32.8 the COPHC model is interprofessional, uses a problem-oriented approach, and mandates community involvement in all phases of the process.

Building professional-community partnerships is an ongoing process. The CDC *Tools and Resources for Public-Private Partnerships* (2017b) at https://www.cdc.gov offers useful information on collaborative and interprofessional initiatives in small and rural communities. At various times, nurses, other health professionals, and community leaders must assume the role of advocate, change agent, educator, expert, or group facilitator to gain both active and passive support from the community. Partnerships involve give-and-take negotiations by all participants to reach consensus. Essentially, the process begins with professionals gaining entrance into a community, establishing rapport and trust with local people, and then working together to empower the community to resolve mutually defined problems and goals. As mentioned previously, and discussed also in Chapter 16, the CDC *Healthy Places Initiative* (2017a) is an excellent resource for developing, defining, and responding to the stated goals. Because of the importance of churches and schools in a rural community, leaders from those institutions often are key players in building provider-community partnerships. The organizational phase is a priority because it forms the foundation for all other activities related to planning, implementing, and evaluating community initiatives.

As was described for case management, professional-community partnerships allow more effective identification of existing informal support systems that are accepted by rural residents. The goal is to integrate community preferences with new or existing formal services. Public input should be encouraged early in the planning process and must continue throughout the process to allow the community to feel that it has ownership in the project. This strategy can go a long way to address local residents' viewing the process as outsiders bringing another bureaucratic program into town. Strategies that nurses can use to enhance the building of partnerships in rural environments are listed in the How To Build Professional-Community-Client Partnerships box.

BOX 32.8 Community-Oriented Primary Health Care (COPHC): A Partnership Process

The steps in the COPHC process include the following:

- Define and characterize the community.
- Identify the community's health problems.
- Develop or modify health care services in response to the community's identified needs.
- Monitor and evaluate program process and client outcomes.

Modified from Centers for Disease Control and Prevention (CDC): *Tools and resources for public-private partnerships*, 2017. Available at https://www.cdc.gov.

HOW TO Build Professional-Community-Client Partnerships

1. Gain the local perspective.
2. Assess the degree of public awareness and support for the cause.
3. Identify special interest groups.
4. List existing services to avoid duplication of programs.
5. Note real and potential barriers to existing resources and services.
6. Generate a list of potential community volunteers and professionals who are willing to assist with the project.
7. Create awareness among target groups of a particular program (e.g., individuals, families, seniors, church and recreation groups, health care professionals, law enforcement personnel, and members of other religious, service, and civic clubs).
8. Identify potential funding sources needed to implement the program.
9. Establish the community's health care priority list, and involve many community members in considering and selecting their health care options.
10. Incorporate business principles in marketing the program.
11. Measure the health system's local economic impact.
12. Educate residents about the important role the local health care system plays in the economic infrastructure of the community and the consequences of a system failure.
13. Develop local leadership and support for the community's health system through training and providing experience in decision making.

Modified from Centers for Disease Control and Prevention (CDC): *Tools and resources for public-private partnerships*, 2017b. Available at https://www.cdc.gov.

Partnership models, such as case management and COPHC, have proven to be highly effective in areas with scarce resources and an insufficient number of health care providers. Individuals and communities who are informed, active participants in planning are more likely to develop consensus about the most appropriate solution for local problems. Subsequently, involved participants are more likely to use and support that system after it is implemented. Partnership models enhance the ability of rural communities to do what they historically have done well (i.e., assume responsibility for the services and institutions that serve their residents). Knowledge about partnership models and the skills to effectively implement them are useful for nurses who coordinate services that are accessible, available, and acceptable for rural populations in their catchment area.

QSEN FOCUS ON QUALITY AND SAFETY EDUCATION FOR NURSES

Targeted Competency: Quality Improvement

Use data to monitor the outcomes of care processes and use improvement methods to design and test changes to continuously improve the quality and safety of health care systems.

Important aspects of quality improvement include:

- **Knowledge:** Explain the importance of variation and measurement in assessing quality of care.
- **Skills:** Use quality measures to understand performance.
- **Attitudes:** Value measurement and its role in good client care.

Quality Improvement Question

Examine health statistics and demographic data in your geographic area to determine which vulnerable groups are predominant. Look on the web for examples of agencies you think provide services to these vulnerable groups. If the agency has a web page, read about the target population they serve, the types of services they provide, and how they are reimbursed for services. Learn about different agencies and share results during class. Based on your findings, identify gaps or overlaps in services provided to vulnerable groups in your community. Which data do these agencies collect to demonstrate the efficacy of their services? How could you deal with these gaps and overlaps to help clients receive needed services?

Modified from Centers for Disease Control and Prevention (CDC): *Performance management and quality improvement,* 2015. Available at https://www.cdc.gov.

PRACTICE APPLICATION

Mrs. Jones, an 89-year-old widow, was diagnosed over 10 years ago with progressive congestive heart failure. She continues to live in her beloved home of 60+ years in spite of being on continuous oxygen the last 3 years. She also has "bad knees" and gets around her house and yard with the use of a walker. Her husband of more than 60 years suddenly died 4 years ago of a heart attack while working on their farm. Their two married daughters live in California and Arkansas. The Midwestern town where she lives has about 1000 residents. The nearest hospital is more than 60 miles away from this town. Mrs. Jones's 82-year-old widowed sister, Lydia Thomas, lives a few blocks from her. Their 76-year-old brother recently entered the county nursing home located in a town 20 miles away.

Even with her dyspnea and physical limitations, Mrs. Jones is able to live alone with her dog and cat, and insists that she will not relinquish her independent lifestyle as has her brother. Yet, in the past year she has been hospitalized three times: for a bad chest cold, for a kidney infection, and after a neighbor found her lying unconscious by the picnic table in her yard. Her doctor says this episode was related to a "heart problem."

Upon being discharged from the hospital, Crystal Moore, the local home health nurse, was assigned to visit Mrs. Jones. Ms. Moore's office is based in the County Senior Center near the nursing home where the brother is a resident. He is also a client of Ms. Moore and she visits him every Wednesday. The nurse provides outreach services to all the residents in the county referred to her by a large home health agency located in the city 70 miles away. As a case manager, she works closely with the hospital's discharge planners to arrange a continuum of care for clients in the county. Nursing-related activities include coordinating formal and informal services for clients, including biomedical supplies, oxygenation, nutrition, hydration, pharmacological care, arranging for personal care, homemaker assistance, writing checks, home maintenance, emergency respite services, and home delivery of meals.

A. Describe the nursing roles that Ms. Moore uses in coordinating a continuum of care for Mrs. Jones in terms of nutrition, oxygenation, pharmaceutical and biomedical equipment, transportation, and homemaker assistance.
B. Identify formal health care and support resources that can be accessed for Mrs. Jones.
C. Identify informal support resources that might be available in the small community that could help to ensure that Mrs. Jones is safe.
D. Identify three outcomes for Mrs. Jones that can be achieved by using nursing care (case) management.
E. Select a rural community in your geographic area. Create hypothetical situations, or select real clients with real health problems (e.g., an older adult with Alzheimer's disease, a middle-aged person with cancer requiring end-of-life care, a child who is dependent on technology as a result of a farm accident). Prepare a list of services and referral agencies in that community that could be used to develop a continuum of care for each of these cases. How are these the same as, or different from, the case described in this chapter?
F. How could a public or home health nurse who is new to the community learn about formal and informal resources that could be accessed to develop a continuum of care for a rural resident for whom she cares?

Answers can be found on the Evolve site.

KEY POINTS

- There is wide diversity in the demography, economy, and geography of rural communities.
- Not all rural communities are based on an agricultural economy; most are not!
- Although many are struggling, not all rural communities are suffering economically. Some rural communities only need more extensive economic development for sustainability.
- Some rural towns are located in urban counties.
- There are wide variations in the health status of rural populations, depending on genetic, social, environmental, economic, and political factors.
- There is a higher prevalence of working poor in rural America than in more populated areas.
- There are rural-urban health disparities. Rural adults 18 years and older overall are in poorer health than their urban counterparts; nearly 50 percent have been diagnosed with at least one major chronic condition. However, they average one less physician visit each year than healthier urban counterparts.
- More than 26 percent of rural families are below the poverty level; more than 40 percent of all rural children younger than 18 years of age live in poverty.
- General practitioners and nurse practitioners are usual providers of care for rural adults and children.
- Rural residents must often travel more than 30 minutes to access a health care provider.
- Nurses must take into consideration the belief systems and lifestyles of a rural population when planning, implementing, and evaluating community services.
- Barriers to rural health care include the lack of availability, affordability, accessibility, and acceptability of services.
- Partnership models, particularly case management and community-oriented primary health care (COPHC), are effective models to provide a comprehensive continuum of care in environments with scarce resources.

CLINICAL DECISION-MAKING ACTIVITIES

1. Compare and contrast the terms *urban, suburban, rural, frontier, farm, non-farm residency,* and *metropolitan* and *micropolitan areas.*
2. Describe residency as a continuum, ranging from farm residency to core metropolitan residency.
3. Discuss economic, social, and cultural factors that affect rural lifestyle and the health care–seeking behaviors of residents who live there.
4. Identify factors that affect the accessibility, affordability, availability, and acceptability of services in the health care delivery system.
5. Compare and contrast the health status and lifestyle behaviors of rural and urban residents.
6. Summarize key nursing concepts in terms of practice in the rural context.
7. Examine the characteristics of rural community nursing practice and describe how these might differ from those of practice in more populated settings.
8. Compare and contrast challenges, opportunities, and benefits of living and practicing as a nurse in the rural environment.
9. Evaluate case management and community-oriented primary care as partnership models that can help nurses enhance the continuum of care for clients living in an environment with sparse resources.
10. Propose potential areas for rural nursing research activities. Specify research questions that focus on the professional and clinical concerns of public health nurses who practice in the rural context.

ADDITIONAL RESOURCES

EVOLVE WEBSITE

http://evolve.elsevier.com/Stanhope/community/

- Answers to Practice Application
- Case Study
- Glossary
- Review Questions

REFERENCES

Agency for Health Care Policy and Research (AHCPR): *National healthcare disparities report*, 2017. Retrieved from https://www.ahrq.gov.

American Nurses Association (ANA): *Public health nursing: scope and standards of practice*, ed 2, Silver Spring, MD, 2013, ANA. Retrieved from https://www.nursingworld.org.

American Nurses Credentialing Center (ANCC): ANCC *Pathway to excellence® program*, 2017. Retrieved from https://www.nursingworld.org.

Bell J, Crawford R, Holloway K: Core components of the rural nurse specialist role in New Zealand, *Rural & Remote Health* 18(2):4260, 2018.

Bigbee J, Crowder E: The Red Cross Rural Nursing Service: an innovative model of public health nursing delivery, *Public Health Nurs* 2(2):109, 1985.

Bolin JN, Bellamy G: *Rural Healthy People: 2020* (vols I–II), 2015. Retrieved from https://srhrc.tamhsc.edu.

Booth L, Graves BA: Service learning initiatives in rural populations: fostering cultural awareness, *Online J Rural Nurs Health Care* 18(1):90–111, 2018.

Bureau of Health Workforce (BHWF): *Supply and demand projections of the nursing workforce: 2014–2030*, 2017. Retrieved from https://bhw.hrsa.gov.

Bureau of Health Workforce (BHWF): *What is shortage designation? Shortage areas*, 2018. Retrieved from https://datawarehouse.hrsa.gov.

Bureau of the Census: *New census data show differences between urban and rural populations*, 2016. Retrieved from https://www.census.gov.

Bushy A: Health disparities in rural populations across the lifespan. In Winters CA, editor: *Rural nursing: concepts, theory, and practice*, ed 4, New York, NY, 2013, Springer Publishing.

Bushy A, Winters C: Nursing workforce development, clinical practice, research and nursing theory: Connecting the dots. In Winters CA, editor: *Rural nursing: concepts, theory, and Practice*, ed 4. New York, NY, 2013, Springer Publishing.

Case T: Work stresses of community health nurses in Oklahoma. In Bushy A, editor: *Rural nursing* (vol 2), Newbury Park, CA, 1991, Sage.

Centers for Disease Control and Prevention (CDC): *Performance management and quality improvement*, 2015. Retrieved from https://www.cdc.gov.

Centers for Disease Control and Prevention (CDC). *Strategies for reducing health disparities*, 2016. Retrieved from https://www.cdc.gov.

Centers for Disease Control and Prevention (CDC): *Healthy places*, 2017a. Retrieved from https://www.cdc.gov.

Centers for Disease Control and Prevention (CDC): *Tools and resources for public-private partnerships*, 2017b. Retrieved from https://www.cdc.gov.

Centers for Disease Control and Prevention (CDC): *Rural health*, 2018a. Retrieved from https://www.cdc.gov.

Centers for Disease Control and Prevention (CDC): *Smoking and tobacco use: fast facts*, 2018b. Retrieved from https://www.cdc.gov.

Council on Linkages between Academia and Public Health Practice: *Core competencies for public health professionals*, 2014. Retrieved from http://www.phf.org.

Davis DJ, Droes NS: Community health nursing in rural and frontier counties, *Nurs Clin North Am* 28:159–169, 1993.

Eisenhauer CM, Pullen CH, Nelson T, Kumm SA, Hunter JL: Partnering with rural farm women for participatory action and ethnography, *Online J Rural Nurs Health Care* 16(1):195–216, 2016.

Hawkins JE, Wiles LL, Karlowicz K, Tufts KA: Educational model to increase the number and diversity of RN to BSN graduates from a resource-limited rural community, *Nurse Educ* 43(4):206–209, 2018.

Institute of Medicine (IOM): *The future of nursing: leading change, advancing health*, 2010. Retrieved from http://www.nationalacademies.org.

Jackman D, Yonge O, Myrick F, Janke F, Konkin J: A rural interprofessional educational initiative: what success looks like, *Online J Rural Nurs Health Care* 16(2):5–26, 2016.

Jakobs L, Bigbee J: The distribution of advanced practice nurses and population health in U.S. frontier counties, 2016, *Online J Rural Nurs Health Care* 16(2):196–218, 2016.

Long KA, Weinert C: Rural nursing: developing the theory base, *Sch Inq Nurs Pract* 3:113–127, 1989.

Meit M, Knudson A, Gilbert T, et al.: *The 2014 Update of the Rural-Urban Chartbook*, 2014. Retrieved from https://ruralhealth.und.edu.

Migrant Clinicians Network (MHN): *FHN Key Resources for Migrant Health*, 2017. Retrieved from https://www.migrantclinician.org.

Molinari D, Bushy A, editors: *The rural nurse: transition to practice*, New York, NY, 2012, Springer Publishing.

Montgomery SR, Sutton AL, Paré J: Rural nursing and synergy, *Online J Rural Nurs Health Care* 17(1):87–99, 2017.

National Advisory Committee on Rural Health and Human Services (NACRHHS): *Social determinants of health: policy brief*, January 2017a. Retrieved from https://www.hrsa.gov.

National Advisory Committee on Rural Health and Human Services (NACRHHS): *Understanding the impact of suicide in rural America: policy brief and recommendations*, 2017b. Retrieved from https://www.hrsa.gov.

National Center for Health Statistics (NCHS): *Data visualization gallery*, 2018. Retrieved from https://www.cdc.gov.

Nelson W, editor: *Handbook for rural health care ethics*, Lebanon, NH, 2009, Dartmouth. Retrieved from http://dms.dartmouth.edu.

Occupational Safety and Health Administration (OSHA)—Department of Labor: *Occupational Health and Safety Administration: Agricultural Operations*, n.d. Retrieved from https://www.osha.gov.

Oosterbroek TA, Yonge O, Myrick F: Rural nursing preceptorship: an integrative review, *Online J Rural Nurs Health Care* 17(1):23–51, 2017.

Ortiz J, Hofle R, Bushy A, Lin Y, Khanijahani A, Bitney A: Impact of nurse practitioner practice regulations on rural population health outcomes, *Healthcare* 6(2):66, 2018.

Paré JM, Sharp DB, Petersen P: A story of emergent leadership: lived experiences of nurses in a critical access hospital, *Online J Rural Nurs Health Care* 17(2):103–125, 2017.

Pavloff M, Farthing PM, Duff E: Rural and remote continuing nursing education: an integrative literature review, *Online J Rural Nurs Health Care* 17(2):88–102, 2017.

Prengaman M, Terry DR, Schmitz D, Baker E: The nursing community apgar questionnaire in rural Australia: an evidence based approach to recruiting and retaining nurses, *Online J Rural Nurs Health Care* 17(2):148–171, 2017.

Quad Council: *Public health nursing competencies*, 2018. Retrieved from http://www.quadcouncilphn.org.

Rural Health Information Hub (RHI-Hub): *Rural Mental Health*, 2017. Retrieved from https://www.ruralhealthinfo.org..

Rural Health Information Hub (RHI-Hub): *What is rural*? 2018. Retrieved from https://www.ruralhealthinfo.org.

U.S. Department of Agriculture (USDA): *Rural America at a glance: 2017 edition*, 2017. Retrieved from https://www.ers.usda.gov.

U.S. Department of Agriculture (USDA): *Rural emergency response*, n.d. Retrieved from https://www.nal.usda.gov.

U.S. Department of Health and Human Services (USDHHS): *Healthy People 2020*, 2013. Retrieved from https://www.healthypeople.gov.

United States Census Bureau: *2010 Census: Apportionment Data Map*. Retrieved from https://www.census.gov.

Williams MA, Andrews JA, Zanni KL, Stewart Fahs PS: Rural nursing: searching for the state of the science, *Online J Rural Nurs Health Care* 12(2):102–117, 2012.

Winters CA, Lee H: *Rural nursing: concepts, theory, and Practice*, ed 3, New York, NY, 2009, Springer Publishing.

Winters CA, editor: *Rural nursing: concepts, theory and practice*, ed 4, New York, NY, 2013, Springer Publishing.

33

Poverty and Homelessness

Mary Kay Goldschmidt, DNP, MSN, RN, PHNA-BC

OBJECTIVES

After reading this chapter, the student should be able to do the following:

1. Analyze the concept of poverty.
2. Understand the historical relationship between race, ethnicity, and poverty.
3. Describe the relationship between poverty, toxic stress, and lifelong adverse health effects.
4. Analyze the concept of homelessness.
5. Discuss the effects of homelessness on the health and well-being of individuals and families across the life span.
6. Discuss the challenges and the unique role of nurses in providing care and advocacy for poor and homeless individuals.

CHAPTER OUTLINE

Defining and Understanding the Concept of Poverty
Poverty and Health: The Impact of Toxic Stress
Defining and Understanding the Concept of Homelessness
Impact of Homelessness on Health Across the Life Span
Unique Role of the Nurse

KEY TERMS

Adverse Childhood Experiences (ACEs), p. 744
affordable housing, p. 743
chronic homelessness, p. 742
Consolidated Health Centers (CHCs), p. 750
Continuum of Care (CoC) programs, p. 743
deep poverty, p. 736
doubling up, p. 743
federal poverty level, p. 736
Housing First, p. 745
Kerner Commission, p. 738
low-income, p. 736
low-income housing, p.749
multidimensional poverty, p. 736
multigenerational poverty, p. 739
racism, p. 738
rapid re-housing, p. 745
relational health, p. 737
Shelter Plus Care, p. 749
safety net, p. 739
social determinants of health, p. 735
social exclusion, p. 737
social interconnection, p. 737
Supplemental Poverty Measure (SPM), p. 736
supportive housing, p. 749
toxic stress, p. 740
trauma-informed care, p. 745
unsheltered homeless, p. 743

Where you are born, live, and work are the most significant factors in determining your health (World Health Organization, 2008, 2018a). The **social determinants of health**, or "social context," are directly linked to the risk of exposure and level of susceptibility, severity, and outcome of disease resulting from infection, metabolic or genetic disorder, degenerative process, or malignancy. If you live in poverty, you are less likely to have access to healthy foods and safe neighborhoods and more likely to have lower levels of education, reduced access to and lower quality health care, engage in unhealthy behaviors, and have worse health outcomes (Centers for Disease Control and Prevention, 2018; Jarrellet al., 2014). Poverty is a foundational component of chronic disease and population health disparities. In order to improve the health of the population, a shift in focus toward addressing the social and environmental factors that contribute to poor health is essential (Levin, 2018).

It is imperative for all health care providers to understand the circumstances that create and deepen poverty, the impact of poverty on health, and how we as nurses can bring all our resources to bear on interrupting the cycle of poverty and homelessness. Caring for these populations involves the development of skills and knowledge beyond that of meeting physiological needs in the health care setting. Nurses must also care for their impoverished and homeless patients at the individual, aggregate, and community level, by advocating for policies which prevent and ameliorate the health effects that arise from these conditions.

DEFINING AND UNDERSTANDING THE CONCEPT OF POVERTY

There are many ways to define and understand poverty. Historically, poverty was defined by measuring household income, the number of individuals living in the home, and a specified income poverty line. Those living below the income poverty line are considered impoverished and those above are not. An example of this approach is the Department of Health and Human Services' **federal poverty level** (FPL), which guides eligibility for federal assistance such as the Supplemental Nutrition Assistance Program (SNAP) and the Children's Health Insurance Program (CHIP). Table 33.1 shows the 2018 poverty guidelines for the 48 contiguous states and the District of Columbia. The method used to calculate the FPL has not fundamentally changed in the 45 years since it was developed, except for accomodating the cost of food inflation. However, families are now far more likely to have two parents working, adding childcare to the cost of living, and housing and transportation are significantly more expensive. Recent studies surmise that families need twice the amount of the FPL in order to meet basic needs. Families living below the 2018 FPL ($25,100 for a family of four) are considered poor. Familes that live at twice (200 percent) the FPL ($50,200 for a family of four) are categorized as "**low-income**" and those who are living at half (50 percent) the FPL ($12,550 for a family of four) are said to be living in "**deep poverty**" (Pascoe et al., 2016; U.S. Department of Health and Human Services, 2018).

Another example is the U.S. Census Bureau poverty threshold, which is used to calculate the number of Americans living in poverty. This calculation does not include non-cash government benefits such as public housing, SNAP, or Medicaid, and uses pre-tax dollars to establish the poverty threshold (U.S. Department of Health and Human Services, 2018). According to the 2017 Poverty Statistics Report issued by the Census Bureau, 12.7 percent of those living in the United States fall below the poverty line (United States Census Bureau, 2017). A state by state representation of individuals living below the poverty line in 2016 is shown in Fig. 33.1.

While both of these federal measures are important for planning and budgetary purposes, they define poverty using an income based, unidimensional, or "headcount ratio." They do not reflect geographic differences in the cost of living or the positive impact of government programs such as the Earned Income Tax Credit (EITC); nutrition program for Women, Infants and Children (WIC); public housing; and energy assistance on lifting families out of poverty. The **Supplemental Poverty Measure (SPM)** was developed in 2010 by the National Academy of Sciences to consider these programs when evaluating poverty and outcomes, as well as adjusting for geographic differences in the cost of living and medical care (Pascoe et al., 2016; United States Census Bureau, 2017). All of these methods provide a "snapshot" of poverty at a given point yet do not measure the impact of poverty over time. The Panel Study of Income Dynamics is an example of a longitudinal, repetitive survey instrument that has been used since 1968 to examine the effects of poverty over time.

In the 1970s, a more comprehensive view of defining poverty was developed which examines how well individuals are able to satisfy their needs. Termed the *direct method* by Amartya Sen, a Nobel prize winning economist, this approach assesses human deprivation by looking at where individuals are unable to meet basic needs. Perhaps most useful for addressing poverty at the public health level, this method measures the capacity of individuals to create their desired living circumstances and fully function in society. The concept behind this method is that poverty cannot be defined by access to economic resources alone. Increased monetary resources may improve standards of living, but only when the necessary resources can be purchased. There are other non-monetary resources needed to fully function in society, such as public education. With the direct method, resources like inner capability and the ability to achieve a desired standard of living are assessed. Individuals or populations can have multiple deprivations across monetary and non-monetary dimensions, which points to more intense levels of poverty. Each dimension is weighted so that it becomes possible to identify the most detrimental deprivations associated with poverty (Callander & Schofield, 2016; United Nations, 2015; Wagle, 2014).

This multidimensional approach to defining poverty was sanctioned by the United Nations Development Programme in 2010, using an adaptation of the Alkire-Foster (2015) counting method (Alkire et al., 2015). The resulting **Multidimensional Poverty** Index (MPI), which looks at poverty across the domains of health, education, and standard of living, provides a composite score which can then be used to compare poverty in other regions or globally. An individual is considered multidimensionally poor if he or she is deprived in 33 percent of MPI indicators. The MPI outcomes can also be sorted by ethnicity,

TABLE 33.1 2018 Poverty Guidelines for the 48 Contiguous States and the District of Columbia

Persons in Family/Household	Poverty Guideline
1	$12,140
2	16,460
3	20,780
4	25,100
5	29,420
6	33,740
7	38,060
8	42,380

For families/households with more than eight persons, add $4320 for each additional person.
From U.S. Department of Health and Human Services, 2018.

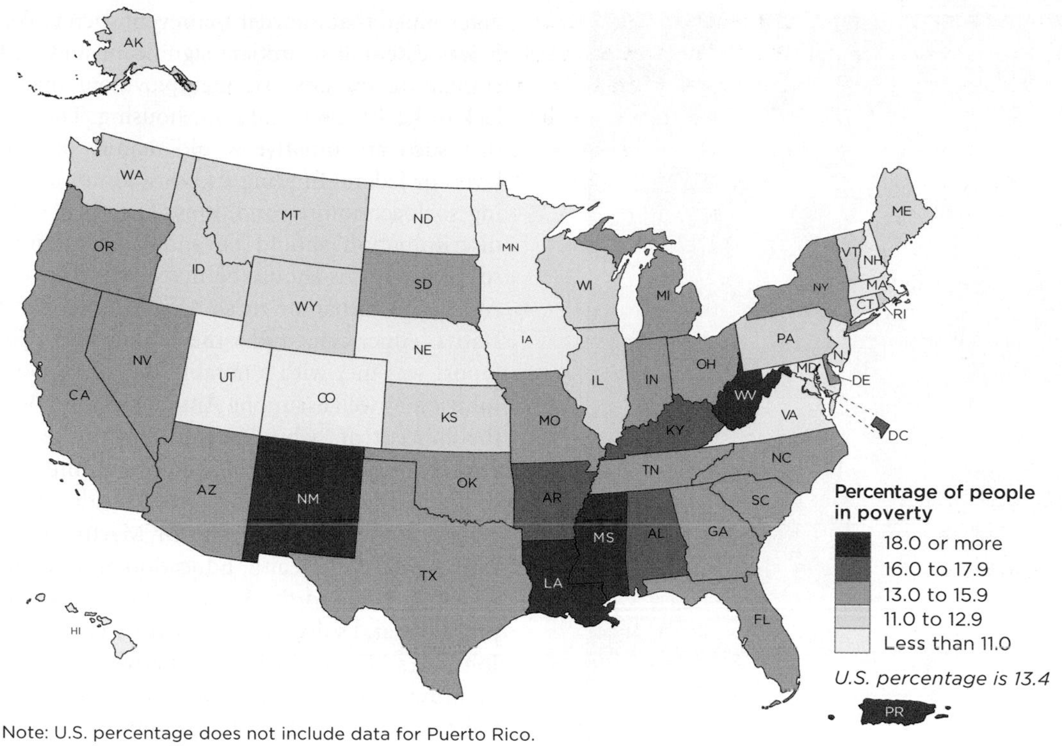

Note: U.S. percentage does not include data for Puerto Rico.

Fig. 33.1 Individuals below the poverty level by state. (From U.S. Census Bureau, 2017. Available at https://www.census.gov.)

religion, age, sex, or other classifications in order to better understand the poverty of a given population (United Nations, 2015).

In 2014, Udaya Wagle surmised that multidimensional approaches to defining poverty tended to overlook the importance of social relationships to a sense of well-being and the capability to function. Wagle points to the connection between social exclusion and poverty and argues for the need to evaluate the level of social interconnectedness when defining poverty. This can be established by determining the level at which "individuals *relate* with others and the broader society or polity in which they live" (Wagle, 2014). One operational indicator used to measure relational resources is to examine active participation in elections. Additional indicators are used to measure the relational dimension, as well as the economic dimension (family income with adjustments for family size) and inner capabilities dimension (educational attainment, educational degree, status of health, and occupational prestige). Wagle applied his method for defining poverty to data contained in the General Social Survey of the United States and demonstrated that a higher number of families/households are deprived of economic and relational resources than of inner capabilities, particularly among minority populations. This suggests that social interconnection (or lack thereof) may play a larger role in poverty than had been previously understood (Wagle, 2014).

It is important for nurses to understand the many ways to define and measure poverty so they can better understand what causes and contributes to poverty and the impact multiple deprivations can have on living a full and functional life. There is an association between multidimensional poverty, self-rated health, and chronic income poverty (Callander & Schofield, 2015; Oshio & Kan, 2014). As these methods for measuring poverty continue to evolve, they may serve as a guide to when, where, and for whom anti-poverty and health care initiatives can be most effective. For example, if a patient has a mental health disorder (health domain deficit), and also has deficits in the social/relational health, education, and income/monetary domains, the nurse may provide assistance by linking him or her to resources such as a mental health support group, a GED class and Temporary Assistance for Needy Families (TANF) benefits. By addressing multiple deprivations in an effective and timely way, the risk of chronic income poverty and worsening health may be interrupted (Callander & Schofield, 2015).

Historical View of Poverty in the United States

In the summer of 1967, intense rioting and looting broke out in a number of America's cities, predominantly in African American communities. The violence was so overwhelming that the National Guard was called in to restore order. Newark and Detroit were among the hardest hit cities. Milwaukee, Cincinnati, Atlanta, and Tampa were among 125 additional cities where significant episodes of violence occurred. Twenty-six people died, including women and children, and property damage was extensive. These events spurred fear, panic, and anger among Americans, and in response President Lyndon Johnson created the National Advisory Commission on Civil Disorders to investigate and report on the causes and solutions to the civil unrest. President Johnson stated: "The only genuine, long-range solution for what has happened lies in an

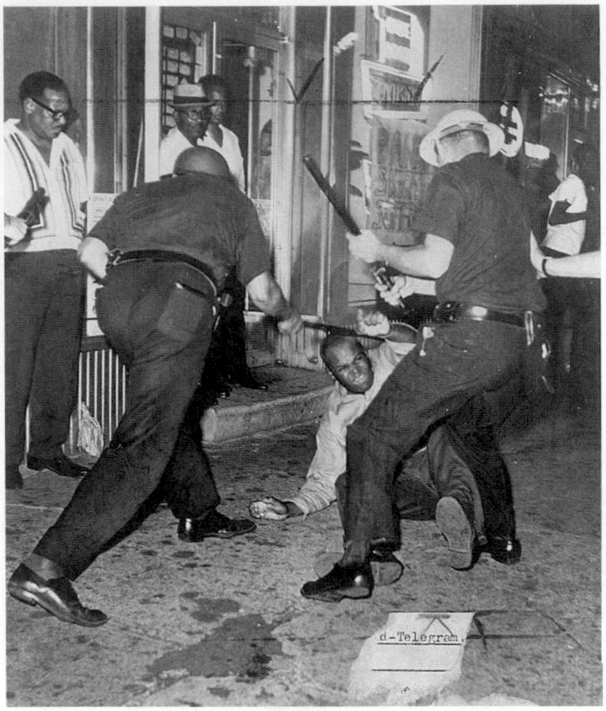

Fig. 33.2 An incident at 133rd Street and Seventh Avenue during the Harlem riot of 1964. (From Library of Congress: https://www.loc.gov.)

attack—mounted at every level—upon the conditions that breed despair and violence. All of us know what those conditions are: ignorance, discrimination, slums, poverty, disease, not enough jobs. We should attack those problems—not because we are fired by conscience. We should attack them because there is simply no other way to achieve a decent and orderly society in America" (Harris & Curtis, 2018) (Fig. 33.2).

The commission, led by David Ginsberg, began their work by holding a series of hearings and hiring staff to conduct field surveys in 23 cities. They conducted interviews and opinion surveys, and commission members visited eight cities that had been the site of rioting. Dubbed the **Kerner Commission**, the group spent an additional 44 days developing a report based on their findings. The Commission concluded that the untenable conditions under which individuals in these cities lived, and institutional **racism**, were the root causes of the violence. They pointed to African Americans migrating to cities in order to escape rural poverty between 1945 and 1965. During that time frame, jobs began moving to the suburbs along with much of the white population, leading to primarily poor and African American inner cities. Confrontation between desperate inner-city residents and majority-white police departments transpired, and hostility continued to escalate until residents erupted in significant, sustained violence in cities across the nation that police were unable to quell.

The Kerner Commission report stated that the United States was moving toward two disparate societies, one African American and one white. Segregation and poverty had created ghettoes the likes of which were unfathomable by whites, though white society was complicit in establishing, condoning, and institutionalizing these conditions. The Commission determined that in order to prevent such violence in the future, it was essential to initiate significant and sustained efforts to combat racism, poverty, unemployment, inadequate education, lack of health care, and poor housing. The Commission noted that such an initiative would require previously unheard of levels of federal funding and should not be limited to improving socioeconomic conditions. They believed that racism and discrimination should be addressed at multiple levels, and social programs should be made available to all impoverished Americans, urban or rural, African American or white, Latino, Native American, and other minorities. The Commission's report was met with a notable lack of support from President Johnson as well as among Americans, who pushed back against the concept of "white racism" and the recommendations for remedying the issues. However, a number of powerful and influential leaders such as Vice President Hubert Humphrey, Senator Robert Kennedy, and Dr. Martin Luther King, as well as the Secretary of Health, Education and Welfare, and Secretary of Labor, believed the Kerner Report accurately portrayed the problems and solutions to violence in the inner cities. President Johnson's "Great Society" initiatives continued forward momentum, and for nearly 10 years America made progress on most of the goals and solutions put forth in the Kerner report.

The Fair Housing Act of 1968 was passed following the release of the Kerner Report and four days after the death of Dr. Martin Luther King. This law prohibited discrimination on the basis of race, religion, or nationality by those selling or renting housing. Increased investment in urban and poor rural schools led to significant improvement in educational inequality, reducing the achievement gap between white and African American 13-year-olds by greater than 50 percent. Latino and African American youth attended college as often as whites by the mid-1970s. The number of Americans living below the poverty line during President Johnson's administration dropped from 22.2 percent to 12.6 percent. Had these improvements continued, the inequality gap in education would have closed by the year 2000.

The Influence of Politics on Poverty

With the advent of the Reagan administration in 1981, federal support for schools, housing, health care, and child welfare was cut, and the gains in educational achievement slowed, then halted, and eventually reversed (Harris & Curtis, 2018). Poverty rates eased upward, spiking at 15.1 percent in 1993 during the administration of President George H. W. Bush, then dropped to a low of 11.3 percent in 2000 under President Bill Clinton, rose sharply again during the George W. Bush administration, topping out in 2010 at 15.1 percent—following the Great Recession (Statista, 2018). During the administration of President Barack Obama (2009-2017), poverty dropped to 12.7 percent, where it remains today. Over the past 50 years, the United States has had a net increase in poverty of 0.1 percent (United States Census Bureau, 2017).

The greatest reductions in poverty followed President Johnson's "War on Poverty" in the mid to late 1960s and during the Clinton administration from 1993 to 2000, both of which included periods of economic expansion. During periods of economic contraction, such as during the Great Recession (December 2007 to June 2009), poverty increases. Federal social **safety net** programs in place at the beginning of the recession reduced the population of those living in poverty by 8.9 percent. By 2012, anti-poverty programs had been expanded, reducing the alternative poverty rate by 12.7 percent (Chaudry et al., 2016).

The Changing Face of Poverty

Today, the face of poverty has changed. Adults over the age of 65 have doubled since 1966, yet the number of seniors who live in poverty has decreased, largely due to Social Security. In 2016, the highest rates of poverty occurred among children under the age of 18, followed by adults aged 18-64, during their prime income producing years. Greater than 26 percent of poor families were headed by females, who also had the lowest median income ($41,027) among family households (United States Census Bureau, 2017). Childhood poverty remains a stubborn problem with rates fluctuating over time, increasing to about 22 percent during the Great Recession and decreasing to 18 percent during the economic expansion that followed (Desilver, 2014; United States Census Bureau, 2017). Since 1966, poverty has decreased among African Americans, though the rate is still double that of whites, and poverty among Hispanics has risen to 19.4 percent (Desilver, 2014). There is significant evidence that higher poverty levels among African Americans and Hispanics are associated with disparities in educational achievement (Stanford Center on Poverty & Inequality, 2017). Americans with lower levels of education, those who are African American or Hispanic, and single mothers with children have consistently experienced higher rates of poverty over time in the United States (Chaudry et al., 2016).

Single Mothers, Women, and Children. Six out of 10 impoverished U.S. children lived in a female-led household in 2016. Of families living in poverty in the United States, those led by a single mother make up the largest group. Over twice as many female householders lived in poverty (26.6 percent) as male householders (13.1 percent) and more than five times as many as "married couple" families. Among single minority women, the rates are even higher with 34.7 percent of Hispanic and 32 percent of African American female householders living in poverty. A number of factors contribute to poverty among single mothers, but figuring centrally are the wage gap between gender and between races and ethnic groups: for women working full-time all year versus men working full-time all year, women make 84 cents for every dollar paid to men, 63 cents for African American women, 57 cents among Native women, and 54 cents on the dollar among Hispanic women. After transitioning to female, transgender women's wages fell by almost 33 percent. The gender income gap has changed little since 2007 and exists among women of all ages, education levels, and nearly all occupations. Mothers incur what is referred to as a "motherhood wage penalty" of about 7 percent lower income for each additional child, while fathers do not. The "motherhood penalty" can significantly impact minimum and low wage workers, which are primarily (58 percent) women. As a result of earning lower wages, women have lower rates of Social Security and retirement income, which can contribute to poverty among the elderly (National Women's Law Center, 2017; Semega et al., 2017).

Minorities. One out of every four African Americans or American Indians living in the United States is poor, as is one out of every five Hispanics. In 2016, poverty rates among racial and ethnic minority groups in the United States were higher for African Americans (22 percent), Hispanics (19.4 percent), and American Indians (25 percent) than they were for whites (11 percent), although the number of whites living in poverty is actually higher, commensurate with the larger population of whites. African Americans and Hispanics living in the rural South, African Americans living in the rural Northeast, and American Indians living in the rural West and urban Midwest have the highest poverty rates in the country. African Americans, Hispanics, and American Indians have historically had lower rates of educational achievement, employment, income, home ownership, and net worth (Goins et al., 2015; Running Strong for American Indian Youth, 2018; Stanford Center on Poverty & Inequality, 2017; United States Census Bureau, 2017). **Multigenerational poverty** is common among African Americans in the South, Hispanics along the border of Mexico, and American Indians who live in states with multiple reservations.

The gap in educational achievement between African Americans, Hispanics, and whites has narrowed in recent years, and high school graduation rates have improved, which is largely attributed to early childhood education programs. However, gaps continue to exist, and it is estimated that it will take 50 years before the level of academic achievement among African Americans and Hispanics is equal to that of whites. The most significant factors contributing to education inequity among these two minority groups are segregration and limited family resources. African Americans and Hispanics are far more likely to live in neighborhoods with higher concentrations of poverty, and parents are less likely to have the resources necessary to support schools, such as higher levels of education and income (Stanford Center on Poverty & Inequality, 2017). American Indians and Alaska Natives (AIAN) have lower rates of high school graduation (72 percent) compared to whites (88 percent) and African Americans (76 percent). Only 17 percent of American Indian students are able to continue their education following high school (Oliff, 2017; U.S. Department of Education, 2018).

The median income in African American and Hispanic households is about 60 percent of that for whites. While the earnings gap between African Americans and whites has decreased 32 percent in the last 40 years, African Americans have seen an overal improvement in income of only 7 percent. Fewer African Americans (41 percent) and Hispanics (45 percent) own their own homes, compared to whites (71 percent), leaving the majority of African American and Hispanic families to rent their homes, thus making them more vulnerable to eviction. The rate of eviction among Hispanic renters is significantly higher (23 percent) than the rate for African Americans (12 percent) or whites (9 percent), which is reflected in the 30 percent increase in the number of Hispanics who were homeless and unsheltered between 2016 and 2017 (Office of Community Planning and Development, 2017; Stanford Center on Poverty & Inequality, 2017).

Housing among AIAN populations is more complex, with about 22 percent living on tribal lands and 77 percent living outside tribal lands, 60 percent of whom live in metropolitan areas. The AIAN home ownership rate overall is 54 percent, though on tribal lands the rate is higher (67 percent). Homelessness among this population is more insidious and rates may be artificially low as AIAN homeless are often sheltered by family members, which can lead to harmful effects such as taxing existing family resources and overcrowding (Pindus et al., 2017; U.S. Department of Health and Human Services, 2017; United States Interagency Council on Homelessness, 2017).

With higher rates of poverty among these three minorities, enrollment in government safety net programs such as SNAP, are generally higher, with a few exceptions. Nearly 26 percent of the AIAN population, 25.3 percent of African Americans, and 20.4 percent of Hispanics receive SNAP benefits. However, American Indians and African Americans are far less likely to enroll in Medicaid. This is referred to as a "double disadvantage effect," meaning these two minorities have higher poverty rates, yet are under-enrolled in Medicaid (Stanford Center on Poverty & Inequality, 2017).

The Elderly. Poverty among those aged 65 and older has decreased overall since 1967, though this demographic saw a statistically significant increase in poverty between 2015 and 2016. The poverty rate rose from 8.8 percent to 9.3 percent, the first such increase since 2010. There is evidence that "near poor" seniors are being pushed into poverty because of medical expenses and because Social Security is keeping fewer seniors out of poverty. A detailed analysis published in 2018 by the U.S. Census Bureau using the SPM, shows that 76 percent of seniors who entered poverty in 2016 did so because of a decrease in Social Security and/or retirement income (about $200) and an increase in medical expenses of about $500 (Fox & Pacas, 2018). Millions of older adults are considered low income because they live above the FPL ($12,140 for one person, $16,460 for two), though they have great difficulty meeting expenses and are one crisis away from sinking into poverty. Some 43 percent of single persons and 21 percent of married couples over the age of 65 rely on Social Security as 90 percent of their income, and the average Social Security benefit is $1,342.00 per month, less than $16,000 per year. The majority of seniors pay an average of $134 per year for Medicare, which is typically deducted directly from Social Security, further reducing their pay. Though a 2 percent cost of living raise has been granted for Social Security for 2018, the increase may be consumed by Medicare Part B costs (Center on Budget and Policy Priorities, 2017). The rate of poverty among seniors increases with age and is higher among women, African Americans, and Hispanics (Kaiser Family Foundation, 2018).

It is clear that the demarcation between poverty and near poverty among those aged 65 and older is fluid and precarious. A serious illness or injury can force a senior to choose between paying for medication and eating and may drop him or her below the poverty line. Food insecurity is an issue for 2.9 million households where a senior is housed, and although three out of five adults are eligible for SNAP, many are not enrolled (National Council on Aging, 2018).

Each of these vulnerable populations faces poverty for a multitude of reasons, and the approach to improving well-being is not uniform. Bringing awareness to those most at risk of poverty, as well as developing an understanding of the appropriate government safety net, faith-based, and privately funded program resources that are available, is essential to understanding the needs of these populations and the substantial link between poverty and health.

POVERTY AND HEALTH: THE IMPACT OF TOXIC STRESS

Health status is included in each of the multidimensional poverty assessment tools because it plays a significant role in the capacity to achieve and maintain a desired standard of living and a sense of well-being. Studies have shown that well-being is associated with a decreased risk of disease, illness, and injury and better immune function, longevity, and productivity. Well-being is reliant upon good health, positive social relationships, and access to basic resources such as food and shelter (National Center for Chronic Disease Prevention and Health Promotion, 2016). Families living in poverty are caught up in a vicious cycle: they are at higher risk of chronic disease, and chronic disease can drag them into a downward spiral of worsening disease and deeper poverty (World Health Organization, 2018b).

High-Risk Populations

The adverse effects of poverty on the health of children are myriad and include increased morbidity and mortality during childhood and a lifelong increased risk of cardiovascular and metabolic disease, much of which can be linked to **toxic stress**. Some 50 percent of African American children and one third of Hispanic children will develop diabetes at some point in their lives, with one in four developing prediabetes as a child (Conway, 2016). Box 33.1 outlines the impact of poverty on the health and well-being of children.

Younger children are more at risk of poverty-related toxic stress because of their vulnerability and the prevalence of poverty among this age group. The high levels of stress experienced by families living in poverty lead to consistently activated stress hormones and inflammatory mediators in children. High levels and/or prolonged exposure to hormones such as cortisol, norepinephrine, and adrenalin, coupled with mediators such as cytokine, affect the entire body and in particular, a child's developing brain. Poor impulse control and self-regulating behaviors may result from this hypervigilant stress response, which may further impair the relational health between a child and a stressed parent and other family members. As young adults, these children may engage in unhealthy behaviors such as smoking or substance abuse, in an effort to provide respite from chronic stress, which can lead to increased morbidity and

BOX 33.1 Impact of Poverty on the Health of Children

- Higher infant mortality
- Low birth weight
- Food insecurity
- Unintentional injury
- Maltreatment
- Increased frequency of asthma
- Poor dental health
- Obesity
- Reduced access to quality health care
- Violence
- Unstable or substandard housing
- Academic underachievement
- Lower quality schools
- Teen pregnancy
- Depression and conduct disorders
- Substance abuse (smoking and alcohol)
- Unsafe or non-existent recreational areas

Data from Impact of poverty on the health of children. From the American Academy of Pediatrics Committee on Psychosocial Aspects of Child and Family Health, Council on Community Pediatrics, 2016.

mortality at a young age. Children who have the benefit of good relational health and a stable family life are better able to minimize the stress response and may not experience the lifelong increased risk of chronic disease. For this reason, interventions that focus on improving parental engagement and good relational health can buffer the harm to a child's developing brain (Pascoe et al., 2016).

EVIDENCE-BASED PRACTICE

Toxic stress among children has been identified as a significant contributor to the development of chronic disease as an adult. Ameliorating the effects of toxic stress among children can be accomplished through stable, supportive relationships with adults during early childhood. Breastfeeding has been suggested as a toxic stress mitigator, beginning with the skin-to-skin contact immediately following birth. This mother-infant contact stimulates a rise in maternal oxytocin and prolactin and decreases cortisol, reducing infant allostatic load and inducing calm. Breastfeeding has been proven to aid in the establishment of maternal-infant attachment and lower the stress response in mothers and infants.

Nurse Use

Interventions that support and promote breastfeeding such as the nurse-family partnership (NFP) address disparities in breastfeeding among communities and work to decrease socioeconomic disparities for mothers and infants. NFP programs have also positively impacted such child/family outcomes as fewer child injuries related to neglect.

Data from Hallowell S, Froh E, Spatz D: Human milk and breastfeeding: an intervention to mitigate toxic stress. *Nurs Outlook* 65(1):58-67, 2017. Available from https://www.nursingoutlook.org.

The American Academy of Pediatrics (AAP) released a policy statement in 2016, outlining factors which mitigate the harmful health effects of childhood poverty. A number of government safety net programs are included in the AAP recommendations such as early identification of families in need of services, tax policies which increase family income, financial aid, comprehensive health care, early childhood education, and home visitation. Programs which provide parental support and build resilience in children are additional ameliorating influences (Pascoe et al., 2016).

Minorities. The higher rates of poverty among racial and ethnic minorities are also associated with chronic disease at an earlier age, at a higher rate, and an earlier death than among whites. Early studies suggest that poverty-related stress can lead to long-term epigenetic changes in gene expression that can impact health as early as pre-birth. African Americans are two to three times more likely to suffer from hypertension and diabetes, have higher rates of cardiovascular disease (CVD), stroke, cancer, asthma, human immunodeficiency virus (HIV)/acquired immunodeficiency syndrome (AIDS) and become victims of homicide, and are two to three times more likely to experience premature death than whites (U.S. Department of Health and Human Services, 2018a). American Indians and Alaska Natives have signficantly higher rates of infant mortality (7.6 per 100,000) than do whites (4.9 per 100,000) (U.S. Department of Health and Human Services, 2017). The major causes of illness, injury, and death are CVD, cancer, unintentional injuries, diabetes, and stroke. The AIAN population has significant risk factors for and a high prevalence of suicide, obesity, substance abuse, liver disease, sudden infant death syndrome (SIDS), and teen pregnancy. Many tribal homes do not have adequate water purification or sewage disposal systems. Access to quality health care on tribal lands is limited because of inadequate funding for Indian Health Services and the geographic isolation of many reservations (U.S. Department of Health and Human Services Office of Minority Health, 2018b).

The Hispanic population has the added difficulty of cultural and language barriers, immigration status, and often lacks insurance, which impacts the ability to access and benefit from health care services. Preventive services in particular are utilized less frequently among this ethnic group. Causes of morbidity and mortality include obesity, diabetes, asthma, CVD, cancer, stroke, chronic obstructive pulmonary disease, unintentional injuries, suicide, HIV/AIDS, and liver disease. One subgroup of the Hispanic population, Puerto Ricans, have disproportionately higher levels of low-birth-weight infants than do whites. Infant mortality, asthma, and HIV/AIDS rates are also higher among this subgroup. Hispanics have higher rates of obesity than whites, and Mexican Americans have higher rates of diabetes than other Hispanic subroups (U.S. Department of Health and Human Services Office of Minority Health, 2018c).

Nursing Intervention: Accessing the Government Safety Net

Historical analyses show that Federal social safety net programs reduce poverty. Social Security cash payments, tax credits such as the Earned Income Tax Credit (EITC), and the SNAP program (formerly known as food stamps) have had the greatest anti-poverty impact (Chaudry et al., 2016). The EITC is a tax credit offered to low-moderate income working individuals, which reduces the tax burden or provides a refund (Internal Revenue Service, 2018). These programs increase income among those who would otherwise fall below the poverty line, and they actually lift more families out of poverty now than when they were created. Nowhere is this more evident than among impoverished children. In the mid-1960s, government policies and programs reduced childhood poverty by 1.1 percent; in the 1970s and 1980s, by 1.6 percent; and in 2016, by 2.3 percent (Chaudry et al., 2016). In 2016, child poverty hit a record low of 15.6 percent, or almost half the 1966 rate. Refundable tax credits and SNAP were the most effective policy programs for easing childhood poverty, lifting some 38 percent of children above the poverty line. These program benefits were equally distributed among African American, white, and Hispanic children.

Other government programs such as Medicaid, CHIP, and the Affordable Care Act (ACA) have proven beneficial to impoverished children by providing health insurance. Ninety-five percent of children in the United States are now insured, and studies that have examined the effect of Medicaid on children's health have shown a significant positive impact, particularly with well child and preventive services (Leininger & Levy, 2015; Shapiro & Trisi, 2017). Among children born after Medicaid was initiated, health care utilization increased, low birth weights decreased, educational outcomes improved, lower rates of poverty were noted, and lower rates of adult mortality occurred. In regions where Medicaid spending was higher and access to health care was initiated at a younger age, outcomes for adults were better and the percent of adults who saw benefit from the program was larger (Stanford Center on Poverty & Inequality, 2017).

Government safety net programs clearly function as they were intended by halting the number of Americans who would otherwise fall below the poverty line and by helping those who live below the poverty line to have a better quality of life. Critics of social safety net programs argue that government assistance disincentivizes working among impoverished individuals, yet the EITC provides benefit to low-income *working* families and the credit increases as the level of income rises—up to the maximum rate (Stanford Center on Poverty & Inequality, 2017).

QSEN FOCUS ON QUALITY AND SAFETY EDUCATION FOR NURSES

Quality and Safety Focus

Targeted Competency: Client-Centered Care

Recognize the client or designee as the source of control and full partner in providing compassionate and coordinated care based on respect for client's preferences, values, and needs.

Important aspects of client-centered care include the following:

- **Knowledge:** Describe how diverse cultural, ethnic, and social backgrounds function as sources of client, family, and community values.
- **Skills:** Provide client-centered care with sensitivity and respect for the diversity of human experience.
- **Attitudes:** Recognize personally held attitudes about working with clients from different ethnic, cultural, and social backgrounds.

Self-awareness is a key component of providing authentic, genuine client-centered care.

In order to clarify their own values and perspectives about poverty, nurses should ask themselves the following questions about poverty and persons living in poverty:

How to Test Values and Beliefs About Poverty

- What do I believe to be true about being poor?
- Do I fully appreciate the impact racism has had on the health and well-being of minorities?
- Do I believe that people are poor because they just don't want to work? Or do I believe that society has a significant influence on one becoming poor?
- What do I personally know about being poor?
- How have family and friends influenced my ideas about being poor?
- Have I ever personally been poor?
- What do I feel when I see a hungry child? A hungry adult?
- What do I really think can be done to prevent poverty and homelessness?
- Can I effectively advocate for a client's needs if it runs counter to my personal beliefs?

Adapted from work by Gail Armstrong, PhD, DNP, ACNS-BC, CNE, Associate Professor, University of Colorado Denver College of Nursing.

DEFINING AND UNDERSTANDING THE CONCEPT OF HOMELESSNESS

The Department of Housing and Urban Development defines "homeless" as "a person who lacks a fixed, regular, and adequate nighttime residence" (Henry et al., 2017). This definition can be expanded to cover categories of homelessness such as "chronically homeless individual" or "chronically homeless people in families," the former referring to an individual who has a disability and has either been homeless at least four times in 3 years—for a minimum of 12 months—or continuously homeless for a total of 1 year, the latter referring to a family where the head of household meets the definition of chronically homeless individual (Henry et al., 2017).

The concept of homelessness encompasses three categories: **chronic homelessness**, transitional, and episodic. The episodic homeless are generally marked by hardship and struggle, including chronic unemployment. These individuals move in and out of homelessness, are younger, and often have mental health and substance abuse problems. Transitional homelessness is typically caused by a catastrophic event which necessitates a short shelter stay, eventually transitioning to permanent housing. This tends to account for the majority of homelessness over time because of the high rates of turnover among this population, which edges the count higher. Finally, the chronically homeless are usually older individuals who are chronically unemployed, have some type of disability or substance abuse problem, and use the emergency shelter system as a long-term housing solution. This group makes up the smallest percent of the homeless population (National Coalition for the Homeless, 2018a).

Those who are homeless sleep at night in shelters that they often must vacate during the day. This means that during the day, they sit or stand on the street; in parks, alleys, shopping centers, and libraries; and in places such as trash bins, cardboard boxes, or under loading docks at industrial sites. Homeless persons may seek shelter in public buildings, such as train and bus stations. Those who do not sleep in shelters may sleep in single-room-occupancy (SRO) hotels, all-night movie theaters, abandoned buildings, and vehicles. Some homeless persons choose to be unsheltered rather than live with family or stay in shelters (Choi et al., 2015; Christian & Mukarji-Connollly, 2018).

The Face of Homelessness in the United States

"On a single night in 2017, 553,742 people were experiencing homelessness in the United States" (Henry et al., 2017). Around two thirds of those people were housed in emergency shelters or transitional programs, and the remaining one third were unsheltered, meaning they slept in non-customary places such as on the street, in parks, or in an automobile. The 2017 Annual Homeless Assessment Report (AHAR) to Congress, published by the U.S. Department of Housing and Urban Development (HUD), reports that a one percent overall increase in homelessness occurred between 2016 and 2017, made up entirely of **unsheltered homeless** individuals (Henry et al., 2017). This represents the first increase in homelessness in seven years and may reflect a higher cost of renting and a lack of market availability for extremely low-income (less than 30 percent of the area median income or below FPL) housing (National Alliance to End Homelessness, 2017; U.S. Department of Housing and Urban Development, 2018a). The high rates of unsheltered homeless in the western part of the United States and in Florida correlate with the low number of units available for rent among extremely low-income households (National Alliance to End Homelessness, 2017). The number of homeless living in shelters and transitional housing declined by three percent between 2016 and 2017, a trend which has continued for the past three years, yet the number of unsheltered homeless rose by 9 percent (Henry et al., 2017).

There are two predominant ways to determine the number of people who are homeless: (1) point-in-time (PIT) counts, where the number of persons who are homeless on a given day or during a given week are counted or (2) period prevalence counts, which examine the number of people who are homeless over a given period of time. The Department of Housing and Urban Development utilizes government designated **Continuum of Care (CoC) programs** to perform an annual PIT count (conducted twice yearly in some locales) to identify and describe the U.S. homeless population. The Housing Inventory Count is used by CoC programs to define the number of beds available to serve the homeless. There were 399 CoC programs as of 2017, covering virtually all of the United States (Henry et al., 2017).

The primary causes of homelessness are a lack of **affordable housing** and insufficient housing assistance. The 2017 Housing Wage necessary to afford housing is $21.21/hour, grossly exceeding minimum wage ($7.25/hour) and well beyond the average hourly wage ($16.38/hour) of a renter. The number of families in the United States who spend greater than 50 percent of their income on housing is growing, and two thirds of those living below the poverty line receive no housing assistance. These factors have led to families becoming homeless and placed others at risk of becoming homeless (Institute for Children, Poverty and Homelessness, 2018a; National Alliance to End Homelessness, 2017; National Coalition for the Homeless, 2018b).

In recent years, questions have been raised regarding whether the PIT count adequately captures the extent of the homeless population in the United States. For example, community-based PIT counts may not include individuals or families that are "**doubling up**" with relatives or friends, or mothers who avoid being counted out of fear it may mean their children could be taken from them. This gap has been partially addressed by a U.S. Department of Education (ED) Data Express survey, which requires schools to report the number of children and families who are homeless, including those that are "doubling up" by housing with another family. These families are not considered homeless by HUD, though they do not have permanent stable housing of their own (Deck, 2017). The ED count shows dramatically higher rates of homeless families; for example, the St. Louis, Missouri, PIT count showed 460 homeless people in families, while the ED count showed 5451 homeless children. Because HUD uses the PIT count to establish the numbers of homeless individuals and families, and the U.S. Interagency Council on Homelessness (USICH) uses HUD data to report on the state of homelessness, the 2016 USICH report reflected a 23 percent decrease in homeless families between 2010 and 2016. The ED count for a similar period (2010-2014) showed a 19 percent increase in homeless students. The 2016 HUD report for 2016 counted 64,197 homeless families in the United States, while the 2016 ED report showed 1.2 million children who were homeless. This would equate to the average family consisting of 20 children! Although families who double up are temporarily housed, their problems have not been solved, and they continue to have challenges in meeting their needs and suffer psychological distress related to a lack of permanent housing (Institute for Children, Poverty and Homelessness, 2018b; National Coalition for the Homeless, 2018f).

Rural communities, despite their peaceful images, are not immune to homelessness. The problem may not be as noticeable in rural areas because homelessness is more concentrated in cities. However, homeless individuals and families living in rural areas suffer from the same issues of poverty and lack of affordable housing and the same health problems as their urban counterparts. The odds of being poor are about 1.2-2.3 times higher for those in nonmetropolitan areas. The extent of homelessness in rural areas may be less apparent because these individuals are hidden from sight, sometimes living in the woods in tents or campers, in barns or ice sheds, or they may crash on a friend's couch. Access to health care becomes more problematic because of fewer resources and transportation issues. HUD calculates the population of rural homeless at 7 percent, and the majority of this population are white, female-led homeless families with higher numbers of children under age 18 (Wiltz, 2015). The homeless in rural areas may be undercounted because estimates of this subgroup rely on service provider counts, which are often fewer in number in rural areas (National Coalition for the Homeless, 2018b).

Homelessness affects psychological, social, and spiritual well-being. Becoming homeless means more than losing a home, or a regular place to sleep and eat; it also means losing friends and family, personal possessions, and familiar surroundings. Homeless persons live in chaos, confusion, and fear. Many describe experiencing loss of dignity, low self-esteem, lack of social support, and generalized despair.

Johnstone et al. (2015) describe discrimination and exclusion of the homeless as having a negative impact on social connection and in turn, their well-being. Turning to others or being part of a cohesive group can help temper the impact of discrimination among disadvantaged groups by strengthening identity and providing social support to better deal with discrimination. A sense of group identity and connection in response to discrimination has been historically demonstrated among African Americans and women. However, even though the homeless face great stigma and discrimination, they may not coalesce around a group identity. They often do not think of themselves as similar to other homeless persons. For example, they may craft an image of being a worker, contrasting themselves with other homeless persons who do not work. In addition, the age variation and reasons for becoming homeless lead to great diversity among this population, making group identity as "homeless" even more difficult. In essence, this disadvantaged group which could derive great benefit from social connectedness and a sense of belonging may be the least likely to experience it (Johnstone et al., 2015).

Who is most likely to be homeless? The number of homeless families with children decreased by 5 percent between 2016 and 2017 and represents 33 percent of the entire homeless population, while individuals who were homeless accounted for 67 percent. The majority of homeless persons were over age 24 (69.6 percent), were more likely to be male (60.5 percent), non-Hispanic (78.4 percent), and white (47.1 percent). Victims of domestic violence and veterans also make up sizable populations within the homeless cohort. Over the past few years, efforts to address the problem of homeless veterans have increased (Henry et al., 2017)

Children and Youth. Homeless children and youth fall into one of two groups: those who are part of a homeless family and those who are "unaccompanied" by homeless family members. As is true for all homeless subpopulations, it is difficult to get an accurate count. According to the 2017 AHAR report, 9.7 percent of the overall homeless population were youth aged 18-24, and 20.7 percent were youth under 18 years of age. Those under age 18 were more likely to be sheltered (28.6 percent) than those aged 18-24 (8.8 percent). About 36,000 youth aged 18-24 were unaccompanied homeless as were 4800 youth under age 18. The majority of unaccompanied youth were male (62 percent), and the rate of unaccompanied female youth (37 percent) was higher than the rate of women among all homeless individuals (28 percent). Unaccompanied youth have a significantly higher rate of living unsheltered (55 percent) than do all homeless persons (35 percent). Causes of homelessness among youth include unstable family life and domestic violence, fractured social supports, substance abuse, mental illness, and sexual orientation and gender identity and expression (SOGIE).

The U.S. Department of Education's ED Data Express provides an estimate of the rates of homelessness among children under the age of 18 that attend public school, but these data do not capture those who are not in the public-school system or those that attempt to hide their homelessness. Adolescents are particularly reticent about identifying as homeless. They do this in an effort to blend in with their peers, or if they are unaccompanied, they may fear entering into the child welfare or criminal justice system (National Network for Youth, 2018). In 2016, there were 1.2 million homeless students in public schools, or 3 percent of the total student population, a rate that has rapidly escalated over prior years. These children are 87 percent more likely to drop out of school, which may in turn, impact graduation from high school, leaving them 4.5 times more likely to become homeless as adults (Institute for Children, Poverty and Homelessness, 2018a).

Another significant factor impacting homelessness among youth is sexual orientation or gender identity expression. An estimated 40 percent of unaccompanied homeless youth are lesbian, gay, bisexual, transgender, and queer (LGBTQ) young adults (Dashow, 2017). Among homeless youth surveyed by human services agencies that worked with LGBTQ youth in 2014, 20 percent identified as lesbian or gay, 7 percent as bisexual, 2 percent as questioning sexuality, and 3 percent as transgender. Youth of color, a subset of LGBTQ homeless who are African American, Latino/Hispanic, American Indian, or Pacific Islander, are overrepresented in the survey, suggesting this group may be at greater risk. The most frequently cited reason for LGBTQ youth homelessness was being forced from their homes or running away because of SOGIE. After addressing the primary housing needs, the second most important need cited by homeless LGBTQ youth in this study was emotional support. Some 60 percent of homeless LGBQ youth and 75 percent of homeless transgender youth have experienced physical, sexual, or emotional abuse, and 10 percent of LGBQ and 25 percent of transgender youth reported intimate partner violence. These experiences contribute to **Adverse Childhood Experiences (ACEs)** that can have lifelong health consequences (Choi et al., 2015).

In 2017, CoC programs began collecting data on homeless unaccompanied youth (under age 25) for the first time, in order to establish baseline data and better understand this population. The inaugural count showed that transgender youth, and those who did not identify as male, female, or transgender, were more likely to be unsheltered than sheltered. A significant portion of this population may choose to live on the streets to avoid harassment and violence at homeless shelters or in foster care (Christian & Mukarji-Connolly, 2018). As the youth counts continue, trends in unaccompanied youth homelessness may be used to inform policy decisions such as determining the amount and type of resources that are needed to prevent homelessness among this population and evaluating which prevention programs are successful (Henry et al., 2017).

Traumatic life events are common not only among LGBTQ homeless youth, but among all homeless youth, and the nurse should consider the use of trauma-screening and trauma-informed care when working with this population (National Coalition for the Homeless, 2018c)

The Mentally Ill. One in five homeless persons has a severe mental illness, with similar rates of chronic substance abuse. Severe mental illness and substance abuse are often associated with chronic homelessness, which may be caused in part, by a lack of adequate engagement with outpatient treatment and long-term follow-up. Historically, the deinstitutionalization of mental health care was thought to be a contributing cause to the high rate of mentally ill persons who are homeless. However, a meta-analysis completed in 2016 showed that other factors may be responsible for the high rate of mentally ill homeless individuals in the United States. These factors include changes in mental health care funding in programs such as Medicaid, restrictions in Social Security and disability payments, a reduction in low-cost housing, and other social and political changes (Winkler et al., 2016).

Many homeless persons were mentally ill before becoming homeless, whereas others develop acute mental distress as a result of being homeless. Although treatment options exist, homeless persons are often unable to access mental health treatment facilities. Barriers to treatment include lack of awareness of treatment options, lack of available space in treatment facilities, inability to pay for treatment, lack of transportation, unsupportive or disrespectful attitudes of care providers, and lack of coordination of services (Roche et al., 2017). Homeless women with mental illness may face additional barriers. For example, in a recent study, women who had a history of substance use disorder (SUD) in the previous year, who also had a minor child, were far less likely to seek treatment (Upshur et al., 2018).

Veterans. A substantial percent (over nine percent) of homeless persons are military veterans. The rate of homelessness among veterans decreased by 33 percent between 2010 and 2016, largely due to a coordinated effort initiated by the U.S. Department of Veterans Affairs (VA) and HUD to engage public and private housing and service providers, and state and federal government agencies to eliminate homelessness among veterans. However, homelessness in this subgroup increased by two percent between 2016 and 2017, primarily consisting of unsheltered veterans in major cities. The majority of homeless veterans (91 percent) are male, though female veteran homelessness also rose by 7 percent during this time frame.

Veterans become homeless for many of the same reasons as non-veterans, but they are overrepresented among the homeless population, and it is thought that the experience of combat and numerous deployments may increase the risk of homelessness. Post-traumatic stress disorder (PTSD), traumatic brain injury with cognitive impairment, and other mental health issues may impair social relational health and/or negatively affect family relationships. In addition, the majority of homeless veterans are unmarried and may be socially isolated, a risk factor for homelessness. About 50 percent of veterans who are homeless have serious mental illness, and 70 percent have substance use issues.

The VA provides universal screening for all veterans who seek services through the VA health system and can be linked with housing and other appropriate services as needed, although some veterans may not be eligible for VA health services, which is dependent upon their discharge status (Henry et al., 2017; National Alliance to End Homelessness, 2018a; United States Interagency Council on Homelessness, 2018a).

A coordinated systems approach that coalesces services community-wide and uses local data to make decisions regarding resource allocation may effectively end homelessness. With this approach, "at-risk" individuals and families are quickly identified, assessed, and referred to services, in order to minimize the negative effects and interrupt a trajectory toward chronic homelessness (National Alliance to End Homelessness, 2018b). Rapid re-housing is one evidence-based approach to quickly re-housing the homeless, through the use of short-term rental assistance. This approach includes the provision of additional support services as needed (National Alliance to End Homelessness, 2018c). Another approach is "Housing First," which quickly re-houses the homeless in order to stabilize the individual/family, rather than requiring that the homeless be stabilized before they are provided housing, which has been the approach of many government and nongovernmental organization (NGO) agencies in the past. With this approach, comprehensive services are provided concurrently in order to stabilize and keep them housed continuously (Fisher, 2015; Gaetz & Dej, 2017).

Nurses may participate as community partners working within the coordinated systems approach, by using a social determinants of health screening tool to quickly identify those at risk and refer them for services (Cox, 2016). The web of causation underlying health issues needs to be addressed by nurses caring for this population. Connecting homeless clients to housing services is important, yet it is only a piece of the puzzle. A wide network of referral agencies and resources are needed to ensure that the scope of the problem is addressed (Institute for Children, Poverty and Homelessness, 2018a).

IMPACT OF HOMELESSNESS ON HEALTH ACROSS THE LIFE SPAN

Poor health is both a cause and an outcome of homelessness. Poor health can lead to work absences, job loss, financial crisis, and subsequent homelessness. Issues related to poor health are a major contributor to homelessness, with over half of personal bankruptcies in the United States due to medical issues (National Coalition for the Homeless, 2018d). Homelessness can also contribute to the risk of developing or worsening chronic disease, leading to higher mortality at a younger age. The homeless often have complex health needs and multiple morbidities, leading to high utilization of acute health services (Roche et al., 2018). They experience illness as much as six times more often than those who are housed, translating to visits at the emergency department at rates three times that of housed individuals. (National Coalition for the Homeless, 2018d; Stevenson & Purpuro, 2018).

Being homeless affects health across the life span. Imagine the effect of homelessness on pregnancy, childhood, adolescence, or older adulthood; each group has different needs. Nurses need to recognize the unique needs of homeless clients and the many factors that lead to homelessness, including joblessness; inability to maintain housing, pay utilities, and buy food; dysfunctional family life; and illness.

Mental health issues, including psychotic disorders, substance use, anxiety, PTSD, and depression, are among the most frequently cited health concerns among the homeless and are also nontraditional factors which are thought to contribute to the higher rate of cardiovascular disease (Baggett et al., 2018; Roche et al., 2018). The homeless suffer a 61 percent to 71 percent higher mortality rate from cardiovascular causes such as hypertension and ischemic heart disease than the general population, though the prevalence of hypertension is similar to those who are housed. Hypertension often goes undiagnosed or untreated, which contributes to higher CVD mortality. The high rate of tobacco use (68-80 percent) and excessive alcohol and illicit drug use add to the risk of CVD and contribute to an increased prevalence of chronic obstructive pulmonary disease, asthma, and bronchitis (Baggett et al., 2018). Diabetes also contributes to the high rates of CVD among the homeless, and lower extremity ulcerations and other foot problems are common, exacerbated by poor disease control. Foot wounds are further complicated by the many hours spent on their feet and the unsanitary conditions in which they live. (Roche et al., 2017; Stevenson & Purpuro, 2018). All of the these chronic conditions are impacted by difficulties encountered with medication adherence among the homeless, including the inability to pay for medications, store them properly, or prevent them from being stolen or lost (Baggett et al., 2018).

Infectious diseases such as HIV/AIDS, hepatitis, sexually transmitted infections (STIs) and tuberculosis are more common among the homeless than the general population. Exposure to the elements, crowded and unsanitary living conditions, malnutrition, lack of sleep, and stress place the homeless at risk for these and other infectious illnesses. Treating the homeless population effectively for these infectious diseases is particularly challenging because of difficulties getting and keeping them engaged in longitudinal treatment (Stevenson & Purpuro, 2018). Preventing infectious disease among this population is also difficult, given that visits to the emergency department or acute care facilities are a primary pathway to medical care. The focus of such care is to stabilize the emergent illness or injury, not on preventive care (Roche et al., 2018).

The HIV infection rate among the homeless ranges between 1.5 percent and 10.5 percent, depending on the subpopulation surveyed (Baggett et al., 2018). The use of intravenous drugs and risky sexual behavior, including unprotected sex and multiple partners, are contributing factors. Suboptimal HIV testing, pre-exposure prophylaxis (PrEP), and antiretroviral medication adherence negatively impact primary and secondary prevention of HIV/AIDS among the homeless (Wenzel et al., 2016).

Prolonged environmental exposure to cold environments can lead to life-threatening hypothermia, particularly when thermoregulation is impaired by age and/or abuse of drugs and alcohol. Homeless persons who lack adequate shelter are at increased risk of hypothermia due to poor mobility, poor nutrition, and mental illness or cognitive impairment. Elevated temperatures during summer can result in heatstroke and dehydration (Lane et al., 2018).

Women and Children. The rate of homeless families decreased by 5 percent between 2016 and 2017. Single, young women with limited education most often head homeless families, and in 2017, 50 percent of these mothers were African American and the remainder were white, and Hispanic (Henry et al., 2017). High rates of SUD, intimate partner violence (IPV), and pregnancy characterize this vulnerable population. In a study conducted in 2015, 62 percent of homeless women had experienced violence in childhood and adulthood, 82 percent were diagnosed with a SUD, 64 percent with major depression, and 50 percent were diagnosed with PTSD. During the study's three-year time frame, 75 percent of women had been victimized (Krahn et al., 2018; Tsaiet al., 2015). Disparities in health are higher for homeless women than for the general population of women; for example, homeless women are substantially more likely to become pregnant and experience poorer birth outcomes. Most often, these pregnancies are unintended and may be related to low levels and correct use of birth control, higher levels of sexual activity, and risky sexual encounters (Krahn et al., 2018; Thompson et al., 2016). Homeless women are less likely to have regular health care, screenings, and appropriate primary or specialty care health (Krahn et al., 2018).

The health problems of homeless children, although similar to those of poor children, are often more significant. There is a continuum of health risks among children, with those who are homeless having poorer health than children living in poverty, and those living in poverty facing greater adversity than those who do not. As with their adult counterparts, minor conditions may go untreated, resulting in higher rates of acute illness such as fever, ear infection, diarrhea, and asthma. Homeless children are at higher risk of exposure to environmental toxins such as lead. They are also at greater risk for inadequate nutrition, which can lead to delayed growth and development, failure to thrive, and conversely, obesity.

Homeless children also experience higher rates of changing schools, school absenteeism and academic progression, all of which may cause or exacerbate learning disabilities and developmental delays (Deck, 2017; Firth, 2014). While only 6.1 percent of children in "doubled up" households changed schools at least one time, 12.2 percent of the "poor but housed" group changed schools at least once, and 34.7 percent of children living in shelters changed schools more than once.

Perhaps the greatest health risk for homeless children and youth is the damaging effect of homelessness on mental health and psychological well-being. In a recent study of homeless youth drawn from the 2013 Minnesota Student Survey, 42 percent had elevated levels of emotional distress, nearly 30 percent reported self-injurious behavior such as self-mutilation, 21 percent had suicidal ideation, and over 9 percent had attempted suicide. Female homeless youth demonstrated higher levels of emotional distress, self-inflicted behavior such as mutilation, suicidal ideation, and suicide attempts than male youth. In this particular study, homeless youth were more likely to be male, youth of color, and living in rural or non-metropolitan areas. Suicide is the second leading cause of death among all youth between ages 10 and 24 but is the leading cause of death among unaccompanied homeless youth. The lifetime prevalence of depression is almost double that of housed youth (Barnes et al., 2018).

Homeless adolescents living on the streets have greater risk-taking behaviors, poorer health status, and decreased access to health care than do teens in the general population. Homeless teens often have histories of runaway behavior and physical and sexual abuse. They are at higher risk of contracting sexually transmitted infections, including HIV, sexual exploitation, traumatic violence/victimization, unintended pregnancy, injury, tuberculosis, asthma, and death. About 25 percent of street youth and 18 percent of youth living in shelters reported a serious health problem in the previous year (Chelvakumar et al., 2016; National Conference of State Legislatures, 2016). Other contributory risk factors for youth homelessness are a poorly functioning child welfare system and adolescents who are aging out of foster care and are at high risk for becoming homeless (National Conference of State Legislatures, 2016).

The health needs of LGBTQ homeless youth are somewhat different than those of non-LGBTQ homeless youth. This population has more public health risks and is less healthy than non-LGBTQ homeless youth. Mental health tends to fare worse with higher levels of depression, anxiety, and internalizing behaviors (tendency to keep problems to oneself). Alcohol and substance abuse is often reported. Homeless transgender youth health fares worse than cis-gender (personal identity corresponds with the sex at birth) youth health, and LGBTQ youth are more likely to have experienced trafficking or sexual exploitation than heterosexual homeless youth (Choi et al., 2015).

Older Adults and the Elderly. Homeless older adults aged 50-62 have a similar level of health care needs as those 10-20 years older who are housed. Common among older homeless adults are cognitive impairments, vision and hearing difficulties, and problems with walking (National Coalition for the Homeless, 2018d). Homeless older adults have an added layer of vulnerability, including "frailty," a constellation of symptoms among the geriatric population that includes physical, psychological, and social components. Predictive of frailty among older homeless adults are age, gender, nutrition, resilience, and utilization of health care. Some 16.4 percent of the homeless adult population meet diagnostic criteria for frailty (Brown et al., 2013; Salem & Ma-Pham, 2015). During a 2015 study of frail and pre-frail homeless women who were primarily over age 50, 70 percent indicated they had fallen over the prior year, with 35 percent having fallen in the previous 30 days. The women also reported that walking on concrete was hard on the hips, and pain medication was necessary if they were going to be able to remain sober. They described a desire to obtain preventive health care such as colonoscopies and other cancer screening tests, while at the same time expressing fear of diagnostic or medical procedures. Many of the study participants had the perception that health care providers possessed an attitude which hindered their responsiveness to the needs of homeless women (Salem & Ma-Pham, 2015).

Until homeless adults reach the age of 62, when they become eligible for social safety net programs for the elderly such as subsidized housing, and at age 65 when they become eligible for Social Security and Medicare, they may not meet criteria for some government assistance programs. Even when they reach the age eligibility requirement for subsidized housing, there is a shortage of affordable housing for the elderly, with nine seniors waiting for every one currently occupied unit. The first step in addressing the health care needs of this population is to provide housing by implementing the rapid re-housing and Housing First approach (National Coalition for the Homeless, 2018d; National Coalition for the Homeless, 2018e).

In summary, homelessness negatively affects the health of persons across the life span. Nurses must be able to identify the precursors to homelessness and anticipate the effects of homelessness on physical and psychological well-being in order to be able to advocate for effective prevention (Fig. 33.3). Innovative responses to serving the health care needs of those who are homeless include nurse practitioner run clinics situated in soup kitchens, emergency night and day shelters, and other mobile health care units that bring health services to where people who are homeless congregate (Stevenson & Purpuro, 2018). Another response has been the development of respite facilities for those discharged from hospitals but are still quite vulnerable, with no

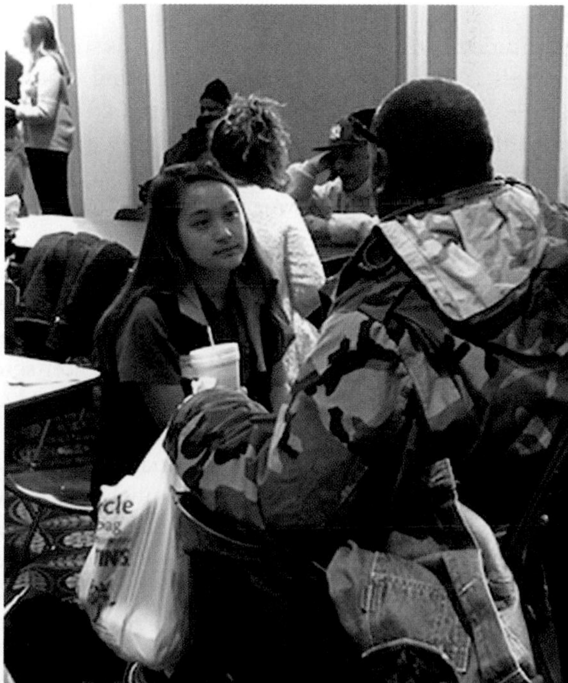

Fig. 33.3 Nurses must be able to communicate therapeutically with homeless individuals to assess their needs, create a plan of care, and effectively advocate for the patient.

home in which to return to recover from surgery or other medical procedures. Research on the effectiveness of respite care has demonstrated positive outcomes for these patients (National Health Care for the Homeless Council, 2018).

Unique Challenges and Barriers to Caring for Homeless Health. Just as people living in poverty have poor access to health care, so do homeless people. One of the topic areas in *Healthy People 2020* discusses access to health care. See the *Healthy People 2020* box for objectives that pertain to poverty and homeless persons. Even though they are at higher risk of physiological problems, homeless persons have greater difficulty accessing and understanding health care services.

HEALTHY PEOPLE 2020

The following is a sampling of goals for addressing social determinants of health among poor and homeless people:

- **AH-5.1:** Increase the proportion of students who graduate with a regular diploma, 4 years after starting 9th grade.
- **AHS-3:** Increase the proportion of persons who are unable to obtain or delay in obtaining necessary medical care, dental care, or prescription medicines.
- **HC/HIT-1.1:** Increase the proportion of persons who report their health care provider always gave them easy-to-understand instructions about what to do to take care of their illness or health condition.
- **EH-19:** Reduce the proportion of occupied housing units that have moderate or severe physical problems.
- **IVP-42:** Reduce children's exposure to violence.

From Office of Disease Prevention and Health Promotion (ODPHP): *HealthyPeople.gov: social determinants of health,* Washington, DC, 2018, ODPHP. Retrieved from https://www.healthypeople.gov.

The attitude of some health care professionals working with the homeless is a significant barrier to accessing health care. The homeless frequently cite the lack of respect and dignity with which they have been treated by providers when accessing care (Salem & Ma-Pham, 2015; Stevenson & Purpuro, 2018). Homeless persons report issues regarding communication and trust with their health care providers, particularly among women seeking gynecologic care, who may be uncomfortable with male providers. The homeless provide accounts of feeling judged and stygmatized, unheard, and rejected. In a 2018 study of homeless women seeking breast and cervical cancer screening in Canada, one woman told of routinely being turned away when seeking a primary care physician. Another reported being told she could not return to see her physician until she completed a series of diagnostic tests. Power imbalances between the homeless patient and the health care provider can be an impediment to therapeutic communication and trust building (Moravac, 2018).

Inadequate self-care is another barrier to addressing health among the homeless as they often give lower priority to health promotion and health maintenance than to obtaining food and shelter (Roche et al., 2018). They spend most of their time trying to survive. Just getting money to buy food is a major chore. In order to gather income, they may pick up odd jobs, beg, sell their blood or plasma, or sell drugs or sex for money.

Consider the case of an insulin-dependent diabetic man who lives on the street and sleeps in a shelter. His ability to get adequate rest and exercise, take insulin on a schedule, eat regular meals, or follow a prescribed diet is virtually impossible. Consider the following issues:

- How does a person buy an antibiotic without money?
- How is a child treated for scabies and lice when there are no bathing facilities?
- How does an older adult with peripheral vascular disease elevate his legs when he must be out of the shelter at 7 AM and is on the streets all day?

Preventive Services: Housing As a Nursing Intervention

The need for comprehensive, affordable, and accessible care for the nation's homeless population is huge. The federal government officially became involved with meeting the needs of the homeless in 1987 with the passage of the Stewart B. McKinney Homeless Assistance Act of 1987 (PL 100-77). Title 11 of the McKinney Act provided funding for outpatient health services; however, these services have often been insufficiently funded, and many needs go unmet. The McKinney Act grants homeless children the same access to education as permanently housed children. This act also created the U.S. Interagency Council on the Homeless (USICH) to coordinate and direct federal homeless activities. Housing assistance is available through the U.S. Department of Housing and Urban Development (2018c), which, along with many other federal agencies, funds programs to help the homeless. In the following section on prevention, an illustration is given of how to access services in a state to assist homeless persons.

The ICH is made up of the heads of 19 federal agencies that sponsor programs or activities for the homeless. The general goals of the ICH are to improve federal programs for the homeless through better coordination and linkages and by decreasing the amount of documentation required to qualify for benefits. By targeting the most vulnerable segments of the homeless population, the ICH intends to influence the problem of homelessness, particularly among children (United States Interagency Council on Homelessness, 2018b).

Essentially, the same government safety net programs available to the poor are also available to those who are homeless. Although some homeless persons are eligible for safety net programs such as Medicaid, TANF, WIC, or Social Security, they may not know they are eligible or how to apply, or they may lack the official identification necessary to apply for these benefits. Utilization rates for safety net programs among poor families and sheltered homeless families are similar, with the exception of WIC, which is underutilized among sheltered homeless families (Burt et al., 2016).

Homeless women with children under the age of five are eligible to receive nutrition assistance from the U.S. Department of Agriculture's WIC program. Persons accessing WIC benefits receive vouchers entitling them to free nutritious foods and infant formulas from local grocers. The Supplemental Nutrition Assistance Program (SNAP) is another source of nutritional assistance for the homeless and is not limited to women with young children. The TANF cash assistance program can be a key source of income for homeless families.

Preventive services related to homelessness are focused on providing affordable, adequate housing. Typically, those who are homeless are housed in emergency shelters that are only open at night and in many cities, only on extremely cold nights. Emergency shelters are an important stopgap measure during a crisis. Those who have been homeless longer may find assistance in permanent **supportive housing**. This type of housing is subsidized by federal, state, or local governments or nonprofit organizations. Supportive housing is typically reserved for vulnerable homeless population groups, such as the chronically homeless, persons with physical and mental disabilities, women and children who are victims of abuse, and those recovering from alcohol and drug use (U.S. Department of Housing and Urban Development, 2016).

Low-income housing, if available, is accessible through Section 8 housing vouchers or through public housing. Both of these subsidized programs generally require the participant to be a U.S. citizen or eligible for immigration status, and applicants are denied housing if they have habits that might be detrimental to the housing community (U.S. Department of Housing and Urban Development, n.d.).

It is difficult to separate services for homelessness into primary, secondary, and tertiary levels of prevention because interventions related to homelessness can be assigned to more than one level. Affordable housing, for example, may qualify as primary prevention, but it could also be an important secondary or tertiary preventive intervention.

Under the public health model of preventing homelessness, strategies are aimed at risk reduction and include primary, selected, and targeted initiatives. Primary preventive services include universal, selected, and targeted prevention strategies. Universal preventive services include poverty reduction, early childhood supports, affordable and subsidized housing, and old age pensions. Selected prevention strategies focus on groups that are at higher risk related to demographic, ethnic, and other inequities. These include school-based programs for youth, and anti-discrimination and anti-oppression strategies to address disparities related to minority populations. Targeted prevention strategies are aimed at populations at higher risk of homelessness because of certain characteristics, for example, LGBTQ youth. Nurses can form networks with other health professionals to educate policy makers and the public about the value of these preventive services. These programs could prevent homelessness from occurring at all, which would prevent many of its devastating sequelae.

Secondary preventive services target persons on the verge of homelessness as well as those who are newly homeless. Examples include rapid re-housing, case management, and shelter services. Nurses can work with the homeless and near-homeless to provide education about existing services and advocate for strategies that move public policy toward providing more comprehensive services for homeless and near-homeless persons.

Tertiary prevention for homelessness focuses on minimizing the impact of homelessness and working to ensure the individual/family never experiences another episode of being homeless. An important prerequisite for population-focused nursing practice is a sound understanding of the sociopolitical milieu in which problems occur. Nurses can influence politicians and other policy makers at the federal, state, and local levels about the plight of vulnerable homeless populations in their community.

Many states have programs that provide a broad spectrum of services that may interrupt the pattern of homelessness. Several follow the guidance of a program called Shelter Plus Care (subsumed in Continuum of Care programs). **Shelter Plus Care** is a program for individuals who need housing and structured social support; the goal is to stabilize those who are homeless and help them transition into permanent housing. The program offers long-term housing and supportive services for those who are homeless and who have mental illness, are in recovery from alcohol and drug abuse, or have HIV/AIDS. It also assists people on the brink of homelessness. Before the creation of Shelter Plus Care, many low-income persons found shelters to be their only resource when faced with a housing crisis. Shelter Plus Care offers an extensive set of neighborhood-based services to help people remain in their housing. The services offered include landlord mediation, budgeting, emergency rental assistance, and job training and assistance (U.S. Department of Housing and Urban Development, 2018b).

Nurses need to understand how to apply the levels of prevention to homeless persons. When nurses advocate for preventive measures for people who are either poor or are homeless, they often do so in the local or state policy arena. Nurses working in communities often need to advocate for affordable housing, community outreach services, health services, and other assistance programs for poor and homeless persons. The HUD Exchange Homelessness Assistance website lists a range of services for homeless persons that are organized by state. Go to the website and look at the topics for homelessness. There are several useful topics in the Populations & Issues drop-down menu. In addition, you can select a state and find contact information about shelters or other assistance. Each state site offers extensive information for homeless persons, beyond housing. Although each state has some unique offerings, they typically provide information about shelters, including special shelters for victims of domestic and sexual violence. The sites generally provide information about services for homeless veterans, persons with disabilities, transitional housing for offenders who are re-entering the community; and about meals, clothing, health care, skills training, counseling, and legal assistance. Although the offerings provided by states are unique, there are three agencies common to all states: Salvation Army, United Way, and Medicaid (U.S. Department of Housing and Urban Development, 2018b).

LEVELS OF PREVENTION

Homelessness

Primary Prevention

Work with a local school district to provide the free breakfast and lunch program to all students.

Secondary Prevention

Screen public school students for homelessness or "doubling up," and connect these students and their families to comprehensive services.

Tertiary Prevention

Connect homeless students with the Summer Food Service program during the summer months when school is not in session.

Accessing Health Care

Unfortunately, health care for homeless persons tends to be fragmented and limited in scope. Health care services are available in every state through Health Care for the Homeless (HCH) services, as well as a variety of privately funded programs, yet care is often sought during an acute health crisis and care is rendered via emergency department visits (Roche et al., 2017; Stevenson & Purpuro, 2018). Safety net hospitals and publicly funded insurance programs such as Medicaid, Medicare, and the Children's Health Insurance Program often cover the costs for these visits.

Following expansion of Medicaid through the Affordable Care Act (ACA), health coverage among HCH program participants rose from 45 percent to 67 percent. However, subsequent changes to the ACA, including a work requirement in some states, may decrease the number of homeless who qualify for Medicaid. The homeless have a number of barriers to employment, including poor mental health and other physical conditions, lack of consistent work history, or a history of incarceration, all of which hinder their ability to obtain and keep work (Center on Budget and Policy Priorities, 2018; Warfield et al., 2016).

Heath Care for the Homeless has been subsumed by the **Consolidated Health Centers (CHCs)** program, which combines federally funded health centers that work with the homeless, migrant and seasonal farmworkers, public housing residents, and young children. By accessing HRSA Find a Health Center, you can explore CHCs that are located in your area and obtain directions and a phone number for the facilities. Once you have identified local facilities, you may determine the array of services available by exploring the individual facility websites.

Some of the most useful health care programs for the homeless began with grants from private funding agencies, such as the Robert Wood Johnson Foundation and the Pew Charitable Trusts. Projects funded by these agencies have followed sound public health principles by encouraging community involvement, public/private partnerships, and commitment to outreach (Institute of Medicine, 1988). Most of these projects rely heavily on nurse practitioners and physician assistants to deliver care in collaboration with physicians, nurses, and social workers. In recent years, many schools of nursing have received funding to establish nurse-managed centers for the homeless. See Chapter 20 for information on nurse managed centers Both faculty and students provide a range of services in these centers.

UNIQUE ROLE OF THE NURSE

Nurses play a critical role in the delivery of care to poor and homeless people. To be effective, nurses need strong physical and psychosocial assessment skills, current knowledge of available resources, and an ability to convey respect, dignity, and value to each person. Nurses need to be able to work with poor and homeless clients to promote, maintain, and restore health. Nurses must be prepared to look at the whole picture: the person, the family, and the community interacting with the environment. The following strategies are important to consider when working with homeless individuals, families, and populations:

- *Show respect, compassion, and concern.* Poor and homeless clients are defeated so often by life's circumstances that they may feel they do not deserve attention. Listen carefully and empathize with clients so they know you believe they are worthy of care. Because clients respond well to nursing interactions that demonstrate respect, it is helpful to use reflective statements that convey acceptance and understanding of their situation. Examples include the following: "I understand you are having difficulty taking your medications regularly because sometimes it comes down to eating instead of buying the medication, is that right?" Or another approach might be "I can see how being unable to cover the co-pay for medications would keep you from taking them regularly. Would you be open to ways in which I can help make sure you are able to do both?"
- *Create a trusting environment.* Trust is essential to the development of a therapeutic relationship with poor or homeless persons. Many clients and families have been disappointed by their interactions with health care and social systems; they become mistrustful and see little hope for change. If you don't know the answer to a question, say, "I don't know the answer, but I will try to find out. Let me make a few phone calls and I will let you know Friday." By following through and doing what they say they will do, nurses can establish trusting relationships with clients. Reliability helps to build the foundation for a trusting relationship.
- *Do not make assumptions.* A comprehensive and holistic assessment is crucial to identifying underlying needs. Just because a young mother with three preschool children misses a clinic appointment does not mean that she does not care about the health of her children. She may not have transportation or the ability to pay for services. Find out the reason for the absence and help solve the problem.
- *Coordinate a network of services and providers.* Working with poor and homeless people is challenging because of their multiple and complex needs. Many services exist, but often the people who could benefit are unaware of their existence. Developing a coordinated network of providers involves conducting a thorough assessment of the service area to identify federal, state, and local services available for poor and homeless clients. Where are the food banks and what are their hours? Where can you get clothing? What programs are available in local churches and schools? How do people access these services? What are the eligibility requirements? How helpful are the people who work at the service agencies? What service is provided to eligible individuals and

families? Nurses can identify these services and help link families with appropriate resources. In addition, a thorough assessment of available services for homeless persons in a nurse's service area can identify significant gaps in essential services. Once these gaps are identified, nurses work with other health care providers and with community members to advocate for necessary services for homeless clients.

- *Advocate for accessible health care services and affordable housing.* Poverty and homelessness create barriers that prevent access to health care services. Nurses can advocate for accessible and convenient locations of health care services. Neighborhood clinics, mobile vans, and home visits can bring health care to people unable to access care. Coordinated services such as primary care and mental health care at a central location often improves client compliance because it reduces the complexity and stress of getting to multiple places. By advocating for affordable housing, nurses are engaging a universal, primary prevention technique designed to help stabilize low-income families and prevent homelessness.
- *Focus on prevention.* Nurses can use every opportunity to provide preventive health care and health promotion teaching. Preventive health care is often overlooked among impoverished or homeless populations. Important health promotion (primary prevention) topics include child and adult immunization, and education regarding sound nutrition, foot care, safe sex, contraception, and prevention of chronic illness. Screening for health problems such as tuberculosis, diabetes, hypertension, foot problems, and anemia is an important form of secondary preventive health care among the homeless population. Knowing what other screening and health promotion services are available in the target area, such as nutrition programs, job-training and educational programs, housing programs, and legal services, is important. All these services may be included in a comprehensive nursing plan of care. See the How To box below to learn ways to evaluate the concept of homelessness.

HOW TO Evaluate the Concept of Homelessness

- What is it like to live on the streets?
- What issues might confront a young, African American, transgender youth inside a homeless shelter?
- What really causes homelessness?
- What goes through your mind when confronted with a person on the street asking for money to buy a sandwich or catch a bus? How do you respond?
- How is your response different (or not) when a young mother with children asks you for money?
- How do you react to the smell of urine in a stairwell or elevator?

- *Know when to walk beside the client and when to encourage the client to move forward on his or her own.* This area is often difficult for the nurse to implement. Nursing interventions range from extensive care activities to minimal support. At times, nursing actions include providing encouragement and support or providing information. At other times, nurses may actually call a pediatrician to set up an appointment for a sick child and may call again to see that the appointment was kept. Nurses assess patients for the presence of strengths, problem-solving and coping ability of an individual or family, while providing information on where and how to gain access to services. For example, a local hospital may provide free mammograms for uninsured women. Women who qualify for this free service may not take advantage of it because they are afraid the procedure will hurt, or they are fearful that they may have breast cancer. Nurses can find out about this important service, inform the women of the service, teach them about the importance of preventive care, and assess and deal with fear and anxiety. The challenge for the nurse becomes choosing whether to schedule the appointment for the woman or to simply provide a referral sheet, knowing that she may not follow through. The choice is not clear, but the goal is to make available a needed screening intervention without taking away the woman's right to have power over the process.
- *Develop a network of support for yourself.* Caring for poor and homeless persons is challenging, rewarding, and at times exhausting. It is important to find a source of personal strength, renewal, and hope. The people you encounter are often looking to you to maintain hope and provide encouragement. Discover for yourself what restores and encourages you. For some nurses it is poetry, music, painting, or reflective practices such as mindful meditation or yoga. For others it is a walk in a peaceful place, a weekend retreat, a good run, a workout at the gym, or meeting with other nurses who are engaged in the same work. Be attentive to your own needs, and create the time and space to restore your spirit.

CHECK YOUR PRACTICE

If you are providing services in a center for homeless families, what resources in your community would you investigate to determine if all services available to this family are being met?

The Linking Content to Practice box describes how to apply selected core public health and public health nursing competencies to the care of poor and homeless people.

LINKING CONTENT TO PRACTICE

When nurses provide care to people who are poor and/or homeless, they use the nursing process that is core to all registered nursing practice. Specifically, nurses assess by gathering a comprehensive set of data on the health status of an individual or population (standard 1); make a diagnosis and set priorities (standard 2); identify expected outcomes and develop a plan based on the population diagnosis and best practices (standard 3), and implement and evaluate the chosen plan (standards 4 and 5) (American Nurses Association, 2017).

Similarly, selected core competencies for public health professionals can be clearly used in providing care to this vulnerable population. For example, use of the ecological perspective to determine health risks of an individual or population is listed as an essential core competency in Domain 1 of the 2018 Quad Council Coalition's Community/Public Health Nursing Competencies. This perspective is used to assess the relationship of multiple determinants of health and health status as well as outcomes for vulnerable populations. In Domain 4, the competencies pertaining to cultural awareness are crucial to working with impoverished and homeless populations. It is essential that the nurse develop strategies to appropriately care for those with diverse backgrounds, taking into consideration socio-cultural and behavioral factors relative to access, availability, acceptability, and delivery of services in public health (Quad Council Coalition, 2018).

PRACTICE APPLICATION

Tonya Sims, a single mother with AIDS, lives in an apartment with seven other family members and her children, who are HIV positive. Ms. Sims does not often keep her children's numerous appointments at the immunology clinic. How do you respond?

A. Make an unsolicited telephone call or visit Ms. Sims and her family to let them know they are important and that you are thinking about them.

B. Call child protective services to report the failure of Ms. Sims to keep her children's appointments; she is noncompliant and neglectful of her children.

C. Do a more thorough assessment to determine why appointments are missed.

Answers can be found on the Evolve website.

KEY POINTS

- The definition of poverty varies depending on the source consulted. The federal government defines poverty on the basis of income and family size. The multidimensional approach takes a more holistic view, defining poverty by considering deficits across health, standard of living, and monetary domains. Newer adaptations of the multidimensional approach consider the significance of social relational health to poverty.
- Racism has played and continues to play a significant role in creating and perpetuating poverty and health inequities among minorities in the United States.
- Factors which impact the prevalence of poor persons in the United States include race and ethnicity; education level; increased substance abuse, including opioids; the number of households headed by women, who also face lower wages than their male counterparts; wage stagnation; reduced Social Security payments; and political reluctance to further advance such anti-poverty initiatives as increasing the minimum wage to a "living wage."
- Poverty affects the health status of people across the life span, and the impacts are disproportionately greater among "at-risk" populations such as single mothers, women, and children; LGBTQ youth; and minorities.
- Poor persons have higher rates of chronic disease and illness and worse outcomes, higher infant mortality, shorter life expectancy, complex multi-morbidity, and lower rates of high school graduation and home ownership.
- The impact of poverty on children is due in large part to the level of toxic stress they encounter as a result of living in poverty, which can harm the developing brain, impair relational health, and leave them at a higher lifetime risk of chronic disease and early mortality.
- Poverty affects both urban and rural communities. The poorer the community, the greater the proportion of residents who are members of a minority. Poverty may be more difficult to identify in rural communities because poor persons may be hidden from view.
- To understand the concepts of poverty and homelessness, consider the historical, political, and social factors that influence poverty and homelessness, and your personal beliefs and attitudes.
- Factors contributing to homelessness include insufficient availability of low-cost housing; poor health; mental illness; substance abuse and in particular, opioid use; lack of consistent, longitudinal treatment for mentally ill persons; intimate partner violence; and family dynamics which cause children and youth to leave home.
- The number of homeless children between 2016 and 2017 decreased by 5 percent, though the rate increased by 6.7 percent among young adults aged 18-24. Nearly 60 percent of homeless people in families were children under age 18, the vast majority of which were sheltered. The number of unsheltered homeless young adults rose by 9 percent.
- The complex health problems of homeless persons include chronic and infectious diseases; exposure to violence and trauma; and mental health problems.
- The homeless face unique challenges in caring for their health, including limited access to and ability to pay for health care, poor self-care, a limited understanding of available treatment options, and the attitude of some health care providers.
- Nurses have a critical role in assessing the health of persons who are poor and homeless and providing access to preventive care, supportive resources, and health care. Nurses bring to each client encounter the ability to assess the client's social determinants of health and to intervene in ways that restore, maintain, or promote health. By intervening early and using a coordinated systems approach, nurses can minimize the effects of poverty and halt a progression to homelessness and/or chronic homelessness.

CLINICAL DECISION-MAKING ACTIVITIES

1. Examine health statistics and demographic data to identify the rate of poverty and homelessness in your geographic area. What programs or services are available to improve social interconnectedness/relational health among impoverished or homeless populations? Parental support? Homeless youth? LGBTQ populations? What resources and agencies are available in your area to support homeless persons? What services are available from federal, state, and local sources? Identify a specific geographic region and assess this target area in terms of services for poor and homeless persons. Do a literature search to identify state-of-the-art, evidence-based interventions for poor and homeless persons. Compare the recommended programs and interventions with those available in your target area. How does your area

measure up? Give some specific recommendations about how you would fill the gaps.

2. Discuss government safety net programs with other students. How does our safety net work to reduce poverty and homelessness? Who receives TANF? Who receives SNAP? Who is eligible for supplemental security income (SSI)? How do people apply for these benefits, and are they difficult to get? What are the strengths and weaknesses of safety net programs in the United States, compared to other first world programs? What do you believe would better address the issues of poverty and homelessness in the United States? Give details of your ideas for changing our anti-poverty systems. Identify federal and state senators and representatives in your districts. Where do they stand on the issues of reducing poverty through tax credits and government safety net programs? What are the financial impacts to the general public of funding these programs? What are the impacts on individuals? What programs are needed in your community, and how could state senators and representatives support such programs?
3. Examine the specific programs identified in the preceding assessment. How and where do those who need services access them? Working with other students, make appointments with key persons in the agencies identified to find out what each agency offers, which particular aggregate is served, how clients access the services, who is eligible, how the agency receives funding, and what methods are used to evaluate the agency's ability to meet the needs of its targeted aggregates. Give some examples.
4. Identify nurses in your community who work with the homeless, medically underserved, or with other vulnerable groups. Invite these nurses to come to a class meeting to share their experiences. What constitutes a typical workday? What are the rewards and challenges of working with vulnerable populations? How do they deal with the frustrations and challenges of their work? What advice might they offer to students working with vulnerable populations? What programs do they recommend? How would they advocate for vulnerable populations in the policy arena? How would you?
5. Imagine yourself as a nurse working in a homeless shelter or making a home visit to a family in an impoverished neighborhood. How have your life experiences and education prepared you (or not) for these situations?

ADDITIONAL RESOURCES

EVOLVE WEBSITE

http://evolve.elsevier.com/Stanhope/community/

- Answers to Practice Application
- Case Study
- Glossary
- Review Questions

REFERENCES

Alkire S, Foster JE, Seth S, Santos ME, Roche JM, Ballon P: *Multidimensional poverty measurement and analysis*, Oxford, UK, 2015, Oxford University Press.

American Academy of Pediatrics Committee on Psychosocial Aspects of Child and Family Health, Council on Community Pediatrics: *Impact of Poverty on the Health of Children*, 2016.

American Nurses Association: *The nursing process*, 2017, American Nurses Association. Retrieved from https://www.nursingworld.org.

Baggett TP, Liauw SS, Hwang SW: Cardiovascular disease and homelessness, *J Am Coll Cardiol* 71(22):2585–2597, 2018.

Barnes AJ, Gilbertson J, Chatterjee D: Emotional health among youth experiencing family homelessness, *Pediatrics* 141(4), 2018.

Brown RT, Kiely DK, Bharel M, Grande LJ, Mitchell SL: Use of acute care services among older homeless adults, *JAMA Intern Med* 173:1831–1834, 2013.

Burt MR, Khadduri J, Gubits D: *Are homeless families connected to the safety net? Homeless Families Research Brief*, 2016, April. Retrieved from U.S. Department of Housing and Urban Development: https://aspe.hhs.gov.

Callander EJ, Schofield DJ: Multidimensional poverty and health status as a predictor of chronic income poverty, *Health Econ* 24(2):1638–1643, 2015.

Callander ES: Pathways into chronic multidimensional poverty amongst older people: a longitudinal study, *BMC Geriatr* 1–8, 2016.

Center on Budget and Policy Priorities: *Social security benefits are modest: benefit cuts would cause hardship for many*, August 7, 2017. Retrieved from https://www.cbpp.org.

Center on Budget and Policy Priorities: *Harm to people experiencing homelessness from taking away medicaid for not meeting work requirements*, May 9, 2018. Retrieved from https://www.cbpp.org.

Centers for Disease Control and Prevention: *Social determinants of health: know what affects health*, January 29, 2018. Retrieved from https://www.cdc.gov.

Chaudry AW, Wimer C, Macartney S, et al.: *Poverty in the United States: 50-year trends and safety net impacts*, Washington, DC, 2016, U.S. Department of Health and Human Services.

Chelvakumar G, Ford N, Kapa HM, Lange H, McRee AL, Bonny AE: Healthcare barriers and utilization among adolescents and young adults accessing services for homeless and runaway youth, *J Community Health* 42:437–443, 2016.

Choi SK, Wilson BDM, Shelton J, Gates G: *Serving our youth 2015: the needs and experiences of Lesbian, Gay, Bisexual, Transgender, and Questioning youth experiencing homelessness*, 2015, The Williams Institute with True Colors Fund.

Christian R, Mukarji-Connolly A: *A new Queer Agenda*, 2018. Retrieved from Scholar & Feminist Online: http://sfonline.barnard.edu.

Conway C: *Poor health: when poverty becomes disease*, January 6, 2016, University of California San Francisco. Retrieved from https://www.ucsf.edu.

Cox K: Nurses and the social determinants of health, *Public Health Nurs* 33(1):1–2, 2016.

Dashow J: *New report on youth homeless affirms that LGBTQ youth disproportionately experience homelessness*, November 15, 2017. Retrieved from Human Rights Campaign: https://www.hrc.org.

Deck SM: School outcomes for homeless children: differences among sheltered, doubled-up, and poor, housed children, *J Child Poverty* 23(1):57–77, 2017.

Desilver D: *Who's poor in America? 50 years into the 'War on Poverty,' a data portrait*, January 13, 2014. Retrieved from Pew Research Center: http://www.pewresearch.org.

Firth P: *Homelessness and academic achievement: the impact of childhood stress on school performance*, September 8, 2014. Retrieved from firesteel: http://firesteelwa.org.

Fisher R: *Homeless prevention: the public health model*, March 15, 2015, Homeless Hub. Retrieved from http://homelesshub.ca.

Fox LP, Pacas J: *Deconstructing poverty rates among the 65 and older population: Why has poverty increased since 2015?* Population Association of America Annual Meeting, April 26-28, 2018, Washington, DC, 2018, U.S. Census Bureau, pp 1–36.

Gaetz S, Dej E: *A new direction: a framework for homelessness prevention*, Toronto, 2017, Canadian Obsrvatory on Homelessness. Retrieved from http://homelesshub.ca.

Goins RT, Schure MB, Crowder J, Baldridge D, Benson W, Aldrich N: *Lifelong disparities among older American Indians and Alaska Natives*, Washington, DC, 2015, AARP Public Policy Institute.

Hallowell SG, Froh EB, Spatz DL: *Human milk and breastfeeding: an intervention to mitigate toxic stress, Nurs Outlook* 65(1):58–67, 2017. Retrieved from https://www.nursingoutlook.org.

Harris F, Curtis A: Introduction and the History of the Kerner Report. In Harris FC, editor: *Healing our divided society: investing in America fifty years after the Kerner Report*, Philadelphia, PA, 2018, Temple University Press, pp 1–8.

Henry M, Watt R, Rosenthal L, Shivji A: *The 2017 Annual Homeless Assessment Report (AHAR) to Congress*, Washington, DC, 2017, U.S. Department of Housing and Urban Development.

Institute for Children, Poverty and Homelessness: *The United States of Homelessness*, 2018a. Retrieved from https://invisiblemillion.org.

Institute for Children, Poverty and Homelessness: *Are we really counting America's homeless families?* 2018b. Retrieved from http://www.icphusa.org.

Institute of Medicine. Homelessness, health, and human needs, Washington, DC, 1988, National Academies Press.

Internal Revenue Service: *Earned Income Tax Credit (EITC)*, 2018, IRS. Retrieved from https://www.irs.gov.

Jarrell K, Ozymy J, Gallagher J, Hagler D, Corral C, Hagler A: Constructing the foundations for compassionate care: how service-learning affects nursing students' attitudes towards the poor, *Nurse Educ Pract* 14(3):299–303, 2014.

Johnstone M, Jetten J, Dingle GA, Parsell C, Walter ZC: Discrimination and well-being amongst the homeless: the role of multiple group membership, *Front Psychol*, 6:739, 2015.

Kaiser Family Foundation: *How many seniors are living in poverty? National and State Estimates Under the Official and Supplemental Poverty Measures in 2016*, Washington, District of Columbia, United States, March 2, 2018.

Krahn J, Caine V, Chaw-Kant J, Singh AE: Housing interventions for homeless, pregnant/parenting women with addictions: a systematic review, *J Soc Distress Homeless* 27(1):75–88, 2018.

Lane K, Ito K, Johnson S, Gibson EA, Tang A, Matte T: Burden and risk factors for cold-related illness and death in New York City, *Int J Environ Res Public Health* 15(4):E632, 2018.

Leininger L, Levy H: Child health and access to medical care, *Future Child* 25:65–90, 2015.

Levin J: Healthcare reform ≠ public health reform: on pathogens, poverty, and prevention, *Glob Adv Health Med* 7:2164957X18756307, 2018.

Moravac CC: Reflections of homeless women and women with mental health challenges on breast and cervical cancer screening decisions: power, trust, and communication with care providers, *Front Public Health* 6:30, 2018.

National Alliance to End Homelessness: *Resources: Unsheltered homelessness: trends, causes, and strategies to address*, July 26, 2017. Retrieved from https://endhomelessness.org.

National Alliance to End Homelessness: *Resources overview: veteran homelessness*, Washington DC, 2018a, National Alliance to End Homelessness.

National Alliance to End Homelessness: *Creating systems that work*, 2018b. Retrieved from https://endhomelessness.org.

National Alliance to End Homelessness: *Rapid Re-Housing*, 2018c. Retrieved from https://endhomelessness.org.

National Center for Chronic Disease Prevention and Health Promotion: *Health-Related Quality of Life*, May 31, 2016. Retrieved from Centers for Disease Control and Prevention: https://www.cdc.gov.

National Coalition for the Homeless: *Types of homelessness*, 2018a. Retrieved from Homelessness in America: http://nationalhomeless.org.

National Coalition for the Homeless: *Building a movement to end homelessness*, 2018b. Retrieved from http://nationalhomeless.org.

National Coalition for the Homeless: *Trauma informed care*, 2018c. Retrieved from https://nationalhomeless.org.

National Coalition for the Homeless: *Health Care*, 2018d. Retrieved from http://nationalhomeless.org.

National Coalition for the Homeless: *Elder homelessness*, 2018e. Retrieved from http://nationalhomeless.org.

National Coalition for the Homeless: *Family homelessness*, 2018f. Retrieved from http://nationalhomeless.org.

National Conference of State Legislatures: *Homeless and runaway youth*, April 14, 2016. Retrieved from http://www.ncsl.org.

National Council on Aging: *Economic security for seniors facts*, Arlington, Virginia, United States, 2018, National Council on Aging.

National Health Care for the Homeless Council: *Medical respite*, 2018. Retrieved from https://www.nhchc.org.

National Network for Youth: *How many homeless youth are in America?* 2018. Retrieved from https://www.nn4youth.org.

National Women's Law Center: *NWLC resources on poverty, income, and health insurance in 2016*, September 12, 2017. Retrieved from https://nwlc.org.

Office of Community Planning and Development: *The 2017 Annual Homeless Assessment Report (AHAR) to Congress*, Washington, DC, 2017, U.S. Department of Housing and Urban Development.

Office of Disease Prevention and Health Promotion (ODPHP): *HealthyPeople.gov: social determinants of health*, Washington, DC, 2018, ODPHP. Retrieved from https://www.healthypeople.gov.

Oliff H: *Graduation Rates and American Indian Education*, May 16, 2017. Retrieved from Partnership with Native Americans: http://blog.nativepartnership.org.

Oshio TK, Kan M: Multidimensional poverty and health: evidence from a nationwide survey in Japan, *Int J Equity Health* 13:128, 2014.

Pascoe J, Wood D, Duffee J, Kuo A: *Mediators and adverse effects of child poverty in the United States*, Itasca, Illinois, 2016, American Academy of Pediatrics Committee on Psychosocial Aspects of Child and Family Health, Council on Community Pediatrics.

Pindus N, Kingsley G, Biess J, Levy D, Simington J, Hayes C: *Housing needs of American Indians and Alaska Natives in Tribal Areas: a report from the Assessment of American Indian, Alaska Native, and Native Hawaiian Housing Needs*, Washington, District of Columbia, United States, January 2017.

Quad Council Coalition: *Community/Public Health Nursing [C/PHN] Competencies*, April 13, 2018. Retrieved from http://www.quadcouncilphn.org.

Roche M, Duffield C, Smith J, et al.: Nurse-led primary health care for homeless men: a multimethods descriptive study, *Int Nurs Rev* 65:392–399, 2018.

Running Strong for American Indian Youth: *The poverty cycle*, 2018. Retrieved from http://indianyouth.org.

Salem BE, Ma-Pham J: Understanding health needs and perspectives of middle-aged and older women experiencing homelessness, *Public Health Nurs* 32:634–644, 2015.

Semega J, Fontenot K, Kollar M: *Income and poverty in the United States: 2016*, Washington, DC, 2017, United States Census Bureau.

Shapiro I, Trisi D: *Child poverty falls to record low, comprehensive measure shows strong government policies account for long-term improvement*, Washington, DC, 2017, Center on Budget and Policy Priorities.

Stanford Center on Poverty & Inequality: *The poverty and inequality report: state of the union 2017*, Stanford, 2017, Pathways Magazine.

Statista Portal: *Poverty rate in the United States from 1990 to 2016*, 2018. Retrieved from https://www.statista.com.

Stevenson E, Purpuro T: Homeless people: nursing care with dignity, *Nursing* 48:58–62, 2018.

Thompson S, Begun S, Bender K: Pregnancy and parenting among runaway and homeless young women. In Colls SJ, editor: *Handbook of missing persons*, Cham, Switzerland, 2016, Springer International, pp 77–91.

Tsai A, Weiser S, Dilworth S, Shumway M, Riley E: Violent Victimization, mental health, and service utilization outcomes in a cohort of homeless and unstably housed women living with or at risk of becoming infected with HIV, *Am J Epidemiol* 181(10):817–826, 2015.

United Nations: *Multidimensional poverty: development issues no. 3*, October 21, 2015. Retrieved from https://www.un.org.

United States Census Bureau: *2017 Current population survey, annual social and economic supplement (CPS ASEC)*, 2017. Retrieved from https://www.census.gov.

United States Census Bureau: *The supplemental poverty measure, 2016*, Washington, DC, September 21, 2017, United States.

United States Interagency Council on Homelessness: *Housing needs of American Indians and Alaska Natives in tribal areas: a report from the assessment of American Indian, Alaska Native, and Native Hawaiian housing needs,* Washington, DC, 2017, United States Interagency Council on Homelessness.

United States Interagency Council on Homelessness: *Homelessness in America: focus on veterans,* Washington, DC, 2018a, USICH.

United States Interagency Council on Homelessness: *USICH Fact Sheet,* May, 2018b. Retrieved from https://www.usich.gov.

Upshur CC, Jenkins D, Weinreb L, Gelberg L, Orvek EA: Homeless women's service use, barriers, and motivation for participating in substance use treatment, *Am J Drug Alcohol Abuse* 44(2):252–262, 2018.

U.S. Department of Education: *National Center for Education Statistics: public high school graduation ratees*, Washington, DC, May, 2018, United States.

U.S. Department of Health and Human Services: *Infant mortality and American Indians/Alaska Natives*, October 6, 2017. Retrieved from https://minorityhealth.hhs.gov.

U.S. Department of Health and Human Services: *2017 Poverty guidelines,* January 18, 2018. Retrieved from https://www.federalregister.gov.

U.S. Department of Health and Human Services Office of Minority Health: *Minority population profile: black/African Americans*, Washington, DC, June 2018a, District of Columbia, United States.

U.S. Department of Health and Human Services Office of Minority Health: *Office of minority health profile: American Indian/Alaska Native*, Washington DC, March 28, 2018b, District of Columbia, United States: U.S. Department of Health & Human Services.

U.S. Department of Health and Human Services Office of Minority Health: *Office of minority health profile: Hispanic/Latino Americans*, Washington DC, September 11, 2018c, District of Columbia, United States: U.S. Department of Health & Human Services.

U.S. Department of Housing and Urban Development: *Notice on prioritizing persons experiencing chronic homelessness and other vulnerable homeless persons in permanent supportive housing,* 25 July, 2016. Retrieved from https://www.hudexchange.info.

U.S. Department of Housing and Urban Development: *Home income limits*, 2018a. Retrieved from https://www.hudexchange.info.

U.S. Department of Housing and Urban Development: *Shelter plus care program*, 2018b. Retrieved from https://www.hudexchange.info.

U.S. Department of Housing and Urban Development: *Homelessness assistance programs*, 2018c Retrieved from https://www.hudexchange.info.

U.S. Department of Housing and Urban Development: *HUD's public housing program,* n.d. Retrieved from https://www.hud.gov.

Wagle UR: The counting-based measurement of multidimensional poverty: the focus on economic resources, inner capabilities, and relational resources in the United States, *Soc Indic Res* 115(1): 223–240, 2014.

Warfield M, DiPietro B, Artiga S: *How has the ACA medicaid expansion affected providers serving the homless population: analysis of coverage, revenues, and costs.* 15 March, 2016. Retrieved from Kaiser Family Foundation: https://www.kff.org.

Wenzel S, Rhoads H, Harris T, Winetrobe H, Rice E, Henwood B: Risk behavior and access to HIV/AIDS prevention services in a community sample of homeless persons entering permanent supportive housing, *AIDS Care Psychological and Socio-medical Aspects of AIDS/HIV* 1–5, 2016.

Wiltz T: *States struggle with 'hidden' rural homelessness*, 26 June, 2015. Retrieved from PEW: http://www.pewtrusts.org.

Winkler P, Barrett B, McCrone P, Csémy L, Janoušková M, Höschl C: Deinstitutionalised patients, homelessness and imprisonment: systematic review, *Br J Psychiatry* 208(5):421–428, 2016.

World Health Organization: *Closing the gap in a generation: health equity through action on the social determinants of health. report from the commission on social determinants of health,* Geneva, Switzerland, 11 June, 2008, World Health Organization. Retrieved from http://www.who.int.

World Health Organization: *Health impact assessment: the determinants of health,* 2018a. Retrieved from http://www.who.int.

World Health Organization: *Part two. the urgent need for action,* 2018b. Retrieved from http://www.who.int.

34

Migrant Health Issues

Candace Kugel, BA, MS, FNP, CNM

OBJECTIVES

After reading this chapter, the student should be able to do the following:

1. Define the terms *migrant farmworker* and *seasonal farmworker,* and discuss the lifestyle and work environments that contribute to their health status.
2. Discuss the difficulties with obtaining epidemiologic and health data on this population.
3. Describe occupational and common health problems of migrant farmworkers and their families and the barriers to securing health care.
4. Evaluate programs to determine effectiveness with encouraging health-seeking and health-promoting behaviors among migrant farmworkers and their families.
5. Analyze the role of the nurse in planning and providing culturally appropriate care to migrant farmworkers and their families.
6. Advocate for legislation and policy that would improve the lives and working conditions of migrant farmworkers and their access to health care services.

CHAPTER OUTLINE

Migrant Lifestyle
Health and Health Care
Occupational and Environmental Health Risks
Common Health Problems
Children and Youth
Cultural Considerations in Migrant Health Care
Nurse-Client Relationship
Health Promotion and Illness Prevention
Role of the Nurse

KEY TERMS

food insecurity, p. 761
health disparities, p. 761
migrant farmworker, p. 756
Migrant Health Act, p. 759
migrant health centers, p. 759
migrant lifestyle, p. 757
occupational health risks, p. 760
pesticide exposure, p. 760
political advocates, p. 768
seasonal farmworker, p. 756
traditional beliefs and practices, p. 765

Migrant and seasonal farmworkers (MSFWs) are essential to the agricultural industry in the United States, especially with the decrease in family farms and the increase in labor-intensive crops such as vegetables, fruit, nuts, and ornamental plants. Although the availability and affordability of food in the United States depend on these individuals, their economic status and social acceptance have not reflected the importance of their work. Estimates of the numbers of MSFWs in the United States vary, with sources identifying about 1.0 to 2.7 million hired farmworkers (U.S. Department of Agriculture, 2017). Numbers vary because of divergent methodologies for estimating numbers and the inherent difficulties in counting mobile populations. Large data sources each have unique limitations prohibiting a clear picture of the MSFW population.

According to the U.S. Department of Labor (2016a), a **migrant farmworker** is a seasonal farmworker who must travel to do farmwork and is unable to return to a permanent residence within the same day. A **seasonal farmworker** returns to his or her permanent residence, works in agriculture seasonally, and does not work year-round exclusively in agriculture. The term *MSFW* also includes migrant food-processing workers, who are defined in the same way as seasonal farmworkers but

The editors of this volume and the second author (CK) wish to acknowledge the significant contributions of Marie Napolitano to the previous edition of this chapter. Even more noteworthy has been her career as an educator and advanced practice nurse working to provide health care services to farmworker families.

work in food processing and are unable to return to a permanent residence on the same day.

The National Agricultural Workers Surveys (NAWS) have been a source of data about the farmworker population since 1989, with their most recent survey of data from 2013-2014 reported in 2016 (U.S. Department of Labor, 2016a). According to the most recent NAWS data, the proportion of migrant crop farmworkers appears to be decreasing by about 25 percent in recent years, whereas that of seasonal farmworkers is increasing (Carroll, 2016). Migrant and seasonal farmworkers share many demographic, cultural, and occupational characteristics. Much of the available information on agricultural farmworkers does not distinguish between migrant and seasonal farmworkers.

The majority of MSFWs are foreign born (72 percent) and predominantly Mexican (67 percent) (Carroll, 2016). The numbers of newly arrived indigenous migrant workers from southern Mexico and Central America are increasing. These individuals are at higher risk for exploitation due to language difficulties, poverty, and fear related to their legal status. Other workers include African Americans, Jamaicans, Haitians, Laotians, and Thais. The composition of the migrant and seasonal population can vary from region to region in the United States. According to the NAWS, 53 percent of MSFWs have legal authorization to work in the United States, and less than 1 percent of farmworkers are in the United States under a guest worker visa. Foreign-born farmworkers have spent an average of 18 years working in the United States, with more than 55 percent for at least 15 years.

According to the most recent NAWS data, MSFWs are typically young, with an average age of 38 years; 18 percent are less than 25 years of age. Interestingly, considering the nature of the work, 32 percent of MSFWs are older than 45 years of age. The majority of MSFWs are male (72 percent); more than 63 percent are married with an average of two children. The proportion of women working in agriculture is gradually increasing, bringing with it additional unique health care challenges. About 39 percent live away from all family members during their agricultural work. Thirty-one percent speak English well and 27 percent cannot speak English at all, though 74 percent report that Spanish is their primary language. The average school grade completed is eighth grade.

CHECK YOUR PRACTICE

Imagine yourself attempting to deliver treatment in a migrant camp to a toddler whose pertussis culture returned positive.

The camp is located in an isolated rural community. The toddler lives in a trailer with her parents and siblings and extended family members (13 individuals). The family must also be treated as contacts. None of these individuals speak English, so you have an interpreter with you. The family has just returned from picking strawberries all day in the fields adjacent to their trailer, and they are tired and hungry.

The family is willing to give medicine to the toddler because she is sick; however, they do not understand why they must take the medicine also, because they are not sick. In addition, the family tells you that they will not be able to take the midday dose because they have no water with them at work. Walking to the drinking barrel will take too long and they will lose income.

As a nurse, what would you do?

MIGRANT LIFESTYLE

Migrant farmworkers traditionally have followed one of three migratory streams: Eastern, originating in Florida; Midwestern, originating in Texas; and Western, originating in California. As workers increasingly travel throughout the country seeking employment, however, these streams are becoming less distinct. Migrant farmworkers are employed in fruit and nut (40 percent), vegetable (21 percent), horticultural (23 percent), field (13 percent), and miscellaneous (3 percent) agricultural venues (Carroll, 2016). Eighty-five percent of farmworkers are hired directly and 15 percent are labor contracted. The cyclic nature of agricultural work, along with its dependence on weather and economic conditions, results in considerable uncertainty for migrant farmworkers. These individuals and families leave their homes with the expectation of work at certain sites. Word of mouth from friends or family, newspaper announcements, or previous employment most often determine their destinations. On arrival, however, migrant farmworkers may find that other workers have arrived first or that the crops are late, leaving the farmworkers unemployed.

Migrant farmworkers are vulnerable to forced labor (labor trafficking). According to the Polaris Project (2018) labor traffickers "use violence, threats, lies, debt bondage, or other forms of coercion to force people to work against their will in many different industries." Trafficked individuals, especially those who are undocumented, need to work but can find themselves in appalling work and housing conditions without means to leave or report, fearful of retaliation. They may owe debt to their employers or recruiters from their home countries. Federal and state legislation exist against human trafficking, but in isolated agricultural areas enforcement is difficult. Although exact numbers are not available, the agricultural sector is recognized as one of the most common labor markets that involves foreign nationals trafficked in the United States (Urban Institute, 2014). The psychological stress of working in a forced labor arrangement can result in physical and mental health problems. Certain questions can identify a victim of forced labor and can be asked as part of a nursing assessment. The National Human Trafficking Hotline (2014) created a set of suggested questions for suspected victims, which includes:

- Do you have a debt to your employer or recruiter that you can't pay off?
- Is your job or work different than you were promised?
- Is there verbal or physical abuse at work?

If a minor is identified, then child protective services and law enforcement should be notified. Richards (2014) recommended involving social workers and others in the plan to assist a trafficked minor. The minor should not be left alone until services arrive. For an adult, obtain permission to contact authorities and get a social worker or agency involved. The National Human Trafficking Resource Center hotline (888-373-7888) should be contacted.

The way of life for any migrant farmworker is stressful. Some of the challenges of the **migrant lifestyle** include leaving one's home every year, traveling, and experiencing uncertainty regarding work and housing, isolation in new communities,

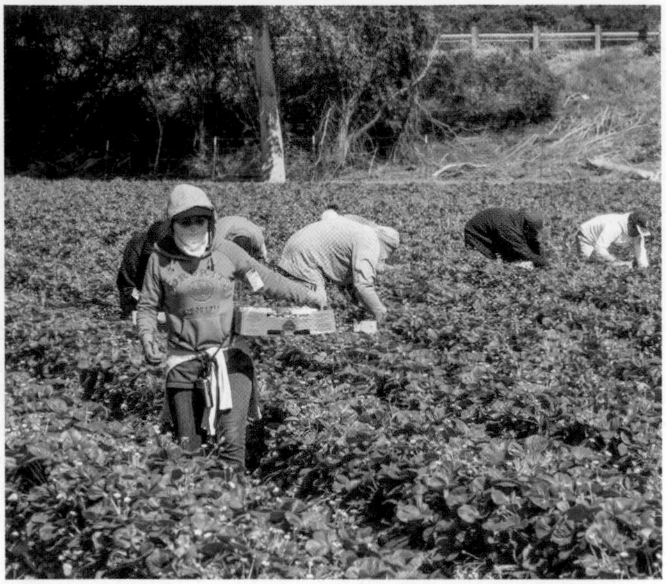

Fig. 34.1 Migrant farmworkers pick and package strawberries in the Salinas Valley of central California. (David Litman/Shutterstock.com.)

and a lack of resources (Fig. 34.1). Farmworkers may be paid an hourly or piece rate, and the specifics for payment differ depending on the location and type of work. Reports of average income for farmworkers have varied. According to the NAWS 2013-2014 statistics, farmworkers reported an average hourly income of $10.19. Although many farmworker families meet the income tests for federal and state assistance programs, undocumented workers are not eligible for most of these programs; for others, changing residence from state to state, lack of knowledge and lack of access to programs impede use of program assistance.

Migrant and seasonal workers often are exempt from the protection of labor laws such as Workers' Compensation as well as from some Occupational Safety and Health Administration (OSHA) protective provisions due to allowances such as small farm exemptions. Where laws do exist to protect agricultural workers, they may be minimally enforced because of lack of staff and resources. Laws have been enacted that intend to protect farmworkers (Farmworker Justice, 2014a). These include the Fair Labor Standards Act that addresses minimum wage, overtime pay, record keeping, and child labor standards. Farms with fewer than seven workers in a calendar quarter are exempt from minimum wage requirements and farmworkers are not included in overtime pay. The Migrant and Seasonal Agricultural Worker Protection Act mandates that farm contractors, employers, and agricultural associations must disclose employment terms, post information about worker protection at the worksite, pay workers what is due and provide itemized statements, and ensure that housing complies with federal and state safety and health standards. Employers and agricultural associations have made multiple attempts to weaken or void the law.

The Occupational Safety and Health Act's Field Sanitation Standards (U.S. Department of Labor, 2008) ensure drinkable water and accessible sanitation facilities. Another set of regulations apply to H-2A guest workers, which allows agricultural employers to hire temporary workers from other countries. These laws are also difficult to enforce and can place workers in a position where they are unable to protect themselves from abusive working conditions (Farmworker Justice, 2018).

As of January 2017, the U.S. Environmental Protection Agency (EPA) implemented revisions to the Agricultural Worker Protection Standard (WPS), regulations that safeguard farmworkers from harmful exposures to pesticides (EPA, 2018). The changes include restrictions related to the age of workers who handle pesticides, training of workers, and other protective practices related to pesticide application (Migrant Clinicians Network, 2017a).

Migrant and seasonal agricultural workers are considered a unique vulnerable population because of the factors cited here, including mobility, the physical demands of their work, social and often geographic isolation, language differences, and high rates of financial impoverishment. Although MSFW problems are numerous and creating solutions is difficult, some progress has been made in improving the condition of the farmworker population. For example, the latest analyzed NAWS data showed improvement in field sanitation conditions such as the provision of drinking water, field toilets, and handwashing facilities.

Housing

Migrant farmworkers often have trouble finding available, decent, and affordable housing. Housing conditions vary among states and localities, and housing arrangements and locations and types of housing differ for migrant and seasonal farmworkers. Housing for migrant farmworkers varies by employer and by region; it can be located in camps with cabins, trailers, or houses and may be near farms. The authors have seen migrant farmworker families living in cars and tents when housing was not available. A recent trend shows that fewer employers provide on-farm housing or labor camps, and farmworkers must rely on private market housing such as apartments or motels. Although research on the current status of farmworker housing is limited, localized studies have revealed numerous violations of housing regulations, including contaminated water, infestations, non-functioning sanitation facilities, and absent fire escapes and alarms (Arcury et al., 2012).

It is widely recognized that crowded conditions, poor sanitation, and proximity to agricultural fields and pesticides are common and contribute to health risks of workers and their family members (Farmworker Justice, 2014b). Because housing may be expensive, many men may live in one house or three families may share one trailer. The health risks of overcrowded housing range from spread of infectious disease to psychosocial effects. While paying for housing during the agricultural season, many farmworker families also support a home-base household. More federal and state programs are seeking to provide private sector housing to farmworker families such as by providing grants to nonprofit agencies serving farmworkers, though insufficient funds are available to meet the demand for farmworker housing.

HEALTH AND HEALTH CARE

Research literature provides only a glimpse into the health status of migrant farmworkers. National data needed to present a clear picture of farmworkers' health status are difficult to obtain because of such factors as high annual turnover, language, mobility, and immigration status. Regional and local cross-sectional health status studies allow some insights, however. In the past, two such reports from California especially highlighted the health issues of this population: *Suffering in Silence: A Report on the Health of California's Agricultural Workers* (California Institute for Rural Studies, 2000) and *In Their Own Words: Farmworker Access to Health Care in Four California Regions* (California Institute for Rural Studies, 2001). These reports showed a population at high risk for chronic disease, poor dental health, and mental health problems; higher rates of certain diseases such as tuberculosis (TB), anemia, diabetes, and hypertension; high levels of work injuries and chemical exposures; and detrimental physical and social environments for the children. Subsequent studies have continued to support the picture of a population with health issues similar to the general population but which are exacerbated by lack of access to services, poor continuity of care, occupational safety issues, poverty, and other social determinants of health (Kugel & Zuroweste, 2010).

Access to Health Care

The **Migrant Health Act**, signed in 1962, provides funds for primary and supplemental health services to migrant workers and their families. As of 2016, these funds are dispersed to 172 community health centers across the United States that serve as models for delivery of services to a difficult-to-reach agricultural worker population. **Migrant health centers** serve almost a million individuals across the country (Health Resources and Services Administration [HRSA], 2017), though estimates show that these clinics serve less than 15 percent of the entire migrant farmworker population. Others receive medical care from private physicians, health departments or emergency departments, or they do not seek help at all.

Migrant farmworkers have limited access to health care. The NAWS findings from 2013-2014 showed that 35 percent of the farmworkers interviewed had accessed health care services in the previous two years, and factors such as gender, immigration status, migrant status, English proficiency, access to transportation, health status, and access to health care services outside of the United States were associated with health care use (U.S. Department of Labor, 2016a).

Factors that limit adequate provision of health care services include the following:

- *Lack of knowledge about services:* Because of their isolation and mobility, migrant farmworkers lack the usual sources for information regarding available services, especially if they are not receiving public benefits.
- *Inability to afford care:* According to the latest NAWS report, 35 percent of farmworkers reported that they had health insurance. The Medicaid program, which is intended to serve the poor, often is not available to migrant farmworkers. Workers may not remain in a geographic area long enough to be considered for benefits, or they may lose benefits when they relocate to a state with different eligibility standards. Their salaries may fluctuate each month, making them ineligible during the times their salaries rise. Employers may not offer health insurance. Undocumented farmworkers are not eligible for Medicaid coverage. Therefore, most migrant farmworkers lack health insurance and state program assistance, which further hinders their access to care. In addition, only 12 states require employers to provide full Workers' Compensation insurance for agricultural workers, while in the remaining states coverage is limited or optional (MCN, 2015b; FJ, 2014a).
- *Affordable Care Act or health insurance subsidies:* Although it is difficult to determine numbers, many farmworkers do not receive employer-sponsored health coverage or subsidies because of the small farm exemption and the exclusion of seasonal workers who are employed less than 120 days in the employer's tax year. Undocumented workers are excluded from any employer and individual insurance mandates.
- *Availability of services:* Immigrants are treated differently, depending on whether they were in the United States before the welfare reform legislation of 1996, and depending on the category of their immigration status. Each state determines whether to fill any or part of the services gap to immigrants. As a result, many legal immigrants and unauthorized immigrants are ineligible for services such as supplemental security income (SSI) and the Supplemental Nutrition Assistance Program (SNAP, or food stamps).
- *Transportation:* Health care services may be located a great distance from work or home, and transportation may not be available or may be too costly.
- *Hours of services:* Many health services are available only during work hours; therefore, seeking health care during work hours leads to loss of earnings and potential loss of employment.
- *Mobility and tracking:* Migrant families move from job to job, but their health care records do not typically travel with them, leading to fragmented services in such areas as TB treatment, chronic illness management, prenatal care, and immunizations. For example, health departments are known to dispense TB medications on a daily or monthly basis, and adequate treatment for TB requires 4 to 12 months of medication. The migrant farmworker who moves for work must locate new health services in order to continue treatment. The Migrant Clinicians Network (MCN) Health Network program assists mobile patients with locating care and transferring medical records when they are enrolled in the program by a health care provider. This "bridge case management" helps maintain continuity of care for TB and other conditions requiring ongoing care for a mobile population (Tschampl et al., 2016).
- *Discrimination:* Although migrant farmworkers and their families bring revenue into the community, they are often perceived as poor, uneducated, transient, and ethnically different. These perceptions foster attitudes and acts of discrimination against them.

- *Documentation:* Unauthorized individuals fear that securing services in a federally funded or state-funded clinic may lead to discovery and deportation.
- *Language:* The majority of migrant farmworkers speaks a language other than English as their first language; most speak Spanish, with a growing number speaking indigenous dialects. Although migrant health centers may hire bilingual Spanish-speaking staff, interpretation services for localized dialects may be more challenging.
- *Cultural aspects of health care:* See the section Cultural Considerations in Migrant Health Care.

OCCUPATIONAL AND ENVIRONMENTAL HEALTH RISKS

The migrant farmworker population is defined by their engagement in agricultural work, and an understanding of the occupational health risks and exposures of that work is therefore critical in understanding the health status and health care needs of this population. Agricultural work ranks as one of the most dangerous industries in the United States. In 2016, the occupational category of agriculture, forestry, fishing, and hunting was reported as having the highest rate of occupational injuries and illnesses (U.S. Bureau of Labor Statistics, 2017).

Heat illness fatalities have been identified as especially significant. Agricultural work is performed in conditions that are particularly high risk for heat-related illness and death (Centers for Disease Control and Prevention [CDC], 2014). In addition, working conditions, such as standing on ladders, exposure to chemicals, and using machinery, produce occupational health risks for farmworkers who may be inadequately protected or educated. The physical demands of harvesting crops 12 to 14 hours a day take their toll on the musculoskeletal system. Stooping to pick strawberries, reaching overhead while on a ladder to pick pears, or lifting heavy crates can all cause musculoskeletal pain (Moyce & Shenker, 2018). Injuries such as sprains and strains, fractures, and lacerations are especially common. Other injuries include falls; amputations; crush injuries from tractors, trucks, or other machinery; injuries related to working with livestock; acute pesticide poisoning; electrical injuries; and drowning in irrigation ponds and trenches. Naturally occurring plant substances or applied chemicals can cause irritation to the skin (contact dermatitis) or to the eyes (allergic or chemical conjunctivitis). Farmworkers also spend considerable time in the sun, which is dangerous to the skin. Infectious diseases caused by poor sanitary conditions at work and home, poor-quality drinking water, and contaminated foods can result in acute gastroenteritis and parasites. Farmworkers are at higher risk for eye injuries because of the lack of eye protection devices; lack of knowledge about prevention of eye injuries; and exposure to chemicals, pollen, and dust. Chronic eye irritation and sun exposure lead to cataracts, pterygium, and cloudy lens (Quandt et al., 2013).

The inherent dangers of farmwork are magnified by the inconsistent and inadequate safety regulations in the industry (Liebman et al., 2013). Lack of a comprehensive surveillance system makes it difficult to know the extent of all injuries within the farmworker population. Because small farms are excluded from governmental annual injury surveys and maintenance of written injury reports, injury statistics for farmworkers are incomplete (Kresge Foundation, 2012). Injuries are often unreported by farmworkers themselves for fear of loss of work and deportation, and workers are inclined to self-treat with over-the-counter remedies for injuries.

Pesticide Exposure

The majority of the North American food supply is treated with pesticides. Organophosphate (OP) pesticides make up the largest group of pesticides in current use. These pesticides are known to be potential hazards. Pesticide exposure risk for farmworkers includes not only the immediate effects of working in fields that are foggy or wet with pesticides, but also the unknown long-term effects of chronic exposure to pesticides. Reported incidents of occupational exposures to pesticides are monitored by the National Institute for Occupational Safety and Health (NIOSH) SENSOR-Pesticides Database (Sentinel Event Notification System for Occupational Risk). A total of 13 states participate in this reporting system, and available data from 1998-2011 reveal that half of the reported occupational pesticide exposures occur in the category of farming, forestry, and fishing (NIOSH, 2017).

The location of the migrant farmworker's dwelling near fields or orchards can also be a major source of contamination for the worker and his or her family. "Take-home exposure" occurs when chemicals on clothes worn at work come into contact with farmworker children as parents embrace or carry their children (American Academy of Pediatrics, 2012). Organophosphate pesticide metabolites have been confirmed in farmworkers and their children.

The EPA Agricultural Worker Protection Standard (WPS) requires that farmworkers be given information about pesticide exposure prevention and safety (EPA, 2018). Due to the challenges of enforcing these regulations, however, migrant farmworkers may not receive this information, they may receive ineffectual training, or they may not understand the information. Also, migrant farmworkers may have preconceived beliefs about pesticides, such as that only weak workers are harmed by them.

The use of personal protection equipment (PPE) is recommended for those who handle pesticides, and the use of such equipment is part of the WPS training. Farmworkers may not have access to protective clothing or they may be unable to afford its purchase; alternatively, they may choose to disregard precautionary procedures and behaviors (such as wearing gloves) that affect their productivity. Although the WPS is in effect to minimize pesticide risk, migrant farmworker families remain at high risk for exposure. Lack of resources for monitoring pesticide exposure, culturally inappropriate educational methods, migrants' fear of reporting violations and being fired, and language differences are just a few barriers that hinder a safer pesticide environment for migrant farmworkers (Farmworker Justice, 2013).

Not all health professionals are educated to recognize and treat pesticide illness and therefore might attribute the farmworkers' symptoms and physical findings to other causes. See the How To box below for ways to recognize the signs and symptoms of acute pesticide exposure. For additional information, see the EPA *Recognition and Management of Pesticide Poisonings* manual (2013).

HOW TO Recognize the Signs and Symptoms of Pesticide Exposure

- Signs and symptoms of acute pesticide exposure vary according to the amount and length of time of exposure. The majority of body systems can be affected by pesticide exposure.
- Acute health effects of pesticide exposure include a wide range of symptoms, including headache, dizziness, confusion, irritability, twitching muscles, muscle weakness, seizures, respiratory symptoms (shortness of breath, difficulty breathing, and nasal and pharyngeal irritation), gastrointestinal symptoms (nausea, vomiting, diarrhea, and stomach cramps), skin rashes, eye or skin irritation, memory loss, flushing, hot sensations, difficulty with concentration, mood changes, and unconsciousness. Symptoms vary depending on whether the pesticide poisoning is mild or severe.
- Effects of chronic exposure are not entirely known but have been related to such illnesses as cancer, Parkinson disease, infertility or sterility, liver damage, and polyneuropathy and neurobehavioral problems.
- If symptoms of pesticide exposure are suspected, the nurse should develop a pesticide exposure history. A good example of an exposure form can be found at https://www.migrantclinician.org.

Data from Environmental Protection Agency (EPA): *Recognition and management of pesticide poisonings,* ed. 6, 2013: Roberts JR, Reigart JR. Available at http://npic.orst.edu.

Effects of chronic pesticide exposure are difficult to study and document, though some research findings point to health impacts related to prolonged or repeated exposure. Of particular concern is exposure of agricultural workers to the widely used insecticides classified as organophosphates (OPs), which can be absorbed through inhalation, ingestion, or skin contact. Research findings of the health impacts of exposure to these products include a wide range of neurological effects, some cancers, reproductive disorders related to endocrine disruption, and developmental disorders in children (Curtis & Sattler, 2018). In spite of these findings, policies regarding the use of these products continue to be under debate at the time of this writing.

COMMON HEALTH PROBLEMS

Migrant and seasonal farmworkers suffer from the same acute and chronic health problems as other populations in the United States. Factors related to their lifestyle and racial or ethnic group membership, however, place them at risk for certain **health disparities** compared with the general population and cause them to have more frequent and more severe health problems than the general population. Health center program data (NCFH, 2016), collected in 2016 from 165 Health Resources and Services Administration health centers serving this population, showed that hypertension, diabetes, otitis media, asthma, depression, and anxiety affected the greatest number of patients identified as agricultural workers.

MSFWs may not know that symptoms such as diarrhea or fever might indicate a more serious health problem, and they often do not seek early treatment. Lack of knowledge and, as discussed earlier, lack of access to health care services, can exacerbate treatable conditions. Undiagnosed health problems in this population such as sexually transmitted infections (STIs), cervical cancer, high blood glucose, high blood pressure, high serum cholesterol, anemia, and untreated dental problems lead to serious health problems such as heart disease, diabetes, and periodontal disease (Kresge Foundation, 2012). For children, many may experience the protective effects of the "healthy immigrant phenomenon" in infancy, though lack of access to health care services and other lifestyle factors later in childhood can lead to a higher incidence of problems such as infectious diseases, asthma, behavioral health issues, ear infections, and skin and dental problems (AAP, 2013). The lack of continuity of care and good record keeping often lead to the children being either over- or under-immunized (McLaurin & Liebman, 2012).

Women who work in agriculture experience reproductive health risks related to occupational health factors, as well as the lack of access to health care and health care information. As a result, farmworker women may experience work-related exposures and may not receive adequate prenatal care. Unfortunately, current data on migrant farmworker women and pregnancy outcomes are limited, although the lack of access to prenatal care for uninsured and undocumented women is a significant concern in the health care community (ACOG, 2015). Loss of Medicaid coverage for prenatal care for migrant women and lack of state coverage through the Children's Health Insurance Program (CHIP) in Nebraska resulted in late entry to prenatal care and an increase in pregnancy complications such as fetal abnormalities (Hopewell, 2011). Study findings have shown associations between pesticide exposures and adverse pregnancy outcomes such as low birth weight, intrauterine growth retardation (IUGR), preterm delivery, and stillbirth (ASRM, 2008). An incident that brought attention to the reproductive health risks of farmworker women occurred in 2004-2005 when four women who worked for the same company in the same fields in North Carolina and Florida during their pregnancies all experienced adverse outcomes. They gave birth within 8 weeks of each other to babies with congenital abnormalities (Calvert el al., 2007). The resulting investigation revealed numerous regulatory violations related to pesticide exposure of the women. Although it was not possible to establish a clear cause and effect relationship, this tragic outcome assisted with a heightened awareness of occupational health risk among those who care for farmworkers. See Box 34.1 for a description of the case management of a pregnant farmworker by MCN's Health Network.

Food insecurity is defined by the U.S. Department of Agriculture (2017a) as lack of access to "enough food for an active, healthy life." Ironically, access to adequate food and nutrition is a more prevalent problem for farmworkers than for the general U.S. population (Fuller, 2016). A variety of factors, including poverty, lack of transportation, and lack of access to a refrigerator and stove, contribute to food insecurity.

BOX 34.1 Case Management of a Pregnant Farmworker

MCN's Health Network is available to health care organizations to provide case management, referral, and record transfer services for patients who are likely to move during treatment. The following case illustrates how this program works for migrant women during pregnancy. Names and other details have been changed to protect patient privacy.

Xiomara was referred to Health Network in May of 2010 by a health department in a southeastern state that sent enrollment forms for this 21-year-old patient for the prenatal arm of Health Network. This referral set into motion a series of interactions that ensured that this young migrant woman would not fall through the cracks in the network of health care services for the underserved.

Once the enrollment paperwork was processed in MCN's Austin, Texas, office, the case was assigned to Gracie Castillo, one of four bilingual Health Network associates. Gracie proceeded to contact the patient, using the telephone numbers provided in the enrollment forms. The patient's sister answered the phone and was able to take a message asking the patient to return the call. Later that day the patient called back, and Gracie was able to establish a better understanding of her situation. Xiomara stated that this was her first pregnancy, she was at about three months, and she was staying temporarily at a motel. She mentioned that she was planning on moving—perhaps to Pennsylvania sometime during the summer—though she did not have an exact address at that point. She expressed concern about the cost of care involved with her pregnancy at her current location and had made an appointment at a different clinic. Gracie provided an overview of Health Network services and gave the patient a direct toll-free number to call in case immediate assistance was required.

The next step was to get medical records from the enrolling clinic. The health department had limited records, however, since they had only performed a pregnancy test and had then referred Xiomara elsewhere for prenatal care. Records were also requested from a secondary site where the patient had been seen. Xiomara called a few days later complaining that she had had some abdominal pain a few days earlier. She had gone to the clinic but was instructed to go to the emergency department since they only had an ob/gyn physician on site one day per week. She admitted that she had not gone because of concern about the cost of a hospital visit and was relieved that she was no longer having pain. Gracie was able to locate a hospital clinic in her area that was willing to work with her financial situation and arranged an appointment for Xiomara.

For two months the patient attended multiple appointments at the new location and touched base regularly with Health Network regarding her progress, and her pregnancy proceeded normally. She received appropriate lab work, an ultrasound, and also completed financial paperwork. Health Network obtained medical records from this site and included these in the patient's file.

When Gracie made a routine follow-up call to Xiomara about a month later, the patient did not answer her phone, despite numerous attempts and voicemails. It was not until three months later that the patient called Health Network reporting she had moved to another state and had recently gone to the emergency department there because of unbearable pain. She did not know her address in the new location and said she would call back when she knew exactly where she was staying. She mentioned that she would only be there for a couple of weeks. She called back with her address, and a clinic was found for her, her medical records were forwarded to this clinic, and an appointment was made. Health Network requested records and lab results for this visit a week after her appointment.

Another month passed when Xiomara did not answer her phone, but she finally returned a call in October, stating that she had just delivered a baby girl by cesarean section. She had returned to her original residence in the southeast and was concerned because of swelling, redness, and general discomfort around her surgical incision. She had attempted to make an appointment at the clinic, but the only one available was a week away. Gracie contacted the clinic to explain the situation and was able to get an appointment for the next day. Despite transportation difficulties and her husband's work demands, she was able to attend the visit and was given treatment. She recovered well and had a six-week postpartum visit, as Gracie had encouraged.

Typically Health Network considers a prenatal case to be completed after the postpartum visit takes place and all records are received. Xiomara provided an unusual opportunity for follow-up when she called Gracie four months after her baby's birth to express her appreciation for Health Network's involvement in her case. She confided that her relationship with her husband had dramatically changed after having her baby, and she was thrilled that she was no longer a victim of abuse.

According to protocol, this case was closed after being reviewed by MCN clinical staff. All notes for interactions with the patient and the various health care organizations involved in Xiomara's care are documented according to HIPAA standards. Through three moves, five health care organizations, and 43 contacts with Health Network, this patient's enrollment in Health Network reveals the impact of "bridge case management," not only through the mechanical services of scheduling appointments and transferring medical records, but also through the more personal avenue of direct communication with patients and their clinicians.

HIPAA, Health Insurance Portability and Accountability Act of 1996; *MCN,* Migrant Clinicians Network.
(Reprinted from Garay R, Kugel C: Pregnancy on the move. *Streamline* Canadian Medical Association Journal, 17(3):5, 2011. © Canadian Medical Association 2011.)

Specific Health Problems

Among the Latino population in the United States, the prevalence of diabetes is estimated to be three to five times greater than that of the general population, with higher rates of end-stage complications. Data specific to MSFWs are limited, and prevalence statistics for the Hispanic/Latino population are used as a proxy; the CDC (2017a) reported the incidence of diabetes in this population to be 8.4 per 1000 individuals, compared to 5.7 per 1000 for non-Hispanic whites. The lifestyle of migrant farmworkers makes it difficult to obtain proper nutrition, adhere to weight control measures, and procure continuity of health care and medication administration necessary for good diabetes control. The MCN Health Network assists providers with accessing information from farmworkers' previous providers who participated in the tracking program, thereby allowing for better continuity of care for diabetes (MCN, 2017b). Box 34.2 provides a brief description of an assessment with a diabetes focus for migrant farmworkers.

Disparities in both primary care and oral health services have been documented with the migrant farmworker population. Dental disease is one of the most common health problems for farmworkers of all ages. According to the CDC (2018a), Hispanic Americans experience higher rates of tooth decay and periodontal disease than do non-Hispanic whites. In an analysis of farmworkers who received care at federally funded health centers (Hu et al., 2016), it was found that 28.43 percent of MSFW patients were unable to get needed dental care, and 32.46 percent were delayed in getting needed dental care. Migrant children also have significantly lower rates of oral health treatment (NCFH, 2018a). Quandt et al. (2007) found

BOX 34.2 Example of Assessment With Migrant Farmworkers

The nurse, working with community partners and migrant camp gatekeepers, visits migrant camps to perform nutrition education (primary prevention) and to screen for diabetes (secondary prevention). If a high glucose level is obtained, the nurse refers the individual to a migrant health center or county health department clinic for a complete assessment. For those individuals in a given camp diagnosed with diabetes, the nurse plans and executes a culturally appropriate educational program on self-care for diabetes (tertiary prevention).

that 80 percent of farmworkers in North Carolina had not received dental care in the last year, and that the few who did receive care returned to Mexico for dental care. Many of the people surveyed had inadequate knowledge of oral health and lack of access to care (and the resources to pay). Funding for increasing access to dental care has been insufficient to meet the needs of this population. Without insurance or personal resources and low Medicaid reimbursement, private dentistry is usually not an option for the farmworker.

Behavioral health issues, including depression, anxiety, post-traumatic stress disorder (PTSD), and stress, are areas of concern for migrants and may be related to isolation, discrimination, trauma, economic hardship, legal status, poor living conditions, and weather conditions that interrupt their work. MSFWs identify themselves as stressed independently of how they rate their physical health (Carvajal et al., 2014). A survey of California farmworker households (O'Connor et al., 2015) found that 22 percent of respondents reported *nervios* (a term used by some Western Hemisphere Hispanics to refer to increased susceptibility to mental stress and symptoms of nervousness). A study in North Carolina by Pulgar et al. (2016) found that almost a third of the farmworker women in their survey reported significant symptoms of depression, markedly higher than in the overall U.S. population. Related factors cited include job conditions, household responsibilities, taking care of children, and poverty. Farmworkers, especially males, are reluctant to seek mental health care.

Female farmworkers, especially the undocumented, are a vulnerable population suffering harassment and sexual abuse (Fig. 34.2). According to a landmark report by Human Rights Watch (2012), harassment and sexual abuse are so common that female farmworkers see no escape from its occurrence and believe it is part of the job. The report identified sexually charged language, unwanted touching, stalking, and rape as common occurrences. Most victims do not report these abuses, often feeling powerless; however, many who have reported have not seen their perpetrators prosecuted (Yeung & Rubenstein, 2013). Recently, the U.S. Equal Employment Opportunity Commission filed lawsuits against employers in the Northwest as a means to address sexual harassment.

Similar to behavioral health issues, drug and alcohol use in migrant communities has been identified as a significant source (or result) of stress, without a clear picture of the scope of the problem in migrant farmworker communities. One study in North Carolina showed a wide variation in drinking patterns,

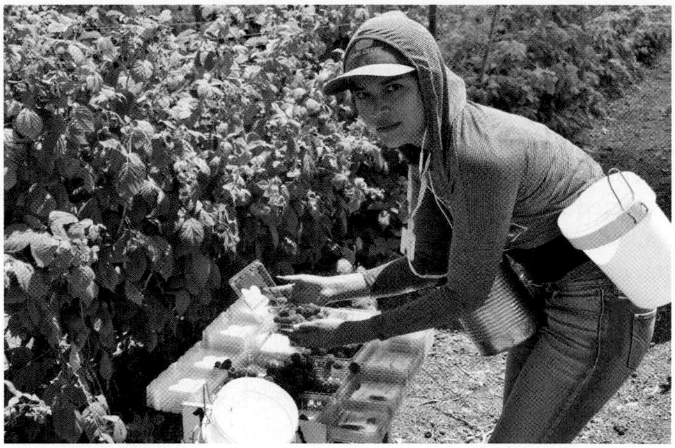

Fig. 34.2 Women working in agriculture face unique challenges, including sexual harassment and reproductive health risks. (David Litman/Shutterstock.com.)

with 26 percent of the farmworkers surveyed abstaining from drinking and 27 percent reporting heavy drinking (Grzywacz et al., 2007). Drinking alcohol poses safety hazards for farmworkers, such as accidents while driving and workplace injuries. Alcohol can also contribute to health problems, greater risk for human immunodeficiency virus (HIV) infection, violence in camps/home sites, domestic violence, and decreased funds for personal and family needs.

The incidence rate for tuberculosis is not known for migrant farmworkers; however, Oren et al. (2016) state that they are "among the highest-risk populations for latent TB infection in the United States." According to CDC statistics (2016), in 2015, Hispanics/Latinos accounted for 28 percent of the U.S. tuberculosis cases and of the TB cases among foreign-born people, Latinos represented 32 percent in 2015. Being born outside of the United States is a significant risk factor for TB; in 2016, foreign-born individuals had a rate of 14.7 per 100,000, or 14 times higher than among native-born individuals (CDC, 2017b). The majority of migrant farmworkers are foreign-born and Hispanic/Latino. MSFWs are thus at increased risk for TB because of higher rates in their countries of origin (Latin America, Haiti, and Southeast Asia), crowded housing, and malnutrition. Required long-term treatment is difficult to complete because of mobility, fear of deportation, language barriers, and lack of access to services. Incomplete treatment contributes to resistant TB (Tschampl et al., 2016). The MCN Health Network TB tracking program fosters continuity and monitoring of TB treatment as migrant farmworkers move to different work and home sites, reporting a treatment completion rate of 83.9 percent of patients enrolled from 2005 to 2013 (MCN, 2015a).

Accurate HIV data for migrant farmworkers is also difficult to obtain; however, in the absence of adequate population-based data on farmworkers, useful inferences may be drawn from statistics collected for Latinos in the United States, a group known to be disproportionately affected and infected by HIV. Latinos make up about 18 percent of the U.S. population, but in 2015, about 23 percent of all newly diagnosed cases in the United States were among Latinos. HIV/acquired immunodeficiency syndrome (AIDS) cases among Latinos increased by 2 percent from 2010 to 2014, according to the CDC (2018b). Risk factors for this population include lack of accurate knowledge, barriers to health care services, limited education, poverty, longer time in the United States, sharing needles for common medications such as vitamins and antibiotics, unprotected sexual activity, isolation and separation from families, available prostitution, migration across borders that results in the spread of HIV, and needle-sharing through amateur tattooing (NCFH, 2018b).

Although there is not a clear statistical picture of the health status of the MSFW population, available data do indicate that this population suffers from challenging health problems that are difficult to address. Since migrant and seasonal farmworkers experience the recognized health risk factors of poverty, stress, occupational exposures, discrimination, and poor access to care, it is clear that this is a highly vulnerable population. Nurses can play a vital role in addressing and changing this situation.

CHILDREN AND YOUTH

Migrant farmworker parents want a better future for their children. In fact, this strong desire is the catalyst for many farmworkers to leave their country of origin. These children often appear to the outsider as happy, outgoing, and inquisitive. They suffer, however, from an array of health problems, including malnutrition (vitamin A and iron deficiencies), infectious diseases (upper respiratory tract infection, gastroenteritis), dental caries (from prolonged bottle-feeding, bottle-propping, and limited access to fluoride and dental care), inadequate immunization status, pesticide exposure, injuries, overcrowding and poor housing conditions, and disruption of their social and school life, which, not surprisingly, lead to anxiety-related problems. A study of migrant farmworker children in Georgia from 2003 to 2011 found an elevated prevalence of obesity, high blood pressure, stunting, and anemia in older children (Nichols et al., 2014). Moving between states and/or being undocumented can affect migrant children's eligibility for Medicaid and the state Children's Health Insurance Program (CHIP). Children living with at least one undocumented parent experience worse health and less access to care and use of public assistance programs. Undocumented parents may be fearful of approaching health services even if their children are eligible for coverage (AAP, 2013).

Children may be separated from their farmworker parents for periods of time when parents leave for work away from the home site. Children experiencing their parents' stress with work, housing, and income when they accompany their parents can result in physical, behavioral, and emotional problems (Fig. 34.3). A survey done by Human Impact Partners (2013) found that, although 82 percent of children of undocumented immigrants in the United States are U.S. citizens themselves, the stress and fear of deportation of their patents had an impact on the mental health of the children. Twenty-nine percent of undocumented parents reported that their child felt afraid all or most of the time over the past month, compared to 12 percent for documented parents.

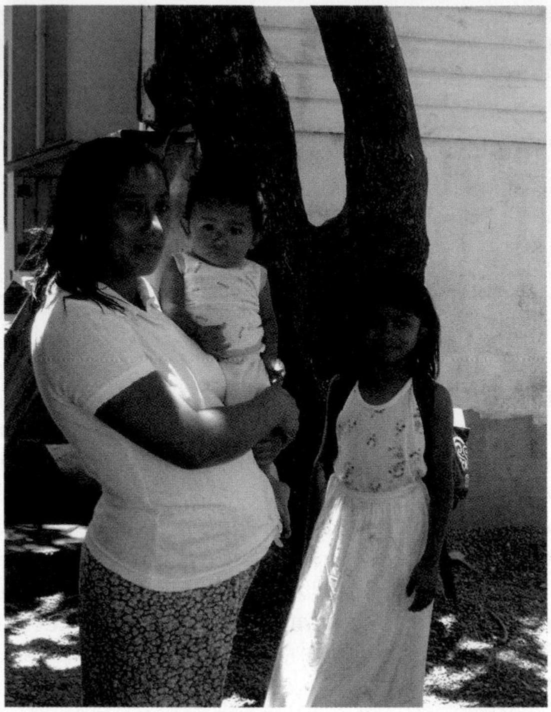

Fig. 34.3 Children of migrant farmworkers experience many hardships. They may have to help with the agricultural work or childcare while trying to maintain their schoolwork. (Diana Mary Jorgenson/Shutterstock .com.)

Since 2014, the United States has experienced surges of unaccompanied minors crossing into the country from Latin America in search of sanctuary and/or work, with over 60,000 arriving in 2014. Although these young people often intend to unite with family members in the United States, they bring with them an array of health concerns that arise from the hardships they have experienced in their travels (Robinson, 2015).

Children of migrant farmworkers may need to work for the family's economic survival. Migrant adolescents who work in agriculture warrant attention. Although the exact number of youth who work in the fields is not known, the National Institute for Occupational Safety and Health estimated that 266,000 youth less than age 20 were employed on U.S. farms in 2014 (NIOSH, 2014). Some adolescents accompany their parents to work or come with others such as an uncle; however, many adolescents migrate alone. Health care providers may believe that they are prohibited from caring for minor unaccompanied youth; however, they should be aware of their state's laws on minors' consent to care that could increase access to care for these youth.

Federal child labor laws have multiple exclusions for agricultural settings. The Fair Labor Standards Act (FLSA) includes restrictions based on age and hours worked. Children younger than 12 years can work on a farm with fewer than seven full-time workers. Children as young as 12 years old can work on a farm if they have parental permission or if their parent is also working on the farm. Children ages 14 or 15 may work in non-hazardous positions in agriculture but not during school hours. Youths age 16 and older may work in any farm job at any time, including performing hazardous work with no restrictions on hours. Some additional protection is provided to children by the majority of states, such as limiting the number of hours per day and week a child can work (U.S. Department of Labor [USDOL], 2016b).

Federal law does not protect children from overworking or by limiting the hours they work outside of school. Therefore, children may work until late in the evenings or very early in the mornings every day of the week if not protected by state law or if inadequately monitored. Personal communication with Marie Napolitano and adolescent farmworkers in Oregon revealed that they were frequently too tired after working to do homework and to attend classes. They may leave school before the end of the term to travel with their families and arrive late to start school in the fall. Child farmworkers may attend three to five different schools each year as they migrate from one farm to another, and these frequent changes in schools and constant fatigue are obvious obstacles to academic success.

Availability of childcare services is a concern for farmworker parents (Liebman et al., 2017). Young children of migrant farmworkers stay home to care for younger siblings and other children. The Migrant Head Start Program is a safe, healthy, and educational option for children six weeks to five years old, though inadequate funding means there are not enough services in all locations for migrant children. The Migrant Education Program is a state- and nationally sponsored summer school program for farmworkers' children more than five years of age. This program is also not available to all eligible migrant youth, especially those living in isolated rural areas.

CULTURAL CONSIDERATIONS IN MIGRANT HEALTH CARE

To provide culturally effective care to migrant farmworkers, nurses need to be knowledgeable about the cultural backgrounds of these individuals. Because the majority of migrant farmworkers are of Mexican descent, this section focuses on Mexican culture. Although certain health beliefs and practices have been identified with the Mexican culture, the nurse must remember that beliefs and practices differ among countries as well as regions and localities of a country, and among individuals. Many of the aspects of Mexican culture described here are similar to Central American countries, though it is a multicultural region and the cultural backgrounds of Mexican and Central American immigrants vary depending on their place of origin and other factors. There are many indigenous groups in the region that speak their own group dialect and may not speak Spanish. Literacy skills may also be limited (36 percent of the NAWS respondents reported attaining a sixth grade education or less). Immigrants who are less educated, have fewer economic resources, and are from rural areas tend to possess more **traditional beliefs and practices** that are unique to their cultural background.

NURSE-CLIENT RELATIONSHIP

The nurse is considered an authority figure in the Latino culture and should show respect (*respeto*) to the individual, be able to relate to the individual on a personal level (*personalismo*), and maintain the individual's dignity (*dignidad*). Mexican individuals prefer polite, non-confrontational relationships with others (*simpatía*). At times, because of *simpatía*, individuals and families may appear to understand what is being said to them (by nodding their heads) when in actuality they do not understand. The nurse should take measures to validate understanding in these situations. The Mexican individual expects to converse about personal matters for the first few minutes of an encounter. They expect the nurse not to appear rushed and to be a good listener. Humor is appreciated, and touching as a caring gesture is seen as a positive behavior. In working with Latino migrant workers, learning some key Spanish words and phrases is an indication of a willingness to connect.

Mexican clients may not seek care with health professionals first. Instead they may consult with trusted and knowledgeable individuals in their family or community (the popular arena of care) or with folk healers (the traditional arena of care). Examples of the members of the popular arena include the *señora*, or wise, older woman living in the community; one's grandmother (*la abuela*); and the local parish priest.

Health Values

Family, in general, is a critical component of a Mexican individual's health care and social support system. In general, the female in the household is considered to be the caretaker, whereas the male is considered to be the major decision maker. Mexican women in certain families, however, have significant influence over most domestic matters, including health decisions. Grandmothers and sisters are highly significant to the wife (female) in the immediate family. They provide advice, care, and support. Not all Mexican immigrants have extended families in the United States. If not present, communication may be maintained with family in Mexico by telephone, though an effective support system for these individuals may be inadequate.

Love of their children, rather than concern for their own health, may encourage MSFW parents to adopt healthier lifestyles. An example is when the parents of a child with asthma choose to stop smoking. In Oregon, when asked if they protected themselves from pesticide exposure, Mexican migrant parents responded negatively in general. They were willing to change their behaviors, however, if their children would be protected from pesticides (Napolitano et al., 2002).

In the experience of the authors, the Mexican client may be more willing to follow the advice of another Mexican individual with a similar health problem rather than the advice of the health professional. For example, Mexican women with type 2 diabetes were more willing to ask and adopt the practices of others with diabetes than follow the redundant advice of physicians to take their medications, watch their diet, and exercise. One woman, who was unable to differentiate the symptoms of hyperglycemia and hypoglycemia, would drink a bottle of grape juice when she felt her "sugar high," as was recommended by her neighbor.

Although the majority of Mexican immigrants may identify themselves as Catholics, many Mexican individuals belong to other religious groups. The individual's religion may influence his or her health practices such as birth control; however, the nurse cannot assume, for example, that a Catholic will not use some method of contraception. The Focus on Quality and Safety Education for Nurses box provides guidelines for client-centered care.

QSEN FOCUS ON QUALITY AND SAFETY EDUCATION FOR NURSES

Targeted Competency: Patient-Centered Care

Recognize the client or designee as the source of control and full partner in providing compassionate and coordinated care based on respect for patient's preferences, values, and needs.

Important aspects of patient-centered interventions include the following:

- **Knowledge:** Discuss principles of effective communication.
- **Skills:** Assess own level of communication skill in encounters with patients and families.
- **Attitudes:** Value continuous improvement of own communication and conflict resolution skills.

Patient-Centered Care Question

To provide patient-centered care, it is important not only to be able to communicate with the person(s) but also to understand the cultural perspectives that influence their health care practices. If you are caring for clients who live in migrant farmworker camps and you observe that they are allowing their children to work several hours both before and after they go to school, how would you approach the situation?

- Would you begin by speaking with the parents?
- Would you speak with the person who owns or manages the farm?
- What would your approach be to those with whom you speak?
- At what point would you consider involving community resources? If you choose this route, what resources would you consider?

Prepared by Gail Armstrong, PhD, DNP, ACNS-BC, CNE, Associate Professor, University of Colorado Denver College of Nursing, based on QSEN Institute: *QSEN competencies*, 2018. Available at http://qsen.org.

Health Beliefs and Practices

In the Mexican culture, good health may be considered a gift from God. Another common perception of health is that a healthy person is one who can continue to work and maintain one's daily activities independent of symptoms or diagnosed diseases. The nurse should understand that a Mexican individual may not return for a clinic appointment because the client felt better or was capable of working that day. Likewise, Mexican immigrants may think illness is a punishment from God and may cite this belief as a rationale for why therapies have not cured them. This more commonly occurs with chronic illnesses.

There are four more common folk illnesses that a nurse may encounter with the Mexican client. These are *mal de ojo* (evil eye), *susto* (fright), *empacho* (indigestion), and *caída de mollera* (fallen fontanelle). Symptoms and treatments may vary depending on the individual's or family's origin in Mexico, and the client may be quite willing to discuss these concerns. Other cultural beliefs related to hot-cold balance, pregnancy, and postpartum behaviors (*cuarentena*) have been documented. When experiencing a folk illness, the traditional Mexican individual would prefer to seek care with a folk healer if possible. The more common healers are the *curanderos, herbalistas,* and *espiritualistas.* The most commonly used herbs are chamomile (*manzanilla*), peppermint (*yerba buena*), aloe vera, cactus (*nopales*), and wormseed or "Mexican tea" (*epazote*). Questioning the client about traditional healing practices related to a current complaint can be a helpful part of an assessment.

HEALTH PROMOTION AND ILLNESS PREVENTION

The same principles of health promotion and illness prevention apply to migrant farmworkers as to other U.S. populations. Health promotion and disease prevention may be difficult concepts for migrant workers to embrace, however, because of beliefs regarding disease causality, irregular and episodic contact with the health care system, and lower educational levels.

Health promotion begins by asking MSFW families which health topics would be of interest to them and whether they are familiar with the available resources to improve their health. Several migrant health programs have recruited current or former migrant workers to serve as outreach workers or community health workers (often referred to as *promotores* or *promotoras*) to assist in outreach and health education of the workers. Nurses can be part of the planning and training of health workers for outreach and educational programs. Evaluation to determine successful outreach educational methods can be undertaken by nurses. Such activities demonstrate the core competencies related to the domain of community dimensions of practice skills for public health nursing (Quad Council Coalition [QCC], 2018). Relevant skills include recognizing community relationships affecting health, collaborating with community partners to promote the health of the population, using group processes to advance community involvement, identifying community assets and resources, and promoting public health programs. The Linking Content to Practice box later in the chapter includes additional discussion of the Quad Council Domains of Public Health Nursing.

ROLE OF THE NURSE

The health of the MSFW population warrants a variety of actions by nurses. Working with this population can be challenging. Insufficient resources, short-term stays in a community, barriers placed by growers, discrimination, and unenforced legislation are just some of the obstacles that confront the nurse. Nurses, however, can make a difference in the health of MSFWs and their families.

In providing health care services, nurses can use primary, secondary, and tertiary prevention actions to help improve the health of migrant farmworkers, as outlined in the Levels of Prevention box. Primary prevention activities include education for the prevention of infectious diseases such as HIV, measures to reduce pesticide exposure, and immunizations in childhood and adulthood. Secondary prevention activities include screening for pesticide exposure, TB skin testing, diabetes screening and monitoring activities, and diagnostic testing done for prenatal care. Tertiary prevention includes rehabilitation for musculoskeletal injury, especially low back pain, and treatments for lead poisoning and anemia.

LEVELS OF PREVENTION

Migrant and Farmworker Health Issues

Primary Prevention

Teach migrant workers how to reduce exposure to pesticides.

Secondary Prevention

Conduct screening for diabetes in adult farmworkers and for anemia in children in camps.

Tertiary Prevention

Educate migrant families regarding appropriate nutrition for an adult with diabetes or a child with anemia.

In this chapter, an overview of the lifestyle and health status of the MSFW population is presented. The public health nurse plays an important role in improving the health of this population. The Linking Content to Practice box reviews the core competencies for public health nursing relevant to working with MSFWs.

LINKING CONTENT TO PRACTICE

Core competencies within five of the Quad Council Coalition Domains of Public Health Nursing guide the nurse in working with migrant farmworkers. These domains are as follows: (1) Assessment/Analytic Skills, which include identifying, describing, and using data obtained from working with migrant individuals, families, and groups; (2) Policy Development/Program Planning Skills, which are directed toward knowing and applying policies, laws, and regulations toward the delivery of health programs and the protection of the migrant population; (3) Communication Skills, which are used to identify health literacy of the migrant farmworker and to communicate in a linguistic and culturally appropriate style; (4) Cultural Competency Skills, which allow the nurse to function in a culturally appropriate manner and to assist the public health organization to become more culturally competent when serving migrant farmworker families; and (5) Community Dimension of Practice Skills, which include use of community resources, establishing linkages between community partners to eliminate redundancy and better serve the migrant population, and maintaining partnerships with migrant leaders and agencies serving this population (QCC, 2018).

Nurses can screen and monitor migrant farmworkers' health. Diseases such as TB, diabetes, and hypertension are often missed in a mobile population without regular access to primary care services. Nurses can create screening programs in migrant camps and other farmworker housing. When problems are identified and treated, nurses can refer for further care and then monitor the success of medication regimens, preventive measures, and follow-up with the health care system. The nurse can provide culturally specific health promotion and disease prevention programs and materials, as well as information about referral sources when needed. The nurse can teach health promotion strategies to lay health promoters who then will educate the migrant community. The Evidence-Based Practice box describes an approach to hypertension screening by community health workers.

EVIDENCE-BASED PRACTICE

The U.S. Preventive Services Task Force (USPSTF) guidelines, as of 2015, recommend screening for high blood pressure in adults aged 18 years or older (*A* recommendation). The USPSTF recommends obtaining measurements outside of the clinical setting for diagnostic confirmation before starting treatment (Siu, 2015). As noted earlier, Latino populations experience disparities in the occurrence of hypertension and other chronic illnesses. With the additional risk factors of mobility, lack of access to care, and lack of continuity of care, the MSFW population should be a high priority for identifying and treating high blood pressure.

Research has demonstrated the value and effectiveness of community health workers in educating and motivating patients. Thompson et al. (2015) demonstrated that trained community health workers were able to assess the risk of MSFWs for diabetes and hypertension comparably to a registered nurse.

Nurse Use

Nurses have the opportunity to be involved in education, screening, and management services related to hypertension for migrant farmworkers. These services can be directed at individuals in a health care setting, in camps or other housing settings, or to groups in community settings. Additionally, nurses can design and support training for community health workers to perform education and screening for cardiovascular disease risk, since this approach has been shown to be effective in addressing the cultural context of farmworkers' knowledge and beliefs related to the benefits of identifying and treating high blood pressure.

Data from Siu AL: Screening for high blood pressure in adults: U.S. Preventive Services Task Force Recommendation statement. *Ann Intern Med* 163:778–786, 2015; Thompson RH, Snyder AE, Burt DR, et al.: Risk screening for cardiovascular disease and diabetes in Latino migrant farmworkers: a role for the community health worker. *J Community Health* 40:131–137, 2015.

Opportunities also exist for nurses to lead or participate in evaluation of the effectiveness of existing programs dedicated to all levels of prevention and treatment for farmworkers. The Clinical Decision-Making Activities at the end of the chapter explore nurses' roles in various health care delivery settings.

The health status of all people is a function of their ecology, or all that "touches" them. The nurse keeps a finger on the pulse of the community by remaining active with political and social issues that involve the client. The nurse can be a catalyst for change to assess farmworker needs continually, to direct efforts to obtain needed health care services, and to evaluate the success of those efforts. Acting as a community educator knowledgeable about how to obtain the latest information and resources, the nurse can work to assess the infrastructure and needs of the community. Follow-up on assessments by the nurse is critical. For example, the needs assessment might indicate inadequate child and adult immunizations in the migrant population, which may best be provided in the fields, camps, and schools. The nurse may instigate and lead in the creation of an immunization tracking system to share information with other counties and states as the farmworkers migrate. Outcome measures relevant to care of MSFWs are listed in the *Healthy People 2020* box.

HEALTHY PEOPLE 2020

Selected Objectives for Migrant Farmworker Populations

This box lists selected *Healthy People 2020* objectives that relate to health promotion and disease prevention in migrant farmworkers. They were selected on the basis of occupational, lifestyle, and socioeconomic factors that place migrant farmworkers and their families at unique risk for suboptimal health.

Environmental Health
- **EH-10:** Reduce pesticide exposures that result in visits to a health care facility.
- **EH-19:** Reduce the proportion of occupied housing units that have moderate or severe physical problems.

Immunization and Infectious Diseases
- **IID-29:** Reduce tuberculosis.
- **IID-30:** Increase treatment completion rate for all tuberculosis patients who are eligible to complete therapy.

Maternal, Infant, and Child Health
- **MICH-10:** Increase the proportion of pregnant women who receive early and adequate prenatal care.

Occupational Safety and Health
- **OSH-2:** Reduce nonfatal work-related injuries.
- **OSH-8:** Reduce occupational skin diseases or disorders among full-time workers.

Data from U.S. Department of Health and Human Services: *Healthy People 2020*, 2018. Available at https://www.healthypeople.gov.

Nurses can also be social and political advocates for the MSFW population. Educating communities about these individuals, collecting necessary data on their lives and health, and communicating with legislators and other policy makers at local, state, and national levels are needed actions that nurses are prepared to undertake. Migrant farmworkers have been a persistently vulnerable population, as discussed throughout this chapter, in spite of the contributions they make to our economy and our food supply. At the time of this writing, however, their status in the United States is particularly precarious due to the potent anti-immigrant climate both politically and socially. Nurses working with farmworkers can serve as a supportive and credible influence on decision makers. Box 34.3 lists selected resources for the nurse working with MSFWs.

BOX 34.3 Resources for the Nurse Working With Migrant Farmworkers

Film
- Edward R. Murrow's *Harvest of Shame:* Access at http://billmoyers.com/2013/07/19/watch-edward-r-murrows-harvest-of-shame.

Written/Online Materials
- Migrant Clinicians Network (MCN) Toolbox and Resource database: This comprehensive online database (https://www.migrantclinician.org) includes downloadable resources as well as links to a wide variety of primary care issues related to migrant farmworkers, links to other organizations, client education tools, clinical guidelines, MCN program materials, research guidelines, and others.
- National Center for Farmworker Health: Factsheets on Migrant Farmworkers http://www.ncfh.org.

Organizations
- Migrant Clinicians Network, Inc.
PO Box 164285
Austin, TX 78716
(512) 327-2017
http://www.migrantclinician.org
- National Center for Farmworker Health
1770 FM 967
Buda, TX 78610
512-312-2700
http://www.ncfh.org
- Farmworker Justice, Inc.
1126 16th St. NW, Suite LL-101
Washington, DC 20036
(202) 293-5420
http://www.farmworkerjustice.org
- Health Outreach Partners
1970 Broadway, Ste. 200
Oakland, CA 94612
510-268-0091
https://outreach-partners.org

PRACTICE APPLICATION

Maricela is 15 years old, and has accompanied her uncle and male cousin to the camp to cook and clean the cabin for them. She also works in the fields picking crops. Maricela has traveled the East Coast for six months with her uncle and cousin. Maricela is originally from Mexico, and Florida is her home base. One evening after finishing her work, Maricela asks to speak with Joan Lewis, the nurse practitioner whose medical van is parked outside the migrant camp where Maricela lives. She tells the nurse that her stomach has been hurting for a while and asks Ms. Lewis for something to stop the pain. While assessing the complaint, Ms. Lewis asks Maricela what she believes has caused the pain. Maricela is very quiet and barely responds to the nurse. She does not make eye contact with Ms. Lewis. Maricela states that she probably ate something hot that upset her stomach. She seems to be in a great hurry and says she does not want her uncle to know she stopped by the van because he would be angry. Ms. Lewis, who speaks fluent Spanish, completes her history, but Maricela does not permit the nurse to examine her abdomen. Maricela also will not talk about her last menstrual period. She asks for medicine again and gets up to leave.

A. What do you see as the important points regarding Maricela's situation?

B. What are cultural considerations that may impact the assessment of Maricela's complaint?

C. What could be the possible causes for Maricela's stomach pain? What is your rationale for each cause?

Answers can be found on the Evolve website.

KEY POINTS

- A migrant farmworker is a laborer whose principal employment involves moving from a home base to another location to plant or harvest agricultural products and lives in temporary housing. Migrant farmworkers may be single or may travel with family members.
- An estimated one to three million migrant farmworkers are in the United States. These numbers are controversial because of the inconsistency in defining farmworkers and limitations in obtaining data.
- Migrant farmworkers are considered a vulnerable population because of their lifestyle and lack of resources.
- Health problems of migrant farmworkers are linked to their work and housing environments, limited access to health services and education, and lack of economic opportunities.
- Migrant farmworkers are faced with uncertainty regarding work and housing, inadequate wages, unsafe working conditions, and lack of enforcement regarding legislation for field sanitation and safety regulations.
- Farmworkers are exposed not only to immediate risk of pesticide exposure in the fields, but also to unknown long-term effects of chronic exposure to pesticides.
- When harvesting is completed, the farmworker becomes simultaneously homeless and unemployed. Forced migration to find employment leaves little time or energy to seek out and improve living standards.
- Children of migrant farmworkers may need to work for the family's economic survival. They are most affected by the disruptive and challenging lifestyle.

CLINICAL DECISION-MAKING ACTIVITIES

1. Interview rural community leaders regarding migrant farmworkers in your area. What do business owners, teachers, clergy, politicians, and other health professionals say about this population? Can you identify misinformation or lack of information on their parts?
2. Outreach workers are personnel generally hired by an agency, such as a health department or health center, to provide services such as education to migrant persons. Lay health promoters, often former farmworkers themselves, also provide community-based education. Find out if these roles exist in your community. Interview these individuals or accompany them in their work. Compare and contrast their roles. How are they complementary? How do they overlap? How can they work together to maximize health? How are their approaches to education different (e.g., does one use a protocol or template, whereas the other uses popular education techniques)? How does the outreach worker role and the lay health promoter role compare with the nursing role? How can the nurse work with the outreach worker and the lay health promoter?
3. Find an agency that visits migrant farmworkers in their housing. Ask to accompany them on subsequent visits. What is the condition of the housing? Are there deficits that could impact the health of the inhabitants?
4. Determine eligibility for Medicaid and Aid to Families with Dependent Children services in your state. You may consult the county health department and the state health department. Do migrant workers in your state qualify for these programs?
5. Design a temporary clinic to provide health care to migrant workers in your area during crop season. What services would you provide? What hours would you operate? How would you staff the clinic? Where would you get funds?
6. Below are a few settings and RN-delivered services for migrant clients. Can you propose others?
   - A. Health department (generally state and/or county funded)—Nurses monitor communicable diseases and provide treatments for outbreaks such as TB and pertussis.
   - B. Migrant camps (generally funded through migrant clinics or health departments)—Nurses assess and triage, screen for disease, dispense medications under protocol, provide education, interview families, and coordinate care in conjunction with health department nurses.
   - C. Migrant clinics (federally funded health centers)—Nurses work with clinics' primary care providers, lead prenatal and diabetes programs (both classes and home visits), educate regarding illnesses, and visit migrant camps to provide services or follow-up on clinic care.

ADDITIONAL RESOURCES

EVOLVE WEBSITE

http://evolve.elsevier.com/Stanhope/community/

- Answers to Practice Application
- Case Study
- Glossary
- Review Questions

REFERENCES

American Academy of Pediatrics (AAP): Policy statement: pesticide exposure in children, *Pediatrics* 130(6):1–7, 2012.

American Academy of Pediatrics (AAP): *Policy statement: providing care for immigrant, migrant, and border children*, 2013. Retrieved from http://pediatrics.aappublications.org.

American College of Obstetricians and Gynecologists (ACOG): Health care for unauthorized immigrants. Committee Opinion No. 627, *Obstet Gynecol* 125:755–759, 2015.

American Society for Reproductive Medicine (ASRM): Proceedings of the summit on environmental challenges to reproductive health and fertility: executive summary, *Fertil Steril* 89: e1–e20, 2008.

Arcury TA, Weir M, Chen H, et al.: Migrant farmworker housing regulation violations in North Carolina, *Am J Ind Med* 55: 191–204, 2012.

California Institute for Rural Studies, Villarejo D, Lighthall D, Williams D III, et al.: *Suffering in silence: a report on the health of California's agricultural workers*, Davis, CA, 2000, California Institute for Rural Studies, pp 1–37.

California Institute for Rural Studies, Ayala M, Clarke M, Kambara K, et al.: *In their own words: farmworker access to health care in four California regions*, Davis, CA, 2001, California Institute for Rural Studies.

Calvert GM, Alarcon WA, Chelminski A, et al.: Case report: three farmworkers who gave birth to infants with birth defects closely grouped in time and place—Florida and North Carolina, 2004–2005, *Environ Health Perspect* 115(5):787–791, 2007.

Carroll D: *Demographic and employment characteristics of California's crop labor force: findings from the national agricultural workers survey 1989–2014* [presentation to the California Agriculture: Water, Labor, and Immigration Conference, U.C. Davis Law School, April 15, 2016]. Retrieved from https://www.doleta.gov.

Carvajal SC, Kibor C, Mcclelland DJ, et al.: Stress and sociocultural factors related to health status among U.S.–Mexico border farmworkers, *J Immigrant Minority Health* 16:1176–1182, 2014.

Centers for Disease Control and Prevention (CDC): *Disparities in oral health*, 2018a. Retrieved from http://www.cdc.gov.

Centers for Disease Control and Prevention (CDC): Heat illness and death among workers—United States, 2012-2013, *MMWR Morb Mortal Wkly Rep* 63(31):661–665, 2014.

Centers for Disease Control and Prevention (CDC): *HIV among hispanics/latinos*, 2018b. Retrieved from https://www.cdc.gov.

Centers for Disease Control and Prevention (CDC): *National diabetes statistics report, 2017; estimates of diabetes and its burden in the United States*, 2017a. Retrieved from https://www.cdc.gov.

Centers for Disease Control and Prevention (CDC): *Trends in tuberculosis, 2016*, 2017b. Retrieved from https://www.cdc.gov.

Centers for Disease Control and Prevention (CDC): *Tuberculosis in hispanics/latinos*, 2016. Retrieved from https://www.cdc.gov.

Curtis AC, Sattler B: Organophosphate insecticide exposure: a clinical consideration of chlorpyrifos regulation, *JAANP* 30: 299–304, 2018.

Environmental Protection Agency (EPA): *Agricultural Worker Protection Standard (WPS)*, 2018. Retrieved from https://www.epa.gov.

Environmental Protection Agency (EPA), Roberts JR, Reigart JR: *Recognition and management of pesticide poisonings*, ed 6, 2013. Retrieved from http://npic.orst.edu.

Farmworker Justice: *Exposed and ignored: how pesticides are endangering our nation's farmworkers*, 2013. Retrieved from https://www.farmworkerjustice.org.

Farmworker Justice: *H2-A Guestworker program*, 2018. Retrieved from https://www.farmworkerjustice.org.

Farmworker Justice: *U.S. Labor law for farmworkers*, 2014a. Retrieved from https://www.farmworkerjustice.org.

Farmworker Justice: *Issue brief: farmworker housing quality and health*, 2014b. Retrieved from https://www.farmworkerjustice.org.

Fuller T: In a California Valley, Healthy Food Everywhere but on the Table, *New York Times* 2016. Retrieved from https://www.nytimes.com.

Garay R, Kugel C: Pregnancy on the move, *Streamline* 17(3):5, 2011.

Grzywacz J, Quandt SA, Isom S, et al.: Alcohol use among immigrant Latino farmworkers in North Carolina, *Am J Ind Med* 50:617–625, 2007.

Health Resources and Services Administration (HRSA): *2016 National health center data: national migrant health centers program grantee data*, 2017. Retrieved from https://bphc.hrsa.gov.

Hopewell J: Access to prenatal care: the case of Nebraska, *Streamline* 17:2–5, 2011.

Hu R, Shi L, Lee DC, Haile GP: Access to and disparities in care among migrant and seasonal farm workers (MSFWs) at U.S. health centers, *J Health Care Poor Underserved* 27(3):1484–1502, 2016.

Human Impact Partners: *Family unity, family health*, 2013. Retrieved from https://www.familyunityfamilyhealth.org.

Human Rights Watch: *Cultivating fear: the vulnerability of immigrant farmworkers in the U.S. to sexual violence and sexual harassment*, 2012. Retrieved from https://www.hrw.org.

Kresge Foundation, Villarejo D: *Health related inequities among hired farm workers and the resurgence of labor-intensive agriculture*, 2012. Retrieved from http://www.cirsinc.org.

Kugel C, Zuroweste EL: The state of health care services for mobile poor populations: history, current status, and future challenges, *J Health Care Poor Underserved* 21:421–429, 2010.

Liebman AK, Simmons J, Salzwedel M, Tovar-Aguilar A, Lee BC: Caring for children while working in agriculture—the perspective of farmworker parents, *J Agromedicine* 22:406–415, 2017.

Liebman AK, Wiggins MF, Fraser C, Levin J, Sidebottom J, Arcury TA: Occupational health policy and immigrant workers in the agriculture, forestry, and fishing sector, *Am J Ind Med* 56(8): 975–984, 2013.

McLaurin JA, Liebman AK: Unique agricultural safety and health issues of migrant and immigrant children, *J Agromedicine* 17:186–196, 2012.

Migrant Clinicians Network (MCN): *Health network*, 2017b. Retrieved from https://www.migrantclinician.org.

Migrant Clinicians Network: A stronger worker protection standard is now in effect. What does it mean for workers? *Streamline* 22:4, 2017a.

Migrant Clinicians Network (MCN): *Updating statistics on TB patients: Q&A with Dr. Ed Zuroweste*, 2015. Retrieved from https://www.migrantclinician.org.

Migrant Clinicians Network (MCN), Farmworker Justice (FJ): *A Guide to workers' compensation for clinicians serving agricultural workers*, 2015. Retrieved from https://www.migrantclinician.org.

Moyce SC, Schenker M: Migrant workers and their occupational health and safety, *Annu Rev Public Health* 39:351–365, 2018.

Napolitano M, Philips J, Beltran M, Philips J, Bryan C, McCauley L: *Un lugar seguro para sus ninos*: development and evaluation of a pesticide education video, *J Immigr Health* 4:35–45, 2002.

National Center for Farmworker Health (NCFH): *Oral health factsheet*, 2018a. Retrieved from http://www.ncfh.org.

National Center for Farmworker Health (NCFH): *HIV/AIDS agricultural worker factsheet*, 2018b. Retrieved from http://www.ncfh.org.

National Center for Farmworker Health (NCFH): *A profile of migrant health: an analysis of the uniform data system,* 2016. Retrieved from http://www.ncfh.org.

National Human Trafficking Hotline: *Labor trafficking victim outreach card,* 2014. Retrieved from https://humantrafficking hotline.org.

National Institute for Occupational Safety and Health (NIOSH): *National estimates of all youth (<20 years) on U.S. farms by type of youth and type of farm,* 2014. Retrieved from https://www .cdc.gov.

National Institute for Occupational Safety and Health (NIOSH): *Pesticide illness & injury surveillance,* 2017. Retrieved from https:// www.cdc.gov.

Nichols M, Stein A, Wold J: Health status of children of migrant farmworkers: farm worker family health program, Moultrie, Georgia, *Am J Public Health* 104:365–370, 2014.

O'Connor K, Stoecklin-Marois M, Schenker MB: Examining *nervios* among immigrant male farmworkers in the MICASA study: sociodemographics, housing conditions and psychosocial factors, *J Immigrant Minority Health* 17:198–207, 2015.

Oren E, Fiero MH, Barrett E, Anderson B, Nuñez M, Gonzalez-Salazar F: Detection of latent tuberculosis infection among migrant farmworkers along the U.S.-Mexico border, *BMC Infectious Diseases* 16:630, 2016.

Polaris Project: *Labor trafficking,* 2018. Retrieved from https:// polarisproject.org.

Pulgar CA, Trejo G, Suerken C, et al.: Economic hardship and depression among women in latino farmworker families, *J Immigr Minor Health* 18, 497–504, 2016.

QSEN Institute: *QSEN competencies,* 2018. Retrieved from http:// qsen.org.

Quad Council Coalition (QCC) of Public Health Nursing Organizations: *Community/public health nursing competencies,* 2018. Retrieved from http://www.quadcouncilphn.org.

Quandt SA, Hiott AE, Grzywacz JG, et al.: Oral health and quality of life of migrant and seasonal farmworkers in the U.S. community/ migrant health centers, *J Agric Saf Health* 13:45–55, 2007.

Quandt SA, Kucera KL, Haynes C, et al.: Occupational health outcomes for workers in the agriculture, forestry and fishing sector: implications for immigrant workers in the southeastern U.S., 2013, *Am J Ind Med* 56(8):940–959.

Richards TA: Health implications of human trafficking, *Nurs Womens Health* 18:155–162, 2014.

Robinson LK: Arrived: The crisis of unaccompanied children at our southern border, *Pediatrics* 135:205–207, 2015.

Siu AL: Screening for High Blood Pressure in Adults: U.S. Preventive services task force recommendation statement, *Ann Intern Med* 163:778–786, 2015.

Thompson RH, Snyder AE, Burt DR, et al.: Risk screening for cardiovascular disease and diabetes in latino migrant farmworkers: a role for the community health worker, *J Community Health* 40:131–137, 2015.

Tschampl CA, Garnick DW, Zuroweste E, Razavi M, Shepard DS: Use of transnational services to prevent treatment interruption in tuberculosis-infected persons who leave the United States, *Emerging Infect Dis* 22(3):417–425, 2016.

U.S. Bureau of Labor Statistics: *2016 Survey of occupational injuries & illnesses,* 2017. Retrieved from https://www.bls.gov.

U.S. Department of Agriculture (USDA): *Food security in the U.S.,* 2017a. Retrieved from https://www.ers.usda.gov.

U.S. Department of Agriculture (USDA): *National agricultural statistics service: farm labor,* 2017. Retrieved from http://usda .mannlib.cornell.edu.

U.S. Department of Health and Human Services: *Healthy people 2020,* 2018. Retrieved from https://www.healthypeople.gov.

U.S. Department of Labor (DOL): *Findings from the National Agricultural Workers Survey (NAWS) 2013–2014,* 2016a. Retrieved from https://www.doleta.gov.

U.S. Department of Labor (DOL): *Child labor bulletin 102: child labor requirements in agricultural occupations under the fair labor standards act,* 2016b. Retrieved from https://www .dol.gov.

U.S. Department of Labor (DOL): *Fact sheet #51: field sanitation standards under the occupational safety and health act,* 2008. Retrieved from http://www.dol.gov.

Urban Institute, Owens, C, Dank, M, Breaux, J, et al.: *Understanding the organization, operation, and victimization process of labor trafficking in the United States,* 2014. Retrieved from https://www .urban.org.

Yeung B, Rubenstein G, Center for Investigative Reporting: *Female workers face rape, harassment in U.S. agricultural industry,* 2013. Retrieved from https://www.revealnews.org.

35

Teen Pregnancy

Sharon K. Davis, DNP, APRN, WHNP-BC

OBJECTIVES

After reading this chapter, the student should be able to do the following:

1. Discuss approaches that could be used in providing care to the adolescent client.
2. Identify trends in adolescent pregnancy, births, abortions, and adoption in the United States.
3. Discuss reasons that may affect whether a teenager becomes pregnant.
4. Explain some of the deterrents to the establishment of paternity among young fathers.
5. Develop nursing interventions for the prevention of pregnancy problems that adolescents are at risk for experiencing.
6. Identify nursing activities that may contribute to the prevention of adolescent pregnancy.

CHAPTER OUTLINE

Adolescent Health Care in the United States
The Adolescent Client
Trends in Adolescent Sexual Behavior, Pregnancy, and Childbearing
Background Factors
Young Men and Paternity
Early Identification of the Pregnant Teen
Special Issues in Caring for the Pregnant Teen
Teen Pregnancy and the Nurse

KEY TERMS

abortion services, p. 774
adoption, p. 776
birth control, p. 773
coercive sex, p. 777
dual protection, p. 776
intimate partner violence, p. 780
long-acting reversible contraception, p. 776
low birth weight, p. 782
paternity, p. 778
peer pressure, p. 776
prematurity, p. 782
prenatal care, p. 780
repeat pregnancy, p. 782
sexual debut, p. 776
sexual victimization, p. 776
statutory rape, p. 777
weight gain, p. 781

Teen pregnancy is an area of public concern because of its significant effect on communities. Resources to support the special needs of pregnant teenagers are decreasing, and the costs of sustaining young families are prohibitive. Many teenagers who become pregnant are caught in a cycle of poverty, school failure, and limited life options. Even under the ideal circumstances of adequate finances, loving and supportive families, and good birth outcomes, a teen mother must circumvent her own necessary developmental tasks to raise her child.

There is neither a uniform reason that teens become pregnant nor a universally acceptable solution. The causes of teen pregnancy are diverse and affected by changing moral attitudes, sexual codes, and economic circumstances. Teen pregnancy places an enormous strain on the health care and social service systems. Social concern is also raised about the lost potential for young parents when pregnancy occurs, and the academic and economic disadvantages that their children will experience. Nurses are in a key position to understand how teen pregnancy affects both the individual and the community. This chapter presents a variety of issues associated with teen pregnancy and proposes nursing interventions to promote healthy outcomes for individuals and communities.

Special thanks go to Dyan Aretakis for her outstanding authoring of several editions of this chapter.

ADOLESCENT HEALTH CARE IN THE UNITED STATES

Adolescents are generally healthy, and when they seek health care it is for reasons different from those of adults or young children. The main causes of teen mortality are high-risk behaviors: motor vehicle accidents (usually including alcohol), homicide, suicide, and accidental injuries (such as falls, fires, or drowning). Teens often engage in behaviors that put them at risk for life-threatening diseases. For example, each year, one fourth of both new human immunodeficiency virus (HIV) infections and newly identified sexually transmitted diseases (STDs) occur among adolescents. During the teen years other behaviors are initiated (e.g., smoking, decreased activity, and poor nutrition) that can ultimately lead to poor health and influence behavior change that can significantly alter a young person's life (Centers for Disease Control and Prevention [CDC], 2018a). National surveys highlight the health issues facing adolescents. There have been some improvements in risk behaviors as well as a worsening of others. Among 9th to 12th graders participating in the 2017 Youth Risk Behavior Surveillance System, fewer teens reported binge drinking or riding in a car with a driver who had been drinking (CDC, 2018b). However, these and other significant risk behaviors continued at high rates. Of 9th to 12th graders, 29.8 percent reported current alcohol use, 35.6 percent had tried marijuana (19.8 percent were current users), 14 percent had taken prescription pain medication without a prescription or differently than instructed, and 39.2 percent of those who drove a car or other vehicle during the 30 days prior to their survey response had texted or emailed while driving (CDC, 2018b).

Mental health issues are also strongly associated with the adolescent years: 19 percent of students had experienced bullying on school property and 31.5 percent reported feeling sad or hopeless for more than 2 weeks; 41.1 percent of females and 21.4 percent of males reported these symptoms. Serious thought of attempting suicide was reported by 17.2 percent of the students nationwide. Suicidal thoughts with a plan existed for 13.6 percent of students, and 7.4 percent attempted suicide nationwide with a higher rate for girls (9.3 percent) than boys (5.1 percent) (CDC, 2018b).

In addition, 30.4 percent of students were either obese or overweight, 15.4 percent had not been physically active for more than 60 minutes total on a single day during the 30 days prior to filling out the survey, 43 percent played video or computer games that were unrelated to school work for three or more hours on a school day, 23.9 percent had been told they had asthma, 10.1 percent used sunscreen when they were in the sun for more than an hour, 8.8 percent had smoked cigarettes, and 13.2 percent had used a vapor product on at least one day during the 30 days prior to filling out the survey. It is the collective impact of these behaviors that not only put adolescents at risk during the teenage years but set the stage for adult morbidity and mortality from heart disease, cancer, and diabetes (CDC, 2018b).

Adolescents may not seek care for these problems for the following reasons: (1) access to health care may be hindered by a lack of transportation or health care facilities, (2) costs of care or availability of insurance, (3) lack of the belief that their visits are confidential, (4) lack of understanding of the need for health care, (5) cultural or language barriers, and (6) a limited number of professionals with expertise in dealing with teenagers who understand that sensitive topics must be broached in a nonjudgmental and supportive manner and demonstrate a desire to work with youth. Nurses who want to promote the health of adolescents by providing anticipatory guidance about peer pressure, assertiveness, and future planning need to understand adolescent behaviors, health risks, and the social context in which they live. Involvement and education of the parents about youth culture and development can promote positive and supportive parenting of teens.

THE ADOLESCENT CLIENT

Adolescents have limited experience in independently seeking health care. When they do seek care, it is often to discuss concerns about a possible pregnancy or to find a **birth control** method. These teens may also need assistance negotiating complex health care systems. Special approaches in both client interview and subsequent client education are often warranted. The behavior of adolescents toward the nurse can range from mature and competent during one visit to hostile, rude, or distant at other times because behavior often reflects intense anxiety over what the teen is experiencing.

Because client interviews usually begin with evaluation of a chief complaint, teens need to know that their concerns are heard. Health care providers may have their own opinions about what teenagers need and may fail to take the chief complaint seriously. For example, when a teen expresses ambivalence about or a desire to become pregnant, this should be discussed in depth even though the nurse may feel uncomfortable when asked to provide information to a teen about how to conceive. During this interview the nurse can provide preconception counseling and emphasize the need to achieve good health and to establish a health-promoting lifestyle before pregnancy. Health risks to the mother, as well as to fetal development, can be discussed. The nurse can encourage a young person to consider lifetime goals and discuss how parenthood might affect them. Not only does information presented this way demonstrate that the nurse has heard what the teen is saying, but it also allows the nurse to provide useful health information that may encourage the teen to examine her plans carefully, seriously, and maturely.

It is also important to pay attention to what the teen *fails* to verbalize. Knowledge of adolescent health care issues is valuable so that the nurse can anticipate other health concerns and provide an environment in which the adolescent feels safe about discussing other issues. By creating a caring and understanding atmosphere, the nurse can encourage the young person to discuss concerns about family violence, drugs, alcohol, or dating.

Discussing reproductive health care is a sensitive matter for both teens and many adults. Teens may have difficulty expressing themselves because of a limited sexual vocabulary or embarrassment resulting from their lack of knowledge. The nurse must recognize this potential deficit and embarrassment and assist teens by anticipating concerns. It is also important to allow teens to express themselves in their own language, which may include crude or offensive words. Nurses must learn about common slang expressions and common misconceptions so they do not miss important concerns that a teenager might have. The nurse can offer more appropriate terms once trust is established.

Teens may have difficulty discussing topics that provoke a judgmental reaction, such as discussing STDs (Box 35.1). The nurse can choose neutral words to evaluate symptoms (e.g., "Has there been a change in your typical vaginal discharge?"). This approach also gives the nurse a chance to educate the young client about normal anatomy and physiology.

Considerable debate exists over whether adolescents should make reproductive health care decisions without their parents' knowledge. As seen in Box 35.2, federal law establishes the adolescent's right for access to contraceptive treatment. Obstacles to services do exist, however, and this may result in a teen not receiving contraceptive information and treatment. Obstacles can include lack of transportation to a health care facility, insufficient money to pay for services, or permission to leave school early to attend an appointment.

BOX 35.1 Sexually Transmitted Diseases and Teen Pregnancy

Sexually transmitted diseases (STDs) affect 25 percent of sexually experienced teenagers each year. STDs are more easily transmitted to women than men. STD infections among women can contribute to infertility, cancer, and ectopic pregnancy. When a young woman is pregnant, these infections can cause premature rupture of membranes, premature labor, and postpartum infection. Also, the baby can be affected by all STDs in several ways: prematurity and low birth weight, febrile infection after delivery, long-term infection, and even death (e.g., exposure to viral infections such as human papillomavirus and herpes simplex virus).

The pregnant adolescent is at high risk for acquiring an STD because she may not be using barrier protection (e.g., condoms). During the pregnancy she will require periodic STD screening. STD education and counseling should accompany this screening. Information given should include ways to reduce risk, such as maintaining a mutually monogamous relationship and using latex condoms.

BOX 35.2 Reproductive Health Care and Adolescents' Rights

No federal regulation requires a young person to have parents involved in decisions on contraception services provided by federal programs. States cannot prohibit an adolescent access to contraception. Several Supreme Court decisions protect this access:

- 1965: *Griswold v. Connecticut*—the right to prevent pregnancy through the use of contraceptives is protected by the right to privacy.
- 1972: *Eisenstadt v. Baird*—the right to privacy in contraceptive use is extended to unmarried individuals.
- 1977: *Carey v. Population Services International*—the right to privacy is specifically extended to minors.

Data from National Abortion and Reproductive Rights Action League Foundation (NARAL): *U.S. Supreme Court decisions concerning reproductive rights: 1927–2016*, Washington, DC, 2017, NARAL. Retrieved from https://www.prochoiceamerica.org.

Although most minor teens can consent to birth control services in the United States, there is great variability in who may access and release their medical records. In recognition of the importance of confidentiality in reproductive health care, federal privacy rules were established in 2002 as follow-up to the Health Insurance Portability and Accountability Act of 1996 (HIPAA). This rule, the HIPAA Privacy Rule (or more correctly, the Standards for Privacy of Individually Identifiable Health Information), established that if a minor consented to care, then only that individual could access and release those medical records. However, the Privacy Rule also deferred to existing state law. In many states the laws specify that parents can legally access all the medical records of their minor children (Guttmacher Institute, 2018), which limits the confidentiality assurances offered to a teen seeking reproductive health care. Nurses who work with teens should be knowledgeable about state and federal laws so that they can accurately inform teenagers of their rights and limitations in seeking reproductive health care.

Abortion services for adolescents are not clearly defined. No federal protection is extended to adolescents requesting abortion services, and the adolescent's right to privacy and ability to give consent varies by state. (See Box 35.3, which describes abortion and adolescent rights. [These were the rights as of 2016. They are changing in some states so learn what is the law in your state. See Prochoice America for the latest information and for the information in your state.]) Confidential care to teenagers may mean the difference in preventing an unwanted pregnancy, an abortion, and a birth. This care can influence whether prenatal visits begin in the first trimester or in the second or third trimester. Teens have various reasons for pursuing confidential care, including seeking independence as well as serious and well-founded concerns about a parent's potential reaction (e.g., abuse or abandonment of the teen). Once nurses recognize the reason for confidential care, they can work with teens to discuss reproductive health care needs with the family. To do so, first clarify family values about sexuality and family communication styles with the teen. In a nonhealthy family, referral to community agencies (e.g., child protective services, Al-Anon) may be necessary. However, the nurse may need to honor the adolescent's need for confidentiality for an unknown period and proceed with the usual interventions, such as pregnancy testing, options counseling, and referral for clinical care.

TRENDS IN ADOLESCENT SEXUAL BEHAVIOR, PREGNANCY, AND CHILDBEARING

In 2016 there were 209,809 births to women under age 20. There was an overall nine percent decline from 2015 with a new low being reached each year since 2009. Teenagers aged 15-19 had a declining birth rate in 40 states from 2015, ranging from a four percent drop in Oklahoma to a 15 percent drop in New Hampshire. Rates were essentially unchanged in 10 states (Connecticut, Delaware, Hawaii, Maine, Montana, North Dakota, Rhode Island, South Dakota, Vermont, and Wyoming) and the District of Columbia (Martin et al., 2018).

BOX 35.3 Abortion and Adolescent Rights

- *Parental consent laws:* One or both parents of a young woman who is under 18 years of age seeking an abortion must give permission to the abortion provider before the abortion is performed. These 25 states have enforceable mandatory consent and notice laws: Alabama, Arizona, Arkansas, California, Idaho, Indiana, Kansas, Kentucky, Louisiana, Maine, Massachusetts, Michigan, Mississippi, Missouri, Montana, Nebraska, New Mexico, North Carolina, North Dakota, Ohio, Pennsylvania, Rhode Island, South Carolina, Tennessee, and Wisconsin.
- *Parental notification laws:* One or both parents of a young woman seeking an abortion must be notified by the abortion provider before the abortion is performed. These laws are in 14 states: Alaska, Colorado, Delaware, Florida, Georgia, Illinois, Iowa, Maryland, Minnesota, Nevada, New Hampshire, New Jersey, South Dakota, and West Virginia.
- *Parental notification and consent laws:* One or both parents of a young woman seeking an abortion must be notified and provide consent before the abortion is performed. These laws are enforced in five states: Oklahoma, Texas, Utah, Virginia, and Wyoming.
- *The following states (12) with parental notification or consent laws permit other trusted adults to stand in for a parent:* Arizona, Colorado, Delaware, Illinois, Iowa, Maine, North Carolina, Nebraska, Pennsylvania, South Carolina, Virginia, and Wisconsin.
- *The following states (five) have laws that have been found unconstitutional and unenforceable:* California, Montana, Nevada, New Jersey, and New Mexico.
- *Judicial bypass:* In a 1979 Supreme Court decision, it was ruled that any mandatory parental consent law must allow the young woman an opportunity to be granted an exception or waiver to the law. A young woman could appeal directly to a judge, who would decide either that she was mature enough to make this decision or that the abortion would be in her best interest.

Data from National Abortion and Reproductive Rights Action League Foundation (NARAL): *Who decides? The status of women's reproductive rights in the United States,* ed. 25, Washington, DC, 2016, NARAL. Retrieved from https://www.prochoiceamerica.org.

Of these births, 17 percent were a repeat birth (Martin et al., 2018). The birth rate in the United States still remains higher than in any other Western industrialized nation (Sedgh et al., 2015). The numbers of teens who become pregnant are generally identified in the following way: by age group (e.g., younger than 15, ages 15-17, ages 18-19, and under age 20), by states, by marital status, by rates (e.g., number of pregnancies, births, and abortions per 1000 young women), and by race/ethnicity (e.g., African American, white, Hispanic/Latino).

Births to teenagers make up 5.3 percent of all births in the United States (U. S. Department of Health and Human Services [USDHHS], 2016a). Teen mothers and their children can have adverse health, economic, and social outcomes, which cost the United States about $9.4 billion annually (Romero et al., 2016). Teen birth rates increase by age, with the highest rates occurring among 19-year-olds. The 2013 U.S. birth rate for teenagers aged 15-19 dropped 57 percent from its highest point in 1991 (Martinez & Abma, 2015). Decreases in pregnancy among teens ages 15 to 17 have been attributed to reduced sexual activity (one fourth of the reduction), and the rest result from improved contraceptive use. Evidence shows that the use of long-acting reversible contraceptives can potentially help more teens avoid an unwanted pregnancy (Guttmacher, 2014). Decline in the teen birth rate varies by race, with the highest birth rates among Hispanic teens (46.3 births per 1000), then African American teens (43.9 births per 1000) and white teens (20.5 births per 1000) (USDHHS, 2016a).

In 2013 there were 448,000 pregnancies to American teens between the ages of 15 and 19 years (Kost et al., 2017). In this same year and age group, 29 percent ended in an abortion, which was a drop from 46 percent in 1985 (Kost et al., 2017). The reasons most teens give for having an abortion is that they are concerned about how a baby would change their lives. They also say that they do not think they could afford to care for a baby, and they do not feel that they are mature enough to raise a child. A sexually active teen who does not use contraceptives has a 90 percent chance of becoming pregnant within one year. Elective abortion rates for teenagers increased from the time of legalization in 1973 until 1988 and then began to decline. This decrease was caused in part by decreases in the pregnancy rate but may also have resulted from laws that required parental notification or consent for minors requesting abortion services in some states. As of July 2018, laws in 37 states required minors seeking abortions to have parental involvement in the decision (Guttmacher Institute, 2018).

HEALTHY PEOPLE 2020

Selected Objectives Related to Adolescent Reproductive Health

Objectives Related to Adolescent Health
- **HIV-13:** Increase the percent of adolescents who have been tested for HIV.

Objectives Related to Family Planning
- **FP-12:** Increase the proportion of adolescents who received formal instruction on reproductive health topics before they are 18 years old.
- **FP-13:** Increase the proportion of adolescents who talked to a parent or guardian about reproductive health topics before they are 18 years old.

Objectives Related to Maternal, Infant, and Child Health
- **MICH-8.1:** Reduce low birth weight (LBW) and very low birth weight (VLBW)
- **MICH-10:** Increase the proportion of pregnant women who receive early and adequate prenatal care.

HIV, Human immunodeficiency virus.
From USDHHS: *Healthy People 2020.* Available at https://www.healthypeople.gov.

BACKGROUND FACTORS

Many adults have difficulty understanding why young people would jeopardize their careers and personal potential by becoming pregnant during the teen years. Adolescents, however, do not view the world in the same way as adults. Teens often feel invincible and therefore do not recognize any risk related to their behaviors or anticipate the consequences. That is, they may not think that sexual activity will lead to pregnancy. When teens become pregnant, they do not believe that the negative outcomes they are advised of could come true. Many teens believe that they are unique and different and that everything will work out fine. The developmental circumstances of adolescence, coupled with potential background disadvantages, can magnify the problems facing the pregnant and parenting teen. Pregnant teens often express the unrealistic attitude that they can do it all: school, work, parenting, and socializing.

Babies born to teenage mothers in the United States are at risk for many of the same problems as their young mothers. These risks include school failure, poverty, and physical or mental illness (USDHHS, 2016b). Specifically, a disproportionate number of teens who give birth are poor, have limited educational achievements, and have limited opportunities within their communities for positive youth experiences (CDC, 2017a). Most teens report that their pregnancy was unplanned. They typically think that a pregnancy should be delayed until people are older, have completed their education, and are employed and married. Several factors that often contribute to pregnancy are discussed next.

Sexual Activity and Use of Birth Control

The **sexual debut**, or first experience with intercourse, for a teen has a significant impact on pregnancy risk. In 2017, among high school students who were surveyed, 39.5 percent had experienced sexual intercourse with 9.7 percent of these having four or more sexual partners (CDC, 2018b). These students answered questions about their sexual contacts, with 45.3 percent identifying contact with only the opposite sex, 1.6 percent had contact with only the same sex, and 5.3 percent had contact with both sexes (CDC, 2018b). From 2005 to 2015 there has been a linear decline in the percent of youth who have initiated sexual intercourse: male students have dropped from 46.8 percent to 41.2 percent, and female students have dropped from 45.7 percent to 39.2 percent. Ethnicity of the students having sexual intercourse was also reported for the same time period: white students dropped from 43 percent to 39.9 percent, black students dropped from 67.6 percent to 48.5 percent, and Hispanic students dropped from 51 percent to 42.5 percent (Ethier et al., 2018). The *Healthy People 2020* goal is to increase the proportion of adolescents who have never engaged in sexual intercourse by age 17 (USDHHS, 2010).

Although more teens have begun using birth control in the past 10 years, there is still progress to be made. *Healthy People 2020* addresses this with goals to increase the proportion of 15- to 19-year-olds who use condoms and a hormonal contraceptive and increase the proportion of teens who receive reproductive health information through formal instruction as well as from their parents or guardians (USDHHS, 2010). Condoms are the most commonly used method of birth control, with 68 percent of adolescent females and 80 percent of adolescent males reporting their use at first voluntary coitus. Great improvement in overall contraceptive use has occurred, with 86 percent and 93 percent of females and males, respectively, reporting that a method of contraception was used at last sex. The current recommendation for greatest protection against pregnancy and sexually transmitted infection (STI) is the use of a hormonal contraceptive, preferably **long-acting reversible contraception** (LARC), and a condom, referred to as **dual protection**. At this time only 20 percent of females and 30 percent of males reported using dual protection the last time they had sex (Guttmacher Institute, 2017). Male teens use condoms with more frequency than female teens, and African American males use condoms more often than any other group, male or female. Overall, 53.8 percent of sexually active teen couples reported that the male partner used condoms the last time they had intercourse, with the greatest use at last intercourse reported by white male teens (761.3 percent) and the lowest use reported by black female teens (47.1 percent). During 1991-2017 there was a significant increase (46.2 percent to 53.8 percent) in the use of condoms at last intercourse (CDC, 2018a).

Inadequate Contraception Knowledge

> **CHECK YOUR PRACTICE**
>
> You are seeing a 16-year-old patient in your office for painful menses and she did not want her mother to be present. The patient says to you, "I make my boyfriend use condoms regularly so I can't get any diseases or get pregnant." What should you ask?

In 2012 the American College of Obstetricians and Gynecologists (ACOG) made a strong recommendation to encourage adolescents to use LARC methods—intrauterine devices and contraceptive implants. These methods are reversible and have the highest rates of continuation and prevention of pregnancy, rapid repeat pregnancy, and abortion in young women. Reports from the Contraceptive CHOICE Project, an observational clinical trial, prompted ACOG to strengthen their recommendation in 2015 when it was reported that LARC methods were 20 times more effective at preventing pregnancy in their participants (American College of Obstetricians and Gynecologists, 2015). Table 35.1 describes hormonal birth control methods and their effectiveness. As noted earlier, the use of alcohol and other substances is common among adolescents and can contribute to unplanned pregnancy. Mood-altering effects may reduce inhibitions about engaging in intercourse and interfere with the proper use of a chosen birth control method.

Peer Pressure and Partner Pressure

Peer pressure among teens is not a new phenomenon, but many of the influences have become more serious. Influence has expanded from fashion and language to cigarettes, substance abuse, sexuality, pregnancy, and sexting. Teens are more likely to be sexually active if their friends are sexually active (Gregg et al., 2018). Peers reinforce teen parenting by exaggerating birth control risks, discouraging abortion and **adoption**, and glamorizing the impending birth of the child.

Both young men and young women may think that allowing a pregnancy to happen verifies one's love and commitment for the other. In addition, young men from socioeconomically disadvantaged backgrounds may be more likely to say that fathering a child would make them feel more manly, and they are less likely to use an effective contraceptive (Farrell et al., 2017).

Other Factors

Other factors influencing teen pregnancy are a history of **sexual victimization**, family structure, parental influences, and diverse

TABLE 35.1 Hormonal Birth Control Methods Recommended for Teenagers

Method	Failure Rate With Typical Use (%/year)	Pattern of Use	Noncontraceptive Benefits
Mirena IUD Paragard IUD Liletta IUD Kyleena IUD Skyla IUD	0.2 0.8	Placed in the uterus; effective continuously for 5 years (Mirena); 10 years (Paragard); 3-5 years (Liletta); 5 years (Kyleena); 3 years (Skyla)	Less menstrual bleeding, often with amenorrhea after initial few months
Nexplanon implant	0.05	Placed subdermally in the upper arm; effective continuously for 3 years	Less menstrual bleeding
Depo-Provera	6	IM injection into either the deltoid or the gluteal muscle every 3 months	• Decreases sickle cell crisis • Decreases the seizure threshold • May become amenorrheic
NuvaRing	9	Vaginal ring inserted for 21 to 32 days; contains estrogen and progestin	For all estrogen/progestin combinations: • Risk of ovarian and endometrial cancer is reduced • May use an extended regimen to reduce menses (except Ortho Evra patch) • May improve acne • Light regular menses (except POP)
Ortho Evra transdermal patch	9	A transdermal patch that is applied to specific skin sites weekly for 3 weeks, and removed for 7 days; contains estrogen and progestin	See above
Birth control pills	9	Take pill daily. COC—estrogen and progestin; POP—progestin only ("mini pill")	See above

COC, Combined oral contraceptive pill; *IM,* intramuscular; *IUD,* intrauterine device; *POP,* progestin-only pill.
(Developed from Planned Parenthood, 2018, learn about birth control. Available at https://www.plannedparenthood.org/learn/birthcontrol.)

sexual orientations. With a history of poverty only, 16.8 percent of teens had been pregnant once by age 17. For teens with a history of poverty and reported child abuse or neglect, 28.9 percent had been pregnant by age 17 (Garwood et al., 2015). Adolescent girls with a history of sexual abuse are at risk for earlier initiation of voluntary sexual intercourse, are less likely to use birth control, are more likely to use drugs and alcohol at first intercourse, and are more likely to have older sexual partners. The prevalence of adolescents experiencing **coercive sex** or **statutory rape** is 11.3 percent (CDC, 2018b). Young women may also become pregnant as a result of forced sexual intercourse. A history of sexual victimization will influence a young woman's ability to exert control over future sexual experiences, which will affect the use of birth control and rejection of unwanted sexual experiences. Teen pregnancy is also more common among sexual minorities compared with heterosexuals, which is thought to be partially due to childhood mistreatment (Charlton et al., 2018). All these factors contribute to an increased risk for becoming pregnant. In addition, young women who have experienced a lifetime of economic, social, and psychological deprivation may think that a baby will bring joy into an otherwise bleak existence. Some mistakenly believe that a baby can provide the love and attention that her family has not provided.

Family structure can influence adolescent sexual behavior and pregnancy. While the number of single-parent families has increased in recent years, it is interesting that recent researchers found that it was not single-parent families with working mothers that had the highest risk for an unplanned teen pregnancy, but that it was adolescents who have girlfriends with early sexual activity who have a 1.63 times greater risk of getting pregnant unintentionally (Vázquez-Nava et al., 2014).

Parenting styles can influence a young woman's risk for early sexual experiences and pregnancy. Parents who are extremely demanding and controlling or neglectful and who have low expectations are least successful in instilling parental values in their children. Parents who have high demands for their children to act maturely and who offer warmth and understanding with parental rules have children more likely to exhibit appropriate social behavior and to delay early sexual experiences and pregnancy. Children of parents who are neglectful are the most sexually experienced, followed by children of parents who are very strict. Furthermore, parents who discuss birth control, sexuality, and pregnancy with their children can positively influence delay of sexual initiation and effective birth control use. Parents who do not communicate about sexuality with their teens may find them more at risk for sexual permissiveness and pregnancy (CDC, 2017b).

YOUNG MEN AND PATERNITY

Although declines among pregnant female teenagers have been seen over the past 27 years, the percent of teenage fathers increased. At first, this may seem contradictory, but it could be explained by several factors: teenage males are partnering with older women, females are partnering with older males, paternity has been more readily ascertained by genetic testing and voluntary establishment, coordinated child support has been reinforcement, and there has been a decrease in stigma (Pirog et al., 2017).

About seven percent of males become fathers before the age of 19. Of this group, two thirds were ages 18 or 19 when they fathered their first child, and one third were less than 18 years old. These numbers may be conservative because not all teen males are aware that a partner became pregnant, nor are they always aware of the outcome of the pregnancy. A review of birth certificate information may not be helpful as many unmarried couples fail to complete the steps required for a father's name to appear. Adolescent males who become fathers are often reported to be second-generation teen parents. Studies demonstrate that they came from poor families, did poorly in school, and engaged in many high-risk behaviors such as gang membership, drugs, and early sexual involvement. These young fathers face special challenges because of concomitant social problems and limited future plans or ability to provide support. There may also be an overlap between young fatherhood and delinquency. Adolescent males who demonstrate law-breaking behaviors, alcohol or substance use, school problems, and aggressive behaviors may have difficulty developing a positive fathering role, yet they are the highest-risk group to become young fathers (Massachusetts General Hospital [MGH], 2016).

Paternity, or fatherhood, is legally established at the time of the birth for a married teen. However, it is more difficult to establish paternity among nonmarried couples. Some of the difficulty lies in the complexity of the specific state system for young men to acknowledge paternity. In some states a young man may have to work with the judicial system outside of the hospital after the birth; if he is under age 18, he may need to involve his parents.

Some young couples do not attempt to establish paternity and prefer a verbal promise of assistance for the teen mother and child. Although a verbal commitment may be acceptable when the child is born, the mother may become more inclined to pursue the establishment of paternity later when the relationship ends or for reasons related to financial, social, or emotional needs of the child. Young women who receive state or federal assistance (e.g., Temporary Assistance for Needy Families, Medicaid) may be asked to name the child's father so the judicial process can be used to establish paternity.

Young men react differently when they learn that their partner is pregnant. The reaction often depends on the nature of the relationship before the pregnancy. Many young men will accompany the young woman to a health care center for pregnancy diagnosis and counseling. A large percent of young men will continue to accompany the young woman to some prenatal visits and may even attend the delivery. These young men may also want, and need, to be involved with their children regardless of changes in their relationships with the teen mother. It is not unusual for a young man to be excluded or even rejected by the young woman's family (usually her mother). He may then begin to act as though he is disinterested when he may really feel that he cannot provide resources for his child or know how to take care of him or her (MGH, 2016) (Fig. 35.1).

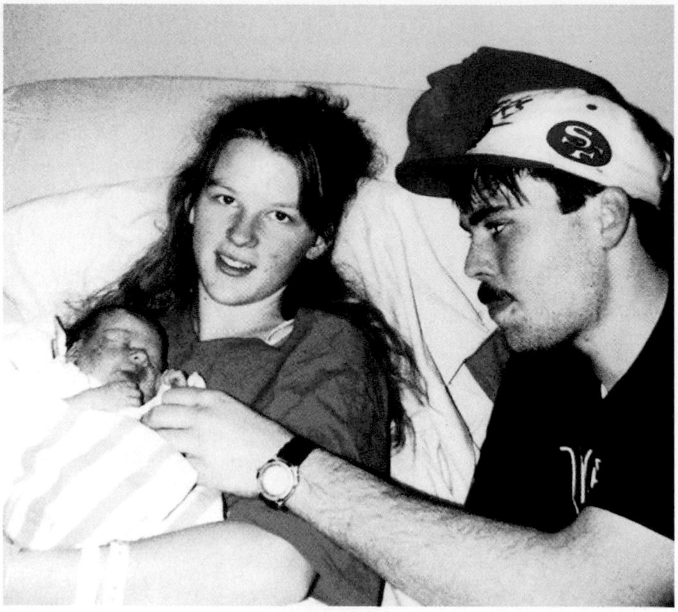

Fig. 35.1 It is important to include both the teen mother and the father in teaching about child development.

Nurses can acknowledge and support the young man as he develops in the role of father. His involvement can positively affect his child's development and provide greater personal satisfaction for him and greater role satisfaction for the young mother. Young mothers who report less social support from their baby's father are more apt to be unhappy and distressed in the parenting role (Dumas et al., 2018). The immediate concerns revolve around his financial responsibility, living arrangements, relationship issues, school, and work. Establishing an opportunity to meet with the young man and both families is helpful to clarify these issues and identify roles and responsibilities. Even if the young father cannot provide financial support, emotional and physical support is still extremely important (Healthy Children Organization [HCO], 2017).

Life experiences for a young man will influence behaviors that can lead to a teen pregnancy or prevent a teen pregnancy. Adverse childhood experiences, including a history of abuse (especially physical and sexual abuse and domestic violence), mental illness and/or substance abuse in the childhood home, criminal behaviors in the home, and separated parents, have been linked to negative behaviors such as early sexual intercourse, multiple partners, and substance use. These behaviors are possible antecedents to male involvement in teen pregnancy (Chilcoat et al., 2016).

Age discrepancy between the pregnant teen and her male partner is an important consideration, even when it is only two years. It raises concern about coercion, potential or actual violence, increase in risk for STI, and exposure to greater substance and alcohol use. The greatest age discrepancies are seen with the youngest pregnant teens. Although these numbers have decreased, the risk is present with more than half of all females ages 15 and younger reporting first sexual intercourse with a male partner who is more than three years older. Protective factors that can reduce the risk of a young teen becoming sexually involved with an older partner include living with both biological parents, greater parental education, and not being born to a teen mother (Masho et al., 2017).

EARLY IDENTIFICATION OF THE PREGNANT TEEN

Some teens delay seeking pregnancy services because they fail to recognize signs such as breast tenderness and a late period, or they are experiencing a variety of other pubertal changes. Most young women, however, suspect pregnancy as soon as a period is late. These young women may still delay seeking care because they falsely hope that the pregnancy will just go away. A teen may also delay seeking care to keep the pregnancy a secret from family members, either fearing an angry or disappointed response or expecting to be forced into a decision that may not be hers.

Nurses must be sensitive to subtle cues that a teenager may offer about sexuality and pregnancy concerns. Such cues include questions about one's fertile period or requests for confirmation that one need not miss a period to be pregnant. Once the nurse identifies the specific concern, information can be provided about how and when to obtain pregnancy testing. The nurse should determine how a teenager would react to the possible pregnancy before completing the test. If the test is negative, the nurse should take the opportunity to assess whether the young woman would consider counseling to prevent pregnancy. A follow up visit is important after a negative test to determine if retesting is necessary or if another problem exists.

In looking at teen pregnancy from the perspective of levels of prevention, several steps could be taken. These are shown in the Levels of Prevention box.

LEVELS OF PREVENTION

Teen Pregnancy

Primary Prevention

Teach young people about sexual practices that will prevent untimely pregnancy.

Secondary Prevention

Provide services for early detection of teen pregnancy.

Tertiary Prevention

Counsel the young person or young couple about available options, including keeping the baby (and making appropriate plans to care for the child), abortion, and adoption.

A young woman with a positive pregnancy test requires a physical examination and pregnancy counseling. It is advantageous to offer these at the same time so that the counseling is consistent with the findings of the examination. The purpose of the examination is to assess the duration and well-being of the pregnancy, as well as to test for STI. The pregnancy counseling should include the following: information on adoption, abortion, and child-rearing; assessment of support systems; assessment of partner violence; and identification of the immediate concerns she might have (Marino, 2016).

The availability of affordable abortion services up to 13 weeks of gestation varies from community to community. Similarly, second-trimester services may be available locally or involve extensive travel and cost. The nurse should know about abortion services and provide information or refer the pregnant teenager to a pregnancy counseling service that can assist.

The pregnant teenager needs information about adoption, such as current policies among agencies that allow continued contact with the adopting family. Also, church organizations, private attorneys, and social service agencies provide a variety of adoption services with which the nurse should be familiar. Box 35.4 lists guidelines for adoption counseling.

Pregnancy counseling requires that the nurse and young woman explore strengths and weaknesses for personal care and responsibility during pregnancy and parenting. Young women vary in their interest in including the partner or their parents in this discussion. Issues to discuss include education and career plans, family finances and qualifications for outside assistance, and personal values about pregnancy and parenting at this time in their life. Often it is difficult to focus on counseling in any depth at the time of the initial pregnancy testing results. A follow-up visit is usually more productive and should be arranged as soon as possible.

As decisions are made about the course of the pregnancy, the nurse can make referrals to appropriate programs such as Women, Infants, and Children (WIC) program (a supplemental

BOX 35.4 Guidelines for Adoption Counseling

1. Assess your own thoughts and feelings on adoption. Do not impose your opinion on the decision-making process of teen mothers.
2. Know about state laws, local resources, and various types of adoption services.
3. Choose language sensitively. Examples follow:
   a. Avoid saying "giving away a child" or "putting up for adoption." It is more appropriate and positive to say "releasing a child for adoption," "placing for adoption," or "making an adoption plan."
   b. Avoid saying "unwanted child" or "unwanted pregnancy." A more appropriate term may be *unplanned pregnancy*.
   c. Avoid saying "natural parents" or "natural child," because the adopted parents would then seem to be "unnatural." The terms *biological parents* and *adoptive parents* are more appropriate.
4. Assess when a discussion of adoption is appropriate. It can be helpful to begin with information on adoption and then explore feelings and concerns over time. Individuals will vary in how much they may have already considered adoption, and this will influence the counseling session.
5. Assess the relationship between the pregnant teen and her partner and what role she expects him to play. Discuss the reality of this.
6. It may be helpful for a pregnant teen to talk with other teens who have been pregnant, are raising a child, have released a child for adoption, or have been adopted themselves.
7. A young woman can be encouraged to begin writing letters to her baby. These can be saved or given to the child when released to the adoptive family.

Modified from Brandsen CK: *A case for adoption*, Grand Rapids, MI, 1991, Bethany.

food program for women, infants, and children), Medicaid, and prenatal services. The young woman and her family also need to know about expected costs of care and, if there is a family insurance policy, whether it will cover the pregnancy-related expenses of a dependent child. For those without insurance, the family can apply for Medicaid or determine whether local facilities offer indigent care programs (e.g., Hill-Burton programs for assistance with hospital expenses). The nurse can also begin prenatal education and counseling on nutrition, substance abuse and use, exercise, and special medical concerns.

SPECIAL ISSUES IN CARING FOR THE PREGNANT TEEN

Pregnant teenagers are considered high-risk obstetric clients. Many of their pregnancy complications result from poverty, late entry into prenatal care, and limited knowledge about self-care during pregnancy. Nursing interventions through education and early identification of problems may dramatically alter the course of the pregnancy and the birth outcome.

Violence

Teens are more likely to experience violence during their pregnancies than adult women. Age may be a factor in their greater vulnerability to potential perpetrators that include partners, family members, and other acquaintances. Violence in pregnancy has been associated with an increased risk for substance abuse, poor compliance with prenatal care, and poor birth outcome. In the case of partner violence, young women may be protective of their partners because of fear or helplessness. Eliciting this history from an adolescent is not easy. Be sure to inquire about violence at every visit. The added risk factor of poverty along with abuse compounds the risk of teenage pregnancy. In one study 16.8 percent of teens with a history of poverty had at least one pregnancy by age 17. If poverty and abuse were reported by the teen, there was a 28.9 percent occurrence of pregnancy by age 17 (Garwood et al., 2015). Violence that began during the pregnancy may continue for several years after, with increasing severity. Teens can be so ingrained in intimate partner violence that they have cannot see symptoms of psychological distress (Bekaert & SmithBattle, 2016). The nurse must observe for physical signs of abuse, as well as for controlling or intrusive partner behavior.

Initiation of Prenatal Care

Pregnant adolescents differ remarkably from pregnant adults in initiation and compliance with prenatal care. Inadequate prenatal care has been associated with increased health risks to both the mother and the fetus. In 2016, 11.2 percent of mothers under the age of 20 years received late or no prenatal care (Martin et al., 2018). Teens have reported barriers to care, which include denial of the pregnancy, fear of telling parents, transportation, dislike of providers' care, and offensive attitudes among clinic staff toward pregnant teens (Heaman et al., 2014).

Once a teen is enrolled in prenatal care, the nurse becomes an important liaison between personnel at the clinical site and the young woman. Confusion and misunderstandings occur easily when teens do not understand what a health care provider says to them. Often these misunderstandings are based on lack of knowledge about basic anatomy and physiology. For example, a teen may be told as she gets close to term that the head of the baby is down and it can be felt. This is an alarming piece of information for a young woman who imagines the entire baby could just pop out at any time!

Cooperation between the nurse and the clinical staff can also maximize the client's compliance with special health or nutritional needs. For example, a teen who has premature contractions may be restricted to bed rest and instructed to increase fluids. The nurse who makes home visits can provide additional assessment of the teen's condition and can solve problems about self-care, hygiene, meals, and schooling.

Low-Birth-Weight Infants and Preterm Delivery

Teens are more likely than adult women to deliver infants weighing less than 5.5 lb or to deliver before 37 weeks of gestation. These low-birth-weight and premature infants are at greater risk for death in the first year of life and are at increased risk for long-term physical, emotional, and cognitive problems (Marvin-Dowle et al., 2018). For example, low-birth-weight and premature infants can be more difficult to feed and soothe. This challenges the limited skills of the young mother and can further strain relations with other members of the household, who may not know how to offer support or assistance.

The risk for low-birth-weight infants and premature births can be averted by the teen's early initiation into prenatal care. Although such births still occur, it is important to work closely with the teen mother as soon as she is identified as pregnant to try to promote compliance with prenatal care visits and self-care during the pregnancy. After the pregnancy these infants and their mothers will benefit from frequent nursing supervision to ensure that their care is appropriate and that everyone in the home is coping adequately with the strain of a small infant.

Nutrition

The nutritional needs of a pregnant teenager are especially important. First, the teen lifestyle does not lend itself to overall good nutrition. Fast foods, frequent snacking, and hectic social schedules limit nutritious food choices. Snacks, which account for about one third of a teen's daily caloric intake, tend to be high in fat, sugar, and sodium and limited in essential vitamins and minerals. Second, the nutritive needs of both pregnancy and the concurrent adolescent growth spurt require the adolescent to change her diet substantially. The growing teen must increase caloric nutrients to meet individual growth needs as well as to allow for adequate fetal growth. Third, poor eating patterns of the teen and her current growth requirement may leave her with limited reserves of essential vitamins and minerals when the pregnancy begins.

The nurse can assess the pregnant teenager's current eating pattern and provide creative guidance. Identifying good choices that a teen can consume "on the run" might include snacks of drinkable yogurt, leftover pizza, string cheese, or energy/granola bars. The teen who often eats out can boost her protein intake at fast-food establishments by ordering milkshakes instead of soft drinks, and cheeseburgers or broiled chicken sandwiches instead of hamburgers. Adding lettuce and tomato or other sliced vegetables to burgers will improve nutrition intake along with fruit smoothies to satisfy a sweet craving (Cornforth, 2018).

Naeye (1981) was the first to introduce the idea that the pregnant teen was in direct competition for nutrients with her fetus at a time when her own nutritional needs are increasing. Improved dairy food intake does have a positive effect on increasing the birth weight for adolescent pregnancies, but more research is needed to determine appropriate dosages of nutritional intake for the best pregnancy outcomes. The nurse and adolescent should collaborate on a reasonable nutritional approach and identify individual health behavior changes that could improve the health of mother and fetus (Soltani et al., 2015).

The nurse, in collaboration with the WIC nutritionist, can determine the nutritional needs of the pregnant teenager to tailor education appropriately. Table 35.2 describes adolescent nutritional needs in pregnancy.

Weight gain during pregnancy is one of the strongest predictors of infant birth weight. Although precise weight gain goals in adolescence are controversial, pregnant adolescents who gain 25 to 35 lb have the lowest incidence of low-birth-weight babies. Babies born to teenagers may be at risk for being small for gestational age despite adequate weight gain if there is very slow gain in the first 24 weeks. Teenagers who begin the pregnancy at a normal weight should be counseled to begin weight gain in the first trimester and to average gains of 1 lb per week for the second and third trimesters. Younger teen mothers (ages 13 to 16), because of their own growth demands, may need to gain more weight than older teen mothers (ages 17 and older) to have the same-birth-weight baby. Table 35.3 shows the recommendations established by the Institute of Medicine for adolescent gestational weight gain by pre-pregnant weight categories.

It is important for the nurse to assess the attitudes of the pregnant teen about weight gain and to monitor her progress, providing feedback on adequate weight gain and counseling if weight gain is excessive. Gaining weight beyond the recommendations raises the risk for infants to be hypoglycemic, to be large for gestational age, and to have a low Apgar score, seizures, polycythemia, and a predisposition to obesity (Restall et al., 2014), Family support of the pregnant teen can be a strong influence in adequate weight gain and good nutrition during

TABLE 35.2 Adolescent Nutritional Needs During Pregnancy

Nutrient	Daily Requirement During Pregnancy[a]	Food Source
Calcium	1000 mg (increase to 1300 mg for <19-year-olds)	Macaroni and cheese; pizza; puddings, milk, yogurt; also fortified juices, water, breakfast bars and fast foods, including Taco Bell's chili cheese burrito, McDonald's Big Mac
Iron	27 mg	Meats; dried beans; peas; dark green, leafy vegetables; whole grains; fortified cereal; absorption of iron from plant foods improved by vitamin C sources taken simultaneously
Zinc	15 mg	Seafood, meats, eggs, legumes, whole grains
Folate (folic acid)	0.6 mg (prenatal vitamins contain 0.4-1.0 mg of folic acid)	Green, leafy vegetables; fruits
Vitamin A	770 mcg RAE per day Age 18 and younger 750 mcg	Dark yellow and green vegetables, fruits
Vitamin B_6	1.9 mg	Chicken, fish, liver, pork, eggs
Vitamin D	600 IU	Fortified milk products and cereals

[a]Higher ranges are especially important for the younger pregnant teen.
(American College of Obstetricians and Gynecologists, 2018. Available at https://www.acog.org/Patients?FAQs/Nutrition-During-Pregnancy.)
RAE, Retinol activity equivalent.

TABLE 35.3 Gestational Weight Gain Recommendations for Adolescents[a]

	RECOMMENDED TOTAL GAIN			
Prepregnant Weight Category[b]	kg	lb	Trimester 1 (lb)	Trimesters 2 and 3 (lb/wk)
Underweight (BMI 19.8)	12.5-18	28-40	5	1.0
Normal weight (BMI 19.9-26)	11.5-16	25-35	3	1.0
Overweight (BMI 26-29)	7.0-11.5	15-25	2	0.66
Very overweight (BMI $\geq$ 29)	5.0-9.1	11-20	1.5	0.5

[a]Very young adolescents (14 years of age or younger, or less than 2 years postmenarche) should strive for gains at the upper end of the range (Soltani, 2015).
[b]BMI (body mass index) is calculated as weight (in kilograms) divided by height (in meters) squared (CDC, 2018c).
From Soltani H, Duxbury A, Rundle R, Chan L: A systematic review of the effects of dietary interventions on neonatal outcomes in adolescent pregnancy, *Evid Based Mdwfry* 13(1):29–34, 2015.

the pregnancy. Nutrition education should emphasize what accounts for weight gain and how fetal growth will benefit.

Globally, iron deficiency anemia is the most common nutritional problem among both pregnant and nonpregnant adolescent females with about 50 percent of the cases being due to inadequate intake. The metabolic processes involved in tissue oxygenation are dependent upon iron (Abu-Ouf & Jan, 2015). The increased maternal plasma volume and increased fetal demands for iron (especially in the third trimester) can further compromise the adolescent. Iron deficiency in pregnancy may contribute to increased fetal **prematurity**, **low birth weight**, and low iron stores for the infant that can last for up to one year. For the mother, iron deficiency may contribute to cardiovascular stress, increased risk of urinary tract infection, sleep difficulties, decreased well-being, postpartum hemorrhage, and slower wound healing (Abu-Ouf & Jan, 2015). The nurse can reinforce the need for the teen to take prenatal vitamins during pregnancy and after the baby's birth. Vitamins should contain 30 to 60 mg of elemental iron daily. The nurse should educate about iron-rich foods and foods that promote iron absorption, such as those containing vitamin C.

Infant Care

Many adolescents have cared for babies and small children and feel confident and competent. Few teens are ever prepared, however, for the reality of 24-hour care of an infant. The nurse can help prepare the teen for the transition to motherhood while she is still pregnant. The trend toward early discharge from the hospital has made prenatal preparation even more important. The nurse can enlist the support of the teen's parents in education about infant care and stimulation. Young fathers-to-be would benefit from this education as well. Family values, practices, and beliefs about childcare may be deeply embedded and require the nurse to work gently and persuasively to challenge any that may be detrimental to an infant (HCO, 2017). For example, a family may believe that corporal punishment is a necessary component of child-rearing.

Adolescents often lack the self-confidence and knowledge required to positively interact with their infants. They may also have unrealistic expectations about their children's development (HCO, 2017). For example, they may expect their children to feed themselves at an early age or think that their children's behavior is more difficult than an adult mother might think. Teen parents often lack knowledge about infant growth and development, as seen in their limited verbal communication with their children, limited eye contact, and the tendency to display frustration and ambivalence as mothers. Over time, adolescents can improve their ability to foster their children's emotional and social growth. Children of adolescent mothers have also been found to be at risk for academic and behavior problems as they enter school. These risks can be reduced when the teen mother receives professional intervention and supervision in the area of infant social and cognitive development (The Urban Child Institute, 2014).

Abusive parenting is more likely to occur when the parents have limited knowledge about normal child development or have been victims of abuse themselves. It may also be more likely to occur among parents who cannot adequately empathize with a child's needs. Younger teens are particularly at risk for being unable to understand what their infant or child needs. This frustration may be exhibited as abusive behavior toward the child. Nurses should continually assess for child abuse risk when dealing with teens who exhibit greater psychological distress or lack social supports (McHugh et al., 2015).

After the birth of the baby the nurse should assess maternal support and observe how the mother responds to infant cues for basic needs and distress. Specific techniques that the new mother can be instructed to use in early childcare are listed in the How To box. Begin parenting education as early as possible. Adolescents who feel competent as parents have enhanced self-esteem, which in turn positively influences their relationship with their child. Recognizing these good parenting skills and providing positive feedback help a young mother gain confidence in her role (Angley et al., 2015).

HOW TO Promote Interactions Between the Teen Mother and Her Baby

The nurse can make the following suggestions to the teen mother:

1. Make eye contact with your baby. Position your face 8 to 10 inches from your baby's face and smile.
2. Talk to your baby often. Use simple sentences, but try to avoid baby talk. Allow time for your baby to "answer." This will help your baby to acquire language and communication skills.
3. Babies often enjoy when you sing to them, and this may help soothe them during a difficult time or help them fall asleep. Experiment with different songs and melodies to see which your baby seems to like.
4. Babies at this age cannot be spoiled. Instead, when babies are held and cuddled, they feel secure and loved.
5. Babies cry for many reasons and for no reason at all. If your baby has a clean diaper, has recently been fed, and is safe and secure, he or she may just need to cry for a few minutes. What works to calm your baby may be different from other babies you have known. You can try rocking, gentle reassuring words, soft music, or remaining quiet.
6. Make feeding times pleasant for both of you. Do not prop the bottle in your baby's mouth. Instead, sit comfortably, hold your baby in your arms, and offer the bottle or breast.
7. When babies are awake, they love to play. They enjoy taking walks and looking at brightly colored objects or pictures and toys that make noises, such as rattles and musical toys.

Repeat Pregnancy

Teen mothers who have a closely spaced second pregnancy, or a **repeat pregnancy**, have poorer birth, educational, and economic outcomes than teens who do not. In 2016, 17 percent of teen births in 15- to 19-year-olds were a repeat birth (USDHHS, 2016a). Teens with more than one child often are unable to finish their education or gain employment. Second children of teen mothers are often born prematurely or too small, often leading to more health problems (CDC, 2013). A *Healthy People 2020* objective is to reduce the proportion of pregnancies conceived within 18 months of a previous birth. Nurses should recognize which teens are at risk for a second teen pregnancy, such as lower educational and cognitive ability, mental health issues, physical trauma, losses (such as death of a loved one), and substance use.

Discussions about family planning should begin during the third trimester of the current pregnancy. Nurses should review contraceptive options and help the young woman identify the methods she is most likely to use. It is helpful to determine at this time the methods she has used in the past, her satisfaction or dissatisfaction, and reasons for use or nonuse. Many teens express unrealistic goals, such as "I am never going to have sex again," or "I need a break from guys," and they may erroneously believe that they are unable to conceive for some time after the delivery. After delivery the nurse should follow up on the young woman's plan. Obstacles to obtaining contraceptives may exist, and the nurse can identify these and help problem-solve with the new mother.

Schooling and Educational Needs

Adolescents who become parents may have had limited school success before the pregnancy. However, coping with the demands of child-rearing coupled with the immaturity of the young mother may make school even less of a priority. Also, the potential for a closely spaced second birth may be lessened by a return to school. Fifty percent of teen mothers earn a high school diploma by the age of 22 years compared with 90 percent of women who did not give birth during the teen years (National Conference of State Legislators [NCSL], 2013). Federal legislation passed in 1975 prohibits schools from excluding students because they are pregnant. Greater emphasis is placed on keeping the pregnant adolescent in school during the pregnancy and having her return as soon as possible after the birth. Several factors may positively influence a young woman's return to school. These include her parents' level of education and their marital stability, small family size, whether there were reading materials at home, whether her mother is employed, and whether the young woman is African American.

A practical challenge for young parents is locating and affording quality childcare; difficulties with this may prevent the highly motivated teenager from returning to high school. In the past 30 years the percent of parenting teens who return to high school and graduate (40 percent) has improved significantly. Attendance in college, now becoming the career requisite, is still less attainable for women who had children as teenagers than for those who delayed childbearing, and less than two percent attain that college degree by the age of 30 (NCSL, 2013).

Young women who have pregnancy complications may seek home instruction. This decision is made according to regulations issued by the state boards of education. Some young women have difficulty attending school because of the normal discomforts of pregnancy or because of social and emotional conflicts associated with the pregnancy. Teens who leave school without parental or medical excuses may face legal problems because of truancy. This increases the potential for them to become school dropouts. The nurse can determine whether this has happened and try to coordinate with the school personnel (and school nurse, if one exists) to tailor efforts for a particular pregnant teen to keep her in school. Specific needs to be addressed include the following: (1) using the bathroom frequently, (2) carrying and consuming more fluids or snacks to relieve nausea, (3) climbing stairs and carrying heavy book bags, and (4) fitting comfortably behind stationary desks. Schools that are committed to keeping students enrolled are generally helpful and will assist in accommodating special needs.

TEEN PREGNANCY AND THE NURSE

Nurses can influence teen pregnancy through appropriate interventions at home and in the community.

Home-Based Interventions

Nurses can identify young women at risk for pregnancy in families currently receiving services. Younger sisters of pregnant teens were 4.8 times more likely to become pregnant themselves with an increase to 5.1 times more likely if both sister and mother had a teen birth (Wall-Wieler et al., 2016). Nurses can offer anticipatory guidance addressing sexuality issues to the parents of all preteens and teens during home visits to increase their knowledge and awareness.

Visiting the pregnant teen in her home allows the nurse to assess the facilities available at home for management of her pregnancy needs and the suitability of the environment for her child. Some specific areas to assess are adequacy of heating and cooling, a source of water, cleanliness of the home, cooking facilities, and food storage. The nurse may find it more convenient for parents and other family members to participate in education and counseling sessions in their own home. Also, the need for financial assistance and other social service support may be more easily identified. Home visiting by nurses during a young woman's pregnancy can be critical in achieving compliance with antepartum goals concerning weight gain, good nutrition, and prenatal medical concerns (Fig. 35.2).

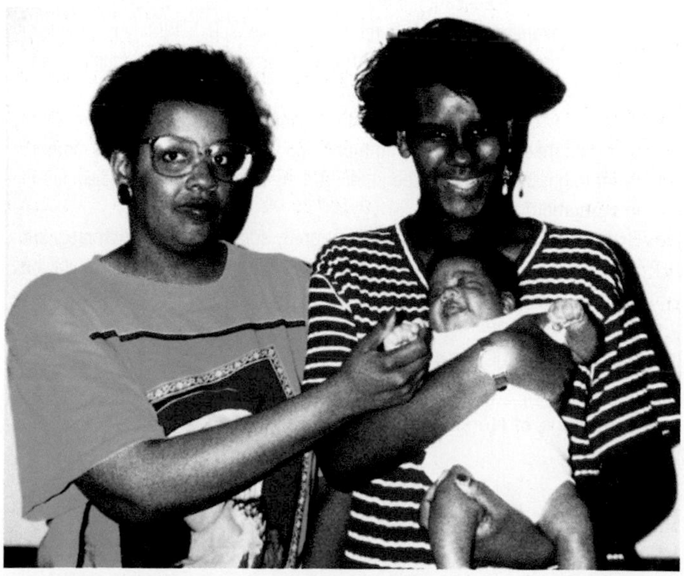

Fig. 35.2 The teen mother and the teen's own mother can be included in health teaching.

A teen pregnancy can shift the family dynamics. Families may go through stages of reactions. First, a crisis stage may occur, characterized by many emotions and conflict. By the third trimester, a honeymoon stage may occur, with greater acceptance and understanding of the teen and the impending birth. Finally, after the infant's birth, reorganization may occur, during which conflict may emerge again over issues of childcare and the young woman's role. The nurse can facilitate family coping and resolution of these stages by treating the family as client and assessing each person's role and strengths. Ultimately, family support for a teen parent can positively influence both mother and infant (Marino et al., 2016). A balance of moderate family guidance and supplementary care supports young mothers in their parenting role rather than replacing it.

QSEN FOCUS ON QUALITY AND SAFETY EDUCATION FOR NURSES

Teen Pregnancy

Targeted Competency: Evidence-Based Practice

Integrate best current evidence with clinical expertise and client/family preferences and values for delivery of optimal health care.

Important aspects of evidence-based practice (EBP) include:

- **Knowledge:** Describe EBP to include the components of research evidence, clinical expertise, and client/family values
- **Skills:** Locate evidence reports related to clinical practice topics and guidelines
- **Attitudes:** Value the need for continuous improvement in clinical practice based on new knowledge

Evidence-Based Practice Question

You are a registered nurse (RN) in a community-based health clinic conducting sports physicals for high-school aged students. You conduct a physical assessment on a female 18-year-old student, Gloria, who has been accompanied to this appointment by her mother. During the physical examination, Gloria confides in you that she is sexually active and is not currently using any form of contraception because her mother is not supportive. You ask Gloria if she would like to be using birth control, and she says that she is not sure. You provide Gloria some educational materials on various contraceptive methods.

After the examination Gloria's mother asks to speak with you privately. Gloria's mother is moderately emotional, worried that her daughter has been sexually active and might be pregnant.

- What are your legal limits around sharing information with Gloria's mother?
- Based on these limits, what information do you share with Gloria's mother?
- What might be your next step in facilitating a mother-daughter dialogue in this situation?
- Find a nursing research article about family communication with pregnant teens. Are there guidelines or outcomes from research that might be applied to this clinical scenario?
- What other patient outcome might you identify that could lead to a successful intervention in this scenario?

Prepared by Gail Armstrong, PhD, DNP, ACNS-BC, CNE, Associate Professor, College of Nursing, University of Colorado.

Community-Based Interventions

Many communities have broad-based coalitions and planning councils that facilitate a comprehensive approach to teen pregnancy. These groups usually include health care professionals, social workers, clergy, school personnel, businessmen, legislators, and members of other youth-serving agencies. Nurses play a significant role on this team by participating in or organizing community assessments, public awareness campaigns, group education (for professionals, parents, and youths), and interprofessional programs for high-risk youths. Community acceptance is more likely when there is a broad base of support for activities directed at the reduction of teen pregnancy or reduction of consequences.

LINKING CONTENT TO PRACTICE

Just as providing care to pregnant teens includes many of the *Healthy People 2020* objectives; this care is also consistent with the standards and competencies for public health professionals, including nurses. Specifically, the nurse assesses the teen population, determines priorities for nursing actions based on the assessment, develops a plan, and implements the plan by coordinating care with many appropriate agencies. In dealing with pregnant teenagers, it is essential to work with schools and many social service agencies in order to provide age-appropriate care and health education for both the teen and the baby. Skills in the core competencies such as assessment, planning, cultural competency, and communication are essential when providing care to this population.

From American Nurses Association: *Scope & standards of practice: public health nursing,* ed. 3, Silver Spring, MD, 2015, ANA; Public Health Foundation Council on Linkages: *Core competencies for public health professionals,* Washington, DC, June 26, 2014, revised and adopted, PHF.

Research has evaluated years of pregnancy prevention programs. As less funding is available, programs must stand out to receive financial support. Research summaries that can be used by communities for strategic planning are available from the Power to Decide organization's national campaign to prevent teen and unplanned pregnancy (https://powertodecide.org), based in Washington, DC. Programs that have been evaluated fall into one of three categories: programs that focus on sexual factors (this includes educational programs addressing sexual behavior and STD/HIV), programs that focus on nonsexual behaviors (service learning that matches volunteerism with a didactic component), and programs that focus on both sexual and nonsexual factors (may bring other risk behaviors and/or protective factors into the curriculum). Because there is diversity available in the programs, communities can match their characteristics and needs with a program.

Health teachers may ask nurses to provide educational materials or assistance with classroom instruction, especially in the areas of family planning, STDs, and pregnancy. Schools that do not have nurses may arrange to have a nurse from the health department available for health consultations with students during school hours. Schools may also request that nurses participate on their health advisory boards.

School-based health care clinics are operating in nearly 2000 elementary, middle, and high schools in the United States (Health Resources and Services Administration, 2017). The services offered may include counseling, referrals, and primary care services. Many middle and high school clinics offer reproductive services, which may include contraception and abstinence counseling, pregnancy and STD testing, dispensing contraceptives, and offering prenatal care. Reproductive health counseling can be vital in efforts to increase the use of contraception, reduce teen pregnancy, and improve student attendance and high school graduation (County Health Rankings and Roadmaps, 2017). The nurse can assist school systems with designing these programs, as well as referring young women in need of reproductive health care services.

Nurses bring their knowledge about youth and reproductive behavior to any organization or group that has teens, their parents, or other professionals working with teens. Churches are becoming increasingly interested in addressing the needs of their youth, especially because teen sexual activity, pregnancy, and parenting are affecting more of their members.

EVIDENCE-BASED PRACTICE

When adolescents become parents they face challenges that set them apart from adult parents. Outcomes for teen parents and their children have been generously studied and clearly stated. What has been lacking in nursing research is a better understanding of the elements of nursing intervention that can improve these outcomes.

Previous studies have identified that pregnant and parenting adolescents can benefit from visiting nursing care on many fronts. This includes decreasing hospitalizations, emergency department visits, and repeat pregnancies; increasing spacing between births; reducing domestic violence; and more. These studies focused more on the improved outcomes rather than informing nursing on the process by which this happens.

This study adds to the data that help us understand how to help teenagers become parents. It focuses on information gathered from 30 public health nurses (PHNs) visiting pregnant and parenting teenagers. These PHNs submitted stories about their young clients, and those were analyzed to understand the basic social psychological problems experienced, as well as the basic social psychological process used by the PHN to help the adolescent attain stronger parenting skills.

Nurse Use

The data that emerged from this study confirmed that adolescents begin parenting with negative life circumstances, a poor knowledge base, and a lack of awareness of how to attain the knowledge. The elements of the PHN interventions that improved the adolescents' role as parents were wide ranging and included case management, health education, counseling, and referral. This greater understanding about the process in which PHN home visiting works is essential for targeted and effective nursing interventions (Atkinson & Peden-McAlpine, 2014).

PRACTICE APPLICATION

A local youth-serving agency requested the assistance of a nurse, Kristen Brown, in the implementation of a new high school–based program for pregnant and parenting teen girls. The primary goal of the program is to keep these teens in school through graduation. The secondary goal is to provide knowledge and skills about healthy pregnancy, labor and delivery, and parenting. After delivery, students enrolled in this program were paid for school attendance, and this money could be used to defray the costs of childcare.

A nurse from the health department was the ideal choice to conduct the educational sessions. The group met weekly during the lunch hour. The curriculum that was developed included topics from early pregnancy through the toddler years. Occasionally, Ms. Brown recruited outside speakers such as a labor and delivery nurse or an early intervention specialist.

She also met individually with each enrolled student to provide case management services. Ideally, she would ensure that each student had a health care provider for prenatal care, that each was visited at home by a nurse, that each had enrolled in WIC and Medicaid if eligible, and that both the pregnant teen and her partner knew about other parenting and support groups.

One educational session that was particularly interesting was the discussion about the postpartum course—the six weeks after delivery. There were many lively discussions about labor experiences as well as some emotional discussions about the reality of coming home with a baby and changes in the relationship with their male partner. Accurate contraception information was provided, which helped to clarify the many myths the girls had heard from friends and older women. Many girls benefited from understanding the normalcy of postpartum blues, but one young woman recognized that she had a more serious and persistent depression and privately approached the nurse for assistance.

At the end of the first school year, the dropout rate for pregnant and parenting teens was reduced by half, and preterm labor rates had also declined. The local school board and a local youth-serving agency joined together to provide financial support to continue this program for an additional two years. Ms. Brown was asked to expand the educational programs and interventions she had developed.

What are some directions in which Ms. Brown might expand the program? List four.

Answers can be found on the Evolve site.

KEY POINTS

- The provision of reproductive health care services to adolescents requires sensitivity to the special needs of this age group. This includes knowing about state laws regarding confidentiality and services for birth control, pregnancy, abortion, and adoption.
- Pregnant teenagers have a substantial percent of the first births in the United States. They are more likely to deliver prematurely and have a low-birth-weight baby. This risk can be reduced by early initiation of prenatal care and good nutrition.

- Factors that can influence whether a young woman becomes pregnant include a history of sexual victimization, family dysfunction, substance use, and failure to use birth control. Several factors may overlap.
- Nutritional needs during pregnancy can be challenged if the teenager has unhealthy eating habits and begins the pregnancy with limited reserves of vitamins and minerals. With education the adolescent can make good food choices while still snacking or eating fast foods. Weight gain during pregnancy is a significant marker for a normal-weight baby.
- Young men need special attention and preparation as they become fathers. The interventions include information about pregnancy and delivery, declaration of paternity, care of infants and children, and psychosocial support in this role.
- The pregnant teen will need support during her pregnancy and in child-rearing. Families may provide most of this support. However, many communities have a variety of services available for adolescents. These services include financial assistance for medical care, nutritional programs, and school-based support groups.
- Adolescent parents often have unrealistic expectations about their children and may not know how to stimulate emotional, social, and cognitive development. The children born to adolescents are at risk for academic and behavioral problems as they become older. Teens who receive education on normal development and childcare are more likely to avert these problems with their children.
- During a pregnancy, teenagers are expected to attend school. Homebound instruction is reserved for those with medical complications. Teen mothers who return to school and complete their education after the birth of their child are less likely to have a repeat pregnancy. Problems finding childcare and the need to have an income can create an obstacle to school return.
- Community coalitions, which include nurses, can have a significant impact on teen pregnancy. These coalitions generally have diverse representation from the community, and therefore their activities meet with more community support.

CLINICAL DECISION-MAKING ACTIVITIES

1. Become familiar with statistics on teen pregnancy, births, miscarriages, and abortions in your area, and collect information on use of prenatal care, low-birth-weight and premature deliveries, high school completion, and repeat pregnancies. Compare the trends in statistics to the impact and costs to the individual, her family, and the community.
2. Call or visit local schools, and interview the school nurse or guidance counselors about teen pregnancy. Determine what resources are available through the schools for pregnancy prevention. Assess the family life education curriculum, and identify a teaching project for nursing students. Can pregnancy prevention and parenting education be incorporated into the learning objectives in the existing school curriculum?
3. Design and offer a childbirth preparation class for pregnant teens and their support persons. Include a plan for identifying potential participants, select a site that is accessible, and develop an evaluation method. Develop teaching tools that acknowledge adolescent development.
4. Assess reproductive health care services for young men in your community. Design an awareness campaign targeting young men on paternity issues and the prevention of pregnancy. Be specific about ways to incorporate male role models and mentors.

ADDITIONAL RESOURCES

EVOLVE WEBSITE

http://evolve.elsevier.com/Stanhope/community/

- Answers to Practice Application
- Case Study
- Glossary
- Review Questions

REFERENCES

Abu-Ouf NM, Jan MM: The impact of maternal iron deficiency and iron deficiency anemia on child's health, *Saudi Med J* 36(2):146–149, 2015.

American College of Obstetricians and Gynecologists: *ACOG strengthens LARC recommendations*, 2015. Retrieved from https://www.acog.org.

American College of Obstetricians and Gynecologists: *Frequently asked questions pregnancy. FAQ001*, 2018. Retrieved from https://www.acog.org.

American Nurses Association: *Scope & standards of practice: public health nursing*, ed 3, Silver Spring, Maryland, 2015, ANA.

Angley M, Divney A, Magriples U, Kershaw T: Social support, family functioning and parenting competence in adolescent parents, *Matern Child Health J* 19(1):67–73, 2015.

Atkinson LD, Peden-McAlpine CJ: Advancing adolescent maternal development: a grounded theory, *J Pediatr Nurs* 29:168–176, 2014.

Bekaert S, SmithBattle L: Teen mothers' experience of intimate partner violence: a metasynthesis, *ANS Adv Nurs Sci* 39(3): 272–290, 2016.

Brandsen CK: *A case for adoption,* Grand Rapids, MI, 1991, Bethany.

Centers for Disease Control and Prevention (CDC): *HIV Among youth*, 2018a. Retrieved from https://www.cdc.gov.

Centers for Disease Control and Prevention (CDC): *Youth risk behavior surveillance — United States, 2017*, 2018b. Retrieved from https://www.cdc.gov.

Centers for Disease Control and Prevention (CDC): *Weight gain during pregnancy*, 2018c. Retrieved from https://www.cdc.gov.

Centers for Disease Control and Prevention (CDC): *Social determinants and eliminating disparities in teen pregnancy*, 2017a. Retrieved from https://www.cdc.gov.

Centers for Disease Control and Prevention (CDC): *Help your teen make healthy choices about sex*, 2017b. Retrieved from https://www.cdc.gov.

Centers for Disease Control and Prevention (CDC): *Preventing repeat teen births*, 2013. Retrieved from https://www.cdc.gov.

Charlton BM, Roberts AL, Rosario M, et al.: Teen Pregnancy Risk Factors among Young Women of Diverse Sexual Orientations, *Pediatrics* 141(4):e20172278, 2018. Retrieved from http://pediatrics.aappublications.org.

Chilcoat D, Pai-Espinosa J, Burton B, Banning S, Prummer M: *Breaking the cycle of intergenerational teen pregnancy using a trauma-informed approach. U.S. Department of health and human services, office of adolescent health*, 2016. Retrieved from https://www.hhs.gov.

Cornforth T: *Healthy eating for pregnant teens. Very well family organization*, 2018. Retrieved from https://www.verywellfamily.com.

County Health Rankings and Roadmaps: *School-based health clinics with reproductive health services*, 2017. Retrieved from http://www.countyhealthrankings.org.

Dumas SA, Terrell IW, Gustafson M: Health and social needs of young mothers, *MCN AM J Matern Child Nurs* 43(3):146–152, 2018.

Ethier KA, Kann L, McManus T: Sexual intercourse among high school students—29 States and United States overall, 2005–2015, *MMWR Morb Mortal Wkly Rep* 66:1393–1397, 2018.

Farrell T, Clyde A, Katta M, Bolland J: The impact of sexuality concerns on teenage pregnancy: a consequence of heteronormativity? *Cult Health Sex* 19(1):135–149, 2017.

Garwood SK, Gerassi L, Jonson-Reid M, Plax K, Drake B: More than poverty—teen pregnancy risk and reports of child abuse reports and neglect, *J Adolesc Health* 57(2):164–168, 2015.

Gregg D, Somers CL, Pernice FM, Hillman SB, Kernsmith P: Sexting rates and predictors from an urban Midwest high school, *J School Health* 88(6):423–433, 2018.

Guttmacher Institute: *Adolescent sexual and reproductive health in the United States*, New York, 2017, Guttmacher Institute. Retrieved from https://www.guttmacher.org.

Guttmacher Institute: *An overview of minors' consent law*, New York, 2018, Guttmacher Institute. Retrieved from https://www.guttmacher.org.

Guttmacher Institute: *Contraception drives decline in teen pregnancy—and expanded access to LARC methods could accelerate this trend*, New York, 2014. Guttmacher Institute. Retrieved from https://www.guttmacher.org.

Health Resources and Services Administration: *School-based health centers*, 2017. Retrieved from https://www.hrsa.gov.

Healthy Children Organization (HCO): *Teen parents*, 2017, American Academy of Pediatrics. Retrieved from https://www.healthychildren.org.

Heaman MI, Moffatt M, Elliott L, et al.: Barriers, motivators and facilitators related to prenatal care utilization among inner-city women in Winnipeg, Canada: a case–control study, *BMC Pregnancy Childbirth* 14:227, 2014.

Kost K, Maddow-Zimet I, Arpaia A: *Pregnancies, births and abortions among adolescents and young women in the United States, 2013: national and state trends by age, race and ethnicity*, New York, 2017, Guttmacher Institute. Retrieved from https://www.guttmacher.org.

Martin JA, Hamilton BE, Osterman MJ, Driscoll AK, Drake P: *Births: Final data for 2016*, Hyattsville, MD, 2018, National Center for Health Statistics. Retrieved from https://www.cdc.gov.

Marino JL, Lewis LN, Bateson D, Hickey M, Skinner SR: Teenager mothers, *Aust Fam Physician* 45(10):712–717, 2016.

Martinez GM, Abma JC: *Sexual activity, contraceptive use, and childbearing of teenagers aged 15–19 in the United States*, NCHS Data Brief, 2015. Retrieved from https://www.cdc.gov.

Marvin-Dowle K, Kilner K, Burley VJ, Soltani H: Impact of adolescent age on maternal and neonatal outcomes in the Born in Bradford cohort, *BMJ Open* 8:e016258, 2018.

Masho SW, Chambers GJ, Wallenborn JT, Ferrance JL: Associations of partner age gap at sexual debut with teenage parenthood and lifetime number of partners, *Perspect Sexl Reprod Health* 49(2):77–83, 2017.

Massachusetts General Hospital (MGH): *Teen dads: the forgotten parent*, 2016. Retrieved from http://www.thefatherhoodproject.org.

McHugh MT, Kvernland A, Palusci V: An adolescent parents' programme to reduce child abuse, *Chld Abuse Review* 26(3):184–195, 2015.

Naeye RL: Teenaged and pre-teenaged pregnancies: consequences of the fetal-maternal competition for nutrients, *Pediatr* 67(1):146–150, 1981.

National Abortion and Reproductive Rights Action League Foundation (NARAL): *U.S. Supreme Court Decisions Concerning Reproductive Rights: 1927–2016*, Washington, DC, 2017, NARAL. Retrieved from https://www.prochoiceamerica.org.

National Abortion and Reproductive Rights Action League Foundation (NARAL): *Who decides? The status of women's reproductive rights in the United States,* ed 25, Washington, DC, 2016, NARAL. Retrieved from https://www.prochoiceamerica.org.

National Conference of State Legislators (NCSL): *Postcard: teen pregnancy affects graduation rates*, 2013. Retrieved from http://www.ncsl.org.

Pirog MA, Jung H, Lee D: The changing face of teenage parenthood in the United States: evidence from NLSY79 and NLSY97, *Child Youth Care Forum* 47:317–342, 2017.

Planned Parenthood: *Birth control*, 2018. Retrieved from https://www.plannedparenthood.org.

Public Health Foundation Council on Linkages: *Core competencies for public health professionals*, Washington, DC, June 26, 2014 revised and adopted, PHF.

Restall A, Taylor RS, Thompson JM, et al.: Risk factors for excessive gestational weight gain in a healthy, nulliparous cohort, *J Obes* 2014:148391, 2014.

Romero L, Pazol K, Warner L, et al.: Reduced disparities in birth rates among teens aged 15–19 years—United States, 2006–2007 and 2013–2014, *MMWR Morb Mortal Wkly Rep* 65:409–414, 2016.

Sedgh G, Finer LB, Bankole A, Eilers MA, Singh S: Adolescent pregnancy, birth, and abortion rates across countries: levels and recent trends, *J Adolesc Health* 56(2):223–230, 2015.

Soltani H, Duxbury A, Rundle R, Chan L: A systematic review of the effects of dietary interventions on neonatal outcomes in adolescent pregnancy, *Evid Based Mdwfry* 13(1):29–34, 2015.

The Urban Child Institute: *How adolescent parenting affects children, families, and communities*, 2014. Retrieved from http://www.urbanchildinstitute.org.

U.S. Department of Health and Human Services: *Healthy people 2020*, Washington, DC, 2010, USDHHS. Retrieved from https://www.healthypeople.gov.

U.S. Department of Health and Human Services (USDHHS): *Office of adolescent health: trends in teen pregnancy and childbearing*, 2016a. Retrieved from https://www.hhs.gov.

U.S. Department of Health and Human Services (USDHHS): *Office of adolescent health: negative impacts of teen childbearing*, 2016b. Retrieved from https://www.hhs.gov.

Vázquez-Nava F, Vázquez-Rodriguez CF, Saldívar-González AH, et al.: Unplanned pregnancy in adolescents: association with family structure, employed mother, and female friends with health-risk habits and behaviors, *J Urban Health* 91(1): 176–185, 2014.

Wall-Wieler E, Roos LL, Nickel NC: Teenage pregnancy: the impact of maternal adolescent childbearing and older sister's teenage pregnancy on a younger sister, *BMC Pregnancy Childbirth* 16:120, 2016.

36

Mental Health Issues

Anita Thompson-Heisterman, MSN, PMHCNS-BC, PMHNP-BC

OBJECTIVES

After reading this chapter, the student should be able to do the following:

1. Describe the history of community mental health and make predictions about the future.
2. Discuss the prevalence of mental illness in the United States and globally.
3. Describe essential mental health services and corresponding national objectives for improving mental health.
4. Evaluate standards, models, concepts, strategies, and research findings for use in community mental health nursing practice to improve community mental health.
5. Describe the role of the community mental health nurse with individuals and with groups at risk for psychiatric mental health problems.
6. Apply the nursing process in community work with clients diagnosed with psychiatric disorders, families at risk for mental health problems, and vulnerable populations.

CHAPTER OUTLINE

Scope of Mental Illness in the United States
Systems of Community Mental Health Care
Evolution of Community Mental Health Care
Deinstitutionalization
Conceptual Frameworks for Community Mental Health
Role of the Nurse in Community Mental Health
Current and Future Perspectives in Mental Health Care
National Objectives for Mental Health Services

KEY TERMS

Americans with Disabilities Act, p. 795
assertive community treatment, p. 797
community mental health centers, p. 793
Community Mental Health Centers Act, p. 794
community mental health model, p. 793
Community Support Program, p. 791
consumer advocacy, p. 791
consumers, p. 795
deinstitutionalization, p. 794
institutionalization, p. 793
intensive case management models, p. 797
managed care, p. 792
mental health problems, p. 790
National Alliance for the Mentally Ill, p. 795
National Institute of Mental Health, p. 794
parity, p. 792
Patient Protection and Affordable Health Care Act, p. 792
recovery, p. 797
reinstitutionalization, p. 795
relapse management, p. 797
serious mental illness, p. 790
severe mental disorders, p. 790
systems theory, p. 796
wellness recovery action plans, p. 804

Because providing community services and nursing care to people suffering from mental illness or emotional distress is complex and influenced by many individual and community factors, it requires a variety of approaches. Complicating factors include (1) the scope of emotional and mental disorders; (2) uncertainty about the specific cause, cure, and treatment for the most severe mental disorders; (3) the severe chronic disabling nature of some mental disorders; and (4) the complexity of the community mental health services sector. The scarcity of resources compounds the problems and presents challenges in community mental health work.

Cultural beliefs and economics influence the amount and types of services and treatment available in various countries. However, two universal truths exist: services for people with mental disorders are inadequate in all countries, and mental illness has a significant effect on families, communities, and nations. Therefore specialized knowledge and skills about severe mental illness and mental health problems are necessary for effective nursing practice in the community. It is helpful to understand both the organization of mental health services from a historical perspective and the trends in current health care demands and delivery. Knowledge about populations at risk for psychiatric mental health problems and understanding illness outcomes in terms of biopsychosocial consequences are even more important. Finally, it is necessary to refine and broaden nursing process skills in treatment planning to include the impact of mental illness on families and communities.

This chapter focuses on the scope of mental disorders, the development of community mental health services, the current health objectives for mental health and mental disorders, and the role of the nurse in community settings. Conceptual frameworks useful in community mental health nursing practice are also presented. Because other chapters in this book are devoted to high-risk groups such as the homeless population and those with substance abuse problems, this chapter's focus is on the variety of **mental health problems** encountered in communities, with an emphasis on populations that have long-term, **severe mental disorders** and groups that are most vulnerable to mental health problems.

SCOPE OF MENTAL ILLNESS IN THE UNITED STATES

Mental health is defined in *Healthy People 2020* (U.S. Department of Health and Human Services [USDHHS], 2010) as encompassing the ability to engage in productive activities and fulfilling relationships with other people, to adapt to change, and to cope with adversity. The World Health Organization (WHO) expands the definition, describing mental health as a state of well-being in which a person can realize his or her potential and notes that mental health is essential if a person is to have health (WHO, 2008). Mental health is an integral part of personal well-being, family and other interpersonal relationships, and contributions to community or society. Mental disorders are conditions that are characterized by alterations in thinking, mood, or behavior that are associated with distress and/or impaired functioning. Mental illness refers collectively to all diagnosable mental disorders. Severe mental disorders are determined by diagnoses and criteria that include degree of functional disability (American Psychiatric Association [APA], 2013).

Mental disorders are indiscriminate. They occur across the life span and affect persons of all races, cultures, genders, and educational and socioeconomic groups. They are a leading cause of disability and even death. One in 10 people suffer from depression and/or anxiety, affecting 676 million people worldwide, and in 2012 there were 800,000 suicides, 86 percent of these in people under age 70 (WHO, 2018). In the United States nearly 18.3 percent of adults (age 18 years and older) have a mental health condition severe enough to impair daily function, and 5.9 percent of these suffer from a **serious mental illness** such as schizophrenia (Substance Abuse and Mental Health Services Administration [SAMHSA], 2015). Nearly half of those with any mental disorder (8.1 percent) meet criteria for two disorders, mental health and substance abuse (SAMHSA, 2017). According to the Centers for Disease Control and Prevention (CDC), there were alarming and increasing rates of opioid abuse, overdoses, and suicide in the United States between 1999 and 2014 (CDC, 2016). The rate of suicide rose from 12.3 to 15.4 per 100,000 people with middle-aged adults ages 45-65 having the largest increase.

Since 2008 prevalence rates of serious mental illness among young adults ages 18-25 have increased from 3.8 to 5.9 percent, yet only half of those received any mental health treatment (SAMHSA, 2017). In 2016 between 7 and 12 percent of youth ages 12-17 had an emotional disturbance serious enough to impair function, and 20 million people over the age of 12 had a substance use disorder (SAMHSA, 2017). Adolescent mental health is a global concern as well (WHO, 2014); 14.5 percent of people over age 50 have a mental disorder, and these rates may rise as the number of older Americans increases over the next two decades. Alzheimer's disease, the primary cause of dementia, is increasing. In 2018 an estimated 5.7 million Americans had Alzheimer's disease. This number includes 5.7 million people who were 65 years or older and about 200,000 individuals under age 65 who had younger-onset Alzheimer's disease (Alzheimer's Association, 2018). The number of cases in the population doubles every 5 years of age after age 60 and is becoming a public health crisis as the baby boomer generation ages. Currently there are 53 million people with Alzheimer's disease, and by 2050 there will be 88 million. Affective disorders include major depression and manic-depressive or bipolar illness. Although bipolar illness may affect only a small proportion of the population, major depression is pervasive and is the leading cause of disability among adults ages 15 to 44. Anxiety disorders, including panic disorder, obsessive-compulsive disorder, post-traumatic stress disorder (PTSD), and phobias, are prevalent, affecting 18 percent of American adults each year. Mental disorders can also be a secondary problem among people with other disabilities. Depression and anxiety, for example, occur more frequently among people with disabilities (NIMH, 2014).

The impact of mental illness on overall health and productivity in the United States and throughout the world is often underrecognized. In the United States mental illness causes about the same amount of disability as heart disease and cancer. Despite the prevalence of mental illness, less than half of persons with a mental disorder obtain help for their illness in any part of the health care system, and the majority of persons with mental disorders do not receive any specialty mental health care. Although 65 percent of persons with the most serious mental illnesses received treatment in 2016, 35 percent did not (SAMHSA, 2017). Sixty percent of youth and 57 percent of adults received no mental health treatment. The WHO (2008) reports the global burden of mental health, substance abuse, and neurological diseases at 14 percent and noted that depression is the main cause of illness and disability in adolescents worldwide (WHO, 2014). In recognition of the lack of resources, the WHO launched a mental health global action program (mhGAP) to begin to address mental health needs (WHO, 2008). Their poster "No Health Without Mental Health" effectively describes the need to integrate physical and mental health services. Given this information, it is critical that nurses recognize and provide health services for those with mental disorders in a variety of nontraditional community settings.

In addition to diagnosable mental conditions, there is growing awareness and concern about the public health burden of stress, especially after terrorist attacks at home and globally; natural disasters, such as hurricanes, tsunamis, tornados, fires, and earthquakes; and human-made disasters such as gun violence in schools, public spaces, and communities. Strengthening the public health sector to respond to these events involves developing community mental health responses, as well as addressing physical health concerns. Community mental health nurses (CMHNs) play an important role in identifying stressful events, assessing stress responses, educating communities, and intervening to prevent or alleviate disability and disease resulting from trauma.

Although all of us are vulnerable to stressful life events and may develop mental health problems, persons with chronic and persistent mental illness have numerous problems. Mental illness is misunderstood, and those who suffer from it often experience stigma and lack of social support, which is so critical to health. Persons with mental illness are often identified by the illness as a schizophrenic instead of a person with the disease of schizophrenia. The disruptive symptoms of this illness often occur just as young persons are attempting to finish schooling and develop a career, shattering lives and driving many into a lifetime of underemployment, poverty, and lack of access to adequate health services, housing, and social supports. Many accessible and coordinated services are needed to enable people with chronic mental illness to live in the community, yet these often are not available. Despite the inadequacy of resources, advances have been made in the treatment of mental illness. Two major movements have influenced these advances: consumer advocacy and a better understanding of the neurobiology of mental illness, requiring a more integrated view of the complexity of factors involved (Macedo, 2017; Pandya & Jän Myrick, 2013). Naturally, the financing of mental health services affects access to care and influences treatment. The system known as managed care significantly affected service delivery for the past 30 years, and passage of mental health parity and national health care reform through the Patient Protection and Affordable Health Care Act have influenced mental health care more recently (Ali et al., 2016; Cowell et al., 2017; Mechanic & Olfson, 2016; Pearlman, 2013).

Consumer Advocacy

Consumer advocacy movements for people with mental illness, like those for other illnesses, came about to fulfill unmet needs and to attempt to decrease the stigma associated with mental illness. Specifically, the National Alliance for the Mentally Ill (NAMI) was the first consumer group to advocate for better services. This consumer advocacy group worked to establish education and self-help services for individuals and families with mental illness. Efforts of the NAMI gained momentum in the early 1980s. Subsequently, political groups and legislative bodies responded with direct support. One example of direct support was funding for the **Community Support Program** (CSP) by the National Institute of Mental Health (NIMH). The CSP provided grant monies to states to develop comprehensive services for persons discharged from psychiatric institutions and invited consumers to participate. These and similar efforts have helped bring consumers, families, and professionals together to work toward improvement in the treatment and care of persons with mental illness.

Neurobiology of Mental Illness

Mental illnesses are complex biopsychosocial disorders. Considerable emphasis in the past 20 years has focused on the biological basis of mental illness. The 1990s were declared the "decade of the brain" as advances in research in neurology, microbiology, and genetics led to understanding the structural and chemical complexity of the brain. Consequently, more is now known about the functions of the brain than at any time in history. We have learned that the brain is not a static organ. The concept of brain plasticity demonstrates that new learning actually changes brain structure. For example, traumatic experiences change brain biochemistry, as do significant positive experiences (Nusslock & Miller, 2016; Rosenzweig et al., 2017). This information supports the thought that both experience and psychosocial factors have effects on the etiology and on the treatment of mental illnesses. Both somatic and psychosocial interventions need to be used to treat mental illness. In addition to research, neuroradiological techniques aid diagnosis and treatment of people with psychiatric disorders. Angiography is used to screen for abnormalities of the vascular system, such as atherosclerosis and brain tumors, that can lead to behavior changes. The use of noninvasive scanning of the brain can help in making diagnoses. Computed axial tomography (CAT) scans provide a cross-sectional view of the brain, whereas nuclear magnetic resonance (NMR) imaging offers the advantage of imaging the brain from different planes. Still other techniques, such as positron emission tomography (PET) and single-photon emission computed tomography (SPECT), provide information about cerebral blood flow and brain metabolism. The information gained from these advanced technologies can lead to better understanding about mental illness and treatment and help scientists study the effects of psychotherapeutic interventions on the brain. Discoveries in psychopharmacology have also revolutionized the treatment of mental illness. New, atypical antipsychotic drugs used in the treatment of schizophrenia can improve the quality of life for many, primarily because of fewer side effects. For example, side effects of antipsychotic drugs include central and peripheral nervous system manifestations. Newer second-generation antipsychotics have reduced some of these side effects, but new adverse effects, including weight gain, insulin resistance, and dangerously high blood glucose levels, collectively known as metabolic syndrome, have created fresh concerns for consumers and providers (Rojo et al., 2015). Although psychopharmacology has dramatically improved the lives of people with severe mental illness, controversies exist about the costs of monitoring treatment. Newer antidepressant medications known as selective serotonin reuptake inhibitors (SSRIs) are now considered the first choice in the treatment of depression as well as for many anxiety disorders because they lead to good responses with fewer side effects. They are now widely prescribed by primary care physicians, as well as psychiatrists, and are some of the most prescribed medications in the United States. Although considered safer than older agents, evidence suggests that the SSRIs may accelerate bone loss, leading to osteoporosis, and they may not be more effective than non-pharmacological interventions, such as exercise, in treating some depression (Holmes, 2016). Future directions suggest the science of pharmacogenetics might enable more individualized treatment of mental illness based on specific, genetically based responses to pharmaceuticals (Rojo et al., 2015).

SYSTEMS OF COMMUNITY MENTAL HEALTH CARE

Managed Care

Managed care is a system of managing health care to ensure access to appropriate and cost-effective services. Managed mental health care grew rapidly during the 1990s, and by 1999 nearly 80 percent of Americans were enrolled in a managed health care plan. Initially a method to control costs and access to mental health care in the private insurance sector, managed care became a significant factor in public mental health, and by the turn of the century more than half of all Medicaid recipients were enrolled in a managed mental health care plan (Mechanic & Olfson, 2016). Consumer outcomes such as health status, quality of life, functioning, and satisfaction are considerations in deciding whether services are effective.

Because one purpose of managed care was to control costs, often by substituting less costly services for more costly ones, the findings about consumer outcomes become critical. The provision of quality comprehensive services needed by persons with serious and persistent mental illness in the community is not inexpensive, but it is generally less costly than hospital care and frequent admissions. Services must fit the needs of the consumer, and outcomes research and consumer satisfaction can help guide care and policy decisions.

Changes continue to take place in mental health funding, and changes in one sector can have far-reaching consequences in many others. Although legislation was passed in 1996 ensuring parity for mental illness coverage in insurance plans, the implementation at the state level and the effects on insurance plans had been rather negligible for a variety of reasons, and further legislation (the Mental Health Parity and Addiction Equity Act) passed in 2008 to improve service access (Mechanic & Olfson, 2016).

The seemingly constant changes in mental health funding present challenges for nurses, who need to make judgments about the positive and negative outcomes of these changes on the people they care for before research findings that can be generalized to the population are readily available.

Patient Protection and Affordable Health Care Act

The Patient Protection and Affordable Health Care Act (ACA, passed in 2010) affected both access to and funding of mental health services and increased the need for CMHNs at the general and advanced practice levels (Mechanic & Olfson, 2016; Pearlman, 2013). The ACA ensured access to mental health services for 27 million more Americans who had no coverage, and an additional 35.5 million were projected to received new or improved mental health services added to existing coverage (Mechanic & Olfson, 2016; Pearlman, 2013). Preventive mental health services, such as depression and behavioral screening, are now required to be offered free of charge, and integration of mental health services into primary care is mandated (USDHHS, 2014). The ACA removed economic and geographic barriers and helped remove the stigma of mental illness through routine screening and treatment within a primary care visit. It was expected that earlier detection and treatment of mental health and substance abuse conditions would occur, thus improving the mental health of the population (Busch et al., 2013). However, despite legislation promoting greater access to care, often substance abuse treatment was not covered (Cowell et al., 2017; Ali et al., 2016). Such a major change in the manner in which services were to be provided along with the expected increase in the number of people seeking mental health care did lead to new challenges and opportunities in the delivery of care. The ACA did increase access to mental health services for many, allowed young people up to the age of 26 to stay on their parent's health plan, prohibited insurers from denying benefits due to pre-existing conditions, and promoted integration of screening and health promotion into primary care. Some provisions of the ACA have recently been changed, and the requirement of enrollment has been discontinued. The future of funding for mental health services remains unclear.

Mental Health Services

Mental health problems and mental disorders are treated by a variety of caregivers who work in diverse and loosely connected facilities. The landmark surgeon general's report on mental health, in an attempt to delineate where Americans receive mental health services, defined four major ways through which people receive assistance: (1) the specialty mental health system, both public and private; (2) the general medical or primary care sector; (3) the human service sector; and (4) the voluntary support network, including advocacy groups (USDHHS, 1999). Nurses need to understand that delivery of mental health services may occur in any of these systems. In fact, most older adults receive mental health services through the primary care sector, whereas most children and adolescents are served through human services that include schools. Those with resources, less severe mental health problems, and access to primary care are more likely to have their mental health needs addressed within the context of a visit to their primary care provider. Because of the initial influence of managed care, access to a specialist, if indicated for psychiatric treatment, had occurred via this route as well. The ACA passed in 2010 now mandates mental health screening and initiation of treatment in primary care and has had an effect on where mental health services are received or at least initiated (Mechanic & Olfson, 2016; Pearlman, 2013). In the 29 states and Washington, DC, where expansion of Medicaid occurred, insurance coverage, access to care, use of preventative services, and self-assessed health increased, particularly among low-income childless adults (Miller & Wherry, 2017; Simon et al., 2017). Integration of behavioral and primary care systems was another benefit (Kim et al., 2017).

The **community mental health model** is the primary method of care for people with serious and persistent mental illness. Components of this model include team care, case management, outreach, and a variety of rehabilitative and recovery approaches to help prevent exacerbations of illness. In most states, services are provided through comprehensive **community mental health centers** (CMHCs). There is great variance in how each state and locality implements mental health service delivery, and each version continues to evolve in this era of health care reform and changing funding sources as the CMHCs react to societal, political, and fiscal pressures. As resources diminish, the focus narrows, and many CMHCs are unable to provide services to populations other than those with serious and persistent mental illness. It is unclear how the growing focus on integration of mental health into primary care, parity in insurance coverage, and the passage of and possible changes in the ACA will continue to impact the community mental health system of care. There has been movement toward more comprehensive, integrated, and less fragmented services and an emphasis on more utilization of mental health nurses as primary providers of care (Mechanic & Olfson, 2016).

EVOLUTION OF COMMUNITY MENTAL HEALTH CARE

Historical Perspectives

How the community has perceived the etiology of mental and emotional illness across the ages has influenced the care and treatment of persons suffering from these disorders. These patterns were often cyclical. In ancient times, mental illness was viewed as resulting from supernatural forces, and those afflicted were sometimes shunned. During the Greco-Roman era, mental and physical illnesses were seen as interrelated and resulting from physical conditions. Treatment was aimed at curing the disease by restoring balance. A return to a belief in supernatural etiologies occurred during the Middle Ages in Europe and continued in the years in which the United States was being formed into a country. These beliefs led to poor treatment of the mentally ill, including incarceration, starvation, and torture. Near the end of the eighteenth century, the revolution in mental health care known as Humanitarian Reform took place. This reform movement, influenced by Philippe Pinel (1759-1820) in France and Benjamin Rush (1745-1813) in North America, led to hospital expansion, medical treatment, and the community mental health movements (Boyd, 2018).

Before the Humanitarian Reform, persons with mental illness were often housed in jails because health and social services had not been developed. Even later, after the development of hospitals as a site of treatment, persons with mental disorders were neglected and mistreated. Although the first psychiatric hospital in the United States was built in Williamsburg, Virginia, in 1773, about 50 years passed before widespread construction of facilities in other states took place. One person in particular, Dorothea Dix, led reform efforts to correct inhumane practices (Boyd, 2018).

Dorothea Lynde Dix (1802-1887) focused attention on criminals, those with mental disorders, and victims of the Civil War. She believed that people with mental disorders needed health and social services, and her efforts influenced the improved organization of mental health services. Her work led to the development of hospitals as the primary site of care, and she influenced standards for hospital administration and nursing care. Because of her lifetime efforts, often through political action, treatment for mentally infirm persons was altered in both North America and Europe (Boyd, 2018).

Hospital Expansion, Institutionalization, and the Mental Hygiene Movement. Psychiatric hospitals constructed during the expansion era were located in rural areas and were intended for small numbers of clients. However, they soon became overcrowded with people who had severe mental disorders, older adults, and immigrants who were poor and unable to speak English. Clients were essentially separated from the community and isolated from their families. Many were institutionalized for the rest of their lives in response to both a continued fear of persons with mental disorders and a lack of community resources. **Institutionalization** of large numbers of people, combined with minimal information about cause, cure, and care, resulted in overcrowded conditions and exploitation of clients.

At the beginning of the twentieth century, institutional conditions were reported publicly in the United States by Clifford Beers, who had been hospitalized both in private and in public mental hospitals (Boyd, 2018). Beers urged reform and influenced the founding of the National Committee for Mental Hygiene. During the mental hygiene movement, attention shifted to ideas about prevention, early intervention, and the influence of social and environmental factors on mental illness. These ideas about treatment also influenced the development of multidisciplinary approaches to treatment. The mental hygiene and community mental health movements increased understanding about mental illness.

Further understanding about the scope of mental illness was gained during the conscription process for the armed services in World War II. Many of the persons screened for military service during World War II were found to have neurological and psychiatric mental health disorders. Even more military personnel required treatment for mental health problems associated with social and environmental stress during and after the war, not only in the United States but also in Europe, Russia, and Pacific Rim countries (Boyd, 2018). At the same time, the community mental health model continued to expand slowly, while populations consisting of individuals with severe mental disorders and older adult persons with dementia grew larger in the state hospitals. Demands for mental health services in communities, combined with concerns about conditions of state psychiatric hospitals, prompted federal legislation that influenced development of the community mental health concept.

Federal Legislation for Mental Health Services. The first major piece of legislation to influence mental health services in

TABLE 36.1 Legislation That Influenced Community Mental Health Services

Year	Legislation	Focus
1946	National Mental Health Act	Education and research for mental health treatment approaches began (NIMH)
1955	Mental Health Study Act	Resulted in Joint Commission on Mental Illness and Health, which recommended transformation of state hospital systems and establishment of community mental health clinics
1963	Community Mental Health Centers Act	Marked beginning of community mental health centers' concept and led to deinstitutionalization of large psychiatric hospitals
1975	Developmentally Disabled Assistance and Bill of Rights Act	Addressed the rights and treatment of people with developmental disabilities and provided foundation for similar action for individuals with mental disorders
1977	President's Commission on Mental Health	Reinforced importance of community-based services, protection of human rights, and national health insurance for mentally ill persons
1981	Omnibus Budget Reconciliation Act	Rescinded much of the 1977 commission's provisions and shifted funds for all health programs from federal to state resources
1986	Protection and Advocacy for Individuals with Mental Illness Act	Legislated advocacy programs for mentally ill persons
1990	Americans with Disabilities Act	Prohibited discrimination and promoted opportunities for persons with mental disorders
1996	Mental Health Parity Act	Attempted to address discrepancy between mental health and medical-surgical benefits in employer-sponsored health plans
2008	Mental Health Parity and Addiction Equity Act	Prohibits discrepancy in coverage between mental health and physical health benefits in employer-sponsored and private insurance plans and added substance abuse as a covered mental health condition
2010	Patient Protection and Affordable Health Care Act	Prohibits discrimination in coverage for pre-existing conditions; prohibits discontinuation of coverage because of illness

NIMH, National Institute of Mental Health.

the United States was the Social Security Act in 1935. This act, created in response to economic and social problems of the era, shifted the responsibility of care for ill people from the state to the federal government. The federal government's role expanded when the demand for mental health services increased during and after World War II. Key points of legislation that influenced the development of community mental health services are summarized in Table 36.1.

In 1946 the National Mental Health Act was passed and the **National Institute of Mental Health** (NIMH) administered its programs. Objectives included development of education and research programs for community mental health treatment approaches. The act also included financial incentives for training grants to increase the number of professional workers, including nurses, in mental health services. Education and research programs materialized readily, along with advances in science and technology and the development of psychotropic medications. In 1955 the Mental Health Study Act was passed, and the NIMH established the Joint Commission on Mental Illness and Health. Members of the commission studied national mental health needs and submitted to Congress a report entitled *Action for Mental Health.* Recommendations of the report included continued development of research and education programs, early and intensive treatment for acute mental illness, and shifting the care of severely mentally ill persons away from the large hospitals to psychiatric wards in general hospitals and to community mental health clinics. Along with prevention and intervention, community services were to include aftercare services following hospitalization for individuals with major mental illness (Boyd, 2018). The shift in the locus of care from state hospitals to community systems was begun.

The **Community Mental Health Centers Act** was passed in 1963, and the CMHC concept was formalized. Federal funds were designated to match state funds to construct CMHCs and start-up programs. CMHCs were mandated to have five basic services: inpatient, outpatient, partial hospitalization, 24-hour emergency services, and consultation/education services for community agencies and professionals. In addition, regulations encouraged states to offer diagnostic and rehabilitative precare and aftercare services (Boyd, 2018). However, many CMHCs, especially those in poor and rural areas, were unable to generate adequate money for continuing their start-up programs. Funding did not follow the client to the community. The deinstitutionalization of persons with severe mental disorders was well underway before some of these shortcomings were recognized.

DEINSTITUTIONALIZATION

Deinstitutionalization involved transitioning large numbers of people from state psychiatric hospitals to communities. The cost of institutional care was perhaps the main reason for the movement; other influences included the discovery of psychotropic medications and civil rights activism (Boyd, 2018). The goal of deinstitutionalization was to improve the quality of life for people with mental disorders by providing services in the communities where they lived rather than in large institutions. To change the locus of care, large hospital wards were closed, and persons with severe mental disorders were returned to the community to live. Many were discharged to the care of family members; others went to nursing homes. Still others were placed in apartments or other types of adult housing; some of these were supervised settings, and others were not.

Not surprisingly, as with any abrupt, dramatic change, problems related to unexpected service gaps between the hospitals and the CMHCs led to continuity-of-care problems. Although deinstitutionalization was a noble idea, resources to support the implementation were inadequate. For example, families were not prepared for the treatment responsibilities they had to assume, and yet few mental health systems offered them education and support programs. Although many older adult clients were admitted to nursing homes and personal care settings, education programs were seldom available for staff members, who often lacked the skills necessary to treat persons with mental disorders. And finally, some clients found themselves in independent settings such as rooming houses and single-room occupancy hotels with little or no supervision and few skills to manage living in the community. Clients, families, communities, and the nation suffered as poor living and social conditions were associated with mental disorders. Homelessness and placement of the mentally ill in jails and prisons also occurred. These conditions may have increased the stigma associated with persons with mental illness. The placement of persons with mental illness in nursing homes, assisted living facilities, and jails was often referred to as "**reinstitutionalization**," because it only shifted people from one institution to another. These issues prompted additional legislation and advocacy efforts.

Civil Rights Legislation for Persons With Mental Disorders

The development of CMHCs was based partially on the principle that persons with mental disorders had a right to treatment in the least restrictive environment (Boyd, 2018). Although CMHCs were less restrictive than institutions, they lacked necessary services. For example, people with severe mental disorders require daily monitoring or hospitalization during acute episodes of illness. Even though hospital services were available, many individuals expressed their rights to refuse treatment and resisted admission. Also, transitional care after discharge for those persons who were admitted to hospitals was not available in most communities. In addition to the right to refuse treatment, advocates for mentally ill individuals focused on such civil rights issues as segregated services, inhumane practices in psychiatric hospitals, and failure to include clients in treatment planning. Activism for minorities and handicapped persons also influenced civil rights legislation for persons with mental disorders. In particular, during the 1970s institutional conditions of persons with developmental handicaps prompted passage of the Developmentally Disabled Assistance and Bill of Rights Act. Other legislation shifted funding from the federal to the state level. The Mental Health Systems Act was passed in 1980 to improve mental health services. However, in 1981 when Ronald Reagan took office, the Act was repealed and replaced with a block grant program reducing the involvement of the federal government (Mechanic & Olfson, 2016). This action limited the federal leadership role, shifted more costs back to the states from the federal government, and further impeded the implementation and provision of community mental health services.

State systems of mental health services developed in unique and diverse ways and were often inadequate. In general, individuals with severe mental disorders were vulnerable and neglected and either lacked or were unable to access health and social services. In an effort to offset these problems, in 1986 the federal Protection and Advocacy for Individuals with Mental Illness Act and the State Comprehensive Mental Health Services Plan Act of 1986 were passed. Advocacy programs for mentally ill persons became part of the same state advocacy systems developed earlier under the Developmentally Disabled Assistance and Bill of Rights Act, and consumer involvement in CMHCs was mandated (Boyd, 2018). In spite of advocacy efforts and legislation, the CMHCs were unable to meet the increased and diverse demands for mental health services in their communities. The lack of services, combined with concerns about discrimination against all people with disabilities, led to additional legislation.

The **Americans with Disabilities Act** (ADA) was passed in 1990. The ADA mandated that individuals with mental and physical disabilities must not be discriminated against and must be brought into the mainstream of American life through access to employment and public services (Boyd, 2018). History reveals that past legislation promoted the rights of persons with mental disorders, but litigation was also responsible for the lack of growth, if not the decline, in community mental health services. In 1996 the Mental Health Parity Act was passed to address discrimination in insurance coverage, and in 2008 the Mental Health Parity and Addiction Equity Act (MHPAEA) was passed, prohibiting differential coverage for mental health (Hargan, 2018). The community mental health and public health nurses can advocate for clients to ensure equality in access to health services, housing, and employment.

Advocacy Efforts

Consumers, defined as persons who are current or former recipients of mental health services, along with their families have had a significant impact on mental health services. As in all areas of health care, the rights and wishes of consumers are important in planning and delivering services. However, consumers of mental health services have traditionally had difficulty advocating for themselves. In the past, treatment programs often fostered passivity in clients and excluded them from the treatment planning process. In addition, family members were responsible for care in the home, but they lacked resources and even information about treatment (Riesser & Schorske, 2013). Like persons with mental illness, family members suffered from the stigma of mental illness and public attitudes that contributed to self-advocacy problems. In contrast, self-advocacy and involvement in treatment planning fosters self-confidence, promotes participation in services, and may have a significant influence on policy decisions (Hyun et al., 2018). Consumer and family groups fostered these objectives.

Family members led self-advocacy efforts in the 1970s, when small groups organized to challenge and change mental health services. These early efforts resulted in the formation of the **National Alliance for the Mentally Ill** (NAMI), which today

BOX 36.1 Advocacy and Self-Help Organizations

- *Community Support Program (CSP):* A program of the U.S. Department of Health and Human Services (USDHHS), Substance Abuse and Mental Health Services Administration (SAMHSA), and the Center for Mental Health Services (CMHS), that developed plans for a model continuum of care, offers grants for demonstration programs including community rehabilitation projects, and provides money to states for development of consumer and family services and advocacy efforts
- *Consumer/Survivor Mental Health Research and Policy Work Group:* An endeavor sponsored by the Mental Health Statistics Improvement Program of the CMHS to initiate consumer representation in activities of the National Association of State Mental Health Program Directors (NASMHPD)
- *Mental Health America (MHA):* An organization aimed at improving mental health in the population at large, emphasizing prevention
- *National Alliance for the Mentally Ill (NAMI):* A family organization that promotes family support groups, education programs, public campaigns to reduce stigma, and advocacy for mental health policy and services at local and national levels
- *NAMI Consumers' Council:* A consumer advocacy group that advocates for improved and effective psychiatric services and consumer empowerment
- *National Mental Health Consumers' Association (NMHCA):* A consumer organization that advocates for improvements in the mental health system

has both state and local affiliates. Soon consumer groups formed to advocate for better services, changes in mental health policy, self-help programs in treatment, and empowerment. Several advocacy groups that support these consumer efforts are summarized in Box 36.1. In their assessment of resources, nurses can identify community advocacy and support groups.

CONCEPTUAL FRAMEWORKS FOR COMMUNITY MENTAL HEALTH

The community mental health principles that are the underpinnings of practice include the right to mental health services delivered in the least restrictive environment, consumer involvement in treatment, advocacy, and rehabilitative and recovery services. Biopsychosocial theories are useful to understand the multidimensional aspects of community mental health nursing. These include theories and models that explain biological processes, systems, personality, life span development, family dynamics, and stress and coping. Focusing on wellness or recovery, relapse prevention, or relapse management and helping the client reach a maximal level of function are useful for nursing practice.

Another helpful framework for community mental health practice is **systems theory**, which emphasizes the relationship between the elements of a unit and the whole. An understanding of the whole occurs through the examination of interactions and relationships that exist between the parts. A holistic view of system and subsystems can be applied in a variety of ways in community mental health practice. One example of a subsystem in a community is its cultural groups. Subsystems of the cultural groups are families; subsystems of the families are individuals. Using systems theory to explore the background, conditions, and context of situations will disclose information about the positive and negative forces that either promote or undermine the well-being of any unit in the system.

The diathesis-stress model is also useful in CMHN practice. This theory integrates the effects of biology and environment, or nature and nurture, on the development of mental illness. Certain genes or genetic combinations produce a predisposition to a disorder. When an environmental stressor challenges a predisposition to a disorder, the mental disorder may be expressed (Edmondson et al., 2014). The integration of psychosocial and neurobiological paradigms is critical to the practice of psychiatric nursing. Nurses must recognize the effects of environment and biology on people and actively work to mitigate psychosocial as well as biological stressors through teaching strategies to promote mental health and reduce stress.

Levels of Prevention

Health promotion and illness prevention are fundamental to community mental health practice as well as to national objectives for mental health (USDHHS, 2010). Therefore the concepts of primary, secondary, and tertiary levels of prevention are useful in community mental health practice (see Levels of Prevention box).

Primary prevention refers to the reduction of health risks. It involves both health promotion and disease prevention. Health promotion strategies aim to enhance the well-being of healthy populations, whereas disease prevention strategies focus on the identification of populations at risk and conditions that may cause stress and illness. Mental health promotion includes providing education about stress reduction techniques to adults in the workplace. An example is to provide mental health information about depression and eating disorders to adolescents in schools.

Secondary prevention activities are aimed at reducing the prevalence or pathological nature of a condition. They involve early diagnosis, prompt treatment, and limitation of disability. Many functions of the practitioner role are aimed at secondary prevention for individuals. These include providing individual and group psychotherapy, case management, and referral. Screening members of a community for depression during National Depression Screening Day is an example of population-based secondary prevention. Counseling, referral, and treatment interventions after traumatic incidents, such as terrorist attacks or natural disasters, are other important community interventions.

Tertiary prevention efforts attempt to restore and enhance functioning. On a community level, tertiary prevention activities might include support of affordable housing, promotion of psychosocial rehabilitation and recovery programs, and involvement in advocacy and consumer groups for persons with mental illness. Many nursing role activities in community mental health are aimed at tertiary prevention with individuals. They include working with individuals to monitor illness symptoms and treatment responses, coordinating transition from the hospital to the community, and identifying respite care options for caregivers.

Relapse management with a focus on recovery is central to many of the programs and activities that enhance coping skills and competence. People are much more than an illness and can, and do, recover from episodes of illness. Nurses often participate in assertive community treatment (ACT) programs, psychosocial rehabilitation (clubhouses), and intensive case management. ACT programs differ from intensive case management approaches in that they are based more on a medical model and team approach and provide crisis and case management services 24 hours a day, 7 days a week. They are sometimes referred to as hospitals without walls (Henwood et al., 2017). Intensive case management models vary across programs but generally include contact with clients several times a week by an individual case manager. Nurses have critical roles in both treatment programs, as they have the knowledge and skills to provide comprehensive biopsychosocial care.

For example, the nurse visits the client at home, checks medication, assesses physical and emotional functioning, and may take the client shopping for nutritional food. The nurse may accompany the consumer to the physician's office and serve as an advocate for the client in this setting.

As case managers, nurses work with consumers, family members, and other caregivers to foster coping and competency aimed at managing illness symptoms. The goal of managing illness symptoms is to offset relapse and promote recovery. Relapse management and promotion of recovery are major goals of intervention in community mental health nursing. Assessment of the frequency, intensity, and duration of symptoms for the purpose of identifying biological, environmental, and behavioral triggers that may lead to illness relapse helps the consumer manage the illness and promotes recovery. Examples of triggers are poor nutrition, poor social skills, hopelessness, and poor symptom management. Once triggers are identified, interventions aimed at fostering effective coping skills can be introduced to offset relapse of symptoms. For example, an intervention that may promote effective coping to offset social isolation is to guide the client to organized consumer group activities available in the community. Another is to promote consumer and family efforts at job training through community vocational agencies. Still another is to promote competency in family members by coordinating services that enhance their understanding of the illness, provide social support, and include respite care when needed. Finally, an alliance with the client to manage medication and side effects is an important component of relapse prevention and recovery promotion (Baker et al., 2013).

As previously discussed, scientific advances that led to the use of medications to treat mental illness revolutionized mental health care and services. Atypical antipsychotics and new antidepressants with fewer side effects have further influenced mental health care in the community. Although these new drugs have dramatically improved the lives of many people with mental disorders, they are not without problems and are not a cure. The nurse has a critical role in monitoring side effects, detecting related health problems such as diabetes, and providing education and intervention. The most effective tertiary prevention is to combine medications with other relapse management and recovery approaches, including culturally sensitive social, behavioral, and psychotherapeutic interventions (Degnan et al., 2018).

LEVELS OF PREVENTION

In Community Mental Health

Primary Prevention

- Educate populations about mental health issues.
- Teach stress reduction techniques.
- Support and provide prenatal education.
- Provide parenting classes.
- Provide support to caregivers.
- Provide bereavement support.

Secondary Prevention

- Conduct screenings to detect mental health disorders.
- Provide mental health interventions after stressful events.

Tertiary Prevention

- Provide health promotion activities to persons with serious and persistent mental illness.
- Promote support group participation for those with mental health disabilities.
- Advocate for rehabilitation and recovery services.

ROLE OF THE NURSE IN COMMUNITY MENTAL HEALTH

The role of the nurse in community mental health was shaped both by the evolution of services and by the work of nursing pioneers. Development of a knowledge base for the nursing discipline and the further expansion of mental health care services to nontraditional community sites called for more advanced community-based practitioners (American Academy of Nursing, 2012). Nursing practice standards reflect the values of the profession, describe the responsibilities of nurses, and provide direction for the delivery and evaluation of nursing care. These standards also describe the roles of nurses in both advanced and basic practice.

Advanced practice psychiatric nurses have graduate-level education. The psychiatric nurse practitioner title and role have been expanded to encompass primary care and specialty knowledge and skills. These nurses provide primary, secondary, and tertiary care to individuals, groups, families, adults, children, and adolescents. Depending on state laws, some prescribe medications and have hospital admission privileges. For example, the advanced practice nurse may see clients individually to provide psychotherapy, may prescribe medications, and may conduct physical examinations or coordinate this care with other providers in primary care settings. The blended nurse practitioner role has been a response to a shift in the health care system away from specialization and toward comprehensive services that address both physical and mental health problems.

Nurses prepared at the undergraduate level provide basic primary, secondary, and tertiary services that are equally valuable. Specific roles and functions of both mental health and

BOX 36.2 Roles and Functions in Psychiatric/Mental Health Nursing Community Practice

Roles
- Clinician
- Educator
- Coordinator

Functions
- Advocacy
- Case finding and referral
- Case management
- Community action and involvement
- Complementary interventions
- Counseling
- Crisis intervention
- Health maintenance
- Health promotion
- Health teaching
- Home visits
- Intake screening and evaluation
- Milieu therapy
- Promotion of self-care activities
- Psychiatric rehabilitation and recovery
- Psychobiological interventions

Modified from American Nurses Association, American Psychiatric Nurses Association, and International Society of Psychiatric Mental Health Nurses: *Scope and standards of psychiatric-mental health nursing,* Washington, DC, 2007, American Nurses Publishing.

community nurses at the basic level (Box 36.2) are based on clinical nursing practice and standards (American Nurses Association [ANA], 2013, 2014). The functions suggest the overlapping roles of clinician, educator, and coordinator.

Clinician

Objectives of the practitioner role are to help the client maintain or regain coping abilities that promote functioning. This involves using the nursing process to guide the diagnosis and treatment of human responses to actual or potential mental health problems (ANA, 2014). Role functions at the basic practitioner level include case management, counseling, milieu therapy, and psychobiological interventions with individuals and with groups. Clinician skills are used with individual clients in a variety of settings, including the home, and often with large groups of people in specific neighborhoods, schools, and public health districts. For example, many clients who have schizophrenia live in personal care homes. These clients require biopsychosocial interventions related to medication management, milieu management for improved social interaction, and assistance with self-care activities for community living such as use of public transportation. Also, the practitioner increasingly coordinates these activities with both the consumer and other staff members in community settings. Therefore coordination of care is often the means for promoting recovery plan outcomes and enhancing quality of life for clients. These activities can support positive outcomes for others in the community at large.

For example, family members are a primary support system for individuals with schizophrenia. Whether the client lives in a personal care home, a family residence, or another setting, counseling family members and the client about the illness may offset the stressors of caregiving. Moreover, educating the public may reduce the stigma and decrease social isolation for both clients and families, lead to public support for needed services, and decrease the costs of health care because of fewer hospitalizations. As suggested in these examples, clinician and educator roles overlap.

Educator

The educator role uses teaching/learning principles to increase understanding about mental illness and mental health. The educator role is foundational to health maintenance, health promotion, and community action. Teaching clients about illness symptoms and the benefits of medications promotes health maintenance and may reduce the risk for illness relapse. Research supports similar education programs for family members to increase their ability to monitor illness symptoms, identify events that lead to relapse, and engage in self-care (Perlick et al., 2018). The nurse may facilitate a combined support and education group for parents of children with schizophrenia or for consumers with major mental illness in weekly sessions at the community mental health center. As seen in Fig. 36.1 the CMHN, both at the basic and at the advanced level, may participate in developing educational groups and programs for consumers, families, and other providers either alone or in collaboration with other organizations such as the local affiliate of Mental Health America or NAMI. The nurse may also teach clients primary prevention skills such as parenting as shown in Fig. 36.2.

At the community level, both formal and informal teaching is important. One important objective for mental health promotion is to teach positive coping skills. Overmedicating is an example of an ineffective individual coping skill. Even when medications are properly used in treatment, the nurse requires specialized knowledge about drug interactions, pharmacokinetics, and pharmacodynamics. Factors that

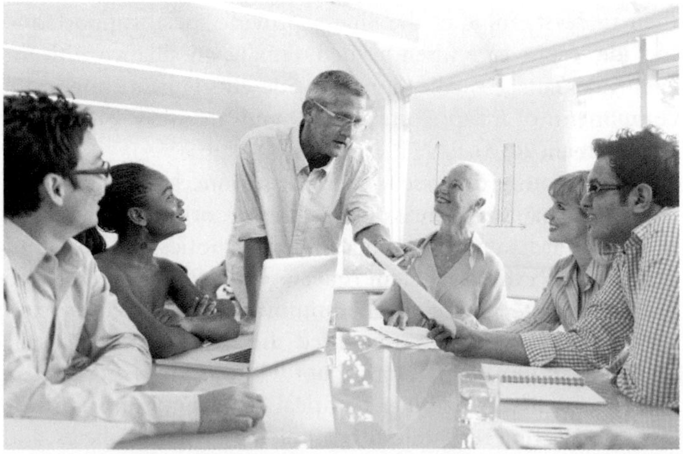

Fig. 36.1 Nurse educator teaching a small group of clients. (Rawpixel Ltd, #489081731, iStock, Thinkstock.)

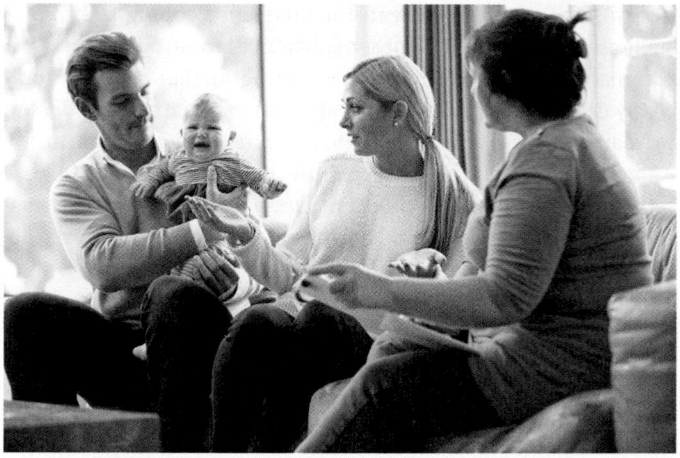

Fig. 36.2 Nurse teaching a young couple parenting skills. (Monkey Business Images, #466375791, iStock, Thinkstock.)

influence pharmacokinetics include anatomical and physiological changes that occur with aging or with coexisting mental and physical conditions. Use of nonprescription medications such as herbal remedies and over-the-counter drugs can influence pharmacokinetics. Because over one third of Americans use nontraditional remedies and many of these are specific for psychiatric conditions, nurses need to assess the use of these substances, be aware of interactions, and share this information with clients (Clarke et al., 2015). For example, people may use herbal remedies such as ginkgo biloba to improve memory, valerian to improve sleep, and St. John's wort to treat depression and these remedies may not be effective.

CHECK YOUR PRACTICE

You are the nurse at a primary care center. You are escorting a 24-year-old man to the examination room for a follow-up visit after starting treatment for depression; his gait is unsteady; and he said he did not sleep well last night but otherwise has felt fine until just now. He is visibly anxious, unable to tell you what medication he is taking and sweating profusely. His pulse is 120 beats per minute, and his blood pressure is 152/88 mm Hg. You do not know what may have caused these symptoms. What should you do?

Coordinator

Coordination of care is a basic principle of the multidisciplinary team approach in community mental health services. Yet there is often a lack of coordination as well as limited services in many communities. Therefore, at a minimum, the role of coordinator must include case finding, referral, and follow-up to evaluate system breakdown and deficits. Because of current system deficits, nurses in community mental health function as coordinators who carry out intake screening, crisis intervention, and home visits. The nurse coordinator also tries to improve the client's health and well-being by promoting independence and self-care in the least restrictive environment. For example, the nurse may teach the client how to fill a medication box or how to use relaxation techniques to reduce stress.

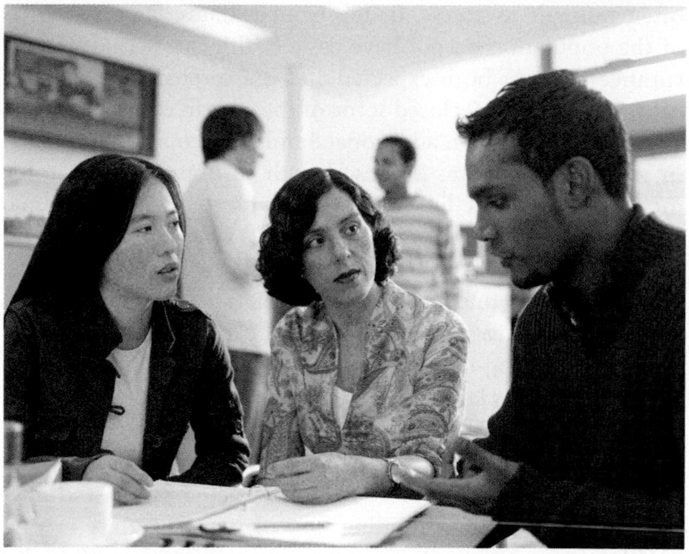

Fig. 36.3 Interdisciplinary mental health planning team meeting. (Digital Vision, #200297936-001, Photodisc, Thinkstock.)

Health teaching related to nutrition, smoking cessation, and sleep promotion is essential for consumers with mental illness. These functions are consistent with descriptions of clinical case management that emphasize continuity of care for individuals who need complex services and with providing information for recovery (Cheng et al., 2018).

To achieve these objectives and improve services, nurses work with a variety of professionals, including advanced practice nurses, social workers, physicians, psychologists, occupational and vocational therapists, and rehabilitation counselors (Fig. 36.3). The nurse is often the advocate for the consumer who needs assistance with making his or her needs clear and accessing both health and social services. Because non-licensed paraprofessionals are frequently involved in direct care activities, their services must be directed, coordinated, and evaluated within the context of treatment planning. Finally, coordination also involves work with individuals who may not have formal preparation but who are essential for positive treatment outcomes. These individuals include family members, shelter volunteers, consumer support groups, and community leaders who can influence development of services. For example, the nurse can teach others about mental illness and effective interventions for times when symptoms become apparent and behaviors become difficult to manage. In the coordinator role, nurses can identify and influence health system effectiveness and ineffectiveness. To assist clients in accessing community resources and services, it is as important to develop positive relationships with other community providers as it is with clients.

CURRENT AND FUTURE PERSPECTIVES IN MENTAL HEALTH CARE

Both nationally and internationally, too few mental health care services exist, and the available services are fragmented and often difficult to access. In the United States, large segments of the population do not have basic health care services or insurance to cover both expected and unexpected illnesses. The ACA passed in 2010 closed some of the gaps in coverage, and as of March 31, 2014, an additional 8 million people had enrolled in an insurance plan. Because health insurance coverage for most Americans is linked to employment, in an economic recession when jobs are lost, insurance is often lost as well, and people are no longer able to afford health care. Also, consumers, family members, and health care providers are concerned about issues of basic treatment, continuity of care, housing, and costs for acute and long-term mental health services for persons with mental illness. As large numbers of baby boomers reach retirement age and Medicare eligibility, there is concern about whether Social Security and Medicare resources will continue to exist for older Americans. Declining state budgets and possible cuts in Medicaid funding may place community mental health services in peril. Therefore implementation of health care reform continues to be a major political, social, and economic issue. Significant alterations in the current health care delivery system are occurring and will continue. Nurses working in communities must understand the models of care, the scope of mental illness, and the national health objectives designed to promote the health and welfare of persons with mental health problems.

Managed care and the ACA, as described previously, will continue to influence the delivery of mental health services. There will be a continued focus on providing services in primary care settings, attempts to reduce inpatient stays, and a more systematic evaluation of the outcomes of the care provided. The massive growth in managed care plans dramatically reduced hospital stays but also limited access to care. Though the passage of the ACA increased access to mental health care through expansion of Medicaid, preventative services, and access for those with a previous illness, it remains unclear how it will continue to impact those with long-term care needs. Because the public mental health system is the only remaining state and federally supported treatment system for persons with serious and persistent mental disorders and Medicaid funds more than half of public mental health services, use of managed care approaches did not always provide for adequate services. The expansion of Medicaid through the ACA did improve access to mental health care for more people and improved delivery and integration of services, but the individual requirement to have insurance was challenged in a Supreme Court ruling and attempts to overturn the ACA continue. Differences in federal and state managed plans and services created barriers to care, and the dismantling of the ACA will lead to gaps in service and large holes in the safety net for vulnerable consumers suffering from mental illness.

Nurses can be important providers in community mental health because of their emphasis on wellness and health promotion, skills at teaching and case management, and lower cost for service. In communities, nurses practice primary, secondary, and tertiary prevention activities by conducting comprehensive client histories to determine health problems and interventions that improve quality of care and cost-effectiveness. In home health settings, nurses screen for ineffective coping techniques such as use of alcohol or other substances to offset the stress of traumatic life events, thereby preventing further problems and costly care. They also screen for signs of psychiatric disorders in primary care and community health care settings. Community mental health services must include access to work and school settings for families and children. These types of nursing assessments and subsequent interventions may offset costly treatment in hospital settings.

Providing the range of community services necessary to handle persistent mental illness is difficult without sufficient funds for health and social services. It is important for nurses and others working in CMHCs to recognize the impact of changes in funding, target populations, restructuring, and disagreements between professions, agencies, and levels of government. Such information enables nurses to advocate for adequate services to meet the needs of individuals with severe and persistent mental illness. The nurse can build relationships with other providers, network with other agencies, and foster interagency collaboration to improve the quality of care for clients and their families.

NATIONAL OBJECTIVES FOR MENTAL HEALTH SERVICES

The goals of the community mental health movement are consistent with the health promotion and disease prevention objectives outlined in *Healthy People 2020* (USDHHS, 2010). The *Healthy People 2020* box illustrates the primary objectives of the national health agenda for mental health promotion and illness prevention. The objectives of *Healthy People 2020* address both settings where people receive care (e.g., primary care, juvenile justice systems) and populations at risk (e.g., children, adults with mental illness, and older adults). Increasing cultural competency and consumer satisfaction with mental health services are further objectives of the national agenda for mental health.

The new millennium brought recognition of the importance of addressing mental health and mental illness as part of disease prevention. Recognition of the burden of mental illness and the status of mental health in the United States was clarified by a landmark report from the surgeon general's office, *Mental Health: A Report of the Surgeon General* (USDHHS, 1999), followed by a report from the Surgeon General's Conference on Children's Mental Health in 2000 (USDHHS, 2000). A national agenda for action described in *Healthy People 2010* and continued in *Healthy People 2020* (USDHHS, 2010) made mental health one of the 10 leading health indicators, which are chosen on the basis of relevance as a broad public health issue. The President's New Freedom Commission on Mental Health further highlighted the need to transform and heal system fragmentation to ensure access to quality mental health services. These goals of a transformed mental health system are found in Box 36.3.

Overall, the national goals of *Healthy People 2020* are to improve mental health and ensure access to quality and

BOX 36.3 New Freedom Commission's Six Goals of a Transformed Mental Health System

1. Americans will understand that mental health is essential to overall health.
2. Mental health care will be consumer and family driven.
3. Disparities in mental health care will be eliminated.
4. Early mental health screening, assessment, and referral will be common practice.
5. Excellent mental health care will be delivered, and research will be accelerated.
6. Technology will be used to access mental health care and information.

From President's New Freedom Commission on Mental Health: *Achieving the promise: transforming mental health care in America,* USDHHS Pub. No. SMA-03-3832, Rockville, MD, 2003, USDHHS.

appropriate mental health services. Approaches emphasize prevention, maintenance, and restoration of mental health and independent functioning. The standards address mental health conditions of concern across the life span and with specific populations. Nurses can (1) promote the standards in the agencies where they are employed, (2) use the standards in community assessment activities, and (3) introduce information about the standards to other groups and agencies, including local consumer and family organizations, to help prioritize mental health concerns. The following box lists selected objectives that pertain to mental health and mental disorders.

HEALTHY PEOPLE 2020

Examples of Targeted National Health Objectives for Mental Health and Mental Disorders

Goal: Improve mental health and ensure access to appropriate, quality mental health services.

- **MHMD-1**: Reduce the suicide rate.
- **MHMD-4**: Reduce the proportion of persons who experience major depressive episode (MDE).
- **MHMD-6**. Increase the proportion of children with mental health problems who receive treatment.
- **MHMD-9**: Increase the proportion of adults with mental disorders who receive treatment.
- **MHMD-10**: Increase the proportion of persons with co-occurring substance abuse and mental disorders who receive treatment for both disorders.

From U.S. Department of Health and Human Services: *Healthy People 2020 objectives,* Office of Disease Prevention and Health Promotion, Washington, DC, 2010, USDHHS.

As indicated in the definitions at the beginning of this chapter, mental health is a dynamic process, influenced by both internal and external factors, that enables and promotes the individual's physical, cognitive, affective, and social functioning. In contrast, threats to mental health create stress that undermines relationships and diminishes the individual's ability to pursue and achieve life's goals. Values and beliefs influence the allocation of resources for neighborhoods and schools and can contribute to or undermine the mental health of people in communities.

Mental health problems are manifested in many ways. Untoward incidents or even anticipated life events can diminish physical, cognitive, affective, and social functioning. For example, in most situations, an anticipated or unexpected death of a family member results in grief that may temporarily interrupt the functioning of surviving family members and produce mental distress. Given adequate support and adaptation, most persons resume their lifestyles after the death of a loved one in spite of the sadness that they are likely to experience. When people do not have adequate resources, or when bereavement is complicated because of the conditions of the situation, there is an increased risk for threats to the mental health of surviving family members. Important interventions with individuals experiencing sorrow and grief are to encourage roles and activities that promote comfort and reduce isolation. Death of a family member can affect survivors of different ages in various ways. Infants and youths may be deprived of significant nurturing and care that will result in long-term emotional deficits, whereas adults are at increased risk for stress related to role changes, and older adults are vulnerable to social isolation as relatives and friends die. In any of these situations, individual or group therapy may be indicated not only for the immediate situation, but also for prevention of longer-term problems.

However, bereavement is not the only cause of diminished mental health. Other causes include, but are not limited to, physical health problems, disabilities resulting from trauma, exposure to violence in the neighborhood, job loss and unstable employment, and unanticipated environmental disasters that result in loss. Because multiple threats to mental health exist across the life span, it is useful to organize the study of problems according to life stages along life's continuum. The box that follows provides suggestions for how nurses can recognize and teach the public the indicators of mental health issues.

HOW TO Recognize Indicators of Mental Health Issues

Community mental health nurses can recognize indicators of mental health issues and educate the public to be aware of:

- Exposure to trauma (abuse, accident, disaster, or violence)
- Withdrawal from social and pleasurable activities
- Exposure to or in temporary stressful living conditions
- Poor work or school performance, unemployment, or school dropout
- Eating or sleeping too much or too little
- Family history of mental illness or substance abuse
- Presence of a substance use disorder

From SAMHSA: *Mental health facts and resources,* 2015. Available at https://www.store.samhsa.gov.

Children and Adolescents

Healthy People 2020 objectives aim to increase the number of children screened and treated for mental health problems. Children are at risk for disruption of normal development by biological, environmental, and psychosocial factors that impair their mental health, interfere with education and social interactions, and keep them from realizing their full potential as adults. For example, children may develop depression after a loss or behavior problems from abuse or neglect. Examples of environmental factors include crowded living conditions, violence, separation from parents, and lack of consistent caregivers. Exposure to community violence can be related to significant stress and depression in children (Sullivan and Simonson, 2016). Types of mental health problems typically diagnosed during childhood are depression, anxiety, and attention-deficit disorders. Examples of chronic disorders commonly seen are Down syndrome and autism. These problems affect growth and development and influence mental health during adolescence.

Suicide is the second leading killer of young persons between ages 15 and 34, and in most cases there was a mental or substance abuse disorder. The second objective of *Healthy People 2020* is to reduce the rate of suicide attempts by adolescents. Some of the risk factors for both adolescents and adults include prior suicide attempts, stressful life events, and access to lethal methods. Increasing the number of adolescents screened for depression in primary health care settings is a new objective of *Healthy People 2020.* Early detection and treatment of depression can help prevent suicide. In addition to depression and substance abuse, adolescent problems include conduct disorders and eating disorders.

Another objective of *Healthy People 2020* is to reduce the proportion of adolescents with eating disorders. Many CMHNs do not directly work with persons with a primary eating disorder; eating disturbances often are a symptom accompanying other conditions. Because most children are not seen in the mental health system, an important role of the CMHN is to educate other community providers, teachers, parents, and children. School nurses are in an ideal position to provide primary, secondary, and tertiary interventions for children with eating disorders. Nutrition education and early recognition, intervention, referral, and follow-up can help prevent eating disorders from becoming severe and can prevent relapses. Nurses can advocate in and beyond their communities for the provision of a nurse in all schools. This can increase the chances of early recognition of and treatment for persons with eating disorders.

Effective service expansion for children, particularly for those with serious emotional disturbances, depends on promoting collaboration across critical areas of support, including schools, families, social services, health, mental health, and juvenile justice. Better services and collaboration for children with serious emotional disturbance and their families will result in greater school retention, decreased contact with the juvenile justice system, increased stability of living arrangements, and improved educational, emotional, and behavioral development. One of the objectives of *Healthy People 2020* is to ensure that children in the juvenile justice system receive access to mental health assessment and treatment (USDHHS, 2010). Children and adolescents require a variety of mental health services, including crisis intervention and both short- and long-term counseling. Nurses working in community settings, well-child clinics, and home health can help to offset this problem through prevention, education, and inclusion of parents in program planning. Because many children and adolescents lack services or access to services, community mental health assessment activities are essential. Assessment activities include identifying types of programs available or lacking in places where children and adolescents spend time. Assessments should be performed in schools and in the homes of clients served, and also in day care centers, churches, and organizations that plan and guide age-specific play and entertainment programs. Assessment data are essential for planning and developing programs that address mental health problems prevalent from the prenatal period through adolescence. Preventing problems during these developmental periods can reduce mental health problems in adulthood.

Adults

Adults suffer from varied sources of stress that contribute to their mental health status. Sources of stress include multiple role responsibilities, job insecurity, and unstable relationships. These and other conditions can undermine mental health and contribute to serious mental illness, depression, anxiety disorders, and substance abuse. *Healthy People 2020* objectives seek to help adults access treatment in order to decrease associated human and economic costs and to reduce suicide rates (USDHHS, 2010).

At some point, virtually all adults will experience a tragic or unexpected loss, a serious setback, or a time of profound sadness, grief, or distress. Major depressive disorder, however, differs both in intensity and in duration from normal sadness or grief. Depression disrupts relationships and the ability to function and can be fatal. In 2016 there were 45,000 reported deaths by suicide. There was a substantial increase in suicide rates among adults aged 45 to 64 years between 1999 and 2014 (CDC, 2016). Many of those who kill themselves have a mental or substance abuse disorder, but in more than half of the suicides in 2015 there was no known mental health condition. Many of these deaths suggested there were relationship problems, substance use, and financial crisis. Other risk factors include prior suicide attempts, stressful life events, and access to lethal methods. Although men are more likely to die by suicide, women are twice as likely to experience depression, and women who are poor, unemployed, or victims of domestic violence are even more at risk (CDC, 2016). Available medications and psychological treatment can help 80 percent of those with depression, yet only a few seek help. Those with depression are more likely to visit a physician for some other reason, and the mental health condition may not be noted. Therefore it is imperative that nurses in all settings recognize and screen for depression. Community health nurses may provide treatment interventions. Nurses can provide mental health screening, support, and education for low-income mothers. Community health nurses at both the generalist and advanced practice levels can be instrumental in designing and developing programs to detect and reduce depression in mothers living in low-resourced communities. These interventions may be critical to ensuring improved mental health of both mothers and their children, as maternal depression is associated with negative emotional outcomes of their children (Beeber et al., 2013; Goodman & Garber, 2017).

Anxiety disorders are common both in the United States and in other countries. An alarming 31.1 percent of the adult population will experience an anxiety disorder at some time in their lives (NIMH, 2018). Anxiety disorders may have an early onset and are characterized by recurrent episodes of illness and periods of disability. Panic disorder and agoraphobia along with depression are associated with increased risks of attempted and completed suicide.

The lifetime rates of co-occurrence of mental disorders and addictive disorders are strikingly high. About one in four persons in the United States experiences a mental disorder in the course of a year, and nearly one in three adults who have a mental disorder in their lifetime also experiences a co-occurring substance (alcohol or other drugs) abuse disorder (SAMHSA, 2017). Individuals with co-occurring disorders are more likely to experience a chronic course and to use services than are those with either type of disorder alone; however, the services are often fragmented, and treatment occurs in different segments of the system.

How can nurses intervene? The general medical sector, including primary care clinics, hospitals, and nursing homes, is typically the initial point of contact for many adults with mental disorders; for some, these providers may be the only source of mental health services. Early detection and intervention for mental health problems can be increased if persons presenting in primary care are assessed for mental health problems. Nurses who work in the general medical sector and in other community settings are in an ideal position to assess and detect mental health problems. Nurses conduct comprehensive biopsychosocial assessments and are often the professional most trusted with sensitive information by clients in these settings. The use of screening tools for depression, anxiety, substance abuse, and cognitive impairment can assist the nurse in early detection and intervention for mental health problems. The Evidence-Based Practice box identifies behavioral interventions for chronic pain, depression, and substance abuse disorders likely to be encountered in primary care.

EVIDENCE-BASED PRACTICE

A systematic review was conducted to identify behavioral interventions targeting chronic pain, depression, and substance use disorders in primary care settings.

The Cumulative Index to Nursing and Allied Health Literature, Medline, PsycInfo, and Google Scholar databases were searched to identify randomized controlled trials using a behavioral intervention with adults with at least two to three conditions.

The search yielded 1862 relevant records, and 6 met final selection criteria. A total of 696 participants were included. Though behavioral interventions varied in content, format, and duration, Mindfulness Oriented Recovery Enhancement, Acceptance and Commitment Therapy, Interpersonal Psychotherapy adapted for pain, and Cognitive Behavioral Therapy showed promising improvements across studies.

Behavioral interventions are effective for assisting patients with pain, depression, and substance abuse in primary care. Integrated delivery of interventions through group sessions, computers, and smart phones may increase patient access to treatment and reduce time, cost, stigma, distress, family burden, and health care fragmentation.

Nurse Use: In order to deliver evidence based nursing care, it is useful to be aware of the above sources to locate studies and other information to use in guiding nursing interventions.

From Barrett K, Chang YP: Behavioral interventions targeting chronic pain, depression, and substance use disorder in primary care. *J Nurs Scholarsh* 48(4):345–353, 2016.

Suicide can be prevented in many cases by early recognition and treatment of mental disorders and by preventive interventions that focus on risk factors. Thus reduction in access to lethal methods and recognition and treatment of mental and substance abuse disorders are among the most promising approaches to suicide prevention. Nurses, long respected as important population-centered providers, can work with legislators for measures to limit access to weapons such as handguns.

LINKING CONTENT TO PRACTICE

This chapter describes the role of the nurse who works with persons with mental illness in the community. The role is diverse and complex and relies on basic nursing knowledge as well as specific knowledge about mental illness. Applying this role in the community draws on many of the recommendations of nursing and public health groups. For example, the core competencies adopted by the Council on Linkages Between Academia and Public Health Practice (2014) include those related to assessment, policy development and program planning skills, communication and cultural competency skills, and involvement with the community in order to provide services effectively. The Quad Council Coalition of Public Health Nursing Organizations (2018) further develops these skills and makes clear application to nursing practice. The American Nurses Association develops and publishes scope and standards of practice documents that identify specific nursing competencies by specialty area (ANA, 2013, 2014).

Adults With Serious Mental Illness

Objectives of *Healthy People 2020* that address tertiary prevention and are targeted to persons with serious mental illness are to reduce the proportion of homeless adults who have serious mental illness, to increase their employment, and to decrease the number of adults with mental disorders who are incarcerated. Brief hospital stays and inadequate community resources have resulted in an increased number of persons with serious mental illness living on the streets or in jail. Though it is difficult to have precise data there is consensus that those with a mental illness are overrepresented. The most precise estimate based on a clinical interview is 14 percent of males and one third of females in jail suffer from a mental illness (Morabito & Wilson, 2015). Some people arrested for nonviolent crimes could be better served if diverted from the jail system to a community-based mental health treatment program with linkage to mental health services. About half of the homeless persons in the United States have a serious mental illness or a substance abuse problem, and on any given night an astonishing 60,000 are veterans (National Coalition for Homeless Veterans, 2014). Most do not have any form of employment. At present, many people with severe mental disorders live in poverty because they lack the ability to earn or maintain a suitable standard of living. Even people who live with family caregivers or in supervised housing are at risk for inadequate services because the long-term care they need often depletes human and fiscal resources. An effective approach for helping persons with serious mental illness is to partner with consumers to facilitate recovery through intensive case management. Persistent client outreach and engagement strategies are effective in helping persons with serious mental illness recover (Fowler et al., 2018).

CMHNs are engaged in all forms of case management activities with persons with serious and persistent mental illness. They provide important case management services, coordinate resources for consumers, and function as important members of ACT programs, which provide continuous assistance to persons with mental illness. Nurses by philosophy and training promote independent living and provide support and encouragement for persons to achieve a maximal level of wellness and function. Nurses recognize the importance of the mental health benefits of meaningful work that improves self-esteem and independence. Nurses can support development of **wellness recovery action plans** at both the individual and agency levels. Nursing health promotion interventions can be provided in shelters, soup kitchens, and other places where homeless persons receive food and protection.

Older Adults

In the United States the population older than 65 years has steadily increased since the year 2000. As the life expectancy of individuals continues to grow, the number experiencing mental disorders of late life will increase. This trend will present society with unprecedented challenges in organizing, financing, and delivering effective preventive and treatment services for mental health in this population. Although many older people maintain highly functional lives, others have mental health deficits associated with normal sensory losses related to aging, failing physical health, difficulty performing activities of daily living, and social deprivation or isolation. Life changes related to work roles and retirement often result in reduced social contacts and support. Other previously described losses are associated with the death of a spouse, other family members, or friends. Reduced social networks and contacts triggered by these life events can influence mood and contribute to serious states of depression. However, depression is not a normal part of aging.

The depression rate among older adults is half that of younger people, but the presence of physical or chronic illness increases rates of depression. Depression rates for older adults in long-term care receiving care either at home or in nursing homes range from five percent to 25 percent (Haigh et al., 2018). Though overall depression rates may be lower in older adults, men over 75 still have the highest suicide rates at 42.4 per 100,000 (CDC, 2016). Alzheimer's disease and vascular conditions can cause a severe loss of mental abilities with behavioral manifestations. Nearly half of those older than age 85 have symptoms of cognitive impairment severe enough to impair function. All these conditions affect the mental health status of individuals and their family caregivers.

Older adults, because they may be dependent on others for care, are at risk for abuse and neglect. Healthy aging activities such as physical activity and establishing social networks improve the mental health of older adults. Older adults underutilize the community mental health system and are more likely to be seen in primary care or to be recipients of care in institutions. The nurse can reach them by organizing health promotion programs through senior centers or other community-based settings. Home health care nurses can assess and intervene to protect those at risk for abuse and neglect, and mental health nurses can provide stress management education for nursing home staff. Stress management for caregivers and respite daycare programs for an older adult family member can increase coping and prevent abuse. Mental health outreach services for older adults have been very effective in reducing depressive symptoms.

Most family caregivers are women who care for a spouse, an aging parent, or a child with a long-term disabling illness. These caregivers are also at risk for health disruption. The risk is particularly great for caregivers of persons with a chronic illness. Caregivers of persons with severely disabling mental disorders often have their mental health threatened by lack of social support, the stigma of the disease, and chronic strain. During stressful life events such as these, it is important for caregivers to know how to manage the many competing demands in their lives.

Activities to improve the mental health status of adults include public education programs, prevention approaches, and provision of mental health services in primary care. Specific approaches to reduce stress include use of community support groups, education about lifestyle management, and worksite programs. Nevertheless, most programs currently available for adults, families, and caregivers with health problems primarily monitor or restore health rather than prevent problems. Therefore the nurse can refer family caregivers and others to organizations such as the local NAMI for group support services. In addition, many national organizations designed for groups with specific problems (Box 36.4) have local chapters or information that can be accessed on the Internet. Some state activities expand mental health services to older adults, and *Healthy People 2020* includes objectives designed to increase services to older adults and cultural competence within the mental health system.

BOX 36.4 Examples of Sources of Information and Help for People With Mental Illness and Mental Health Problems

- Alcoholics Anonymous
- Al-Anon
- Alzheimer's Association
- American Anorexia/Bulimia Association
- American Association of Suicidology
- Anxiety Disorders Association of America
- Attention Deficit Information Network
- Children and Adults with Attention-Deficit/Hyperactivity Disorder
- Gamblers Anonymous
- National Center for Post-Traumatic Stress Disorder (it is a government agency)
- National Center for Learning Disabilities
- International OCD Foundation
- Overeaters Anonymous
- Schizophrenics Anonymous

QSEN FOCUS ON QUALITY AND SAFETY EDUCATION FOR NURSES

Quality and Safety Focus

Targeted Competency: Safety

Minimizes risk of harm to clients and providers through both system effectiveness and individual performance.

Important aspects of safety include:

- **Knowledge:** Examine human factors and other basic safety design principles, as well as commonly used unsafe practices (such as workarounds and dangerous abbreviations)
- **Skills:** Use national client safety resources for own professional development and to focus attention on safety in care settings
- **Attitudes:** Value the contributions of standardization/reliability to safety

Safety Question

Nurses engage in patient-specific interventions to keep patients safe. Nurses also regularly contribute to the development of safety approaches at the systems level. System-level approaches to safety ensure standardization of processes and a consistent methodology to addressing recurring safety concerns.

You are working as a registered nurse (RN) in home care. Your home care agency has had three patients admit to suicidal ideation and intention in the last three months. In all three situations the home care nurses handled the situations very differently, with varied success. Your manager asks you to participate in a task force to develop a standard operating procedure that all home care nurses can employ to respond to a suicidal patient in the home.

- What health care team members would be helpful in addressing the development of this standardized operating procedure?
- What evidence might you look to in developing this standardized procedure?
- How might you envision most effectively training home care nurses in this standardized approach?

Prepared by Gail Armstrong, PhD, DNP, ACNS-BC, CNE, Associate Professor, University of Colorado Denver College of Nursing.

Cultural Diversity

To work effectively, health care providers need to understand the differences in how various populations in the United States perceive mental health and mental illness and treatment services. These factors affect whether people seek mental health care, how they describe their symptoms, the duration of care, and the outcomes of the care received. Various populations use mental health services in different ways. People may not seek mental health services in the formal system, they may drop out of care, or they may seek care at much later stages of illness, which typically costs more. This pattern of use may be the result of a community-based mental health service system that is not culturally relevant, responsive, or accessible to select populations. Although all socioeconomic and cultural groups have mental health problems, low-income groups are at greater risk because they often lack minimal resources for meeting basic physical and mental health needs.

In an effort to describe and remedy mental health disparities based on culture, a supplemental report was published to the landmark surgeon general's report on mental health (USDHHS, 2001). Caution is needed, however, when discussing differences among racial and ethnic groups in the rates of mental illness. Studies of the number of cases of mental health problems among racial and ethnic populations, while increasing in number, remain limited and often inconclusive. Discussion of the rates of existing cases must consider differences in how persons of different cultures and racial and ethnic groups perceive mental illness. Behavioral problems, often viewed in Western medicine as signs of mental illness, may be assessed differently by individuals in various racial and ethnic groups. The manner in which people of different cultures describe emotional distress may affect the detection and treatment of mental illness. With this caution in mind, along with the recognition that sample sizes for racial and ethnic groups may be limited, examination of existing large-scale studies for mental health trends and disparities among racial and ethnic groups remains important. According to the surgeon general's landmark report on culture, race, and ethnicity, the predominant minority populations in the United States are African Americans, Hispanics, Asian and Pacific Islander Americans, and American Indians, including Alaska Natives (USDHHS, 2001). A notable omission from this landmark federal report is Middle Eastern Americans, and little information could be found either in the literature or through national websites, although there is a significant and growing population, particularly in the upper Midwest. Great diversity exists among people from the Middle East, although they may share some cultural traditions with Asians, Africans, or Europeans and in some cases have been included in those classifications. However, within each of the groups identified in the federal report, there is also much diversity, as each group consists of subgroups with unique cultural differences. Therefore it is important to avoid simplification and overgeneralization in discussions about the characteristics and problems of minorities and to examine both individual and national bias. It is critical to conduct community assessments to determine unique characteristics and factors that contribute to mental health needs within specific aggregates of the population. The information presented here is intended to stimulate thinking and awareness for developing nursing activities in individual communities. Community assessments that include data about specific populations from organized agencies such as the Indian Health Service (2014) are important because assessment data can help guide role activities during all steps of the nursing process. However, the most important data comes from the individual communities.

Nurses provide a variety of primary, secondary, and tertiary prevention interventions with populations at risk that help meet the objectives for improving mental health. Consumers have historically influenced mental health services, and the health care industry increasingly is using consumer opinion to gain information on service needs and changes. Objectives of *Healthy People 2020* are to increase state tracking of consumer satisfaction with mental health services and to increase the number of states that incorporate plans addressing cultural competence. Nurses working within broad-based coalitions of consumers, families, other providers, and community leaders can help to achieve the goals of accessible, culturally sensitive, quality mental health services for all people.

African Americans. African Americans are the second largest minority population in the United States. In 2015, 25.4 percent of African Americans compared to 10.4 percent of non-Hispanic whites were living at the poverty level (USDHHS, 2016a). Ethnic and racial minorities in the United States may live in an environment of social and economic discrimination and inequality, which takes a toll on mental health and places them at risk for associated mental problems. African Americans are more likely to be exposed to, or to become victims of, violence, placing them at risk for the development of PTSD. They are overrepresented both in the homeless and correctional system populations, further increasing the risk of developing mental health problems. Although they were less likely to commit suicide, the suicide rate of young African American men rose in the previous two decades (CDC, 2016). Despite these issues, African Americans are less likely to use mental health services and may have significant negative expectations about mental health services. Nurses can promote the mental health of African Americans by integrating mental health care into primary care settings, providing services in community centers, collaborating with African American faith communities, providing education to decrease the stigma, working toward the provision of safer communities, and recruiting African Americans to work as community mental health providers.

Hispanic Americans. Hispanic Americans are the second largest minority group in America, representing 17.6 percent of the population, and by 2050 they are projected to make up 25 percent of the population (USDHHS, 2016b). Although they live primarily in the southwestern regions of the country, many have migrated to states in the Southeast and Midwest. Migrant farmworkers are also an important subpopulation among Latinos. As discussed in Chapter 34, migratory living patterns that are marked by low income, poor education, and lack of health services contribute to stressful living conditions. Nurses and nurse practitioners may be primary health care providers for migrant laborers and new immigrants. Their roles expand beyond traditional practice to encompass case management and interagency collaboration. Collaboration includes networking and referral to community mental health agencies and to advanced practice psychiatric nurses when either drug or alcohol abuse or mental illness is the primary health problem.

Hispanic Americans living in low-income urban areas are subject to many of the conditions described for low-income and disadvantaged African American families. Initially, it was reported that recent Hispanic immigrants had lower rates of depression than those born in the United States, but evidence from the CDC (2016) found suicide to be 50 percent higher than whites among young Hispanic women in grades 9-12. There are significant relationships between suicide and having a family history of suicide, physical or sexual abuse, and environmental stress. These findings suggest serious stressful living conditions for both individuals and families. Nurses working with Hispanic families need knowledge and skill in both the language and cross-cultural therapies, and they also need to include consumers in planning and evaluating mental health service delivery. Focus groups can be held to involve community members in the planning and implementation of culturally relevant mental health services.

Asian and Pacific Islander Americans. Asian and Pacific Islander Americans are a diverse and rapidly increasing population, currently representing 5.4 and 1.3 percent of the population, respectively (USDHHS, 2016c). This group includes both settled citizens and new refugees. The largest segment of this population lives in California. Whereas Asian and Pacific Islander Americans, like other minority groups, are represented in all socioeconomic strata, the lower-income groups include refugees and recent immigrants who are dealing with the displacement issues of loss, adjustment, and adaptation. Losses often involve forfeiture of family, traditions, and lifestyles for cultures that may seem alien. Adjustments and adaptations include those basic to daily living: learning new languages, laws, and monetary systems, and locating support systems. Finding support systems includes becoming acquainted with the health care delivery system. Though the suicide rate of Asian Americans is half that of white Americans, it is the ninth leading cause of death in this population (USDHHS, 2016c). Our knowledge of the mental health needs of this population is limited, because they do not seek mental health services compared to other groups. This avoidance of mental health care needs further exploration to understand the perceptions of mental health disorders. Assessment, planning, and interventions with members of this diverse group must include information about their health beliefs, a key component in any program.

Population-focused mental health nurses need to understand existing cultural barriers and help to design culturally sensitive approaches for vulnerable populations. Nurses can work to decrease the stigma of mental illness by educating minorities about the biological basis of many mental disorders. Recruitment of a culturally diverse nursing workforce may increase use of mental health services.

American Indians. American Indians represent two percent of the U.S. population. Although this is a small group, it is also diverse, with more than 573 recognized tribes and more than 200 languages. American Indians also appear to have significant rates of substance abuse, depression, and suicide particularly among the young aged 10-34. In 2014 suicide was the leading cause of death among young women and the second leading cause of death among young men. Exposures to unintentional injury, violence, and homicide are high, which results in significant rates of PTSD (Indian Health Service, 2014; USDHHS, 2016d). Use of mental health services has been difficult to determine, because only a small percent of American Indians use those provided by the Indian Health Service.

A promising intervention to address the needs of this diverse group is to build on the traditions of the specific tribe culture to foster identity and integration and enhance protective factors. A return to traditional values of community and group support has been shown to be effective in reducing rates of substance abuse (Indian Health Service, 2014). Nurses working with American Indians, as with all population groups, need to learn the culture of the specific group and to mutually plan culturally sensitive mental health interventions at levels of primary, secondary, and tertiary prevention.

PRACTICE APPLICATION

Mr. B. is an 81-year-old white widowed man living in a rural area 20 miles from a small city. The nurse practitioner who treated Mr. B. for sinusitis referred him to the outreach nurse for an evaluation. The nurse practitioner was concerned when she noted that Mr. B. had lost weight and started to cry when talking about his wife who had died several years before. During the initial visit the nurse noted that Mr. B. weighed only 110 lb., was not sleeping, had stopped going to church, and was quite anxious and sad about his finances, his limitations from arthritis, his relationship with his 27-year-old stepson, Bart, and the possibility of nursing home placement.

The nurse conducted a suicide assessment, knowing that Mr. B. was at high risk because of his age, his mood, and the presence of guns in the home. Mr. B. stated that he had considered shooting himself, but he was reluctant to have the rifles removed at the nurse's suggestion because Bart used the guns for hunting. Mr. B. agreed to a family meeting with his stepson, and Bart agreed to remove the guns from the house. Both Mr. B. and Bart needed significant education about the biological basis of depression and the efficacy of using a new antidepressant along with support to treat his condition. Mr. B., like many older adults, did not wish to see a psychiatrist or use the community mental health system. He did agree to a trial of antidepressants, however.

The nurse, through the primary care nurse practitioner, arranged for a prescription of an antidepressant (an SSRI) that is safe for use with older adults, and Mr. B. started the medication within two weeks of the initial visit. In addition to medication and counseling, Mr. B. needed help with nutrition. Because Bart was away 10 hours a day, at work in the city, Mr. B. was alone all day. Mr. B. was not able to prepare meals because of his arthritis. The nurse arranged with the local board for aging to provide home-delivered meals. This not only helped with nutrition, but also gave Mr. B. a visit from the volunteer twice a week.

Mr. B. and Bart needed help with financial planning, as they did not want to lose the farm should Mr. B. need more assistance or nursing home placement in the future. The nurse arranged for them to talk with a social worker regarding long-term care planning.

In addition to addressing the immediate concerns, the nurse continued to provide weekly visits to Mr. B. for support and counseling, medication monitoring, and case management activities. Family meetings with Bart and Mr. B. to discuss mutual concerns were arranged every two months and as needed. The significant improvement of depressive symptoms (that is, sleep, appetite, weight, and mood) in Mr. B. was monitored both clinically and through use of a depression rating scale.

Psychological, physical, and social problems of older adults are closely intertwined and are best evaluated and treated by a multidisciplinary team. Psychiatric illness often presents first with physical symptoms, and physical limitations create further psychological distress. Older adults often prefer not to use formal mental health services, so careful assessment in primary care settings is critical to detect their mental health problems.

A. In addition to his stepson and the nurse, who else might notice if Mr. B.'s condition began to deteriorate?

B. What nursing measures are important in monitoring Mr. B.'s response to the antidepressant?

C. What secondary prevention measures did the nurse use?

D. What resources might be available for Bart should he need more information about depression?

Answers can be found on the Evolve site.

KEY POINTS

- Reform movements and subsequent federal legislation influenced the development of the current community mental health model that includes team care, case management, prevention, and rehabilitation and recovery components of service.
- During the past two decades, federal legislation in the United States focused on mainstreaming persons with mental disabilities into American life by legislating access to employment, services, and housing.
- Prevalence rates for mental health problems are very high, and people are at risk for threats to mental health at all ages across the life span. Low-income and minority groups are often at increased risk because they lack access to services and because programs may lack cultural sensitivity.
- National health objectives to promote health and services for persons who have mental health problems and severe mental disorders illustrate the scope of mental illness and provide direction for community mental health practice.
- Guidelines for attaining national health objectives were designed to help individuals at regional and local levels establish health priorities that include those for mental illness.
- The American Nurses Association standards provide a framework for the roles and functions of community mental health nurses.
- Frameworks that are useful in community mental health nursing include primary, secondary, and tertiary levels of prevention; biological theories including the effects of psychosocial factors on the brain, growth, and development; and rehabilitation and recovery models.

CLINICAL DECISION-MAKING ACTIVITIES

1. For one week, keep a list of incidents related to mental health problems that you learn about in the local media. Categorize the incidents according to age, sex, and socioeconomic, ethnic, or minority status. Which populations seem to have the most mental health problems?
2. Visit a local shelter or organization that offers temporary protection for persons with mental disorders. Determine services that are available or lacking for children, women, and men. Describe a nursing intervention that would improve services.
3. Visit with representatives of your local self-help organizations for consumers to determine their needs and the adequacy of resources for people with severe mental disorders and their caregivers; determine gaps in services. Develop a list of the agencies in your community that provide direct or indirect services for those with mental illness and their families.
4. Interview a school nurse, an occupational health nurse, an emergency department nurse, or a hospice nurse in your community to discuss types of mental health problems they see with clients in their practice settings. Determine resources that are available or lacking for primary, secondary, and tertiary prevention. Design a primary prevention intervention.
5. Interview a nurse working in a local community mental health agency to discuss roles, functions, programs, and resources available or lacking for primary, secondary, and tertiary prevention. Compare findings about prevention programs with information obtained from the preceding interview.
6. Visit a consumer-operated program or a psychosocial rehabilitation program. Interview members to learn how they view services and resources available or lacking in this setting. Describe how your attitudes about persons in recovery from mental illness changed after your visit.
7. Accompany a community mental health nurse on home visits to clients enrolled in an assertive community outreach program, and then accompany a psychiatric nurse in a home care agency. Compare and contrast how the services, funding, populations served, and philosophies of treatment differ.
8. As a class activity, arrange for a panel of speakers representing the minority populations described in this chapter. Discuss their views about the way culture shapes thinking about mental illness, and determine types of culturally sensitive services that are available or lacking in your community.
9. Review articles in at least four research journals to determine current research findings about mental disorders and mental health problems, and compare nursing care in the United States with that of other countries. Discuss the differences in mental health care between countries.

ADDITIONAL RESOURCES

EVOLVE WEBSITE

http://evolve.elsevier.com/Stanhope/community/

- Answers to Practice Application
- Case Study
- Glossary
- Review Questions

REFERENCES

Ali MM, Chen J, Mutter R, et al.: The ACA's dependent coverage expansion and out of pocket spending by young adults with behavioral health conditions, *Psy Ser* 67(9):977–982, 2016.

Alzheimer's Association: *Alzheimer's disease facts and figures*, 2018. Retrieved from alz.org.

American Academy of Nursing Psychiatric Mental Health Substance Abuse Expert Panel: Essential psychiatric mental health and substance use competencies for the registered nurse, *Arch Psychiatr Nurs* 26:80–110, 2012.

American Nurses Association (ANA): *Public health scope and standards of nursing practice*, Washington, DC, 2013, American Nurses Publishing. Retrieved from http://www.nursesbooks.org.

American Nurses Association, American Psychiatric Nurses Association, International Society of Psychiatric Mental Health Nurses: *Scope and standards of psychiatric–mental health nursing,* Washington, DC, 2014, American Nurses Publishing.

American Psychiatric Association (APA): *Diagnostic and statistical manual of mental disorders*, ed 5, Washington, DC, 2013, APA.

Baker E, Fee J, Bovingdon L, et al.: From taking to using medication: recovery-focused prescribing and medicines management, *Adv Psychiatr Treat* 19:2–10, 2013. Retrieved from http://apt.rcpsych.org.

Barrett K, Chang YP: Behavioral interventions targeting chronic pain, depression, and substance use disorder in primary care, *J Nurs Scholarsh* 48(4):345–353, 2016.

Beeber LS, Schwartz TA, Holditch-Davis D, Canuso R, Lewis V, Hall HW: Parenting enhancement, interpersonal psychotherapy to reduce depression in infants and toddlers: a randomized trial, *Nurs Res* 62:82–90, 2013.

Boyd MA: Mental health care in contemporary society. Psychiatric nursing and evidence based practice. In Boyd MA, editor: *Psychiatric nursing: contemporary practice,* ed 6, Philadelphia, 2018, Lippincott, Williams & Wilkins, pp 2–12.

Busch SH, Meara E, Huskamp HA, Barry CL: Characteristics of adults with substance use disorders expected to be eligible for Medicaid under the ACA, *Psychiatr Serv* 64:520–526, 2013.

Centers for Disease Control and Prevention (CDC): *Increase in suicide in the United States, 1999–2014*, 2016. Retrieved from https://www.cdc.gov.

Cheng JF, Huang XY, Lin MC, Wang YH, Yeh TP: A mental health home visit service partnership intervention on improving patients' satisfaction, *Arch Psychiatr Nurs* 32(4):610–616, 2018.

Clarke TC, Black LI, Stussman BJ, Barnes PM, Nahin RL: Trends in the use of complementary health approaches among adults: United States, 2002–2012, *National Health Stats Report* 10(79): 1–16, 2015.

Council on Linkages between Academia and Public Health Practice: *Core competencies* for *public health professionals,* Washington, DC, 2014, Public Health Foundation, Health Resources and Services Administration.

Cowell AJ, Prakash S, Jones E, et al.: Behavioral health coverage in the individual market increased after ACA parity requirements, *Health Affairs* 37(7), 2017.

Degnan A, Baker S, Edge D, et al.: The nature and efficacy of culturally-adapted psychosocial interventions for schizophrenia: a systematic review and meta-analysis, *Psychol Med* 48(5): 714–727, 2018.

Edmondson D, Kronish IM, Wasson LT, Giglio JF, Davidson KW, Whang W: A test of the diathesis-stress model in the emergency department: who develops PTSD after an acute coronary syndrome? *J Psychiatr Res* 53:8–13, 2014. Retrieved from http://www.ncbi.nlm.nih.gov.

Fowler D, Hodgekins J, French P, et al.: Social recovery therapy in combination with early intervention services for enhancement of social recovery in patients with first-episode psychosis (SUPEREDEN3): a single-blind, randomized controlled trial, *Lancet Psychiatry*, 5(1):41–50, 2018.

Goodman SH, Garber J: Evidence-based interventions for depressed mothers and their young children, *Child Dev* 88(2):368–377, 2017.

Haigh EAP, Bogucki OE, Sigmon ST, Blazer DG: Depression among older adults: a 20-year update on five common myths and misconceptions, *Am J Geriatr Psychiatry* 26(1):107–122, 2018.

Hargan ED: *Release of the HHS mental health and substance use disorder parity action plan*, 2018. Retrieved from https://www.hhs.gov.

Henwood, BF, Siantz, E, Hrouda, DR, et al.: Integrated primary care in assertive community treatment, *Psy Serv* 69(2):133-135, 2017.

Holmes D: Bone: Dual mode of action of SSRIs on bone remodeling, *Nat Rev Endocrinol* 12(12):688, 2016.

Hyun MS, Nam KA, Kim H: Effects of a brief empowerment program for families of persons with mental illness in South Korea: a pilot study, *Issues in Men Health Nur* May 30:1–7. 2018.

Indian Health Service (IHS): *IHS fact sheet: indian health disparities,* 2014. Retrieved from http://ihs.gov.

Kim JY, Higgins TC, Esposito D, Hamblin A: Integrating health care for high-need Medicaid beneficiaries with serious mental illness and chronic physical health conditions at managed care, provider and consumer levels, *Psychiatr Rehabil J* 40(2):207–215, 2017.

Macedo, AF: Neurobiology of mental illness from reductionism to integration, *Intern J of Clin Neurosci and Ment Health* 4(Suppl 3):S01, 2017.

Mechanic D, Olfson M: The relevance of the Affordable Care Act for improving mental health care, *Annu Rev Clin Psychol* 12:515–542, 2016.

Miller S, Wherry LR: Health and access to care during the first 2 years of the ACA Medicaid expansions, *N Engl J Med* 376:947–956, 2017.

Morabito MS, Wilson AB: Selecting a method of case identification to estimate the involvement of people with mental illnesses in the criminal justice system: a research note, *Int J Offender Ther Comp Criminol* 61(8):919–937, 2015.

National Coalition for Homeless Veterans: *Background & statistics*, 201, 2014. Retrieved from http://www.nchv.org.

National Institute of Mental Health (NIMH), National Institutes of Health (NIH), U.S. Department of Health and Human Services (USDHHS): *Any anxiety disorder,* Washington, DC, 2018, NIMH. Retrieved from https://www.nimh.nih.gov.

National Institute of Mental Health (NIMH), National Institutes of Health (NIH), U.S. Department of Health and Human Services (USDHHS): *Statistics from the WHO*, Washington, DC, 2014, NIMH. Retrieved from: http://www.nimh.nih.gov.

Nusslock R, Miller GE: Early-life adversity and physical and emotional health across the lifespan: a neuroimmune network hypothesis, *Biol Psychiatry* 80(1):23–32, 2016.

Pandya A, Jän Myrick K: Wellness recovery programs: a model of self-advocacy for people living with mental illness, *J Psychiatr Pract* 19:242–246, 2013.

Pearlman SA: The Patient Protection and Affordable Health Care Act: impact on mental health services demand and provider availability, *J Am Psychiatr Nurses Assoc* 19:327–334, 2013.

Perlick DA, Jackson C, Grier S, et al.: Randomized trial comparing caregiver-only family-focused treatment to standard health education on the 6-month outcome of bipolar disorder, *Bipolar Disord* 20(7):622–633, 2018.

President's New Freedom Commission on Mental Health: *Achieving the promise: transforming mental health care in America,* USDHHS Pub No SMA-03-3832, Rockville, MD, 2003, USDHHS.

Quad Council Coalition of Public Health Nursing Organizations: *Quad council competencies for public health nurses*, 2018. Retrieved from www.achne.org.

Riesser GG, Schorske BJ: Relationships between family caregiver and mental health professionals: the American experience. In Lefley H, Wasow M, editors: *Helping families cope with mental illness*, vol 2, New York, 2013, Routledge, pp 3–26.

Rojo LE, Gaspar PA, Silva H, et al.: Metabolic syndrome and obesity among users of second generation antipsychotics: a global challenge for modern psychopharmacology, *Pharmacol Res* 101:74–85, 2015.

Rosenzweig JM, Jivanjee P, Brennan EM, et al.: *Understanding neurobiology of psychological trauma: tips for working with transition-age youth*, Portland OR, 2017, Research & Training Center. Retrieved from www.pathwaysrtc.pdx.edu.

Substance Abuse and Mental Health Services Administration (SAMHSA): *2016 National survey on drug use and health (NSDUH) Report, America's behavioral health changes and challenge. Key Substance use and mental health indicators in the United States, [USDHHS Publication No.SMA17-5044]*. Rockville, MD, 2017, SAMHSA.

Substance Abuse and Mental Health Services Administration (SAMHSA): *Mental health facts and resources*, 2015. Retrieved from https://www.store.samhsa.gov.

Simon K, Soni A, Cawley J: The impact of health insurance on preventative care and health behaviors: evidence from the first two years of the ACA Medicaid expansions, *J Pol Anal Manag* 36(2):390–417, 2017.

Sullivan AL, Simonson GR: A systematic review of school-based social emotional interventions for refugee and war traumatized youth, *Rev Ed Res* 86(2):503–530, 2016.

U.S Department of Health and Human Services (USDHHS): *Mental health: a report of the surgeon general*, Rockville, MD, 1999, USDHHS.

U.S. Department of Health and Human Services: U.S. Department of education; U.S. Department of Justice: *Report of the surgeon general conference on children's mental health: a national action agenda,* Washington, DC, 2000, U.S. Department of

Health and Human Services. Retrieved from http://www.ncbi.nlm.nih.gov.

U.S. Department of Health and Human Services (USDHHS): *Mental health: culture, race, and ethnicity—supplement to mental health: a report of the surgeon general*, Rockville, MD, 2001, USDHHS.

U.S. Department of Health and Human Services (USDHHS): *Healthy people 2020: mental health and mental disorders*, Washington, DC, 2010, Office of Disease Prevention and Health Promotion. Retrieved from http://healthypeople.gov.

U.S. Department of Health and Human Services (USDHHS) Office of Minority Health: *Mental health of African Americans*, Washington, DC, 2016a, USDHHS. Retrieved from https://minorityhealth.hhs.gov.

U.S. Department of Health and Human Services (USDHHS) Office of Minority Health: *Mental health and hispanics*, Washington, DC, 2016b, USDHHS. Retrieved from https://minorityhealth.hhs.gov.

U.S. Department of Health and Human Services (USDHHS) Office of Minority Health: *Mental health and Asian Americans*, Washington, DC, 2016c, USDHHS. Retrieved from https://minorityhealth.hhs.gov.

U.S. Department of Health and Human Services (USDHHS) Office of Minority Health: *Mental health and American Indians/Alaska Natives*, Washington, DC, 2016d, USDHHS. Retrieved from https://minorityhealth.hhs.gov.

U.S. Department of Health and Human Services (USDHHS): *Patient protection and affordable health care act*, 2014. Retrieved from http://www.hhs.gov.

World Health Organization (WHO): *mhGAP, mental health action programme: scaling up care for mental, neurological and substance use disorders*, Geneva, Switzerland, 2008, WHO.

World Health Organization (WHO). *World health statistics 2018: monitoring health for sustainable development goals*, 2018. Retrieved from http://www.who.int.

World Health Organization (WHO): *Health for the world's adolescents: a second chance in the second decade*, Geneva, Switzerland, 2014, WHO. Retrieved from www.who.int.

37

Alcohol, Tobacco, and Other Drug Problems

Mary Lynn Mathre, RN, MSN, CARN and Amber M. Bang, RN, BSN

OBJECTIVES

After reading this chapter, the student should be able to do the following:

1. Analyze personal attitudes toward alcohol, tobacco, and other drug problems.
2. Differentiate among these terms: *substance use, abuse, dependence*, and *addiction*.
3. Discuss the differences among the major psychoactive drug categories of depressants, stimulants, marijuana, hallucinogens, and inhalants.
4. Explain the role of the nurse in primary, secondary, and tertiary prevention of alcohol, tobacco, and other drug problems as it relates to individual clients, their families, and special populations.
5. Evaluate the role of the nurse in primary, secondary, and tertiary prevention of alcohol, tobacco, and other drug problems as it relates to the community and national policies on drug control.

CHAPTER OUTLINE

Alcohol, Tobacco, and Other Drug Problems in Perspective
Psychoactive Drugs
Predisposing/Contributing Factors
Primary Prevention and the Role of the Nurse
Secondary Prevention and the Role of the Nurse
Tertiary Prevention and the Role of the Nurse
Outcomes

KEY TERMS

addiction treatment, p. 828
Alcoholics Anonymous (AA), p. 830
alcoholism, p. 814
biopsychosocial model, p. 814
blood alcohol concentration, p. 816
brief interventions, p. 831
codependency, p. 826
cross-tolerance, p. 829
denial, p. 823
depressants, p. 815
detoxification, p. 827
drug addiction, p. 814
drug dependence, p. 814
enabling, p. 827
fetal alcohol syndrome, p. 816
hallucinogens, p. 815
harm reduction, p. 813
mainstream smoke, p. 817
people who inject drugs, p. 825
polysubstance use or abuse, p. 821
prohibition, p. 812
psychoactive drugs, p. 814
set, p. 820
setting, p. 820
sidestream smoke, p. 817
stimulants, p. 815
substance abuse, p. 814
tolerance, p. 816
withdrawal, p. 814

Substance abuse is the number one national health problem, causing more deaths, illnesses, and disabilities than any other health condition. Substance abuse affects not only the health of the individual user but also the health and safety of family members, coworkers, as well as the broader health of the community.

Substance abuse and addiction permeate all segments of society. As seen in *Healthy People 2020* (USDHHS, 2010), tobacco use and substance abuse are two major topic areas, with the aim of addressing numerous objectives and subobjectives both directly and indirectly related to these areas. The newer phrase *alcohol, tobacco, and other drug (ATOD) problems* rather than *substance abuse* reminds us that alcohol and tobacco represent the major drugs of abuse when discussing substance abuse, drug addiction, or chemical dependency.

This chapter begins by providing a broad perspective of ATOD problems to clarify the relevant issues. A historical overview of ATOD problems and attitudes toward ATOD users and addicted persons is examined. Relevant terms are defined to decrease confusion caused by frequent misuse of terms. The major substance categories are described in the chapter, including information on commonly used substances and current ATOD use trends. The remainder of the chapter examines the role of the nurse in primary, secondary, and tertiary prevention and describes how the nurse can improve outcomes for individuals, families, and various populations with ATOD problems when using a harm reduction model. It is important to apply nursing strategies to the *Healthy People 2020* objectives for ATOD problems.

TABLE 37.1 Caffeine Content in Commonly Consumed Substances

Drink/Food/ Supplement	Amount of Drink/Food	Amount of Caffeine
Jolt cola	12 oz	71.2 mg
Mountain Dew	12 oz	55 mg
Coca-Cola	12 oz	34 mg
Diet Coke	12 oz	45 mg
Pepsi	12 oz	38 mg
7-Up	12 oz	0 mg
Brewed coffee (drip method)	5 oz	115 mg[a]
Iced tea	12 oz	70 mg[a]
Cocoa beverage	5 oz	4 mg[a]
Chocolate milk beverage	8 oz	5 mg[a]
Dark chocolate	1 oz	20 mg[a]
Milk chocolate	1 oz	6 mg[a]
Cold relief medication	1 tablet	30 mg[a]
Vivarin	1 tablet	200 mg
Excedrin extra strength	2 tablets	130 mg

[a]Denotes average amount of caffeine.
Data from U.S. Food and Drug Administration, National Soft Drink Association, Center for Science in the Public Interest. Available at http://kidshealth.org.

ALCOHOL, TOBACCO, AND OTHER DRUG PROBLEMS IN PERSPECTIVE

ATOD abuse and addiction can cause multiple health problems for individuals, their families, and the community. Heavy ATOD use has been associated with many problems, including overdose; neonates with low birth weight and congenital abnormalities; accidents, homicides, and suicides; chronic diseases, such as cardiovascular diseases, cancer, lung disease, hepatitis, human immunodeficiency virus (HIV)/acquired immunodeficiency syndrome (AIDS), and mental illness; violence; and family disruption. Factors that contribute to the substance abuse problem include lack of knowledge about the drug use; the emphasis on illicit drugs and law enforcement rather than the prevention and treatment of abuse and addiction of ATODs; overprescription; lack of quality control of illegal drugs; and punitive drug laws that label certain drug users as criminals, encouraging negative attitudes and stigma toward these persons.

Historical Overview

Psychoactive drug use has been deeply ingrained in most cultures since the beginning of humanity. Often a culture encourages use of some drugs while discouraging the use of others. Caffeine, alcohol, and tobacco are socially acceptable drugs in the United States and Canada, whereas other cultures prohibit their use. People often do not recognize the amount of caffeine in the drinks that they may consume. It is generally not considered a drug, but it is important to recognize that its use should be limited (see Table 37.1). Conversely, cannabis, cocaine, and heroin use have not traditionally been accepted in mainstream U.S. society, although these substances are considered sacred or beneficial and their use is accepted in various other cultures. As a result, such cultural viewpoints concerning substances have been translated into law accordingly.

The United States' primary solution to various "drug problems" has been **prohibition**. During alcohol prohibition from 1920 to 1933, the United States experienced a sharp increase in violent crime and corruption among law officials as a result of the illicit marketing of alcohol. Use of distilled beverages was encouraged because of the higher profit margin per bottle of liquor than for beer or wine. The high alcohol content in illicit moonshine caused severe health problems and deaths across the United States. The alcohol prohibition was eventually recognized as a failure and repealed (Rose, 1996).

Similar problems continue to occur with the current "War on Drugs" and the more recent prohibition on cannabis, cocaine, and other drugs. The War on Drugs was coined during the Nixon administration in the 1970s as a catchphrase for the U.S. federal government's series of anti-drug policies to address drug abuse as "public enemy number one." It was during this time as well that the Controlled Substances Act was initiated and the Drug Enforcement Administration was created, launching the new era of drug control in the United States. Today, North America's rates of drug consumption and drug-related death and morbidity surpass that of any region in the world (UNODC, 2015).

Prohibitionist policies inherently support an illicit market for illegal drugs. A large body of evidence indicates that such policies additionally do little to reduce drug consumption or production. Increased law enforcement of drug prohibition has in fact contributed to increased gun violence and high homicide rates (Werb et al., 2011). Additionally, drug prohibition laws have created mandatory sentences for drug offenders and violated civil liberties, resulting in the United States having the highest rate of incarceration in the world (World Prison Brief, 2018). As the drug war budget grows each year, most of that budget goes to law enforcement and punishment, leaving less than half for prevention and treatment (USONDCP, 2017). Furthermore, the 2018 national drug control budget reduced funding allocated for prevention, increasing funding for law enforcement and efforts to disrupt illicit drug markets. Controversially, President Trump's 2019 budget request includes a 95 percent budget cut for the Office of National Drug Control as part of the administration's strategy for addressing the national opioid crisis, shifting resources largely to the DEA to continue drug control efforts (USOMB, 2018). How this manifests for public health efforts concerning substance abuse remains to be seen.

Attitudes and Myths

Attitudes are developed through cultural learning and personal experiences. Attitudes toward ATOD problems are influenced by the way society arbitrarily categorizes drugs as either "good" or "bad." In the United States, good drugs are typically over-the-counter (OTC) drugs or those prescribed by a health care provider as *medicine*, but this makes them no less problematic or addictive. Bad drugs are the illegal drugs, and persons who use these drugs are considered criminals regardless of whether the drug has caused any problems. This harmful, arbitrary practice of moralizing certain substances has come under question in the recent shift in attitude toward cannabis as demonstrated in its legalization for recreational use in nine states and the District of Columbia.

Americans rely heavily on prescription and OTC drugs to relieve, or mask, anxiety, tension, fatigue, and physical or emotional pain. Rather than learning holistic, nonmedicinal methods of coping, many people rely on the "quick fix" and take pills to cope with their problems or difficult feelings.

Addicted persons are often viewed as immoral, weak-willed, or irresponsible persons who should try harder to help themselves. Although alcoholism was recognized as a disease by the American Medical Association in 1954 and drug addiction was recognized as a disease some years later, much of the public and many health care professionals have failed to change their attitudes to accept addicted persons as individuals suffering from illness requiring health care.

It is important for nurses to examine their attitudes toward ATOD use, abuse, and addiction before working with this health problem. To be therapeutic, the nurse must develop a trusting, nonjudgmental relationship with the client. Systematic assessment in patients for ATOD problems is based on awareness that there may be problems with both legal and illegal drugs. If the nurse's attitude toward a client with a drug abuse problem is negative or punitive, the issue may never be directly addressed or the client may be avoided. If the client senses the negative attitude of the health care provider, either by words or from tone of voice, communication may cease and information may be withheld. As always, to engage in therapeutic communication, nurses need to engage in self-awareness of their own preexisting judgments and reconcile them with the duty to provide care. It is important for nurses to realize any drug can be abused, that anyone may develop drug dependence, and that drug addiction can be successfully treated.

Myths develop over years, and if myths are not questioned, many attitudes may be formed solely on the basis of fiction rather than fact. Some common myths are as follows:

- "An alcoholic is a skid row bum"—less than 5 percent of persons with addictions fit this description.
- "If you teach people about drugs, they will abuse them"—although it is true that people may choose to use drugs if they have knowledge about them, it is more likely that people without knowledge about them will abuse them.
- "Addiction is a sin or moral failing"—addiction is recognized as a health problem involving biopsychosocial factors, and persons who use drugs do not do so with the intent to become addicted.

Paradigm Shift

We can hope to see a major shift in how the United States conceptualizes ATOD problems. The old criminal justice model is based on stereotypes, misinformation, and punishment, and it uses war tactics to fight the drug users, addicted persons, and suppliers. Campaigns have been launched using the slogans "zero tolerance" for drug users, "just say no" to drugs, and striving for a "drug-free America"—all of which vilify the drug user or drug-addicted person. However, there are still divergent opinions on the best approaches to substance abuse problems, both nationally and globally. While the Obama administration's approach to the nation's drug problem was to approach it as a public health problem rather than a criminal justice problem, the Trump administration has diverted a large portion of the drug control funding in the 2019 budget request to the Department of Justice rather than increasing funding for the Department of Health and Human Services, which focuses efforts on prevention and treatment. Meanwhile, on the international level, experts suggest that national drug policies need to be focused on health of the individual and the community rather than on law enforcement strategies. Still, many countries continue to rely on criminal justice as the main approach to substance use issues.

The **harm reduction** model is a public health approach to ATOD problems initially used in Great Britain, The Netherlands, Germany, Switzerland, and Australia, and interest in it is spreading throughout Europe and in Canada. This approach is supported by a variety of organizations, including the International Drug Policy Consortium and the World Health Organization. This public health model recognizes the following:

- Addiction is a health problem.
- Any psychoactive drug can be abused.
- Accurate information can help people make responsible decisions about drug use.
- People who have ATOD problems can be helped.

This approach accepts the reality that psychoactive drug use is endemic, and it focuses on pragmatic interventions, especially education, to reduce the adverse consequences of drug abuse and get treatment for addicted persons. The United States has already taken a harm reduction approach with tobacco and alcohol, legally sanctioned drugs. Educational campaigns are used to inform the public about the health risks of tobacco use. Warnings have appeared on tobacco product labels since 1967 as a result of the surgeon general's 1964 report on the dangers of smoking. In 1971, a ban on television and radio cigarette advertising was imposed. Consequently, cigarette smoking declined from 42 percent in 1965 to 15.5 percent in 2016; 37.8 million Americans continue to smoke (CDC, 2018a). Smoking is on the decline among 8th to 12th graders. According to *Results From the 2016 National Survey on Drug Use and Health*, past month use of any tobacco product among persons aged 12 or older decreased from 26.0 percent in 2002 to 19.1 percent in 2016, and past month tobacco use among 12- to 17-year-olds fell from 13.0 percent to 3.4 percent in that same period (SAMHSA, 2017). Similarly, education continues to address the dangers of alcohol abuse and establish guidelines for safe alcohol use. Accordingly, the percent of adolescents aged 12–17 with an alcohol use disorder dropped from 5.9 percent in 2002 to 2 percent in 2016 (SAMHSA, 2017).

Nurses need to seek the underlying roots of various health problems and plan action that is realistic, nonjudgmental, holistic, and positive. A harm reduction model for ATOD problems facilitates such an approach. See www.harmreduction.org for more resources and information concerning harm reduction (see Box 37.1 for principles for an effective drug policy).

Definitions

The terms *drug use* and *drug abuse* have virtually lost their usefulness because the public and government have narrowed the term *drug* to include only illegal drugs rather than including prescription, OTC, and legal recreational drugs. The current phrase *alcohol, tobacco, and other drugs* (ATODs) is a reminder that the leading drug problems involve alcohol and tobacco.

BOX 37.1 High-Level Principles for an Effective Drug Policy

We propose that national drug strategies should always be based on five core principles:

1. Drug policies should be developed through a structured and objective assessment of priorities and evidence.
2. All activities should be undertaken in full compliance with international human rights law.
3. Drug policies should focus on reducing the harmful consequences rather than the scale of drug use and markets.
4. Policy and activities should seek to promote the social inclusion of marginalized groups.
5. Governments should build open and constructive relationships with civil society in the discussion and delivery of their strategies.

Modified from the drug policy guide created by the International Drug Policy Consortium (IDPC), published in March 2012. Available at https://idpc.net. Each chapter of the guide fully integrates the above five core principles.

The term *substance* broadens the scope to include alcohol, tobacco, legal drugs, and even foods. **Substance abuse** is the use of any substance that threatens a person's health or impairs social or economic functioning. This definition is more objective and universal than the government's definition of drug abuse, which is the use of a drug without a prescription or any use of an illegal drug. *Misuse* of a drug refers to using prescribed drugs different from directed use. Although any drug or food can be abused or misused, this chapter focuses on **psychoactive drugs**—drugs that affect mood, perception, and thought.

Drug dependence and drug addiction are often used interchangeably, but they are not synonymous. **Drug dependence** is a state of neuroadaptation (a physiological change in the central nervous system [CNS]) caused by the chronic, regular administration of a drug; in drug dependence, continued use of the drug becomes necessary to prevent withdrawal symptoms. For example, when a person is given an opiate such as morphine on a regular basis for pain management, the amount of morphine administered needs to be gradually tapered down rather than abruptly stopped, to prevent physiological symptoms of **withdrawal**.

Drug addiction is a pattern of abuse characterized by a compulsive preoccupation with the use of a drug, securing its supply, and a high tendency to relapse if the drug is removed. This definition approximates to a severe substance use disorder as defined in the *Diagnostic and Statistical Manual of Mental Disorders,* fifth edition (DSM-5). Frequently, addicted persons are physically dependent on a drug, but there is also an added psychological component that causes the intense cravings and subsequent relapse. Furthermore, addiction is linked to physiological changes in the reward, stress, and self-control brain circuits, which may continue long after use of the drug of addiction (Goldstein et al., 2011). In general, anyone can develop drug dependence as a result of regular administration of drugs that alter the CNS; however, only a small percent of these individuals will develop an addiction. The process of becoming addicted is complex and related to several factors, including the addictive properties of the substance, family and peer influences, personality, age of first use, cultural and social factors, existing psychiatric disorders, and genetics.

Alcoholism is addiction to the drug called alcohol—increasingly referred to as a severe alcohol use disorder. Alcohol and drug addictions are recognized as illnesses under a **biopsychosocial model**. Simply stated, the disease concept of addiction identifies it as a chronic and progressive disease in which a person's use of a drug or drugs continues despite problems it causes in any area of life—physical, emotional, social, economic, or spiritual.

The DSM-5 employs the catchall phrase *substance use disorder*. This umbrella diagnosis for individuals is defined as mild, moderate, or severe and identified by the substance, such as "alcohol use disorder—moderate." The severity of the disorder for a given individual is determined by the number of diagnostic criteria that are met, which vary by substance The DSM-5 uses nine substance use disorder categories: Alcohol; Caffeine; Cannabis; Hallucinogens; Inhalants; Opioids; Sedatives, hypnotics, or anxiolytics; Stimulants; and Tobacco (American Psychiatric Association, 2013).

PSYCHOACTIVE DRUGS

Psychoactive drugs, which can alter emotions, are used for enjoyment in social and recreational settings and for personal use to self-medicate physical or emotional discomfort. Psychoactive drugs are divided into categories according to their effect on the CNS and the general feelings or experiences the drugs may induce. There are numerous ways in which drugs are categorized, as seen in the DSM-5 categories. The Internet or a pharmacology text can provide detailed information on these drug categories (e.g., **depressants**, **stimulants** [as shown in Box 37.2], **hallucinogens**, inhalants [as shown in Box 37.3], and cannabis, and a drug chart of commonly abused drugs is provided on the Evolve site for this book. This chapter focuses on alcohol, tobacco, cannabis, and opioids, since these drugs cause the greatest harm and cannabis is the most commonly used illicit drug.

BOX 37.2 Stimulants

Commonly used stimulants include caffeine, amphetamines, and cocaine. Caffeine is one of the most widely used psychoactive drugs in the world, with a U.S. daily per capita consumption of 211 mg. As seen in Table 37.1, caffeine is found in coffee, tea, chocolate, soft drinks, and various medications. Moderate doses of caffeine from 100 to 300 mg per day increase mental alertness and probably have little negative effect on health. Higher doses can lead to insomnia, irritability, tremulousness, anxiety, cardiac dysrhythmias, gastrointestinal (GI) disturbances, and headaches. Regular use of high doses can lead to physical dependence, and the withdrawal symptoms may include headaches, slowness, and occasional depression (Mayo Clinic Staff, 2017). Treating afternoon headaches with analgesics containing caffeine may in reality be preventing a withdrawal symptom from heavy morning coffee consumption.

The most commonly used illicit stimulants include cocaine and amphetamines (not prescribed). Cocaine comes from the coca shrub cultivated by South American indigenous peoples for thousands of years. Purified cocaine can be snorted, smoked, or injected. Crack is a cheap form of smokable cocaine that produces an intense high but lasts for a short period. Street cocaine ranges in purity from 50 to 60 percent and may be cut with other drugs, such as procaine or amphetamine, or any white powder, such as sugar or baby powder. High doses can cause extreme agitation, paranoid delusions, hyperthermia, hallucinations, cardiac dysrhythmias, pulmonary complications, convulsions, and possibly death (O'Malley & O'Malley, 2018c).

Amphetamines are a class of stimulants similar to cocaine, but the effects last longer and the drugs are cheaper. Amphetamines have a chemical structure similar to adrenaline and noradrenaline and are generally used to decrease fatigue, increase mental alertness, suppress appetite, and create a sense of well-being. Legally manufactured amphetamines are most commonly prescribed for attention-deficit/hyperactivity disorder (ADHD), narcolepsy, and obesity. They are popular with people who abuse these drugs to stay awake for long hours to work or study. They can be taken as pills, injected, snorted, or smoked. "Ice," the smokable form of crystal methamphetamine, is easy to manufacture on the illicit market, and its effects can last up to 24 hours (O'Malley & O'Malley, 2018b).

Chronic administration of these stimulants can lead to a neurotransmitter depletion (especially of dopamine), which results in an extreme dysphoria characterized by apathy, sadness, and anhedonia (lack of joy). Thus, these users can get caught up in a dangerous cycle of gaining an extreme high followed by an extreme low. To avoid that low, the person consumes more of the stimulant. Addicted persons who use these drugs soon are overwhelmed by their cravings and may engage in criminal activities such as theft or prostitution to get more drugs. In addition, chronic frequent use of methamphetamine can lead to "meth mouth," which describes dental caries and decay that result from dry mouth and poor oral hygiene. Individuals who abuse methamphetamine are four times as likely to have dental caries, and twice as likely to have multiple decayed, missing, or filled teeth, compared to non-abusers (Shetty et al., 2016).

BOX 37.3 Inhalants

Inhalants are often among the first drugs that young children use. The primary abusers of most inhalants are adolescents who are 12 to 17 years of age. The 2016 National Survey on Drug Use and Health found that 526,000 persons aged 12 or older had used inhalants for the first time within the past 12 months and 54.6 percent of them were under the age of 18 (SAMHSA, 2017). Use often ends in late adolescence.

Inhalants are breathable chemicals, which include gases and solvents, and they do not fit neatly into other categories. The four categories of inhalants are volatile organic solvents, aerosols, volatile nitrites, and gases. These substances are inhaled ("huffed") from bottles, aerosol cans, or soaked cloth or put into bags or balloons to increase the concentration of the inhaled fumes and decrease the inhalation of other substances in the vapor (e.g., paint particles). (See www.inhalants.org for examples of products in these categories and specific drug information.) Inhalant users can get high several times in a short period, since the inhalants are short acting and have a rapid onset. Users are predominately white. Experimental use is about equal for males and females, but males are more likely to engage in chronic use.

Depending on the dose, the user may feel slight stimulation, less inhibition, or even lose consciousness. Signs of use include paint or stains on clothes or the body; spots or sores around the mouth; red or runny eyes or nose; chemical breath odor; a drunk, dazed, or dizzy appearance; nausea and loss of appetite; and finally anxiety, excitability, and irritability. Users can die from "sudden sniffing death" syndrome, and this can occur from the 1st to the 100th time he or she uses the inhalant. This death appears to be related to acute cardiac dysrhythmia. Dangers with administration of gases increase when inhaling directly from pressurized tanks because the gas is very cold and can cause frostbite to the nose, lips, and vocal cords. Also, if a gas such as nitrous oxide is not mixed with oxygen, the user may die from asphyxiation (NIDA, 2017).

Alcohol

Alcohol (ethyl alcohol or ethanol) is the oldest and most widely used psychoactive drug in the world. In 2016, a national survey found that young people between the ages of 12 and 20 are more likely to use alcohol than to use tobacco or illicit drugs, including cannabis (SAMHSA, 2017). Youth tend to drink less often than adults, but they consume more alcohol per occasion. Nearly 90 percent of all alcohol consumed by adolescents occurs as binge drinking (Levy, 2018). In 2016, 62.5 percent of underage current drinkers were binge alcohol users. Binge drinking is defined here as having five or more drinks on one occasion for males and four or more drinks for females (SAMHSA, 2017). Alcohol abuse contributes to illness in each of the top three causes of death in the United States: heart disease, cancer, and stroke. In 2016, an estimated 20.1 million persons were classified with a substance use disorder in the past year based on criteria specified in the DSM-5. Of these, 15.1 million people aged 12 or older had an alcohol use disorder. While this number seems high, this outcome actually reflects a decrease from 2002-2014 (SAMHSA, 2017).

Alcohol abuse costs billions of dollars in lost productivity, property damage, medical expenses from alcohol-related illnesses and accidents, family disruptions, alcohol-related violence, and neglect and abuse of children. Chronic alcohol abuse leads to profound metabolic and physiological effects on all organ systems. Gastrointestinal (GI) disturbances include inflammation of the GI tract, malabsorption, ulcers, liver problems, and cancers. Cardiovascular disturbances include cardiac dysrhythmias, cardiomyopathy, hypertension, atherosclerosis, and blood dyscrasias. CNS problems include depression, sleep disturbances, memory loss, organic brain syndrome, Wernicke-Korsakoff syndrome, and alcohol withdrawal syndrome. Neuromuscular problems include myopathy and peripheral neuropathy. Males may experience testicular atrophy, sterility, impotence, or gynecomastia, and females who consume alcohol during pregnancy may reproduce neonates with **fetal alcohol syndrome** (FAS) or fetal alcohol effects (FAE). Some of the metabolic disturbances include hypokalemia, hypomagnesemia, and ketoacidosis. Also, endocrine disturbances may result in pancreatitis or diabetes (O'Malley & O'Malley, 2018a).

The concentration of alcohol in the blood is determined by the concentration of alcohol in the drink, the rate of drinking, the rate of absorption (slower in the presence of food), the rate of metabolism, and a person's weight and sex. The amount of alcohol the average liver can metabolize per hour is equal to about ¾ oz of whiskey, 4 oz of wine, or 12 oz of beer. Fig. 37.1 shows the effects on the CNS as the **blood alcohol concentration** (BAC) increases. However, with chronic consumption, tolerance will develop, and a person can reach a high BAC with minimal CNS effects.

Alcohol use in moderation may provide health benefits by providing mild relaxation and lowering the serum cholesterol level. Controlled drinking organizations such as Moderation Management (http://www.moderation.org) provide guidelines for persons who want to have alcohol in their lives. See Box 37.4 for safe limits of alcohol consumption and Table 37.2 for standard drink equivalents.

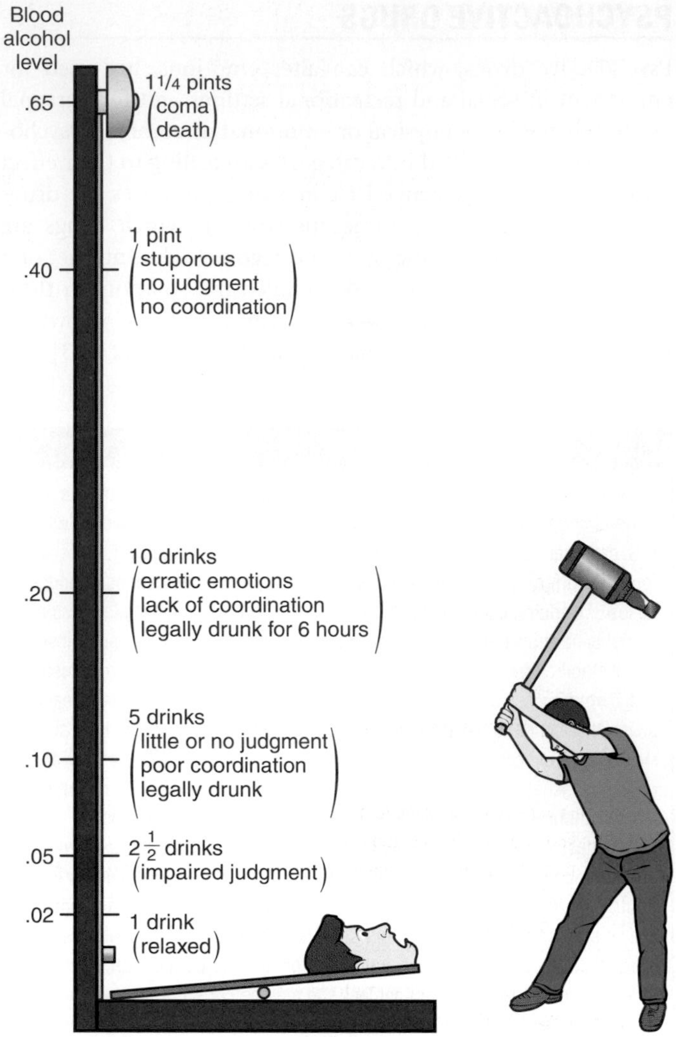

Fig. 37.1 Blood alcohol level and related central nervous system effects of a normal drinker (160-lb man) according to the number of drinks consumed in one hour. (From Kinney J: *Loosening the grip: a handbook of alcohol information,* ed. 10, New York, 2011, McGraw-Hill.)

BOX 37.4 What Are the Recommended Safe Limits for Alcohol Consumption?

For healthy men up to age 65:
- No more than 4 drinks in a day AND
- No more than 14 drinks in a week

For healthy women (and healthy men over age 65):
- No more than 3 drinks in a day AND
- No more than 7 drinks in a week

From National Institute on Alcohol Abuse and Alcoholism: *Helping patients who drink too much: a clinician's guide (update),* NIH Pub. No. 07-3769, Rockville, MD, 2005, USDHHS.

Tobacco

Smoking is the most preventable cause of death and disease in the United States, with one in five deaths attributed to cigarettes. For every person who dies from tobacco use, another 30 will suffer from at least one serious tobacco-related illness (USDHHS, 2014). Table 37.3 shows cigarette smoking–related mortality in the United States. It is estimated that more than 480,000 deaths per year are caused by complications of cigarette smoking (USDHHS, 2014). In 2016, an estimated 63.4 million Americans aged 12 or older were current (past month) users of a tobacco product. This represents 23.5 percent of the population in this age range. In addition, 51.3 million persons (19.1 percent of the population) were current cigarette smokers; 12.3 million (4.6 percent) smoked cigars; 8.8 million (3.3 percent) used snuff and chewing tobacco; and 2.3 million (0.8 percent) smoked tobacco in pipes. Young adults ages 18 to 25 reported the highest rate of current tobacco use at 23.5 percent (SAMHSA, 2017).

The economic toll from tobacco use in the United States is enormous. Cigarette smoking is responsible for more than $300 billion in annual health-related losses, with $170 billion in direct medical costs and $156 billion in lost productivity (CDC, 2018b).

Nicotine, the active ingredient in the tobacco plant, is a particularly toxic drug. To protect itself, the body quickly develops tolerance to the nicotine. If a person smokes regularly, **tolerance** to nicotine develops within hours, compared with days for heroin or months for alcohol. Pipes and

TABLE 37.2 What Is a Standard Drink?

A standard drink in the United States is any drink that contains about 14 g of pure alcohol (about 0.6 fluid oz or 1.2 tbsp). The U.S. standard drink equivalents shown here are approximate, since different brands and types of beverages vary in their actual alcohol content.

12 oz of beer or cooler	8-9 oz of malt liquor 8.5 oz shown in a 12-oz glass that, if full, would hold about 1.5 standard drinks of malt liquor	5 oz of table wine	3-4 oz of fortified wine (such as sherry or port) 3.5 oz shown	2-3 oz of cordial, liqueur, or aperitif 2.5 oz shown	1.5 oz of brandy (a single jigger)	1.5 oz of spirits (a single jigger of 80-proof gin, vodka, whiskey, etc.) Shown straight and in a highball glass with ice to show level before adding mixer[a]

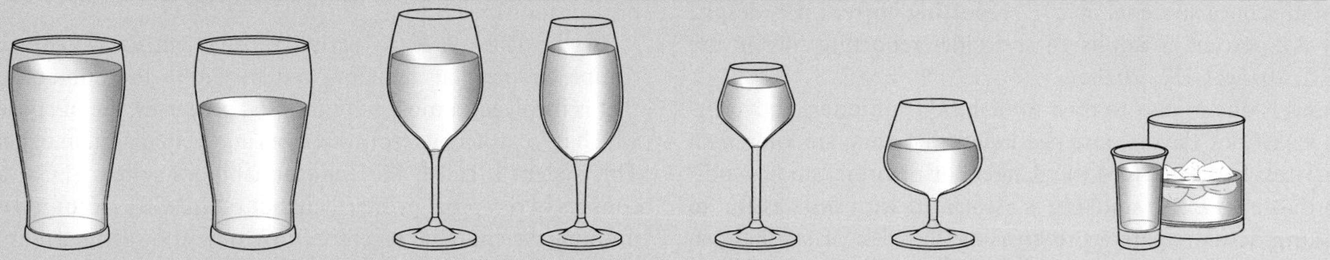

12 oz	8.5 oz	5 oz	3.5 oz	2.5 oz	1.5 oz	1.5 oz

Many people do not know what counts as a standard drink and so they do not realize how many standard drinks are in the containers in which these drinks are often sold. Some examples:

For beer, the approximate number of standard drinks in

12 oz = 1	22 oz = 2
16 oz = 1.3	40 oz = 3.3

For malt liquor, the approximate number of standard drinks in

12 oz = 1.5	22 oz = 2.5
16 oz = 2	40 oz = 4.5

For table wine, the approximate number of standard drinks in a standard 750 mL (25 oz) bottle = 5

For 80-proof spirits, or "hard liquor," the approximate number of standard drinks in

a mixed drink = 1 or more[a]	a fifth (25 oz) = 17
a pint (16 oz) = 11	1.75 L (59 oz) = 39

[a]*Note:* It can be difficult to estimate the number of standard drinks in a single mixed drink made with hard liquor. Depending on factors such as the type of spirits and the recipe, a mixed drink can contain from one to three or more standard drinks.

TABLE 37.3 Cigarette Smoking–Related Mortality

Disease	Men	Women	Overall
Cancers			
Lung	74,300	53,400	127,700
Other	26,000	10,000	36,000
Subtotal	100,300	63,400	163,700
Cardiovascular Diseases and Metabolic Diseases			
Coronary heart disease	61,800	37,500	99,300
Other heart disease	13,400	12,100	25,500
Cerebrovascular disease	8,200	7,100	15,300
Other vascular disease	6,000	5,500	11,500
Diabetes mellitus	6,200	2,800	9,000
Subtotal	95,600	65,000	160,000
Respiratory Diseases			
Pneumonia/influenza	7,800	4,700	12,500
COPD	50,400	50,200	100,600
Subtotal	58,200	54,900	113,100
Total	**254,100**	**183,300**	**437,400**

COPD, Chronic obstructive pulmonary disease.
Modified from Centers for Disease Control and Prevention: *Annual cigarette smoking-related mortality in the United States.* Available at http://www.cdc.gov.

cigars are less hazardous than cigarettes because the harsher smoke discourages deep inhalation. However, pipes and cigars increase the risk of cancer of the lips, mouth, and throat.

Smoke can be inhaled directly by the smoker (**mainstream smoke**), or it can enter the atmosphere from the lit end of the cigarette and be inhaled by others in the vicinity (sidestream smoke). **Sidestream smoke** or secondhand smoke contains higher concentrations of toxic and carcinogenic compounds than mainstream smoke. Exposure to sidestream tobacco smoke has been causally linked to cancer, respiratory and cardiovascular diseases, and adverse effects on the health of infants and children (USDHHS, 2014). Sidestream smoke is only about 20 percent less dangerous than actually smoking, and most of the toxic effects occur within the first five minutes of exposure (Barnoya & Glanz, 2005). Smoking bans continue to be adopted to reduce the discomfort and health hazards among nonsmokers.

Nicotine is also used as chewing tobacco or snuff. Marketed as "smokeless tobacco," a wad is put in the mouth and the nicotine is absorbed sublingually. Higher doses of nicotine are delivered in the smokeless forms because the nicotine is not destroyed by heat. Nevertheless, this form is less addictive because nicotine enters the bloodstream less directly. Smokeless tobacco users are 20 percent more likely to die of heart disease than nonusers, and they are at a higher risk for cancers of the mouth, pharynx, esophagus, stomach, and pancreas (Barry, 2007).

More recently, electronic cigarettes, or e-cigarettes, have gained popularity in the United States, especially among adolescents. E-cigarettes contain liquid nicotine, which is heated into a vapor and inhaled. They are the most commonly used form of tobacco among youth in the country, with 11.7 percent of high school students in 2017 reporting current use, despite only 3.2 percent of adults 18 and older reporting current use (CDC, 2017c; CDC, 2018c).

This is due in part to their availability, unhindered advertising, variety of flavors, and the belief that they are safer than cigarettes. In addition to the dangers of nicotine, studies indicate that e-cigarette smoking is associated with progression to smoking actual cigarettes, increasing the risk of smoking in vulnerable populations like adolescents (Soneji et al., 2017). While the long-term health effects of e-cigarettes are still unknown, many e-cigarette products have been found to contain known carcinogens and toxic chemicals (Hess et al., 2017).

Cannabis (Marijuana)

Cannabis (*Cannabis sativa* or *C. indica*) is the most widely used illicit drug in the United States. In 2016, a national survey found that an estimated 24 million Americans aged 12 or older were current users of cannabis (SAMHSA, 2017). Compared with other psychoactive drugs, cannabis has little toxicity and is one of the safest therapeutic agents known. Psychological dependence can occur with chronic use, but little is known about any potential physical dependence. Users enjoy a mild euphoria, a relaxed feeling, and an intensity of sensory perceptions. Some call the effect a dreamy state of consciousness in which ideas seem disconnected, unanticipated, and free flowing. Time, color, and spatial perceptions may be altered (O'Malley & O'Malley, 2018d). Side effects include dry and reddened eyes, increased appetite, dry mouth, drowsiness, and mild tachycardia. Adverse reactions include anxiety, disorientation, and paranoia.

Although the vast majority of cannabis users do not experience serious negative physical side effects, emergency departments have started to see an increase of patients suffering from cannabinoid hyperemesis syndrome. This manifests as cyclic episodes of nausea and vomiting in frequent users, resolving spontaneously within 48 hours without cannabis use and relieved only by hot baths (Lu & Agito, 2015). This phenomenon may be explained by frequent use of cannabis extracts and concentrates, which contain exponentially larger dosages of cannabinoids than traditional plant material.

In general, the greatest physical concern for chronic users is possible damage to the respiratory tract from smoking the drug, though even daily smokers do not develop obstructive airway disease. For chronic users, tolerance can develop, as well as physical dependence; however, withdrawal symptoms are benign. As with any euphoria-inducing drug, addiction can occur for some chronic users and is difficult to treat because the progression tends to be subtle.

Despite its widely accepted therapeutic effects, especially in treating chronic pain (Mucke et al., 2018), the federal government continues its total prohibition efforts. By 2018, 30 states and the District of Columbia had laws broadly legalizing marijuana in some form (see map). Additionally, several state nurses associations, the American Nurses Association, and the American Public Health Association, among other health care organizations, support access to the medicinal use of cannabis. See www.medicalcannabis.com for a full list of supporting organizations.

In the late 1980s to early 1990s, scientists discovered a complex molecular signaling system within the human body that is involved in most physiological processes, the purpose of which is to protect us from stressors and help maintain balance. This system is called the endocannabinoid system (ECS) and consists of receptors primarily in our brain (CB1 receptors) and immune system (CB2 receptors). We now know that all animals have an ECS and that we make cannabinoids (endogenous cannabinoids) that are similar in structure to the phytocannabinoids found in the cannabis plant. This new science is shedding light on human physiology and helps explain how and why cannabis has such a wide margin of safety and is helpful for such a wide array of health problems (Pacher et al., 2006; Werner, 2011). Research efforts to further elucidate the beneficial properties of Cannabidiol (CBD) continue to increase, and safer therapeutic uses of CBD have become more well-known in recent years. CBD is a cannabinoid compound found in cannabis that is not psychoactive and has been found to have antiinflammatory, anti-pain, and potentially antipsychotic properties (Burstein, 2015; Leweke et al., 2012). In light of these findings, more evidence is needed to further elucidate the beneficial properties of cannabinoids in order to harness their potential for therapeutic use in health care (Box 37.5).

Opioids

President Trump declared a public health emergency in October 2017 concerning the opioid epidemic in the United States. Opioids are the number one cause of drug overdose deaths in the country. On average, 115 Americans die every day from an opioid overdose (CDC, 2017b). Drug overdose death rates have more than tripled in the United States since 1999. In 2016, drug

BOX 37.5 Synthetic Cannabinoids

While dronabinol (Marinol) is synthetic tetrahydrocannabinol (THC) in sesame oil and approved as a Schedule III drug by the Food and Drug Administration (FDA), numerous "synthetic cannabinoids" have started to appear on the market. These synthetic cannabinoids are much stronger than the FDA-approved medication and are usually smoked or inhaled as a vapor. In the past decade, these have become an increasingly popular substance of abuse globally. There are many different formulations of synthetic cannabinoids in existence, some of which have become illegal. Many formulations, however, remain available on the legal market and are sold under names such as K2, Spice, and Black Mamba. Individuals often use synthetic cannabinoids due to the belief that they are safer because they are legal. While some report effects similar to cannabis, effects are inconsistent and may even be dangerous and fatal, depending on formulation and use (NIDA, 2018b).

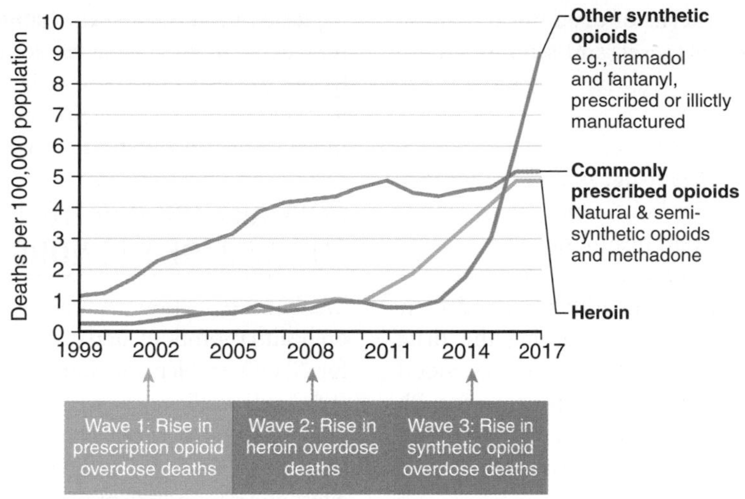

Fig. 37.2 Three waves of the rise in opioid overdose deaths. (From https://www.cdc.gov.)

overdose was the leading cause of injury death, and the third overall cause of death in the United States (CDC, 2017f). People aged 12 or older who misused prescription pain relievers in 2016 reported the most common source was from a friend or relative (53 percent) (SAMHSA, 2017). From 1999 to 2016, the drug overdose rate more than tripled, leading to 63,600 drug overdose deaths in 2016. Of these deaths, 66.4 percent involved an opioid (CDC, 2017a). It is estimated that the total economic burden of prescription opioid misuse is $78.5 billion in health care, lost productivity, addiction treatment, and criminal justice costs (Florence et al., 2016).

Opioids are primarily used for pain management by acting on opioid receptors on nerve cells to decrease pain and produce euphoria and drowsiness. Tolerance and physical dependence develop quickly, requiring a tapering down in therapy to avoid withdrawal symptoms after several days' use (O'Malley & O'Malley, 2018e).

The opioid epidemic began in 1999, primarily with the misuse of common prescription opioid drugs used to treat pain, which include hydrocodone (Vicodin), oxycodone (OxyContin, Percocet), codeine, fentanyl, and morphine (Kadian, Avinza), among others. This was in large part due to inappropriate physician prescription of these drugs, buoyed by improper marketing, lobbying, and pharmaceutical kickbacks (Dasgupta et al., 2018). In 2010, heroin overdose deaths saw a sharp increase, with the CDC reporting heroin deaths had doubled from 2010 to 2012 (CDC, 2014b). This spike occurred in part due to increasing dependency and tolerance to prescription opioids and desiring a cheaper and more potent alternative. In fact, multiple studies in 2013 found that about 80 percent of heroin users first misused prescription opioids before using heroin, which has steadily decreased in cost over the years (Muhuri et al., 2013). Yet even with this increase, still more than twice as many died from prescription opioid overdoses than heroin in 2012 (CDC, 2014a). It should also be noted that while 21-29 percent of patients prescribed opioids for chronic pain misuse them, only 8-12 percent develop an opioid use disorder, and an estimated 4–6 percent transition to heroin use (NIDA, 2018a).

The third phase of the opioid epidemic began in 2013 with the increased use of synthetic opioids (other than methadone) including tramadol, fentanyl, and fentanyl analogs such as carfentanil, which have been responsible for the bulk of opioid-related deaths since that time. Deaths from synthetic opioids doubled from 9580 in 2015 to 19,413 in 2016 (Seth et al., 2018). Fentanyl is a synthetic opioid that is 50 times more potent than heroin and 100 times more potent than morphine. Carfentanil is 5000 times more potent than heroin. Although fentanyl is produced and used legally, illegal production of fentanyl/fentanyl analogs has soared, such that most synthetic opioid overdoses today involve illicitly manufactured fentanyl, often added into counterfeit prescription opioid tablets, heroin, cocaine, or methamphetamine without the user's knowledge. While synthetic opioids were the most common drug involved in overdose deaths in 2016, 80 percent of these overdose deaths involved alcohol or another drug—most commonly another opioid (Jones et al., 2018) (Fig. 37.2).

In 2016, 35.6 percent of the population aged 18 and older reported using prescription pain relievers in the past year, although only 4.5 percent of the population reported misusing opioids, including heroin and other illicit opioids (SAMHSA, 2017). The proportion of persons who misuse opioids to the number of overdose deaths resulting from their use highlights the lethal potential of these drugs when misused. The CDC released a guideline for prescribing opioids for chronic pain to better ensure appropriate prescribing practices to reduce potential for misuse. The three main areas of focus are (1) determining when to initiate or continue opioids for chronic pain; (2) opioid selection, dosage, duration, follow-up, and discontinuation; and (3) assessing risk and addressing harms of opioid use. Increasingly, efforts are transitioning to emphasis on nonopioid pharmacological and nonpharmacological treatments for chronic pain (CDC, 2016a).

PREDISPOSING/CONTRIBUTING FACTORS

In addition to the specific drug being used, two other major variables influence the particular drug experience: set and setting. To understand various patterns of drug use and abuse by individuals, all three factors (drug, set, and setting) should be considered.

Set

Set refers to the individual using the drug, as well as that person's expectations, including unconscious expectations, about the drug being used. A person's current health may alter a drug's effects from one day to the next. Some people are genetically predisposed to alcoholism or other drug addiction, and their chemical makeup is such that simply consuming the drug triggers the disease process. Persons with underlying mood disorders or other mental illness may try to self-medicate with psychoactive drugs. Sometimes the choice of drug exacerbates symptoms; for example, a depressed person might consume alcohol and become more depressed.

Setting

Setting is the influence of the physical, social, and cultural environment within which the use occurs. Social conditions influence the use of drugs. The fast pace of life, competition at school or in the workplace, and the pressure to accumulate material possessions are daily stressors. Pharmaceutical, alcohol, and tobacco companies are continuously bombarding the public with enticing advertisements pushing their products as a means of feeling better, sleeping better, having more energy, or just as a "treat." People grow up believing that most of life's problems can be solved quickly and easily through the use of a drug. For persons of a lower socioeconomic background, with minimal education or employment possibilities, many of life's opportunities can seem out of reach. Rather than seeking relief through holistic means or behavioral health treatment, the use of psychoactive drugs may offer a way to numb the pain or escape from a hopeless reality. They may rely on alcohol or illicit drugs, which are more readily available. For some, selling illicit drugs may appear to be the only way to support themselves and their loved ones in avoiding a future of poverty and unemployment.

Biopsychosocial Model of Addiction

Many theories have been proposed to explain the etiological factors of addiction, and no consensus exists on specific causes. These theories include the belief that addiction is a disease, a moral failing, a psychological disturbance, a personality disorder, a social problem, a dysbehaviorism, or a maladaptive coping mechanism. Different people develop addiction in different ways. For example, some alcohol-addicted persons say, "I knew I was an alcoholic from my first drink; I drank differently than others." Others have no family history of addiction, but when stressed (such as from chronic pain, significant losses, abusive relationships that lead to low self-esteem, or trauma resulting in post-traumatic stress disorder), they find that drugs may temporarily relieve their stress. Over time, heavy use of one or more drugs to cope with the stress may lead to a substance use disorder. As discussed earlier, current research focuses on the neurochemistry of addiction, which shows brain chemistry changes among addicted persons. The "just say no" approach neglects the fact that such changes to the brain's reward system may make it impossible for some already addicted individuals to do so. The biopsychosocial model provides a framework for understanding addiction as the result of the interaction of multiple factors involved in drug, set, and setting.

PRIMARY PREVENTION AND THE ROLE OF THE NURSE

The harm reduction approach to substance use disorders focuses on health promotion and disease prevention. Primary prevention for ATOD problems includes (1) the promotion of healthy lifestyles and resiliency factors and (2) education about drugs and guidelines for their use. Nurses are ideally prepared to use health promotion strategies such as promoting and facilitating healthy alternatives to indiscriminate, careless, and often dangerous drug use practices and providing education about drugs to decrease harm from irresponsible or unsafe drug use practices.

Promotion of Healthy Lifestyles and Resiliency Factors

It is possible to teach clients to have more agency in their relationships with others and how to make more beneficial decisions by looking carefully at the pros and cons of each option and the related consequences. People may turn to medications, especially psychoactive drugs, when they have persistent health problems such as difficulty sleeping, muscle tension, lack of energy, chronic stress, and mood swings. Nurses can help clients understand that medications may mask problems rather than solve them. Stress reduction and relaxation techniques along with a balanced lifestyle may be more effective than medications. Lack of sleep, improper diet, and insufficient exercise contribute to many health complaints. Assisting clients to balance their need for rest, nutrition, and exercise on a daily basis can reduce these complaints. Nurses can provide useful information to groups, assisting in the development of community recreational resources or facilitating stress reduction, relaxation, or exercise groups. Nurses can help people learn about drug-free community activities. The How To box lists community activities in which the nurse may become involved.

HOW TO Set Up Community-Based Activities Aimed at Substance Abuse Prevention

- Increase involvement and pride in school activities.
- Facilitate a peer mentorship program to discourage youth from joining gangs.
- Establish a support group for veterans.
- Organize substance-free promoting events for youth at skate parks.
- Organize a Students Against Drunk Driving (SADD) chapter.
- Mobilize parental awareness and action groups (e.g., Mothers Against Drunk Driving [MADD]).
- Establish an Al-Anon or Alateen meeting.
- Increase availability of recreational facilities.
- Curtail media messages that glamorize drug and alcohol use.
- Support and reinforce anti-drug use peer-pressure skills.
- Collaborate with community leaders to address problems related to crime, housing, jobs, and access to health care.

Lack of educational opportunities, job training, or both can contribute to socioeconomic stress and poor self-esteem, which can lead to drug use to escape the situation. Nurses can help clients identify community resources and address problems to meet basic needs rather than avoid them.

In addition to decreasing risk factors associated with ATOD problems, it is important to increase protective or resiliency factors. Prevention guidelines to teach parents and teachers how to increase resiliency in youths include the following strategies:

- Help them develop an increased sense of responsibility for their own success.
- Help them identify their talents.
- Encourage them to find inspiration in helping society rather than in consumerism.
- Provide realistic appraisals and feedback; stress multicultural competence; encourage and value education and skills training.
- Increase cooperative solutions to problems rather than competitive or aggressive solutions.

Drug Education

ATOD problems include more than abuse of psychoactive drugs. Today more than 450,000 different drugs and drug combinations are available by prescription or over the counter. Nurses have knowledge about medication administration, the benefits of drugs, and their shortcomings. Nurses can influence the health of clients by destroying the myth of good drugs versus bad drugs. This means (1) teaching clients that no drug is completely safe and that any drug can be abused, (2) helping persons learn how to make informed decisions about their drug use to minimize potential harm, and (3) teaching them to always tell their health care provider what supplements they are taking.

Drug technology is growing, yet the public receives little information about how to safely use this technology. Harm reduction as a goal recognizes that people consume drugs and that they need to know about the use of drugs and risks involved in order to make safer decisions about their drug use. Drug education should begin on an individual basis by reviewing the client's prescription medications. Clients often presume little risk is involved because a physician or nurse practitioner has prescribed the medication.

Is the client aware of any untoward interactions this drug may have with other drugs being used or with food? A common occurrence with drug users is taking drugs from different categories together or at different times to regulate how they feel, known as **polysubstance use or abuse**. For example, a person may drink alcohol when snorting cocaine to "take the edge off"; or some intravenous drug users combine cocaine with heroin (speedball) for similar reasons. Polysubstance use can cause drug interactions that can have additive, synergistic, or antagonistic effects. Indiscriminant polysubstance abuse may lead to serious physiological consequences and can be complicated for the health care professional to assess and treat. It is important to encourage clients to ask questions about their drug use. The How To box lists key information that clients should obtain before taking a drug or medication to decrease the possible harm from unsafe medication consumption.

HOW TO Determine the Relative Safety of a Drug for Personal or Client Use

Before using a drug/medication, always determine the following:

- The chemical being taken
- How and where the drug works in the body (main effects, side effects, and adverse reactions)
- The correct dosage and route of administration
- Whether there will be drug interactions, including interactions with herbal remedies or foods
- Awareness of the symptoms of a potential allergic reaction and knowing when to seek help
- If there will be drug tolerance
- If the drug will produce physical dependence

Purity of the chemical and potential for unknown additives also should be determined.

Nurses can identify references and community resources available to provide the necessary information, and they can clarify the information. User-friendly reference texts and online resources are available that describe drug interactions among medications, other drugs (including alcohol, tobacco, marijuana, and cocaine), and other substances (food and beverages); they serve as excellent guides for nurses and their clients. (See http://www.drugs.com for more information.) Clients should learn and ask questions about their prescription medications, self-administered over-the-counter drugs, including supplements and herbal remedies, and recreational drugs. This does not mean that nurses should encourage other drug use, but rather that the potential harm from self-medication can be reduced if clients have the necessary information to make more informed decisions.

Parents should seek information about their use of medications so they can act as role models for their children. It can be confusing for children and adolescents to be told to "just say no" to drugs when they see their parents trying drugs or they see drug advertisements offering to "quick fix" every health complaint or feeling of stress, anxiety, or depression with a medication. The simple "just say no" approach does not help young people for several reasons. First, children are naturally curious, and drug experimentation is often a part of normal development. Second, children from dysfunctional homes may use drugs to get attention, to escape an intolerable environment, or because a family member introduced certain drugs to them. And finally, the "just say no" approach does not address the powerful influence of peer pressure.

Drug education moved into school curriculum with Project DARE (Drug Abuse Resistance Education) in the 1980s, the most widely used school-based drug-use prevention program in the United States. This abstinence-based program uses law enforcement officers to teach the material, but studies have found that it is less effective than other interactive prevention programs and may even result in increased drug use (Pan & Bai, 2009). DARE has since added to their program a curriculum targeting elementary and middle school students called *keepin' it REAL*, which is supported by the 2016 U.S. surgeon general's report on addiction (USDHHS, 2016).

Basic ATOD prevention programs for young people should combine efforts to increase resiliency factors with drug education. Nurses can serve as educators or as advisors to the school systems or community groups to ensure that all of these areas are addressed. Role-playing and peer facilitation is useful in teaching many of these skills.

As with much of the public health field, more online and mobile phone apps have been introduced to educate people, especially youth, about drugs and drug use. Young people are the most likely to be receptive to such mobile health (mHealth) efforts, as they may feel more comfortable using such technology than older populations. In addition, mHealth preventive interventions have the ability to reach large numbers of individuals at their convenience in comparison to in-person interventions. Although the use of such technology is still quite new in substance abuse prevention, early research points to the effectiveness of such interventions when applied in real-life, real-time contexts (Kazemi et al., 2017).

CHECK YOUR PRACTICE

As a public health nurse who works one day a week in a middle school, you are developing a program and fact sheet for eighth grade students. What are some of the age-appropriate items you would include in order to help these students know where to locate resources about alcohol and other drugs?

SECONDARY PREVENTION AND THE ROLE OF THE NURSE

Screening for health problems has long been a basic tool used by public health nurses when working with various populations. There are numerous screening tools for ATOD problems that can be used independently or integrated with broader health screening tools. When drug abuse, dependence, or addiction is identified, nurses must assist clients to understand the connection between their drug use patterns and the negative consequences on their health, their families, and the community. Brief interventions include effective strategies nurses can initiate for early intervention before a person needs more extensive or specialized treatment.

One such intervention is called Screening, Brief Intervention, and Referral to Treatment (SBIRT). SBIRT is an evidence-based practice used to identify, reduce, and prevent problematic use, abuse, and dependence on alcohol, tobacco, and other drugs. The SBIRT model was incited by an Institute of Medicine recommendation that called for community-based screening for health risk behaviors, including substance use. Primary care centers, hospital emergency departments, trauma centers, and other community settings provide opportunities for early intervention with at-risk substance users before more severe consequences occur.

- *Screening* quickly assesses the severity of substance use and identifies the appropriate level of treatment.
- *Brief intervention* focuses on increasing insight and awareness regarding substance use and motivation toward behavioral change.
- *Referral to treatment* provides those identified as needing more extensive treatment with access to specialty care.

A key aspect of SBIRT is the integration and coordination of screening and treatment components into a system of services. This system links a community's specialized treatment programs with a network of early intervention and referral activities that are conducted in medical and social service settings (http://www.integration.samhsa.gov.). Some apps have also been developed to aid health care professionals in employing SBIRT in their interactions with clients. Research points to the effectiveness of the universal application of SBIRT in the school setting for all adolescents, even outside of the clinic setting, demonstrating that it promotes continued abstinence and reduces substance use (Maslowsky et al., 2017). For example, the prevention program Brief Alcohol Screening and Intervention for College Students (BASICS) is an evidence-based intervention that has been found to return $17.61 for each dollar spent (USDHHS, 2016).

Assessing for Alcohol, Tobacco, and Other Drug Problems

In addition to the SBIRT, there are many other screening tools that can be used in order to assess for substance abuse problems. The National Institute on Drug Abuse has developed a compilation of resources for clinicians through a Physicians' Outreach Initiative called NIDAMED, including tools and resources for screening. These screening and assessment tools are available at https://www.drugabuse.gov. Of note, the Alcohol Use Disorders Identification Test (AUDIT) and Drug Abuse Screening Test (DAST) are helpful, commonly used screening instruments for health professionals.

Self-assessment screening tools are available online at http://www.alcoholscreening.org and www.drugscreening.org. These screening tools are based on the Alcohol, Smoking, and Substance Involvement Screening Test (ASSIST) developed by the World Health Organization and allow for immediate feedback. People can participate in this screening anonymously.

During any health assessment, the nurse should assess for substance abuse problems, including both self-medication practices and recreational drug use when taking a medication history. Thus, all relevant drug use history is collected and aids in the assessment of drug use patterns. Note any changes in drug use patterns over time. After obtaining a medication history, follow-up questions can determine if problems exist. The following are examples:

- If using a prescription drug, is the client following the directions correctly?
- Has the client increased the dosage or frequency above the prescription level?
- Is the person using any other prescribed or recreational psychoactive drugs, including alcohol and tobacco?
- If so, for how long and what is the dosage?

One useful assessment tool is the five A's when screening for ATOD problems: (1) Ask about use; (2) Assess amount and pattern of use; (3) Advise about safe use as appropriate; (4) Assist with identifying help or resources; (5) Arrange for follow-up as needed.

When assessing self-medication and recreational or social drug use patterns, determine the reason the person uses the drug. Some underlying health problems (e.g., pain, stress, weight, insomnia) may be relieved by nonpharmaceutical interventions. The amount, frequency, duration of use, and the route of administration of each drug should be determined. To establish the presence of a substance abuse problem, it is necessary to determine if the drug use is causing any negative health consequences or problems with relationships, employment, finances, or the legal system. The How To box lists examples of questions to ask to determine the presence of socioeconomic problems that are often a result of substance abuse. If a pattern of chronic, regular, and frequent use of a drug exists, nurses should assess for a history of withdrawal symptoms to determine if there is physical dependence on the drug. A progression in drug use patterns and related problems warns about the possibility of addiction. **Denial** is a primary symptom of addiction. Methods of denial include the following:

- Lying about use
- Minimizing use patterns
- Blaming or rationalizing
- Intellectualizing
- Changing the subject
- Using anger or humor
- "Going with the flow" (agreeing that a problem exists, stating the behavior will change, but not demonstrating any behavior changes)

A problem should be suspected if the client becomes defensive or exhibits other behavior indicating denial when asked about alcohol or other drug use.

HOW TO Assess Socioeconomic Problems Resulting From Substance Abuse

If the client admits to use of alcohol, tobacco, or other drugs, ask the following questions:

- Do your parents, spouse, or friends worry or complain about your drinking or using drugs?
- Has a family member sought help about your drinking or using drugs?
- Have you neglected family obligations as a result of drinking or using drugs?
- Have you missed work because of your drinking or using drugs?
- Does your boss complain about your drinking or using drugs?
- Do you drink or use drugs before or during work?
- Have you ever been fired or quit because of drinking or using drugs?
- Have you ever been charged with driving under the influence (DUI) or being drunk in public (DIP)?
- Have you ever had any other legal problems related to drinking and using drugs, such as assault and battery, breaking and entering, or theft?
- Have you had any accidents while intoxicated, such as falls, burns, or motor vehicle accidents?
- Have you spent your money on alcohol or other drugs instead of paying your bills (e.g., telephone, electricity, rent)?

The Levels of Prevention box shows the levels of prevention related to substance abuse that can be used by nurses.

LEVELS OF PREVENTION

Substance Use Disorders

Primary Prevention

Provide community education to teach healthy lifestyles; focus on how to resist getting involved in substance abuse; engage individuals in activities and interests they can be passionate about.

Secondary Prevention

Institute early detection programs in schools, the workplace, and other areas in which people gather to determine the presence of substance abuse; educate individuals on how to recognize substance abuse in friends/family/coworkers.

Tertiary Prevention

Develop programs to help people reduce or end substance abuse; educate individuals who abuse drugs on safe drug use.

Drug Testing

During the 1980s, pre-employment or random drug testing in the workplace gained popularity. A person's urine, blood, saliva, or hair can be examined to test for the use of drugs. The breath can be tested for alcohol. Urine testing is the most common method of drug screening. Urine testing indicates only past use of certain drugs, not current intoxication. Thus, persons can be identified as having used a certain drug in the recent past, but the degree of intoxication and extent of performance impairment cannot be determined with urine testing. Also, most drug-related problems in the workplace are related to alcohol, and alcohol is not always included in a urine drug screen.

When is drug testing appropriate? Drug testing that follows documented impairment may help substantiate the cause of the impairment, thus serving as a backup rather than the primary screening method. It is also useful for recovering addicted persons. If part of their treatment is to abstain from psychoactive drug use, a urine test yielding positive results for a drug indicates a relapse.

Blood, breath, and saliva drug tests can indicate current use and relative amount. Any of these tests can help determine alcohol intoxication, and they are often used to substantiate suspected impairment. A serum drug screen can be useful to determine the specific drug ingested when overdose is suspected. The testing of hair is gaining attention because the results can provide a long history of drug use patterns.

Alcohol and other drug testing should be used as a clinical and public health tool, but not for harassment and punishment. For example, many people seen in trauma centers were drinking at the time of their injuries. Hence, it is recommended that breath alcohol testing should be routinely done for clients admitted to the emergency department for traumatic injuries.

Employee assistance programs (EAPs) are a beneficial service in many work settings. EAP programs can identify personal and/or work-related problems among employees and offer short-term counseling or referral to other health care providers as necessary. Such programs also offer services to employees to reduce stress and provide other forms of support to prevent substance abuse problems from developing. Nurses frequently develop and run these programs.

Often, a sizeable number of EAP clients have substance use problems, since most adults with these problems are employed. The 2016 National Survey on Drug Use and Health found that of the about 19 million adults classified with dependence or abuse, 54.5 percent were employed full time (SAMHSA, 2017).

High-Risk Groups

Identifying high-risk groups helps nurses design programs to meet specific needs and to mobilize community resources.

Adolescents. The younger a person is when beginning intensive experimentation with drugs, the more likely dependence will develop. Underage drinking is considered the most serious drug problem for youth in the United States. Findings from the 2016 National Survey on Drug Use and Health found that 19.3 percent of individuals aged 12 to 20 had used alcohol in the past month, and that 12.1 percent of those had engaged in binge alcohol use. This survey also notes these past-year drug use patterns among 12- to 17-year-olds: 15.8 percent had used illicit drugs in the past year, with 12 percent using cannabis, 0.5 percent cocaine, 0.1 percent heroin, 1.8 percent hallucinogens (including LSD, PCP, and ecstasy), 2.2 percent inhalants, 0.1 percent methamphetamine, and 5.3 percent psychotherapeutic drugs nonmedically (with 3.5 percent using pain relievers) (SAMHSA, 2017).

People who misuse illicit prescription drugs are at risk of abuse and addiction as well as overdose deaths. Many teens and college youth steal drugs from their family members or are given them by friends and family, and others buy them off the Internet. The most commonly abused opioids among teens are hydrocodone (Vicodin) and oxycodone (OxyContin), and these are sometimes crushed and snorted or injected. Friends in school share their amphetamine salts (Adderall) or methylphenidate (Ritalin) with other students, who often use them to help them study. Benzodiazepines such as diazepam (Valium) and alprazolam (Xanax) are the depressants of choice.

Students say that prescription drugs are often cheaper and easier to obtain, and some believe that they are "cleaner" or safer than illicit drugs such as cannabis or cocaine. This is increasingly untrue as synthetic opioids have made their way into counterfeit OxyContin tablets and Xanax bars. Young people generally have no idea of the toxic effects when these drugs are taken in high doses or combined.

Although risk-taking and trying new things is a normal part of adolescent development, heavy drug use during adolescence can interfere with normal brain development. Note that *Healthy People 2020* objectives SA-2 and TU-3 reduce the initiation of the use of tobacco, alcohol, and other drugs (see *Healthy People 2020* box) (U.S. Department of Health and Human Services, 2010). Family-related factors (genetics, family stress, parenting styles, child victimization) appear to be the greatest variable that influences substance abuse among adolescents. The co-occurrence with psychiatric disorders (especially mood disorders) and behavioral problems is also associated with substance abuse among adolescents, leaving peer pressure as a less influential factor. Research suggests that successful social influence-based prevention programs may be driven by their ability to foster social norms that reduce an adolescent's social motivation to begin using ATODs. One particularly effective treatment approach for adolescents is the use of family-oriented therapy (NIDA, 2014). The Quality and Safety in Nursing Education box provides information about using information management tools to develop ATOD prevention programs in a school.

Lobbying and policy changes are an important factor in primary prevention for youth as well. For example, in an attempt to limit the number of youth who use tobacco, six states and 340 localities have raised the minimum legal sale age for tobacco products to 21 years old as a result of successful campaigning ("States and Localities," 2018).

HEALTHY PEOPLE 2020

Objectives Related to Substance Abuse

- **SA-2:** Increase the proportion of adolescents never using substances.
- **SA-8:** Increase the proportion of persons who need alcohol and/or illicit drug treatment and received specialty treatment for abuse or dependence in the past year.
- **SA-14:** Reduce the proportion of persons engaging in binge drinking of alcoholic beverages.
- **SA-17:** Decrease the rate of alcohol-impaired driving (0.08+ blood alcohol content [BAC]) fatalities.

Objectives Related to Tobacco Use

- **TU-3:** Reduce initiation of tobacco use among children, adolescents, and young adults.
- **TU-11:** Reduce the proportion of nonsmokers exposed to secondhand smoke.
- **TU-14:** Increase the proportion of smoke-free homes.
- **TU-18:** Reduce the proportion of adolescents and young adults in grades 6 through 12 who are exposed to tobacco marketing.

From U.S. Department of Health and Human Services: *Healthy People 2020:* national health promotion and disease prevention objectives. Washington, DC.

QSEN FOCUS ON QUALITY AND SAFETY EDUCATION FOR NURSES

Targeted Competency: Informatics

Use information technology to communicate, manage knowledge, mitigate error, and support decision making.

Important aspects of informatics to include:

- **Knowledge:** Identify essential information that must be available in a common database to support client care.
- **Skills:** Use information management tools to monitor outcomes of care processes.
- **Attitudes:** Value technologies that support clinical decision making, error prevention, and care coordination.

Informatics Question

You are the school nurse at a large high school in a rural, impoverished area. There has been a recent tragedy involving a senior from this high school drinking and doing other drugs while driving with friends in the car, resulting in one student death, and significant injury to the driver and another passenger. You have been asked to address use of alcohol, tobacco, and other drugs (ATOD) at this high school.

- What data should you collect to assess the scope of the ATOD problem at this school? How does the community environment impact ATOD use culture for students at the school?
- Who are some key informants you want to interview? What information will you seek from them?
- You decide that a drug and alcohol education social media campaign is needed. What data will you want to track over time to assess the effectiveness of this intervention?

Older Adults. Older adults (65 years of age and older) represent 15.2 percent of the U.S. population and are the fastest-growing segment of U.S. society, expected to represent 21 percent by the year 2030 (Ortman et al., 2014). Older adults use more prescription drugs than any other age group; 65 percent of adults aged 65 or older take three or more prescriptions drugs, and 39 percent take five or more prescription drugs (Charlesworth et al., 2015).

Alcohol and prescription drug misuse affects as many as 17 percent of adults age 60 and older. Problems with alcohol consumption, including interactions with prescribed and OTC drugs, far outnumber any other substance abuse problem among older adults (SAMHSA, 2009). A Substance Abuse and Mental Health Services Administration (SAMHSA) comprehensive screening and brief interventions guide to preventing older adult alcohol and psychoactive medication misuse/abuse is available at https://www.ncoa.org.

The increased use of prescription drugs and alcohol by older adults may be related to coping problems. Problems of relocation, loss of independence, retirement, illness, death of friends/family, and lower levels of achievement contribute to feelings of sadness, boredom, anxiety, and loneliness. Factors such as slowed metabolic turnover of drugs, age-related organ changes, enhanced drug sensitivities, a tendency to use drugs over long periods, and a more frequent use of multiple drugs (polypharmacy) all contribute to greater negative consequences from drug use among older adults. Alcohol abuse may not be identified because its effects on cognitive abilities may mimic changes associated with normal aging or degenerative brain disease. Also, depression may simply be attributed to more frequent losses rather than the depressant effects of alcohol, and the older adult may subsequently receive medical treatment for depression rather than alcoholism. Of note, it is recommended that both men and women aged 60 and older consume no more than one standard drink per day and no more than seven standard drinks per week. For older adult women, three or more drinks in a day is considered binge drinking (SAMHSA, 2012).

People Who Inject Drugs. In addition to the problem of addiction, people who inject drugs (intravenously or subcutaneously) (PWID) are at risk for other health complications. Intravenous (IV) administration of drugs always carries a greater risk of overdose because the drug goes directly into the bloodstream. With illicit drugs, the danger is increased because the exact dosage is unknown. In addition, the drug may be contaminated with other chemicals, such as sugar, starch, or quinine, or other drugs that can cause negative consequences. Often PWID make their own solution for IV administration, and any particles present can result in complications from emboli.

PWID often share needles. HIV, hepatitis C, and other bloodborne diseases can be transmitted through contaminated needles. Infections and abscesses may develop as a result of dirty needles or poor administration techniques. Although HIV incidence in PWID decreased 48 percent from 2008 to 2014, PWID continue to represent 1 in 10 new HIV diagnoses. In a change of statistical trends, fewer African Americans than whites are becoming new PWID, and whites are more likely to share needles (CDC, 2016b). Emphasis is being placed on reducing the transmission of this disease through contaminated needles. Abstinence is ideal but unrealistic for many addicted persons. Using the harm reduction model, the nurse should provide education on cleaning needles with bleach between uses and on needle exchange programs to decrease the spread of bloodborne disease. See more about this later in Safer Substance Use in Tertiary Prevention and the Role of the Nurse.

Drug Use During Pregnancy

Most drugs can negatively affect a fetus. Thus, the use of any drug during pregnancy should be discouraged unless medically necessary. *Healthy People 2020* objectives address this issue under the Maternal, Infant and Child Health topic area with several objectives that describe recommendations to improve the health of infants, such as reducing the occurrence of fetal alcohol syndrome (FAS) (MICH-25), and increasing abstinence from alcohol, cigarettes, and illicit drugs among pregnant women (MICH-11). FAS is considered the leading preventable birth defect, causing mental and behavioral impairment. In 2016 about 4.3 percent of pregnant women reported binge drinking and 0.9 percent reported heavy drinking in the past month. These low rates may be due to the extensive information available about the effects of alcohol on the fetus. With the opioid epidemic in full swing, the rates of babies born with neonatal abstinence syndrome (NAS) are also on the rise. In 2000, babies born with NAS represented 1.2 of 1000 hospital births, and by 2012 the rate had risen to 5.8 per 1000. This is equivalent to one baby born with NAS every 25 minutes (NIDA, 2015).

In 2016, the rate of past-month illicit drug use during pregnancy for women aged 15 to 44 was 6.3 percent. Tobacco remains the most-used addictive substance during pregnancy, with about 10 percent of pregnant women smoking (SAMHSA, 2017). In some states, pregnant women who are using illicit drugs are reported to child protective services because of the potential harm to the fetus.

Despite the increased focus on drug abuse interventions, many pregnant women with drug problems do not receive the help they need. This may be a result of ignorance, poverty, lack of concern for the fetus, lack of available services, and fear of the punitive consequences of revealing drug use. The fear of criminal prosecution may push addicted women farther away from the health care system, cause them to conceal their drug use from medical providers, and cause them to avoid the critical treatment and medical care that they need (Brady & Ashley, 2005).

Persons Who Use Illicit Drugs. The strategy of "just say no" to drugs is both simplistic and misleading. Indiscriminant use of "good" drugs has caused more health problems from adverse reactions, drug interactions, dependence, addiction, and overdoses than use of "bad" drugs. However, the war on drugs focuses on illicit drugs and punishes illicit drug users. The black market associated with illicit drug use puts otherwise law-abiding citizens in close contact with criminals, prevents any quality control of the drugs, increases the risk of HIV and hepatitis as a result of needle sharing, and hinders health care professionals' accessibility to the drug user. Lack of quality control (unknown strength and purity) can cause unexpected overdoses or secondary effects of the impurities; for example, a synthetic analog of fentanyl (3-methylfentanyl) marketed as "heroin" is 6000 times as potent as morphine. Unsafe administration (contaminated needles) leads to local and systemic infections. The high cost of drugs on the black market leads to crime to support the addiction. In 2016, the highest rate of current illicit drug use was among 18- to 20-year-olds at 23.8 percent, with the next highest rate occurring among 21- to 25-year-olds at 22.8 percent (SAMHSA, 2017). See Table 37.4 for illicit drug use by race/ethnicity.

Codependency and Family Involvement

Drug addiction is often a family disease. One in four Americans experiences family problems related to alcohol abuse. People in a close relationship with the addicted person often develop unhealthy coping mechanisms to continue the relationship. This behavior is known as **codependency**—a stress-induced preoccupation with the addicted person's life, leading to extreme dependence and excessive concern with the addicted person.

Strict rules typically develop in a codependent family to maintain the relationships: don't talk, don't feel, don't trust, don't lose control, and don't seek help from outside the family. Codependents try to meet the addicted person's needs at the expense of their own. Codependency may underlie many of the

TABLE 37.4 Past Month Illicit Drug Use Among Persons Aged 12 or Older, by Age Group and Demographic Characteristics, 2015 and 2016

Demographic Characteristic	Aged 12+ (2015)	Aged 12+ (2016)	Aged 12-17 (2015)	Aged 12-17 (2016)	Aged 18+ (2015)	Aged 18+ (2016)	Aged 18-25 (2015)	Aged 18-25 (2016)	Aged 26+ (2015)	Aged 26+ (2016)
TOTAL GENDER	17.8	18.0	17.5[b]	15.8	17.9	18.2	37.5	37.7	14.6	15.0
Male	20.5	20.7	16.8[a]	15.4	20.9	21.3	41.1	40.4	17.3	18.0
Female	15.3	15.5	18.1[a]	16.3	15.1	15.4	33.9	35.0	12.0	12.3
Hispanic Origin and Race										
Not Hispanic or Latino	18.0	18.4	17.3[a]	15.8	18.0	18.6	38.3	38.9	14.9	15.6
White	17.9	18.5	17.6[b]	15.7	17.9	18.7	39.4	40.8	14.9	15.7
Black or African American	20.7	20.1	17.6	17.0	21.0	20.4	38.4	38.0	17.4	16.8
American Indian or Alaska Native	22.9	23.6	16.6	21.0	23.7	23.8	42.5	*	19.9	19.2
Native Hawaiian or Other Pacific Islander	20.5	16.0	*	*	19.5	16.5	*	*	*	12.5
Asian	9.2	9.2	8.6	10.2	9.3	9.1	22.5	20.1	6.9	7.0
Two or More Races	27.1	30.2	22.5	22.5	28.1	31.7	51.0	48.8	21.6	27.7
Hispanic or Latino	17.2	16.0	18.1[a]	15.8	17.0	16.1	34.7	33.2	12.7	11.9
Education										
< High School	da	da	da	da	16.9	16.1	35.1	35.4	13.6	12.8
High School Graduate	da	da	da	da	18.1	18.4	36.2	37.3	14.3	14.6
Some College/ Associate's Degree	da	da	da	da	21.1	21.4	39.7	39.5	16.6	17.0
College Graduate	da	da	da	da	14.8	15.7	36.9	35.4	13.4	14.4
Current Employment										
Full-Time	da	da	da	da	18.9	19.2	39.1	38.9	16.0	16.5
Part-Time	da	da	da	da	22.5	23.6	39.2	40.8	16.2	16.8
Unemployed	da	da	da	da	30.2	31.2	41.1	43.0	25.3	26.2
Other[1]	da	da	da	da	12.7	12.9	31.1	29.6	10.7	11.2

* = low precision; — = not available; da = does not apply.

NOTE: Illicit Drug Use includes the misuse of prescription psychotherapeutics or the use of marijuana, cocaine (including crack), heroin, hallucinogens, inhalants, or methamphetamine.

NOTE: Misuse of prescription psychotherapeutics is defined as use in any way not directed by a doctor, including use without a prescription of one's own; use in greater amounts, more often, or longer than told; or use in any other way not directed by a doctor. Prescription psychotherapeutics do not include over-the-counter drugs.

[a]The difference between this estimate and the 2016 estimate is statistically significant at the .05 level. Rounding may make the estimates appear identical.

[b]The difference between this estimate and the 2016 estimate is statistically significant at the .01 level. Rounding may make the estimates appear identical.

[1]The Other Employment category includes students, persons keeping house or caring for children full time, retired or disabled persons, or other persons not in the labor force.

From Substance Abuse and Mental Health Services Administration: *Results from the 2016 National Survey on Drug Use and Health: detailed tables,* NSDUH Series H-52, USDHHS Pub. No. SMA 17-5044, 2017, Rockville, MD. See Table 1.30B at https://www.samhsa.gov.

medical complaints and emotional stress seen by health care providers, such as ulcers, skin disorders, migraine headaches, chronic colds, and backaches.

When the addicted person refuses to admit the problem, the family continues to adapt to emotionally survive the stress of the addicted person's irrational, inconsistent, and unpredictable behavior. Family members consequently develop various roles that tend to be gross exaggerations of normal family roles, and they cling irrationally to these roles, even when they are no longer functional.

One of the most significant roles a family member may assume is that of an enabler. **Enabling** is the act of shielding or preventing the addicted person from experiencing the consequences of the addiction. As a result, the addicted person does not always understand the cost of the addiction and thus is "enabled" to continue to use. Although codependency and enabling are closely related, a person does not have to be codependent to enable. Anyone can be an enabler: a police officer, a boss or coworker, and even a drug treatment counselor. Health care professionals who do not address the negative health consequences of the drug use with the addicted person are enablers.

The nurse can help families recognize the problem of addiction and help them confront the addicted member in a caring manner. Whether or not the addicted family member is agreeable to treatment, the family members should be given some guidance about the literature and services that are available to help them cope more effectively. The nurse can help identify treatment options, counseling assistance, financial assistance, support services, and (if necessary) legal services for the family members. Children of ATOD abusers or addicted persons are themselves at greater risk for developing addiction and must be targeted for primary prevention.

TERTIARY PREVENTION AND THE ROLE OF THE NURSE

The nurse is in a key position to help the addicted person and his or her family. The nurse's knowledge of community resources and how to mobilize them can significantly influence the quality of care clients receive.

Safer Substance Use

Harm reduction is key in providing interventions for persons who abuse substances. There are a number of ways in which nurses can help support safer use of substances. It is important to educate clients who use drugs on how to safely use them to prevent overdose, infection, or mental health disorders. With the increase of synthetic heroin-adulterated opioids, cocaine, and methamphetamine, drug testing kits can help drug users identify when they have received a product of very low purity, meaning it contains very little of the substance they intend to use. Conversely, a person who regularly uses low-purity product may unintentionally overdose upon receiving a very high-purity product. It is also necessary to educate friends and family of drug users to recognize the signs of overdose. Public alerts concerning dangerous new formulations of substances are also significant in educating drug users so that they may make better-informed decisions.

> **BOX 37.6 Naloxone**
>
> Naloxone (Narcan) is a fast-acting opioid overdose reversal drug. It is available in nasal spray and injection (intramuscular and intravenous) form. Naloxone effectively removes opioids from the user's opioid receptors until it is metabolized from the system. It may be necessary to administer naloxone more than once until the individual can receive more acute medical interventions. Even in the event that naloxone is available, the Good Samaritan law protects individuals and opioid overdose victims from prosecution for drug possession charges if medical help is called.

For PWID, safe needle use prevents transmission of bloodborne disease and reduces incidence of injection-related injury and infection. Public health nurses can educate and provide resources to help PWID engage in safe needle use. Syringe exchange programs are also hugely beneficial for PWID. Such programs provide free sterile needles and syringes and safe disposal of used injection equipment. They reduce new HIV and hepatitis infections by decreasing shared syringes and needles, as well as reduce overdose deaths. Furthermore, PWID are five times as likely to enter treatment for substance use disorder when they use a syringe services program, as these sites also function as public health outreach locations. Most programs provide access to naloxone (an opioid overdose reversal drug) education, referrals, screenings, and other medical services (CDC, 2017e). See Box 37.6.

Detoxification

Detoxification is the clearing of one or more drugs from the person's body and managing the withdrawal symptoms. Depending on the particular drug and the degree of dependence, the time required may range from a few days to several weeks. Because withdrawal symptoms vary (depending on the drug used) and range from uncomfortable to life threatening, the setting for and management of withdrawal depend on the drug used.

Drugs such as stimulants or opiates may produce withdrawal symptoms that are uncomfortable but not life threatening. Detoxification from these drugs does not require direct medical supervision, but medical management of the withdrawal symptoms increases comfort to help individuals through the process. On the other hand, drugs such as alcohol, benzodiazepines, and barbiturates can produce life-threatening withdrawal symptoms. These clients should be under close medical supervision during detoxification and should receive medical management of the withdrawal symptoms to ensure a safe withdrawal. Of those who develop delirium tremens from alcohol withdrawal, 15 percent may not survive despite medical management; therefore close medical management is initiated as the blood alcohol level begins to fall.

A general rule in detoxification management is to wean the person off the drug by gradually reducing the dosage and frequency of administration. Thus, a person with chronic alcoholism could be safely detoxified by a gradual reduction in alcohol consumption. In practice, however, the switch to another drug, usually a benzodiazepine, often offers a safer withdrawal from alcohol as well as an abrupt end to the intoxication from the drug of choice. For example, chlordiazepoxide (Librium) is commonly used for alcohol detoxification. Outpatient or home detoxification for persons requiring medical detoxification for alcohol withdrawal can be a cost-effective treatment. Nurses can monitor and evaluate the client's health status in the home environment to reduce the risk of medical complications related to alcohol withdrawal, and to provide encouragement and support for the client to complete the detoxification.

Addiction Treatment

Addiction treatment differs from the management of negative health consequences of chronic drug abuse, overdose, and detoxification. **Addiction treatment** focuses on the addiction process. The goal is to help clients view addiction as a chronic disease and assist them to make lifestyle changes to halt the progression of the disease. According to the disease theory, addicted persons are not responsible for the symptoms of their disease; they are, however, responsible for treating their disease. In 2016, 20.1 million persons aged 12 or older needed treatment for an illicit drug or alcohol use problem (7.5 percent of the persons aged 12 or older). Of these, 3.8 million persons aged 12 or older received treatment for alcohol or illicit substance use problems (SAMHSA, 2017). Fig. 37.3 shows the common reasons persons do not receive treatment.

Most treatment facilities are multidisciplinary because the intervention strategies require a wide range of approaches. Their programs involve interactions between the addicted person, family, culture, and community. Strategies include medical management, education, counseling, vocational rehabilitation, stress management, and support services. In addition, specific programs address the needs of various populations such as adolescents, pregnant women, specific ethnic groups, lesbian/gay/bisexual/transgender/queer and a plus sign to designate those not included (LGBTQ+) individuals, as well as health care professionals. The key to effective treatment is to match individual clients with the interventions most appropriate for them. Box 37.7 lists 13 fundamental principles for effective addiction treatment.

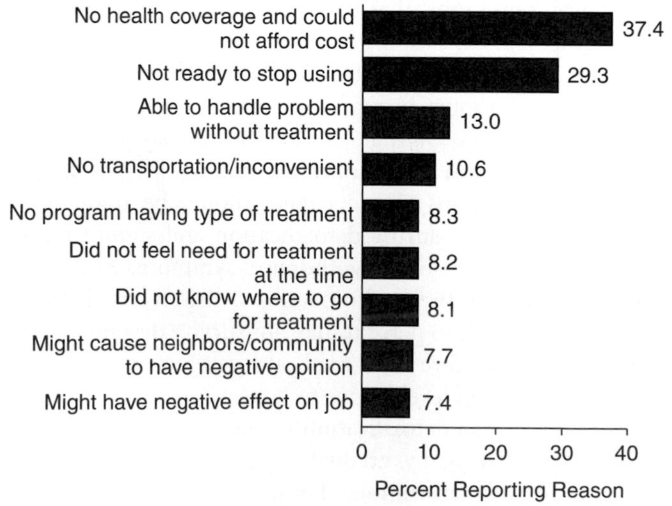

Fig. 37.3 Reasons for not receiving substance use treatment in past year among persons aged 12 or older who needed treatment but did not receive treatment and felt they needed treatment, 2016. (See Table 5.53B at https://www.samhsa.gov.) (From Substance Abuse and Mental Health Services Administration: *Results from the 2016 National Survey on Drug Use and Health: detailed tables,* NSDUH Series H-52, USDHHS Pub. No. SMA 17-5044, Rockville, MD, 2017.)

BOX 37.7 Principles of Drug Addiction Treatment

More than three decades of scientific research have yielded 13 fundamental principles that characterize effective drug abuse treatment. These principles are detailed in the National Institute on Drug Abuse's (NIDA's) *Principles of Drug Addiction Treatment: A Research-Based Guide* (2018c).

1. No single treatment is appropriate for all individuals. Matching treatment settings, interventions, and services to each client's problems and needs is critical.
2. Treatment needs to be readily available. Treatment applicants can be lost if treatment is not immediately available or readily accessible.
3. Effective treatment attends to multiple needs of the individual, not just his or her drug use. Treatment must address the individual's drug use and associated medical, psychological, social, vocational, and legal problems.
4. At different times during treatment, a client may develop a need for medical services, family therapy, vocational rehabilitation, and social and legal services.
5. Remaining in treatment for an adequate period of time is critical for treatment effectiveness. The time depends on an individual's needs. For most clients, the threshold of significant improvement is reached at about 3 months in treatment. Additional treatment can produce further progress. Programs should include strategies to prevent clients from leaving treatment prematurely.
6. Individual and/or group counseling and other behavioral therapies are critical components of effective treatment for addiction. In therapy, clients address motivation, build skills to resist drug use, replace drug-using activities with constructive and rewarding non–drug-using activities, and improve problem-solving abilities. Behavioral therapy also facilitates interpersonal relationships.
7. Medications are an important element of treatment for many clients, especially when combined with counseling and other behavioral therapies. Buprenorphine, methadone, and levo-alpha-acetylmethadol (LAAM) help persons addicted to opiates stabilize their lives and reduce their drug use. Naltrexone is effective for some opiate addicts and some clients with co-occurring alcohol dependence. Nicotine patches or gum, or an oral medication, such as bupropion, can help persons addicted to nicotine.
8. Addicted or drug-abusing individuals with coexisting mental disorders should have both disorders treated in an integrated way.
9. Medical detoxification is only the first stage of addiction treatment and by itself does little to change long-term drug use. Medical detoxification manages the acute physical symptoms of withdrawal. For some individuals it is a precursor to effective drug addiction treatment.
10. Treatment does not need to be voluntary to be effective. Sanctions or enticements in the family, employment setting, or criminal justice system can significantly increase treatment entry, retention, and success.
11. Possible drug use during treatment must be monitored continuously. Monitoring a client's drug and alcohol use during treatment, such as through urinalysis, can help the client withstand urges to use drugs. Such monitoring can also provide early evidence of drug use so that treatment can be adjusted.
12. Treatment programs should provide assessment for human immunodeficiency virus (HIV)/acquired immunodeficiency syndrome (AIDS), hepatitis B and C, tuberculosis and other infectious diseases, and counseling to help clients modify or change behaviors that place them or others at risk of infection. Counseling can help clients avoid high-risk behavior and help people who are already infected manage their illness.
13. Recovery from drug addiction can be a long-term process and frequently requires multiple episodes of treatment. As with other chronic illnesses, relapses to drug use can occur during or after successful treatment episodes. Participation in self-help support programs during and following treatment often helps maintain abstinence.

Total abstinence is the most recommended treatment goal for ATOD addiction. People who are addicted to a particular drug (e.g., cocaine) are advised to abstain from the use of all psychoactive substances. The use of another drug may simply reinforce the craving for the original drug and cause relapse. More commonly, the addiction merely transfers to the replacement substance.

Treatment may be on an inpatient or outpatient basis. In general, the more advanced the disease is, the greater the need for inpatient treatment. Inpatient treatment programs usually range from less than 1 week to as long as 90 days. Once a person has completed detoxification (considered the first phase of the treatment process), the programs use counseling and group interaction to help the client stay clean long enough for the body chemistry to rebalance. This is often a difficult time for persons recovering from addictions because they may experience mood swings and difficulty sleeping and dealing with emotions.

The goal of the educational part of the programs is to provide information about the disease and how drugs affect a person physically and psychologically. Clients are informed of the various lifestyle changes that are recommended, and they learn about tools to assist them in making these changes. Discharge planning continues throughout treatment as clients build the support systems that they will need when they leave the controlled environment of a treatment center where they will face pressures and temptations (triggers) that may lead to relapse.

Long-term residential programs, also called halfway houses, have been developed to ease the person recovering from an addiction back into society. These facilities provide continued support and counseling in a structured environment for persons needing long-term assistance in adjusting to a drug-free lifestyle. The residents are expected to secure employment and take responsibility in managing their financial obligations.

Outpatient programs are similar in the education and counseling offered, but they allow the clients to live at home and continue to work while undergoing treatment. This method is effective for persons in the earlier stages of addiction who feel confident that they can abstain from drug use and have established a strong support network. Some ways of finding an appropriate treatment program include:

1. Call SAMHSA's National Helpline for treatment referral and information at 1-800-662-HELP (4357). This service is a free, confidential, 24/7, 365 days a year helpline available in both English and Spanish for individuals and families needing help with mental and/or substance use disorders.
2. Look it up on the SAMHSA website. Their Substance Abuse Treatment Facility Locator Internet-based service provides an easy-to-use directory to help you locate (including road maps to each facility) and contact public and private treatment programs (http:/findtreatment.samhsa.gov).

For those addicted individuals unwilling or unable to completely abstain from psychoactive drugs, other medications can assist them in abstaining from their drug of choice. Currently there are three commonly used types of medication-assisted treatment (MAT) for treating opioid addiction: methadone, buprenorphine, and naltrexone. Methadone, when administered in moderate or high daily doses, produces a **cross-tolerance** to other opioids, thereby blocking their effects and decreasing the craving for the drug of choice. The advantages of methadone are that it is long acting, does not produce a "high," and is inexpensive. The oral use of methadone eliminates the danger of the spread of HIV and other bloodborne infections that commonly occur among PWID. Buprenorphine acts similarly to methadone, but is a shorter acting drug. Suboxone is a popular combination drug of buprenorphine and naloxone, preventing most users from being able to abuse it through IV use, as naloxone is poorly absorbed orally, but works well once in the bloodstream to block opioid receptors. Naltrexone is a non-opioid drug that works by inhibiting drug-induced euphoria, thereby reducing drug cravings by tapping into the reward circuit in the brain. It is also used in alcohol use disorder treatment. Although not recognized as a cure for heroin (or other opioid) addiction, MAT maintenance is a harm reduction intervention because it reduces deviant behavior and introduces addicted persons to the health care system (Volkow et al., 2014).

Recovery from addiction involves a lifetime commitment and may include periods of relapse. The addicted person must realize that modern medicine has not found a cure for addiction; therefore returning to drug use may ultimately reactivate the disease process.

EVIDENCE-BASED PRACTICE

Scavone et al. (2013) examined the use of cannabis prior to and during methadone maintenance treatment (MMT) for opioid dependence via a chart review of 91 patients undergoing MMT in Pennsylvania. They found that those opioid addicts with a history of cannabis use reported "significantly less daily expenditure on acquisition of opiates." In addition they found that those who used cannabis during induction had lower ratings of opiate withdrawal symptoms. The researchers concluded that these findings point to novel interventions for the treatment of opioid dependence that specifically target cannabinoid-opioid system interactions. This study supports earlier work by Reiman (2009), who found that many patients in a California cannabis dispensary reported using cannabis to help them get off and stay off of problematic drug use with alcohol, opioids, and other drugs of abuse. There is a marked reduction in prescriptions and dosages of opioids, as well as opioid overdose deaths, in states with medical cannabis programs, especially where dispensaries are permitted (Bachhuber et al., 2014; Liang et al., 2018; Wen et al., 2018). As of July 2018, New York, New Jersey, and Pennsylvania have allowed the use of medical cannabis to treat opioid use disorders.

Nurse Use

With the emerging understanding of the endocannabinoid system and its overall role of maintaining homeostasis, the research supports the healing properties of cannabis as it relieves withdrawal symptoms from dangerous, addictive drugs and helps addicted persons reach stabilization. This is not to say that a person may not have a problem with cannabis, but rather it is important to assess the reasons for drug use and the consequences of that use to determine whether or not the person has a substance use disorder.

Scavone JL, Sterling RC, Weinstein SP, et al.: Impact of cannabis use during stabilization on methadone maintenance treatment. *Am J Addict* 22(4):344-351, 2013.

Smoking Cessation Programs

Nearly 35 million Americans try to quit smoking each year. Fewer than 10 percent of those who try to quit on their own are able to stop for a year, and fewer than one-third of smokers who tried to quit used evidence-based cessation treatment. Interventions that involve medications and behavioral treatments allow individuals to be more successful (USDHHS, 2014). For example, nicotine replacement therapy can be used to help smokers withdraw from nicotine while focusing their efforts on breaking the psychological craving or habit. Five types of nicotine replacement products are available: nicotine gum, lozenges, and skin patches are available over the counter, and nicotine nasal spray and inhalers are available by prescription. These products are about equally effective and can almost double the chances of successfully quitting. Other treatments include smoking cessation clinics, hypnosis, acupuncture, and mobile phone apps/messaging services. The most effective way to get people to stop smoking and prevent relapse involves multiple interventions and continuous reinforcement, and most smokers require several attempts at cessation before they are successful. Many resources are available on smoking cessation programs and support groups, including those listed in Box 37.8. There is a website developed specifically for nurses to help nurses quit smoking: http://www.tobaccofreenurses.org. Smoking cessation efforts have proven to be successful for many—since 2002, the number of former smokers has been greater than the number of current smokers (CDC, 2017d).

LINKING CONTENT TO PRACTICE

Using the tools of primary, secondary, and tertiary prevention with individuals, families, and communities in whom alcohol and other drug use is an issue incorporates both public health and public health nursing guidelines and competencies. Specifically, the core competencies of the Council on Linkages Between Academia and Public Health Practice (2014) begin by identifying the analytic and assessment skills needed by public health professionals. The 12 skills in this competency category are used in providing services to the population described in this chapter. For example, you begin by assessing the "health status of populations and their related determinants of health and stress." You next move to skill #2, which is describing the "characteristics of a population-based health problem." These competencies are described through a set of eight domains. Each domain can be used with populations dealing with alcohol and other drug problems.

Similarly, the Intervention Wheel, which is the subject of Chapter 11, has many applications with this population. Many of these interventions have application with the populations described in this chapter. For example, case finding, referral and follow-up, health teaching, counseling, and policy development and enforcement are selected examples of ways in which public health nurses intervene in serving a vulnerable population with alcohol- and drug-related problems.

Support Groups

The founding of Alcoholics Anonymous (AA) in 1935 began a strong movement of peer support to treat a chronic illness. AA groups have developed around the world. Their success has led to the development of other support groups such as the following:

- Narcotics Anonymous (NA) for persons with narcotic addiction
- Pills Anonymous for persons with polydrug addictions
- Overeaters Anonymous
- Gamblers Anonymous

AA and NA help addicted people develop a daily program of recovery and reinforce the recovery process. The fellowship, support, and encouragement among members provide a vital social network for the person recovering from an addiction.

Al-Anon and Alateen are similar self-help programs for spouses, parents, children, or others involved in a painful relationship with an alcoholic. Nar-Anon is a support group for those in relationships with persons with narcotic addictions. Al-Anon family groups are available to anyone who has been affected by their involvement with an alcoholic person. The

BOX 37.8 Smoking Cessation Resources

The following organizations have a range of helpful information:

American Cancer Society
"How to Quit Smoking or Smokeless Tobacco" and more
http://www.cancer.org.

American Heart Association
"Quit Smoking Tobacco"
http://www.americanheart.org.

American Lung Association
"Freedom From Smoking Plus"
http://www.lung.org.

Centers for Disease Control and Prevention: Office on Smoking and Health
www.cdc.gov/tobacco.

The Foundation for a Smoke-Free America
"Quitting Tips" and more
http://www.tobaccofree.org.

National Cancer Institute (NCI)
http://www.cancer.gov.
Quitting information, cessation guide, and counseling is offered, as well as information on state telephone-based quit programs

Smokefree.gov
"Smokefree Apps"
http://www.smokefree.gov.
Excellent source created by Tobacco Control Research Branch of NCI

Smokefree Women
http://women.smokefree.gov.
NCI collaborated with:
Centers for Disease Control and Prevention—Office on Smoking and Health
Centers for Disease Control and Prevention—Division of Reproductive Health
Health Canada
American Legacy Foundation
The Robert Wood Johnson Foundation

SmokEnders
"The Quit Kit," an 11-week program
http://www.smokenders.com.

purposes of Alateen include providing a forum for adolescents to discuss family stressors, learn coping skills from one another, and gain support and encouragement from knowledgeable peers. Adult Children of Alcoholics (ACA) groups are also available in most areas to address the recovery of adults who grew up in alcohol use disorder homes and are still carrying the scars and retaining dysfunctional behaviors.

For some persons, the AA program places too much emphasis on a higher power or focuses too much on the negative consequences of past drinking. Women for Sobriety focuses on rebuilding self-esteem, and this is often a core issue for many women with alcohol problems. (See www.womenforsobriety.org for additional information.) Rational Recovery has a cognitive orientation and is based on the assumption that ATOD addiction is caused by irrational beliefs that can be understood and overcome. See www.rational.org for additional information on this approach.

Nurse's Role

Many people with alcohol and drug addiction become lost in the health care system. If satisfactory care is not provided in one agency or the waiting list is months long, the person may give up rather than seek alternative sources of care. The nurse who knows the client's history, environment, support systems, and the local treatment programs can offer guidance to the most effective treatment modality. Brief interventions by health care professionals who are not treatment experts can be effective in helping people who abuse ATOD and addicted persons change their risky behavior. **Brief interventions** may convince these individuals to reduce substance consumption or follow through with a treatment referral. Box 37.9 describes six elements commonly included in brief interventions, using the acronym FRAMES. Strategies used with clients can vary depending on their readiness for change. Understanding the stages of change listed in Box 37.10 and recognizing which stage a client is in are important factors for determining which interventions and programs may be most helpful to the client.

After the client has received treatment, the nurse can coordinate aftercare referrals and follow up on the client's progress. The nurse can provide additional support in the home as the client and family adjust to changing roles and the stress involved with such changes. The nurse can support addicted persons who have relapsed by reminding them that relapses may well occur, but that they and their families can continue to work toward recovery and an improved quality of life.

BOX 37.9 Brief Interventions Using the FRAMES Acronym

Feedback. Provide the client direct feedback about the potential or actual personal risk or impairment related to drug use.

Responsibility. Emphasize personal responsibility for change.

Advice. Provide clear advice to change risky behavior.

Menu. Provide a menu of options or choices for changing behavior.

Empathy. Provide a warm, reflective, empathetic, and understanding approach.

Self-efficacy. Provide encouragement and belief in the client's ability to change.

From Center for Substance Abuse Treatment: *Brief interventions and brief therapies for substance abuse,* TIP 34, DHHS Pub. No. (SMA) 99-3353, Rockville, MD, 1999, USDHHS.

BOX 37.10 Stages of Change

Pre-Contemplation

At this stage, the person does not intend to change in the foreseeable future. The person is often unaware of any problem. Resistance to recognizing or modifying a problem is the hallmark of pre-contemplation.

Contemplation

At this stage, the individual is aware that a problem exists and is seriously thinking about overcoming it but has not yet made a commitment to take action. The nurse can encourage the individual to weigh the pros and cons of both the problem and the solution to the problem.

Preparation

Preparation was originally referred to as *decision making.* At this stage, the individual is prepared for action and may reduce the problem behavior but has not yet taken effective action (e.g., reduces amount of smoking but does not abstain).

Action

At this stage, the individual modifies the behavior, experiences, or environment to overcome the problem. The action requires considerable time and energy. Modification of the target behavior to an acceptable criterion and significant overt efforts to change are the hallmarks of action.

Maintenance

In this stage, the individual works to prevent relapse and consolidate the gains attained during action. Stabilizing behavior change and avoiding relapse are the hallmarks of maintenance.

Modified from DiClemente CC, Schlundt D, Gemmell L: Readiness and stages of change in addiction treatment. *Am J Addict* 13(2): 103-119, 2004.

OUTCOMES

Health promotion and risk reduction are basic concepts in nursing. Promoting a healthy environment in the home and local community provides individuals and families a nurturing environment in which to achieve optimal health. Individuals with high self-esteem and access to health care and information about the health risks related to drug use can be responsible for their personal health and make informed decisions about drug use. Nurses can assess the health of the community and its citizens, prioritize the needs, and identify local resources to collaborate with others to develop strategies that will improve the underlying health of the community.

Early identification and intervention for persons with ATOD problems can prevent many of the harmful physical, emotional, and social consequences that may occur if abuse continues and may also prevent abuse patterns from developing into addiction. The nurse needs to assess individual and community ATOD problems and target at-risk groups to develop strategies to increase assessment and provide appropriate interventions. Review the national health objectives (refer back to the *Healthy*

People 2020 box) for the tobacco and substance abuse areas and note how many can be achieved with secondary prevention strategies.

Besides saving taxpayers' money, treatment helps addicted individuals and their families recover from the devastating effects of addiction. Addicted persons and their families often become hopeless and helpless. The nurse can offer hope in affirming the addicted person's self-worth and can be the bridge to community resources to assist in treatment and recovery.

Many of these expected outcomes for ATOD problems have been lessened because a lack of funding has resulted from federal strategies that focus on law enforcement and punishment rather than on education and treatment. The greatest challenge for nurses is to influence policy makers to put the emphasis on health care for this major health problem.

PRACTICE APPLICATION

Ann Greene is a 25-year-old mother of two. Ann lives in an urban impoverished, low-income housing area where resources are limited and crime is a daily concern. Ann is a widow and has two sons, ages three and five. Her husband, who had an alcohol use disorder, was killed while driving under the influence of alcohol. Ann, who was a passenger in the accident, suffered a neck injury at the time, leaving her in severe pain. She left the hospital with a prescription for oxycodone, which she took as directed. However, as her tolerance increased, she found the prescribed amount did not sufficiently manage her pain anymore. She began to take more than the prescribed amount to adequately manage her pain, and when she returned to the emergency department to ask for a refill, she was denied and accused of being drug seeking. When she told her sister, Elise, about this, Elise offered Ann the rest of her Percocet prescription from when she had broken her ankle. At this point, Ann was taking twice as much twice as often to control the pain. She soon began buying painkillers from someone introduced to her by a friend of a friend.

During this time, Ann continued to work full time as a night-shift security guard at a factory in town, but her income could not support her obligations as a single mother in addition to her increasing demand for pills. Eventually, she found herself supplementing by smoking heroin she would get from her upstairs neighbor to take the edge off. This soon progressed to IV use. At this point, her friends and family started to notice changes in Ann's behavior. She would ask them to watch her kids but return much later than she had said she would. Her kids started to tell Elise that Ann was sleeping all the time. She would have inexplicable reasons for being unable to meet responsibilities and would leave for long periods of time to meet vague obligations.

Elise, suspecting Ann's behavior changes might be related to opioid use, confronted her about it. Ann denied it at first, but eventually confessed to letting her drug use get a little out of hand. When Elise tried to convince her to seek treatment, Ann was unwilling to go. Elise goes in to talk to a public health nurse at her local public health department to get advice on how to deal with this problem.

A. What interventions should the nurse provide for Elise?

B. What harm reduction interventions can the nurse offer Ann, knowing that she is unwilling to seek treatment at this time?

C. Knowing that there is a genetic link to addiction and being aware of the high rate of drug problems in their environment, how can the nurse help prevent Ann's children from developing substance abuse problems?

D. What are some things the prescriber should have considered before sending Ann home with a strong opioid prescription?

Answers can be found on the Evolve site.

KEY POINTS

- Substance abuse is the number one national health problem, linked to numerous forms of morbidity and mortality.
- Harm reduction is an approach to ATOD problems that deals with substance abuse primarily as a health problem rather than as a criminal problem.
- All persons have ideas, opinions, and attitudes about the use of drugs that influence their actions.
- Social conditions such as a fast-paced life, excessive stress, and the availability of drugs influence the incidence of substance use disorders.
- Important terms to understand when working with individuals, groups, or communities for whom substance abuse is prevalent are *drug dependence, drug addiction, alcoholism, psychoactive drugs, depressants, stimulants, cannabis, hallucinogens,* and *inhalants.*
- Primary prevention for substance use disorders includes education about drugs and guidelines for use, as well as the promotion of healthy alternatives to drug use either for recreation or to relieve stress.
- Nurses can help develop community prevention programs.
- Secondary prevention depends heavily on careful assessment of the client's use of drugs. Such assessment should be part of all basic health assessments.
- High-risk groups include pregnant women, young people, older adults, intravenous drug users, and illicit drug users.
- Drug addiction is often a family, not merely an individual, problem.
- Codependency describes a companion illness to the addiction of one person in which the codependent member is addicted to the addicted person.
- Brief interventions by a nurse can be as effective as treatment.
- Nurses are in ideal roles to assist with tertiary prevention for both the addicted person and the family.

CLINICAL DECISION-MAKING ACTIVITIES

1. Read your local newspaper or online news for four days and select stories that illustrate the effects of substance abuse on individuals, families, and the community. What interventions would you use? Who would you involve in your work? Are the interventions primary, secondary, or tertiary in nature? How would you evaluate your work?
2. For each of the stories in the news related to substance abuse, describe preventive strategies that a nurse might have tried before the problem reached such a dire state.
3. Looking at your local community resources directory or the Internet, identify agencies that might serve as referral sources for individuals or families for whom substance abuse is a problem.
4. Review popular magazine, television, and/or social media advertisements for alcohol, tobacco, cannabis, and other medicines (e.g., sleep aids, analgesics, laxatives, stimulants). In small groups, discuss the messages conveyed in the advertisements, and discuss the implications of client education to reduce possible harm from misuse and abuse of these substances.
5. Attend an open AA or NA meeting and an Al-Anon meeting. Go alone if possible or with an alcohol- or drug-addicted friend. As the members introduce themselves, give your first name and state, "I am a visitor." Plan to listen and do not attempt to take notes. Respect the anonymity of the persons present. Write a statement about your experience and what you learned from others at the meeting.
6. In groups of four or five, review the national health objectives in *Healthy People 2020* (see www.healthypeople.gov) under Tobacco Use and under Substance Abuse. Pick an objective from each section and brainstorm about possible community efforts a nurse could initiate to reach that objective.

ADDITIONAL RESOURCES

EVOLVE WEBSITE

http://evolve.elsevier.com/Stanhope/community/

- Answers to Practice Application
- Case Study
- Glossary
- Review Questions

REFERENCES

American Psychiatric Association: *Diagnostic and statistical manual of mental disorders*, ed 5, Arlington, VA, 2013, American Psychiatric Publishing.

Bachhuber MA, Saloner B, Cunningham CO, et al: Medical cannabis laws and opioid analgesic overdose mortality in the United States, 1999-2010, *JAMA Intern Med* 174(10):1668–1673, 2014.

Barnoya J, Glanz SA: Cardiovascular effects of secondhand smoke nearly as large as smoking, *Circulation* 111:2684–2698, 2005.

Barry M: *Health Harms from Secondhand Smoke*, 2007, National Center for Tobacco-Free Kids. Retrieved from http://tobaccofreekids.org/.

Brady TM, Ashley OS, editors: *Women in substance abuse treatment: results from the Alcohol and Drug Services Study (ADSS), Office of Applied Studies. DHHS Pub No SMA* 04-3968, Analytic Series A-26, Rockville, MD, 2005, SAMHSA.

Burstein S: Cannabidiol (CBD) and its analogs: a review of their effects on inflammation, *Bioorg Med Chem* 23(7):1377–1385, 2015.

Centers for Disease Control and Prevention: *Heroin Overdose Deaths Increased in Many States Through 2012*, 2014a. Retrieved from https://www.cdc.gov.

Centers for Disease Control and Prevention: *Increases in Heroin Overdose Deaths – 28 States, 2010 to 2012*, 2014b. Retrieved from https://www.cdc.gov.

Centers for Disease Control and Prevention: *CDC Guideline for Prescribing Opioids for Chronic Pain – United States, 2016*, 2016a. Retrieved from https://www.cdc.gov.

Centers for Disease Control and Prevention: *HIV and Injection Drug Use*, 2016b. Retrieved from https://www.cdc.gov.

Centers for Disease Control and Prevention: *Drug Overdose Deaths in the United States, 1999-2016*, 2017a. Retrieved from https://www.cdc.gov.

Centers for Disease Control and Prevention: *Opioid overdose: Understanding the Epidemic*, 2017b. Retrieved from https://www.cdc.gov.

Centers for Disease Control and Prevention: *QuickStats: Percentage of Adults Who Ever Used an E-cigarette and Percentage Who Currently Use E-cigarettes, by Age Group – National Health Interview Survey, United States, 2016*, 2017c. Retrieved from https://www.cdc.gov.

Centers for Disease Control and Prevention: *Smoking & Tobacco Use: Quitting Smoking*, 2017d. Retrieved from https://www.cdc.gov.

Centers for Disease Control and Prevention: *Reducing Harms from Injection Drug Use & Opioid Use Disorder with Syringe Services Programs*, 2017e. Retrieved from https://www.cdc.gov.

Centers for Disease Control and Prevention: *Web-based Injury Statistics Query and Reporting System (WISQARS) Nonfatal Injury Date*, 2017f. Retrieved from https://www.cdc.gov.

Centers for Disease Control and Prevention: *Current Cigarette Smoking Among Adults – United States, 2016*, 2018a. Retrieved from https://www.cdc.gov.

Centers for Disease Control and Prevention: *Economic Trends in Tobacco*, 2018b. Retrieved from https://www.cdc.gov.

Centers for Disease Control and Prevention: *Tobacco Product Use Among Middle and High School Students – United States, 2011-2017*, 2018c. Retrieved from https://www.cdc.gov.

Charlesworth CJ, Smith E, Lee DSH, et al: Polypharmacy among adults aged 65 years and older in the United States: 1988-2010, *J Gerontol A Biol Sci Med Sci* 70(8):989–995, 2015.

Council on Linkages Between Academia and Public Health Practice: *Core competencies for public health professionals*, Washington DC, 2014, Public Health Foundation/Health Resources and Services Administration.

Dasgupta N, Beletsky L, Ciccarone D: Opioid crisis: no easy fix to its social and economic determinants, *AJPH* 108(2):182–186, 2018.

DiClemente CC, Schlundt D, Gemmell L: Readiness and stages of change in addiction treatment, *Am J Addict* 13(2):103–119, 2004

Florence CS, Zhou C, Luo F, et al: The economic burden of prescription opioid overdose, abuse, and dependence in the United States, 2013, *Medical Care* 54(10):901–906, 2016.

Goldstein RZ, Volkow ND: Dysfunction of the prefrontal cortex in addiction: neuroimaging findings and clinical implications, *Nat Rev Neurosci* 12(11):652–669, 2011.

Hess CA, Olmedo P, Navas-Acien A, et al: E-cigarettes as a source of toxic and potentially carcinogenic metals, *Environ Res* 152: 221–225, 2017.

Jones CM, Einstein EB, Compton WM: Changes in synthetic opioid involvement in drug overdose deaths in the United States, 2010-2016, *JAMA* 319(17):1819–1821, 2018.

Kazemi DM, Borsari B, Levine MJ, et al: A Systematic Review of the mHealth Interventions to Prevent Alcohol and Substance Abuse, *J Health Commun* 22(5):413–432, 2017.

Kinney J: *Loosening the grip: a handbook of alcohol information,* ed 10, New York, 2011, McGraw-Hill.

Levy S: Drug and substance use and abuse in adolescents. In Porter RS, Kaplan JL, editors: *The merck manual online*, 2018. Retrieved from https://www.merckmanuals.com.

Leweke FM, Piomelli D, Pahlisch F, et al: Cannabidiol enhances anandamide signaling and alleviates psychotic symptoms of schizophrenia, *Transl Psychiatry* 2(3):e94, 2012.

Liang D, Bao Y, Wallace M, et al: Medical cannabis legalization and opioid prescriptions: Evidence on US Medicaid enrollees during 1993-2014, *Addiction research report* 2018.

Lu ML, Agito MD: Cannabinoid hyperemesis syndrome: marijuana is both antiemetic and proemetic, *Cleve Clin J Med* 82(7):429–434, 2015.

Maslowsky J, Capell JW, Moberg DP, et al: Universal school-based implementation of screening brief intervention and referral to treatment to reduce and prevent alcohol, marijuana, tobacco, and other drug use: Process and feasibility, *Subst Abuse* 11:1178221817746668, 2017.

Mayo Clinic Staff: *Caffeine: How Much Is too Much?* March 8, 2017. Retrieved from https://www.mayoclinic.org.

Mothers Against Misuse and Abuse: *Drug Consumer Safety Rules*, Mosier, OR. Retrieved from http://mamas.org, n.d.

Mucke M, Phillips T, Radbruch L, et al: Cannabis-based medicines for chronic neuropathic pain in adults, *Cochrane Database Syst Rev* 3:CD012182, 2018.

Muhuri PK, Gfroerer JC, Davis MC: Associations of nonmedical pain reliever use and initiation of heroin use in the United States, *CBHSQ Data Rev* 2013.

National Institute on Alcohol Abuse and Alcoholism: *Helping patients who drink too much: a clinician's guide (Update). NIH Pub No 07-3769*, Rockville, MD, 2005, USDHHS. Retrieved from https://pubs.niaaa.nih.gov.

National Institute on Drug Abuse: *Dramatic Increases in Maternal Opioid Use and Neonatal Abstinence Syndrome*, 2015. Retrieved from https://www.drugabuse.gov.

National Institute on Drug Abuse: *Inhalants*, 2017. Retrieved from https://www.drugabuse.gov.

National Institute on Drug Abuse: *Opioid Overdose Crisis*, 2018a. Retrieved from https://www.drugabuse.gov.

National Institute on Drug Abuse: *Principles of Adolescent Substance Use Disorder Treatment: A Research-Based Guide*, 2014. Retrieved from https://www.drugabuse.gov.

National Institute on Drug Abuse: *Principles of Drug Addiction Treatment: A Research Based Guide, NIH Pub No* 09-4180, Revised January 2018, ed 3, 2018. Retrieved from https://www.drugabuse.gov.

National Institute on Drug Abuse: *Synthetic Cannabinoids (K2/Spice)*, 2018b. Retrieved from https://www.drugabuse.gov.

O'Malley GF, O'Malley R: Alcohol toxicity and withdrawal. In Porter RS, Kaplan JL, editors: *The merck manual online*, 2018a. Retrieved from https://www.merckmanuals.com.

O'Malley GF, O'Malley R: Amphetamines (Methamphetamine). In Porter RS, Kaplan JL, editors: *The merck manual online*, 2018b. Retrieved from https://www.merckmanuals.com.

O'Malley GF, O'Malley R: Cocaine (Crack). In Porter RS, Kaplan JL, editors: *The merck manual online*, 2018c. Retrieved from https://www.merckmanuals.com.

O'Malley GF, O'Malley R: Marijuana (Cannabis). In Porter RS, Kaplan JL, editors: *The merck manual online*, 2018d. Retrieved from https://www.merckmanuals.com.

O'Malley GF, O'Malley R: Opioid toxicity and withdrawal. In Porter RS, Kaplan JL, editors: *The merck manual online*, 2018e. Retrieved from https://www.merckmanuals.com.

Ortman JM, Velkoff VA: *An Aging Nation: The Older Population in the United States*, 2014, U.S. Census Bureau. Retrieved from https://www.census.gov.

Pacher P, Bátkai S, Kunos G: The endocannabinoid system as an emerging target of pharmacotherapy, *Pharmacol Rev* 58(3): 389–462, 2006.

Pan W, Bai H: A multivariate approach to a meta-analytic review of the effectiveness of the D.A.R.E program, *Int J Environ Res Public Health* 6(1):267–277, 2009.

Reiman A: Cannabis as a substitute for alcohol and other drugs, *Harm Reduct J* 6:35, 2009.

Rose KD: *American women and the repeal of prohibition*, New York, NY, 1996, New York University Press.

Scavone JL, Sterling RC, Weinstein SP, et al: Impact of cannabis use during stabilization on methadone maintenance treatment, *Am J Addict* 22(4):344–351, 2013.

Seth P, Rudd RA, Noonan RK, et al: Quantifying the epidemic of prescription opioid overdose deaths, *AJPH* 108(4):500–502, 2018.

Shetty V, Harrell L, Clague J, et al: Methamphetamine users have increased dental disease: A propensity score analysis, *J Dent Res* 95(7):814–821, 2016.

Soneji S, Barrington-Trimis JL, Wills TA, et al: Association between initial use of e-cigarettes and subsequent cigarette smoking among adolescents and young adults: a systematic review and meta-analysis, *JAMA Pediatr* 171(8):788–797, 2017.

Substance Abuse and Mental Health Services Administration: *A Guide to Preventing Older Adult Alcohol and Psychoactive Medication Misuse/Abuse: Screening and Brief Interventions*, 2012, SAMHSA. Retrieved from https://www.ncoa.org.

Substance Abuse and Mental Health Services Administration: *Key Substance Use and Mental Health Indicators in the United States: Results from the 2016 National Survey on Drug Use and Health. NSDUH Series H-52, HHS Publication No. (SMA) 17-5044*, Rockville, MD, 2017, SAMHSA. Retrieved from https://www.samhsa.gov.

Substance Abuse and Mental Health Services Administration, Office of Applied Studies: *Treatment episode data set (TEDS). Highlights—2007, National Admissions to Substance Abuse Treatment Services. DASIS Series: S-45, DHHS Pub No (SMA) 09–4360*, Rockville, MD, 2009.

States and localities that have raised the minimum legal sale age for tobacco products to 21, August 2018. Retrieved from https://www.tobaccofreekids.org.

United Nations Office on Drugs and Crime (UNODC): *World Drug Report*, Vienna, 2015. Retrieved from https://www.unodc.org.

U.S. Department of Health and Human Services: Center for Substance Abuse Treatment: *Brief interventions and brief therapies for substance abuse.* TIP 34, DHHS Pub No (SMA) 99-3353, Rockville, MD, 1999, USDHHS.

U.S. Department of Health and Human Services: *Healthy people 2020: national health promotion and disease prevention objectives*, Washington, DC, 2010, U.S. Government Printing Office. Retrieved from http://www.healthypeople.gov.

U.S. Department of Health and Human Services: *Facing addiction in america: the surgeon general's report on alcohol, drugs, and health*, Washington, DC, 2016. Retrieved from https://addiction.surgeongeneral.gov.

U.S. Department of Health and Human Services: *The health consequences of smoking—50 years of progress: a report of the surgeon general*, Atlanta, 2014, USDHHS, CDC, National Center for Chronic Disease Prevention and Health Promotion, Office on Smoking and Health.

U.S. Office of Management and Budget: *An american budget: budget of the U.S. Government: 22. Federal Drug Control Funding*, Washington, DC, 2018. Retrieved from https://www.whitehouse.gov.

U.S. Office of National Drug Control Policy: *National drug control budget: FY 2018 funding highlights*, Washington, DC, 2017. Retrieved from https://www.whitehouse.gov.

Volkow ND, Frieden TR, Hyde PS, et al: Medication-assisted therapies—tackling the opioid-overdose epidemic, *N Engl J Med* 370:2063–2066, 2014.

Wen H, Hockenberry JM: Association of medical and adult-use marijuana laws with opioid prescribing for Medicaid enrollees, *JAMA Intern Med* 178(5):673–679, 2018.

Werb D, Rowell G, Guyatt G: Effect of drug law enforcement on drug market violence: a systematic review, *Int J Drug Policy* 22(2): 87–94, 2011.

Werner C: *Marijuana gateway to health: how cannabis protects us from cancer and Alzheimer's Disease*, San Francisco, 2011, Dachstar Press.

World Prison Brief: *Highest to Lowest – Prison Population Rate*. 2018. Retrieved from http://www.prisonstudies.org.

38

Violence and Human Abuse

Jeanne L. Alhusen, PhD, CRNP, RN, FAAN, Gerard M. Jellig, EdD, and Jacquelyn C. Campbell, PhD, RN, FAAN

OBJECTIVES

After reading this chapter, the student should be able to do the following:

1. Discuss the scope of the problem of violence in American communities.
2. Examine at least three factors existing in most communities that influence violence and human abuse.
3. Define the four general types of child abuse: neglect, physical, emotional, and sexual.
4. Discuss elder abuse as a crucial community health problem.
5. Discuss the principles of nursing intervention with violent families.
6. Describe specific nursing interventions with women experiencing intimate partner violence.

CHAPTER OUTLINE

Social and Community Factors Influencing Violence
Violence Against Individuals or Oneself
Family Violence and Abuse
Nursing Interventions

KEY TERMS

assault, p. 839
child abuse, p. 844
child neglect, p. 846
elder abuse, p. 850
emotional abuse, p. 846
emotional neglect, p. 846
forensic, p. 842
homicide, p. 839
incest, p. 847
intimate partner violence, p. 843
passive neglect, p. 846
physical abuse, p. 844
physical neglect, p. 846
post-traumatic stress disorder, p. 840
rape, p. 840
sexual abuse, p. 844
sexual assault nurse examiner, p. 842
sexually transmitted disease, p. 840
spouse abuse, p. 847
suicide, p. 842
survivors, p. 842
violence, p. 837
wife abuse, p. 847

Violence is a serious problem in the United States. It is a leading cause of death and disability that disproportionately affects youth, low-income populations, and people of color. An estimated 65,000 individuals die each year in the United States as a result of violence-related injuries. While homicide rates have decreased over the last 20 years, homicide is the third leading cause of death for individuals 15 to 34 years of age, and the fourth leading cause of death for individuals 1 to 14 years of age (Centers for Disease Control and Prevention [CDC], 2016). Intimate partner homicide accounts for a substantial proportion of female homicide victimization. The Centers for Disease Control and Prevention (CDC) examined homicides from 18 states from 2003 to 2014 and found that over half (55.3 percent) of the homicides committed against women involved an intimate partner (Petrosky et al., 2017). Suicide is one of the top 10 leading causes of death in the United States, and the rate in the United States trended upward from 1999 through 2014. During this time period, increases in suicide rates occurred for both males and females in every age group but the oldest age group (aged 75 and older). The largest rate increases were noted among females aged 10 to 14 and males aged 45 to 64 (Curtin et al., 2016). These statistics do not account for the significant morbidity associated with interpersonal violence. For every person who dies as a result of violence, many more are injured and suffer lasting physical, sexual, and mental health sequelae. As the World Health Organization has reported, when interpersonal violence results in large numbers of deaths, the issue is a significant public health concern necessitating attention from researchers, policy makers, health care providers, and the public (Krug et al., 2002).

Violence is an important public health nursing issue. Violence leads to significant mortality and morbidity. Communities across the United States are concerned about crime and violence rates. Medical, nursing, psychology, and social service professionals have been slow to develop an integrated response to violence that is part of their daily professional lives. As a result, the estimated 3.5 million victims of violence annually may not receive the best care possible. Nurses are in a unique position to develop community responses to violence, to influence public policy regarding violence, and to provide individuals, families, and communities with the necessary resources to mitigate violence and its consequences. Nurses represent a large group of health care providers who have an ethic of caring and value early intervention and health promotion. This can optimize individual, familial, community, and societal health outcomes.

This chapter examines violence as a public health problem and discusses how nurses can help individuals, families, groups, and communities cope with and reduce violence and abuse. Nurses work with clients in a wide variety of settings, including the home. Because nurses are in key positions to detect and intervene in community and family violence, an understanding of how community-level influences can affect all types of violence is necessary. The *Healthy People 2020* box as follows lists five objectives for reducing violence in communities.

HEALTHY PEOPLE 2020

Objectives for Reducing Violence

- **IVP-29:** Reduce homicides.
- **IVP-35:** Reduce bullying among adolescents.
- **IVP-37:** Reduce child maltreatment deaths.
- **IVP-39:** Reduce violence by current or former intimate partners.
- **IVP-40:** Reduce sexual violence.

U.S. Department of Health and Human Services (USDHHS): *Healthy People 2020: objectives,* Washington, DC, 2010, Office of Disease Prevention and Health Promotion, USDHHS.

SOCIAL AND COMMUNITY FACTORS INFLUENCING VIOLENCE

The ultimate goal is to stop violence before it begins. Identifying the factors that protect individuals or place them at a higher risk for experiencing or perpetrating violence can help focus prevention efforts. The Centers for Disease Control and Prevention uses a four-level social-ecological model to better understand violence and the complex interplay between individual, relationship, community, and societal factors. At each level, there are varied factors that increase one's risk for violence or protect an individual from experiencing or perpetrating violence. However, just as the presence of risk factors does not guarantee that an individual will experience violence, the presence of protective factors does not eliminate one's risk of violence. The overlapping rings within the model illustrate how factors at one level may influence risk and protective factors at another level (Fig. 38.1). The following section includes a discussion of selected factors that may influence violence. The Linking Content to Practice box discusses how public health nurses can collaborate in the community to prevent violence.

LINKING CONTENT TO PRACTICE

According to the Quad Council Domains of Public Health Nursing Practice (Swider et al., 2013) and the American Public Health Association (2017), public health nurses must collaborate in partnership with communities to identify and assess community needs; plan, implement, and evaluate community-based programs; and assist in the setting of policy that will contribute to the needs of the community in relationship to all types of interpersonal violence. The Quad Council competencies in the analytic assessment domain direct nurses to conduct thorough health assessments of individuals, families, communities, and populations and to develop diagnoses for the population being assessed (Swider et al., 2013). Public health nurses can help the community in many ways, as is described throughout this chapter.

Individual

The first level of the social-ecological model identifies biological and personal history factors that may increase the likelihood of an individual becoming a victim or perpetrator of violence. Demographic characteristics such as age, socioeconomic status, employment status, and educational attainment are associated with violence risk. Research also supports witnessing interparental violence, and a history of child maltreatment as risk factors for violence. Mental health disorders, including depression, anxiety, and post-traumatic stress disorder, as well as substance use disorders, are positively related to violence perpetration (Giancola, 2015; Harford et al., 2018; Jolliffe et al., 2016; Van Dorn et al., 2012).

Relationship

The second level of the social-ecological model explores how close social relationships, including relationships with peers, intimate partners, and family members, increase one's risk for violent victimization and perpetration of violence. In the cases of partner violence and child maltreatment, for example, frequent interactions or sharing a home with an abuser may increase the opportunity for violent encounters. With regard to violence among youths, research demonstrates that adolescents are significantly more likely to engage in negative activities when peers accept these behaviors (Garthe et al., 2017). Peer-based social networks are significantly related to both healthy and violent relationships. Specific to youth violence, research has demonstrated that low hyperactivity, low parental stress, strong parental supervision, positive attitude to school, and quality housing are risk-based protective factors (Jolliffe et al., 2016). Peers, intimate partners, and family members are all key influences on an individual's behavior and potential exposure to violence.

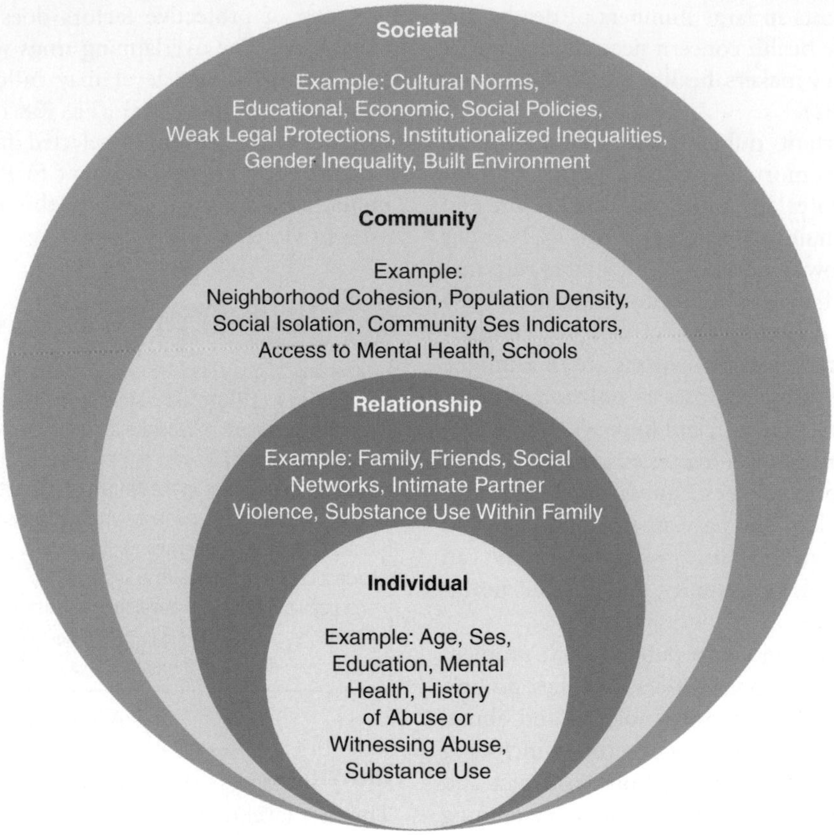

Fig. 38.1 The social-ecological model: a framework for violence prevention. (Modified from Heise LL: Violence against women: an integrated, ecological framework. *Violence Against Women* 4:262-290, 1998.)

Community

The third level of the social-ecological model examines how community contexts (e.g., schools, places of employment, neighborhoods) are associated with being victims or perpetrators of violence. With regard to neighborhoods, a high level of residential mobility, low level of neighborhood cohesion, and high population density are associated with higher levels of violence (Beyer et al., 2015). Communities with higher levels of drug trafficking or widespread social isolation are also more likely to experience violence. Community- or neighborhood-level indicators most frequently associated with violence are related to community socioeconomics such as unemployment rate, per capita income, and poverty rate. However, this also means that community protective factors may reduce one's risk of experiencing violence. Factors that increase peoples' and communities' resilience to violence include:

- Coordination of resources and support services among community agencies
- Access to mental health and substance abuse treatment services
- Support and connectedness, including connectedness to one's community, family, pro-social peers, and school

Schools are important settings for positively influencing our youth. Schools serve as a central community place of socialization, and while they can be safe havens for some youth, they can be stressful places for others. Using a nationally representative sample from 2015, 22.6 percent of youth in high school reported being involved in a physical fight over the previous year and 16.2 percent reported carrying a weapon at least once in the prior month (Centers for Disease Control and Prevention, 2016). Youth living in urban areas, particularly ethnic minority youth, are at a heightened risk for experiencing violence (McMahon et al., 2013). The importance of school climate (e.g., safety, relationships, teaching and learning practices, institutional environment) has been well established in the literature with a recent meta-analysis of 13 longitudinal studies of 5th-12th grade students demonstrating a significant relation between perceived school climate and student problem behaviors across time (Reaves et al., 2018). Thus schools represent an opportune vehicle to effect social change.

Societal

The fourth and final level of the ecological model examines the broader societal factors that influence rates of violence. These include factors that contribute to a culture that accepts violence, those that reduce inhibitions against violence, and those that both create and perpetuate disparities between different segments of society. Broader societal factors may include but are not limited to:

- Cultural norms that support violence as an acceptable means for resolving conflict
- Societal attitudes that regard suicide as an individual's choice instead of a preventable act of violence

- Cultural norms that support male dominance over women and children
- Educational, economic, and social policies that foster high levels of inequality between its citizens
- Norms that support political conflict

VIOLENCE AGAINST INDIVIDUALS OR ONESELF

The potential for violence against individuals (e.g., murder, robbery, rape, assault) or oneself (e.g., suicide) is directly related to the level of violence in the community. Persons living in areas with high rates of crime and violence are more likely to become victims than those in more peaceful areas. The major categories of violence addressed in this chapter are described in terms of the scope of the problem in the United States and underlying dynamics.

Homicide

Homicide is defined as a death resulting from the use of force against another person when a preponderance of evidence indicates that the use of force was intentional (Parks et al., 2014). Age-specific homicide rates are highest (11.7 deaths per 100,000 population) among those aged 20 to 24 years, followed by those aged 25 to 29 years (10.7 deaths per 100,000 population). Importantly, the homicide rate for males is nearly four times that of females (7.7 and 2.1 per 100,000, respectively). Non-Hispanic African Americans account for nearly half (49.6 percent) of homicide deaths and have the highest rate (15.2 deaths per 100,000 population), followed by American Indians/Alaska Natives (10.0) and Hispanics (5.1) (Parks et al., 2014). Rates of homicide for infants under the age of one year were highest among non-Hispanic African Americans and American Indians/Alaska Natives (Parks et al., 2014). Parents perpetuate the majority of homicides of children. Strangers cause 15 percent of male and 9 percent of female homicides in the United States (Catalano et al., 2009). When strangers are involved, many of these homicides are related to the illegal substance abuse network. The majority of homicides are perpetrated by a friend, acquaintance, or family member. Therefore prevention of homicide is at least as much an issue for the public health system as for the criminal justice system.

Firearm violence is a major public health issue in the United States, a country with the highest levels of firearm homicide incidences compared to other high-income countries (Richardson & Hemenway, 2011). In 2015, 72.9 percent of homicides were firearm homicides and, about 90 percent were committed with a handgun (CDC, 2016). Multiple studies have demonstrated a significant relationship between higher gun ownership at the state level and higher overall state-specific rates of firearm homicide (Fleegler et al., 2013; Siegel et al., 2013). Research has recently demonstrated that a higher proportion of household gun ownership at the state level is associated with statistically significant increased rates of nonstranger total firearm homicides. By contrast, there was not a statistically significant relationship between household gun ownership and stranger homicides, challenging the argument that gun ownership deters violent crime, particularly homicides (Siegel et al., 2014). Importantly, the number of nonfatal firearm injuries is more than double the number of deaths (CDC, 2017). While much attention has been given to the mass shootings that have occurred in the United States recently, the 88 deaths per day due to firearm-related homicides, suicides, and unintentional deaths highlight the magnitude of the issue (Hoyert & Xu, 2012).

In 2015, about 55 percent of homicides of women and 6 percent of homicides of men were committed by intimate partners, and about 55 percent of all intimate partner homicides were committed with guns (U.S. Department of Justice, 2015). Across studies, major risk factors for intimate partner homicide include previous violence, unemployment, access to firearms, estrangement, threats to kill, threats with a weapon, and a stepchild in the home (if the victim is female) (Campbell et al., 2000, 2003; Smith et al., 2014). Importantly, the risk of intimate partner homicide increases by 500 percent when a violent intimate partner has access to a firearm (Campbell et al., 2003). Many victims of intimate partner homicide are parents, and due to the nature of intimate partner homicide, which often occurs in the home, children are frequent witnesses (Lewandowski et al., 2004). Not only has one parent died; the other parent is incarcerated, has fled, or has committed suicide (Steeves & Parker, 2007). These children are confronted with significant trauma, loss, and hardship and require critical support systems.

Homicide is the leading cause of death for pregnant and postpartum women, and research has shown an overall pregnancy-associated violent death mortality rate of 4.9 per 100,000 births. Nearly two-thirds of pregnancy-associated violent deaths occur during pregnancy with the remaining occurring in the first year post partum (Palladino et al., 2011). Indeed, pregnancy-associated homicide and suicide each account for more maternal deaths than many other obstetric complications, commonly thought of as more "traditional" causes of maternal mortality. Nurses working in perinatal care environments are uniquely positioned to screen for intimate partner violence (IPV) and provide the necessary supports and referrals for those women screening positive.

Assault

The death toll from violence is staggering, yet the physical injuries and emotional costs of **assault** are equally important issues in terms of the acute health care system. Twenty-two percent of females compared with 7.4 percent of males reported injury related to physical assault. Age is the greatest risk factor for an individual's victimization through violence, and youths are at significantly higher risk. Although more males than females are victims of homicide and assault, women are more likely to be victimized by a relative, especially a male partner (Catalano et al., 2009). In some instances the response time of emergency services and the quality of treatment facilities determine whether an assault will end as a homicide. The same community measures used to address homicide are useful to combat assault. Also, nurses often care for the long-term health problems associated with assaults such as head injuries, spinal cord injuries, and stomas from abdominal gunshot wounds in a home health care setting. In addition to providing physical care, nurses must also address the emotional trauma resulting from a violent attack by helping victims talk through their traumatic experience to try to make some sense of the violence, and by referring them for further counseling if anxiety, sleeping problems, or depression persists after the assault.

Rape

In the United States, an estimated 19.3 percent of women and 1.7 percent of men have been raped in their lifetimes (Breiding et al., 2014). The lifetime and 12-month prevalence of rape by an intimate partner for women was an estimated 8.8 percent and 0.8 percent, respectively. Among female victims of rape, an estimated 78.7 percent experienced this form of sexual violence before 25 years of age, and an estimated 40.4 percent before the age of 18 (Breiding et al., 2014). From 1995 to 2005, the rate of completed rape or sexual assault declined from 3.6 per 1000 females to 1.1 per 1000 females. The rate of sexual violence against females declined with age. In 2005-2010, sexual violence was committed against females aged 12 to 34 at a rate of about 4 victimizations per 1000, compared to a rate of 1.5 victimizations per 1000 for females aged 35 to 64 and 0.2 per 1000 for females age 65 or older. For all racial and ethnic groups, the rate of sexual violence was lower in 2005-2010 than it was in 1994-1998 (Planty et al., 2013). Based on data from the Bureau of Justice Statistics' National Crime Victimization Survey (NCVS), non-Hispanic white females and African American and Hispanic females had a similar rate of sexual violence over time. However, Hispanic females (1.4 per 1000) had lower rates of sexual violence than African American females (2.8 per 1000) in 2005-2010. While American Indians and Alaska Natives (4.5 per 1000) appeared to experience rape or sexual assault victimization at higher rates than females in other racial and ethnic groups, the NCVS cautions that rates are based on small sample sizes and thus should be interpreted with caution (Planty et al., 2013). From 1995 to 2010, about nine percent of all rape or sexual assault victimizations involved male victims. In 2010, the rate of rape or sexual assaults was 0.1 per 1000 for males as compared to a rate of 2.1 per 1000 for females. In 2005-2010, most rape or sexual assault victims (78 percent) knew the perpetrator, and about one-third of all rapes or sexual assaults were committed by an intimate partner (Planty et al., 2013). Because the majority of violence against women is IPV and women are raped more often by someone they know rather than by strangers, health care providers must be alert for date and marital rape. An estimated 65 percent of rapes in the United States between 2006 and 2010 went unreported to law enforcement, making rape the most underreported violent crime in the country (Langton et al., 2012).

College women are at particularly high risk for sexual victimization in the United States; an estimated 20 to 25 percent of college-aged females experience attempted rape or completed rape during their college career, yet these rates of victimization vary from campus to campus (Moynihan et al., 2011). A recent study demonstrated that female undergraduate students were more likely to be victimized than graduate students, and the vast majority of students who experienced sexual violence were victimized when they were incapacitated due to intoxication or asleep (Campbell et al., 2017). Data from the Bureau of Justice Statistics demonstrate that despite arrest rates for sexual assault remaining stable, twice as many women reported a sexual assault by an intimate partner in 2010 as compared with 1994 (Catalano, 2013). The health impact of sexual assault is highly significant. Health issues include high-risk sexual behavior, substance abuse, unintended pregnancy, depression, post-traumatic stress disorder (PTSD), suicidal ideation, and eating disorders (Silverman et al., 2001). Nurses are well positioned to provide victims with comprehensive care, including mental health services. Nurses can identify and refer clients who have experienced sexual assault. Advanced practice nurses are often providers of primary health care on college campuses, placing them in a unique position to educate and support students on the issue of dating violence.

Another form of rape is forced sexual initiations, with as many as 21 percent of young women in the United States whose first sexual experience is below the age of 14 reporting that this initiation was physically forced, usually by a date or boyfriend (Stockman et al., 2010). These early sexual experiences are associated with unplanned, adolescent pregnancies as well as human immunodeficiency virus (HIV)/sexually transmitted disease (STD) risk behaviors.

Prevention of rape, like that of other forms of human abuse, requires a broad-based community focus for educating both the community as a whole and key groups such as police, health providers, educators, and social workers. Rape rates and community-level variables such as community approval and legitimization of violence (e.g., violent network television viewing and permitting corporal punishment in schools) appear related and underscore the need for community-level intervention (Casey & Lindhorst, 2009).

Human Trafficking

Human trafficking is a significant public health issue globally, including in the United States. Human trafficking is an umbrella term that includes activities involved in recruiting, harboring, transporting or providing an individual for forced service or commercial sex acts through the use of force, deception or coercion (United Nations Office on Drugs and Crime, 2019). Due to the secretive nature of human trafficking, accurate prevalence estimates are difficult to obtain yet an estimated 50,000 women and children may be trafficked into the United States each year (Siskin & Sun, 2013). Human trafficking is the fastest growing and one of the most lucrative crimes in the United States, thus it is imperative that nurses and other health care professionals are trained in the identification, care, and supports needed for these individuals (United Nations Office on Drugs and Crime, 2019).

Human trafficking affects all races, ages, and genders; yet, women and children under the age of 18 are at heightened risk (United Nations Office on Drugs and Crime, 2019). Children are often targeted due to their earning potential, with runaway and homeless youth at greatest risk (United Nations Office on Drugs and Crime, 2019). The majority of individuals experiencing human trafficking in the United States are women or girls, and the majority of these individuals are forced into the sex service industry (United Nations Office on Drugs and Crime, 2019).

Most trafficked individuals will come in contact with a health care provider, often through the emergency department setting, for treatment of an illness or injury at some point during their captivity. Yet, they are seldom appropriately identified as victims of trafficking (Peters, 2013). Victims are not likely to identify themselves as such for a number of reasons including fear of captor, distrust of available support systems (e.g., medical, legal, social services), uncertainty about available supports, unfamiliarity with regional language or culture, or feelings of shame about their situation (Becker & Bechtel, 2015).

Victims of human trafficking will often present to the health care system accompanied by their trafficker who may identify themselves as a family member or trusted support person. The trafficker may be male or female, and may appear to be supportive, caring, and sympathetic to the individual (Becker & Bechtel, 2015). Thus identifying trafficked individuals may be difficulty but there are "red flags" in their presentation that can be useful. A "family member" or "friend" who doesn't allow the individual to answer the health care provider's questions or consistently answers for them should raise suspicion. The individual may appear to be reluctant in describing symptoms or the events leading up to the presenting complaint; they may be vague in their responses or report inconsistencies in their responses. Individuals may not be able to provide a home address, have no identification documents, and may be unaware of the city or state in which they are receiving services.

The signs and symptoms of trafficking are multifaceted, and may occur in isolation or in combination. Physical symptoms may include, but are not limited to, unexplained bruises, burns, lacerations, bite marks, vaginal or anal tearing, sexually transmitted infections, unintended pregnancy, nutritional deficits, and substance use disorder (De Chesnay, 2013; Isaac et al., 2011; Richards, 2014). With regards to mental health issues, victims of human trafficking are at increased risk for depression, posttraumatic stress disorder, suicidal ideation or suicide attempts (Richards, 2014).

Caring for a potential victim of human trafficking requires a trauma-informed, empowering, nonjudgmental manner. The goal of the interaction should be to create a safe space and empowerment. It is critical that the health care provider can interview the patient alone thereby facilitating disclosure. Explaining that it is routine practice in a particular health care setting to interview patients alone may decrease suspicion in the captor. However, if it is difficult to obtain a one-on-one interview, it can be helpful to accompany the patient to a restroom or to a private setting for a particular reason, such as the laboratory or x-ray. If the victim does not speak English, it is critical to use a professional interpreter to assure accuracy in the assessment.

There are no validated screening questions for human trafficking, yet there are a number of questions that have been useful for health care providers to ask. These include:

- Can you come and go from your home (or job) whenever you please?
- Has anyone at home or work ever physically harmed you?
- Have you been threatened for trying to leave your job?
- Is anyone forcing you to do things you do not want to do?
- Do you have to ask permission to eat, sleep, or use the bathroom?
- Are there locks on your doors and windows that keep you from leaving?
- Have you ever been denied food, water, sleep, or medical care?
- Has anyone ever threatened your family?
- Has anyone taken away your identification papers or cards? (Crane, 2013)

If the health care provider suspects that a patient is a victim of human trafficking, it is essential to engage the assistance of a social worker or victim advocate early in the patient's care. For patients under the age of 18, a call to the state's child protective services agency is necessary. If the health care provider feels that the patient is in immediate danger, law enforcement should be contacted. If the patient isn't believed to be in immediate danger, the health care provider should notify the patient prior to engaging law enforcement on their behalf. Involving the patient may improve trust, and facilitate disclosure by the victim.

There are a number of resources available for providing care to victims of human trafficking. The National Human Trafficking Resource Center hot line (1-888-373-7888) is available to anyone with a suspicion of trafficking. It is toll free, available 24 hours/day and available in 180 languages. The Center can provide guidance on interview questions as well as indicators of potential trafficking. Importantly, it can provide access to safety resources including shelters, as well as other critical safety resources. Another helpful resource is https://polarisproject.org. This site includes an interactive map of the United States with updated listings of local organizations and resources for victims, as well as state laws regarding human trafficking.

Human trafficking is a significant issue in the United States. The physical and mental health sequelae for victims of trafficking is significant and sustained. It is critical that health care providers recognize the warning signs, acknowledging that engagement with the health care system may be one of the few opportunities for victims to escape their situations. An understanding of this issue, and supports available is key to saving lives.

Attitudes. The first priority is to change attitudes about rape and about victims or survivors. Rape is a crime of violence, not a crime of passion. The underlying issues are hostility, power, and control rather than sexual desire. The defining issue is lack of consent of the victim. When a woman or man refuses any sexual activity, that refusal means "no." People have the right to change their mind, even when they seemed initially agreeable. Pressure from physical contact, threats, or deliberate inducement of drug or alcohol intoxication is a violation of the law. The myths that women say "no" to sex when they really mean "yes" and that the victims of rape are culpable because of the way they dress or act must end.

Pornography. Although there is evidence of a relationship between the viewing of pornographic material showing violence against women and aggressive sexual behavior, it is not clear if the relationship is causal. In other words, our current research does not yet show that viewing pornography occurs before sexual aggressiveness or that young men who are sexually violent tend to watch pornography. The current research tends to minimize the relationship between sexual assault and pornography (Ferguson & Hartley, 2009). However, there is some evidence that claims that early exposure to pornography as a child may be related to sexual offense in the future (Seto & Lalumière, 2010). Prevention programs, or more accurately labeled risk reduction or avoidance programs, also involve providing information to women about self-protection, including using self-defense procedures, avoiding high-risk locations, and safeguarding one's home against unwanted entry. Most rape prevention programs have been oriented toward women. However, men are increasingly becoming involved in rape prevention education via anti-rape websites (Masters, 2010). Many of these websites are community-based programs that promote education about violence against women and promote a positive male role model of gender equity. They often depict examples of consensual and nonconsensual sexual behaviors.

Victim or Survivor? During the act of rape, survivors are often hit, kicked, stabbed, and severely beaten. It is this violence that is most traumatic because of the survivors' fear for their lives, helplessness, lack of control, and vulnerability.

People react to rape differently, depending on their personality, past experiences, background, and support received after the trauma. Some cry, shout, or discuss the experience. Others withdraw and fear discussing the attack. During the immediate as well as the follow-up stages, victims tend to blame themselves for what happened. When working with rape victims, help them identify the issues behind self-blame. While not placing fault on survivors, teach them to take control, learn assertiveness, and therefore believe that they can take certain actions to prevent future rapes. Survivors need to talk about what happened and to express their feelings and fears in a nonjudgmental atmosphere. Survivors of drug- or alcohol-facilitated/incapacitated (DAFR/IR) rape are substantially less likely to seek health care, rape crisis, or law enforcement services compared with survivors of forcible rape. Recent research suggests that women with forced rape were nearly three times more likely than women with DAFR/IR-only to report seeking support services (Walsh et al., 2016). Public service campaigns designed to increase awareness that DAFR/IR constitutes rape, even if force is not present, may help reduce evident disparities in rape-related service seeking (Walsh et al., 2016).

In any psychological trauma, victims should be given privacy, respect, and assurance of confidentiality. They should also be told about health care procedures conducted immediately after the rape and should be linked with proper resources for ease of reporting the crime. Nurses often provide continuous care once the victim enters the health care system. Because many victims deny the event once the initial crisis is past, a single-session debriefing should be completed during the initial examination. Specially trained providers should perform the physical assessment, examination, and debriefing.

As discussed in Chapter 44, in most states, nurses trained as sexual assault nurse examiners (SANEs), a subspecialty of forensic nursing, perform the physical examination in the emergency department to gather evidence (e.g., hair samples, skin fragments beneath the victim's fingernails, evidence from pelvic examinations obtained by colposcopy) for criminal prosecution of sexual assault (Sheridan, 2004). This is an important nursing intervention because physicians may not be able to take the time required for this procedure; nurses can take advantage of this opportunity to provide therapeutic communication and support. Nurses can be trained to conduct the examination either in SANE trainings or in forensic nursing programs in many schools of nursing, and their evidence is credible and effective in resultant court proceedings (Campbell et al., 2006, 2008; Houmes et al., 2003). Nurses can lobby for changes in hospital policies and state laws to make this strategy a reality in all states.

Rape is a situational crisis for which advance preparation is rarely possible. Therefore nursing efforts are directed toward helping victims cope with the stress and disruption of their lives caused by the attack. Counseling focuses on the crisis and the concomitant fears, feelings, and issues involved. Nurses can help survivors learn how to regroup personal strengths. If PTSD occurs, professional psychological or psychiatric treatment is indicated.

Many communities have developed multidisciplinary teams, sexual assault response teams (SARTs), to coordinate response between the health care system, criminal justice system, and victim advocacy organizations to sexual assault victims. The purpose of SARTs is two-fold: to provide comprehensive, timely care and to support engagement with community services, and to collect high-quality forensic evidence (Cole, 2016). Limited evidence suggests that there are benefits of a coordinated model, including improved communication between service providers, decreased wait times at hospitals, and improved forensic evidence collection (Greeson & Campbell, 2013). Nurses must be aware of the services within their communities to assure a timely and appropriate referral to necessary service providers.

Suicide

According to the National Violent Death Reporting System (NVDRS), suicide accounted for the highest rate of violent death in 2007, taking the lives of 9245 people. Firearms accounted for 50.7 percent, hanging/strangulation/suffocation for 23.1 percent, and poisoning for 18.8 percent of suicides. Firearms (56 percent) or hanging/strangulation/suffocation (24.4 percent) were the most common form of suicide for men. Women used poisoning (40.8 percent) most frequently, followed by firearms (30.9 percent). Precipitating factors for suicide were mental health (45 percent), IPV (30 percent), and physical health problems (21.4 percent) (CDC, 2014a). The risk for death by suicide is greater than for death by homicide. Rates of completed suicide are higher for men, especially older adults, non-Hispanic whites, and Alaska Natives/American Indians (Karch et al., 2010). Affluent and educated people often have higher rates of suicide than do the economically and educationally disadvantaged except for Alaska Native/American Indian populations, who are often poor and yet commit suicide in alarming numbers. The presence of a gun in the home is an important risk factor for both suicide and homicide (Campbell, 2007).

Suicide is the third-leading cause of death among young people ages 15 to 24. During 2005 to 2009, the highest suicide rates were among American Indian/Alaska Native males, with 27.61 suicides per 100,000, and non-Hispanic white males, with 25.96 suicides per 100,000. Of all female race/ethnicity groups, the American Indians/Alaska Natives and non-Hispanic whites had the highest rates with 7.87 and 6.71 suicides per 100,000, respectively. For American Indian youth, adverse childhood experiences, particularly witnessing a mother being abused, and historical trauma are salient risk factors for suicidality (Brockie et al., 2015). Boys and young men between the ages of 15 and 19 were five times more likely to commit suicide than females and four times more likely if between the ages of 20 and 24 (Karch et al., 2010). Attempted suicide was more prevalent for white, African American, and Hispanic females than for males of the same racial background. Leading risk factors for adolescent suicide are mental health, unintended pregnancy, and STD, especially HIV (Eaton et al., 2010). An important risk factor for actual and attempted suicide in adult women is IPV.

The majority of individuals who complete suicide have visited a health care provider in the previous month of their suicide; therefore health care providers are key for screening and intervening for individuals at risk. On a community level, nurses can be involved in a coordinated response to the prevention of suicide and the care of attempted suicides. Through their roles in public health and school nursing, they can help develop policies and protocols for suicide across the life span. Nursing care may focus on family members and friends of suicide victims. The loss of a person by suicide can arouse different feelings of grief among relatives and close friends of those who have committed suicide than the emotions they experience when death occurs from natural causes. Communicating one's feelings is an integral part of the healing process, and support groups play an important role in this healing.

FAMILY VIOLENCE AND ABUSE

Intimate partner violence (IPV), defined as physical, sexual, or psychological harm caused by a former or current intimate partner, is a major public health problem in the United States. Data from the 2011 National Intimate Partner and Sexual Violence Survey (NISVS) suggests that over 10 million women and men experience physical violence each year by a current or former intimate partner (Breiding et al., 2015). Importantly, more than one in five women (22.3 percent) and nearly one in seven men (14.0 percent) have experienced severe physical violence by an intimate partner in their lifetime (Breiding et al., 2015). The recognition of IPV is critical given it is one of the most well-established predictors of attempted or completed intimate partner homicide. The Centers for Disease Control and Prevention recently analyzed homicides from 18 states between 2003 and 2014, finding that over half (55.3 percent) of homicides committed against females in the United States involved an intimate partner (Petrosky et al., 2017).

The majority of IPV is directed at women, with the majority of IPV perpetrated by a male partner or ex-partner (Black et al., 2011). A recent integrative review synthesized results from 42 studies that examined IPV and sexual violence among sexual minorities between 1989 and 2015 (Brown & Herman, 2015). Results demonstrated that bisexual women were 1.8 times more likely to experience IPV than heterosexual women, and 2.6 times more likely to report having experienced sexual violence as compared to heterosexual women. Bisexual men were noted to also be at increased risk for IPV. A limited number of studies examined transgender people, finding they were at higher risk of IPV, with lifetime prevalence estimates ranging from 31.1 percent to 50.0 percent (Brown & Herman, 2015). Lesbian, gay, bisexual, transgender, queer (LGBTQ) IPV generally follows similar dynamics as heterosexual IPV (emotional, verbal, physical, and/or sexual violence, threats, isolation, and intimidation, in a context of one partner maintaining power and control over another) and results in similarly adverse health outcomes. As with heterosexual IPV, dynamics of power and control caused by race, gender expression, ability, immigration status, age, and class are methods of control in same-sex IPV (National Coalition of Anti-Violence Programs, 2017). LGBTQ people face many of the barriers to help seeking that non-LGBTQ people do, but they face additional barriers that are related to their sexual orientation or gender identity. These may include but are not limited to:

- Legal definitions of intimate partner violence that exclude same-sex couples
- The risks associated with "outing" oneself when seeking help and the potential for negative response from family, friends, and society
- A lack of knowledge about resources specific for LGBTQ survivors
- Potential discrimination from service providers or non-LGBTQ survivors of IPV
- Lack of knowledge or sensitivity on behalf of law enforcement officials and courts for LGBTQ people (Brown & Herman, 2015)

Recognizing the IPV survivor in the emergency department may be simple after the fact. It is unfortunate that, by the time medical care is sought, serious physical and emotional damage may have been done. Nurses are in a key position to predict and deal with abusive tendencies. By understanding factors contributing to the development of abusive behaviors, nurses can identify incidents of IPV.

Development of Abusive Patterns

Perpetrators of IPV often believe that violence within an interpersonal relationship is a normal behavior pattern (Stover et al., 2010). Factors that characterize people who become involved in IPV include upbringing, living conditions, and increased stress. Understanding how these factors influence the development of abusive behavior can help the nurse manage abusive families.

Upbringing. The most predictable factor in the background of an abuser is previous exposure to some form of violence (Whiting et al., 2009). As children, abusers were often beaten or witnessed the beating of siblings or a parent. These children learn that violence is a suitable way to manage conflict. For both men and women, witnessing abuse as a child was associated with abuse of their children. Being financial solvent and having support tended to decrease the incidence of child abuse (Dixon et al., 2009; Whiting et al., 2009). Childhood physical punishment teaches children to use violent conflict resolution as an adult. A child may learn to associate love with violence because a parent is usually the first person to hit a child. Children may think that those who love them are also those who hit them. The moral rightness of hitting other family members thus may be established when physical punishment is used to train children, especially when it is used more than occasionally. These experiences predispose children ultimately to use violence with their own children.

As well as having a history of child abuse themselves, people who become abusers tend to have hostile personality styles and be verbally aggressive. They have often learned these characteristics from their own childhood experiences. Their parents may have set unrealistic goals, and when the children failed to perform accordingly, they were criticized, demeaned, punished, and denied affection. These children may have been told how to act, what to do, and how to feel, thereby discouraging the development of normal attachment, autonomy, problem-solving skills, and creativity (Dixon et al., 2005). Children raised in this way grow up feeling unloved and worthless. They may want a child of their own so that they will feel assured of someone's love.

Because of their experiences of trauma and to protect themselves from feelings of worthlessness and fear of rejection, abused children form a protective shell and grow increasingly hostile and distrustful of others. The behavior of potential abusers reflects a low tolerance for frustration, emotional instability, and the onset of aggressive feelings with minimal provocation. Because of their emotional insecurity, perpetrators of abuse often depend on a child or spouse to meet their needs of feeling valued and secure. When their needs are not met by others, they become overly critical. Critical, resentful behavior and unrealistic expectations of others lead to a vicious cycle. The more critical these people become, the more they are rejected and alienated from others. Abusive individuals tend to perceive that the target of their hostility is "out to get" them. These distorted perceptions can be detected when parents talk about an infant crying or keeping them up at night "on purpose" (Dixon et al., 2005).

Increased Stress. A perceived or actual crisis may precede an abusive incident. Because a crisis reinforces feelings of inadequacy and low self-esteem, a number of events often occur in a short time to precipitate abusive patterns. Unemployment, strains in the marriage, or an unplanned pregnancy may precipitate violence, especially in people with other risk factors such as a history of trauma themselves.

The daily hassles of raising young children, especially in an economically strained household, intensify an already stressed atmosphere for which an unexpected and difficult event may provoke violence. Stressful life events, poverty, and cultural values and social isolation are often associated with family violence. Crowded living conditions may also precipitate abuse. The presence of several people in a small space heightens tensions and reduces privacy; tempers flare because of the constant stimulation from others.

A significant amount of research has demonstrated the links between social support and optimal health. Conversely, social isolation is linked to poor mental and physical health and is associated with a higher risk of violence in families (Thompson, 2015). Social isolation is associated with increased stressors, less socialization of healthy parenting practices, and limited interpersonal and material resources for support. The problem may be intensified if an abusive family member tries to keep the family isolated to avoid detection. Therefore when a family chronically misses clinic or home visit appointments, nurses need to keep in mind that abuse may be present. Nurses can encourage involvement in community activities and can help neighbors reach out to neighbors to help prevent abuse.

Frequent moves disrupt social support systems, are associated with an overall increased stress level, and tend to isolate people, at least briefly. Mobility can have a serious negative effect on the abuse-prone family. These families do not readily initiate new relationships; they rely on the family for support. Resources may be unfamiliar or inaccessible to them. Because frequent moving may be both a risk factor for abuse and a sign of an abusive family trying to avoid detection, nurses should assess such families carefully for abuse.

Types of Intimate Partner and Family Violence

Because various forms of family violence and violence outside the home often occur together, nurses who detect child abuse should also suspect other forms of family violence. When older adult parents report that their (now adult) child was abused or has a history of violence toward others, the nurse should recognize the potential for elder abuse. **Physical abuse** of women is frequently accompanied by **sexual abuse** both inside and outside the marital relationship. Severe wife abusers may have a history of other acts of violence. Families who are verbally aggressive in conflict resolution (e.g., using name calling, belittling, screaming, and yelling) are more likely to be physically abusive. Although the various forms of family violence are discussed separately, they should not be thought of as totally separate phenomena.

No member of the family is guaranteed immunity from abuse and neglect. Spouse abuse, child abuse, abuse of older adults, serious violence among siblings, and mutual abuse by members all occur. Although these examples are not inclusive, they demonstrate the scope of family violence.

Child Abuse. **Child abuse** is an important cause of pediatric morbidity and mortality and is associated with significant physical and mental health sequelae that can extend into adulthood. A national survey estimated that in 2011, there were 742,000 unique reports of children and adolescents who were subjected to neglect, medical neglect, physical and sexual abuse, and emotional maltreatment. Of these children, 78 percent were victims of neglect, 18 percent were victims of physical abuse, 10 percent were sexually abused, and 8 percent were psychologically maltreated. Except for sexual abuse, which is four times as high for girls as for boys, victims are equally distributed among abused male and female children (U.S. Department of Health and Human Services [USDHHS], 2016). Fatal cases of abuse, although less common, disproportionally affect the youngest children, with 71 percent of fatalities occurring in children less than three years of age (USDHHS, 2016).

The effects of child exposure to IPV have been recognized with research demonstrating significant associations with social, emotional, and behavioral problems (Levendosky et al., 2013). Children who are exposed to IPV are at an increased risk for depression, anxiety, and attachment disorders. Further, they exhibit more behavioral problems, including aggression and delinquency (Kimball, 2016). The consequences may last into adulthood with difficulties establishing and maintaining healthy relationships and an increased risk for perpetrating IPV. A recent systematic review demonstrated that childhood abuse and witnessing IPV in childhood and adolescence were consistent predictors of IPV perpetration and victimization for males and females (Costa et al., 2015). These findings highlight the need for resources targeting at-risk families early in life.

Poverty is a well-known risk factor for child maltreatment, and the important role of community-level poverty on nonfatal child maltreatment is increasingly recognized (Leventhal & Gaither, 2012). In 2016, the American Academy of Pediatrics published a policy statement on poverty and child health in the United States, highlighting the salient role of poverty in health disparities, including infant mortality and injury (Council on Community Pediatrics, 2016). An analysis of CDC mortality files of child abuse fatalities in U.S. children aged 0 to 4 years from 1999 to 2014 revealed that counties with the highest poverty concentration had more than three times the rate of child abuse fatalities compared with counties with the lowest poverty concentration (Farrell et al., 2017). These findings highlight that child abuse prevention efforts must recognize community poverty and related factors in contributing to violence. Child characteristics that increase one's risk of maltreatment include those that make a child more difficult to care for. Examples include children living with special health care needs, chronic illnesses, or physical or developmental disabilities (Hibbard & Desch, 2007). A child born prematurely may have unique needs, and early and prolonged separation may contribute to an increased risk of maltreatment (Wu et al., 2004). Physical aggression, difficulty following parental direction, and antisocial behaviors are more common among maltreated children. The box that follows lists ways to recognize actual or potential signs of child abuse. The How To box below lists ways to identify potentially abusive parents.

HOW TO Identify Potentially Abusive Parents

The following characteristics in couples expecting a child constitute warning signs of actual or potential abuse:

- Denial of the reality of the pregnancy, as seen in a refusal to talk about the impending birth or to think of a name for the child
- An obvious concern or fear that the baby will not meet some predetermined standard: sex, hair color, temperament, or resemblance to family members
- Failure to follow through on the desire for an abortion
- An initial decision to place the child for adoption and a change of mind
- Rejection of the mother by the father of the baby
- Family experiencing stress and numerous crises so that the birth of a child may be the last straw
- Initial and unresolved negative feelings about having a child
- Lack of support for the new parents
- Isolation from friends, neighbors, or family
- Parental evidence of poor impulse control or fear of losing control
- Contradictory history
- Appearance of detachment
- Appearance of misusing drugs or alcohol
- Shopping for hospitals or health care providers
- Unrealistic expectations of the child
- Verbal, physical, or sexual abuse of mother by father, especially during pregnancy
- Child is not biological offspring of male stepfather or mother's current boyfriend
- Excessive talk of needing to "discipline" children and plans to use harsh physical punishment to enforce discipline

From an ecological perspective, interactions among and between children, parents, family members, and the broader community may all increase the likelihood of maltreatment. Parents or caregivers with mental health concerns, limited social support, limited knowledge of normal childhood development, low sense of parenting competence, experiencing IPV, or who have non biologically related adults in the home may be at increased risk (Farrell et al., 2017; Lane, 2014). Some of the risk factors are identified in Box 38.1 (USDHHS, 2013; Zimmerman & Mercy, 2010). Importantly, several protective factors should also be noted. Social support is a key protective factor; families with higher levels of social support demonstrate lower rates of child

BOX 38.1 Determining Risk Factors for Child Abuse

Ask the following questions or observe the following behaviors to determine whether risk factors are present.

1. Are the parents unemployed?
2. Do the parents have the financial resources to care for a child?
3. Is there a support network that is willing to offer assistance?
4. Do one or both parents have a history of child abuse?
5. Is a parent a victim or perpetrator of intimate partner violence?
6. Do the parents have knowledge about child development?
7. Do one or both parents have problems with substance abuse?
8. Are the parents overly critical of the child?
9. Are the parents communicative with each other and the nurse?
10. Does the mother of the child seem frightened of her partner?
11. Does the child suffer from recurrent injuries or unexplained illnesses?

Data from Rodriguez CM: Personal contextual characteristics and cognitions: predicting child abuse potential and disciplinary style. *J Interpers Violence* 25(2):315-335, 2010; U.S. Department of Health and Human Services, Administration for Children and Families, Administration on Children, Youth and Families, Children's Bureau: *Child maltreatment, 2008*, 2010. Available at http://www.acf.hhs.gov.; Zimmerman F, Mercy JA: A better start: child maltreatment prevention as a public health priority. *Zero Three* 30(5):4-10, 2010.

maltreatment and greater use of effective parenting practices other than corporal punishment (McCurdy, 2005). A parent's sense of competence in child care practices may enable him or her to more successfully cope with the challenges associated with child rearing. Thus successfully linking parents to specific programs for the prevention of child maltreatment or referring families to community-based programs can help parents meet their children's needs.

Parents who have inadequate parenting skills or resources have more difficulty providing the care and nurturing that is needed for children to have safe, nurturing relationships. There is substantial evidence that parenting programs or behavioral family interventions that target influencing children's behavior through positive reinforcement are effective at influencing the child-rearing practices of families (Kaminski et al., 2008; Lundahl et al., 2006). Some evidence suggests that these types of support programs may also reduce or prevent physical abuse and neglect (Whitaker et al., 2005).

Foster care. When child abuse is discovered, the child is often placed in a foster home. It is the legal responsibility of the nurse to report all cases of child abuse. Ideally, the initial report begins a process in which both the child and the family can receive the care needed. Although the focus of care should be on the best interests of the child and the parents, the primary attention should be on the health and safety of the child. While in foster care the abused child should receive continuous nursing care. The nurse is often the one consistent person abused children can relate to as they are transferred from their home to foster care and hopefully back to their home. Abused children generally want to return to their parents, and the goal of most agencies is to help natural families stay together as long as it is safe for the child. However, a family preservation approach may not always keep children safe (O'Reilly et al., 2010). Often the nurse's role is to help monitor a family in which a formerly abused child is returned from foster care. Keen judgment and close collaboration with social services are necessary in these situations. The nurse must ensure the safety of the child while working with the parents in an empathetic way. The nurse's goal is to enhance parenting skills through education on child care and development, communication, and principles of social learning theory. Parents must also be given positive support and reassurance about their ability to provide proper care to their child.

One of the most distressing outcomes of child abuse is depression and other mental health problems, especially suicide. Adolescents who have been placed in the social service system many times or who move from one foster home to another are at risk for delinquency, severe depression, alcohol and substance abuse, and suicide. Nurses need to understand the dynamics of adolescent suicide and substance abuse (Fletcher, 2010; Ford et al., 2010).

Indicators of child abuse. It is essential that nurses recognize the physical and behavioral indicators of abuse and neglect. Child abuse ranges from violent physical attacks to passive neglect. Violence such as beating, burning, kicking, or shaking may lead to severe physical injury. **Passive neglect** may result in insidious malnutrition or other problems. Abuse is not limited to physical maltreatment but includes **emotional abuse** such as yelling at or continually demeaning and criticizing the child. Children who come from a family where IPV occurs are at greater risk for physical and psychological abuse and child neglect (Fletcher, 2010; Hines & Malley-Morrison, 2005; Whiting et al., 2009). The How To box provides information about ways to recognize actual or potential child abuse.

HOW TO Recognize Actual or Potential Child Abuse

Be alert to the following:

- An unexplained injury
- Skin: burns, old or recent scars, ecchymosis, soft tissue swelling, human bites
- Fractures: recent, or older ones that have healed
- Subdural hematomas
- Trauma to genitalia
- Whiplash (caused by shaking small children)
- Dehydration or malnourishment without obvious cause
- Provision of inappropriate food or drugs (alcohol, tobacco, medication prescribed for someone else, foods not appropriate for the child's age)
- Evidence of general poor care: poor hygiene, dirty clothes, unkempt hair, dirty nails
- Unusual fear of nurse and others
- Considered to be a "bad" child
- Inappropriate dress for the season or weather conditions
- Reports or shows evidence of sexual abuse
- Injuries not mentioned in history
- Seems to need to take care of the parent and speak for the parent
- Maternal depression
- Maladjustment of older siblings
- Current or history of intimate partner violence in the home

Emotional abuse involves extreme debasement of feelings and may lead the child to feel inadequate, inept, uncared for, and worthless. These children learn to hide their feelings to avoid more scorn. They may act out by performing poorly in school, becoming truant, and being hostile and aggressive. Children who are abused or who witness domestic violence can suffer developmentally (Kletter et al., 2009; Rodriguez, 2010). Major responses of adolescents to physical and sexual abuse are substance abuse, severe depression, and running away from home (Fletcher, 2010; Ford et al., 2010).

Physical symptoms of physical, sexual, or emotional stress may include hyperactivity, withdrawal, overeating, dermatological problems, vague physical complaints, stuttering, enuresis (bladder incontinence), and encopresis (bowel incontinence). Ironically, bedwetting is often a trigger for further abuse, thereby creating a vicious cycle. When a child displays physical symptoms without clear physiological origin, the nursing assessment should rule out the possibility of abuse.

Child neglect. **Child neglect** occurs when a child's basic needs are not adequately met. Basic needs include adequate nutrition, clothing, stable housing, adult supervision, protection, health care, education, love, and nurturance. The four categories of child neglect include physical, emotional, medical, and educational neglect. **Physical neglect** is failure to provide adequate food, proper clothing, shelter, hygiene, or necessary medical care and is most often associated with extreme poverty. In contrast, **emotional neglect** is the lack of the basic nurturing, acceptance, and caring essential for healthy personal development. These children are largely ignored or treated as nonpersons, which affects the development of self-esteem. A neglected child has difficulty feeling self-worth because the parents have not shown that they value the child. Medical and educational neglect consist of the failure to provide for a child's basic medical and educational needs. Medical neglect may be due to an inability to buy basic drugs needed for common diseases. All forms of neglect may be involved when a parent fails to teach children about risky behaviors such as smoking and substance abuse (Hines & Malley-Morrison, 2005). Extreme cases of neglect are easily identified, but the majority of neglect cases are complex and lack precise identification.

Prevention and treatment of child maltreatment is challenging. In addition to addressing the consequences of poverty, substance abuse, poor mental health, and other common issues confronting families involved with child welfare, effective interventions must address the parent–child relationship. According to a national panel of child maltreatment experts, Abuse Focused Cognitive Behavioral Therapy (AF-CBT) and Parent-Child Interaction Therapy (PCIT) are two interventions that may be effective for the treatment of child maltreatment. Both are dyadic interventions, focused on altering specific patterns of interaction found in parent–child relationships (Schilling & Christian, 2014).

Sexual abuse. Child abuse also includes sexual abuse. About 1 in 4 female children and 1 in 10 males in the United States experience some form of sexual abuse by the time he or she reaches 18 years of age. It is difficult to determine the exact prevalence because not all children have the cognitive ability to describe these experiences. Rates based on reports to child protective services estimate that 50 in every 1000 children suffer from child abuse and/or neglect (USDHHS, 2016). This abuse ranges from unwanted sexual touching to intercourse. The child generally knows and trusts the person who perpetrates the sexual abuse. One-third to one-half of all sexual abuse involves a family member (Hines & Malley-Morrison, 2005; USDHHS, 2016). A child's risk for abuse is highest with parents, immediate family members, and nonrelated caregivers, although coaches, scout leaders, and even priests and other church workers have been reported as sexual abusers. The long-term effects of sexual abuse include depression, sexual disturbances, suicide, and substance abuse. Individuals with a history of both physical and sexual abuse tend to experience more severe symptoms than children who experience one form of abuse (Fletcher, 2010; Stevenson, 2009). Physically and sexually abusive parents share many of the same characteristics, including unhappiness, loneliness, and rigidity. However, sexually abused children have more gastrointestinal symptoms and post-traumatic stress disorders than physically abused children (Drossman, 2011).

Father–daughter **incest** is the type of incest most often reported; however, mothers do engage in child sexual abuse. In recent years more males have discussed their experiences of child sexual abuse. It is estimated that one in five children is a victim of child sexual abuse. Cases of father–daughter, father–son, mother–daughter, and mother–son incest have been reported (Hines & Malley-Morrison, 2005). Many cases of parental sexual abuse go unreported because victims fear punishment, abandonment, rejection, or family disruption if the problem is acknowledged. Although stepfathers are considered the most common perpetrator of father–daughter incest, we know little about female perpetrators. Incest occurs in all races, religious groups, and socioeconomic classes. Incest is receiving greater attention because of mandatory reporting laws, yet all too often its incidence remains a family secret.

Nurses must be aware of the incidence, signs and symptoms, and psychological and physical trauma of incest. Symptoms include low self-esteem, depression, anxiety, and somatic symptoms of headaches, eating and sleeping disorders, menstrual problems, and gastrointestinal distress (Drossman, 2011). Sexually abused children often exhibit premature sexual behavior, such as masturbation. Children often try to avoid or escape the abusive behavior. Avoidance can be through either behavioral or mental reactions, such as dressing to cover one's body or pretending that the abuse is not taking place. The child can escape either physically by running away or emotionally by withdrawing into other activities and thereby placing the sexual abuse in the background (Stevenson, 2009).

Adolescents may display inappropriate sexual activity or truancy or may run away from home. Running away is usually considered a sign of delinquency; however, an adolescent who runs away may be exhibiting a healthy response to a violent family situation. Therefore the assessment should include questions about sexual and physical abuse at home and a plan for appropriate intervention.

The effects of childhood sexual abuse can be mitigated by continual professional support. At different developmental stages, children may need assistance to overcome negative feelings about their own sexuality (Stevenson, 2009). Adult survivors of sexual abuse often are socially isolated and have significant health problems that need to be addressed in terms of the ongoing effects of their childhood and adult experiences (Mapp, 2006).

Abuse of Female Partners. Neither the term **wife abuse** nor the term **spouse abuse** takes into account violence in dating or cohabitating relationships or violence in same-sex relationships. IPV, a more inclusive term, refers to all kinds of violence between partners. IPV is not a rare event, with one in three women and one in four men reporting physical violence, rape, and/or stalking by a current or former intimate partner at some point in their life (Black et al., 2011). However, these figures do not include psychological forms of IPV, which also could have severe consequences. Recently, more attention has been given to female-perpetrated IPV and bidirectional violence (i.e., male-to-female violence concurrent with female-to-male violence), especially in the context of teen dating violence. Nevertheless, female victims of IPV are more likely to report severe IPV and experience more negative individual, family, and community consequences than their male counterparts, and a greater potential for intimate partner homicide (Black et al., 2011; Campbell, 2007).

IPV appears early in life. In fact, about 22 percent of victims of rape, physical abuse, and/or stalking by an intimate partner report their first experience when they were between the ages of 11 and 17. Nearly half (47 percent) report their first incident between the ages of 18 and 24 (Black et al., 2011). As in adulthood, IPV experienced by adolescents and young adults is associated with poor mental health outcomes such as depression and suicidality, is linked to risky behaviors such as substance abuse and risky sexual behaviors, and contributes to the intergenerational transmission of interpersonal violence (Reyes et al., 2016). Adolescence is an important developmental period that should be effectively targeted to prevent violence, thus mitigating its effects into adulthood.

Signs of abuse. Abused women often have bruises and lacerations of the face, head, and trunk of the body. Attacks are often carefully inflicted on parts of the body that are disguised by clothing. This pattern of proximal location of injuries (e.g., breasts, abdomen, upper thighs, and back) rather than distal and patterned injuries (in various stages of healing, in particular configurations matching the body part or object used as a weapon) is characteristic of abuse (Campbell & Sheridan, 2004; Sheridan & Nash, 2009). When a woman has a black eye or bruises about the mouth, the nurse should ask, "Who hit you?" rather than, "What happened to you?" The latter implies that the nurse is neither knowledgeable nor comfortable with violence, and this may prompt the woman to fabricate a more acceptable cause of her injury.

Once abused, women tend to exhibit low self-esteem and depression, and even PTSD (Humphreys & Campbell, 2010). They have more physical health problems than other women, such as chronic pain (back, head, abdominal), neurological problems, problems sleeping, gynecological symptoms, urinary tract infections, and chronic gastrointestinal problems (Campbell, 2002). Victims of IPV are also at greater risk for HIV and other sexually transmitted infections (STIs), which appear to be both a risk factor and consequence of the abuse (Coker et al., 2009). In addition, female victims of IPV are more at risk for chronic diseases such as cardiovascular disease, atherosclerosis, and autonomic nervous system disorders (Symes et al., 2010). Although the focus tends to be on the victim of the abuse, it is important to note that there are health consequences to the perpetrator and children witnessing the abuse as well. These physical and mental health consequences incur health care costs that are preventable (Rivara et al., 2007).

Abuse as a process. Nursing research by Ford-Gilboe et al. (2010) suggests that there is a process of response to battering over time wherein the woman's emotional and behavioral reactions change. At first there is a great need to minimize the seriousness of the situation. The violence usually starts with a slight shove in the middle of a heated argument. If there is any physical aggression, both the man and the woman tend to blame the incident on something external such as a stressful day at work or drinking too much. The male partner usually apologizes for the incident, and as with any problem in a relationship, the couple tries to improve the situation. Although marital counseling may be useful at this early stage, it is generally contraindicated at all other stages because of the risk to the woman's safety. Unfortunately, abuse tends to escalate in frequency and severity over time, often leading to severe physical injuries and even death (Piquero et al., 2006), and the man's remorse tends to lessen. Similar power and control dynamics and risks have been documented in same-sex relationships, yet these dynamics may be more difficult to assess because screening and services for IPV are often designed for heterosexual relationships (Alhusen et al., 2010).

Because women have often been taught to take responsibility for the success of a relationship, they usually go through a period in which they try to change their behavior to end the violence. They may even blame themselves for infuriating their partner. Women who blame themselves for provoking the abuse are more likely to have low self-esteem and be depressed than those who do not blame themselves. Some women experience a moral conflict between their need to leave an abusive relationship and their sense that it is their responsibility to maintain a relationship (Edwards et al., 2015). A woman is also typically concerned about her children, which may create barriers to a woman's ability to leave or to remain out of the relationship. The frequency of abuse, severity of power and control tactics used by the perpetrator, feelings of guilt, and social and financial responsibility are additional influences on a woman's decision about how she responds to the abuse and whether she stays or leave the relationship (Rhodes et al., 2010; Sonis & Langer, 2008).

Although leaving the abusive partner may ultimately contribute to a decrease in the woman's risk for further victimization, the moment in which she leaves the relationship is the time in which there is the greatest risk for intimate partner homicide (Campbell, 2007). This creates a Catch-22 situation, in which the woman feels she will die whether she stays or leaves. Consequently, battered women often try several times to leave a relationship. The safety of the woman and her children is a nursing priority during these attempts.

EVIDENCE-BASED PRACTICE

Sharps et al. (2016) conducted a multistate longitudinal study testing the effectiveness of a structured intimate partner violence (IPV) intervention integrated into health department perinatal home visitation programs in rural and urban locations. All women (n = 239) enrolled in the randomized clinical trial were pregnant at the time of enrollment and reported a positive history of IPV in the perinatal period. The research partners included individuals from two schools of nursing, an urban East Coast health department, and 13 rural Midwestern health departments. The Domestic Violence Enhanced Home Visitation (DOVE) intervention, based on an empowerment model, combined two evidence-based interventions: a 10-minute brochure-based IPV intervention and perinatal nurse home visitation. Quantitative and qualitative data revealed that women in both the intervention group and control group demonstrated a significant decrease in IPV over time. However, women receiving the DOVE intervention had significantly lower levels of IPV than did women randomized to usual care at 24 months. Home visitors in both groups (e.g., intervention and control) were taught how to screen for IPV and how to coordinate appropriate referrals, ensuring that each woman received basic safety information.

Nurse Use

Nurses need to be able to work with survivors of IPV as well as providers within communities who work with abused women. Community-based partnerships are essential to most effectively develop and implement evidence-based IPV interventions such as DOVE. To best address IPV in a community, nurses must understand cultural differences among women who experience IPV as well as among community advocates who may also be assisting abused women. Public health nurses are well positioned to forge such partnerships and take an active role in planning, implementing, and evaluating programmatic change.

Partnering with the community. Nurses need to be able to work to address IPV on various levels of intervention. Community-based partnerships are essential collaborative actions that will assist in the reduction of IPV. To do so, nurses must understand cultural differences related to IPV, as well as the needs and strengths of the communities with which they partner. Public health nurses can take an active role in leading groups and planning, implementing, and evaluating programmatic change. There are various examples of nurse-led community partnerships to prevent and address IPV. For example, both Belknap and VandeVusse (2010) and Gonzalez-Guarda et al. (2013) partnered with community agencies, schools, and community members to identify needs and preferences for IPV prevention and services for the Hispanic/Latino community. This work has led to the development, implementation, and evaluation of dating violence prevention programs for Hispanic/Latino youth.

The CDC has launched an initiative called Dating Matters. The purpose of this program is to teach parents and adolescents about healthy relationships and to give them tools to deal with unhealthy relationships such as teen dating violence (CDC, 2014b). Dating Matters focuses on 11- to 14-year-olds in high-risk, urban communities, and includes prevention strategies for individuals, peers, families, schools, and neighborhoods. The Migrant Clinicians Network, an organization to help migrant and other poor transient workers, has developed a natural helper model for migrant workers, to work within their own community to identify and teach about IPV (Kugel et al., 2009). On the basis of models developed in the 1980s, communities are developing a coordinated response in which multiple agencies work together to assist with preventing IPV.

Screening. Given the high prevalence of IPV and the negative physical, psychological, social, and economic consequences associated with this public health problem, adolescents and adults should be screened for violence in their primary intimate relationship. The U.S. Preventive Services Task Force recommends screening women of childbearing age for IPV and referring or providing women who disclose abuse to intervention services (U.S. Preventive Services Task Force, 2013). The use of effective screening protocols, institutional support for implementing screening, initial and ongoing staff training, and access to services onsite or through a strong referral system are recommended as part of a comprehensive screening program (O'Campo et al., 2011).

Safety planning. Victims of IPV are at high risk for severe injuries and homicide, especially at the moment they decide to leave an abusive relationship (Campbell, 2007). As such, nurses should work with women victims in creating a safety plan. This plan may include the following: (1) an order of protection (a legal document to keep the abuser away from her); (2) help in getting to a safe place, such as a domestic violence shelter in an anonymous location; (3) access to individual advocacy and support groups/or the criminal justice system (Harding & Helweg-Larsen, 2009); and (4) a carefully calculated plan for escape that includes keeping a bag with a copy of important documents and other resources (e.g., keys, phone, contact information) for emergencies. Although leaving an abusive relationship has been shown to be protective in the long term (Campbell, 2007), it is important to avoid pushing women into actions they are not ready to take. Cultural factors that influence responses to IPV are also important to consider in the development of interventions addressing the safety of victims (Belknap & VandeVusse, 2010; Ward & Wood, 2009).

Batterer's interventions. The male partner may attend a program for batterers as an alternative to ending the relationship. These programs appear to be effective for some individuals. These programs are most effective if they are part of a coordinated community response, involve appropriate risk assessment and management practices, are of adequate structure (e.g., duration), are court-mandated and closely monitored, and involve training and close supervision of the staff implementing the program (Salcido Carter, 2009).

Intimate partner sexual abuse. Abused women are often forced into sexual encounters. This sexual abuse is usually but not always accompanied by physical abuse. Women who are sexually abused are at risk for STDs (Coker et al., 2009). Sexual abuse increases the risk for mental health problems for all women who are involved in physically abusive relationships. Women who experience child abuse are at even greater risk for depression than those not exposed to abuse as a child (Fogarty et al., 2009).

The belief that men have a right to force their wives to have sex comes from traditional English law that said a woman gave irrevocable and perpetual consent to her husband on marriage to have sex whenever and however he wanted. Marital rape was not considered a crime in the United States until 1993 (Yllo, 1999). Marital rape leads to serious physical and emotional damage. Women who suffer from IPV may not consider forced sex a form of abuse. It is essential when women come to the emergency department with injuries that they are assessed for the presence of both physical and sexual abuse (Bazargan-Hejazi et al., 2014).

To assess for sexual assault, the following question should be used in all nursing assessments to determine whether marital rape, date rape, or rape of a male has occurred: "Have you ever been forced into sex you did not wish to participate in?"

Abuse During Pregnancy. Abuse during pregnancy has serious implications for the health of women and their children. As a conservative estimate, 3to 8 percent of pregnant women in the United States are physically abused during pregnancy, with a larger proportion of women abused during the year before pregnancy. Even more (up to 20 percent) adolescents are abused during pregnancy than adult women (Lewis et al., 2017). IPV during pregnancy is associated with depression and PTSD both during pregnancy and in the postpartum period (Alhusen et al., 2015). The effects of IPV extend to the consequent health of the infant. There is a significant association between IPV during pregnancy and increased risk of spontaneous abortion, preterm birth, low birth weight, and small-for-gestational-age infants (Alhusen et al., 2013). Experiencing IPV in the perinatal period is associated with delayed entry into prenatal care, and inadequate prenatal care. Poor nutrition and inadequate gestational weight gain have also been associated with abuse during pregnancy (Alhusen et al., 2015). Further, women experiencing abuse during pregnancy are more likely to smoke tobacco, drink alcohol, and use illicit substances during pregnancy as compared to their non abused counterparts (Alhusen et al., 2015). A man's control of contraception, a form of abusive controlling, may lead to unintended pregnancy and subsequent abuse. In addition, a man's refusal to use a condom places a woman at increased risk of sexually transmitted infections, including infection with HIV (Stockman et al., 2010).

All pregnant women should be screened for abuse at each prenatal care visit, and postpartum home visits should include assessment for child abuse and partner abuse. The U.S. Preventive Services Task Force updated its recommendations on screening women for IPV and concluded that screening instruments accurately identify women experiencing IPV and screening could reduce IPV and improve outcomes depending on the population screened and outcome measured (Nelson et al., 2012). Prenatal care presents a unique window of opportunity in which nurses can foster trusting relationships with pregnant women, thereby increasing the likelihood of IPV detection and mitigating its related negative consequences to both mother and child.

CHECK YOUR PRACTICE

A 23-year-old woman presents for her first prenatal care appointment. She is at 22 weeks' gestation, and her chart indicates she has missed three previously scheduled appointments. She is visibly upset during the appointment, provides short responses to your questions, and hesitates when you provide her a gown to change into. She tells you, "I am accident prone so I have a lot of bruises on my arms and abdomen." You sense that she is in an unsafe relationship.

What should you do?

Elder Abuse. The World Health Organization defines elder abuse broadly, as "a single or repeated act or lack of appropriate action, occurring within any relationship where there is an expectation of trust which causes harm or distress to an older person" (World Health Organization, 2002, p. 29). Research findings regarding the prevalence of elder abuse vary widely, depending on the population that is studied (e.g., community-dwelling elders versus those who are institutionalized), the study methods (e.g., review of service provider and protective service records versus population-based surveys of elders themselves), and the specific definition of elder abuse that was used in the research (Acierno et al., 2010; Mysyuk et al., 2013). Even the definition of who may be considered an "elder" is not consistent across research studies (Acierno et al., 2010) or across cultures (Mysyuk et al., 2013). Large, longitudinal national studies that describe the prevalence of elder abuse, its risk and protective factors, and its consequences to health over time are needed (Dong & Simon, 2011).

Regardless, it is clear that elder abuse is common. In a random-digit dial survey of 5777 community-dwelling U.S. elders at least 60 years of age, 1 in 10 reported past-year emotional, physical, or sexual mistreatment or potential neglect (i.e., an identified need for assistance that no one was addressing) (Acierno et al., 2010). Elder abuse has significant implications for public health, as it is associated with significant consequences to mental and physical health; increasing risk of physical injury; gastrointestinal, gynecological, and musculoskeletal issues; delusions, dementia, anxiety, and depression; and mortality (Daly, 2011). Elder abuse is underreported across virtually all cultures and constitutes a violation of elders' basic human rights (World Health Organization, 2002).

Types of elder abuse. Specific types of elder abuse include the following (Daly, 2011):

- *Physical abuse:* The use of physical force, potentially resulting in injury, pain, or impairment
- *Sexual abuse:* Nonconsensual sexual contact of any kind
- *Emotional abuse:* Verbal or nonverbal acts that inflict psychological anguish, pain, or distress
- *Financial or material abuse:* Illegal or improper use of the elder's money, property, or assets
- *Neglect:* Refusing or failing to fulfill one's obligations or duties to an elder
- *Abandonment:* Desertion by a caregiver or custodian

Perpetrators of elder abuse may include family members, caregivers in home or institutional settings, and intimate partners. In addition, "resident-to-resident" verbal, sexual, and/or physical aggression within long-term care settings has been described (Daly, 2011). Although resident-to-resident aggression may not clearly fall under the World Health Organization definition of elder abuse (which implies a trusting or caregiver relationship), this type of violence also has obvious potential for harm to vulnerable elders.

Prevention of elder abuse. Effectively addressing elder abuse requires the involvement of multiple sectors and disciplines. Increasing awareness and recognition of elder abuse among professionals and the public, and training of service providers, are key areas for intervention (Daly, 2011; World Health Organization, 2002), as is improving education for health professionals on management and reporting guidelines for elder abuse (Dong & Simon, 2011).

Screening for elder abuse. The U.S. Preventive Services Task Force (USPSTF) has recommended that clinicians routinely screen all women of childbearing age for IPV. In the same report, the USPSTF concluded that there is insufficient evidence to support universal screening of elders for abuse. However, the Task Force also noted that elder abuse is both common and underreported, suggesting potential benefits for universal screening, and that the existing evidence regarding the lack of harm resulting from IPV screening suggests that screening for elder abuse may also represent a small risk of harm (U.S. Preventive Services Task Force, 2013). More research is needed in this area. In the absence of support for universal screening, evidence-based guidelines for nurses published in 2010 indicate that certain groups of elders are particularly likely to benefit from assessment for abuse or risk for abuse (Daly, 2011). A systematic review of studies of community-dwelling elders by Johannesen and LoGiudice (2013) suggested that living with others (versus living alone) was correlated with overall abuse but not financial abuse; this may be another factor that warrants added attention to risk assessment.

For nurses, in-depth evidence-based guidelines for the prevention of elder abuse and numerous risk assessment tools for elder abuse are available from the University of Iowa College of Nursing's Hartford/Csomay Center for Gerontological Excellence. See https://nursing.uiowa.edu/csomay. If a nurse is working with an elder and abuse or risk of abuse is identified, the nurse should create an individualized plan of care and service, using such evidence-based practice guidelines. To be effective, these plans should focus on both the elder and his or her caregiver (Daly, 2011).

Nurses also can play a key role in facilitating primary and secondary prevention interventions. More research is needed regarding the effectiveness of such interventions, including evaluation of outcomes related to mandatory reporting laws. However, evidence to date suggests that there are a number of promising interventions, including educational programs (for elders, the general public, care providers including nursing assistants, or for mandatory reporters), home visitation, caregiver skill-building, counseling or social support interventions, respite care, and batterer intervention (for intimate partners who are violent) (Daly, 2011; U.S. Preventive Services Task Force, 2013). Nurses can also play a role in advocating for vulnerable elders with policy makers, working to ensure adequate funding of state and federal legislation that addresses elder abuse; in the United States these include the Older Americans Act, the Violence Against Women Act, and the Elder Justice Act (Dong & Simon, 2011).

NURSING INTERVENTIONS

Primary Prevention

Public health strategies for the prevention of violence, such as education, behavior change, policy implementation, and environmental support, are guided by the social-ecological model that outlines how strategies should be implemented across individual, relationship, community, and societal levels. Public health nurses can help the community in the following areas.

First, the community can take a stand against violence and make sure their elected officials and the local media consider nonviolence a priority. Public education programs can educate communities about various forms of violence and ways to get help and intervene to best support those impacted. Nurses, as community advocates, should be integral in this process. Nurses are well-positioned to advocate for legislative reform aimed at reducing violence. According to the U.S. Bureau of Justice Statistics the number of intimate partner homicides of women decreased by 26 percent between 1993 and 2008. Many experts in violence-related research attribute this decline, in large part, to the Violence Against Women Act (VAWA), first authorized by Congress in 1994, which provides funding for programs targeting interventions to reduce violence (Modi et al., 2014). Nurses are often the first people to identify survivors of violence and refer them to organizations for needed resources. Thus it is critical that nurses understand current legislation and advocate for policies that improve the health and well-being of those impacted by violence.

Communities have long been recognized as critical partners in violence prevention. High levels of collective efficacy within neighborhoods can reduce the risk of violence presumably through informal policing of community members. Nurses can work with advocacy groups to make sure law enforcement personnel deal with assault within marriage as swiftly, surely, and severely as assault between strangers (Stover et al., 2010). School nurses play a vital role in violence prevention in the school setting. School nurses work to create safe environments by collaborating with school personnel, parents, and community members. They are ideally positioned to implement educational programs about violence prevention because they are non disciplinary members of the academic team and can often establish unique rapport with students that facilitates disclosure of violence (King, 2014; National Association of School Nurses, 2018).

QSEN FOCUS ON QUALITY AND SAFETY EDUCATION FOR NURSES

Quality and Safety Focus

Targeted Competency: Teamwork and Collaboration

Function effectively within nursing and interprofessional teams, fostering open communication, mutual respect, and shared decision making to achieve quality client care.

Important aspects of teamwork and collaboration include:

- **Knowledge:** Recognize contributions of other individuals and groups in helping client/family achieve health goals.
- **Skills:** Assume role of team member or leader, based on the situation.
- **Attitudes:** Respect the unique attributes that members bring to a team, including variations in professional orientations and accountabilities.

Teamwork and Collaboration Question

If you learned, after careful assessment of your community, that family violence is a significant community health problem, what plan of action could you take to intervene? Remember that the goal is to promote health. Are there other individuals in the community whose collaboration you could enlist? Might there be insights and assistance that could be offered by leaders in church organizations, educators in schools, primary care providers, or social workers? Outline a plan of action with objectives, timetables, implementation strategies, and evaluation plans for intervening in family violence in your community. Include the unique contributions of other team members.

Prepared by Gail Armstrong, PhD, DNP, ACNS-BC, CNE, Associate Professor, University of Colorado Denver College of Nursing.

Second, people can take measures to reduce their vulnerability to violence by improving the physical security of their homes and learning personal defense measures. Nurses can encourage people to keep windows and doors locked, trim shrubs around their homes, and keep lights on during high-crime periods. Many neighborhoods organize crime watch programs and post signs to that effect. One sign, often posted in a window, shows a hand and indicates that people in this home will assist children who need help. Also, many neighbors informally agree to monitor one another's property and safety, and many law enforcement agencies evaluate homes for security and teach individual or neighborhood safety programs.

Unfortunately, handguns are far more likely to kill family members than intruders (Azrael et al., 2018). Firearm accidents are a leading cause of death for young children, and handguns kept in the home are easy to use when people are either depressed or very angry. A handgun is used in the majority of homicides between family members and in most suicides. Nursing assessments should include a question about guns kept in the home. The family should be made aware of the risk that a handgun holds for family members. If the family thinks that keeping a gun is necessary, safety measures should be taught, such as keeping the gun unloaded and in a locked compartment, keeping the ammunition separate from the gun and also locked away, and teaching children about the dangers of firearms. Lobbying for handgun control laws is a primary prevention effort that can significantly decrease the rate of death and serious injury caused by handguns in the United States.

Assessment for Risk Factors. Identification of risk factors is an important component of primary prevention. Although abuse cannot be predicted with certainty, several factors influence the onset and support the continuation of abusive patterns. Nurses can identify potential victims of abuse because they care for clients in a variety of settings. Factors to include in an assessment for individual or family violence, or the potential for family violence, are identified in Fig. 38.2. Both individual and familial factors must be assessed within the context of the larger community (Straus et al., 2009). Factors that must be included are found in Box 38.2.

Individual and Family Strategies for Primary Prevention. Primary prevention of violence can take place through community, family, and individual interventions (Box 38.3). Nurses, in their work with schools, community groups, employee groups, daycare centers, and other community institutions, can foster healthy developmental patterns and identify signs of potential abuse. For example, nurses may take part in media campaigns that identify risk factors for abuse. Nurses can lead in developing after-school programs and late-night programs that support young people to work toward positive goals and to develop a constructive support network. These primary prevention efforts should be broad-based, to include vulnerable youth populations such as sexual minorities, that is, a group whose sexual orientation and practices are different from the majority in a given society (Walters et al., 2013). Nurses can identify community needs and resources by capacity mapping. The identification of strengths and weaknesses can assist in determining future goals and needed interventions for the good of the community.

Primary prevention of abuse includes strengthening individuals and families so they can cope more effectively with multiple life stressors and demands, and mitigating the risk factors in the community that increase the risk of violence. Providing support and psychological enrichment to at-risk individuals and families often prevents the onset of health disruption. For example, nurses can strengthen and teach parenting abilities. A class, clinic, or home visiting services can include basic skills such as diapering, feeding, quieting, and even holding and rocking. Parents also need to learn acceptable and effective ways to discipline children so that limits are maintained without causing the child emotional or physical harm. Home visiting interventions are the most widely used parenting intervention in the United States, and their adoption is growing globally. The Nurse-Family Partnership (NFP) provides intensive prenatal and postnatal home visitation, ideally to the child's second birthday. The intervention is delivered by registered nurses to low-income first-time mothers. Research on the NFP demonstrated that there was a reduced rate of verified cases of child maltreatment among program participants during the first two years of their children's lives. Additional research has demonstrated that these effects were sustained for when the children were 15 years of age, with families in the intervention (i.e., NFP) group having significantly fewer verified child maltreatment reports over that 15-year period (Eckenrode et al., 2017).

Mutual support groups are valuable for new parents, families of children with special needs, or abused people themselves. Such groups have variable formats and can provide information, support, and encouragement to facilitate positive outcomes. Nurses can help establish such groups, refer clients, or serve as group leaders. Chapter 19 describes the role of the nurse in working with community groups.

LEVELS OF PREVENTION

Violence

Primary Prevention
Strengthen individual and family by teaching parenting skills.

Secondary Prevention
Reduce or end abuse by early screening; teach families how to deal with stress and how to have fun and enjoy recreation.

Tertiary Prevention
When signs of abuse are evident, refer client to appropriate community organizations.

Secondary Prevention

When abuse occurs, nurses can initiate measures to reduce or end further abuse. Both developmental and situational crises present opportunities for abusive situations to develop. On a community level, nurses must form collaborative relationships to provide health services for battered women (McFarlane et al., 2005). There is a critical lack of appropriate services and resources available for many violence survivors, such as LGBT persons (Walters et al., 2013); nurses are key change agents in reaching vulnerable subpopulations. Researchers must work effectively with community agencies to use current research to screen for domestic violence and to use model treatments that have a positive effect on decreasing domestic violence (Humphreys & Campbell, 2010).

Nurses can be primary leaders in the development of screening practices in the health care arena (Alhusen et al., 2013). The development of training programs for health care providers can be an effective step in identifying and treating victims of

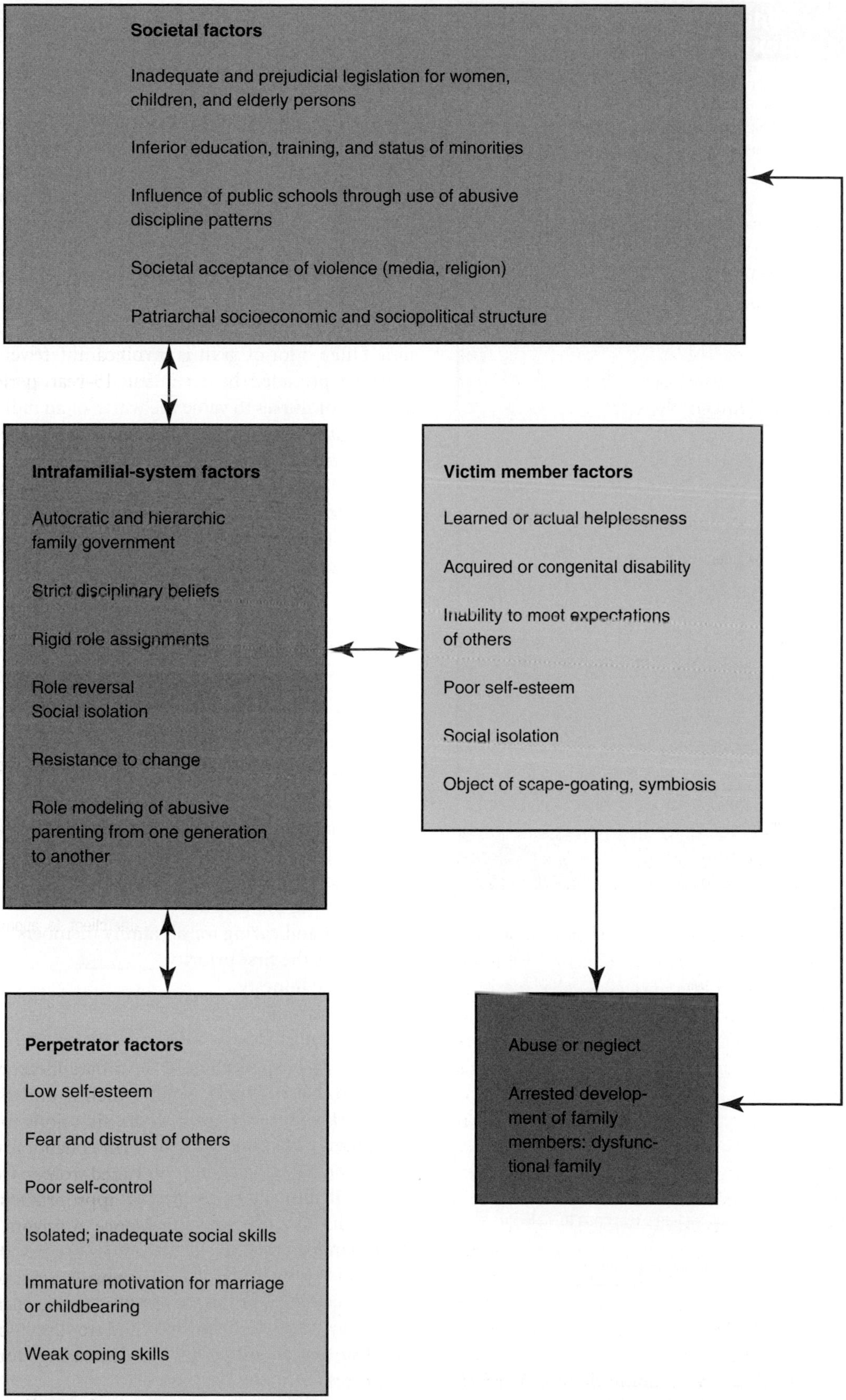

Fig. 38.2 Factors to include when assessing an individual's or a family's potential for violence.

BOX 38.2 Assessing for Violence in a Community Context

Individual Factors

- Signs of physical abuse (e.g., abrasions, contusions, burns)
- Physical symptoms related to emotional distress
- Developmental and behavioral difficulties
- Presence of physical disability
- Social isolation
- Decreased role performance within the family, and in job- or school-related activities
- Mental health problems such as depression, low self-esteem, and anxiety
- Fear of intimate others
- Substance abuse

Familial Factors

- Economic stressors
- Presence of some form of family violence
- Poor communication
- Problems with child rearing
- Lack of family cohesion
- Recurrent familial conflict
- Lack of social support networks
- Poor social integration into the community
- Multiple changes of residence
- Access to guns
- Homelessness

Community Characteristics

- High crime rate
- High levels of unemployment
- Lack of neighborhood resources and support systems
- Lack of community cohesiveness

BOX 38.3 Prevention Strategies for Violence

Individual and Family Levels

- Provide education on developmental stages and needs of children (primary).
- Teach parenting techniques (primary).
- Teach stress-reduction techniques (primary).
- Provide assessment during routine examination (secondary).
- Assess for marital discord (secondary).
- Provide counseling for at-risk parents (secondary).
- Encourage assistance with controlling anger (secondary).
- Provide treatment for substance abuse (tertiary).

Community Level

- Develop policy.
- Conduct community resource mapping.
- Collaborate with community to develop systemic response to violence.
- Develop media campaign.
- Develop resources such as transition housing and shelters.

violence. Nurses can work closely with domestic violence shelters in identifying the needs of individuals who seek sanctuary from abusive situations.

On a family level, nursing intervention can help family members discuss problems and seek ways to deal with the tension that led to the abusive situations. Injured persons must be temporarily or permanently placed in a safe location. Secondary preventive measures are most useful when potential abusers recognize their tendency to be abusive and seek help. For children, there is often a need for 24-hour child protection services or caregivers who can take care of the child until the acute family or individual crisis is resolved. Respite care is extremely important in families with frail older adult family members. Telephone crisis lines can be used to provide immediate emergency assistance to families.

Effective communication with abusive families is important. Typically, these families do not want to discuss their problems and many are embarrassed to be involved in an abusive situation. Often a lot of guilt is involved. Effective communication must be preceded by an attitude of acceptance. It is often difficult for nurses to value the worth of an individual who willfully abuses another. The behavior, not the person, must be condemned.

In addition, families do not always know how to have fun. Nurses can assess how much recreation is integrated into the family's lifestyle. Through community assessment, nurses know what resources and facilities are available and how much they cost. Families may need counseling about the value of recreation and play in reducing tension and appropriately channeling aggressive impulses.

Tertiary Prevention: Therapeutic Intervention With Abusive Families

Although it may be difficult for abusive families to form trusting relationships with health care providers, nurses can act as a case manager, coordinating the other agencies and activities involved. Principles of giving care to families who are experiencing violence include the following:

- Intolerance for violence
- Respect and caring for all family members
- Safety as the first priority
- Absolute honesty
- Empowerment

Nurses must clearly indicate that any further violence, degradation, and exploitation of family members will not be tolerated, and that all family members are respected, valued human beings. However, everyone must understand that the safety of every family member is the first priority.

Abusers often fear they will be condemned for their actions, making it difficult to maintain contact with abusive families. Although nurses convey an attitude of caring and concern for them, families may doubt the sincerity of this concern. They may avoid being home at the scheduled visit time out of fear of the consequences of the visit or an inability to believe that anyone really wants to help them. If the victim is a child, parents may fear that the nurse will try to remove the child.

Nurses are mandatory reporters of child abuse, even when only suspected, in all states. They are also mandatory reporters of elder abuse and abuse of other physically and cognitively dependent adults as well as of felony assaults on anyone in most states. The mandatory reporting laws also protect reporters from legal action on cases that are never substantiated. Even so, physicians and nurses are sometimes reluctant to report abuse. They may be more willing to report abuse in a poor family than in a middle-class one, or they may think that an older adult or child is better off at home than in a nursing home or foster home. Referral to protective service agencies should be viewed as enlisting another source of help, rather than as an automatic step toward removal of the victim or criminal justice action. This same attitude can be communicated to families, so that reporting is done with families rather than without their knowledge and prior input. Absolute honesty about what will be reported to officials, what the family can expect, what the nurse is entering into records, and what the nurse is feeling is essential.

To further empower the family, the nurse needs to recognize and capitalize on the violent family's strengths, as well as to assess and deal with its difficulties. The nurse must use a nurse-family partnership rather than a paternalistic or authoritarian approach. Families can often generate many of their own solutions, which tend to be more culturally appropriate and individualized than those the nurse generates. Victims of direct attack need information about their options and resources, and they need reassurance that abuse is unfortunately rather common and that they are not alone in their dilemma. They also need reassurance that their responses are normal and that they do not deserve to be abused. Continued support for their decisions must be coupled with nursing actions to ensure their safety.

Nursing Actions. The nurse can meet the family's therapeutic needs in a variety of ways. Besides referral to appropriate community agencies, nurses can act as role models for the family. During clinic and home visits, nurses can demonstrate constructive adult-child interactions. Nurses often teach mothers childcare skills such as proper feeding, calming a fretful child, effective discipline, and constructive communication.

Nurses can demonstrate good communication skills and discipline by teaching both parents and children in a calm, respectful, and informative manner. Caregivers, especially those caring for children, people with special needs, or older adults, may need to learn age-appropriate expectations. It is unreasonable to expect a 14-month-old infant to differentiate between right and wrong. Children at this age do not deliberately annoy caregivers by breaking delicate pieces of china. Likewise, a person with poor sphincter control does not willingly soil clothes or bedding.

Role modeling can be used with abuse victims of all ages. When providing nursing care to abused spouses or to older adults, nurses can demonstrate communication skills, conflict resolution, and skill training. For example, adult children often become abusive toward their older parents when they become frustrated in trying to care for them. During home visits, nurses can show how to physically and psychologically care for the relative. The nurse can work with caregivers to help them develop approaches that are acceptable to the individual older adult. Assessment, creativity, and critical thinking help the nurse, family, and client learn how to meet client and family needs without causing undue stress and frustration.

BOX 38.4 Common Community Services

- Child protective services
- Child abuse prevention programs
- Adult protective services
- Parents Anonymous
- Domestic violence shelters
- Programs for children of battered women
- Community support groups
- 24-hour hotline
- Legal advocacy or information
- State/county coalition against domestic violence
- Batterer treatment
- Victim assistance programs
- Sexual assault programs
- Transition housing

Working with abusers and victims of abuse can be emotionally intensive and physically draining. Abusers present difficult clinical challenges because they are often reluctant to seek help or to remain actively involved in the helping process.

Referral is an important part of tertiary prevention. Nurses should know about available community resources for abuse victims and perpetrators. Some of these resources are listed in Box 38.4. If community attitudes and resources are inadequate, it is often helpful to work with local radio and television stations and newspapers to provide information about the nature and extent of human abuse as a community health problem. This also helps acquaint people with available services and resources. Frequently, people do not seek services early in an abusive situation because they simply do not know what is available to them. Ideally, a program or plan for abused people begins with a needs assessment to identify potential clients and to determine how to effectively serve this group. Nurses can help get programs started and provide public education.

Nursing Interventions Specific to Female Partner Abuse. Women experiencing IPV are often unlikely to voluntarily disclose their experiences unprompted. Even when women do recognize their experiences as abusive, only a small proportion seek specialized IPV services. Often, the presentation of IPV may not be obvious; rather, women may present with other complaints that could be indicators of abuse such as chronic gastrointestinal symptoms, headaches, chronic pelvic pain, sexually transmitted infections, or mental health conditions, including anxiety, depression, sleep disorders or substance use. It is therefore critical that health care providers are screening all women for IPV (Valpied & Hegarty, 2015). Despite the overall prevalence of IPV and its resultant physical and emotional health problems for women, health professionals, even those working in emergency departments, often fail to identify abused women. Some health care professionals are perceived as paternalistic, judgmental, insensitive, and less effective and helpful than they could be (Alhusen et al., 2010).

Because of the stigma and unease involved, women and health care providers may hesitate to initiate discussion about abuse. However, the majority of battered women claim they would have liked to talk about the issue with a health care professional if they were asked (Alhusen et al., 2013). Because abuse typically develops slowly, starting with minor psychological abuse and building to more severe physical incidents, victims and health care providers alike may not recognize the abuse until a severe episode occurs.

The quality of health care that a battered woman receives often determines whether she follows through with referrals to legal, social service, and health care agencies. The emergency department is the point of entry for many women in abusive relationships. Care in the emergency department is often fragmented and necessarily oriented toward addressing the most acute illness or injury. Therefore women may not be adequately assessed and often receive little or no support or referral to services to assist in dealing with the abuse. The initial response to disclosure of IPV should be one that validates her experience and provides support for her safety. It is imperative that women feel that they are believed and are not to be blamed. Nurses and other health care providers should also discuss that IPV is not an acceptable behavior and review its impact on the physical and mental health of the woman and any children. Finally, nurses should demonstrate their commitment to supporting the woman in whatever decision she makes. Even if a woman is not ready to leave an abusive relationship, a nurse's initial response will be critical in the likelihood of an abused woman returning for help (Valpied & Hegarty, 2015).

Managed care and clinic settings may be the best places to routinely screen for IPV. Ideally a clinical nurse specialist who is an expert in screening for IPV is available to coordinate efforts in the different health care settings. If battered women can be identified, perhaps effective interventions can be provided that will prevent the kind of serious injury that later results in emergency department visits or even a homicide.

However, some abused women hesitate to identify themselves as victims of domestic violence for several reasons. They may fear that revelation will further jeopardize their safety by increasing the violence, and they may also think that it will increase their sense of shame and humiliation. In addition, the nature of the systems in which victims of violence introduce themselves can be barriers. Emergency departments, clinics, managed care settings, and health departments are busy places. Staff members work hard to maintain the functioning of these facilities. Sometimes it is difficult in such chaotic settings for staff members to realize their importance as the first or only health provider to recognize violence in their clients' lives, and that women need them to take the time to deal with this issue (Straus et al., 2009).

Assessment. Assessment for all forms of violence against women should therefore take place for all women entering the health care system. The assessment should be ongoing and confidential. A thorough assessment gathers information on physical, emotional, and sexual trauma from violence, risk for future abuse, cultural background and beliefs, perceptions of the woman's relationships with others, and stated needs. Conduct the assessment in private and direct other adults who are present to the waiting area and tell them that it is policy that initially women are seen alone. Women should be asked directly if they were in an abusive relationship as a child or are currently in an abusive relationship as an adult. They should also be asked whether they have ever been forced into sex. Shame and fear often make disclosure difficult. Verbal acknowledgment of the situation and emotional and physical support assist women in talking about past or current circumstances (Valpied & Hegarty, 2015).

Women can be categorized into three groups: no, low, or moderate to high risk. Women with no signs of current or past abuse are considered at no risk. However, every future visit should include questioning a woman about whether there have been any changes in her life or whether she has additional information or questions about topics discussed at previous visits. If there is a new intimate partner in her life, she should again be screened for abuse. The Abuse Assessment Screen (AAS) is a four-question screen that has been successfully used in almost every kind of health care setting and can be downloaded from the Nursing Network on Violence Against Women International (NNVAWI) website (http://www.nnvawi.org).

Women at low risk show no evidence of recent or current abuse. Education that helps a woman gain perspective on her situation and her needs should be discussed. Resource materials including group and individual formats can be suggested. The risk level should be recorded and preventive measures and teaching should be documented.

Assessment of moderate to high risk includes evaluation of a woman's fear of both psychological and physical abuse. Lethality potential should be assessed and can be done with the Danger Assessment (DA), an instrument designed to assess the likelihood of lethality or near lethality occurring in a case of IPV (Campbell et al., 2009). The DA was developed based on data from a sample of women whose partners or ex-partners tried to kill them. The first portion of the DA assesses severity and frequency of abuse by presenting the woman with a calendar over the past year. The second part is a "yes/no" dichotomous response format of risk factors associated with intimate partner homicide such as:

- Has the physical violence increased in severity or frequency over the past year?
- Does he own a gun?
- Is he unemployed?
- Does he threaten to kill you?
- Does he ever try to choke you?
- Does he threaten to harm your children?
- Do you believe he is capable of killing you?

Based on the score, a woman's risk for intimate partner homicide is classified as low (8 or less); moderate (9-13); high (14-17), or extremely high (18 or higher). Based on the woman's score, health care providers can tailor counseling and provision of support services. The Danger Assessment is available at https://www.dangerassessment.org/ and is also available at the NNVAWI website (https://www.nnvawi.org/). In all cases, a history of abuse and alcohol and drug use should be collected and carefully documented. The determined risk level should also be documented along with any past or present physical evidence of abuse from prior or current assault; this evidence should be photographed, shown on a body map, or described narratively. It is important that the assailant be identified in the record; this can take the form of either quotes from the woman or subjective information. These records can be very important for women in future assault or child custody cases, even if the woman is not ready to make a police report at the present time.

Many women are not ready to leave an abusive relationship at the time of screening for violence. It is important that health care providers are comfortable discussing strategies to promote a woman's safety while remaining in the abusive relationship. The discussion should also include her plan for leaving if that is what she ultimately decides; leaving an abusive relationship without a safety plan can increase a woman's danger. Strategies to consider may include keeping copies of vital records (e.g., birth certificates, Social Security cards, passports, medical information) and money hidden or with a trusted individual, discussing ways to protect any children involved, and understanding the steps for obtaining a restraining order (Paterno & Draughon, 2016). Women should also be provided with local resources such as advocacy groups, domestic violence specialists, or a local shelter. If the woman resides in an area with limited resources, such as a rural area, resources such as the National Domestic Violence Hotline (1-800-799-SAFE) and the National Sexual Assault Hotline (1-800-656-HOPE) should be made available. Determining the timing of the last abusive episode and whether sexual assault occurred is important as the jurisdictions have evidence collection time limits, often between 72 and 120 hours (Paterno & Draughon, 2016). Lists of resources such as rape crisis clinics and support groups for survivors of physical and emotional abuse should be made available.

Prevention. Prevention, public policy, and social attitudes are intertwined. Our society has taken a major step toward the secondary prevention of abuse through the establishment of programs that encourage women and children to speak about their experiences. Nurses need to support these programs further by supporting individuals and families confronted with violence. In the development of laws that punish perpetrators of child and women abuse, society has given some support to the victims of abuse. Often, however, the victims are again victimized by disbelief of their experiences, a devaluing of the effects of these assaults, and a focus on assisting the perpetrators of the crimes. Primary prevention includes a social attitudinal change. Both girls and boys need to be taught human values of interdependence, respect for human life, and a commitment to empathy and strength in the development of the human species regardless of sex, race, or socioeconomic status. We must urge continued progress toward eliminating the feminization of poverty and ensuring gender parity in economic resources. In addition, local communities must make it clear that violence against women is not tolerated. Examples of what communities can do include eliminating pornography, mandating arrests of abusers, and creating a general climate of non violence.

Abused women need assistance in making decisions and taking control of their lives. Public health nurses, prenatal nurses, Planned Parenthood, primary care, and emergency department nurses are involved with women when they can be screened for the presence or absence of abuse. There are mechanisms for routinely asking women who are either abused or at risk for abuse (Sharps et al., 2016). To intervene effectively, nurses must understand abuse as a cumulative process that must be examined as a continuum within the context of a relationship. During this process, the abuse, the relationship, and a woman's view of changes within herself require time-specific interventions. Women are often blamed and held responsible for the abuse inflicted on them by their male partners (Kennedy & Prock, 2018). When this happens, either they are assisted in a way that discounts their feelings and further devalues them, or the abuse is ignored.

Strategies for addressing education for health professionals. Various strategies have been reported that address the knowledge deficit of health practitioners on abuse issues. The National March of Dimes Birth Defects Foundation has sponsored a variety of training sessions for health professionals and produced an excellent training manual that addresses violence against women and battering during pregnancy (McFarlane & Parker, 2005). The program covers the assessment and planning of interventions to assist pregnant women in abusive relationships.

More and more nursing programs are implementing courses on how to intervene with IPV. Wallace (2009) developed and implemented a two-credit elective course focusing on attitudes, knowledge, and interventions in a structured learning environment to help nursing students acquire the expertise needed to work with women in abusive relationships. Organizations such as Futures Without Violence (https://www.futureswithoutviolence.org/) have numerous resources to support nurses in screening, and intervening in IPV. These include safety cards and other printed display material for health care settings as well as resource cards for nurses on how to assess safety, make referrals, and document findings. Additionally, there are many webinars and archived recordings on all aspects of violence that can be very helpful to health care providers caring for women, children, and families dealing with violence.

Nurses are also joining in community-based efforts to prevent and intervene with IPV and child abuse. Nurses work in public health collaborating with shelters for women, community mental health centers, criminal justice and advocacy institutions, and community-based health care. Bloom et al. (2009) developed a program to assist Latinas experiencing IPV. The program was developed specifically for the cultural and linguistic needs of the population. Emphasis was placed on assisting the Hispanic community in developing the knowledge and background to deal with the issue. At the same time, community efforts focused on expanding the knowledge base of the community at large about IPV.

PRACTICE APPLICATION

Mrs. Smith, a 75-year-old bedridden woman, became consistently rude and combative when her daughter Mary attempted to bathe her and change her clothes each morning. During a home visit, Mary told the nurse, Mrs. Jones, that she had become so frustrated with her mother on the previous morning that she had hit her. Mary felt terrible about her behavior. She stressed that her mother's incontinence made it essential that she be kept clean; her clothes had to be changed every day for her own safety and physical well-being.

A. How should Mrs. Jones respond to this disclosure?
B. What specific nursing actions should be taken?
C. What ongoing services does the nurse need to provide?

Answers can be found on the Evolve site.

KEY POINTS

- Violence and human abuse are not new phenomena, but they have increasingly become public health concerns.
- Communities throughout the United States are angry and frustrated about increasing levels of violence.
- Nurses can evaluate and intervene in incidents of community and family violence; to intervene effectively, the nurse must understand the dynamics of violence and human abuse.
- Factors influencing social and community violence include changing social conditions, economic conditions, population density, community facilities, and institutions within a community, such as organized religion, education, the mass communication media, and work.
- The potential for violence against individuals or against oneself is directly related to the level of violence in the community. Identification and correction of factors affecting the level of violence in the community constitute one way of reducing violence against family members and other individuals.
- Violence and abuse of family members can happen to any family member: spouse, older adult, child, or developmentally disabled person.
- People who abuse family members were often themselves abused and react poorly to real or perceived crises. Other factors that characterize the abuser are the way the person was raised and the unique character of that person.
- Child abuse can be physical, emotional, or sexual. Incest is a common and particularly destructive form of child abuse.
- Spouse abuse is usually wife abuse. It involves physical, emotional, and, frequently, sexual abuse within a context of coercive control. It usually increases in severity and frequency and can escalate to homicide of either partner.
- Nurses are in an excellent position to identify potential victims of family abuse because they see clients in a variety of settings, such as schools, businesses, homes, and clinics. Treatment of family abuse includes primary, secondary, and tertiary prevention and therapeutic intervention.

CLINICAL DECISION-MAKING ACTIVITIES

1. For one week, keep a log or diary related to violence.
   A. Make a note of each time you feel as though you are losing your temper. Consider what it might take to cause you to react in a violent way.
   B. Think back. When was the last time you had a violent outburst? What precipitated it? What were your thoughts? What were your feelings? How might you have handled the situation or those feelings without reacting in a violent way?
   C. During this same week, make note of the episodes of violent behaviors you observe. For example, do parents hit children in the supermarket? What seems to precipitate such outbursts? What alternatives might exist for reacting in a less violent way?
2. If you learned, after a careful assessment of your community, that family violence is a significant community health problem, what plan of action might you take to intervene? Remember that the goal is to promote health. Outline a plan of action with objectives, timetables, implementation strategies, and evaluation plans for intervening in family violence in your community.
3. Complete a partial community assessment to determine the actual incidence and types of violence in your community.
4. What resources are available in your community for victims of violence? Interview a person who works in an agency that seeks to aid victims of violence. What is the role of the agency? Do its services seem adequate? Who is eligible? Is there a waiting list? What is the fee scale?
5. Cut out all stories about violence that you find in your local newspaper every day for 2 weeks. Note the patterns. Is the majority of the violence perpetrated by strangers or family members? How are the victims portrayed? What kinds of families are involved? What kinds of stories and families get front-page treatment rather than a few lines in the back of the paper?

ADDITIONAL RESOURCES

EVOLVE WEBSITE

http://evolve.elsevier.com/Stanhope/community/

- Answers to Practice Application
- Case Study
- Glossary
- Review Questions

REFERENCES

Acierno R, Hernandez MA, Amstadter AB, et al: Prevalence and correlates of emotional, physical, sexual, and financial abuse and potential neglect in the National Elder Mistreatment Study, *Am J Public Health* 100:292–297, 2010.

Alhusen JL, Baty M, Glass N: Perceptions of and experiences with system responses to female same-sex intimate partner violence, *Partner Abuse* 1:443–462, 2010.

Alhusen JL, Lucea M, Bullock L, et al: Intimate partner violence and adverse neonatal outcomes among urban women, *J Pediatr* 163:471–476, 2013.

Alhusen JL, Ray E, Sharps P, et al: Intimate partner violence during pregnancy: maternal and neonatal outcomes, *J Womens Health (Larchmt)* 24:100–106, 2015.

American Public Health Association: *10 Essential Public Health Services*, 2017. Retrieved from https://www.cdc.gov.

Azrael D, Cohen J, Salhi C, et al: Firearm storage in gun-owning households with children: results of a 2015 national survey, *J Urban Health* 95:295–304, 2018.

Bazargan-Hejazi S, Kim E, Lin J, et al: Risk factors associated with different types of intimate partner violence (IPV): An emergency department study, *J Emerg Med* 47:710–720, 2014.

Becker HJ, Bechtel K: Recognizing victims of human trafficking in the pediatric emergency department, *Pediatric Emergency Care* 2:144–147, 2015.

Belknap RA, VandeVusse L: Listening sessions with Latinas: documenting life contexts and creating connections, *Public Health Nurs* 27:337–346, 2010.

Beyer K, Wallis AB, Hamberger LK: Neighborhood environment and intimate partner violence: a systematic review, *Trauma Violence Abuse* 16:16–47, 2015.

Black MC, Basile KC, Breiding MJ, et al: *The National Intimate Partner and Sexual Violence Survey (NISVS): 2010 Summary Report*, Atlanta, GA, 2011, National Center for Injury Prevention and Control, Centers for Disease Control and Prevention.

Bloom T, Wagman J, Hernandez R, et al: Partnering with community-based organizations to reduce intimate partner violence, *Hisp J Behav Sci* 31:244–257, 2009.

Breiding MJ, Smith SG, Basile KC, et al: Prevalence and characteristics of sexual violence, stalking, and intimate partner violence victimization- national intimate partner and sexual violence survey, United States, 2011, *MMWR Surveill Summ* 63:1–18, 2014.

Brockie TB, Dana-Socco M, Wallen GR, et al: The relationship of Adverse Childhood Experiences to PTSD, depression, poly-drug use and suicide attempt in reservation-based Native American adolescents and young adults, *Am J Community Psychol* 55: 411–421, 2015.

Brown TNT, Herman JL: *Intimate partner violence and sexual abuse among LGBT people: A review of existing research*, Los Angeles, CA, 2015, Williams Institute.

Campbell JC: Health consequences of intimate partner violence, *Lancet* 359:1331–1336, 2002.

Campbell JC: *Assessing Dangerousness: Violence by Batterers and Child Abusers*, ed 2, New York, NY, 2007, Springer.

Campbell R, Patterson D, Adams AE, et al: A participatory evaluation project to measure SANE nursing practice and adult sexual assault patients' psychological well-being, *J Forensic Nurs* 4:19–28, 2008.

Campbell JC, Sharps PW, Glass NE: Risk assessment for intimate partner homicide. In Pinard GF, Pagani L, editors: *Clinical Assessment of Dangerousness: Empirical Contributions*. New York, NY, 2000, Cambridge University Press, pp 136–157.

Campbell JC, Sheridan DJ: Assessment of intimate partner violence and elder abuse. In Jarvis C, editor: *Physical Assessment for Clinical Practice*. Philadelphia, PA, 2004, Elsevier Science, pp 74–82.

Campbell R, Townsend SM, Long SM, et al: Responding to sexual assault victims' medical and emotional needs: a national study of the services provided by SANE programs, *Res Nurs Health* 29: 384–398, 2006.

Campbell JC, Webster DW, Glass NE: The Danger Assessment: validation of a lethality risk assessment instrument for intimate partner femicide, *J Interpers Violence* 24:653–674, 2009.

Campbell JC, Webster D, Koziol-McLain J, et al: Risk factors for femicide in abusive relationships: results from a multi-site case control study, *Am J Public Health* 93:1089–1097, 2003.

Campbell JC, Sabri B, Budhathoki C, et al: Unwanted sexual acts among university students: correlates of victimization and perpretration, *J Interpers Violence*. doi:10.1177/0886260517734221, 2017. [Epub ahead of print].

Casey EA, Lindhorst TP: Toward a multi-level, ecological approach to the primary prevention of sexual assault: prevention in peer and community contexts, *Trauma Violence Abuse* 10:91–114, 2009.

Catalano S: *Intimate Partner Violence: Attributes of Victimization, 1993-2011*, Washington, DC, 2013, Bureau of Justice Statistics. Retrieved from http://www.bjs.gov.

Catalano S, Smith E, Snyder H, et al: *Female Victims of Violence*, Washington, DC, 2009, Bureau of Justice Statistics Selected Findings. Retrieved from https://www.bjs.gov.

Centers for Disease Control and Prevention (CDC): *Youth Risk Behavior Surveillance System (YRBSS) United States, 2015*, 2016. Retrieved from https://www.cdc.gov.

Centers for Disease Control and Prevention (CDC): *Web-Based Injury Statistics Query and Reporting System (WISQARS)*, 2017. Retrieved from http://www.cdc.gov.

Centers for Disease Control and Prevention (CDC): *National Suicide Statistics at a Glance*, 2014a. Retrieved from http://www.cdc.gov.

Centers for Disease Control and Prevention (CDC): *Dating Matters Initiative*, 2014b. Retrieved from http://www.cdc.gov.

Coker AL, Hopenhayn C, DeSimone CP, et al: Violence against women raises risk of cervical cancer, *J Womens Health* 18: 1179–1185, 2009.

Cole J: Structural, organizational, and interpersonal factors influencing interprofessional collaboration on sexual assault response teams, *J Interpers Violence*. doi:10.1177/0886260516628809, 2016. [Epub ahead of print].

Costa BM, Kaestle CE, Walker A, et al: Longitudinal predictors of domestic violence perpetration and victimization: a systematic review, *Aggression and Violent Behavior* 24:261–272, 2015.

Council on Community Pediatrics: Poverty and child health in the United States, *Pediatrics* 137(4):e20160339, 2016.

Crane P: A Human trafficking toolkit for nursing intervention. In: De Chesnay M: Sex Trafficking: A clinical guide for nurses. New York, NY, 2013, Springer.
Curtin SC, Warner M, Hedegaard H: Increases in suicide in the United States, 1999-2014, *NCHS Data Brief 241*, 2016.
Daly JM: Elder abuse prevention: evidence-based practice guidelines, *J Gerontol Nurs* 37:11–17, 2011.
De Chesnay M: Sex trafficking: A clinical guide for nurses. New York, NY, 2013, Springer.
Dixon L, Browne K, Hamilton-Giachritsis C: Patterns of risk and protective factors in the intergenerational cycle of maltreatment, *J Fam Viol* 24:111–122, 2009.
Dixon L, Hamilton-Giachritsis C, Browne K: Risk factors of parents abused as children: a mediational analysis of the intergenerational continuity of child maltreatment, *J Child Psychol Psychiatry* 46: 59–68, 2005.
Dong X, Simon MA: Enhancing national policy and programs to address elder abuse, *JAMA* 305:2460–2461, 2011.
Drossman AD: Abuse, trauma, and GI illness: is there a link? *Am J Gastroenterol* 106:14–25, 2011.
Eaton DK, Kann L, Kinchen S, et al: Youth risk behavior surveillance—United States, 2009, *MMWR Surveill Summ* 59:1–42, 2010.
Eckenrode J, Campa MI, Morris PA, et al: The prevention of child maltreatment through the Nurse Family Partnership Program: Mediating effects in a long-term follow-up study, *Child Maltreatment* 22:92–99, 2017.
Edwards KM, Gidycz CA, Murphy MJ: Leaving an abusive dating relationship: a prospective analysis of the Investment Model and Theory of Planned Behavior, *J Interpers Violence* 30:2908–2927, 2015.
Farrell CA, Fleegler EW, Monuteaux MC, et al: Community poverty and child abuse fatalities in the United States, *Pediatrics* 139(5):e20161616, 2017.
Ferguson CJ, Hartley RD: The pleasure is momentary . . . the expense damnable? The influence of pornography on rape and sexual assault, *Aggress Violent Behav* 14:323–329, 2009.
Fleegler EW, Lee LK, Monuteaux MC, et al: Firearm legislation and firearm-related fatalities in the United States, *JAMA Intern Med* 173:732–740, 2013.
Fletcher J: The effects of intimate partner violence on health in young adulthood in the United States, *Soc Sci Med* 70:130–135, 2010.
Fogarty CT, Fredman L, Heeren TC, et al: Synergistic effects of child abuse and intimate partner violence on depressive symptoms in women, *Prev Med* 46:463–469, 2009.
Ford JD, Elhai JD, Connor DF, et al: Poly-victimization and risk of posttraumatic, depressive, and substance use disorders and involvement in delinquency in a national sample of adolescents, *J Adolesc Health* 46:545–552, 2010.
Ford-Gilboe M, Varcoe C, Wuest J, et al: Intimate partner violence and nursing practice. In Humphreys J, Campbell JC, editors: *Intimate Partner Violence and Nursing Practice*, New York, NY, 2010, Springer, pp 115–153.
Garthe RC, Sullivan TN, McDaniel MA: A meta-analytic review of peer risk factors and adolescent dating violence, *Psychology of Violence* 7:45–57, 2017.
Giancola PR: Development and evaluation of theories of alcohol-related violence: covering a 40-year span, *Subst Use Misuse* 50:1182–1187, 2015.
Gonzalez-Guarda RM, Cummings AM, Becerra M, et al: Needs and preferences for the prevention of intimate partner violence among Hispanics: a community's perspective, *J Prim Prev* 34:221–235, 2013.
Greeson MR, Campbell R: Sexual response teams (SARTs): an empirical review of their effectiveness and challenges to successful implementation, *Trauma Violence Abuse* 14:83–95, 2013.
Harding H, Helweg-Larsen M: Perceived risk for future intimate partner violence among women in a domestic violence shelter, *J Fam Violence* 24:75–85, 2009.
Harford TC, Yi HY, Chen CM, et al: Substance use disorders and self- and other-directed violence among adults: Results from the National Survey on Drug Use and Health, *J Affect Disord* 225: 365–373, 2018.
Heise LL: Violence against women: an integrated, ecological framework, *Violence Against Women* 4:262–290, 1998.
Hibbard RA, Desch LW, American Academy of Pediatrics Committee on Child Abuse and Neglect: Maltreatment of children with disabilities, *Pediatrics* 119:1018–1025, 2007.
Hines DA, Malley-Morrison K: *Family Violence in the United States*, Thousand Oaks, CA, 2005, Sage.
Houmes BV, Fagan MM, Quintana NM: Violence: recognition, management and prevention: establishing a Sexual Assault Nurse Examiner (SANE) program in the emergency department, *J Emerg Med* 25:111–121, 2003.
Hoyert DL, Xu J: Deaths: preliminary data for 2011, *Natl Vital Stat Rep* 61:1–51, 2012.
Humphreys JC, Campbell JC: *Family violence and nursing practice*, New York, NY, 2010, Springer.
Isaac R, Solak J, Giardino A: Health care providers' training needs related to human trafficking: Maximizing the opportunity to effectively screen and intervene, *J Appl Res Child* 2:1–32, 2011.
Johannesen M, LoGiudice D: Elder abuse: a systematic review of risk factors among community-dwelling elders, *Age Ageing* 42:292–298, 2013.
Jolliffe D, Farrington DP, Loeber R, et al: Protective factors for violence: Results from the Pittsburgh Youth Study, *J Crim Justice* 45:32–40, 2016.
Kaminski JW, Valle LA, Filene JH, et al: A meta-analytic review of components associated with parent training program effectiveness, *J Abnorm Child Psychol* 36:567–589, 2008.
Karch DL, Dahlberg LL, Patel N: Surveillance for violent deaths—National Violent Death Reporting System, 16 states, 2007, *MMWR Surveill Summ* 59:1–50, 2010.
Kennedy AC, Prock KA: "I still feel like I am not normal" A review of the role of stigma and stigmatization among female survivors of child abuse, sexual assault and intimate partner violence, *Trauma Violence Abuse* 19(5):512–527, 2018. oi:10.1177/ 1524838016673601.
Kimball E: Edleson revisited: Reviewing children's witnessing of domestic violence 15 years later, *J Fam Violence* 31:625–637, 2016.
King KK: Violence in the school setting: A school nurse perspective, *Online J Issues Nurs* 19(1):Manuscript 4, 2014.
Kletter H, Weems CF, Carrion VG: Guilt and posttraumatic stress symptoms in child victims of interpersonal violence, *Clin Child Psychol Psychiatry* 14:71–83, 2009.
Kugel C, Retzlaff C, Hopfer S, et al: Familias con Voz: community survey results from an Intimate Partner Violence (IPV) Prevention Project with migrant workers, *J Fam Viol* 24:649–660, 2009.
Krug EG, Dahlberg LL, Mercy JA, et al: *World Report on Violence and Health*, Geneva, Switzerland, 2002, World Health Organization.
Lane W: Prevention of child maltreatment, *Pediatr Clin North Am* 61:873–888, 2014.
Langton L, Berzofsky M, Krebs CP et al: *Victimizations not reported to the police, 2006-2010*. U.S. Department of Justice National Crime Victimization Survey, 2012.

Levendosky A, Bogat G, Martinez-Torteya C: Symptoms in young children exposed to intimate partner violence, *Violence Against Women* 19:187–201, 2013.

Leventhal JM, Gaither JR: Incidence of serious injuries due to physical abuse in the United States: 1997 to 2009, *Pediatrics* 130:847–852, 2012.

Lewandowski L, McFarlane J, Campbell JC, et al: "He killed my mommy!" Murder or attempted murder of a child's mother, *J Fam Violence* 19:211–220, 2004.

Lewis JB, Sullivan TP, Angley M, et al: Psychological and relational correlates of intimate partner violence profiles among pregnant adolescent couples, *Aggress Behav* 43:26–36, 2017.

Lundahl B, Risser HJ, Lovejoy MC: A meta-analysis of parent training: moderators and follow-up effects, *Clin Pyschol Rev* 26:86–104, 2006.

Mapp SC: The effects of sexual abuse as a child on the risk of mothers physically abusing their children: a path analysis using systems theory, *Child Abuse Negl* 30:1293–1310, 2006.

Masters NT: "My strength is not for hurting": men's anti-rape websites and their construction of masculinity and male sexuality, *Sexualities* 13:33–46, 2010.

McCurdy, K: The influence of support and stress on maternal attitudes, *Child Abuse Negl* 29:251–268, 2005.

McFarlane JM, Groff JY, O'Brien JA, et al: Prevalence of partner violence against 7,443 African American, white, and Hispanic women receiving care at urban public primary care clinics, *Public Health Nurs* 22:98–107, 2005.

McFarlane J, Parker B: *Abuse during pregnancy: a protocol for prevention and intervention*, White Plains, NY, 2005, March of Dimes Birth Defects Foundation.

McMahon SD, Todd NR, Martinez A, et al: Aggressive and prosocial behavior: community violence, cognitive, and behavioral predictors among urban African American youth, *J Community Psychol* 51:407–421, 2013.

Modi MN, Palmer S, Armstrong A: The role of violence against women act in addressing intimate partner violence: a public health issue, *J Women's Health* 23:253–259, 2014.

Moynihan MM, Banyard VL, Arnold JS, et al: Sisterhood may be powerful for reducing sexual and intimate partner violence: an evaluation of the Bringing in the Bystander in-person program with sorority members, *Violence Against Women* 17:703–719, 2011.

Mysyuk Y, Westendorp RG, Lindenberg J: Added value of elder abuse definitions: a review, *Ageing Res Rev* 12:50–57, 2013.

National Association of School Nurses: *School violence: the role of the school nurse (position statement)*, Silver Spring, MD, 2018, Author.

National Coalition of Anti-Violence Programs: *A crisis of hate: A mid year report on Lesbian, Gay, Bisexual, Transgender and Queer Hate Violence Homicides*. 2017. Retrieved from http://avp.org.

Nelson HD, Bougatsos C, Blazina I: Screening women for intimate partner violence: a systematic review to update the U.S. Preventive Services Task Force recommendation, *Ann Intern Med* 156: 796–808, 2012.

O'Campo P, Kirst M, Tsamis C, et al: Implementing successful intimate partner violence screening programs in health care settings: evidence generated from a realist-informed systematic review, *Soc Sci Med* 72:855–866, 2011.

O'Reilly R, Wilkes L, Luck L, et al: The efficacy of family support and family preservation services on reducing child abuse and neglect: what the literature reveals, *J Child Health Care* 14:82–94, 2010.

Palladino CL, Singh V, Campbell J, et al: Homicide and suicide during the perinatal period: findings from the National Violent Death Reporting System, *Obstet Gynecol* 119:1056–1063, 2011.

Parks SE, Johnson LL, McDaniel DD, et al: Surveillance for violent deaths—National Violent Death Reporting System, 16 States, 2010, *MMWR Surveill Summ* 63:1–33, 2014.

Paterno M, Draughon J: Screening for intimate partner violence, *J Midwifery Womens Health* 61:370–375, 2016.

Peters K: The growing business of human trafficking and the power of emergency nurses to stop it, *J Emerge Nurs* 39:280–288, 2013.

Petrosky E, Blair JM, Betz CJ, et al: Racial and ethnic differences in homicides of adult women and the role of intimate partner violence- United States, 2003-2014, *MMWR Morb Mortal Weekly Report* 66:741–746, 2017.

Piquero AR, Brame R, Fagan J, et al: Assessing the offending activity of criminal domestic violence suspects: offense specialization, escalation and de-escalation evidence from the Spouse Assault Replication Program, *Public Health Rep* 121:409–418, 2006.

Planty M, Langton L, Krebs C, et al: *Female Victims of Sexual Violence, 1994-2010* [Bureau of Justice Statistics Bulletin], 2013. Retrieved from https://www.bjs.gov.

Reaves S, McMahon SD, Duffy S, et al: The test of time: A meta-analytic review of the relation between school climate and problem behavior over time, *Aggress Violent Behav* 39:100–108, 2018.

Reyes HLM, Foshee, VA, Niolon PH, et al: Gender role attitudes and male adolescent dating violence perpetration: Normative beliefs as moderators, *J Youth Adolescence* 45:350–360, 2016.

Richards T: Health implications of human trafficking, *Nurs Womens Health* 18:155-162, 2014.

Rhodes K, Cerulli C, Dichter M, et al: "I didn't want to put them through that": the influence of children on victim decision-making in intimate partner violence cases, *J Fam Violence* 25: 485–493, 2010.

Richardson EG, Hemenway D: Homicide, suicide, and unintentional firearm fatality: comparing the United States with other high-income countries, *J Trauma* 70:238–243, 2011.

Rivara FP, Anderson ML, Fishman P, et al: Intimate partner violence and health care costs and utilization for children living in the home, *Pediatrics* 120:1270–1277, 2007.

Rodriguez CM: Personal contextual characteristics and cognitions: predicting child abuse potential and disciplinary style, *J Interpers Violence* 25:315–335, 2010.

Salcido Carter L: *Batterer intervention: doing the work and measuring the progress: a report on the December 2009 expert round table*, 2009. Retrieved from https://www.futureswithoutviolence.org.

Schilling S, Christian CW: Child physical abuse and neglect, *Child Adolesc Psychiatr Clin N Am* 23:309–319, 2014.

Seto MC, Lalumière ML: What is so special about male adolescent sexual offending? A review and test of explanations through meta-analysis, *Psychol Bull* 136:526–575, 2010.

Sharps P, Bullock LF, Campbell JC, et al: Domestic Violence Enhanced Perinatal Home Visits: The DOVE randomized clinical trial, *J Womens Health* 25:1129–1138, 2016.

Sheridan D: Legal and forensic nursing responses to family violence. In Humphreys J, Campbell JC, editors: *Family Violence and Nursing Practice*, Philadelphia, PA, 2004, Lippincott, Williams & Wilkins, pp 385–406.

Sheridan DJ, Nash KR: Acute injury patterns of intimate partner violence victims, *Trauma Violence Abuse* 8:281–289, 2009.

Siegel M, Ross CS, King C: The relationship between gun ownership and firearm homicide rates in the United States, 1981-2010, *Am J Public Health* 103:2098–2105, 2013.

Siegel M, Negussie Y, Vanture S, et al: The relationship between gun ownership and stranger and nonstranger firearm homicide rates in the United States, 1981-2010, *Am J Public Health* 104: 1912–1919, 2014.

Silverman JG, Raj A, Mucci LA, et al: Dating violence against adolescent girls and associated substance use, unhealthy weight control, sexual risk behavior, and suicidality, *JAMA* 286:572–579, 2001.

Siskin A, Sun WL: *Trafficking in persons: U.S. policy and issues for Congress*. Washington, DC: Congressional Research Service, 2013.

Smith SG, Fowler KA, Niolon PH: Intimate partner homicide and corollary victims in 16 states: National Violent Death Reporting System, 2003-2009, *Am J Public Health* 104:461–466, 2014.

Sonis J, Langer M: Risk and protective factors for recurrent intimate partner violence in a cohort of low-income inner-city women, *J Fam Violence* 23:529–538, 2008.

Steeves RH, Parker B: Adult perspectives on growing up following uxoricide, *J Interpers Violence* 22:1270–1284, 2007.

Stevenson M: Perceptions of juvenile offenders who were abused as children, *J Aggress Maltreat Trauma* 18:331–349, 2009.

Stockman J, Campbell J, Celentano D: Sexual violence and HIV risk behaviors among a nationally representative sample of heterosexual American women: the importance of sexual coercion, *J Acquir Immune Defic Syndr* 53:136–143, 2010.

Stover CM, Berkman M, Desai R, et al: The efficacy of a police-advocacy intervention for victims of domestic violence: 12 month follow-up data, *Violence Against Women* 16:410–425, 2010.

Straus H, Cerulli C, McNutt LA, et al: Intimate partner violence and functional health status: associations with severity, danger, and self-advocacy behaviors, *J Womens Health* 18:625–631, 2009.

Swider SM, Krothe J, Reyes D, et al: The Quad Council practice competencies for public health nursing, *Public Health Nurs* 30:519–536, 2013.

Symes L, McFarlane J, Frazier L, et al: Exploring violence against women and adverse health outcomes in middle age to promote women's health, *Crit Care Nurs Q* 33:233–243, 2010.

Thompson RA: Social support and child protection: lessons learned and learning, *Child Abuse Negl* 41:19–29, 2015.

U.S. Bureau of Justice Statistics: Retrieved from https://www.bjs.gov.

U.S. Department of Health and Human Services (USDHHS): *Healthy people 2020: objectives*, Washington, DC, 2010, Office of Disease Prevention and Health Promotion, USDHHS.

U.S. Department of Health and Human Services, Administration for Children and Families, Administration on Children, Youth and Families, Children's Bureau: *Child maltreatment 2012*, 2013. Available at: http://www.acf.hhs.gov.

U.S. Department of Health and Human Services, Administration for Children and Families, Administration on Children, Youth and Families, Children's Bureau: *Child Maltreatment 2014*, 2016. Retrieved from https://www.acf.hhs.gov.

United Nations Office on Drugs and Crime: *Human trafficking*, 2019. Retrieved from https://www.unodc.org.

U.S. Department of Justice, Federal Bureau of Investigation: *Uniform crime reporting program data: supplementary homicide reports*, 2013. Retrieved from https://www.icpsr.umich.edu.

U.S. Preventive Services Task Force: *Screening for intimate partner violence and abuse of elderly and vulnerable adults* [U.S. Preventive Services Task Force Recommendation Statement], 2013. Retrieved from http://www.uspreventiveservicestaskforce.org.

Valpied J, Hegarty K: Intimate partner abuse: identifying, caring for and helping women in healthcare settings, *Women's Health* 11:51–63, 2015.

Van Dorn R, Volavka J, Johnson N: Mental disorder and violence: Is there a relationship beyond substance use? *Soc Psychiatry Psychiatr Epidemiol* 47:487–503, 2012.

Wallace CM: *Measuring changes in attitude, skill and knowledge of undergraduate nursing students after receiving an educational intervention in intimate partner violence [doctoral dissertation]*. College of Saint Mary, 2009.

Walters ML, Chen J, Breiding MJ: *The national intimate partner and sexual violence survey (NISVS): 2010 findings on victimization by sexual orientation*, Atlanta, GA, 2013, National Center for Injury Prevention and Control, Centers for Disease Control and Prevention.

Walsh K, Zinzow HM, Badour CL, et al: Understanding disparities in service seeking following forcible versus drug- or alcohol-facilitated/incapacitated rape, *J Interpers Violence* 31:2475–2491, 2016.

Ward C, Wood A: Intimate partner violence: NP role in assessment, *Am J Nurs Pract* 13:9–15, 2009.

Whitaker DJ, Lutzker JR, Shelley GA: Child maltreatment prevention priorities at the Centers for Disease Control and Prevention, *Child Maltreat* 10:245–259, 2005.

Whiting JB, Simmons LA, Havens JR, et al: Intergenerational transmission of violence: the influence of self-appraisals, mental disorders and substance abuse, *J Fam Viol* 24:639–648, 2009.

World Health Organization: *Active ageing: a policy framework*, Geneva, 2002, World Health Organization.

Wu SS, Ma C, Carter RL, et al: Risk factors for infant maltreatment: a population-based study, *Child Abuse Negl* 28:1253–1264, 2004.

Yllo K: Wife rape, *Violence Against Women* 5:1059–1063, 1999.

Zimmerman F, Mercy JA: A better start: child maltreatment prevention as a public health priority, *Zero Three* 30:4–10, 2010.

39

Advanced Nursing Practice in the Community

Sallie J. Shipman, EdD, MSN, RN, CNL, NHDP-BC, Melanie Gibbons Hallman, DNP, CRNP, CEN, FNP-BC, ACNP-BC, FAEN, and Patricia M. Speck, DNSc, APN, APRN, FNP-BC, DF-IAFN, FAAFS, FAFN, FAAN

OBJECTIVES

After reading this chapter, the student should be able to do the following:

1. Discuss the historical development of the roles of the public health nurse in advanced nursing practice and the advanced nurse practitioner in public health.
2. Describe the educational requirements for population-focused advanced practice nurses.
3. Discuss certification/credentialing mechanisms in nursing as they relate to the roles of the advanced public health nurse and the advanced practice nurse.
4. Compare and contrast the various role functions and practice arenas of population-focused advanced public health nurses and advanced practice nurses in public health.
5. Explore current issues and concerns related to public health nursing practice.
6. Identify five stressors that affect nurses in expanded roles whether advanced public health nurses or nurse practitioners in public health.

CHAPTER OUTLINE

Historical Perspective
Competencies
Educational Preparation of Advanced Nursing Practice—NP Versus APHN
Credentialing
Advanced Practice Roles
Arenas for Practice
Issues and Concerns
Role Stress
Trends in Advanced Practice Nursing

KEY TERMS

administrator, p. 869
advanced nursing practice in public health, p. 864
advanced practice nurse, p. 864
advanced public health nurse, p. 866
certification, p. 867
clinical nurse leader, p. 865
clinical nurse specialist, p. 865
clinician, p. 868
competencies, p. 873
consultant, p. 870
educator, p. 869
faith community nursing, p. 871
***Healthy People 2020*, p. 872**
independent practice, p. 871
institutional privileges, p. 874
interprofessional collaborative practice, p. 875
liability, p. 875
nurse practitioner, p. 864
nursing centers, p. 871
parish nursing, p. 871
portfolios, p. 874
prescriptive authority, p. 868

Continued

The authors want to acknowledge the legacy of Kellie A. Smith, RN, EdD, posthumously for the many contributions to this chapter in edition 9 of the text.

KEY TERMS—cont'd

primary health care, p. 865
professional isolation, p. 875
protocols, p. 868
researcher, p. 870
retail clinics, p. 871
third-party reimbursement, p. 865

This chapter explores the advanced nursing practice roles of both the clinical specialist in advanced public health nursing, and the advanced practice nursing specialties in the community. Why, one might ask, is this chapter in the text? For a few good reasons. One is the intent to provide the bachelor of science in nursing (BSN) student with an understanding of career opportunities that are available when continuing one's education to the graduate level. Another is for the nurse in a graduate program. The chapter provides an in-depth understanding of advanced nursing practices of both clinical specialties and advanced practice nurse roles in public health settings. The advanced nursing practice roles described in this chapter often collaborate, whether an advanced public health nurse or an advanced practice nurse. The role delineation offers excellent opportunities for two exciting careers that highlight potentials for major contributions impacting health outcomes of individuals and improving health rankings of populations of patients.

Advanced nursing practice (ANP) is broadly defined by the American Association of Colleges of Nursing (AACN) (2006) as:

> *any form of nursing intervention that influences health care outcomes for individuals or populations, including the direct care of individual patients, management of care for individuals and populations, administration of nursing and health care organizations, and the development and implementation of health policy. (p. 2)*

The **advanced nursing practice in public health** is a licensed professional nurse prepared at the master's or doctoral level to assume leadership roles by applying the nursing process and public health sciences to achieve specific public health outcomes for the community; this nurse is often referred to as an advanced public health nurse (APHN). Both the American Nurses Association (ANA, 2013) and the Association of Community Health Nursing Educators (ACHNE, 2007) refer to this specialized role as APHN; therefore APHN is the title that is used in this chapter. The APHN in the community may be an **advanced practice nurse** (APN) or a **nurse practitioner** (NP). An NP is generally a nurse with a master's or doctoral degree, who autonomously and in collaboration with health care professionals and other individuals provides a range of primary, acute, and specialty health care services (American Association of Nurse Practitioners [AANP], 2014b). The APHN and NP often work in similar settings. However, the client focuses differ. The NP's client is an individual or family, usually in a fixed setting, identifying individual or community trends in their practices, such as an outbreak of a sexually transmitted infection (STI). The NP works closely with the APHN (e.g., notifying of the STI outbreak), whose clients are individuals, families, groups at risk, or communities. The APHN's final goal is the health of the whole community (ANA, 2013; RWJF, 2017) (e.g., stopping the outbreak in the population). The APHN always has a population focus and obtains knowledge from nursing, social, and public health sciences to achieve goals of promoting and protecting the health of populations by creating conditions in which people optimize their health (ACHNE, 2007; ANA, 2013). Table 39.1 compares the functions taught to the APHN and the NP in their educational programs.

TABLE 39.1 How to Distinguish Similarities and Differences in Functions of Advanced Public Health Nurses and Nurse Practitioners

Function	NP Program	APHN Program
Comprehensive assessment	Always	Often
Physiology and pharmacology	Almost always	Often
Diagnosis and management	Always	Often
Systems	Individual/family focus	More systems focused
Leadership	Usually	Almost always
Program planning and evaluation	Less often	Always in community and public health
Research	Generally	Generally

APHN, Advanced public health nurse; *NP,* nurse practitioner.
From Association of Community Health Nursing Educators (ACHNE): *Graduate education for advanced practice in community/public health nursing: at the crossroads,* Latham, NY, 2007, ACHNE; American Nurses Association (ANA): *Public health nursing: scope and standards of practice,* ed 2, Washington, DC, 2013, ANA.

The chapter also provides a history of the educational preparation of the advanced practice nurse. The authors discuss the functions in advanced nursing practice and settings for practices, as well as issues and concerns, role negotiation, and areas of role stress relative to the APHN and the NP in the community.

HISTORICAL PERSPECTIVE

A shift in societal demands and needs resulted in changes in health care systems and nursing over the past few decades.

Trends influencing the roles of the APHN and NP include a shift from institution-based health care to population-focused health care (RWJF, 2017), improvements in technology, self-care, cost-containment measures, accountability to the client, **third-party reimbursement**, and demands for making technology-related care more responsive and client (patient) centered. Reversal of the Affordable Care Act (ACA) tax mandate in 2017 did not diminish the need for ANPs but did reverse self-reported insurance coverage trends. Rising health care costs for reduced coverage continue, and higher deductibles remain under current mandatory ACA rules.

The **clinical nurse specialist** (CNS) role began in the early 1960s and grew out of a need to improve client care. In addition to providing direct patient care, CNSs influence care outcomes by providing expert consultation for nursing staffs and by implementing improvements in health care delivery systems (National Association of Clinical Nurse Specialists, 2018). Concurrently, there was a shortage of physicians and an increasing tendency among physicians to specialize. The reduction in the number of physicians providing general medical care across the nation became a trend that continues today. Consequently, a serious and growing gap in **primary health care** (PHC) services developed, widening each decade. PHC includes both public health and primary health care services. The barriers to PHC include "(a) needed service delivery reforms to build a PHC-oriented system, (b) reforms to integrate public health initiatives into PHC settings, and (c) leadership to promote dialogue among stakeholders" (Gauld et al., 2012).

In 1965 at the University of Colorado, Dr. Loretta Ford, a nurse, and Dr. Henry Silver, a pediatrician, thought that the morbidity among medically deprived children might be decreased by nurses educated to provide well-child and sick care to children of all ages. The nursing practice for early pediatric nurse practitioners in Colorado included the identification, assessment, and management of common acute and chronic health problems, with appropriate referral of more complex problems to physicians (Silver et al., 1967). The nurse practitioner role in pediatric practice aligned with the priorities of the traditional nursing profession, which are to care for and support the well, the worried well, and the ill, offering physical care services previously provided only by physicians. Preparing nurses in the Colorado style, as primary health care providers, was responsive to the "fundamental shift in society's critical need for primary health care services," including health promotion and illness prevention (Institute of Medicine, 2011; RWJF, 2017).

Simultaneously in 1965, Duke University initiated the physician assistant (PA) role. The intent of the PA program was to attract former military corpsmen for training as "physician extenders" (Cooper et al., 1998). Often lumped with other nonphysician providers into a single category of "physician extenders," nurse practitioners and others promised to relieve the physician shortages (Wallen et al., 1982). Dr. Loretta Ford challenges the medicalization of the APN role as a physician extender by physicians in this excerpt:

> *As conceptualized, the nurse practitioner was always intended to be a nursing model focused on the promotion of health in daily living, on growth and development of children in families, and on the prevention of disease and disability. Nursing as a discipline and a profession evolved not because there was a shortage of physicians but because of societal needs. The early plans did not include preparing nurses to assume medical functions. The interests were in health promotion and disease prevention for aggregate populations in community settings, including underserved groups. These were the hallmarks of community-oriented nursing. (Ford, 1986, p. 6)*

When challenged as a threat to medical care, Wallen reported, "Patient acceptance and the quality of care rendered by these providers appear to be high" (Wallen et al., 1982). Early studies supported the report issued by the U.S. Department of Health, Education, and Welfare (now the U.S. Department of Health and Human Services [USDHHS]), *Extending the Scope of Nursing Practice* (1971), and helped convince Congress about the value of NPs as primary health care providers. The Nurse Training Act of 1971 (PL 92-158) and the comprehensive Health Manpower Training Act of 1971 (PL 92-157) provided education funding for many NP and PA programs through the 1970s and into the 1980s. Similarly, the concept of an expanded practice role for nurses was garnering interest in Canada in the 1970s. The United Kingdom followed suit in the 1980s and increased the number of advanced practice nurse programs available to educate and monitor the role's development. The number of NPs in the United States grew to a quarter million in 2018 (AANP, 2018), and while growing in numbers worldwide, the NP roles continue to experience barriers to practice and population barriers to health (Kleinpell et al., 2014).

Monitoring the roles in a variety of disciplines, graduate education for nursing began to change in the early 2000s. In 2007, the AACN called for the creation of a new nursing role—the clinical nurse leader (CNL) (AACN, 2017; AACN 2018). The **clinical nurse leader** is defined as a nurse who is a master's degree–prepared generalist who functions at the institution's microsystem level and assumes accountability for health care outcomes for a specific group of clients within a unit or area (AACN, 2018b; Commission on Nurse Certification, 2018; Foster et al., 2011). A prelicensure or licensed registered professional nurse, with graduate preparation (earned master's) from a CNL program, is an advanced nursing practice generalist, working at point of care facilitates providing direct patient care and focuses on "evidence-based practice, safety, quality, risk reduction, and cost containment" (Mohr & Coke, 2018, p. 141). The CNL is a clinical leader who, at the point of care, focuses on care coordination, outcome measurement, transitions of care, interprofessional communication, team leadership, risk assessment, implementation of best-practices based on evidence, and quality improvement.

In the 1990s, the seeds for doctoral preparation for the practicing nurse took root and early academic institutions' programs of study graduated the first practice doctorates in 1999 and 2000. By 2007, the AACN determined that the preferred preparation for advanced practice nurses' specialties should be the doctor of nursing practice (DNP) (AACN, 2017). Autonomous or freestanding schools were the first to offer a BSN-to-DNP and admit a small proportion of their applicants, who were typically part of a health professions school with doctoral research programs. Nurses with the doctor of philosophy (PhD) degree developed the first practice doctorates, and many continue to struggle with the differences between the two nursing doctorates—PhD (new knowledge) and DNP (quality improvement). Today, structural characteristics correlate with the consensus decisions to offer the BSN-to-DNP (Auerbach et al., 2015, pp. 23–24). There are stark differences between schools offering the BSN-to-DNP and those without the program of study, and many of the differences relate to capacity to offer the program of study. As more DNPs graduate, schools enlist their clinical expertise to teach in the DNP programs of study. Others offer faculty tenure tract positions to DNP graduates who demonstrate their national impact through scholarship.

COMPETENCIES

The Quad Council of Public Health Nursing Organizations, now the Quad Council Coalition, in 2003 developed a set of national public health competencies specific for public health nursing practice that reflect the *Core Competencies for Public Health Professionals* authored by the Council on Linkages Between Academia and Public Health Practice. The design for the core competencies served as a starting point for academic and practice organizations to understand, assess, and meet educational and workforce needs for health professionals practicing in public health; they were updated in 2018 (Quad Council Coalition [QCC], 2018). The Quad Council Coalition competencies are more specific to public health nursing, and the design of the tool assists agencies with language to describe workforce minimal competency for beginning positions and maximum competency needed for advancement in the employment of public health nurses. Academic settings benefit by using the competencies to prepare nurses with minimal skills as public health nurses. The competencies also are used to facilitate graduate education, agency orientation, on-the-job training, and lifelong learning (QCC, 2018) (see the Linking Content to Practice box).

The ANA, in 2013, revised and published *Public Health Nursing: Scope and Standards of Practice,* which includes population-focused standards of care in the following areas: assessment, population diagnosis and priorities, outcome identification, planning, implementation, evaluation, and standards for professional performance in ethics, education, evidence-based practice and research, quality of practice, communication, leadership, collaboration, professional practice evaluation, and resource utilization, environmental health, and advocacy. The basis of the document arose from the collaboration between the American Nurses Association and the American Public Health Association (APHA)-Public Health Nursing Section (2013). The document provided a definition and described the role of public health nursing practice. It minimally answered the following questions asked by ANA scope and standards of practice:

- **Who:** Registered Nurses (RN) and Advanced Practice Registered Nurses (APRN) comprise the "who" constituency and have been educated, titled, and maintain active licensure to practice nursing.
- **What:** Nursing is the protection, promotion, and optimization of health and abilities; prevention of illness and injury; facilitation of healing; alleviation of suffering through the diagnosis and treatment of human response; and advocacy in the care of individuals, families, groups, communities, and populations.
- **Where:** Wherever there is a client in need of care.
- **When:** Whenever there is a need for nursing knowledge, compassion, and expertise.
- **Why:** The profession exists to achieve the most positive client outcomes in keeping with nursing's social contract and obligation to society (ANA, Scope of Practice, 2018, items 1–5).

This second edition required the same rigor as the first, published in 2007. This revised edition "looks to the future of public health nursing and provides essential guidance in the form of standards and competencies for public health nurse generalist and the advanced public health nurse" (ANA, 2013). The document now includes competencies for the **advanced public health nurse** that appear at the end of each of the standards of practice. For example, under Standard 1: Assessment, additional competencies for the advanced practice nurse include the following: gathers data from multiple interdisciplinary sources as well as synthesizes qualitative and quantitative data during data analysis for a comprehensive population assessment (ANA, 2013).

EDUCATIONAL PREPARATION OF ADVANCED NURSING PRACTICE—NP VERSUS APHN

Educational preparation for the APHN includes a minimum of a master's degree and is based on a synthesis of current knowledge and research in nursing, public health, and other scientific disciplines. In addition to performing the functions of the generalist in population-focused nursing, the specialist possesses clinical experience in interprofessional planning, organizing, community empowerment, delivering and evaluating service, political and legislative activities, and assuming a leadership role in interventions that have a positive effect on the health of the community. ACHNE recommendations for graduate nursing education for the public health nurse specialty are guided by the report *Who Will Keep the Public Healthy?* (Institute of Medicine, 2003), the ANA's *Public Health Nursing: Scope and Standards of Practice* (2013), and the AACN's *Essentials of Doctoral Education for Advanced Practice Nursing* (2006). ACHNE has also identified five role characteristics of APHNs: (1) population-level health care focus; (2) ecological view; (3) responsibility for health outcomes for populations; (4) partnership and collaboration, using an interprofessional approach; and (5) leadership in practice. The identified curriculum areas for the APHN are population-centered nursing theory and practice, interprofessional practice, leadership, systems thinking, biostatistics, epidemiology, environmental health sciences, health policy and management, social and behavioral sciences, public health informatics, genomics, health communication, cultural competence, community-based participatory research, global health, policy, and law, and public health ethics. In addition to didactic content, graduate education for the APHN includes practicum experience that takes place at the population level, is grounded in the ecological perspective, and includes the measurement of outcomes (ACHNE, 2007; RWJF, 2017).

In contrast to the APHN, educational preparation of the NP has not always been at the graduate level. Early NP programs were continuing education and certificate programs, and the baccalaureate degree was not easily attained, nor was it a requirement. At present, however, NPs are required to hold master's degrees and encouraged to obtain a practice doctorate (e.g., DNP) (AACN, 2017). The curriculum prepares NPs to perform a wide range of professional nursing functions, including assessing and diagnosing, conducting physical examinations, ordering laboratory and other diagnostic tests, developing and implementing treatment plans for some acute and chronic illnesses, prescribing medications, monitoring client status, educating and counseling clients, and consulting and collaborating with and referring to other providers (American Nurses Credentialing Center [ANCC], 2014).

In 2006, an AACN position statement supported advanced DNP education for ANPs and nurses seeking top systems and organizational roles. The eight foundational essentials for DNP programs are knowledge with a scientific underpinning, organizational and systems leadership, clinical scholarship, information systems, policy, collaboration, prevention and population health, and advanced nursing practice (AACN, 2006; AACN, 2015). Future recommendations for doctoral programs in nursing continue to be reviewed and discussed (Ketefian & Redman, 2015). The Academic Partnerships to Improve Health (APIH) is a collaborative between the AACN and the Centers for Disease Control and Prevention to help build capacity in the public health nursing workforce. The program supports faculty development in population health and connects nursing students with hands-on experiences at the community level to enhance their preparation for professional practice (AACN, 2018a; RWJF 2017).

CREDENTIALING

The American Nurses Credentialing Center (ANCC) and the American Association of Nurse Practitioners (AANP) offer certification examinations for a variety of specialties in advanced practice nursing. The purpose of professional certification is to confirm knowledge and educational expertise, but also provide recognition of professional achievement in a defined area of nursing. **Certification** is a means of assuring the public that nurses who claim to be competent at an advanced level have credentials verified through examination (ANCC, 2018). Although certification itself is not mandatory, many state boards of nursing require nurses in advanced practice, particularly those in an NP role, be nationally certified to practice.

The ANA began its certification program in 1973 and has continued to offer NP certification examinations since 1976. The ANA certification programs transitioned in 1984–1985, and ANCC began to offer certifications in 1991 in a variety of nursing specialties, primarily advanced practice nursing. Until 2009, a nurse was also certified as a generalist or as a BSN-prepared specialist in community health, and until 2017, a nurse could certify as an advanced public health nurse. However, ANCC closed both programs and currently no other certification programs exist for the APHN or PHN. Public health nursing was not the only casualty, because all rare non-NP advanced nursing practice certifications ended. Those holding non-NP certifications may maintain their certifications. In summary, since 1985, the basic qualifications for certification as an NP is a baccalaureate degree in nursing and successful completion of a formal NP program. As of 1992, a master's or higher degree in nursing is required for NP certification through the ANCC and AANP. NPs are required to maintain certification by renewing every five years.

Several nurse practitioner certifications are available at the ANCC. The examination topics vary, based on the specialty area (ANCC, 2018). The AANP also has national competency-based certification examinations in three areas: family, adult, and adult-gerontology primary care nurse practitioners (AANP, 2018a).

The certification examination for CNS in public/community health nursing was first offered in October 1990 and required a master's or higher degree in nursing with a specialization in community/public health nursing practice. Effective in 1998, eligibility requirements included holding a master's or higher degree in nursing with a specialization in community/public health nursing or holding a baccalaureate or higher degree in nursing and a master's degree in public health with a specialization in community/public health nursing. In 2009, the ANCC Commission changed the certification examination from clinical nurse specialist in public/community health to either advanced public health nursing or public health clinical nurse specialist. However, as of December 31, 2013, these examinations are no longer available. If one already holds these certifications through examination, they are renewed with professional development and practice hours. Effective January 1, 2014, an advanced public health nurse-board certified (APHN-BC) credential is obtained by the "certification through portfolio assessment" method (ANCC, 2018). However, in 2017, the APHN-BC, along with others, was no longer offered to new graduates; if certification is current, renewal is possible (ANCC, 2018). Certification is not a requirement for practice in public health nursing or advanced practice public health nursing.

ADVANCED PRACTICE ROLES

APNs holding a master's degree in nursing or DNP and specializing in public health nursing, in community health nursing, or as a nurse practitioner have many roles, which are described here. It should be noted that the "nursing role in APPHN [advanced practice public health nursing] is not distinguished by the sites at which nurses practice, but rather by the perspective, knowledge base, and principles that focus on care of populations" (ACHNE, 2007, p. 16). The APHN's role characteristics include a focus on population health such as population and community assessment; advocacy and policy setting at the organizational, community, and state levels; ecological view for large-scale program planning and project management; and leadership and partnership building. APHNs deliver population-focused services, programs, and research (ACHNE, 2007; APHA, 2013).

Clinician

Most of the differences between the roles of the APHN and the NP are seen in clinical practice. Although the APHN's practice includes nursing directed at individuals, families, and groups, the primary responsibility is to take a leadership role in the overall assessment, planning, development, coordination, and evaluation of innovative programs to meet identified community health needs. The APHN provides the direction for population-focused health care by identifying and documenting health needs and resources in a community and in collaborating with population-focused nurse generalists, other health professionals, and consumers (ACHNE, 2007; APHA, 2013). Practicing within the role of **clinician**, the APHN involvement is in conducting community assessments; identifying needs of populations at risk; and planning, implementing, and evaluating population-focused programs to achieve health goals, including health promotion and disease prevention activities. The APHN ultimately works toward the goals of promoting and protecting the health of populations by creating conditions for optimal health (ANA, 2013; APHA, 2013).

The NP applies advanced practice nursing knowledge and physical, psychosocial, and environmental assessment skills to manage common health and illness problems of clients of all ages and genders. The NP's primary client is the individual and family. In the direct role of clinician, the NP assesses health risks and health and illness status, as well as the response to illness of individuals and families. The NP also diagnoses actual or potential health problems; decides on treatment plans jointly with clients; intervenes to promote health, to protect against disease, to treat illness, to manage chronic disease, and to limit disability; and evaluates with the client and other primary care team members about how effective and comprehensive the nursing intervention may be in providing continuity of care (AACN, 2011). Despite the setting, the practice of the nurse practitioner can be population focused. Common interventions often include community assessment and analysis, case finding, an emphasis on prevention, and participation in public policy. An advanced practice nurse in the community works in agencies or settings where the caseload consists of individuals who present themselves for services. The APHN goal is to identify others in the community who are at risk and in need of the services. Outreach activities accomplish these goals while also trying to accomplish the goals and objectives of *Healthy People 2020* (Box 39.1). Currently, planning is underway for *Healthy People 2030.*

BOX 39.1 Example of a *Healthy People 2020* Objective and Selected Advanced Practice Nursing Activities

Objective

- MHMD-1: Reduce suicide rate to no more than 10.2 suicide deaths per 100,000 people.

Activities

- Review recent literature and epidemiology of suicide.
- Provide in-service education programs to groups of health professionals related to groups at risk for suicide and related assessment and screening tools for early detection and treatment of depression.
- Become active in legislation activities related to firearm access.
- Assess individual clients for depression and suicide risk.

U.S. Department of Health and Human Services: *Healthy People 2020,* Washington, DC, 2014, U.S. Government Printing Office. Retrieved from https://www.healthypeople.gov/.

The ability of NPs to diagnose and treat increased the access to health care, teaching, and client compliance with treatment plans. State legislation guides the amounts of physician involvement in the NP's practice (AANP, 2018b). In states requiring relationships between the physician and nurse practitioner, the NP uses **protocols** or algorithms previously agreed on by the physician and the NP. The documents serve as standing orders for the management of certain illnesses. As of 2010, all states passed legislation, either partial or full, granting NPs supervisory, collaborative, or independent authority to practice. Each state has differing regulatory and legislative mandates regarding NP areas of practice authority, reimbursement, and **prescriptive authority** (Phillips, 2017). The most up-to-date information on state nurse practitioner practices and laws is available through the American Association of Nurse Practitioners (AANP) website (https://aanp.org/).

An important area for both APHNs and NPs to include in their advanced practice is health promotion/disease prevention. Within the past several decades, there has been a growing belief that the most effective way of dealing with major health problems is through prevention. Refocusing toward prevention requires the health care system to identify aggregates (populations) at risk, introduce risk reduction interventions, teach people that they control their own health, and encourage health promotion and disease prevention behaviors. The Patient Protection and Affordable Care Act (PPACA, 2010) goals continue at this printing and include improvement of the individual health care experience, reduction of the cost of health, and improvement of the health of populations; these create the potential for new public health nursing roles and responsibilities. Regardless of the outcome, public health nurses in the community (through their assessment skills, primary care focus, and system-level perspectives) are vital to the interprofessional teams necessary to ensure that all people have equitable access to high-quality care and healthy environments through health systems (APHA, 2013). The USDHHS (2014a) develops national objectives for promoting health and preventing disease.

Since 1997, this initiative, called *Healthy People* in 2000, 2010, 2020, and planning for 2030, has set and monitored national health objectives to meet a broad range of health needs, encourage collaboration across sectors, guide individuals toward making informed health decisions, as well as measure the impact of prevention activities. The *Healthy People* campaign is essential to measure outcomes for APHNs and NPs working toward the goal of a healthier nation. Nurses and advanced practice nurses also use *The Guide to Clinical Preventive Services* to address health promotion and disease prevention and 2018 *Preventive Health Care Guidelines* (CDC, 2018; USDHHS/AHRQ/USPSTF, 2014). APHNs and NPs are especially involved in helping meet the proposed objectives in equity in health care services, including access, educational and community-based programs, and public health infrastructure domains.

Population-Focused Intervention

The following example illustrates a population-focused intervention. An APHN was recently hired at a community hospital in the hospital's community health department. Traditionally, the department provided excellent health education and screening programs to individuals in the surrounding communities. However, outreach activities did not occur. After reviewing the data on attendance at community health events, the APHN developed and implemented a needs assessment in three neighboring communities not attending the events. In one neighborhood, consisting of 1800 apartments, 85 percent of the population was middle-income African Americans of all ages. The needs assessment revealed a strong interest in health promotion and disease prevention but nevertheless a lack of participation. The APHN developed a collaborative relationship with churches and community groups in the neighborhood. Health fairs and events were initiated (see the Levels of Prevention box).

LEVELS OF PREVENTION

Population-Focused APHN Activities

Primary Prevention

- Flu immunizations at churches
- Classes on breast self-examination
- Education on the need for early detection of breast cancer

Secondary Prevention

- "Men's Night Out" event with screenings for blood pressure and cholesterol (at neighborhood sites)
- Health fair at neighborhood sites with screenings

Tertiary Prevention

- Identified need and follow-up at clinics for groups with chronic diseases (diabetes, cancer, hypertension)

Educator

Nurses in advanced practice function in several indirect nursing care roles, including that of **educator**. The role of the APHN and NP includes health education within a nursing framework (as opposed to health educators, who do not have a nursing background) and professional nurse educator (faculty) roles.

The APHN identifies groups at risk within a community and implements, for example, health education interventions. The APHN and NP increase wellness and contribute to maintaining and promoting health by teaching the importance of good nutrition, physical exercise, stress management, and a healthy lifestyle. Health educators also provide education about disease processes and the importance of following treatment regimens. In addition, they provide anticipatory guidance and educate clients on the use of medications, diet, birth control methods, and other therapeutic procedures (ACHNE, 2007; ANA, 2013; APHA, 2013). They also counsel clients, families, groups, and the community on the importance of assuming responsibility for their own health. The health educators provide education to individuals, families, or groups at institutional and ambulatory levels, or home settings, or it occurs in the community with vulnerable at-risk populations. As professional nurse educators, the APHN and NP also provide formal and informal teaching of staff nurses and undergraduate and graduate students in nursing and other disciplines (Fig. 39.1). They also serve as role models by instructing (or being a preceptor to) students in advanced nursing practice in the clinical setting.

Administrator

The APHN and NP function in administrative roles. As a health **administrator**, they are responsible for all administrative matters within an agency setting. They are responsible for and have direct or indirect authority and supervision over the organization's staff and client care. In this capacity, nurses in advanced practice serve as decision makers and problem solvers. They are also involved in other business and management aspects such as supporting and managing personnel; budgeting; establishing quality control mechanisms; program planning and influencing policies; public relations; and marketing (ACHNE, 2007; Drennan, 2012; Quad Council Coalition, 2018).

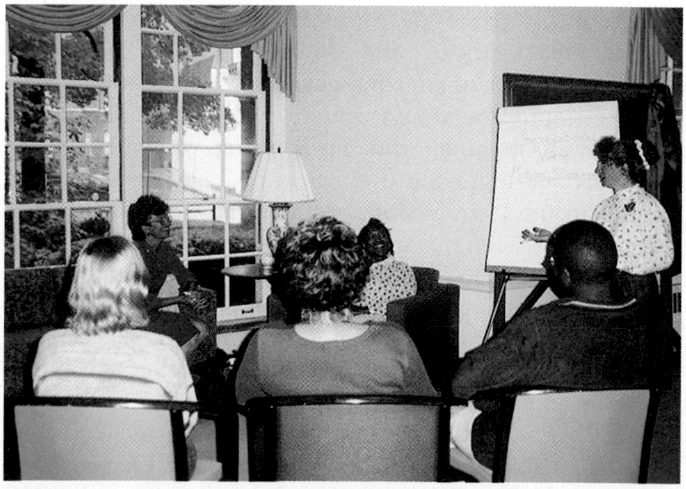

Fig. 39.1 An advanced practice public health nurse leads a training session for a group of congregational nurses.

Consultant

Consultation is an important part of practice for APHNs and NPs. The consultant solves problems for and with individuals, families, or communities to improve health care delivery. Steps followed throughout the consultation process include assessing the problem, determining the availability and feasibility of resources, proposing solutions, and assisting with implementing a solution, if appropriate (AACN, 2011; APHA, 2013). The APHN and NP serve as a formal or informal **consultant** to other nurses, providing them with information on improving client care. Consultants counsel physicians and other health care providers and organizations or schools to improve the health care of clients. For example, nurse consultants are often used at the district or state level of public health departments. APHNs and NPs work closely with nurse supervisors, other NPs, and staff public health nurses to develop programs and improve the services provided to clients at clinics and in the home. Nurse consultants in the public health arena work with all other public health nurses or work in departments as members of an interprofessional team such as maternal–child health, chronic diseases, or family planning (University of Michigan Center of Excellence, 2013).

Researcher

Improvement in nursing practice depends on the commitment of nurses to developing new knowledge and refining practice improvements through application to research. Government and other funding sources now encourage research–practice partnerships, collaborating with stakeholders, for funding in the community of interest. Researchers may be academicians or may be nurses with dual PhD and practice doctorates, as well as being a practicing NP or APHN! Practicing APHNs and NPs are in ideal positions to identify researchable nursing problems for researchers that relate to the communities they serve. Collaborations are encouraged in community-based participatory research applications for funding, and when complete, the community of providers apply their research findings to the community health practice setting of interest.

All APHNs and most NPs have training in the research process and, as **researchers**, conduct their own improvement science investigations and collaborate with doctorate-prepared nurses, answering questions related to nursing practice improvement and primary health care. The acts of identifying, defining, and investigating clinical nursing problems and reporting findings encourages peer relationships with other professions and contributes to health care policy and decision making (Harne-Britner & Schafer, 2009). For example, APHNs in administrative, consultant, or practitioner roles encounter situations daily that need improvement and further investigating (e.g., noncompliance with certain public health regimens or immunization schedules). They, anecdotally or through needs assessments, identify a trend for which, if examined, population-based strategies can be implemented (see the Evidence-Based Practice box). APHNs and NPs collaborate with population-focused nurses at all levels to develop the research design, collect and analyze the data, and determine the implications for further use of nursing interventions identified and are co-authors in dissemination. APHNs play a critical role in ensuring that evidence-based research is shared and integrated into health care practice (APHA, 2013; Harne-Britner & Schafer, 2009; Issel et al., 2011).

EVIDENCE-BASED PRACTICE

Although cancer incidence and mortality are declining, cancer remains among the leading causes of death in the United States. Research shows that cancer morbidity and mortality can be reduced by early detection. However, both cancer risks and screening behavior remain understudied in the homeless population. A cross-sectional survey of homeless individuals ($n = 201$) was conducted. The analysis describes the demographic, psychosocial, and behavioral associations with cancer screenings and knowledge of the lung cancer screening recommendation among homeless populations

The study participants' mean age was 51.7 years; the group was largely African American (77.3 percent) and male (67.9 percent). Among women, the breast and cervical cancer screening rates were 46.5 percent (breast) and 85.1 percent (cervical). Among men, the prostate cancer screening rate was 34.2 percent. Among all participants, the colon cancer screening rate was 44 percent. Lung cancer screening knowledge was low (23.0 percent). Cancer risk behaviors were high with participation in cancer screening below national benchmarks and was associated with age, income, health status, obesity, tobacco use, and physical activity.

Nurse Use

To improve cancer survival among disparate populations, sustained community outreach is necessary to increase awareness of screening recommendations, to identify high-risk individuals, and to guide them to available resources.

Williams LB, McCall A, Looney SW, et al.: Demographic, psychosocial, and behavioral associations with cancer screening among a homeless population. *Public Health Nurs* 35(4):281-290, 2018.

ARENAS FOR PRACTICE

Regardless of where public health nurses work (e.g., schools, homes, clinics, jails, shelters, mobile vans, or after a disaster), the core interventions to accomplish the goals of promoting and protecting the health of populations are similar across all practice arenas. Positions for APHNs and NPs vary greatly in terms of scope of practice, degree of responsibility, power and authority, working conditions, and innovation. The factors and the impact on practice are influenced by nurse practice acts and other legislation (e.g., reimbursement and prescriptive privileges) that govern the legal practice in each state (Phillips, 2017). The following areas include traditional as well as alternative practice settings for APHNs and NPs.

Primary Care

Research indicates that the opportunities for APNs in primary care settings is increasing, and the trend is expected to continue (APHA, 2013; Fairman et al., 2011). Primary care settings such as private practices, large health systems, community health centers, patient-centered medical homes, and others provide various roles for the advanced practice nurse. For example, many practices employ NPs, physician's assistants, RNs, licensed practical nurses, pharmacists, behavioral health providers, community health workers, and physicians to provide care in formal or informal team structures (Flinter et al., 2017). Over 40 years of evidence demonstrates that nurses in rigorous education programs of study in primary care from accredited academic settings produce the same high-quality providers and care, achieving equally positive health outcomes for the patient as physicians. In general, preliminary research found no appreciable differences between physicians and nurses in health outcomes for clients, process of care, resource utilization, or cost (Laurant et al., 2018).

Independent Practice

Nurses form an **independent practice** for several reasons. Reasons vary and include personal goals of access to care in remote areas, not served by others, or a professional desire to break new ground for nursing in meeting the health care needs within all communities. Today, some enter the profession for the independence, job security, and pay. It is important to investigate the state's nurse practice act to determine the limitations and laws related to the practices available for NPs. For example, NPs provide a comprehensive array of health services in states where they have legislative authority to prescribe drugs. Nurses in many states successfully lobbied for third-party reimbursement for all RNs who provide direct care services to individual clients (Phillips, 2017). The independent practice option is more likely to be chosen by APHNs and NPs in states that have established legislation to provide structure to guide their nursing practices.

Another option for APHNs and NPs interested in an entrepreneurial independent practice is to contract with physicians or organizations to provide certain services for their clients or staff. Nurses need to define a service package and market it attractively. An example for APHNs is providing a home visit to new parents after two weeks to assess the newborn, respond to parental concerns, and provide counseling and anticipatory guidance about nutrition, development, and immunization needs. This service may be marketed to pediatricians and family practice physicians who would offer or recommend the service to their clients as an option. An NP negotiates with a local school board to provide preschool children with health examinations or physical assessments before the children participate in sports. Under a contract, APHNs develop and implement health and safety programs on accident prevention and health promotion activities for small companies.

Nursing Centers

Nursing centers or nurse-managed health clinics, a type of joint practice developed by advanced practice nurses to address vulnerable populations, provide opportunities for collaborative relationships for APHNs, NPs, baccalaureate-prepared nurses, other health care professionals, and community members (National Nursing Centers Consortium, 2018). Primary health services are provided by NPs, depending on state legislation. Community APHNs, along with nurses and nursing students, focus on the neighborhood level and understand community needs. A central mission of nurse-managed clinics is community development such as health care accessibility and resources; public involvement; interprofessional practice; and health promotion and disease prevention supported by the principles of primary health care (National Nursing Centers Consortium, 2018). Nursing center models are discussed in more detail in Chapter 20.

Retail Clinics

Retail clinics are staffed primarily by NPs with convenient hours. The first retail clinic opened in Minneapolis in 2000, but their growth between 2006 and the present is substantial. They offer routine preventive and acute care services, usually covered by a protocol for consistent care between agencies. Although still generally operated by large retail pharmacies, involvement of hospital systems in retail clinic ownership is a more recent phenomenon (IOM, 2018; RAND Corp., 2016).

Faith Community Nursing/Parish Nursing

Faith community nursing, also known as **parish nursing**, is a concept that began in the late 1960s in the United States when increasing numbers of churches employed registered nurses to provide holistic, preventive health care to congregation members. Faith community nursing is a model of care that uses nurses based within faith communities such as churches and synagogues to provide health services to the members of those communities. Faith community nursing is a practice specialty that focuses on the intentional care of the spirit, promotion of an integrative model of health, and prevention and minimization of illness within the context of a faith community. Although primarily for faith community nurses and the nursing profession, it is also aimed at other health care providers, spiritual leaders, families, and members of faith communities (ANA, 2017).

The activities are complementary to the population-focused practice of APHNs, and faith community nurses either have a strong public health background or work directly with both baccalaureate-prepared nurses and APHNs. Faith community nurses positively affect client outcomes by providing health services in health promotion and disease prevention, chronic disease management, and culturally sensitive services (Roberts, 2014). See Chapter 45 for further discussion about faith community/parish nursing.

Institutional Settings

Ambulatory/Outpatient Clinics. APHNs and NPs have employment in the primary care unit of an institution (e.g., the ambulatory center or outpatient clinic). The centers/clinics generally provide hospital referral, hospital follow-up care, and health maintenance and management for nonemergency problems. The population served is usually culturally and economically diverse and represents a larger geographic area than patients served by private practices. In the outpatient settings, NPs typically practice jointly with physicians to provide acute and chronic primary care. Hospital acute care outpatient services include clinics for general medicine or family practice, or specialty-oriented clinics, such as pediatric, obstetrical-gynecological, and ear, nose, and throat clinics. Outpatient clinics organized for chronic care are problem-oriented (e.g., hypertension, diabetes, or acquired immunodeficiency syndrome [AIDS] clinics).

Emergency Departments. Persons without access to health care, such as the medically uninsured and the homeless, often do not seek health care services until they become ill. Hospital emergency departments (EDs) are increasingly used for nonemergency primary care. Although use of an emergency department is an inappropriate use of expensive health services, it is a result of the current system, which limits access to routine and preventive health care. Emergency department care is one of the most expensive services offered in health care today (Wood et al., 2010).

Emergency services often require long waits for persons who have nonemergency problems. Fast-track/nonemergency zones or areas (sometimes called urgent care) of EDs have become commonplace to accommodate these situations. NPs in these settings see clients with nonemergent problems and provide necessary treatment and applicable counseling. APHNs also educate clients about the importance of health care and methods to gain access to the preventive health care system. APHNs, with their knowledge of community health resources, help ensure that psychosocial needs are assessed and met. APHNs often act as liaisons or mediators for community programs that serve the needs of special populations.

Long-Term Care Facilities. The elderly age group represents the fastest-growing population (especially those over 85 years of age) in the United States (Administration on Aging, 2017). The data reveal a long-anticipated trend that we are living longer, resulting in a higher percent of elderly Americans. By 2040, it is projected that 82.3 million people will be age 65 or older, twice the number of older Americans in 2000. Past statistics revealed a shortage of advanced practice nurses specializing in gerontological nursing to care for the growing older adult population (Donald et al., 2013).

Gerontology is an increasingly important field of study, and many courses are available on the health needs of older adults. APHNs and NPs with an interest in geriatrics need to continue their education in this area to increase their knowledge and skills specific to this at-risk aggregate (Donald et al., 2013). Many APHNs and NPs view long-term care facilities as exciting areas for practice and a way of increasing quality of care while containing costs for older adults and the disabled. U.S. federal legislation provides reimbursement for APHNs and NPs to provide care to clients in Medicare-certified nursing homes and to recertify eligible clients for continued Medicare coverage. In long-term care facilities where clients are not ambulatory, APHNs and NPs make regular nursing home rounds, assess the health status of clients, and provide care and counseling as appropriate. In long-term care facilities in which the residents are more ambulatory, APHNs and NPs also provides health maintenance and other primary health care services to the nursing home clients.

Industry/Occupational Health. The *Healthy People 2020* (USDHHS, 2018a) objectives include a section on occupational health and safety with goals to reduce work-related injuries and deaths. Thousands of new cases of disease and death occur each year from occupational exposures.

APHNs and NPs are increasingly useful in occupational health programs as business and industry seek ways to control their health care costs and to provide preventive and primary on-site care services. The services help reduce absences from work and increase productivity of workers. The APHN or an occupational health nurse in an industrial/occupational setting assesses the health needs of the organization based on claims data, cost-benefit health research, results of employee health screening, and the perceived needs of employee groups (Levin et al., 2013). The APHN working as an occupational health nurse can receive certification in the specialty as a Certified Occupational Health Nurse (COHN) or Certified Occupational Health Nurse-Specialist (COHN-S) (AAOHN, 2018). With their advanced administrative and clinical skills, APHNs plan, implement, and evaluate company-wide health programs. The role of the occupational health nurse is discussed in Chapter 43.

Government

U.S. Public Health Service. The U.S. Public Health Service operates the National Health Service Corps (NHSC), which places health providers in federally designated areas with shortages of health workers; and the Indian Health Service, which provides health services to American Indians.

During the 1970s, both the Corps and the Indian Health Service offered to pay to educate RNs to become nurse practitioners if they promised to work for a designated period with the Public Health Service. These programs were discontinued during the 1980s when more emphasis was placed on physician recruitment. In 1988, Congress reauthorized two loan repayment programs for the education of NPs—one with the Corps and one with the Indian Health Service. In 2009, the American Recovery and Reinvestment Act invested an additional $300 million into the Corps, hoping to double its field strength by providing more scholarships and loan repayment options for health care providers. Depending on the needs of the area, an NP employed by the Public Health Service is the only health care provider in the setting or practices with a group of providers to serve a rural, an urban underserved, or an American Indian population (USDHHS, 2018b).

Armed Services. The increased availability of physicians reduced the active recruitment of nurses to advanced degree programs by the armed forces during the 1980s. NPs are used in ambulatory clinics serving active duty and retired personnel and their dependents. Care of the war veterans with post-traumatic stress disorder, amputation, and multiple rehabilitation needs, along with integration into the community, is ongoing and essential (Military Health System, 2018). APHNs use their skills with needs assessment and program planning/evaluation to develop programs aimed at improving the health of the aggregate military population. In 2016, the U.S. Department of

Veterans Affairs (VA) granted full practice authority to NPs (U.S. Department of Veterans Affairs, 2016).

Public Health Departments. Public health departments are increasingly employing advanced practice nurses with master's degrees. These APHNs and NPs have administrative and clinical skills to work collaboratively with physicians and to manage and implement clinical services provided by the health departments. Home care and hospice services are nursing sections in many public health departments and require the services of population-oriented nurse clinical specialists.

Health departments also provide primary care services in well-child clinics, family planning clinics, and general adult primary health care clinics. A public health department uses NPs and APHNs, depending on the size of the department, the department's health priorities in the community, and financial constraints.

APHNs possess basic competencies for responding to disasters whether the health threats are natural, intentional, or technological (mass casualty incidents, unfolding infectious disease outbreaks, bioterrorism, or evolving environmental disasters). APHNs are well positioned to collaborate with leaders of the community to develop and implement systems-level preparedness and response plans for populations before, during, and after an event (Aiken, 2011; University of Michigan Center of Excellence, 2013).

CHECK YOUR PRACTICE

You have recently graduated from the BSN program at the local university. You have accepted a position as a school nurse and you are going to be working with an advanced practice public health nurse. What is the difference in your practice in the school system and the APHNs? Where will you go to find the differences in practice in your state? What do you see as your role in improving the health of the population of school children?

Schools. School health nursing, discussed in Chapter 42, involves comprehensive assessment and management of care, with emphasis on health education, to promote healthy behaviors in children and their families. Innovative practice occurs in school nursing (RWJF, 2013). APHNs and NPs are employed as school health nurses by school boards or county health departments to provide specific services to schools, such as confirming that immunization status is current; performing hearing and vision screenings; and providing many organizational, community assessment, and political functions. School-based health services are staffed by APHNs and/or nurses prepared as school, pediatric, or family nurse practitioners. Services provided by these advanced nurse practitioners include not only basic health screening but also monitoring of children with chronic health problems and finding health care for children with limited access to medical care. The nurses work collaboratively with parents, community leaders, educators, and physicians to ensure that each child within the school community receives needed services. APHNs and NPs are well suited to manage school health services if they meet specific criteria developed by individual states.

Other Arenas

Home Health Agencies. Major legislative changes in Medicare and third-party reimbursement for hospital services resulted in unprecedented growth in the home health care industry through the 1990s. Home health care is less expensive than extended hospital care and thus is an attractive option for third-party payers (Riggs et al., 2011). In addition, equipment and drug companies are developing products for home use, physicians and hospitals are exploring the development of home services, and consumers are demanding more services. Advanced practice nurses have traditionally been involved in home care in many capacities. Because of their knowledge and skills in the following areas, APHNs and NPs are well qualified to provide home health care that yields positive outcomes for clients and their families. Home health APNs engage in holistic health assessments and coordinate services with an interprofessional team for clients with complex health needs; are involved in coaching, consultation, evaluating, and using research findings; provide leadership in both the clinical and professional arenas; and collaborate interprofessionally to accomplish client goals and outcomes (Levin et al., 2013). The role of the nurse in home health is discussed in Chapter 41.

Many APNs today are practicing in telehealth environments. Telehealth is the practice of health care delivery, diagnosis, consultation, treatment, and transfer of medical data and education using interactive video, visual, audio, and data telecommunication (Kvedar et al., 2014).

Correctional Institutions. Residents of prisons and jails are a population with health needs that are met by APHNs and NPs. APHNs are an asset within prison systems, planning and implementing coordinated health programs that include health education as well as health services. Where personnel resources are limited, APHNs provide health education and counseling for inmates and/or their families to prepare prison clients for going back into the community on their release. NPs often practice in on-site health clinics at correctional institutions, providing both primary care services and health education programs (Almost et al., 2013).

ISSUES AND CONCERNS

Legal Status

The legal authority of nurses in advanced practice is determined by each state's nurse practice act and, in some states, by additional rules and regulations for practice (Phillips, 2017). In the 1970s, regulations for the direct care role performed by NPs, including diagnosis and treatment, were less defined in state nursing laws than they are today, and the legal status of NPs was being questioned. Since 1971, when Idaho revised its nurse practice act to include the practice of NPs, all 50 states have amended their nurse practice acts or revised their definitions of nursing to reflect the new nursing roles. NPs are regulated by their state boards of nursing through specific regulations (Phillips, 2017). Legislative authority to prescribe has changed dramatically in the last several years. By 2002, NPs in all states (including the District of Columbia) had prescriptive authority, some with independent authority to prescribe and some dependent on physician collaboration (Phillips, 2017).

Reimbursement

The third-party reimbursement system in the United States, both public and private, is complicated. To practice independently or work collaboratively with physicians, NPs need to be reimbursed adequately. Because states regulate the insurance industry, available third-party private reimbursement depends in large part on state statute. Advanced practice nurses want direct access to third-party payers. The most common mechanism by which NPs get access to direct payment is through benefits-required laws. Laws also include the right to practice without being discriminated against by another provider or a health care agency (Phillips, 2014).

The Rural Health Clinic Services Act of 1977 (PL 95-210) was the first breakthrough in third-party reimbursement for nurses in primary care roles (Box 39.2). The law authorized Medicare and Medicaid reimbursement to qualified rural clinics for services provided by NPs and PAs, regardless of the presence of a physician (Wasem, 1990). The intent of the act was to improve access to health care in some of the nation's underserved rural areas; however, its use from state to state has varied dramatically. Recent legislative changes to include the coverage of services by certified nurse midwives, clinical psychologists, and social workers have improved the effectiveness of the Rural Health Clinic Services Act for reimbursement options.

In 1989, Congress mandated reimbursement for services furnished to needy Medicaid clients by a certified family nurse practitioner or certified pediatric nurse practitioner, whether or not under the supervision of a physician. With the 1997 passing of the Balanced Budget Act, NPs were directly reimbursed, regardless of geographic setting, at 85 percent of physician pay (if the service is covered under Medicare part B) (Pearson, 1998).

BOX 39.2 Landmark U.S. Legislation for Advanced Practice Nurses

- 1977: Rural Health Clinic Services Act authorized NP and PA services to be directly reimbursed when provided in a rural area.
- 1989: As part of the Omnibus Budget Reconciliation Act (OBRA), Congress recognized NPs as direct providers of services to residents of nursing homes.
- 1990: Congress established a new Medicare benefit through federally qualified health centers, where services of NPs are directly reimbursed when provided in these centers.
- 1997: Passage of the Balanced Budget Act of 1997 (PL 105-33). NPs are now be directly reimbursed, regardless of geographic setting, at 85 percent of physician pay (if the service is covered under Medicare part B).
- 2003: Individuals applying for Medicare provider numbers, such as NPs, must possess a master's degree from an NP program, as well as national certification and state licensure.
- 2010: Passage of the Patient Protection and Affordable Care Act. As a result, there will be a higher demand for primary care providers, such as NPs, with an emphasis on prevention, chronic care management, and cost-effective quality care.

NP, Nurse practitioner; *PA,* physician assistant.

Since January 1, 2003, individuals applying for Medicare provider numbers as NPs must possess a master's degree from an NP program, as well as national certification and state licensure. Once an NP has a provider number, he or she submits bills, using the standard government form, to the local Medicare insurance carrier agency for each visit or procedure.

Institutional Privileges

NPs in the community are more concerned than APHNs about **institutional privileges**. Historically, NPs experienced difficulty in obtaining hospital privileges within institutions where their patients are admitted. However, with the broadening scope of practice and professional responsibilities, more nurse practitioners are obtaining hospital privileges (often referred to as credentialing). An application process is generally required and reviewed by a credentialing board typically composed of physicians, administrators, and in some cases advanced practice providers (NPs, PAs). The criteria for nurse practitioners wishing to obtain hospital privileges vary by hospital and state; however, most hospitals require that nurse practitioners have national certification.

Employment and Role Negotiation

For APHNs and NPs to collaboratively provide comprehensive primary health care, they must understand and develop negotiating skills. Positive working relationships with health professionals, organizations, and clients require role negotiation, particularly when few guidelines exist for a role or a role is new and undeveloped. APHNs and NPs need to assess the internal politics of the organization as part of their role negotiation. Networking is another necessary skill. Forums, joint conferences, collaborative practice, and research provide opportunities to expand their functions.

Because APHNs and NPs in some locations often seek employment, as opposed to being sought by employers, assertiveness is needed. Increased financial constraints have reduced the number of job opportunities. APHNs and NPs should feel comfortable about marketing their skills. Marketing strategies should be designed to project an image that shows a nurse's individual achievement. In assessing and analyzing the needs of target markets, nurses must consider professional and institutional goals, and the target client group's goals. Methods of obtaining positions and negotiating future roles include providing **portfolios** of credentialed documents and samples of professional accomplishments such as audiovisual materials, program plans, and evaluations conducted, client education packets, and history and physical assessment tools developed. Portfolios are physical packets or web-based files that contain all these documents to showcase the nurse's abilities. APHNs and NPs should keep current portfolios containing examples of their professional activities. Names, addresses, and telephone numbers of professional and personal references should be furnished in the portfolios (but only after the referring persons have granted permission). In an electronic portfolio, or e-portfolio, information is housed on the Internet and is easily updated and shared/transmitted to employers and others. Many websites provide e-portfolio management and services, such as Decision Critical website (https://www.healthstream.com/).

ROLE STRESS

Factors causing stress for advanced practice nurses include legal issues (as discussed previously), **professional isolation**, **liability**, collaborative practice, conflicting expectations, and professional responsibilities. APHNs and NPs want to identify self-care strategies to cope with predictable stressors, some of which are discussed here.

Professional Isolation

Professional isolation is a source of conflict for APHNs and NPs. Because they practice across all age groups, APHNs and NPs are likely to be hired in remote practice employment sites. Rural communities unable to support a physician, for example, find the NP an affordable and logical alternative for primary care services. The autonomy of practice in these sites attracts many APHNs and NPs, who fail to consider the disadvantages of isolated practice. Long drives, long hours, lack of social and cultural activities, and lack of opportunity for professional development are often experienced by these rural practitioners. These sources of stress, which leads to job dissatisfaction, can be reduced or eliminated by negotiating the employment contract to include educational and personal leaves.

Liability

All nurses are liable for their actions. Because more legal action is appearing in the judicial system, specifically concerning NPs, the importance of liability and/or malpractice insurance cannot be overemphasized (AANP, 2018b). Although malpractice insurance is not required to function as an APHN or an NP, most nurses carry their own liability insurance. It is in the best interest of APHNs and NPs to thoroughly investigate the coverage offered by various companies rather than to assume that the coverage is adequate. Practitioners who function without a physician on site are particularly vulnerable. The scope of individual APHN and NP authority determines the liability standards applied. The limits of each practitioner's authority are legislated by individual states (Phillips, 2017).

Interprofessional Collaborative Practice

The future of APHNs and NPs depends on whether they make a recognized difference in the health of families and communities, and on their ability to practice collaboratively with physicians. **Interprofessional collaborative practice** defines a peer relationship with mutual trust and respect. Working out a collaborative practice takes a considerable amount of time and energy. Until such practice relationships evolve within joint practice situations, the quality health care that nursing and medicine collaboratively provides will not be achieved. The arrangement demands the professional maturity to work together without territorial disputes, and the structure and philosophy of the organization must support joint practice as a mechanism for health care delivery. The growing pains of establishing such a practice produce stress for all involved; however, the results and benefits to clients and professionals are worth the effort (Interprofessional Education Collaborative Expert Panel, 2011).

Interprofessional collaborative practice for APHNs and NPs involves more disciplines than just medicine. Advanced practice nurses work with baccalaureate-prepared nurses and other nurses, social workers, public health professionals, nutritionists, occupational and physical therapists, and community leaders and members to meet their goals for the health of individuals, families, groups, and communities. To work toward the *Healthy People 2020* objectives, collaboration of multidisciplinary groups is essential. APHNs, NPs, and baccalaureate-prepared nurses provides leadership in attaining this collaborative effort.

Conflicting Expectations

Services provided by APHNs and NPs in health promotion and maintenance are often more time consuming and complex than just the management of clients' health problems. APHNs and NPs frequently experience conflict between their professional practice goals in health promotion and the need to see a required number of clients to maintain the worksite's financial goals. The problem is worsened if a facility administrator or physician views APHNs and NPs only as medical extenders and limits reimbursement to the nurse provider. A practice model that assists nurses in including health promotion and maintenance activities as well as medical case management into each client visit uses (1) flexible scheduling, (2) health maintenance flow sheets, and (3) problem-oriented recording with nursing goals and plans prominently displayed in the health record. For APHNs, program planning and evaluation based on systematic needs assessments conducted with communities are methods to show the needs and benefits of health promotion/disease prevention. Being an educator and role model in carrying out *Healthy People 2020* objectives emphasizes the importance of health promotion and disease prevention in the health care system.

Professional Responsibilities

Professional responsibilities contribute to role stress. Most states require APHNs and NPs in expanded roles to be nationally certified and to maintain certification. Recertification requires documentation of continuing education hours with composition of subject matter defined by the certifying body and often requires a prescribed minimum number of work hours in certification specialty. There are not many nurse practitioners in an area, and continuing education may not be locally available and requires travel and lodging expenses in addition to time away from the practice site. Anticipating professional responsibilities and travel expenses in financial planning decreases these concerns. Negotiating contracts with the employer for educational leave and expenses helps divert financial stress.

Quality of client care, however, cannot be measured or ensured by continuing education or the nurse's credentials.

Professional responsibility includes monitoring one's own practice according to standards established by the profession and protocols, if used, and a personal feeling of responsibility to the community. Continuous quality improvement is another professional responsibility for APHNs and NPs. This process should evaluate need, cost, and effectiveness of care in relation to client outcomes (Kelly et al., 2014).

TRENDS IN ADVANCED PRACTICE NURSING

Advanced practice nurses are prominent in multiple health care arenas today, and this is unlikely to change in the future (National Advisory Council, 2016; Van Vleet & Paradise, 2015). With the goals of the Patient Protection and Affordable Care Act (PPACA, 2010) and *Healthy People 2020* objectives, a substantial need for health care providers exists. The prominence of interprofessional education and practice, along with team-based and patient-centered care, is congruent with the PPACA and *Healthy People 2020*. APHNs and NPs have the knowledge and skills base to lead the health care team in both individual- and population-based outcomes in prevention and population health.

APHNs and NPs, in collaboration with nurses, community agencies and members, and other disciplines, have the potential to make an impact on health promotion and disease prevention at the individual, family, group, and community levels. Population-focused APHNs and NPs are in excellent positions to use the *Healthy People 2020* National Health Promotion and Disease Prevention objectives and the Healthy People in Healthy Communities model in planning their advanced practice nursing interventions

QSEN FOCUS ON QUALITY AND SAFETY EDUCATION FOR NURSES

The Advanced Practice Nurse in the Community

Targeted Competency: Informatics

Use information and technology to communicate, manage knowledge, mitigate error, and support decision making.

Important aspects of informatics include:

- **Knowledge:** Describe examples of how technology and information management are related to the quality and safety of patient care.
- **Skills:** Use information management tools to monitor outcomes of care processes.
- **Attitudes:** Value nurses' involvement in design, selection, implementation, and evaluation of information technologies to support patient care.

Informatics Question

You are an adult/geriatric NP who has just been hired at a nursing center, where that targeted patient population is patients over the age of 65, covered by Medicare insurance. Because your nursing center provides primary care for a substantial portion of your community's Medicare population, you have been approached by the local hospital and home care agency to help them track ED visits (not resulting in admission) and hospital readmission rates, within 30 days of a hospitalization.

- What data points will you want to track to establish a preintervention baseline for these data?
- Assuming you are involved in developing an educational module for at-risk patients, families, and home care nurses, what data points will you want to track after implementing this educational module?
- Which EHR (hospital, home care, nursing center) might contain these data points?
- How might you envision shared documentation/communication among the hospital, home care agency, and nursing center to effectively manage the targeted patients?

ED, Emergency department; *EHR,* electronic health record; *NP,* nurse practitioner.
Prepared by Gail Armstrong, PhD, DNP, ACNS-BC, CNE, Associate Professor, University of Colorado Denver College of Nursing.

LINKING CONTENT TO PRACTICE

In this chapter, emphasis is placed on the role of the advanced public health nurse (APHN) in the community and how advanced nursing practice relates to the generalist public health nurse. The Community/Public Health Nursing Competencies (Quad Council Coalition, 2018) were developed by four organizations:

Alliance of Nurses for Healthy Environments (AHNE)
Association of Community Health Nursing Educators (ACHNE)
Association of Public Health Nurses (APHN)
American Public Health Association—Public Health Nursing Section (APHA-PHN)

The competencies are categorized into eight domains and are applied to three tiers of community/public health nursing practice:

- Tier 1: Generalist community/public health nurses (C/PHN) who carry out day-to-day functions in community organizations or state and local public health organizations, including clinical, home visiting, and population-based services, and who are not in management positions
- Tier 2: Community/public health nurses with an array of program implementation, management, and/or supervisory responsibilities, including responsibility for clinical services, home visiting, and community-based and population-focused programs
- Tier 3: Community/public health nurses at an executive/senior management level and leadership levels in public health or community organizations

The domains are core areas of analytic and assessment skills, policy development/program planning, communication, cultural competency, community dimensions of practice, public health science, financial planning, evaluation and management, and leadership and systems thinking skills (Quad Council Coalition, 2018). The latter tiers include a higher-level mastery of skills and competencies. As an example, their fifth domain, Community Dimensions of Practice Skills, lists a Tier 1 competency as use formal and informal relational networks among community organizations and systems conducive to improving the health of individuals, families, and groups within communities; a Tier 2 competency as use formal and informal relational networks among community organizations and systems conducive to improving the health within programs, communities, and populations; and a Tier 3 competency as create internal and external organizational relationships, processes, and system improvements to enhance the health of populations (QCC, 2018). The Tier 2 and Tier 3 competencies/skills are clearly consistent with the APHN role and are at an advanced mastery level. This is in contrast to the generalist/staff public health nurse, where the expected level of performance mastery for this domain is more at providing care for individuals, families, and groups. Thus if an agency planned to conduct health education programs within a community, the APHN would take leadership roles in developing, implementing, and evaluating a needs assessment and interacting with community stakeholders to assist with conducting the health education programs that would be most relevant and accessible to the community.

PRACTICE APPLICATION

APHN

Martha Corley is an APHN who coordinates the aftercare services for a community hospital's early discharge clients. Martha has worked with the nursing staff to develop a nursing history form to identify family and social supports available to clients who are likely to need nursing or supportive care for a limited time after discharge. With this and additional information from head nurses, Martha visits selected clients to begin discharge planning. She consults with each client and family to validate assessed needs. The physician is also consulted about medical therapies to be continued at home. Martha has access to nurses and other resources throughout the community that accept cases on contract. She outlines the initial care plan with nurse case managers assigned to the client and receives regular progress reports. An essential aspect of her practice is to evaluate outcomes of her interventions.

Which of the following is the best example of evaluation of Martha's nursing care?

A. Assessment of client and family satisfaction with her services
B. Reported medical complications of her caseload
C. Review of related literature about home care programs
D. Collected data on hospital readmissions of her clients

Case 2: Family Nurse Practitioner

Answers can be found on the Evolve site.

KEY POINTS

- Changes in the health care system and nursing have occurred in the past few decades because of a shift in society's demands and needs.
- Trends such as a shift of health care from institution-based sites to the community, an increase in technology, self-care, cost-containment measures, accountability, third-party reimbursement, and demands for humanizing technical care have influenced the new roles of the APHN and NP.
- Educational preparation of the APHN has always been at the graduate level, whereas this has not been true of the NP; however, there are implications that both the APHN and NP have educational preparation at the Doctor of Nursing Practice level.
- Specialty certification began through the ANA in 1976 for NPs, and through the ANCC in 1990 for APHNs but is no longer available. It is not required for APHN practice at this time.
- The major role functions of the APHN and NP in community health are clinician, consultant, administrator, researcher, and educator; typically, the NP spends a greater amount of time in direct care clinical activities and less time in indirect activities than the APHN.
- Major arenas for practice for APHNs and NPs in community health include primary care practice, institutional settings, industry, government, public health agencies, schools, home health, correctional health, nursing centers, retail clinics, and health ministry settings.
- Legal status, reimbursement, institutional privileges, and role negotiation are important issues and concerns to nurses who practice in an advanced role in public health nursing.
- Major stressors for APHNs and NPs include professional isolation, liability, collaborative practice, conflicting expectations, and professional responsibilities.
- The use of *Healthy People 2020* objectives is important in emphasizing health promotion and disease prevention in advanced practice nursing and in improving the health of the nation.

CLINICAL DECISION-MAKING ACTIVITIES

1. Explore the development of the APHN and NP in the community. Give details about the differences in the roles.
2. Investigate graduate programs in public health in a state or region to determine the requirements for admission, the type of degree awarded, and whether or not APHN and/or NP preparation is available. Do the similarities and differences make sense to you? Why?
3. Review your state's nurse practice act and any rules and regulations governing advanced practice roles. Are rules different for APHNs and NPs? Give examples.
4. Negotiate a clinical observation experience with an APHN and a NP in community and public health and compare and contrast their roles. Discuss the roles as you see them with the APHN and NP. When you consider your thoughts about the roles, have you considered what the APHN and NP have told you about their roles? How has their input changed your views?

ADDITIONAL RESOURCES

EVOLVE WEBSITE

http://evolve.elsevier.com/Stanhope/community/

- Answers to Practice Application
- Case Study
- Glossary
- Review Questions

REFERENCES

Administration on Aging: *A Profile of Older Americans*, 2017. Retrieved from https://www.acl.gov.

Almost J, Doran D, Ogilvie L, et al: Exploring work-life issues in correctional settings, *J Forensic Nurs* 9:3–13, 2013.

American Association of Colleges of Nursing (AACN): *The essentials of doctoral education for advanced practice nursing*, Washington, DC, 2006, AACN.

American Association of Colleges of Nursing (AACN): *The essentials of master's education in nursing*, Washington, DC, 2011, AACN.

American Association of Colleges of Nursing (AACN): *DNP Fact Sheet*, 2017. Retrieved from http://www.aacnnursing.org.

American Association of Colleges of Nursing (AACN): *AACN Announces CDC Funding Opportunities in Population Health AACN and CDC Partner to Advance the Public Health Nursing Workforce*, 2018a. Retrieved from http://www.aacnnursing.org.

American Association of Colleges of Nursing (AACN): *Clinical Nurse Leader*, 2018b. Retrieved from http://www.aacnnursing.org.

American Association of Colleges of Nursing (AACN): *The Doctor of Nursing Practice: Current Issues and Clarifying Recommendations Report from the Task Force on the Implementation of the DNP*, August 2015. Retrieved from http://www.aacnnursing.org.

American Association of Nurse Practitioners (AANP): *Certification*, 2018a. Retrieved from http://www.aanpcert.org.

American Association of Nurse Practitioners (AANP): *State Practice Environment*, 2018b. Retrieved from https://www.aanp.org.

American Nurses Association (ANA): *Faith community nursing: Scope and standards of practice*, Washington, DC, 2017, ANA.

American Nurses Association (ANA): *Public health nursing: scope and standards of practice*, ed 2, Washington, DC, 2013, ANA.

American Nurses Association (ANA): *Recognition of a Nursing Specialty, Approval of a Specialty Nursing, Scope of Practice Statement, Acknowledgment of Specialty Nursing Standards of Practice, and affirmation of Focused Practice Competencies*, 2017. Retrieved from https://www.nursingworld.org.

American Nurses Credentialing Center (ANCC): *Advanced practice certification information*, Washington, DC, 2018, ANA. Retrieved from https://www.nursingworld.org.

American Public Health Association (APHA), Public Health Nursing Section: *The definition and practice of public health nursing*, Washington, DC, 2013, APHA, Public Health Nursing Section.

American Nurses Association: *Scope of practice*, 2018. Retrieved from https://www.nursingworld.org.

American Association of Occupational Health Nurses (AAOHN). *Becoming certified*, 2018. Retrieved from http://aaohn.org.

Association of Community Health Nursing Educators (ACHNE): *Graduate education for advanced practice in community/public health nursing: at the crossroads*, Latham, NY, 2007, ACHNE.

Centers for Disease Control and Prevention (CDC): *Preventive Health Care Guidelines*, 2018. Retrieved from http://www.cdc.gov.

Auerbach DI, Martsolf GR, Pearson ML, et al: The DNP by 2015: A Study of the Institutional, Political, and Professional Issues that Facilitate or Impede Establishing a Post-Baccalaureate Doctor of Nursing Practice Program, *Rand Health Q* 5:3, 2015.

Commission on Nurse Certification: *Clinical nurse leader career resource guide*, Washington, DC, 2018, AACN. Retrieved from http://www.aacnnursing.org.

Donald F, Martin-Misener R, Carter N, et al: A systematic review of the effectiveness of advanced practice nurses in long-term care, *J Adv Nurs* 69:2148–2161, 2013.

Drennan J: Master's in nursing degrees: an evaluation of management and leadership outcomes using a retrospective pre-test design, *J Nurs Manage* 20:102–112, 2012.

Flinter M, Hsu C, Cromp D, et al: Registered Nurses in Primary Care: Emerging New Roles and Contributions to Team-Based Care in High-Performing Practices, *J Ambul Care Manage*, 40(4):287–296, 2017.

Ford LC: Nurses, Nurse Practitioners: The Evolution of Primary Care [book review], *Image J Nurs Scholar* 18:177, 1986.

Foster J, Clark AP, Heye ML, et al: Differentiating the CNS and CNL roles, *Nurs Manage* 42:51–54, 2011.

Gauld R, Blank R, Burgers J, et al. The World Health Report 2008 – Primary Healthcare: How Wide Is the Gap between Its Agenda and Implementation in 12 High-Income Health Systems? *Healthcare Policy* 7(3):38–58, 2012.

Harne-Britner S, Schafer D: Clinical nurse specialists driving research and practice through research roundtables, *Clin Nurse Spec* 23:305–308, 2009.

Institute of Medicine: *Who will keep the public health?* Washington, DC, 2003, National Academies Press.

Institute of Medicine: *The future of nursing: leading change, advancing health*, Washington, DC, 2011, National Academies Press.

Institute of Medicine (US): *Committee on the Robert Wood Johnson Foundation initiative on the future of nursing, at the institute of medicine*, Washington, DC, 2011, National Academies Press (US).

Interprofessional Education Collaborative Expert Panel: *Core competencies for interprofessional collaborative practice: report of an expert panel*, Washington, DC, 2011, Interprofessional Education Collaborative.

Issel LM, Bekemeier B, Baldwin KA: Three population-patient care outcome indicators for public health nursing: results of a consensus project, *Public Health Nurs* 28:24–34, 2011.

Ketefian S, Redman RW. A critical examination of developments in nursing doctoral education in the United States, *Revista Latino-Americana de Enfermagem*, 23(3):363–371, 2015.

Kleinpell R, Scanlon A, Hibbert D, et al. Addressing Issues Impacting Advanced Nursing Practice Worldwide, *OJIN: Online J Issues Nurs* 19(2), May 31, 2014.

Kvedar J, Coye MJ, Everett W: Connected health: a review of technologies and strategies to improve patient care with telemedicine and telehealth, *Health Aff (Millwood)* 33:194–199, 2014.

Laurant M, Reeves D, Hermens R, et al: Featured review: Nurses as substitutes for doctors in primary care, *Cochrane Database Syst Rev*, Hoboken, New Jersey, July 2018, John Wiley and Sons.

Levin PF, Swider SM, Breakwell S, et al: Embracing a competency-based specialty curriculum for community-based nursing roles, *Public Health Nurs* 30:557–565, 2013.

Mohr LD, Coke LA. Distinguishing the Clinical Nurse Specialist from other Graduate Nursing Roles, *Clin Nurse Spec* 32(3):139–151, 2018.

National Advisory Council on Nurse Education and Practice: *Preparing nurses for new roles in population health management*, USDHHS, HRSA, 2016. Retrieved from http://www.hrsa.gov.

National Association of Clinical Nurse Specialists: *History*, 2018. Retrieved from http://nacns.org.

National Nursing Centers Consortium: *NNCC: Nurse-Led Care Policy*, 2018. Retrieved from https://nurseledcare.org.

Patient Protection and Affordable Care Act, Public Law No. 111-148, Section 2702, 124 Stat 119, 318–319, 2010.

Phillips SJ: 29th Annual APRN Legislative Update, *Nurse Pract* 42(1):18–46, 2017.

Quad Council of Public Health Nursing Organizations: *Quad Council Public Health Nursing Competencies*, 2018. Retrieved from http://www.quadcouncilphn.org.

RAND Corporation: *The evolving role of retail clinics*, Santa Monica, CA, 2016. Retrieved from https://www.rand.org.

Riggs JS, Madigan EA, Fortinsky RH: Home health nursing visit intensity and heart failure patient outcomes, *Home Health Care Manag Pract* 23:412–420, 2011.

Robert Wood Johnson Foundation: *CATALYSTS FOR CHANGE Harnessing the Power of Nurses to Build Population Health in the 21st Century*, 2017. Retrieved from https://www.rwjf.org.

Robert Wood Johnson Foundation: *School Nurse Shortage May Imperil Some Children, RWJF Scholars Warn*, December 12, 2013. Retrieved from http://www.RWJF.org.

Roberts ST: Parish nursing: providing spiritual, physical, and emotional care in a small community parish, *Clin Nurs Studies* 2: 118–122, 2014.

Silver HK, Ford LC, Stearly SA: A program to increase health care for children: the pediatric nurse practitioner program, *Pediatrics* 39:756, 1967.

University of Michigan Center of Excellence in Public Health Workforce Studies: *Enumeration and characterization of the public health nurse workforce: findings of the 2012 public health workforce surveys*, Ann Arbor, MI, 2013, University of Michigan.

Van Vleet A, Paradise J: *Tapping Nurse Practitioners to Meet Rising Demand for Primary Care*, Jan 20, 2015, Kaiser Family Foundation. Retrieved from http://www. KFF.org.

Military Health System: *Access to health care*, 2018. Retrieved from https://www.health.mil.

U.S. Department of Veterans Affairs: *VA Grants Full Practice Authority to Advance Practice Registered Nurses*, 2016. Retrieved from https://www.va.gov.

U.S. Department of Health, Education, and Welfare: *Extending the scope of nursing practice*, Washington, DC, 1971, U.S. Government Printing Office.

U.S. Department of Health and Human Services, Agency for Healthcare Research and Quality, U.S. Preventive Services Task Force (USDHHS/AHRQ/USPSTF): *The Guide to Clinical Preventive Services*, 2014. Retrieved from https://www.ahrq.gov.

U.S. Department of Health and Human Services (USDHHS): *Healthy People 2020*, Washington, DC, 2018a, U.S. Government Printing Office. Retrieved from https://www.healthypeople.gov.

U.S. Department of Health and Human Services (USDHHS): *National Health Service Corps About us*, 2018b. Retrieved from https://nhsc.hrsa.gov.

Wallen J, Davidson SM, Epstein D, Connelly JP: Nonphysician health care providers in pediatrics, *Paediatrician* 11(3-4). 225–239, 1982.

Wasem C: The Rural Health Clinic Services Act: a sleeping giant of reimbursement, *J Am Acad Nurse Pract* 2:85–87, 1990.

Wood C, Wettlaufer J, Shaha SH, et al: Nurse practitioner roles in pediatric emergency departments: a national survey, *Pediatr Emerg Care* 26:406–407, 2010.

40

The Nurse Leader in the Community

*Lisa M. Turner, PhD, RN, PHCNS-BC**

OBJECTIVES

After reading this chapter, the student should be able to do the following:

1. Explain why nurses need effective leadership, management, and consultation skills in today's public health care environment.
2. Explore what is meant by partnership and interprofessional practice and describe how these concepts are related to nursing leadership, management, and consultation.
3. Analyze what is meant by systems thinking in community-based and public health settings.
4. Describe the major competencies required to be effective as a nurse leader, manager, and consultant in community-based and public health settings.
5. Examine nursing leadership strategies to enhance client safety and reduce health care errors in community settings.
6. Explain how nurses provide leadership in care coordination in the community.

CHAPTER OUTLINE

Major Trends and Issues
Definitions
Leadership and Management Applied to Population-Focused Nursing
Consultation
Competencies for Nurse Leaders
Future of Nursing Leadership

KEY TERMS

alliances, p. 887
budget, p. 893
business plan, p. 892
coaching, p. 891
coalitions, p. 887
collaborative, p. 882
complex adaptive systems, p. 884
conflict resolution, p. 892
consultation, p. 883
consultation contract, p. 886
contracting, p. 886
cost-effectiveness analysis, p. 893
delegation, p. 888
distribution effects, p. 884
empowerment, p. 888
external consultant, p. 885
internal consultant, p. 887
leadership, p. 882
learning organizations, p. 884
managed care organizations, p. 881
management, p. 882
microsystems, p. 884
negotiation, p. 886
partnerships, p. 881
political skills, p. 882
power dynamics, p. 892
process model consultation, p. 885
seamless system of care, p. 881
service delivery networks, p. 881
supervision, p. 891
systems thinking, p. 884
variance analysis, p. 893
vertical integration, p. 881

*Dr. Turner would like to acknowledge the author of this chapter in edition 8 of the text, Dr. Juliann G. Sebastian, PhD, RN, FAAN, for her many contributions that continue to appear in this chapter.

The profession of nursing has consistently ranked highly in public surveys as the most trusted profession (Gallup Inc., 2017). As such, the general public looks to nurses to act as leaders, providing guidance on health care choices. With nearly three million nurses employed in the United States (Bureau of Labor Statistics [BLS], 2018), the nursing profession has the potential to greatly influence the health of the nation. It is therefore imperative that nurses understand how to be leaders, not only with their professional colleagues, but also within their communities. Leadership as a role for nurses began to emerge as the profession became more structured in the mid-1800s, moving from a loosely defined trade to an organized, educated profession (Forrester, 2016). Florence Nightingale (1912), the founder of modern nursing, devoted a chapter in her book, *Notes on Nursing,* to what she called "petty management," defining the importance of a nurse being able to think critically, act proactively, and take charge of a situation in an efficient manner, all essential leadership skills. Since then, the concept of nursing leadership has evolved to include such qualities as developing relationships, facilitating communication between individuals and groups, providing guidance and direction, inspiring groups and organizations, and demonstrating vision (Huber, 2018). Agencies, localities, and professional organizations increasingly recognize the need for effective leadership in public health and community life.

Population-focused nurses have a responsibility to provide leadership in creating a new future for healthier communities. Members of the public ask whether better approaches to health care delivery might be developed that will ensure that all people around the world live in health-promoting communities and have access to quality health care as well as to health promotion and illness prevention services. Population-focused nurses practice in a variety of settings, including public health departments, community-based clinics, occupational health settings, schools, and **managed care organizations**. Leadership, management, and consulting skills are important to the success of client outcomes that depend heavily on cost-effective, efficient delivery of care. Care coordination and managing care transitions throughout the community, including acute and long-term care settings, are important to promoting a healthy community. Nurses need effective skills in communication, negotiation, and interprofessional practice and good leadership, management, and consultation skills, even if they do not have formal positions as managers or consultants.

Nurses must focus attention not only on the populations that are served by their organizations but also on those that are not. Because they concern themselves with the total public, their focus is always on the future and on the interacting factors that influence the health of the public. Nurses work with partnerships of community members and community organizations. **Partnerships** can be complex and require time and thoughtful attention. This chapter examines the roles and functions of nurse leaders, managers, and consultants in the twenty-first century. It emphasizes nursing leadership in public health and community-based nursing practice, personnel management, and consultation with groups and individuals.

MAJOR TRENDS AND ISSUES

Ensuring client safety and quality of care, performing evidence-based practice, eliminating disparities in health care access and outcomes, and focusing on consumer participation in and satisfaction with care are key trends in health care.

The Institute of Medicine (IOM) (2000) report titled *To Err Is Human* focused attention on the incidence of health care errors. The IOM (2001) followed this report with another one, titled *Crossing the Quality Chasm,* which offered strategies for improving the health care system. The most recent report from the IOM (2015a), titled *Improving Diagnosis in Health Care*, is a continuation of the previous landmark reports, brings attention to the need to address the occurrence of diagnostic errors to improve quality and safety in health care. The issue of reducing health care errors continues to be a topic of interest for health leaders. A 2016 study conducted by patient safety experts at Johns Hopkins found that medical errors are the third leading cause of death in the United States, noting that most of the errors represent systemic problems, including poorly coordinated care, fragmented insurance networks, the absence or underuse of safety nets, and other protocols, in addition to unwarranted variation in physician practice patterns that lack accountability (Makary & Daniel, 2016). This is a concern in the community just as in hospitals and long-term care agencies. For example, studies show that older adults living in the community are at high risk for medication errors. Sometimes this is because they are taking high-risk medications, or because they cannot read instructions for medications, or because of medication complexity (polypharmacy) and not understanding how to take medications that have been prescribed for them (Hanlon et al., 2017; Miller et al., 2017; Shade et al., 2017).

Evidence-based practice is another trend important for public health nurses. Basing clinical practice patterns and community programs on research and other forms of evidence such as best practice data is a key strategy for ensuring high-quality care. One example of evidence-based practice in a community setting is examining the impact of community-based nurse-led clinics (Randall et al., 2017). In this systematic review, the researchers evaluated the impact nurse-led clinics have on patient outcomes, patient satisfaction, patient access to services, and cost-effectiveness. The researchers concluded that the nurse-led clinics have shown a positive impact on each of the study variables, with mixed results on cost-effectiveness.

The health system in some local areas has been reorganized to provide a full continuum of services in a **seamless system of care**. Large, vertically integrated systems are able to do this. **Vertical integration** means that the system owns all of the services that clients might need (e.g., clinics, hospitals, and home health agencies). In other cases, free-standing agencies collaborate and contract with one another to achieve seamlessness. The goal is to reduce fragmentation, which should be helpful for vulnerable populations. Nurses coordinate clients' care across agencies, but this new trend in the health care system places added emphasis on relationships, such as alliances, agency partnerships, joint programs, and participation in **service delivery networks** (Allen, 2017; Berry et al., 2013).

Nurses actively participate in these groups and need good negotiating and **political skills** to be effective.

Another important trend is related to the movement toward more community partnerships (Cutts et al., 2017; Johnston & Finegood, 2015). Partnerships with community members and community agencies are essential to effective public and community health practice. The public has an increasing interest in becoming involved in planning for health services and in being active partners in their own care. Partnerships succeed when strong communication mechanisms are in place to ensure definition of needs and problems, timely problem resolution, and ongoing development of shared visions. In public and community health, the development of shared visions and goals and the operational mechanisms to make those goals a reality is the key to success. Nurses need to be able to listen well and collaborate with lay community members, whose goals and ideas may differ from those of health care professionals. Faith and community partnerships have been effective in reaching underserved populations (Cipriano, 2014). For example, in Harlem, nurses and faith leaders come together to offer health screenings, education, and improve access to health care services through the Community Health Nursing-Faith Based Partnership Program (Cipriano, 2014).

The public is increasingly using the Internet, a wide variety of publications, and lay support groups to obtain health information. People need help deciding which information is good and how best to work with their health care providers to adapt information to their own health profiles. Those with low health literacy (see Chapter 19) need special help in obtaining the health information necessary to be effective partners in health care (Batterham et al., 2016; World Health Organization, 2013).

To know whether an agency is performing as expected, nurses must be familiar with their professional standards of care, the standards held by accrediting bodies, such as The Joint Commission, and guidelines for practice, such as those published by the federal Agency for Healthcare Research and Quality and the U.S. Preventive Services Task Force (2014). Nurse leaders also need to know how to use electronic health records and management information systems to link client outcomes with clinical and administrative processes. Registries are examples of clinical databases dedicated to certain population groups, such as people with cancer, diabetes, injuries, or population groups such as women. Nurses should know how to work with the taxonomies for nursing diagnoses, interventions, and outcomes of nursing actions (Butcher et al., 2019) because these are being included in electronic health records and will help nurses identify changing health needs (Englebright et al., 2014; Gottlieb et al., 2015).

One trend that combines the idea of partnerships with a structured method for rapid performance improvement is the use of collaboratives. A **collaborative** is a group of similar organizations that agree to use common processes for providing clinical care and share certain types of data so all may learn. A well-known example is the Health Care Disparities Collaboratives (HDCs) used by the Federal Bureau of Primary Health Care. The HDCs are a nationwide initiative to improve care for people with chronic conditions (Bureau of Primary Health Care, 2014). Community health centers may apply to participate in HDCs that target certain chronic health problems, such as diabetes or cardiovascular disease.

A major trend in public health is a stronger focus on implementing the core functions of public health and providing the essential services of public health (Council on Linkages Between Academia and Public Health Practice, 2014). Competencies have been identified for generalist public/community health nurses that build on the core function and essential services (Association of Community Health Nurse Educators Education Committee, 2009; Quad Council Coalition Competency Review Task Force, 2018).

EVIDENCE-BASED PRACTICE

Spano-Szekely et al. (2016) examined the relationship between emotional intelligence (EI) and transformational leadership (TL) in nurse managers. Previous nursing studies showed that TL style managers had greater commitment from their followers than other leadership styles and that EI is a potential characteristic of TL managers. The researchers found that EI was significantly positively correlated with TL and with followership outcome measures of extra effort, effectiveness, and satisfaction. EI was significantly negatively correlated with laissez-faire leadership. Furthermore, a positive relationship was found between TL and nurse managers with advanced education and administrative certification.

Nurse Use

Nurse leaders need to consider EI characteristics when hiring nurse managers. Development and improvement of EI skills in nurses may lead to more effective leadership styles.

Spano-Szekely L, Quinn Griffin MT, Clavelle J, et al.: Emotional intelligence and transformational leadership in nurse managers, *J Nurs Admin* 46(2):101-108, 2016.

DEFINITIONS

Leadership can be defined as the process of influence that occurs between a leader and an individual, group, organization, community, or society, often by inspiring, enlivening, and engaging others to participate in the achievement of goals (Weiss & Tappen, 2015). Therefore nursing leadership refers to the influence that nurses exert on improving client health, whether clients are individuals, families, groups, or entire communities. **Management**, on the other hand, focuses on achieving organizational goals by using the managerial tasks of planning, organizing, commanding, coordinating, and motivating employees to work (Weiss & Tappen, 2015). For nurses, these resources might be people, as when a nurse coordinates an interprofessional team, or financial resources. An example of managing financial resources is when a nurse monitors the budget for an immunization program to make sure that personnel time, supplies, and equipment are being used efficiently. Nurses also manage time. For example, home health nurses must manage their time in order to provide clients with direct and indirect nursing services, such as health education and making referrals, respectively.

It is important to point out that leadership and management are two different skills. Leadership sets the direction, and management ensures that goals will be achieved. Nurses must possess strong clinical leadership and management skills to be effective, whether or not they hold management positions.

Consultation in nursing refers to the process that occurs when a nurse works with an individual, group, organization, or community with the specific purpose of assisting them to solve actual or potential problems related to the health status of patients or to the health care organization (Franks, 2014; Ridge, 2015). Clinical consultation increasingly focuses on ways to better coordinate the care delivery process across sites of care. Population-focused nurses have a breadth of knowledge that makes them desirable consultants for colleagues both inside and outside the organizations in which they work. For example, a nurse working in a home health agency might be called on by a school nurse to give suggestions about the most effective way to intervene for a child using a respirator. Another example that occurs frequently is the informal consultation provided by nurses in the community, who help nurses working in hospitals make effective community referrals. At the population level, nurses who consult with a local health department about developing a program for obesity prevention in school-age children are focusing their efforts on a particular target population. An example would be the nurse leader of a community-based diabetes program who works with clinical colleagues in a hospital to improve the self-management education for people with diabetes.

Consultation is closely linked with the ideas of empowerment and self-management. When consultants help clients identify and work through problems and learn new skills that clients see as most important, they are enabling clients to solve more of their own problems. This is very similar to the traditional nursing philosophy of helping people solve their own problems, whether they are individuals, families, groups, or communities. Empowerment is consistent with Jean Watson's theory of human caring (Watson, 2008), in which the nurse may advocate for the client but also may assist the client to advocate for themselves (Sitman & Watson, 2018; Smith, Turkel, & Wolf, 2013).

LEADERSHIP AND MANAGEMENT APPLIED TO POPULATION-FOCUSED NURSING

Goals

Emphasizing the importance of the nurse leaders in addressing the health and well-being of populations, the Robert Wood Johnson Foundation (2017) report titled *Catalysts for Change* states that, "The key to implementing a population-focused vision of the future is strong nursing leadership, which will drive the monumental culture change required to improve health and reduce costs in our country" (p. 4). Nursing leaders work with others to ensure a healthy community. They serve as an advocate for vulnerable and high-risk populations and work toward achieving health equity, eliminating disparities, and improving the health of all groups. Nurse leaders also participate in establishing public and organizational policies and programs that promote a healthy living and working environment, and they work with interprofessional teams to design ways to coordinate care across sites and over time, in order to evaluate and continually improve health care outcomes.

One way nurses lead is by participating in advocacy and policy development at the local level. Working with others to develop policies for smoke-free public spaces is an example of promoting healthy living and working environments. Another example is collaborating with consumers and professionals from other disciplines to evaluate root causes of medication errors in home-bound elders and design a process improvement strategy to reduce errors.

Nursing managers use a systems perspective to achieve agency and professional goals for client services and clinical outcomes. Managers help personnel perform their responsibilities effectively and efficiently, and they mentor other staff members and foster lifelong learning. Furthermore, nurse managers develop new services that will enable the agency to respond to emerging community health needs, monitor health outcomes for particular population groups, and identify changes or variances suggesting new problems.

An example of how nurses show management abilities occurs when they develop plans for broad-based immunization clinics, such as smallpox vaccination clinics. Doing this in advance of confirmed bioterrorism is a way of preparing to meet an emerging community health need that achieves goals of protecting the public's health and helping personnel work effectively and efficiently. Table 40.1 shows examples of ways population-focused nurse leaders and managers facilitate primary, secondary, and tertiary preventive services.

Theories of Leadership and Management

Leadership and management theories help explain individual and group behavior as well as organizational and system dynamics. Theories that help explain and predict individual behavior often focus on employee motivation and job satisfaction. Some theories address interpersonal issues such as leadership, communication, conflict resolution, and group dynamics. Working with consumers, staff members, and other health professionals in an adult daycare facility to design a memory improvement program for participants highlights the use of these theories. This type of project requires knowledge of motivation and leadership, teamwork, change theory, and project planning, management, and evaluation. Organizational and systems theories explain issues at a broader agency or community level. These theories focus on the best ways to organize work, on how to obtain the resources necessary to accomplish agency goals, on organizational level change, on power dynamics, and understanding systems. Systems theories help explain the dynamics of rapid, interconnected change and the emergence of patterns of activity (Crowell, 2016).

Good leadership skills are essential for nurse leaders and are among the key competencies for generalist public/community health nurses recommended by the Quad Council Coalition Competency Review Task Force (2018) and for entry level public health professionals by the Council on Linkages Between Academia and Public Health Nursing Practice (2014).

The transformational leader is able to transform, or change, the situation to one that differs from the status quo

TABLE 40.1 Examples of Levels of Prevention and Population-Focused Nursing Leadership and Management

Levels of Prevention	Nursing Leadership (Sets Goals)	Nursing Management (Directs Use of Resources)
Primary (prevention of illnesses or problems before they begin)	Works with a community coalition to design a broad-based strategy for ensuring health and social needs of uninsured and underinsured populations are met. Works with nurses and interprofessional colleagues to develop goals related to preventing health care errors and ensuring client safety	Develops policies and procedures for a referral program for low-income mothers and children to obtain nutrition services. Ensures that individuals and families understand care routines to promote adherence and reduce chances of health care error
Secondary (screening for illness and treatment of health problems before they worsen)	Works with local government and health department to design lead screening and abatement programs in high-risk census tracts. Monitors data about a caseload of clients to determine whether patterns are developing that might indicate a health problem or issue needs to be resolved	Designs protocols for lead-screening program and hires staff to implement program. Works with other members of care team to design protocols to improve specific health outcomes
Tertiary (treatment of health problems to foster stabilization or delay exacerbation)	Participates on a planning commission with local health department, hospitals, police, and political leaders to update a community-wide disaster response plan that accounts for bioterrorism. Collaborates with interprofessional teams to set goals for performance improvement and rapid changes in quality of care problems	Serves as chair of a committee that organizes, staffs, and monitors budget for a smallpox vaccination program. Monitors implementation of performance improvement activities to ensure timely and appropriate completion or revision as necessary

Table developed by J. Sebastian (2010) for the eighth edition of *Public Health Nursing*.

(Fischer, 2016). Transformational leaders are sometimes found in **learning organizations**, or agencies that create cultures that support ongoing learning, experimentation, and creation of new knowledge (Roussel, Thomas, & Harris, 2016). Transformational leadership is essential to promoting a culture of safety and positive work environments for others (IOM, 2011).

Systems theories and **systems thinking** emphasize the interdependence of multiple parties. Nurses often recognize interdependence of units within an agency but may be less aware of agency interdependence. Economists analyze how distribution of resources affects policies, which players in a system will be influenced by policies, and how they will be influenced. These are called **distribution effects**. For example, if the federal government reduces money for health and social services, the clients of those services may be negatively affected. Employees of service agencies are also affected because agencies are likely to downsize to manage the reduced funding. Consequently, employees may either lose their jobs or experience wage cuts. Others likely to be affected include voluntary agencies and religious groups, which might be expected to provide more services.

Roy's adaptation model of nursing has been extended to include nursing management (Alligood, 2018). Roy argues that agencies are composed of interdependent systems. The role of nurse managers is to help the agency adapt to changing circumstances in the most effective way possible. Roy's model is particularly helpful for explaining and predicting how nurse managers and consultants can help agencies adapt to change. Nurse leaders should analyze how well interdependent units function to achieve agency goals. Furthermore, nurse leaders function as change agents because they foster agency adaptation. Complexity leadership theory accounts for the unpredictability of the behavior of people and organizations (Crowell, 2016). The combination of unpredictability and interdependence leads to disequilibrium and potentially to adaptation and growth. Communities exemplify **complex adaptive systems**. Nurse leaders must understand the analytical, political, and communication skills needed to work effectively in these systems.

Clinical **microsystems** are the systems, people, information, and behaviors that take place at the point of client care (Likosky, 2014). Evidence-based clinical improvements can be implemented quickly in a clinical microsystem that has sufficient data about the practice, information systems that support clinical decision making, and a well-functioning team. For example, nurses working in a mobile health unit are part of a clinical microsystem. The team can make rapid changes in responses to quality problems if team members work well together and the mobile health clinic has an information system that makes it possible to track population health outcomes and clinical practice patterns.

Population-focused nurse leaders should assess the systems within which they work to evaluate risks to client safety. In the community these risks might be related to communication problems, inadequate follow-up, or lack of continuity of care. Nurses should maintain accountability for the outcomes of individuals, families, and groups and should do their best to ensure that complete care is provided across the continuum and that clients feel empowered to manage their own care.

Nurse Leader and Manager Roles

First-line nurse managers may be team leaders or program directors (e.g., director of a satellite occupational health clinic or director of a small migrant health clinic), whereas mid- or executive-level nurse managers may be division directors (including multiple programs or departments), local or state commissioners of health, or directors of large home health agencies with multiple offices. They function as coaches, facilitators, role models, evaluators, advocates, visionaries, community health program planners, teachers, and supervisors. Population-focused nurse leaders have ongoing responsibilities for the health of clients, groups, and communities, as well as for personnel and fiscal resources under their supervision. Nurse leaders may have positions as managers or they may be excellent clinicians and change agents who are seen as opinion leaders.

CONSULTATION

Goal

The goal of consultation is to help others empower themselves to take more responsibility, feel more secure, deal with their feelings and with others in interactions, and use flexible and creative problem-solving skills (Hamric et al., 2014). The functions of a consultant differ from those of a manager because consultation is typically a temporary and voluntary relationship between a professional helper and a client. The similarities between consultants and leaders are in the emphasis on empowerment and helping others develop. Consulting relationships are based on cooperation and respect between consultants and clients, who share equally in problem solving (Hamric et al., 2014).

The nurse's job responsibilities may include internal and external consultation. Internal consultants are members of the organization who work in a temporary capacity to help the client create or sustain change. For example, a nurse may be employed to consult with other nurses in the agency about client care problems or, as an employee of the health department, may serve as a consultant to a local community retirement center about the public health care needs of its residents. If the nurse is an internal consultant, the nurse is employed on a full-time salaried basis by a community agency in which the consultation takes place. If the nurse is an **external consultant**, the nurse is employed temporarily on a contractual basis by the client. The client of the external nurse consultant may be a colleague, another health provider, or a community group or agency. Consulting may occur informally when a staff nurse asks a colleague for advice or help in solving a problem. The nature of the consultation relationship, whether it is internal or external, should not change the goal of consultation.

Theories of Consultation

Several models of consultation have been developed. Although nurses often consult with individuals about their own health care, or with another nurse or health professional about the needs of an individual client, this section emphasizes population-based consultation. At this level, the nurse focuses on the needs of a group, organization, or community. The client in this case is an organization or group. Content models emphasize the role of consultant as the expert who provides specific answers to problems or issues identified by the client. This approach has the advantage of being relatively quick and often responsive to client requests, but it does not help engage the client in problem solving and learning how to address similar issues in the future (Schein, 1969, 1999, 2011, 2016). This chapter focuses on Edgar Schein's (1969, 1999) model of process consultation because it is consistent with the nursing process and with nursing values of empowering clients and collaboratively working as partners with clients. The **process model consultation** focuses on the process of problem solving and collaboration between consultant and the client. The major goal of the process model is to help the client assess both the problem and the kind of help needed to solve it (Schein, 1969, 1999, 2011). Process consultation includes assessing the underlying agency culture that influences the problem and its solution (Schein & Schein, 2016). Both consultant and client participate in the problem-solving steps that lead to changes or to actions for problem solution.

Although consultants should emphasize process consultation, they should be willing to share their expert knowledge when appropriate. Because process consultation is collaborative, Schein (2011) recommends that consultants be willing to offer opinions and advice at all stages of the consultation process. Thus although the major emphasis should be on process consultation, consultants may find it effective to integrate both context and process. Furthermore, Schein (2016) notes that for complex problems, an open, trusting relationship with the client is vital. Thus the consultant needs to be aware of the client's own view of what is going on and be adaptive to those needs.

In the process model, the consultant is a resource person whose primary goal is to provide the client with choices for decision making. Process consultation includes the same steps as the nursing process: establishing a nurse–client relationship based on trust to assess the problem, planning and implementing actions, and evaluating the outcomes of nursing interventions. Nursing interventions may be described as direct client care or as consultation activities, depending on the goal of the intervention.

Consultation may occur before a problem occurs or after a problem exists. For example, a parent–teacher council developing a school-based family center contacts the nurse to assist with options for future nursing and health care for the students and their families. The board wishes to be proactive and plan for the needs of high-risk students and families. The administrator of a minimum-security prison has found that inmates are missing work for minor health problems and that health costs are skyrocketing. The nurse is asked to help explore solutions to the problem. Prison administration is reacting to an existing problem requiring immediate intervention.

The client is identified by determining who in the situation has the problem and needs to change. The following vignette illustrates this point:

Barry Henderson, RN, has been asked by the pastor of his congregation to consult with the parish council regarding the potential establishment of a health ministry. Barry decides that the consultation contract needs to include representatives of the parish council and parishioners themselves to find effective answers to the question. He realizes that time would be wasted and resistance to change would still be present if the focus were on only one group at a time. If he met separately with the parish council, they may decide such a program should include only one set of services. The parishioners either may want a different set of services or may desire to have services and programming organized in a very different manner. For example, the parish council may be especially interested in blood pressure screening, whereas the parishioners may be interested in wellness classes to keep the congregation healthy and in-home visiting for those who are ill. After spending much energy meeting with both groups separately, Barry believes that by being a messenger between the two groups rather than a facilitator for problem solving, the consultant role has been diluted. On the other hand, by meeting with both groups together, Barry could serve as a resource, helping them explore all viewpoints and alternatives for developing the new program.

In this case, both the parish council and the parishioners are Barry's clients.

Consultation Contract

The consultation relationship is based on expectations. The consultant has expectations concerning time, money, resources, and the participation of the client in the process. Clients have expectations about what they will gain from the consultation relationship. Discussing the terms of a **consultation contract** makes expectations explicit, lessens the likelihood of violations of contract terms, and reduces the risk of additional demands being made on either party. **Contracting** involves identifying expectations and responsibilities by both parties. Some contracts are informal, verbal agreements between individuals, whereas others (such as the consulting contract) are formal, written agreements. Areas to include in the written consultation contract are as follows:

- Client and consultant goals
- The identified problem
- The time commitment
- Limitations of the contract
- Cost
- Conditions under which the contract may be broken or renegotiated
- Intervention strategies suggested
- Expected benefits for the client
- Methods of data collection to be used
- Potential interventions
- Evaluation methods to be used
- Confidentiality

Writing a contract for consultation relationships has a number of advantages. The contract terms assist the consultant in determining the number of hours that must be devoted to the interaction and in identifying needed resources and out-of-pocket expenses required to complete the interaction. **Negotiation** of the contract assists the client in identifying realistic expectations of the consultant and firmly establishes what the consultant will and will not do. The client has the opportunity during the negotiation to place limits on what the consultant can do, and the contract allows for future renegotiation of terms. Pricing methods for consultation services vary with the nature of the services. Consultants may price their services on the basis of the actual number of billable hours required to perform the service, or they may set a flat fee during the contract negotiation phase. Flat fees are more attractive to clients because they reduce uncertainty over the total cost of the consultation. They create an incentive for consultants to be efficient and to use an accurate method of estimating their services before the contract negotiation meeting.

The initial contact is made when the client or someone in a family, group, agency, or community communicates with the nurse about a potential problem that requires intervention. The communication may be a person-to-person contact during a home visit, may be written, or may occur by telephone. On initial contact, the client and the nurse have an exploratory meeting to define the problem, assess the nurse's interest and ability to help, and formulate future actions. If the nurse has little experience with the type of problem presented, the client may wish to seek assistance elsewhere. The nurse may also conclude that the situation is not within the nurse's expertise and will want to recommend someone else to work with the client.

Next, the terms of the relationship are discussed. The nurse consultant finds out what the client expects to gain from the relationship and develops terms for the interaction. Finally, in the initial exploratory meeting, the setting for the consultation is decided, the time schedule is set, the goals of the interaction are established, and the mode of intervention is chosen.

When the terms of the contract are agreed on, the data-gathering methods will be part of the agreement. Data-gathering methods used by consultants include direct observation, individual and group interviews, use of questionnaires or surveys, and tape recordings. While data are being gathered and after the diagnosis has been finalized, the nurse implements the intervention. After fulfilling the terms of the contract, the nurse must disengage or reduce the amount of involvement with the client. Decreased contacts allow each side to evaluate the effectiveness of the intervention. During disengagement, the nurse reassures the client that future interactions are possible at the client's discretion. When the agreed-on period of disengagement has passed, the relationship is terminated. The nurse typically provides the client with a written summary of the findings and recommendations resulting from the interactions during the disengagement and termination phases (Duffy et al., 2016).

An example of an internal consultative intervention follows:

The director of nursing in a local health department telephoned the state public health nursing consultant for alcohol and other substance abuse prevention and requested a meeting at the local health department. The purpose of the meeting was to help staff analyze the evidence base and develop the protocols for a community-wide substance abuse prevention program they wished to provide. Several departments within the health department had been providing different aspects of substance abuse prevention but a coordinated effort was not in place. The nurse consultant,

Paula, met with the client, Maggie, and reviewed her findings, sharing her analysis of the current situation and contributing factors. The central issue was defined as an organizational culture that did not promote interprofessional teamwork. This resulted in difficulties providing comprehensive and coordinated substance abuse prevention initiatives. Maggie then spoke with the other department directors to identify barriers and facilitators to interprofessional teamwork. Each director agreed to speak with staff in their departments to obtain their input on barriers and facilitators. One suggestion made by staff members was to hold an off-site retreat for team-based planning related to transitional care programs such as this one. Paula worked with Maggie to help develop suggestions for the agenda and logistics that Maggie shared with the other directors. The directors asked Paula to facilitate the retreat. After revision of the program plan during the retreat, Paula met with Maggie and the other directors to help them develop additional strategies to foster an organizational culture that promoted interprofessional teamwork. She maintained contact with Maggie until the updated evidence base and program plan had been approved by the health department board and termination of the consultation occurred.

QSEN FOCUS ON QUALITY AND SAFETY EDUCATION FOR NURSES

Targeted Competency: Teamwork and Collaboration

Function effectively within nursing and interprofessional teams, fostering open communication, mutual respect, and shared decision making to achieve quality patient care.

Important aspects of teamwork and collaboration include the following:

- **Knowledge:** Describe own strengths, limitations, and values in functioning as a member of a team.
- **Skills:** Initiate plan for self-development as a team member.
- **Attitudes:** Acknowledge own potential to contribute to effective team functioning.

Teamwork and Collaboration Question

You have been selected to lead a task force aimed at reducing obesity rates in your community. Although you feel you are knowledgeable about obesity prevention and have several ideas for nursing interventions to reduce the obesity rate, you feel somewhat overwhelmed to be the person in charge of the task force. What can you do to feel more confident in your new leadership role?

Answer

First, reflect on what knowledge, values, and skills you bring to the task force that are strengths and identify areas that you feel less confident in. For example, you may feel you have a good understanding of obesity prevention but lack experience in team building and conflict resolution. Next, make a plan for how you can improve your weaknesses. For example, you could attend a continuing education workshop about team building or read the current literature on strategies for conflict resolution. Consider inviting people and organizations to join your taskforce who are proficient in the areas you feel weakest in. By reminding yourself of your strengths and actively working to improve your weaknesses, you are taking the steps to seeing your potential as an effective leader on the task force.

Nurse Consultant Role

An agency whose delivery of care is similar to that of an official public health service will most likely employ a nurse who provides traditional or nursing consultation for a broad range of community health activities (e.g., a community or public health nurse clinical specialist). A community health agency that provides a program approach to the delivery of community health services, such as family planning, maternity, child health, handicapped children's services, school health, or home health, will tend to employ specialist consultants. These consultants may have skills and training in specific clinical areas (e.g., a nurse with expertise in maternal and child health). Agencies providing primary health care require a consultant with both general knowledge of public health practice and specialized knowledge in a primary care clinical area. This is also a requirement in agencies involved in long-term and home health care.

The nurse consultant employed in an official public health agency functions as an **internal consultant** to the employing agency. As a representative of the agency, the nurse provides nursing and consultation to colleagues, other disciplines, agency administration, and other health and human service agencies and/or community groups. Two primary roles of the internal consultant are resource person and facilitator.

With knowledge of available resources, the nurse consultant can identify gaps in service, identify the critical services provided by the health care delivery system, and promote services for meeting health or social needs of the population. The consultant facilitates staff nurse problem solving about individual client and family needs, health needs of a group of clients, or professional concerns and attitudes. The consultant may assist managers and administrators in solving problems about personnel, program needs, organizational goals, community relationships, and client population needs. The consultant may also facilitate communication across agencies by working with interagency **coalitions** or **alliances**.

Consultants from federal agencies are often used as external nurse consultants. The nurse consultant from the federal agency may come to the local or state agency to serve on request as facilitator or resource person helping with program planning, development, and implementation. The primary role function of this consultant is to serve as a resource person, although the consultant may facilitate movement toward identifying actual program objectives.

An example of a vital role nurse consultants can play is in helping a community agency or a coalition conduct community needs assessments and develop strategic plans and associated action plans for achieving *Healthy People 2020* goals (see the *Healthy People 2020* box) (USDHHS, 2010).

COMPETENCIES FOR NURSE LEADERS

Nurses should watch for opportunities to participate in leadership development institutes or consider ongoing formal education through advanced public health nursing degree programs. Leadership development programs are available at various levels and are provided by civic and professional organizations. Civic programs introduce participants to the full range of

HEALTHY PEOPLE 2020

Objectives Related to the Four Overarching Goals

The following are examples of some of the proposed objectives related to leadership, management, and consultation by public health nurses:

- **AHS-2:** (Developmental) Increase the proportion of persons with coverage of appropriate evidence-based clinical preventive services.
- **HC/HIT-11:** (Developmental) Increase the proportion of meaningful users of health information technology.
- **PHI-1:** Increase the proportion of federal, tribal, state, and local public health agencies that incorporate core competencies for public health professionals into job descriptions and performance evaluations.
- **PHI-14:** Increase the proportion of national and local public health jurisdictions that conduct a public health system assessment based on national performance standards.

AHS, Access to health services; *HC/HIT,* health communication/health information technology; *PHI,* public health infrastructure.
From U.S. Department of Health and Human Services: *Healthy People 2020,* Washington, DC, 2010. Available at www.healthypeople.gov.

leadership and quality-of-life issues in a community, including health, education, politics, the arts, and business. This breadth of concerns is consistent with nurses' understanding that health results from the interaction of many facets of social and economic influences. Other leadership development opportunities are provided by professional organizations (e.g., the International Honor Society for Nursing, the American Public Health Association), continuing education, and local groups. Graduate degree programs in public health nursing provide systematic academic development of public and leadership competencies and prepare nurses to sit for advanced nursing certification through the American Nurses Credentialing Center, such as the Nurse Executive Certification. Nurses should take advantage of opportunities such as these for lifelong learning and the strengthening of leadership skills.

The following section describes essential competencies that nurses must master in order to become effective leaders in the community.

Leadership Competencies

Nurses need effective leadership, interpersonal, political, organizational, fiscal, analytical, and information competencies. Some competencies are similar to those required for leadership in other clinical areas, such as good communication skills and the ability to delegate effectively. Working in the community means being able to work with populations and groups, to build coalitions and work with partnerships. Leadership essential to these roles involves identifying a shared vision and influencing others to achieve the vision, emphasizing that client needs are the basis for health services, empowering others, delegating tasks and managing time appropriately, and making decisions effectively. Public health nurse managers should be involved in developing agency-level vision, mission, and goal statements.

Empowerment. Leaders help others empower themselves to make organizations more responsive to client needs. This means removing barriers to decision making and allowing staff nurses the authority to make client decisions in "real time," as needs demand, rather than requiring nurses to obtain numerous approvals. **Empowerment** is more than simply increasing nurses' authority—it includes ensuring that they have the necessary knowledge, skills, and resources to effectively make the decisions for which they are held accountable. For example, nurse managers who are responsible for preparing their own department or program budgets and for approving program spending must be given the opportunity to learn budgetary concepts. Nurses are likely to feel more empowered to do their work in a less bureaucratic environment that supports clinical autonomy and collaborative professional relationships (Cordo & Hill-Rodriguez, 2017).

The concept of empowerment underpins the consulting process. Consultants assist others in identifying solutions to problems and, more importantly, in developing the ability to manage problems independently in the future.

Delegation. Effective delegation is a key competency of public health nurses. The Association of Community Health Nurse Educators Education Committee (2009) listed delegation among the basic competencies for community/public health nurses. This group noted that delegation is part of ensuring that care is appropriately coordinated within an interprofessional health care team. It has become increasingly necessary because of the complexity of care in public health and community settings (Schaffer et al., 2016).

Agency efficiency increases when tasks are assigned to the first level in the hierarchy where employees possess the necessary skills and knowledge to complete the task and where the task is related to the goals of those positions. **Delegation** develops others' talents and can contribute to job satisfaction. Asking a nurse in a nursing clinic for homeless families to develop a booklet describing community resources for this population helps the staff nurse learn more about community resources, the gaps that exist in local resources, and where opportunities exist for interagency collaboration. The nurse is also likely to learn about visual presentation, layout and brochure design issues, and how to present material at the appropriate reading level. Finally, delegation is an important tool in time management. A school nurse may delegate locating resources for a screening clinic to the parent-teacher association, and the time saved can be spent on developing a teaching plan for volunteers who will help with the actual screening. Strategies for delegating responsibilities are listed in Box 40.1. Fig. 40.1 provides a

BOX 40.1 Delegating Responsibility

Nurse managers share responsibility for any tasks they delegate to others. The nurse manager delegates responsibility for a task but retains final accountability for the safe, effective outcome of the task (ANA, 2016). It is critical, then, that nurse managers know that the individuals to whom they are delegating responsibility are both prepared and capable of effectively performing the tasks. Nurse managers should provide clear guidelines and plan specific times to obtain progress reports on task completion. This will allow the opportunity to manage problems as they arise and to provide staff with helpful feedback or instruction if needed.

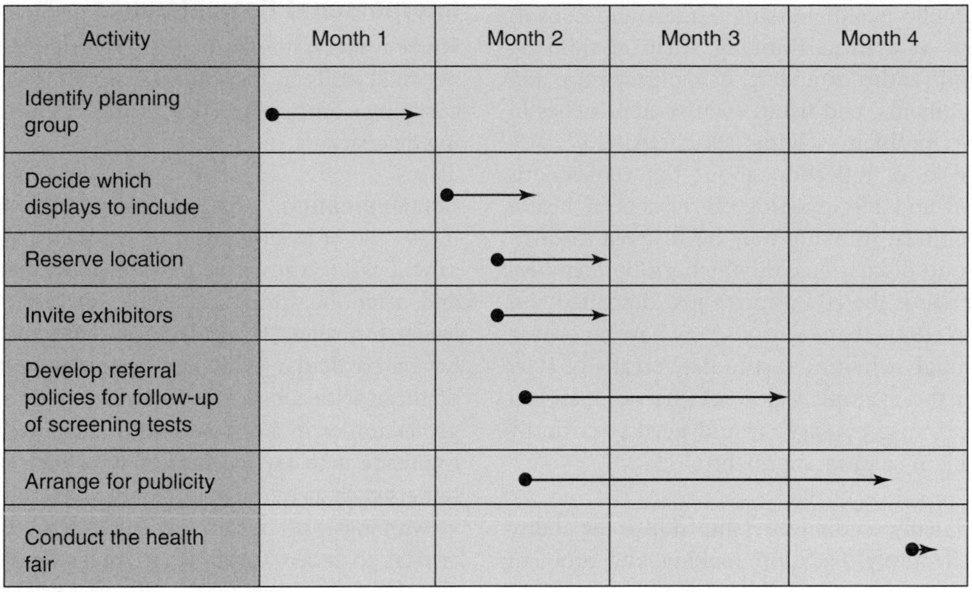
Activity
Month 1
Month 2
Month 3
Month 4
Identify planning group
Decide which displays to include
Reserve location
Invite exhibitors
Develop referral policies for follow-up of screening tests
Arrange for publicity
Conduct the health fair

Fig. 40.1 Sample timetable for conducting a health fair.

sample timetable for conducting a health fair, showing how the nurse might decide which activities need to be completed and suggesting those that might be delegated.

Delegation has become an increasingly important skill for nurses, whether they have official roles as managers or not. As more agencies increase their use of unlicensed assistive personnel and lay community workers, nurses are increasingly delegating selected aspects of practice to others and supervising the completion of those tasks. In the National Council of State Boards of Nursing's (NCSBN's) (2016) Delegation Model, responsibilities of the employer/nurse leader, the licensed nurse, and the delegatee are outlined. Sometimes nurses mistakenly think that they are not accountable for tasks that are indirectly delegated through agency policies (e.g., policies for cross-training). However, if nursing care has been delegated, then nurses and their organizations are accountable for the safe and effective completion of that care (NCSBN, 2016). When delegating, the licensed nurse determines if the activity is appropriated based on the Five Rights of Delegation: right task, right circumstance, right person, right directions and communication, and right supervision and evaluation (NCSBN, 2016).

The first source of guidance for delegating tasks to unlicensed individuals is the state nurse practice act (NCSBN, 2016). The next source of assistance comes from specialty professional organizations. For example, the National Association of School Nurses and the ANA included care coordination and working with students, family, staff, and community members (ANA, 2017) in the standards of professional performance for school nurses. Related responsibilities include ensuring optimal outcomes and quality of care.

To delegate effectively, public health nurses must understand the differences between responsibility, accountability, and authority (NCSBN, 2016). The nurse may have the authority to delegate certain tasks to another individual or group. That individual or group accepts the responsibility to complete the task, but the nurse retains accountability to ensure the safety and quality of the outcome.

For example, a school nurse has the responsibility to assess a child with physical disabilities and develop a plan of care for that child. Selected aspects of that plan of care, such as assisting with feeding or emptying a catheter bag and recording output, could be delegated to an assistant, provided that person had received appropriate training and was competent to perform the task. This means that it is not adequate that the nurse know the individual has been certified as a nursing assistant; the nurse also needs to know that the individual is competent to safely perform the delegated task. It is important to ensure that those to whom certain tasks have been delegated have been trained to accept the responsibility and carry it out effectively. Public health nurses must also provide adequate time to plan the delegation process and to communicate with the person or group to whom a task is being delegated (NCSBN, 2016). Communication should occur throughout the process to allow for feedback and clarifications when needed. The nurse retains the legal accountability for safe client care. This responsibility may be shared with the person to whom one is delegating, but accountability is never transferred (ANA, 2016; NCSBN, 2016).

CHECK YOUR PRACTICE

You are a school nurse assigned to two elementary schools. At school A, you have four students with daily scheduled medications for attention-deficit/hyperactivity disorder, two students with prn inhalers for asthma, and one third grade student with newly diagnosed type 1 diabetes. At school B, you have three students with daily scheduled medications for attention deficit disorder, two students with severe peanut allergies with prn EpiPens, and one fourth grade student with type 1 diabetes who has an insulin pump. The schools are too far apart for you to be able to administer all scheduled medications and insulin at both schools.

- What would you do?
- What can you delegate to unlicensed assistive personnel? How will you ensure proper delegation is followed? How will you prioritize care?

Critical Thinking. Public health nursing leaders and consultants must be adept at critical thinking. Critical thinking includes analyzing and synthesizing data, using knowledge and values in making judgments, and using creative approaches in decision making and problem solving (Michelangelo, 2013; Solman, 2017). It includes reflection about the connections between sociocultural and biophysiological aspects of health status and services. Critical thinking may be fostered through the use of guided group discussions, in which group members are assisted to think about the connections just described and about the distribution effects that decisions may have on others. It is also fostered through activities to stimulate creativity, such as brainstorming. In the example below of the occupational wellness program, the nurse manager would need to critically think about ways to increase program quality.

Decision Making. Finally, a core leadership skill is the ability to make decisions effectively. Decision making and problem solving are critical aspects of nursing practice in complex clinical environments (Michelangelo, 2013; Solman, 2017). This is a two-stage process in which the nurse first must decide how much input to seek from others and second must generate alternatives for the decision and choose among the alternatives. Including others in the decision-making process is beneficial in part because others may have information and ideas that would lead to a better decision and also because others may support the decision more if they are involved in making it. This also fosters team building and collaboration, which are two competencies for public health nurses (Council on Linkages Between Academia and Public Health Practice, 2014; Quad Council Coalition Competency Review Task Force, 2018).

A decision tree can be used for selecting a leadership style that varies from a unilateral, independent decision process, to progressively more participative styles, with the most participative style involving delegating authority to a group that will be responsible for making the decision. Although many assume that autocratic decision making is not effective, in fact it may be both effective and efficient under certain circumstances, such as emergencies. In other situations, it is better to seek input from others, individually or as a group, to seek suggestions for solutions from the group, or to simply turn a problem over to a group to solve on their own.

The next stage of the decision-making process is to generate alternative solutions and to choose among those solutions. Both risk and cost are important dimensions in most situations. The goal involves low cost and low risk to clients and staff. Other dimensions might be unique to the situation. For example, if the nurse is trying to decide whether to develop an in-house wellness program for an occupational setting or to contract with a consulting group for that service, the nurse could compare the risks and benefits of both alternatives. The occupational health nurse might decide that the advantages of an in-house wellness program are that (1) it allows for staff participation in identifying key dimensions and goals and brainstorming creative solutions, (2) participants' values are built into the dimensions and goals, and (3) it allows for both creative and logical thinking processes.

Interpersonal Competencies

Nurse leaders, managers, and consultants need effective interpersonal skills in communicating, motivating, appraising and coaching, contracting, supervising, team building, and promoting diversity.

Communication. Good communication skills, including skills in the use of assertiveness techniques and conflict resolution, as well as communicating through the media and professional and scientific literature, are essential to being effective in leadership roles (Foronda et al., 2016; Vertino, 2014). Nurses have a particular challenge in communicating because many of those with whom they work may be in a different health profession or in a different field altogether. Nurses often communicate with lay workers or with the public through media outlets such as newspaper columns, television and radio interviews, blogs, and public service announcements. It is especially critical to listen carefully, to make underlying assumptions clear, and to speak in the other's language. This may mean avoiding the use of professional jargon and speaking in more commonly shared language or speaking in the listener's primary language. It is increasingly important for nurses to be bilingual or multilingual, depending on the ethnic composition of the community.

Communication must be culturally competent to be effective. Because communication involves words, tone of voice, posture, eye contact, and spatial relationships, cultural norms often influence the meanings given to different aspects of body language. For example, whereas most advise direct eye contact when communicating, in some cultures this may be viewed as aggressive, especially when the eye contact is prolonged. Some cultures prefer the closer-space relationships that may make others feel they are being crowded. Other aspects of communication are important as well, such as the appropriate place for reprimands. It is never appropriate to reprimand or criticize in public, although public praise is usually an excellent idea. Nurse managers and consultants should be sensitive to the power of written communication and be aware that, although putting a message in writing is a good way to avoid confusion, it also may be seen as aggressive, distrustful, or a bid for power. The key is to make certain that the message that is communicated is the message that was intended. Effective communication skills are listed in Box 40.2.

BOX 40.2 Effective Communication Skills

- Listen actively.
- Restate the main points.
- Speak in the listener's language.
- Maintain culturally appropriate eye contact and body language.
- Provide an appropriate environment.
- Be aware of the power of written communication.
- Use simple, direct words.
- Use "I" statements and say how you feel.
- Provide frequent feedback.
- Reflect on the meaning of the message.

Creating a Motivating Workplace. One of the more difficult skills to master is motivating other people; in fact, one cannot ever really motivate others, because motivation is internal. However, the skillful leader can create a motivating environment, working to make certain that both individual and agency goals are met to the extent possible. Sometimes individual motivation may be low because employees do not believe they have the skills necessary to achieve their goals, or they believe that the system will not allow them to do so. The effective nurse leader identifies which perceptions are inaccurate and helps individuals develop plans for improving their personal capacities for achieving goals. Although adequate salaries are important, compensation is not the only way to create a motivating environment for professionals. One home health aide supervisor is known for the high level of morale among her staff and the unusually low level of turnover. She makes a point of being available for discussion before the aides leave the agency in the morning and on their return in the afternoon. She always gives each person a birthday card, and thanks them for a job well done. For the long-term good, leaders should work with others in the community to increase salaries if they are not competitive.

Appraisal and Coaching. Employee appraisal and coaching are closely related to motivation and individual development (Mackenzie, 2013; Mone & London, 2018; Okello & Gilson, 2015). The purpose of performance evaluation is to assist employees to more effectively meet the objectives of their roles and to help them develop their potential in ways that facilitate achieving agency goals. Performance evaluation should not take place just before an annual appraisal interview is scheduled. It should be a regular part of the job, with the manager providing regular feedback on employee progress toward goals. Performance appraisal is particularly challenging for nurse managers because so many community health workers practice independently in the field. For example, nurse managers in home health must plan either to make visits with the nursing staff on a regular basis or to obtain other forms of input on employee performance, such as planning telephone or office conferences with staff.

Coaching involves working one-on-one with others to improve clinical care delivery (Westcott, 2016). With coaching, managers retain responsibility for decisions but request input and explain decisions. They support progress by helping the employee break the tasks into manageable parts, providing resources for accomplishing tasks and for acquiring the necessary skills, and praising task accomplishment. Coaching is most useful with people who may not yet be skillful in a particular area and who are not confident about their skills.

Supervision. Nurse managers who delegate tasks to others must supervise the completion of those tasks and build in mechanisms to make certain that the tasks are completed safely and effectively (ANA, 2016; NCSBN, 2016). Supervision means decision making and implementation of activities in an ongoing relationship. It may occur either on site when the nurse manager is present and while the activity is being performed, or off site when the nurse is providing care in a community setting. It is important for nurse managers to build effective means of providing off-site supervision because so many community health activities do not take place within a single agency (e.g., home health care occurs in individual homes, and school health services are provided in individual schools).

Handling criticism is a difficult skill that involves both the giving and the taking of criticism related to job performance. Nurse managers should provide constructive critique as close as possible to the time they observe a problem with an employee's job performance. Constructive criticism focuses on the behaviors necessary to meet the job expectations and helps identify sources of problems, resources for managing problem behavior, and feedback. For example, if an employee is chronically tardy, the nurse manager should speak privately with the employee about the job expectation for promptness, identify why the employee is frequently tardy, establish a behavioral goal with time frames and consequences of achieving or not achieving the goal, and assist the employee to develop a plan for achieving the goal. The employee may be unaware of the importance of being punctual and can easily change the behavior. On the other hand, a behavior modification plan may be useful to help change the behavior. Behavioral consequences may include both positive reinforcers, such as praise, and disciplinary measures, such as oral and written warnings, limited raises, suspension, and termination. Suspension and termination are normally used only with problems related to safety, inability to perform job duties, breach of confidentiality, and illegal acts; they are detailed in agency policies and procedures.

Team Building. Finally, team building and managing diversity are group-level skills needed by nurse leaders, managers, and consultants (LeBlanc, 2014; Phillips, 2016). Interprofessional teams increasingly are used to assess clients, plan client care or services, and manage quality improvement activities. Teams may include members of multiple health disciplines as, for example, with community health coalitions. They also may include people from other backgrounds, including lay community health workers. Nurse managers and consultants can facilitate team building by assisting the team to develop goals and ground rules, identifying who will fill various roles and determining how to share leadership, developing strategies for ongoing cooperation and recognition of contributions of each member, and resolving conflict.

Promoting Diversity. A key challenge to nurse managers is promoting and managing diversity in positive ways that value different perspectives and provide insights into culturally competent strategies to eliminate disparities. By 2060, the U.S. population is expected to be older (nearly one in five over the age of 65 by 2030) and more diverse, with significant increase in the number of immigrants than previous years (U.S. Census Bureau, 2018). Nurse leaders must work with others to create workplaces that build on the strengths of a diverse workforce to provide excellent health care and eliminate disparities in outcomes. Nurses should partner with schools, faith communities, health care agencies, and universities to encourage minority group members who are interested in nursing careers. This will help build a community nursing workforce that better reflects the population as a whole (Craft-Blacksheare, 2018; Kowlowitz et al., 2018). Nurse managers must understand cultural values and norms to communicate effectively and interpret behavior accurately. They must know how to prevent any form of racial, sexual, or ethnic harassment and ensure a positive and welcoming environment in the workplace.

Power Dynamics and Conflict Resolution

Power imbalances can occur within groups, community organizations, and policy-making bodies, and affect health care professionals and community members. Managing power dynamics effectively requires that public health nurses understand community systems, collaboration, and strategies for providing information to empower others to work on their own behalf. Public health nurses work closely with community groups to build capacity for assessing strengths and needs, developing solutions to community health problems and promoting health and wellness, and managing long-term approaches for healthier communities. This is particularly important when working with vulnerable populations (Kyounghae et al., 2016; Ray, 2016).

Effective conflict resolution requires negotiation skills as well as skills in recognizing and managing power dynamics. Principled negotiation (McKibben, 2017; Rosenstein, Dinklin, & Munro, 2014) emphasizes collaborative problem solving and development of mutually agreeable ways of achieving goals. Conflict resolution strategies can result in win-win, win-lose, or lose-lose outcomes. Strategies most likely to create win-win situations include collaborating, confronting problems directly, building consensus, and ensuring that all parties have an adequate opportunity for input (McKibben, 2017; Rosenstein et al., 2014).

Population-focused nurse leaders must understand power dynamics. Because nurses possess altruistic values, they may believe that being powerful is not necessary. However, it is impossible to create health-promoting public health services without some legitimacy in decision-making arenas. Membership on community agency boards and advisory committees puts nurse managers in the position to influence service delivery.

Consultants' advice may be followed because the client feels that the consultant possesses superior knowledge or skills and is trustworthy and credible. Internal nurse consultants may have power resulting from their roles in the organization. The client may not feel obligated to implement the recommendations of external consultants. On the other hand, external consultants may be viewed as influential because of an affiliation with other well-known consultants or a national organization. The consultant's ability to persuade clients by offering reasons, new techniques, or methods of problem solving may motivate clients to follow the consultant's advice.

Organizational Competencies

Nurses use organizational skills, such as planning, organizing, implementing, and coordinating as well as monitoring, evaluating, and improving quality. Nurses use these skills when managing programs and projects and when coordinating care for individuals, families, and groups.

Planning. Planning includes prioritizing daily activities to achieve goals. It also includes long-range planning, such as working with nurses in a department to plan a new program. Planning is a collaborative activity that can involve interprofessional teams, community groups, and policy makers. Developing a shared vision, goals, and measurable objectives provides the foundation for a plan. Nurses must be able to anticipate the cost of providing nursing services to a certain population over a period of time and to develop a proposal (or a business plan) for a contract to provide the services. Because planning is primarily a cognitive activity, nurse managers and consultants may tend to lessen its importance and allow little time for adequate planning. However, planning is the basis for direct nursing services and it is an essential competency for population-focused nurse care (ANA, 2013; Quad Council Coalition Competency Review Task Force, 2018), so it is important to make adequate time for planning.

Several resources are available to help nurse managers and consultants plan nursing services. *Healthy People 2020* (USDHHS, 2010) defines the national health goals for the United States by the year 2020 and should be the basis for program planning. The Community Preventive Services Task Force (2018) maintains *The Community Guide* to provide evidence-based strategies for community health planning. The KU Center for Community Health Development developed and manages the *Community Tool Box* (2018a), which provides free online resources for those working to build healthier communities and bring about social change.

Organizing. Organizing involves determining appropriate sequencing and timelines for the activities necessary to achieve goals and arranging for the appropriate people to carry out the plan. Flow sheets and timetables are helpful tools that allow nurse managers and consultants to visualize how tasks are organized and to identify gaps in the planning. Fig. 40.1, as shown earlier, illustrates a timetable for conducting a health fair.

Implementing and Coordinating. Implementing and coordinating a plan includes not only following the timelines but also making certain that the relevant regulations and policies are adhered to, that activities are appropriately documented, and that the work of all team members is coordinated. One strategy that helps ensure coordination is use of an action plan (Community Tool Box, 2018b). This is a table that includes the program goals and objectives, activities to meet the objectives, identification of those responsible for each activity, the time frame for completing the activities, and the plan for evaluating achievement of the objectives. Team members should review the action plan at regular meetings and make changes as necessary. Action plans are also used to coordinate care for people with chronic illnesses such as obesity (see, e.g., Waldecker, Malpass, King, & Ridd, 2018). Nurse managers and consultants should give sufficient attention to the change process by helping those involved identify the need for change, keeping them informed, soliciting their input, and making modifications in the plan as necessary.

Monitoring, Evaluating, and Improving. Monitoring, evaluating, and making improvements are critical to nursing services. Nurses should monitor nursing services on a regular basis and make improvements as soon as the need for improvements becomes apparent. Professional standards and the standards of various accrediting bodies guide the focus of monitoring and evaluating. The Joint Commission standards for home health and ambulatory care clinics (http://www.jointcommission.org/) provide detailed and explicit minimal standards that all such agencies should be expected to meet.

In addition to professional standards of practice available from the ANA and specialty nursing organizations, the Agency for Healthcare Research and Quality has published clinical guidelines for prevention and treatment of selected health problems, such as wound care, pain, and tobacco cessation. Using evidence-based clinical guidelines is a key way to improve the quality of care. Finally, nurses should evaluate and monitor changes in client health outcomes. Effective outcomes management programs using information systems can be applied for ongoing planning and program improvements for target populations such as women and children (Olds et al., 2014).

Fiscal Competencies

Forecasting Costs. Nurse leaders must be skilled in the area of fiscal management. Nurse managers and consultants must be able to project the cost of public health nursing services. This is especially important in today's tight economic environment because the forecast should include an assessment of the risk rating of the likely health and illness experiences of a target population. Combining community health assessment skills, epidemiologic projections, and consultation are key steps in this process and make it possible to design health programs to reduce health risks among various populations. After developing a profile of the anticipated health and illness experiences of a target population, the next step is anticipating the amount and kind of nursing resources needed by the population. These skills are basic to the development of proposals for new nursing services and contracts with external groups.

Develop and Monitor Budgets. Nurse managers have taken on more responsibility for developing and monitoring their own department budgets as agencies have decentralized. They must be able to develop a justifiable budget and monitor how actual spending compares with planned spending. Expenses commonly included in an operating budget are salaries and benefits, equipment, supplies, travel, and overhead. It is helpful to obtain staff input when developing a budget in order to make financial projections as realistic as possible. Nurse managers should review program action plans with staff to determine the resources necessary to implement the program. Combining anticipated volume, revenues, and expenses allows the nurse manager to anticipate a breakeven point for new services (i.e., determining when a new program can be expected to be financially self-sufficient).

Variance analysis means identifying the difference between actual and planned results, determining the cause of the variation, and correcting problems when they exist. Spending more than anticipated is not always negative; it may simply indicate that client or service volume was higher than anticipated. This could, however, be of concern in an agency that is fully capitated and receives a set amount of money to see a client for usually a year, regardless of the cost of the services the client needs. Additional services do not bring in additional revenues. Nurses in fully capitated environments have more opportunity than ever before to focus on health promotion and illness prevention services.

Higher expenses than planned are not always under the control of the nurse manager. For example, if the prevailing wage increases because of changes in the labor market, an agency may spend more than expected on salaries. On the other hand, spending less than predicted does not always indicate that a program is running efficiently; client volume may be down, or staff may not be providing adequate services. The most important thing for a public health nurse to do initially is to monitor expenses carefully and analyze why expenses might differ from the original plan.

For example, if a nurse manager observes that more has been spent on salaries and supplies than originally budgeted, and less on travel, should he or she think this is desirable or undesirable? To analyze the variance, the nurse should ask if the prices for labor and supplies were higher than expected or if the agency has used more nursing time or supplies than planned (Jones et al., 2018; Lim & Noh, 2015; Talley, Thorgrimson, & Robinson, 2013). The answers to these questions will help determine whether the variance resulted from factors under the manager's control, such as inefficiency, or from factors outside of the manager's control, such as higher wages or higher prices than expected. The answers will also help determine whether the variance resulted from an increase in client volume or an alteration in case mix, with the agency serving sicker clients.

Conduct Cost-Effectiveness Analysis. Regardless of the type of reimbursement system in place, nurses should be able to conduct a simple cost-effectiveness analysis of their interventions. Such analyses are not measurements of the efficiency of a program (see Chapter 23 for a discussion of this distinction) but are comparisons of the money spent for the outcomes across two or more interventions. Cost-effectiveness analyses compare alternative approaches for achieving the same goals. The nurse should measure the full costs and benefits (or savings) of each alternative intervention and construct ratios to compare the alternatives. The final result might be stated as the number of people who were able to achieve a desired health outcome (e.g., losing weight or adhering to an exercise program) for each additional dollar spent. The results of cost-effectiveness analyses sometimes raise new questions that must be analyzed. For example, in a study of the cost-effectiveness of nurse practitioner/community health worker care management intervention to reduce cardiovascular health disparities, investigators found the patients in the intervention group had significant improvements in low-density lipoprotein (LDL) cholesterol, systolic and diastolic blood pressure (BP), and hemoglobin A1c (HbA1c) compared to those receiving usual care (Allen et al., 2014). Although Allen et al. (2014) concluded that the nurse practitioner (NP)/community health worker (CHW) care management teams were a cost-effective strategy to reduce cardiovascular risk, they also reported that those in the intervention group had higher laboratory costs and medication costs than those in the comparative group receiving usual care. What would you recommend to management in a primary care setting, based on those results?

Analytical and Information Competencies

It is increasingly important for nurses to have excellent analytical competencies and competencies in the use of information. For example, access to useful and needed data helps nurses and other health professionals monitor clinical outcomes, identify systems issues that can result in health care errors, and plan to better meet the health needs of their populations. Population-focused nurses need a good understanding of descriptive and clinical epidemiology as well as the ability to analyze graphical data displays such as histograms, flowcharts, and line graphs. Use of aids such as checklists, reminders, and clinical decision support are all good ways to improve the quality of care and prevent errors (Kihlgren et al., 2016; Massarweh et al., 2017). Because nurses are interested in identifying patterns of health problems, care delivery, and outcomes in community settings, more nurses are including nursing taxonomies (or languages) in electronic client records. Nursing leaders who participate in incorporating electronic records and information systems should have a conceptual framework to guide the project (Englebright et al., 2014; Jones & Seckman, 2018).

FUTURE OF NURSING LEADERSHIP

As noted at the beginning of this chapter, as the most trusted profession, nursing is in a position of influence. Using that power in a responsible and effective way is the task of the nurse leader.

In 2010, the IOM released its landmark report, *The Future of Nursing: Leading Change, Advancing Health.* In this report sponsored by the Robert Wood Johnson Foundation (RWJF), the committee described a vision of a transformed health care system in which quality care is accessible to the diverse populations of the United States, wellness and disease prevention are promoted, health outcomes improve, and compassionate care is provided across the life span (IOM, 2011). To achieve this health care system, the IOM (2011) recommends that the nursing workforce become prepared to "assume leadership positions across all levels" and suggests that nursing have representatives on boards, executive management teams, and in other key leadership positions. The 2015 IOM report assessing progress made on *The Future of Nursing* recommendations noted significant progress in many areas and called for more focus and attention on removing barriers to practice and care, transforming education, continued collaborating and leading by nurses, promoting diversity, and improving data sets (IOM, 2015b).

The Future of Nursing: *Campaign for Action* (2018) was convened to address the IOM's (2011) recommendations by mobilizing Action Coalitions in every state and Washington, DC, working with policy makers, health care professionals, educators, and business leaders. The *Campaign for Action* (2018) currently ties its work with the Robert Wood Johnson Foundation's (2015) *Culture of Health* vision. Convened in 2014 in response to *The Future of Nursing* report, the *Nurses on Boards Coalition* (2018) raises awareness that all boards would benefit from the nursing perspective and works towards its goal of at least 10,000 nurses on boards by 2020. By working with policy makers, government leaders at all levels, and advocacy organizations, nurse leaders have the power to change the health care system to provide accessible, quality, evidence-based care to individuals and populations. With the passage and implementation of the Affordable Care Act of 2010 (ACA), nurses have the opportunity to take a pivotal leadership role in leading the nation in transforming the health care system (Wakefield, 2013). In 2013, Kathleen G. Sebelius, Secretary of the U.S. Department of Health and Human Services, expressed the vital role nurses can play in whether or not the ACA is successful, stating nurses are "at the heart of our healthcare system" (Nurse.com News, 2013). A national survey of public health nurses (PHNs) regarding their knowledge, perceptions, and practices under the ACA concluded that PHNs are making a substantial contribution to the implementation of the health care reform act, particularly in the integration of primary care and public health, provision of clinical prevention services, care coordination, patient navigation, establishment of private-public partnerships, population health strategies, and population health data assessment and analysis (Edmonds et al., 2016). Nurse leaders are needed to provide education to individuals and communities about the ACA and assist them in navigating the health insurance marketplace. Furthermore, nurse leaders are needed to address these potential influences and to develop innovative solutions to the challenges that arise.

The Association of Public Health Nurses (APHN) released a position paper in 2016 titled *The Public Health Nurse—Necessary Partner for the Future of Healthy Communities.* This position paper acknowledges the vital role the public health nursing workforce plays in delivering essential services and impacting successful population-based outcomes. Furthermore, the report notes the important role PHN leaders have had historically in positively influencing community health and the need for PHNs to continue to provide leadership in an ever-changing health system environment, evolving and strengthening their practice with community systems.

LINKING CONTENT TO PRACTICE

This chapter emphasizes the use of leadership, management, and consultative skills and knowledge in public health nursing practice, whether one has an official leadership or consulting role or not. Use of the theories and principles of leadership, management, and consultation with public health and nursing science is key to promoting healthy communities and achieving the goals of *Healthy People 2020* (USDHHS, 2010). Entry-level public health nurses are expected to possess competencies in these areas, including communication, collaboration, team building, analysis, program planning and management, managing budgets, and understanding and implementing policies (Council on Linkages Between Academia and Public Health Practice, 2014; Quad Council Coalition Competency Review Task Force, 2018). Public health nurses focus on working with communities in addition to other staff members and colleagues, and work with broad problems and issues that require systems thinking, leadership, and building coalitions (Bekemeier et al., 2015; Olson, 2013). When a public health nurse thinks about empowerment, for example, he or she considers how to provide information and foster skill development for empowerment of other staff members and of community members. Thinking about working in partnership with community groups and policy makers influences a public health nurse's use of theories and principles of leadership, management, and consultation.

PRACTICE APPLICATION

The nurse manager of a nursing clinic in a residential facility for frail older adults approached the local college of nursing for assistance with health promotion and health monitoring activities for the residents. The facility was undergoing renovation and was expected to more than triple its capacity by the time the renovation was completed. The nurse manager thought the health promotion activities that were already in place would be inadequate to serve the growing needs. Most of the residents were more than 70 years of age and had several chronic illnesses. The residential complex was 10 to 15 miles away from health care facilities.

Shirley, the nurse manager, supervised a staff of three nurses and one homemaker aide. She contracted with a local physical therapy firm for services as needed for the residents. Shirley had asked the staff if they thought they could realistically expand their services, and they suggested consultation. The staff commented that residents needed nurses who could provide health monitoring and skilled nursing services in their apartments, because so many were increasingly homebound. Staff members were hesitant about expanding into home care themselves because they feared it would mean a cutback in the health promotion activities they currently offered. They thought the needs, and the resources that would be required to meet the needs, should be evaluated before making any final decision.

What should the staff do to complete the evaluation of the problem?

A. Call a meeting of persons affected by the problem and decide on using an internal or external consultant to help evaluate the problem.
B. Write a contract and indicate how they want the evaluation to be done.
C. Develop a plan to implement home health services because the plan would include an analysis of needs and resources.
D. Continue with their health promotion activities and decide about home health services when more resources could be identified.

Answers can be found on the Evolve site.

KEY POINTS

- Nurse leaders may function in formal roles as managers or consultants, or they may use managerial and consulting skills in their everyday clinical practice.
- Nurse leaders, managers, and consultants should work with organizations, coalitions, and community groups to design local strategies that will help achieve the *Healthy People 2020* goals.
- The goals of nursing leadership and management are (1) to achieve organization and professional goals for client services and clinical outcomes, (2) to empower personnel to perform their responsibilities effectively and efficiently, (3) to develop new services that will enable the organization to respond to emerging community health needs, and (4) to work with others for a healthy community.
- Systems thinking promotes sensitivity to the interdependence of parts of a system and the potential causes and consequences of organizational actions.
- Nurse managers may be team leaders or program directors, directors of home health agencies or community-based clinics, or commissioners of health. They function as visionaries, coaches, facilitators, role models, evaluators, advocates, community health and program planners, and teachers. They have ongoing responsibilities for clients, groups, and community health and for personnel and fiscal resources under their direction.
- The goal of consultation is to stimulate clients to take responsibility, feel more secure, deal constructively with their feelings and with others in interaction, and internalize skills of a flexible and creative nature.
- Consultation models can be categorized as content or process models. Process model consultation helps the client assess both the problem and the kind of help needed to solve the problem.
- Consultation involves seven basic phases: initial contact, definition of the relationship, selection of setting and approach, data collection and problem diagnosis, intervention, reduction of involvement and evaluation, and termination.
- Nurse consultants may function as internal consultants within an organization or external consultants outside the client organization.

- Nurse managers and consultants need a wide variety of competencies, including leadership, interpersonal, organizational, and political skills. Leadership skills include abilities to influence others to work toward achieving a vision, empower others, delegate tasks, manage time, and make decisions effectively.
- Interpersonal skills include communication, motivation, appraisal and coaching, contracting, team building, and diversity management skills.
- Organizational skills include planning, organizing, and implementing community nursing services; monitoring and evaluating services; quality improvement; and managing fiscal resources.
- Political skills are those used in negotiation and conflict management and managing power dynamics among health care teams and within the community.
- Population-focused nurses need analytical and informatics skills to be able to identify and monitor trends, improve health care safety, and evaluate outcomes.
- In general, both nurse managers and consultants must hold a minimum of a baccalaureate degree in nursing. Organizations employing nurses without this credential should help them obtain additional education in the areas of community or nursing, management theories and principles, and theories and principles of consultation.
- By working with policy makers, government leaders at all levels, and advocacy organizations, nurse leaders have the power to change the health care system to provide accessible, quality, evidence-based care to individuals and populations.

CLINICAL DECISION-MAKING ACTIVITIES

1. Discuss with your class members the implications that managed care and discounted fee-for-service preferred provider organizations have for nurse managers and consultants in community-based organizations and in the public health departments. What other implications can you think of in addition to those described in the text?
2. Draft a vision and mission statement for a nursing clinic with your classmates. Develop goals and objectives that follow the vision and mission you selected. What type of employees would you need to hire? List some of the policies and procedures you would need to have in such a clinic on the basis of your vision, mission, goals, and objectives.
3. Have several class members obtain the vision, mission, and philosophy statements from agencies in which students have community health clinical experiences. Compare these statements in terms of the agencies' target populations, basic values, and essential functions.
4. Interview one or more practicing staff nurses working with populations. Ask them to describe the activities of their jobs that could be categorized as consultation. During the interview, attempt to determine the following:
   A. How they define consultation
   B. The goals they are attempting to achieve with their consulting activities
   C. The model they seem to be applying in their consulting activities
   D. The intervention strategies they use
   E. Whether their activities are of a generalist or a specialist nature and of an internal or external consultative nature
   F. The strengths and limitations they perceive in themselves regarding their consultative functions (e.g., education, experiential, organizational, relational, economic)
5. Interview one or more nurse consultants. During the interview, attempt to determine the answers to the preceding questions. Compare the responses of the two groups (public health nurse consultants and population-focused staff nurses). Analyze the factors you think account for the similarities and differences.
6. Visit a nurse-managed clinic for underserved populations. Talk with nurses and other staff members about how they work together as a team and what they do to promote client involvement in determining needed clinic services. Develop a case analysis of the microsystem within the clinic and how clinical care delivery is continuously monitored, evaluated, and improved within the system. What recommendations might you have for strengthening the clinical information system in the clinic?

ADDITIONAL RESOURCES

EVOLVE WEBSITE

http://evolve.elsevier.com/Stanhope/community/

- Answers to Practice Application
- Case Study
- Glossary
- Review Questions

REFERENCES

Allen JK, Dennison Himmelfarb CR, Szanton SL, Frick KD: Cost-effectiveness of nurse practitioner/community health worker care to reduce cardiovascular health disparities, *J Cardiovasc Nurs* 29(4):308–314, 2014.
Allen PM: Strategic partnering to gain competencies for future healthcare delivery, *Front Health Serv Manage* 34(1):41–47, 2017.
Alligood MR: *Nursing theorists and their work*, ed 9, St. Louis, 2018, Elsevier.

American Nurses Association (ANA): *Public health nursing: scope and standards of practice*, ed 2, Silver Spring, MD, 2013, ANA.
American Nurses Association (ANA): *Nursing administration – scope and standards of practice*, ed 2, Silver Spring, MD, 2016, ANA.
American Nurses Association (ANA): *School nursing - scope and standards of practice*, ed 3, Silver Spring MD, 2017, American Nurses Association and the National Association of School Nurses.
Association of Community Health Nurse Educators Education Committee: *Essentials of baccalaureate nursing education for entry-level community/public health nursing*, Wheat Ridge, CO, 2009, ACHNE.
Association of Public Health Nurses: *The public health nurse – necessary partner for the future of healthy communities*, 2016, APHA. Retrieved from http://phnurse.org.
Batterham RW, Hawkins M, Collins PA, Buchbinder R, Osborne RH: Health literacy – applying current concepts to improve health services and reduce health inequalities, *Public Health* 132:3–12, 2016.
Bekemeier B, Walker Linderman T, Kneipp S, Zahner SJ: Updating the definition and role of public health nursing to advance and guide the specialty, *Public Health Nurs* 32(1):50–57, 2015.
Berry LL, Rock BL, Smith Houskamp B, et al: Care coordination for patients with complex health profiles in inpatient and outpatient settings, *Mayo Clin Proc* 88:184–194, 2013.
Bureau of Labor Statistics (BLS): *Occupational Handbook – Registered Nurses*, 2018, US Department of Labor. Retrieved from https://www.bls.gov.
Bureau of Primary Health Care: Report to Congress: *Efforts to expand and accelerate health center program quality improvement*, Washington, DC, 2014, U.S. Department of Health and Human Services. Retrieved from https://bphc.hrsa.gov.
Butcher HK, Bulechek GM, Dochterman JM, Wagner C: *Nursing interventions classification*, ed 7, St. Louis, 2019, Mosby.
Campaign for Action: *About us*, 2018, AARP Foundation, AARP, Robert Wood Johnson Foundation. Retrieved from https://campaignforaction.org.
Cipriano PF: Faith, community, and health: partnerships with good neighbors, *Am Nurse Today* 9(2), 2014.
Community Preventive Services Task Force: *The community guide*, Atlanta, GA, 2018, USDHHS. Retrieved from https://www.thecommunityguide.org.
Community Tool Box: *About the tool box*, 2018a, KU Center for Community Health and Development. Retrieved from https://ctb.ku.edu.
Community Tool Box: *Developing an action plan*, 2018b, KU Center for Community Health and Development. Retrieved from https://ctb.ku.edu.
Cordo J, Hill-Rodriguez D: The evolution of a nursing professional practice model through leadership support of clinical nurse engagement, empowerment, and shared decision making, *Nurse Leader* 15(5):325–330, 2017.
Council on Linkages between Academia and Public Health Practice: *Core competencies for public health professionals*, Atlanta, GA, 2014, Centers for Disease Control and Prevention, Health Resources and Services Administration, and the Public Health Foundation. Retrieved from http://www.phf.org.
Craft-Blacksheare M: New careers in nursing—an effective model for increasing nursing workforce diversity, *J Nurs Educ* 578(3): 178–183, 2018.
Crowell DM: *Complexity leadership – nursing's role in health-care delivery*, ed 2, Philadelphia, 2016, F. A. Davis Company.
Cutts T, Gunderson G, Carter D, et al: From the Memphis Model to the North Carolina Way: lessons learned from emerging health system and faith community partnerships, *N C Med J* 78(4): 267–272, 2017.
Duffy M, Dresser S, Fulton JS: *Clinical nurse specialist toolkit—a guide for new clinical nurse specialist*, New York, 2016, Springer Publishing Company, LLC.
Edmonds JK, Campbell LA, Gilder RE: Public health nursing practice in the Affordable Care Act era: a national survey, *Public Health Nurs* 34(1):50–58, 2016.
Englebright J, Aldrich K, Taylor CR: Defining and incorporating basic nursing care actions into the electronic health record, *J Nurs Scholarsh* 46:50–57, 2014.
Fischer SA: Transformational leadership in nursing—a concept analysis, *J Adv Nurs* 72(11):2644–2653, 2016.
Foronda C, MacWilliams B, McArthur E: Interprofessional communication in healthcare – an integrative review, *Nurse Educ Pract* 19:36–40, 2016.
Forrester DA: *Nursing's greatest leaders*, ed 1, New York, 2016, Springer Publishing Company.
Franks H: The contribution of nurse consultants in England to the public health leadership agenda, *J Clin Nurs* 23(23/24):3434–3448, 2014.
Gallup Inc: *Nurses keep healthy lead as most honest, ethical profession*, 2017, Brenan M. Retrieved from https://news.gallup.com.
Gottlieb LM, Tirozzi KJ, Manchanda R, Burns AR, Sandel MT: Moving electronic medical records upstream, *Am J Prev Med* 48(2):251–218, 2015.
Hamric AB, Hanson CM, Tracy MF, et al: *Advanced practice nursing: an integrative approach*, ed 5. St. Louis, 2014, Elsevier.
Hanlon JT, Perera S, Newman AB, et al: Potential drug-drug and drug-disease interactions in well-functioning community-dwelling older adults, *J Clin Pharm Ther* 42(2):228–233, 2017.
Huber D: *Leadership and nursing care management*, ed 6, St. Louis, 2018, Elsevier.
Institute of Medicine (IOM): *To err is human: Building a safer health system*. In Kohn L, Corrigan J, Donaldson M, editors: Washington, DC, 2000, National Academy Press.
Institute of Medicine (IOM): *Crossing the quality chasm: a new health system for the 21st* century, Committee on Quality and Health Care in America, Washington DC, 2001, National Academy Press.
Institute of Medicine (IOM): *The future of nursing: leading change, advancing health*, 2011, Committee on the Robert Wood Johnson Foundation Initiative on the Future of Nursing. Washington, DC, 2011, National Academies Press.
Institute of Medicine (IOM): In Balogh EP, Miller BT, Ball JR, editors: *Improving diagnosis in health care*, Washington, DC, 2015a, National Academy Press, pp. 1–276.
Institute of Medicine (IOM): *Assessing progress on the Institute of Medicine Report the future of nursing*, 2015b. Retrieved from http://www.nationalacademies.org.
Johnston LM, Finegood DT: Cross-sector partnerships and public health: challenges and opportunities for addressing obesity and noncommunicable diseases through engagement with the private sectors, *Annu Rev Public Health* 36:255–271, 2015.
Jones C, Finkler SA, Kovner CT: *Financial management for nurse managers and executives*, ed 5, St. Louis, 2018, Saunders.
Jones NT, Seckman C: Facilitating adoption of an electronic documentation system, *CIN: Comput Inform Nurs* 36(5): 225–231, 2018.
Kihlgren A, Svensson F, Lovbrand C, Gifford M, Adolfsson A: A decision support system (DSS) for municipal nurses encountering health deterioration among older people, *BMC Nursing* 15(63): 1–10, 2016.
Kowlowitz V, Woods-Giscombe C, Kneipp SM, Page J, Gray TF: Careers beyond the bedside—an effective program to increase diversity in nursing, *J Cult Divers* 25(2):41–48, 2018.

Kyounghae K, Choi JS, Choi E, et al: Effects of community-based health worker interventions to improve chronic disease management and care among vulnerable populations—a systematic review, *Am J Public Health* 106(4):e3–e38, 2016.

LeBlanc P: Leadership by design—creating successful 'TEEAMS', *Nurs Manage* 45(3):49–51, 2014.

Likosky DS: Clinical microsystems—a critical framework for crossing the quality chasm, *J Extra Corpor Technol* 46(1):33–37, 2014.

Lim JY, Noh WN: Key components of financial-analysis education for clinical nurses, *Nurs Health Sci* 17(3):293–298, 2015.

Mackenzie R: Supervision and appraisal: how to support staff performance, *Nurs Resid Care* 15:452–454, 2013.

Makary MA, Daniel, M: Medical error—the third leading cause of death in the US, *BMJ (Online)*, 353:i2139, 2016. doi:10.1136/bmj.i2139.

Massarweh LJ, Tidyman T, Luu DH: Starting the shift out right—the electronic eAssignment sheet using clinical decision support in a quality improvement project, *Nursing Economics* 35(4):194–200, 2017.

Michelangelo L: *Emotional intelligence, emotional competency, and critical thinking skills in nursing and nursing education [doctoral dissertation]*, 2013, Walden University. Full text retrieved from CINAHL website.

Miller GE, Sarpong EM, Davidoff AJ, Yang EY, Brandt NJ, Fick DM: Determinants of potentially inappropriate medication use among community-dwelling older adults, *Health Serv Res* 52(4): 1534–1549, 2017.

Mone EM, London M: *Employee engagement through effective performance management—a practical guide for managers*, ed 2, New York, 2018, Taylor & Francis.

National Council of State Boards of Nursing (NCSBN): National guidelines for nursing delegation, *J Nurs Regul* 7(1):5–14, 2016.

Nightingale F: *Notes on Nursing. 1859*, Reprint, 1912, New York, D. Appleton and Company.

Nurse.com News: *Sebelius Lauds Nurses, Pledges Continued Support*, 2013. Retrieved from https://www.nurse.com.

Nurses on Boards Coalition: *About our story*, 2018. Retrieved from https://www.nursesonboardscoalition.org.

Olds DL, Kitzman H, Knudtson MD, Anson E, Smith JA, Cole R: Effect of home visiting by nurses on maternal and child mortality—results of a 2-decade follow-up of a randomized clinical trial, *JAMA Pediatr* 169(9):800–806, 2014.

Olson LG: Public health leadership development: factors contributing to growth, *J Public Health Manag Pract* 19:341–347, 2013.

Okello DR, Gilson L: Exploring the influence of trust relationships on motivation in the health sector—a systematic review, *Hum Resour Health* 13(16):1–18, 2015.

Phillips M: Embracing the multigenerational nursing team, *MEDSURG Nursing* 25(3):197–198, 2016.

Quad Council Coalition Competency Review Task Force: *Community/Public Health Nursing Competencies,* 2018. Retrieved from http://www.quadcouncilphn.org.

Randall S, Crawford T, Currie J, River J, Betihavas V: Impact of community-based nurse-led clinics on patient outcomes, patient satisfaction, patient access and cost effectiveness—a systematic review, *Int J Nurs Stud* 73:24–33, 2017.

Ray MA: *Transcultural caring dynamics in nursing and health care*, ed 2, Philadelphia, 2016, F. A. Davis Company.

Ridge RA: A look at nurse consultancy, *Nurs Manage* 46(8):52–54, 2015.

Robert Wood Johnson Foundation: *From vision to action: a framework and measures to mobilize a culture of health*, 2015. Retrieved from https://www.rwjf.org.

Robert Wood Johnson Foundation: *Catalysts for change: harnessing the power of nurses to build population health in the 21st* century, *executive summary*, 2017, RWJF. Retrieved from https://www.rwjf.org.

Rosenstein AH, Dinklin SP, Munro J: Conflict resolution—unlocking the key to success, *Nurs Manage* 45(10):34–39, 2014.

Roussel LA, Thomas PL, Harris JL: *Management and leadership for nurse administrators*, ed 7, Burlington, 2016, Jones & Bartlett Learning, LLC.

Schaffer MA, Anderson LJW, Rising S: Public health interventions for school nursing practice, *J Sch Nurs* 32(3):195–208, 2016.

Schein EH: *Process consultation*, Reading MA, 1969, Addison-Wesley.

Schein EH: *Process consultation revisited,* Englewood Cliffs, NJ, 1999, Prentice-Hall.

Schein EH: *Helping: how to offer, give, and receive help*, San Francisco, 2011, Berrett-Koehler.

Schein EH: *Humble consulting—how to provide real help faster*, Oakland CA, 2016, Berrett-Koehler Publishers, Inc.

Schein EH, Schein P: *Organizational culture and leadership*, ed 5, Hoboken, 2016, John Wiley & Sons.

Shade MY, Berger AM, Chaperon C, Haynatzki G, Sobeski L, Yates B: Factors associated with potentially inappropriate medication use in rural, community-dwelling older adults, *J Gerontol Nurs* 43(9):21–30, 2017.

Sitman K, Watson J: *Caring science, mindful practice: implementing Watson's Human Caring Theory*, ed 2, New York, 2018, Springer Publishing Company, LLC.

Smith MC, Turkel MC, Wolf ZR: *Caring in nursing classics—an essential resource*, ed 1, New York, 2013, Springer.

Solman A: Nursing leadership challenges and opportunities, *J Nurs Manag* 25(6):405–406, 2017.

Talley LB, Thorgrimson DH, Robinson NC: Financial literacy as an essential element in nursing management practice, *Nurs Econ* 31:77–82, 2013.

U.S. Census Bureau, Vespa J, Armstrong DM, Medina L: *Demographic turning points for the United States: Population Projections for 2020 to 2060*, P25–1144, 2018,Washington, DC, U.S. Department of Commerce, Economics and Statistics Administration, U.S. Census Bureau. . Retrieved from https://www.census.gov.

U.S. Clinical Preventive Services Task Force: *Guide to clinical preventive services*, 2014, Recommendations of the U.S. Preventive Services Task Force. AHRQ Publication No. 14-05158. Rockville, MD, 2014, Agency for Healthcare Research and Quality. Retrieved from https://www.ahrq.gov.

U.S. Department of Health and Human Services (USDHHS): *Healthy People 2020*, Washington, DC, 2010, Office of Disease Prevention and Health Promotion. Retrieved from www.healthypeople.gov.

Vertino KA: Effective interpersonal communication—a practical guide to improve your life, *OJIN: Online J Issues Nurs* 19(3):1, 2014.

Wakefield M: Nurses and the Affordable Care Act: a call to lead. *Reflect Nurs Leadersh* 39(3), 2013.

Waldecker A, Malpass A, King A, Ridd MJ: Written action plans for children with long-term conditions—a systematic review and synthesis of qualitative data, *Health Expectations* 21(3):585–596, 2018.

Watson J: *Nursing - the philosophy and science of caring,* (Rev. ed), Boulder, 2008, University Press of Colorado.

Weiss SA, Tappen RM: *Essentials of nursing leadership and management*, ed 6, Philadelphia, 2015, F. A. Davis Company.

Westcott L: How coaching can play a key role in the development of nurse managers, *J Clin Nurs* 25(17/18):2669–2677, 2016.

World Health Organization: In Kickbusch I, Pelikan JM, Apfel F, Tsouros AD, editors: *Health literacy: the solid facts,* UN City, 2013, Regional Office for Europe, WHO, pp. 1–80.

41

The Nurse in Public Health, Home Health, Hospice, and Palliative Care

Karen S. Martin, RN, MSN, FAAN and
Kathryn H. Bowles, RN, PhD, FAAN

OBJECTIVES

After reading this chapter, the student should be able to do the following:

1. Compare different practice models for home and community-based services.
2. Summarize the basic roles and responsibilities of public health, home health, hospice, and palliative care nurses.
3. Explain the professional standards and educational requirements for nurses in public health, home health, hospice, and palliative care.
4. Describe the three components of the Omaha System.
5. Analyze how nurses in public health, home health, hospice, and palliative care use best practices, evidence-based practice, and quality improvement strategies to improve the care they provide.
6. Cite examples of trends and opportunities in public health, home health, hospice, and palliative care involving technology, informatics, and telehealth.

CHAPTER OUTLINE

Home Health Care
Hospice and Palliative Care
Additional Nurse-Led Models
Population Health
Scope and Standards of Practice
Omaha System
Practice Guidelines
Practice Linkages
Accountability and Quality Management
Professional Development and Collaboration
Legal, Ethical, and Financial Issues
Trends and Opportunities
Summary

KEY TERMS

accreditation, p. 915
benchmarking, p. 915
client outcomes, p. 909
consumer engagement, p. 900
documentation, p. 907
electronic health record (EHR), p. 907
evidence-based practice, p. 900
family caregiver, p. 901
home health care, p. 901
home health nursing, p. 902
hospice and palliative care, p. 903
hospice care, p. 903
information management, p. 907
interoperability, p. 919
interprofessional collaboration, p. 900
Medicare-certified, p. 902
Merit-based Incentive Payment System (MIPS), p. 919
nursing practice, p. 907
nursing process, p. 907
Omaha System, p. 907
Omaha System Intervention Scheme, p. 908
Omaha System Problem Classification Scheme, p. 908
Omaha System Problem Rating Scale for Outcomes, p. 909
Outcome and Assessment Information Set (OASIS), p. 903
Outcome-Based Quality Improvement (OBQI), p. 915
palliative care, p. 903
population health, p. 900
practice settings, p. 900
regulations, p. 902
skilled nursing care, p. 921
skilled nursing services, p. 902
telehealth, p. 918
transitional care, p. 906

Public health, home health, hospice, and palliative care nursing are rapidly expanding specialties under the broad umbrella of public health, community-oriented, and population-focused practice. When nurses practicing these specialties provide comprehensive assessment, planning, intervention, and evaluation services, they contribute to the total health of the general public as noted on the first page of this book and Chapter 1. Two additional nurse-led models are summarized in this chapter, the Nurse-Family Partnership and transitional care. Although the practice of these nurses is very diverse, **evidence-based practice** should be the goal. More details will be described later in the chapter.

For the purposes of this chapter, public health, home health, hospice, and palliative care nursing refer to a wide variety of **practice settings** and holistic services typically provided to clients of all ages by these nurses in their residences, noninstitutional settings, and some institutional settings. In general, public health and home health providers offer intermittent, skilled supportive care, treatments, and/or assistance with activities of daily living so that elders and others who are ill or have disabilities remain safe and avoid unnecessary hospitalization. Hospice and palliative care services are intended to provide comfort and meet physical, emotional, and spiritual needs to all ages. Hospice services are provided at end of life and do not include curative treatment according to Medicare rules. In contrast, palliative care is a wider range of services, is not limited to the days or weeks prior to end of life, and may include curative treatment.

A number of agencies have agreements with diverse settings, including residential and acute care facilities, so that nurses provide services in locations in addition to clients' homes. The settings include community or senior centers, libraries, corrections facilities, and work sites. As will be described later, public health, home health, hospice, and palliative care nurses and their interprofessional colleagues are employed by diverse organizations such as public health departments and voluntary, hospital-based, and proprietary organizations. Mergers, buyouts, and collaborative agreements are increasing rapidly and causing practice boundaries to blur. It is very important to note that an organization's name does not predict the types of programs and services provided.

Numerous references in this chapter describe research, finances, client personal preference, and new technology suggesting that the home is the optimal location for diverse health and nursing services (Ansberry, 2018; Buhler-Wilkerson, 2002; Gao, Maganti, & Monsen, 2017; Gorski, 2017; Marrelli, 2018a; Milone-Nuzzo & Hollars, 2017; NFP, 2017; NHPCO, 2018; Reddy, 2018; Wright, 2018). Client residences include houses, apartments, trailers, boarding and care homes, hospice houses, assisted living facilities, shelters, and cars. Home health, hospice, and palliative services are provided by formal caregivers who include nurses, social workers, physical and occupational therapists, home health aides, licensed practical nurses, chaplains, physicians, and others. Because of the nature of the practice, a team approach and **interprofessional collaboration** are required. The specific disciplines involved vary with the program, the intensity of the client and family's needs, the location of the program and home, and reimbursement.

The Triple Aim model for health care was published in 2008 (Berwick, Nolan, & Whittington, 2008). However, the primary concepts of the model have been the foundation and core values of public health, home health, and related community-based services from their inception: improve the health of populations, enhance the experience of care for individuals, and reduce the per capita cost of health care. The Triple Aim is a good strategy to encourage health promotion, prevention, and healthier lifestyles regardless of the program or setting, although all illness, including chronic illness, cannot be prevented or cured. Because the population is aging rapidly in this country and internationally, the need for services is increasing dramatically. In 2015, less than 50 million Americans were 65 years and older compared to about 98 million projected for 2060. Almost 20 million Americans may be 85 years and older in 2060 (Ansberry, 2018; Kerr et al., 2019; MedPAC, 2018; U.S. Census Bureau, 2017). Although a related concept, **population health**, is older than the Triple Aim, the term was not widely used in this country until more recently. Population health is the health status of a population of individuals, including the distribution of health status within the group (Kindig & Stoddart, 2003). According to Storfjell, Winslow, and Saunders (2017), nurses must become a well-utilized population health resource and full partner in bringing solutions to the national high cost/poor health dilemma.

Access to other health care professionals, resources, and equipment is very different when home and institutional care settings are compared. Many nurses find public health, home health, hospice, and palliative practice very rewarding because they observe the impact of their services and practice with a high degree of autonomy. Nurses who make home visits need to have good organizational, communication, critical thinking, and documentation skills. They need to understand ever-changing reimbursement regulations. Competence, integrity, adaptability, good judgment, and creativity are essential characteristics. Public health, home health, hospice, and palliative nurses need to watch for risks in the physical environment and to be savvy about their own safety as well as the safety of their clients. The Agency for Healthcare Research and Quality (AHRQ, 2017) provides rich resources about client and patient safety. It is important to stay alert and change the plan of action quickly if trouble arises when using cars or public transportation, and when inside, entering, or leaving clients' residences (Marrelli, 2018a; Milone-Nuzzo & Hollars, 2017; Schoon, Porta, & Schaffer, 2018).

When entering a residence, the public health, home health, hospice, or palliative care nurse is a guest and needs to earn the trust of the family and establish a partnership with the client and family (Fig. 41.1); more details are described later in the Practice Guidelines section. It is essential that clients and families are involved in making decisions for home-based services to be efficient and effective; this team approach may be referred to as **consumer engagement**.

Family is defined by the individual client and includes any caregiver or significant other who assists the client with care at

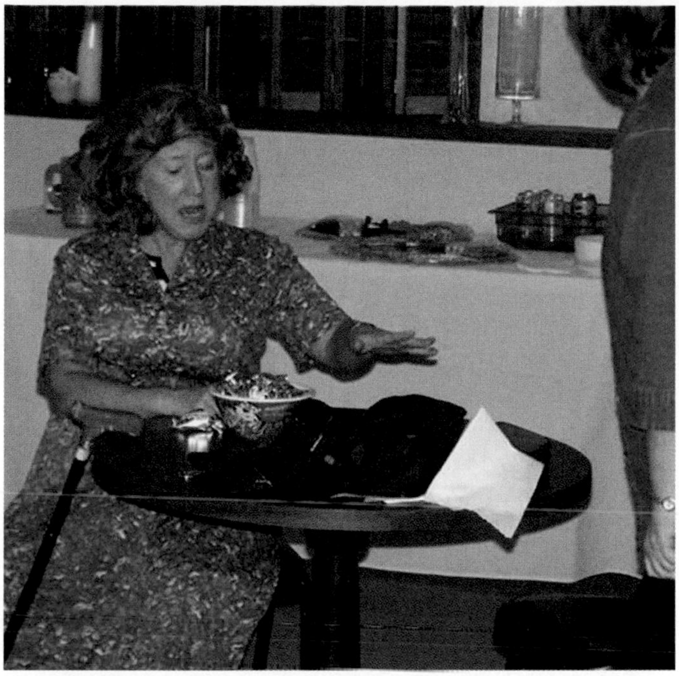

Fig. 41.1 Nurses are guests in clients' homes. (From www.omahasystem.org/photogallery.html. Used with permission from Karen S. Martin, RN, MSN, FAAN.)

home. Family caregiving involves transportation, helping clients meet their basic needs, and providing care such as personal hygiene, meal preparation, medication administration, and simple as well as complex treatments. Today's clients and family caregivers provide many aspects of care in the home that were previously provided in hospitals or in home by professional caregivers. Care can be confusing, challenging, stressful, burdensome, and frightening for family caregivers; many are not well-prepared for their new roles. Clients need to be monitored regularly, and some require 24-hour care. Many family caregivers need assistance to identify diverse support services that enable them to provide care while maintaining their own physical and emotional health (Ansberry, 2018; Chow & Dahlin, 2018; Diefenbeck, Klemm, & Hayes, 2017; Gao et al., 2017; Gasper et al., 2018; Gorski, 2017; Izumi, 2017; Marrelli, 2018a; Milone-Nuzzo & Hollars, 2017; NHPCO, 2018; Reddy, 2018; Wright, 2018).

HOME HEALTH CARE

Evolution of Home Health Care

Home health care provided by formal caregivers in the United States originated in the nineteenth century. In many communities, the initial programs evolved into nonprofit visiting nurse agencies and health departments. The movement expanded rapidly in the United States, resulting in the formation of 71 home health agencies prior to 1900, and 600 organizations by 1909. Additional historical details are described in Chapter 2 and other publications (Buhler-Wilkerson, 2002; Donahue, 2011).

Home health services were included as a major benefit when Medicare and Medicaid legislation was passed in 1965 and implemented in 1966. (See Chapter 5, Economics of Health Care Delivery.) Both resulted in significant changes nationally. The Medicare benefit was designed to provide intermittent, shorter visits with temporary lengths of stay to people age 65 and older who were homebound. Medicaid covered a wider range of services than Medicare and included children, pregnant women, parents of certain Medicaid-eligible children, and persons with certain disabilities. For clients who qualified for Medicare or Medicaid services, the home health agency was required to develop a plan of care for clients and obtain the signature of a physician.

During the next 30 years, the number of Medicare-certified agencies grew rapidly as a result of the aging population and prospective payment legislation that decreased the length of hospital stays. This trend changed when the Balanced Budget Act of 1997 was enacted, changing the home health payment system from a fee-for-service model to prospective payment based on a standardized assessment completed at admission. The Act prompted the closure of more than 30 percent of the country's Medicare-certified home health agencies and a dramatic decline in the number of clients served. Between 2004 and 2015, the number of agencies grew by more than 60 percent, a dramatic increase. Although the number of agencies fell slightly in 2016, the general trend is increasing growth (MedPAC, 2018; U.S. Census Bureau, 2017; Wright, 2018).

Description of Home Health Care

Home health care is a broad concept and approach to services and is at the top of the list of the fastest growing, service-providing industries in this country (BLS, 2017a). It includes a focus on primary, secondary, and tertiary prevention; the primary focus can involve aggregates, similar to those provided by other population-focused nurses. (See the Levels of Prevention box.) Initiatives involving primary and secondary prevention have always been important to home health care.

LEVELS OF PREVENTION

Home Health

Primary Prevention

The nurse (1) administers seasonal and newer strains of flu vaccine or (2) provides case management interventions so clients obtain the vaccines at convenient locations.

Secondary Prevention

The nurse monitors clients in their homes for early signs of new health problems in order to initiate prompt treatment. When the nurse works collaboratively with the physician and/or nurse practitioner, effective interventions can be provided. An example is monitoring clients for medication side effects.

Tertiary Prevention

The nurse provides instruction about dietary modifications and insulin injections to clients with new diagnoses of diabetes. Clients and their families implement the therapeutic plan to identify signs of infection, prevent complications, and maintain the highest possible level of health and self-care.

Home health nursing is "a specialty area of nursing practice that promotes optimal health and well-being for patients, their families, and caregivers within their homes and communities. Home health nurses use a holistic approach aimed at empowering patients/families/caregivers to achieve their highest levels of physical, functional, spiritual, and psychosocial health. Home health nurses provide nursing services to patients of all ages and cultures and at all stages of health and illness, including end of life" (ANA, 2014, p. 7). Home health nurses include generalist nurses, public health nurses, clinical nurse specialists, and nurse practitioners. They and their interprofessional team members provide diverse services to target populations such as new parents; clients recovering from injuries, acute illness, and surgery; frail elders; and clients managing disabilities, and chronic health problems. Some home health agencies include wellness programs, health fairs, school nurses, communicable disease prevention, and other programs that are similar to those offered by public health departments.

Home health nurses and their team members help clients and their families achieve improved health and independence in a safe environment. In addition to nursing care, the following are available to those who are Medicare eligible: physical therapy, occupational therapy, speech and language pathology, home health aide, and medical social services. Skilled nursing and **skilled nursing services** are the Medicare terms that describe the duties of the registered nurse, refer to the requirement of professional nursing judgment, and include diverse assessment, teaching, case management, and other interventions (CMS, 2016, 2018b, 2018c). Using Omaha System terms that are introduced later in this chapter, assessment involves Environmental, Psychosocial, Physiological, and Health-Related Behaviors concerns, while interventions are categorized as Teaching, Guidance, and Counseling; Treatments and Procedures; Case Management; and Surveillance (Martin, 2005; Monsen, 2018; Omaha System, 2018).

According to MedPAC (2018), about 3.4 million individuals received **Medicare-certified** home health services in 2016 that were reimbursed by the Centers for Medicare and Medicaid Services (CMS). The total number of visits exceeded 114 million, and beneficiaries averaged 33 visits during the year. About 51 percent of the visits included skilled nursing, 39 percent therapy, 10 percent home health aides, and 1 percent medical social services (MedPAC, 2018). An unknown number of additional clients received services from non-Medicare-certified agencies. The majority of home health clients were 65 years and older; more were women than men; and many had diagnoses of circulatory disease, diabetes, neurological conditions, and depression (CMS, 2016; MedPAC, 2018).

Home health agencies can be divided into the following five general categories (Fazzi, 2018; MedPAC, 2018) (Fig. 41.2).

- Official or public agencies receive tax revenue and are operated by state, county, city, or other local government units, such as health departments. Typically, official agencies also offer well-child clinics, immunizations, health education programs, and home visits for preventive health care.
- Voluntary and private agencies are nonprofit home health agencies and usually receive some funds from United Way, donations, and endowments. Currently, there are about the same number of voluntary and private agencies. Visiting Nurse Associations, AS EXAMPLE, are usually freestanding, voluntary, nonprofit organizations governed by a board of directors, and usually financed by earnings, donations, and tax-deductible contributions. Sometimes they are categorized with combination agencies because of their similar characteristics.

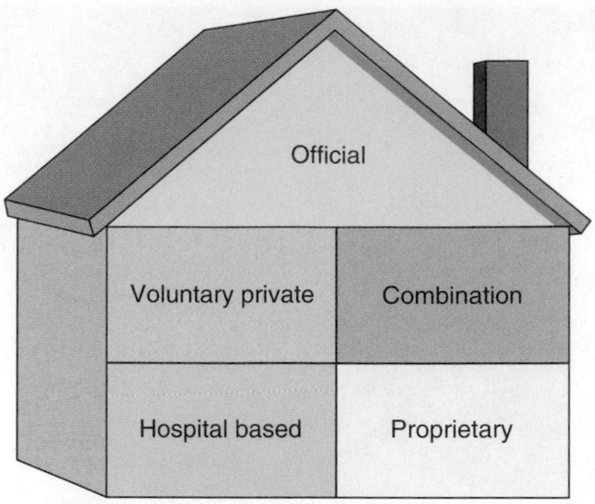

Fig. 41.2 Types of home health agencies.

- Combination agencies have characteristics of both governmental and voluntary agencies. The number of combination agencies continues to decrease, although some are large agencies.
- Hospital-based agencies grew rapidly during the 1970s and 1980s when the advent of diagnosis-related groups led to earlier hospital discharges and Medicare reimbursement was encouraging. Since then, some hospitals and their home health agencies separated because of changes in reimbursement and other pressures.
- Proprietary agencies are freestanding, for-profit agencies that are required to pay taxes. Many are part of large chains. Proprietary agencies now dominate the industry and represent about 80 percent or more of all agencies. Almost all new providers are proprietary agencies.

In 2018, about 12,200 agencies provided Medicare services (MedPAC, 2018). Texas has more than 2000 agencies, while California and Florida have just over 1000 agencies (Fazzi, 2018). The size of individual agencies varied from those that employ a few nurses to the Visiting Nurse Service of New York with its 1525 nurses, more than 13,000 employees, 48,500 daily client census, and 1,363,488 annual visits (VNSNY, 2017, Sockolow, 2018).

Although agencies vary as to programs offered, size, administration, ownership, organization, and board structures, they must meet ever-changing licensure, certification, and accreditation **regulations** established by national and state groups. The primary source of those regulations is CMS (CMS, 2017b, 2017c, 2018b, 2018c). To be Medicare-certified and reimbursed, CMS requires that home health agencies complete a rigorous certification process, follow the rules of the Conditions of Participation (CoPs), and provide intermittent, skilled professional services

(CMS, 2017c). The rule book that agencies must follow is referred to as the Conditions of Participation (CoPs); key criteria are (1) the client must be home-bound or are unable to leave home without considerable effort; (2) services must be intermittent and include a skilled service provided by a nurse, physical therapist, or speech and language pathologist; (3) a plan of care must be initiated and followed; and (4) Medicare forms, physician orders, and client records must be completed on a timely basis.

The Conditions of Participation are lengthy, complex, and subject to change. For example, in 1999, CMS mandated the Outcome and Assessment Information Set (OASIS); it has been updated several times. The current version is described later in this chapter as are other Medicare regulations, reimbursement, and accreditation details (CMS, 2017c). Beginning in 2011, physicians or allowed non-physician practitioners (nurse practitioners and physician assistants) must have a face-to-face encounter with clients prior to signing orders and initiating care (CMS, 2017c). Home health nurses must be well-informed about Medicare regulations to determine the visit frequency and timing based on their clients' conditions and communicate with physicians. Frequently, clients and their families ask nurses to help them understand their Medicare benefits.

Annual national expenditures for home health care in 2016 were $18.1 billion (Fazzi, 2018; MedPAC, 2018). During the same year, home health accounted for about 3 percent of the country's total Medicare expenditures in contrast to 49 percent for hospitals and 11 percent for skilled nursing facilities. Medicare is the largest payer for home health services. In addition to Medicare, state and local governments accounted for 15 percent of home health reimbursement, Medicaid for 24 percent, private insurance for 8 percent, out-of-pocket or private pay 10 percent, and other sources 2 percent (CMS, 2016).

HOSPICE AND PALLIATIVE CARE

Evolution of Hospice and Palliative Care

Hospice care was introduced in the United States in the 1970s by Florence Wald, often referred to as the mother of the hospice movement. Before establishing Connecticut Hospice in 1974, Dr. Wald collaborated with Dame Cicely Saunders, a British nurse, physician, and social worker who founded St. Christopher's Hospice in England in 1967 (ANA/HPNA, 2014; Wright, 2018; Zerwekh, 2006). During the same era, Dr. Elisabeth Kübler-Ross, a physician, published *On Death and Dying* (1969), a book that was widely read by the public and health care professionals. Dr. Ross described the inhumanity of a death-denying society such as the United States, the need to provide sensitive end-of-life care and involve clients in choices, and an emphasis on the quality of life (ANA/HPNA, 2014; Perry & Parente, 2017; Zerwekh, 2006).

Medicaid reimbursement for hospice care began in 1980 and Medicare in 1983; reimbursement determines many aspects of the programs, including the types and length of services. The number of Medicare-certified hospices grew from 31 in 1984 to 2323 in 2002 and to 4199 in 2015. In 2016, 1.4 million Medicare beneficiaries were enrolled in hospice care (NHPCO, 2018). Because the time of death is difficult to predict and many people in this country are reluctant to acknowledge a terminal prognosis, hospice care often begins late in the disease process. Barriers and stigmas continue to be associated with hospice for some clients, families, and physicians; because they equate hospice with hopelessness and giving up, they are reluctant to consider hospice. A number of the same people are receptive to the concept of palliative care and will accept those services (Buch & Nies, 2015; CMS, 2018c; Gasper et al., 2018; Marrelli, 2018b; NHPCO, 2018; Perry & Parente, 2017; Stober, 2017; Wright, 2018; Zerwekh, 2006).

In 1987, the first comprehensive, integrated palliative care program was established in the United States at the Cleveland Clinic. The focus was specialized care for those living with signs and symptoms and the stress of serious illness. Similar palliative care programs originated earlier in England (Etkind et al., 2017). In 1999, the Robert Wood Johnson Foundation funded the Center to Advance Palliative Care (CAPC) to stimulate the development of high-quality palliative care programs in hospitals and other health care settings. In 2010, the CAPC convened a consensus panel to establish criteria for palliative care assessment components at hospital admission and during the hospital stay (CAPC, 2018; Weissman & Meier, 2011). Assessment items include recent history of the illness, pain and symptom assessment, patient-centered goals of care, and transition of care plans; the goal is to help clinicians identify those individuals and their families who need palliative care. CAPC reports that the number of palliative care programs in U.S. hospitals increased from 658 in 2000 to 1831 in 2016 (CAPC, 2018).

Description of Hospice and Palliative Care

Hospice and palliative care are similar and, yet, very different. Similarities that are described throughout this chapter include a client-focused/consumer engagement approach, holistic and evidence-based practice, emphasis on ethics, communication skills, interprofessional collaboration, care coordination, focus on transitions of care, and caregiving skills that include symptom management, pain relief, and comfort. The following differences are primarily related to reimbursement requirements in this country and include the length of care and frequency and intensity of services. The goal of the hospice movement is to humanize the end-of-life experience. For hospice services, physicians need to indicate that clients have six months or less to live, and clients acknowledge that they have a terminal prognosis and select care that is comfortable, not life-extending. In contrast, the goal of palliative care is quality of life. Palliative services are not restricted based on the disease or progress and may be appropriate for those with a serious, complex illness regardless if they are expected to recover fully, live with a chronic illness for an extended time, or experience serious disease progression (ANA/HPNA, 2014; CMS, 2017b; 2018b, 2018c; Chow & Dahlin, 2018; Etkind et al., 2017; HPNA/ANA, 2007; Perry & Parente, 2017; Slipka & Monsen, 2018; U.S. Census Bureau, 2017).

The Hospice and Palliative Nurses Association (HPNA) and others suggest that palliative care is a broad term occurring over a longer period of time, and hospice is a subset with a short time period. The HPNA developed an illustration referred to as the Trajectories of Palliative Care and included it in their 2014 publication (ANA/HPNA, 2014). The title of the illustration is palliative care and represents an extended continuum of chronic serious illness to acute serious illness during which stabilization and exacerbations may occur. Services and treatment vary during this time. The continuum encompasses three segments: a longer segment that is referred to as diagnosis, limited signs and symptoms, and increasing severity of signs and symptoms; a relatively short period of hospice care and death; and a period of bereavement care for family members.

The HPNA is an umbrella organization that represents hospice and palliative nurses and other members of the team employed in home-based organizations as well as acute and long-term care, outpatient, and other settings (ANA/HPNA, 2014; ANA/HPNA, 2017). The organization's mission is to advance expert care during serious illness; it is based on four pillars of education, advocacy, leadership, and research. Nurses who are members of hospice and palliative care teams "provide evidence-based physical, emotional, psychosocial, and spiritual or existential care to individuals and families experiencing life-limiting, progressive illness" (HPNA/ANA, 2007, p. 1). The definition of hospice focuses on comfort for individuals and their families at the end of life and does not include curative treatment. The HPNA did not define their specialty in their new 2014 publication, but, instead, endorsed the National Consensus Project of Palliative Care's (NCP) definition. "Palliative care means patient and family-centered care that optimizes quality of life by anticipating, preventing, and treating suffering. Palliative care throughout the continuum of illness involves addressing the physical, intellectual, emotional, social, and spiritual needs and [facilitating] patient autonomy, access to information, and choice" (NCP, 2013, p. 9; NCP, 2018.

Both the interprofessional hospice and palliative care teams work closely together to provide comprehensive care in partnership with clients and their families. The teams include nurses, physicians, social workers, therapists, chaplains, counselors, aides, pharmacists, and volunteers; volunteers are essential team members. The Bureau of Labor (2017b) suggests that the need for employees and volunteers is increasing dramatically. Most agencies and team members consider conferences and continuing education essential to develop and renew their skills involving topics such as advance care planning, end-of-life comfort measures, new medications and treatments, therapeutic communication, compassion fatigue, spirituality, complex family dynamics, and cultural awareness. Working with clients who are dying involves unique emotional stress; hospice and palliative care programs usually address the team's well-being as well as that of the clients and families (ANA/HPNA, 2014, 2017; Buch & Nies, 2015; Diefenbeck et al., 2017; Hinds et al., 2005; Izumi, 2017; NHPCO, 2018; Slipka & Monsen, 2018; Wright, 2018; Zerwekh, 2006).

Clients and their families and friends are at the center of the hospice and palliative care teams and will be involved in advance care planning, symptom and medication management, personal care, and the use of supplies. Death produces intense emotions even when family members have prepared for it. Bereavement services that are part of hospice involve attending the funeral or other services for the deceased client, and contact at anniversaries of death, holidays, and the client's birthday for 13 months after the client's death. Hospice organizations usually offer support group opportunities for families or refer them to support groups in the area.

Palliative care has no specific federal designation as a specialty; rather it exists as a consultative discipline delivering a philosophy of care. Palliative care programs in hospitals have been growing steadily. As of 2016, 75 percent of hospitals were able to support inpatient palliative care programs, an increase from 25 percent in 2000 (Center to Advance Palliative Care [CAPC], 2018).

Palliative care clinicians must meet certain regulatory requirements when they practice in home health or other community agencies (ANA/HPNA, 2014). There are many predictions and publications that support the need for palliative care programs in the home, but very few articles or studies published about actual programs outside of acute care settings. Health care professionals, educators, researchers, organizations, and the media are making slow progress to introduce palliative care in the home without Medicare, Medicaid, or other funding sources that are available for hospice (ANA/HPNA, 2017; Chow & Dahlin, 2018; Etkind et al., 2017; Izumi, 2017; Stober (2017) conducted a literature review and found nine articles published in the last ten years; palliative care at home improved the quality of care and client outcomes including the reduction of 30-day hospital readmissions. Gasper et al. (2018) designed and conducted a quality improvement project for 13 subjects admitted to a home health care organization in Pennsylvania with a diagnosis of heart failure. Providers' skills improved with education and training, and 30-day hospital readmissions were reduced.

Hospice is a formalized, funded program in hospice and home health agencies with extensive data. For that reason, it is the focus of the following paragraphs. Initially, cancer was the primary diagnosis of most clients in hospice programs. More recently, cancer is the diagnosis of about 20-30 percent of hospice clients, and dementia, cardiac and circulatory, neurological, respiratory, and other end-stage diseases make up 70-80 percent of the diagnoses (NHPCO, 2018). More than one million clients received Medicare-certified hospice services in 2017 with an average stay of 87.8 days (MedPAC, 2018). The average length of stay will rise if home health nurses and others provide information about end-of-life hospice care to clients and families, and hospice becomes more widely accepted by the public. Most agencies are educating their nurses to recognize clients in need of hospice or palliative care and have discussions with clients and families as a strategy to decrease the hospice stigma that results in late referrals or missed opportunities. Even when nurses, physicians, and others discuss quality of life and encourage the transition from palliative services to hospice, clients and/or families may continue in denial and not accept hospice until the last several days of life. Late referrals resulting in brief hospice stays make it difficult for the hospice team to provide comprehensive, expert, cost-effective services to clients and families. For many in this country, death is not viewed as a normal or natural part of the life cycle (Buch & Nies, 2015; Izumi, 2017; Marrelli, 2018b; NHPCO, 2018; Perry & Parente, 2017; Wright, 2018; Zerwekh, 2006).

Hospice providers can be divided into four general categories. Freestanding facilities are the most common followed by home health agencies and hospital-based facilities. Skilled nursing facilities are the least common. Many freestanding facilities are for-profit providers, similar to home health agencies. The average length of hospice service in 2016 was 71 days, and the median length was 24 days (NHPCO, 2018).

After the client acknowledges a terminal prognosis and selects comforting care rather than life-extending or curative care, hospice organizations coordinate services in partnership with the client and family and provide financial case management. According to Zerwekh (2006), hospice addresses four foci: (1) attention to the body, mind, and spirit; (2) death is not a taboo topic; (3) health care technology should be used with discretion; and (4) clients have a right to truthful discussion and participation in treatment decisions. The four types of care and the percent used are (1) routine home care with intermittent visits, 92.3 percent; (2) continuous home care when condition is acute and death is near, 1.3 percent; (3) general inpatient/hospital care for symptom relief, 6.1 percent; and (4) respite care in a nursing home of no more than 5 days at a time to relieve family members, 0.3 percent (NHPCO, 2018).

Hospice is the only Medicare benefit that includes medications, medical equipment, 24-hour/seven-day-a-week access to care, and support for family members after death. Those who receive Medicare-certified hospice services are evaluated during the 6-month period to determine if they are eligible to continue. The time period is divided into two 90-day certification periods, and is followed by an unlimited number of subsequent 60-day periods. Authorization by physicians is required for the certification periods (CMS, 2017b, 2018c; Perry & Parente, 2017).

Hospice programs are usually operated and staffed as independent entities or corporations even when they are part of a larger organization because of the specialized nature of the practice and the complex Medicare regulations and financial requirements. Similarly to home health, hospice nurses must be familiar with regulations and financial requirements; however, the OASIS is not a requirement for hospice programs as it is for home health.

Medicare, Medicaid, U.S. Department of Veterans Affairs (VA), managed care, private insurance, and private donations fund most hospice services. Medicare provides the most funds and spent 16.9 billion dollars in 2016. Hospice services account for about 6 percent of the total Medicare budget, about twice as much as home health services (CMS, 2016, 2017b, 2018c; NHPCO, 2018).

Home Care of Dying Children. "The death of a child alters the life and health of others immediately and for the rest of their lives" (Hinds et al., 2005, p. S70). The needs of dying children and their families are unique because of the degree of emotional impact, and because the young are not expected to die or precede the death of their parents. Nurses need to recognize the child's physical, cognitive, psychosocial, and spiritual development as well as the family's dynamics, cultural heritage, and spiritual beliefs. That recognition is essential to provide appropriate pain management, assist the child and family to communicate with each other, advocate for their needs in the community, and provide case management and continuity of care (Hinds et al., 2005; Kaye et al., 2015; Levine et al., 2017; Weaver et al., 2016).

Bereavement programs as described for hospice programs are especially important for families who have lost a child. Parents, grandparents, and siblings can participate in a variety of support groups offered by the hospice program or other bereavement organizations (Levine et al., 2017; Weaver et al., 2016).

HOW TO Use a Hospice Approach to Care in Any Setting

The hospice philosophy of care means providing comfort measures to individuals before death and support for their families before and after death. Individuals may be any age. Death may occur in the individual's home, a hospital setting, or an uncontrolled setting such as the community. How does one adapt nursing care in any situation? What basic skills can professional caregivers use that can be applied in any situation or setting? How do professional caregivers adapt to the death of a hospice client, inpatient death, or a sudden, unexpected death where, for example, many people have died as a result of a natural disaster or a terrorist act?

- Be prepared. Consider your own philosophy of death so that you can assist others without distraction when that time comes.
- Cultures vary in their beliefs about and responses to death. Know the differences in cultural responses so that you can effectively help people in their time of need.
- Death events cannot be totally controlled even in a hospice environment where the eventual death has been illustrated to family and friends and the dying individual before the death. Expect the unexpected and take cues from the client and the loved ones regarding their needs.
- Shock, disbelief, and crisis reactions occur even with prepared, hospice deaths. Ask family and caregivers what they need; provide them with the basics such as food or blankets; provide comfort; if it is not contraindicated, provide the family/friends with personal effects or mementos of the individual; give sensitive, caring support. Sit with them and listen.

Modified from Mistovich JJ, Karren KJ: *Prehospital emergency care*, ed. 10, Upper Saddle River, NJ, 2014, Pearson Education; Mistovich JJ, Karren, KJ: *Prehospital emergency care*, ed. 11, Upper Saddle River, NJ, 2018, Pearson Education.

ADDITIONAL NURSE-LED MODELS

The Nurse-Family Partnership and transitional care are focused on interprofessional collaboration as well as care coordination, critical thinking, best practices, and evidence-based practice. Best practices suggest using credible, established evidence from a variety of sources including research, experience, and expert clinicians; evidence-based practice suggests increased emphasis on programs of research that demonstrate consistently good outcomes (Melnyk & Fineout-Overholt, 2015; Melnyk & Gallagher-Ford, 2015). With both models, nurses have essential roles in the provision of care, documentation of services, program development and management, outcome measurement and effectiveness analysis, and public education.

Nurse-Family Partnership

The Nurse-Family Partnership (NFP) was initiated in 1977 by a researcher, David Olds, and a nurse, Harriet Kitzman; it is probably the best known and well-funded nurse home visit specialty program in the United States (Enoch et al., 2016; NFP, 2017; Olds et al., 1997). The Partnership is a network of nurses, families, and policy makers. Nurses receive extensive orientation and provide structured education and case management during regularly scheduled home visits to pregnant women; visits continue until the children's second birthday. The goals of the program are to improve pregnancy outcomes, child health and development, and economic self-sufficiency of the families. Many rigorous studies and longitudinal, randomized controlled trials have documented numerous lifelong improvements in health outcomes that were statistically significant and economically sound. Mothers had fewer children, were more likely to become employed, and were less likely to enter the criminal justice system. Children were less likely to be abused, experience behavioral and intellectual problems by age 6, to be arrested by age 15, or to be obese. Both mothers and children demonstrated improved health and development. More fathers were present in the households. Initial recipients of care were ethnically diverse, low-income, first-time mothers and their families who lived in New York, Tennessee, and Colorado. In 2017, nurses visited more than 50,000 families in 42 states. Federal and private funding continues to increase as the program maintains successful outcomes and grows. NFP had revenues of more than 36.9 million dollars in 2017 (Enoch et al., 2016; Miller, 2015; NFP, 2017; Olds et al., 1997; Thorland et al., 2017).

Transitional Care

As a result of a fragmented health care system, increasing complexity of client care, and rising costs, transitional care has gained much needed attention in this country and internationally (Meadows et al., 2014). Transitional care is defined as "a set of actions designed to ensure the coordination and continuity of health care as clients transfer between different locations and different levels of care in the same location" (Coleman & Berenson, 2004, p. 1). Challenges to quality care originate from a lack of depth, accuracy, and timeliness of information received from the referring site; the need for complex medication reconciliation; and difficulties with communication and coordination among community-based providers.

Transitional care programs that involve home health have emerged as low- and high-intensity interventions that include, but vary from, traditional home health interventions. Low-intensity interventions include coaching, telephone follow-up, and specific disease management programs. High-intensity transitional care programs are designed for populations who have complex or high-risk health problems. An example is the Transitional Care Model, where advanced practice nurses perform transitional care from hospital to home providing in-hospital visits and discharge planning followed with home visits, primary care office visits, and telephone follow-up for one to three months after discharge (Naylor et al., 2017). Numerous studies have been conducted to test the Transitional Care Model with high-risk groups such as heart failure and dementia (Naylor et al., 2016). The research model is currently implemented in practice settings in collaboration with major insurance companies and home care agencies (Naylor et al., 2013).

Outcomes achieved with the Transitional Care Model consistently show cost savings and improvements in clinical and quality outcomes for clients receiving the intervention compared with usual care (Naylor et al., 2013). The most common outcome across all populations is a consistent reduction in readmissions to a hospital. The Transitional Care Model strategies emphasize screening in acute care for high-risk clients; engaging the elder/caregiver in designing personalized goals and the plan of care; managing symptoms; educating and promoting self-management; and collaborating with the multidisciplinary team members to assure continuity and a team approach. Both the low- and high-intensity transitional care programs have spread rapidly into practice as hospitals seek ways to avoid the financial penalties associated with higher than the national average 30-day readmission rates. The penalties are instituted through the Readmission Reduction Program enacted through the 2010 Patient Protection and Affordable Care Act (CMS, 2018e).

CHECK YOUR PRACTICE

You are working with a home health agency that is interested in defining the populations they serve. You have been asked to suggest and approach to accomplish this task. What approach would you suggest and how can you help with the task? What would you do?

POPULATION HEALTH

Population health is the health status of a population of individuals, including the distribution of health status within the group as mentioned early in this chapter and in Chapter 1. The field or emerging specialization of population health includes health status, determinants of the population's health, and policies and interventions that link those two (Kindig & Stoddart, 2003). Although the concept of population health was discussed for some years, dissemination was limited. After the concepts of the Triple Aim were widely embraced, population health began appearing more frequently in practice, education, research, health care literature, and the public press. The speed increased when CMS and private insurers began to move away from fee-for-service reimbursement and toward value-based care.

Nurses are educated to consider health issues in a large context. Nurses who work in community practice settings are involved in population health each day as they make home visits and provide care to clients and families in diverse settings. Aspects of population health are related to community assessment and windshield surveys, projects and assignments that nurses have used in community health practice and academic settings for years (Kerr et al., 2016, 2019). Models are described elsewhere in this book (see Chapter 17). Social science professionals described a four-step approach and the associated functions, key questions, and key challenges to improve population health. The steps are reflect, assess, specify changes, and implement and evaluate (Wendel et al., 2018). Notice how similar these problem-solving steps are to the nursing process described in the next section of this chapter.

Storfjell et al. (2017) conducted a project for the Robert Wood Johnson Foundation and published an excellent report entitled *Catalysts for Change: Harnessing the Power of Nurses to Build Population Health in the 21st Century.* Their purpose was to "describe how nurses can best promote the health of the US population and reverse current health declines. The paper explores population-health related nursing roles and skills, and identifies their implications for nursing practice, education, research, and policy" (p. 2). "A population-focused nurse will move beyond the individualistic, downstream approach, viewing individuals and families in the context of their environment, and assessing how their community affects them" (p. 3). Nurses should identify and address social determinants of health, discern patterns across populations, link individuals and families to community resources, and develop broad-based interventions. Focusing on social determinants of health offers an upstream focus and offers opportunities for data mining, big data analysis, and quantifying outcomes of care (Gao et al., 2017; Gao et al., 2018; Monsen et al., 2016). According to Susan Swider (Storfjell et al., 2017), "If you think about population health and nursing practice, there is a role for nursing caring for individuals to better understand care coordination and how to assess for and address the social determinants of health. That is very much in the bailiwick of individual nursing practice. It doesn't require you to do big picture planning across large numbers of people, but it requires [the RN] to practice a bit differently" (p. 4).

Other authors have suggested practical ways that nurses can improve the health of their communities. Ross (2018) states that nurses can take action and make a difference where they learn, pray, work, and live and suggests that nurses become involved with schools, faith-based organizations, workplaces, neighborhoods, and advocacy. Duke University and the Duke University School of Nursing have developed a comprehensive, long-term plan to involve students and faculty in population health (Duke Nursing, 2018). An example of a population health approach will be described in the Medication Management section later in this chapter.

SCOPE AND STANDARDS OF PRACTICE

Nursing is a theory and practice-based profession that incorporates art and science. Examples of nursing, family, and systems theories are mentioned and summarized in other chapters of this book. Chapter 8 focuses on cultural diversity, and includes many references. In addition, Smith (2017a, 2017b) published articles that are students' and nurse educators' guides to cultural competence. Chapter 10 addresses evidence-based practice; the concept is addressed frequently in this chapter, and one example is included. Melnyk is one of the most prolific authors on this topic (Melnyk & Fineout-Overholt, 2015; Melnyk & Gallagher-Ford, 2015). Several chapters of this book describe the Quad Council Coalition's (2018) eight domains of practice; those domains are linked to information in this chapter in the Linking Content to Practice box.

The **nursing process** is the theoretical framework used by the American Nurses Association (ANA), which notes that the nursing process is the essential methodology by which client goals are identified and achieved. Their scope and standards publications, including those for home health nursing and palliative nursing, are organized according to the nursing process and contain two sections: the Standards of Care and the Standards of Professional Performance (ANA, 2013, 2014; ANA/HPNA, 2014). Publications include the six steps of the nursing process: assessment, diagnosis, outcomes identification, planning, implementation, and evaluation; the steps are linked to standards and more specific measurement criteria that are stated in behavioral objectives. The standards address quality of care, performance appraisal, critical thinking skills, education, collegiality, ethics, collaboration, research, and resource use.

OMAHA SYSTEM

The **Omaha System** was initially developed to operationalize the nursing process and provide a practical, easily understood, computer-compatible, quantifiable guide for daily use in diverse community settings. It is the only ANA-recognized terminology developed inductively by and for nurses who practice in the community (ANA, 2018).

As early as 1970, the nurses, other staff, and administrators of the Visiting Nurse Association (VNA) of Omaha, Nebraska, began addressing **nursing practice**, **documentation**, and **information management** concerns. Information management is the integration of clinical, demographic, financial, administrative, and staffing data; manipulation or processing of these data; and production of various reports that transform data into meaningful information for decision making (Martin, 2005). At that time, clinicians were not using computers, and there was no systematic nomenclature or classification of client problems and concerns, interventions, or client outcomes to quantify and measure clinical data and integrate with a problem-oriented record system.

More than 22,000 multiprofessional clinicians, educators, and researchers use Omaha System point-of-care **electronic health records (EHRs)** across the health care continuum in the United States and other countries, far beyond the initial use in community settings in the United States. About 2000 more use paper-and-pen records. EHRs are longitudinal collections of clinical and demographic client-specific data that are stored in a computer-readable format. By 2005, 85 percent of all counties in Minnesota had one or more public health or home care agencies or schools/colleges of nursing using Omaha System software. That number continues to increase as clinicians, providers, and funders want to measure the outcomes of care. During 2014, Minnesota became the first state to recommend that the Omaha System be used as a standardized terminology in the EHRs of all community health care settings in the state. Details about Omaha System application, users, case studies, inclusion in reference terminologies, research, best practices/evidence-based practice, and listserv are described in publications and on the website (Eardley et al., 2018; Martin, 2005; Martin & Kessler, 2017; Monsen, 2018; Monsen et al., 2018; Omaha System, 2018; Topaz, Golfenshtein, & Bowles, 2014).

Description of the Omaha System

Between 1975 and 1993, the VNA of Omaha staff conducted four extensive, federally funded development and refinement research studies that established reliability, validity, and usability of the Omaha System. The result of the research was the Problem Classification Scheme, the Intervention Scheme, and the Problem Rating Scale for Outcomes. These three components of the Omaha System were designed to be used together, be comprehensive, relatively simple, hierarchical, multidimensional, and computer compatible. The Omaha System has existed in the public domain since the initial research in 1975. Because it is not held under copyright, software companies can use it as the foundation of their software without obtaining licenses or paying fees. They are expected to replicate the structure, terms, and codes as presented and cite their source (Eardley et al., 2018; Martin, 2005; Martin & Kessler, 2017; Omaha System, 2018).

As depicted in Fig. 41.3, the Omaha System conceptual model is based on the dynamic, interactive nature of the nursing or problem-solving process, the practitioner-client relationship, and concepts of diagnostic reasoning, critical thinking, and quality improvement. The client as an individual, a family, or a community appears at the center of the model. This location suggests the range of Omaha System application, client-centered care, and the essential partnership between clients and practitioners that Omaha System developers and users have embraced from the onset. The term *consumer engagement* has been used to describe this partnership, especially in acute care practice. Most nurses and other clinicians employed in community settings recognized that partnership was essential from the beginning of their employment. The outer circle is the practitioner-client relationship. Additional details about the conceptual model are described in the following paragraphs (Gao et al., 2018; Martin, 2015; Monsen et al., 2016; Omaha System, 2018).

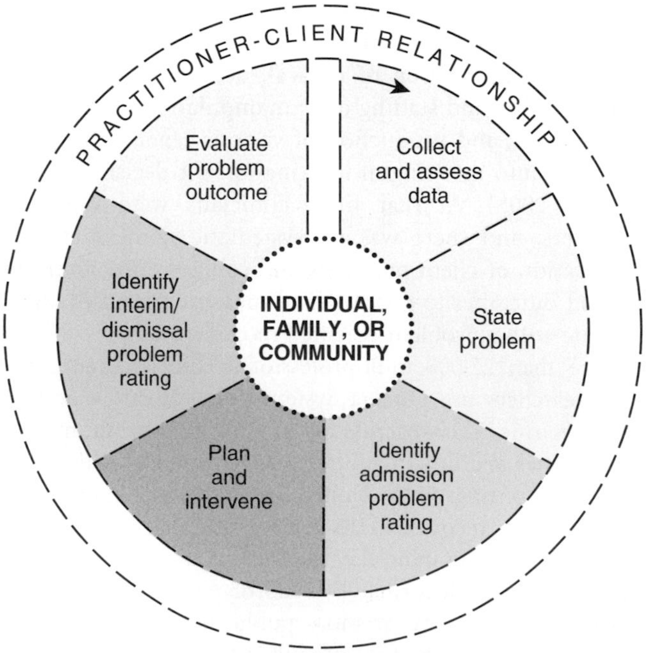

Fig. 41.3 Omaha System model of the problem-solving process. (From Martin KS: *The Omaha System: a key to practice, documentation, and information management,* reprinted ed. 2, Omaha, NE, 2005, Health Connections Press.)

Early Omaha System practice, education, and research use focused on individuals and families. The focus on the community or population level is increasingly rapidly as changes occur throughout the health care system and reimbursement (Kerr et al., 2016; Kerr et al., 2019; Monsen, 2018; Monsen et al., 2016; Monsen et al., 2018; Schoon et al., in press)

The Omaha System was intended for use by nurses and all members of the health care delivery team. The goals of the research were to (1) develop a structured and comprehensive system that could be both understood and used by members of various disciplines, and (2) foster collaborative practice. Therefore the Omaha System was designed to guide practice decisions, sort and document pertinent client data uniformly, and provide a framework for an agency-wide, multidisciplinary clinical information management system capable of meeting the daily needs of clinicians, managers, and administrators (Eardley et al., 2018; Martin, 2005; Martin & Kessler, 2017; Monsen et al., 2018; Omaha System, 2018; Quad Council Coalition, 2018).

Problem Classification Scheme. The Omaha System Problem Classification Scheme is a comprehensive, orderly, nonexhaustive, mutually exclusive taxonomy designed to identify diverse clients' health-related concerns. Its simple and concrete terms are used to organize a comprehensive assessment, an important standard of nursing practice. The Problem Classification Scheme consists of four levels. Four domains appear at the first level and represent priority areas. Forty-two terms, referred to as client problems or areas of client needs and strengths, appear at the second level. The third level consists of two sets of problem modifiers: health promotion, potential and actual, as well as individual, family, and community. Clusters of signs and symptoms describe actual problems at the fourth level. The content and relationship of the domain and problem levels depicted in Box 41.1 are further illustrated by the case example at the end of this chapter. Understanding the meaning of and relationships among the terms is a prerequisite to using the scheme accurately and consistently to collect, sort, document, analyze, quantify, and communicate client needs and strengths.

Intervention Scheme. The Omaha System Intervention Scheme is an important standard of nursing practice in providing

BOX 41.1 Domains and Problems of the Omaha System Problem Classification Scheme

Environmental Domain

Material resources and physical surroundings both inside and outside the living area, neighborhood, and broader community:

- Income
- Sanitation
- Residence
- Neighborhood/workplace safety

Psychosocial Domain

Patterns of behavior, emotion, communication, relationships, and development:

- Communication with community resources
- Social contact
- Role change
- Interpersonal relationship
- Spirituality
- Grief
- Mental health
- Sexuality
- Caretaking/parenting
- Neglect
- Abuse
- Growth and development

Physiological Domain

Functions and processes that maintain life:

- Hearing
- Vision
- Speech and language
- Oral health
- Cognition
- Pain
- Consciousness
- Skin
- Neuro-musculo-skeletal function
- Respiration
- Circulation
- Digestion-hydration
- Bowel function
- Urinary function
- Reproductive function
- Pregnancy
- Postpartum
- Communicable/infectious condition

Health-Related Behaviors Domain

Patterns of activity that maintain or promote wellness, promote recovery, and decrease the risk of disease:

- Nutrition
- Sleep and rest patterns
- Physical activity
- Personal care
- Substance use
- Family planning
- Health care supervision
- Medication regimen

From Martin KS: *The Omaha System: A key to practice, documentation, and information management*, reprinted ed. 2, Omaha, NE, 2005, Health Connections Press.

interventions. Four broad categories of interventions appear at the first level of the Intervention Scheme. An alphabetical list of 75 targets or objects of action and 1 "other" appear at the second level. Client-specific information generated by clinicians is at the third level. The contents of the category and target levels are depicted in Boxes 41.2 and 41.3, respectively. The Intervention Scheme provides the terms for care plans and services. It enables clinicians to describe, quantify, and communicate their practice, including improving or restoring health, describing deterioration, or preventing illness.

Problem Rating Scale for Outcomes. The Omaha System Problem Rating Scale for Outcomes consists of three five-point, Likert-type scales for measuring the entire range of severity for the concepts of Knowledge, Behavior, and Status. Each of the subscales is a continuum providing a framework for measuring and comparing problem-specific client outcomes at regular or predictable times, because evaluation is an important standard of nursing practice. Suggested times include admission, specific interim points, and discharge. The content and relationships of the scale are depicted in Table 41.1. Using the Problem Rating Scale for Outcomes with the Problem Classification Scheme and the Intervention Scheme creates a comprehensive problem-solving model for practice, education, and

BOX 41.2 Categories of the Omaha System Intervention Scheme

Teaching, Guidance, and Counseling

Activities designed to provide information and materials, encourage action and responsibility for self-care and coping, and assist the individual, family, or community to make decisions and solve problems.

Treatments and Procedures

Technical activities such as wound care, specimen collection, resistive exercises, and medication prescriptions that are designed to prevent, decrease, or alleviate signs and symptoms for the individual, family, or community.

Case Management

Activities such as coordination, advocacy, and referral that facilitate service delivery; promote assertiveness; guide the individual, family, or community toward use of appropriate community resources; and improve communication among health and human service providers.

Surveillance

Activities such as detection, measurement, critical analysis, and monitoring intended to identify the individual, family, or community's status in relation to a given condition or phenomenon.

From Martin KS: *The Omaha System: a key to practice, documentation, and information management*, reprinted ed. 2, Omaha, NE, 2005, Health Connections Press.

BOX 41.3 Targets of the Omaha System Intervention Scheme

anatomy/physiology	medication administration
anger management	medication coordination/ordering
behavior modification	medication prescription
bladder care	medication set-up
bonding/attachment	mobility/transfers
bowel care	nursing care
cardiac care	nutritionist care
caretaking/parenting skills	occupational therapy care
cast care	ostomy care
communication	other community resources
community outreach worker services	paraprofessional/aide care
continuity of care	personal hygiene
coping skills	physical therapy care
daycare/respite	positioning
dietary management	recreational therapy care
discipline	relaxation/breathing techniques
dressing change/wound care	respiratory care
durable medical equipment	respiratory therapy care
education	rest/sleep
employment	safety
end-of-life care	screening procedures
environment	sickness/injury care
exercises	signs/symptoms-mental/emotional
family planning care	signs/symptoms-physical
feeding procedures	skin care
finances	social work/counseling care
gait training	specimen collection
genetics	speech and language pathology care
growth/development care	spiritual care
home	stimulation/nurturance
homemaking/housekeeping	stress management
infection precautions	substance use cessation
interaction	supplies
interpreter/translator services	support group
laboratory findings	support system
legal system	transportation
medical/dental care	wellness
medication action/side effects	other

From Martin KS: *The Omaha System: a key to practice, documentation, and information management*, reprinted ed. 2, Omaha, NE, 2005, Health Connections Press.

research; the model operationalizes the nursing or problem-solving process.

PRACTICE GUIDELINES

Nursing practice is based on education, experience, and evidence. Because home health and hospice and palliative care nurses usually work with clients and their families in their homes, they must develop skills to conduct home visits efficiently, effectively, and safely (Box 41.4). A positive attitude about client-centered care, the nurse-client partnership, and consumer engagement is essential. Critical thinking skills are also essential. Effective care coordination requires familiarity with community resources. Knowledge and skills involving medications, treatments, documentation, and equipment are necessary. Excellent strategies include accompanying skilled home health, hospice, and palliative care nurses when they make home visits as well as having expert mentors. However, novice nurses also need a commitment to lifelong learning, practice, and self-evaluation (Buch & Nies, 2015; Marrelli, 2018a; Milone-Nuzzo & Hollars, 2017; Radhakrishnan et al., 2016; Schoon et al., in press; Zerwekh, 2006). The following is a brief summary of steps included in a home visit; these steps can be modified slightly for other noninstitutional settings:

- Review client data, including the referral from the intake department, hospital discharge summary, orders, and plan of care to become familiar with the client's history, purpose of the visit, and expectations.
- Contact the client or family by calling the telephone number listed on the referral information to obtain agreement for the visit, schedule the day and time, and discuss the address.
- Gather agency and Medicare forms, a nursing bag, cellular phone or pager, portable computing device, teaching materials, and supplies; understand the client's location; follow the agency policy when checking-out for the visit.
- Observe the neighborhood for resources and safety when approaching the client's home.
- Greet the client/family to begin developing a positive, appropriate professional relationship; involve them as much as possible during the visit and post-visit activities.

TABLE 41.1 Omaha System Problem Rating Scale for Outcomes

Concept	1	2	3	4	5
Knowledge: Ability of client to remember and interpret information	No knowledge	Minimal knowledge	Basic knowledge	Adequate knowledge	Superior knowledge
Behavior: Observable responses, actions, or activities of client fitting occasion or purpose	Not appropriate behavior	Rarely appropriate behavior	Inconsistently appropriate behavior	Usually appropriate behavior	Consistently appropriate behavior
Status: Condition of client in relation to objective and subjective defining characteristics	Extreme signs/ symptoms	Severe signs/ symptoms	Moderate signs/ symptoms	Minimal signs/ symptoms	No signs/symptoms

From Martin KS: *The Omaha System: a key to practice, documentation, and information management,* reprinted ed. 2, Omaha, NE, 2005, Health Connections Press.

BOX 41.4 Guidelines for Public Health, Home Health, and Hospice

- You are a guest in your client's home and neighborhood. Your behavior and your manners must convey that you recognize this role.
- Respect the client's cultural, religious, and ethnic heritage. Hesitate before contradicting that heritage. Clients are more likely to follow their heritage than your advice.
- The client may not respect your cultural, religious, and ethnic heritage. If you are a male nurse, the client may expect, and even request, a female nurse. Develop interpersonal skills—and a tough skin.
- Almost every client has family members, significant others, or friends who offer advice and can serve as either your advocate or your foe. Try to enlist them as your advocate.
- The client "owns" the health-related problem that initiated your services. That problem is just one portion of the client's past, present, and future. Thus it is the client who experiences, learns to understand, and ultimately solves the problem. It is your goal to help clients and their families become independent as quickly as possible. Talk to your peers and supervisors if you sense that you may be losing that perspective.
- Enjoy the unique autonomy and challenges of providing highly complex care in the home and community setting. Practice requires integration of high-technology skills, teaching, case management, and monitoring. Remember the need and benefits of collaboration with other members of the health care team. The nurse is usually responsible for judging whether or not the client can safely remain at home. However, data and information to support this and other decisions need to be communicated with team members orally and through the electronic health record.
- Maintain your sense of humor. You will need it!

Modified from Black JM, Hawks JH: *Medical surgical nursing*, ed. 8, St. Louis, 2009, Saunders, p. 94.

- Obtain signatures and complete needed forms.
- Provide care by completing a comprehensive assessment, identifying client problems, providing interventions, and evaluating client outcomes. Interventions may include teaching, guidance, and counseling; treatments and procedures; case management; and surveillance (Martin, 2005).
- Discuss the plan of care with the client and family during informal or formal conferences; modify as needed.
- Document some or all of the visit details in the home, preferably while using a portable computing device and an EHR.
- Discuss the next visit as well as follow-up activities and referrals.
- Proceed to the next scheduled visit after checking in, according to the agency policy.
- Complete remaining visit documentation, submit forms, coordinate referrals to other community resources, and communicate with agency colleagues, the referral source, physicians, and others as appropriate. Obtain revised orders if needed.
- Revisit to reassess the client and provide care.

Clinical Example From Community-Focused Practice

The example describes an innovative and collaborative community-focused program developed in Tucson, Arizona, by the Pima County Health Department and the Pima County Public Library. Since this program was initiated, other communities have involved nurses in their libraries (Innes, 2012; RWJF, 2013, 2018). The Pima County Public Library requested that the Health Department hire a social worker to increase safety and a welcoming environment in five high-risk libraries. Concerns included loitering, behavioral health concerns, encampment, and abandonment. Many patrons were homeless and/or had chronic diseases that were not being managed. Children and elders were left at the library by family members while they completed errands or went to work.

After a root-cause analysis was conducted and a logic model developed, the decision was made by Kathleen Malkin, Public Health Nursing Division Manager, and the Health Department and Library management staff to hire one full-time public health nurse in January 2012, a first in this country. It was decided that a nurse could better meet the identified needs of the patrons and library staff. In addition to increasing safety and a welcoming environment, a goal was to coordinate with community resource agencies to provide nutritious snacks for children and reduce hunger concerns.

During the first year, the program expanded to include five public health nurses working in six high-risk libraries. They made 180 visits to the libraries and had 2181 patron encounters. Client problems and clinician interventions were documented. The most frequently identified problems were health care supervision, nutrition, circulation, hearing, personal care, and cognition. The nurses instructed the library staff on communicable disease prevention topics. During the first year, calls made to the police and 911 were reduced by 6 percent and calls to 911 for medical emergencies were reduced by 20 percent.

In the second year, the program expanded to 13 library sites, including 2 bookmobile sites serving rural communities. Student nurses assisted the public health nurses as they completed community assessments and tailored services to the needs of each library. Working with library patrons, nurses completed 3746 encounters and 1160 assessments; 1420 health education sessions; and 192 referrals for services. They also provided health education to 76 library staff members. During the third year, nurses provided diverse health education and services to patrons. Services include assistance applying for public or private insurance, diabetes education, flu vaccine, and health education for library staff.

Using the Omaha System and an automated documentation system to capture community-level data had numerous benefits. Included were communication between the nurses and between the nurses and their health department; an evidence-based approach to practice; a standardized method of assessment, care planning, services, and evaluation; and a process that generated accurate and consistent data capable of conversion to information and useful reports.

PRACTICE LINKAGES

There are no limits to the diversity of clients who live in the community, their problems, and their strengths; the interventions that nurses provide; and the client outcome data that are generated. Although many examples are diverse, as can be seen in the practice application, and in Box 41.7, they represent a small fraction of the actual roles and responsibilities of public health, home health, hospice, and palliative care nurses. The examples illustrate fundamental principles of professional practice: (1) a holistic approach to the steps of the nursing or problem-solving process; (2) consumer engagement or a partnership with clients as unique individuals, families, and communities; and (3) a focus on outcomes.

The following sections of the chapter are designed to increase the reader's understanding about the links between systematic best practices, evidence-based practice, and other aspects of the public health, home health, hospice, and palliative milieu. The typical nurse will not be involved with the theme of each section daily, but will over a period of months.

Setting short- and long-term goals provides criteria for evaluation and increases continuity of care and the potential for improved outcomes. Research has shown that goals set with the client rather than for the client are more successful regarding self-motivation, adherence, and attainment (Curtis et al., 2018; Zhang et al., 2015).

Outcome and Assessment Information

In 1999, the CMS mandated the collection of the Outcome and Assessment Information Set (OASIS) from all adult, nonmaternity home health clients as part of the Conditions of Participation for Medicare-certified home health agencies (CMS, 2017c). Completion of the OASIS provides a systematic, comparative measurement of client outcomes at two or more points in time. The completed OASIS improves communication about the clients' conditions among the agency's clinicians, other agency staff, and external groups; improves reimbursement; and demonstrates improved, cost-effective client outcomes as a result of home health services. CMS provides agencies with reports of their process quality (how well they follow best practices), risk-adjusted outcomes (physical and functional improvement or stabilization), and potentially avoidable events (hospitalization, new wounds). OASIS also provides data for calculating the agency's reimbursement for a particular client's episode, and promotes a standardized approach to assessment within the home care industry (Fig. 41.4) (2018a). OASIS results are publicly reported by CMS on Home Health Compare to provide comparisons of agency performance on select OASIS items such as improvement in managing daily activities and pain, treating symptoms, and preventing unplanned hospitalization (Medicare, n.d.).

The OASIS has had several revisions to improve its comprehensiveness, ease of use, reliability, and validity. The current version, OASIS-C2, was implemented on January 1, 2017, and the OASIS-D collection became available January 2019 to meet requirements within the IMPACT Act of 2014 (CMS, 2018d). Major sections include functional, physical, and service-related items each followed by a list of choices or fill-in-the-blanks (CMS, 2017c). (See Resource Tool 41.A on the Evolve website for an example of this assessment.

The OASIS is a complex and important component of home health practice. While providing care in the home, a nurse or therapist (physical, occupational, or speech and language) collects and completes the OASIS with the client and their caregivers at the start of care, after hospitalization, at the 60-day recertification date following admission, at discharge, or if transferred to a facility. It is important for clinicians to complete the OASIS accurately and consistently to reflect a client's actual status and integrate the OASIS with other portions of the agency's comprehensive assessment. They or their colleagues compare initial data to future versions as do Medicare surveyors and reimbursement reviewers. Final data from the OASIS must be submitted to CMS electronically.

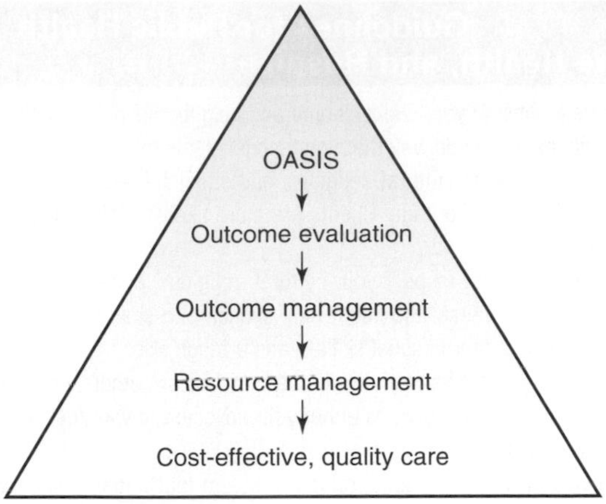

Fig. 41.4 The outcome model. *OASIS,* Outcome and Assessment Information Set. (From Centers for Medicare and Medicaid Services: *Outcome-based quality improvement [OBQI] implementation manual,* August 2010, pp. 2-9.)

The OASIS offers a challenging assignment for those who provide direct care, and one that requires extensive orientation and review. In many agencies, nurse experts serve as compliance officers to help ensure accurate and consistent completion. Not only is evidence of the quality of care related to OASIS, but so is agency reimbursement and a publicly available comparison of their client outcomes to those of other agencies. Agencies may receive sanctions or be denied payment by CMS for services provided based on claims data, audits, or surveys that reflect responses on OASIS. More recently, agencies have received Additional Development Requests (ADRs) generated by CMS. ADRs require agencies to submit extensive verification that the services they provided were essential; if verification is not adequate, agencies must initiate a legal appeal or return funds to CMS.

Target areas for emphasis on OASIS mirror clients' health challenges identified by nurses and home health agencies. Included are diabetic foot care, fall prevention, depression intervention, pain, pressure ulcers, safety, medication management, and infection control.

Box 41.5 illustrates M2001 from OASIS, one of the items related to medication management. Although all target areas are important, the latter two are of special concern to many nurses employed in hospice and palliative programs as well as diverse public health and other health care settings; they are summarized below.

BOX 41.5 Example of an Item From OASIS-C2

M2001 Drug Regimen Review: Does a complete drug regimen review indicate potential clinically significant medication issues (for example: adverse drug reactions, ineffective drug therapy, significant side effects, drug interactions, duplicate therapy, omissions, dosage errors, or noncompliance [non-adherence])?

0 No—No issues found during review [Go to M2010]

1 Yes—Issues found during review

9 NA—Patient is not taking any medications [Go to M2040]

OASIS, Outcome and Assessment Information Set.
From Centers for Medicare and Medicaid Services (CMS): *Outcome and Assessment Information Set OASIS-C2 guidance manual,* 2017. Available at http://www.cms.gov.

Medication Management

Medication management is an important component of home health practice. The goal is to assist clients and family caregivers to become independent and reliable in managing medication administration at home, and prevent adverse drug events, side effects, inadequate symptom control, and hospitalizations. However, home health clients experience many challenges, including the complexity of their chronic conditions, impaired cognitive status, inadequate coordination of their medical care, drug-drug interactions and side effects of medications, and cost. A systematic review on the frequency and causes of medication errors committed by patients or their caregivers at home revealed an incidence rate between 19 percent and 59 percent (Mira et al., 2015). Between 1988 and 2010 the median number of prescription medications used among adults aged 65 and older doubled from two to four, and the average proportion taking five or more medications tripled from 12.8 percent to 39.0 percent (Charlesworth et al., 2015). Too often, the number of medications is more than is clinically indicated, known as *polypharmacy* (Riker & Setter, 2013). This can result in side effects such as increased confusion, urinary incontinence, increased weakness, dizziness, and changes in sleeping patterns. Riker and Setter (2012, 2013) discuss how to assess for polypharmacy, its causes, and the interprofessional management of polypharmacy with emphasis on the role of the home care nurse.

Home health nurses expect to spend considerable time with medication reconciliation and management. They address medications during the initial and subsequent home visits. Unlike clients in residential settings, home health clients may or may not have all of their medications, may not take them as ordered, and may not store them appropriately. When nurses ask to see medications, they are often given a box or bag that includes current medications and ones that are extremely outdated, discontinued, or prescribed for other family members. Corbett et al. (2010) found that medication discrepancies were astoundingly widespread during the transition from hospital to home. In their study of 101 subjects, 94 percent had at least 1 discrepancy, most had an average of 3.3, and some had more; discrepancies were identified in almost all classes of medications, including those considered high risk. Reidt et al. (2014) conducted a study to explore the benefit of a pharmacist serving as a home health agency team member; findings included a positive clinical impact on clients. An excellent, comprehensive resource is the Medication Adherence Educators Toolkit, the product of a competition by schools of pharmacy (AACP/NCPA, 2013). It consists of four sections: assessing medication adherence, improving medication adherence through the use of aids, empowering patients to improve medication adherence, and resolving barriers to medication adherence. The toolkit includes evidence-based detailed information that addresses literacy, e-reminders, interprofessional practice, and cultural awareness.

Many tools are available in addition to those specific for home health nurses to assess and manage medication administration (Riker & Setter, 2013). Teaching clients to use a medication organizer for oral medications is frequently an initial intervention. However, that alone does not ensure that medications will be taken appropriately; subsequent teaching, return demonstrations, and surveillance are essential. Often the medication administration is complex with multiple drugs, in repeated dosages throughout the day, by various routes of administration.

A population health approach to medication management, for example, might be for providers to screen the medication regimen of all heart failure patients for complexity and polypharmacy. They would then work with their interdisciplinary partners (physicians and pharmacists) to simplify the medication regimen. This is also an area in need of further research and innovation. The Garfinkel "poly-de-prescribing" method shows promise. In a longitudinal, nonrandomized study of 122 older adults, they achieved significant reductions in the number of medications, and significantly less deterioration in functional, mental and cognitive status, sleep quality, appetite, sphincter control, and the number of major complications (Garfinkel, 2018).

Nurses must also understand the impact of medication management on the client and seek clients' perspectives, voices, and needs around medication adherence and management. (Zullig & Hayden, 2017) Self-efficacy, or the person's belief in their ability to manage their medications, is associated with medication adherence (Huang, Shiyanbola, & Smith, 2018) In addition, clients and caregivers need comprehensive materials about medication benefits, interactions, and side effects as well as the steps they should take to communicate that information to others (Vandermause et al., 2016). Materials need to be simple, understandable, and in the appropriate language. Clients who cannot read need graphic materials.

Another growing medication-related challenge is the management of opioid medications and overdose risk in home and community settings. A survey of community dwelling adults in the United States reported long-term opioid use in 76.9 percent of the cases (Shmagel et al., 2018). Clinicians must be aware of addiction issues; know how to safely administer antidote or direct its administration by others; and teach clients and caregivers how to safely administer, store, and dispose of narcotics (McAuley, Munro, & Taylor, 2018).

Home care agencies have policies on the safe disposal of narcotics and other pharmaceutical products. Proper disposal is important for client, child, and environmental safety, and the nurse has a role in teaching safe disposal by the client. The Food and Drug Administration provides guidance on where and how to dispose of unused medicines through drug take-back programs or self-disposal through the trash or down the sink or toilet (FDA, 2017). Under current law, unless there is local legislation that allows disposal, home health and hospice staff are not legally permitted to handle or destroy controlled substances in the home. Pending legislation regarding the disposal of unused medication will permit disposal by clinicians if passed (NAHC, 2018).

Infection Prevention

Infection prevention is an important priority in home health and hospice practice. Infection prevention usually focuses on wound care, and invasive devices such as urinary and intravenous catheters as well as chest, tracheostomy, gastrostomy, and other tubes. Preventing infection by promoting appropriate vaccinations such as flu and pneumonia is also a priority. Most importantly, nurses need to assume that every client is potentially infected or colonized with an organism that can be transmitted, and recognize that all blood and body secretions may contain transmissible agents. They need to be familiar with the infectious process, research evidence and best practices, bag technique, personal protective equipment, cleaning equipment, medical waste management, and infection control programs. Nurses need to practice sound technique during each and every client encounter (see How To box).

HOW TO Promote Infection Prevention Standards

The practice of standard precautions means that all blood and body fluids must be treated as potentially infectious. Standard precautions are implemented to prevent exposure and infection of family caregivers and health care providers.

- Hand hygiene is the single most important practice in preventing infections. Hand hygiene should be performed before and after providing client care and before and after preparing food, eating, feeding, or using the bathroom.
- Use extreme care to prevent injuries when handling needles, scalpels, and razors. Do not recap, bend, break, or remove needles from syringes before disposal. Discard needles and syringes in puncture-resistant containers made of plastic or metal and dispose of them as directed by agency policy or community guidelines.
- Wear barrier precautions such as gloves, masks, eye covering, and gowns when contact with blood and body fluids is expected. Use masks in combination with eye protection to eliminate contact with respiratory secretions or sprays of blood or body fluids during invasive respiratory procedures or wound irrigations.
- Use aseptic technique with all sterile injection equipment.
- Double bag and discard soiled dressings or other materials contaminated with body fluids in polyethylene garbage bags.
- Clean kitchen counters, dishes, and laundry with warm water and detergent after use. Clean bathrooms with a household disinfectant.
- For clients with multidrug resistant organisms, limit the amount of non-disposable equipment brought into the home; use disposable stethoscopes, etc., when possible.

Nurses need to become familiar with evidence-based practice literature specific to infection prevention. Nurses are increasingly called upon to have a role in antibiotic stewardship (Carter et al., 2018; CDC, 2017). Guidelines exist for long-term care, but not for community-based care, providing an opportunity for nursing leadership in this area (CDC, 2017). The Centers for Disease Control and Prevention (CDC) offers a variety of materials, including guidelines to prevent the most frequent infections (CDC, 2018). Russell et al. (2018) describe home health and hospice infection prevention and control programs, lessons learned, and knowledge and attitudes toward infection control. Shang et al. have an active research agenda on infection prevention in home health care (Shang et al., 2018). Gorski (2017) is a home infusion therapy expert who has published extensively about central venous access devices (CVADs). Gorski states that infections are preventable when four topics are implemented consistently: attention to hand hygiene, site assessment and care, use of aseptic technique with all infusion-related procedures, and thorough education for the client and family. In 2014, the American Society for Parenteral and Enteral Nutrition (ASPEN) published a comprehensive set of recommendations about parenteral nutrition safety, and a publication by Ayers et al. (2014) is another good resource. Specific details about parenteral nutrition infusion and blood samples are described in the Evidence-Based Practice box.

EVIDENCE-BASED PRACTICE

The question "What practices maintain patient safety during the infusion of parenteral nutrition?" is included in ASPEN's parenteral nutrition safety publication. One of the 18 recommendations for this question is vascular access devices used for parenteral nutrition administration should not be used to obtain blood samples for laboratory tests unless no peripheral access is available. Evidence indicates that vascular access devices are a leading cause of serious adverse complications, in particular, central-line associated bloodstream infection. In addition, blood specimens drawn from vascular access devices have resulted in incorrect values and inappropriate treatment. When the recommendation was followed in recent years, infection rates were reduced substantially. Many home care organizations have added this recommendation to their protocols; all should do so.

Nurse Use

Nurses who provide parenteral nutrition care in the home should also become familiar with this comprehensive publication.

ASPEN, American Society for Parenteral and Enteral Nutrition.
From Ayers P, Adams S, Boullata J, et al.: A.S.P.E.N. parenteral nutrition safety consensus recommendations. *JPEN J Parenter Enteral Nutr* 38:296-333, 2014.

ACCOUNTABILITY AND QUALITY MANAGEMENT

Evidence-Based Quality/Performance Improvement

All providers, whether they are within community-based settings, hospitals, long-term care, or private practices, are accountable to their clients, reimbursement sources, and professional standards. Accountability is directly linked to quality or the degree to which health services for individuals, families, and communities increase the likelihood of desired health outcomes and are consistent with current professional knowledge. Florence Nightingale is often credited with establishing standards of care, demonstrating the value of evidence-based practice, and analyzing health-related outcome data successfully.

Most public health, home health, hospice, and palliative care providers have a long history of evaluating the quality of care they provided to their clients. Often, agencies use a systematic, triangulated approach in their pursuit of excellence that includes hiring qualified personnel, new employee orientation, mentoring programs, case conferences, supervisory shared visits, record audits, utilization reviews, quality studies, client satisfaction surveys, in-service education, recognition for outstanding performance, and annual evaluations. Some agencies became accredited as a way to distinguish themselves from other providers.

The sophistication of quality and performance improvement strategies used in home health, hospice, and palliative care has dramatically improved in recent years. Changes were prompted by the interest in research-based practice that has evolved into programs of research and evidence-based practice, use of computers and the Internet, guidelines developed by the National Quality Forum (2014), and the mandate from Medicare to use the OASIS and Outcome-Based Quality Improvement. Nurses should have access to current research literature, know how to critique that research, and apply it to their practice. Frameworks have been described to guide evidence-based practice projects (Levin et al., 2010; Melnyk & Fineout-Overholt, 2015).

Evaluating the quality of care professionally and legally should be done in many ways, but documentation is of special significance. The steps of the nursing process must be documented and include communication with team members, physicians, and community resources. It is through the clinical record that nurses demonstrate that they are delivering quality care and identifying strategies to improve the quality of care.

Outcome-Based Quality Improvement

Outcome measurement and cost control are the focus of the CMS **Outcome-Based Quality Improvement (OBQI)** program. Their definition of outcomes is (1) health status changes between two or more time points, where the term *health status* encompasses physiological, functional, cognitive, emotional, and behavioral health; (2) changes that are intrinsic to the client; (3) positive, negative, or neutral changes in health status; and (4) changes that result from care provided or natural progression of disease and disability, or both (CMS, 2012).

Data from OASIS-C2 are part of the two-stage CMS OBQI framework to produce various reports. The first stage, outcome analysis, enables an agency to compare its performance to a national sample, note factors that may affect outcomes, and identify final outcomes that show improvement in or stabilization of a client's condition. Comparing agency data and trends to a national sample is also known as **benchmarking**, an analysis process that has been used by many businesses but is relatively new to health care. The second stage, known as outcome enhancement, enables the agency to select specific client outcomes and determine strategies to improve care. Reports include agency–client-related characteristics (case mix), potentially avoidable events (adverse event outcomes), and end-result and utilization outcomes. The reports are for a 12-month period, the agency's previous 12-month period, and national reference or comparative data. Comparisons are risk adjusted for client differences, both over time for the agency and between the agency and the reference group. Similar to OASIS, a detailed manual describes the OBQI program; the most recent manual was published in 2012 (CMS, 2012). Due to the importance of the OASIS measures to provide information for describing the epidemiology of home health clients, reimbursement, publicly reported quality of care measures, and clinical care planning, accurate completion of the OASIS is critical. Clinicians must balance extensive documentation requirements, often using electronic devices, with building the therapeutic relationship with clients (Yang et al., 2019).

Accreditation

Home health and hospice providers participate in several different continuous quality improvement options. They may elect to meet the **accreditation** standards of one of the following groups and complete the Medicare survey according to their guidelines: the Joint Commission, the Community Health Accreditation Partner, or the Accreditation Commission for Health Care. If providers do not seek accreditation, Medicare surveyors will conduct regular reviews. In 2007, the Public Health Accreditation Board was established to offer national public health accreditation. Because some home health and hospice programs are integrated with health departments, they will participate in public health accreditation (PHAB, 2018).

After an agency applies for accreditation, a lengthy self-study must be completed that addresses all aspects of the agency's operation, and an accreditation team schedules a site visit. All three accrediting organizations review agencies' organizational structure, compliance with Medicare Conditions of Participation, care provided during home visits and documentation of those visits, and the outcomes of client care with a focus on improved health status. Site visitors accompany nurses and other clinicians on home visits to observe the steps of the problem-solving process in action. To maintain accreditation, agencies must follow guidelines and undergo periodic reviews. Some futurists predict that accreditation may become a requirement for licensure of all home health agencies.

PROFESSIONAL DEVELOPMENT AND COLLABORATION

Education, Certification, and Roles

Nurses are employed in public health, home health, hospice, and palliative care from a variety of educational and practice backgrounds. They should be educated to function at a high level of competency so that they can be relied on not only by their professional colleagues but also by the community. They have diverse roles and responsibilities in their practice settings; autonomy is a fundamental characteristic that was mentioned earlier in this chapter. Nurses are responsible for basing their practice on research evidence. A growing number of public health, home health, hospice, and palliative care nurses are conducting research; some are members of interprofessional research teams. Their studies add to the body of knowledge for evidence-based practice, especially when the focus is on outcomes of care. The application of existing evidence and generation of new research must be priorities to increase the quality and cost-effectiveness of care (ANA, 2014; ANA/HPNA, 2014). A high-quality resource is the Alliance for Home Health Quality and Innovation, a not-for-profit organization focused on leading and sponsoring research and education on the value home health provides to clients and the entire U.S. health system (AHHQI, 2018).

The educational preparation of the 179,310 nurses employed in home health agencies varies greatly (BLS, 2017b). According to the ANA (2014), a baccalaureate degree in nursing should be the minimum requirement for entry into professional practice, and the Home Health Nursing Scope and Standards states that completion of a baccalaureate degree is the appropriate and preferred educational preparation. Roles for nurses include care management and coordination of care, education, advocacy, administration, supervision, and quality improvement. The nurse with a baccalaureate degree functions in the role of a generalist, providing skilled nursing and coordinating care for a variety of clients. Nurses with graduate degrees are prepared for roles as clinical specialists, nurse practitioners, researchers, administrators, or educators. Educational programs are increasing to prepare nurses for advanced practice roles in home health. As home health continues to expand, the need for specialized nurse clinicians will also increase to meet the highly technological and complex care needs of individuals, families, and communities. In managed care, more clinical specialists will be needed to provide a case management or population health focus and to develop programs to meet the needs of the populations served by the managed care network. For example, nurse practitioners can provide primary care to frail older adults and other homebound clients in the home.

The Hospice and Palliative Nurses Association (HPNA) offers many conferences, certification examinations, and credentialing (ANA/HPNA, 2014). There are about 14,000 credentialed registered hospice and palliative nurses. Licensed registered nurses may qualify for two levels of specialty practice certification that are differentiated by education, complexity of practice, and performance of certain nursing functions. Similar to home care, generalists provide direct care, function as educators, case managers, nurse clinicians, administrators, and other roles. The roles of the advanced practice nurse in hospice and palliative care include expert clinician, leader and facilitator of interprofessional teams, educator, researcher, consultant, collaborator, advocate, case manager, or administrator.

Interprofessional Collaboration

Typically, public health, home health, hospice, and palliative care nurses are members of interprofessional teams. The primary goal of the team is to help populations and individual clients achieve their maximum level of health, self-care, and independent functioning in a safe environment. Medicare regulations, professional organizations, and state licensing boards influence team composition and functions.

Box 41.6 and Fig. 41.5 illustrate successful interprofessional collaboration that depends on the knowledge, skills, and attitudes of each team member. When team members work collaboratively in partnership with clients, families, volunteers, and community resources, the plan of care can be implemented effectively and reinforced by all. Although each team member has a specific responsibility, any overlap in responsibilities can be beneficial for reinforcement. Team members communicate through email, phone calls, video calls, and face-to-face case conferences to review the plan of care, client progress, and team effectiveness (Marrelli, 2018a; Martin, 2005; Milone-Nuzzo & Hollars, 2017; Wright, 2018).

BOX 41.6 Factors for Successful Interprofessional Collaboration

Knowledge

1. Understand how the group process can be used to achieve group goals.
2. Understand problem solving.
3. Understand role theory.
4. Understand what other professionals do and how they view their roles.
5. Understand the differences between client levels of acuity across levels of care, including acute care, home care, ambulatory care, and long-term care.

Skills

1. Use principles of group process effectively.
2. Communicate clearly and accurately.
3. Communicate without using the profession's jargon.
4. Express self clearly and concisely in writing.

Attitudes

1. Feel confident in role as a professional.
2. Trust and respect other professionals.
3. Share tasks with other professionals.
4. Work effectively toward conflict resolution.
5. Be flexible.
6. Adopt an attitude of inquiry.
7. Be timely.

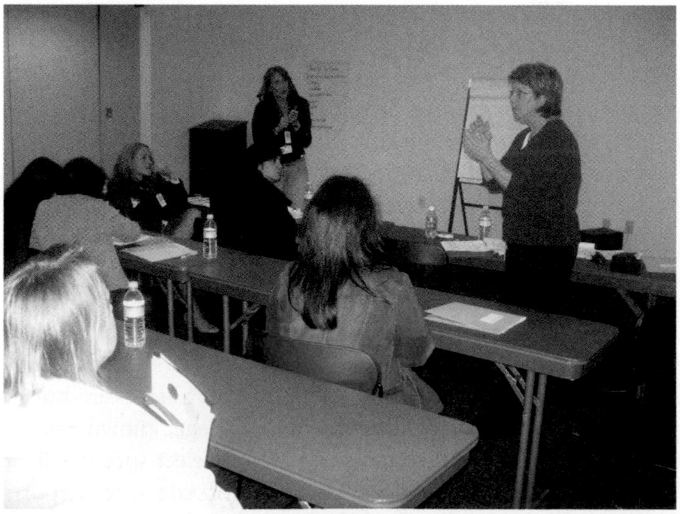

Fig. 41.5 Interprofessional team. (From www.omahasystem.org/photogallery.html. Used with permission from Karen S. Martin, RN, MSN, FAAN.)

Details about the role of nurses have been described in other sections of this chapter. Nurses often serve as the team leader or care manager in part because nursing service may be the client's primary need. Larger agencies may expand their nursing services to include wound and ostomy, intravenous, psychiatric/mental health, nurse practitioner, and other nursing specialists.

Physicians are an integral part of interprofessional teams; they submit initial and interim orders and review and sign the initial and updated plan of care. Many agencies hire a physician on a part-time basis or have an agreement with a physician who serves as a voluntary consultant. Because state laws are changing rapidly, nurse practitioners are increasingly involved and may have responsibilities similar to physicians. In addition, agencies may have specialized services such as podiatrists, pharmacists, registered dietitians, respiratory therapists, music therapists, psychologists, and chaplains.

The services of physical therapists, occupational therapists, speech and language pathologists, social workers, and home health aides are available in most agencies. They may be employed by the agency or hired through contractual agreements. Their roles are summarized below.

- Physical therapists: Provide maintenance, and preventive and restorative treatment that includes strengthening muscles, restoring mobility, controlling spasticity, gait training, and teaching active and passive resistive exercises.
- Occupational therapists: Focus on upper extremities to restore muscle strength and mobility for functional skills and performance of activities of daily living.
- Speech and language pathologists: Evaluate speech and language abilities, develop a plan of care, and teach clients to improve their communication involving speech, language, or hearing.
- Social workers: Help clients and families manage social, emotional, and environmental factors that affect their well-being through identification and referral to appropriate community resources.
- Home health aides: Provide personal care and assist with activities of daily living under the supervision of nurses or physical therapists. Home health aides or homemakers may also help with light housekeeping, laundry, meal preparation, and shopping.

LEGAL, ETHICAL, AND FINANCIAL ISSUES

The potential for human error as well as illegal and unethical activity exists in every health care organization. Examples of Medicare fraud and abuse in home health and hospice include inappropriate use of services, excessive payments to administrative staff or owners, "kickbacks" for referrals, and billing for visits and/or medical supplies that are not authorized or not provided. In addition, the complex regulations of CMS are difficult to understand and have not been interpreted consistently by Medicare surveyors.

Nurses are confronted with legal and ethical issues regularly. They need to be familiar with the living will, power of attorney for health care, and do-not-resuscitate documents. In addition, they need to be informed about local, state, and federal regulations that govern their profession and nursing license; and those that govern their employers. They need to be alert for potential problems or violations and identify solutions in a proactive manner. The privacy guidelines of the Health Insurance Portability and Accountability Act of 1996 ensure protection of clients' personal health information, include provisions about informed consent, and allow clients full access to their health care records (USDHHS, 2017).

Nurses are expected to follow professional, legal, and ethical standards to deliver care to clients, develop trusting relationships, act as client advocates, and help clients and families increase their self-advocacy skills. Because these responsibilities can produce tension, nurses need to recognize their personal values and biases to make certain they do not interfere with those of clients and families. Nurses should continually reassess client and family needs to avoid inappropriate use and overuse of services. This will become even more challenging because recent legislation has decreased an episode of home care from 60 days to 30 days (CMS, 2017a). Nurses will need to plan well and make sure clients understand the time-limited nature of their services.

The safety of clients who live alone as well as family caregiver neglect and/or abuse are ethical concerns. If the clients' needs are greater than what reimbursement allows, nurses need to talk to the clients, their families, and agency personnel to consider alternatives. In addition, many agencies have established ethics committees to assist with ethical dilemmas.

Reimbursement for home health, hospice, and palliative care is complex and tenuous; historical milestones are described earlier in this chapter, and more details about economics and reimbursement are included in Chapter 5. Medicare, state and local governments, Medicaid, and managed care are the principal funding sources for home health and hospice (NHPCO, 2016). If clients meet the eligibility criteria for the Conditions of Participation, Medicare is used as their primary payment source. When clients no longer meet those criteria and still require care, their services may be reimbursed by Medicaid, private insurance, donations, or the agency's United Way and other special needs funds. As mentioned earlier, value-based purchasing programs with bundled payments are the newest innovations in reimbursement models to affect community-based care. These innovations make partnering with acute care and other referral sources even more important, and effective collaboration among the interprofessional team is critical to achieve positive outcomes.

Nurses who work in public health, home health, hospice, and palliative care are involved with financial aspects of care to a greater extent than most other nurses. Nurses and their social work colleagues must be well informed about services available in the communities, and those that are covered by Medicare and other funding sources, and recognize how tenuous those funding sources are. Clients and families often ask for help to understand decisions about care and the numerous notices and bills that they receive. Nurses participate directly in decisions about the frequency, length, and type of client services, and their documentation needs to accurately support those decisions (Irani et al., 2018). Nurses must be knowledgeable about the reimbursement of medical supplies and should discuss problematic situations with clients, families, and agency personnel.

TRENDS AND OPPORTUNITIES

National Health Objectives

The overarching goals of the *Healthy People 2020* objectives (USDHHS, 2014) are as follows:

- Attain high-quality, longer lives free of preventable disease, disability, injury, and premature death.
- Achieve health equity, eliminate disparities, and improve the health of all groups.
- Create social and physical environments that promote good health for all.
- Promote quality of life, healthy development, and healthy behaviors across all life stages.

Nurses who work with clients and families in the home and community have opportunities to promote achievement of key objectives. They can assess client status, identify available resources and gaps to meet client needs, encourage clients and families to use resources, and coordinate care with other providers and community agencies. They can participate in numerous population-level projects and campaigns.

The *Healthy People 2020* box highlights objectives relevant to home health and hospice nurses. Note that many objectives relate to lifestyle issues. With appropriate health education, referral to community resources, and follow-up, there is a potential to reduce morbidity and mortality and decrease chronic disabilities. Nurses can make important contributions on one-to-one and population-focused levels.

HEALTHY PEOPLE 2020

Examples of National Health Objectives for the Year 2020

- **AOCBC-11:** Reduce hip fractures among older adults.
- **C-1:** Reduce the overall cancer death rate.
- **C-13:** Increase proportion of cancer survivors beyond 5 years.
- **CKD-9:** Reduce kidney failure due to diabetes.
- **HD-3:** Reduce stroke deaths.
- **HDS-1:** (Developmental) Increase overall cardiovascular health in the U.S. population.
- **HDS-5:** Reduce the proportion of persons in the population with hypertension.
- **IID-4:** Reduce invasive pneumococcal infections.

From U.S. Department of Health and Human Services: *Healthy People 2020: 2020 topics and objectives-objectives A-Z,* 2014. Available at http://www.healthypeople.gov.

Organizational and Professional Resources

It is increasingly important for nurses to be involved in political, economic, and regulatory issues at the local, state, and national levels before they affect practice and services to clients. Joining organizations, reviewing the Internet, networking with colleagues, reading professional literature, and serving on expert panels provide opportunities to become informed and influence decisions.

Nationally, several prominent home health organizations have extensive resources and websites. The National Association for Home Care & Hospice (NAHC) is a trade organization formed in 1982. A few years later, the Hospice Association of America (HAA) and NAHC developed an organizational partnership. Many agencies join as members, but nurses can also participate in the nursing section after joining as individual members. Lobbying is NAHC's primary focus; it also schedules an annual meeting and offers educational opportunities. The Visiting Nurse Association of America (VNAA), formed in 1983, has a similar focus, but membership is limited to community-based, nonprofit home health and hospice providers. Recently the VNAA and Alliance for Home Health Improvement formed an umbrella organization referred to as ElevatingHome to increase their collective influence nationally. *Home Healthcare Nurse, Home Healthcare Now, Home Health Care Management and Practice, Family and Community Health, Journal of Community Health Nursing,* and *Home Health Care Services Quarterly* are the leading journals for home health administrators, clinicians, managers, and researchers.

Hospice and palliative care organizations also have extensive resources and websites. The National Hospice and Palliative Care Organization was formed in 1978 to stimulate public and professional interest. The Hospice Foundation of America was founded in 1982; its initial mission was fundraising. The Hospice Nurses Association was formed in 1986. About 12 years later, the organization expanded and became the Hospice and Palliative Nurses Association (HPNA), and also changed the name of its national certification board. HPNA now has more than 11,000 members (HPNA, 2018). The organization schedules conferences, publishes the *Journal of Hospice and Palliative Nursing,* and offers certification and credentialing. The *American Journal of Hospice and Palliative Care, Journal of Pediatric Oncology Nursing, International Journal of Palliative Nursing, Journal of Palliative Medicine,* and other related journals address nursing practice, pain control, oncology, and medical practice.

Home health, hospice, and palliative care nurses belong to a variety of specialty organizations such as Infusion Nurses Society; Wound, Ostomy, and Continence Nurses Society; American Public Health Association; and Healthcare Information and Management Systems Society along with nurses employed in diverse settings. It is important that they share their knowledge about community-focused practice by being active members, speaking, and writing for publication.

Technology, Informatics, and Telehealth

Technology. Advances in technology, informatics, and **telehealth** are pervasive in health care and nursing practice. They are changing the ways in which care is provided. Many home health and hospice nurses have developed specialized technical skills with the following: wound management, parenteral nutrition, chemotherapy, intravenous therapy for hydration and antibiotics, intrathecal pain management, ventilators, ventricular assist devices, and apnea monitors. As mentioned earlier in the chapter, clients and family caregivers must learn to complete procedures and manage equipment frequently. It is the responsibility of the nurse and fellow team members to determine if such procedures and equipment can be used safely; when the answer is yes, team members must provide sufficient education, demonstrations, and monitoring so that care continues safely and effectively. Advances in technology, informatics, and telehealth are not replacements for nurses and team members, but are tools to improve the quality and effectiveness of their practice. The tools are evolving rapidly, influencing community-based practice, and transforming home health operations.

Nursing Informatics. Nursing informatics (NI), defined as the "science and practice (that) integrates nursing, its information and knowledge, with information and communication technologies to promote the health of people, families, and communities worldwide." (Nelson & Staggers, 2018). NI is one of the most important new tools for nurses in all settings as they face urgent information management challenges, including the need for timely, reliable, and valid quantified data and information about clients, the services they receive, and their outcomes of care (Eardley et al., 2018; Monsen, 2018). They also need verbal and automated methods to communicate with other nurses and health care providers wherever they are in the community. The majority of agencies require clinicians to document care during the visit using electronic devices, rather than in their office or other location (Martin, 2005, Martin & Utterback, 2018; Monsen, 2018; Monsen et al., 2018; Yang et al., 2019).

The ANA anticipated the impact of information technology on the profession and took the first step to integrating nurse-generated data into the EHR early in the 1990s. They began to recognize standardized terminologies that could be used by nurses and other health care disciplines to describe, document, and quantify their daily practice accurately and consistently (ANA, 2014, 2018; Omaha System, 2018). The Omaha System and 11 more interface or point-of-care and reference terminologies have been recognized by the ANA. The Omaha System is an interface or point-of-care terminology; clinicians see it imbedded in their clinical documentation systems and need to learn to use it accurately and consistently.

Successful integration of nurse-generated data involves **interoperability**—the exchange of coded data and ability to use those data for multiple purposes such as quality measurement, reimbursement, and research (ANA, 2018; Bowles et al., 2013). SNOMED CT and Logical Observation Identifiers, Names, and Codes (LOINC) are examples of reference terminologies that facilitate interoperability by sharing data generated by the interface terminologies. Minnesota is the first state to recommend that health care providers use both ANA-recognized standardized point-of-care and reference terminologies. In 2014, Minnesota released their decision that the Omaha System should be the point-of-care terminology for the software used by all public health, home health, and other community-based providers (Omaha System, 2018).

Now that electronic data sets are more available and can be linked to national claims data and other rich sources of health information to form large data sets, data science is a growing methodology nurse scientists may use to capitalize on this resource (Brennan & Bakken, 2015). A form of data science, data mining is the process of discovering useful information in large data repositories (Tan et al., 2019). Through data mining, prediction models and clinical decision support systems are developed to alert clinicians of risk, changing clinical parameters, and progress and needs of their clients (Gao et al., 2018). Public health, home health, and hospice are ripe with opportunities for data science research especially when standardized data sets are used for clinical operations (Monsen et al., 2018). The OASIS data set provides a national, standardized data set to examine clients' conditions over time. OASIS linked with CMS claims data and other national data sets provide rich insights into home care practice and effectiveness (Murtaugh et al., 2017; O'Connor et al., 2014).

The sharing of information from one health care setting or provider to another is critical for community-based care, especially as clients make the transition between hospital and home. Safe, high-quality care is dependent on the sharing of information, goals of care, and care plans. Health information exchanges (HIEs) support this need and are growing in number and functionality. HIEs give care providers access to patient records from hospitals, emergency departments, skilled nursing facilities, and laboratories across the state, saving valuable time and costs associated with searching paper records, faxing, making phone calls, or re-collecting information.

The concept of meaningful use has evolved as one component of the **Merit-based Incentive Payment System (MIPS)**. MIPS combines meaningful use and other CMS quality programs, including Physician Quality Reporting System and the Value-Based Payment Modifiers into a single program to improve quality of care. MIPS promotes the use of certified EHRs that support care coordination, quality measurement, and improved patient-clinician relationships (Office of the National Coordinator for Health Information Technology, 2017b). This suggests that better health care does not come solely from the adoption of technology itself, but through the exchange and use of electronic health information to best inform clinical decisions at the point-of-care. Public health and other community-based practitioners play an important role in identifying critical information needed to conduct care and to communicate with clients, families, interprofessional team members, policy makers, and payers. They also must support the development and seek the purchase of certified EHRs that meet documentation and interoperability standards and meaningful use criteria.

Health care providers throughout the United States are rapidly converting to EHRs. The 2009 American Recovery and Reinvestment Act (ARRA), and the Health Information Technology for Economic and Clinical Health (HITECH) Act, provided reimbursement incentives for eligible professionals and hospitals to become "meaningful users" (Friedman, Parrish, & Ross, 2013). Although home health agencies were not able to obtain funding through AARA, their adoption of EHRs has also increased.

Personal health records (PHRs) are another important development (U.S. National Library of Medicine, 2018). A PHR is an electronic collection of health-related information, managed and controlled by the client rather than by clinicians and agencies. Typically, a PHR includes a health history, medications, allergies, and results from laboratory and other tests.

The Blue Button is a PHR initiative that began in 2010 by the Department of Veterans Affairs (Office of the National Coordinator for Health Information Technology, 2017a; The Blue Button, 2017). Soon after an online patient portal was launched. While their initiative is limited to veterans, many other groups use the Blue Button symbol. Usage of the Blue Button logo and brand is free but must conform to user guidelines. The goal is to encourage as many people as possible to use a Blue Button site to download their own health information.

Increasingly, individuals and families served by public health, home health, hospice, and palliative care nurses have information technology skills. They may use the Internet frequently and be well informed about diagnoses, treatments, and medications. They may also use smartphones, other mobile devices, and social media. Nurses need to inquire about their clients' skills rather than make assumptions based on their age or other factors.

Telehealth. Telehealth supports long-distance health care, client and professional health-related education, and public health and health administration using electronic information, medical devices, and telecommunications technologies (Schlachta-Fairchild et al., 2018). The technology used varies to include live videoconferencing, the Internet, store-and-forward imaging, streaming media, satellite, wireless communications, and plain old telephone systems. Telehealth equipment and program components include telephone triage and advice, and biometric telemonitoring equipment to measure vital signs, weight, cardiac function, and point-of-care diagnostics. The system may or may not include video technology for live interaction (Schlachta-Fairchild et al., 2018).

The increased availability of telehealth coincides with trends described in this and other chapters in this book: an aging population, increased chronic illness and costs, and changes in health care reimbursement by CMS and other payers. The Center for Connected Health Policy (Center for Connected Care, 2018) provides a concise overview of the current reimbursement mechanisms for telehealth. Currently, Medicare only reimburses for live-video conferencing under very specific circumstances and has restricted the types of sites that may conduct telehealth for reimbursement. To date, home health and hospice telehealth services do not qualify. However, a new chronic care management billing code provides for non–face-to-face consultation, which can include remote monitoring of chronic conditions, opening the way for collaborative management of chronic illness between home health and hospice and community-based physicians and other providers. In addition, Medicare Advantage plans (managed Medicare) do provide reimbursement under Medicare Part B for telehealth services and several bills are pending approval in Congress. Accountable care organizations and bundled payment initiatives are also able to obtain reimbursement. Medicaid plans also cover telehealth services but vary by state. These new trends promote new opportunities: public health, home health, hospice, and palliative care nurses can increasingly use innovations such as telehealth in combination with in-person visits to effectively and efficiently manage chronic conditions. They can monitor health status and symptom recognition, provide education, increase communication, and enable clients to become active partners in their own care (Madigan et al., 2013; Schlachta-Fairchild, et al., 2018).

Older adults are increasingly accepting of information technologies to help them manage their complex chronic conditions, and this information is being used for population health management. Focus groups reveal seven conditions that play an important role in acceptance of telehealth by consumers: perceived usefulness, effort expectancy, social influence, perceived security, computer anxiety, facilitating conditions, and physicians' opinions (Cimperman et al., 2013). Patients with chronic obstructive pulmonary disease reported a general satisfaction and they found the telemonitoring systems useful to help them manage their disease. Some reported difficulties in their use, which affected compliance in using the technology as prescribed (Cruz, Brooks, & Marques, 2014).

Numerous studies have confirmed that telehealth is used successfully to improve physical, emotional, and financial health outcomes for diverse home health clients. Telehealth is most commonly used and studied with heart failure patients. Fifteen systematic reviews of heart failure research published between 2003 and 2013 reported significant reductions in mortality and heart failure–related hospitalizations when using telehealth compared to usual care. However, more research is needed because the quality of studies varies, and only automated device based monitoring and mobile telemonitoring were effective (Kitsiou, Paré, & Jaana, 2015).

Telemonitoring is increasingly being used with infants, women with high-risk pregnancies, and adults with various health problems, including mental health. Smart homes are emerging to help the older adult to "age in place" (Rantz et al., 2013). Sensors can monitor activities and detect adverse events such as a fall or lack of movement and trigger a call for help. Medication management devices remind clients to take their medications, dispense medications, and send alerts to providers if devices are not accessed as expected (Marek et al., 2013). The next generation of devices is taking advantage of handheld devices such as smartphone and tablet technologies, making telemonitoring even more ubiquitous.

SUMMARY

Public health, home health, hospice, and palliative care continue to evolve with changing national policies and innovations. The need for nurses prepared to practice in these specialties is growing as the public becomes more interested in prevention, the population ages, chronic illness increases, and more care is delivered in the community. Practice will become ever more complex and diverse as individuals live longer with multiple chronic conditions and they and their families are more engaged in their care and request more choices and personalized care. Practice in this challenging environment requires a strong educational background, critical thinking skills, and a commitment to lifelong learning. The autonomy afforded by community-based practice requires strong interpersonal, communication, technological, and clinical skills. It is a good time to celebrate the past, embrace the present, and look forward to the future.

QSEN FOCUS ON QUALITY AND SAFETY EDUCATION FOR NURSES

Targeted Competency: Client-Centered Care

Recognize the client or designee as the source of control and full partner in providing compassionate and coordinated care based on respect for client's preferences, values, and needs.

Important aspects of client-centered care include:

- **Knowledge:** Demonstrate comprehensive understanding of the concepts of pain and suffering, including physiological models of pain and comfort.
- **Skills:** Elicit expectations of client and family for relief of pain, discomfort, or suffering.
- **Attitudes:** Recognize that client expectations influence outcomes in management of pain or suffering.

Client-Centered Care Question

Visit a community-based hospice or palliative care unit. Spend time observing the care provided in this setting.

1. How is care provided in this setting different from care you have seen in the acute care setting? In the home health setting?
2. Notice how nurses and nursing assistants assess pain in this environment.
3. Discuss with the nurses how they address concerns around pain and suffering with clients and families in this environment. How do nurses evaluate clients' and families' expectations around pain?
4. Discuss with the nurses differences in care approaches between a community-based hospice or palliative care versus care approaches for home hospice and palliative care. Is there additional education that is required for the client and family, because the family often provides some aspects of care for home hospice and palliative care?

Prepared by Gail Armstrong, PhD(c), DNP, ACNS-BC, CNE, Associate Professor, University of Colorado Denver College of Nursing.

LINKING CONTENT TO PRACTICE

The Nurse in Public Health, Home Health, Hospice, and Palliative Care

The individuals, families, and communities served by public health, home health, palliative, and hospice nurses are described throughout this chapter as are the knowledge, skills, and attitudes of nurses who function well in those settings. The descriptions are evident in the text, clinical examples, boxes/figures/tables, references, and other parts of the chapter. The competencies in this chapter are congruent with the following core competencies of the Quad Council Coalition's Domains of Public Health Nursing (2018): (1) assessment analytic skills, (2) policy development and program planning skills, (3) communication skills, (4) cultural competency skills, (5) community dimensions of practice skills, (6) public health sciences skills, (7) financial planning and management skills and planning skills, and (8) leadership and systems thinking skills. Students and new graduates cannot be expected to have developed all of these skills when they begin to practice (Milone-Nuzzo & Hollars, 2017; Schoon et al., 2018, Smith, 2017a, 2017b; Wright, 2018). However, as nurses proceed in their career development and gain valuable work experience, they will progress along the novice to expert continuum.

PRACTICE APPLICATION

The first example is an individual who lives alone, the second is an individual whose family includes an involved spouse, and the third is a community client that is described in the Omaha System section of this chapter. Ideally, the student who visits Martha P. and the home health nurse who visits Mr. and Mrs. Jones use portable computing devices and document in the EHRs in the home. The public health nurses who are part of the Library Nurse Project use laptops for documentation.

Martha P. is an older woman who lives in a deteriorating home. She is a relatively typical client for a student or home health nurse to visit.

Box 41.7 consists of a story and answers designed to promote independent learning and group discussion. Note that the story and answers should be congruent: all pertinent data in the story should be reflected in the answers and all answers should match pertinent details in the story.

Mr. Jones, the second clinical example, is also a relatively typical client. After reading the example, identify the Omaha System problems, interventions, and ratings that are illustrated in the story. Discuss key characteristics of practice during this visit and an appropriate care plan for the next visit.

Mr. Jones, 70 years old, was discharged from the hospital yesterday after heart surgery for coronary artery disease and was referred to the local home health agency. Today, the home health nurse admitted him for **skilled nursing care** services. The nurse assessed Mr. Jones' cardiovascular status, the healing of his incisions, adjustment to his postsurgical status, and level of self-care. The nurse talked to Mr. and Mrs. Jones about exercise, nutrition, the signs and symptoms of possible postoperative cardiac problems, and their coping. Together, they looked at his medications. Mrs. Jones indicated that they were getting along well, but were concerned about the high cost of his new medications. They reviewed Mr. Jones' discharge packet. The nurse emphasized the need to maintain close communication with his physician and nurse practitioner, and the need to participate in the local exercise and nutrition rehabilitation program that they had prescribed. Mr. and Mrs. Jones indicated that they would do so. Before the visit ended, the nurse completed the necessary forms, documented the visit, and offered to call a local social service agency about financial assistance for medications. They made an appointment for the nurse's return visit.

The third clinical example was described previously in the Omaha System section of this chapter.

The home visit is the hallmark of nursing in home health and hospice. Nurses are guests when they enter a client's home and must recognize that their services can be accepted or rejected. The interpersonal relationship established during the

BOX 41.7 Martha P.: Older Woman Living in a Deteriorating Home

Joan B. Castleman, RN, MS, Clinical Associate Professor
College of Nursing, University of Florida
Gainesville, Florida

Information Obtained During the First Visit/Encounter

Martha P. was a 93-year-old woman who lived by herself in a deteriorating house. She had kyphosis and arthritis that contributed to her unsteady gait. Martha rarely used her cane in her house, but steadied herself by holding on to furniture.

When a student nurse arrived, Martha was shivering under a thin blanket. Boxes filled with old papers were stacked along the walls. The student nurse asked Martha if she had wood for the stove that heated the house. She replied that she ran out of wood yesterday and said, "I don't know what I'm going to do, but I'm not leaving this house." She reported that people from a church had brought the last load of wood. The student asked permission to contact Concerned Neighbors, a volunteer organization that could provide firewood. Martha was pleased. The student expressed concern that the boxes of paper, especially those near the stove, were a fire hazard. "Those boxes have been there for years, and I use them to light the stove," Martha said. When the student asked if she could help Martha move the four boxes near the stove to the other wall, she grudgingly agreed.

The student nurse noted that Martha was wearing a "Lifeline necklace," a fall alert system, and asked about her history of falls. Martha described how she moved around her home and fell in the bathroom last week when she was trying to take a sponge bath. She pushed the button, and "two nice gentlemen from the fire department came to pick me up." The student and Martha walked around her house. They talked about where she fell in the past, how fortunate she was not to have injuries, and ways to decrease her risk of falling in the future. Martha was willing to have a personal care assistant visit weekly to help her with a bath and shampoo as long as there was no charge. Before leaving, the student took Martha's vital signs and blood pressure and noted that they were within normal limits. The student called Concerned Neighbors and arranged for firewood to be delivered that day; the student also telephoned a local health assistance organization to schedule a home health aide to provide personal care for the next week. Although Martha sounded grumpy, she asked the student to return.

Application of the Omaha System Problem: Residence (High Priority)

Problem Classification Scheme

Modifiers: Individual and Actual
Signs/symptoms of Actual:
- Inadequate heating/cooling
- Cluttered living space
- Unsafe storage of dangerous objects/substances

Intervention Scheme

Category: Teaching, Guidance, and Counseling
Targets and Client-specific Information: Safety (moved boxes away from stove; Martha unwilling to dispose of papers)
Category: Case Management
Targets and Client-specific Information: Other community resources (referred to Concerned Neighbors; arranged delivery of firewood)
Category: Surveillance
Targets and Client-specific Information: Home (needed wood)

Problem Rating Scale for Outcomes

Knowledge: 2—minimal knowledge (not aware/unwilling to recognize fire hazards)
Behavior: 2—rarely appropriate behavior (unable/unwilling to make changes)
Status: 2—severe signs/symptoms (residence was livable but needed changes)
Domain: Physiological

Problem: Neuro-Musculo-Skeletal Function (High Priority)

Problem Classification Scheme

Modifiers: Individual and Actual
Signs/symptoms of Actual:
- Limited range of motion
- Decreased balance
- Gait/ambulation disturbance

Intervention Scheme

Category: Teaching, Guidance, and Counseling
Targets and Client-specific Information: Mobility/transfers (ways to decrease risk of falling, absence of injuries, continue wearing "Lifeline necklace")
Category: Surveillance
Targets and Client-specific Information:
- mobility/transfers (how, when falls occurred)
- signs/symptoms—physical (falls/injuries; vital signs, blood pressure)

Problem Rating Scale for Outcomes

Knowledge: 2—minimal knowledge (knew few options to decrease falls)
Behavior: 2—rarely appropriate behavior (had not used cane in house; did wear and use "Lifeline necklace")
Status: 3—moderate signs/symptoms (activities restricted, fell last week)
Domain: Health-Related Behaviors

Problem: Personal Care (High Priority)

Problem Classification Scheme

Modifiers: Individual and Actual
Signs/symptoms of Actual:
- Difficulty with bathing
- Difficulty shampooing/combing hair

Intervention Scheme

Category: Teaching, Guidance, and Counseling
Targets and Client-specific Information: Personal hygiene (needed help with bathing, shampoo)
Category: Case Management
Targets and Client-specific Information: Paraprofessional/aide care (referred to health assistance organization for home health aide)

Problem Rating Scale for Outcomes

Knowledge: 3—basic knowledge (knew she needed to bathe, but not aware of assistance)
Behavior: 3—inconsistently appropriate behavior (tried to take a sponge bath)
Status: 3—moderate signs/symptoms (cannot bathe safely without help)

This case illustrates use of the Omaha System with a client in the home. Talk with your classmates and other colleagues about how use of the Omaha System can guide your practice and documentation and can generate aggregate data to promote high-quality home health service. Identify Martha P.'s strengths and how to maximize those when providing care.

From Martin KS: *The Omaha System: a key to practice, documentation, and information management*, Omaha, NE, 2005, Health Connections Press.

first visit is critical, as is the initial assessment of the client, support system, and environment.

A. What strategies should the nurse use to develop a positive relationship during the first visit?
B. What are the most important elements to assess in the home environment?
C. What should the nurse do to establish a partnership with the client?
D. What is necessary for the nurse to include in the client contract?
E. How can the nurse determine the client's preferred learning style?

Answers can be found on the Evolve site.

KEY POINTS

- Public health, home health, hospice, and palliative care nursing practice provided in the client's home differ from care in institutional settings. The home setting affects practice in unique ways, including establishing trust, developing care partnerships (consumer engagement), selecting interventions, collecting outcomes and data, ensuring client safety, and promoting quality.
- Family members, including caregivers and significant persons who provide assistance and/or care, are essential members of the health care team.
- Home health has its roots in public health nursing, with an emphasis on health promotion, illness prevention, and caring for people in their communities.
- Home health and hospice practice and reimbursement changed when they became major Medicare benefits.
- Five models of care are described in this chapter: public health, home health, hospice, palliative care, Nurse-Family Partnership, and transitional care. All nurses should become familiar with these models to inform clients, their families, and their communities about options and educate providers who are potential referral sources.
- Medicare-certified home health and hospice agencies are divided into various types of administrative and organizational structures. However, many aspects of nursing practice are the same in the various types.
- Standards of public health, home health, and hospice/palliative care nursing practice originate from the ANA in partnership with specialty organizations, and encourage adoption of evidence-based practice.
- Consistently demonstrating professional competency is essential for public health, home health, hospice, and palliative care nurses.
- Interprofessional collaboration is inherent in public health, home health, hospice, and palliative care.
- The Omaha System was developed and refined through a process of research. Reliability, validity, and usability were established for the entire system.
- The Omaha System is unique in that it is the only comprehensive vocabulary developed initially by and for nurses practicing in the community.
- The Omaha System consists of the Problem Classification Scheme (assessment), Intervention Scheme (care plans and services), and Problem Rating Scale for Outcomes (client change/evaluation).
- The Omaha System is designed to enhance practice, documentation, and information management. These areas are of concern to community health educators and students as well as clinicians and administrators.
- Interprofessional clinicians employed in Medicare-certified home health agencies use OASIS-C2 at designated intervals; it is the outcome measurement tool mandated by the Centers for Medicare and Medicaid Services' Conditions of Participation.
- Evidence-based quality/performance improvement is important in all home health and hospice agencies. Currently, Medicare's Outcome-Based Quality Improvement program is used for outcome measurement and cost control.
- Exciting trends and opportunities are pervasive in public health, home health, hospice, and palliative care. Many nurses are developing skills using technology, informatics, and telehealth; a commitment to lifelong learning is necessary.

CLINICAL DECISION-MAKING ACTIVITIES

1. Make a home visit with an experienced public health, home health, or hospice nurse and do the following:
   A. Evaluate the process and content of the nurse-client interaction to determine what aspects of the visit were based on evidence-based practice; describe the process of the visit.
   B. Compare actual roles and functions with the ANA scope and standards or other specialty standards as appropriate for the client population.
   C. Observe and discuss whether that nurse uses a client problem/nursing diagnosis, intervention, or outcome measurement system or framework. Is it important to use a system or framework approach? Explain.
   D. Consider the information about consumer engagement, strengths-based practice, social determinants of health, and population health described in this chapter. What examples did you observe?
2. Work with a partner or in a small group. Select a client you have visited or invent a fictitious client, and list data for a typical referral and initial visit. Independently apply the three parts of the Omaha System to the client data. Compare each portion of your selections with that of your partner or group members.
3. Make a joint home visit with another health care professional and assess as in the preceding activity. Attend a

client/family-provider conference and write a summary of the group process. Has your attitude changed after you listened to the opinions expressed by family members?
4. Review a client record. What client outcomes were met through home health care? What specific outcomes showed an improvement or a stabilizing condition?
5. Interview a public health, home health, or hospice nurse who uses electronic health records (EHRs). Ask about the advantages of EHRs and challenges associated with them. How can aggregate clinical data generated by EHRs help nurses better understand the needs of their clients? How might knowing the needs of their clinical population assist in reviewing the research literature and planning new interventions?
6. Review your state's laws governing advance directives. Consider the legal and ethical advantages and disadvantages of having such directives. How would you write an advance directive for yourself?
7. Participate in a telehomecare visit using video technology or observe the analysis of data from remote monitoring. Trace the nurse's decision making and changes in the plan of care based on the telemonitoring data. Determine what outcomes might be expected from this type of care.

ADDITIONAL RESOURCES

EVOLVE WEBSITE

http://evolve.elsevier.com/Stanhope/community/

- Answers to Practice Application
- Case Study
- Glossary
- Review Questions

REFERENCES

Agency for Healthcare Research and Quality (AHRQ): *Patient Safety Measure Tools and Resources*, 2017. Retrieved from http://www.ahrq.gov.

Alliance for Home Health Quality and Innovation (AHHQI): *About the Alliance*, 2018. Retrieved from http://ahhqi.org/about/.

American Association of Colleges of Pharmacy and National Community Pharmacists Association (AACP/NCPA): *Medication Adherence Educators Toolkit*, 2013. Retrieved from http://www.aacp.org.

American Nurses Association (ANA): *Home health nursing: scope and standards of practice*, ed 2, Silver Spring, 2014, Nursesbooks.org.

American Nurses Association (ANA): *Inclusion of Recognized Terminologies Supporting Nursing Practice within Electronic Health Records and Other Health Information Technology Solutions*, 2018. Retrieved from https://bit.ly/21673bj.

American Nurses Association (ANA): *Public health nursing: scope and standards of practice (ebook)*, ed 2, Silver Spring, MD, 2013, Nursesbooks.org.

American Nurses Association, Hospice and Palliative Nurses Association (ANA/HPNA): *Palliative nursing: scope and standards of practice—an essential resource for hospice and palliative nurses*, Silver Spring, MD, 2014, Nursesbooks.org.

American Nurses Association, Hospice and Palliative Nurses Association (ANA/HPNA): *Call for Action: Nurses Lead and Transform Palliative Care*, 2017. Retrieved from https://bit.ly/2Lut4vb.

Ansberry C: U.S. is running out of caregivers, *Wall St J* 10(7):21–22, 2018.

Ayers P, Adams S, Boullata J, et al: A.S.P.E.N. parenteral nutrition safety consensus recommendations, *JPEN J Parenter Enteral Nutr* 38:296–333, 2014.

Berwick DM, Nolan TW, Whittington J: The Triple Aim: care, health, and cost, *Health Aff (Millwood)* 27:759–769, 2008.

Black JM, Hawks JH: *Medical surgical nursing*, ed 8, St. Louis, MO, 2009, Saunders, p 94.

Bowles KH, Potashnik S, Ratcliffe SJ, et al: Conducting research using the electronic health record across multi-hospital systems: semantic harmonization implications for administrators, *J Nurs Adm* 43:355–360, 2013.

Brennan PF, Bakken S: Nursing needs big data and big data needs nursing, *J Nurs Scholarsh* 47(5):477–484, 2015.

Buch CL, Nies MA: Home health and hospice. In Nies MA, McEwen M, editors: *Community/public health nursing: promoting the health of populations*, ed 6, St. Louis, MO, 2015, Elsevier, pp 645–657.

Buhler-Wilkerson K: No place like home: a history of nursing and home care in the U.S., *Home Healthc Nurse* 20:641–647, 2002.

Bureau of Labor Statistics (BLS): *Projections of Industry Employment*, 2016-26, 2017a. Retrieved from https://stats.bls.gov.

Bureau of Labor Statistics (BLS): *Occupational Employment Statistics*, 2017b. Retrieved from https://www.bls.gov.

Carter EJ, Greendyke WG, Furuya EY, et al: Exploring the nurses' role in antibiotic stewardship: a multisite qualitative study of nurses and infection preventionists, *Am J Infect Control* 46(5):492–497, 2018.

Center for Connected Care: *Fact Sheet: Telehealth Reimbursement*, 2018. Retrieved from http://www.cchp.org.

Center to Advance Palliative Care (CAPC): *Growth of Palliative Care in U.S. Hospitals: 2018 Snapshot*, 2018. Retrieved from https://media.capc.org.

Centers for Disease Control and Prevention (CDC): *The Core Elements of Antibiotic Stewardship for Nursing Homes*, 2017. Retrieved from https://www.cdc.gov.

Centers for Disease Control and Prevention (CDC): *Healthcare-Associated Infections*, 2018. Retrieved from https://www.cdc.gov.

Centers for Medicare and Medicaid Services (CMS): *Outcome-Based Quality Improvement (OBQI) Manual*, 2012. Retrieved from https://www.cms.gov.

Centers for Medicare and Medicaid Services (CMS): *2016 CMS Statistics*, 2016. Retrieved from https://www.cms.gov.

Centers for Medicare and Medicaid Services (CMS): *CMS Announces Proposed Payment Changes for Medicare Home Health Agencies for 2018 and 2019*, 2017a. Retrieved from https://www.cms.gov.

Centers for Medicare and Medicaid Services (CMS): *Hospice Payment System*, 2017b. Retrieved from https://www.cms.gov.

Centers for Medicare and Medicaid Services (CMS): *Outcome and Assessment Information set OASIS-C2 Guidance Manual*, 2017c. Retrieved from https://www.cms.gov.

Centers for Medicare and Medicaid Services (CMS): *Home Health Quality Reporting Program*, 2018a. Retrieved from https://www.cms.gov.

Centers for Medicare and Medicaid Services (CMS): *Home Health Providers*, 2018b. Retrieved from https://www.cms.gov.

Centers for Medicare and Medicaid Services: *Hospice*, 2018c. Retrieved from https://www.cms.gov.

Centers for Medicare and Medicaid Services (CMS): *IMPACT Act Spotlights and Announcements*, 2018d. Retrieved from https://www.cms.gov.

Centers for Medicare and Medicaid Services (CMS): *Hospital Readmissions Reduction Program (HRRP)*, 2018e. Retrieved from https://www.cms.gov.

Charlesworth CJ, Smit E, Lee DS, Alramadhan F, Odden MC: Polypharmacy among adults aged 65 years and older in the United States: 1988-2010, *J Gerontol A Biol Sci Med Sci* 70(8): 989–995, 2015.

Chow K, Dahlin C: Integration of palliative care and oncology nursing, *Semin Oncol Nurs* 34(3):192–201, 2018.

Cimperman M, Brenčič MM, Trkman P, Stanonik Mde L: Older adults' perceptions of home telehealth services, *Telemed J E Health* 19(10):786–790, 2013.

Coleman EA, Berenson RA: Lost in transition: challenges and opportunities for improving the quality of transitional care, *Ann Intern Med* 141:533–536, 2004.

Corbett CF, Setter SM, Daratha KB, Neumiller JJ, Wood LD: Nurse identified hospital to home medication discrepancies: implications for improving transitional care, *Geriatr Nurs* 31: 188–196, 2010.

Cruz J, Brooks D, Marques A: Home telemonitoring in COPD: a systematic review of methodologies and patients' adherence, *Int J Med Inform* 83(4):249–263, 2014.

Curtis JR, Downey L, Back AL, et al: Effect of a patient and clinician communication-priming intervention on patient-reported goals-of-care discussions between patients with serious illness and clinicians: a randomized clinical trial, *JAMA Intern Med* 178(7):930–940, 2018.

Diefenbeck CA, Klemm PR, Hayes ER: "Anonymous meltdown": content themes emerging in a nonfacilitated, peer-only, unstructured, asynchronous online support group for family caregivers, *Comput Inform Nurs* 35:630–638, 2017.

Donahue MP: *Nursing, the finest art*, ed 3, St. Louis, MO, 2011, Elsevier.

Duke Nursing: Bringing population health into focus, *Duke University School of Nursing* 14:4–7, 15, 2018

Eardley DL, Krumwiede KA, Secginli S, et al: The Omaha System as a structured instrument for bridging nursing informatics with public health nursing education: a feasibility study, *Comput Inform Nurs* 36:275–283, 2018.

Enoch MA, Kitzman H, Smith JA, et al: A prospective cohort study of influences on externalizing behaviors across childhood: Results from a nurse home visiting randomized controlled trial, *J Am Acad Child Adolesc Psychiatry* 55: 376–382, 2016.

Etkind SN, Bone AE, Gomes B, et al: How many people will need palliative care in 2040? Past trends, future projections and implications for services, *BMC Med* 15:102, 2017.

Fazzi: *Home Health & Hospice Data*, 2018. Retrieved from https://www.fazzi.com.

Friedman DJ, Parrish RG, Ross DA: Electronic health records and US public health: current realities and future promise, *Am J Public Health* 103:1560–1567, 2013.

Gao G, Maganti S, Monsen KA: Older adults, frailty, and the social and behavioral determinants of health, *Big Data Inf Anal* 2:191–202, 2017.

Gao G, Kerr MJ, Lindquist RA, et al: A strengths-based data capture model: mining data-driven and person-centered health assets, *JAMIA Open* 1(1):11–14, 2018.

Garfinkel D: Poly-de-prescribing to treat polypharmacy: efficacy and safety, *Ther Adv Drug Saf* 9(1):25–43, 2018.

Gasper AM, Magdic K, Ren D, Fennimore L: Development of a home health-based palliative care program for patients with heart failure, *Home Healthc Now* 36:84–92, 2018.

Gorski LA: Infection prevention concepts. In Gorski LA, editor: *Fast facts for nurses about home infusion therapy: the expert's best-practice Guide in a Nutshell*, New York, NY, 2017, Springer Publishers, pp 27–42.

Hinds PS, Schum L, Baker JN, Wolfe J: Key factors affecting dying children and their families, *J Palliat Med* 8(Suppl 1):S70–S78, 2005.

Hospice and Palliative Nurses Association (HPNA): *About Us*, 2018. Retrieved from https://advancingexpertcare.org.

Hospice and Palliative Nurses Association, American Nurses Association (HPNA/ANA): *Hospice and palliative nursing: scope and standards of practice*, Silver Spring, MD, 2007, Nursesbooks.org.

Huang YM, Shiyanbola OO, Smith PD: Association of health literacy and medication self-efficacy with medication adherence and diabetes control, *Patient Prefer Adherence* 12:793–802, 2018.

Innes S: Library nurses look after those in need, *Arizona Daily Star*, Tucson, AZ, 2012. Retrieved from https://tucson.com.

Irani E, Hirschman KB, Cacchione PZ, Bowles KH: Home health nurse decision-making regarding visit intensity planning for newly admitted patients: a qualitative descriptive study, *Home Health Care Serv Q* 37(3):211–231, 2018.

Izumi S: Advance care planning: the nurse's role, *Am J Nurs* 117: 56–61, 2017.

Kaye EC, Rubenstein J, Levine D, Baker JN, Dabbs D, Friebert SE: Pediatric palliative care in the community, *CA Cancer J Clin* 65:316–333, 2015.

Kerr MJ, Flaten C, Honey ML, et al: Feasibility of using the Omaha System for community-level observations, *Public Health Nurs* 33:256–263, 2016.

Kerr MJ, Gargantua-Aguila SDR, Glavin K, et al. Feasibility of describing community strengths relative to Omaha System concepts, *Public Health Nurs* 36(2):245–256, 2019.

Kindig D, Stoddart G: What is population health? *Am J Public Health* 93:380–383, 2003.

Kitsiou S, Paré G, Jaana M: Effects of home telemonitoring interventions on patients with chronic heart failure: an overview of systematic reviews, *J Med Internet Res* 17(3):e63, 2015.

Kübler-Ross E: *On death and dying*, New York, NY, 1969, McMillan.

Levin RF, Keefer JM, Marren J, Vetter M, Lauder B, Sobolewski S: Evidence-based practice improvement: merging 2 paradigms, *J Nurs Care Qual* 25:117–126, 2010.

Levine DR, Mandrell BN, Sykes A, et al: Patients' and parents' needs, attitudes, and perceptions about early palliative care integration in pediatric oncology, *JAMA Oncol* 3:1214–1220, 2017.

Madigan E, Schmotzer BJ, Struk CJ, et al: Home health care with telemonitoring improves health status for older adults with heart failure, *Home Health Care Serv Q* 32:57–74, 2013.

Marek KD, Stetzer F, Ryan PA, et al: Nurse care coordination and technology effects on health status of frail older adults via enhanced self-management of medication: Randomized clinical trial to test efficacy, *Nurs Res* 62;269-278, 2013.

Marrelli TM: *Handbook of home health standards: quality, documentation, and reimbursement*, ed 6, Venice, FL, 2018a, Marrelli & Associates.

Marrelli TM: *Hospice and palliative care handbook: quality, compliance, and reimbursement*, ed 3, Venice, FL, 2018b, Marrelli & Associates.

Martin KS: *The Omaha System: a key to practice, documentation, and information management, reprinted*, ed 2, Omaha, NE, 2005, Health Connections Press.

Martin KS, Kessler PD: The Omaha System: improving the quality of practice and decision support. In Harris MD, editor: *Handbook of home health care administration*, ed 6, Burlington, MA, 2017, Jones & Bartlett, pp 235–248.

Martin KS, Utterback KB: Home health and related community-based systems. In Nelson R, Staggers N, editors: *Health informatics: an interprofessional approach*, ed 2, St. Louis, MO, 2018, Elsevier, pp 153–169.

McAuley A, Munro A, Taylor A: "Once I'd done it once it was like writing your name": lived experience of take-home naloxone administration by people who inject drugs, *Int J Drug Policy* 58:46–54, 2018.

Meadows CA, Fraser J, Camus S, Henderson K: A system-wide innovation in transition services: transforming the home care liaison role, *Home Healthc Nurse* 32:78–86, 2014.

Medicare: *What is Home Health Compare?* n.d. Retrieved from https://www.medicare.gov.

Medicare Payment Advisory Commission (MedPAC): *Hospice Services*, 2018. Retrieved from http://www.medpac.gov.

Melnyk BM, Fineout-Overholt E: *Evidence-based practice in nursing and healthcare: a guide to best practice*, Philadelphia, PA, 2015, Lippincott, Williams & Wilkins.

Melnyk BM, Gallagher-Ford L: Implementing the new essential evidence-based practice competencies in real-world clinical and academic settings: moving from evidence to action in improving healthcare quality and patient outcomes, *Worldviews Evid Based Nurs* 12(2):67–69, 2015.

Miller TR: Projected outcomes of Nurse-Family Partnership home visitation during 1996–2013, *USA, Prev Sci* 16:765–777, 2015.

Milone-Nuzzo P, Hollars ME: Transitioning nurses to home care. In Harris MD, editor: *Handbook of home health care administration*, ed 6, Burlington, MA, 2017, Jones & Bartlett, pp 455–466.

Mira JJ, Lorenzo S, Guilabert M, Navarro I, Pérez-Jover V: A systematic review of patient medication error on self-administering medication at home, *Expert Opin Drug Saf* 14(6):815–838, 2015.

Mistovich JJ, Karren KJ, Hafen B: *Prehospital emergency care*, ed 10, Upper Saddle River, NJ, 2014, Pearson Education.

Mistovich JJ, Karren KJ: *Prehospital emergency care*, ed 11, Upper Saddle River, NJ, 2018, Pearson Education.

Monsen KA, Martinson B, Lawrence EC, et al: Toward population health literacy, wellbeing, consumer engagement, and information exchange: developing Omaha System icons for digital platforms, *Int J Healthc* 2:71–81, 2016.

Monsen KA: *Intervention effectiveness research: quality improvement and program evaluation*, Cham, Switzerland, 2018, Springer.

Monsen KA, Kelechi TJ, McRae ME, Mathiason MA, Martin KS: Nursing theory, terminology, and big data: data-driven discovery of novel patterns in archival randomized clinical trial data, *Nurs Res* 67:122-132, 2018.

Murtaugh CM, Deb P, Zhu C, et al: Reducing readmissions among heart failure patients discharged to home health care: effectiveness of early and intensive nursing services and early physician follow-up, *Health Serv Res* 52(4):1445–1472, 2017.

National Association for Home Care & Hospice (NAHC): *NAHC Supports Bill to Permit Disposal of Unused Hospice Meds in the Home*, 2018. Retrieved from https://www.nahc.org.

National Consensus Project for Quality Palliative Care (NCP): *Clinical practice guidelines for quality palliative care*, ed 3, Pittsburgh, PA, 2013, Author.

National Consensus Project for Quality Palliative Care (NCP): *2018 Clinical practice guidelines for quality palliative care*, ed 4, Pittsburgh, PA, in press, Author.

National Hospice and Palliative Care Organization (NHPCO): *Facts and Figures Hospice Care in America Revised*, 2018. Retrieved from https://www.nhpco.org.

National Hospice and Palliative Care Organization (NHPCO): *Hospice Policy Compendium: The Medicare Hospice Benefit, Regulations, Quality Reporting, and Public Policy*, 2016. Retrieved from https://www.nhpco.org.

National Quality Forum: *About Us*, 2014. Retrieved from http://www.qualityforum.org.

Naylor MD, Bowles KH, McCauley KM, et al: High-value transitional care: translation of research into practice, *J Eval Clin Pract* 19:727–733, 2013.

Naylor MD, Hirschman KB, Hanlon AL, et al: Effects of alternative interventions among hospitalized, cognitively impaired older adults, *J Comp Eff Res* 5(3):259–272, 2016.

Naylor MD, Shaid EC, Carpenter D, et al: Components of comprehensive and effective transitional care, *J Am Geriatr Soc* 65(6):1119–1125, 2017.

Nelson R, Staggers N: *Health informatics: an interprofessional approach*, ed 2, St. Louis, MO, 2018, Elsevier.

Nurse-Family Partnership (NFP): *Annual Report 2017*, 2017. Retrieved from https://www.nursefamilypartnership.org.

O'Connor M, Bowles KH, Feldman PH, et al: Frontloading and intensity of skilled home health visits: a state of the science, *Home Health Care Serv Q* 33(3):159–175, 2014.

Office of the National Coordinator for Health Information Technology: *2017*, 2017a. Retrieved from http://www.healthit.gov.

Office of the National Coordinator for Health Information Technology: *Advanced Alternative Payment Model*, 2017b. Retrieved from https://www.healthit.gov.

Olds DL, Eckenrode J, Henderson CR Jr, et al: Long-term effects of home visitation on maternal life course and child abuse and neglect: fifteen-year follow-up of a randomized trial. *JAMA* 278:637–643, 1997.

Omaha System: *Is it There?* 2018. Retrieved from http://www.omahasystem.org.

Perry KM, Parente CA: Integrating palliative care into home care practice. In Harris MD, editor: *Handbook of home health care administration*, ed 6, Burlington, MA, 2017, Jones & Bartlett, pp 767–782.

Public Health Accreditation Board (PHAB): *Welcome to PHAB*, 2018. Retrieved from http://www.phaboard.org.

Quad Council Coalition: *Community/Public Health Nursing Competencies*, 2018. Retrieved from http://quadcouncilphn.org.

Radhakrishnan K, Martin KS, Johnson KE, Garcia AA. Effective teaching-learning strategies for the Omaha System, *Home Healthc Now* 34:86–92, 2016.

Rantz MJ, Skubic M, Miller SJ, et al: Sensor technology to support aging in place, *J Am Med Dir Assoc* 14:386–391, 2013.

Reddy S: A tech test to keep seniors in their homes longer, *Wall St J*, A12, July 26, 2018.

Reidt SL, Larson TA, Hadsall RS, Uden DL, Blade MA, Branstad R: Integrating a pharmacist into a home healthcare agency care model: impact on hospitalizations and emergency visits, *Home Healthc Nurse* 32:146–152, 2014.

Riker GI, Setter SM: Polypharmacy in older adults at home: what it is and what to do about it—implications for home healthcare and hospice, *Home Healthc Nurse* 30(8):474–485, 2012.

Riker GI, Setter SM: Polypharmacy in older adults at home: what it is and what to do about it—implications for home healthcare and hospice, Part 2, *Home Healthc Nurse* 31(2):65–77, 2013.

Robert Wood Johnson Foundation (RWJF): *Public Health Nurses Bringing Care to Libraries*, 2013. Retrieved from https://www.rwjf.org.

Robert Wood Johnson Foundation (RWJF): *Creating a Shared Vision to Help Restore Atlantic City*, 2018. Retrieved from https://www.rwjf.org.

Ross B: What RNs can do to improve the health of their communities, *Am J Nurs* 118:11, 2018.

Russell D, Dowding DW, McDonald MV: Factors for compliance with infection control practices in home healthcare: findings from a survey of nurses' knowledge and attitudes toward infection control, *Am J Infect Control*, 46(11):1211–1217, 2018.

Schlachta-Fairchild L, Rocca M, Cordi V, et al: Telehealth and applications for delivering care at a distance. In Nelson R, Staggers N, editors: *Health informatics: an interprofessional approach*, ed 2, St. Louis, MO, 2018, Elsevier, pp 131–152.

Schoon P, Porta C, Schaffer M: *Population-based public health nursing clinical manual: the henry street model for nurses*, ed 3, 2018, Sigma Theta Tau International.

Shang J, Dick AW, Larson EL, Stone PW: A research agenda for infection prevention in home healthcare, *Am J Infect Control* 46(9):1071–1073, 2018.

Shmagel A, Ngo L, Ensrud K, Foley R: Prescription medication use among community-based U.S. adults with chronic low back pain: a cross-sectional population based study, *J Pain* 19(10):1104–1112, 2018.

Slipka AF, Monsen KA: Toward improving quality of end-of-life care: encoding clinical guidelines and standing orders using the Omaha System, *Worldviews Evid Based Nurs* 15:26–37, 2018.

Smith LS: Cultural competence: a nurse educator's guide, *Nursing* 47:18–21, 2017a.

Smith LS: Cultural competence: a guide for nursing students, *Nursing* 47:18–20, 2017b.

Sockolow P, Wojciechowicz C, Holmberg A, et al: Home care admission information: what nurses need and what nurses have. A mixed methods study, *Stud Health Technol Inform* 250:164–168, 2018.

Stober M: Palliative care in home health: a review of the literature, *Home Healthc Now* 35:373–377, 2017.

Storfjell JL, Winslow BW, Saunders JSD: *Catalysts for Change: Harnessing the Power of Nurses to Build Population Health in the 21st Century*, 2017. Retrieved from https://www.rwjf.org.

Tan PN, Steinbach M, Karpatne A, Kumar V: *Introduction to data mining*, ed 2, London, UK, 2019, Pearson.

The Blue Button: *Medicare's Blue Button*, 2017. Retrieved from http://www.mymedicare.gov.

Thorland W, Currie D, Wiegand ER, Walsh J, Mader N: Status of breastfeeding and child immunization outcomes in clients of the Nurse-Family Partnership, *Matern Child Health J* 21:439–445, 2017.

Topaz M, Golfenshtein N, Bowles KH: The Omaha System: a systematic review of the recent literature, *J Am Med Inform Assoc* 21: 163–170, 2014.

U.S. Census Bureau: *Profile American Facts for Features*. CB17-FF 08, April 10, 2017. Retrieved from https://www.census.gov.

U.S. Department of Health and Human Services (USDHHS): *Healthy People 2020: 2020 Topics and Objectives-Objectives A-Z*, 2014. Retrieved from http://www.healthypeople.gov.

U.S. Department of Health and Human Services (USDHHS): *HIPAA for Professionals*, 2017. Retrieved from https://www.hhs.gov.

U.S. Food & Drug Administration (FDA): *Where and How to Dispose of Unused Medicines*, 2017. Retrieved from https://www.fda.gov.

U.S. National Library of Medicine: *Personal Health Records*, 2018. Retrieved from https://medlineplus.gov.

Vandermause R, Neumiller JJ, Gates BJ, et al: Preserving self: medication-taking practices and preferences of older adults with multiple chronic medical conditions, *J Nurs Scholarsh* 48(6): 533–542, 2016.

Visiting Nurse Service of New York (VNSNY): *Our Services*, 2017. Retrieved from http://www.vnsny.org.

Weissman DE, Meier DE: Identifying patients in need of a palliative care assessment in the hospital setting: a consensus report from the Center to Advance Palliative Care, *J Palliat Med* 14:17–23, 2011.

Wright E: Clients receiving home health and hospice care. In Rector C, editor: *Community and public health nursing*, ed 9, Philadelphia, PA, 2018, Wolters Kluwer, pp 1166–1189.

Weaver MS, Heinze KE, Bell CJ, et al: Establishing psychosocial palliative care standards for children and adolescents with cancer and their families: an integrative review, *Palliat Med* 3:212–223, 2016.

Wendel ML, Garney WR, Castle BF, Ingram CM: Critical reflexivity of communities on their experience to improve population health, *Am J Public Health* 108:896–901, 2018.

Yang Y, Bass EJ, Bowles KH, Sockolow PS: Impact of home care admission nurses' goals on electronic health record documentation strategies at the point of care, *Comput Inform Nurs* 37(1): 39–46, 2019.

Zerwekh JV: *Nursing care at the end of life: palliative care for patients and families*, Philadelphia, PA, 2006, F.A. Davis.

Zhang KM, Dindoff K, Arnold JM, Lane J, Swartzman LC: What matters to patients with heart failure? The influence of non-health-related goals on patient adherence to self-care management, *Patient Educ Couns* 98(8):927–934, 2015.

Zullig LL, Hayden B: *Engaging Patients to Optimize Medication Adherence*, 2017. Retrieved from https://catalyst.nejm.org.

42

The Nurse in the Schools

Erin G. Cruise, PhD, RN

OBJECTIVES

After reading this chapter, the student should be able to do the following:

1. Discuss the history of school nursing and describe, compare, and contrast the professional standards and scope of practice of school nursing with those of public health nursing
2. Differentiate the roles, responsibilities, and activities of school nurses from those of nurses in other settings.
3. Describe various frameworks and models that provide the foundation for school nursing practice.
4. Discuss common health problems of children and adolescents seen in the school setting and the school nurse's support of education for children with illness and disabilities
5. Analyze the nursing care given in schools in the context of primary, secondary, and tertiary levels of prevention.
6. Anticipate future trends in school nursing.

CHAPTER OUTLINE

History of School Nursing
Federal Legislation Affecting School Nursing Practice
Standards of Practice for School Nurses
Educational and Licensure Credentials of School Nurses
Roles and Functions of School Nurses
School Health Services
School Nurses and *Healthy People 2020*
The Levels of Prevention Applied in Schools
Controversies in School Nursing
Ethics in School Nursing
Future Trends in School Nursing

KEY TERMS

advanced practice nurses, p. 933
case manager, p. 934
Child Nutrition Act, p. 932
community outreach, p. 935
consultant, p. 935
counselor, p. 934
crisis teams, p. 940
direct caregiver, p. 934
do-not-attempt-resuscitation orders, p. 950
Education for All Handicapped Children Act, p. 931
emergency plan, p. 940
Every Student Succeeds Act (ESSA), p. 932
Family Education Rights and Privacy Act (FERPA), p. 932
health educator, p. 934
Health Insurance Portability and Accountability Act (HIPAA), p. 932
Healthy, Hunger-Free Kids Act, p. 932
individualized education plans (IEPs), p. 931
individualized health plans (IHPs), p. 931
Individuals with Disabilities Education Act (IDEA), p. 931
Individuals with Disabilities Education Improvement Act of 2004 (IDEIA) p. 931
National Association of School Nurses, p. 933
No Child Left Behind Act, p. 932
primary prevention, p. 937
researcher, p. 935
school-based health centers, p. 953
School Health Policies and Practices Study, p. 936
school-linked program, p. 953
school nursing, p. 929
secondary prevention, p. 937
Section 504 of the Rehabilitation Act, p. 931
tertiary prevention, p. 937

School nursing is a specialty practice focused on providing health care and illness prevention to school-age children with the goal of facilitating their participation in educational opportunities (American Nurses Association [ANA] & National Association of School Nurses [NASN], 2017). School nursing services are provided to individuals within the school setting, including children, staff, and teachers. School nursing is also population focused, utilizing many of the concepts of public health nursing to prevent illness and injury and to stop the spread of disease within the school, family, and community. While school nursing has required a comprehensive approach to health care and health promotion since its inception, the practice continues to evolve and increase in complexity (Wolfe, 2013). School nurses provide leadership and coordinate health and safety programs in their schools and communities.

According to the National Center for Education Statistics, there were an estimated 50.7 million children in more than 98,000 U.S. public schools in 2017 (Institute of Education Sciences [IES]: National Center for Education Statistics [NCES], 2017). Of these, 35.6 million attended preschool, elementary, and middle schools and 15.1 million were in grades 9 through 12. In the 34,600 U.S. private schools, enrollment was predicted to be an additional 5.2 million students. School nurses provide care to these children in all school settings, as well as in their homes, correctional settings, hospitals, and during field trips, athletic competitions, and other extracurricular events (ANA & NASN, 2017).

U.S. public and private schools employ about 3.6 million teachers as well as other adult school administrators and staff such as administrative assistants, custodians, food service workers, and bus drivers (Institute of Education Sciences: National Center for Education Statistics [IES: NCES], 2017). In addition to care for children, school nurses are often asked to provide health services for these adult school staff members. This requires school nurses to have expertise in a wide variety of adult health care issues, including nutrition, medication, communicable diseases, and chronic illness (Wolfe, 2013).

This chapter will consider the history of school nursing and examine the evolving roles and activities of school nurses in modern times. Frameworks for evidence-based school nursing practice will be explained, as well as professional scope and standards of the specialty. The impact of federal regulations on the education of children and the practice of school nursing will be investigated. This chapter will also assess the relationship of public health nursing and school nursing. Different types of school health services will be examined and the levels of care required for a variety of children's health problems most commonly found in schools will be discussed. The chapter ends with a discussion of the ethical dilemmas that may arise for school nurses, and the future of nursing in the schools is predicted for ever-changing communities.

HISTORY OF SCHOOL NURSING

Origins of School Nursing

The earliest organized school health services were implemented in France in the 1830s where policies were passed to require health services and a sanitary environment for children in schools (Zaiger, 2013, p. 4). In 1874, Brussels, Belgium, employed physicians to conduct health inspections throughout the city's schools. In the 1880s and 1890s in England, a variety of volunteer nursing services were provided in the schools in London and Liverpool, with the purpose of addressing contagious disease, minor illnesses and injuries, and assessing the nutritional status of low-income children (Zaiger, 2013). While charitable funding only supported five nurses to cover the 500 elementary schools in London, the activities of these nurses significantly reduced absences. This led the London County Council to take over the funding of school nurse services by 1904 (Brainard, as cited in Zaiger, 2013, p. 5).

In the 1890s in the United States, Boston, Chicago, and New York City instituted medical inspection programs in schools to address rising levels of absenteeism due to communicable diseases, especially among immigrant and low-income populations (Rogers, 1905). Inspections were conducted by physicians without the assistance of nurses, who excluded affected children from school to prevent the spread of serious communicable and parasitic diseases among their classmates (Baker, Wald, as cited in Houlahan, 2018). However, many children were not treated due to their parents' inability to read the physicians' instructions or afford the required medications. Thus thousands of children never returned to school, yet could be found playing with their non-excluded classmates after school (Houlahan, 2018). This program did little to stem the tide of contagious disease or reduce absenteeism in New York City schools.

By 1902, the failure of the medical inspections program became more conspicuous and controversial. Lillian Wald, well known among public health authorities and charitable organizations as a strong advocate for the poor, was consulted for ideas to address plummeting school attendance in the city's poor, immigrant neighborhoods (Houlahan, 2018). Ms. Wald agreed to provide the services of Lina Rogers in the schools to assist the physicians on an experimental basis for one month.

Ms. Rogers was assigned to four schools with a total student population of 8671 students (Rogers, 1905). She conducted a thorough assessment of the schools, surrounding community, and affected families and found a lack of communication between physicians, parents, students, and school personnel (Rogers, 1905). This often led to children being readmitted to school before they had been cured of their contagious diseases, or a revolving door of returning and being sent home again (Houlahan, 2018).

Ms. Rogers worked to improve children's health by working with the physicians to screen for illness in the schools each day, providing treatment for some ailments at school, and making daily home visits to address issues that fostered the development and persistence of illness among the students. In many cases, the home environment was unsanitary or other family members were ill. Ms. Rogers educated the children and their families, administered treatments in the home, assisted with cleaning, and obtained resources for those who could not afford medications, physician visits, or cleaning supplies (Rogers, 1905).

The goal of Ms. Rogers' school nursing practice was to facilitate children's attendance at school by intervening in a timely, effective, and holistic manner to eradicate disease. As Rogers (1908) stated, these children "could least afford to lose their schooling, as they belong, almost all, to that class of wage earners who are legally allowed to work [and leave school] at the age of fourteen" (p. 967).

After the first month, Ms. Rogers' interventions were deemed so successful that the New York City Department of Health and the Department of Education agreed to provide funding to expand the program. A team of 12 school nurses, working under Ms. Rogers' direction, reduced school exclusions of children from more than 10,000 in September 1902, to 1100 in September 1903, a decrease of 98 percent in only one year (Rogers, 1905, 1908). By February 1903, the number of school nurses was increased to 27 (Houlahan, 2018).

Evolution of School Nursing Practice

Within a few years, many large cities in the United States had implemented school nurse programs, though these varied from state to state and within each state. In some communities, nurses were hired directly by the school districts. In others, local and state health department nurses provided services in schools, as well as in children's homes (Zaiger, 2013). In rural areas, services were provided by the American Red Cross Visiting Nurse Associations, the Frontier Nursing Service, and other private or charitable groups. The greatest impetus for instituting school nurse services was prevention of communicable diseases and decreasing absenteeism in schools, but health education and addressing family health needs were always part of the approach to achieving these goals.

In the early years of U.S. school nursing, services were primarily targeted at elementary-aged children and their families. However, in the 1930s, some states began to expand health programs to include high school students. Speaking at the 1936 National Organization for Public Health Nursing Convention, Foeller (1936) emphasized the importance of school nurses being qualified to deliver health education to this age group, conduct physical assessments, teach anatomy and physiology, and provide mental health services and counseling. She also promoted collaboration between the school nurse, physical education teachers, and the local health department and the importance of a thorough medical examination for all new students.

Throughout the Depression and World War II, school nursing evolved from its focus on public and community health to being mostly confined within the school walls (Apple, 2017). Some of this was due to budget constraints and some was due to changes in society. Despite evidence that school nurses' interventions decreased absenteeism and improved student engagement, thereby reducing the overall cost of educating children, many school administrators declined to pay for public health nurses to make home visits and serve the broader community. Some school districts chose to eliminate school nurses altogether. U.S. society was also evolving during this time. More women entered the workforce, requiring children to spend longer hours in school. School nurses had less time to make home visits or become involved in the community's health, as they were administering medications and providing more direct health care services to children throughout the school day (Apple, 2017).

In the 1940s and into the second half of the twentieth century, school and public health nursing experts wrestled with defining the roles, practice, and educational requirements of school nurses, as well as meeting the complex health needs of students (Zaiger, 2013). Variations in state regulations, school nurse preparation, numbers of schools and students covered by each nurse, and expectations of school administrators and parents fostered inconsistency in the practice of school nursing throughout the country. The introduction of antibiotics and immunizations meant that fewer children were attending school with communicable diseases, yet emphasis on screening, health education, supporting children with disabilities, and mental health counseling was intensified (School Nurses Branch, 1961). Teachers were increasingly expected to provide health education and first aid to students, as a way of minimizing interruptions in the classroom and maximizing the number of schools one nurse could cover. School health councils were developed in some communities to enhance collaboration among physicians, teachers and other school personnel, school nurses, public health departments, and families and address the multifaceted expectations of school health programs (Zaiger, 2013).

In 1960, the School Nurses Branch of the American Nurses Association (ANA) developed a detailed position statement that delineated functions and educational preparation of school nurses. This statement proposed a comprehensive and leadership role for school nurses in the delivery and oversight of school health programs. According to these experts, school nurses should:

- Function as the administrators of their schools' health programs.
- Identify and address health problems that may interfere with students' education.
- Foster holistic growth and development of children.
- Support children and families in obtaining the full range of health services.
- Develop policies and procedures to prevent or intervene in communicable disease outbreaks, including immunization programs.
- Collaborate with teachers in the creation and evaluation of the school's curriculum for health education.
- Engage in development of the budget for school health services.
- Serve as equal members of the faculty.
- Provide leadership in community health issues.
- Assist in researching best practices for school nursing and interventions for school health problems.
- Assist in the education of nursing students and nurses entering the field of school nursing (School Nurses Branch, 1961).

Additional functions were outlined for school nurse administrators in hiring, training, and supervising school nursing staff, as well as overseeing the school program's operations, budget, and facility improvement to enhance the effectiveness of school nursing practice. Finally, the School Nurses Branch (1961) recommended that school nurses be prepared at the baccalaureate level with additional training, experience, or graduate education specific to the field. Interestingly, this position statement aligns closely with the original 1983 *Standards of School Nursing Practice,* which have been regularly updated in

TABLE 42.1 High Points In School Nursing History

Decade	Major Events in School Nursing
1890s	English and American nurses are used in schools to examine children for infectious diseases and to teach about alcohol abuse.
1900s	Henry Street Settlement in New York City sends nurses into schools and homes to investigate children's overall health.
1910s	School nursing course added to Teachers College nursing program. School nursing spreads throughout the country.
1920s and 1930s	School nurses are employed by community health departments.
1940s	School districts employ school nurses.
1950s	Children are screened in schools for common health problems.
1960s	Educational preparation for school nurses is debated.
1970s	School nurse practitioner programs began. Increased emphasis put on mental health counseling in schools.
1980s	Children with long-term illness or disabilities attend schools. Introduction of *School Nursing: Scope and Standards of Practice* by ANA and NASN.
1990s	School-based and school-linked clinics are started. Total family and community health care is offered.
2000s	School nurses give comprehensive primary, secondary, and tertiary levels of nursing care. *The Framework for 21st Century School Nursing Practice* is adopted.

Data from Apple R.: School health is community: school nursing in the early twentieth century in the USA. *History of Education Review* 46(2):136-149, 2017; Zaiger D: Historical perspectives of school nursing. In Selekman J, editor: *School nursing: a comprehensive text*, ed. 2, Philadelphia, 2013, F.A. Davis Company, pp. 2-24.

the intervening decades, most recently in 2017 (ANA & NASN, 2017). Contemporary school nursing practice continues to evolve but remains focused on meeting the complex needs of school-age children, school staff, families, and the community.

Table 42.1 gives the highlights of school nursing history over the last century.

FEDERAL LEGISLATION AFFECTING SCHOOL NURSING PRACTICE

Federal legislation requiring that schools educate children with medical needs and disabilities has had a substantial impact on the practice of school nursing since the latter part of the twentieth century. Survival of children born prematurely increased significantly during that time. This can be correlated with an increase in children with physical, behavioral, and learning disabilities (American Academy of Pediatrics [AAP], Council on School Health, 2016). The number of children with chronic diseases, such as asthma and diabetes, is also on the rise. In the past, children with these conditions did not often survive past infancy. If they did survive, they were likely to be institutionalized rather than cared for at home and would probably not have been educated in public schools as they are now.

In 1954, the U.S. Supreme Court declared that racial segregation of schools was unconstitutional. In 1964, the Civil Rights Act strengthened laws against discrimination on the basis of race, gender, religious affiliation, or ethnic background. This trend toward equality opened the door for parents to demand civil rights for their children with disabilities under the 14th Amendment of the U.S. Constitution (Gibbons et al., 2013). In 1973, **Section 504 of the Rehabilitation Act** required that public schools and other entities receiving federal funding could not be discriminated against and children could not be denied the benefits of an education (U.S. Department of Education Office for Civil Rights [DOE-OCR], 2010).

In 1975, the **Education for All Handicapped Children Act** was passed. This law further specified the requirements for special education approaches and school health services to allow children with disabilities to reach their full potential (Yonkaitis & Shannon, 2017). This law was amended several times over the next decade, increasing eligibility for services to children ages birth to 21 years and providing financial incentives to states for early intervention programs. States were also encouraged to provide transition to work and adult life programs for disabled children as they aged out of the school system (Gibbons et al., 2013).

The **Individuals with Disabilities Education Act (IDEA)** was reauthorized in 1990 and the Americans with Disabilities Act (ADA) was also passed in 1990, further ensuring the protection of civil rights for those with disabilities, including the right to a "free and appropriate education" (FAPE) for children ages birth to 21 years of age (Gibbons et al., 2013). FAPE is interpreted to mean services are free and meet the needs of disabled children in order to promote their highest achievable level of learning and development in the least restrictive educational environment (DOE-OCR, 2010). IDEA was renamed the **Individuals with Disabilities Education Improvement Act (IDEIA)** in 2004 and extended coverage till the child turns 22 (Gibbons et al., 2013). **Individualized education plans (IEPs)** and **individualized health plans (IHPs)** are among the processes that school nurses participate in to ensure that any specialized health care needs required for disabled children to participate in FAPE are met. According to the *2016 School Health Policies and Practice Study,* 71.5 percent of states require that school nurses participate on teams developing IEPs (Centers for Disease Control and Prevention [CDC], 2016d).

IDEA is reviewed and amended periodically to determine whether it is meeting its intended goals, to strengthen access, and clarify regulations. However, in 2017, Congress found that while 40 percent of the funding for IDEA is supposed to come from the federal government, only 8 percent federal funding is currently being provided to school districts throughout the country (U.S. Government Printing Office [GPO], 2017). While Congress acknowledged the burden this places on school districts in trying to comply with the law, the amount of federal money needed to fully fund IDEA services was $10 billion annually, an amount that Congress had stated should be provided "as soon as reasonably possible, through the reallocation of non-education funds within the current budget monetary constraints" (GPO, 2017, p. 1215). In order to provide education to these medically fragile children, they must rely on the assistance of school nurses to oversee and deliver higher-level health care than was needed before the enactment of these laws. The lack of funding from the federal government makes it difficult for schools to provide adequate special educational and health care services to students covered by these laws.

Several other federal laws impact the education and health services of children in public schools. In 2015, the Every Student Succeeds Act (ESSA) replaced the 2001 No Child Left Behind Act (NCLB). NCLB required that accommodations be made to promote academic achievement for children with disabilities and those living in poverty, having limited English proficiency (LEP), or who were homeless (DOE, 2008). ESSA strengthens and clarifies these requirements but also includes regulations requiring that states must allocate a percentage of their federal funds toward "activities to support safe and healthy students" (DOE, 2018, p. 219). These activities must include education on drug use and violence prevention; comprehensive mental and behavioral health services; prevention of bullying, harassment, and suicide; and integration of health, nutrition, and safety into physical education programs. School nurses are specifically named in the ESSA as being responsible for providing instruction in healthy lifestyles and chronic disease management (DOE, 2018).

The Child Nutrition Act (CNA) was originally passed in 1964 to combat malnutrition and hunger among disadvantaged children and pregnant women. This law funds the National School Lunch Program, breakfast and summer food programs in schools and preschools, and food supplements for pregnant and breastfeeding women and their preschool children (U.S. Congress, 2010). The Act also establishes minimum standards for nutrition content of meals, requires decreased student access to non-nutritious foods on school grounds, and the inclusion of nutrition education, physical activity, and school wellness programs. This law has been reauthorized every five years, with the last reauthorization in 2010 as the Healthy, Hunger-Free Kids Act (HHFK) (U.S. Congress, 2010). By continuing to reauthorize the CNA in its various iterations, Congress and presidents have acknowledged the importance of nutrition in promoting child health, which in turn improves children's ability to engage in educational opportunities. The HHFK Act expired in 2015 due to differences between the House and Senate on policy, including nutrition standards (Food Research and Action Center, 2018). However, the HHFK/CNA programs continue as permanent law so long as Congress continues to fund them.

Health information of students in schools is protected under both the Family Education Rights and Privacy Act (FERPA) of 1974 and the Health Insurance Portability and Accountability Act (HIPAA) of 1996. FERPA covers educational records of any child in an educational setting that receives federal funding from the U.S. Department of Education (Caldart-Olson & Thronson, 2013). This includes student health records maintained by all public schools and many private schools in the United States. In general, FERPA restricts the disclosure of any information that could be used to identify the student without written permission of the parents, except within the school to school officials or teachers who have a legitimate right to know. The focus of sharing this information should be considered only to protect the health and safety of the school. On the other hand, HIPAA restricts the sharing of individual students' health information but specifically allows discussions and electronic transmission about treatment and medication between the school nurse and the child's health care providers, as long as reasonable efforts are made to protect the privacy of the student's information (Caldart-Olson & Thronson, 2013).

School nurses should stay abreast of laws and regulations that affect their practice and the health of the children in their care. Just as the School Nurses Branch recommended in 1961, school nurses must provide leadership in all health and safety-related activities in their schools. Knowing these legal requirements can help them advocate for students and their rights to a healthy and safe school environment.

Table 42.2 summarizes the effects of these laws on school nurses and schoolchildren.

TABLE 42.2 Federal Legislation Affecting School Nursing

Law	Effect on School Nurses and Children
1954 Desegregation of Schools; 1964 Civil Rights Act	Schools can no longer be segregated by race. Expanded civil rights open the door for children with disability to attend schools.
1973: PL 39-112, Section 504 of Rehabilitation Act	Children cannot be excluded from schools because of a handicap. The school must provide health services that each child needs.
1975: PL 94-142, Education for All Handicapped Children Act	All children should attend school in least restrictive environment. Requires school district's committee on handicapped to develop individualized education plans (IEPs) for children.
1992: Americans with Disabilities Act	Persons with disabilities cannot be excluded from activities.
1997: PL 105-17, Individuals with Disabilities Education Act (IDEA) with updates in 2004	Educational services must be offered by schools for all disabled children from birth through age 22 years.
2001: No Child Left Behind Act of 2001 (NCLB); 2015 Every Student Succeeds Act (ESSA)	NCLB requires all children must receive standardized education in a healthy environment. ESSA includes provisions for health and safety in schools.
2004: Child Nutrition and WIC Reauthorization Act of 2004	Every local education agency (LEA) participating in federal school meal programs must establish a local school wellness policy.
2010: Healthy, Hunger-Free Kids Act of 2010	Reform of the National School Lunch Program and National School Breakfast Program through increased funding and setting policy on nutritional quality of foods served on school grounds. Also opens eligibility requirements to improve access to the free and reduced-price lunch program.

WIC, Women, Infants, and Children program.

Data from Gibbons LJ, Lehr K, Selekman J: Federal laws protecting children and youth with disabilities in the schools. In Selekman J, editor: *School nursing: a comprehensive text,* ed. 2, Philadelphia, 2013, F.A. Davis Company, pp. 257-283; U.S. Department of Education: *The Every Student Succeeds Act: P.L. 115-224,* 2018; U.S. Department of Education, Office for Civil Rights: *Free appropriate public education for students with disabilities: requirements under section 504 of The Rehabilitation Act of 1973,* 2010.

STANDARDS OF PRACTICE FOR SCHOOL NURSES

The professional organization for school nurses is the National Association of School Nurses (NASN), headquartered in Washington, DC. The mission of the NASN is "To optimize student health and learning by advancing the practice of school nursing" (NASN, 2018a, para. 3). NASN advances school nursing practice through education, state and national conferences, access to legal and school health resources, lobbying efforts on behalf of children and school nurses, and establishment of the *School Nursing: Scope and Standards of Practice,* which were most recently updated in 2017 (ANA & NASN, 2017). These standards "are professional expectations that guide the practice of school nursing" (ANA & NASN, 2017, p. xi). They delineate the roles, activities, ethical requirements, and standards of professionalism and practice for which school nurses are held accountable to the public.

Within the *Scope and Standards of Practice,* the *Standards of Practice* follow the nursing process: assessment, diagnosis, outcomes identification, planning, implementation, and evaluation. The *Standards of Professional Performance for School Nursing* describe the professional competencies that school nurses are responsible for. These include:

- Ethical practice
- Ensuring confidentiality of student health information
- Cultural competence
- Effective communication and interprofessional collaboration
- Continuing education to ensure current, quality, and evidence-based nursing practice
- Ongoing self-evaluation
- Appropriate and responsible utilization of resources
- School health services program management and policy development with accountability for student health
- Leadership within the school health program and community (ANA & NASN, 2017).

EDUCATIONAL AND LICENSURE CREDENTIALS OF SCHOOL NURSES

The practice of school nursing is highly complex and requires a great deal of autonomy and clinical judgment. School nurses may be required to train and supervise others and to delegate certain health care tasks to unlicensed assistive personnel. Registered nurses (RNs) can be licensed at either the bachelor of science in nursing (BSN) or associate's degree level (ADN) or in a diploma program, as long as they can pass their state board's licensure examination. The BSN curriculum includes all of the same coursework that an associate's degree or diploma does, in addition to education on leadership, management, population health, health promotion, nursing theory, health policy, and quality improvement (American Association of Colleges of Nursing, 2017). Extensive research has demonstrated that patient outcomes are improved in acute care settings when a higher percentage of nurses is prepared at the BSN level (Institute of Medicine, 2011). However, there is limited research on this specifically related to school health outcomes. Experts in the field of pediatrics and school health recommend that school nurses have a minimum licensure of RN and a minimum education level of BSN for entry into the school nursing specialty (AAP, 2016; NASN, 2016). The American Nurses Association (2013) asserts that public health nursing requires a minimum of a BSN to practice. Because school nurses care for groups of children and school personnel whose health issues may affect the greater community population, this practice is considered to be a type of public health nursing (NASN, 2016).

The NASN also recommends school nurse certification, which requires training beyond that provided in most bachelor's degree preparation (NASN, 2016). While individual states may have various requirements or pathways for certification of school nurses, certification at the national level requires licensure as an RN and a bachelor's degree in a health-related field, not necessarily nursing (National Board for Certification of School Nurses, 2018).

Despite these recommendations, school nurses across the United States vary widely in their educational preparation for assuming this critical role. According to the *Results From the School Health Policies and Practices Study* (SHPPS) (CDC, 2016), 20.7 percent of districts in the United States have no requirements related to the educational preparation of newly hired school nurses. A minimum of an ADN was required in 23.6 percent of school districts. A BSN was required in 26 percent of school districts, a significant increase from the 2012 study, which found that only 5.4 percent of newly hired school nurses were required to have a BSN (Brener et al., 2013).

Many school districts (27 percent) allow nurses with minimal education, such as licensed practical nurses (LPNs), to practice in schools (CDC, 2016d). The percentage of districts requiring RN licensure for newly hired school nurses has declined to 79 percent from about 86 percent in 2012 (Brener et al., 2013). Only 39 percent of school districts require state school nurse certification, and only 7.3 percent require national certification (CDC, 2016d). These numbers are concerning in light of the expert recommendations discussed earlier, the increasing complexity of school nursing practice, and the rising numbers of vulnerable children and families in school communities (NASN, 2016).

A 2018 study by Willgerodt, Brock, and Maughan found about 1200 advanced practice nurses (APNs) practicing in U.S. schools. These APNS may be clinical nurse specialists or nurse practitioners with specialization in pediatrics, family nursing, school nursing, or public health nursing (ANA & NASN, 2017). Some of these APNs are providing school health services at the conventional level, or they may be providing primary care services in school-based clinics (Proctor, 2013). Having APNs provide primary care may improve access to health care for families who lack a provider or health insurance, as well as minimize barriers such as transportation for families without a vehicle or employer restrictions on parents leaving work. These advanced practice nurses may be certified by professional organizations such as the ANA or their own professional organization. Most hold master's degrees in nursing (ANA & NASN, 2017).

Just as with educational and certification requirements, there is little consistency in the minimal requirements for years or types of work experience for newly hired nurses across the United States. While it is common that school nurses come to the field with prior nursing experience, it is possible for newly graduated nurses to work in the schools, depending on the entry criteria of their state and local health departments and schools. Ideally, the less experienced nurses should complete an extended orientation period until they feel comfortable practicing alone (Proctor, 2013). The *School Nursing: Scope and Standards of Practice* can provide guidance to school districts, administrators, and school nurse managers in the development of position descriptions for recruitment of new school nurses and competencies for orientation and ongoing evaluation of school nurse employees (ANA & NASN, 2017; Proctor, 2013).

ROLES AND FUNCTIONS OF SCHOOL NURSES

School nurses function in many roles within their practice. They serve as educators, counselors, consultants, case managers, and direct caregivers to children and school staff. They must coordinate the health care of many students in their schools with the health care that the children receive from their personal health care providers.

In order to ensure that school nurses can provide safe and effective care for their students, the *Healthy People 2020* Objective ECBP-5 recommends an increase in the proportion of schools that have a minimum of one full-time registered nurse for every 750 students (U.S. Department of Health and Human Services, 2018). However, as of 2016, only 10.9 percent of schools have a required minimum school nurse-to-student ratio (CDC, 2016d). The NASN (2015) supports increasing the proportion of schools served by full-time school nurses and states that "every student needs direct access to a school nurse so that all students have the opportunity to be healthy, safe, and ready to learn" (para. 10). Only one-third of schools in the United States require a full-time nurse, and fewer than 80 percent of school districts employed any school nurses as of 2016, a decline of 14 percent since 2000 (CDC, 2016d). The proportion of schools meeting the *Healthy People 2020* recommendations of one full-time nurse for every 750 students has increased from 40.6 percent in 2006 to 51.1 percent in 2014, a hopeful sign that school administrators recognize the benefits of having a school nurse provide care to their students (USDHHS, 2018). NASN (2015) and the AAP (2016) assert that there is no standardized ratio that would fit every school in every district. They propose determining school nurse-to-student ratios using a multifaceted approach, including assessment of students' health needs, social determinants of health affecting each school community, and use of evidence-based research on safe staffing and workload assignment. This is the best way to ensure that students receive the care they need and that school health programs are coordinated and implemented by qualified professionals (AAP, 2016; NASN, 2015c).

School Nurse Roles

Direct Caregiver. The school nurse functioning in the role of direct caregiver is expected to give immediate nursing care to ill or injured children or school staff members. While many people envision the school nurse caregiver role as providing minor interventions such as bandages and ice packs, nothing could be further from the truth in the majority of U.S. schools (Anderson et al., 2017). Whenever a child comes into the clinic, the school nurse must first assess the seriousness of their complaint or symptoms and then determine possible causes. Some causes are obvious, such as an injury from a fall, and some less so, such as respiratory symptoms, which could be due to communicable disease, allergies, etc. The school nurse intervenes to alleviate symptoms, provide first aid in the event of an injury, stabilize the child in an emergency situation, provide ongoing care for chronic illnesses, such as diabetes or asthma, and prevent the spread of communicable diseases (AAP, 2016). As stated earlier, many children now attend school with even more complex medical needs, requiring procedures such as intermittent catheterization, tube feeding, tracheostomy suctioning and care, and ventilator management (Shannon & Minchella, 2016; Toothaker & Cook, 2018). Some children's care needs are so time-consuming, they require the assignment of a personal or private duty nurse during the school day. This nurse assumes care for that child alone, rather than the entire student body.

Although most school nurses are in public or private schools and give care only during school hours, the nurse in boarding schools, summer camps, and detention centers provides nursing care to children 24 hours a day and seven days a week. In these residential programs, children live on the premises and may only go home for vacations or not at all if they are incarcerated. In some settings, the nurse also lives at the school and may be on call at all times. School nurses in these residential settings can impact students' academic outcomes by partnering with administrators, teachers, and families to promote a healthy school environment, adequate rest, good nutrition, regular physical activity, and comprehensive, high-quality health care services (Wernette & Emory, 2017). The nurse makes many of the health care decisions for the child and has a referral system to contact parents or guardians and other health care providers, such as physicians and psychological counselors, if needed.

Health Educator. The school nurse in the health educator role may be asked to teach children both individually and in the classroom. School nurses may provide education about disease process and management to parents and children, especially if they don't understand instructions from the primary provider (Anderson et al., 2017). School nurses provide health education to groups of children about injury and communicable disease prevention, dental hygiene, puberty, substance abuse, and nutrition, among others (AAP, 2016; Rebmann, Weaver, et al., 2018). They may be required by state or local school board policies to teach specific subjects or develop health education based on the needs of the school and parent requests.

Case Manager. The school nurse is expected to function as a case manager, helping coordinate the health care for children with complex health problems (AAP, 2016). School nurses may collaborate with the family, teachers, and administrators to ensure that health care services promote the child's ability to learn and participate in the academic environment to the greatest extent possible. Care may be provided in the schools by physical therapists, occupational therapists, speech therapists, or other health care providers during the school day. The nurse may need to develop health care plans for children that clearly explain procedures and treatments needed for their conditions, as well as provide referrals and reports to other health care providers about children's response to treatments and interventions provided in the school (ANA & NASN, 2017).

Consultant. The school nurse is the person best able to provide health information to school administrators, teachers, and parent-teacher groups. As a consultant, the school nurse can provide professional information about proposed changes in the school environment and their impact on the health of the children. The nurse can also recommend changes in the school's policies or engage community organizations to help make the children's schools healthier places (Schaffer et al., 2016). This is a population-level role for the school nurse; the population consists of all children, families, staff, and the surrounding community.

Counselor. School nurses are reported to spend nearly one-third of their time assisting students with mental health needs (Government Accountability Office, as cited in Bohnenkamp et al., 2015). School nurses are familiar and trusted members of the school community. Children often see the nurse as a safe person in whom they may confide about problems such as bullying, physical abuse, substance abuse, grief, and suicidal thoughts. School nurses should always be alert to the potential for such problems when children come to their clinic, especially those who visit frequently with vague complaints or frequent requests to go home (Bohnenkamp et al., 2015). It is important for nurses to be honest with the child about the need to report dangerous situations to their parents, school officials, social services, and/or legal authorities. The nurse should emphasize that the child's confidentiality and privacy are central and reporting is only done as needed to protect them from harm.

Community Outreach. When participating in community outreach, nurses can be involved in community health fairs or festivals in the schools, using that opportunity to promote health through education, screenings, and immunization programs. They may be able to engage local providers, such as dentists and ophthalmologists, to provide free screenings at the school (Schaffer et al., 2015). School nurses should collaborate with area schools of nursing to provide clinical experiences for nursing students, as well as involve those future nurses in providing various health promotion and education events for the children. School nurses should attend meetings of parent-teacher associations, so they get to know the families of their students and offer education on health concerns these families raise. Attendance at school board meetings may also provide school nurses with opportunities to be seen as experts available to answer questions about school health needs, as well as concerned and engaged members of the school community.

Nurses can participate in coalitions focused on addressing a multitude of school and community health concerns from bullying and violence prevention to poverty and teenage pregnancy (Shaffer et al., 2016). They may be able to engage community faith-based and service organizations in providing food and other supplies for children living in poverty. Some school nurses coordinate weekend backpack food relief for children who only eat regularly on school days.

EVIDENCE-BASED PRACTICE

Because of the obesity epidemic in the United States, interventions to increase physical activity and reduce sedentary behaviors have become a priority for public health practitioners. This research study evaluated the feasibility and efficacy of a school nurse–delivered intervention aimed at improving diet and activity and reducing body mass index (BMI) among overweight and obese adolescents. This study used a pair-matched cluster-randomized controlled school-based trial. Six high schools were randomized into either the six-session counseling intervention or the control group. The intervention, "Lookin' Good Feelin' Good," consisted of six one-on-one school nurse–led counseling sessions conducted over 2 months during school hours. Those in the control group had six one-on-one visits with the school nurse over 2 months to be weighed and review informational pamphlets on weight management. Although there was no significant difference in BMI, activity, or caloric intake between the groups at 2 months, those in the intervention group ate breakfast on more days of the week and had a lower intake of sugar than the control group.

Nurse Use

This study indicates that a school nurse–delivered obesity intervention is feasible and may improve select behaviors that may result in obesity.

Pbert L, Druker S, Gapinski MA, et al.: A school nurse-delivered intervention for overweight and obese adolescents. *J Sch Health* 83(3):182-193, 2013.

Researcher. Research on school nursing practice and impact has grown steadily over the past couple of decades. Current, ongoing research can be found on school nursing practice, staffing and workloads, educational preparation and professional development of school nurses, and the use of evidence-based practice for a host of health conditions addressed by school nurses (Allen-Johnson, 2017; NASN, 2018b; Willgerodt et al., 2018). School nurses are responsible for providing nursing care that is based on solid, evidence-based practice. School nurses can, and should, be involved in research as participants by completing surveys and questionnaires from reputable researchers and professional organizations (Maughan et al., 2016; NASN, 2018b). School nurses may also function as researchers if they are properly educated to conduct ethical and scientifically founded research, provide human subject protections if applicable, and obtain institutional review board approval from their school system or an affiliated health care or educational institution.

SCHOOL HEALTH SERVICES

School health services vary in their scope throughout the United States. However, there are common parts to the programs.

CHECK YOUR PRACTICE

While working as a student in school health you have been asked to participate in the development of a school health program for your community that emphasizes the development of healthy schools. What would you do?

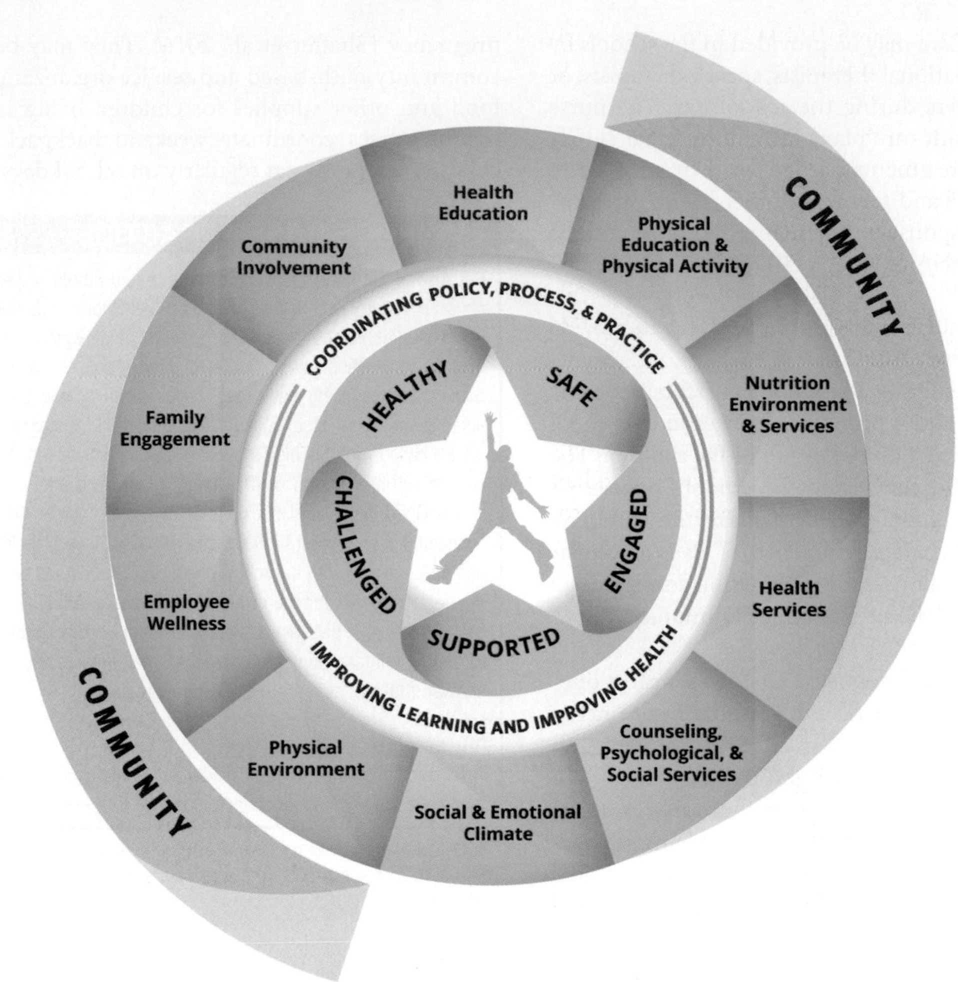

Fig. 42.1 WSCC model for school health practice. *WSCC,* Whole School, Whole Community, Whole Child. (Available at https://www.cdc.gov.)

Federal School Health Programs

The federal government, through the coordination of the CDC, with an emphasis on the health of the population of children and the school community, has developed the Healthy Schools initiative, which utilizes the Whole School, Whole Community, Whole Child (WSCC) model as a framework that school health programs are encouraged to follow (CDC, 2018a) (Fig. 42.1).

CDC Healthy Schools provides funding, training, and other resources that support schools in promoting health and adopting the components of the WSCC framework. CDC Healthy Schools provided more than $15 million to the nation's schools in 2016 with the goals of eliminating health disparities, providing evidence-based health education and services, and utilizing epidemiologic surveillance and research to prevent chronic disease and decrease the spread of communicable disease (CDC, 2016a). Between 2000 and 2014, CDC Healthy Schools funding, education, and technical support significantly improved the nutritional quality of school meals. Between 2013 and 2015, CDC Healthy Schools resources helped achieve significant increases in schools that avoid selling non-nutritious foods and beverages to students and provide physical education classes one or more days a week. Nearly 100 percent of schools track chronic health problems in their students due to the support provided by this federal program (CDC, 2016a).

School Health Policies and Practices Study 2016

Since 1994, the School Health Policies and Practices Study (SHPPS) has been conducted periodically (at least every 6 years) in all 50 states and the District of Columbia to evaluate the 10 components of the WSCC model. The study also measures progress in achieving *Healthy People 2020* goals and objectives in the area of health education, disease prevention, and health promotion (CDC, 2016d). The 2016 SHPPS assessment of achievement of *Healthy People 2020* objectives for school nurse-to-student ratios and school district requirements for nurse qualifications and licensure were discussed earlier in this chapter.

The 2016 study found that the number of school districts with arrangements for school-based or off-site health centers to provide health services such as primary care, dental services, or counseling/mental health services to students decreased significantly in recent years. This is concerning because school-based health centers (SBHCs) provide a variety of health services to children who may not have access to other community resources (Price, 2017). Having these services located at the school allows children to receive timely care and decreases time missed from class. Children whose health problems are not addressed may not be able to take full advantage of academic opportunities (Price, 2017). Having services on site may also help parents avoid missing work in order to take their children to an off-site provider. Some employers do not allow time off for such activities. School nurses can more easily assist families to get health care for their children when an SBHC is available.

According to the SHPPS (CDC, 2016d), most students in the United States were found not to be participating in the recommended 60 minutes a day of physical activity. Fewer than half of school districts had an indoor air quality management program, though more than 75 percent had policies requiring regular inspections of ventilation, heating and cooling systems, and other aspects of building integrity that could promote mold growth and other environmental contamination within school buildings. On the positive side, the SHPPS found that around 80 percent of districts prohibited all tobacco use, including vaping and e-cigarettes, by students, employees, or visitors during the school day or at school events (CDC, 2016d). Furthermore, a majority of school districts have enhanced security and safety measures in their schools, instituted disaster/crisis preparedness plans, and established programs to prevent bullying and address issues related to aggressive behaviors.

SCHOOL NURSES AND *HEALTHY PEOPLE 2020*

Many *Healthy People 2020* proposed objectives are directed toward the health of children. In addition, several point directly at the care that nurses give to children in the schools. The *Healthy People 2020* box lists the objectives that involve school-age children. These objectives are concerned with the children with disabilities in the schools, the number of children with major health problems, and the ratio of nurses to children in the schools. Nurses can accomplish the goals using the three levels of prevention, as discussed next.

THE LEVELS OF PREVENTION APPLIED IN SCHOOLS

The three levels of prevention—primary, secondary, and tertiary—have always been a part of health care in the schools (Wold & Selekman, 2013). **Primary prevention** provides health promotion and education to prevent health problems in children. **Secondary prevention** includes the screening of children for various illnesses, monitoring their growth and development, and caring for them when they are ill or injured. **Tertiary prevention** in the schools is the continued care of children who need long-term health care services, along with education within the community (Fig. 42.2).

HEALTHY PEOPLE 2020

Objectives Related to School Health and School Nursing

- **ECBP-2:** Increase the proportion of elementary, middle, and senior high schools that provide comprehensive school health education to prevent health problems in the following areas: unintentional injury; violence; suicide; tobacco use and addiction; alcohol or other drug use; unintended pregnancy, HIV/AIDS and STD infection; unhealthy dietary patterns; and inadequate physical activity.
- **ECBP-4:** Increase the proportion of elementary, middle, and senior high schools that provide school health education to promote personal health and wellness in the following areas: hand washing or hand hygiene; oral health; growth and development; sun safety and skin cancer prevention; benefits of rest and sleep; ways to prevent vision and hearing loss; and the importance of health screenings and checkups
- **ECBP-5:** Increase the proportion of elementary, middle, and senior high schools that have a full-time registered school nurse-to-student ratio of at least 1:750.
- **IID-10:** Maintain vaccination coverage levels for children in kindergarten.
- **IID-11:** Increase routine vaccination coverage levels for adolescents.
- **NW-2:** Increase the percentage of schools that offer nutritious foods and beverages outside of school meals.
- **TU-3:** Reduce the initiation of tobacco use among children, adolescents, and young adults.
- **TU-15:** Increase tobacco-free environments in schools, including all school facilities, property, vehicles, and school events.

AIDS, Acquired immunodeficiency syndrome; *HIV,* human immunodeficiency virus; *STD,* sexually transmitted disease.
From U.S. Department of Health and Human Services: *Healthy People 2020 topics and objectives*, 2018. Available at https://www.healthypeople.gov.

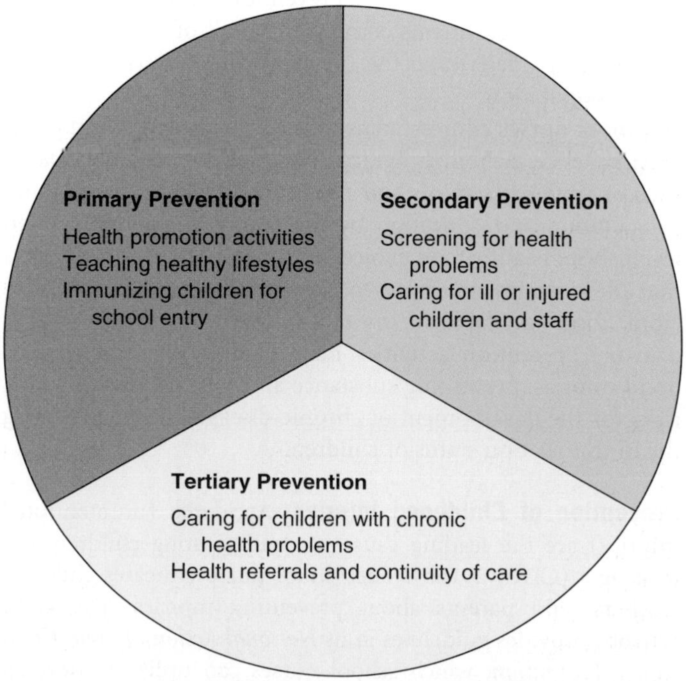

Fig. 42.2 Prevention levels in schools.

Primary Prevention in Schools

Primary prevention encompasses activities that are intended to prevent the development of illness, disease, and injury in those who are currently healthy (Wold & Selekman, 2013). The strategies for achieving primary prevention are health promotion and implementation of measures that protect people from agents that may cause disease or injury.

Health education is the most commonly used approach in health promotion. Historically, health teaching was considered "the fundamental basis of all school health work" (Struthers, as cited in Wold & Selekman, 2013). The school nurse may have the opportunity to go into the classroom to teach health promotion concepts, such as hand-washing or dental hygiene skills. This is population-level primary prevention.

School nurses also provide individual education to children who come to the school clinic for various health concerns or questions. Individual education about disease prevention may also be provided to school employees and parents (Wold & Selekman, 2013).

HOW TO Teach Young Children in School

When teaching children in preschools and elementary schools:

- Keep the lesson to no more than 10 minutes.
- Use a lot of examples, pictures, and stuffed animals in the talk.
- Always remember the developmental stage of the children when teaching them.

School nurses use the nursing process while they care for children in the schools. In their primary prevention efforts, they assess children and families to determine their level of knowledge about various health issues. Finding out whether children are at risk for preventable disease is also important. Decisions about where to focus primary prevention efforts are made by analyzing the assessments completed on all of the children in the school to determine the most pressing priorities for the school population.

School nurses address many areas of primary prevention in their practice. School programs designed to promote health, such as nutritious meals and physical education, may require consultation and education by the school nurse. Nurses can teach about healthy food choices and encourage school districts that allow vending machines to have nutritious foods instead of "junk food" available in the machines (CDC, 2016a). Other primary prevention activities may include preventing childhood injuries, preventing substance abuse behaviors, reducing risks for the development of chronic diseases, and monitoring the immunization status of children.

Prevention of Childhood Injuries. Accidents (unintentional injuries) are the leading cause of death among children and teenagers (CDC, 2016b). The school nurse educates children, teachers, and parents about preventing injuries. The CDC (2016b) provides guidelines in its *National Action Plan for Child Injury Prevention,* which school nurses can utilize to develop evidence-based educational programs to encourage children to use their seat belts or bicycle helmets to prevent injuries. Other classes can be on crossing the street, water safety, and fire safety. The school nurse, as a trusted health care provider at school, is able to quickly give information to help prevent injuries from occurring, since most injuries are preventable (Rebmann, Weaver, et al., 2018).

School nurses also provide health promotion to prevent playground injuries, which number over 200,000 injuries to children under age 14 per year (CDC, 2016c). School nurses can utilize guidelines published by the U.S. Consumer Product Safety Commission (2015) to assess their school playgrounds for equipment safety.

School sports also have the potential to cause injuries to children. The school nurse is often involved in deciding with parents and coaches on how to best prevent injuries when children are engaged in athletic activities (Rebmann, Weaver, et al., 2018). From 2015 to 2016, more than 150,000 children were seen in emergency departments from injuries sustained while riding scooters, hoverboards, or skateboards (Bandzar et al., 2018). Injuries included fractures and head injuries. School nurses can also promote the use of helmets and knee pads and work with communities to provide safe places, such as skateboard parks, for children to engage in these activities. Educating parents, children, and school personnel on safety measures to prevent any type of injury can decrease the incidence of these injuries, as well as decrease emergency department visits (Bandzar et al., 2018; Salam et al., 2016). This makes the entire community safer and decreases health care costs for all.

Substance Abuse Prevention Education. Research has found that the percentage of adolescents who report never having used substances such as alcohol, tobacco, and drugs increased between 1976 and 2014, as did the percentage of adolescents who report not having used substances in the preceding 30 days (Levy et al., 2018). However, early use of alcohol, tobacco, and drugs can lead to a plethora of health problems and carries a higher risk for addiction due to the development of the adolescent brain (National Institute on Drug Abuse, 2014). Primary prevention interventions by the school nurse include educating children and adolescents about the effects of tobacco, drugs, and alcohol on their bodies. School nurses should start early with education of children about the negative effects of street drugs (such as marijuana, cocaine, crack, and heroin), tobacco, and alcohol on their bodies and how to avoid them (NASN, 2015b).

Despite the overall decrease in use of substances, misuse of some illegal and legal drugs has remained steady or increased. Providers are seeing an increase in the use of "club drugs" such as lysergic acid (LSD), ketamine, gamma hydroxybutyrate (GHB), Rohypnol, and Ecstasy (MDMA). The school nurse can provide instruction about the serious side effects of Ecstasy, especially that it causes a very high body temperature that can lead to death. Marijuana and alcohol use have leveled off in recent years, rather than decreasing as with many other substances. Researchers postulate that this is related to easier accessibility of these substances to youth, especially with the legalization of marijuana in many states and marketing of these substances as safe and enjoyable by their powerful lobby groups (Levey et al., 2018). Students may find these substances in their homes being used by their parents. In the past decade, the abuse of opioids has reached epidemic proportions. The 2013

Partnership Attitude Tracking Study found that 23 percent of teenagers had taken prescription pain medication for nonmedical reasons at least once in their lifetimes and 16 percent had done so in the past year (Feliz, as cited in NASN, 2015b). Teaching children about the dangers of all drugs is an important responsibility of the school nurse. In addition, the school nurse can teach parents and other members of the community about the risks of substance use, ways to secure their own prescriptions and model safe use of legal substances, and how to recognize warning signs of substance abuse in their children so that early intervention can occur. Increasing everyone's awareness of these dangerous trends may lead to a decrease in abuse of those substances that is on the rise in the United States and subsequently improve the overall health of the population (NASN, 2015b).

Disease Prevention Education. The nurse has the opportunity to teach children healthy lifestyles to reduce their risk of disease later in life. For example, children can be taught ways to reduce their risk of becoming obese by teaching and reinforcing healthy nutrition and exercise (CDC, 2018d). Health education may also include ways to promote cardiovascular health, oral health, and prevent the spread of communicable diseases. The school nurse should collaborate with teachers to create evidence-based health education plans.

Dissemination of health promotion information to the parents of the children is often a challenge for the school nurse. There are many ways to increase accessibility of health information, such as providing a website or newsletter that parents can read outside of school hours without interfering with their work schedules. School nurses may consider presenting information during a parent-teacher association meeting. They could survey families for health issues they have questions or concerns about and arrange a guest speaker if the nurse is not well versed on the topic. Providing babysitters, food, and transportation to these meetings could remove barriers for families with low incomes and long workdays. By educating parents and children, the school nurse is able to promote the health of not only the schoolchildren but also the community.

Vaccinations for Schoolchildren. All states have laws that require that children receive immunizations, or vaccinations, against communicable diseases before they attend school (CDC, 2017c). School nurses must be up to date on the latest laws on immunizations for children in their own state and actively educate parents about the benefits of vaccinating their children. The CDC (2017c) provides recommendations for vaccinations, but it is up to each individual state to determine which immunizations are required for enrollment and attendance at a school or childcare facility. Vaccine requirements and exemptions laws vary from state to state (CDC, 2017c). Depending on the state's law, children may be prevented from enrolling in or attending school if they have not had the required immunizations or have not provided the required paperwork for exemptions (either for medical, religious, or philosophical/conscientious belief reasons) (CDC, 2017c). Some parents may request that their child be exempted from the required immunizations because of their belief that not all immunizations are good for their children, for medical reasons, or for religious or philosophical reasons (NASN, 2015a). The school nurse should be aware of the laws in the state regarding acceptable reasons for immunization exemption. At the same time, the nurse has the opportunity to teach parents and the rest of the community about the overall benefits to society and to their children from the use of immunizations (NASN, 2015a).

For children entering kindergarten, most state-required vaccinations include diphtheria, pertussis, and tetanus (the DTaP series); measles, mumps, and rubella (the MMR series); polio; and others. Chapters 14 and 15 have a more complete discussion of communicable diseases and immunizations in children.

The school nurse must keep a complete file of all of the children's vaccination records in order to meet the state's laws. These files will contain the student's name, date of birth, address and telephone number, parents'/guardians' names, and contact information. They will also include the student's primary health care provider's name, telephone number, and address. Most important, the information should include all the vaccinations with the dates the child received booster shots, as well as any immunizations the child may be exempted from based on medical or religious reasons (NASN, 2015a). This makes it easier for the school nurse to find out which children still need immunizations or boosters or, in the event of a vaccine preventable disease outbreak, to notify parents about the signs and symptoms of the disease, when to seek care, and the potential need to keep their children home from school until the outbreak is resolved.

The HIPAA of 1996 requires that all health information be private. This Act can present a challenge for the school nurse and personnel within the school and the school system. Teachers and school administrators as well as interprofessional health care partners may feel they have the right to know about health issues of their students. Thus they may challenge the school nurse if the nurse declines to share information to protect the child's privacy (Caldart-Olson & Thronson, 2013).

There is conflicting information on whether sharing of information about the immunization status of children between providers and school nurses is covered by HIPAA. However, the USDHHS published a statement in 2008 that protected health information may be shared between school nurses and primary providers when needed to make decisions about treatment of children in the schools (USDHHS, 2008).

The nurse will need to contact the parents to get the immunization history for the child. Written notes will need to be sent to each child's home at least one year before each new immunization is needed so that the parents have time to get the child to his or her health care provider for the shots. If the parents or guardians do not speak English, these notes will need to be translated into the family's language. If the parents have lost the information that gives the child's immunization history, they should be encouraged to contact their physician or nurse practitioner to get it.

Many problems with children not being immunized or having incomplete vaccination records may arise in families who have moved a great deal, such as those serving in the armed services or experiencing homelessness, or those who do not have a regular physician. The parents may have no idea whether the child has even received the recommended or required vaccines. Some parents are not aware that, since the implementation of the Affordable Care Act, insurance is required to pay for certain preventive care, including childhood immunizations (Hahn, 2016). Families may also believe that, if they do not have health insurance, they will have to pay for their children's immunizations out of pocket, which can be expensive. Certain low-income families without health care insurance may qualify for federal programs that provide free immunizations to children (CDC, 2017b). Most states have their own programs to fund childhood immunizations, many through state and local public health departments, so school nurses will want to become familiar with what their state provides.

School nurses can also play an important role in immunizing children against seasonal flu. The CDC (2018e) recommends that everyone six months of age and older receive an annual seasonal influenza vaccination, especially children younger than five years of age and all children with chronic medical conditions. Vaccination against influenza should begin as soon as that season's vaccine becomes available (CDC, 2018e). During the 2009 H1N1 influenza outbreak, school nurses were at the front line of the epidemic. In fact, it was a school nurse in Queens, New York, who first notified the CDC that the influenza epidemic had reached U.S. soil (Robert Wood Johnson Foundation, 2010). School nurses were challenged to reduce the spread of this epidemic among school-age children. School nurses may administer the influenza vaccine to children at the school or work with the local public health department to do so, with the parents' permission. This has the potential to promote health within the entire community, as well as decrease costs and missed work time for parents (Fiorivant & Ward, 2018).

Secondary Prevention in Schools

Because secondary prevention involves early intervention for children when they need health care, this is the largest responsibility for the school nurse (Wold & Selekman, 2013). This includes caring for ill or injured students and school employees. It also involves screening and assessing children and referral to appropriate health agencies or providers. The school nurse uses the nursing process during secondary prevention activities. When an ill or injured child comes to the school's health office, the nurse must immediately assess the child for the degree of illness or injury.

Children seek out the school nurse for a variety of different needs:

- Headaches
- Stomachaches
- Diarrhea
- Anxiety over being separated from the parents
- Cuts, bruises, or other injuries

In addition, children may seek reassurance from the school nurse or even appear to hide in the nurse's office. This may be a result of harassment or bullying from other children in the school (John & Chewey, 2013).

Once the assessment data are gathered, the nurse determines the course of action and follows it through the implementation and evaluation phases. This occurs for direct care as well as for screening children for other health problems. If assessment indicates the child has a health problem, the school nurse continues to follow the nursing process to intervene within his or her scope of practice or to refer the child to providers who can provide the most appropriate health care.

Nursing Care for Emergencies in the School. Events that occur in or near schools may cause a crisis for children, teachers, and staff. The school nurse must have an **emergency plan** in place so that a routine can be followed when emergencies occur. Disaster planning in the schools includes becoming prepared for natural disasters (such as fire or severe weather), man-made disasters (such as school shooting or structure collapse), as well as health condition emergencies (such as asthma attack or seizure) (Rebmann, Elliott, et al., 2016). The NASN recommends that school nurses provide leadership to schools in all phases of emergency preparedness and management (Tuck et al., 2014).

The following summarizes the NASN's recommendations of the role of the school nurse during each phase of disaster planning (Tuck et al., 2014):

- Prevention/Mitigation: perform an ongoing assessment to identify hazards
- Preparedness: serve on planning groups, establish emergency response plans, provide training to school personnel
- Response: perform triage, coordinate the first-aid response team, provide direct hands-on care to victims, act as a counselor to help everyone cope with the emotional aspects of this serious event (Box 42.1)
- Recovery: provide direct support, act as liaison between community resources and those in need; school may become an emergency shelter for community-at-large

The U.S. Department of Education et al. (2013) recommend that all schools have crisis plans in place to help the children, teachers, parents, and community cope with the sudden event. **Crisis teams** are prepared to help everyone respond quickly to the crisis, to ensure the safety of the school, and to follow up on the effects of the crisis on the members of the school (Tuck et al., 2014). The crisis plan includes an administrative policy made either for the entire school district or, if the schools are large, for each individual school. The plan includes the names of the persons on the crisis team: the superintendent of the school district, the school nurse, the guidance counselor, the school psychologist or social worker, teachers, police or school

BOX 42.1 Dealing With a Disaster: Responsibilities of the School Nurse

- Provide triage.
- Communicate with emergency medical personnel.
- Assess the school community for the presence of shock and stress.
- Recommend reduced television viewing of the disaster.
- Provide grief counseling.
- Communicate with the children, parents, and school personnel.
- Follow up with assessment of children for anxiety, depression, regression, and post-traumatic stress disorder.

Modified from Doyle J.: Emergency management, crisis response, and the school nurse's role. In Selekman J, editor: *School nursing: a comprehensive text,* ed. 2, Philadelphia, 2013, F.A. Davis Company, pp. 1216-1244.

security, clergy from the community, and parents. Plans to obtain and share information can be made quickly (U.S. Department of Education et al., 2013).

The nurse can help the crisis team make a checklist for everyone to follow that explains what to do in every possible crisis situation. Then, at the end of the crisis, the crisis team will want to take time to counsel all of the people who helped in the crisis, including the teachers, emergency personnel, and parents, as well as the children. That way everyone can talk about the crisis. The crisis plan should be reviewed every year to see what parts of the plan need updating. Drills take place to act out the plan to see how it works and how it can be revised to make it more workable (Tuck et al., 2014; U.S. Department of Education et al., 2013).

Individualized emergency plans are made for all students who may have a health problem that could result in an emergency situation in the school (Tuck et al., 2014). This plan could be for the child with food allergies (e.g., to peanuts), one who has sensitivity to insect bites that could result in anaphylactic shock, or those with chronic illnesses such as asthma, diabetes, or hemophilia. The individualized emergency plan should include the student's medical history, list of medications, location of emergency medication, and list of personnel trained to administer emergency medication. It is important that the school nurse communicate with school personnel about students requiring emergency medication to ensure quick access to emergency medications at all times.

The nurse may not always be at the school and the emergency may have to be handled by a teacher, administrator, secretary, custodian, or coach (U.S. Department of Education et al., 2013). This issue is especially applicable to school nurses in rural settings, who may have several schools for which they are responsible when such schools may be far apart (Rebmann, Elliott, et al., 2016). Therefore all emergency procedures must be clearly spelled out and easily accessible to anyone in the school. Along with the procedures and an emergency manual written or obtained by the school nurse, an injury or illness log should be available for personnel to fill out so that there is an accurate record of what happened. Along with this form, procedures for notifying the parents or legal guardians about the emergency are explained. Information must be provided to parents about any actions taken for the child and where the child was sent if transfer to a hospital or other medical agency was required (Tuck et al., 2014). Good communication with parents is important to decrease their anxiety and assist them in reuniting with their children. School nurses are uniquely qualified to provide this information because they may have ongoing relationships with parents due to providing day-to-day care for their children.

Because the school nurse may have to give nursing care to a child or adult in respiratory or cardiac arrest, the nurse must have current certification in cardiopulmonary resuscitation (CPR) and the use of the automated external defibrillator (AED), which should be available to all school nurses. All 50 states have passed laws requiring that public gathering places have AEDs available, some requiring them in the schools (AED Brands, 2015). Other education in the area of emergency response would also be helpful to the school nurse, including pediatric advanced life support (PALS) or emergency nursing for pediatrics (ENPC) certification (Doyle, 2013).

Emergency Equipment in the School Nurse's Office. The school nurse needs a great deal of equipment to deal with emergencies in the school. These needs are based on the guidelines of the NASN (Doyle, 2013). The school office will need to have basic emergency items on hand (Box 42.2). Additional equipment may be obtained if a nurse is present in the school every day (see Box 42.2). Various sizes of these items are needed since children may be of different ages in the school. Another recommended item for the nurse's office includes an epinephrine auto injector kit (EpiPen auto injector) in case a child goes into anaphylactic shock after exposure to an allergen (Wahl et al., 2015). This should be locked in a medication cabinet

BOX 42.2 Emergency Items for Schools With and Without a School Nurse Present

Supplies for Schools WITHOUT a School Nurse Present

- Accessible keys to locked supplies
- Accessible list of phone resources
- Automated external defibrillator (AED) if school meets the AHA guidelines
- AED supplies stored with AED (razor, alcohol pads, dry towel, scissors, electrode pads)
- Biohazard waste bags
- Blunt scissors
- Clock with a second hand
- CPR trained staff on-site when students are on the premises
- Disposable blankets
- Emergency cards on all staff
- Emergency cards on all students
- Established relationship with local EMS personnel
- Eye protection (full peripheral glasses or goggles, face shield)
- Ice (not cold packs)
- Individual care plans/emergency plans for students with specialized needs
- First aid tapes
- Nonlatex gloves
- One-way resuscitation mask
- Cell phone or other two-way communication device
- Posters with CPR/abdominal or chest thrusts instructions
- Refrigerator or cooler
- Resealable plastic bags
- School-wide emergency operations/response plan
- Sharps container
- Soap and source of water/hand sanitizer for hand and wound cleansing
- Source of oral glucose (i.e., frosting gel, glucose tablets, juice box)
- Splints
- Staff names who have received basic first aid training
- Variety of bandages and dressings
- Water source/normal saline for wound/eye irrigation

Additional Supplies for Schools with a School Nurse Present

- C-spine immobilizers of different sizes
- Glucose monitoring device[a]

Continued

BOX 42.2 Emergency Items for Schools With and Without a School Nurse Present—cont'd

- Medications[b]
- Albuterol
- Epinephrine (auto injector preferred)
- Oxygen
- Nebulizer
- Penlight
- Self-inflating resuscitation device in two sizes (500 ml and 1 liter) with appropriate sized masks to meet needs of population being served
- Stethoscope
- Sphygmomanometer and cuffs in pediatric, adult regular, and adult large sizes
- Suction equipment (minimal source, does not have to be electric, i.e. bulb suction or v-vac type device)

AHA, American Heart Association; *CPR,* cardiopulmonary resuscitation; *EMS,* emergency medical services.
[a]Committee acknowledges challenges with maintenance and expense of test strips. Monitoring of machine must also be in compliance with CLIA (Clinical Laboratory Improvement Amendments).
[b]All medications including oxygen should be in accordance with state laws, pharmacy, and nurse practice acts.
From Tuck CM, Haynie K, Davis C: *Emergency preparedness and response in the school setting—the role of the school nurse (NASN Position Statement),* 2014. Available at https://www.nasn.org.

because of the needle in the kit. The school nurse will need to teach other school personnel how to use the EpiPen auto injector in an emergency (Wahl et al., 2015).

Gloves to meet standard precautions guidelines and a telephone available for calling emergency personnel and parents are essential. Next to the telephone, paper and pen should be available so that instructions from the emergency personnel can be written down (Doyle, 2013). The AED should be located in a central location in the school for easy access in an emergency. It should not be locked in the nurse's office but available for school staff to obtain in case the nurse is off site that day.

Giving Medication in School. The school nurse, as part of secondary prevention, may be responsible for giving medications to children during the school day (Hinkson, et al., 2017). These may include prescribed medications, over-the-counter medications that parents have asked the school's nurse to give (such as cold remedies), or vitamins (CDC, 2018b). The two most commonly administered medications in schools are those for attention-deficit/hyperactivity disorder (ADHD) and asthma (Maughan, McCarthy, et al., 2017). In all instances, the nurse should collaborate with school district administration to develop a series of medication administration policies and guidelines that allow children to receive care they need to perform well in school while following the laws and nurse practice act of the state. As part of the assessment of the health history and needs of children enrolled in the school, the school nurse should inquire of parents whether the child is taking any medications (Hinkson et al., 2017). A current, signed parental consent form, with primary care provider's approval and directions, must be provided before administering medication to any student (Hinkson et al., 2017). HIPAA requires that all of this information be kept confidential, but the consent form should include permission for the school nurse to discuss the medication and treatment plan with the prescribing provider to ensure the safety of the child (Caldart-Olson & Thronson, 2013). Nurses may also need to request permission to discuss the medication with the child's teachers so they are aware of potential side effects or adverse reactions and can alert the nurse immediately if there are any problems.

The prescribed drug must have the original prescription label on it and be in the original container to decrease the risk of errors and securely stored (Maughan, McCarthy, et al., 2017). Over-the-counter medications should also be stored securely in their original and labelled containers. Having a current drug reference in the nurse's office is important so that it can be consulted for information about any medication, or if the medication appears different, it can be matched to photographs in this reference. Nurses are expected by state law to know the mechanism of action, side effects, and implications prior to administering any medication. The child's pharmacist may also need to be contacted if there is any question about the medication appearance, dosage, or potential adverse reactions.

Delegation. Some states allow school nurses to delegate medication administration to unlicensed assistive personnel (UAP) or to a licensed practical nurse (Hinkson et al., 2017). There are several benefits and challenges associated with delegation in the school setting. On the positive side, delegation allows services to be provided in the absence of a school nurse, which is especially helpful if a nurse is covering multiple schools (Cagginello et al., 2014). Also, delegation allows children with more complex medical needs to attend school more safely, as UAPs can be trained to provide one-on-one care for some procedures. The challenge with delegation is ensuring the UAPs receive adequate training and regular supervision and monitoring of the UAP (Cagginello et al., 2014). Delegation can be done safely in the school environment provided the nurse has clear policies and procedures to follow, understands the "Five Rights of Delegation," understands the scope of practice and procedures allowed to be delegated under the state's nurse practice act, and has a trusting relationship with the UAP and school administrators (Cagginello et al., 2014).

Assessing and Screening Children at School. Children should receive screening for vision, hearing, height and weight, oral health, tuberculosis (TB), and scoliosis in the schools (Wold & Selekman, 2013). For each of these areas, the school nurse must keep a confidential record of all of the screening results for the children in the school according to HIPAA requirements. In addition, each state has different laws regarding screenings requirements, and the nurse will need to be aware of these laws.

Screening for TB in schoolchildren is required in several states prior to school entry (Wold & Selekman, 2013). It may be difficult to administer screening at school because the nurse cannot read the Mantoux test, or the TST test, until three days after

QSEN FOCUS ON QUALITY AND SAFETY EDUCATION FOR NURSES

Targeted Competency: Safety

Safety minimizes risk of harm to patients and providers through both system effectiveness and individual performance.

Important aspects of safety include:

- **Knowledge:** Describe factors that create a culture of safety (such as open communication strategies and organizational error reporting systems).
- **Skills:** Communicate observations or concerns related to hazards and errors to patients, families, and the health care team.
- **Attitudes:** Value own role in preventing errors.

Safety Question

Imagine you are working as a nurse in an elementary school. Due to budget cuts, you are only at the school two days a week. Juan, a student in the third grade, is newly diagnosed with asthma and will have an inhaler at school for emergencies. Your state allows nurses to delegate the administration of inhaler medications to unlicensed personnel. You decide to delegate the administration of Juan's emergency inhaler to his classroom teacher, Mr. Smith. What steps would you take to ensure you safely delegated this medication?

Answer

First, you would need to establish open communication between Mr. Smith and yourself. After providing the initial medication training, you should maintain open communication by checking in with Mr. Smith on a regular basis to assess his knowledge and comfort level in administering Juan's inhaler. Second, in the event that Mr. Smith gives Juan a dose from the inhaler, have a system in place to document when and why the medication was given. Emphasize the importance of such documentation to avoid medication errors/overdose and to track Juan's health condition and response to treatment. Periodically review the records to ensure that everything was documented correctly and that the medication was given for appropriate reasons. Last, in the event of a medication error, report to the proper authorities, evaluate the circumstances that led to the error, and determine what can be done differently to prevent future errors. In some circumstances, delegation may need to be withdrawn if it is determined that Mr. Smith is not capable of properly and safely administering Juan's medication.

it is administered. Often nurses are part time and may not be at the school on the day the child's test needs to be read. In some states, school nurses are required to participate in a training program to read the tests. It may be more efficient to have children screened for TB at their pediatrician's office or the local health department or prior to admission to the school (Bobo et al., 2013). If the school nurse is trained to read the test, he or she sends the results to the health clinic for follow-up. If the site is positive, it is possible the child has been exposed to TB and needs further health screening, including a chest x-ray, and treatment. A determination will need to be made about whether the child has active TB and could have spread it to other children or staff at school. In that case, the health department must be notified so that screening and prophylactic medications can be administered to all exposed individuals (Bobo et al., 2013).

The school nurse can also screen children and adolescents for hypertension, or high blood pressure. Children who develop high blood pressure are more likely to have this condition in adulthood (Cassidy-Bushrow et al., 2015). Identifying and treating hypertension early can prevent many serious, long-term health conditions. One study of more than 300 adolescents found that 14.2 percent had elevated blood pressures (Cassidy-Bushrow et al., 2015). These findings indicate the importance of the school nurse in providing effective prevention strategies related to screening, follow-up, and treatment.

Physical examinations prior to participation in a school sport are required by all 50 states (Johnson et al., 2018). While students may also obtain these physicals from their primary provider, an urgent care clinic, or a community health center, some children may not have access to a regular physician or other primary health care provider because they are uninsured or the agency is not open during hours that parents are off from work. School nurses can assist by arranging for sports physicals at school, conducting part of the screenings within their scope of practice and monitoring or assisting with the portions of these examinations being done by the school's physician or nurse practitioner. The school nurse's presence during these screenings can facilitate health education, case finding, and referrals to community resources or specialists for health problems (Johnson et al., 2018). The AAP (2016) recommends that children have regular health and developmental screenings in the school setting. The school nurse can collaborate with other school professionals to provide or facilitate such screenings as obtaining information on children's language skills, motor abilities, social skills, and behavioral health. As the children grow up, their level of physical growth can be noted as well as their sexual maturation. Dental screenings in school can also be beneficial to children to determine whether they have good oral health (Griffin et al., 2016). School nurses may arrange for dentists to provide group oral health screenings in the schools. In some states, school nurses may be able to conduct these screenings and refer children to a dentist for follow-up of suspected problems with oral health.

Screening Children for Pediculosis (Lice). School nurses are frequently called upon to screen children in their schools for pediculosis or lice infestation. Many myths abound related to risks of transmission of head lice, leading to unnecessary panic and exclusion of children from school, despite the fact that pediculosis is frequently misdiagnosed even by experienced nurses and primary care providers (Pontius, 2014). Lice do not spread disease, even though they may cause irritating symptoms, such as itching, sleep disturbance (due to itching), and sores from scratching (Smith et al., 2016). Children determined to have lice or lice eggs in their hair miss an average of four days per school year in schools with "no-nit" (no lice eggs) policies. Besides the loss to children of academic opportunity, such absenteeism costs schools hundreds of millions of dollars in annual funding and parents thousands of dollars in lost wages and treatment expenses per occurrence (Pontius, 2014).

Prevalence of lice is impossible to establish, as it is not a reportable disease and is so frequently misdiagnosed (Pontius, 2014). NASN, AAP, the Harvard School of Public Health, and the CDC recommend against no-nit policies because it is impossible for nits to be transmitted from one person to another. Nits firmly adhere to the hair shaft when they are laid by the louse, making them unlikely to come off without significant effort to remove them. Lice require human hosts to live, so if they fall off and are not deposited on a person's head within 24 hours, they will die. Nits require the warmth of the human body to hatch. The idea that lice are a sign of poverty and poor hygiene is also a myth. Lice are found in all socioeconomic groups and are just as likely to be seen in clean hair as unwashed.

Due to the inaccuracy of results, the lack of impact on the incidence of head lice in a school, and the significant loss of educational time, the NASN, AAP, and CDC recommend against routine screening for head lice or after a case has been identified (Pontius, 2014). There is significant risk of violation of privacy rights when conducting a classroom screening. The stigma and shame associated with even false identification of head lice and subsequent exclusion from school can be emotionally and socially devastating for students and caregivers (Smith et al., 2016). Frequent or incorrect use of pediculosis treatments, especially in misdiagnosed children, can have side effects from localized irritation of the scalp, eyes, and skin to allergic reactions and neurological repercussions in susceptible persons. School nurses have a responsibility to educate parents, teachers, and school administrators about the lack of effectiveness of mass school screenings for lice and to encourage and practice evidence-based approaches to prevent or treat any cases that are found.

In the case of a suspected case of lice, the school nurse should privately screen the child and be absolutely sure that he or she is seeing live lice before recommending treatment (Pontius, 2014). When lice are seen, they have likely been on the hair for as long as a month, so to insist on immediate exclusion from the classroom will not effectively prevent transmission. School nurses should teach children, parents, and teachers how to properly prevent lice and treat cases of infestation. The nurse can do this by teaching children not to share combs and hats, and teaching parents to follow package directions exactly when treating their child with pediculocidal medications (Pontius, 2014). Parents should also remove as many nits as possible from the head with a fine-toothed comb and repeat this every few days to continue removal of any remaining nits and live lice that hatch out. Family members and other close contacts should be screened, but treatment should only be provided in the case of a definitive finding of live lice. It may be advisable to wash any bed linens and clothing worn in the past day, but spraying the house with insecticides and whole house cleaning are not currently recommended. If live lice are seen a week or more after treatment with an over-the counter product, a repeat treatment may be advisable. If live lice are still found after the second treatment, children should be referred to a primary care provider for possible prescription treatments (Pontius, 2014).

Identification of Child Abuse or Neglect. Child abuse and neglect are a serious public health concern in this country. In 2014, more than six million children were reported to authorities as suspected victims of maltreatment, with nearly half a million of these turning out to be substantiated cases and nearly 1500 children killed as a result of their abuse (Jordan, et al., 2017). Victims of child abuse have a higher risk for health issues in adulthood, such as obesity, hypertension, and mental health problems.

Child abuse and neglect often go unrecognized and are seriously underreported. Research has shown that failure to report is often due to a lack of confidence about suspicions of abuse, lack of knowledge about the effects of child maltreatment, fear of repercussions for the child, family, or reporter, and reluctance to engage with law enforcement or social services (Jordan et al., 2017). School nurses are mandated by state laws to report suspected cases of child abuse or neglect, so they may need education and training to properly recognize signs of child maltreatment and report them to the proper authorities in a timely manner. Laws for reporting differ from state to state, as do school system policies on assessment of children for injuries. School nurses must be familiar with the particular requirements for reporting in their state and school district.

When the nurse identifies a child who may be abused, or receives information from a teacher or other staff member that leads to the belief that a child has been abused, the nurse must contact the appropriate legal authorities as well as the school's principal. The nurse should be careful about asking the child too many questions or suggesting possible answers for the signs, symptoms, and complaints the child is having. A confidential file with objective assessment information should be made about the incident in case the nurse is called to testify. The nurse should contact government authorities directly and in a timely manner, usually the state or county child protection department, who will look into the suspected case (Jordan et al., 2017). In all cases, the child must be protected from harm, and those who have no right to know that child abuse or neglect is suspected should not be given any information.

Communicating With Health Care Providers. The school nurse often makes an assessment of a child that requires referral to the child's family physician or other health care provider. The findings from these assessments must be communicated accurately to the child's parent and the provider (Caldart-Olson & Thronson, 2013). The nurse must be able to disseminate the information quickly and accurately to the child's parents. Again, HIPAA privacy rules must be followed.

HOW TO Develop Good Relationships With Families

School nurses need to have good relationships with families. The school nurse can make this possible by doing the following:

- Being visible at school events.
- Sending home invitations for parents and guardians to call the nurse at any time.
- Inviting parents to visit the school health office.
- Calling parents or guardians to ask about ill children.
- Offering to help families cope with children who have long-term illnesses.
- Acting as a referral source for families with health care needs.
- Including parents and members of the community in health education activities.

One way to do this is to write a detailed report about the findings. This information can be given to the child to take home to the parents, but there may also be issues related to parental literacy (Pontius, 2013). If the concern is not an emergency, the best way to communicate with parents may be to speak to them directly by phone or meet with them if they come to pick up their child at the end of the day. If the nurse expresses concern for the child's well-being, most parents will appreciate this personal interaction (Cornell & Selekman, 2013). Explain to the parents why the child needs to see the physician or nurse practitioner and that the child will be bringing the information home that day so they can ask the child for it at the end of the day. Verbal explanations will help in the case of low health literacy, as well as give the parent the opportunity to ask questions. The nurse may also pick up on the need for assistance during the conversation and can refer the family to community resources if they do not have a primary care provider.

Efforts to Prevent Suicide and Other Mental Health Problems. Among teenagers, more than 17 percent have considered suicide and more than 8 percent have actually attempted to take their own lives (Substance Abuse and Mental Health Services Administration [SAMHSA], 2017). Suicide is caused by complex interactions of multiple factors, such as social and environmental problems, gender identity confusion, academic problems, mental illness, bullying, and exposure to violence (Nolta, 2014). Protective factors for suicide prevention include strong family relationships, supportive religious connections, and interest in hobbies and other activities.

Suicide prevention must be addressed by school nurses. Government and professional organizations provide recommendations for reducing the incidence of suicide in teenagers. A suicide prevention program developed in one school district (see later discussion) contains ideas for the school nurse to use. Nurses can lead educational programs within the schools to emphasize coping strategies and stress management techniques for children and adolescents who have problems, and to teach about the risk factors. The school nurse can teach faculty members to look for warning signs that a student may be considering suicide. These signs include children talking about wanting to die, feelings of isolation and hopelessness, feeling anxious or depressed, giving away possessions and saying good-bye to loved ones, and demonstrating mood swings and extreme anger (National Institute of Mental Health [NIMH], 2017). The school nurse can also help organize and train peer counselors to help teenagers cope with school stresses.

Students who are expressing feelings associated with suicide risk or threaten suicide at school must be taken seriously. They should be asked directly if they are contemplating suicide, referred to mental health services within the school, encouraged to talk about their feelings, denied access to any methods of self-harm, and monitored for increasing symptoms and other risk factors (NIMH, 2017). Many states require that schools notify parents if children express intent to harm themselves. Students threatening to commit suicide should be immediately removed from any situation that is contributing to their despair. While the parents are being called, the nurse and available mental health professionals in the school should monitor and assess the student for having already made their attempt using medications or other method and if so, call for immediate emergency first responders.

In the unfortunate instance that a student commits suicide, the school nurse is called upon to help the school population, both students and teachers, cope with the death. Grief counseling should be set up and coordinated by the school nurse, usually in collaboration with guidance counselors and school administrators. In addition, further assessments can be made regarding the suicide potential among the deceased teenager's friends, since suicide clusters have been noted.

Other mental health problems may affect students. Adolescents may have early signs of mental or emotional problems such as behavioral problems in class or severe class or test anxiety. Families may be in crisis, which can translate into problems for their children. Sometimes, children with mental health issues come to the school nurse with somatic complaints and nothing can be found on assessment (Bohnenkamp et al., 2015). The nurse should be alert to the possibility that the child is experiencing emotional problems, hunger, or family problems in such cases and investigate further to find the source of the complaints.

Children who are homeless have special problems. Because these children do not have a stable address, they may have moved frequently from school to school. School nurses may need to provide assistance for obtaining medical records, make sure children are eating at school in case they are not getting meals away from school, and make referrals to community resources for financial and other assistance. Children whose parents are addicted to drugs or alcohol can also benefit from support from the school nurse, such as referrals to mental health counselors. The lack of a stable environment may increase chances that children will develop a mental or emotional problem (Bohnenkamp et al., 2015). The school nurse should be an advocate for these children and their families.

Violence at School. Results of the 2015 National Youth Risk Behavior Survey demonstrated that 6 percent of students were threatened with a weapon at school, 6 percent stayed home from school due to fears of violence, and 23 percent were in a physical fight at school (Flynn et al., 2018, p. 263). Hundreds of students reported carrying a weapon onto school grounds, and nearly two-thirds of schools reported the occurrence of at least one violent crime during the previous school year. In the past several years, there has been an increase in school shootings by students or other attackers against other students and teachers.

Bullying is at the center of attention among child and adolescent advocates. In 2015, about 20 percent of U.S. high school students experienced bullying while on school property and 16 percent were bullied online ("cyberbullying") (Wheeler et al., 2018). Bullying is defined as repetitious, unwanted, aggressive behavior intended to cause harm to another. Students with disabilities, academic problems, and speech impairments, as well as those who are lesbian, gay, bisexual, transgender, or questioning (LGBTQ) are most frequently targeted. Physical injury, social and emotional distress, suicide attempts, and even death can result from bullying. Affected students may come to the school nurse complaining of psychosomatic illnesses, such as headaches and stomachaches, due to bullying (Wheeler et al., 2018). The school nurse needs to be knowledgeable about bullying, take students' concerns seriously, and work to protect them from aggression. School nurses should provide leadership to implement bullying prevention strategies in their schools and communities, such as increased supervision and anti-bullying policies. In an effort to reduce the prevalence of bullying, 49 states now have anti-bullying laws (USDHHS, 2017).

The school nurse's primary goal is to prevent violence from occurring and prioritize the safety of everyone on the school's campus (Flynn et al., 2018). Interventions that the nurse can implement to prevent violence include:

- Facilitate student connectedness to the school community.
- Engage parents in school activities that promote connections with their children, and foster communication, problem solving, limit setting, and monitoring of children.
- Support activities and strategies to help establish a climate that promotes and practices respect for others and for the property of others.
- Support policies of zero tolerance for weapons on school property, including school buses.
- Advocate for adult monitoring in the hallways between classes and at the beginning and end of the school day, and the assignment of staff to monitor the playground, cafeteria, and school entrances before and after school.
- Serve as positive role models, developing mentoring programs for at-risk youth and families.
- Educate students and their parents about gun safety (Flynn et al., 2018; Wheeler et al., 2018).

If violence occurs, the school nurse should do the following:

- Coordinate emergency response until rescue teams arrive;
- Provide nursing care for injured students;
- Apply crisis intervention strategies that help de-escalate a crisis situation and help resolve the conflict;
- Identify and refer those students who require more in-depth counseling services; and
- Participate in crisis intervention teams (Doyle, 2013).

By helping identify the student who might be considering school violence or by teaching students and teachers about these warning signs in students, the school nurse may be able to help prevent violent actions through education and follow-up of children who need help. The U.S. federal government has many agencies and resources that can help school nurses develop programs in their schools (U.S. Department of Education et al., 2013).

Tertiary Prevention in Schools

Using the nursing process, the school nurse gives nursing care related to tertiary prevention when working with children who have long-term or chronic illnesses or special needs. The goal of tertiary prevention is to assist children to return to their highest level of function possible after injury or illness, as well as to prevent complications (Wold & Selekman, 2013). As prevalence of chronic conditions such as asthma and diabetes increases among children, today's school nurse faces a school population that is more medically diverse than ever seen in the past (Shannon & Minchella, 2016; Toothaker & Cook, 2018; Wolfe, 2013). The school nurse should be part of the team that develops an individual education plan (IEP for students with long-term health needs that may affect their learning abilities and needs (Box 42.3).

BOX 42.3 States That Require School Nurses to Participate in Individualized Education Plans for Students

• Alabama	• Maryland	• Rhode Island
• Arizona	• Massachusetts	• South Carolina
• Colorado	• Minnesota	• Tennessee
• Delaware	• Mississippi	• Texas
• District of Columbia	• Nevada	• Utah
• Hawaii	• New Jersey	• Vermont
• Illinois	• New Mexico	• Virginia
• Indiana	• New York	• Washington
• Iowa	• North Carolina	• West Virginia
• Louisiana	• Oklahoma	• Wisconsin

Compiled from Centers for Disease Control and Prevention: *State level school health policies and practices: a state-by-state summary from the School Health Policies and Programs Study 2006,* Atlanta, 2006, CDC, USDHHS.

As discussed earlier, school nurses must have information about children's medications that need to be administered during school hours. They also need to know if children need any type of procedure, such as tracheostomy suctioning or intermittent catheterization, or therapy during the school day, such as physical or occupational therapy (Shannon & Minchella, 2016; Toothaker & Cook, 2018). If the child has a hearing or vision problem, the nurse may need to ask the teacher to seat the child in the best place in the classroom so the child can see or hear better. If a child is in a wheelchair or uses crutches, federal regulations may require that the school building itself accommodates the child's ability to get around the school and use the restrooms. It is the responsibility of the nurse to tell the school's administrators about any needs such as these.

Children With Allergies. Food and insect allergies that result in anaphylaxis are being diagnosed more frequently (Pistiner & Mattey, 2017). Anaphylaxis is a severe allergic reaction that occurs quickly and can be life-threatening. In 2017, 10,704 high school students reported having to avoid foods due to the risk of allergy (CDC, 2017a). Milk, eggs, fish, shellfish, wheat, soy, peanuts, and tree nuts account for 90 percent of serious allergic reactions in the United States (CDC, 2018d). Insect allergies may be to stinging insects, such as bees and wasps; household pests, such as cockroaches and dust mites; or biting insects, such as bedbugs and some flies (Asthma and Allergy Foundation of America, 2015).

The school nurse must take a leadership role in coordinating care for these students. The AAP has developed an allergy and anaphylaxis care plan that provides guidance for planning for and responding to allergic reactions in the school (Pistiner & Mattey, 2017). The CDC (2018c) and NASN (2014) provide toolkits, checklists, and guidelines that school nurses can utilize in planning for care of children with allergies. The school nurse must develop a plan for preventing exposure to a known allergen and responding to an allergy emergency, collaborating with the student, the student's parents, and school personnel to determine the best plan of action (Pistiner & Mattey, 2017). Some students may have to eat at a separate table in the cafeteria that is designated allergen-free. Food and snacks in these children's classrooms may have to be restricted to items without the allergenic substance. This can result in communication challenges from parents whose children do not have allergies. The school nurse may need to help these parents understand the risks and rationale for these restrictions (Asthma and Allergy Foundation of America, 2015). Most states have laws that allow students to carry emergency medication and, if developmentally appropriate, self-administer as needed (Pistiner & Mattey, 2017). School nurses should assess children's understanding of criteria for self-administering emergency medications, ability to correctly self-administer, safe handling of needles, and when to seek help. Some states allow trained unlicensed assistive personnel to administer the emergency medication if the student is unable to do so and a nurse is not available. The school nurse must provide annual training to school personnel who are involved with the student or possibly responding to an emergency reaction (Pistiner & Mattey, 2017).

Children With Asthma. Asthma is the leading cause of children being absent from school because of a chronic illness (Cicutto et al., 2017). Children may be hospitalized with an asthma attack or they may have just returned home from the hospital. Time missed from class, either for treatment or because of absenteeism, can interfere with a child's educational progress. Asthma can also be caused by allergic triggers that affect children in the school. Possible culprits are chalk dust from the blackboards, molds or mildew in the school, or dander from pets that live in some classrooms (CDC, 2018c).

There may also be concerns about the quality of the air in the school building because many doors are shut. Indoor air pollution within schools can occur as a result of materials used in art class, woodworking, or cooking, perfumes and other scented body products, air fresheners, exhaust fumes from buses and delivery vehicles that idle near open doors or ventilation systems, outdated ventilation systems and those lacking proper maintenance, radon, mold, and secondhand smoke (U.S. Environmental Protection Agency [EPA], n.d.). The school nurse should keep track of the indoor air quality (IAQ) of the school and student complaints potentially related to IAQ so that school administrators have data about what can affect the children. Surveillance of the numbers of asthma and allergy exacerbations will help the school nurse recognize potential problems. Fig. 42.3 contains the questions developed by the EPA that the school nurse should answer regarding the air quality of the school.

The nurse uses tertiary prevention when helping children who have asthma. This includes administering, or helping them use, their inhalers or other asthma rescue medications (Cicutto et al., 2017). It also includes instructing administrators, teachers, children, and parents about asthma and ways to reduce allergens in the classroom (Asthma and Allergy Foundation of America, 2015). The nurse should determine the types of cleaning solutions used in schools. Many school systems are going with non-toxic cleaners, but many still use chemicals, such as bleach-based solutions, that can be dangerous to children if not properly stored and used (EPA, n.d.). School nurses should advocate for a transition to safer cleaning solutions and assess safe storage as part of regular school IAQ inspections (CDC, 2018e).

Children With Diabetes Mellitus. Diabetes is one of the most prevalent chronic diseases in children and adolescents, its long-term impact and the cost of treatment make it vitally important to be addressed by school nurses (Miller et al., 2016). About 132,000 people below the age of 18 years were diagnosed with diabetes as of 2015 (National Center for Chronic Disease Prevention and Health Promotion, 2017). While most of these children have type 1 diabetes, in the last couple of decades, type 2 diabetes (formerly known as adult-onset diabetes) has been reported among U.S. children and adolescents with increasing frequency (Miller et al., 2016). Case management and coordination of care are critical roles for the school nurse in caring for diabetic students (Siminerio, 2015). The school nurse must work with students' primary care provider, parents, and school personnel to establish a plan of care for managing diabetes. This includes methods of monitoring blood glucose levels and administering insulin or other medications during the school day, as well as how to respond in the event of hyperglycemic or hypoglycemic reactions (Siminerio, 2015). Emergency medications, such as glucagon, should be readily available, and staff involved with the student should be trained to administer them in case the nurse is not present in the school during an emergency. Special nutritional needs also need to be discussed with parents, teachers, and cafeteria staff. There may be significant challenges getting the child's nutritional restrictions met due to the institutional nature of most school food services and lack of education of staff about nutrition-related health concerns. The family, school nurse, and other school personnel may benefit from consultation and/or training by a diabetes educator or registered dietitian/nutritionist (Siminerio, 2015).

Children With Autism or Attention Deficit/Hyperactivity Disorder. "Autism, or autism spectrum disorder (ASD), refers to a broad range of conditions characterized by challenges with social skills, repetitive behaviors, speech and nonverbal communication" (Autism Speaks, 2018, para. 1). Autism may also be associated with medical problems such as gastrointestinal disorders and seizures. Because most children are expected to attend some school regardless of their illness, children with autism are legally entitled to attend public schools (DOE-OCR, 2010). Children with autism are more likely to experience fragmented services leading to unmet health care needs, as well as difficulty with school accommodations for their medical, sensory, social, and educational challenges (Russell & McCloskey, 2016). Parents caring for children with special needs such as autism report a sense of guilt, emotional strain, financial hardship, social isolation, and marital difficulties. They expressed dissatisfaction and frustration with providers and schools for not collaborating with the family to meet their child's needs (Russell & McCloskey,

Health Officer/School Nurse

This checklist discusses three major topic areas:
Student Health Records Maintenance
Public Health and Personal Hygiene Education
Health Officer's Office

Instructions:
1. Read the IAQ *Backgrounder.*
2. Read each item on this Checklist.
3. Check the diamond(s) as appropriate or check the circle if you need additional help with an activity.
4. Return this checklist to the IAQ Coordinator and keep a copy for future reference.

Name: ______________________

Room or Area: ______________________

School: ______________________

Date Completed: ______________________

Signature: ______________________

MAINTAIN STUDENT HEALTH RECORDS

There is evidence to suggest that children, pregnant women, and senior citizens are more likely to develop health problems from poor air quality than most adults. Indoor Air Quality (IAQ) problems are most likely to affect those with preexisting health conditions and those who are exposed to tobacco smoke. Student health records should include information about known allergies and other medically documented conditions, such as asthma, as well as any reported sensitivity to chemicals. Privacy considerations may limit the student health information that can be disclosed, but to the extent possible, information about students' potential sensitivity to IAQ problems should be provided to teachers. This is especially true for classes involving potential irritants (e.g., gaseous or particle emissions from art, science, industrial/vocational education sources). Health records and records of health-related complaints by students and staff are useful for evaluating potential IAQ-related complaints.

Include information about sensitivities to IAQ problems in student health records
- Allergies, including reports of chemical sensitivities.
- Asthma.

◇ Completed health records exist for each student.
◇ Health records are being updated.
○ Need help obtaining information about student allergies and other health factors.

Track health-related complaints by students and staff
- Keep a log of health complaints that notes the symptoms, location and time of symptom onset, and exposure to pollutant sources.
- Watch for trends in health complaints, especially in timing or location of complaints.

◇ Have a comprehensive health complaint logging system.
◇ Developing a comprehensive health complaint logging system.
○ Need help developing a comprehensive health complaint logging system.

Recognize indicators that health problems may be IAQ
- Complaints are associated with particular times of the day or week.
- Other occupants in the same area experience similar problems.
- The problem abates or ceases, either immediately or gradually, when an occupant leaves the building and recurs when the occupant returns.
- The school has recently been renovated or refurnished.
- The occupant has recently started working with new or different materials or equipment.
- New cleaning or pesticide products or practices have been introduced into the school.
- Smoking is allowed in the school.
- A new warm-blooded animal has been introduced into the classroom.

◇ Understand indicators of IAQ-related problems.
○ Need help understanding indicators of IAQ-related problems.

HEALTH AND HYGIENE EDUCATION

Schools are unique buildings from a public health perspective because they accommodate more people within a smaller area than most buildings. This proximity increases the potential for airborne contaminants (germs, odors, and constituents of personal products) to pass between students. Raising awareness about the effects of personal habits on the well-being of others can help reduce IAQ-related problems.

Obtain *Indoor Air Quality: An Introduction for Health Professionals*
- Contact IAQ INFO, 800-438-4318.

◇ Already have this EPA guidance document.
◇ Guide is on order.
○ Cannot obtain this guide.

Inform students and staff about the importance of good hygiene in preventing the spread of airborne contagious diseases
- Provide written materials to students (local public health agencies may have information suitable for older students).
- Provide individual instruction/counseling where necessary.

◇ Written materials and counseling available.
◇ Compiling information for counseling and distribution.
○ Need help compiling information or implementing counseling program.

Provide information about IAQ and health
- Help teachers develop activities that reduce exposure to indoor air pollutants for students with IAQ sensitivities, such as those with asthma or allergies (contact the American Lung Association [ALA], the National Association of School Nurses [NASN], or the Asthma and Allergy Foundation of America [AAFA]). Contact information is also available in the IAQ Coordinator's Guide.
- Collaborate with parent-teacher groups to offer family IAQ education programs.
- Conduct a workshop for teachers on health issues that covers IAQ.

◇ Have provided information to parents and staff.
◇ Developing information and education programs for parents and staff.
○ Need help developing information and education program for parents and staff.

Establish an information and counseling program regarding smoking
- Provide free literature on smoking and secondhand smoke.
- Sponsor a quit-smoking program and similar counseling programs in collaboration with the ALA.

◇ "No Smoking" information and programs in place.
◇ "No Smoking" information and programs in planning.
○ Need help with a "No Smoking" program.

HEALTH OFFICER'S OFFICE

Since the health office may be frequented by sick students and staff, it is important to take steps that can help prevent transmission of airborne diseases to uninfected students and staff (see your IAQ Coordinator for help with the following activities).

Ensure that the ventilation system is properly operating
- Ventilation system is operated when the area(s) is occupied.
- Provide an adequate amount of outdoor air to the area(s). There should be at least 15 cubic feet of outdoor air supplied per occupant.
- Air filters are clean and properly installed.
- Air removed from the area(s) does not circulate through the ventilation system into other occupied areas.

◇ Ventilation system operating adequately.
○ Need help with ventilation-related activities.

☐ **No Problems to Report.** I have completed all the activities on this checklist, and I do not need help in any areas.

Fig. 42.3 Environmental Protection Agency indoor air quality checklist. (From U.S. Environmental Protection Agency: *School and child care-based asthma education programs,* 2010. Available from http://www.epa.gov.)

2016). Because many children with autism have communication problems, the school nurse can advocate for the child and collaborate with the parents to learn the most effective ways to determine and meet the child's needs. The nurse should participate on IEP teams to plan care and accommodations for children with autism. The nurse should educate teachers and other school personnel to be sure they understand how to appropriately interact with the child and what, if any, limitations autism may place on his or her participation in class or physical education activities (Rutkowski & Brimer, 2014). The nurse can give the child prescribed medications for mood or prevention of seizures. The nurse may recommend the use of sign language, picture boards, or other types of communication devices that are used by the child. In addition, the nurse can teach the parents about autism. The nurse can also help parents work with others in the health care system, such as speech-language therapists and developmental specialists, so that the child can have a positive learning experience at school (Rutkowski & Brimer, 2014).

Children with attention-deficit/hyperactivity disorder (ADHD) also attend school. In 2016, there were an estimated 6.1 million children ages 2 to 17 diagnosed with ADHD in the United States (CDC, 2018). Of these, two-thirds had another mental health or behavioral problem. Children with ADHD often have trouble sitting still, may be forgetful, have difficulty focusing on tasks or instructions, and may exhibit poor impulse control. Causes are unknown, though children exposed to environmental toxins, such as lead, and those with brain injury, prematurity, and low birth weight are more likely to be diagnosed with ADHD. School nurses may administer medications at school and may need to monitor the child for adverse reactions (Heuer & Williams, 2016). Due to their difficulty focusing, children with ADHD may need reminders to take their medications. Some medications can decrease appetite, so the school nurse can partner with parents and teachers to ensure that children do not experience nutritional deficits. Because of the behaviors common in children with ADHD, school personnel may become frustrated with them. The school nurse must advocate for the child, work with him or her to facilitate behavioral and time management skills, and encourage good communication with parents, providers, and school personnel (Heuer & Williams, 2016). Referral to mental health providers within or outside the school may be needed if the child's behaviors interfere with their ability to function and learn.

Children With Special Needs in the Schools. As discussed earlier in this chapter, children who need urinary catheterization, dressing changes, peripheral or central line intravenous catheter maintenance, tracheotomy suctioning, gastrostomy or other tube feedings, or intravenous medication also attend schools (Toothaker & Cook, 2018). The school nurse may supervise a health aide or personal care nurse who is assigned to the child to assist with complex nursing needs. In all these cases, the school nurse provides tertiary care to maintain the child's health. The nurse has the skills needed to assess the child's well-being. In addition, the nurse may have to teach another person in the school how to care for the child in case the nurse is not in the building when the child needs help (Cagginello et al., 2014). It is the responsibility of the school nurse to keep up to date with the latest health care information through in-service and continuing education programs, as well as regularly reading journals in the fields of pediatrics and school nursing.

An example of how a school nurse can help an injured child return to school after long absences follows. Enrique, a sixth-grade boy who had received serious facial burns, is preparing to return to school. Enrique is afraid of how the children will respond to the pressure mask he wears to minimize future scarring. The nurse has a meeting with Enrique's mother and the school's principal and also contacts nurses from the hospital's burn unit to determine a plan for Enrique's reentry to school. According to their plan, the school nurse first teaches a lesson to the boy's classmates about burns and their treatment. After the lesson, Enrique joined the class with the nurse and showed his classmates his face with and without his pressure mask. With the parents' and Enrique's permission, both Enrique and the nurse answered the children's questions. In addition to the education provided, changes were made in Enrique's schedule so he could be out of the sun during the school day and physical education class. The nurse found that Enrique's burns were soon forgotten and he was accepted by his friends.

Children can contract human immunodeficiency virus (HIV) from their mother before or during birth. In 2014, there were about 10,000 children diagnosed with HIV in the United States (CDC, as cited in Rasberry et al., 2017). Children with HIV or acquired immunodeficiency syndrome (AIDS) attend school and may require care from the school nurse to manage their illness and prevent complications. Because of privacy and confidentiality laws, the school nurse may not even know that the child has this disease. In some cases, the nurse may be directly notified of the child's HIV status either by the parents or physician or may suspect the diagnosis due to HIV medications being administered during the school day (Selekman, et al., 2013). In all cases, the nurse must maintain confidentiality. This means that information cannot be released to anyone, including teachers, other health professionals, other students, or staff.

School nurses should ensure that universal precautions are practiced by all personnel handling blood or body fluids of anyone at school. Most school districts are required to provide employees with bloodborne pathogens training and protective equipment under Occupational Safety and Health Administration (OSHA) (2000) regulations. These precautions can protect employees from exposure to HIV, as well as other bloodborne diseases such as hepatitis B and C. As part of regular health education in the school, the school nurse can provide education about HIV/AIDS prevention and risks to the children, school employees, and community (Rasberry et al., 2017). The school nurse should also be part of the school health advisory committee to develop an HIV/AIDS health curriculum that teaches about HIV/AIDS prevention and transmission so that children know how to protect themselves and are not afraid to go to school with children who have the disease. Nearly one-third of children report sexual activity by the time they are in high school, and more than 40 percent report not using a condom during intercourse (Rasberry et al., 2017). School nurses should refer children who report sexual activity or sexual abuse to testing for sexually transmitted diseases, including HIV/AIDS. This requires knowing about available community resources for free or confidential testing and transportation if students do not wish to involve their parents. The nurse may be required to report to the parents and legal authorities if sexual abuse is suspected. The school nurse can encourage and assist the child in disclosing sexual activity to the parents if required by state law.

Children With DNAR Orders. As part of tertiary prevention, the school nurse cares for children with highly complex conditions and terminal diseases who attend school. The numbers of children receiving only palliative care is rising (Begley et al., 2018). These children benefit from participation in school activities, socialization with their peers, and following a daily routine. The IDEIA, as discussed earlier in this chapter, requires that children be allowed to attend school in the "least restrictive environment" (DOE-OCR, 2010). Therefore children with terminal illnesses may have **do-not-attempt-resuscitation orders** (DNAR orders) at school, and some may die at school, though this is not common (Begley et al., 2018). DNAR orders are signed by the parents and the physician according to their state's law. In some states, the courts have found that the school nurse and other school staff are bound to obey the DNAR order; however, state and local laws and school district policies vary, so school nurses should determine what is required or allowed, as well as consult legal counsel for the school district to verify support for the family's decisions.

The AAP's committees on school health and bioethics reaffirmed a set of guidelines to help school health providers and the schools decide what to do when a child with a DNAR order attends the school (AAP, 2010/2016). A formal request to the school and the school board from the parents and physician is a must regarding the written DNAR order. The school nurse should be involved in discussions regarding when to use the DNAR order. The decision not to do anything for a dying child, and how to function if the child were to suddenly face death, can be emotionally and ethically difficult. As an advocate for the child and family, school nurses should coordinate ongoing communication with parents, providers, school staff, and administrators well in advance of such an event (Begley et al., 2018).

When a child dies in school, the nurse is responsible for helping the children who witnessed the death. The nurse becomes a grief counselor and helps the children and teachers cope with the death. Further education about death and dying given by the school nurse would also help the school community cope with death in the schools (Begley et al., 2018).

Homebound Children. Even though the laws regarding disabled persons state that all children should go to school, some children cannot. Instead, they may be taught in the home or in another institutional setting such as the hospital. In these situations, the school nurse should be a liaison between the child's teacher, physician, school administrators, parents, and any nurses and other health care providers caring for the child in the home regarding the child's needs (Shannon & Minchella, 2016). The nurse participates with the child's IEP team so that it is appropriate for the child and does not remove necessary learning from the plan. The child should be allowed to go to school when he or she is able, at which point the school nurse coordinates the child's care to facilitate a smooth transition between the two settings and ensure that health care needs are met.

Pregnant Teenagers and Teenage Mothers at School. In 2015, nearly 230,000 babies were born to teenage girls between the ages of 15 and 19 (CDC, 2017b). While this is a decline of 8 percent since 2014, the United States still has a higher rate than other industrialized countries. Many teenage girls who are pregnant attend school and are protected from discrimination by Title IX of the 1972 Education Amendment Act (Disney et al., 2015). Therefore the school nurse may provide ongoing care to the mother as well as coordination of care outside the school system, including visits to the physician or nurse practitioner and assistance with setting up home school until the teen is released from medical restrictions following birth (Disney et al., 2015). Some schools provide on-site child care to encourage teen mothers to return to finish their schooling. Although this may appear to be primary prevention, it is tertiary prevention because adolescent pregnancies are considered to be high risk. Teen fathers may also require advocacy from the school nurse if they are involved with their child's care. Teen pregnancy is discussed in more detail in Chapters 28 and 35.

CONTROVERSIES IN SCHOOL NURSING

School nursing has evolved into a complex health care role, and some areas of the field still cause controversy, such as providing education on family planning and providing birth control to students in the schools where it is allowed. Although differences in opinion exist relating to sex education, reproductive services, and screening for sexually transmitted diseases in the schools, the literature supports a comprehensive approach to sexual health education (Kern et al., 2016). The school nurse should educate community members, the school board, teachers, parents, and students about the benefits of different types of services in the schools to the health of students and school personnel.

ETHICS IN SCHOOL NURSING

The school nurse may be faced with ethical issues in the schools. For example, a child may have a DNAR order that the parents wish to be used if the child dies at school (see earlier text), but following the DNAR order may be against the nurse's personal beliefs. Perhaps a girl asks the nurse where she can get an abortion and wishes to talk to the school nurse about how she feels, but the nurse is against abortions. Alternatively, a teenager asks for emergency contraception, which conflicts with the nurse's religious beliefs or the nurse is not allowed to provide with his or her scope of practice, state laws, or school district regulations. In these cases, as in any other setting, the nurse must give nursing care to the student client according to the *School Nursing: Scope and Standards of Practice* (ANA & NASN, 2017) and the state's nurse practice act. However, if the nurse feels so strongly that he or she cannot work with the situation, another school nurse should be called for help, or the student should be referred to other health providers who can give the care the student needs. Care should never be denied or ignored; referral is a good option.

FUTURE TRENDS IN SCHOOL NURSING

The future of school nursing is strong. The amount of health care being given in the schools is increasing. In the future, school nursing may coordinate primary health care and specialist consultations for students in rural areas with limited access to care. Telecommunication may also be utilized to teach health education or to facilitate care coordination and make meetings more accessible for collaboration with other school nurses (Haynie, et al., 2017). Online resources are listed in Table 42.3. The school nurse is responsible for keeping up with the latest changes in health care and health practice so that the health of children in the schools can be enhanced by new trends in health care.

The National Association of School Nurses is looking to the future through development of the *Framework for 21st Century School Nursing Practice* (Maughan et al., 2018). This framework (Fig. 42.4) was developed by the NASN board of directors and an advisory group including school nurses and school nurse leaders. This framework integrates various models and principles that have been utilized to guide school nursing practice through the years. As the health needs of children become more complex and expectations of schools and parents grow, this framework "... provides guidance for the practicing school nurse to reach the goal of supporting student health and academic success by contributing to a healthy and safe school environment" (Maughan et al., p. 219).

TABLE 42.3 Online Resources for School Nurses

Organization	Internet Address
The American Academy of Child and Adolescent Psychiatry	http://www.aacap.org
American Academy of Pediatrics	http://www.aap.org
National Association of School Nurses	http://www.nasn.org
Center for Health and Health Care in the Schools	http://www.healthinschools.org
National Youth Violence Prevention Centers	https://www.cdc.gov
U.S. Department of Education Emergency Preparedness	https://www.fema.gov
Healthy Schools Network	http://www.healthyschools.org
U.S. Environmental Protection Agency	https://www.epa.gov

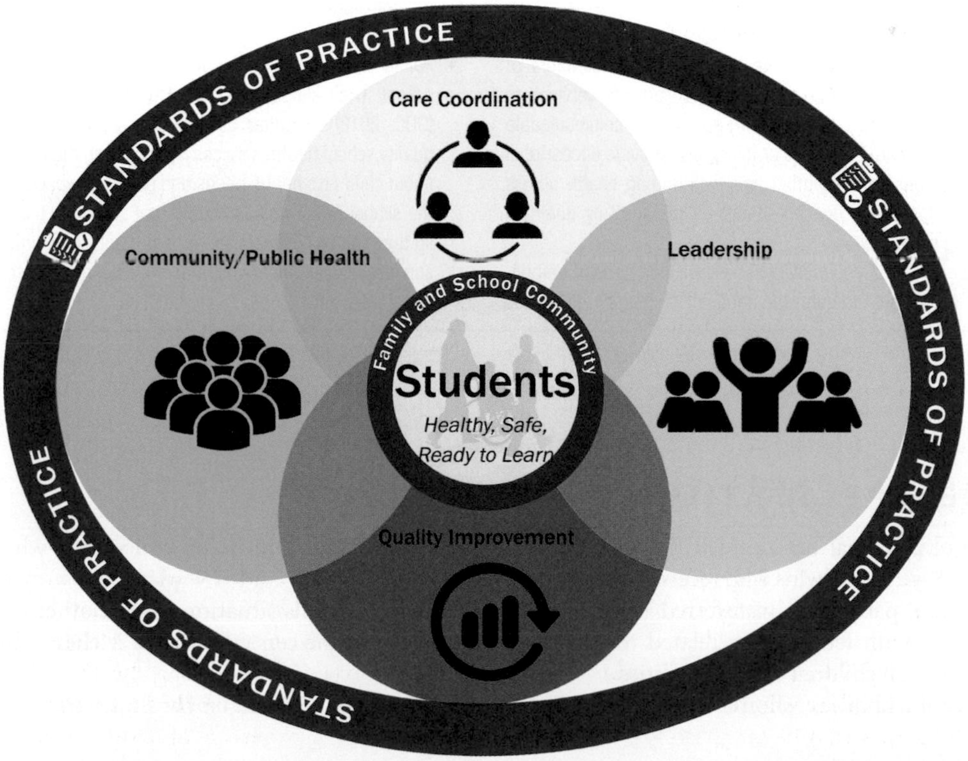

Fig. 42.4 Framework for 21st Century School Nursing Practice. (Reprinted with permission by the National Association of School Nurses. Available at https://www.nasn.org/nasn/nasn-resources/professional-topics/framework.)

LINKING CONTENT TO PRACTICE

School nurses play a primary role in the development and implementation of the CDC's WSCC model components. These components are described below and addressed throughout this chapter. The emphasis in this program design is working with the school as a population or community. This plan has 10 parts:

- *Physical education and physical activity*—The CDC (2018e) recommends that schools follow the national comprehensive physical activity framework, which includes support for regular physical activity during and outside of the school day, coordination with community, families, and school staff, and a curriculum throughout the child's school career that teaches health behaviors, sportsmanship, and other important skills related to health. Teachers of this curriculum should be licensed and certified in physical education (CDC, 2018f).
- *Nutrition environment and services*—The entire school environment should promote healthy eating, which has been shown to support student learning (CDC, 2018f). Information on nutrition and diet should be taught to all children. In addition, schools should provide healthy food choices for students in their meal programs (both breakfast and lunch). School nutrition staff should be educated to prepare food in ways that are both healthy and appetizing to encourage nutritious eating habits among staff and students. Nutrition staff should also be trained annually on safe food handling practices to decrease the risk of communicable disease outbreaks. Vending machines, school celebrations, and concession stands should offer healthy choices, following the Smart Snacks in Schools initiative, or be off limits to children, especially during the school day (CDC, 2018f). School employees, including school nurses, should model healthy eating behavior.
- *Health education*—This component includes teaching children about how to stay healthy and how to avoid becoming ill or being injured. The health education should be offered in a planned, sequential, K-12 curriculum that addresses all dimensions of health, following the National Health Education Standards (CDC, 2018f).
- *Health services*—School health services should be designed to prevent illness, promote health, and intervene in the event of illness or injury of students and school staff. Specifically, the schools can provide services to ensure access or referral to primary care, prevent and control communicable disease, provide emergency care for illness or injury, and provide educational and counseling opportunities for promoting and maintaining health across all settings (CDC, 2018f). Health services should be provided by qualified professionals, including school nurses.
- *Counseling, psychological, and social services*—This component emphasizes prevention and intervention to meet the needs of students in the areas of behavioral and mental health. School counselors, psychologists, and social workers should be qualified to provide guidance for children and their family, to alleviate barriers for children with learning needs, and provide referrals to community mental health and social services when needed (CDC, 2018f).
- *Physical environment*—The physical environment includes the school building and grounds, as well as environmental influences within and outside of the school that may impact the health of school staff and students. Indoor air quality, safe handling and use of chemicals (including pesticides and cleaning supplies), temperature and noise levels, and lighting are all addressed under this component (CDC, 2018f). This component also addresses violence and crime prevention in the schools.
- *Social and emotional school climate*—This component encompasses a safe and supportive environment for students and staff. A supportive environment fosters healthy growth and development, as well as academic achievement and healthy relationships among students.
- *Employee wellness*—Nurses often provide health care for teachers and other staff members in the schools. Staff can ask nurses about their health and obtain health education at school during their workday. This component also covers worksite safety for employees (CDC, 2018f). Nurses should be familiar with Occupational Safety and Health Administration (OSHA) guidelines for personal protective equipment, bloodborne pathogen prevention education, and healthy school environment (available from www.osha.gov). Healthy school employees are less likely to miss work and to be more productive, thereby reducing costs of finding replacements and decreasing health insurance costs for everyone.
- *Community involvement*—The school health program should contact families and community leaders to find out what health services are needed the most and how they can work together to emphasize health education, promote health in the school and community, and thereby support student learning (CDC, 2018f). Coalition building with school community partners is an important role for the school nurse, as discussed earlier in this chapter.
- *Family engagement*— Families should be made to feel welcome in the school. Their support is critical to the health and learning of their children (CDC, 2018f). Families can provide support for adequate, safe, and high-quality school health services by educating their school board representatives about children's health needs and parents' expectations for health care during the school day. Families should feel confident that privacy will be protected so they can comfortably share health and social information, as well as bring supplies and medications that may be needed to support their children's health at school.

CDC, Centers for Disease Control and Prevention; *WSCC,* Whole School, Whole Community, Whole Child.

PRACTICE APPLICATION

The elementary school principal has notified the school nurse that Melissa and John, 8-year-old twins who receive daily physical therapy for mild cerebral palsy, have transferred to the school. The nurse must comply with federal laws related to providing education and services to all children with disabilities.

A. What nursing responsibilities should the school nurse carry out?

B. What factors must be considered when the nurse coordinates the IEP and IHP plans?

C. How will this situation impact other children at school?

D. What is the central focus of Melissa's and John's education?

Answers can be found on the Evolve site.

KEY POINTS

- School nurses provide health care for children and families.
- In the early 1900s school nurses screened children for infectious diseases and educated families on prevention and treatment.
- School nursing practice has grown in complexity, becoming more holistic and adhering to professional practice standards.
- The National Association of School Nurses (NASN) is the professional organization for school nurses.
- School nurses have varying educational levels depending on state laws.
- The U.S. government supports **school-based health centers, school-linked programs**, and full-service school-based health centers.
- *Healthy People 2020* has objectives to enhance the health of children in schools and increase school nurse-to-student ratios.
- Primary prevention in schools includes health promotion and education to prevent childhood injuries, disease, and substance abuse.
- The school nurse monitors the children for all of their state-mandated immunizations for school entry.
- HIPAA privacy rules regarding the health information of children apply in schools.
- Secondary prevention involves screening children for illnesses and providing direct nursing care.
- School nurses develop plans for emergency care in the schools.
- Giving medications to children in the school must be monitored carefully to prevent errors.
- School health nurses are mandated reporters of suspected cases of child abuse and/or neglect.
- Disaster-preparedness plans should be set up for all schools with the school nurse as a member of the crisis response team.
- Tertiary prevention includes caring for children with long-term health needs, such as asthma, diabetes, and disabling conditions.
- School nurses carry out catheterizations, suctioning, gastrostomy feedings, and other complex clinical skills in schools.
- Some ethical dilemmas in the schools are related to women's health care.
- Some school nurses utilize telecommunications to coordinate health care for children and their families.

CLINICAL DECISION-MAKING ACTIVITIES

1. For the state where you live, make a list of the immunizations required for children attending schools. Then contrast this to the immunizations you received when in school. How has this changed over the years?
2. Contact the nurse in your former high school. Interview the nurse, focusing on the major focus of the role. Describe what the nurse likes best and least about the role. What changes could be made to help the nurse provide care more effectively?
3. Arrange to visit an elementary school health office during screening activities. Observe the interaction between the nurse and the children. Describe how the nurse is using the nursing process during the screening process.
4. Organize a group of nursing students to volunteer at a school health fair. Develop a health education booth for the fair. Describe how the health information can be used by the children, families, and the community.
5. Attend the annual school board meeting that discusses the budget for the next year. Analyze the budget for health services. Determine whether this will be adequate to care for the children. What issues influence the budgetary process?
6. Search the Internet to learn more about your state's health department. What trends do you see relating to health in the schools?
7. Volunteer as a participant in your school district's emergency response drill. How did the school nurse's responsibilities work to help reduce confusion and increase the provision of emergency care?

ADDITIONAL RESOURCES

EVOLVE WEBSITE

http://evolve.elsevier.com/Stanhope/community/

- Answers to Practice Application
- Case Study
- Glossary
- Review Questions

REFERENCES

AED Brands: *AED State Laws & Legislation*, 2015. Retrieved from https://www.aedbrands.com.

American Academy of Pediatrics, Council on School Health: Role of the school nurse in providing school health services, *Pediatrics* 137(6):1–6, 2016.

American Academy of Pediatrics, Council on School Health and Committee on Bioethics: Honoring do-not-attempt-resuscitation requests in schools, *Pediatrics* 125(5):1073–1077, 2010/reaffirmed 2016.

American Association of Colleges of Nursing: *Fact sheet: The Impact of Education on Nursing Practice,* 2017. Retrieved from http://www.aacnnursing.org.

American Nurses Association: *Public Health Nursing: Scope and Standards of Practice,* ed 2, Silver Spring, MD, 2013, Author.

American Nurses Association and National Association of School Nurses: *School nursing: scope and standards of practice,* ed 3, Silver Spring, MD, 2017, Authors.

Anderson LJW, Schaffer MA, Hiltz C, O'Leary SA, Luehr RE, Yoney EL: Public health interventions: School nurse practice stories, *J Sch Nurs* 34(3):192–202, 2017.

Apple RD: School health is community: School nursing in the early twentieth century in the USA, *His Educ Rev* 46(2): 136–149, 2017.

Asthma and Allergy Foundation of America: *Insect Allergies,* 2015. Retrieved from http://www.aafa.org.

Autism Speaks: *What is Autism?* 2018. Retrieved from https://www.autismspeaks.org.

Bandzar S, Funsch DG, Hermansen R, Gupta S, Bandzar A: Pediatric hoverboard and skateboard injuries, *Pediatrics* 141(4):e20171235, 2018.

Begley C, Cowan T, Crowe D, Allsbrook P, Graf K: *Do not Attempt Resuscitation—The Role of the School Nurse* (NASN Position Statement), 2018. Retrieved from https://higherlogicdownload.s3.amazonaws.com.

Bobo N, Kimel L, Bleza S: Promoting health at school. In Selekman, J, editor: *School nursing: a comprehensive text,* ed 2, Philadelphia, 2013, F.A. Davis Company, pp 440–472.

Bohnenkamp JH, Stephan SH, Bobo N: Supporting student mental health: The role of the school nurse in coordinated school mental health care, *Psychol Sch* 52(7):714–727, 2015.

Brener ND, Vernon-Smiley M, Leonard S, Buckley R: *Health services: Results from the school health policies and practices study 2012,* Atlanta, GA, 2013, Centers for Disease Control and Prevention.

Cagginello J, Blackborow M, Porter J, Disney J, Andresen K, Tuck C: *Nursing Delegation to Unlicensed Assistive Personnel in the School Setting (NASN Position Statement),* 2014. Retrieved from https://www.nasn.org.

Caldart-Olson L, Thronson, G: Legislation affecting school nurses. In Selekman, J, editor: *School nursing: a comprehensive text,* ed 2, Philadelphia, 2013, F.A. Davis Company, pp 225–256.

Cassidy-Bushrow AE, Johnson DA, Peters RM, Burmeister C, Joseph CL: Time spent on the internet and adolescent blood pressure, *J Sch Nurs* 31(5):374–384, 2015.

Centers for Disease Control and Prevention: *At a Glance, 2016: Healthy Schools: The Right Place for a Healthy Start,* 2016a. Retrieved from https://www.cdc.gov.

Centers for Disease Control and Prevention: *National Action Plan for Child Injury Prevention,* 2016b. Retrieved from https://www.cdc.gov.

Centers for Disease Control and Prevention: *Playground Safety,* 2016c. Retrieved from https://www.cdc.gov.

Centers for Disease Control and Prevention: *Results from the School Health Policies and Practices Study,* 2016d. Retrieved from https://www.cdc.gov.

Centers for Disease Control and Prevention: *High School YRBS, 2017 Results,* 2017a. Retrieved from https://nccd.cdc.gov.

Centers for Disease Control and Prevention: *Reproductive Health: Teen Pregnancy,* 2017b. Retrieved from https://www.cdc.gov.

Centers for Disease Control and Prevention: *School Vaccination Requirements and Exemptions,* 2017c. Retrieved from https://www.cdc.gov.

Centers for Disease Control and Prevention: *About CDC Healthy Schools,* 2018a. Retrieved from https://www.cdc.gov.

Centers for Disease Control and Prevention: *Attention Deficit/Hyperactivity Disorder: Data and Statistics,* 2018b. Retrieved from https://www.cdc.gov.

Centers for Disease Control and Prevention: *Controlling Asthma in Schools,* 2018c. Retrieved from https://www.cdc.gov.

Centers for Disease Control and Prevention: *Food Allergies in School,* 2018d. Retrieved from https://www.cdc.gov.

Centers for Disease Control and Prevention: *Key Facts about Seasonal Flu Vaccine,* 2018e. Retrieved from https://www.cdc.gov.

Centers for Disease Control and Prevention: *Whole School, Whole Community, Whole Child,* 2018f. Retrieved from https://www.cdc.gov.

Cicutto L, Gleason M, Haas-Howard C, Jenkins-Nygren L, Labonde S, Patrick K: Competency-based framework and continuing education for preparing a skilled school health workforce for asthma care: the Colorado experience, *J Sch Nurs* 33(4): 277–284, 2017.

Cornell M, Selekman J: Collaboration with the community. In Selekman J, editor: *School nursing: a comprehensive text,* ed 2, Philadelphia, 2013, F.A. Davis Company, pp 163–194.

Disney JA, Jordan A, Wheller J, Porter J, Lambert P, Blackborow M, Zacharski S: *Pregnant and Parenting Students – The Role of the School Nurse* (NASN Position Statement), 2015. Retrieved from https://www.nasn.org.

Doyle, J: Emergency management, crisis response, and the school nurses's role. In Selekman J, editor: *School nursing: a comprehensive text,* ed 2, Philadelphia, PA, 2013, F.A. Davis Company, pp 1216–1244.

Fiorivant, M, Ward C: *School-Located Vaccination (NASN Position Statement),* 2018. Retrieved from https://www.nasn.org.

Foeller, H: The nurse in the high school, *Public Health Nurs* 28(9):617–619, 1936.

Food Research and Action Center: *Child Nutrition Reauthorization (CNR),* 2018. Retrieved from http://www.frac.org.

Flynn K, McDonald CC, D'Alonzo BA, Tam V, Wiebe DJ: Violence in rural, urban, and suburban schools in Pennsylvania, *J Sch Nurs* 34(4):263–269, 2018.

Gibbons LJ, Lehr K, Selekman J: Federal laws protecting children and youth with disabilities in the schools. In Selekman J, editor: *School nursing: a comprehensive text,* ed 2, Philadelphia, 2013, F.A. Davis Company, pp 257–283.

Griffin SO, Wei L, Gooch BF, Weno K, Espinoza L: Vital signs: Dental sealant use and untreated tooth decay among U.S. school-aged children, *Morb Mortal Wkly Rep,* 65:1141–1145, 2016.

Hahn J: The Affordable Care Act at the 6 Yr. mark: A policy update, *Virginia Nurses Today* 24(3):6–7, 2016.

Haynie KM, Lindahl B, Simons-Major K, Meadows L, Maughan ED: *The Role of School Nursing in Telehealth* (Position Statement), 2017. Retrieved from https://www.nasn.org.

Hinkson E, Mauter E, Wilson L, Johansen A, Maughan ED: *Medication Administration in Schools (NASN Position Statement),* 2017. Retrieved from https://www.nasn.org.

Houlahan B: Origins of school nursing, *J Sch Nurs* 34(3):203–210, 2018.

Heuer B, Williams S: Collaboration between PNPs and school nurses: Meeting the complex medical and academic needs of the child with ADHD, *J Pediatr Health Care* 30(1):88–93, 2016.

Institute of Education Sciences: National Center for Education Statistics: *Fast Facts: Back to School Statistics,* 2017, Author. Retrieved from https://nces.ed.gov.

Institute of Medicine: *The future of nursing: leading change, advancing health,* Washington, DC, 2011, National Academies Press.
John R, Chewey L: Common complaints. . In Selekman J, editor: *School nursing: a comprehensive text,* ed 2, Philadelphia, 2013, F.A. Davis Company, pp 578–640.
Johnson KE, Morris M, McRee AL: Full coverage sports physicals: School nurses' untapped role in health promotion among student athletes, *J Sch Nurs* 34(2):139–148, 2018.
Jordan KS, MacKay P, Woods SJ: Child maltreatment: optimizing recognition and reporting by school nurses, *NASN Sch Nurse* 32(3):192–199, 2017.
Kern L, Emge G, Reiner K, Rebowe D: *Sexual Health Education in Schools* (NASN Position Statement), 2016. Retrieved from https://www.nasn.org.
Levy S, Campbell MD, Shea CL, DuPont R: Trends in abstaining from substance use in adolescents: 1975–2014, *Pediatrics* 142(2):e20173498, 2018.
Maughan ED, Bobo N, Butler S, Schantz S: Framework for 21st century school nursing practice, *NASN School Nurse* 31(1): 45–53, 2018.
Maughan ED, McCarthy AM, Hein M, Perkhounkova Y, Kelly MW: Medication management in schools: 2015 survey results, *J Sch Nurs* 1–12, 2017.
Miller GF, Coffield E, Leroy Z: Prevalence and costs of five chronic conditions in children, *J Sch Nurs* 32(5):357–364, 2016.
National Association of School Nurses: *About: NASN Mission*, 2018a, Author. Retrieved from https://www.nasn.org.
National Association of School Nurses: *Research Priorities: NASN Research Priorities* 2018-2019. 2018b, Author. Retrieved from https://www.nasn.org.
National Association of School Nurses: *Education, Licensure, and Certification of School Nurses:* (Position statement), 2016, Author. Retrieved from https://higherlogicdownload.s3.amazonaws.com.
National Association of School Nurses: *Food Allergies & Anaphylaxis,* 2014, Author. Retrieved from https://www.nasn.org.
National Association of School Nurses: *Immunizations* (Position Statement), 2015a: Author. Retrieved from https://www.nasn.org.
National Association of School Nurses: *Naloxone Use in the School Setting: The Role of the School Nurse* (Position Statement), 2015b, Author. Retrieved from https://www.nasn.org.
National Association of School Nurses: *School Nurse Workload: Staffing for Safe Care: Position Statement*. 2015c, Author. Retrieved from https://www.nasn.org
National Board for Certification of School Nurses: *Eligibility to Take the NCSN Exam,* 2018, Author. Retrieved from https://www.nbcsn.org.
National Institute on Drug Abuse: *Principles of Adolescent Substance Use Disorder Treatment: a Research-Based Guide,* 2014. Retrieved from https://www.drugabuse.gov.
National Institute of Mental Health: *Suicide Prevention*, 2017. Retrieved from https://www.nimh.nih.gov.
Nolta K: A school-based suicide risk assessment strategy, *NASN Sch Nurse* 29(6):295–298, 2014.
Occupational Safety and Health Administration: *Bloodborne Pathogens and Needlestick Prevention,* 2000. Retrieved from https://www.osha.gov.
Pistiner M, Mattey B: A universal anaphylaxis emergency care plan: introducing the new allergy and anaphylaxis care plan from the American Academy of Pediatrics, *NASN Sch Nurse* 32(5): 283–286, 2017.
Pontius DJ: Demystifying pediculosis: School nurses taking the lead, *Pediatric Nursing* 40(5):226–235, 2014.
Pontius DJ: Health literacy part 2: Practical techniques for getting your message home, *NASN Sch Nurse* 29(1):30–42, 2014.
Price OA: Strategies to encourage long-term sustainability of school-based health centers, *Am J Med Res* 4(1):61–83, 2017.
Proctor S: Standards of practice. In Selekman J, editor: *School nursing: a comprehensive text,* ed 2, Philadelphia, 2013, F.A. Davis Company, pp 48–78.
Rasberry CN, Liddon N, Adkins SH: The importance of school staff referrals and follow-up in connecting high school students to HIV and STD testing, *J Sch Nurs* 33(2):143–153, 2017.
Rebmann T, Elliott MB, Artman D, VanNatta M, Wakefield M: Impact of an education intervention on Missouri K-12 school disaster and biological event preparedness, *J Sch Health* 86(11):794–802, 2016.
Rebmann T, Weaver NL, Elliott MB, DeClue RW, Patel NJ, Schulte L: Factors related to injury prevention programming by Missouri school nurses, *J Sch Nursg* 34(4):292–300, 2018.
Robert Wood Johnson Foundation: Unlocking the potential of school nursing: Keeping children healthy, in school, and ready to learn, *Charting Nursing's Future* 14:2–5, 2010.
Rogers LL: The nurse in the public school, *Am J Nurs* 5:764–769, 1905.
Rogers LL: 1908 Some phases of school nursing. Rogers LL: Some phases of school nursing. *Am J Nurs* 8:966–974, 1908.
Russell S, McCloskey CR: Parent perceptions of care received by children with an autism spectrum disorder, *J Pediatr Nurs* 31(1):21–31, 2016.
Rutkowski EM, Brimer D: Physical education issues for students with autism: school nurse challenges, *J Sch Nurs* 30(4):256–261, 2014.
Salam RA, Arshad A, Das JK, et al: Interventions to prevent unintentional injuries among adolescents: A systematic review and meta-analysis, *J Adolesc Health* 59(Suppl 4):S76–S87, 2016.
Schaffer MA, Anderson LJ, Rising S: Public health interventions for school nursing practice, *J Sch Nurs* 32(3):195–208, 2016.
School Nurses Branch: Functions and qualifications of school nurses, *Am J Nurs* 61(5):93–97, 1961.
Selekman J, Bochenek J, Lukens M: Children with chronic conditions. In: Selekman J, editor: *School nursing: a comprehensive text*, ed 2, Philadelphia, 2013, F.A. Davis Company, pp 700–783.
Shannon RA, Minchella L: Students requiring personal nursing care at school: Nursing care models and a checklist for school nurses, *NASN Sch Nurse* 30(2):76–80, 2015.
Siminerio LM: Diabetes education and support, *NASN Sch Nurse* 30(6):320–321, 2015.
Smith S, Bobo N, Strasser KM, Haynie KM: *Head Lice Management in the School Setting* (NASN Position Statement), 2016. Retrieved from https://www.nasn.org.
Substance Abuse and Mental Health Services Administration: *Suicide Prevention*, 2017. Retrieved from https://www.samhsa.gov.
Toothaker R, Cook P: A review of four health procedures that school nurses may encounter, *NASN Sch Nurse* 33(1):19–22, 2018.
Tuck CM, Haynie K, Davis C: *Emergency Preparedness and Response in the School Setting - The Role of the School Nurse (NASN Position Statement),* 2014. Retrieved from https://www.nasn.org.
U.S. Congress: *Public Law* 111-296: Healthy hunger free Kids act of 2010, 2010, Author. Retrieved from https://www.congress.gov.
U.S. Consumer Product Safety Commission: *Public playground safety handbook,* 2015, Author. Retrieved from https://www.cpsc.gov.
U.S. Department of Education: *The every student succeeds act: P.L.* 115-224, 2018, Author. Retrieved from https://legcounsel.house.gov.

U.S. Department of Education: *Final title I regulations to strengthen NCLB: Title I—Improving the academic achievement of the disadvantaged, final regulations, 34 CFR Part 200.* 2008: Author. Retrieved from https://www2.ed.gov.

U.S. Department of Education, Office for Civil Rights: *Free appropriate public education for students with disabilities: requirements under section 504 of the rehabilitation Act of 1973*, 2010, Author. Retrieved from https://www2.ed.gov.

U.S. Department of Education, U.S. Department of Health and Human Services, U.S. Department of Homeland Security, U.S. Department of Justice, Federal Bureau of Investigation, & Federal Emergency Management Agency: *Guide for developing high-quality school emergency operations plans*, 2013, Author. Retrieved from https://www.fema.gov.

U.S. Environmental Protection Agency: *Indoor air quality tools for schools action kit*, n.d. Retrieved from https://www.epa.gov.

U.S. Government Printing Office: *Funding for individuals with disabilities education Act*, 2017, Author. Retrieved from https://www.gpo.gov.

U.S. Department of Health and Human Services: *Stopbullying.gov: Laws & policies*, 2017, Author. Retrieved from https://www.stopbullying.gov.

U.S. Department of Health and Human Services: *Health information privacy: FAQ*, 2008, Author. Retrieved from https://www.hhs.gov.

U.S. Department of Health and Human Services: *Healthy People 2020: Educational and community-based programs, ECBP 5*, 2018, Author. Retrieved from https://www.healthypeople.gov.

Wahl A, Stephens H, Ruffo M, Jones AL: The evaluation of a food allergy and epinephrine autoinjector training program for personnel who care for children in schools and community settings, *J Sch Nurs* 31(2):91–98, 2015.

Wernette MJ, Emory J: Student bedtimes, academic performance, and health in a residential high school. *J Sch Nurs* 33(4):264–268, 2017.

Wheeler, J. M., Ward, C., Rebowe D: *Bullying and Cyberbullying—Prevention in Schools (NASN Position Statement)*, 2018. Retrieved from https://higherlogicdownload.s3.amazonaws.com.

Willgerodt MA, Brock DM, Maughan ED: Public school nursing practice in the United States, *J Sch Nurs* 34(3):232–244, 2018.

Wold SJ, Selekman J: Frameworks and models for school nursing practice. In Selekman J, editor: *School nursing: a comprehensive text*, ed 2, Philadelphia, 2013, F.A. Davis Company, pp 79–108.

Wolfe L: The profession of school nursing. In Selekman J, editor: *School nursing: a comprehensive text*, ed 2, Philadelphia, 2013, F.A. Davis Company, pp 25–47.

Yonkaitis CF, Shannon RA: The role of the school nurse in the special education process: Part 1 student identification and evaluation, *NASN School Nurse* 32(3):179–184, 2017.

Zaiger D: Historical perspectives of school nursing. In Selekman J, editor: *School nursing: a comprehensive text*, ed 2, Philadelphia, 2013, F.A. Davis Company, pp 2–24.

43

The Nurse in Occupational Health

Bonnie Rogers, DrPH, COHN-S, LNCC, FAAN

OBJECTIVES

After reading this chapter, the student should be able to do the following:

1. Describe the nursing role in occupational health.
2. Discuss current trends in the U.S. workforce.
3. Use the epidemiologic model to explain work–health interactions and give examples of work-related illness, injuries, and hazards.
4. Complete an occupational health history.
5. Differentiate between the functions of the Occupational Safety and Health Administration (OSHA) and the National Institute for Occupational Safety and Health (NIOSH).
6. Explain an effective disaster plan in occupational health.

CHAPTER OUTLINE

Definition and Scope of Occupational Health Nursing
History and Evolution of Occupational Health Nursing
Roles and Professionalism in Occupational Health Nursing
Workers as a Population Aggregate
Application of the Epidemiologic Model
Organizational and Public Efforts to Promote Worker Health and Safety
Nursing Care of Working Populations
***Healthy People 2020* Document Related to Occupational Health**
Legislation Related to Occupational Health

KEY TERMS

agents, p. 962
biological agents, p. 963
chemical agents, p. 965
enviromechanical agents, p. 965
environments, p. 957
Hazard Communication Standard, p. 973
host, p. 962
National Institute for Occupational Safety and Health (NIOSH), p. 973
National Occupational Research Agenda (NORA), p. 973
occupational and environmental health nursing, p. 958
occupational health hazards, p. 970
occupational health history, p. 968
physical agents, p. 965
psychosocial agents, p. 965
work–health interactions, p. 958
workers' compensation acts, p. 973
worksite walk-through, p. 970

Work can be both fulfilling and hazardous or risky. Many changes have occurred in the nature of work and workplace risks, the work environment, workforce composition and demographics, and health care delivery mechanisms. An analysis of the trends suggests that work–health interactions will continue to grow in importance, affecting how work is done, how hazards are controlled or minimized, and how health care is managed and integrated into workplace health delivery strategies. Although some workers may never face more than minor adverse health effects from exposures at work, such as occasional eyestrain resulting from poor office lighting, every industry has grappled with serious hazards (USDHHS, NIOSH, 2018). Nurses provide care to individuals to help them achieve optimal health; yet, at the same time in the course of their work, nurses face numerous hazardous substances such as blood, body fluids, or chemicals and often must lift heavy loads.

In America, work is viewed as important to one's life experiences, and most adults spend about one-third of their time at work (Rogers, 2019). Work—when fulfilling, fairly compensated, healthy, and safe—can help build long and contented lives and strengthen families and communities. No work is completely risk free, and all health care professionals should have some basic knowledge about workforce populations, work and related hazards, and methods to control hazards and improve health.

Important developments are occurring in occupational health and safety programs designed to prevent and control work-related illness and injury and to create environments that foster and support health-promoting activities. Occupational health nurses have performed critical roles in planning and delivering worksite health and safety services, which must continue to grow as comprehensive and cost-effective services. In addition, the continuing increase in health care costs and the concern about health care quality have prompted the inclusion of primary care and management of non–work-related health problems in the health services' programs. In some settings, family services are also provided.

Health at work is an important issue for most individuals for whom the nurse provides care. With many individuals spending so much time working, the workplace, regardless of setting, has significant influence on health and can be a primary site for the delivery of health promotion and illness prevention. The home, the clinic, the nursing home, and other community sites, such as the workplace, will become the dominant areas where health and illness care will be sought.

This chapter describes the nurse's role in occupational health—working with employees and the workforce population. The focus is on the knowledge and skills needed to promote the health and safety of workers through occupational health programs, recognizing work-related health and safety, and the principles for prevention and control of adverse **work–health interactions**. The prevalence and significance of the interactions between health and work underscore the importance of including principles of occupational health and safety in nursing practice. The types of interactions and the frequent use of the general health care system for identifying, treating, and preventing occupational illnesses and injuries require nurses to use this knowledge in all practice settings. The epidemiologic triangle is used as one model for understanding these interactions, as well as risk factors, and effective nursing care for promoting health and safety among employed populations.

DEFINITION AND SCOPE OF OCCUPATIONAL HEALTH NURSING

Adapted from the American Association of Occupational Health Nurses (AAOHN) (2016), **occupational and environmental health nursing** is the specialty practice that provides for and delivers health and safety programs and services to workers, worker populations, and community groups. The practice focuses on the promotion and restoration of health, prevention of illness and injury, and protection from work-related and environmental hazards. Occupational and environmental health nurses have a combined knowledge of health and business that they blend with health care expertise to balance the requirement for a safe and healthful work environment with a healthy bottom line.

The foundation for occupational and environmental health nursing is research-based. Recognizing the legal context for occupational health and safety, this specialty practice derives its theoretical, conceptual, and factual framework from a multidisciplinary base including, but not limited to:

- Nursing science
- Medical science
- Public health sciences such as epidemiology and environmental health
- Occupational health sciences such as toxicology, safety, industrial hygiene, and ergonomics
- Social and behavioral sciences
- Management, administration, and financial principles

Guided by an ethical framework made explicit in the AAOHN *Code of Ethics* (2016), occupational and environmental health nurses encourage and enable individuals to make informed decisions about health care concerns. Confidentiality of health information is integral and central to the practice. Occupational and environmental health nurses are advocates for client(s), fostering equitable and quality health care services and safe and healthy environments in which to work.

HISTORY AND EVOLUTION OF OCCUPATIONAL HEALTH NURSING

Nursing care for workers began in 1888 and was called industrial nursing. A group of coal miners hired Betty Moulder, a graduate of the Blockley Hospital School of Nursing in Philadelphia (now Philadelphia General Hospital), to take care of their ailing coworkers and families (AAOHN, 1976). Ada Mayo Stewart, hired in 1885 by the Vermont Marble Company in Rutland, Vermont, is often considered the first industrial nurse. Riding a bicycle, Miss Stewart visited sick employees in their homes, provided emergency care, taught mothers how to care for their children, and taught healthy living habits (Felton, 1985). In the early days of occupational health nursing, the nurse's work was family centered and holistic.

Employee health services grew rapidly during the early 1900s as companies recognized that the provision of worksite health services led to a more productive workforce. At that time, workplace accidents were seen as an inevitable part of having a job. However, the public did not support this attitude, and a system for workers' compensation arose that remains today (McGrath, 1945).

Industrial nursing grew rapidly during the first half of the twentieth century. Educational courses were established, as were professional societies. By World War II there were about 4000 industrial nurses (Brown, 1981). The American Association of Industrial Nursing (AAIN) (now called the American Association of Occupational Health Nurses) was established as the first national occupational nursing organization in 1942. The aim of the AAIN was to improve industrial nursing education and practice and to promote interprofessional collaborative efforts (Rogers, 1988). Passage of several laws in the 1960s and 1970s to protect workers' safety and health led to an increased need for occupational health nurses. In particular, the passing of the landmark Occupational Safety and Health Act in 1970, which created the Occupational Safety and Health Administration (OSHA) and the National Institute for Occupational Safety and Health (NIOSH), discussed later in this chapter, resulted in a great need for nurses at the worksite to meet the demands of the many standards being implemented. Under OSHA, the Act focuses primarily on protecting workers from work-related hazards. NIOSH focuses on education and research. In 1988 the first occupational health nurse was hired by OSHA to provide technical assistance in standards development, field consultation, and occupational health nursing expertise. In 1993 the Office of Occupational Health Nursing was established within the agency. In addition to direct health care delivery, nurses are more engaged than ever in policy making and management of occupational health services. In addition, in 1998, the AAOHN adopted the concept of environmental health as a significant component of the practice field. To this end, AAOHN has incorporated the term "environmental," as in occupational and environmental health nurse, in its documents and publications. In 1999, AAOHN published its first set of competencies in occupational health nursing, which have been updated, and established the AAOHN Foundation to support education, research, and leadership activities in occupational health nursing. Role expansion includes environmental health, total worker health, and forging sustainable relationships in the community to better improve worker health.

ROLES AND PROFESSIONALISM IN OCCUPATIONAL HEALTH NURSING

As U.S. industry has shifted from agrarian to industrial to highly technological processes, the role of the occupational health nurse has continued to change. The focus on work-related health problems now includes the spectrum of human responses to multiple, complex interactions of biopsychosocial factors that occur in community, home, and work environments. The customary role of the occupational health nurse has extended beyond emergency treatment and prevention of illness and injury to include the promotion and maintenance of health, overall risk management, care for the environment, efforts to reduce health-related costs in businesses, and total worker health. The interprofessional nature of occupational health nursing has become more critical, as occupational health and safety problems require more complex solutions. The occupational health nurse frequently collaborates closely with multiple disciplines and industry management, as well as with representatives of labor.

Occupational health nurses constitute the largest group of occupational health professionals. The most recent national survey of registered nurses indicates that there are about 19,000 licensed occupational health nurses (Health Resources and Services Administration, 2010). Occupational health nurses hold positions as nurse practitioners, clinical nurse specialists, managers, supervisors, consultants, educators, and researchers, and many occupational health nurses are employed in single-managed occupational health nurse units in a variety of businesses. The occupational health nursing role requires the nurse to adapt to an organization's needs as well as to the needs of specific groups of workers.

The professional organization for occupational health nurses is the American Association of Occupational Health Nurses. The AAOHN's mission is comprehensive. It supports the work of the occupational health nurse and advances the specialty. The AAOHN also does the following:

- Promotes the health and safety of workers
- Defines the scope of practice and sets the standards of occupational health nursing practice
- Develops the code of ethics for occupational health nurses with interpretive statements
- Promotes and provides continuing education in the specialty
- Advances the profession through supporting research
- Responds to and influences public policy issues related to occupational health and safety

The AAOHN (2012) provides the Standards of Occupational and Environmental Health Nursing Practice to define and advance practice and provide a framework for practice evaluation. The AAOHN Code of Ethics lists eight code statements based on the goal of occupational and environmental health nurses to promote worker health and safety (AAOHN, 2016). Both documents can be obtained from the AAOHN at http://www.aaohn.org.

Occupational health nurses have many roles, such as clinician, case manager, coordinator, manager, nurse practitioner, corporate director, health promotion specialist, educator, consultant, and researcher (Rogers, 2019). The majority of occupational health nurses work as solo clinicians, but additional roles are being included increasingly in the specialty practice. In many companies, the occupational health nurse has assumed expanded responsibilities in job analysis, safety, and benefits management. Many occupational health nurses also work as independent contractors and consultants or have their own businesses that provide occupational health and safety services to industry. Specializing in the field is often a requirement.

Ethical conflict is nothing new in occupational and environmental health nursing practice. Traditional concerns about confidentiality of employee health records, hazardous workplace exposures, issues of informed consent, risks and benefits, and dual duty conflicts (workers versus management) are now married with newer concerns of genetic screening, worker literacy and understanding, work organization issues, and untimely return to work (Rogers, 2019). With the current changes in health care delivery and the movement toward managed care, occupational health nurses will need increased skills in primary care, health promotion, and disease prevention. The aim of the occupational health nurse will be to devote much attention to keeping workers and, in some cases, their families healthy and free from illness and worksite injuries.

Academic education in occupational health and safety is generally at the graduate level. Training grants from NIOSH support master's and doctoral-level education with emphases in occupational health nursing, industrial hygiene, occupational medicine, and safety. These programs, shown in the resource section, are offered through NIOSH funded Occupational Safety and Health Education and Research Centers throughout the country. Certification in occupational health nursing is provided by the American Board for Occupational Health Nurses (ABOHN). ABOHN offers two basic certifications: the COHN (Certified Occupational Health Nurse) and COHN-S (Certified Occupational Health Nurse–Specialist). Eligibility for the COHN requires licensure as a registered nurse, whereas the COHN-S requires RN licensure plus a baccalaureate degree. Certification is achieved through experience, continuing education, professional activities, and examination. Those interested in certification can view the requirements on the ABOHN website (www.abohn.org).

WORKERS AS A POPULATION AGGREGATE

The population of the United States is expected to increase from about 326 million people in 2018 to an estimated 404 million by the year 2060 (U.S. Census Bureau, 2018). In the United States in 2050, the population greater than 65 years of age is projected to reach an estimated 83.7 million people, almost double the about 43 million in 2012 (Ortman et al., 2014). In 2016, nearly 20 percent (ninc million) of Americans over 65 were employed compared to about 12 percent in 2000 (Desilver, 2018). Bureau of Labor Statistics (BLS, 2018) data show total workforce projection to increase by 7.4 percent from 2016 to 2026 with workers aged 65 to 74 experiencing the fastest growth rate.

By 2024, the BLS projects the labor force will grow to 164 million civilian wage and salary workers employed in the United States (Toossi & Torpey, 2017). More than 91 percent of those who are able to work outside of the home do so for some portion of their lives. These statistics do not indicate the number of individuals who are at risk of exposure to work-related health hazards. Although some individuals may currently be unemployed or retired, they continue to bear the health risks of past occupational exposures. The number of affected individuals may be even larger, as work-related illnesses are found among spouses, children, and neighbors of exposed workers. In addition, more than seven million individuals report that they work multiple jobs (BLS, 2018).

Americans are employed in diverse industries that range in size from one to tens of thousands of employees. Types of industries include traditional manufacturing (e.g., automotive and appliances), service industries (e.g., banking, health care, and restaurants), agriculture, construction, and high-technology firms, such as computer chip manufacturers. Although some industries are noted for the high degree of hazards associated with their work (e.g., manufacturing, mines, construction, and agriculture), no worksite is free of occupational health and safety hazards. In addition, the larger the company, the more likely it is that there will be health and safety programs for employees. Smaller companies are more apt to rely on external community resources to meet their needs for occupational health and safety services.

Characteristics of the Workforce

The U.S. workplace has been changing rapidly. Jobs in the economy continue to shift from manufacturing to service. Longer hours, compressed workweeks, shift work, reduced job security, and part-time and temporary work are realities of the modern workplace. New chemicals, materials, processes, and equipment are developed and marketed at an ever-increasing pace.

As the population increases, the U.S. workforce is expected to grow as well and will become older and more racially diverse (BLS, 2018b). These changes will continue to present new challenges to protecting worker safety and health.

The demographic trends in the U.S. workforce describe a changing population aggregate that has implications for the prevention services targeted to that group. Major changes in the working population are reflected in the increasing numbers of women, older individuals, and those with chronic illnesses who are part of the workforce. Because of changes in the economy, extension of life span, legislation, and more working women, the proportion of the employed population that these three groups represent will probably continue to grow.

For example, in the late 1990s, while nearly 60 percent of all women were employed, women were predicted to account for 67 percent of the increase in the labor force in the twenty-first century (BLS, 2018). These workers tended to be married, with children and aging parents for whom they were responsible. This aggregate of workers presents new issues for individual and family health promotion, such as childcare and elder care, which can be addressed in the work environment. In 1990 more than half of the female labor force was concentrated in three areas: administrative support/clerical (26 percent), service (14 percent), and professional specialty (14 percent). Twelve percent were employed in fields such as labor, transportation and moving, machine operation, precision products, crafts, farming, construction, forestry, and fishing. In the male labor force, nearly 20 percent worked in precision production, crafts, or repair occupations, 13 percent in executive positions, 11 percent in professional specialty occupations, and 10 percent in sales. Other trends shaping the profile of the workforce include more education and mobility.

Future employment trends projected to 2026 are shown in Figs. 43.1 and 43.2. Of the 20 fastest-growing occupations in the economy, 10 are related to health care (BLS, 2018a). Health care is experiencing rapid growth, due in large part to the aging of the Baby Boomer generation, who will require more medical care. In addition, some health care occupations will be in greater demand for other reasons. As health care costs continue to rise, work is increasingly being delegated to lower-paid workers in order to cut costs. For example, tasks that were previously performed by doctors, nurses, dentists, or other health care professionals increasingly are being performed by physician assistants, nursing and medical assistants, dental hygienists, and physical therapist aides. In addition, clients increasingly are seeking home care as an alternative to costly stays in hospitals or residential care facilities, causing a significant increase in demand for home health aides. Although not classified as health care workers, personal and home care aides are being affected by this demand for home care as well.

Characteristics of Work

There has been a dramatic shift in the types of jobs held by workers. Following the evolution from an agrarian economy to a manufacturing society and then to a highly technological workplace, the greatest proportion of paid employment was in the occupations of trade, transportation, and utilities.

The nature of work has been accompanied by many new occupational hazards, such as complex chemicals, nanotechnology, nonergonomic workstation design (requiring the adaptation of the workplace or work equipment to meet the employee's

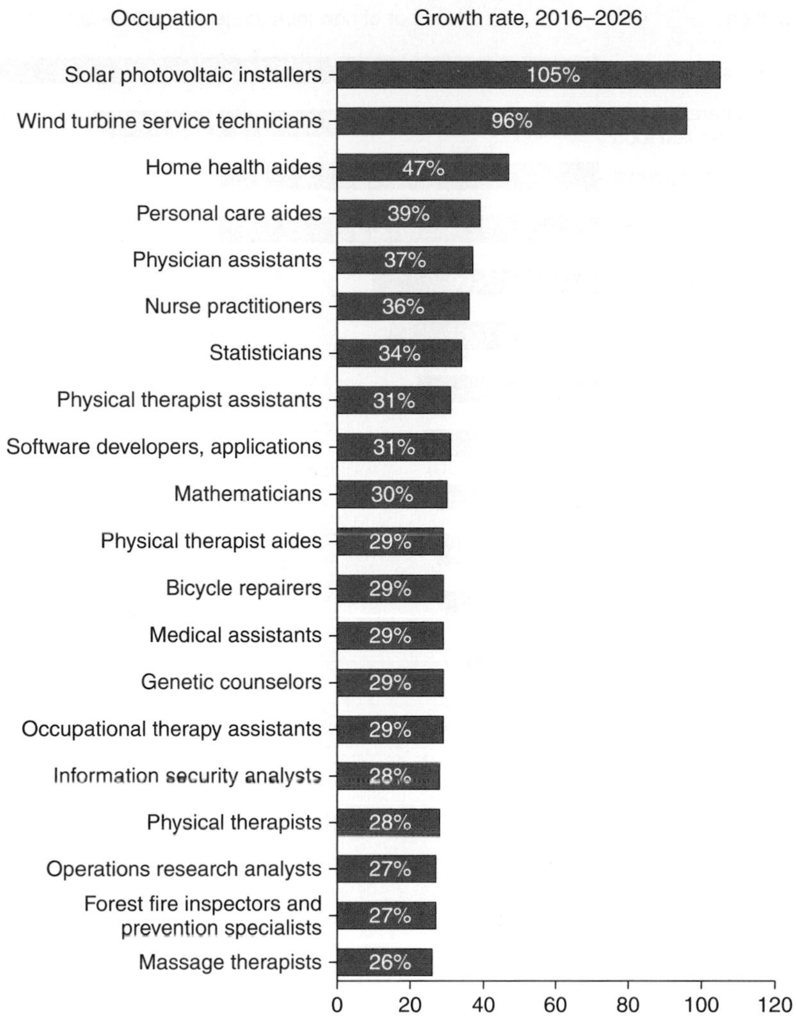

Fig. 43.1 Fastest growing occupations 2016–2026. (From Bureau of Labor Statistics, 2018. Available at https://www.bls.gov.)

health and safety needs), and many issues related to work organization such as job stress, burnout, and exhaustion. In addition, the emergence of a global economy with free trade and multinational corporations presents new challenges for health and safety programs that are culturally relevant.

Work–Health Interactions

The influence of work on health, or work–health interactions, is shown by statistics on illnesses, injuries, and deaths associated with employment.

As reported by the Census of Fatal Occupational Injuries (CFOI) (BLS, 2017s), there were 5190 fatal work injuries recorded in the United States in 2016, a seven-percent increase from the 4836 fatal injuries reported in 2015. This is the third consecutive increase in annual workplace fatalities and the first time more than 5000 fatalities have been recorded by the CFOI since 2008. The fatal injury rate increased to 3.6 per 100,000 workers from 3.4 in 2015, the highest rate since 2010. Fatal work injuries from falls, slips, or trips continued a general upward trend from 2011, increasing 6 percent in 2016 and 25 percent overall since 2011. Overdoses from the nonmedical use of drugs or alcohol while on the job increased from 165 in 2015 to 217 in 2016, a 32-percent increase. Overdose fatalities have increased by at least 25 percent annually since 2012.

Employers reported 2.9 work injuries and occupational illnesses per 100 workers in 2016 (BLS, 2017a) with 2.9 million incidents reported. Occupational injuries alone are reported to cost over $100 billion in lost wages and lost productivity, administrative expenses, health care, and other costs. This figure does not include the cost of occupational diseases. These figures are often described as the "tip of the iceberg," because many work-related health problems go unreported. However, even the recorded statistics are significant in describing the amount of human suffering, financial loss, and decreased productivity associated with workplace hazards. In 2016, there were 892,270 occupational injuries and illnesses resulting in days away from work with a median of 8 days absent (BLS, 2017b).

The high number of work injuries and illnesses can be drastically reduced. In fact, significant progress has been made in improving worker protection since Congress passed the 1970 Occupational Safety and Health Act. For example, vinyl chloride–induced liver cancers and brown lung disease (byssinosis) from

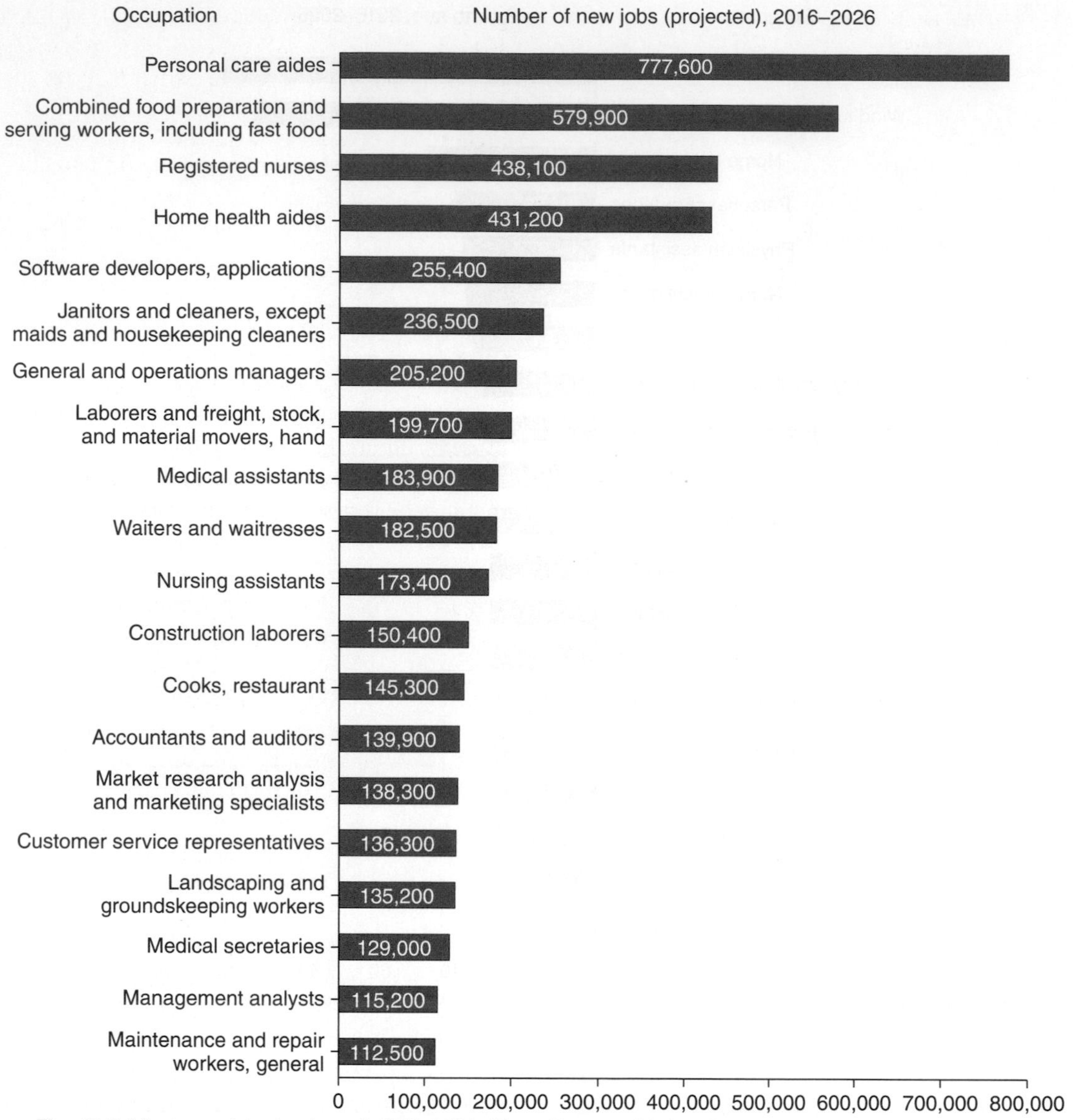

Fig. 43.2 Most new jobs (projected) 2016–2026. (From Bureau of Labor Statistics, 2018. Available at https://www.bls.gov.)

cotton dust exposure have been almost eliminated. Reproductive disorders associated with certain glycol ethers have been recognized and controlled. Fatal work injuries have declined substantially through the years. Notably, from 1970 to 1995, fatal injury rates in coal miners were reduced by more than 75 percent, and the disease prevalence was reduced by 90 percent. However, since 1995 there has been a doubling of the disease incidence (NIOSH, 2014).

The U.S. workplace is rapidly changing and becoming more diverse. Major changes are also occurring in the way work is organized, with increased shift work, reduced job security, and part-time and temporary work as realities of the modern workplace. In addition, new chemicals, materials, processes, and equipment (such as nanotechnology and fermentation processes in biotechnology) continue to be developed and marketed at an accelerating pace, creating new work-related hazards.

APPLICATION OF THE EPIDEMIOLOGIC MODEL

The Epidemiologic Triangle can be used to understand the relationship between work and health (Fig. 43.3). The reader is referred to Chapter 13, Epidemiology, for a fuller description. With a focus on the health and safety of the employed population, the **host** is described as any susceptible human being. Because of the nature of work-related hazards, nurses must assume that all employed individuals and groups are at risk of being exposed to occupational hazards. The **agents**, factors associated with illness and injury, are occupational exposures that are classified as biological, chemical, enviromechanical, physical, or psychosocial (Box 43.1). The environment includes all external conditions that influence the interaction of the host and agents. These may be workplace conditions such as temperature extremes, crowding, shift work, and inflexible management styles. The basic principle of epidemiology is that health

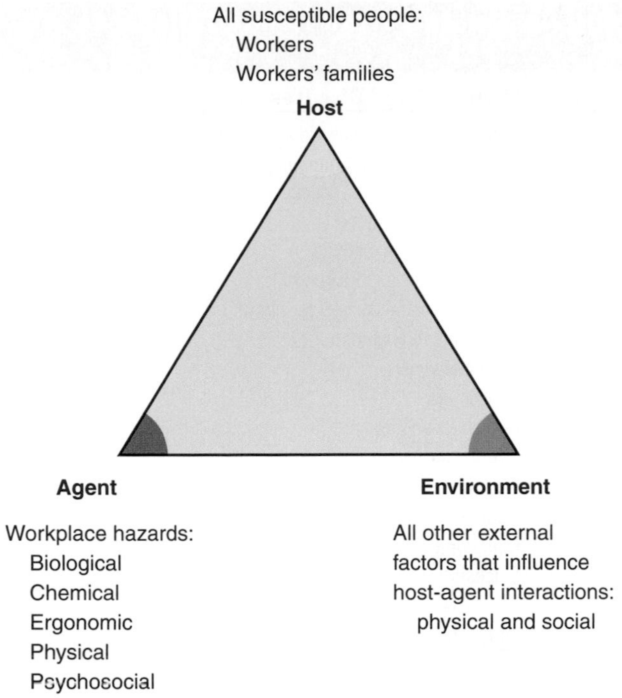

Fig. 43.3 The epidemiologic triangle.

BOX 43.1 Categories of Work-Related Hazards

Biological and infectious hazards—Infectious/biological agents, such as bacteria, viruses, fungi, or parasites, that may be transmitted via contact with infected clients or contaminated body secretions/fluids to other individuals

Chemical hazards—Various forms of chemicals, including medications, solutions, gases, vapors, aerosols, and particulate matter, that are potentially toxic or irritating to the body system

Enviromechanical hazards—Factors encountered in the work environment that cause or potentiate accidents, injuries, strain, or discomfort (e.g., unsafe/inadequate equipment or lifting devices, slippery floors, workstation deficiencies)

Physical hazards—Agents within the work environment, such as radiation, electricity, extreme temperatures, and noise, that can cause tissue trauma

Psychosocial hazards—Factors and situations encountered or associated with one's job or work environment that create or potentiate stress, emotional strain, or interpersonal problems

From Rogers B: *Occupational health nursing: concepts and practice.* In press, 2019.

status interventions for restoring and promoting health are the result of complex interactions among these three elements. To understand these interactions and to design effective nursing strategies for dealing with them in a proactive manner, nurses must look at how each of these elements influences the others.

Host

Each worker represents a host within the worker population group. Certain host factors are associated with increased risk of adverse response to the hazards of the workplace. These include age, sex, health status, work practices, ethnicity, and lifestyle factors (Rogers, 2019). For example, the population group at greatest risk for experiencing work-related accidents with subsequent injuries is new workers with less than one year of experience on the current job. Most nonfatal injuries and illnesses involving days away from work occur among new workers (the highest percentages were in mining [44 percent]; agriculture, forestry, and fishing [43 percent]; construction [41 percent]; and wholesale and retail trade [34 percent]). Thirty-five percent of injury and illness cases with days away from work occurred among workers with 5 or fewer years of service with their employer (BLS, 2017b). The host factors of age, sex, and work experience combine to increase this group's risk of injury because of characteristics such as risk taking, lack of knowledge, and lack of familiarity with the new job.

Older workers may be at increased risk in the workplace because of diminished sensory abilities, the effects of chronic illnesses, and delayed reaction times. Another population group that may be very susceptible to workplace exposure is women in their childbearing years. The hormonal changes during these years (along with the increased stress of new roles and additional responsibilities) and transplacental exposures are host factors that may influence this group's response to potential toxins.

In addition to these host factors, there may be other, less well-understood individual differences in response to occupational hazard exposures. Even if employers maintain exposure levels below the level recommended by occupational health and safety standards, 15 percent to 20 percent of the population may have health reactions to the "safe" low-level exposures (Levy et al., 2017). This group has been termed *hypersusceptible.* A number of host factors appear to be associated with this hypersusceptibility: light skin, malnutrition, compromised immune system, glucose-6-phosphate dehydrogenase deficiency, serum alpha1-antitrypsin deficiency, chronic obstructive pulmonary disease, sickle cell trait, and hypertension. Individuals who have known hypersusceptibility to chemicals that are respiratory irritants, hemolytic chemicals, organic isocyanates, and carbon disulfide may also be hypersusceptible to other agents in the work environment (Levy et al., 2017). Although this has prompted some industries to consider preplacement screening for such risk factors, the associations between these individual health markers and hypersusceptible response are speculative and require further research.

Agent

Work-related hazards, or agents (see Box 43.1), present potential and actual risks to the health and safety of workers in the millions of business establishments in the United States. Any worksite commonly presents multiple and interacting exposures from all five categories of agents. The following paragraphs discuss each of these five agents in more detail. Table 43.1 lists some of the more common workplace exposures, their known health effects, and the types of jobs associated with these hazards.

Biological Agents. Biological agents are living organisms whose excretions or parts are capable of causing human disease, usually by an infectious process. Biological hazards are common in workplaces such as health care facilities and clinical laboratories, where employees are potentially exposed to a variety of infectious agents, including viruses, fungi, and bacteria. Of particular

TABLE 43.1 Selected Job Categories, Exposures, and Associated Work-Related Diseases and Conditions

Job Categories	Exposures	Work-Related Diseases and Conditions
All workers	Workplace stress	Hypertension, mood disorders, cardiovascular disease
Agricultural workers	Pesticides, infectious agents, gases, sunlight	Pesticide poisoning, "farmer's lung," skin cancer
Anesthetists	Anesthetic gases	Reproductive effects, cancer
Automobile workers	Asbestos, plastics, lead, solvents	Asbestosis, dermatitis
Butchers	Vinyl plastic fumes	"Meat wrappers' asthma"
Caisson workers	Pressurized work environments	Caisson disease ("the bends")
Carpenters	Wood dust, wood preservatives, adhesives	Nasopharyngeal cancer, dermatitis
Cement workers	Cement dust, metals	Dermatitis, bronchitis
Ceramic workers	Talc, clays	Pneumoconiosis
Demolition workers	Asbestos, wood dust	Asbestosis
Drug manufacturers	Hormones, nitroglycerin, etc.	Reproductive effects
Dry cleaners	Solvents	Liver disease, dermatitis
Dye workers	Dyestuffs, metals, solvents	Bladder cancer, dermatitis
Embalmers	Formaldehyde, infectious agents	Dermatitis
Felt makers	Mercury, polycyclic hydrocarbons	Mercurialism
Foundry workers	Silica, molten metals	Silicosis
Glass workers	Heat, solvents, metal powders	Cataracts
Hospital workers	Infectious agents, cleansers, radiation	Infections, latex allergies, unintentional injuries
Insulators	Asbestos, fibrous glass	Asbestosis, lung cancer, mesothelioma
Jack-hammer operators	Vibration	Raynaud's phenomenon
Lathe operators	Metal dusts, cutting oils	Lung disease, cancer
Office computer workers	Repetitive wrist motion on computers	Tendonitis, carpal tunnel syndrome, tenosynovitis, eye strain

concern in occupational health is the infectious agent transmitted by humans (e.g., from client to worker or from worker to worker) in a variety of work settings. Bloodborne and airborne pathogens represent a significant class of exposures for U.S. health care workers at risk. Occupational transmission of bloodborne pathogens (including the hepatitis B and C viruses and the human immunodeficiency virus [HIV]) occurs primarily by means of needlestick injuries as well as through exposures to the eyes or mucous membranes (Dupler et al., 2013). The risk of hepatitis B virus infection following a single needlestick injury with a contaminated needle varies from 2 percent to greater than 40 percent, depending on the antigen status of the source person and the nature of the exposure. The risk of hepatitis C virus transmission depends on the same factors and ranges from 3.3 percent to 10 percent (Dupler et al., 2013).

While the number of cases and reports of tuberculosis has decreased in the United States, transmission of tuberculosis (TB) within health care settings (especially multidrug-resistant TB) continues as a major public health problem (Stewart et al., 2017). Since 1989 outbreaks of this type of TB have been reported in hospitals, and some workers have developed active drug-resistant TB. In addition, among workers in health care, social service, and correctional facilities who work with populations at increased risk of TB, hundreds have experienced tuberculin skin test conversions. Reliable data are lacking on the extent of possible work-related TB transmission among other groups of workers at risk for exposure. Many workers in these settings were employed as maintenance workers, security guards, aides, or cleaning people, who were not well protected from inadvertent exposure. Education should be provided to all health care workers, including those not having direct client care, in the proper handling and disposal of potentially contaminated linens, soiled equipment, and trash containing contaminated dressings or specimens (Gonzalez & Conlon, 2013) (see Evidence-Based Practice box).

EVIDENCE-BASED PRACTICE

The aim of this study was to investigate occupational exposures of health care workers to blood and body fluids in eastern Ethiopia (Reda et al., 2010). Health care workers still fail to adhere to standard precaution guidelines despite evidence that such a failure increases the risk of mucocutaneous blood and body fluid exposure resulting in bloodborne infection. The major infectious occupational hazards in the health care sector are hepatitis B and C viruses (HBV, HCV) and human immunodeficiency virus (HIV).

A total of 475 health care workers were surveyed working in 10 hospitals in eastern Ethiopia with an 84.4 percent response rate. Lifetime needlestick risk was 30.5 percent, and lifetime blood/body fluid exposure risk was 28.8 percent. Only 80.8 percent followed standard precautions regularly, while 46.9 percent recapped and 5.9 percent reused syringes; 44.8 percent of health care workers reported they were dissatisfied by the supply of personal protective equipment (PPE), and 70.9 percent perceived they were at risk in the workplace.

Nurse Use

Training programs and better provision of PPE are critically needed. Compliance with PPE must be emphasized along with effective teaching in infection control and safe work practice behavior.

Modified from Reda AA, Fisseha S, Mengistie B, et al.: Standard precautions: occupational exposure and behavior of health care workers in Ethiopia. *PLoS One* 5(12):e14420, 2010. doi:10.1371/journal.pone.0014420.

Chemical Agents. More than 300 billion pounds of chemical agents are produced annually in the United States. Of the about 2 million known chemicals in existence, less than 0.1 percent have been adequately studied for their effects on humans. Of those chemicals that have been linked to carcinogens, about half test positive as animal carcinogens. Most chemicals have not been studied epidemiologically to determine the effects of exposure on humans (Levy et al., 2017). As a consequence of general environmental contamination with chemicals from work, home, and community activities, a variety of chemicals have been found in the body tissues of the general population. These tissue loads may result in part from the accidental release of chemicals into the environment, such as that which occurred in Love Canal when chemicals leached out from buried industrial wastes.

In many workplaces, significant exposure to a daily, low-level dose of workplace chemicals may be below the exposure standards but may still create a potentially chronic and perhaps cumulative assault on workers' health. Predicting human responses to such exposures is further complicated because multiple chemicals often combine and interact to create a new chemical agent. Human effects may be associated with the interaction of these agents rather than with a single chemical. Another concern about occupational exposure to chemicals is reproductive health effects. Workplace reproductive hazards have become important legal and scientific issues. Toxicity to male and female reproductive systems has been demonstrated from exposure to common agents such as lead, mercury, cadmium, nickel, and zinc, as well as in antineoplastic drugs. Because data for predicting human responses to many chemical agents are inadequate, workers should be assessed for all potential exposures and cautioned to work preventively with these agents. High-risk or vulnerable workers, such as those with a latex allergy—a widely recognized health hazard—should be carefully screened and monitored for optimal health protection (Levy et al., 2017). To accurately assess and evaluate the exposure and recommend changes for abatement, it is essential that the nurse have a good understanding of the basic principles of toxicology, including routes of exposure (i.e., inhalation, skin absorption, and ingestion), dose-response relationships, and differences in effects (i.e., acute versus chronic toxicity).

Enviromechanical Agents. Enviromechanical agents are those that can potentially cause injury or illness in the workplace. They are related to the work process or to working conditions, and they can cause postural or other strains that can produce adverse health effects when certain tasks are performed repeatedly. Examples are repetitive motions, poor or unsafe workstation-worker fit, slippery floors, cluttered work areas, and lifting heavy loads. Severity of illness or injury can be estimated from the number of days away from work. In 2016 (BLS, 2017b), sprains and strains, bruises/contusions, cuts/lacerations, fractures, and multiple injuries accounted for more days away from work than for all types of injury and illness, accounting for 30 percent of total injury and illness cases.

Back pain/injury is one of the most common and significant musculoskeletal problems in the world. In 2011, back injuries and disorders accounted for 36 percent of all nonfatal occupational injuries and illnesses involving days away from work in the United States. Although the exact cost of back disorders is unknown, the estimates are staggering and in the billions per year. Regardless of the estimate used, the problem is large both in health and economic terms. Moreover, workers in six occupations accounted for 26 percent of musculoskeletal cases: nursing assistants; laborers; janitors and cleaners; heavy and tractor-trailer truck drivers; registered nurses; and stock clerks (BLS, 2011). The research on these hazards, related human responses, and prevention is evolving. The most productive strategy in preventing these exposures is redesigning the workplace and the work machinery or processes.

Physical Agents. Physical agents are those that produce adverse health effects through the transfer of physical energy. Commonly encountered physical agents in the workplace include temperature extremes, vibration, noise, lasers, radiation, and electricity. For example, vibration, which accompanies the use of power tools and vehicles such as trucks, affects internal organs, supportive ligaments, the upper torso, and the shoulder-girdle structure. Localized effects are seen with handheld power tools; the most common is Raynaud's phenomenon. The control of worker exposure to these agents is usually accomplished through engineering strategies such as eliminating or containing the hazardous agent. In addition, workers must use preventive actions, such as practicing safe work habits and wearing personal protective equipment when needed. Examples of safe work habits include taking appropriate breaks from environments with temperature extremes and not eating or smoking in radiation-contaminated areas. Personal protective equipment includes hearing protection, eye guards, protective clothing, and devices for monitoring exposures to agents such as radiation.

Psychosocial Agents. Psychosocial agents are conditions that create a threat to the psychological and/or social well-being of individuals and groups (Rogers, 2019). A psychosocial response to the work environment occurs as an employee acts selectively toward the environment in an attempt to achieve a harmonious relationship. When such a human attempt at adaptation to the environment fails, an adverse psychosocial response may occur. Work-related stress or burnout has been defined as an important problem for many individuals (Rogers, 2019). Responses to negative interpersonal relationships, particularly those with authority figures in the workplace, are often the cause of vague health symptoms and increased absenteeism. Epidemiologic work in mental health has pointed to environmental variables such as these in the incidence of mental illness and emotional disorder.

The psychosocial environment includes characteristics of the work itself, as well as the interpersonal relationships required in the work setting and shift work. About 10 percent of U.S. workers do some form of shift work that has the potential to lead to a variety of psychological and physical problems, including exhaustion, depression, anxiety, and gastrointestinal disturbance (BLS, 2018). Strategies to minimize the adverse effects of shift work are beneficial. For example, a rotating shift allows the employee to move through a cycle of working the day shift, then the evening shift, and then the night shift over the course of several weeks, with the goal of the workforce sharing the stress of the least desirable shifts. Job characteristics such as low autonomy, poor job satisfaction, and limited control over the pace of work have been associated with an increased risk of heart disease among clerical and blue-collar workers.

Interpersonal relationships among employees and coworkers or bosses and managers are often sources of conflict and stress. Another aspect is organizational culture. This refers to the norms and patterns of behavior that are sanctioned within a particular organization. Such norms and patterns set guidelines for the types of work behaviors that will enable employees to succeed within a particular firm. Examples include following organizational norms for working overtime, expressing constructive dissatisfaction with management, and making work a top priority (USDHHS/NIOSH, 2002). These factors and the employee's response to them must be assessed if strategies for influencing the health and safety of workers are to be effective.

Nonfatal violence in the health care worker's workplace is a serious problem that is underreported. Much of the study of health care worker violence has been in psychiatric settings; however, reports in other areas such as the emergency department have been provided. Risk factors associated with this type of violence must be identified and strategies implemented to reduce the risk (Rogers et al., 2018).

Environment

Environmental factors influence the occurrence of host-agent interactions and may direct the course and outcome of those interactions. The physical environment involves the geological and atmospheric structure of an area and the source of such elements as water, temperature, and radiation, which may serve as positive or negative stressors. Although aspects of the physical environment (e.g., heat, odor, ventilation) may influence the host-agent interaction, the social and psychological environment can be equally important (Gordis, 2013).

New environmental problems continue to arise, such as an increase in industrial wastes and toxins and indoor and outdoor environmental pollution, which present opportunities for significant health threats to the working and general population. The social aspects of the environment encompass the economic and political forces affecting society and its health. This includes factors such as sanitation and hygiene practices, housing conditions, level and delivery of health care services, development and enforcement of health-related codes (e.g., occupational health and safety, pollution), employment conditions, population crowding, literacy, ethnic customs, extent of support for health-related research, and equal access to health care. In addition, addictive behaviors such as alcohol and substance abuse and various forms of psychosocial stress may be an outgrowth of negative social environments.

Consider an employee who is working with a potentially toxic liquid. Providing education about safe work practices and fitting the employee with protective clothing may not be adequate if the work must occur in a very hot and humid environment. As the worker becomes uncomfortable in the hot clothing, protection may be compromised by rolling up a sleeve, taking off a glove, or wiping the face with a contaminated piece of clothing. If the norms in the workplace condone such work practices (e.g., "Everyone does it when it's too hot"), the interventions that address only the host and agent will be ineffective; strategies to address the environment itself must be considered, such as cooling fans or minimization of exposure through job rotation. The epidemiologic triangle can be used as the basis for planning interventions to restore and promote the health of workers. These efforts are influenced by society and by organizational activities related to occupational health and safety (Rogers, 2019).

The occupational environment, within the context of the social environment, is represented by the workplace and work setting and the interactive effects of this environment on the worker. The nurse must consider the hazards and threats posed by this environment and the commitment of the employer to providing a safe and healthful workplace through use of preventive strategies and controls (e.g., engineering, substitution) (Rogers, 2019).

ORGANIZATIONAL AND PUBLIC EFFORTS TO PROMOTE WORKER HEALTH AND SAFETY

Promotion of worker health and safety is the goal of occupational health and safety programs. These programs are offered primarily by the employer at the workplace, but the range of services and the models for delivering them have been changing dramatically over the past few years. In addition to specific services, legislation at the federal and state levels has had a significant effect on efforts to provide a healthy and safe environment for all workers. Under the Occupational Safety and Health Act and because of increased public concern about worker health and safety, companies are cited for not meeting minimal occupational health and safety standards. Criminal charges have been filed against business owners when preventable work-related deaths occurred. These events have redirected an emphasis on preventive occupational health and safety programming.

Unless they have OSHA-regulated exposures, business firms are not required to provide occupational health and safety services that meet any specified standards. With few exceptions, there is no legal recourse for specific services or level of personnel provided by employers to protect worker health and safety. Therefore the range of services offered and the qualifications of the providers of occupational health and safety vary widely across industries. An important stimulus for health and safety programs is avoiding cost that can be attributed to the effectiveness of prevention services, as well as the need to support occupational health and safety and health promotion at the worksite.

On-Site Occupational Health and Safety Programs. Optimally, on-site occupational health and safety services are provided by a team of occupational health and safety professionals. The core members of this team are the occupational health nurse, occupational physician, industrial hygienist, and safety professional. In addition, more and more ergonomists are playing an important role in the occupational health and safety team. The largest group of health care professionals in business settings is occupational health nurses; therefore the most frequently seen model is that of the one-nurse unit. This nurse collaborates with a community physician or occupational medicine physician who provides consultation and accepts referrals when medical intervention is needed. The collaboration may occur primarily through telephone contact, or the physician may be under contract with the company to spend a certain amount of on-site time each week. As companies become larger, they are likely to hire additional nurses, safety professionals, industrial hygienists, and physicians, the latter usually on a part-time or consultant basis. An increasingly popular option is to contract some health, safety, and industrial hygiene work to external providers. The largest firms often have corporate occupational health and safety professionals who set policy and participate in company decision making at the corporate level. These professionals work with the nurses employed at the individual sites within the company. Depending on the needs of the company and the workers, additional professionals may be on the occupational health and safety team, including employee assistance counselors, physical therapists, health educators, physical fitness specialists, and toxicologists.

The services provided by on-site occupational health programs range from those focused only on work-related health and safety problems to a wide scope of services that includes primary health care (Box 43.2). Increasingly employers supporting health promotion programs are offering employees incentives to stay healthy, such as gym memberships, on-site exercise facilities, or massage therapists during work hours.

BOX 43.2 Scope of Services Provided Through an Occupational Health and Safety Program

Health/medical surveillance
Workplace monitoring/surveillance
Health assessments
Preplacement
Periodic, mandatory, voluntary assessments and services
Transfer of clients/services
Retirement/termination
Executive
Return to work
Health promotion
Health screening
Employee assistance programs
Case management
Primary health care for workers and dependents
Worker safety and health education related to occupational hazards
Job task analysis and design
Prenatal and postnatal care and support groups
Safety audits and accident prevention
Workers' compensation management
Risk management, loss control
Emergency preparedness
Preretirement counseling
Integrated health benefits programs

In industries that have exposures regulated by law, certain programs are required, such as respiratory protection or hearing conservation. The ability of a company to offer additional programs depends on employee needs, management's attitudes and understanding about health and safety, acceptance by the workers, and the economic status of the company. A significant increase in the number of health promotion and employee assistance programs offered in industry has occurred over the past few years. Health promotion programs focus on lifestyle choices that cause risks to health (e.g., job stress, obesity, smoking, stress responses, or lack of exercise) (O'Donnell, 2017). Employee assistance programs are designed to address personal problems (e.g., marital/family issues, substance abuse, or financial difficulties) that affect the employee's productivity. Since such efforts are cost-effective for businesses, they should continue to increase.

Similar types of occupational health and safety programs are available on a contractual basis from community-based providers. These may be offered by free-standing occupational health clinics, health maintenance organizations, hospitals, emergency clinics, and other health care organizations. In addition, consultants in each discipline work in the private sector (self-employed, in group practice, or in insurance companies) and in the public sector (in local and state health departments or departments of labor and industry). These services may be provided on-site, delivered at a specific location in the community, or offered through a mobile van that visits companies. These multiple resources have increased the options for companies that need occupational health and safety services, and they have also broadened the employment opportunities for health and safety professionals.

NURSING CARE OF WORKING POPULATIONS

The nurse is often the first health care provider seen by an individual with a work-related health problem. Consequently, nurses are in key positions to intervene with working populations at all levels of prevention (see the Levels of Prevention box). Prevention may be accomplished in the prepathogenesis period by measures designed to promote general optimal health, by protection against specific disease agents, or by the establishment of barriers against agents in the environment. These procedures have been termed *primary prevention.*

LEVELS OF PREVENTION

Occupational Health

Primary Prevention
Nurse provides education on use of personal protective equipment in the workplace to prevent injury/exposure.

Secondary Prevention
Nurse screens for hearing loss resulting from noise levels in the plant.

Tertiary Prevention
Nurse works with chronic diabetic workers to ensure appropriate medication use and blood glucose screening to avoid lost work days.

Secondary prevention may be accomplished by early diagnosis and prompt and adequate treatment. When the process of pathogenesis has progressed and the disease has advanced beyond its early stages, secondary prevention may be accomplished by means of adequate treatment to prevent sequelae and limit disability. Later, when defect and disability have been resolved, tertiary prevention may be accomplished by rehabilitation.

The occupational health nurse practices all levels of prevention (Rogers, 2019). Delivery of primary prevention services to employees is directed toward promoting health and averting a problem. In the occupational health setting, the purpose of health promotion is to maintain or enhance the well-being of individuals or groups of employees, and the company in general. This may include programs designed to enhance coping skills or good nutrition and knowledge about potential health hazards both inside and outside of the workplace.

Health protection (i.e., taking primary prevention measures) is designed to eliminate or reduce the risk of disease in order to prevent the development of an illness or injury. Walk-throughs by the occupational health nurse and/or other team members to identify workplace hazards are aimed at health protection. Specific protection programs or interventions often require active participation on the part of the employee. Participation in an immunization program, employment of personal protective equipment such as respirators or gloves, and cessation of smoking are examples of specific health protection measures.

CHECK YOUR PRACTICE

As a senior nursing student, you have been asked by the occupational health nurse to help develop a secondary prevention approach to detect the most common health problem shared by the workers at the auto plant in the local community. What would you do?
END

Secondary prevention occurs after a disease process has already begun. It is aimed at early detection, prompt treatment, and prevention of further limitations. For employees, early detection involves health surveillance and periodic screening to identify an illness at the earliest possible moment in its course, and elimination or modification of the hazard-producing situation. Interventions aimed at disability limitation are intended to prevent further harm or deterioration, and they include referral for counseling and treatment of an employee with an emotional or mental health problem whose work performance has deteriorated, as well as removal of workers from heavy-metal exposure who manifest neurological symptoms.

Tertiary prevention is intended to restore health as fully as possible and assist individuals to achieve their maximum level of functioning. Rehabilitation strategies such as return-to-work programs after a heart attack or limited duty programs after a cumulative trauma injury are examples of tertiary prevention.

Worker Assessment

The initial step of assessment involves the traditional history and physical assessment, emphasizing exposure to occupational hazards and individual characteristics that may predispose the client to the increased health risk of certain jobs. The **occupational health history** is an indispensable component of the health assessment of individuals (Rogers et al., 2018). Because work is a part of life for most people, including an occupational health history in all routine nursing assessments is essential. Many workers in the United States do not have access to health care services in their workplaces, yet it is not unusual to find health care providers in the community who have little or no knowledge about workplaces or expertise in occupation-related illnesses and injuries. Because of the large number of small businesses that do not have the resources for maintaining on-site health care, injured and ill workers are first seen in the public and private health care sector (e.g., in clinics, emergency departments, physicians' offices, hospitals, health maintenance organizations, and ambulatory care centers). Nurses are often the first-line assessors of these individuals and perhaps the only contact for education about self-protection from workplace hazards.

Identifying workplace exposures as sources of health problems may influence the client's course of illness and rehabilitation and may also prevent similar illnesses among others with potential for exposure (Levy et al., 2017). Including occupational health data into client assessments begins with recognizing the possible relationship between health and occupational factors. The next step is to integrate into the history-taking procedure some routine assessment questions that will provide the data necessary to confirm or rule out occupationally induced symptoms.

Symptoms of hazardous workplace exposures may be indicated by vague complaints involving any body system. These complaints are often similar to common medical problems. Three points that occupational health histories should include are a list of current and past jobs the client has held; questions about exposures to specific agents and relationships between the symptoms and activities at work, job titles, or history of exposures; and other factors that may influence the client's susceptibility to occupational agents (e.g., lifestyle history such as smoking, underlying illness, previous injury, or disabling condition).

Questions about the employee's occupational history can be included in existing assessment tools. The more complete the data collected, the more likely the nurse is to notice the influence of work–health interactions. All employees should be questioned about their employment history. To describe only a current status of "retired" or "housewife" may lead to the omission of needed data. The nurse should be aware that not all workers are well informed about the materials with which they work or about potential hazards. For this reason, the nurse must develop basic knowledge about all of the types of jobs held by clients and the possible hazards associated with them. Because there is an increased likelihood of multiple exposures from other environments such as the home and the community that may interact with workplace exposures, the nurse should extend the questioning to include this information.

Identifying work-related health problems should be an integrated focus of any assessment effort. A systematic approach for evaluating the potential for workplace exposures is the most effective intervention for detecting and preventing occupational health risks. Fig. 43.4 shows one short assessment tool

I. Present Job

A. What is your job title? ______

B. What do you do for a living? ______

C. How long have you had this job? ______

D. Describe the specific tasks of this job: ______

E. What product or service is produced by the company where you work? ______

F. Are you exposed to any of the following on your present job?

Metals	Radiation	Stress
Vapors, gases	Vibration	Others: ______
Dusts	Loud noise	
Solvents	Extreme heat or cold	

G. Do you feel you have any health problems that may be associated with your work?
If yes, describe: ______

H. How would you describe your satisfaction with your job? ______

I. Have any of your coworkers complained of illness or injuries that they associate with their jobs?
If yes, describe: ______

II. All Past Work

Starting with your first job, please provide the following information:

Job title	Years held	Description of work	Exposures	Injuries/Illnesses	Personal protection equipment used

III. Other Exposures

A. Do you have any hobbies that involve exposure to chemicals, metals, or any of the other agents mentioned before? If yes, describe: ______

B. Are any other members of your household exposed to any of the substances listed above? If yes, describe: ______

C. Do you live near any factories, dump sites, or other sources of pollution? If yes, describe: ______

Fig. 43.4 Occupational health history form.

that can be incorporated into routine history taking. Similar questions can be included in the assessment of workers' spouses and dependents, who may receive secondhand or indirect exposure to occupational hazards.

QSEN FOCUS ON QUALITY AND SAFETY EDUCATION FOR NURSES

Targeted Competency: Evidence-Based Practice

Integrates the best current clinical evidence with client and family preferences and values to provide optimal client care.

- **Knowledge:** Explain the role of evidence in determining best clinical practice.
- **Skills:** Read original research and evidence reports related to area of practice.
- **Attitudes:** Appreciate the importance of reading relevant professional journals.

Evidence-Based Practice Question

The public health nursing Quad Council competency of leadership and systems thinking skills recommends the beginning public health nurse identify organizational quality improvement initiatives that provide opportunities for improvement in public health nursing practice (2018). You are working as an occupational health nurse. You have noticed there are a lot of work days lost because of work-related injuries or exposure to some type of hazard in the workplace. In this chapter you will see which of the injuries and exposures are more likely to occur in industry. Choose one of the hazard categories and read the evidence available about this hazard category. What does the evidence suggest in terms of organizational changes that could help reduce the risk for this hazard? How can the occupational health nurse promote changes in practice using the evidence available?

Prepared by Gail Armstrong, PhD(c), DNP, ACNS-BC, CNE, Associate Professor, University of Colorado Denver College of Nursing (updated August 2018).

During these health assessments, the nurse has the opportunity to teach about workplace hazards and prevention measures the worker can use. At the same time, the nurse is obtaining information that will be valuable in optimizing the fit between the job and the worker. Such assessments can be done during preplacement examinations before the client begins a job, on a periodic basis during employment, or when a work-related health problem or exposure becomes apparent. One important group to consider are the nearly 15 million truck drivers who face health hazards from long work hours and fatigue, shift work, sleep deprivation, chemical exposure, and sedentary work and lifestyle. Life expectancy for these workers is only 61 years, which is 16 years less than the national average (Patton, 2012). The occupational health nurse can help identify physical and psychosocial health and life-threatening issues for this workforce and develop interventions to mitigate the risk. Work-related health assessments should also be conducted when an employee is being transferred to another job with different requirements and exposures. The goal of these assessments is to identify agent and host factors that could place the employee at risk and to determine prevention steps that can be taken to eliminate or minimize the exposure and potential health problem.

When the health data from such assessments are considered collectively, the nurse may determine some patterns in risk factors associated with the occurrence of work-related injuries and illnesses in a total population of workers. For example, a nurse practitioner in a clinic noted a dramatic increase in the number of dermatitis cases among her clients. When she looked at factors in common among these individuals, she determined that they all worked at a company with solvent exposure commonly associated with dermal irritations. She worked with the union and the company to assess the environment/agent exposure to the employees and design mitigation strategies. This nursing intervention led to a safer work environment and a decrease in dermatitis in this population group. Such an approach can be used at the company, industry, and community levels. The initial collection of data and the questioning about workplace exposures are vital steps for any intervention.

Workplace Assessment

The nurse may conduct a similar assessment of the workplace itself. The purpose of this assessment, known as a **worksite walk-through** or survey, is to become knowledgeable about the work processes and the materials, the requirements of various jobs, the presence of actual or potential hazards, and the work practices of employees (Rogers et al., 2018). Fig. 43.5 shows a brief outline that can be used to guide a worksite assessment. More complex surveys are performed by industrial hygienists and safety professionals when the purpose of the walk-through is environmental monitoring using sampling techniques or a safety audit. However, most occupational health nurses have developed expertise in these areas and include such tasks as part of their functions. For all health care providers who assess workers, this information makes an important database. In addition, for the on-site health care provider, worksite walk-throughs assist the professional in developing rapport with and being seen as a credible worker among the employees.

A worksite survey begins with an understanding of the type of work that occurs in the workplace. All business organizations are classified within the North American Industry Classification System (NAICS) with a numerical code. This code, usually a two- to four-digit number, indicates a company's product and, therefore the possible types of **occupational health hazards** that may be associated with the processes and materials used by its employees. NAICS codes are used to collect and report data on businesses. For example, illness and injury rates of one company are compared with the rates of other companies of similar size with the same code to determine whether the company is having an excess of illness or injury. In addition, by knowing the NAICS code of a company, a health care professional can access reference books that describe the usual processes, materials, and by-products of that kind of company.

The nurse will want to review the work processes and work areas by jobs or locations in the workplace. These preliminary data provide clues about what hazards may be present and an understanding of the types of jobs and health requirements that may be involved in a particular industry. A description of the work environment is next and provides an overall picture of

Name of company: ______________________ Date: __________
Address: ______________________
Telephone: ______________________
Parent company (if any): ______________________
Location of corporate offices: ______________________
SIC code: __________

The Work

Major products: ______________________
Major processes and operations, raw materials, by-products: ______________________
____
Type of jobs: ______________________
____
Potential exposures: ______________________
____

Work Environment

General conditions: ______________________
Safety signs: ______________________
Physical environment: ______________________

Worker Population

Employees
Total number: __________ Number in production: __________ Others: __________
% Full-time: __________ % Men: __________ % Women: __________
% First shift: __________ % Second shift: __________ % Third shift: __________
Age distribution: __________
% Unionized: __________ Names of unions: __________

Human Resources Management

Corporate commitment to health
Personnel
Policies/procedures
Input/surveys/committees
Record keeping

Health Data

Work-related illnesses, injuries, deaths per annum: ______________________
OSHA recordable: __________ Workers' compensation: __________
Other: __________ Most frequent complaints: __________
Average number of monthly calls to the health unit: ______________________
Absenteeism rate: ______________________

Occupation Health and Safety Services

Examinations
Employee assistance
Treatment of illness/injury
Health education
Physical fitness, health promotion activities
Mandatory programs
Safety audits
Environmental monitoring
Health risk appraisal
Screenings
Health promotion

Control Strategies

Engineering
Work practice
Administrative
Personal protective equipment

Fig. 43.5 Worksite assessment guide. *OSHA*, Occupational Safety and Health Administration; *SIC*, Standard Industrial Classification.

general appearances, physical layout, and safety of the environment. Are safety signs posted and readable where needed? Is there clutter or dampness on the floor that could cause slips or falls?

A description of the employee group is necessary information to understand the demographics and the work distribution in the company. Knowing about shift work and productivity can be helpful in pinpointing potential stressors. Human resources' management and corporate commitment to health and safety are needed to develop a supportive culture for effective and efficient programming. Reviewing the status of policies and procedures and assessing opportunities for input into improving service are important to establish the organization's strength in occupational health and safety management. Gathering data about the incidence and prevalence of work-related illnesses and injuries and the cost patterns for these conditions provides useful epidemiologic trend data and helps target high-cost areas. The types of occupational safety and health services and programs are important to know. This will show whether required programs are being offered and includes health promotion and disease prevention strategies.

HOW TO Assess a Worker and the Workplace

Assessing the worker for a work-related problem is a critical practice element. You need to do the following:

- Complete general and occupational health history-taking with emphasis on workplace exposure assessment, job hazard analysis, and list of previous jobs.
- Conduct a health assessment to identify agent and host factors that interact to place workers at risk.
- Identify patterns of risk associated with illness/injury.

Assessing the work environment is necessary to determine workplace exposures that create worker health risk. You need to do the following:

- Understand the work being done.
- Understand the work process.
- Evaluate the work-related hazards.
- Gather data about incidence/prevalence of work-related illness/injuries and related hazards.
- Conduct a walk-though of the work environment.
- Examine prevention and control strategies in place for eliminating exposures.

Finally, examining control strategies that are effective in eliminating or reducing exposure is important in determining risk reduction. Control strategies follow a hierarchical approach. Engineering controls can reduce worker exposure by modifying the exposure source, such as putting needles in a puncture-proof container. Work practice controls include good hygiene and proper waste disposal and housekeeping. Administrative controls reduce exposure through job rotation, workplace monitoring, and employee training and education. Finally, personal protective control is the last resort and requires the worker to actively engage in strategies for protection such as use of gloves, masks, and gowns to prevent exposures (Rogers et al., 2018).

The more information that can be collected before the walk-through, the more efficient the process of the survey will be. After the survey is conducted, the nurse can use the information with the aggregate health data to evaluate the effectiveness of the occupational health and safety program and to plan future programs.

HEALTHY PEOPLE 2020 DOCUMENT RELATED TO OCCUPATIONAL HEALTH

In an attempt to meet the goal of attaining high-quality, longer lives free of preventable disability, injury, and premature death for Americans, health promotion and protection strategies are proposed to address the needs of large population groups such as the American workforce. As part of the *Healthy People 2020* document (USDHHS, 2010), occupational safety and health objectives were identified to promote good health and well-being among workers, including the elimination and reduction of elements in occupational environments that cause death, injury, disease, or disability. In addition, this document promotes the minimizing of personal damage from existing occupationally related illness.

HEALTHY PEOPLE 2020

Objectives Related to Occupational Health

- **OSH-1:** Reduce deaths from work-related injuries.
- **OSH-2:** Reduce nonfatal work-related injuries.
- **OSH-3:** Reduce the rate of injuries and illness cases.
- **OSH-4:** Reduce pneumoconiosis deaths.
- **OSH-5:** Reduce deaths from work-related homicides.
- **OSH-6:** Reduce work-related assault.
- **OSH-7:** Reduce the proportion of persons who have elevated blood lead concentrations from work exposures.
- **OSH-8:** Reduce occupational skin diseases or disorders among full-time workers.
- **OSH-10:** Reduce new cases of work-related noise-induced hearing loss.

Data from U.S. Department of Health and Human Services: *Healthy People 2020.* Washington, DC, 2010, U.S. Government Printing Office.

LEGISLATION RELATED TO OCCUPATIONAL HEALTH

The occupational health and safety services provided by an employer are influenced by specific legislation at federal and state levels. Although the relationship between work and health has been known since the second century (Ramazzini, 1713), public policy that effectively controlled occupational hazards was not enacted until the 1960s. The Mine Safety and Health Act of 1968 was the first legislation that specifically required certain prevention programs for workers. This was followed by the Occupational Safety and Health Act of 1970, which established two agencies, OSHA and NIOSH, each with discrete functions (Box 43.3) to carry out the Act's purpose of ensuring "safe and healthful working conditions for working men and women" (PL 91-596, 1970). The reader is also referred to Chapters 3 and 5, the Affordable Care Act, for additional information on employer mandates.

In the context of the Occupational Safety and Health Act, OSHA, a federal agency within the U.S. Department of Labor, was created to develop and enforce workplace safety and health standards and regulations on workers' exposure to potentially

BOX 43.3 Functions of Federal Agencies Involved in Occupational Safety and Health

Occupational Safety and Health Administration (OSHA)

Determines and sets standards and permissible exposure limits (PELs) for hazardous exposures in the workplace.

Enforces the occupational health standards (including the right of entry for inspection).

Educates employees and employers about occupational health and safety.

Develops and maintains a database of work-related injuries, illnesses, and deaths.

Monitors compliance with occupational health and safety standards.

National Institute for Occupational Safety and Health (NIOSH)

Conducts research and reviews findings to recommend exposure limits for occupational hazards to OSHA.

Identifies and researches occupational health and safety hazards.

Educates occupational health and safety professionals.

Distributes research findings relevant to occupational health and safety.

From U.S. Department of Health and Human Services, National Institute for Occupational Safety and Health: *National Occupational Research Agenda.* Cincinnati, OH, 2018, USDHHS.

toxic substances, enforcing these at the federal and state levels. Specific standards and information about compliance can be obtained from federal, regional, and state OSHA offices, which can be found on the OSHA website.

The **National Institute for Occupational Safety and Health (NIOSH)** was established by the Occupational Safety and Health Act of 1970 and is part of the Centers for Disease Control and Prevention (CDC). In 1996 NIOSH and its partners unveiled a 10-year **National Occupational Research Agenda (NORA)**, a framework to guide occupational safety and health research into the following decade. The NIOSH agency identifies, monitors, and educates about the incidence, prevalence, and prevention of work-related illnesses and injuries and examines potential hazards of new work technologies and practices (USDHHS, NIOSH, 2018). Subsequently, the NORA has been updated and is focused on targeted sectors to reduce the still significant toll of workplace illness and injury.

Many standards have been established by OSHA and promulgated to protect worker health. One example is the **Hazard Communication Standard**. This standard is based on the premise that while working to reduce and eliminate potentially toxic agents in the work environment, an important line of defense is to provide the work community with information about hazardous chemicals in order to minimize exposures. The Hazard Communication Standard, which was first established in 1983, requires that all worksites with hazardous substances inventory their toxic agents, label them, and provide information sheets, called safety data sheets (SDSs), for each agent. In addition, the employer must have in place a hazard communication program that provides workers with education about these agents. This education must include agent identification, toxic effects, and protective measures. Numerous standards have been established by OSHA for specific chemicals and programs. A standard familiar to all health care professionals is the *Bloodborne Pathogens Standard.*

Workers' compensation acts are important state laws that govern financial compensation to employees who suffer work-related health problems. These acts vary by state, and each state sets rules for the reimbursement of employees with occupational health problems for medical expenses and lost work time associated with the illness or injury. Workers' compensation claims and the experience-based insurance premiums paid by industry have been important motivators for increasing the health and safety of the workplace.

LINKING CONTENT TO PRACTICE

Disaster Planning and Management

Although disaster planning and management have been functions of occupational health and safety programs, this is an area of legislation that affects businesses and health professionals. The legislation of the Superfund Amendment and Reauthorization Act (SARA) requires that written disaster plans be shared with key resources in the community, such as fire departments and emergency departments. Concern about disasters—such as the terrorist attacks on the World Trade Center and Pentagon on September 11, 2001; the methyl isocyanate leak in Bhopal, India; effects of hurricanes such as Katrina and Sandy; or the community exposure to chemicals at Times Beach, Missouri, and exposure to radiation from crippled nuclear plants in Japan—has mandated more attention to disaster planning.

In occupational health, the goals of a disaster plan are to prevent or minimize injuries and deaths of workers and residents, minimize property damage, provide effective triage, and facilitate necessary business activities. A disaster plan requires the cooperation of different personnel within the company and community. The nurse is often a key person on the disaster planning team, along with safety professionals, physicians, industrial hygienists, the fire chief, and company management. The potential for disaster (e.g., explosions, floods, fires, leaks) must be identified, and this is best achieved by completing an exhaustive chemical and hazard inventory of the workplace. The safety data sheet and plant blueprints are critical for correctly identifying substances and work areas that may be hazardous. Worksite surveys are the first step to completing this inventory. The reader is also referred to Chapter 21 on the public health nurse (PHN) and disaster management.

Effective disaster plans are designed by those with knowledge of the work processes and materials, the workers and workplace, and the resources in the community. Specific steps must be detailed for actions to be put in place by specific individuals in the event of a disaster. The written plan must be shared with all who will be involved. Employees should be prepared in first aid, cardiopulmonary resuscitation, and fire brigade procedures. Plans must be clear, specific, and comprehensive (i.e., covering all shifts and all work areas) and must include activities to be conducted within the worksite and those that require community resources. Transportation plans, fire response, and emergency response services should be coordinated with the agencies that would be involved in an actual disaster. The disaster plan, emergency and safety equipment, and the first response team's abilities should be tested at least annually with a drill. Practice results should be carefully evaluated, with changes made as needed.

Continued

LINKING CONTENT TO PRACTICE—cont'd

Disaster Planning and Management

Hospitals and other emergency services, such as fire departments, should be involved in developing the disaster plan and should receive a copy of the plan and a current hazard inventory. It is imperative that the plan and hazard inventory be periodically updated. The occupational health nurse or another company representative should provide emergency health care providers with updated clinical information on exposures and appropriate treatment. It should never be presumed that local services will have current information on substances used in industry. Representatives of these agencies should visit the worksite and accompany the nurse on a worksite walk-through so that they are familiar with the operations.

In disaster planning, the nurse is often assigned or assumes the responsibility for coordinating the planning and implementing efforts, working with appropriate key people within the company and in the community to develop a workable, comprehensive plan. Other tasks include providing ongoing communication to keep the plan current; planning the drills; educating the employees, management, and community providers; and assessing the equipment and services that may be used in a disaster.

In the event of a disaster, the nurse should play a key role in coordinating the response. Principles of triage may be used as the response team determines the extent of the disaster and the ability of the company and community to respond. Post-disaster nursing interventions are also critical. Examples include identifying the ongoing disaster-related health needs of workers and community residents, collecting epidemiologic data, and assessing the cause and the necessary steps to prevent a recurrence.

Occupational health nursing is a broad, dynamic specialty practice. The Public Health Foundation provides the basis for practice, supporting a health promotion and protection and prevention model. The occupational health nurse must have interprofessional skills and linkages to provide the most effective care and service. Occupational health nurses are involved in all levels of prevention in their practice.

PRACTICE APPLICATION

An insurance company recently renovated its claims processing office area and fitted the workstation with new computers. The company's occupational health nurse noticed an increase in visits to the health unit for complaints of headaches, stiff neck muscles, and visual disturbances consistent with computer usage.

To conduct a complete investigation of this problem, the nurse assessed the workers, the agent (computer), previously existing potential agents, and the work environment. Interventions focused on designing the health hazard out of the work process, if possible. In the present example, the first level of intervention was to refit the workstation for better worker use of the computer.

Minimizing the possible hazards of the agent involved recommendations for desks, chairs, and lighting designs that would accommodate the individual worker and allow shielding of the monitor. The nursing interventions included strengthening the resistance of the host by prescribing appropriate rest breaks, eye exercises, and relaxation strategies. Recognizing that previous cervical neck injury or impaired vision may increase the risk of adverse effects from computer work, the nurse would include assessment for these factors in employees' preplacement and periodic health examinations.

For the environmental concerns, the nurse educated the manager about the health risks of paced, externally controlled work expectations and recommended alternatives.

This case is an example of which of the following?

A. The application of the occupational health history
B. A worksite assessment or walk-through
C. A work–health interaction
D. The use of the epidemiologic triangle in exploring occupational health problems

Answers can be found on the Evolve site.

KEY POINTS

- Occupational health nursing is an autonomous practice specialty.
- The scope of occupational health nursing practice is broad, including worker and workplace assessment and surveillance, case management, health promotion, primary care, management/administration, business and finance skills, and research.
- The workforce and workplace are changing dramatically, requiring new knowledge and new occupational health services.
- The type of work has shifted from primarily manufacturing to service and technological jobs.
- Workplace hazards include exposure to biological, chemical, enviromechanical, physical, and psychosocial agents.
- The Occupational Safety and Health Act of 1970 states that workers must have a safe and healthful work environment.
- The interprofessional occupational health team consists of the occupational health nurse, occupational medicine physician, industrial hygienist, and safety specialist.
- Work-related health problems must be investigated and control strategies implemented to reduce exposure.
- Control strategies include engineering, work practice, administration, and personal protective equipment.
- The Occupational Safety and Health Administration enforces workplace safety and health standards.
- The National Institute for Occupational Safety and Health is the education and research agency that provides grants to investigate the causes of workplace illness and injuries.
- Workers' compensation acts are important laws that govern financial compensation of employees who suffer work-related health problems.
- The occupational health nurse should play a key role in disaster planning and coordination.
- Academic education in occupational health nursing is generally at the graduate level.

CLINICAL DECISION-MAKING ACTIVITIES

1. Arrange to visit a local industry to observe work processes and discuss working conditions. See if you can identify the work-related hazards and make recommendations for eliminating them.
2. Interview the occupational health nurse in an industry setting and ask questions about scope of practice, job functions, and contributions to the business. Compare and contrast what you have learned about this nurse role to that of the school health nurse.
3. Contact the American Association of Occupational Health Nurses and ask what the most pressing trends are in the specialty. What are some of the complex issues related to these trends?
4. Obtain a proposed standard from the Occupational Safety and Health Administration, critique it, and submit your comments.
5. Attend a workers' compensation hearing, analyze the problem, and critique the outcome. How is your critique affected by what you thought the outcome should be?

ADDITIONAL RESOURCES

EVOLVE WEBSITE

http://evolve.elsevier.com/Stanhope/community/

- Answers to Practice Application
- Case Study
- Glossary
- Review Questions

REFERENCES

American Association of Occupational Health Nurses: *The nurse in industry*, New York, NY, 1976, AAOHN.

American Association of Occupational Health Nurses: *Standards of occupational and environmental health nursing practice*, Chicago, IL, 2016, AAOHN.

American Association of Occupational Health Nurses: *Code of ethics*, Chicago, IL, 2016, AAOHN.

American Association of Occupational Health Nurses: *OHN fact sheet*, Chicago, IL, 2016, AAOHN.

Brown M: *Occupational health nursing*, New York, NY, 1981, MacMillan.

Bureau of Labor Statistics: *Census of fatal occupational injuries summary*, 2017a. Retrieved from https://www.bls.gov.

Bureau of Labor Statistics: *Employer – Reported Workplace Injury and Illnesses*, 2017b. Retrieved from https://www.bls.gov.

Bureau of Labor Statistics: *Fastest growing occupations 2016-2026, occupational outlook handbook*, Washington, DC, 2018a, U.S. Department of Labor.

Bureau of Labor Statistics: *Non-fatal occupational injuries and illnesses requiring days away from work, 2011*, Washington, DC, 2012, U.S. Department of Labor.

Bureau of Labor Statistics: *Labor force statistics for current population*, Washington, DC, 2018, U.S. Department of Labor.

Desilver D: *More older Americans working more than they used to*, Washington, DC, 2018, Pew Research Center.

Dupler AE, Postma J, Sanders A: Minimizing nurses' risks for needlestick injuries in the hospital setting, *Workplace Health Saf* 61(5):197–2023, 2013.

Felton J: The genesis of American occupational health nursing, part 1, *Occup Health Nurs* 33:615, 1985.

Gonzalez M, Conlon H: Updating a tuberculosis surveillance program: Considering all of the variables, *Workplace Health Saf* 61(6):271–278, 2013.

Gordis L: *Epidemiology*, ed 4, St Louis, MO, 2013, Elsevier.

Health Resources and Services Administration: *The Registered Nurse Population: Findings from the 2008 National Sample Survey of Registered Nurses*, 2010. Retrieved from http://bhpr.hrsa.gov.

Levy BS, Wegman DH Baron SL, Sokas RK: *Occupational health: recognizing and preventing occupational disease*, Philadelphia, PA, 2017, Lippincott Williams & Wilkins.

McGrath B: Fifty years of industrial nursing, *Public Health Nurs* 37:119, 1945.

National Institute for Occupational Safety and Health: *Occupational Respiratory Disease Surveillance*, 2014. Retrieved from www.cdc/niosh.gov.

O'Donnell M: *Health promotion in the workplace*, Troy, MI, 2017, Art & Science of Health Promotion Institute.

Ortman, Velkoff, and Hogan: An aging nation: *The older population in the United States*, US Census Department, 2014, U.S. Census Bureau.

Patton O: *FMCSA Answers questions about driver life expectancy statistics*, 2012. Retrieved from www.truckinginfo.com.

Public Law 91-596: *The occupational safety and health act*, Washington, DC, 1970, U.S. Department of Labor.

Quad Council Coalition Competency Review Task Force: Community/Public Health Nursing Competencies, 2018.

Ramazzini B: *De Morbis Artificum [Diseases of Workers], 1713, Translated by Wright WC*, Chicago, IL, 1940, University of Chicago Press.

Reda AA, Fisseha S, Mengistie B, et al: Standard precautions: occupational exposure and behavior of health care workers in Ethiopia, *PLoS One* 5(12):e14420, 2010.

Rogers B: Perspectives on occupational health nursing, *AAOHN J* 36:100–105, 1988.

Rogers B, Randolph S, Mastroianni K: *Occupational health nursing guidelines for primary clinical conditions*, Beverly, MA, 2018, OEM Press.

Rogers B: Occupational Health Nursing: *Concepts and Practice*. In Press, 2019.

Stewart RJ, Tsang CA, Pratt RH, Price SF, Langer AJ: Tuberculosis – United States, 2017, *MMWR Morb Mortal Wkly Rep* 67:317–323, 2017.

Toossi M, Torpey E: *Older Workers: Labor Force Trends and Career Options*, 2017. Retrieved from https://www.bls.gov.

U.S. Census Bureau: 2018. US Department of Commerce, Washington, DC. Retrieved from http://www.census.gov/.

U.S. Department of Health and Human Services: *National institute for occupational safety and health: the changing organization of work and the safety and health of working people, Pub No 2002-116*, Cincinnati, OH, 2002, USDHHS.

U.S. Department of Health and Human Services: *Healthy people 2020*, Washington, DC, 2010, U.S. Government Printing Office.

U.S. Department of Health and Human Services: *National institute for occupational safety and health: National occupational research agenda*, Cincinnati, OH, 2018, USDHHS.

44

Forensic Nursing in the Community

Laura Suzuki, PhD(c), MPH, BSN, RN, Natalie McClain, PhD, RN, CPNP, and Melissa A. Sutherland, PhD, FNP-BC

OBJECTIVES

After reading this chapter, the student will be able to do the following:

1. Describe the specialized competencies and skills of the forensic nurse within the nursing process.
2. Discuss the relationship of the forensic nurse with public health professionals in addressing injury as a public health concern.
3. List the health risks that result from incidents of injury.
4. Identify how forensic nurses deal with injuries in the three levels of prevention.
5. Discuss the health disparities that contribute to the occurrence and poor outcomes in marginalized groups who experience injury.
6. Explain the contribution of theoretical underpinnings to current models of forensic nursing practice.
7. Identify client populations and clinical arenas in the community where forensic nurses practice.
8. Define the key terms and concepts within forensic nursing theory.
9. Identify professionals who commonly work in collaboration with the forensic nurse in addressing injury care and prevention.

CHAPTER OUTLINE

Perspectives on Forensics and Forensic Nursing
Injury Prevention
***Healthy People 2020* Goals, Prevention, and Forensic Nursing**
Forensic Nursing as a Specialty Area That Provides Care in the Community
Current Perspectives
Ethical Issues
Future Perspectives

KEY TERMS

adjudication, p. 979
forensic, p. 977
forensic nurse examiner, p. 977
forensic nursing, p. 977
injury, p. 977
justice, p. 981
legal nurse consultants, p. 979
perceptivity, p. 981
sexual assault nurse examiner (SANE), p. 977
victimization, p. 982

PERSPECTIVES ON FORENSICS AND FORENSIC NURSING

Injuries resulting from crime and victimization cause pain and suffering and may cause disability, economic failure, and "distress of the human spirit" (Lynch, 2011, p. 15). However, such injuries have often taken a back seat to treatment of disease and infection. Today forensic nurses expertly care for victims of injuries, largely as a community-based specialty, from a medical as well as a legal perspective. Whether the injury is caused by intentional violence or unintentional accident, forensic nurses are involved with not only the treatment but also the prevention of injury, the leading cause of death in the first four decades of life (Centers for Disease Control and

Special thanks goes to Dr. Susan Patton who authored this chapter in the eighth edition of the textbook. Appreciation is given to Drs. Karen Landenburger and Jacquelyn Campbell for providing some content related to forensic nursing that was moved from Chapter 38, which discusses violence in the community.

Prevention [CDC], 2016). The burden of injuries to individuals ranges from minimal and brief to debilitating or fatal. The economic burden worldwide is tremendous. Each year in the United States more than 3 million people are hospitalized and 27 million people receive treatment in emergency departments as a result of violence and injuries (CDC, 2015). The total costs, for both fatal and nonfatal injuries and violence, are estimated to be more than $671 billion in medical care and lost productivity each year (CDC, 2015). Because injuries result from a wide variety of physical, environmental, and behavioral causes, risk reduction comes from a variety of approaches. Forensic nurses have a unique set of skills for dealing with injury, and these skills will be discussed in this chapter.

Forensic means pertaining to the law. **Forensic nursing** synthesizes the biopsychosocial and spiritual aspects of nursing care with an expert understanding of forensic science and the criminal justice process (International Association of Forensic Nurses, 2017). Forensic nursing has a unique body of knowledge and set of skills. It also has unique practice arenas and the client population served. The skill set is defined by the scope and standards of practice, which includes skills such as collection, documentation, and preservation of evidence and other findings that may later be used in the prosecution of a crime. Practice standards reflect care given to both the living and the dead, victims of trauma and perpetrators of crime, as well as families and affected groups within a community. Forensic nurses often have experience in emergency and trauma services and can provide an expert analysis of wounding patterns and physiological response to injury. They are able to compassionately care for individuals and families who experience emotional reactions to trauma from a variety of causes. While the majority of forensic nurses in the United States are **sexual assault nurse examiners (SANEs)**, other roles exist to care for survivors of other violent crimes, liability-related injury, and deaths. These include the clinical forensic nurse, **forensic nurse examiner** or investigator, forensic psychiatric nurse, forensic correctional nurse, legal nurse consultant, nurse attorney, and nurse coroner or death investigator (Bauman & Stark, 2015). Arenas of care include but are not limited to emergency departments and community-based urgent care clinics, offices of the medical examiner and coroner, investigative units of law enforcement and criminal justice agencies, and governmental programs of safety prevention.

Forensic nursing care largely occurs in collaboration with professionals, both within and outside of nursing, including public health professionals, epidemiologists, law enforcement and corrections officers, emergency department providers, and psychiatric practitioners. Forensic nurses may also work in conjunction with public health nurses who bring a population focus to injury prevention programs. As part of a public health approach to crime prevention and response, forensic nurses may serve as content experts, clinician advisors, and/or the clinical managers of care facilities that may contribute to a community response to injury prevention.

INJURY PREVENTION

Not surprisingly, the health determinants of injury as identified in *Healthy People 2020* mirror disease occurrence in a community. The rate of injury and crime is lower in communities that promote good health. Where inequities of resources and education exist, health disparity, violence, and other crimes rise and accidental injuries occur more often (Jackson & Vaughn, 2018). Trauma victims are overrepresented in minority, disenfranchised, and disadvantaged groups. Disparity can also be seen in the prosecution, conviction, and incarceration of individuals of minority groups in many countries. In the United States, African Americans are more than five times as likely and Hispanics twice as likely to be incarcerated as whites (Sakala, 2014). Populations that experience more disease also experience more violent as well as accidental injury and more events that lead to prosecution. The measures that improve overall health, lower risk, and reduce disparity also reduce physical and emotional injury. **Injury** now joins certain categories of disease, disability, and premature death as a major preventable health state. Reducing injury reflects the goals of *Healthy People 2020* as well as goals of other organizations such as the U.S. Public Health Service, the Centers for Disease Control and Prevention (CDC), the World Health Organization (WHO), and the International Association of Forensic Nurses (IAFN).

The National Center for Injury Prevention and Control (NCIPC), within the CDC, was established in 1997 to coordinate prevention of injuries, violence, and their consequences. NCIPC provides grants that fund prevention programs, aids in the dissemination of research findings, and maintains a website and other electronic information such as blogs, podcasts, and electronic newsletters. The NCIPC website includes a wide variety of information on injury and violence prevention, home and recreational safety, traumatic brain injury, injury data and statistics, motor vehicle safety, and opioid overdose prevention (CDC, 2018). The efforts described on this website help inform the public of the epidemiology of injury and provide resources for professionals. The database of the International Association of Forensic Nurses (http://www.iafn.org) lists over 900 facilities that provide sexual assault services in the United States, Canada, and Australia. Forensic nurse death investigators serve as trainers for the CDC's national Sudden Unexplained Infant Death Investigation program.

HEALTHY PEOPLE 2020 GOALS, PREVENTION, AND FORENSIC NURSING

The *Healthy People 2020* goals that deal with reducing injury and violence in the United States reflect the breadth of concerns and problems that result in injury, both intentional and unintentional, in communities. Objectives related to safety, violence, injury, and sexual assault are incorporated throughout the *Healthy People 2020* document. These objectives relate to injuries that are both intentional and unintentional. The box that follows lists selected objectives related to violence.

HEALTHY PEOPLE 2020

Objectives Pertaining to Injury

The following proposed objectives are examples that pertain to injury and are relevant in forensic nursing:

- **IVP-29:** Reduce homicides.
- **IVP-30:** Reduce firearm-related deaths.
- **IVP-33:** Reduce physical assaults.
- **IVP-34:** Reduce physical fighting among adolescents.
- **IVP-36:** Reduce weapon carrying by adolescents on school property.
- **IVP-40:** Reduce sexual violence (U.S. Department Health and Human Services, 2010).

From U.S Department of Health and Human Services: Healthy People 2020. Available at http://www.healthypeople.gov.

Nurses who work in the area of forensics use all three levels of prevention. For example, forensic nurses (FNs) promote safety in their involvement with projects that aim to prevent domestic violence, sexual assault, child abuse, and accidental injuries before they occur (primary prevention) and in program development and management of care centers. Community awareness of violent crimes is achieved in concert with certain programs and the community-based professionals who work there. Secondary prevention is practiced following the occurrence of injuries and crime. Forensic nurses provide direct care to both victims and perpetrators. Their expertise serves the individual as well as the community in the collection of evidence for the legal justice system. Goals of compassionate holistic care are to minimize the spiritual, psychological, physical, and social trauma, as well as the financial burden. Although the World Health Organization (WHO) guidelines recommend against routine intimate partner screening at all health encounters (WHO, 2013), the 2013 U.S. Preventive Services Task Force recommends, "that clinicians screen women of childbearing age for intimate partner violence such as domestic violence . . . . " (Feder et al., 2013; Moyer, 2013). Worth noting is that the WHO does recommend that health care providers ask about intimate partner violence (IPV) exposure in situations involving injuries or that may have been caused or complicated by IPV. FNs are often the first providers to assess a patient's medical situation and to have contact with victims.

If disability, incarceration, or death occurs, FNs provide tertiary care in settings appropriate to address rehabilitation or identify factors that have put individuals at risk. Evidence should be collected in such a way that the collection itself protects rather than destroys or alters the evidence.

LEVELS OF PREVENTION

Intentional Injury

Primary Prevention

Develop programs that promote safety and avoidance of violence, including both intentional violence and unintentional accidents.

Secondary Prevention

Provide timely, sensitive, direct care to both victims of injury and perpetrators of crime and violent behavior.

Tertiary Prevention

When injury has occurred, refer clients to appropriate community services for appropriate follow-up care and rehabilitation of the effects of trauma.

FORENSIC NURSING AS A SPECIALTY AREA THAT PROVIDES CARE IN THE COMMUNITY

Within communities, the growing prevalence of "criminal and negligence-based trauma" indicates a need for health professionals who can intercede with skills that address social justice as well as care for social offenders (Lynch, 2011, p. 17). Thus forensic nurses respond to sexual assault, drug- and alcohol-related crimes, incidents of human trafficking, elder mistreatment, child abuse, gang violence, as well as mass disaster, automobile crashes, and work-related injuries (Harris, 2013; Scannell et al., 2018). In each situation, forensic nurses look for historical, behavioral, and physical indicators that a crime has been committed and intentional injury has occurred. For example, children who are abused may have cigarette burns, bite marks, pressure sores, and other physical signs that parents may claim to be the result of accidents. Munchausen syndrome by proxy is a form of child abuse in which the primary caregiver induces or fabricates illness or clinical symptoms in a child leading to attention from medical professionals and unnecessary and at times invasive tests and interventions (Squires & Squires, 2013).

A client who is admitted to a hospital with traumatic injuries should be evaluated as to the potentially forensic nature of the injuries (Pasqualone & Michel, 2015; Filmalter, et al, 2018). Additionally, a comprehensive trauma assessment should be done, which can be used to provide teaching, referrals, and access to appropriate resources (Amar, 2016). The response to victims of assault includes a number of steps, as outlined in Box 44.1. The nurse most often comes in contact with police, victims, and perpetrators of violence or crime in the emergency department. The nurse provides a vital link between the investigative process, health care, and the court (Campbell et al., 2012; Malmgren & Leahy, 2016). Nurses should take specific actions when they come in contact with victims to ensure potential evidence is properly preserved, collected, and documented. It is important that evidence be collected in a manner that adheres to legal standards, including chain of custody requirements, in order to establish the reliability and integrity of evidence for use in court cases (Pagliaro, 2013).

BOX 44.1 Emergency Response to Assault Victims

1. Use standardized medical treatment and forensic protocols.
2. Assess for sexual assault using "forced sex" terminology rather than "rape" or "sexual assault," and call a sexual assault nurse examiner if appropriate.
3. Support privacy of assault victim.
4. Explain procedures clearly to the assault victim.
5. Document location, date, and time of assault.
6. Collect evidence in a systematic format; take pictures if necessary.
7. Take care not to destroy evidence while giving care.
8. Maintain chain of evidence.
9. Maintain evidence integrity.
10. Document the following:
    a. Injuries
    b. Emotional state
    c. Medical history
    d. Victim's account of assault
11. Identify and refer to resources that can be used after the assault.

One example of appropriate forensic care is avoid cutting through the bullet hole in the shirt when cutting a shirt off a victim who has been shot in the chest. Rather, it should be cut to the side of the hole to protect the point of origin of the bullet for later criminal investigation. The collection of DNA is a primary function of the forensic nurse and can play a significant role in criminal investigations including sexual assault (Menaker et al., 2017). It is essential that DNA be collected correctly and that elimination samples of DNA be collected from authorized people at the crime scene and from the victim (USDOJ/Office on Violence Against Women, 2013).

The most common types of evidence encountered when conducting a forensic assessment of victims of violence, including those who are raped, are clothing, footwear, bullets, bloodstains, and trace evidence such as hairs, fibers, tissue, and small pieces of metal, glass, paint, wood, or plant material (Pagliaro, 2013). In the investigation of sexual assault, an evidence kit should be used within 72 hours of the assault with specimens collected and preserved according to jurisdictional and state crime lab protocols. Only the victim or a nurse wearing protective gloves should handle the clothing. Throughout the collection process, the nurse should remain sensitive to the psychological trauma that the patient may be experiencing after an assault and maintain objectivity in recording observations and conducting the forensic exam (Jamerson & Turvey, 2014).

Amar et al. (2016) provide a useful guide to assessment of all forms of violence, including child abuse and neglect, elderly abuse, and intimate partner violence. Documentation can include written descriptions, drawings, diagrams, body charts, as well as forensic photography (Cabelus & Spangler, 2013). Written forms of documentation should be as factual, complete, and prompt as possible, avoiding the use of jargon, abbreviations, and unclear statements. Digital imaging is the most common way to take the necessary photographs. The photographs should be taken in context, using the "rule of three" guideline to capture the overall scene, a medium-range shot, and a close-up shot of the injury or potential piece of evidence (Zercie & Penders, 2013). Injuries should also be depicted on diagrams and recorded in the nurses' notes. The How To box describes how to label photographs taken after the injury.

HOW TO Label Photos

All photos should be clearly labeled with the following information:

- Client's name
- Client's medical identification number
- Client's date of birth
- The date and time of the photograph
- The name of the photographer
- The body location of the injury
- The forensic case number

From Sheridan, DJ: Legal and forensic nursing responses to family violence in Humphrey J, Campbell JC, editors: Family violence and nursing practice, Philadelphia, 2004, Lippincott Williams & Wilkins.

Forensic nurses may have expertise in alternative specialties that are combined to serve special populations. Advanced practice nurses (APNs) such as psychiatric, pediatric, geriatric, and acute care nurse practitioners bring to forensic nursing skills that allow them to provide advanced assessment and prescription of medications and treatments needed by forensic clients. Notably, forensic psychiatric nurses treat both victims of post-traumatic stress disorder and seriously emotionally disturbed clients incarcerated for violent crimes. APNs in correctional facilities may identify themselves as forensic nurses when they manage acute and chronic illness, promote wellness, and work within these systems to develop policies around legal and ethical issues.

The specialty also incorporates three subspecialties of nursing practice within the criminal justice system: forensic nurse, nurse attorney, and legal nurse consultant. Forensic nurses employed in the criminal justice arena generally provide care to individuals who are either victims of injury or perpetrators of a crime that is under investigation. **Legal nurse consultants** provide expert consultation regarding health care to attorneys in either civil or criminal court cases but do not render direct client care in that setting. Some of these situations might include medical malpractice, personal injury, workers' compensation, and probate. Nurse attorneys hold a license to practice law from a state bar association in addition to a nursing license and generally use their nursing knowledge for adjudication. **Adjudication** refers to a judicial decision or a sentence.

Finally, forensic nurses are advocates for programs that prevent injuries, which occur as a result of both intentional injury and health hazards related to environments that create injury. Relying on an understanding of epidemiology, these nurses have knowledge of occurrence as well as the mechanisms of injury in a community. Forensic nurses partner with public health professionals, including nurses, to design, implement, and evaluate projects and programs that have a forensic focus.

History of Forensic Nursing

Early writings about the evolution of modern nursing, particularly with regard to care given to victims of war, mental illness, and abuse, lay a foundation for the advent of forensic nurses in the twentieth century (Nutting & Dock, 1907). Chapter 2 discusses the history of public health nursing; this section emphasizes nursing history's linkages to forensic nursing. With public health nurses, forensic nurses celebrate the early pioneers working in communities that brought medical care to the most vulnerable and marginalized. They worked to develop national and international organizations such as the National Organization for Public Health Nursing (1912), National Society of Nurses (later the American Nurses Association [ANA], 1912), the International Congress of Nursing (1912), and the WHO (1948). These organizations were designed to give structure and standards for care and education regarding issues of violence and neglect. These issues pertain to public health, mental health, and forensic nurses who are experts in dealing with the effects of trauma, and who advocate for care of the wounded, both physically and emotionally.

Contemporary practice of forensic nursing in the United States was largely propelled by early efforts to identify and prevent child abuse and neglect and sexual assault of women. In the 1940s through the 1960s, radiologists identified fractures that they linked to assault and pediatricians began describing indicators of "battered child syndrome" (Crane, 2015). Subsequently, nurses became aware of their role in identifying indicators of assault. In emergency departments, forensic nurses assisted in "rape" kit collection. The nurses showed compassion and competence in preserving crucial evidence and had a strong understanding of the "rape trauma syndrome" first described by Burgess in 1973. Burgess and other advanced practice nurses initiated previously undescribed care with forensic clients. The first nurse-run sexual assault clinics opened in Memphis and Minneapolis in 1974 (Speck, n.d.) with subsequent development of the first protocols for sexual assault care (Ledray, 1998). In 1985, the U.S. Surgeon General identified violence as a health care issue, and health care providers such as nurses working with victims and perpetrators of crimes, as key agents in ameliorating the effects of violence in our communities (USDHHS, HRSA, 1986). In 1990 Virginia Lynch published her dissertation on the role description and Integrated Practice Model of Forensic Nursing care of both living and deceased victims of trauma and perpetrators of crime (Lynch, 1990). By 1992, The Joint Commission began to require hospitals to develop protocols for the treatment of victims of sexual assault. At the present time, most victims of sexual assault go to emergency departments. The lack of availability of trained providers and recognition of the need for uniformity in collection and processing of evidence spurred the development of SANE programs (Simmons, 2014).

Today, the Integrated Practice Model of Forensic Nursing Science is recognized internationally as the basis for practice as well as education of forensic nurses. Following efforts to describe the unique contribution of forensic nursing (Lynch, 1986), the specialty was recognized by the American Academy of Forensic Science in 1991. The following year SANEs from the United States and Canada established the International Association of Forensic Nurses (IAFN). In 1995, the ANA designated forensic nursing as a specialty, and it is now recognized as one of the fastest growing specialties in nursing. IAFN boasts a membership of over 3700 nurses worldwide and has members in 27 countries (IAFN, 2018).

Educational Preparation

Historically, forensic nurses refined and developed their forensic skills through clinical practice and continuing education. Today, there are three primary routes for training in forensic nursing. First, nurses can gain additional skills and knowledge through continuing education courses or basic concepts introduced in generalist education. Second, certificate programs include specific content and entrance requirements, and many have clinical opportunities. Third, graduate nursing academic programs are offering minors or concentrations in forensic nursing.

Formal graduate course work on forensic nursing began at the University of Texas, Arlington, in 1986. To begin a specialty by starting with graduate preparation is both uncommon and courageous; more often content is introduced in the undergraduate studies, and graduate study assists in refining and developing the content until it is formalized in courses and majors. By 2000 there were 12 graduate programs preparing clinical nurse specialists and nurse practitioners with a focus on forensic nursing. The development of the scope and standards of practice and a core curriculum for graduate study in 2004 facilitated the development of new programs of study and formed the basis for advanced practice credentialing of students and practicing clinicians. A forensic focus in research became more prevalent in both master's and doctoral studies, which facilitated the opening of the first doctor of nursing practice (DNP) program focused on forensic nursing in 2002 at the University of Tennessee Health Science Center in Memphis. Now, new DNP programs are opening based on this model of advanced nursing practice.

The inclusion of forensic nursing content into undergraduate generalist education remains controversial. The American Association of Nurse Attorneys (TAANA) and the IAFN have recommended coursework regarding public and private legal proceedings. Students need to develop a working understanding of laws and procedures applicable to nursing practice and certain client situations, such as mandated reporting of child abuse (IAFN, 2017). In addition, nurses are prepared to care for families experiencing trauma. Many educators in the United States believe the complexity of forensic content has evolved so that the skills and competencies required to differentiate the specialty are not appropriate in a generalist educational curriculum.

Theoretical Foundations of Forensic Nursing

Humans seek stability; they seek safety from physical trauma and emotional wounding from violent relationships; and they seek protection of their finances and freedom from fears that threaten their very understanding of human existence. Theories that contribute to our understanding of what constitutes safety and well-being have been extrapolated from a variety of sources outside of nursing. Maslow, an American psychologist, developed a hierarchy of needs and desires that are seen as influencing the development of an individual toward high levels of "self-actualization" and satisfaction (Maslow, 1943). Nursing has embraced his conceptualization of the hierarchy of human need attainment. Specifically, for this chapter, it is important to consider the need for safety and the desire for security that may be threatened by injury.

In examining methods to identify the risk of injury, William Haddon, a physician and expert on automobile injury, developed a matrix that looks at factors related to personal attributes, vector or agent attributes, and environmental attributes before, during, and after an injury or death. He demonstrated that by using this framework, a person can evaluate the relative importance of different factors and design interventions (Haddon, 1972; O'Neill, 2002). Subsequently, community-based nurses such as those who work in public health and forensic nursing and, increasingly, hospital-based nurses have used the matrix to develop programs to prevent a wide variety of injuries, including burns, falls, firearm injuries, and, most recently, critical incidents from medical error.

More recently, forensic science has informed and continues to inform forensic nursing practice. This is particularly true in terms of the intricacies of evidence collection and the growing body of knowledge within criminalistics (James & Nordby, 2014). In addition, the influence of law, including structure of the court system, federal rules of evidence, principles of witness testimony, expert opinions, and rights of citizens, has shaped the unique body of knowledge that guides the specialty from outside of nursing. Criminal justice principles and law inform practice and form the boundaries of many aspects of practice such as client consent, rules of evidence, and expert courtroom testimony.

Professional organizations outside of nursing that address large-scale health concerns such as the CDC and the WHO have contributed to nursing's understanding of injury. At the turn of the twenty-first century these organizations began a global campaign toward violence prevention that had a tremendous influence on developing a primary prevention approach within the forensic community (WHO, 2014, 2015, 2016). For example, in 2002, the CDC Injury Center developed a state-based surveillance system, the National Violent Death Reporting System (NVDRS), that compiles data on violent deaths from multiple sources. It includes all types of homicides and suicides, including child maltreatment fatalities, intimate partner homicides, deaths of law enforcement occurring in the line of duty, unintentional firearm injury deaths, and deaths of undetermined intent (CDC, 2017). Subsequently, a task force was formed to uniformly prepare individuals to conduct sudden unexplained infant death investigations. Forensic nurses practicing as death investigators served in the development of training programs that are now used nationwide. Today, the NVDRS operates in 40 states, the District of Columbia, and Puerto Rico. The system is designed to provide states and agencies with valuable data that can be used to make decisions about violence intervention and prevention activities within their communities (CDC, 2017).

In nursing, the conceptualizations that have contributed the most to forensic nursing include holism through caring; ways of knowing, including intuition and suspicion; human reaction to trauma, including the rape trauma syndrome; and models specific to forensic nursing. Hammer et al. (2013) examined the connection between the construct of caring and the unique relationship between forensic nurses and their clients. Although caring was previously recognized as the "hallmark of professional nursing" by theorists in the 1980s, Hammer et al. recognized that part of what makes forensic nursing a specialty is the manner in which caring is translated.

The caring component addresses caring for both clients and for one's self. A sense of self-worth must be cultivated and nurtured to the degree that caring is conscientious, objective, and demanding of the scientific truth. Caring must also be curious and questioning; it should be directed toward colleagues, and finally, caring should be about firm and valued concepts that inform practice (Hammer et al., 2013).

In that regard, questioning and ways of knowing, particularly intuition, are viewed as vital for a successful practice. Winfrey and Smith (1999) have described the concept of knowing as, more accurately, being suspicious in forensic nursing. Questioning also led to a greater understanding of what most would consider the unexplainable and the unimaginable: the manifestations of rape trauma syndrome (Burgess & Holmstrom, 1974), behaviors of the seriously emotionally disturbed offender (Mason & Mercer, 1998), and widespread occurrence of intimate partner violence (Campbell & Humphreys, 2011). Lynch's Integrated Practice Model of Forensic Nursing Science, as previously discussed, depicts the biopsychosocial and spiritual dimensions of nursing care with the legal expertise needed when trauma results in court-related issues. Lynch and Duval (2011) have credited several nursing theorists—including Paterson and Zderad; Conway and Hardy; Leininger, Giger, and Davidhizar; Chinn and Kramer; and Brenner—in the development of forensic nursing theory and practice. Subsequent to Lynch's efforts, Hufft (2013) described forensic nursing within the domains of nursing and delineated the theoretical foundations for advanced forensic practice. Together, these role descriptions have informed the scope and standards of practice of the forensic nurse as well as the subroles within the specialty. Knowledge, observation, and intuition are aspects of all types of forensic nursing.

Key Concepts in Forensic Nursing

The core concepts or conceptual metaphors that underlie forensic and other nursing models are not unique to nursing. Concepts when applied to the nursing process guide knowledge, skills, and attitudes found in practice. Concepts in forensic nursing theory include, but are not confined to, safety, injury, presence, perceptivity, victimization, truth, and justice.

Safety is among the five basic needs of humans identified by Maslow in his theory of self-actualization (Maslow, 1943). Maslow describes the first basic need as meeting one's physiological needs. This need is followed by safety needs, which can be affected by levels of security. The need for safety can become acute during periods of emergent trauma or chronic during periods of collective violence or chronic abuse. Until an individual is safe and wounding has healed, he or she cannot move on to higher levels of understanding and satisfaction.

Injury involves trauma or damage that is physiological, emotional, financial, spiritual, intellectual, and societal. Injury may be intentional, often known as violence, or may be unintentional. The cause may be a single source or multifaceted; it may be of human etiology or of natural causes. Making the distinction between the causes of injury is key to forensic practice. **Justice** is the concept of moral rightness based on ethics, rationality, law, natural law, fairness, and equity. As such, justice is viewed in the context of bioethics of the health care professions and the prevailing law of a particular society and culture. Therefore the fact that justice is an important goal in forensic nursing care must be viewed in the context of the environment in which the care is given.

Presence is used by nurses as a part of the humane, holistic approach to both victims of trauma and perpetrators of crime. Lynch (2011) has defined presence as "the invisible quality that commands and comforts while directing attention away from one's self and into the being of another, instilling confidence and respect in the self of that being" (p. 12).

Perceptivity, as an element of intuitiveness, is one tool the forensic nurse uses to investigate injury. Perceptivity involves an increased awareness of human behavior and environment that is interpreted by knowledge and lived experience in making expert decisions.

Truth is conceptualized as an agreement with fact or reality but also reflects characteristics such as honesty and sincerity on the part of the truth teller. Conceptualization of truth is influenced by philosophies that view it as subjective, objective, relative, or absolute. Forensic nurses hold the ideal that the results of scientific inquiry form the basis for their interactions with clients, health care systems, and the judicial system, which interact with their care; they are not influenced by personal bias or outside influence.

Victimization occurs when individuals or groups are exploited or treated unfairly, generally when there is an imbalance of power. The harm may be systematic when groups are mistreated or witness violence or it may be the result of individual attacks. Psychological responses to victimization include heightened feelings of vulnerability, depression, and anger. Juxtaposed to victimization is client empowerment, often through advocacy.

Scope and Standards of Practice

The scope and standards of practice for forensic nursing that identify the "expectations for the role and practice of the forensic nurse" were first published in 1997 and updated in 2009. The standards are delineated in each of the recognized areas: Scientific Process, Quality of Practice, Education, Professional Practice, Evaluation, Collaboration, Ethics, Research, Resource Utilization, and Leadership. Although each of these parameters helps differentiate forensic nursing from other specialties (ANA, 2017), competencies related to the scientific process, or nursing process, are perhaps the most indicative of the specialized nature of the specialty. For example:

- Assessment includes the collection of forensic data, which may involve interviewing the client for evidentiary purposes, reviewing medical legal documents, and collecting trace evidence to be used in a criminal investigation.
- Formulating a diagnosis or impression regarding the differentiation of intentional and unintentional injury is a skill that involves a unique understanding of mechanisms of injury and correlation of this with the history of the event. The impression of the forensic clinician has extraordinary legal implications beyond the realm of the health-related diagnosis.
- The identification of realistic outcomes of care is most commonly performed in collaboration with a team that frequently consists of professionals outside of nursing, including law enforcement, criminal justice, community advocates, and social service agencies. Care may reflect a decision that is humane and ensures community safety, but may not necessarily be reflective of the client's wishes.
- Formulation of the care plan involves collaboration with a team and should support the integration of clinical, human, social, and financial resources with medical-legal parameters to complete the decision-making processes.
- Implementation of the plan involves skills and techniques that are derived from sound evidence related to the applied science of both nursing and forensics. Current knowledge of both is mandated.
- Coordination of care relevant to forensic outcomes often involves including education and other strategies to prevent injuries well after the occurrence, perhaps after the death of an individual who has been injured.
- Evaluation of outcomes, particularly when viewed in aggregate, may involve dissemination of the results not only to the client and others involved in the care or situation but also to local, national, and international agencies as appropriate, for the development of laws and regulations to protect individuals in a community.

LINKING CONTENT TO PRACTICE

This chapter discusses the role of forensic nurses in the prevention and treatment of victims of violence. In addition to using the ANA competencies for practice, the forensic nurse includes the public health competencies as described in the Council on Linkages Domains and Core Competencies (2014). For example, the analytic/assessment skills that discuss assessment, data collection, and use of ethical principles are integral to this nursing role. In regard to applying ethical principles, the nurse would use them in the collection, maintenance, use, and dissemination of data and information. Clearly this skill is a part of forensic nursing.

CURRENT PERSPECTIVES

Evidence-Based Practice and Research

Evaluation of competency is required of all professions. Evaluation of nurses begins in school and continues through testing for entry-level licensure, certification examination, peer review, and personal reflection. Reflection should be on practice as well as during practice. As part of professional expectations and standards, forensic nurses are encouraged to participate in continuous quality improvement using the best evidence for practice or promising practice methods under evaluation (Meunier-Sham et al., 2013). Scientific research in forensic nursing is in its infancy. Although a large majority of the published research consists of descriptive studies of the forensic nursing role and the client populations (Orr, 2016; Valentine, 2014), there are a growing number of studies examining forensic practice and outcomes. For example, research on sexual assault response teams supports the use of these approaches to practice and recommends outcome measurement of both short-term outcomes such as client satisfaction and long-term outcomes such as prosecution rates (Campbell et al., 2014; DuMont et al., 2014). Studies in collaboration with other disciplines are currently under way to test the basis for distinctions among injuries such as bruising (Lombardi et al., 2015; Pollitt et al., 2016). Forensic nurses are producing valuable information regarding DNA sampling (Eldredge et al., 2012). Scholarly contributions to forensic nursing practice have increased since professional journals such as the *Journal of Forensic Nursing* have increased publication of forensic specific content. The following Evidence-Based Practice example describes the ways in which DNA evidence can be accurately obtained.

EVIDENCE-BASED PRACTICE

An essential step in a forensic evaluation following an alleged sexual assault is the collection of trace evidence including DNA. In addition to the history of the assault, alternative light sources (ALSs) have been used to assist examiners in identifying areas of potential DNA evidence. A common ALS used is the Wood's lamp. The goal of this project was to determine the best practice using an ALS to aid in the identification of trace DNA evidence in sexual assault forensic exams.

The authors reviewed the limited data available on this topic (seven studies) and concluded that the Wood's lamp should no longer be used as the ALS. However, ALS with wavelengths able to detect DNA should be used. Most importantly, examiners must be educated about the advantages and disadvantages and proper use of ALS. Further research is necessary on the use of ALS in forensic evaluations along with development of new techniques to assist in identification of semen in forensic exams.

Nurse Use

SANEs play a key role in providing care for victims of sexual assault. The training to become a SANE is specialized and growing in importance and the recognition of its value to victims, their families, and the criminal justice system (IAFN, 2014). Evidence-based practice ensures patients receive the highest quality of care supported by research.

SANE, Sexual assault nurse examiner.
Data from Eldredge K, Huggins E, Pugh LC: Alternate light sources in sexual assault examinations: an evidence-based practice project. *J Forensic Nurs* 8:39-44, 2012.

Certification

The scope and standards of forensic nursing practice have been used for the development of the certification examination and other credentials that are intended to demonstrate competence of the practitioner. Credentialing within forensic nursing, as with all new professional specialties, has become an increasingly important issue. Different types of credentials pertain to nursing, both within and outside the discipline. While all nurses should have an understanding of credentialing and the implications and responsibilities that accompany such a designation, it is uniquely important for FNs who maintain close relationships to both the medical and the legal communities. FNs provide care when health and the law intersect and must therefore have credentials that speak to their unique qualifications to give that specialized care (Pasqualone, 2015).

Certification examination for pediatric (SANE-P) and adolescent/adult sexual assault nurse examiners (SANE-A) is available through the International Association of Forensic Nurses. This certification along with the Legal Nurse Consultant, Corrections Nurse, Death Investigator, and Forensic Examiner are offered by other organizations to registered nurses meeting entry criteria and generally do not require a graduate degree. Forensic Nurse Examiners are most often referred to as Forensic Examiners, Medicolegal Death Investigators and Coroners, Sexual Assault Nurse Examiners, or Advanced Forensic Nurses. Advanced forensic nurse certification (AFN-BC) previously offered by the American Nurses Credentialing Center through the portfolio review method was discontinued in 2017. Graduate and undergraduate certificate programs in forensic nursing are offered at various universities as well as the American Institute of Health Care Professionals, but currently there is not a profession-wide standard certification.

ETHICAL ISSUES

Ethical considerations in the practice of forensic nursing are unique because of the implications to not only a client's health but, in some cases, his or her freedom. Practice outcomes affect individuals and families, as well as communities and society as a whole. Ethics and law are closely tied but are not equivalent. Ethical nursing practice involves adherence to law in most cases, but also to the ethics of nursing and the dictates of one's conscience (Constantino et al., 2013). Nurses maintain a different code of conduct than do other professionals. For example, law enforcement personnel answer singly to the law for their standard. Knowledge and understanding of these considerations is core to the specialty of forensic nursing (International Association of Forensic Nurses Ethics Committee, 2008).

Olsen (2013) organized ethical principles into five categories: respect for person, beneficence, distributive justice, respect for community, and contextual caring. Each of these categories reflects examples of the tension that may arise when the forensic nurse faces a dilemma imposed by conflicting interests. An overriding consideration is the need to respect each person and to develop contextual caring within the art of nursing. Respect for person means respect for autonomy while protecting vulnerable persons. The right of each human to self-determination is recognized within nursing but may not be respected by all societies. Therefore respect for human rights may involve advocacy to some degree. Laws, cultural norms, and considerations of safety, which limit the liberty of an individual, may constrain the nurse's ability to fully exercise a therapeutic relationship. Questions raised pose dilemmas in a variety of medical and psychiatric settings.

Forensic environments include courtrooms, jails, prisons, and psychiatric facilities for the criminally insane. When criminal action or trauma to an individual requires care, the need for coercion is likely. Certain situations may make medical coercion necessary. These situations include incapacity (or inability) to make decisions and making decisions that could result in harm to self or harm to others in the absence of interventions. Paternalism has been defined as "the principle that allows one person to make decisions for another" (Williams, 2007, p. 93). This may be necessary in the case of minors or older adults. Paternalistic intervention was viewed by the U.S. Supreme Court as lawful in the case of *Washington v Harper* (1990), when it ruled that mentally ill inmates could be compelled to take psychotropic medications against their will if the mental disorder is serious, the inmate is dangerous to himself, and the medication prescribed is in the inmate's best medical interest. Therefore the ability of a psychiatric forensic nurse practicing in an advanced role to make a determination of rational autonomy is crucial in questions of coercion: to make judgments without being judgmental (Martin et al., 2013).

Beneficence (care) and the complementary principle of nonmaleficence (without harm) go beyond autonomy in the responsibility of the nurse not only to support an individual's choices but to perform actions that enhance the health of others. Nurses provide care without prejudice of the circumstance or individual characteristics. They provide care to the injured, marginalized, and poor whether the individuals are victims or offenders. Nurses who care for pregnant teens in a youth facility or collect evidence from drug addicts each hold the same ethical responsibility as described previously (Dhaliwal & Hirst, 2016; Ferszt et al., 2013). Questions may arise when the resources to achieve adequate health are not plentiful enough for all to receive adequate care. When economic restraints limit funds to process sexual assault evidentiary kits, treat victims of assault, and provide dental care to methamphetamine addicts in prison, where should the funds be applied? Principles of distributive justice address such questions in deciding what goods will be distributed to which persons in what proportions. Forensic nurses may find themselves in a policy-making position to answer such questions to ensure that their clients, given similar circumstances, are treated no better or worse than others in the application of protection and medical care. Also, when there are questions of retribution, whether withholding provisions or threatening harm, forensic nurses never participate in the punishment, however subtle, of another being.

Ethical decisions can be exceedingly difficult when the safety of a society is at risk. One approach to making decisions with respect for the community is utilitarianism, which appeals exclusively to outcomes or consequences in determining which choice to make. Williams (2009) explains:

> *Utilitarianism, with its mandate for the general good, rather than a specific interest, would place the safety of the community above the rights of any one individual. The forensic nurse expert, hired by the court to evaluate a client, as an example, testifies on behalf of society, not the individual. To that end, it may be argued that the nurse expert uses a utilitarian perspective that may not serve the interests of the client but instead, serves the interests of society. Traditional nursing mandates that the correct focus (and therefore the right moral choice) be placed on the individual. However, the burden of responsibility often shifts in forensic nursing from the individual to the community, a correct moral choice under utilitarianism (p. 50).*

During a forensic examination, the potential exists for withholding vital information in the investigation of wrongdoing. The temptation to "assist" the perceived victim's case may be justified by a desired outcome for that individual as well as the ultimate safety of a community. This dilemma of information can be carried to situations of privacy protection. The entitlement to privacy may be changed when someone's safety is at stake. If a specimen for DNA is collected during the investigation of a crime, should that information remain in the Combined DNA Index System (CODIS) for use in future crimes, regardless of the outcome of prosecution of that case and when there is the potential for repeat offense (Williams & Wienroth, 2017)? Do hospitals have the right to videotape parents who are suspected of Munchausen syndrome, or is this a violation of Fourth Amendment rights (Morrison, 1999)? When victims give information to sexual assault examiners, are they informed that records may be released to law enforcement and attorneys? Should they consent to the release of photographs that depict intimate areas of their body for anyone in law enforcement, attorneys, and juries to see, even in the name of full disclosure (Ledray, 2008)?

Finally, there are always questions regarding the relationship between forensic clients and nurses. Caring is the essence and core value of nursing (Watson, 2008). Olsen (2013) recognized that caring as well as ethics is influenced by the context of relationships and that nurses' "emotion is inextricably bound to moral good" (p. 51). Contextual caring is not synonymous with beneficence but "entreats the forensic nurse to interact with each client, whether criminal or victim, as a person within an ethical relationship of caring concern grounded in the nurse's personal values" (Olsen, 2013, p. 51). The care goes beyond the "obligatory dictates" of client rights. Unique problems are posed when the client is in denial about the role he or she plays in the problem or poses a safety risk to the nurse. In addition, forensic nurses must overcome the societal bias of establishing relationships with individuals believed to have injured another, perhaps intentionally. Finally, when personal bias or issues of conscience impair the ability to prescribe or participate in particular medical interventions, objections may be raised. Examples of situations at risk for bias in forensics include collection of trace evidence from individuals who have impaired consciousness or are coerced into consent (Constantino, et al., 2014), prescription of birth control following sexual assault, participation in capital punishment, and the use of unnecessary physical or medical restraint. Nurses and other health care professionals have well-established codes of ethics and other examined statements to guide practice and inform care (ANA, 2015; IAFN, 2008; Martin et al., 2013). It is imperative to view these statements that guide practice as a basis for conduct as well as for reflective dialogue in real client situations.

CHECK YOUR PRACICE

A mother and her seven- year -old son come to the clinic for a routine check up and for immunizations. While examining the boy, the nurse notices that he has several scratches and bruises on his upper thighs and genital area. The mother avoids eye contact with the nurse during the examination.

What actions should the nurse take?

The following two case studies demonstrate some of the aspects of forensic nursing care.

Case #1: Tamara Lynch is a six-year-old child who lives in a busy household of four children, her grandmother, mother, and stepfather. She is a client of the local pediatric clinic and has an appointment today for a school-related examination. She has been very interested in school in the past but recently her grades have declined and her mother describes her behavior as withdrawn. Shirley Meres is the pediatric nurse practitioner who has seen Tamara for her most recent health care. She too has noted the change in Tamara's affect. Based on the health history, Ms. Meres uses

CHECK YOUR PRACICE—cont'd

developmentally appropriate questions to ask Tamara about situations in which she may not feel safe or situations with adults that have made her feel uncomfortable about her body. Tamara describes repeated episodes with her stepfather during which she was inappropriately touched and fondled. The nurse meets with Tamara's mother and explains her role as a forensic nurse. She explains that Tamara will need a specialized physical examination with collection of evidence, including laboratory specimens and photographs. After obtaining permission from the mother, the evaluation is performed using enhanced lighting and visualization equipment to collect photographic evidence, and body fluids for diagnostic and forensic testing. The nurse tells Tamara and her mother that the examination is normal for her age; no indications of trauma are noted. All evidence is packed for preservation according to crime lab protocols. Following the interview and examination, Ms. Meres counsels the child and mother about predictable psychological reactions to child sexual assault and disclosure even though no evidence of abuse was found in the nurse's examination. The mother is given information on advocacy, the legal process that follows a report to law enforcement agencies, and mental health counseling that is available locally. Tamara is given an appointment at the clinic in two weeks. The nurse makes contact with law enforcement to report the child's disclosure and make arrangements for transfer of all evidence. Ms. Meres continues to follow the health care of the family in the months to follow for evaluation and prevention of common problems that present to families who experience child abuse.

Case #2: Mike Post is an 18 year-old male who is taken to the emergency department by ambulance for what appeared to be a motor vehicle collision. His condition is considered serious. Following resuscitative measures, he is pronounced dead. Staff members at the emergency department contact the medical examiner's office to report the death. Sean Miller is the forensic nurse investigator on duty who receives the call. When Mr. Miller arrives at the emergency department, he interviews paramedics and emergency department clinicians about the accident site and the appearance of the decedent on arrival. He photographs the body, clothing, and other sources of trace evidence, including items in the decedent's pockets. Mr. Miller performs a thorough examination of Mike Post and discovers a small bullet hole in the left postauricular tissue. All items are individually bagged, sealed, and labeled for further analysis by the crime laboratory. The nurse then meets with the family to explain the need for investigation of all sudden, unexpected deaths. He describes the process involved in the investigation and preparation of the body prior to transfer to a funeral home. Copies of the medical record and x-rays obtained at the facility are transported with the body for autopsy. Mr. Miller reports his findings to the forensic pathology team and law enforcement officers. The autopsy is performed and the ballistics analysis of the recovered bullet leads to the arrest of the alleged assailant. When the case goes to court, the nurse is subpoenaed to testify about the investigation and collection of evidence. The nurse maintains contact with the family to keep them informed of the progress of the case and the resources for legal and family grief counseling available in their community. See the Quality and Safety in Nursing Education box that follows to learn ways in which nurses partner with families to coordinate care.

QSEN FOCUS ON QUALITY AND SAFETY EDUCATION FOR NURSES

Quality and Safety Focus

Targeted Competency: Client-Centered Care

Recognize the client or designee as the source of control and full partner in providing compassionate and coordinated care based on respect for client's preferences, values, and needs.

Important aspects of client-centered care include:

- **Knowledge:** Describe strategies to empower clients or families in all aspects of the health care process.
- **Skills:** Assess level of client's decisional conflict and provide access to resources.
- **Attitudes:** Value active partnership with clients or designated surrogates in planning, implementation, and evaluation of care.

Client-Centered Care Question

You are an RN at a correctional facility, where system-focused updates have recently been implemented to ensure provider safety. A metal detector has been implemented that all inmates must pass through before entering the clinic. A standardized frisk procedure has also been implemented. The presence of a security guard has been standardized for all clinic visits. The clinic environment has been modified so that all sharp objects or potentially dangerous objects have been locked up. Extra surveillance cameras have been added to each clinical examination room, and panic buttons have been added as extra security for providers in each exam room.

- Which system updates might impact patients' experience of care?
- Amidst all of the identified heightened security approaches, how do you communicate client-centered care to your clients?
- How do you address client safety in this new environment?
- How do you protect client confidentiality and privacy in this new environment?

RN, Registered nurse.

Prepared by Gail Armstrong, PhD, DNP, ACNS-BC, CNE, Associate Professor, University of Colorado Denver College of Nursing.

FUTURE PERSPECTIVES

Forensic nursing is predominantly a community-oriented specialty. Practice arenas are associated with health care facilities such as private clinics and emergency departments, criminal justice centers for victims of crime, medical examiner offices, police departments, correctional facilities, and mental health centers. What is consistent in each of these practice sites is the care of individuals who have experienced the effects of injury, either intentional or unintentional. Increasingly it is being recognized that hospitals need forensic nursing services. Clients routinely enter hospitals with conditions that have overlying legal implications (Amar, 2016). In addition, injuries occur as a result of medical incidents and errors. Forensic nurses use their expert understanding of cause and effects of trauma and are in a position to investigate the circumstances in order to design a plan of care for individual as well as special groups of clients. They serve as a liaison between the hospital and the medical-legal community to reduce the effects of trauma.

PRACTICE APPLICATION

A 26-year-old woman arrived unaccompanied to the emergency department of an academic medical center with cuts on her face, hands, legs, and pelvic area. She was crying and said that she had been attacked and was afraid to have an examination or to provide the name of her attacker. What is the first action that the nurse should take?

A. Explain to her the importance of reporting this crime immediately.
B. Listen closely to her and reflect back to her the fear, anger, and other feelings you hear in her voice.
C. Immediately call law enforcement officials yourself.

Once you select the first action that you would take, explain your rationale and outline your exact actions.

Answers can be found on the Evolve site.

KEY POINTS

- Forensic nursing is a community-oriented specialty that addresses the prevention and treatment of accidental injury and violent crimes.
- The specialty reflects an integration of nursing, forensic science, and the law.
- Forensic nursing is needed whenever injury has legal implications.
- Forensic nurses need to maintain objectivity in rendering care to both victims of injury and perpetrators of crime.
- The scope and standards of forensic nursing practice guides forensic nurses with unique skills of the specialties such as expert courtroom testimony and documentation and security of evidence.
- Forensic nurses work in cooperation with public health professionals, including nurses, in developing programs of prevention such as automobile safety and intimate partner violence prevention.
- Educational programs for forensic nurses are offered through continuing education offerings and formal graduate degree programs.
- Credentialing for forensic nurses include pediatric and adolescent/adult sexual assault nurse examiners (SANE-A and SANE-P).

CLINICAL DECISION-MAKING ACTIVITIES

1. Think about injuries you have experienced and answer the following questions:
   A. How did the injury affect my ability to perform normal activities of my daily routine?
   B. What injury patterns did I have that would lead me to conclude it was violent or accidental?
   C. What could I have done to prevent the injury from occurring?
2. Discuss the effects of violence in your community with a fellow student. What situations exist that increase the risk that someone will be assaulted?
3. Write a list of the types of evidence that can be collected at a crime scene or in an emergency department based on a scenario of crime involving a young woman who is the victim of sexual assault.
4. In a short paragraph, explore how you might feel toward someone who commits a crime and needs nursing care. What ethical standards of nursing will influence your treatment of this individual?

ADDITIONAL RESOURCES

EVOLVE WEBSITE

http://evolve.elsevier.com/Stanhope/community/

- Answers to Practice Application
- Case Study
- Glossary
- Review Questions

REFERENCES

American Nurses Association: *Recognition of a Nursing Specialty, Approval of a Specialty Nursing Scope of Practice Statement and Acknowledgement of Specialty Nursing Standards of Practice, and Affirmation of Focused Practice Competencies*, August 2017.

American Nurses Association: *Code of ethics for nurses with interpretive statements*, Silver Spring, MD, 2017. Retrieved from www.nursingworld.org.

Amar A: Response to victimization. In Amar A, Sekula LK, editors: *A practical guide to forensic nursing*, Indianapolis, IN, 2016, Sigma Theta Tau International.

Bauman R, Stark S: The role of forensic death investigators interacting with the survivors of death by homicide and suicide, *J Forensic Nursing* 11(1):28–32, 2015.

Burgess AW, Holmstrom LL: Rape trauma syndrome, *Am J Psychiatr* 131(9):981–986, 1974.

Cabelus NB, Spangler K: Evidence collection and documentation. In Hammer R, Moynihan B, Pagliaro E, editors: *Forensic nursing: a handbook for practice*, Burlington, MA, 2013, Jones-Bartlett.

Campbell R, Bybee D, Townsend SM, Shaw J, Karim N, Markowitz J: The impact of sexual assault nurse examiner programs on criminal justice case outcomes, *Violence Against Women* 20(5):607–625, 2014.

Campbell R, Patterson D, Bybee D: Prosecution of adult sexual assault cases: a longitudinal analysis of the impact of a Sexual Assault Nurse Examiner program, *Violence Against Women* 18(2):223–244, 2012.

Campbell JC, Humphreys JC, editors: *Family violence and nursing practice*, New York, NY, 2011, Springer Publishing Company.

Centers for Disease Control and Prevention: Estimated lifetime medical and work-loss costs of emergency-department treated injuries, United States, 2013, *MMWR Morb Mortal Wkly Rep* 2015;64(38):1078-1082.

Centers for Disease Control and Prevention: *National Center for Injury Prevention and Control* website, 2015. Retrieved from https://www.cdc.gov.

Centers for Disease Control and Prevention: *National Center for Injury Prevention and Control, National Violent Death Reporting System website*, 2017. Retrieved from https://www.cdc.gov.

Centers for Disease Control and Prevention: *National Center for Injury Prevention and Control: Web-based Injury Statistics Query and Reporting System (WISQARS)*, 2016: Retrieved from http://www.cdc.gov.

Constantino RE, Zalon ML, Young, SE: The ethical, legal, and sociocultural issues in forensic nursing. In Constantino R, Crane P, Young, S, editors: *Forensic nursing: evidence-based principles and practice*, Philadelphia, PA, 2013, F.A. Davis Company.

Constantino R, Stewart C, Campbell P, et al: Evidence collection for the unconscious and unconsented patient, *Open J Nursing* 4(4):287–295, 2014.

Council on Linkages Between Academia and Public Health Practice: *Core Competences for Public Health Professionals: Tier*, 2012. Retrieved from http://www.phf.org.

Crane J: 'The bones tell a story the child is too young or too frightened to tell': the battered child syndrome in post-war Britain and America, *Soc Hist Med* 28(4):767–788, 2015.

Dhaliwal K, Hirst S: Caring in correctional nursing: a systematic search and narrative synthesis, *J Forensic Nursing* 12(1):1–12, 2016.

DuMont J, MacDonald S, White M, et al: Client satisfaction with nurse-led sexual assault and domestic violence services in Ontario, *J Forensic Nursing* 10(3):122–134, 2014.

Eldredge K, Huggins E, Pugh LC: Alternate light sources in sexual assault examinations: an evidenced-based practice project, *J Forensic Nursing* 8:39–44, 2012.

Feder G, Wathen CN, MacMillian HL: An evidence-based response to intimate partner violence, WHO guidelines, *JAMA* 310(5): 479–480, 2013.

Ferszt GG, Hickey JE, Seleyman K: Advocating for pregnant women in prison: the role of the correctional nurse, *J Forensic Nursing* 9(2):105–110, 2013.

Filmalter CJ, Heyns T, Ferreira R: Forensic patients in the emergency department: who are they and how should we care for them? *Intl Emerg Nurs*, in press, 2018;40:33-36.

Haddon W: A logical framework for categorizing highway safety phenomena and activity, *J Trauma* 12:193–207, 1972.

Hammer RM, Moynihan B, Pagliaro E: *Forensic nursing: a handbook for practice*, Sudbury, MA, 2013, Jones and Bartlett.

Harris C: Occupational injury and fatality investigation, *J Forensic Nursing* 9(4):193–199, 2013.

Hufft AG: Theoretical foundations for advanced practice nursing. In Hammer RH, Moynihan B, Pagliaro EM, editors: *Forensic nursing: a handbook for practice*, Sudbury, MA, 2013, Jones and Bartlett.

International Association of Forensic Nurses: Joint position statement: Care of prepubescent pediatric sexual abuse patients in the emergency care setting, *J Forensic Nursing* 13(3):150–153, 2017.

International Association of Forensic Nurses (IAFN): *History of IAFN*, 2018, IAFN website. Retrieved from https://www.forensicnurses.org.

International Association of Forensic Nurses (IAFN): *Forensic nursing: scope and standards of practice*, ed 2, 2017, American Nurses Association.

International Association of Forensic Nurses (IAFN): *Position Statement, Adult/Adolescent SANE Education and Certification*, 2014. Retrieved from https://cdn.ymaws.com.

International Association of Forensic Nurses: *Vision of Ethical Practice*, 2008. Retrieved from http://www.forensicnurses.org.

Jackson DB, Vaughn MG: Promoting health equity to prevent crime, *Prev Med* 113:91–94, 2018.

James SH, Nordby JJ, editors: *Forensic science: an introduction to scientific and investigative techniques*, ed 4, Boca Raton, FL, 2014, Taylor & Francis.

Jamerson CM, Turvey BE: Forensic nursing: objective victim examination. *In forensic victimology: examining violent crime victims in investigative and legal contexts*, Amsterdam, 2014, Elsevier.

Ledray L: *SANE development and operation guide*, Washington, DC, 1998, Sexual Assault Resource Service, U.S. Department of Justice, Office of Justice Programs, and Office of Victims of Crime.

Ledray LE: Consent to photograph: how far should disclosure go? *J Forensic Nurs* 4(4):188–189, 2008.

Lombardi M, Cantor J, Patrick PA, Altman R: Is fluorescence under an alternate light source sufficient to accurately diagnoses subclinical bruising? *J Forensic Sci* 60(2):444–449, 2015.

Lynch VA: Forensic Nursing: *A New Field for the Profession*. Paper presented at the 38th Annual Meeting of the American Academy of Forensic Science, 1986.

Lynch VA: *Clinical forensic nursing: a descriptive study in role development*, Arlington, TX, 1990, University of Texas.

Lynch VA: Concepts and theory of forensic nursing science. In Lynch VA, Duvall JB, editors: *Forensic nursing science*, ed 2, St Louis, MO, 2011, Elsevier.

Lynch VA, Duval JB, editors: *Forensic nursing science*, ed 2, St Louis, MO, 2011, Elsevier.

Malmgren J, Leahy C. Overarching issues: Testifying. In Price B, Maguire K, editors: *Core curriculum for forensic nursing*, Philadelphia, PA, 2016, Wolters Kluwer.

Martin T, Maguire T, Quinn C, Ryan J, Bawden L, Summers M: Standards of practice for forensic mental health nurses—identifying contemporary practice, *J Forensic Nursing* 9(3): 171–178, 2013.

Maslow AH: A theory of human motivation, *Psychol Rev* 50:370–396, 1943. Retrieved from http://psychclassics.yorku.ca.

Mason T, Mercer D, editors: *Critical perspectives in forensic care: inside out*, Hampshire, London, 1998, Macmillan.

Menaker TA, Campbell BA, Wells W: The use of forensic evidence in sexual assault investigations, *Violence Against Women* 23(4):399–425, 2017.

Morrison CA: Cameras in hospital rooms: the fourth amendment to the constitution and Munchausen syndrome by proxy, *Crit Care Nurs Q* 22(1):65–68, 1999.

Moyer VA: U.S. Preventive Services Task Force, Screening for intimate partner violence and abuse of elderly and vulnerable adults: U.S. preventive services task force recommendation statement, *Ann Intern Med* 158(6):478–486, 2013.

Meunier-Sham J, Cross TP, Zuniga L: The seven pillars of quality care in a statewide pediatric sexual assault nurse examiner program, *J Child Sexual Abuse* 22(7):777–795, 2013.

Nutting MA, Dock LL: *A history of nursing: the evolution of nursing systems from the earliest times to the foundation of the first English and American training schools for nurses,* vol 1, New York, NY, 1907, G.P. Putnam's Sons.

O'Neill B: Accidents or crashes: highway safety and William Haddon Jr, *Contingencies* 24(1):30–32, 2002.

Olsen D: Ethical considerations in forensic nursing. In Hammer RH, Moynihan B, Pagliaro EM, editors: *Forensic nursing: a handbook for practice*, ed 2, Sudbury, MA, 2013, Jones and Bartlett, pp 45–71.

Orr JL: The role of the forensic SANE nurse in pediatric sexual assault, *J Leg Nurs Consult* 27(4):16–20, 2016.

Pagliaro EM: Evidence: Collection, preservation, databases, and cold cases. In Constantino RE, Crane PA, Young, SE, editors: *Forensic nursing: evidence-based principles and practice*, Philadelphia, PA, 2013, F. A. Davis and Company.

Pasqualone GA: The relationship between forensic nurses in the emergency department and law enforcement, *Crit Care Nurs Q* 38(1):36–48, 2015.

Pasqualone G, Michel C: Forensic patients hiding in full view, *Crit Care Nurs Q* 38(1):3–16, 2015.

Pollitt EN, Anderson JC, Scafide KN, Holbrook D, D'Silva G, Sheridan DJ: Alternate light source findings of common topical products, *J Forensic Nurs* 12(3):97–103, 2016.

Sakala L: *Breaking down mass incarceration in the 2010 Census: State-by-State incarceration rates by race/ethnicity*, 2014, Prison Policy Initiative. Retrieved from https://www.prisonpolicy.org.

Scannell M, MacDonald AE, Berger A, Boyer N: Human trafficking: how nurses can make a difference, *J Forensic Nursing* 14(2): 117–121, 2018.

Simmons, B: Graduate forensic nursing education: how to better educate nurses to care for this patient population, *Nurse Educator* 39(4): 184–187, 2014.

Speck PM: The Lived History of Forensic Nursing, PowerPoint presentation, Memphis, n.d.

Squires JE, Squires RH: A Review of Munchausen syndrome by proxy. *Pediatr Ann* 42(4):e67–e71, 2013.

U.S. Department of Justice/Office on Violence Against Women: *A national protocol for sexual assault medical forensic examinations adult/adolescents*, ed 2, 2013. Retrieved from https://www.ncjrs.gov.

U.S. Department of Health and Human Services, Office of Disease Prevention and Health Promotion: *Healthy People 2020*, 2010. Retrieved from http://www.health.gov.

U.S. Department of Health and Human Services, Health Resources and Services Administration: *Surgeon General's Workshop on Violence and Public Health Report*. DHHS Publication No. HRS-D-MC-86-1, 1986.

Valentine JL: Why we do what we do: a theoretical evaluation of the integrated practice model for forensic nursing science, *J Forens Nursing* 10(3):113–119, 2014.

Washington v Harper, 494 U.S., 1990.

Watson J: Social justice and human caring: a model of caring science as a hopeful paradigm for moral justice for humanity, *Creative Nurs* 14(2):54–61, 2008.

Williams D: Forensic nursing and utilitarianism: the quest for being right, *J Forensic Nurs* 5(1):49–50, 2009.

Williams DL: Is there a case for paternalism in forensic nursing? *J Forensic Nurs* 3(2):93–94, 2007.

Williams R, Weinroth M: Social and ethical aspects of forensic genetics: a critical review, *Forensic Sci Rev* 29(2):145–169, 2017.

Winfrey ME, Smith AR: The suspiciousness factor: critical care nursing and forensics, *Crit Care Nurs Q* 22(1):1, 1999.

World Health Organization: *Responding to Intimate Partner Violence and Sexual Violence Against Women:* WHO Clinical and Policy Guidelines, 2013. Retrieved from http://apps.who.int.

World Health Organization: *Global Status Report on Violence Prevention*, 2014. Retrieved from http://www.who.int.

World Health Organization: *Preventing Youth Violence: An Overview of the Evidence*, 2015. Retrieved from http://apps.who.int.

World Health Organization: *Global Action Plan to Prevent Interpersonal Violence*, 2016. Retrieved from http://www.who.int.

Zercie K, Penders, P: Photography in forensic nursing. In Hammer R, Moynihan B, Pagliaro E, editors: *Forensic nursing: a handbook for practice*, Burlington, MA, 2013, Jones-Bartlett.

45

The Nurse in the Faith Community

Lisa M. Zerull, PhD, RN-BC

OBJECTIVES

After reading this chapter, the student should be able to do the following:

1. Define faith community nursing and holistic health promotion.
2. Differentiate between spirituality and religiosity.
3. Examine the historical roots of faith community nursing.
4. Discuss scope and standards of practice for faith community nursing.
5. Develop awareness of the nurse's role within faith communities for spiritual care, health promotion, and disease prevention.
6. Apply the nursing process in a faith community to assess, implement, and evaluate programs for healthy congregations using *Healthy People 2020* leading health indicators.

CHAPTER OUTLINE

Perspectives on Faith Community Nursing
History of Faith Community Nursing
Rationale for Faith Community Nursing as a Viable Community Health Model
Definitions in Faith Community Nursing
Faith Community Nursing Practice
Issues in Faith Community Nursing Practice
National Health Objectives and Faith Communities
Conclusion

KEY TERMS

congregants, p. 995
congregation, p. 993
congregational model, p. 1000
faith communities, p. 993
faith community nurse, p. 993
faith community nurse coordinator, p. 996
faith community nurse transitional care, p. 993
faith community nursing, p. 990
healing, p. 990
health cabinet, p. 995
health ministries, p. 994
holistic or whole person care, p. 995
holistic health center, p. 990
institutional model, p. 1000
parish, p. 993
parishioner, p. 1001
parish nurse, p. 993
parish nursing, p. 990
partnership, p. 992
pastoral care staff, p. 998
polity, p. 1001
religiosity, p. 990
religious care, p. 995
specialization, p. 992
spirituality, p. 990
wellness committee, p. 995

PERSPECTIVES ON FAITH COMMUNITY NURSING

With increased incidence of chronic diseases such as hypertension and diabetes along with health concerns of obesity, substance abuse, and depression, there is a need for creative wellness initiatives in the community. One such community setting of care is the congregation or faith community as an ideal location for screening, education, and compassionate support. It is in this setting where wellness promotion efforts focus on much more than the physical needs of individuals. Rather, nursing care out of the congregation provides a comprehensive whole person approach involving care of the physical, emotional and spiritual. Faith community nurses have the knowledge, skills, and experience to offer whole person care to the wide array of persons across the life span who gather together for the purpose of worship, fellowship, and participating in specific rituals of faith.

Faith community nursing, previously call **parish nursing**, is a recognized nursing specialty practice, yet is frequently overlooked when creative strategies are needed for improving the health of individuals and the larger community. Not surprising when only 11.7 percent of nurses reported receiving adequate spiritual care training as part of their nursing education, yet 92.4 percent of nurses feel strongly that spiritual care is a legitimate part of the profession (Delgado, 2015). Nurses often confuse religious practice or religiosity with spirituality and may neglect patients' spiritual needs (O'Brien, 2017). Whereas **religiosity** relates to "a person's beliefs and behaviors associated with a specific religious tradition or denomination" (O'Brien, 2017), **spirituality** is "an individual's attitudes and beliefs related to transcendence (God) or to the nonmaterial forces of life and nature" (O'Brien, 2017). Thus additional education in spiritual care is needed to distinguish between the two and to provide an understanding of faith community nursing (Delgado, 2015).

Registered nurses working out of a faith community or congregation establish close relationships with individuals, families, and often, the larger community to coordinate programs and services that significantly affect health, healing, and wholeness (ANA/HMA, 2017; Butler & Diaz, 2017; Callaghan, 2016; Gotwals, 2016, 2018; Laming & Stewart, 2016; Young, 2016; Ziebarth, 2015, 2016). Faith community nurses balance knowledge and skill in their role to facilitate the faith community as it becomes a caring place—a place that is a source of health and **healing** for its members. Many nurses are drawn to faith community nursing because it encourages the expression of spirituality as a part of health and healing. Others are drawn to this specialty practice out of vocational calling (O'Brien, 2017).

Faith community nurses address health concerns of individuals, families, and groups of all ages (Callaghan, 2015). Like other communities, the members of faith communities experience birth and death; acute and chronic illness; growth and development; stress or dependency concerns; challenges from life transitions; and decisions regarding healthy lifestyle choices. Serving as good stewards of resources, faith community nurses encourage partnering with community health agencies as well as lay and professional church leaders to arrive at creative responses to health issues and to develop health-promoting and spiritually healing activities. The nurse serves the faith community by focusing on the needs of the individual parishioner and the overall faith community with special attention given to spiritual care support.

HISTORY OF FAITH COMMUNITY NURSING

Faith community nursing has its historical roots in the Judeo-Christian tradition with early Biblical references to women providing care to the sick and persons in need. For centuries, Catholic Sisters and Protestant women specialty trained as nurses have promoted health and cared for the sick, the poor, the fallen, and the unbelieving (Doyle, 1929; Fliedner, 1870). Likewise, parish nurses, now called faith community nurses, have followed this same tradition for more than three decades by working out of the congregation to promote whole person health—ministering to body, mind, and spirit of parishioners from the time of birth through the end of life.

In 1984, the concept of parish nursing was introduced to churches in the Chicago, Illinois, area by Lutheran chaplain Granger Westberg (1913-1999) as way of expanding existing health ministries and providing another link between faith and health (see Box 45.1, Timeline of Faith Community Nursing). Westberg described parish nursing as a way for the church to reclaim its traditional role in healing (1990). Having previous experience with setting up **holistic health centers** out of churches, Westberg fully understood that hospitals and

BOX 45.1 Timeline of Faith Community Nursing

- 1983 Pilot program with a nurse running a wellness clinic out of the congregation setting—Our Saviour Lutheran Church, Tucson, AZ.
- 1984 Parish Nurse Program partnership begun with six congregations and Lutheran General Hospital, Park Ridge, IL.
- 1986 Lutheran General Hospital establishes a Parish Nurse Resource Center to share information about health ministry and parish nursing with others.
- 1987 First Westberg Parish Nurse Symposium is held and Granger Westberg publishes book *The Parish Nurse*. Parish Nurse Resource Center becomes the *National* Parish Nurse Resource Center.
- 1989 Health Ministries Association began in Iowa.
- 1991 Marquette University offers eight-day parish nurse education program titled the *Wisconsin Model*, a curriculum later modified to become the *Foundations of Faith Community Nursing* course.
- 1995 Lutheran General merges with Evangelical Health Systems Corporation to create Advocate Health Care. National Parish Nurse Resource Center becomes the *International* Parish Nurse Resource Center.
- 1997 American Nurses Association recognizes parish nursing as a specialty practice.
- 1998 ANA/HMA publish first Scope and Standards for parish nursing. Parish Nurse Preparation Curriculum is published.
- 1999 Parish Nurse Coordinator Curriculum is published. Death of Granger Westberg (July 1913-February 1999).
- 2002 IPNRC transfers assets from Advocate Health System, Chicago, IL, to Deaconess Foundation, St. Louis, MO.
- 2004 World Forum for Faith Community Nursing is formed with 22 members from Australia, Canada, South Korea, Swaziland, and United States.
- 2005 ANA/HMA revised and published scope and standards. Nurse title changed from parish nurse to faith community nurse.
- 2011 IPNRC transfers assets from Deaconess Foundation, St. Louis, MO, to the Church Health Center, Memphis, TN. The 25th Annual Westberg International Parish Nurse Symposium is held.
- 2012 ANA/HMA publish second edition faith community nurse scope and standards.
- 2014 American Nurses Credentialing Center (ANCC) launches faith community nursing certification through portfolio. *Foundations of Faith Community Nursing* curriculum revised.
- 2016 IPNRC renamed Westberg Institute. The 30th anniversary of the Annual Westberg International Parish Nurse Symposium held in Chicago, IL.
- 2017 ANA/HMA publish third edition faith community nurse scope and standards. ANCC ends FCN certification by portfolio.
- 2018 Thirty-one countries active with faith community nursing.

ANA, American Nurses Association; *FCN,* faith community nurse; *HMA,* Health Ministries Association; *IPNRC,* International Parish Nurse Resource Center.

physicians deal with illness, yet there is a need for preventive medicine and wellness in the community and churches fit right in (1990). He also recognized that it was nurses who could have the largest impact on the delivery of whole person care within a congregation, using the nurse's broad background of health promotion, education, spiritual care, and social work (Westberg, 1985).

Westberg's rejuvenation of parish nursing in the 1980s built on the strengths of his previous work and focused on the nurse-clergy team working with individuals and their families. Nurses used their professional knowledge, skills, and experience to listen to the spoken and unspoken concerns of individuals, resulting in whole person care provision with spiritual care central to the relationship. By 1984, Westberg partnered with Lutheran General Hospital (Park Ridge, Illinois—now known as Advocate Health) on a pilot project within six Chicago-area churches (Solari-Twadell & McDermott, 2006). These partnerships established the first institutionally based paid parish nurse program between **a health system** and churches in the United States (Westberg & McNamara, 1987).

As the contemporary parish nurse movement grew, information was spread by advocates of whole person health. This resulted in the establishment of a Resource Center (International Parish Nurse Resource Center [IPNRC]) in 1986 to provide information, printed literature, and news of emerging parish nurse programs across the United States, both paid and unpaid. Through the collaborative efforts of the health system, educators, and the IPNRC, a foundational course was designed to provide basic education to prepare nurses in parish nursing. As noted in the timeline, the IPNRC moved from Illinois to Missouri and now its current home with Church Health in Memphis, Tennessee.

The need of a membership organization for a growing number of parish nurses served as a catalyst for the founding of the Health Ministries Association (HMA) 1989. The HMA provided networking and communications for nurses along with others active in health ministry. Through HMA's leadership, the American Nurses Association (ANA) recognized parish nursing as a professional nursing specialty in 1997 with the first scope and standards of practice published in 1998 (ANA/HMA 2017). The title of parish nurse was changed to faith community nurse with the 2005 revisions to the scope and standards reflective of the need to be inclusive of nurses in all faith traditions (ANA/HMA 2005). Another milestone was reached in 2014 when the American Nurses Credentialing Center (ANCC) released a nurse specialty certification by portfolio for faith community nurses; however, due to low applicant volumes combined with administrative costs, the certification was discontinued after three years (ANCC, 2017).

Another key contributor to faith community nursing is the IPNRC, whose name was changed to Westberg Institute in 2016 for a variety of reasons (Campbell, 2016). First was to honor contemporary faith community nurse founder Granger Westberg and also to support its parent organization Church Health's branding and planning future marketing strategies (Campbell, 2016). Throughout the resource center's history, the focus has remained on the provision and promotion of quality education,

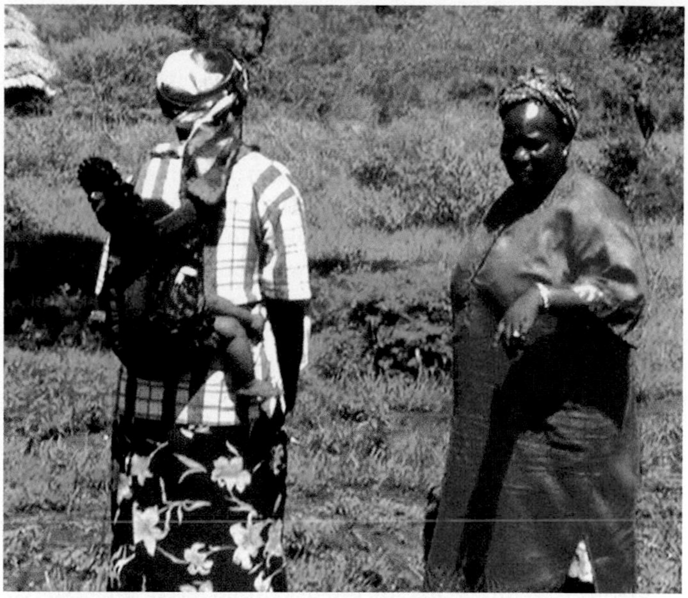

Fig. 45.1 Parish nurse in rural Swaziland, Africa, making a home visit.

research, and support through curriculum, resources and continuing education opportunities.

Today, faith community nursing continues to be a recognized specialty practice by the ANA complete with scope and standards to guide nursing practice and an ever increasing body of research and evidence-based practice literature. There are more than 17,000 faith community nurses across the United States and in at least 31 countries around the world such as Australia, Canada, New Zealand, Germany, Swaziland (Fig. 45.1), Ukraine, and Pakistan (Bana, 2018; Glaser, 2018; Izang, 2018; Mansour, 2018; Nicholson & Dlamini, 2018; Van Loon, 2018; Vaughan, 2018; Wordsworth, 2018; Zerull, 2018). Most countries have established resource centers, educational preparation programs, and active networks for support. The number of faith community nurses is a conservative estimate based on the number of nurses who report taking foundations courses and does not reflect the numbers of nurses who provide some form of health ministry to congregations without formal education in the specialty area (Daniels, 2016). Faith community nursing continues to evolve as a nursing specialty practice offering creative strategies for whole person health.

RATIONALE FOR FAITH COMMUNITY NURSING AS A VIABLE COMMUNITY HEALTH MODEL

Early chapters in Parts 1 and 2 of this text familiarize the reader with the historical, economic, social, political, environmental, and ethical perspectives and influences on health care. The health care delivery system is challenged to work within parameters of tighter financial constraints while addressing patients' complex health concerns and also responding to federal mandates for expensive automated systems (i.e., electronic health records) that span the continuum of care. Current health care reform reflects a shift in health care delivery from hospital to community for more comprehensive wellness-focused programs (Briggs et al., 2017; Callaghan, 2016; Garrett Wright et al., 2015; Meyer & Holland, 2016; Sturgeon et al., 2016) and transitional care models to reduce hospital readmissions (Munning & Owen, 2018; Ziebarth, 2015, 2016; Ziebarth & Campbell, 2016). Transitional care models are defined as "care provided by a faith community nurse in a faith community to support the patient's experience of transition from one level of care to another" (Ziebarth & Campbell, 2016).

Faith community nurses are well positioned to provide lower cost and wholistic community-based care for vulnerable and underserved populations as well as collaborate with other care providers (McLean & Habicht, 2016; Young, 2016; Ziebarth, 2016).

After major hospitalizations, clients may return to their homes very sick with few, if any, care providers available. Caregivers are faced with the multiple tasks of managing finances, maintaining family responsibilities, and learning caregiving skills. Fragmented care and inadequate caregiver training and availability are problems for the disenfranchised, underserved, and uninsured, as well as for economically well-situated and better-educated persons. Families are challenged to seek the best ways to meet the multiple demands of young children, teens, and aging parents whether living in metropolitan, suburban, or rural areas.

Consumer demand for involvement in health care decisions continues to increase, and society emphasizes individual responsibility for health. Simultaneously, consumers have increased interest in their own well-being and have expressed needs for health information to be available in a variety of formats (McLean & Habicht, 2016). In addition to consumer interest and a heightened awareness of responsibility for one's own health, health care providers and managed care systems have found it financially advantageous for individuals to remain healthy and minimize unnecessary access to care. Consumers struggle to cope with the challenges of rising costs of care, decreasing reimbursement, and the complex health system demands on individuals and families.

The traditional health care delivery model will not meet the burgeoning needs of the future (Chase-Ziolek, 2015). The skills of professional nurses, such as faith community nurses, will become more important with the provision of health care services in nontraditional settings (O'Brien, 2017; Ziebarth, 2017). It is important to differentiate the unique practice of faith community nursing from other community-based specialty practices. Faith community nursing shares many similarities with home health, hospice, and public health nursing—promoting health in the community setting; however, it is set apart from other community-based nurses by its whole person health approach and care of the spirit. Nursing care is also shaped and guided by the faith community's traditions, rites, and rituals.

A primary focus of all nurses in the last few decades has been to coordinate care and to link health care providers, groups, and community resources as the client tries to understand complicated health plans. Negotiating with individuals, agencies, and community **partnerships** within the complex maze of the broader health care environment demands a knowledgeable and seasoned professional. Nurses are aware of the necessity of collaborative practices and the formation of partnerships to care for groups and individuals across the life span. These nurses recognize the need for identifying strategies to address health promotion and disease prevention at all levels. They advocate for healthy lifestyle choices in exercise, nutrition, substance use, and stress management. Nurses realize that information and guidance must be available via media, in schools, workplaces, faith communities, and residential neighborhoods. Faith community nurses partner with others such as faculty in academic settings, health care institutions, and federal agencies as they serve populations in faith communities (Opalinski et al., 2017; Power et al., 2016; Young & Smothers, 2018; Ziebarth, 2016) to help improve health outcomes.

DEFINITIONS IN FAITH COMMUNITY NURSING

The ANA describes the development of a specialty practice in nursing as nurses expanding their practice to include the knowledge and skills necessary to meet the needs of patients requiring specialty care. Faith community nursing is defined by the ANA as a specialized practice of professional nursing that focuses on the intentional care of the spirit as well as the promotion of whole person health and the prevention or minimization of illness within the context of a faith community and the wider community (ANA/HMA, 2017).

Requirements for the faith community nurse include (1) an active registered nurse license in the state in which he or she practices; (2) minimum diploma or associate degree in nursing; however, a minimum of baccalaureate degree in nursing preferred; (3) completion of an educational course to prepare for this nursing specialty practice (and ministry); (4) experience in nursing with community nursing experience preferred; (5) specialized knowledge of the spiritual beliefs and practices of the faith community served; (6) reflection of personal spirituality maturity in his or her practice; and (7) being organized, flexible, a self-starter, and a good communicator (ANA/HMA, 2017; Westberg Institute, 2018). Variation in the depth and breadth of nursing practice results from the nurse's education, experience, practice setting, and populations cared for by the nurse. For example, a nurse experienced in gerontology may seek out other nurses or health professionals in the congregation to assist with initiatives designed to support care of a teen population. Thus the faith community nurse is not required to be an expert with all populations and settings, rather is able to identify and coordinate additional resources to meet the needs.

Specialization involves focusing on nursing practice in a specific area, identified from within the whole field of professional nursing and in collaboration with specialty nursing organizations. For example the Health Ministries Association (HMA) and Faith Community Nurses International (FCNI) are identified as the two professional membership organizations for faith community nurses. Additionally, the ANA delineates the components of professional nursing practice that are essential for any particular specialty. As the specialty continues to evolve, the valuable contributions of nurses begin to distinguish them from other care providers.

This has been true for the evolution of parish nursing. Early on, nurses involved with spiritual care struggled to find a workable definition for the role. Concerns were raised about nurses calling themselves parish nurses without any formal education—simply a nurse license and a willingness to serve their congregation. In order to validate the ministry of parish nurses to that of a recognized nursing specialty, additional education with a defined curriculum including spiritual care was created. Following much dialogue and work to validate the specialty practice, parish nursing was recognized as a nursing specialty in 1997 by the American Nurses Association (ANA/HMA, 2017).

With the 2005 revision of the *Scope and Standards of Practice,* the nurse title changed from parish nurse to faith community nurse (ANA/HMA 2005). The new title was more inclusive of diverse faith traditions and in response to international considerations (ANA/HMA 2017). **Parish nurse** was the original title chosen by Granger Westberg in the 1980s as a theological choice because it connoted service to the **congregation** and also the wider community within a geographical area. A congregation also refers to a variety of faith institutions, including churches, synagogues, temples, and mosques or other faith-based organizations (ANA/HMA 2017; Mattern, 2016). The word **parish** can mean *congregation* and also *geographical area served by a congregation.* Additional titles for nurses working out of faith communities include parish nurse, congregational nurse, health ministry nurse, crescent nurse, or health and wellness nurse (ANA/HMA, 2012, p. 7).

The **faith community nurse** is a licensed registered nurse "with well-developed clinical and interpersonal skills, a strong personal religious faith, and a desire or felt call to serve the needs of a faith community" (O'Brien, 2017, p. 335). With additional education in spiritual care of self, individuals, and groups, the faith community nurse works out of the congregational setting. It is expected that the professional registered nurse possesses competence in practice resulting from his or her application of knowledge, skills, and experience, functions with a deep understanding of the faith community's traditions, and fully integrates *care of the spirit* with care of the body and mind (ANA/HMA, 2017; O'Brien, 2017). The assumptions that underlie faith community nursing are as follows:

1. Health and illness are human experiences.
2. Health is the integration of the spiritual, physical, psychological, and social aspects of the health care consumer to create a sense of harmony with self, others, the environment, and a higher power.
3. Health may be experienced in the presence of disease or injury.
4. The presence of illness does not preclude health nor does optimal health preclude illness.
5. Healing is the process of integrating the body, mind, and spirit to create wholeness, health, and a sense of well-being when the health care consumer's illness is not cured.

QSEN FOCUS ON QUALITY AND SAFETY EDUCATION FOR NURSES

The Nurse in the Faith Community

Targeted Competency: Quality Improvement

Use data to monitor the outcomes of care processes and use improvement methods to design and test changes to continuously improve the quality and safety of health care systems.

Important aspects of safety include:

- **Knowledge:** Describe approaches for changing processes of care.
- **Skills:** Design a small test of change in daily work (using an experiential learning method such as plan-do-study-act).
- **Attitudes:** Value measurement and its role in good patient care.

Quality Improvement Question

You are a paid faith community nurse at a busy, urban church that partners with a regional hospital on a transitional care project to decrease readmission rates for chronically ill older adults. **Faith community nurse transitional care** is defined as *care provided by a nurse working out of the faith community to support the patient's experience of transition from one level of care to another* (Ziebarth, 2016). An alarmingly high percent of your congregation is over the age of 65 and challenged with chronic diseases of congestive heart failure (CHF) and type 2 diabetes.

As the faith community nurse you obtained additional training in transitional care at the local hospital and developed a relationship with the discharge planning team. Accepting one or two referrals every six months, you work closely with the discharge planning team and the referred individual to create the best plan of care. Beginning interventions include a wholistic assessment; medication and diabetes management review with teach-back; signs and symptoms of acute exacerbations of chronic disease; and spiritual care interventions requested by the individual such as healing presence, prayer, or scripture reading. You also accompanied the individual to primary care provider appointments for clarification of information. You want to evaluate the effectiveness of these interventions.

Step 1: What is the problem or issue that the transitional care nurse program addresses?

Step 2: Identify both short-term and long-term goals for transitional care.

Step 3: How would you document the specific program outcomes?

Step 4: Are there best practices that might inform your whole person care interventions or your collaboration with the local hospital and discharge planning team?

Step 5: How would you evaluate the short-term and long-term goals of the transitional care program?

Faith communities are organizations of groups, families, and individuals who share common values, beliefs, religious doctrine, and faith practices that influence their lives, such as a church, homeless shelter, synagogue, temple, or mosque, and that function as a patient system, providing a setting for faith community nursing (ANA/HMA, 2017). Faith communities are found all over the world wherever individuals gather for the common purpose of worship, fellowship, the giving and receiving of love, grace, and hope, as well as the invitation, not obligation, to participate in the rites and rituals of a faith tradition (Fig. 45.2). Some common examples include baptism, devotions, communion, reading of scripture, prayer, and singing. The important role of the faith community in a person's life is amplified with the recognition that it is one of the only institutions with a connection to an individual from birth through

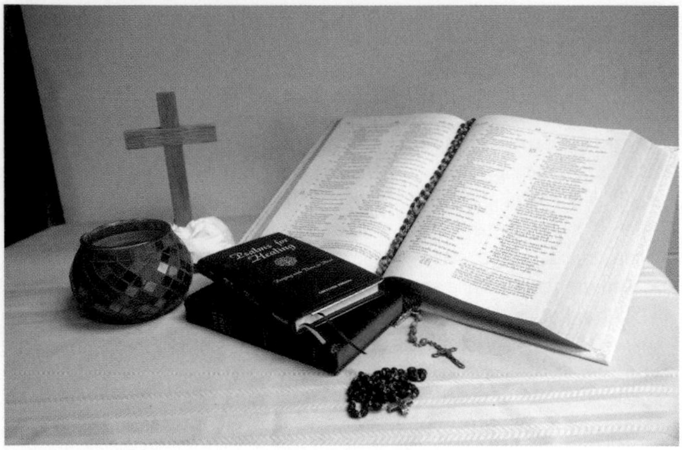

Fig. 45.2 Religious symbols, images, rituals, and sacred places are significant to ministry.

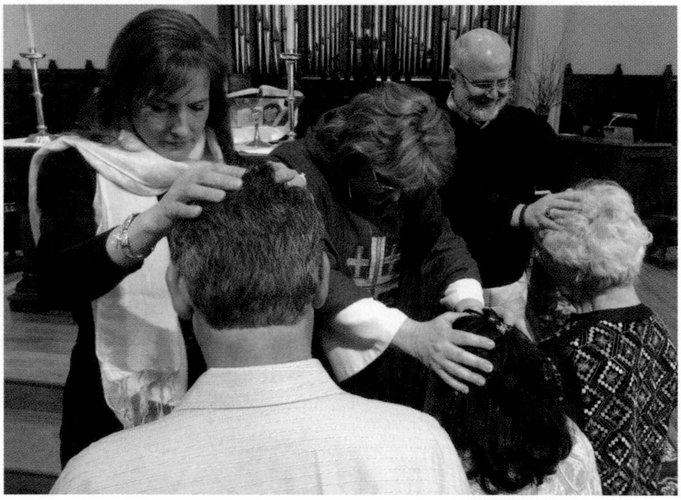

Fig. 45.3 Prayers for healing service with ritual of laying on of hands.

death. While many recognize and receive spiritual care support in the congregation, there may not be a conscious awareness of the church being an ideal place for health promotion of body and mind.

Health ministries are visible activities, programs, and rituals of faith organized around health and healing of the congregation's membership and offered by the faith community nurse, clergy, layperson, or community resource. Health ministries may be informal or more specifically planned and encompass a gamut of activities, including home visitation, providing meals for families in crisis or upon return home after hospitalization, quilting circles, grief support groups, and prayers for healing services (Fig. 45.3) to name a few (Church Health, 2018; Patterson, 2012, 2013). Evidence suggests that health ministries potentially improve the health outcomes of all members of the faith community, including various ethnicities at higher risk for chronic disease (Asomugha et al., 2011; Horton et al., 2014). As an active member of the health ministry team, the faith community nurse emphasizes health promotion and models a visible healing presence to members of the congregation.

Faith community nurses respond to health and wellness needs of individuals, groups, and populations in fulfilling the mission of health ministry and intentional spiritual care. Services may also extend to those beyond the congregational setting, such as a food pantry, blood pressure screenings, transportation, and warm meals for those in need (Butler & Diaz, 2017; Chase-Ziolek, 2015; Garrett Wright et al., 2015). Additionally, the faith community nurse may work out of an adult daycare center, an immigrant community, a homeless shelter, an amusement park, a crisis center (Callaghan, 2015; Opalinski et al., 2017; Parker, 2018; Power et al., 2016).

According to the ANA *Scope and Standards of Practice* for all nurses (ANA/HMA, 2012), spiritual care is part of all nursing practice and acknowledges a person's sense of meaning and purpose in life, which may or may not be expressed through formal religious beliefs and practices. It is also described as a distinct type of care defined by acts of listening, compassionate presence, open-ended questions, prayer, use of religious objects, talking with clergy, guided visualization, contemplation, meditation, conveying a benevolent attitude, or instilling hope (O'Brien, 2017). Spiritual care is helping the patient make meaning out of his or her experience or find hope (Ziebarth, 2016). Unique to faith community nursing as a specialty nursing practice is the primary focus on care of the spirit, with *spirit* defined as the core of a person's being. Box 45.2 provides a detailed listing of the core interventions for care of the spirit performed by faith community nurses. The compassionate and intentional healing presence of a spiritually mature nurse with individuals or groups is vital to addressing spiritual care needs.

BOX 45.2 Nursing Interventions Classification Core Interventions for Faith Community Nursing

- Abuse Protection Support
- Active Listening
- Anticipatory Guidance
- Caregiver Support
- Coping Enhancement
- Crisis Intervention
- Culture Brokerage
- Decision-Making Support
- Emotional Support
- Environmental Management: Community
- Family Integrity Promotion
- Family Support
- Forgiveness Facilitation
- Grief Work Facilitation
- Guilt Work Facilitation
- Health Care Information Exchange
- Health Education
- Health Literacy Enhancement
- Health System Guidance
- Hope Inspiration
- Humor
- Listening Visits
- Medication Management
- Presence
- Referral
- Religious Addiction Prevention
- Religious Ritual Enhancement
- Relocation Stress Reduction
- Self-Care Assistance: IADL
- Socialization Enhancement
- Spiritual Growth Facilitation
- Spiritual Support
- Surveillance
- Sustenance Support
- Teaching: Group
- Teaching: Individual
- Telephone Consultation
- Touch
- Values Clarification

IADL, Instrumental activities of daily living.

From Bulechek G, Dochterman J, Butcher H, et al.: Core interventions for nursing specialty areas: faith community nursing. In *Nursing Interventions Classification (NIC)*, ed. 7, St. Louis, 2018.

Spiritual care is much different from **religious care**. Whereas religious care stems from the doctrine, rites, and rituals of a specific denomination or set of beliefs, spiritual care is unique to the individual's purpose in life, the fulfilling of that purpose, and living it wholeheartedly. In most denominations, religion creates a nurturing environment where groups gather for worship or defined activity and in which spirituality emerges and grows. Nurses in secular health care may not give priority to spiritual care due to lack of time (Delgado, 2015) or a reluctance to address spiritual care for fear of "stirring things up that they will not know how to address" (Jackson, 2011, p. 4), or crossing professional boundaries. With faith community nursing, intentional spiritual care is invited, expected, and appreciated.

One nurse differentiated her experiences in providing hospital care versus faith community nursing care: "I have always thought of my nursing care as being whole person in nature; however in secular settings, I had to *ask permission* to care for the spiritual needs of my patients, whereas in the congregational setting, spiritual care *is expected*. It is a rare interaction with a parishioner where prayer, a gentle touch or warm embrace are not a part of my nursing care!" (Erbach, 2005).

Holistic or whole person care relates to the relationship between body, mind, and spirit in a constantly changing environment and involves caring for the soul in a special kind of engagement that goes beyond seeing the physical patient but includes observation of the entire patient (Dossey & Keegan, 2016). The faith community nurse, supported by members of the congregation, assesses, plans, implements, and evaluates holistic care programs. The process of operationalizing holistic care is enhanced by an active **wellness committee** or **health cabinet** composed of congregation members or congregants who may or may not be health professionals (e.g., doctors, therapists, social workers) and who are fully engaged in health ministry (Patterson, 2003; Westberg, 1990). The committee is most effective when members represent the broad spectrum of the life of the church. An active wellness committee provides leadership and influence throughout the faith community; ideas come not from one individual but are generated out of a committee structure (McNamara, 2006; Patterson, 2003; Westberg, 1990). The faith community nurse uses the collective knowledge and skills of this collaborative group to provide comprehensive and effective services. The outcome is a caring congregation that understands the strong link between faith and health and supports healthy, spiritually fulfilling lives. Resources for faith community nursing can be found on this book's Evolve website.

FAITH COMMUNITY NURSING PRACTICE

Similar to public health nurses in the United States, faith community nurses identify the need for health promotion services across the life span, particularly in underserved urban and rural areas. Nurses are adept at creatively addressing gaps in the delivery of service. The congregation provides an ideal setting of care for **congregants** to benefit from health counseling and health promotion services at all levels of prevention. The following provides an overview of levels of prevention for older adult health.

LEVELS OF PREVENTION

Older Adult Health

Primary Prevention

- Hold classes for older adults on healthy eating, including food selection, preparation, and increasing socialization opportunities at mealtimes for widows/widowers.
- Promote and encourage age-appropriate activities that include daily physical exercise with increased focus on improved balance related to muscle strength, proprioception, and coordination.
- Encourage a variety of activities of individual and group interest and discourage extended inactivity.
- Encourage healthy snacks and meals for older adult gatherings and activities.
- Write faith community newsletter articles targeting topics of interest to older adults (e.g., recommended annual screenings, signs and symptoms of heart attack and stroke, medication management, Medicare benefits). Place the same health information on a bulletin board located in a high traffic area of the congregation.
- Provide an eyeglasses drive for missions, reminding older adults to get vision checks by an eye doctor at least every 1 to 2 years, and update glasses or contact lenses when vision changes.
- Provide support groups based on needs and interests (e.g., grief support/bereavement; low vision; transitions to long-term care/retirement community; Alzheimer caregivers; adults living with disabilities).
- Coordinate medication management opportunities such as inviting a pharmacist to assist in a medication review after worship.
- Initiate a walk for fun program (e.g., Walk to Emmaus)
- Host a community health fair offering resources related to whole person health.

Secondary Prevention

- Provide health assessment and counseling during home visits for health promotion such as visits after a hospitalization.
- When making home visits, identify safety concerns and make suggestions such as eliminating throw rugs, decreasing clutter, decreasing use of extension cords, and moving heat sources from flammable products such as oxygen.
- Using an attitudinal/behavioral risk survey, identify factors influencing health behaviors.
- Be available for health counseling for older adults before and after activities.

Tertiary Prevention

- Collaborate closely with ministerial team about sessions that deal with healthy nutrition, exercise with injury prevention guidelines, health concerns related to being overweight, and advantages of maintaining a healthy weight, and support, stress management, and improved quality-of-life sessions.
- Follow up and monitor health care provider's plan of care for older adults challenged with chronic disease such as diabetes, hypertension, and depression; provide education, support, and spiritual care.
- Facilitate a faith-based activities program for aging in place.
- Discuss in older adult gatherings the need for loving, caring friends and the support needed for mental health and overall well-being.

Faith community nurse services emphasize whole person health promotion and disease prevention within a supportive and caring faith community. Nurses acknowledge the inner strength and spirituality of persons and groups to enhance healing. Faith community nurses draw on knowledge and skills with communication, negotiation, collaboration, and leadership. Working with the congregation as the population group, faith community nurses attempt to include in the wellness programs those persons who are less vocal or visible in the community of faith. The spiritual dimension of health is optimized by complementing pastoral care with faith community nursing care.

Profile of the Faith Community Nurse

The practice of the faith community nurse is governed by (1) the Nurse Practice Act of the state in which the nurse practices; (2) *Nursing: Scope and Standards of Practice* (ANA, 2015); (3) *Faith Community Nursing: Scope and Standards of Practice* (ANA/HMA 2017); and (4) *Code of Ethics with Interpretive Statements* (for nurses) (ANA, 2015). According to the International Parish/Faith Community Nurse Resource Center located in Memphis, Tennessee (Church Health, 2018), the suggested requirements to be a faith community nurse include the following:

- Active registered nurse license in the state of practice
- Baccalaureate degree or higher in nursing with experience in community nursing preferred
- Completion of a foundational education course in faith community nursing
- Specialized knowledge of the spiritual beliefs and practices of the faith community
- Personal spirituality maturity in practice
- Organized, flexible, a self-starter, and a good communicator

The majority of nurses choosing to become specialized in faith community nursing are experienced and have been in practice for several years. A large survey of faith community nurses (n = 1161) across the United States yielded the following description:

- Average age = 55 years
- 89 percent female
- 32 percent prepared at baccalaureate level in nursing, 24 percent prepared at the diploma level, 14 percent prepared at the associate's level, 12 percent hold a master's in nursing
- 68 percent serve as unpaid staff in towns (47 percent), cities (42 percent), and metro areas (11 percent)
- Majority are from Christian faith traditions with only 2 percent of the sample Jewish; 25 percent, Lutheran; 23 percent, Roman Catholic; 16 percent, Methodist
- 17 percent have had membership in the American Nurses Association (Solari-Twadell, 2006)

Because many faith community nurses practice within their own congregation, they are considered to be a known and trusted resource. By virtue of relationship, congregants access the services of the faith community nurse with a high comfort level and awareness that information shared will be kept confidential by the nurse professional. Faith community nurses are well aware of the beliefs, faith practices, and level of spiritual maturity of the members served and link these with health and healing.

Many faith community nurses function in a part-time capacity and serve as salaried or unpaid staff. Some nurses are responsible for services for several faith communities, whereas others engage in faith community nursing as part of a full-time commitment in other capacities. For example, a nurse might be employed part-time as a public health nurse and part-time as a faith community nurse in the same community. Alternatively, a nurse employed full-time in an acute care setting may spend time serving in an unpaid capacity working in a faith community with a group of other nurses. Depending on the practice model, the nurse has a narrowly defined or a wider realm of responsibility. Faith community nurse practices may be integrated into a health care system or into practices that collaborate with related professional practice areas such as health departments or colleges of nursing. Health care systems employ **faith community nurse coordinators**, who facilitate different arrangements with several faith communities of varying backgrounds (Zerull & Solari-Twadell, 2006). Practices in which several faith community nurses are supervised by a coordinator have built-in opportunities for networking, partnering, and mentoring (Durbin et al., 2013).

As advanced practice nurse and faith community nurse practices increase in numbers and varieties of arrangements, evaluation of practice trends within the health care delivery system and the needs of society is necessary. Nursing must be accountable and responsive to those being served, as well as to those who provide opportunities to serve.

The goals for a faith community are clearly defined in the 2017 scope and standards for practice (ANA/HMA, 2017). First is the protection, promotion, and optimization of health and abilities of the congregants. Next is the prevention of illness and injury and facilitation of healing. The faith community nurse works to alleviate suffering through the diagnosis, referral, and treatment. Lastly, the faith community nurse advocates for all persons in the context of the values, beliefs, and practices of the congregation. Nurses work with a health cabinet or wellness committee to evaluate assets and areas of need in order to plan services that will attain outcomes congruent with goals established by the congregation and faith communities served.

Characteristics of Faith Community Nurse Practice

Since the early 1990s, five characteristics have been identified as central to the philosophy of faith community nursing by nursing educators and practitioners (Solari-Twadell, 2006):

1. The spiritual dimension is central to the practice. Nursing embodies the physical, psychological, social, and spiritual dimensions of clients into professional practice. Although parish nursing includes all four, it focuses on intentional and compassionate care, which stems from the spiritual dimension of all humankind.
2. The roots of the role balance both knowledge and skills of nursing, using nursing sciences, the humanities, and theology. The nurse combines nursing functions with pastoral care functions. Visits in the office, home, hospital, or nursing home often involve prayer and may include a reference to scripture, symbols, sacraments, and liturgy of the faith

community represented by the nurse. The values and beliefs of the faith community are integral to the supportive care given. Nurses also assist with worship services as appropriate within the faith community.

3. The focus of the specialty is the faith community and its ministry. The faith community is the source of health and healing partnerships, which result in creative responses to health and health-related concerns. Partnerships may be among individuals, groups, and health care professionals within the congregation. They may also be among various congregations or community agencies, institutions, or individuals. Partnerships also evolve as the congregation visualizes its health-related mission beyond the walls, stones, and steeples of its own place of worship.
4. Parish nurse services emphasize the strengths of individuals, families, and communities. Parish nurses endorse this fourth characteristic in their practice. As congregations realize the need for care and care for one another, their individual and corporate relationship with their Creator is often enhanced. This provides additional coping strength for future crisis situations within the family and community.
5. Health, spiritual health, and healing are considered an ongoing, dynamic process. Because spiritual health is central to well-being, influences are evident in the total individual and noted in a healthy congregation. Well-being and illness may occur simultaneously; spiritual healing or well-being can exist in the absence of cure.

CHECK YOUR PRACTICE

At the conclusion of the worship service you notice a long-time member of the congregation sitting alone in a back pew with her head down. Mrs. E is an 84-year-old widow whose husband died one month ago. She is well-known to you as you visited the couple's home many times over the course of his lengthy battle with cancer. She is visibly sad and withdrawn from other congregants leaving the sanctuary. You do not know if she wants to be left alone or desires the healing presence of a faith community nurse. What should you do?

Faith Community Nurse Interventions and Programs

Faith community nurses provide care to individuals, families, congregations, and communities across the life span. The practice includes the full cultural and geographic community regardless of ethnicity, lifestyle, gender, sexual orientation, or creed. The nurse incorporates faith and health, uses the nursing process in providing services to the faith community, and facilitates collaborative health ministries as an important component of the practice.

One of the first tasks of a new faith community nurse is to explore the social demographics and identify the health needs of the congregation (O'Brien, 2017). This is accomplished by selecting a congregational health needs survey available online or in print for public use (Durbin et al., 2013). In collaboration with the ministry team, the faith community nurse determines actionable priorities and then applies his or her knowledge, skills, and experience to plan health promotion and spiritual care initiatives. Often, due to limited congregational resources, the faith community nurse must conduct a resource assessment to determine feasibility when matching need with time and financial resources.

Since limited resources in faith communities often challenge program development, the faith community nurse must match need with available resources. The following set of questions helps determine what is possible to consider in advance of carrying out health promotion projects (Solari-Twadell & McDermott, 2006, p. 104):

1. What resources are needed?
2. What resources are available?
3. Which of the available resources are accessible to the nurse for the accomplishment of a specific effort or project?
4. Can the work of the project or program be accomplished with what is available and accessible?

Several images of the faith community nurse in practice highlight varying settings and professional activities. Central to all interactions is intentional care of the spirit and the healing presence of the faith community nurse. Healing presence and prayer are frequently offered in most interactions. Bulletin board displays are helpful to promote health topics of interest in hallways with high visibility. Blood pressure screenings offer therapeutic touch as well as assessment for cardiac status, social health, and overall well-being as the individual spends time with the nurse (Fig. 45.4). Informal pew-side consultations take place after worship when individuals ask health-related questions or request resource or referral information (Fig. 45.5). Young families require comprehensive support with diverse needs related to age, supportive relationships, childcare support, and parenting (Fig. 45.6). The health educator role requires creative and differing teaching strategies for the nurse based on the ages of individuals or groups being taught (Fig. 45.7). Faith community nurses may organize an annual health fair inviting community partners and service agencies to share resources and promote health ministries to parishioners

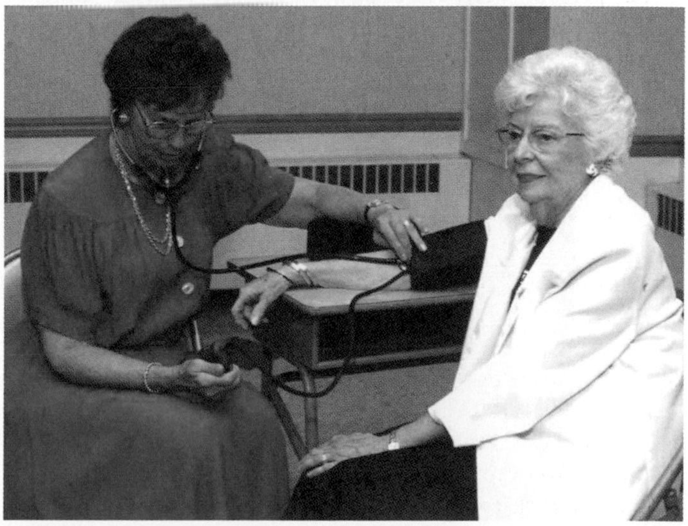

Fig. 45.4 Blood pressure screening in the faith community.

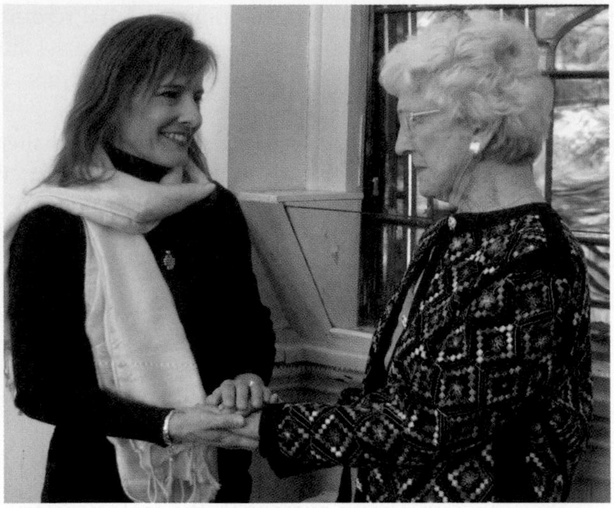

Fig. 45.5 Faith community nurse provides informal pew-side health consultation.

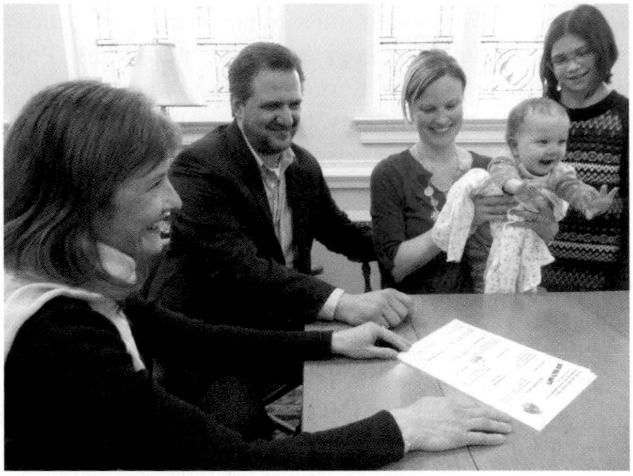

Fig. 45.6 Offering education and support to families.

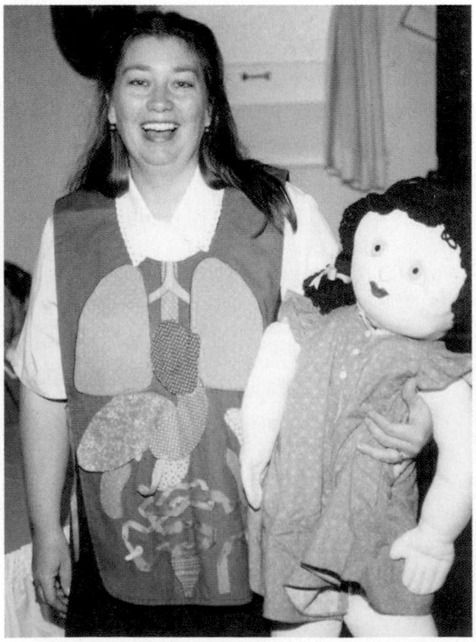

Fig. 45.7 Faith community nurse as educator using visual art as clothing for health education.

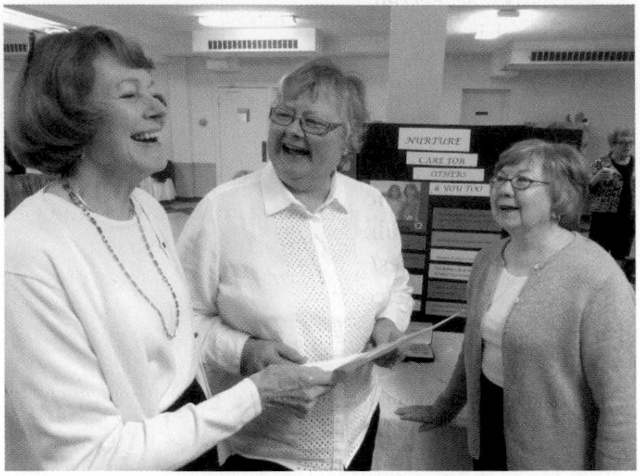

Fig. 45.8 Health fair for the congregation and community.

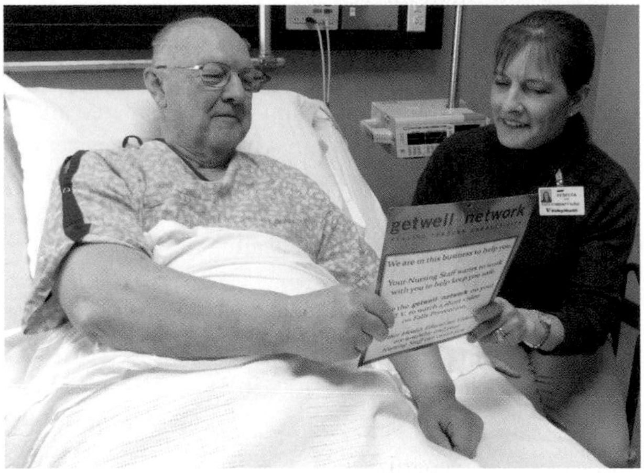

Fig. 45.9 Hospital visitations include care of the spirit.

of all ages (Fig. 45.8). Hospital and institutional care visits provide spiritual and emotional support when unexpected illness and health crisis may challenge coping skills and raise questions about faith and denominational theology (Fig. 45.9). In congregations with older adults, an organized bereavement/grief support group for widows and widowers may or may not be led by the faith community nurse. Depending on social ministries in place, the faith community nurse may interface with homeless persons accessing congregational resources of food or financial support. Other interventions, services, or programs provided by the faith community nurse are determined by taking into consideration specific congregation needs; the mission, vision, and strategic plan of the congregation matched with the knowledge, skills, and experience as well as time availability of the faith community nurse.

As one of the trusted members of the **pastoral care staff**, the faith community nurse will find it helpful to develop ease in inquiring about a person's spiritual journey. Assessments, whether physical or spiritual, are used to gather data for planning nursing care. Because care of the spirit is central to faith community nursing, spiritual assessment instruments are useful tools and applicable to diverse populations (Puchalski,

2018, Puchalski & Ferrell, 2010). One widely used spiritual assessment tool is constructed with sample questions and the acronym FICA:

F-Faith or beliefs: What are your spiritual beliefs? Do you consider yourself spiritual? What things do you believe in that give meaning to life?

I-Importance and influence: Is faith/spirituality important to you? How has your illness and/or hospitalization affected your personal practices/beliefs?

C-Community: Are you connected with a faith center in the community? Does it provide support/comfort for you during times of stress? Is there a person/group/leader who supports/assists you in your spirituality?

A-Address: What can I do for you? What support/guidance can health care provide to support your spiritual beliefs/practices? (Puchalski, 2018).

In addition to assessment data, history of family relationships and past association with faith communities provides background information. The nurse needs to be comfortable with questions that lead parishioners to expand on their faith beliefs. Compassionate, careful listening involves being still, reflecting, and being intentionally in the present. Being sensitive to the differing needs of personal spirituality during various points along life's journey is important to consider while guiding persons through the spiritual assessment. The nurse then also helps individuals share necessary information about spirituality needs with other health care providers and clergy as appropriate.

Faith Community Nurse Education

The registered nurse choosing to serve a faith community in a formal role should obtain additional education in the nursing specialty practice recognizing that most undergraduate nurse programs offer limited content on spiritual care. A variety of educational programs and curricula are available through health care institutions, colleges and universities, seminaries, or faith-based denominations. Education offered in classroom or online formats range from weekend to week-long curricula which may or may not award continuing education contact hours, to academic courses awarding three to six credit hours of study. Depending on the course or education sponsor, additional content may include denomination specific topics, regional community resources, complementary therapies, and transitional care to name a few.

The most widely used continuing education curriculum around the world is published by the Westberg Institute supported by Church Health in Memphis, Tennessee. Guided by the scope and standards for faith community nursing and incorporating the latest evidence in research and practice, the curriculum provides comprehensive education organized around four core values of spiritual formation, professionalism, whole person health, and community (Church Health Center, 2014). A list of available courses using this curriculum is found at https://westberginstitute.org.

Westberg Institute offers curriculum for two courses—Foundations and the Coordinator/Advanced. The Foundations course offers topics within content areas to include theology of health and healing; the nurse's role in spiritual care; use of prayer; the history, philosophy, and models of care; advocacy; assessment; beginning your ministry; working with a congregation; care coordination; communication and collaboration; documentation, ethical and legal issues; family violence; grief and loss; healing and wholeness; health promotion; and self-care (IPNRC, 2014). The Coordinator/Advanced course is designed to build on the Foundations course and offers administrative and program management content: (1) coordinator self-care; (2) working with diverse faith traditions; (3) documentation; (4) the role of the coordinator; (5) human resource management; (6) utilizing research; (7) professional development; (8) emerging trends and issues; (9) new program development; (10) growing and sustaining; (11) marketing and promoting; (12) program funding and grant writing; and (13) working with faith communities. The Advanced course equips the faith community nurse with the tools necessary to coordinate a group of faith community nurses within a congregation or a larger regional or denomination-based network.

Ongoing education for faith community nurses may be obtained locally, regionally, or internationally. At the local level, education programs are often coordinated through established networks and are institution based or university sponsored. Regionally, networks of faith community nurses may gather monthly or annually for one day or weekend program retreats. Larger conferences such as the Westberg International Symposium offered by the Westberg Institute and the annual Health Ministries Association conference provide comprehensive sessions and forums for nurses to gain new knowledge, network with others, and stay abreast of current resources, trends, and issues in the specialty practice. Additionally, there are educational programs offered by faith community resource centers around the globe such as in Germany, the United Kingdom, and Australia (Glaser, 2018; Van Loon, 2018; Wordsworth, 2018). Information about accessing faith community nursing resource centers can be found on this book's Evolve website.

Advanced practice opportunities also enrich a specialty practice. Master's-prepared nurses (with specialization in congregational leadership, congregational health, public health nursing, or holistic nursing) and nurse practitioners have found niches in faith community nursing. Universities and seminaries have developed creative and unique partnerships to provide educational opportunities for faculty and students at the undergraduate and graduate levels.

Formal educational preparation and continuing education options must continue to include the basics and enrichment courses in nursing practice, research, theology, and pastoral care (see the following How To box). In addition, the specialty practice nurse benefits from updates in the areas of public health, medicine, technology, and sensitivity awareness with the lesbian/gay/bisexual/transgender/queer (LGBTQ) community or bariatric population. Enhancing collaboration, negotiation, and coordination skills, as well as consultation, leadership, and research skills, is essential. Faith community nurses accept responsibility for ongoing professional education within nursing and ministry arenas (ANA/HMA, 2017).

HOW TO Work With Baccalaureate Nursing Students and Nursing Faculty

Baccalaureate students benefit from the integration of whole person and spiritual care in courses throughout a curriculum (Johnson et al., 2014). Additionally, a clinical practicum experience in the faith community setting provides a greater understanding of community and population-focused care. Nursing students assess community needs, plan, implement, and assist in the evaluation of programs to promote health and wellness within faith communities. When exploring the possibility of using a faith community as a clinical site for nursing students, consider the following aspects:

- *Curricular aspects:* What is the academic level of the nursing student? How are content and methods for teaching spiritual care integrated throughout the program of study, specifically in courses of assessment, health promotion, community and public health, maternal–child health, and population management? What are the course objectives? Specific unit objectives? Student learning objectives?
- *Understanding:* Nursing faculty should explore the student's knowledge of faith community nursing. What specific information about the faith community denomination and the religious rites and rituals are needed prior to the start of the student experience? Has the student reviewed the scope and standards of practice for faith community nursing?
- *Time/Students:* Consider the number of hours available for this experience and the flexibility of the student's hours with the availability of the faith community nurse. Based on the faith tradition, when will worship services (e.g., Sunday or Saturday) and planned activities take place? Can the setting accommodate one or multiple students?
- *Supervision and Evaluation:* Who will provide overall supervision of the student's activities? In what ways will the faith community nurse have input in the evaluation of the student's activities? How will the student evaluate the faith community nurse and community experience?
- *Guidelines:* Consider the guidelines needed for student safety, in-home or institutional visitation, confidentiality, and documentation. What documentation from the student and academic institution is required by the faith community?
- *Activities:* Formulate activities that include all aspects of the nursing process for the student(s) to actively participate. Identify areas from various stages of the life cycle and with varying cultural backgrounds, if possible. If required for the clinical practicum, identify a project that is feasible and realistic for the student given his or her education level, course and student learning objectives matched with the needs of the faith community.

Modified from Johnson EJ, Testerman N, Hart D: Teaching spiritual care to nursing students: an integrated model. *J Christ Nurs* 31(2): 94-199, 2014.

Models of Faith Community Nursing

Models of faith community nursing consider the organizational mission along with the influencing factors of economics, infrastructure, available personnel, and willingness of stakeholders to take some risks. Four primary models for faith community nursing are found in practice. The models are differentiated by employer and remuneration wherein the nurse is paid or unpaid.

A paid **institutional model** is supported by a health care institution (e.g., hospital, health department, or long-term care facility) where nurses are paid (salary or hourly) either by the institution or a shared salary with the congregation over time. Second is the unpaid institutional model where an institution provides soft support in the form of continuing education and spiritual development; however, the nurse is not paid a salary and is governed by the congregation who budgets for some expenses such as mileage and health education materials. Many nonprofit hospitals provide soft support to a network of faith community nurses as a partnership for promoting wellness to residents in the community and to meet requirements for tax-exempt status (Butler & Diaz, 2017). Third is the paid **congregational model** where the nurse is governed and paid by the congregation with no contractual support from any sponsoring health care institution. Fourth is the unpaid congregational model where the nurse is governed by the congregation with no contractual support from any sponsoring health care institution. When unpaid, the nurse may negotiate financial support for expenses such as gas/mileage, postage, and health promotion literature.

Pros and cons exist for each model. Paid faith community nurses tend to work more hours, more fully develop the role, and provide a stronger presence within the congregation than the unpaid parish nurse. Often with outside health care organization sponsorship, faith community nurse initiatives typically disappear during congregation transitions of transfer, retirement, or leave of absence. In all models, nurses work closely with health care professionals, pastoral care and health ministry staff, and lay volunteers.

The pursuit of faith community nursing as a specialty practice has been somewhat hindered by the larger number of unpaid nurses practicing a few hours per week or preferring to serve in a volunteer yet professional role. The ongoing question of pay is similar to the evolution of paid congregation staff for youth education and music ministry. The trend for older nurses to call themselves faith community nurses "after retirement" also sent the message of a volunteer ministry versus a professional nurse engaged in a specialty practice of nursing. Yet as faith community nurses wanting to do more in their churches can attest, financial constraints of smaller churches have prevented the creation of a paid position or increasing hours from part-time to full-time status. Regardless of the selected model, the faith community nurse uses knowledge, skills, and experience to promote whole person health of body, mind, and spirit. The ideal outcome is a caring congregation that supports healthy, spiritually fulfilling lives. Resources for faith community nursing can be found on this book's Evolve website.

Holistic Health Care

Holistic health practices emphasize nurses' and clients' commitment to optimal wellness. Such practices focus nurses and clients on seeking the meaning of wellness for the individual or situation, and on considering options from an array of therapies. Harmony between the physical, emotional, psychological, and spiritual self is sought. In addition to sharing backgrounds and functions similar to those of public health nursing, faith community nursing also parallels and benefits from commonalities and distinct practices of holistic nursing. Regardless of specialty or practice setting, nurses who practice in a holistic manner acknowledge wholeness as more than the sum of the individual parts (Dossey et al., 2016). The philosophy of holistic nursing practice (also a specialty in nursing) embraces concepts of presence, healing, and holism. The interconnectedness of body, mind, and spirit is basic to holistic nursing and is embedded in the practice of faith community nurses. Like faith community nursing, holistic nursing emphasizes wholeness of persons across the life span.

Faith community nurses use some of the interventions commonly found in holistic nursing. Additional exploration by faith community nurses enhances practice possibilities to promote wellness and healing for practitioner and client (ANA, 2013). Both faith community nurses and holistic nurses share the skill of creating a healing environment (Dossey et al., 2016). Listening coupled with intentional compassion is basic to effective interventions. Selected interventions that are often used in both specialties of nursing are prayer, meditation, counseling, guided imagery, health promotion guidance, journaling, therapeutic touch, healing presence, and massage. Information about accessing the American Holistic Nurses Association (AHNA) can be found on this book's Evolve website.

ISSUES IN FAITH COMMUNITY NURSING PRACTICE

As a specialty practice of nursing, the faith community nurse must be alert to issues of accountability to populations served, as well as to those who entrust the nurse with the responsibility to serve a designated population. Because the role involves professional, legal, ethical, theological, and relational issues, the nurse will need to review, understand, and apply all professional parameters involved. The potential for conflicts can be reduced by the following:

- Negotiations with the pastoral staff, congregations, institutions, and the wider community must be involved in job description preparation and program planning.
- Provision of care for individuals and groups is documented and remains confidential.
- Issues such as privacy, confidentiality, group concerns, access, and record management must be discussed with the pastoral staff or the contracting agency at the outset of any program agreement.
- Discussions of health promotion activities may include the individual, the family, and the faith community leadership.

Professional Issues

A position description is a necessary tool for the defining faith community nursing practice. The description should accurately reflect the qualifications, skills, accountabilities, and responsibilities of the position. Annual and periodic evaluations of faith community nurse practice, as well as assessments and evaluations of services needed, are certainly indicated. Evaluations should include input from self, peer, congregational staff, and institutional evaluations as applicable for constructive feedback and to enhance practice.

Professional appraisal, or a portfolio, is becoming a standard in nursing practice and therefore is needed within faith community nursing. The appraisals guide the nurse's professional development as well as program development. Because the scope of faith community nursing practice is broad and focuses on the independent practice, the nurse must consider a wide variety of topics to be used in the appraisal, such as position description, professional liability, professional educational and experiential preparation, collaborative agreements, and the ability to work with lay volunteers as well as practicing and retired professionals. Abiding by the professional nursing code is understood and must be reflected in the appraisal. The nurse must also be assessed in the application of skills related to the **polity**, expectations, and mission of the particular faith community.

Nurses advocate for the health and well-being of **parishioners** and thus are in unique positions to highlight justice issues influencing local and national legislation. As the faith community reflects on the implications of legislation on their congregation and the larger denomination, the nurse contributes information to policy makers about the implications for health and well-being for the congregation, for the local community, and for the global community. Active participation in political activities contributes to health care policy changes and potential financial support for health promotion and health screening programs.

Faith community nurses face many of the same ethical issues as other nurses in different practice settings. The nurse must respect the parishioner's expectations for veracity and truth telling, advocacy, and privacy and confidentiality unless the client is in danger or laws mandate reporting of certain circumstances. However, the nurse must be keenly aware of the communal nature of the faith community—a setting where there is a commitment to pray for others, and a setting where joys and struggles are sometimes openly shared.

Documentation Issues

An ongoing challenge for faith community nurses is documenting care provision and reporting trends and outcomes. Extracting meaningful data from traditional, handwritten notes is cumbersome and labor intensive, and paper records were not designed with the accountable care requirements of today's health care system (Mayernik, 2013). Technology offers an alternative option to paper records. With advances in electronic health records, both online and stand-alone databases are widely available, though often at considerable expense that prevents many smaller faith communities from using them. Several automated documentation systems allow faith community nurses and health ministers to document, analyze, and report individual interactions, group interactions, and perceived cost savings or avoidance of interventions. Automated documentation can be accessed from any Internet capable device, including smartphones, tablets, and computers. Envision a faith community nurse visiting a parishioner at home with laptop in hand to document assessment, interventions, and plan of care or after worship service at the end of a pew looking up a medication or community resource via cell phone in answer to a health question. (See Fig. 45.5 on pew-side consultations.) As a nursing specialty practice, it is imperative that nurses document care to maintain and enhance quality of preparation and services offered, engage in evidence-based practice, network within professional organizations, and become involved in outcomes-oriented research.

According to the American Nurses Association scope and standards of practice for faith community nurses (2017), documentation should contribute to the quality of nursing practice and be kept confidential and secure while also being easily retrievable for those with permission to access. One example of an automated documentation tool for faith-based care delivery is the Henry Ford Macomb Faith Community Nursing and Health Ministry Documentation and Reporting System. The system was initially developed in 2000 to address the sponsoring health care institution's goals: (1) provide network partners (congregations and faith community nurses [FCNs]) with an easy and efficient automated documentation system; (2) meet documentation standards for professional practice; (3) allow for aggregation of data; and (4) report outcomes of faith community and health ministry initiatives with anticipated demonstration of wise and appropriate stewardship of the institutions' resources (Brown & Yore, 2013).

Legal Issues

Although the provision of nursing care in the congregational setting carries lower risk for litigation than other settings, faith community nurses engage in autonomous practice and may be involved in a legal suit. Within the legal system, the courts find no difference in the actions of nurses working in a hospital versus an alternative setting because both must adhere to the same standards of practice (ANA/HMA 2017). Therefore it is strongly recommended that the faith community nurse carry individual malpractice insurance. In addition, the faith community nurse must maintain an active nursing license, abide by the laws and regulations set forth by the state's nurse practice act, and adhere to the ANA's scope and standards for registered nurse and for specialty nurse practice (ANA, 2015; ANA/HMA, 2017). Additional legal concerns pertain to institutional contractual agreements, health records management, release of information, and volunteer liability. Resources to address legal issues of faith community practice include the faith community's legal consultant, the position statements for faith community nursing practice, and guidelines of any institutional partner (ANA/HMA, 2017).

As required by law, nurses advocate for individuals and groups. The nurse is also expected to identify and report cases of neglect, abuse, and illegal behaviors to the appropriate legal sources. The faith community nurse appropriately refers members to pastoral or community resources if the scope of the problem is not within the professional realm of the nurse. Referral is also indicated if conflict between nurse and parishioner is such that no further progress is possible. The faith community nurse who has a positive relationship that values open dialogue with the pastoral team will be supported in efforts to select the most appropriate community resource for clients.

Financial Issues

Most congregations are dependent on the contributions of their members and often operate with a limited budget for operations, salaries, and expenses. While larger congregations can support larger budgets and expanded ministries, smaller congregations are often challenged to meet expenses for operations and clergy salary. Thus there may not be sufficient funds available for a paid faith community nurse. Regardless of paid status, the faith community nurse is challenged to be creative in identifying sustainable financial support for programs as well as in finding low-cost or free resources. Considerations for planning budget may include educational and promotional materials, equipment, travel expenses, postage, continuing education, and malpractice insurance. Money, time, and human resources may limit what services or programs are offered within a faith community. Nonetheless as evidenced by the literature, faith community nurses can offer much to a congregation without additional non-salary expenses in the form of assessment, screening, health promotion, and healing presence (Alexander & Branstetter, 2017; Callaghan, 2016; Laming & Stewart, 2016; Meyer & Holland, 2016).

Future Growth

Faith community nurses can develop comprehensive, population-focused practices. They may also implement programs at beginning levels of community-based practices to ensure comprehensive care for individuals and families. The continuing challenge for nurses, other health care providers, and the communities will be to garner government, foundation, and private funding and combine it with support from volunteer activities, family involvement, and community groups to create the unique mix needed for each community. Nurses are asked to partner with community members where they live, work, attend school, and gather for worship; to closely partner with these same members to advocate for those who are powerless; to identify health and health-related needs; to detect and address those needs to prevent costly use of the health care system; and to be closely aligned with those who can implement visionary policy that improves health care for community members across the life span.

Uncovering and understanding the intricacies of the work of faith community nurses is a difficult task because minimal research on the outcomes of faith community nursing interventions has been conducted (Callaghan, 2016). The following How To box provides a general guide to program evaluation for faith community nurses. Comprehending the distinctiveness of the role of faith community nursing is important to the maturation of the specialty because it allows for a clear recognition of the work done (Solari-Twadell, 2006). Early groundbreaking research was conducted in 2002 by Solari-Twadell using the Nursing Interventions Classification (NIC) system (McCloskey & Bulechek, 2000). With data from more than 1000 parish nurses, essential or core nursing interventions were named that help differentiate the practice. A more recent review of literature conducted by Ziebarth in 2016 identified five essential attributes of faith community nursing to include (1) faith integrating; (2) disease managing and health promoting; (3) coordinating; (4) empowering; and (5) accessing health care. The research confirms that spiritual care is the hallmark of the faith community nurse's practice. Other primary interventions used daily and weekly include active listening, presence, spiritual support, emotional support, spiritual growth facilitation, humor, and hope instillation (Solari-Twadell, 2006).

HOW TO Evaluate Program Outcomes in Faith Communities

Faith community nurses plan and provide health-promotion and disease-prevention activities within faith communities. The nurses often must provide these services with limited resources of money, time, and equipment. The following model for program development and evaluation is useful in the creation of high-quality and cost-effective programs:

Step 1: What problem or issue is the program designed to address? Be specific about the problem as it guides the search for evidence-based information.

Step 2: Identify program partnerships such as regional faith community nurses, hospital, chronic disease management centers.

Step 3: Identify both short- and long-term goals. The goals help prioritize what needs to be documented, tracked, and reported.

Step 4: Document the specific program outcomes. This may include numbers of attendees, participation rates, desired changes in measurements, and any unexpected outcomes.

Step 5: Develop and implement the interventions for the program, as determined by best practices, to achieve the goals identified in Step 4.

Step 6: Evaluate the short- and long-term goals and the specific program outcomes. Share the outcome results with individuals or in aggregate form to the faith community. Disseminate findings to other faith community nurses at local, national, and international levels.

Data from Callaghan DM: Implementing faith community nursing interventions to promote healthy behaviors in adults. *International Journal of Faith Community Nursing* 2(1), 2016. Available at https://digitalcommons.wku.edu.

NATIONAL HEALTH OBJECTIVES AND FAITH COMMUNITIES

Healthy People 2020 provides evidence based national objectives for improving the health of all Americans. The *Healthy People 2020* indicators encourage communities to support individuals and families to make informed decisions, retain a high quality of life free of preventable diseases across the life span, reduce health disparities across groups, and create environments or access to settings that promote health. Faith communities offer an ideal setting for health promotion and have long-held positions of esteem and influence in communities and where strong partnerships can be established with health care institutions and community agencies. For example, the Carter Center in Atlanta and the Park Ridge Center for Health, Faith, and Ethics in Chicago collaborated with health care professionals and leaders of faith traditions to identify the key roles faith communities have in addressing national health objectives and approaches to improving overall public health.

On a national level, multiple partnerships have been established between faith communities and federal agencies as well as high-profile not-for-profit organizations. The U.S. Department of Health and Human Services established a Center for Faith-Based and Neighborhood Partnerships, recognizing that faith communities are an ideal setting for education and health promotion initiatives (CDC, 2017). A well-known organization, the National Heart, Lung and Blood Institute, created a faith-based toolkit to promote heart health for women (Box 45.3). Notably, the American Heart Association (2016) created the *EmPowered to Serve* program designed to bring organizations together in partnership to make a positive impact around health in the faith-based community with special focus on increased physical activity, increased consumption of fruits and vegetables, reduction or limitation of sodium and sugar sweetened beverages, and improving the health of the entire family leading to improved health of the overall community.

Recognizing that older adults are one of the fastest growing age groups in the community, including baby boomers (adults born between 1946 and 1964), a new goal was added to *Healthy People 2020—improve the health, function, and quality of life of older adults.* It is estimated that more than 37 million people in this older adult group (60 percent) will manage more than one chronic condition by 2030 (CDC, 2017). Thus older adults are at high risk for developing chronic illnesses and related disabilities such as diabetes mellitus, arthritis, congestive heart failure, and dementia. Infectious disease combined with chronic conditions is the leading cause of death among older adults (CDC, 2017). Often, acute exacerbations from one or more

BOX 45.3 Example of Online Faith-Based Resources

National Heart, Lung and Blood Institute Faith-Based Toolkit

This faith-based activities toolkit contains ideas and resources you can use to conduct activities to promote *The Heart Truth®* for women in your faith community. Campaign background information, faith-based resources, and other promotional and educational materials, as well as the activity ideas contained in this kit can help you formulate a plan for your own faith-based program.

Activity Ideas

Consider these ideas for planning an event to promote the heart health of women in your faith community.

- Organize a "*Red Dress* Sunday" or "*Red Dress* Sabbath" event for your place of worship. You can put a notice in the bulletin, hold an educational session, and distribute brochures and fact sheets. Also see the Ten Commandments for a Healthy Heart and Talking Points for *Red Dress* Sunday/Sabbath.
- Ask the female leader of your place of worship to become an ambassador for heart disease awareness for women in your congregation.
- Ask your ministry leader to deliver *The Heart Truth* messaging from the pulpit. Consider using Talking Points for *Red Dress* Sunday/Sabbath.
- Organize a session using *The Heart Truth for Women: A Speaker's Kit*, during a women's ministry or health ministry meeting.
- Organize a health-themed Bible study.
- Form partnerships with retail/clothing outlets to stage a *Red Dress* fashion show that donates a percent of the profit for every red dress sold to a nonprofit heart disease organization. (Sample partner outreach letter available online.)
- Incorporate a *Red Dress* theme for your women's ministry brunch or Mother's Day event.
- Organize a heart health screening event and health fair for women at your place of worship.
- Distribute *Red Dress* pins.
- Place a link to *The Heart Truth* Web pages (www.hearttruth.gov) on your place of worship's website.
- Include an article on heart disease and *The Heart Truth* in the church's newsletter/magazine.
- Consider including Ten Commandments for a Healthy Heart.
- Organize a heart healthy meal for your community.

From National Heart, Lung and Blood Institute: *Faith-based toolkit*, 2016. Available at http://www.nhlbi.nih.gov.

illnesses require hospitalizations, frequent access to health care services, and nursing home admissions. Ultimately, the older adult may lose the ability to live independently at home. Congregations with large numbers of older adults present special needs for the faith community nurse to address in order to improve the health and well-being of this vulnerable population (see *Healthy People 2020* box).

HEALTHY PEOPLE 2020

Objectives Related to Older Adult Health in Faith Communities

Prevention

- **OA-1:** Increase the proportion of older adults who use the Welcome to Medicare benefit.
- **OA-2:** Increase the proportion of older adults who are up to date on a core set of clinical preventive services.
- **OA-6:** Increase the proportion of older adults with reduced physical or cognitive function who engage in light, moderate, or vigorous leisure-time physical activities.

Long-Term Services and Supports

- **OA-8:** Reduce the proportion of noninstitutionalized older adults with disabilities who have an unmet need for long-term services and supports.

From U.S. Department of Health and Human Services: *Healthy People 2020: older adult objectives.* Washington, DC, 2013, USDHHS.

National health objectives from *Healthy People 2020* provide a framework for health education opportunities within a faith community. These objectives, coupled with a congregational health assessment, help identify the specific health needs of a faith community. Additional considerations to determine health priorities include sociodemographic data of the membership combined with the mission, vision, polity, and strategic plan for the faith community. Often there is a wellness committee or health cabinet established in the congregation with the faith community nurse as one member. Together the team can regularly review health status objectives, make comparisons with national and specific state objectives, and prioritize initiatives to promote health, reduce risk, and prevent illness. Some examples are as follows:

- Offer regular blood pressure screening and monitoring activities focused on heart disease and stroke prevention.
- Lead age-appropriate discussion of illness prevention activities (e.g., immunizations; breast and prostate self-exam; smoking cessation; accident-free living spaces).
- Teach signs and symptoms of heart attack and stroke through newsletters, flyers placed in bathroom areas for a captive audience, and bulletin board displays in prominent well-traveled hallways.
- Coordinate healthy low-fat meals at congregation functions.
- Encourage individuals to choose healthy fruit and vegetables as snacks.
- Coordinate a series of classes for families of adolescents on stress management and sessions on the use and misuse of alcohol, tobacco, and other drugs.
- Encourage or lead a faith-based exercise program for individuals as a part of ongoing faith community activity.

EVIDENCE-BASED PRACTICE

Because of the increasing numbers of people having diabetes worldwide, interventions to increase improved glycemic control and reduction of overall health care costs have become a priority in community settings. Type 2 diabetes poses a significant health concern due to the many complications resulting from uncontrolled blood glucose levels. Community-based diabetes education provides much-needed information for individuals to better manage the disease. This research study addressed the clinical question: Following a faith-based community diabetes education program, does health coaching increase self-efficacy in people with type 2 diabetes in comparison to no additional intervention? The study utilized an experimental pre-test/post-test format for a small population of persons from several community churches. A certified diabetes educator and certified health coach collaborated with faith community nurses to provide diabetes education. Two evidence-based valid and reliable instruments were used to identify diabetes knowledge and diabetes self-efficacy. Participants were randomized into two groups with one receiving diabetes education interventions and the second receiving no intervention. Although the intervention of health coaching did not lead to significant increases in self-efficacy, the individual knowledge and self-efficacy scores improved, which may result in better self-care management of diabetes.

Nurse Use

Faith community nurses working out of the congregation setting and having additional training in diabetes management are in a unique position to assist congregants with improved glucose management. As a known and trusted health professional he or she is in a unique position to educate, support, and make appropriate referrals. As faith community nurses reach out to their surrounding community, creative strategies and collaboration with other care providers positively influence health attitudes and behaviors with resultant cost-effective strategy for screening and enhanced disease management.

Data from Meyer JL, Holland BE: Health coaching in faith-based community diabetes education. *International Journal of Faith Community Nursing* 2(1), 2016. Available at http://digitalcommons.wku.edu.

CONCLUSION

In a span of more than 30 years, parish/faith community nursing went from pilot project to recognized nursing specialty practice complete with scope and standards. The role of the faith community nurse was clearly defined, incorporating holistic health promotion and care of body, mind, and spirit to individuals and groups out of a congregational setting. A standardized curriculum for foundational and advanced preparation of faith community nurses is now widely available to help assure minimum knowledge and skills for practice. In addition, the ANCC recognizes faith community nursing as a specialty practice. Screening, monitoring, wellness education, and referrals to appropriate services are combined with a spiritual component of care to promote health and healing and fulfill the church's historic role in health and healing. Ongoing research documents favorable outcomes associated with intentional holistic health promotion to individuals, groups, and faith communities. Successful faith community nurse networks, whether institutional or congregation-based models, continue to be established in the United States and around the world. Schools of nursing faculty are engaging in academic practice collaboration with congregations, as well as providing nursing students with exceptional community learning experiences out of the congregation. Hospitals and health systems, particularly if nonprofit, partner with faith community nurses to strengthen community connections. Careful examination of faith community nursing provides the opportunity for leaders in nursing and health policy to identify successful strategies that could improve the health and well-being of a community.

LINKING CONTENT TO PRACTICE

This chapter described individual, group, and population health out of the congregational setting. The faith community is instrumental in providing the structure, place, and resources and may intentionally seek out the vulnerable and marginalized to receive support from other community or denominational organizations closely aligned with mission and outreach activities for a common purpose. The organizations may include a health care institution, a childcare or adult daycare center, an immigrant community, a homeless shelter, an amusement park, a crisis center, a preschool, or local public schools. Depending on desired outcomes, the faith community nurse combines knowledge, skills, and experience in collaboration with others to make a difference for a larger population.

To illustrate, a faith community partners with a hospital, the local agency on aging, and a retirement community to promote older adult health. Key stakeholders gather for discussions on priorities identified from a community needs assessment completed by the hospital. The stakeholders also review suggested prevention and services objectives for older adult health from *Healthy People 2020*. The group considers baseline data and identifies desired outcomes. From discussions, activities and programs are planned, drawing from the collective human and financial resources. In this example, the faith community nurse works with hospital staff to coordinate screenings and health promotion programs held in the congregation setting and at various locations using a mobile health vehicle. Participating older adults requested additional services such as medication reviews and educational health talks on topics of depression, advance directives, and Medicare enrollment benefits. Successful disease management programs for diabetes and congestive heart failure were extended beyond the walls of the hospital into the community to reach a larger population. Hospital readmission within 30 days data were reviewed with the faith community nurses to identify creative strategies to reduce future readmissions. All services were evaluated for content and quality, as well as to track, trend, and report outcomes. As with most collaborative initiatives, more was accomplished through partnership with the congregation, and the faith community nurse was instrumental in bringing the partners together.

PRACTICE APPLICATION

The nursing process is a method that can be used for program planning and evaluation in the faith community setting. Such an approach involves congregants and faith community nurses in a dynamic endeavor to jointly learn about the members' individual health status, as well as that of the faith community, local community, and broader geographic community. Faith community nurse programs are derived in various ways. Initially, the impetus for faith community nursing may stem from an unmet health need, from members' concern about caring for vulnerable individuals or groups within the congregation, or from committee recommendations related to health and wellness issues.

Which of the following activities is most likely to increase the interest and involvement of the faith community's members?

A. Writing a contract for the services of the faith community nurse
B. Exploring the faith community's environment
C. Offering a multiple week Bible study on the topics of health, healing, and wholeness
D. Gathering information on leaders and valued activities in the congregation through focus groups of pastoral staff
E. Conducting a congregational health needs assessment survey
F. Holding a health fair
G. Attending a regional faith community nursing network meeting.

Answers can be found on the Evolve site.

KEY POINTS

- Faith community nurse services respond to health, healing, and wholeness within the context of the faith community. Although the emphasis is on health promotion and disease prevention across the life span, the central focus of practice is on the "intentional care of the spirit."
- Spiritual care is different from religious care and is an expected and welcomed component of faith community nursing care.
- Note that spiritual assessment and care can also be provided outside of a congregational setting in the larger community. Faith community nurses may work in other settings of retirement communities, faith-based amusement parks, senior centers, food pantries, and day shelters.
- Faith community nursing evolved from the historical roots of healing traditions in faith communities; early public health nursing efforts with individuals, families, and populations in the community; and more recently the professional practice of nursing.
- The faith community nurse partners with the congregational wellness committee and volunteers to plan programs that address health-related concerns within faith communities.
- The usual functions of the faith community nurse include health counseling and teaching for individuals and groups, facilitating linkages and referrals to congregation and community resources, advocating and encouraging support resources, and providing spiritual care.

- Faith community nurses collaborate to plan, implement, and evaluate health promotion activities considering the faith community's beliefs, rituals, and polity. *Healthy People 2020* objectives and health indicators offer effective frameworks for health ministry efforts of wellness committees and basic to partnering for programs.
- Nurses in congregational or institutional models enhance health ministry programs of faith communities when carefully chosen partnerships are formed within the congregation, with other faith communities, and with local health and social community organizations.
- Nurses working as faith community nurses must obtain foundational and ongoing educational and skill preparation to be accountable to those served.
- Faith community nurses document care interventions offered to individuals and groups, in addition to tracking and reporting program statistics and outcomes to validate and sustain the professional practice.
- Faith community nurses may offer additional resources to hospitals and health systems challenged to reduce 30-day hospital readmissions.
- Nurses are encouraged to consider innovative approaches to creating caring communities. These may be in individual faith communities; among several faith communities in a single locale, regionally or internationally; or in partnership with other organizations and institutions.
- To sustain oneself as a faith community nurse who provides spiritual care to support individuals, families, and communities in the healing and wholeness process, the nurse must be intentional about self-care, spiritual formation, and renewal.

CLINICAL DECISION-MAKING ACTIVITIES

1. Contact the local organization of faith communities (such as the Council of Churches or health system) to see if there is a faith community nursing network in your area. If so, make contact and arrange to spend a day with a nurse.
2. Interview the nurse about the faith community nurse role functions. Compare and contrast the nurse's answers to what you learned in this chapter.
3. Ask how the faith community nurse standards of practice are integrated into the practice. How can you verify the answer?
4. Interview the faith community nurse coordinator for a regional nurse network. Identify key questions of interest such as regional network demographics; current evidence-based practice or research; organizational and community priorities; and outcomes to name a few.
5. If possible, spend time in a variety of faith communities. Compare and contrast urban and rural settings, different faith traditions, and nontraditional settings.
6. Discuss with classmates the similarities and differences between home health care nursing, school nursing, public health nursing, and faith community nursing. Compare your answers.
7. Choose a *Healthy People 2020* indicator to implement in a faith community setting. Discuss plans for implementing the objective and evaluating the outcomes with the faith community nurse and wellness committee. What data did you use to develop a plan for implementation? How did you choose your population? How did you evaluate the outcomes of your goals and activities?
8. Interview a clergy member of a local church, temple, synagogue, or mosque in your area (preferably someone with a different background than your own). Ask the individual to elaborate on traditions of faith, health, and healing connections. Consider how you might be able to meet the unique needs of that faith community.
9. Visit a senior citizen daycare center and speak with participants about important events in their lives. Do they refer to rituals from faith traditions? Ask them about their connections to faith communities during their lives.
10. With classmates, interview a youth group leader and nurse in a local faith community about the concern of preventing risky behaviors among youths. What perspectives of this concern would the faith community nurse staff need to consider?

ADDITIONAL RESOURCES

EVOLVE WEBSITE

http://evolve.elsevier.com/Stanhope/community/

- Answers to Practice Application
- Case Study
- Glossary
- Review Questions

REFERENCES

Alexander L, Branstetter ML: General nutrition knowledge and perceived stress in a rural female faith community, *International Journal of Faith Community Nursing* August 2017. Retrieved from https://digitalcommons.wku.edu.

American Heart Association: *EmPowered to Serve –End Stroke*, 2015. Retrieved from https://www.empoweredtoserve.org.

American Nurses Association: *Code of Ethics with Interpretive Statements (for nurses)*, 2015. Retrieved from https://www.nursingworld.org.

American Nurses Association: *Higher Education: Learning What it Means to Provide Spiritual Care*, 2016. Retrieved from http://www.theamericannurse.org.

American Nurses Association: *Holistic nursing: scope and standards of practice*, ed 2, Silver Spring, MD, 2013, ANA.

American Nurses Association: *Nursing: scope and standards of practice*, ed 3, Silver Spring, MD, 2015, ANA.

American Nurses Association and Health Ministries Association (ANA/HMA): *Scope and standards of practice of parish nursing practice*, Washington DC, 1998, American Nurses Publishing.

American Nurses Association and Health Ministries Association (ANA/HMA): *Faith community nursing: scope and standards of practice*, Silver Spring, MD, 2005, ANA.
American Nurses Association and Health Ministries Association (ANA/HMA): *Faith community nursing: scope and standards of practice*, ed 2, Silver Spring, MD, 2012, ANA.
American Nurses Association and Health Ministries Association (ANA/HMA): *Faith community nursing: scope and standards of practice*, ed 3, Silver Spring, MD, 2017, ANA.
American Nurses Credentialing Center: *Faith community nurse certification no longer available*, October 2017, Retrieved from http://www.nursecredentialing.org.
Ferrell K: *Nurses legal handbook*, ed 6, Philadelphia, PA, 2015, Lippincott Williams & Wilkins.
Banas AT: Philippines: For unto us, In *Perspectives* 17(2), Church Health, 11, 2018.
Briggs M, Morzinski JA, Ellis J: Influences of a church-based intervention on falls risk among seniors, *Wisconsin Medical Society* 2017. Retrieved from https://www.wisconsinmedicalsociety.org.
Brown A, Coppolla P, Giacona M, et al: Faith community nursing demonstrates good stewardship of community benefit dollars through cost savings and cost avoidance, *Fam Community Health* 32(4):330–338, 2009.
Brown AR, Yore J: Documenting health ministry using available technology: the Henry Ford Macomb FCN/health ministry documentation and reporting system, *Perspectives* 12(3):8–9, 2013.
Bulechek G, Dochterman J, Butcher H, et al: Core interventions for nursing specialty areas: faith community nursing. In *Nursing interventions classification (NIC)*, ed 6, St. Louis, MO, 2013, Mosby.
Butler S, Diaz C: *Nurses as Intermediaries in the Promotion of Community Health: Exploring their Roles and Challenges*, 2017. Retrieved from https://www.brookings.edu.
Callaghan DM: Implementing faith community nursing interventions to promote healthy behaviors in adults, *International Journal of Faith Community Nursing* February 2016. Retrieved from https://digitalcommons.wku.edu.
Callaghan DM: The development of a faith community nursing intervention to promote health across the life span, *International Journal of Faith Community Nursing* July, 2015. Retrieved from https://digitalcommons.wku.edu.
Campbell Katora P: IPNRC becomes the Westberg Institute, *Perspectives* 15(2):1, 2016.
Centers for Disease Control and Prevention: *Chronic Diseases and Health Promotion*, June 28, 2017. Retrieved from http://www.cdc.gov.
Centers for Disease Control and prevention: *Resources for Faith-Based and Community Organizations*, 2018. Retrieved from https://www.dhs.gov.
Chase-Ziolek M: Reclaiming the church's role in promoting health: A practical framework, *J Christ Nurs* 32(2):101–107, 2015.
Church Health Center: *Foundations in faith community nursing-participant*, Memphis, 2014.
Church Health Center: FCNS active around the world, *Perspectives* 17(2):8–9, 2018.
Church Health Center: Health promoters lead congregations into healing, *Church Health Reader* 3(1):14, 2013.
Crisp CL: Faith, hope and spirituality: supporting parents when their child has a life-limiting illness, *J Christ Nurs* 33(1), 2016.
Daniels M: Faith community nursing—It can appear a small thing, but then …! *Perspectives* 15(2):12–13, 2018.
Delgado C: Nurses' spiritual care practices: becoming less religious, *J Christ Nurs* 32(2):116–122, 2015.
Dossey BM, Keegan L: *Holistic nursing: A handbook for practice*, ed 7, Burlington, MA, 2016, Jones & Bartlett Learning.
Doyle A: Nursing by religious orders in the United States: part VI—Episcopal sisterhoods 1845–1928, *Am J Nurs* 29(12): 1466–1484, 1929.
Durbin N: Interview, January 11, 2006, interview DS 2013, transcript, Lisa Zerull Private Papers, Winchester, Virginia.
Durbin NLR, Cassimere M, Howard C, et al: *Faith community nurse coordinator manual: a guide to creating and developing your program*, Memphis, TN, 2013, Church Health Center.
Erbach M: Interview, October 10, 2005, transcript, Lisa Zerull Private Papers, Winchester, Virginia.
Nevergall M: *An ELCA Congregation Discovers That Having a Disaster Plan Works*, 2008. Retrieved from http://www.elca.org.
Catholic Health Association of the United States: *Faith Community Nursing: Advocating Greater Partnerships to Care for Elderly*, 2016. Retrieved from https://www.chausa.org.
Fliedner T: *Some account of the deaconess work in the Christian church*. Kaiserswerth, Germany, 1870, Sam Lucas, p 26.
Garrett-Wright DM, Main ME, Branstetter ML: *Practice Matters: Screening and Caring for those with Hypertension*, Spring 2015. Retrieved from https://digitalcommons.wku.edu.
Gotwals B: Self-efficacy and nutrition education: a study of the effect of an intervention with faith community nurses, *J Relig Health* February 2018. Retrieved from https://link.springer.com.
Glaser A: Germany: Vis-à-vis parish nurses, *Perspectives* 17(2): 3, 2018.
Izang IA: Nigeria: Education is growing the numbers of FCNs, *Perspectives* 17(2):5, 2018.
Jackson C: Addressing spirituality: a natural aspect of holistic care, *Holist Nurs Pract* 25(1):3–7, 2011.
Johnson EJ, Testerman N, Hart D: Teaching spiritual care to nursing students: an integrated model, *J Christ Nurs* 31(2): 94–199, 2014.
Laming E, Stewart A: Parish nursing: an innovative community service, *Nursing Standard* 30(46):46–51, 2016.
Mansour R: Palestine: A focus on elder care, *Perspectives* 17(2), Church Health, 10, 2018.
Mattern LA: A day in the life of a wellness nurse at a retirement community, *Home Healthcare Now [serial online]* November/December 2016. Retrieved from https://www.nursingcenter.com.
Mayernik D: Faith community nursing in the accountable care era: documentation of interventions demonstrates improved health outcomes, *Perspectives* 12(3):6–7, 2013.
Meyer JL, Holland BE: Health coaching in faith-based community diabetes education, *International Journal of Faith Community Nursing* 2(1), 2016. Retrieved from http://digitalcommons.wku.edu.
McCloskey JC, Bulechek GM: *Nursing interventions classification (NIC): Iowa interventions project*, St Louis, MO, 2000, Mosby.
McLean E, Habicht L: Perceptions of advance care planning among latino adults in the community setting, *Creative Nursing* 22(2):106–113, 2016.
McNamara JW: *Health & wellness: what your faith community can do*, Cleveland, OH, 2006, Pilgrim Press.
Munning S, Owen L: Care transitions navigators in a rural setting: Identifying barriers, finding solutions, *Perspectives* 17(1):6–7, 2018.
National Heart, Lung and Blood Institute: *Faith-based Toolkit*, 2016. Retrieved from https://www.nhlbi.nih.gov.

Nicholson A, Dlamini T: Swaziland: holistic care making a difference with the HIV/AIDS Epidemic, In *Perspectives* 17(2), Church Health, 4, 2018.

O'Brien ME: *Spirituality in nursing: standing on holy ground*, ed 6, Sudbury, MA, 2017, Jones and Bartlett.

Opalinski A, Dyess SM, Stein N, Saiswick K, Fox V: *Broadening Practice Perspective by Engaging in Academic-Practice Collaboration: A Faith Community Nursing Exemplar*, August 2017. Retrieved from https://digitalcommons.wku.edu.

Patterson DL: *The essential parish nurse*, Cleveland, OH, 2003, The Pilgrim Press.

Patterson D: *Get my people going: On a journey toward wellness*, Memphis, TN, 2012, Church Health Center.

Patterson D: Top ten ways to improve the health of a congregation, *Church Health Read* 3(1):5, 2013.

Power R, Toone AR, Deal B: Nurse educator perceptions of faith-based organizations for service-learning, *Nursing Faculty Publications and Presentations* Paper 18, 2016.

Puchalski C: *FICA Spiritual History Tool of the George Washington Institute for Spirituality and Health*, 2018. Retrieved from https://smhs.gwu.edu.

Schnorr M, Hardecopf K: Parish nurse newsletter: coping with life's transitions, Lutheran *Church Missouri Synod*, Summer 2018. Retrieved from https://blogs.lcms.org.

Solari-Twadell PA: The emerging practice of parish nursing. In Phyllis Ann Solari-Twadell PA, McDermott MA, editors: *Parish nursing: promoting whole person health within faith communities*, Thousand Oaks, CA, 1999, Sage Publications, pp 3–24.

Solari-Twadell PA: Uncovering the intricacies of the ministry of parish nursing practice through research. In Solari-Twadell PA, McDermott MA, editors: *Parish nursing: development, education, and administration*, St Louis, MO, 2006, Elsevier, p 22.

Solari-Twadell PA, Hackbarth DP: Evidence for a new paradigm of the ministry of parish nursing practice using the Nursing Intervention Classification System, *Nurs Outlook* 58(2):69–75, 2010.

Solari-Twadell PA, McDermott MA, editors: *Parish nursing: development, education, and administration*, St Louis, MO, 2006, Mosby.

Sturgeon LP, Underwood TM, Blankenship M: *Practice matters: prevention and care of individuals with type 2 diabetes*, February 2016. Retrieved from https://digitalcommons.wku.edu.

The Joint Commission: *Comprehensive accreditation manual for hospitals: the official handbook*, Chicago, IL, 2017, Joint Commission Resources.

U.S. Department of Health and Human Services: *Healthy People 2020*, Washington, DC, 2013, USDHHS.

Van Loon A: Australia: A snapshot from "Down Under", *Perspectives* 17(2), Church Health, 6, 2018.

Vaughan H: New Zealand: Connecting the Holy Trinity to the Work and Ministry, *Perspectives* 17(2), Church Health, 7, 2018.

Westberg GE: *Presentation on 12 September 1985, Westberg Collection*, Loyola University at Chicago University Archives, Box 1, folder 3, 1.

Westberg GE: *The parish nurse: providing a minister of health for your congregation*, Minneapolis, 1990, Augsburg Press.

Westberg GE, McNamara JW: *The parish nurse: How to start a parish nurse program in your church*, Park Ridge, IL, 1987, Parish Nurse Resource Center.

Westberg Institute: *What is faith community nursing*, 2017. Retrieved from https://westberginstitute.org.

Westberg Institute: *Position paper: Faith community nursing (FCN): Direct care or "hands-on" practice and glucose testing*, Memphis, 2018, Church Health.

Wordsworth H: United Kingdom: organizing, expanding, and educating, *Perspectives* 17(2):1, 2018.

Young S, Urban parish nurses: a qualitative analysis of the organization of work in community-based practices, *Journal of Nursing Education and Practice* 6(2):19–26, 2016.

Young S: Smothers: Partnership for faith community nurse practice: a model of nursing faculty practice within a faith community, *Perspectives* 17(1):4–5, 2018.

Zerull LM: FCNs active around the world, *Perspectives* 17(2), Church Health: 8–9, 2018.

Zerull LM: *Nursing Out of the Parish: A History of the Baltimore Lutheran Deaconesses 1893–1911*, Dissertation 2010.

Zerull LM, Solari-Twadell PA: Administration of parish nursing: describing the roles. In Solari-Twadell PA, McDermott MA, editors: *Parish nursing: development, education, and administration*, St Louis, MO, 2006, Mosby.

Ziebarth D: Factors that lead to hospital readmissions and interventions to reduce them: moving toward a faith community nursing intervention, *International Journal of Faith Community Nursing*, Spring, 2015. Retrieved from https://digitalcommons.wku.edu/.

Ziebarth DJ: Transitional care interventions as implemented by faith community nurses, *Dissertation*, Philadelphia, PA, 2016, LWW Journals.

Ziebarth D, Campbell KP: A transitional care model: using faith community nurses, *J Christ Nurs* 33(2):112–118, 2016.

46

Public Health Nursing at Local, State, and National Levels

Lois A. Davis, RN, MSN, MA

OBJECTIVES

After reading this chapter, the student should be able to do the following:

1. Define public health, public health system, public health nursing, and local, state, and national roles.
2. Identify trends in public health nursing.
3. Provide examples of public health nursing roles.
4. Differentiate the emerging public health issues that specifically affect public health nursing.
5. Describe the principles of partnerships.
6. Identify educational preparation of public health nurses and competencies necessary to practice.

CHAPTER OUTLINE

Roles of Local, State, and Federal Public Health Agencies
History and Trends in Public Health
Scope, Standards, and Roles of Public Health Nursing
Issues and Trends in Public Health Nursing
Models of Public Health Nursing Practice
Education and Knowledge Requirements for Public Health Nurses
National Health Objectives
Functions of Public Health Nurses

KEY TERMS

federal public health agencies, p. 1010
incident commander, p. 1021
local public health agencies, p. 1011
partnerships, p. 1009
public health, p. 1009
public health nursing, p. 1010
public health programs, p. 1009
state public health agency, p. 1011

All of public health is built on **partnerships**. **Public health programs** are designed with the goal of improving a population's health status. They go beyond the administration of health care of individuals to a primary focus on the health of populations. Public health programs include community health assessment and interventions based on assessment results, analysis of health statistics, public education, outreach, case management, advocacy, professional education for providers, disease surveillance and investigation, emergency preparedness and response, compliance to regulations for some institutions/agencies and school systems, and follow-up of populations. Examples of follow-up care include communicating with persons with active, untreated tuberculosis, pregnant women who have not kept prenatal visits, and parents of underimmunized children. Public health programs are frequently implemented by the development of partnerships or coalitions with other providers, agencies, and groups in the location being served. Community-Campus Partnerships for Health (CCPH) defines partnerships as "a close mutual cooperation between parties having common interests, responsibilities, privileges and power." Partnerships are built on trust, mutual respect, and the sharing of power. CCPH further emphasizes partnership approaches to health that focus on changing the conditions and environments in which people live, work, study, pray, and play (CCPH, 2018).

Box 46.1 presents principles of partnership within a public health system (CCPH, 2018). Public health nurses are skilled at developing, sustaining, and evaluating community-wide partnerships. Public health nurses are involved in these activities in various ways depending on the public health agency (local, state, or federal) and the identified needs. Public health nurses may be the partnership facilitator or a member of the partnership representing their agency.

Public health is not a branch of medicine; it is an organized community approach designed to prevent disease, promote health, and protect populations. It works across many disciplines and is based on the scientific core of epidemiology (IOM, 2003). Governmental agencies at the local, state, and federal levels are partners in the public health system that must work together to develop and implement solutions that will improve a community's health. Fig. 46.1 represents the diverse and complex network of individuals and agencies making up the public

BOX 46.1 Principles of Partnership

Community-Campus Partnerships for Health (CCPH) involved its members and partners in developing the following "principles of good practice" for community partnerships:

1. The Partnership forms to serve a specific purpose and may take on new goals over time.
2. The Partnership agrees upon mission, values, goals, measurable outcomes and processes for accountability.
3. The relationship between partners in the Partnership is characterized by mutual trust, respect, genuineness, and commitment.
4. The Partnership builds upon identified strengths and assets, but also works to address needs and increase capacity of all partners.
5. The Partnership balances power among partners and enables resources among partners to be shared.
6. Partners make clear and open communication an ongoing priority in the Partnership by striving to understand each other's needs and self-interests, and developing a common language.
7. Principles and processes for the Partnership are established with the input and agreement of all partners, especially for decision making and conflict resolution.
8. There is feedback among all stakeholders in the Partnership, with the goal of continuously improving the Partnership and its outcomes.
9. Partners share the benefits of the Partnership's accomplishments.
10. Partnerships can dissolve, and when they do, need to plan a process for closure.
11. Partnerships consider the nature of the environment within which they exist as a principle of their design, evaluation, and sustainability.
12. The Partnership values multiple kinds of knowledge and life experiences.

From Community-Campus Partnerships for Health (CCPH) Board of Directors: Position statement of authentic partnerships. *Community-Campus Partnerships for Health, 2013.* Available at https://ccphealth.org.

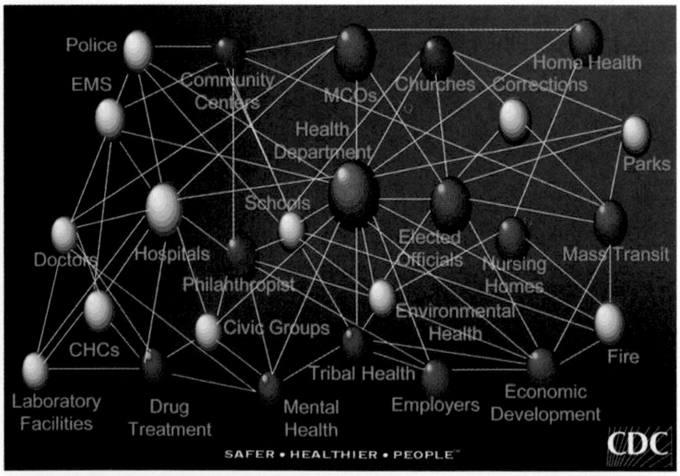

Fig. 46.1 The diverse and complex network of individuals and agencies making up the public health system. *CHC*, Consolidated Health Center; *EMS*, emergency medical services; *MCO*, managed care organization. (From Centers for Disease Control and Prevention (CDC): *The National Public Health Performance Standards, an overview, slide 9,* 2005. Available at http://www.cdc.gov.)

health system (CDC, 2017). This public health system may include public, private, and voluntary entities such as the local health department, businesses, and civic associations. Public health nurses partner with interprofessional teams of people within the public health areas (Fig. 46.2), in other human services and public safety agencies, and in community-based

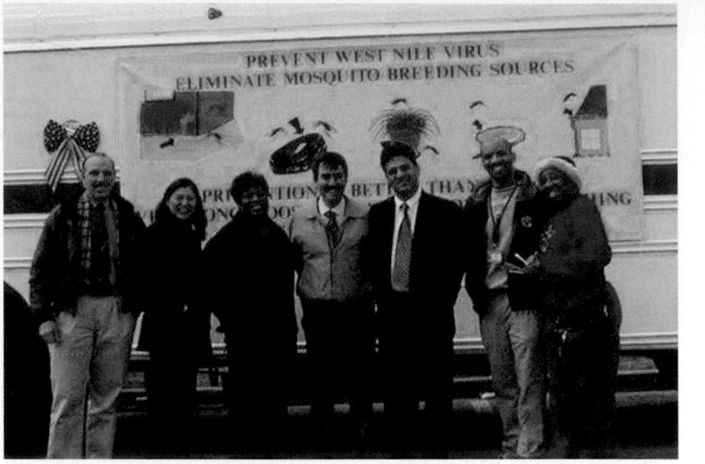

Fig. 46.2 Public health nurses work on multidisciplinary teams that include environmental health specialists to increase public awareness about strategies to prevent transmission of West Nile virus. (Courtesy Arlington County Department of Human Services/Public Health Division, Arlington, VA.)

organizations. The health of communities is a shared responsibility that requires a variety of diverse and often nontraditional partnerships. A critical partnership that shapes **public health nursing** practice in the United States is the interaction of local, state, and federal public health agencies.

ROLES OF LOCAL, STATE, AND FEDERAL PUBLIC HEALTH AGENCIES

In the United States, the local–state–federal partnership includes federal agencies, the state, tribal and territorial public health agencies, and the 2500 local public health agencies (Association of State and Territorial Health Officials [ASTHO]). The interaction of these agencies is critical to effectively leverage precious resources, both financial and personnel, and to protect and promote the health of populations. Public health nurses employed in all of these agencies work together to identify, develop, and implement interventions that will improve and maintain the nation's health.

Federal public health agencies develop regulations that implement policies formulated by Congress, provide a significant amount of funding to state and territorial health agencies for public health activities, survey the nation's health status and health needs, set practices and standards, provide expertise that facilitates evidence-based practice, coordinate public health activities that cross state lines, and support health services research (IOM, 2003). The U.S. Department of Health and Human Services (USDHHS) and the Environmental Protection Agency (EPA) are the federal agencies that most influence public health activities at the state and local levels (see Chapter 3 and 9). The USDHHS includes the Centers for Disease Control and Prevention (CDC), the Health Resources and Services Administration (HRSA), the Agency for Healthcare Research and Quality (AHRQ), and the Food and Drug Administration (FDA). The USDHHS is the agency that facilitates development of the nation's *Healthy People* objectives (USDHHS, 2018).

In the United States, states hold primary responsibility for protecting the public's health. Each of the states and territories has a single identified official **state public health agency** that is managed by a state health commissioner. The structure of state public health agencies varies. Some states require that the state health commissioner be a physician. A growing number of states do not limit the position to physicians but rather require specific public health experience. California, Maryland, Iowa, Oregon, Washington, and Michigan are examples of states that focus on public health experience as a requirement for the state health commissioner position. Public health nurses have been appointed to the state health commissioner positions in a number of states: California, Oregon, Washington, and Michigan. The Association of State and Territorial Health Officials defines the state public health agency as the organizational unit of the state health officer, who works in partnership with other government agencies, private enterprises, and voluntary organizations to ensure that services essential to the public's health are provided for all populations. State public health agencies are responsible for monitoring health status and enforcing laws and regulations that protect and improve the public's health. In addition to state funds appropriated by state legislatures, these agencies receive funding from federal agencies for the implementation of public health interventions, such as communicable disease programs, maternal and child health programs, chronic disease prevention programs, and injury prevention programs. The agencies distribute federal and state funds to the local public health agencies to implement programs at the community level, and they provide oversight and consultation for local public health agencies. State health agencies also delegate some public health powers, such as the power to quarantine, to local health officers.

Local public health agencies have responsibilities that vary depending on the locality, but they are the agencies that are responsible for implementing and enforcing local, state, and federal public health codes and ordinances and providing essential public health programs to a community. The goal of the local public health department is to safeguard the public's health and to improve the community's health status. The health department's authority is delegated by the state for specific functions. The duties of local health departments vary depending on the state and local public health codes and ordinances and the responsibilities assigned by the state and local governments. Usually, the local public health department provides for the administration, regulatory oversight, public health, and environmental services for a geographic area. The National Association of County and City Health Officials' (NACCHO's) operational definition of a local health department provides a description of the basic public health protections people in any community, regardless of size, can expect from their local health department. The description of local health departments includes the systems, competencies, frameworks, relationships, and resources that enable public health agencies to perform their core functions and essential services. Infrastructure categories encompass human, organizational, informational, legal, policy, and fiscal resources (NACCHO, 2014). A sample of these standards can be found in Box 46.2. As with state health departments, some states require that local health directors be physicians, whereas other states focus on public health experience. For example, public health nurses in Maryland, Kentucky, Illinois, Washington, Wisconsin, and California have held local health director positions.

BOX 46.2 Local Public Health Agency Functions

The following are selected standards by selected essential public health service performed by local public health agencies:

Essential Public Health Service 1: Monitor Health Status to Identify Community Health Problems

- Obtain data that provide information on the community's health.
- Develop relationships with local providers and others in the community who have information on reportable diseases and other conditions of public health interest and facilitate information exchange.
- Conduct or contribute expertise to periodic community health assessments in order to develop a comprehensive picture of the public's health.
- Integrate data with other health assessment and data collection efforts conducted by the public health system.
- Analyze data to identify trends and population health risks.

Essential Public Health Service 4: Mobilize Community Partnerships to Identify and Solve Health Problems

- Engage the local public health system in an ongoing, strategic, community-driven, comprehensive planning process to identify, prioritize, and solve public health problems; establish public health goals; and evaluate success in meeting the goals.
- Promote the community's understanding of, and advocacy for, policies and activities that will improve the public's health.
- Develop partnerships to generate interest in and support for improved community health status, including new and emerging public health issues.

Essential Public Health Service 7: Link People to Needed Personal Health Services and Ensure the Provision of Health Care When Otherwise Unavailable

- Engage the community to identify gaps in culturally competent, appropriate, and equitable personal health services, including preventive and health promotion services, and develop strategies to close the gaps.
- Support and implement strategies to increase access to care and establish systems of personal health services, including preventive and health promotion services, in partnership with the community.
- Link individuals to available, accessible personal health care providers.

From National Association of County and City Health Officials: *Operational definition of a functional local health department*, 2014. Available at http://www.naccho.org.

The majority of local, state, and federal public health agencies will be involved in the following:

- Collecting and analyzing vital statistics (Chapter 13)
- Providing health education and information to the population served (Chapter 19)
- Receiving reports about and investigating and controlling communicable diseases (Chapter 14)
- Planning for and responding to natural and man-made disasters and emergencies (Chapter 21)
- Protecting the environment to reduce the risk to health (Chapter 6)
- Providing some health services to particular populations at risk or with limited access to care (local public health agencies, guided by state and federal policies and goals and community needs) (Chapters 26-38)

- Conducting community assessments to identify community assets and gaps (Chapter 17)
- Identifying public health problems for at-risk and high-risk populations (Chapter 17)
- Partnering with other organizations to develop and implement responses to identified public health concerns (Chapters 16-18 and 23)

Public health nurses practice in partnership with each other at the local, state, and federal levels and with other public health staff, other governmental agencies, and the community to safeguard the public's health and to improve the community's health status. Public health agency staffs include physicians, nutritionists, environmental health professionals, health educators, various laboratory workers, epidemiologists, health planners, and paraprofessional home visitors and outreach workers. Community-based organizations include the American Red Cross, free clinics, Head Start programs, daycare centers, community health centers, hospitals, senior centers, advocacy groups, churches, academic institutions, and businesses. Other governmental agencies include the fire/emergency services department, law enforcement agencies, schools, parks and recreation departments, and elected officials. Changes in local, state, and federal governments affect public health services, and public health nursing has to develop strategies for dealing with these changes. Public health nurses facilitate community assessments to identify emerging public health concerns within communities and, based on results of community assessments, help develop programs to provide needed services.

HISTORY AND TRENDS IN PUBLIC HEALTH

A person born today can expect to live 30 years longer than a person born in 1900. Medical care accounts for 5 years of that increase. Public health practice, resulting in changes in social policies, community actions, and individual and group behavior, is responsible for the additional 25 years of that increase (USDHHS, 2010). Historically, public health nurses were valued by and important to society and functioned in an autonomous setting. They worked with populations and in settings that were not of interest to other health care disciplines or groups. Much public health service was delivered to the poor and to women and children, who did not have political power or voice. During the course of the twentieth century, public health responsibilities expanded beyond communicable disease prevention, occupational health, and environmental health programs to include reproductive health, chronic disease prevention, and injury prevention activities. As a result of Medicaid-managed care, many public health agencies were no longer providing personal health care services. Public health agencies began to shift emphasis from a focus on primary health care services to a focus on core public health activities such as the investigation and control of diseases and injuries, community health assessment, community health planning, and involvement in environmental health activities. As the twentieth century came to a close, developments in genetic engineering, the emergence of new communicable diseases, prevention of bioterrorism and violence, and the management and disposal of hazardous waste were emerging as additional public health issues (CDC, 1999). The Institute of Medicine (IOM, 2003) identified the following seven priorities for public health in the twenty-first century:

- Understand and emphasize the broad determinants of health.
- Develop a policy focus on population health.
- Strengthen the public health infrastructure.
- Build partnerships.
- Develop systems of accountability.
- Emphasize evidence-based practice.
- Enhance communication.

In supporting the 2003 IOM priorities, the National Academy of Medicine (NAM) released *Public Health 3.0: A Call to Action for Public Health to Meet the Challenges of the 21st Century* and recommended actions for public health as follows:

- Public health leaders should take on the role of chief health strategists in their communities.
- Health departments should work with private and public stakeholders in their communities to form partnerships to guide health initiatives.
- Accreditation of public health departments by the Public Health Accreditation Board (PHAB) should be encouraged and supported to assure all citizens are served by a nationally accredited health department.
- Timely, reliable, and actionable data should be accessible to communities, and clear metrics should be developed to document success of public health's practice to guide, focus, and assess the impact of prevention initiatives, which include targeting the social determinants of health and enhancing health equity.
- Public health funding should be enhanced and substantially modified by using innovative funding models to expand financial support for both infrastructure and community level work (NAM, 2017).

Public health activities at the beginning of the twenty-first century were shaped by the September 11, 2001, terrorist attacks of the World Trade Center, the Pentagon, and a field in Pennsylvania, in which thousands were murdered. However, public health nursing activities at the federal, state, and local levels were even more dramatically affected by a series of anthrax exposures that occurred shortly after the terrorist attacks. In addition to anthrax exposures in Florida and New York, one month after the attacks of September 11, thousands of workers at the Brentwood Post Office and the Senate Building in Washington, DC, were exposed to an especially virulent strain of anthrax from a contaminated letter. These exposures required public health nurses to rapidly establish mass medication distribution clinics, while also responding to frightened calls from community members and requests for information from the media.

The anthrax exposures alerted policy makers to the weakening public health infrastructure required to respond to bioterrorism events. As society grapples with the upheaval created by the reality of a bioterrorism event and an increase in violence, public health nurses learn to leverage existing authority and expertise to ensure that all critical issues threatening the public's health are addressed. The shift of funding to support bioterrorism response efforts has the potential of weakening existing important public health programs. Nurses are well positioned to actively participate in policy decisions that will ensure that a public health infrastructure able to prevent and respond to bioterrorism will be strengthened and maintained within the context of general communicable disease surveillance and response. Public health nurses are facing issues such as unprecedented influenza, tetanus, and childhood vaccine shortages and emerging infections, such as severe acute respiratory syndrome (SARS) and the influenza A virus (H1N1) pandemic, that compete with bioterrorism activities for resources. One of these issues presented itself in the fall of 2009 and spring of 2010 when the world grappled with the lack of enough vaccine to prevent the virus from spreading across the world. (See later discussion.)

During the twentieth century, public health nurses were a major force in the nation, achieving immunization rates that accounted for the dramatic decrease in measles. A policy brief issued by All Kids Count (2000, p. 1) stated, "in 1941, more than 894,000 cases of measles were reported in the U.S. In 2013, preliminary data indicated that just 159 cases were reported—a reduction of 99.9%." Measles is still common in many parts of the world, and travelers continue to bring the disease into the United States. There have been a few measles outbreaks in recent years in the United States, primarily from unvaccinated individuals. In 2017, there were only 118 cases from 15 states reported (CDC, 2018). However, the general public is not well informed about how this immunization activity was accomplished or about its effect on improving health and lowering health care costs.

Public health nurses' difficulty in explaining the value of ongoing prevention activities can result in a decrease in resources required to ensure adequate surveillance and containment of communicable disease outbreaks. For public health services to receive adequate funding, it is necessary for the public and the government to be aware of the benefits provided to a community by public health nurses. Public health nurses must be at the table, as advocates and experts, when issues are being discussed and decisions are being made to make certain that public health programs are provided for the populations at risk. For example, as the incidence of active tuberculosis (TB) cases decreases, officials will consider shifting funds for TB control to other efforts. Public health nurses at the national, state, and local levels work together to educate officials about the importance of continuing funding for surveillance and containment efforts if the lower TB incidence rates are to be maintained. A recent public health concern is the unaccompanied immigrant children crossing the Mexican borders with no medical records. Efforts are being made to provide TB tests and to start immunizations at clinics near the border before the children migrate to other states and enter school. Public health nurses working in schools are challenged with surveillance of the immigrant students to assure the health and safety of the indigenous students and the population of the community.

The twenty-first-century public health nurse is working to develop a public health system able to monitor and detect suspicious trends and respond rapidly to prevent widespread exposure, whether the result of a deliberate or a natural epidemic. A prime example of emerging infectious diseases is severe acute respiratory syndrome (SARS), caused by a virus that brought illness and death to many in 2003. The disease spread quickly from China to other countries, being transported by airline passengers traveling internationally. The novel H1N1 influenza A virus pandemic provides another example of a natural epidemic that required a rapid, intensive, long-term response from public health nurses at the federal, state, and local levels. In 2009, the world was alerted to a new rapidly spreading influenza A virus (H1N1) when Mexico declared a state of emergency and closed schools and congregations in public settings in response to outbreaks of respiratory illness and increased reports of clients with influenza-like illness in several areas of the country (CDC, 2009). The first U.S. human cases of H1N1 were identified in April 2009 in California and Texas. On October 24, 2009, President Barack Obama declared H1N1 a national emergency in the United States. Public health nurses throughout the country shifted their activities to support the response to H1N1. Public health nurses who usually worked in areas such as family health services or school health services rapidly had to shift their focus to the H1N1 response. Family health service clinics and home-visiting services were either cancelled or scaled back to free up public health nurse time to respond to the emerging pandemic. More recent examples of diseases that have been monitored closely by public health nurses and officials are Middle Eastern respiratory syndrome (MERS) and Ebola virus. In the spring of 2014, the United States confirmed its first case of MERS-CoV, a corona virus, first reported in Saudi Arabia in 2012 (CDC, 2014a). The Ebola virus epidemic in African countries is being watched carefully by public health officials, and preventive measures are being taken to protect populations (see Chapter 14 for more on the Ebola virus outbreak in the United States).

More recently public health nurses and officials have had to educate and implement preventive measures for the Zika virus, which is contracted through mosquito bites and can be transmitted by pregnant women to their babies and additionally through sexual contact with an infected person (CDC, 2018).

SCOPE, STANDARDS, AND ROLES OF PUBLIC HEALTH NURSING

In 1920 C. E. A. Winslow defined public health as "the science and art of preventing disease, prolonging life and promoting health and efficiency through organized community effort" (Turnock, 2010, p. 10). This definition is still used in public health textbooks because it focuses on the relationship between social conditions and health across all levels of society. The IOM defines public health practice as "what we as a society do collectively to assure the conditions in which people can be healthy" (IOM, 2003, p. 28). Reflecting these definitions, the Public Health Nursing Section of the American Public Health Association defined public health nursing as "the practice of promoting and protecting the health of populations using knowledge from nursing, social and public health sciences"

(APHA, 2013, p. 1). The American Nurses Association (ANA) adds that public health nursing is a population-focused practice that works to promote health and prevent disease for the entire population. Public health nursing is a specialty practice of nursing defined by scope of practice and not by practice setting (APHA, 2013).

Additional knowledge, skills, and aptitudes are necessary for a nurse to go beyond focusing on the health needs of the individual to focusing on the health needs of populations (see Chapters 1 and 19). This additional knowledge distinguishes the public health nurse from other nurses who are practicing in the community setting. Public health nursing practices arise from knowledge gained from the physical and social sciences, psychological and spiritual fields, environmental areas, political arena, epidemiology, economics, community organization, public health ethics, community-based participatory research, and global health. The Quad Council of Public Health Nursing Organizations identified eight principles (Box 46.3) that distinguish the public health nursing specialty from other nursing specialties. Although other nurses may practice some or all of these eight principles, they are not incorporated as a core foundation of the practice in other specialties. Public health nurses adhere to all eight principles of public health nursing (APHA, 2013).

A variety of settings and a diversity of perspectives are available to nurses interested in developing a career in public health nursing. Public health nurses working at the federal, state, and local levels integrate community involvement and knowledge about the entire population with clinical understandings of the health and illness experiences of individuals and families in the population. They translate and articulate the health and illness needs of diverse, often vulnerable individuals and families in the population to planners and policy makers. As advocates, public health nurses help members of the community voice their problems and aspirations. Public health nurses are knowledgeable about multiple evidence-based strategies for intervention, from those applicable to the entire population, to those for the family and the individual. Public health nurses are directly engaged in the interprofessional activities of the core public health functions of assessment, assurance, and policy development. In any setting, the role of public health nurses focuses on the prevention of illness, injury, or disability, as well as the promotion and maintenance of the health of populations (APHA, 2013).

Public health nurses deliver services within the framework of ever-constricting resources coupled with emerging and complex public health issues. This requires the efficient, equitable, and evidence-based use of resources. The *Guide to Community Preventive Services* is a resource used by public health nurses to help determine which interventions to use (CDC, 2014b). This guide provides recommendations about the effectiveness of selected health promotion/disease prevention guidelines. Box 46.4 presents selected Task Group recommendations.

BOX 46.3 Tenets of Public Health Nursing

The following eight tenets of public health nursing distinguish public health nursing from other nursing specialties and are included in the *Scope and Standards of Public Health Nursing Practice* of the American Nurses Association (2013).

1. Population-based assessment, policy development, and assurance processes are systematic and comprehensive.
2. All processes must include partnering with representatives of the people.
3. Primary prevention is given priority.
4. Intervention strategies are selected to create healthy environmental, social, and economic conditions in which people can thrive.
5. Public health nursing practice includes an obligation to reach out to all who might benefit from an intervention or service.
6. The dominant concern and obligation is for the greater good of all the people or the population as a whole.
7. Stewardship and allocation of available resources supports the maximum population health benefit gain.
8. The health of the people is most effectively promoted and protected through collaboration with members of other professions and organizations.

Data from American Public Health Association, Public Health Nursing Section: *The definition and practice of public health nursing: a statement of Public Health Nursing Section,* Washington, DC, 2013, American Public Health Association.

BOX 46.4 How to Use Evidence to Determine Interventions

Selected Task Force on Community Preventive Services Recommendations: Vaccine-Preventable Diseases

Recommendation	Interventions
Enhancing Access to Vaccination Services	
Recommended (strong evidence)	Expanding access in medical offices or public health clinics
Recommended (strong evidence)	Reducing out-of-pocket expenses
Recommended (sufficient evidence)	Vaccination programs in WIC settings
Recommended (sufficient evidence)	Home visits
Recommended (sufficient evidence)	Vaccination programs in schools
Insufficient evidence to determine effectiveness	Vaccination in childcare centers
Increasing Community Demand for Vaccines	
Recommended (strong evidence)	Client reminder/recall systems
Recommended (strong evidence)	Multicomponent interventions that include education
Recommended (sufficient evidence)	Vaccination requirements for childcare, school, and college attendance
Insufficient evidence to determine effectiveness	Clinic-based education only
Insufficient evidence to determine effectiveness	Client or family incentives
Insufficient evidence to determine effectiveness	Client-held medical records
Insufficient evidence to determine effectiveness	Community-wide education only

WIC, Women, Infants, and Children.

From Centers for Disease Control and Prevention: *The guide to community preventive services*, 2014b. Available at http://www.thecommunityguide.org.

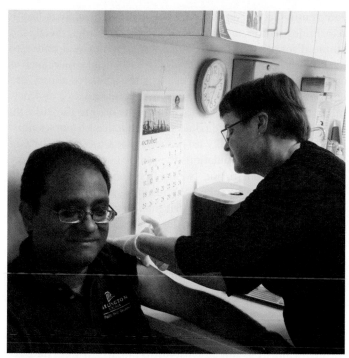

Fig. 46.3 Public health nurses protect the population's health by providing immunizations. (Courtesy Arlington County Department of Human Services/Public Health Division, Arlington, VA.)

The *National Public Health Performance Standards* program (CDC, 2015), a federal, state, and local partnership, has developed evaluation instruments that can be used to collect and analyze data on the programs provided through state and local public health systems. The instruments link with the 10 essential services of public health that define the core functions of public health (see Chapter 1) and help public health nurses at state and local health departments identify which essential services are met and which need additional resources.

Public health nurses make a significant difference in improving the health of a community by monitoring and assessing critical health status indicators such as immunization levels (Fig. 46.3), infant mortality rates, and communicable diseases. On the basis of their assessment and in partnership with the community, public health nurses advocate for evidence-based interventions to respond to negative health status indicators. For example, a community assessment may indicate that a significant percent of children have hemoglobin levels below 11 mg/dL. The public health nurse will know that additional information such as blood lead levels will be needed in order to implement an appropriate intervention. Public health accreditation is being encouraged at the federal level by the Public Health Accreditation Board (PHAB, 2018) for local and state health departments to meet specific standards of practice. Community health assessments and community health improvement plans are required components for each local health department. Community partnerships are imperative for the community health assessment and plan to be a meaningful and effective tool. Public health nurses are knowledgeable about resources and agencies within the community that can be partners in the accreditation process. Public health nurses can lead the accreditation process in their communities.

Public health's shift from being the primary care provider of last resort to developing partnerships to meet the health promotion and disease prevention needs of populations has raised concerns about available health care for the uninsured and underinsured. The public health nurses' role in this ongoing shift in health care delivery is still being developed for many agencies. Public health nurses retain responsibility for assuring that all populations have access to affordable, quality health care services. They accomplish this by advocating for legislation that promotes universal health care, such as increased funding for community health centers and expansion of Medicaid eligibility criteria; and by forming partnerships with hospitals, free clinics, and other organizations to guarantee health care for all populations in the community. Case management at the community level is a renewed effort in public health nursing. Through case management activities, public health nurses link populations with needed health care providers, as well as social services providers (see Chapter 25).

Uninsured individuals seek services on a sliding payment scale from such sources as university or public hospital clinics, neighborhood health centers, nurse-managed clinics, or community-based free clinics. Public health nurses serve as a bridge between these populations and the resource needs for this at-risk group by approaching health care providers on behalf of individuals seeking medical/health services and by keeping the needs of this population on the political agenda. Frequently, low-income populations or populations with multiple chronic illnesses lack the knowledge and skills to negotiate the complex health care system. This population needs education and training in identifying their problems, approaches to self-care, and illness prevention strategies and lifestyle choices that will have an effect on their health. The public health nurse understands barriers these populations confront, such as transportation issues, language barriers, cultural differences, and difficulty understanding and following health care provider instructions.

Although vulnerable populations have always benefited from public health nursing services, the populations that are most acutely in need of public health nursing services have changed dramatically over the last couple of decades. Of particular concern are the number of young women and their partners who are substance abusers and have risky behaviors that put their pregnancy or children at high risk of injury or abuse. Public health nurses at the federal, state, and local levels have developed innovative, collaborative approaches to prepare staff to work effectively with this population. Public health nurses can cultivate community partnerships to help address the needs of this population. Needle exchange programs are an example of a community effort promoted by public health nurses that can decrease the spread of bloodborne infections for this population and provide opportunities to connect with community resources that can assist individuals who have addiction problems.

CHECK YOUR PRACTICE

Disease Prevention

A client confides that she is worried about increased violence and vandalism in her neighborhood. She suspects a group of teenagers is involved in some of these unlawful activities. She has notified the police on several occasions about fights and gunshots. A local newspaper reported an increase in bloodborne infections from intravenous drug use and unprotected sexual activity. She has found needles at the park where her children play and has observed what appear to be drug deals. She is concerned that the adolescents may be:

- Smoking marijuana or using illegal intravenous drugs
- Involved in gang activity
- Having multiple sexual partners to obtain drugs

What actions can the public health nurse take?

EVIDENCE-BASED PRACTICE

The Kentucky Health Access Nurturing Development Services (HANDS) program is a voluntary home visiting program targeting first-time pregnant mothers or parents with infants (up to 3 months old), who may have challenges such as low income, single parenthood, substance abuse problems, or have been victims of abuse or domestic violence. HANDS is designed to facilitate positive pregnancy and child health outcomes and maximize child growth and development, as well as prevent child maltreatment and improve family functioning. A trained paraprofessional or professional home visitor, such as a public health nurse or social worker, conducts prenatal and postnatal home visits with parents, performs assessments, provides parenting information, problem-solving techniques, parenting skill development; and addresses basic needs.

An analysis compared a group of 2253 prenatal mothers who were referred to the HANDS program and received at least one home visit to a group of 2253 demographically similar mothers who did not participate in HANDS. HANDS participants had lower rates of preterm delivery and low-birth-weight infants. HANDS participants also were significantly less likely to have a substantiated report of child maltreatment compared to controls. Participants in the HANDS program also had an increase in adequate prenatal care and a reduction in maternal complications during pregnancy. An additional conclusion showed pregnancy outcomes improved as the number of prenatal home visits increased. The rate of preterm births among those receiving seven or more prenatal home visits was 9.4 percent lower than the state-wide rate.

Nurse Use

HANDS program participation appears to result in significant improvements in maternal and child health outcomes, most specifically for those receiving seven or more prenatal home visits. As a state-wide, large scale home visiting program, this has significant implications for the continued improvement of maternal and child health outcomes in Kentucky (Williams et al., 2017).

ISSUES AND TRENDS IN PUBLIC HEALTH NURSING

The discovery and development of antibiotics in the 1940s, coupled with immunization programs and improvements in sanitation, contributed to the decrease in infectious disease–related morbidity and mortality during the twentieth century (CDC, 1999). Twenty-first-century issues facing public health nursing include increasing rates of drug resistance to community-acquired pathogens, societal issues such as health reform legislation, access to affordable housing, racial and ethnic disparities in health outcomes, and unequal access to health care. Additionally, behaviorally influenced issues (such as chronic diseases, violence in society, and substance abuse) and emerging infections (for example, SARS, hepatitis C, and new influenza strains, such as the H3N2 virus during the 2017 flu season [CDC, 2018]) are issues that public health nurses must help control. Community assessments need to reflect the factors that affect the populations the public health nurse serves.

For example, a major twenty-first-century public health challenge is emerging infections resulting from drug resistant organisms. The widespread, often inappropriate use of antimicrobial drugs has resulted in loss of effectiveness for some community-acquired infections such as gonorrhea, pneumococcal infections, and tuberculosis and in increasing rates of drug resistance in community-acquired pathogens such as *Streptococcus pneumoniae, Escherichia coli,* and *Salmonella* spp. The rise in antimicrobial resistance in community and health care settings is causing alarm among public health leaders, nurses, and infectious disease experts. "Staph" infections caused by methicillin-resistant *Staphylococcus aureus* (MRSA) have received increasing attention in recent years. MRSA is a type of staph bacteria that has developed resistance to certain antibiotics, including methicillin and other more common antibiotics such as oxacillin, penicillin, and amoxicillin (CDC, 2018). Public health nurses are building partnerships, providing education, and making surveillance a top priority to prevent the spread of antimicrobial-resistant infections. Public health nurses can influence this trend by objecting to inappropriate use of antibiotics by providers and educating individuals, families, health care providers, elected officials, and the community about the dangers of misuse and overuse of antibiotics (CDC, 2018).

Societal issues such as welfare and health insurance reform will influence a population's ability to obtain preventive health services either because of limited health care providers accepting government-sponsored health care coverage or because the low-wage jobs they take do not allow time off for health care. When childcare is an issue for the welfare mother returning to work, consideration must be given to effects on the individual, family, community, and population. Public health nurses assess the problem and determine what is wrong with a system that forces parents to go to work so they can be removed from welfare rolls but that does not provide for childcare. The question to be answered by a nurse is, "What will it take to change the system?"

Partnerships and collaboration among groups are much more powerful in making change than the individual client and public health nurse working alone. As another example, the depressed, nonfunctional mother in need of counseling is a significant public health concern because the mother's, children's, and family's needs are not being met. Frequently, the problem may not be obvious to the health professional who sees this woman for the first time. Public health nurses have special preparation to help them both identify the individual's problem and look at its effects on the broader community. In this example, the children may grow to be adults with mental health problems, and the community mental health services will need to be able to handle the increase in this population. Children may become violent adults, resulting in a need for more correctional facilities. Mothers may need additional mental health services. Children may be absent from school often and may not be able to contribute to society. They may be nonproductive in the workplace because absence from school leads to lack of skills. One problem of the single individual can place great burdens on the community.

The IOM (2002) reported that disparities in health care treatment accounted for some of the gaps in health outcomes between racial and ethnic groups. This report found that minorities received lower-quality health care than white people, regardless of insurance status, income, and severity of the condition. In 2016, the Agency for Healthcare Research and Quality released a report that includes various indicators of health care access and quality for disparate populations. The report shows areas of improvement, areas of no change, and areas that have worsened for disparate populations (AHRQ, 2016).

Public health nurses work as case managers and at the policy level to promote equal access to health care, including health literature and spoken services that reflect the community in which the services are being delivered (see Chapter 25). The public health nurse working directly as a case manager or in a clinic setting or in the community can promote ethnicity-friendly services by partnering with other community agencies such as interpreter services. Identifying and alerting the community to gaps in available services can facilitate equal access to health care. For example, some communities may appear to have an adequate number of pediatricians to meet the community's needs. However, a community assessment may reveal that the community is home to a high number of children who rely on Medicaid as payment for services or to families whose primary language is not English. Matching this information with the pediatrician population may reveal that none of the pediatricians accept Medicaid as payment for services, or they all deliver services in English only.

HOW TO Educate Nurses for Roles in Public Health: Curriculum Objectives for Public Health Nursing

The nurse should be able to do the following:

- Articulate similarities and differences between individual-focused and population-focused nursing practice.
- Describe the history and current perspectives of public health nursing practice.
- Demonstrate skills used to apply key nursing contributions to public health practice (core functions and essential services) in a community.
- Apply principles and skills of population health to practice in the public health agency.
- Use current information and communication technology in all public health agencies.
- Communicate the benefits of public health and public health nursing practice.
- Develop community partnerships that will assist in meeting the health needs of the community.

Developed by Downing, Diane: Public health nursing at local, state, and national levels. In Stanhope and Lancaster: *Public health nursing: population-centered health care in the community*, ed. 8, St. Louis, MO, 2012, Elsevier.

Population-focused public health nursing requires that public health nurses consider social determinants of health, including social and environmental factors that influence the health of communities, families, and individuals. For example, a public health nurse providing communicable disease control services for the homeless population or the refugee population will also work for policies that ensure affordable housing. A public health nurse providing case management services for a new teen mother will include ensuring that the mother returns to school; has safe, affordable housing; and has safe childcare available while she attends school. The Kentucky HANDS program is an example of a model program that considers the social determinants of health (Williams et al., 2017).

MODELS OF PUBLIC HEALTH NURSING PRACTICE

In response to the IOM (1988) report that described public health in a state of disarray and the need for all federal public health agencies to work to identify core public health functions, public health nurses have worked to develop models of practice that will operationalize the role of public health nursing. This section presents examples of models developed by local and state departments of health. These models also serve as examples of the important work that can be accomplished by local, state, and federal partnerships.

In Virginia, a statewide committee led an examination of the role of public health nursing in the context of increasing public expectation of accountability and the shift of public health nursing emphasis from clinical services to population-focused services. Their work resulted in a document that identifies public health nursing roles within the framework of the core public health functions (see Chapter 1). The work identifies the educational needs of staff that would prepare them to function effectively in the changing public health arena. Essential elements of the role were identified. These essential elements are being implemented through multiprofessional public health teams. The document includes a matrix that demonstrates the relationship of the public health functions defined by the essential elements to the public health nursing roles at the local level, as well as the role of the state in this responsibility (see Appendix F.1).

The Public Health Nursing Section of the Minnesota Department of Health (2001) developed a framework called the Intervention Wheel that defines public health nursing interventions by level of practice (see Chapter 11). Public health nurses deliver services within a framework of core interventions. The three levels of public health nursing practice are systems, community, and individual/family. The model identifies 17 population-based public health interventions delivered by public health nurses. It also identifies population-based interventions as those that do the following:

- Focus on entire populations possessing similar health concerns or characteristics
- Are guided by an assessment of health status
- Consider the broad determinants of health, such as housing, income, education, cultural values, and community capacity

- Consider all levels of prevention, with primary prevention a priority
- Consider all levels of practice (community, system, and individual/family) (see Appendix F.1)

The public health nursing practice model of Los Angeles County Department of Health describes public health nursing practice as population based. It synthesizes the 10 essential services of public health practice, principles identified by the Quad Council of Public Health Nursing Organizations and the Minnesota Department of Health, PHN Section, and tenets of the ANA *Scope and Standards of Public Health Nursing Practice*. It includes the following criteria:

- Focuses on entire populations possessing similar health concerns or characteristics
- Relies on an assessment of population health status
- Considers the broad determinants of health
- Considers all levels of prevention, with a preference for primary prevention
- Considers all levels of practice: individual/family-focused practice, community-focused practice, and systems-focused practice
- Reaches out to all who might benefit, not focusing on just those who present themselves
- Demonstrates a dominant concern for the greater good of all the people (the interest of the whole taking priority over the best interest of the individual or group)
- Creates healthy environmental, social, and economic conditions in which people can thrive (Los Angeles County Department of Public Health/Public Health Nursing, 2007)

EDUCATION AND KNOWLEDGE REQUIREMENTS FOR PUBLIC HEALTH NURSES

The Council on Linkages Between Academia and Public Health Practice (2014) examined a decade of work to identify a list of core public health competencies that represent a set of skills, knowledge, and attitudes necessary for the broad practice of public health. Initially adopted in 2001, the core competencies were revised and adopted unanimously by the Council in June 2009. The accomplishments of the Council on Linkages include not only developing the Core Competencies for Public Health Professionals to guide curriculum and workforce development but also promoting public health systems research to increase understanding of and improve public health infrastructure, as well as focusing the field on evidence-based strategies to improve worker recruitment and retention and combat emerging worker shortages. The Council is located in Washington, DC, and is staffed by the Public Health Foundation. A list of member organizations is located at http://www.phf.org.

The competencies are built around the Essential Public Health Services. This is the only consensus set of core competencies in public health that apply to all practicing public health professionals. They capture the cross-cutting competencies necessary for all disciplines that work in public health, including public health nurses, physicians, environmental health specialists, health educators, and epidemiologists. The competencies are applied to three tiers as follows: generalist, supervisor, and executive level. A detailed list of core competencies by job category and skill level is available. The core public health competencies have been applied to public health nursing (see the appendix).

LINKING CONTENT TO PRACTICE

In April 2018, the Quad Council Coalition of Public Health Nursing Organizations (QCC, 2018) released the 2018 Community/Public Health Nursing (C/PHN) Competencies. The core public health competencies are divided into the following eight domains. These eight domains are guidelines for public health departments to use in meeting standards for the public health accreditation process, which begins with a community assessment and plan conducted through collaboration with community partners.

The content related to the domains can be found in the chapters noted.

1. Analytic assessment skills: Chapters 1, 10, 11, 17 18, and 26 to 38
2. Basic public health sciences skills: Chapters 3, 6, 7, 11, 12 to 16, 21 to 25, 32
3. Cultural competency skills: Chapters 4 and 8
4. Communication skills: Chapters 19 and 25
5. Community dimensions of practice skills: Chapters 16, 17, 22, and 42 to 46
6. Financial planning and management skills: Chapter 5
7. Leadership and systems thinking skills: Chapter 40
8. Policy development/program planning skills: Chapters 9 and 23

In addition to being skilled in the areas of epidemiology, analytic assessment skills, environmental health, health services administration, cultural sensitivity, and social and behavioral science, the twenty-first-century public health nurse must be competent in areas such as community mobilization, risk communication, genomics, informatics, community-based participatory research, policy and law, global health, and public health ethics (ANA, 2013).

Many of these core public health competencies are provided by public health nurses who have learned these skills in the workplace while gaining knowledge through years of practice. Rapid changes in public health represent a challenge to public health nurses in that there is neither the time nor the staff to provide the on-the-job training needed to learn and upgrade skills and knowledge of staff. Nurses with baccalaureate or master's preparation are needed to provide a strong public health system (see Chapter 1). In 2007 and again in 2013, the ANA revised the 1999 *Scope and Standards of Public Health Nursing Practice* to reflect the increasing complexity and rapid changes faced by public health nurses. The revised standards include those that are expected of all baccalaureate degree nurses, the entry level into public health nursing practice, and the standards of the advanced practice public health nurse prepared at the master's level (APHA, 2013).

NATIONAL HEALTH OBJECTIVES

Since 1979 the U.S. Surgeon General has worked with local, state, and federal agencies, the private sector, and the U.S. population to develop objectives for preventing disease and promoting health for the nation. These objectives are revisited every 10 years. In 2009 the proposed *Healthy People 2020* objectives were released for public comment (see the *Healthy People 2020* box).

HEALTHY PEOPLE 2020

Selected National Health Objectives Related to the Public Health Infrastructure

- **PHI-1:** Increase the proportion of federal, tribal, state, and local public health agencies that incorporate core competencies for public health professionals into job descriptions and performance evaluations.
- **PHI-4:** Increase the number of public health or related graduate degrees, post-baccalaureate certificates, and bachelor's degrees awarded.
- **PHI-13:** Increase the proportion of tribal, state, and local public health agencies that provide or assure comprehensive epidemiology services to support essential public health services.
- **PHI-14:** Increase the proportion of state and local public health jurisdictions that conduct a public health system assessment using national performance standards.
- **PHI-15:** Increase the proportion of tribal, state, and local public health agencies that have developed a health improvement plan and increase the proportion of local health jurisdictions that have a health improvement plan linked with their state plan

From U.S. Department of Health and Human Services: *Healthy People 2020: national health promotion and disease prevention objectives*, 2010. Available at http://www.healthypeople.gov.

State health departments help set local goals using the *Healthy People 2020* objectives as a framework. Knowing that public health departments do not have the resources to accomplish these goals independently, collaboration is essential to quality nursing practice and is encouraged at the local level with existing groups. New partnerships are developed related to specific goals. Communities develop coalitions to address selected objectives, based on community needs, to include all of the local community stakeholders such as social services, mental health, education, recreation, government, and businesses. Membership varies from community to community depending on that community's formal and informal structure. The groups join the coalition for a variety of reasons. For example, businesses see the value of developing a productive workforce that will be of importance to them and the community in the future. Emphasis is being placed on national accreditation for state and local public health departments. The Healthy People indicators, along with the National Public Health Performance Standards, are used as guidelines for accreditation. The Public Health Accreditation Board (PHAB) is the accrediting agency.

Public health nurses help clients identify unhealthy behaviors and then help them develop strategies to improve their health. Some of the behaviors addressed by public health nurses are tobacco use, physical activity, and obesity, all of which affect quality and years of healthy life. Public health nurses also organize the community to conduct community health assessments to identify where health disparities exist and to target interventions to address those disparities. For example, community health assessments may disclose that certain populations are at higher risk for asthma, diabetes, low immunization rates, high cigarette smoking behavior, or exposure to environmental hazards.

Some *Healthy People 2020* communicable disease areas of focus are vaccine-preventable infectious diseases, emerging antimicrobial resistance, tuberculosis infection and disease, and levels of human immunodeficiency virus (HIV), acquired immunodeficiency syndrome (AIDS), and sexually transmitted infections. To help clients reduce their risk of acquiring a communicable disease, public health nurses provide clients with instructions on the use of barrier methods of contraception and information on the hazards of multiple sexual partners and street drug use. Obtaining a complete sexual history on all clients coming to the health department for services takes special skills but is essential to determine the behaviors that have brought the client to the local health department. Education of young persons before they become sexually active has helped reduce the incidence of some sexually transmitted diseases in this population.

FUNCTIONS OF PUBLIC HEALTH NURSES

Public health nurses have many functions depending on the needs and resources of an area (Fig. 46.4). Advocate is one of the many roles of the public health nurse. As an advocate, the public health nurse collects, monitors, and analyzes data and works with the client to identify and prioritize needed services, whether the client is an individual, a family, a community, or a population. The public health nurse and the client then develop the most effective plan and approach to take, and the nurse helps the client implement the plan so that the client can become more independent in making decisions and obtaining the services needed. At the community and population levels, public health nurses promote healthy behaviors, safe water and air, and sanitation. They advocate for healthy policies at the local, state, and federal levels that will develop healthy communities (see Chapter 9).

Legislation is a public health tool used to ensure the health of populations. Implemented with extreme concern for the balance between individual rights and community rights, public policy is a critical function for the public health nurse. Examples of legislation that has successfully improved the health of populations are required immunizations for school entry, seat belt use, smoke-free environments, and bicycle and motorcycle helmet use.

Case management is a major role for public health nurses (see Chapter 25). The 2010 health reform legislation will increase the importance of the case management role as newly insured clients attempt to link with health care providers and the Nurse-Family Partnership program (2018) is expanded. Public health nurses use the nursing process of assessing, planning, implementing, and evaluating outcomes to meet clients' needs. Clear and complex communications are frequently an important component of case management. Other health and social agency providers may not be familiar with the home and community living conditions that are known to the public health nurse. It is the nurse who sees the living conditions and who can tell the story for the client or assist the individual,

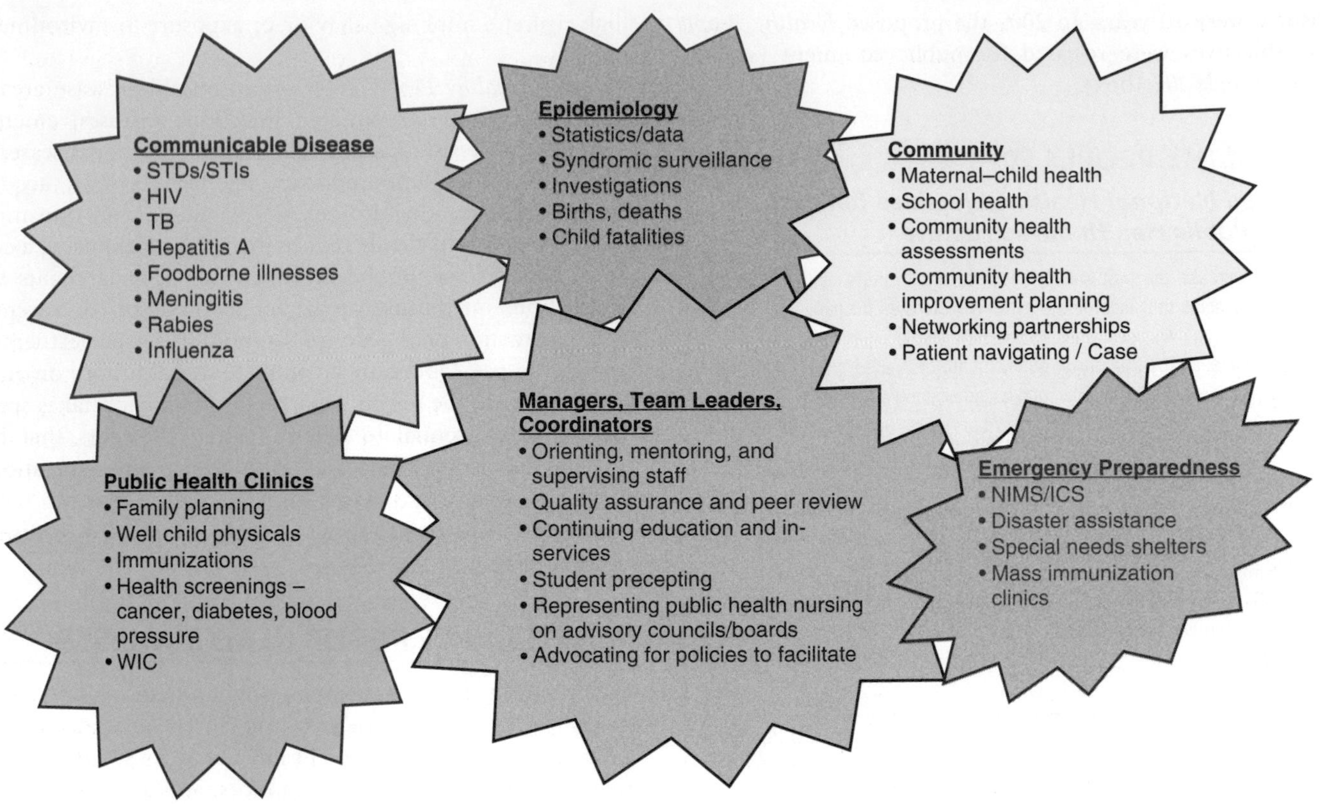

Communicable Disease
• STDs/STIs
• HIV
• TB
• Hepatitis A
• Foodborne illnesses
• Meningitis
• Rabies
• Influenza
Epidemiology
• Statistics/data
• Syndromic surveillance
• Investigations
• Births, deaths
• Child fatalities
Community
• Maternal–child health
• School health
• Community health assessments
• Community health improvement planning
• Networking partnerships
• Patient navigating / Case
Public Health Clinics
• Family planning
• Well child physicals
• Immunizations
• Health screenings – cancer, diabetes, blood pressure
• WIC
Managers, Team Leaders, Coordinators
• Orienting, mentoring, and supervising staff
• Quality assurance and peer review
• Continuing education and in-services
• Student precepting
• Representing public health nursing on advisory councils/boards
• Advocating for policies to facilitate
Emergency Preparedness
• NIMS/ICS
• Disaster assistance
• Special needs shelters
• Mass immunization clinics

Fig. 46.4 Public health nursing roles. *HIV,* Human immunodeficiency virus; *ICS,* Incident Command System; *NIMS,* National Incident Management System; *STD,* sexually transmitted disease; *STI,* sexually transmitted infection; *TB,* tuberculosis; *WIC,* Women, Infants, and Children.(Prepared by Lois Davis, RN, MSN, MA, public health clinical instructor, University of Kentucky College of Nursing, Lexington, KY.)

family, or community with the telling of their story. Case managers assist clients in identifying the services they need the most at the least cost. They also assist communities and populations in identifying and linking with services that will increase the overall population health status.

Public health nurses are a major referral resource. They maintain current information about health and social services available within the community. They know what resources will be acceptable to the client within the social and cultural norms for that group. The nurse educates clients to enable them to use the resources and to learn self-care. Nurses refer to other services in the area, and other services refer to the public health nurse for care or follow-up. For example, the mother and new baby may be referred to the public health nurse for postnatal care with postpartum home visit follow-up. School nurses often function as public health nurses because they are aware of the students' needs, have knowledge about resources in the community for referrals, and focus on preventive services.

Assessment of literacy is a large part of public health nursing. Many individuals are limited in their ability to read, write, and communicate clearly. The public health nurse has to be culturally sensitive and aware of the specific areas of unique problems of clients, such as financial limitations that may in turn limit educational opportunities. Frequently, when a person goes to a physician's office, clinic, or hospital, they are clean and neatly dressed. The assumption is made that when they nod at the health care provider it means that they understand what has been said. This is frequently not the case, but the client is embarrassed to admit that he or she does not understand what has been said. Being illiterate does not mean a person is mentally slow. It is important for the public health nurse to follow up on the many contacts the individual or family has with medical, social, and legal services to clarify what is understood and to find an answer to the questions that have not been asked by the client or answered by the services.

The public health nurse is an educator, teaching to the level of the client so that information received is information that can be used. Patience and repetitions over time are necessary to develop trust and to enable the client to use the relationship with the nurse for more information. As educator, the public health nurse identifies community needs (e.g., playground safety, hand hygiene, pedestrian safety, safe-sex practices) and develops and implements educational activities aimed at changing behaviors over time.

Public health nurses are direct primary caregivers in many situations, both in the clinic and in the community. Where the public health nurse provides primary care is determined by community assessment and is usually in response to an identified gap to which the private sector is unable to respond, coupled with an assessment of the impact of the gap in services on the health of the population. Examples include prenatal services for uninsured women, free or low-cost immunization services for targeted populations, directly observed therapy for clients with active tuberculosis, and treatment for sexually transmitted infections.

Public health nurses ensure that direct care services are available in the community for at-risk populations by working with the community to develop programs that will meet the needs of those populations. Currently, no system of outreach service in the medical models of care addresses the multiple needs of high-risk populations. High-risk populations frequently do not understand the medical, social, educational, or judicial system and the professional languages, codes of behavior, or expected outcomes of these services. Clients need a case manager, a health educator, an advocate, and a role model to enable them to benefit from these services and to teach them how to avoid complex and expensive problems in the future. The local public health nurse fills these roles and many more for this population. These are examples of the difficult clinical issues that public health nurses face in making ethical and professional decisions.

The public health nurse's role is unique and essential in many situations. Access to homes gives the nurse information that usually cannot be gathered in the hospital or clinic setting. The public health nurse learns to ask intimate questions creatively and to seek information that will facilitate case management and provide the clinical and social care needed, including other community resources. Careful attention must be paid to privacy and confidentiality in delivering public health nursing services. The credibility of the nurse and the agency depends on the professional handling of the public health information of each and every staff member.

When a disaster (see Chapter 21) occurs, public health nurses at the local, state, and federal levels have multiple roles in assessing, planning, implementing, and evaluating needs and resources for the different populations being served. Whether the disaster is local or national, small or large, natural or man-made, public health nurses are skilled professionals essential to the team. As a health care facility, the local public health department has a disaster plan, as well as a role in the local, regional, and state disaster plans. Public health nurses' roles include providing education that will prepare communities to cope with disasters and professional triage for local shelters, conducting enhanced communicable disease surveillance, planning and implementing mass dispensing sites, working with environmental health specialists to ensure safe food and water for disaster victims and emergency workers, and serving on the local emergency planning committee. Their presence may be required in other regions of the state or country to provide official public health nursing duties in a time of crisis, such as a hurricane, that requires a lengthy period of recovery. Each governmental jurisdiction has an emergency plan. The public health agency is expected to provide planning and staffing during a disaster. These local emergency preparedness plans may be multigovernmental, which requires coordination between communities. Public health nurses have a critical role in ensuring that emergency preparedness plans address the special needs of vulnerable populations such as those with disabilities or low-income populations who lack the resources to maintain the recommended three- to five-day supply of food and medication.

Essential and unique roles for public health nurses exist in the area of communicable disease control. Public health nursing skills are necessary for education, prevention, surveillance, and outbreak investigation. Public health nurses can find infected individuals; notify contacts; refer; administer treatments; educate the individual, family, community, professionals, and populations; act as advocates; and in general be state-of-the-art resources to reduce the rate of communicable disease in the community (see Chapters 14, 15, and 22). The communicable disease role is one of the most important roles for public health nursing during disasters. During the terrorist attacks on September 11, 2001, the SARS outbreak, and the novel H1N1 pandemic, public health nurses at the federal, state, and local levels immediately implemented active enhanced surveillance activities and prepared for implementation of mass dispensing sites. Information about communicable diseases seen at the local level was passed on to the state public health agency and finally to the CDC. At each step, the data were analyzed for evidence of unusual disease trends.

When October 2001 alerts from the CDC began presenting information about a photo editor in Florida who had been hospitalized with inhalation anthrax, public health nurses and hospital infection control practitioners throughout the nation increased activity. Public health response to disasters requires that resources be redirected temporarily from other programs while maintaining programs that will prevent additional outbreaks. Therefore public health nurses not normally involved in communicable disease activities can be shifted to this function. The exposures resulting from the anthrax-tainted letters presented unprecedented public health challenges. The Washington, DC, anthrax exposures resulted in thousands of possible work-related exposures, five cases of inhalation anthrax in the region, and two deaths over a period of months. Public health at the federal, state, and local levels was looked to for coordinated leadership and answers to a situation in which experience was limited and answers were uncertain.

With the first Ebola virus outbreak in the United States in Dallas, public health workers were case finding, that is, identifying contacts with the person presenting with Ebola virus. After contacts were identified, they were visited to assess them for symptoms of Ebola virus. In addition, public health workers were going door to door to see if anyone had been exposed to the virus through the identified contacts of the patient. The purpose in case finding is to be able to treat all who have symptoms to reduce the risk of a massive outbreak of a disease (CDC, June 2018).

Although communicable disease control is a core public health service, the role of the public health nurse as **incident commander** in a widespread public health emergency is a new role (see Fig. 46.5). Issues such as how to conduct mass treatment in response to a bioterrorism event, which jurisdiction is in charge, how to communicate uncertain information to the public, and who should take antibiotics for how long had to be rapidly resolved across jurisdictional and agency lines. Public health nurses often complete the Federal Emergency Management Agency (FEMA) National Incident Management System (NIMS) courses to learn about the chain of command, and participate in public emergency events (U.S. Department of Homeland Security, 2017). The anthrax exposures are typical of the nature of public health emergencies. They unfold as the communicable disease moves through communities.

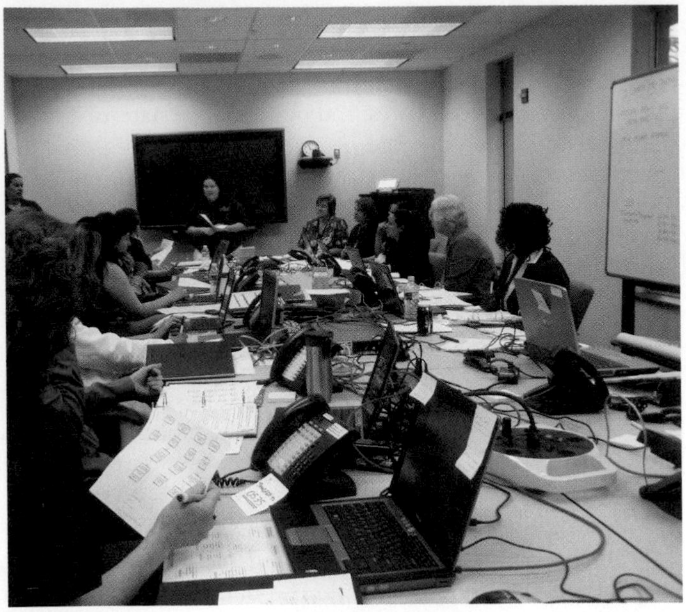

Fig. 46.5 Public health nurses respond to community-wide disease outbreaks within the framework of the incident command structure. (Courtesy Arlington County Department of Human Services/Public Health Division, Arlington, VA.)

Public health nurses are essential partners in disaster drills. In Virginia, an electrical company has a nuclear plant that requires annual multijurisdictional disaster drills. These disaster planning and practice sessions are an opportunity for local public health nurses to get to know other agencies' representatives and to let them know what public health nursing can offer. Because public health nurses are out in the communities and have assessment skills, they are essential in evaluating how the disaster was handled and making suggestions about how future events might be managed. To be most effective as disaster responders, public health nurses have to be a part of the team *before* an emergency. Knowing what type of disaster is likely to occur in a community is essential for planning. Types of disasters vary from place to place, but there is a history of past events and how they were handled, as well as resources and training from regional, state, and federal agencies. Public health nurses can help educate the public about the individual responsibilities and preparations that can be in place both for the person and for the community. The Levels of Prevention box presents additional examples of public health nurses' functions by level of prevention. Public health nurses at the local, state, and federal levels work in partnership to accomplish each function.

LEVELS OF PREVENTION

Primary Prevention

- Partnering with the community to conduct a community health assessment to identify community assets and gaps
- Partnering with the community to develop primary prevention programs in response to identified gaps
- Providing information about safe-sex practices
- Providing individual and community-based education to increase knowledge and modify perceptions of risks
- Educating daycare centers and families about the dangers of lead-based paint
- Educating daycare centers, schools, and the general community about the importance of hand hygiene to prevent transmission of communicable diseases
- Inspecting daycare centers, nursing homes, and hospitals to ensure client safety and quality of care
- Providing immunizations
- Advocating for issues such as mandatory seat belt legislation, smoke-free environments, and universal access to health care
- Providing no-charge infant car seats accompanied by classes in use of safety seats
- Identifying environmental hazards such as housing quality, playground safety, pedestrian safety, and product safety hazards, and working with the community and policy makers to mitigate the identified hazards
- Developing social networking interventions to modify community norms related to sexual risk behaviors, condom use, and abstinence
- Larvaciding against mosquitoes in areas frequented by populations 55 years of age and over
- Working with communities to develop citizen emergency preparedness plans

Secondary Prevention

- Identifying and treating clients in a sexually transmitted disease clinic
- Identifying and treating clients with TB infection and disease in a TB clinic
- Providing directly observed therapy (DOT) for clients with active TB
- Conducting lead screening activities for children
- Conducting contacting/tracing for individuals exposed to a client with an active case of TB or a sexually transmitted disease
- Conducting ongoing disease surveillance for communicable diseases and implementing control measures when an outbreak is identified
- Implementing screening programs for genetic disorders/metabolic deficiencies in newborns; breast, cervical, and testicular cancer; diabetes; hypertension; and sensory impairments in children, and ensuring follow-up services for clients with positive results
- Conducting syndromic surveillance to ensure early identification of victims of an influenza epidemic or bioterrorism event
- Providing low-cost antibiotics for treatment of Lyme disease
- Conducting enhanced surveillance for novel influenza virus infection among travelers with severe unexplained respiratory illness returning from affected countries
- Establishing mass dispensing clinics for antibiotic distribution in response to a bioterrorism event or influenza pandemic

Tertiary Prevention

- Providing case management services that link clients with chronic illnesses to health care and community support services
- Providing case management services that link clients identified with serious mental illnesses to mental health and community support services
- Educating at rehabilitation centers to help clients with stroke optimize their functioning
- Establishing an alternative treatment site for victims of a smallpox epidemic

TB, Tuberculosis.

From U.S. Department of Health and Human Services: *Healthy People 2020: national health promotion and disease prevention objectives*, 2010. Available at http://www.healthypeople.gov.

QSEN FOCUS ON QUALITY AND SAFETY EDUCATION FOR NURSES

Public Health Nursing at Local, State, and National Levels

Targeted Competency: Teamwork and Collaboration

Function effectively within nursing and interprofessional teams, fostering open communication, mutual respect, and shared decision making to achieve quality patient care.

Important aspects of teamwork and collaboration include:

- **Knowledge:** Describe scopes of practice and roles of health care team members.
- **Skills:** Integrate the contributions of others who play a role in helping patient/family achieve health goals.
- **Attitudes:** Respect the unique attributes that members bring to a team, including variations in professional orientations and accountabilities.

Teamwork and Collaboration Question

Your state has recently been awarded funding from the Centers for Disease Control and Prevention to prevent the spread of viral hepatitis through increased testing, improving access to care, and strengthening surveillance to detect viral hepatitis transmission and disease. You are the Director of Nursing for the State Public Health Department and currently serve on the Infectious Disease Prevention (IDP) committee. The IDP committee has been given the responsibility to determine how to best utilize this new funding to effectively meet the objectives of the grant. Consider the following:

- As the Director of Nursing for the State Public Health Department, what is your role in addressing this initiative at the state level? How would your role change if you were a public health nurse working at the local health department?
- In addition to nursing, give examples of other professionals who likely serve on the IDP committee with you. Describe the role for each professional for this committee.
- Identify local and state organizations in your community that you would recommend that the IDP committee collaborate with to develop and implement a response to the identified health issue
- Through this grant, your state is addressing several objectives in the *Healthy People 2020* focus area of Immunization and Infectious Diseases. Go to the *Healthy People 2020* website and identify which specific objectives would apply to this initiative.

Prepared by Lisa Turner, PhD, RN, PHCNS-BC, Assistant Professor, Berea College Nursing Program, Berea, Kentucky.

PRACTICE APPLICATION

A retirement community in a small town reported to the local health department 24 cases of severe gastrointestinal illness that had occurred among residents and staff of the facility during the past 24 to 36 hours. It was determined that the ill clients became sick within a short, well-defined period, and most recovered within 24 hours without treatment. The communicable disease outbreak team, composed of public health nurses, public health physicians, and an environmental health specialist, was called to respond to this possible epidemic.

How should they respond to this situation? (Refer to Chapter 13 for help in answering this question.)

A. Call the Centers for Disease Control and Prevention and ask for help with surveillance.
B. Send all the ill persons in the retirement community to the hospital.
C. Evaluate the agent, host, and environmental relationships to determine the cause of the problem.
D. Close the dining room and find another source to provide food to the residents.

Answers can be found on the Evolve site.

KEY POINTS

- Local public health departments are responsible for implementing and enforcing local, state, and federal public health codes and ordinances while providing essential public health services.
- The goal of the local health department is to safeguard the public's health and improve the community's health status.
- State health departments hold primary responsibility for promoting and protecting the public's health.
- Public health nursing is the practice of promoting and protecting the health of populations using knowledge from nursing and social and public health sciences.
- Public health is based on the scientific core of epidemiology.
- Marketing of public health nursing is essential to inform both professionals and the public about the opportunities and challenges of populations in public health care.
- A driving force behind public health nursing changes is globalization that allows rapid transmission of emerging infections and the expectation that public health nurses will be active partners in emergency preparedness activities.
- Some of the roles public health nurses function in are advocate, case manager, referral source, counselor, educator, outreach worker, disease surveillance expert, community mobilizer, and disaster responder.
- Public health nurses have an important role in conducting community assessments, including partnering with the community to collect and analyze data, developing community diagnosis, and implementing evidence-based interventions.
- Public health nurses base interventions on identified health status of populations and their related determinants of health.

CLINICAL DECISION-MAKING ACTIVITIES

1. What are some of the various roles of the public health nurse in the local, state, and federal public health systems? Contrast the roles. Explain why they may be different from one another.
2. How can public health nurses prepare themselves for change? Illustrate what you mean.
3. What can today's public health nurses learn from the past practice of public health nurses? How can you verify your answer?
4. Describe collaborative partnerships that public health nurses have developed. How do partnerships help solve public health problems?
5. What are some external factors that have an effect on public health nursing? How can you deal with the complexities of these factors?
6. What are core functions used by public health nurses as they plan interventions? Do these functions make sense to you? Explain.
7. If you were a public health nurse for a day, what would you like to accomplish? Why? Is your answer supported by evidence? Be specific.
8. How would you determine the most pressing public health issue in your community? Gather several points of view from key leaders in the community.
9. Give an example of a policy change or an effect from the work of public health nurses. How did this policy make a difference in client health outcomes?

ADDITIONAL RESOURCES

EVOLVE WEBSITE

http://evolve.elsevier.com/Stanhope/community/

- Answers to Practice Application
- Case Study
- Glossary
- Review Questions

REFERENCES

Agency for Healthcare Research and Quality: *2016 National Healthcare Quality and Disparities Report*, 2016. Retrieved from https://www.ahrq.gov.

All Kids Count: *Policy brief – sustaining financial support for immunization registries*, Decatur, GA, 2000, All Kids Count.

American Nurses Association: *Public health nursing: scope and standards of practice*, Silver Springs, MD, 2007/2013, ANA.

American Public Health Association, Public Health Nursing Section: *The definition and practice of public health nursing: a statement of public health nursing section*, Washington, DC, 2013, American Public Health Association.

Centers for Disease Control and Prevention (CDC): Achievements in public health, 1900-1999, *MMWR* 48:621–629, 1999.

Centers for Disease Control and Prevention (CDC): *The National Public Health Performance Standards, An Overview, slide 9*, 2005. Retrieved from http://www.cdc.gov.

Centers for Disease Control and Prevention: Outbreak of swine-origin influenza A (H1N1) virus infection—Mexico, March–April 2009, *MMWR* 58(17):467–470, 2009. Retrieved from http://www.cdc.gov.

Centers for Disease Control and Prevention: *Influenza (Flu), New Flu Information for 2017-2018,* June 2019. Retrieved from https://www.cdc.gov.

Centers for Disease Control and Prevention: *MRSA*, 2010a. Retrieved from http://www.cdc.gov.

Centers for Disease Control and Prevention: *Antibiotic/Antimicrobial Resistance Campaign*, 2010b. Retrieved from https://www.cdc.gov.

Center for Disease Control and Prevention: Control of infectious diseases-measles, *MMWR* 2013. Retrieved from https://www.cdc.gov.

Centers for Disease Control and Prevention: *MERS-CoV*, 2014a. Retrieved from http://www.cdc.gov.

Centers for Disease Control and Prevention: *The Guide to Community Preventive Services*, 2014b. Retrieved from http://www.thecommunityguide.org/.

Centers for Disease Control and Prevention: *Cases of Ebola Diagnosed in the United States*, 2014c. Retrieved from http://www.cdc.gov.

Centers for Disease Control and Prevention: *About Zika,* March 2019. Retrieved from https://www.cdc.gov.

Centers for Disease Control and Prevention: *The National Public Health Performance Standards (Homepage)*, 2015. Retrieved from http://www.cdc.gov.

Community-Campus Partnerships for Health (CCPH) Board of Directors: *Position Statement of Authentic Partnerships. Community-Campus Partnerships for Health*, 2013. Retrieved from https://www.ccphealth.org.

Council on Linkages Between Academia and Public Health Practice: *Core competencies for public health professionals*, Washington, DC, 2014, PHF. Retrieved from http://www.phf.org.

Institute of Medicine: *The future of public health*, Washington, DC, 1988, National Academies Press.

Institute of Medicine: Unequal Treatment: *Confronting racial and ethnic disparities in health care*, Washington, DC, 2002, National Academies Press.

Institute of Medicine: *The future of public health in the 21st century*, Washington, DC, 2003, National Academies Press.

Los Angeles County Department of Public Health-Public Health Nursing: *Public Health Nursing Practice Model*, 2007. Retrieved from http://publichealth.lacounty.gov.

National Academies of Sciences, Engineering, and Medicine, Health and Medicine division: *Public Health 3.0: A Call to Action for Public Health to Meet the Challenges of the 21st Century*, 2017. Retrieved from https://nam.edu.

National Association of County and City Health Officials: *Operational Definition of a Functional Local Health Department*, 2014. Retrieved from http://www.naccho.org.

Nurse Family Partnership: *Helping First Time Parents Succeed*, 2018. Retrieved from http://www.nursefamilypartnership.org.

Public Health Accreditation Board: *Public Health Accreditation Standards*, 2014. Retrieved from http://www.phaboard.org.

Public Health Nursing Section, Minnesota Department of Health: *Public health interventions—applications for public health nursing practice*, St. Paul, MN, 2001, Department of Health, APHA.

Quad Council Coalition: *Community/ Public Health Nursing Competencies,* 2018. Retrieved from http://www.quadcouncilphn.org.

Turnock BJ: Public Health: *What It Is and How It Works*, ed 3, Sudbury, MA, 2010, Jones and Bartlett.

U.S. Department of Health and Human Services: *Healthy People 2020: National Health Promotion and Disease Prevention Objectives*, 2010. Retrieved from http://www.healthypeople.gov.

U.S. Department of Homeland Security, Federal Emergency Management Agency: *National Incident Management System (NIMS)*, 2017. Retrieved from https://training.fema.gov.

Williams CM, Cprek S, Asaolu I, et al: Kentucky Health Access Nurturing Development Services Home Visiting Program Improves Maternal and Child Health, *Matern Child Health J* 21(5):1166–1174, 2017.

A APPENDIX

Program Planning and Design

Program planning is a process of outlining, designing, contemplating, and deliberating to develop actions to accomplish desirable goals and attain desirable outcomes.

PLANNING PROCESS

The successful program requires a lot of planning before implementation. The following need to be considered:

1. Who is in charge?
2. Who should be involved?
3. When is the best time to plan?
4. What data are needed?
5. Where should planning occur?
6. Will there be resistance?
7. Where will resistance come from?
8. Who will be early adopters?

Failing to plan can result in the inability to have a program that is viable and that will attain the goals and outcomes.

TIMETABLE

Timetables are very important to the success of planning. Two methods often used by planners are the following:

- Program Evaluation and Review Techniques (PERT)
- GANTT

PERT

The PERT method requires the planner to do the following:

- State the goal.
- List in sequence all the steps and activities for each step to accomplish the goal.
- Target dates for accomplishing each step are set.
- Diagram the process for easy use.

Student Activity

1. Go to literature and find a PERT application and diagram.
2. Draw a diagram of your program plan or a hypothetical one.
3. Be prepared to submit with end-of-module assignment.

GANTT

A GANTT chart is also a flow diagram that can be used to map out the activities needed to be accomplished so that one can maintain a timeline to achieve the goal. The GANTT chart looks much like a calendar.

Student Activity

1. Go to the literature and find a GANTT chart that has been applied to a project.
2. Complete a GANTT chart of the activities related to each objective in your project that are stated to meet the goal or do a hypothetical one.
3. Be prepared to submit at the end of the module.

PEOPLE PLANNING

To have a successful plan, one needs to involve the clients who are to be served by the program. Others to be involved are the following:

- Administrators
- Staff (providers)
- Other key stakeholders

REASONS

- Develop ownership
- Develop commitment
- Develop pride
- Develop understanding of problems
- Brainstorm
- Generate ideas

DATA PLANNING

To have a successful program, one must collect data on the following:

- Demographics of clients
- Disease statistics
- Vital statistics
- Existing similar programs
- Successes and barriers of similar programs
- Socioeconomic/environmental support
- Political issues

Student Activity

1. Find a source of data for one of the above categories.
2. Explain why it is a good data source for your program.

PERFORMANCE PLANNING

Some programs, called projects, are planned for a one-time-only event. Most programs are planned to be ongoing.

1. Question: Are problems that programs address usually solved?
   a. Explain your answer and give an example.
2. The following should be considered in planning for performance:
   a. Staff is the most expensive resource in planning.
   b. For efficiency, programs should be planned as ongoing activities.
   c. A 6-month start-up and a 5-year budget should be developed.
   d. Long-term commitment of resources to a program is essential.
   e. Planners must develop marketing tools, policies and procedures, and job descriptions before implementation.
   f. Organizational structures including committees need to be drafted.
   g. Community partners and advisory board should be planned and contacted for agreement to serve.

Priority Planning

1. Plan programs for the greatest need and the best potential for making a difference.
2. Available resources to accomplish goal no. 1 must be sought. If resources are not available, the program plan is time wasted.
3. Be a comprehensive planner.
4. Complete ongoing needs assessments to determine community changes.
5. Prioritize the greatest needs.
6. Plan new programs or change existing ones for goal no. 5.

Plan for Measurable Outcomes

1. Collect baseline data on the problem and the target population.
2. Analyze needs assessment.
3. Look at incidence and prevalence of problems.
4. Look at available services currently addressing the problem.
5. Determine the impact of the current services, using SWOT.

Evaluation Planning

1. This must begin with the needs assessment.
2. Plan for process evaluation.
3. Plan for summative evaluation.
4. Develop a timeline for evaluation to occur.
5. Develop systems for records and data collection and choose evaluation instruments.

Questions to Be Answered

1. Do you have the right people doing the planning?
2. Do you have the essential data for planning?
3. Is this the right time to plan this program?'
4. Why should evaluation occur?
5. Who should do it?
6. What data should be gathered?
7. Should evaluation occur?

Planning Models

1. Choose a model for planning your program.
2. Two models developed for program planning by the Centers for Disease Control and Prevention are PATCH and APEX.

Student Activity

1. Read about these two models.
2. Briefly explain how these models can be applied to program planning.
3. Briefly explain the model you have chosen for planning. Include the following:
   a. Definition
   b. Goal
   c. Model elements
   d. Planning process

MISSION

All programs will want to have a Mission Statement. Elements of a Mission Statement should include the following:

- Name of agency
- Name of program
- Who program serves
- Purpose of program
- Program goal
- Services offered

Student Activity

Write a Mission Statement for your program.

VISION

A Vision Statement is a brief one- or two-sentence statement that expresses the impact this program will have.

Student Activity

Write a Vision Statement for your program.

WORKSHEET FOR WRITING THE PHILOSOPHY

Questions for Discussion

What are our community's values and beliefs about health?

What is the purpose of our program?

What is our position on community involvement and responsibility for health?

What is our role in providing leadership?

Worksheet for Finding and Overcoming Obstacles

Goal:

Forces working against reaching goal (barriers/obstacles/challenges):

Forces working for reaching goal (existing resources/strengths):

Approaches to overcome obstacles:

WORKSHEET FOR WRITING OBJECTIVES

Health Issue:

Goal:

Objectives (write the most important objectives first):

1.

2.

3.

4.

CHECKLIST FOR PROGRAM PLANNING AND IMPLEMENTATION

1. Have you established a community advisory group with:
   ___ Representation of your targeted groups
   ___ The ability to provide valuable links with the community
   ___ Skills and resources that will be useful to the program
2. Have you identified community needs and concerns by way of:
   ___ Surveys/questionnaires
   ___ Focus groups
   ___ Public meetings or forums
   ___ Interested party analysis
3. Have you determined the community's priorities, taking into account:
   ___ Historical conditions
   ___ Traditional practices
   ___ Political and economic conditions
4. Have you developed program goals and objectives?
   ___ Yes
   ___ No
5. Have you decided on program strategies that:
   ___ Fit with the resources and needs of the community
   ___ Consider the beliefs, values, and practices of the community
   ___ Reflect field testing
   ___ Dispel health misconceptions
   ___ Change behavior
   ___ Change the environment
6. To implement your program, have you:
   ___ Prepared a timeline for program implementation
   ___ Listed people to be involved, and resources needed
   ___ Hired staff (preferably from the community)
   ___ Developed linkages with other community agencies, as appropriate
   ___ Planned to carry out an evaluation
7. Have you chosen appropriate methods and questions for:
   ___ Process evaluation
   ___ Outcome evaluation

REFERENCES

Green LW, Kreuter M: *Health Program Planning: an Education and Ecological Approach,* ed 4. New York, 2004, McGraw-Hill.

Issel LM, Wells R: *Health Program Planning and Evaluation: a Practical, Systematic Approach for Community Health,* ed 4. Boston, 2018, Jones and Bartlett.

Linfield K, Posavac EJ: *Program Evaluation: Methods and Case Studies,* ed 9. Boston, 2019, Prentice Hall, Routledge, NY.

Veney J, Kaluzny A: *Evaluation and Decision Making for Health Service Programs.* Englewood Cliffs, NJ, 2005, Prentice Hall.

Flu Pandemics

INTRODUCTION

A pandemic is a global disease outbreak. An influenza pandemic occurs when a new influenza virus emerges for which there is little or no immunity in the human population, begins to cause serious illness, and then spreads easily from person to person worldwide.

NEW FLU VIRUSES

There are four types of influenza viruses: A, B, C, and D. Human influenza A and B viruses cause seasonal influenza epidemics almost every winter in the United States. Influenza epidemics occur when there is an emergence of a new and different influenza A virus infecting people. Influenza type C infections generally cause a mild respiratory illness and are not thought to cause epidemics. Influenza D viruses predominately affect cattle and are not known to infect or cause illness in people.

Influenza viruses are constantly changing. They can change in two ways. One way they change is called *antigenic drift,* which occurs as a result of small changes in the virus as it replicates itself. The drifting is frequently enough to make a new strain of the virus unrecognizable to the human immune system as the antigenic drift accumulates, resulting in the person getting sick more than one time. For this reason, a new flu vaccine must be produced each year to combat that year's prevalent strains.

Type A influenza also undergoes infrequent and sudden changes called *antigenic shift.* Antigenic shift occurs when two different flu strains infect the same cell and exchange genetic material. The novel assortment of HA or NA proteins in a shifted virus creates a new influenza A subtype; their appearance tends to coincide with a very severe flu epidemic or pandemic.

CHARACTERISTICS AND CHALLENGES OF A FLU PANDEMIC

1. **There Will Be Rapid Worldwide Spread**
   - When a pandemic influenza virus emerges, its global spread is considered inevitable.
   - Preparedness activities should assume that the entire world population would be susceptible.
   - Countries might, through measures such as border closures and travel restrictions, delay arrival of the virus but cannot stop it.
2. **Health Care Systems Will Be Overloaded**
   - Most people have little or no immunity to a pandemic virus. Infection and illness rates soar. A substantial percentage of the world's population will require some form of medical care.
   - Nations are unlikely to have the staff, facilities, equipment, and hospital beds needed to cope with large numbers of people who suddenly fall ill.
   - Death rates are high, largely determined by four factors: the number of people who become infected, the virulence of the virus, the underlying characteristics and vulnerability of affected populations, and the effectiveness of preventive measures.
   - Past pandemics have spread globally in two and sometimes three waves.
3. **Medical Supplies Will Be Inadequate**
   - The need for vaccine is likely to outstrip supply.
   - The need for antiviral drugs is also likely to be inadequate early in a pandemic.
   - A pandemic can create a shortage of hospital beds, ventilators, and other supplies. Surge capacity at nontraditional sites such as schools may be created to cope with demand.
   - Difficult decisions will need to be made regarding who gets antiviral drugs and vaccines.
4. **There Will Be Economic and Social Disruption**
   - Travel bans, closings of schools and businesses, and cancellations of events could have major impact on communities and citizens.
   - Care for sick family members and fear of exposure can result in significant worker absenteeism.

Seasonal Flu Versus Pandemic Flu

	Seasonal Flu	Pandemic Flu
How often does it happen?	Happens annually and usually peaks between December and February	Rarely happens (three times in 20th century)
Will most people be immune?	Usually some immunity from previous exposures and influenza vaccination	Most people have little or no immunity because they have no previous exposure to the virus or similar viruses
Who is at risk for complications?	Certain people are at high risk for serious complications (infants, elderly, pregnant women, and persons with extreme obesity and certain chronic medical conditions)	Healthy people also may be at high risk for serious complications
Where can I get medical care?	Health care providers and hospitals can usually meet public and patient needs	Health care providers and hospitals may be overwhelmed Alternate care sites may be available to meet public and patient needs
Will a vaccine be available?	Vaccine available for annual flu season Usually, one dose of vaccine is needed for most people	Although the US government maintains a limited stockpile of pandemic vaccine, vaccine may not be available in the early stages of a pandemic Two doses of vaccine may be needed
Will antivirals be available?	Adequate supplies of antivirals are usually available	Antiviral supply may not be adequate to meet demand
How many people could get sick and suffer complications?	Rates of medical visits, complications, hospitalizations (https://www.cdc.gov/flu/about/disease/2014-15.htm), and death can vary from low to high CDC estimates that flu-related hospitalizations since 2010 ranged from 140,000 to 710,000, while flu-related deaths are estimated to have ranged from 12,000 to 56,000.	Rates of medical visits, complications, hospitalizations, and death can range from moderate to high Number of deaths could be much higher than seasonal flu (e.g., the estimated U.S. death toll during the 1918 pandemic [https://www.cdc.gov/flu/pandemic-resources/basics/past-pandemics.html] was approximately 675,000)
What impact will it have on schools and workplaces?	Usually causes minor impact on the general public, some schools may close, and sick people are encouraged to stay home Manageable impact on domestic and world economies	May cause major impact on the general public, such as travel restrictions and school or business closings Potential for severe impact on domestic and world economies

From Centers for Disuse Control and Prevention: How is pandemic flu different from seasonal flu? 2018. Available at https://www.cdc.gov.

PARENT FACT SHEET

The Centers for Disease Control and Prevention has developed an excellent fact sheet for parents entitled *The Flu: A Guide for Parents,* which can be retrieved from https://www.cdc.gov.

COMMUNICATIONS AND INFORMATION ARE CRITICAL COMPONENTS OF PANDEMIC RESPONSE

Education and outreach are critical to preparing for a pandemic. Understanding what a pandemic is, what needs to be done at all levels to prepare for pandemic influenza, and what could happen during a pandemic helps us make informed decisions both as individuals and as a nation. Should a pandemic occur, the public must be able to depend to its government to provide scientifically sound public health information quickly, openly, and dependably.

BIBLIOGRAPHY

Centers for Disease Control and Prevention: *Types of influenza*, 2017. Retrieved from https://www.cdc.gov.

Chandler RC: *Pandemic: a unique crisis communication category*. Retrieved from http://go.everbridge.com.

Los Angeles Unified School District: *Pandemic influenza: characteristics and challenges*. Retrieved from http://www.lausd-oehs.org.

Friedman Family Assessment Model (Short Form)

Before using the following guidelines in completing family assessments, two words of caution. First, not all areas included below will be germane for each of the families visited. The guidelines are comprehensive and allow depth when probing is necessary. The student should not feel that every sub-area needs to be covered when the broad area of inquiry poses no problems to the family or concern to the health worker. Second, by virtue of the interdependence of the family system, one will find unavoidable redundancy. For the sake of efficiency, the assessor should try not to repeat data, but to refer the reader back to sections where this information has already been described.

IDENTIFYING DATA

1. Family Name
2. Address and Phone
3. Family Composition (see table)
4. Type of Family Form
5. Cultural (Ethnic) Background
6. Religious Identification
7. Social Class Status
8. Family's Recreational or Leisure-Time Activities

DEVELOPMENTAL STAGE AND HISTORY OF FAMILY

9. Family's Present Developmental Stage
10. Extent of Developmental Tasks Fulfillment
11. Nuclear Family History
12. History of Family of Origin of Both Parents

ENVIRONMENTAL DATA

13. Characteristics of Home
14. Characteristics of Neighborhood and Larger Community
15. Family's Geographic Mobility
16. Family's Associations and Transactions with Community
17. Family's Social Support Network (Ecomap)

FAMILY STRUCTURE

18. Communication Patterns
    - Extent of Functional and Dysfunctional Communication (Types of recurring patterns)
    - Extent of Emotional (Affective) Messages and How Expressed
    - Characteristics of Communication Within Family Subsystems
    - Extent of Congruent and Incongruent Messages
    - Types of Dysfunctional Communication Processes Seen in Family
    - Areas of Open and Closed Communication
    - Familial and External Variables Affecting Communication
19. Power Structure
    - Power Outcomes
    - Decision-Making Process
    - Power Bases
    - Variables Affecting Family Power
    - Overall Family System and Subsystem Power
20. Role Structure
    - Formal Role Structure
    - Informal Role Structure
    - Analysis of Role Models (Optional)
    - Variables Affecting Role Structure
21. Family Values
    - Compare the Family to American or Family's Reference Group Values and/or Identify Important Family Values and Their Importance (Priority) in Family
    - Congruence Between the Family's Values and the Family's Reference Group or Wider Community
    - Congruence Between the Family's Values and Family Member's Values
    - Variables Influencing Family Values
    - Values Consciously or Unconsciously Held
    - Presence of Value Conflicts in Family
    - Effect of the Above Values and Value Conflicts on Health Status of Family

FAMILY FUNCTIONS

22. Affective Function
    - Family's Need-Response Patterns
    - Mutual Nurturance, Closeness, and Identification
    - Separateness and Connectedness
23. Socialization Function
    - Family Child-Rearing Practices
    - Adaptability of Child-Rearing Practices for Family Form and Family's Situation
    - Who Is (Are) Socializing Agent(s) for Child(ren)?
    - Value of Children in Family
    - Cultural Beliefs That Influence Family's Child-Rearing Patterns

Social Class Influence on Child-Rearing Patterns
Estimation About Whether Family Is at Risk for Child-Rearing Problems and, if so, Indication of High-Risk Factors
Adequacy of Home Environment for Children's Needs to Play

24. Health Care Function
    Family's Health Beliefs, Values, and Behavior
    Family's Definitions of Health-Illness and Their Level of Knowledge
    Family's Perceived Health Status and Illness Susceptibility
    Family's Dietary Practices
    Adequacy of Family Diet (recommended 24-hour food history record)
    Function of Mealtimes and Attitudes Toward Food and Mealtimes
    Shopping (and its planning) Practices
    Person(s) Responsible for Planning, Shopping, and Preparation of Meals
    Sleep and Rest Habits
    Physical Activity and Recreation Practices (not covered earlier)
    Family's Drug Habits
    Family's Role in Self-Care Practices
    Medically Based Preventive Measures (physicals, eye and hearing tests, and immunizations)
    Dental Health Practices
    Family Health History (both general and specific diseases—environmentally and genetically related)
    Health Care Services Received
    Feelings and Perceptions Regarding Health Services
    Emergency Health Services
    Source of Payments for Health and Other Services
    Logistics of Receiving Care

FAMILY STRESS AND COPING

25. Short- and Long-Term Familial Stressors and Strengths
26. Extent of Family's Ability to Respond, Based on Objective Appraisal of Stress-Producing Situations
27. Coping Strategies Utilized (present/past)
    Differences in Family Members' Ways of Coping
    Family's Inner Coping Strategies
    Family's External Coping Strategies
28. Dysfunctional Adaptive Strategies Utilized (present/past; extent of usage)

FAMILY COMPOSITION FORM

Name (Last, First)	Gender	Relationship	Date and Place of Birth	Occupation	Education
1. (Father)					
2. (Mother)					
3. (Oldest child)					
4.					
5.					
6.					
7.					
8.					

Comprehensive Occupational and Environmental Health History

WORK HISTORY

1. List your current and past longest held jobs, including the military:

Company	Dates Employed	Job Title	Known Exposures

2. Do you work full time? NO ___ YES ___ How many hours per week? ___

3. Do you work part time? NO ___ YES ___ How many hours per week? ___

4. Please describe any health problems or injuries that you have experienced in connection with your present or past jobs:

5. Have you ever had to change jobs because of health problems or injuries? YES ___ NO ___
   If yes, describe: Did any of your co-workers experience similar problems?

6. In what type of business do you currently work?

7. Describe your work (what you actually do):

8. Have you had any current or past exposure (through breathing or touching) to any of the following?

__acids	__alkalies	__arsenic	__benzene	__cadmium
__chlorinated naphthalenes	__chloroprene	__coal dust	__dichlorobenzene	__ethylene dichloride
__halothane	__isocyanates	__lead	__mercury	__nickel
__PBBs	__perchloroethylene	__phenol	__radiation	__silica powder
__styrene	__TDI or MDI	__trichloroethylene	__vibration	__welding fumes
__alcohols	__ammonia	__asbestos	__beryllium	__carbon tetrachloride
__chloroform	__chromates	__cold (severe)	__ethylene dibromide	__fiberglass
__heat (severe)	__ketones	__manganese	__methylene chloride	__noise (loud)
__PCBs	__pesticides	__phosgene	__rock dust	__solvents
__talc	__toluene	__trinitrotoluene	__vinyl chloride	__x-rays

9. Did you receive any safety training about these agents? YES ___ NO ___
   Explain:

10. Are you involved in any work processes such as grinding, welding, soldering, or polishing that create dust, mists, or fumes?
    YES ___ NO ___
    If yes, describe:

11. Did you use any of the following personal protective equipment when exposed?

__boots	__respirator	__welding mask
__gloves	__sleeves	__glasses/goggles
__shield	__earplugs/muffs	
__coveralls	__safety shoes	

12. Is your work environment generally clean? YES ___ NO ___
    If no, describe:

13. What ventilation systems are used in your workplace?

14. Do they seem to work? Are you aware of any chemical odors in your environment (if so, explain)?

15. Where do you eat, smoke, and take your breaks when you are on the job?

16. Do you use a uniform or have clothing that you wear only to work? YES ___ NO ___

17. How is your work clothing laundered (at home, by employer, etc.)?

18. How often do you wash your hands at work and how do you wash them (running water, special soaps, etc.)?

19. Do you shower before leaving the worksite? YES ___ NO ___

20. Do you have any physical symptoms associated with work? YES ___ NO ___
    If yes, describe:

21. Are other workers similarly affected? YES ___ NO ___

HOME EXPOSURES

1. Which of the following do you have in your home?
   __air conditioner __fireplace __electric stove
   __central heating (gas or oil) __air purifier __woodstove

2. In approximately what year was your home built?

3. Have there been any recent renovations? YES ___ NO ___
   If yes, describe:

4. Have you recently installed new carpet, purchased new furniture, or refinished existing furniture? YES ___ NO ___
   If yes, explain:

5. Do you use pesticides around your home or garden? YES ___ NO ___
   If yes, describe:

6. What household cleaners do you use? (List most common and any new products you use.)

7. List all hobbies done at your home:

8. Are any of the agents listed earlier for work exposures encountered in hobbies or recreational activities?
   YES ___ NO ___

9. Is any special protective equipment or ventilation used during hobbies? YES ___ NO ___
   Explain:

10. What are the occupations of other household members?

11. Do other household members have contact with any form of chemicals at work or during leisure activities?
    YES ___ NO ___
    If yes, explain:

12. Is anyone else in your home environment having symptoms similar to yours? YES ___ NO ___
    If yes, explain briefly:

COMMUNITY EXPOSURES

1. Are any of the following located in your community?
   __industrial plant __major source of air pollution __waste site
   __landfill __toxic spill __other______________

2. What is your source of drinking water?
   __private well __public water source __other

3. Are neighbors experiencing any health problems similar to yours? YES ___ NO ___
   If yes, explain:

KEY OCCUPATIONAL AND ENVIRONMENTAL HEALTH QUESTIONS TO BE ASKED WITH ALL HISTORIES

1. What are your current and past longest-held jobs?

2. Have you been exposed to any radiation or chemical liquids, dusts, mists, or fumes? YES ___ NO ___

3. Is there any relationship between current symptoms and activities at work or at home? YES ___ NO ___

From Pope AM, Snyder MA, Mood LH, editors: *Nursing, health, and environment: strengthening the relationship to improve the public's health*, Washington, DC, 1995, National Academy Press.

E APPENDIX

Essential Elements of Public Health Nursing

EXAMPLES OF PUBLIC HEALTH NURSING ROLES AND IMPLEMENTING PUBLIC HEALTH FUNCTIONS

This document is intended to clearly present the role of public health nurses in Virginia as members of the multidisciplinary public health team in a changing health care environment. The following matrices present the role of public health nursing in Virginia. The following definitions were used to develop these matrices.

Essential Element is taken from the National Association of City and County Health Officials' (NACCHO's) document *Blueprint for a Healthy Community.* The following public health essential elements are used as a framework to present the role of public health nursing in Virginia:

- Conducting Community Assessments
- Preventing and Controlling Epidemics
- Providing a Safe and Healthy Environment
- Measuring Performance, Effectiveness, and Outcomes of Health Services
- Promoting Healthy Lifestyles
- Providing Targeted Outreach and Forming Partnerships
- Providing Personal Health Care Services
- Conducting Research and Innovation
- Mobilizing the Community for Action

Public Health Function is defined as a broad public health activity needed to ensure a strong, flexible, accountable public health structure. It may require a multidisciplinary team to carry out.

Public Health Nurse Role is the activity the public health nurse is responsible for, either alone or as a member of a team, to accomplish the stated public health function. This can be the public health nurse at the local level or at the state level.

State Role is what public health nurses need from the state level to do their jobs (e.g., policy, aggregate data, training). This refers to any Central Office program or staff, not just nurses.

A process was implemented that would involve all public health nurses in Virginia. Although this lengthened the timeline to completion, it will ensure that the final document represents a consensus developed through creative open dialogue.

From National Association of City and County Health Officials: Blueprint for a healthy community: a guide for local health departments, Washington, DC, 1994, The Association.

ESSENTIAL ELEMENT 1: Conduct Community Assessment: Systematically collecting, assembling, analyzing, and making available health-related data for the purpose of identifying and responding to community- and state-level public health concerns and conducting epidemiologic and other population-based studies.

Public Health Function	PHN Roles	State Roles
Develop frameworks, methodologies, and tools for standardizing data collection and analysis and reporting across all jurisdictions and providers.	• Provide, review, and comment on proposed methodologies and tools for data collection. • Field-test tools and methods.	• Collaborate with professional organizations and academic and governmental institutions to develop and test tools and methods. • Provide educational opportunities in areas of and use of tools. • Work with local-level agencies to standardize definitions, data collected, etc., across jurisdictions and among all stakeholders (schools, community-based organizations, and private providers).
Collect and analyze data.	• Collaborate with the community to identify population-based needs and gaps in service. • Analyze data and needs, knowledge, attitudes, and practices of specific populations. • Identify patterns of diseases, illness, and injury and develop or stimulate development of programs to respond to identified trends.	• Provide aggregated data to the local level in a timely and accurate manner. • Provide census tract–level aggregated data to the local level. • Provide national and state comparisons to be used with local data to obtain trends and assist localities in documenting need, progress, etc., to attain standard outcomes.

ESSENTIAL ELEMENT 2: Preventing and Controlling Epidemics: Monitoring disease trends and investigating and containing diseases and injuries.

Public Health Function	PHN Roles	State Roles
Develop programs that prevent, contain, and control the transmission of diseases and danger of injuries (including violence).	• Provide community-wide preventive measures in the form of health education and mobilization of community resources. • Ensure isolation/containment measures when necessary. • Ensure adequate preventive immunizations. • Implement programs that control the transmission of diseases and danger of injuries during disasters.	• Work with local jurisdictions to develop tools such as videos, PSAs, and/or posters that local jurisdictions can use. • Work with local jurisdictions to develop disaster plans for the control of the transmission of diseases and danger of injuries during disasters. • Facilitate state-level partnerships that promote health, healthy lifestyles, and wellness (individual and family).
Develop regulatory guidelines for the prevention of targeted diseases.	• Implement regulatory measures. • Implement OSHA Guidelines for Blood Borne Pathogens and the Prevention of the Transmission of TB in Health Care Settings.	• In partnership with localities, develop regulatory guidelines. • Serve as clearinghouse or source of information.

ESSENTIAL ELEMENT 3: Providing a Safe and Healthy Environment: Maintaining clean and safe air, water, food, and facilities both in the community and in the home environment.

Public Health Function	PHN Roles	State Roles
Develop methods/tools for collection and analysis of health-related data (occurrence of mortality and morbidity relating to both communicable and chronic diseases, injury registries, sentinel event establishment, environmental quality, etc.).	• Provide reporting guidelines and consultation regarding disease prevention, diagnosis, treatment, and follow-up of cases/contacts to physicians and institutions (emergency department, university and secondary school student health, prisons, industries, etc.). • Conduct/participate in community needs assessments to determine customer/provider knowledge deficits and perceptions of need. • Provide education to individuals, providers, targeted populations, etc., in response to knowledge deficits, disease outbreaks, toxic waste emissions, etc. • Provide individual follow-up/case management of communicable diseases that are transmitted by air, water, food, and fomites (TB, hepatitis A, salmonella, staphylococcus, etc.).	• Develop standard methodology and tools for collection and analysis of health-related data. • Provide training in area of data collection and analysis. • Evaluate activities and outcomes of interactions. • Work in partnership with localities to develop program based on data analysis needs.
Develop programs that promote a safe environment in the home.	• Provide childhood lead poisoning screenings and follow-up. • Teach clients to inspect homes for safety violations and toxic substances and to practice safe behaviors; assist families to access/use available resources/safety devices. • Assess/teach regarding safe food selection, preparation, and storage. • Train/supervise volunteers/auxiliary personnel in performance of the above tasks. • Teach families that all men, women, and children have a right to a safe environment free of physical or mental abuse.	• Provide consultation and technical assistance to state/local organizations regarding laws and regulations that protect health and ensure safety. • In partnership with localities, develop and evaluate educational programs.
Develop programs that promote a safe environment in the workplace.	• Provide consultation in implementation of OSHA regulations relating to occupational exposure to diseases. • Provide educational program related to healthy lifestyles (smoking cessation, back protection, etc.). • Ensure provision of screenings for individuals to determine baselines and occurrence of infectious diseases and preventable deterioration of health and function: hearing, back soundness, lung capacity, RMS indicators, PPDs, etc. • Assist in policy/practice development to address prevention of the above. • Provide immunizations.	• Monitor and assist localities to implement prevention activities. • Assist localities in developing and evaluating educational programs. • Monitor outcomes of screening activities and evaluate interventions.

Continued

ESSENTIAL ELEMENT 3: Providing a Safe and Healthy Environment—cont'd

Public Health Function	PHN Roles	State Roles
Develop programs that promote a safe environment in the school setting.	• Provide consultation on implementation of OSHA regulations relating to occupational exposure to diseases. • Provide educational programs related to healthy lifestyles (smoking cessation, etc.). • Ensure provision of screenings for students to determine baselines and occurrence of infectious disease and preventable deterioration of health and function. • Assist in policy/practice development to address prevention of the above. • Provide immunizations.	• Develop guidelines that ensure accountability in meeting standards set forth. • Ensure that policy is developed to protect children in the school environment. • Monitor immunization status of children and provide immunizations during outbreaks and evaluate activities.
Develop programs that promote a safe environment in the community.	• Identify population clusters exhibiting an unhealthy environment; provide consultation/group education regarding preventive measures. • Participate in development of local disaster plans to ensure provision of safe water, food, air, and facilities. • Respond in time of natural disasters such as floods, tornadoes, and hurricanes. • Participate in developing plans for shelter management during disasters, especially "Special Needs" shelters that may require nursing staff.	• In times of disaster, facilitate availability of resources across jurisdictions. • Have a statewide plan. • Ensure that localities have developed plans to protect the public in time of national and/or other disasters. • Coordinate efforts statewide. • Assist localities in responding. • Evaluate efforts.
Develop and issue standards that guide regulations and mandate policy and program development.	• Survey worksites, schools, institutions, etc., for compliance to regulations that protect health and ensure safety.	• Develop a systematic evaluation tool for collection of data to measure trends.
Develop protocols to ensure accountability of all health care providers, public and private.	• Provide technical assistance (i.e., interpretation, implementation, and evaluation processes).	• Assist localities in developing standards to mandate accountability.
Provide inservice to all providers of health care services.	• Share and implement knowledge gained in inservices.	• Provide consultation/technical assistance to localities.

ESSENTIAL ELEMENT 4: Measuring Performance, Effectiveness, and Outcomes of Health Services: Monitoring health care providers and the health care system to identify gaps in service, deteriorating health status indicators, effectiveness of interventions, and accessibility and quality of personal and population-wide health services.

Public Health Function	PHN Roles	State Roles
Promote competency in public health issues throughout the health delivery system.	• Provide educational and technical assistance in areas such as case management and appropriate treatment and control of communicable diseases to the community.	• Develop appropriate regulatory, educational, and technical assistance programs. • Provide technical assistance and training to local health department for local forecasting and interpretation of data.
Collect data.	• Participate in data collection with a target population. • Ensure that the data collection system supports the objectives of programs serving the community by participating in the design and operation of data collection systems. • Collect data via surveys, polls, interviews, focus groups that will enable assessment of the community's perception of health status and understanding how the system works and how to obtain service needs.	• Work with localities (health districts, private providers, other state and local agencies) to develop standard data elements and definitions across jurisdictions and among all stakeholders, especially for consistency in coding of population-based data. • Identify data collection and analytic issues related to monitoring the impact of health system changes such as costs and benefits of record linkage, strategies for ensuring confidentiality, and strategies for analyzing trends in health within a broader social and economic context. • Advocate for uniform data collection from all managed care plans so that outcomes and health trends can be analyzed and tracked and sentinel events reported.

ESSENTIAL ELEMENT 4: Measuring Performance, Effectiveness, and Outcomes of Health Services—cont'd

Public Health Function	PHN Roles	State Roles
Analyze data to ensure accurate diagnosis of health status, identification of threats to health, and assessment of health service needs.	• Participate in a systematic approach to convert data into information that will identify gaps in service at the local and state level and will lead to action. • Monitor health status indicators to identify emerging problems and facilitate community-wide response to identified problems. • Facilitate data analysis as part of a local collaborative effort.	• Develop a systematic, integrated statewide approach to converting data into information that directs action. • Ensure that resources, such as hardware and software, to analyze data are available at the local level. • Work with localities (health districts, private providers, other state and local agencies) to address issues related to variable access to technology, confidentiality issues. • Educate and train currently employed public health nurses in areas of epidemiology and population-based services.
Monitor health status indicators for the entire population and for specific population groups and/or geographic areas.	• Identify target populations that may be at risk for public health problems such as communicable diseases, unidentified and untreated chronic diseases. • Conduct surveys or observe targeted populations such as preschools, childcare centers, and high-risk census tracks to identify health status. • Monitor health care utilization of vulnerable populations at the local and regional level.	• Develop methodology for identification, measurement, and analysis of key indicators of health care utilization of vulnerable populations.
Monitor and assess availability, cost-effectiveness, and outcomes of personal and population-based health services.	• Identify gaps in services (e.g., a neighborhood with deteriorating immunization rates may indicate lack of available primary care services). • Ensure that all receive the same quality of care, including comprehensive preventive services. • Monitor the impact of health system reforms on vulnerable populations. • Evaluate the effectiveness and outcomes of care. • Plan interventions based on the health of the overall population, not just for those in the health care system. • Identify interventions that are effective and replicable.	• Develop analyses that demonstrate the cost-effectiveness of investment in public health services. • Develop protocols and technical assistance for ensuring accountability of Medicaid managed care plans and other government-funded plans for service delivery and overall health status of their covered populations. • Identify standard theoretical, methodological, and measurement issues that are specific to population subgroups for monitoring the impact of health system changes on vulnerable populations.
Disseminate information.	• Disseminate information to the public on community health status, including how to access and use services appropriately. • Disseminate information to other health care providers regarding gaps in services or deteriorating health status indicators.	• Ensure a mechanism for public accountability of performance and outcomes through public dissemination of information and in particular ensure that underservice, a risk inherent in capitated plans, is measurable through available data. • Ensure that information is provided to communities, local health departments, managed care plans, and other appropriate state agencies.

ESSENTIAL ELEMENT 5: Promoting Healthy Lifestyles: Providing health education to individuals, families, and communities.

Public Health Function	PHN Roles	State Roles
Promote informed decision making of residents about things that influence their health on a daily basis.	• Exert influence through contact with individuals and community groups. • Accept and issue challenge of healthy lifestyles to all contacts. • Reinforce and reward positive informed decisions made for healthy lifestyles.	• Develop and monitor standards for the changes to determine changes in behavior.
Promote effective use of media to encourage both personal and community responsibility for informed decision making.	• Be a resource for the community. • Gather data and address findings as appropriate. • Work with community groups to promote accurate information for healthy lifestyle through the media. • Use current information and other agency's resources to maximize information accessible to the public.	• Assist localities to provide current information to community organizations and other state organizations. • Serve as a resource for localities and work with media.
Develop a public awareness/marketing campaign to demonstrate the importance of public health to overall health improvement and its proper place in the health delivery system.	• Provide education to special groups (e.g., local politicians, school boards, PTAs, churches, civic groups, news media) regarding the benefits of preventive health.	• Develop training activities to assist localities in marketing.
Develop public information and education systems/programs through partnerships.	• Provide educational sessions/programs to public regarding components of healthy lifestyles. • Access grants/other funding sources to promote healthy lifestyle decisions (e.g., cervical and breast cancer prevention, bike helmets, hypertension). • Provide/promote teaching for individuals and families at every opportunity (home, clinic, community settings).	• Assist localities in developing and evaluating educational programs. • Assist localities in funding. • Hold regional/state training sessions. • Evaluate outcomes and plan ongoing educational systems/programs.

ESSENTIAL ELEMENT 6: Providing Targeted Outreach and Forming Partnerships: Ensuring access to services, including those that lead to self-sufficiency, for all vulnerable populations and ensuring the development of culturally appropriate care.

Public Health Function	PHN Roles	State Roles
Ensure accessibility to health services that will improve morbidity, decrease mortality, and improve health status outcomes.	• Provide family-centered case management services for high-risk and hard-to-reach populations that focus on linking families with needed services. • Improve access to care by forming partnerships with appropriate community individuals and entities. • Increase influence of cultural diversity on system design and on access to care, as well as on individual services rendered. • Ensure that translation services are available for the non–English-speaking population. • Participate in ongoing community assessment to identify areas of concern and above needs for rules. • Provide outreach services that focus on preventing epidemics and the spread of disease, such as tuberculosis and sexually transmitted diseases.	• Provide funds in cooperation with locality. • Ensure policy development that includes case management and is culturally sensitive. • Provide adequate ongoing continuing education for staff (especially in areas common to all localities). • Participate in state-level contract development to ensure that contracts with health plans require and include incentives for health plans to offer and deliver preventive health services in the minimum benefits package. • Educate financing officials about the roles of public health both in performing core public health services and in ensuring access to personal health services.

ESSENTIAL ELEMENT 7: Providing Personal Health Care Services: Providing targeted direct services to high-risk populations.

Public Health Function	PHN Roles	State Roles
Provide direct services for specific diseases that threaten the health of the community and develop programs that prevent, contain, and control the transmission of infectious diseases.	• Plan, develop, implement, and evaluate: • Sexually transmitted disease services • Communicable disease services • HIV/AIDS services • Tuberculosis control services • Develop and implement guidelines for the prevention of the above targeted diseases.	• Establish standards/criteria for personal health care. • Work with local health departments to assist in developing infrastructure and management techniques to facilitate record-keeping and appropriate financial monitoring and tracking systems, which enable local health departments to enter into contractual arrangements for preventive health and primary care services.
Provide health services, including preventive health services, to high-risk and vulnerable populations (e.g., the uninsured working poor), and in geographic areas where primary health care services are not readily accessible or available in a privatized setting.	• Provide coordination, follow-up, referral, and case management as indicated. • Integrate supportive services (such as counseling, social work, nutrition) into primary care services. • Assess existing community medical capacity for referral and follow-up.	• Continue to work at the state and local level to build capacity of primary and preventive health services, particularly in traditionally underserved areas, to ensure availability to providers and primary care sites essential to primary care access.

ESSENTIAL ELEMENT 8: Conducting Research and Innovation: Discovering and applying improved health care delivery mechanisms and clinical interventions.

Public Health Function	PHN Roles	State Roles
Ensure ongoing prevention research relating to biomedical and behavioral aspects of health promotion and prevention of disease and injury.	• Develop outcome measures. • Identify research priorities for target communities and develop and conduct scientific and operations research for health promotion and disease/injury prevention.	• Provide training in area of measuring program effectiveness.
Implement pilot or demonstration projects.	• Develop and implement linkages with academic centers, ensuring that clients and populations who participate in research projects benefit as a result of the research.	• Support evaluations and research that demonstrate the benefits of public health, as well as the consequences of failure to support public health interventions.

ESSENTIAL ELEMENT 9: Mobilizing the Community for Action: Providing leadership and initiating collaboration.

Public Health Function	PHN Roles	State Roles
Provide leadership to stimulate development of networks or partnerships that will ensure the availability of comprehensive primary health care services to all, regardless of ability to pay.	• Advocate for improved health. • Disseminate health information. • Build coalitions. • Make recommendations for policy implementation or revision.	• Facilitate the establishment and enhancement of statewide high-quality, needed health services. • Administer quality improvement programs.
Initiate collaboration with other community organizations to ensure the leadership role in resolving a public health issue.	• Facilitate resources that manage environmental risk and maintain and improve community health. • Provide information for a community group working on impacting policy at the local, state, or federal level. • Use results of community health assessments to stimulate the community to develop a plan to respond to identified gaps in service.	• Use information-gathering techniques of assessment to assist policy/legislature activities to develop needed health services and functions that require statewide action or standards. • Recommend programs to carry out policies.

F APPENDIX

American Public Health Association Definition of Public Health Nursing

THE DEFINITION AND PRACTICE OF PUBLIC HEALTH NURSING

2013

Acknowledgments

This statement was developed by the Public Health Nursing Definition Document Task Force under the direction of the leadership of the Public Health Nursing Section of the American Public Health Association. The statement was adopted by the Public Health Nursing Section Council at the American Public Health Association Annual Meeting on November 5, 2013. The Task Force gratefully acknowledges the valuable assistance of individuals who contributed comments and recommendations throughout the development of this document.

Public Health Nursing Definition Document Task Force

Betty Bekemeier, Co-chair

Tessa Walker Linderman, Co-chair

Jo Anne Bennett

Shawn Kneipp

Martha Bergren

Kirk Koyama

Janet Braunstein Moody

Pam Kulbok

Marjorie Buchanan

Lauren Lawson

Laura Debiasi

Kathlynn Northrup-Snyder

Joyce Edmonds

Sue Stroschein

Alexandra Garcia

Recommended citation:

American Public Health Association, Public Health Nursing Section (2013). The definition and practice of public health nursing: A statement of the public health nursing section. Washington, DC: American Public Health Association.

November 11, 2013

THE DEFINITION AND PRACTICE OF PUBLIC HEALTH NURSING

A Statement of the APHA Public Health Nursing Section

2013

This document updates the 1996 American Public Health Association Public Health Nursing Section definition statement and affirms the original definition.[1] This statement addresses some of the evolving economic, health, political, and societal trends that shape the context of public health nursing practice.

Definition

Public health nursing is the practice of promoting and protecting the health of populations using knowledge from nursing, social, and public health sciences.

Public health nursing is a specialty practice within nursing and public health. It focuses on improving population health by emphasizing prevention, and attending to multiple determinants of health. Often used interchangeably with community health nursing, this nursing practice includes advocacy, policy development, and planning, which addresses issues of social justice. With a multi-level view of health, public health nursing action occurs through community applications of theory, evidence, and a commitment to health equity. In addition to what is put forward in this definition, public health nursing practice is guided by the American Nurses Association *Public Health Nursing: Scope & Standards of Practice* [2] and the Quad Council of Public Health Nursing Organizations' *Core Competencies for Public Health Nurses.*[3]

Elements of Practice

Key characteristics of practice include 1) a focus on the health needs of an entire population, including inequities and the unique needs of sub-populations; 2) assessment of population health using a comprehensive, systematic approach; 3) attention to multiple determinants of health; 4) an emphasis on primary prevention; and 5) application of interventions at all levels—individuals, families, communities, and the systems that impact their health.[4]

Public Health Nursing Perspective

Public health nursing aims to improve the health outcomes of all populations. Applying their clinical knowledge and expertise in health care from an ecological perspective, public health nurses acknowledge the complexity of public health problems and the contextual nature of health—including cultural, environmental, historical, physical, and social factors. Public health nurses apply systems-level thinking[5,6] to assess the potential or actual assets, needs, opportunities, and inequities of individuals, families, and populations and translate this assessment into action for public good.

Public Health Nursing Activities and Practice Settings

Public health nursing activities comprise the domains depicted by the *Public Health Intervention Wheel* and the *10 Essential Public Health Services.* [7,8] These activities include community collaboration, health teaching, and policy development, in response to priorities derived from ongoing, comprehensive population focused assessment. Public health nurses are members and leaders of interprofessional teams in diverse settings and in many different types of agencies and organizations including all levels of government, community-based and other nongovernmental service organizations, foundations, policy think tanks, academic institutions and other research settings. Increasing numbers of public health nurses work in global health in an effort to promote global responsibility and connectivity. Public health nurses that work with individuals and families do so within the context of a population focus—applying a systems perspective to factors that impact health.

Determinants of Health
Eliminating population health disparities by addressing multiple determinants that lead to poor health is a national goal.[9] Public health nurses are in a position to provide leadership through public policy reform efforts, community-building, and system-level change.[10] Environmental, physical, and social determinants explain most health disparities in the United States.[11,12,13,14,15] Socioeconomic disadvantages such as poverty, low levels of education, and belonging to a racial or ethnic minority group, are more robust risk factors of poor health than a lack of access to health care or predominantly genetic factors of disease.[16,17,18] While the discipline of nursing was founded on improving environmental conditions to facilitate health at the bedside,[19] public health nurses focus on improving population health in the environments where people live, work, learn, and play.

Opportunities & Challenges
Adherence to public health nursing's key characteristics requires that the practice must evolve to address current societal needs. Public health nursing has faced multiple challenges over its history while engaging in leadership opportunities that have shaped nursing practice, addressing environmental and social justice issues, affecting population health, and exploring health promotion concepts. One example is the Patient Protection and Affordable Care Act (ACA).[20] The ACA has greatly altered the landscape for health care and health improvement in the U.S., creating the potential for new public health nursing roles and responsibilities. The ACA includes goals to 1) improve the individual health care experience; 2) reduce the cost of health care; and 3) improve the health of populations. With their positions embedded within communities, public health nurses are vital to the interprofessional teams needed to assure that all people have equitable access to high quality care and healthy environments through health system reform.[21] Their assessment skills, primary prevention focus, and system-level perspectives can assure that local and state needs are met, services and programs are coordinated, and communities are engaged.

Public health nurses are prepared to lead efforts that align emerging systems of care for population health improvement, health promotion, risk reduction, and disease prevention efforts that are within the nucleus of a reformed health system. Fewer public health nursing positions and decreased public health funding influence leadership roles and access to health care in communities.[22] Within the context of health care reform these challenges offer opportunities to emphasize a strong, well-educated public health nursing workforce to lead and carry out system coordination and change at local, state, national, and international levels.[23]

An emerging health care model that requires public health nursing leadership is the integration of primary care and public health.[24] Primary care and public health share a focus on prevention, population health, transitional care, and care coordination across settings to promote health through collaboration. With a unique focus from individuals and families to populations and systems, public health nurses are well positioned to integrate new health system models and meet the demands of an ever-changing health system.[25]

Public Health Nursing Education

The baccalaureate degree in nursing (BSN) is recommended for entry-level public health nurses.[26] *The Essentials of Baccalaureate Education for Professional Nursing Practice* emphasize fundamental concepts for public health nursing practice such as clinical prevention, population health, health care policy, finance, and regulatory environments, and interprofessional collaboration.[27] The graduate is prepared to conduct community assessments and apply the principles of epidemiology among other competencies.

Nurses with a master's degree or higher, and with specialization in population health, demonstrate the knowledge and skills required for leadership positions. Competencies include mastery of interprofessional collaboration, health policy and advocacy, population assessment, prevention strategies, and program planning and evaluation.[28] The doctor of nursing practice (DNP) degree, with a public health emphasis, has emerged in the last decade, and provides the foundation for advanced practice in executive leadership, systems development, and the translation of research into practice. The doctor of philosophy (PhD) and other research-focused doctoral degrees remain the preparation for public health nurses to develop the science relevant to public health nursing and to generate the evidence needed to guide practice. In some states a public health nursing certification is needed to signify a nurse's specific competence and expertise in public health nursing. National advanced public health nursing certification is available via portfolio assessment through American Nurses Credentialing Center.

Summary

Public health nurses provide leadership for emerging advances in population health and health care—particularly in terms of addressing health inequities. Equipped with a baccalaureate degree or higher, public health nurses are prepared to address multiple determinants of health and participate fully in the challenges of attaining and maintaining population health. With a scope of practice that includes community-building, health promotion, policy reform, and system-level changes to promote and protect the health of populations; public health nurses have an essential role and responsibility as leaders in health improvement and promoting health equity.

---

[1] American Public Health Association, Public Health Nursing Section. (1996). Definition and role of public health nursing: A statement of the public health nursing section. Washington, DC; Author.

[2] American Nurses Association. (2013). *Public health nursing: Scope and standards of practice. (2nd ed.),* Washington, DC: American Nurses Publishing.

[3] Quad Council of Public Health Nursing Organizations. (2011). Core competencies for public health nurses. Washington, DC: Quad Council of Public Health Organizations.

[4] Keller, L.O., Schaffer, M., Lia-Hoagberg, B., Strohschein, S. (2002). Assessment, program planning, and evaluation in population-based public health practice. *Public Health Management Practice,* 8 (5), 31-32.

November 11, 2013

[5] Leischow, S., Milstein, B. (2006) Systems thinking and modeling for public health practice. *AJPH 96*(3): 403-404

[6] Swider, S., Krothe, J., Reyes, D., Cravetz, M. (2013). The Quad Council practice competencies for public health nursing. *Public Health Nursing*. doi: 10.1111/phn.12090

[7] Public Health Nursing Section (2001). Public health interventions–applications for public health nursing practice. St. Paul: Minnesota Department of Health.

[8] Centers for Disease Control and Prevention. (2010). National public health performance standards program, 10 essential public health services. Retrieved from: cdc.gov/nphpsp/essentialservices.html

[9] U.S. Department of Health and Human Services. Office of Disease Prevention and Health Promotion. (2011). Healthy People 2020. Washington, DC. Retrieved from: http://www.healthypeople.gov/2020/default.aspx.

[10] United States Department of Health and Human Services, Healthy People 2020. (2012). *Public health infrastructure*: *Overview*. Retrieved from: http://www.healthypeople.gov/2020/topicsobjectives2020/overview.aspx?topicid=35

[11] Marmot, M. (2000). Multilevel approaches to understanding social determinants. In Berkman LF, Kawachi I (Eds), *Social Epidemiology (*347-367). New York, NY: Oxford University Press.

[12] Braveman, P. (2011). Accumulating knowledge on the social determinants of health and infectious disease. *Public Health Reports*, 126 (3), 28-30.

[13] Braveman, P., Egerter, S., Williams, D.R.(2011). Determinants of health: Coming of age. *Annual Review of Public Health,* 32, 381-98.

[14] Woolf, S.H., Braveman, P. (2011). Where health disparities begin: the role of social and economic determinants--and why current policies may make matters worse. *Health Affairs*, 30, 1852-1859.

[15] Marmot, M., Wilkinson, R.G. (2000). *Social Determinants of Health*. Oxford: Oxford University Press.

[16] Blane, D., Brunner, E., Wilkinson, R. (1996). *Health and Social Organization: Towards a Health Policy for the Twenty-First Century*. London: Routledge.

[17] Krieger, N. (2005). *Embodying Inequality: Epidemiologic Perspectives*. Amityville, NY: Baywood Publishing Company, Inc.

[18] Berkman, L.F., Kawachi, I. (2000) *Social Epidemiology*. Oxford: Oxford University Press.

[19] Buhler-Wilkerson, K. (1993). Bringing care to the people: Lillian Wald's legacy to public health nursing. *American Journal of Public Health*, 83,1778-86.

[20] Patient Protection and Affordable Care Act, Pub. L. No. 111-148, §2702, 124 Stat. 119, 318-319 (2010).

November 11, 2013

[21] American Public Health Association. (2013). ACA basics and background. Retrieved from: http://www.apha.org/advocacy/Health+Reform/ACAbasics/

[22] Robert Wood Johnson Foundation. (2011) Recession Takes Bite Out of Nation's Public Health Nursing Infrastructure. Retrieved from: http://www.rwjf.org/newsroom/product.jsp?id=73642

[23] Institute of Medicine. (2010). The future of nursing: leading change, advancing health. Washington, D.C.: The National Academies Press. Retrieved from: http://books.nap.edu/openbook.php?record_id=12956

[24] Institute of Medicine. (2012). *Primary Care and Public Health: Exploring Integration to Improve Population Health.* Washington, DC: The National Academies Press.

[25] Robert Wood Johnson Foundation. (2012) *RWJF Fellow Works to Push Public Health Nursing Forward.* Retrieved from: http://www.rwjf.org/en/about-rwjf/newsroom/newsroom-content/2012/04/rwjf-fellow-works-to-push-public-health-nursing-forward.html

[26] American Nurses Association. (2013). *Public health nursing: Scope and standards of practice. (2nd ed.),* Washington, DC: American Nurses Publishing.

[27] American Association of Colleges of Nursing (2008). *The essentials of baccalaureate education for professional nursing practice*, Washington, DC: American Association of Colleges of Nursing.

[28] American Association of Colleges of Nursing (2011). *The essentials of master's education in nursing*, Washington, DC: American Association of Colleges of Nursing.

November 11, 2013

G APPENDIX

American Nurses Association Scope and Standards of Practice for Public Health Nursing

STANDARDS OF CARE

Standard 1: Assessment

The public health nurse collects comprehensive data pertinent to the health status of populations.

Standard 2: Population Diagnosis and Priorities

The public health nurse analyses the assessment data to determine the diagnoses or issues.

Standard 3: Outcomes Identification

The public health nurse identifies expected outcomes for a plan specific to the population or situation.

Standard 4: Planning

The public health nurse develops a plan that prescribes strategies and alternatives to attain expected outcomes.

Standard 5: Implementation

The public health nurse implements the identified plan.

Standard 5A: Coordination of Care. The public health nurse coordinates care delivery.

Standard 5B: Health Teaching and Health Promotion. The public health nurse employs multiple strategies to promote health and a safe environment.

Standard 5C: Consultation. The public health nurse provides consultation to influence the identified plan, enhance the abilities of others, and effect change.

Standard 5D: Prescriptive Authority. Not applicable

Standard 5D: Regulatory Activities. The public health nurse participates in applications of public health laws, regulations, and policies.

Standard 6: Evaluation

The public health nurse evaluates progress toward the attainment of outcomes.

STANDARDS OF PROFESSIONAL PERFORMANCE

Standard 7: Ethics

The public health nurse practices ethically.

Standard 8: Education

The public health nurse attains knowledge and competency that reflect current practice.

Standard 9: Evidence-Based Practice and Research

The public health nurse integrates evidence and research findings into practice.

Standard 10: Quality of Practice

The public health nurse contributes to quality nursing practice.

Standard 11: Communication

The public health nurse communicates effectively in a variety of formats in all areas of practice.

Standard 12: Leadership

The public health nurse demonstrates leadership in the professional practice setting and the profession.

Standard 13: Collaboration

The public health nurse collaborates with the population and others in the conduct of nursing practice.

Standard 14: Professional Practice Evaluation

The public health nurse evaluates her or his own nursing practice in relation to professional practice standards and guidelines, relevant statutes, rules, and regulations.

Standard 15: Resource Utilization

The public health nurse utilizes appropriate resources to plan and provide nursing and public health services that are safe, effective, and financially responsible.

Standard 16: Environmental Health

The public health nurse practices in an environmentally safe, fair, and just manner.

Standard 17: Advocacy

The public health nurse advocates for the protection of the health, safety, and rights of the population.

APPENDIX H

The Health Insurance Portability and Accountability Act (HIPAA): What Does It Mean for Public Health Nurses?

Public Health Nursing Practice—definition: a specialty practice within nursing and public health. Practice focuses on improving population health by emphasizing prevention and attending to multiple determinants of health. Practice includes advocacy, policy development, and planning, which addresses issues of social justice. With a multilevel view of health, public health nursing action occurs through community applications of theory, evidence, and a commitment to health equity. The goal is to prevent disease and disability and promote and protect the health of the community as a whole.

EXPLANATION

- Federal privacy standards were created by the Department of Health and Human Services (USDHHS) to protect patients' medical records and other health information provided to health plans, doctors, hospitals, and other health care providers.
- These standards took effect on April 14, 2003.
- Standardization of electronic transactions, and the elimination of inefficient paper forms, will save the health care industry more than $29 billion in the next 10 years.

PRIVACY RULE

- Protects the confidentiality of individually identifiable health information, whether it is on paper, in computers, or communicated orally.
- Protected health information (PHI) is the name for this individually identifiable health information.
- Limits the ways that health plans, pharmacies, hospitals, and other covered entities can use patients' personal medical information.

PATIENT PROTECTIONS

- Patients should be able to see, obtain copies, and make corrections to their medical records.
- Patients should receive a notice from health care providers regarding how their personal medical information may be used by them and their rights under the privacy regulation. Patients can restrict this use.
- Limits have been set on how health care providers can use individually identifiable health information. Doctors, nurses, and other providers can share information needed to treat a patient. For purposes other than medical care, personal health information generally may not be used.
- Pharmacies, health plans, and other covered entities must obtain an individual's authorization before disclosing patient information for marketing purposes.

PUBLIC HEALTH SERVICES AND PHI

Overview: Although protection of health information is important, PHI is used for the public good by health officials to identify, monitor, and respond to disease, death, and disability among populations. Examples of ways PHI is used include public health surveillance, program evaluation, terrorism preparedness, outbreak investigations, direct health services, and public health research. Public health authorities have taken precautions in the past to protect the privacy of individuals and will continue to do so under HIPAA. The privacy rule, however, still permits PHI to be shared for important public health purposes.

PERMITTED PHI DISCLOSURES TO A PUBLIC HEALTH AUTHORITY

Without Authorization

- Reporting of disease, injury, and vital events
- Conducting public health surveillance, investigations, and interventions
- Reporting child abuse or neglect to a public health or other government authority legally authorized to receive such reports
- To a person subject to jurisdiction of the Food and Drug Administration (FDA) concerning the quality, safety, or effectiveness of an FDA-related product or activity for which that person has responsibility
- To a person who may have been exposed to a communicable disease or may be at risk for contracting or spreading a disease or condition, when legally authorized to notify the person as necessary to conduct a public health intervention or investigation
- To an individual's employer, under certain circumstances and conditions, as needed for the employer to meet the requirements

of the Occupational Safety and Health Administration, Mine Safety and Health Administration, or similar state law

HIPAA AND NURSING RESEARCH

Definitions

Covered entity: a health plan, a health care clearinghouse, or a health care provider who transmits any health information in electronic form.

Individually Identifiable Health Information (IIHI): information about an individual regarding his or her physical or mental health; the provision of health care; or the payment for the provision of health care; and which identifies the individual.

It is the covered entity's obligation not to disclose the information improperly when a researcher seeks data that includes PHI.

A covered entity can disclose IIHI for research purposes under any of the following conditions:

1. The IIHI pertains only to deceased persons.
2. The IIHI can be examined for reviews preparatory to research if it is not removed from the covered entity.
3. Information that has been de-identified can be disclosed; this information is no longer considered IIHI and thus not covered by HIPAA.
4. Data must be disclosed as part of a limited data set if the researcher has a data use agreement with the covered entity.
5. The researcher has a valid authorization from the research subject to disclose IIHI.
6. An IRB or privacy board has waived the authorization requirement.

Creating Data

Researchers may also be creating IIHI. If the researcher is part of a covered entity, any PHI obtained by any means is covered by HIPAA, and the researcher and his or her institution are bound by HIPAA regulations. Most universities with nursing schools will be hybrid entities (i.e., some parts of the university are a covered entity and some are not). Researchers should check their institution's policies.

Disclosing Data

Nurse researchers should be aware that sharing data with colleagues and students may constitute disclosures of IIHI and they should conform to HIPAA regulations. In this case, the researcher is the holder of the IIHI and can disclose it only under appropriate conditions:

1. Patients agree to specific disclosures in the initial authorization.
2. Former patients sign an additional authorization.
3. An IRB or privacy board waives the need for authorization.
4. The holder allows the colleague to review the data to prepare a research protocol if the colleague takes no information away.
5. A holder enters the data in a limited data set and signs a data use agreement with the recipient.
6. A holder de-identifies the data and shares it freely.

INDEX

A

AACN *see* American Association of Colleges of Nursing
AAOHN *see* American Association of Occupational Health
AAOHN Code of Ethics, 959
AAOHN Foundation, 958–959
AAP *see* American Academy of Pediatrics
AAPCC *see* Adjusted average per capita cost
ABC-X model, 611
ABOHN *see* American Board for Occupational Health Nurses
Abortion, 779
Abortion services, 774
Abrams, Sarah, 40b
Abuse
  child, 844–847, 845b, 846b
  elder, 850–851
  emotional, 846
  family violence and, 843–851
  physical, 844
  during pregnancy, 849–850, 850b
  sexual, 844
  spouse, 847–849
  wife, 847–849
Abusive head trauma (AHT), 640
ACA *see* Affordable Care Act
Acceptability of care, 725
Access to health care
  current U.S. system and, 49, 49b
  migrant farmworkers and, 759–760
  and rationing, 98–99
  status of children, 628
Accommodating, 565b
Accountability, 525
  and quality management, 914–915
Accountable care organizations (ACOs), 523, 547
Accreditation, 527
  home health/hospice nursing and, 915
  voluntary approach to, 527
ACHIEVE *see* Action Communities for Health, Innovation, and EnVironmental ChangE
Acquired immunity, 303
Acquired immunodeficiency syndrome (AIDS), 78–79, 334
  adult health concerns and, 663
  directly observed therapy and, 352–353
  epidemic of, 271
  global health care, 79b
  homelessness and, 741
  migrant farmworkers and, 763–764
  rural communities and, 719–720
  in school nursing, 949
Action Communities for Health, Innovation, and EnVironmental ChangE (ACHIEVE), 360
Action for Mental Health, 794
Action steps, 508
Active immunization, 303
Active participation, 373
Active surveillance, 284
Active system, as surveillance systems, 489
Activities of daily living (ADL), 682
Acute infectious disease, 101–102
Acute watery diarrhea, 80
ADA *see* Americans with Disabilities Act
Addiction treatment, 828–829, 828b, 828f, 829b
Adenine, 257
Adequacy, 511–512
Adjudication, 979
Adjusted average per capita cost (AAPCC), 6b
Administration of Developmental Disabilities (ADD), 693–694
Administration on Aging, health policy and, 656
Administrator, 869
Adolescents
  see also Teen pregnancy
  as client, 773–774
  developmental considerations and, 638
  with disabilities, 684, 686
  health and, 626–652
  health care for, 773
  health effects of poverty on, 741
  homelessness and, 747
  hormonal birth control methods for, 777t
  mental health objectives for, 801–802
  migrant farmworkers and, 764–765
  risk-taking behaviors and, 629
  role of population-centered nursing for, 648–649
  trends in sexual behavior, pregnancy, childbearing and, 774–775
Adoption, 776
  pregnant teens and, 779, 779b
Adult
  disabled, 685
    effects on community of, 686–687
  incarcerated, 670
Adult day health, 672
Adult health
  community-based models of care for, 671–673
    community care settings and, 672–673
    nursing roles and, 671–672
Adult health *(Continued)*
  concerns of, 659–664
  disparities among special groups of, 669–671
  environmental impact and, 657, 657b
  ethical and legal issues and legislation for, 656–657
  health issues and chronic disease management of, 653–677, 672–673b
  health policy and legislation, 654–657, 655f
  health status indicators for, 657–659
  historical perspective on, 654
  linking content to practice, 673b
  mental health objectives for, 802–803
  prevention strategies for, 668b
Adults of color, 670
Advanced Forensic Nurse (AFN), 983
Advanced medical directives, 656–657
Advanced nursing practice, in the community, 863–879, 864t
  advanced practice roles, 867–870
    administrator, 869
    clinician, 868–869, 868b
    consultant, 870
    educator, 869, 869f
    population-focused intervention, 869, 869b
    researcher, 870, 870b
  arenas for practice, 870–873
    faith community nursing/parish nursing, 871
    government, 872–873, 873b
    independent practice, 871
    institutional settings, 871–872
    nursing centers, 871
    other arenas, 873
    primary care, 870–871
    retail clinics, 871
  competencies, 866, 876b
  credentialing, 867
  educational preparation of, NP *versus* APHN, 866–867
  historical perspective, 864–866
  issues and concerns, 873–875
    employment and role negotiation, 874–875
    institutional privileges, 874
    legal status, 873–874
    reimbursement, 874, 874b
  role stress, 875–876
    conflicting expectations, 875
    interprofessional collaborative practice, 875
    liability, 875
    professional isolation, 875
    professional responsibilities, 875–876
  trends in, 876, 876b
Advanced practice nurse (APN), 864
  direct reimbursement of, 209
  as director, 443–444
  forensic nursing and, 979
  multilevel interventions, 440
  in nurse-led health centers, 442f
  primary health care and, 48
  school nurses as, 933
  title protection of, 211
Advanced practice psychiatric nurses, 797
Advanced practice registered nurses (APRNs), 721
Advanced public health nurse, 866
Adverse childhood experiences (ACEs), 703, 744
Advisory board, as nurse-led health center staff, 444
Advisory Committee on Immunization Practices (ACIP), 314
Advocacy, 151b, 180
  codes and standards of practice for, 159–160
  conceptual framework for, 160
  definition of, 245
  and ethics, 159–161
  health care reform and, 161
  levels of intervention and, 241t
  mental illness and, 791
  for persons with disabilities, 690
  practical framework for, 161b
  public health nursing process and, 251
  self-help organizations and, 796b
  in skills for case managers, 560–561
    allocation and, 564
    impact of, 563–564
    linking content to practice in, 562b
    process of, 561–563
    skill development, 563
    systematic problem solving in, 563
  vulnerable populations and, 704, 711
Advocate role, 560
AED *see* Automated external defibrillator
Affective disorder, 790
Affective domain, 417
Affective function, 579
Affirming, in advocacy process, 562–563
Affordability, 725
Affordable Care Act (ACA) of 2010, 49, 57–58, 374–375, 598, 605, 621, 628, 656, 742
  features of, 57t
  and public health support, 112, 112t
Affordable housing, lack of, 743
African American nurses, 31

African Americans
health disparities with, 287
health risks to, 723–724t
HIV and, 336t
mental health and, 806
sickle cell anemia and, 259
After Discharge Care Management of Low Income Frail Elderly (AD-LIFE), 559b
Age
cultural and ethnic backgrounds, 422
as mortality predictor, 286–287
vulnerability and, 702
Age adjustment, methods for, 286
Age-related risk, 609–612
Agency for Healthcare Research and Quality (AHRQ), 522
evaluating evidence and, 223b, 224
federal agency and, 1010
federal system and, 203–204
genetic testing and, 260
Agent
categories of, 303, 303b
in communicable disease transmission, 302–303, 303f
epidemiologic triangle and, 127, 278, 279b, 279f
as workplace hazards, 963–966, 963b, 963f, 964t
Aggregate
see also Population
definition of, 10–11, 19, 371
nurse advocate's role for, 560–561
population, workers as, 960–962
in rural communities, 723–724t
Aging population, 106
Agreements, nursing centers and, 446–447
Agricultural Workers Health Study, 757
AIDS *see* Acquired immunodeficiency syndrome
AIDS Drug Assistance Programs (ADAPs), 334
Aikenhead, Mary, 26
Air Carrier Access Act of 198, 694
Air pollution
children with asthma, 947
environmental health and, 132–133, 132b, 133f
Al-Anfal genocide, 85
Al-Gasseer, Dr. Naeema, 201
Alcohol, 815–816, 816b, 816f, 817t
Alcohol, tobacco, and other drug problems, 811–835, 812t
attitudes and myths, 813
definitions, 814, 814b
historical overview, 812–813
outcomes, 831–832
paradigm shift, 813–814
predisposing/contributing factors, 819–820
biopsychosocial model of addiction, 820
set, 820
setting, 820
Alcohol, tobacco, and other drug problems *(Continued)*
primary prevention and role of nurse, 820–822
drug education, 821–822, 821b, 822b
promotion of healthy lifestyles and resiliency factors, 820–821, 820b
psychoactive drugs, 814, 815–819, 815b
alcohol, 815–816, 816b, 816f, 817t
cannabis (marijuana), 818, 818b
opioids, 818–819, 819f
tobacco, 816–818, 817t
secondary prevention and role of nurse, 822–827
assessment, 822–823, 823b
codependency and family involvement, 826–827
drug testing, 823–824
drug use during pregnancy, 825–826, 826t
high-risk groups, 824–825, 824b
tertiary prevention and role of nurse, 827–831
addiction treatment, 828–829, 828b, 828f, 829b
detoxification, 827–828
nurse's role, 831, 831b
safer substance use, 827, 827b
smoking cessation programs, 830, 830b
support groups, 830–831
Alcoholics Anonymous (AA), 830
Alcoholism, 814
Algorithms, 484
All Kids Count, 1013
Allergies, children with, 946–947
Alliances, 887
Allocation, and advocacy, 564
Allowable costs, 115
Alternate care centers, 474
Alternatives, generation of, in systematic problem solving, 563
Alzheimer's disease, 790
Ambulatory/outpatient clinics, 871–872
Ambulatory payment classes (APCs), 115
American Academy of Forensic Science, 980
American Academy of Nursing (AAN), 260
American Academy of Pediatrics (AAP)
immunization and recommendations by, 632
school nurses and, 943
social determinants of health and, 405
American Association of Colleges of Nursing (AACN)
accreditation and, 527
nursing shortage and, 213
American Association of Industrial Nursing (AAIN), 958–959
American Association of Nurse Attorneys (TAANA), 980
American Association of Occupational Health Nurses (AAOHN)
Code of Ethics (2009), 958
history of, 958
mission, 959
Standards of Occupational and Environmental Health Nursing Practice, 959
American Board for Occupational Health Nurses (ABOHN), 959–960
American Cancer Society (ACS), children's environmental health and, 136
American Community Survey, disability determination and, 679
American Heart Association, *EmPowered to Serve* from, 1003
American Indian/Alaskan Native, cultural competence and, 168
American Indians
hantavirus pulmonary syndrome and, 307
health disparities with, 287
mental health and, 806–807
American Journal of Hospice and Palliative Care, 918
American Lung Association, 133
American Medical Association (AMA), history of nursing and, 26
American Nurses Association (ANA), 201
definition of nursing and, 270
definition of public health nursing and, 1018
on ethics in nursing education, 150
faith community nursing and, 991, 992, 1002
forensic nursing history and, 979
forensic nursing scope and standards of practice and, 982
genomic health care ethics and, 261
history of, 35
House of Delegates, on nursing Code of Ethics, 151
informatics and, 919
Intervention Wheel adoption and, 245–247
nurse-led health center, 438, 438b
and nursing reimbursement, 116
precautionary principle and, 138–139
school nursing and, 933
American Nurses Credentialing Center (ANCC), 983
faith community nursing and, 991
American Public Health Association (APHA)
advocacy and, 159–161
Code of Ethics and, 153
American Public Health Association *(Continued)*
Model Standards of, 531
nursing history and, 30
in public health nursing, 9–10
Public Health Nursing Section of, 375
American Red Cross
direct nursing service and, 35
disaster facts from, 455, 456t
disaster work, volunteer opportunities and, 462b
history of, 28, 33
nursing scholarships and, 30
Town and Country Nursing Service and, 29
American Society of Hematology, 83
Americans with Disabilities Act (ADA), 655, 678
civil rights for persons with mental disorders and, 795
components of, 692b
disability definition and, 680
legislation and, 692–693
Americans with Disabilities Act in 1992, school nursing and, 931
Americans with Disabilities Act of 1990, AIDS in the community and, 338–339
Amplifying, 561
ANA *see* American Nurses Association
Analytic epidemiology, 288–291
case-control studies and, 290–291, 290f
cohort studies and, 288–290, 289f
cross-sectional studies and, 291
definition of, 271
ecologic studies and, 291
Analytical competencies, 894
Andragogy, 422
Anemia, iron deficiency, 82–83
Angiography, 791–792
Angola Mosquito Net Project, 79
Annual implementation plan, 540
Annual summary, 540
Anonymous testing, 337–338
Anorexia, 664
Anthrax, 311–312
Antibiotic-resistant infections, gonorrhea and, 342
Antigenic shift/drift, type A influenza and, 317
Antimalarial interventions, 79
Antiretroviral therapies (ARTs), opportunistic infections and, 327
Anxiety disorder, 790
APEXPH in Practice, 531
APHA *see* American Public Health Association
APN *see* Advanced practice nurse
Appraisal, 891
in faith community nursing, 1001
Appropriate technology, 359
Armed services, 872–873
Army and Navy Nurse Corps, 33
Artemisinin-based combination therapies (ACTs), 79

Arthritis, 681
Asian, mental health and, 806
Assault, 839–840
forensic nursing and, 979–980
response to victims of, 978, 978b
Assertive community treatment (ACT), 797
Assertiveness, 565
Assess a Worker and the Workplace, 972b
Assessment
common elements of, 375b
community, 374–376
core functions and, 4f, 18b
definition of, 3
of environmental health, 129–132
ethics and, 156–157
of genetic/genomic knowledge, 263–264
instruments, family, 592–595
ecomap as, 593–595, 595f
genogram as, 593, 593f, 594b, 594f, 595b
key points on, 19
of migrant farmworkers, 763b
of need, 502 503, 502b
community assessment and, 502, 502b
population assessment and, 502–503
plan for family, 591b
public health nurses and, 1020
vulnerable population groups and, 709–710b, 709–713
Assessment Protocol for Excellence in Public Health (APEXPH), 514t, 515
Assisted living, 673
Association for Community Health Improvements, 361
Association of Collegiate Schools of Nursing, 35
Association of Community Health Nursing Educators (ACHNE), 375
policy process and, 208
Scope and Standards of Public Health Nursing Practice and, 9–10
Association of Occupational and Environmental Clinics (AOEC), 143–144
Association of Public Health Nurses (APHN), 375
Association of State and Territorial Directors of Public Health Nursing, 9–10
Association of State and Territorial Health Officials, 1011
Assumptions
intervention wheel and, 234–239
vulnerable populations and, 710
Assurance
core function and, 4f, 13, 18b
definition of, 4, 19
ethics and, 157
Assurance activities, 526
case management and, 552
Asthma, in children, 947
At-risk population, public health nurse and, 1021
Attack rate, 277
Attention deficit/hyperactivity disorder (ADHD), schoolchildren with, 947–949
Attrition, 225
Audit process, 533, 533f
Autism, schoolchildren with, 947–949
Autistic spectrum disorders (ASD), 688
Automated external defibrillator (AED), 941
Autonomy, 158b, 568
Availability, 725
Avian influenza A (H5N1), 300, 318–319
Avoiding, 565b

B

Baby boomer population, 49
Baccalaureate Nursing Students and Nursing faculty, in faith community, 1000b
Bachelor's prepared nurse, 444–445
Bacille Calmette-Guérin (BCG) vaccine, 78
Back pain/injury, 965
"Back to Sleep" campaign, 642–643
Balanced Budget Act of 1997
APN reimbursement and, 209
health care system and, 103
home health and, 901
Medicare SNFs and, 110
Balanced families, 585
Barefoot doctors, 74
Bargaining, 564
Barriers
to access, 702
educator-related, 423–424
health care
overcoming distance and, 103
primary reasons for, 99
in rural communities, 733
learner-related, 424–425
low literacy levels, 424–425, 425b
"Battered child syndrome," 979–980
Beers, Clifford, 793
Behavior
change evaluation of, 426–427
and primary prevention, 99
Behavioral health, 440
Behavioral risk, 609, 614
health risk assessment of, 615
Behavioral Risk Factors Surveillance Survey (BRFSS), 377t
Benchmarking, 915
Beneficence, 154, 154b, 568, 983–984
Benefits, distributive justice and, 154
Bereavement, 801, 905
Best practice health care map (BPHM), 556
Betts, Virginia Trotter, 201
Bias
case-control studies and, 290
causality and, 293
Bilateral organizations, 69
Bioaccumulated, 143
Bioecological systems theory, 589–590, 590f
Bioethics, 150, 151b, 154–156
Bioethics movement, 151
Biological agents, 963–964
Biological risk, health risk assessment and, 612
Biological variations, cultural competence and, 171, 171b
Biomonitoring, 125
Biopsychosocial model, 814
BioSense, 466–467
BioSense Platform, 489
Bioterrorism, 84–85, 455, 482
agents of, 311–313
anthrax and, 311–312
health care professionals and, 85
plague and, 313
public health system and, 205, 1012–1013
smallpox and, 312–313
surveillance for agents of, 304–305
BioWatch, 466–467
Birth, family demographics and, 582–583
Birth control method, teens and, 773, 776
Blended family households, 583
Blinding, 225
Block grant, state health care and, 198
Blockley Hospital School of Nursing, 958
Blood alcohol concentration (BAC), 816
Blood pressure screenings, in faith community, 997–998, 997f
Bloodborne pathogen
biological agents, 963–964
hepatitis B and, 345
Bloody diarrhea, 80
BLS *see* Bureau of Labor Statistics
Blue Cross insurance, 34
Blue Cross system, 112
Blue Shield, 112
Blue wedge, 238f, 239
Board of directors, as nurse-led health center staff, 444
Boarding school, nursing in, 934
Boardman, Mabel, 716–717
Boards of nursing, 206
Body mass index (BMI), 634, 663–664, 663t
childhood obesity and, 249–250
Bolton Act of 1943, 33
Bosnian genocide, 85
Boston Dispensary, 28
Bottom-up approach, 360
Boundaries, program planning model and, 504
Bovine spongiform encephalopathy (BSE), 300
Brainstorming, 529, 563
Breast cancer, 666
Breckinridge, Mary, 31
Brewster, Mary, 28
Brief interventions, 831
Broad-based inclusive process, 361–362
Brown, Esther Lucile, 35
Brownfield sites, 134
Brush family genogram, 597f
Budget limits, 94–95
Budgeting, fiscal competencies and, 893
Building Healthy Communities, 364
Built environment, 632–637
see also Built food environment
digital media and, 635–637
injuries and accidents in, 637–641, 637f
nutrition assessment and, 634, 635t
obesity and, 408–409, 408t, 632–634, 633f
physical activity and, 635
schools and, 635
social determinants of health and, 405
Built food environment, 634
Bulimia, 664
Bull's-eye lesion, 322
Bullying, 644, 688
Burden of chronic disease, 681
Burdens, distributive justice and, 154
Bureau of Labor Statistics (BLS), 960
and health care employment, 103
migrant farmworkers and, 760
Bureau of Primary Health Care (BPHC), 441
Bureau of the Census, population shift and, 718
Burnout, workplace, 965–966
Bush, President George W., 205
Business and Labor Resource Service, 339
Business cycle, 96
Business plan, 445–446, 445b, 892
Butterfield, Patricia, 128

C

Cadet Nurse Corps, 33
California Endowment Building Healthy Communities fund, 364
California Healthy Cities and Communities, 364
California Institute for Rural Studies (CIRS), 759
Call to Action, 66
Campbell Collaboration, 222, 223b
Canada
NAFTA and, 66
population health and, 66
Canadian Medical Association Journal, 219–220
Cancer
adult health concerns and, 662–663, 662t
cervical
herpes simplex virus and, 343
human papillomavirus infection and, 343

Cancer *(Continued)*
hereditary syndromes and, 258
case example on, 258–259
migrant farmworkers and, 761
screening for, 257b
unique to men, 668–669
Cannabis (marijuana), 818, 818b
Capacity building model, 590
Capitation, 116
definition of, 17
Cardiac bypass surgery, case management of, 558
Cardiovascular disease (CVD), 660–661
CARE, 71
Care
community-based culturally competent, 439
coordination, 551
culturally competent, 167
guidance formats, critical paths and, 556
nursing models of, 438
transitions of, 551–552
Care management, 548
Care maps, 556
Caregiver, 655–656
Caregiver burden, 655–656
Caring, forensic nursing and, 984
Carnegie Foundation, 71
Carondelet Health, 557–558
Carter Center, 1003
Cartographic data, 285–286
Case-control studies, 289t, 290–291, 290f
Case definitions, 488
criteria for, 488
examples of, 488
Case fatality rate (CFR), 278
Case finding
Intervention Wheel and, 233f, 238f
levels of intervention and, 241t
Navajo Wheel and, 246f
public health interventions and, 244
vulnerable populations and, 708
Case law, 206
Case management, 244, 546–574, 713
characteristics and roles in, 552–553, 554b
as a competency, 551
concepts of, 551–557
essential skills for case managers in, 560–567
evidence-based examples of, 557–560
contemporary evidence as, 558–560
historical evidence as, 557–558
issues in, 567–569
ethical, 568–569
legal, 567–568
knowledge and skill requisites in, 553, 555b, 555f
levels of prevention in, 564b
linking content to practice, 569b
Case management *(Continued)*
model, 550f
nursing process and, 552, 553t
PHN implementation process and, 249
plans, 555, 556
public health nurses and, 1019–1020
resources for, 568t
in rural settings, 730–731
websites for, 569t
Case management services, 709
Case Management Society of America, 547, 554f
Case managers
credentialing resources for, 568t
disease management and, 549
essential skills for, 560–567
advocacy as, 560–561
collaboration as, 565–567, 565b, 566f
conflict management as, 564–565, 565b
HIV with, 558
liability concerns of, 567
as mediator, 560
as promoter, 560
roles of, 552–553
school nurses as, 934–935
tools of, 553–557, 558
Case register, 517, 517b
Categorical funding, 205
Categorical program, 200
Catholic Relief Services (CRS), 71
Catholic Sisters, nurses from, 990
Cats, *Toxoplasma gondii* and, 327
Causality, 292–293
assessing for, 293
bias and, 293
clinical trials and, 292
criteria for, 293b
statistical associations and, 292–293
CBRNE threats (chemical, biological, radiological, nuclear, and explosive), 458
CDC *see* Centers for Disease Control and Prevention
Cell phone ownership, 386, 387f
Census Bureau, disability determination and, 679
Center for an Accessible Society (CAS), 685
Center for Civic Partnerships, 364
Center for Ethics and Human Rights, 151
Center for Faith-Based and Neighborhood Partnerships, 1003
Center for Reviews and Dissemination (CRD), 222, 223b
Center to Advance Palliative Care (CAPC), 903
Centers for Disease Control and Prevention (CDC), 633t
biomonitoring and, 125
burden of chronic disease and, 681
County Health Rankings, 377t
Centers for Disease Control and Prevention *(Continued)*
definition of childhood obesity and, 632–633
Emerging Infectious Diseases, 308
Environmental Hazards and Effects Program (EHEP), 657
evidence-based practice resources and, 223b
federal health agencies and, 202–203, 203f
federal school health programs and, 936
food safety, 321b
foodborne illnesses and, 301, 319
FoodNet and, 319
Framework for Preventing Infectious Disease: Sustaining the Essentials and Innovating for the Future, 308
genetic testing oversight and, 260
genomic competencies for nurses, 263
Healthy Communities Initiative of, 730
Healthy Communities Program, 360
healthy place, definition by, 359
Morbidity and Mortality Weekly Report by, 481–482
National Center for Injury Prevention and Control and, 977
National Center on Birth Defects and Developmental Disabilities and, 680
obesity and, 271–272, 408–409
reportable disease list and, 305–306, 305–306b
rubella and, 315–316
social determinants of health, 377t
Task Force on Community Preventive Services of, 6
tick-borne disease prevention/control and, 323
tools for community action and, 360
vaccine information statements and, 632–633
WBDO and, 322
Wonder, 377t
Centers for Medicare and Medicaid Services (CMS)
federal agencies and, 204
genetic testing oversight and, 260
and health care spending, 105
home-based primary care, 902
Outcome and Assessment Information Set and, 912
and public support, 109–112
safety and, 50
CERT *see* Community Emergency Response Team
Certificate of need (CON), 499–501
Certification, 867
for forensic nursing, 983
home health/hospice nurses and, 915–916
quality management and, 528
Certification in cardiopulmonary resuscitation (CPR), 941
Certified Occupational Health Nurse (COHN), 959–960
Certified Occupational Health Nurse-Specialist (COHN-S), 959–960
Change, 416
Charge method, 115
Charity Organization Society, 29
Charter, 528
Chemical Abstracts Service number, 130
Chemical agents, 965
Chemical emergency, 85
Chemical exposure, 125
Chemical Safety Information, Site Security, and Fuels Regulatory Act (Amendment to Section 112 of Clean Air Act), 141–142b
Chemical terrorism, 482–483
Chemicals
"families" of, 127
industrialization and, 77
Chemotherapy
for malaria, 79
for tuberculosis, 78
Chickenpox, 312b
Child abuse, 844–847, 845b, 846b
forensic nursing and, 979–980
identification of, 944
indicators of, 846
Child development, 629–631
developmental screening, 630–631, 630t
growth and, 629–630, 630f
theories of, 630
Child feeding practices, 634
Child Labor Act of 1938, 764–765
Child maltreatment, 640, 640f
Child neglect, 846–847
identification of, 944
Child Nutrition and WIC Reauthorization Act of, 932
Child Protective Service, 640
Childbearing, adolescents and, 774–775
Childhood
acute illnesses and, 642
chronic health conditions and, 643–644
disability, 682–683, 683b
environmental health and, 644–647, 645t
environmental tobacco smoke and, 646–647
mental health and, 644
oral health and, 643
Children
acute illnesses and, 642
built environment and, 632–637
bullying and, 644
development of, 629–631
disabilities in
effects on community of, 686–687
effects on family of, 685–686
disaster, stress and, 468, 469f

Children *(Continued)*
environmental health of, 136–137, 136b, 137b
under 5
anemia in, 83
diarrhea and, 80
infant mortality and, 64
mortality in less developed countries, 75–76
WHO and, 70
health and, 626–652
linking content to practice and, 648b
health problems and, 642–647
hepatitis A and, 344
with HIV infection, 339
homeless, 744–745, 746–747
health problems of, 746
immigrant, 627–628
immunizations and, 631–632
infectious diseases and, 301–302
learning strategies for, 422
mental health objectives for, 801
of migrant farmworker, 764f, 769
models for health care delivery to, 647
obesity and, 249–250
population-focused nursing and, 627
poverty and, 752
rural and urban community health of, 722
status of, 627–629
access to care and, 628
infant mortality and, 628–629
poverty, 627, 627f
risk-taking behaviors, 629
Children with special health care needs (CSHCN), 680
Children's Bureau, 31
Children's Health Insurance Program (CHIP), 113
status of children and, 628
China
health care systems in, 74–75
Healthy Cities movement in, 67b
nursing education system in, 74–75
nursing role in, 68
CHIP *see* Children's Health Insurance Program
Chlamydia, 340–341t, 582
Choi, Mona, 127
Chromosomes, 257
Chronic Care Model (CCM), 659–660
Chronic disease, 654
adult health concerns and, 659–660
burden of, 681
community nursing approach to, 644b
disability and, 680
and health care cost, 107
prevention of, 360
rural communities and, 719–720, 720b
during twenty-first century, 103–104
Chronic disease self-management (CDSMP), 660
Chronic homelessness, 742
Chronic liver disease, 346
Chronic stress, vulnerability and, 702
Chronosystems, 590
Church Health, 991, 999
Church World Service, 71
Cities Readiness Initiative, 466–467
CITYNET-Healthy Cities, 363
Civil immunity, 208
Civil Rights of Institutionalized Persons Act of 1997, 694
Civil Works Administration (CWA), 32
Clarifying, 561–562
Classification bias, 293
Classism, 184–185
Clean Air Act, 132, 141–142b
Clean Water Act (CWA), 141–142b
Cleveland Visiting Nurse Association, 29–30
Client-based outcomes, 444
Client-centered care, 417b
definition of, 18b
Client engagement, advocacy and, 563–564
Client-focused models, for case management, 558
Client outcome, 909–910
Client satisfaction, 536–537, 536f
malpractice litigation and, 537
Client system, 407
Climate change, 129
Clinical medicine, golden age of, 102
Clinical nurse leader (CNL), 443, 865
Clinical nurse specialist (CNS), 865
Medicare part B and, 116
postindustrial era, 102
Clinical paths, 556
Clinical record, 540
Clinical trials, 292
Clinician, 868–869, 868b
nurse as mental health, 798
Clinton, President Bill, 501
"Club drugs," 938–939
Clusters, event-related, 288
Clusters of illness, 482
CMS *see* Centers for Medicare and Medicaid Services
Coaching, 891
Coalition building
definition of, 245
levels of intervention and, 241t
Coalitions, 373, 887
Cochrane Library, 222
Code for Professional Nurses, 151
Code of Ethics, 151, 151b
advocacy and, 160
genomics and, 261
population-centered nurses and, 159
Code of Ethics for Nurses
ethical issues and, 568
ICN, 151
Public Health Code of Ethics and, 159
Code of Ethics for Nurses with Interpretative Statements, 151
Code of Professional Conduct for Case Managers, 568
Codependency, 826
Coercive sex, 776–777
Cognitive development, 630
Cognitive domain, 416–417
Cohabitation
effects on children of, 582
family structure and, 581
Cohesion, 427–428
Cohort studies, 288–290, 289f, 289t
Collaboration, 241t, 244–245, 249
community, 438
conflict management and, 565b
definition of, 18b
and developing healthy communities, 362
home health/hospice nurses and, 916–917, 916b
interorganizational and interprofessional, 439
in skills for case managers, 565–567, 565b, 566f
goal of, 565
stages of, 566b
Collaborative, 882
Collaborative team
roles of, 443
staff, 443, 443b
Collective system, 74
College Settlement, 28
Columbus Regional Hospital, 364
Commercial reimbursement, private insurers and, 446
Commission on Collegiate Nursing Education (CCNE), 527
Committee on Rural Nursing, 716–717
Committee on the Costs of Medical Care, 112
Commodification, 71
Common law, 206
Common source, 490
Common vehicle, 304
Communicable diseases, 76–79, 299–300
bioterrorism agents and, 311–313
emerging infectious diseases and, 306–308
foodborne/waterborne diseases and, 319–322
healthcare-associated infections and, 327–328
historical and current perspectives on, 300–302
and infectious diseases, 299–332, 333–356, 334b
surveillance of, 304–306
transmission of, 302–304
travelers diseases and, 323–324
universal precautions and, 328
vaccine-preventable diseases and, 313–319
vector-borne diseases and, 322–323
zoonoses and, 324–325
Communicable diseases *(Continued)*
linking content to practice, 328b
parasitic diseases and, 325–327
prevention and control of, 299–311
multisystem approach to, 311, 311t
primary, secondary, and tertiary, 310, 310b
role of nurses in, 310–311
preventive care for, nurse's role in, 347–353
primary prevention and assessment and, 347–353
evaluation, 351
interventions and, 349
secondary prevention and partner notification and contact tracing, 352, 352b
testing and counseling for HIV and, 351–352, 351b, 352b
tertiary prevention and directly observed therapy and, 352–353
standard precautions and, 353
public health nurse and, 1021
transmission of
agent, host and environment in, 302–303
disease development and, 304
disease spectrum and, 304
modes of, 304
Communicable period, 304
Communication
collaboration and, 565
community systems and, 386–387
of information in transitions of care, 577
interpersonal competencies and, 890–892, 890b
with legislators, 209, 209b, 211b
Communities Putting Prevention to Work (CPPW), 360
Community, 400–401, 400b
assessment of, 366, 374–380
as client, 371–374
definition of, 235, 371
geographic location, interests, or values, 371
disaster affecting
stress reactions and, 468–469, 470f
stress reactions in individuals and, 467–468, 467b, 468b, 468f, 469f
effect of teen pregnancy on, 772
effects of disabilities on, 686–687
families as resources in, 620–623
forensic nursing in, 976–988
key points of, 392–393
nurse leader in, 880–898, 887b
competencies for, 887–894
consultation and, 885–888
definitions for, 882–883
future of, 894–895
introduction of, 881

Community *(Continued)*
leadership and management applied to, 883–885, 884t
linking content to practice, 895b
major trends and issues of, 881–882
orientation, 365
as partner, 380–381
of place, 371
poverty and, 745
Community advocates, as nurse-led health center staff, 444
Community-as-partner model, 380–381
Community assessment, 374–376, 440, 502
case management and, 552
conduct of, 375–376t, 381–392, 381b
disaster recovery and, 475
evidence-based practice and, 505b
model of, 380, 382f
public health nursing process and, 248
Community Assessment for Public Health Emergency Response (CASPER), 471
toolkit, 380
Community assessor(s), 381
Community Builders of New South Wales, Australia, 361
Community-Campus Partnerships for Health (CCPH), 1009
Community care settings, 672–673
adult day health as, 672
assisted living as, 673
home health, palliative care, and hospice as, 672–673
long-term care and rehabilitation as, 673
senior centers as, 672
Community collaboration, 439–440
Community Commons, 361–362
Community education, communicable diseases and, 351
Community Emergency Response Team (CERT), 52, 461–462
Community engagement, principles of, 366b
Community Guide, 100
Community health, 372–373
integrative model for promotion of, 407–408
Intervention Wheel assumptions and, 235
Community Health Accreditation Partner (CHAP), 527, 915
Community Health Assessment and Group Evaluation (CHANGE) Tool, 381t
Community health assessment models, 380
Community health education
levels of prevention, 415b
population considerations based on, 422
Community Health Improvement Process (CHIP), 6
Community Health Needs Assessment (CHNA), 381t
Community health nurse, community as client and, 372
Community health nurse specialists, 15
Community health nursing, history of, 22–44
Community health planning, 499
Community health profile, 6, 6b
indicators used for, 6b
Community health promotion, 396
key points in, 410
models and frameworks of, 401–404
Community Health Promotion Model, 365, 404
steps of, 365–366
Community Health Promotion Process, 363
Community health report card, 523
Community Health Status Indicator (CHSI) Project, 523
Community health workers (CHWs), 374, 440
nurse case manager and, 559–560
Community-level practice, 236
goal of, 240
Community mental health care
evolution of, 793–794
federal legislation for services and, 793–794, 794t
historical perspectives of, 793–794
hospital expansion, institutionalization, mental hygiene movement and, 793
Community mental health center (CMHC)
community mental health models and, 793
eating disorders and, 802
Community Mental Health Centers Act of l963, 794
Community mental health models, 793
Community mental health nurse (CMHN)
diathesis-stress model and, 796
as educator, 798
Community organizing, 241t, 245
Community-oriented care, 15
Community-oriented nursing practice, 15b
Community outreach
communicable diseases and, 350–351
school nurses as, 935
Community participation, 54–55, 359
Community partnerships
for assessment, 373–374
nursing models of care and, 439
Community practice
assumptions about, 360
personal safety in, 382b
Community preparedness, disaster and, 462–464, 463b, 463f
Community preventive service
develop guide to, 223b
evidence-based practice guide to, 223b
Community/Public Health Nursing Competencies, 375, 375–376t
Community rate, 113
Community resilience, 457, 464
disaster recovery and, 475
Community Support Program (CSP), 791
Community systems
in place, 384–387, 387f, 388b
potential measures of, 388b
Community trials, 292
Community-based care, 15
Community-based models, for care of adults, 671–673
Community-based nursing
nursing models of care and, 439
public health nursing *versus,* 14–15, 14f, 15b
Community-based participatory research (CBPR), 396, 406
Comparison groups, 286
Compassion, vulnerable populations and, 710
Compendium of Animal Rabies Prevention and Control, 325
Competency, 873
ethical tenets and, 156–157
for forensic nursing, 982, 983b
Competing, 565b
Complementary and alternative therapy, menopausal symptoms and, 665, 666b
Complex adaptive systems, 884
Compliance, 142
Comprehensive Environmental Response, Compensation, and Liability Act (CERCLA or Superfund), 141–142b
Comprehensive primary health care centers, types of nursing centers and, 440–441
Comprehensive services, 707
Comprehensive support, in faith community, 997–998, 998f
Compromising, 565b
Computed axial tomography (CAT) scans, 791–792
Computerized systems, 444
Computers, corporate era, 103
Conceptualizing, program planning model and, 505
Concern, vulnerable populations and, 710
Concurrent audit, 533
Concurrent utilization review, 533–534
Conditions of Participation, 902–903
OASIS and, 912
Condom, female, 349–350, 350f
Conduct and Utilization of Research in Nursing Project (CURN), 219
Conflict resolution, 892
Confounding variables, 225
Congenital syphilis, 342
Congregants, 995
Congregation, 993
nursing care in, 989
Congregational model
nurse consultant role and, 887–888
Congregational model, of faith community nursing, 1000
Consensus Conference on the Essentials of Public Health Nursing Practice and Education, 10
Consequentialism, 153
Consolidated Health Centers (CHCs), 750
Consultant, 870
school nurses as, 935
Consultation, 883
contract, 886–887
goal of, 885
public health nursing process and, 251
theories of, 885–886
Consumer advocacy, mental illness and, 791
Consumer confidence reports, 135
Consumer engagement, 900
Consumers, in mental health, 795
Contact tracing, communicable diseases and, 352
Contemplation, 403
Contextual caring, 984
Contingency contract, 618–619
Continuous quality improvement (CQI)
definition of, 522
model program for, 537–540, 537f
using QA/QI in, 532, 532t
Continuous source, 490
Continuum of Care (CoC) programs, 743
Contract, nursing centers and, 446–447
Contracting, 886
process of, 619, 619t
Cooperation, 565
Coordinate, 551
Coordination
organizational competencies and, 892–893
vulnerable populations and, 710–711
Coordinator, nurse as mental health, 799, 799f
Coordinator/Advanced course, for faith community nurse, 999
Core-based statistical area (CBSA), 717–718
Core Competencies of Public Health Professionals, 7, 7b
literacy assessment and, 424–425, 425b
Core Functions Project, 4f, 5–6
Coronary heart disease
cross-sectional studies and, 291

Coronary heart disease *(Continued)*
prospective cohort studies and, 288–289
Correctional health, laws influencing, 208
Correctional institutions, 873
Cost
current U.S. system and, 48–49
evidence-based practice and, 226
of HIV/AIDS, 334
teen pregnancy and, 772
Cost-benefit analysis (CBA), 97
Cost-effectiveness, 449
Cost-effectiveness analysis (CEA), 97, 97b, 893–894
Cost-plus reimbursement, 110
Cost-shifting, 115
Cost studies, 509
Cost-utility analysis (CUA), 97
Cottage industry, definition of, 17
Council on Linkages
Core Competencies and, 7
cultural competency and, 189b
rural health settings and, 731b
Council on Linkages Between Academia and Public Health Practice
description of, 524
population health concepts and, 271b
vulnerable populations and, 708b
Counseling
definition of, 244
levels of intervention and, 241t
steps for intervention of, 245b
Counselor, school nurses as, 935
County Health Rankings model, 699, 699f
Covered lives, 17, 115
Covert intentional prejudice/racism, 186b
Covert unintentional prejudice/racism, 186b
CQI *see* Continuous quality improvement
Craven, Florence Sarah Lees, 27
Credentialing, 527
for forensic nursing, 983, 986
Crick, Francis, 256
Crimean War, 27, 150
Crisis standards of care, 465
Crisis teams, 940–941
Critical appraisal, 219–220
Critical pathways, 549
Critical thinking, 890
Cross-sectional studies, 289t, 291
Cross-tolerance, 829
Crossing the Quality Chasm, 881
Cultural accommodation, 187–188
Cultural assessment, 190–191
Cultural awareness, 169b, 181–184
Cultural blindness, 186
Cultural competence
barriers to developing, 184–189
cultural conflict as, 186–187
cultural imposition as, 186
Cultural competence *(Continued)*
culture shock as, 187
ethnocentrism as, 185–186
prejudice as, 184–185
racism as, 185, 186b
stereotyping as, 184
cultural awareness and, 169b, 181–184
cultural desire and, 183–184
cultural encounter and, 183f, 184
cultural immersion and, 184
cultural knowledge and, 182
cultural skill and, 182–183
definition of, 166
developing, 181, 181t
diversity on, 170–178
biological variations in, 171, 171b
communication, 172–173
cultural diversity, 170–171
cultural variations, 171–178
environmental control, 172
foreign born, 175–178, 175f, 177f
immigrant issues, 174–175
nutritional practices, 173–174, 173b
personal space in, 171
religion, 174
social organization, 172
time perception, 172
evidence-based practice for, 182b
in health care, 165–195
issues affecting, 178–180
health disparities, 179–180, 180b
health equity, 180
health literacy, 179
marginalization, 179
social determinants of health, 178
social justice, 180
socioeconomic status, 178–179, 178t
linking content to practice and, 189b
nursing interventions for, 187
nursing standards for, 167b
organizational, developing, 191
quality and safety education for, 189b
Cultural conflict, 186–187
Cultural desire, 183–184
Cultural diversity
and health disparities, 170–171
mental health care and, 805–807
African Americans, 806
American Indians, 806–807
Asian and Pacific Islander Americans, 806
Hispanic Americans, 806
Cultural encounter, 183f, 184
Cultural immersion, 184
Cultural imposition, 186
Cultural knowledge, 182
Cultural nursing assessment, 190–191
Cultural preservation, 187
Cultural racism, 185
Cultural relativism, 186
Cultural repatterning, 188
Cultural Revolution, 74–75
Cultural skill, 182–183
Culture, 168–170, 168b, 169b, 169f
Culture brokering, 188
Culture of health, 395–413
Culture shock, 187
Cumulative incidence rate, 275–276
Cumulative risks, 713
Cumulative trauma, 968
Curve-shifting principle, 405
Cutaneous anthrax, 311–312
Cutpoint, 283–284
Cycle to vulnerability, 703
Cyclical patterns, 288
Cyclones, 84
Cytosine, 257

D

DALY *see* Disability-adjusted life-years
Dana Farber Cancer Institute, 69
Danger assessment, "DARN-CAT" mnemonic, 420
Dartmouth Atlas of Health Care, 377t
Darwin, Charles, 256
Dashboard functions, 555
Data, 374
analysis of, 388–389
primary sources of, 377–379
secondary sources of, 377, 377b
Data collection, pre-encounter, 590–591
Data collection phase, of cultural assessment, 190
Data manager program coordinator, 444
Data operations personnel, 444
Data sources, 284–286, 376–380
data collected for other purposes and, 285
epidemiologic data and, 285
routinely collected data and, 285
Death rate, calculation of, 275
Decision making, 890
Decision trees, 505, 506f
Declaration of Alma-Ata, 45
"Deep poverty," 736
Definition and Role of Public Health Nursing in the Delivery of Health Care, 9–10
Degradation, water quality, 133
Dehumanization, 85
Dehydration, and diarrhea, 80
Deinstitutionalization, 745, 794–796
Delano, Jane, 716–717
Delegated functions, 241t, 244, 249
Delegation, 888–889, 888b, 889b, 889f
Demand curve, 95
Demand management, 549
Democratic leadership, 430
Demographic data, 388–389
Demographic trends, of workforce, 46–47
Demographics
employee group, 972
for migrant and seasonal farmworkers, 757
Demonstration, 421b
Denial, 823
Denominator, 275
Dental disease, migrant farmworkers and, 761
Deontology, 151b, 153–154, 160b
Deoxyribonucleic acid (DNA)
collection of, 979
genetic testing and, 258–259
relationship of genomics and genetics to, 257–259
replication of, 257
Department of Agriculture, 204
Department of Defense, 204
Department of Justice
federal non-health agencies and, 204
Voting Accessibility for the Elderly and the Handicapped Act of 1984 and, 694
Department of Labor, 204
Depressants, 815
Depression
of 1930, and health insurance, 112
men's health concerns and, 669
migrant farmworkers and, 761
public health issues and, adults and, 802
in rural communities and, 722
Descriptive epidemiology, 286–288
definition of, 271
personal characteristics and, 286–287
place and, 287
time and, 287–288
Detailing phase, 505–506, 506f
Determinants of health, 699–700
definition of, 271
factors of, 235
Intervention Wheel assumptions and, 234–235, 235f
population conditions and, 66
Detoxification, 827–828
Deutsch, Naomi, 32
Developed country, 64
Development, definition of, 629
Developmental Disabilities Act and Bill of Rights Act of 2000, 693–694
Developmental disability, 680
Developmental screening, 630–631, 630t
Devolution, 198
Diabetes mellitus
adult health concerns and, 661–662
children with, 947
migrant farmworkers and, 761
Diagnosis, community nursing, 389–391, 391b

Diagnosis-related groups (DRGs), 110, 110–111b, 110b
Diarrheal diseases, 80–81
travelers and, 324
Diathesis-stress model, 796
Dichlorodiphenyltrichloroethane (DDT), and malaria prevention, 79
Digital media, built environment and, 635–637
Direct age-adjusted rate, 286
Direct caregiver, 934
Direct cultural encounter, 183
Direct services, 198–199
Directly observed therapy (DOT), 78, 281, 352–353
Director, of nurse-led health centers, 443–444
Disabilities
children and, 680, 684, 686
effects of, 683–687, 683b
on family, 685–686, 685f
on individual, 683–685
federal agencies and, 694b
legislation and, 691–694, 692b
quality and safety education for, 691b
role of nurse and, 690–691
scope of problem with, 681–683
additional causes in, 681–682, 682f
burden of chronic disease and, 681
mental illness and, 683
number of disabled in, 681
selected issues and, 687–690
types, 679b
understanding, 679–681
additional definitions for, 680–681
Americans with Disabilities Act and, 680
census determination in, 679
definition in, 679
functional, 680
linking content to practice and, 681b
models in, 679
social security disability in, 679–680
Disability-adjusted life-years (DALY)
global burden of disease and, 75–76, 75b
malnutrition and, 83
psychiatric disorders and, 75–76
top 20 conditions in, 76t
Disability Determination Services, 680
Disabled Americans, 681
Disadvantaged position, 703
Disaster
affecting communities, 467–469
definition of, 455, 455b, 455f
facts of, 455–456
Healthy People 2020 objectives and, 457–458, 458b
management of, future, 476
Disaster *(Continued)*
national disaster planning and response, 457
natural/man-made, 83–87
nurse care delivery during, 68
surveillance systems in, 86–87
public health nurse and, 1021
types of, 455b
Disaster communication, nursing role in, 471–473, 473b
Disaster exercise, 465b
Disaster management cycle
nursing role for, 458–476, 458f
preparedness and, 459–465
prevention (mitigation and protection), 458–459
public health nursing practice and, 454–480
recovery and, 474–476
Disaster Medical Assistance Team (DMAT), 461–462
Disaster medicine, core competencies for, 460–461, 461b
Discrimination, 184–185
migrant farmworkers and, 759
Disease, 304
development of, 304
global
communicable diseases and, 76–79
acquired immunodeficiency syndrome, 78–79
malaria, 79
tuberculosis and, 77–78
diarrheal disease and, 80–81
influence of place on, 287
notifiable, 486–488, 487b
national, 486, 487b
state, 486–488
patterns of, 274–275
spectrum of, 304
surveillance of, 482–486
collaboration among partners and, 483–484
data sources for, 485–486, 486b
definitions and importance of, 482–483
nurse competencies in, 484–485
purposes of, 483
uses of, 483
vaccine-preventable, 313–319
childhood immunization and, 314
influenza, 317–319
measles and, 314–315
pertussis, 316–317
rubella and, 315–316
Disease and health event investigation
definition of, 244
levels of intervention and, 241t
Disease management, 549
case managers and, 549
components of, 556
Disease prevention, primary health care and, 45–46
Disenfranchisement, 703
Disillusionment phase, 469
Disparities
in health, 700–701
in quality, 525
Disseminated intravascular coagulation (DIC), 79
Distinguishing process, 206
Distribution, 271
effects, 884
Distributive justice, 154, 154b, 158b, 372
Distributive outcomes, 564
District nursing, 27
Diversity
on cultural competence, 170–178
biological variations in, 171, 171b
communication, 172–173
cultural diversity, 170–171
cultural variations, 171–178
environmental control, 172
foreign-born, 175–178, 175f, 177f
immigrant issues, 174–175
nutritional practices, 173–174, 173b
personal space in, 171
religion, 174
social organization, 172
time perception, 172
promotion of, 891–892
Division of Nursing, evidence-based practice and, 219
Divorce, 581–582
Dix, Dorothea Lynde, 793
DNA *see* Deoxyribonucleic acid
DNP *see* Doctor of Nursing Practice
Do-not-attempt-resuscitation orders (DNAR orders), 656–657, 950
"Do nothing" decision, 505
Doctor of Nursing Practice (DNP)
barriers to public health nursing and, 16–17
education for, 10
forensic nursing and, 980
Doctors Without Borders, 71, 83
Documentation, Omaha system and, 907, 908f
Documentation issues, in faith community nursing practice, 1001–1002
Donabedian's model, 509
Donut hole, 107
Double ABC-X model, 611
Double-blind study, 292
"Doubling up," 743
"Doughnut effect," 718
Droughts, 83–84
Drug addiction, 814
Drug dependence, 814
Drug-resistant organism, 1016
Drugs
migrant farmworkers and, 763
substance use and, 614
toxicology of, 125–127, 126t
Dual diagnosis, 683
Dual protection, 776
Durable medical power of attorney, 656–657
Dysfunctional families, 585

E

Early Head Start, 441–442
Early Periodic Screening and Developmental Testing (EPSDT), 200
Earthquakes, 83–84
East Side Village Health Worker Partnership (ESVHWP), 406
Eating disorders, mental health objectives and, 802
Ebola, 300–301, 306–307
public health nurse and, 1021
Ecologic fallacy, 291
Ecologic studies, 289t, 291
Ecological approach, 270–271
community health promotion, 404–405
population health and, 404–407
social determinants of health, 405–406, 405b
Ecomap
as assessment instrument, 593–595, 595f
environmental risk assessment and, 612–614
Economic and Social Council, 69–70
Economic function, 579
Economic growth
definition of, 96
measurement of, 96
Economic Opportunity Act, 36
Economic prevention strategies, 99b
Economic risk, 612
Economics
analysis tools for, 97–98
community systems and, 385
definition of, 93
principles of, 94–98
public health and, 93–94
Ecosocial or social-ecological perspective, 397–398
Ectoparasites, 325
Ecuador, health care systems in, 73–74
Education
community systems and, 385
definition of, 416
disease prevention, 939
for faith community nurse, 993b, 999–1000
forensic nurse and, 980, 986
for genetic/genomic nursing assessment, 264
home health/hospice nurses and, 915–916
issues in, 421–427
barriers to learning, 423–425
population considerations, 422
use of technology in learning, 422–423

Education *(Continued)*
in the least restrictive environment (LRE), 693
process, 418–421
for public health nursing, 10, 10b
quality and safety, 18b
vulnerability and, 700
Education for All Handicapped Children Act, 931
Educational methods, 418–419, 419b
Educational plan, implementing, 432–433
Educational product, 426
health behavioral change evaluation and, 426
long-term evaluation, 426
short-term evaluation, 426
Educator, 869, 869f
core competencies for communication skills of, 432b
evaluation of, 426
nurse as mental health, 798–799, 798f, 799f
as nurse-led health centers staff, 444
public health nurse and, 1020
skills of effective, 419
Effectiveness, 95–96, 96b, 512
Efficiency, 512
and microeconomics, 95–96, 96b
Egalitarian, 155t
Egg sensitivity, 317
Ehrlichiosis, 300
EHRs *see* Electronic health records
Elder abuse, 850–851
prevention of, 850
reporting laws and, 208
screening for, 850–851
types of, 850
Elderly
abuse and neglect of, 687–688
homeless, 747–748, 747f
poverty and, 747–748, 747f
Electric wave sources, 134
Electronic health records (EHRs)
case management and, 553
Omaha system and, 907–908
technology and, 48
Electronic nicotine delivery systems (ENDS), 646
Electronic prescribing, 104
Electronic records, 448
Elementary and Secondary Education Act of 1965, 693
Elimination, of infectious disease, 308
Emergency departments, 872
Emergency equipment, in school nurse's office, 941–942, 941–942b
Emergency housing, 749
Emergency Maternity and Infant Care Act of 1943, 33
Emergency nursing for pediatrics certification (ENPC), 941
Emergency Operations Center (EOC), 465
Emergency plan, 940–941
Emergency Planning and Community Right to Know Act (EPCRA), 141–142b
Emergency shelters, 749
Emergency Support Function 8: Public Health and Medical Services, 457
Emerging infectious diseases, 306–308
emergence factors of, 306–308, 308t
examples of, 308, 309f, 309t
Emerging Infectious Diseases, 308
Emotional abuse, 846
Emotional neglect, 846–847
Employers, and health insurance, 113–114
Employment, trends of, 960
EmPowered to Serve, 1003
Empowerment
of family, 619–620
nurse leaders and, 888
Enabling, 827
nurse-led health centers and, 442
Endemic, 304, 490
Endocannabinoid system (ECS), 818
Energized family, 606
Energy, 134
Enhanced Nurse Licensure Compact (NLC), 527
Enviromechanical agents, 965
Environment, 966
in communicable disease transmission, 302–303, 303f
epidemiologic triangle and, 278, 279b, 279f
epidemiology and, 127
factor, 303
Environmental control, cultural competence and, 172
Environmental exposure, 122
by media, 132–134
Environmental health, 121–148
assessment of, 129–132
childhood and, 644–647, 645t
lead poisoning and, 646
mercury and, 644
plasticizers and, 644
climate change and, 129
competencies for nurses, 124b
disparities in, 143
epidemiology of, 127
historical context of, 124–125
linking content to practice and, 124b
migrant farmworkers and, 760–761
multidisciplinary approaches to, 128, 128b
nursing process and, 130–131
policy and advocacy, 142–143
referral resources, 143–144, 144b
risk assessment of, 135
Environmental health *(Continued)*
risk reduction and, 139–140, 139b
roles for nurses in, 144–145
sciences of, 125–128
vulnerable populations and, 135–138
Environmental justice, 125, 143
Environmental laws, 141–142b
Environmental pollution, reduction of, 139b
Environmental protection
governmental, 141–142b, 141–142
primary prevention and, 280–281
Environmental Protection Agency (EPA), 758
cigarettes and, 646–647
indoor air quality and, 133
local and state influence of, 1010
Environmental risk, 612
assessment of, 612–614
Environmental sanitation, 77
primary care and, 67
Environmental standards, 142
Environmental tobacco smoke (ETS), 646–647
Environmental Working Group (EWG), 125
Enzyme-linked immunosorbent assay (ELISA), 284
HIV testing and, 337
EPA *see* Environmental Protection Agency
Epidemic, 84–85, 304, 490
definition of, 271–272
HIV/AIDS and, 335–336
preindustrial era and, 101
Epidemiologic methods, formation of, 272
Epidemiologic model, application of, 962–966, 963b
Epidemiologic triangle, 278–279, 279b, 279f
application of, 962–963, 963b
causal factors of, 490–491, 490b
communicable disease transmission and, 302–303, 303f
concepts of, 127
work/health relationship and, 963f
Epidemiology, 269–298
application in nursing of, 293–295, 294b
basics concepts in, 274–282
community-oriented, 294
definitions and descriptions of, 271–272
evidence-based practice on, 295b
historical perspectives of, 272–273, 272t, 273–274f
of HIV/AIDS, 335–337, 336f, 336t
methods in, 284–286
quality and safety education for, 294b
Epigenetics, 126–127, 266b
EpiPen auto injector, 941–942
Equality, 698
Equity, 359
Eradication, of infectious disease, 308
Erectile dysfunction, 669
Escherichia coli, 300, 307
enterohemorrhagic, 321
Essential Public Health Services, 4f, 1018
Established group, 430, 430f
Ethical decision making, 152, 160b
frameworks for, 152, 152t
Ethical dilemma, 151b, 152
Ethical issues, 152
case management and, 568–569
in faith community nursing, 1001
for forensic nursing, 983–985
home health/hospice nurses and, 917
Ethical terms, 151b
Ethics, 151b, 415
advocacy and, 159–161
application of
Code of Ethics for, 158–159
in community, 149–164, 159b
core functions of population-centered nursing practice and, 156–157
ethical decision making and, 152–153
evidence-based practice for, 154b
history of, 150–151
levels of prevention in, 159b
linking content to practice and, 161b
public health code of ethics and, 159
QSEN, 156b
virtue, caring, and feminist ethical theories and, 155
of care, 155–156, 156b
caring and ethic of care, 155–156
definition, theories and principles of, 153–154
disaster response, nursing role in, 473
feminist, 156
key terms in, 151b
of public health, 150
in school nursing, 950–951
Ethnicity, 170
poverty rates and, 178t
Ethnocentrism, 185–186
Evaluating phase, 506
organizational competencies and, 893
Evaluation, 425–427
definition of, 499
of health and behavioral changes, 426–427
educational outcome, 426
educational product, 426
process evaluation, 426
of process standards, 539–540

Evaluation models, and techniques, 517
case register as, 517, 517b
structure-process-outcome evaluation as, 517
tracer method as, 517
Evaluation of Genomic Applications in Practice and Prevention Working Group (EGAPP), 262–263
Evaluative studies, 535
Event, 274–275
Event outbreak patterns, 482
Event-related clusters, 288
Every Student Succeeds Act (ESSA), 932
Evidence
approaches to finding, 222–224
collection of, 978b
evaluation of, 224–225, 225b, 225t
types of, 221
Evidence-based medicine, 219
Evidence-Based Medicine Working Group, 219
Evidence-based nursing, 219, 223b
Evidence-based practice
after discharge care, of low income frail elderly, 559b
finding evidence and, 222–224
approaches to implementing, 225–226
barriers to, 221–222
on childhood immunization, 313–314b
community assessment and, 505b
community health promotion models and, 404b
conceptualizing process and, 505
for cultural knowledge, 182b
current perspectives of, 226–227
definition of, 18b
effectiveness of nursing intervention and, 611–612b
environmental health and, 136b
ethical dilemmas in vulnerable groups and, 708b
evaluating evidence and, 224–225, 225t
examples of
chronic disease and, 219b
how to develop guide to community preventive service, 223b
factors leading to change, 221
in faith communities, 1004b
family use and, 579b
forensic nursing and, 982–983
health promotion and, 657–658b
history of, 219–220
homeless women and, 741b
immigrant children and, 628b
individual differences, 226–227
levels of prevention, 226b
linking content to practice and, 227b
migrant farmworkers and, 767b
Evidence-based practice *(Continued)*
model of
Health Insurance Portability and Accountability Act (HIPAA) and, 448–449
nursing centers and, 448b
in occupational health, 964b, 967b, 968b, 970b
SANEs and, 983b
mothers with intellectually disabled child and, 684b
nurse leader and, 882b
nursing informatics and, 247b
older adults psychiatric services and, 803b
practice models of, 900
process of, 222–225
public health emergencies and, 473b
to public health nursing, 228
public health surveillance and, 484b
quality improvement and, 534b
resources for, 223b
rural nursing practice and, 726b
sedentary behavior in schools and, 935b
sexually transmitted diseases, 348b
state health insurance and, 199b
steps in process of, 222–225
teen pregnancy and, 785b
use of technology in learning, 423b
Evidence-based protocol, developing, 224b
Evidence-based public health, 219, 223b
Evidence-based quality/ performance improvement, for home health, 914–915, 914b
Evidence-based strategies, case management and, 548, 550f
Exceptional Medical Expenses Act (AWBZ), 73
Executive branch, federal government, 197
Exosystems, 590
Expanded Program on Immunization, 76–77
Experience rate, 113
Experimental studies, 291–292
clinical trials and, 292
community trials and, 292
Experimental treatment and technology, 567
External consultant, 885
External locus of control, vulnerable population groups and, 702
Extrapolation, 125

F

Fair Housing Act of 1988, 694
Fair Labor Standards Act, 758, 764–765
Faith communities
definition of, 993–994
evidence-based practice in, 1004b
goals for, 996
Faith communities *(Continued)*
national health objectives and, 1003–1004
nurse in, 989–1008
characteristics of, 996–997
definition of, 993
education, 999–1000
interventions and programs for, 997–999, 997f, 998f
linking content to practice of, 1005b
profile of, 996
quality and safety education for, 993b
requirements for, 992, 996
spiritual assessment tool for, 998–999
transitional care, 993b
objectives related to older adult health, 1004b
perspective on, 989–990
program outcomes in, 1003b
Faith community nurse coordinators, 996
Faith Community Nurses International (FCNI), 992–993
Faith community nursing, 990
assumptions in, 993
characteristics of, 996–997, 997b
core interventions for, 994b
definitions in, 992–995
essential attributes of, 1002
history of, 990–991, 990b
issues in practice of, 1001–1003
documentation, 1001–1002
financial, 1002
future growth as, 1002
legal, 1002
professional, 1001
levels of prevention in, 995b
models of, 1000
practice, 995–1001
rationale for, as viable community health mode, 991–992
Faith community nursing/parish nursing, 871
False negatives, 283–284
Families with strengths, 585
Family, 591
as client, 587
as component of society, 587
as context, 585–587
contracting with, 618–619
crisis, 608–609, 609t
definition of, 604
demographics, 580–585
births and, 582–583
caregivers and, 584–585
immigration and, 584
marriage, divorce, and cohabitation, 581–582
parenting and, 583–584
developmental and life cycle theory and, 588–589
traditional stages, 589, 589t
effects of disabilities on, 685–686
empowering, 619–620
genogram, 613f
Family *(Continued)*
health of, 606, 610b
life cycle stages, 610t
structures of, 579–580, 580b, 580f
as system, 587
Family and Community Health, 918
Family and Medical Leave Act (FMLA), 655–656
Family caregiver, 900–901
Family-centered medical home, 647
Family cohesion, 585
Family contracting, 618–619
advantages and disadvantages of, 619
process of, 619, 619t
purposes of, 618–619
Family crisis, 608–609, 609t
Family Education Rights and Privacy Act (FERPA), 932
Family flexibility, 585
Family health, 585
characteristics of, 585b
concepts in, 607–608, 607b
definition of, 585
family health care policy and, 605
genomics/genetics and, 257
history of, 264b
Family health literacy, 595
Family health nursing, legal issues and, 208
Family health risks, 604–625
appraisal and, 609–615, 610b
behavioral risk and, 614
behavioral risk assessment and, 615
biological and age-related risk and, 609–612
biological health risk assessment, 612
environmental risk and, 612
environmental risk assessment and, 612–614
community resources of, 620–623
concepts in, 607–609
early approaches to, 606–607
nursing interventions and, family health risk appraisal and, 609–615
reduction, 615–620
Family interview, 592b
Family level of practice, 241
Family Medical Leave Act (FMLA), 621
Family nursing
definitions of, 576
designing family interventions and, 595–598, 596b, 596f, 597f
family appointment and, 591
determine where to meet the family, 591
planning for safety and, 591–592
family demographics and, 580–585
family functions and structure and, 579–580
family health and, 585

Family nursing *(Continued)*
family health literacy and, 595
four approaches to, 585–587, 586f, 587f
Healthy People, 576b
interviewing the family and, 592, 592b
working for family outcomes, assessment instruments, 592–595
levels of prevention and, 579b
linking content to practice and, 576b
living arrangements and, 581
pre-encounter data collection, 590–591
social and family policy challenges and, 598–600
theories of, 587–590, 587f
bioecological systems theory, 589–590, 590f
developmental and life cycle theory and, 588–589
family systems theory and, 588
Family nursing assessment, 585
Family planning, teen pregnancy and, 783
Family policy, 598, 621
Family stress theory, 611
Family structure, 579–580, 580b, 580f
teen pregnancy and, 777
Family violence and abuse, 843–851
development of abusive patterns, 843–844
types of intimate partner and family violence, 844–851, 845b, 848b
Famines, 84
Farm residency, 717, 717b
Farm stress, 722–723
Feasibility study, 445
Fecal pollution, industrialization and, 77
Federal Drug Administration (FDA), genetic testing oversight and, 260
Federal Emergency Management Agency (FEMA), 462
Federal Emergency Relief Administration (FERA), 32
Federal health agencies
Environmental Protection Agency (EPA) and, 201
Occupational Safety and Health Administration, 201
U.S. Department of Health and Human Services and, 201–202
Federal Insecticide, Fungicide, and Rodenticide Act (FIFRA), 141–142b
Federal Medical Stations (FMS), 474b
Federal poverty guideline, 703
Federal poverty level (FPL), 627, 736
Federal public health agencies, 1010
Federal school health programs, 936, 936f
Federal system, 51–52, 51f
Federal tax status, nurse-led health centers and, 440
Federal Tort Claim coverage, 441
Federal Trade Commission (FTC), genetic testing advertisement and, 260
Federally qualified health centers (FQHCs), 440
Fee-for-service
health care practitioners payment and, 116
nursing centers and, 446
primary prevention and, 100
Feedback loops, 362
Female condoms, 349–350, 350f
Feminist ethics, 156, 156b
Feminists, 156
Fertility rates, 582
Fetal alcohol syndrome (FAS), 815–816
Fidelity, 568
Financial exploitation, 656
Financial issues
in faith community nursing practice, 1002
home health/hospice nurses and, 917
Financial records, 540
Financial support, instructive district nursing and, 28
Financing, government health care function and, 199
First International Sanitary Conference, 69–70
First response, nursing role in, 470–471, 472f
Fiscal competencies, 893–894
cost effectiveness analysis and, 893–894
developing/monitoring budget and, 893
forecasting costs and, 893
Flat-rate premium, 73
Flexner Report, 102
Fliedner, Pastor Theodor, 26–27
Floods, 84
Flu immunizations, 317
Focus group, 379
Focus of care, 407
Follow-up, length of, 225
Food, 134, 134b
safe preparation of, 320, 321b
Food deserts, 634
Food insecurity, 627
migrant farmworkers and, 761
Food labeling, 122
Food landscape, 634
Food poisoning, 320
Food Quality Protection Act (FQPA), 141–142b
Food safety, goals in achieving, 320
Food stamps, 741–742
Foodborne diseases, 319–322, 320t
enterohemorrhagic *Escherichia coli* and, 321
parasitic infections and, 325–327
safe food preparation and, 320, 321b
salmonellosis and, 321
travelers and, 323–324
Foodborne Diseases Active Surveillance Network, 319
FoodNet, 319
Ford Foundation, 71
Forensic, 977
Forensic environments, 983
Forensic Nurse Death Investigators, 977
Forensic nurse examiner, 977
Forensic nurses, 978
education of, 980, 986
Forensic nursing, 842
in community, 976–988
concepts of, 981–982
current perspectives of, 982–983
educational preparation for, 980
ethical issues in, 983–985
examination, 984–985b
future perspectives of, 985–986
Healthy People 2020 and, 977
history of, 979–980
injury prevention and, 977
perspectives on, 976–977
scope and standards of practice of, 982, 986
theoretical foundations of, 980–981
Forensic photography, 979
Formal groups, 427
Formative evaluation, 499
Formulating, 503–505
Foster care, 846
Foundations course, for faith community nurse, 999
Fracking sites, 127
Frail elderly, health disparities, 671
Framework, conceptual
community mental health and, 796–797
evidence-based process and, 233f
Framework for 21st Century School Nursing Practice, 951–952, 951f
Frankel, Dr. Lee, 31
Fraud, 567
Free and appropriate public education (FAPE), 693
Front line staff/entry level, 681b
Frontier, 717b, 722
Frontier Nursing Service (FNS), 31
Fry, Elizabeth, 26–27
Function, community, 371
Functional disability, 680
Functional families, 585
Functional health literacy, 595
Functional limitations, 680
Functional Needs Support Services (FNSS), 473–474
Fund-raising, 446
Funding, categorical approach to, 32–33
Future growth, of faith community nursing practice, 1002
Future of Nursing, Leading Change, Advancing Health, 18
Future of Public Health, IOM on, 37, 270–271

G

Galton, Francis, 256
Gardner, Mary, 29–30
Gastrointestinal anthrax, 311–312
Gatekeepers, 374
Gates Foundation, 71
GDP *see* Gross domestic product
Gebbie, Christine, 13
General model, 365
General population shelter, 473–474
Genes, 257
Genetic information, 257
Genetic Information Nondiscrimination Act (GINA), 258
ethical/legal considerations and, 261
Genetic red flags, 266b
Genetic testing, 258–259
Genetically modified organisms (GMOs), 134
Genetics
biological family health risks and, 609–615
current issues in, 259–262
definition of, 256
DNA and, 257–259
ethical and legal considerations for, 261
evidence-based practice, 266b
future of, 266–267
linking content to practice and, 266b
nursing application of knowledge in, 263–264
in public health nursing practice, 263–264
Genital herpes, 340–341t, 343
Genital warts, 340–341t, 343
Genocide
biopsychological changes and, 85
definition of, 85
perpetrators of, 85
restoration after, 85
Genogram
assessment instruments and, 593, 593f, 594b, 594f, 595b
biological health risk assessment, 612
brush family, 597f
Genome, 255–256
Genomics
competencies for nurses, 263
current issues in, 259–262
definition of, 256
DNA and, 257–259
future of, 266–267
Healthy People 2020, 263b
history of, 256–257
linking content to practice and, 266b

Genomics *(Continued)*
nursing application of knowledge in, 263–264
personalized health care and, 262–263
in public health nursing, 255–256
in public health nursing practice, 263–264
quality and safety education for, 262b
Geographic information systems (GIS), 380
disease distribution patterns and, 274–275
environmental health studies and, 127
epidemiologic data and, 285–286
German measles, 315
Gestational diabetes mellitus (GDM), 665
GI bill, 33
Gilligan, Carol, 155–156
Global burden of disease (GBD), 75–76
Global Burden of Disease Study, 681
Global development, 71–72
Global Giving for Africa, 79
Global health
evidence-based practice in, 63b
global development and, 71–72, 72f
health care systems and, 73–75
iron deficiencies and, 82–83
linking content to practice in, 86–87b
major organizations in, 69–71
major problems, burden of disease and, 75–87
nursing and, 67–69, 68f
overview and historical perspective of, 63–66
perspectives in, 62–90
primary health care and, 67
staying current about, 81b
Global health diplomacy, 71–72
Global HIV/AIDS Epidemic fact sheet, 76
Global Outbreak Alert and Response Network, 86
Global Polio Eradication Initiative, 310
Global positioning system (GPS), 285–286, 380
Global TB Drug facility, 77–78
Global Tuberculosis Program (GTB), 78
Global warming, 84
GNP *see* Gross domestic product
Goals and objectives
of education, 418
of process evaluation, 426
program planning and, 507–509, 508b
Gold standard, 283
Gonorrhea *(Neisseria gonorrhoeae),* 339, 340–341t
Good relationships with families, 944b
Goodrich, Annie, 716–717
Government, 872–873, 873b
community systems and, 385
funding by, 94
health care functions of, 198–200
direct service and, 198–200
financing, 199
information, 199–200, 199t
policy setting, 200
public protection, 200
U.S. health care system and, 197–200
Grading the strength of evidence, 224
Graduate Medical Education funds, 199
Grant writing, 518
Grants, 446
"Great Recession," 48
"Green areas," 358
"Green" spaces, 132
Green wedge, 238f, 239
Gross domestic product (GDP)
health care costs and, 48
health care spending and, 105
as measure of economic growth, 96
Gross national product (GNP), as measure of economic growth, 96
Group
concepts of, 427–429
definitions of, 427
developmental stages of, 429–430
for health change, 430–432, 430f
managing the community, 432
as tool for health education, 427–433
Group culture, 429
Group purpose, 427–429
Growth, definition of, 629
Guanine, 257
Guide to Community Preventive Services, choice of intervention and, 1014–1015
Guide to District Nurses, 27
Guide to the Code of Ethics for Nurses, advocacy and, 560
Guinea worm disease, eradication of, 308
Gulf of Mexico, Deepwater Horizon Oil Spill in, 84
Gull Lake Conference, 35–36
Gun violence, reducing, 640–641
Guyatt, Gordon, 219

H

H1N1, novel influenza A, 300, 318
H5N1, avian influenza A, 300, 318–319
Haddon, William, 980
Hahn, Ellen, 13
Haiti, earthquake in, 83–84
Hallucinogens, 815
Hamburger, *E. coli* and, 321
Handicapped, 680–681
Handwashing, teach families about, 642b
Hantavirus pulmonary syndrome, 300, 307
Happening, 274–275
Hard reduction model, 813
Haven Hill Conference, 35–36
Hawes, Bessie B., 31
Hazard Communication Standard, 973
HBM *see* Health belief model
Healing, 990
Healing service, 994, 994f
Health, 45
of adult population, 654
and behavior and lifestyle, 99
community-wide, 366
culture of, 395–396
definition of, 270–271, 371, 396–397, 397b
determinants of, 396, 699–700
disease oriented *versus* process and environmentally oriented, 400
of families, 606, 610
historical perspectives on, 396–397, 397b
of migrant children, 762–763
of nation, 606–607
older adult, 995b
prerequisites for, 358
social inequalities in, 279
at work, 957, 958
Health Access Nurturing Development Services (HANDS) program, 1016b
Health assets and challenges, identification of, 389
Health behavior
Milio's propositions for improving, 401b
rural-urban disparities and, 720b
societal resources and, 401
Health belief model (HBM), 403, 425
Health beliefs and practices, migrant farmworkers and, 766
Health cabinet, 995
Health care
availability and access of, 721
demand for, forces stimulating in, 46–48
demographic trends, 46–47
health workforce trends, 47–48
social and economic trends, 47
technological trends, 48
ethical protections in, 261–262
financing of, 109–115
government role in, 197–200
Human Genome Project and, 256
the law and, 205–206
migrant farmworkers and, 759–760
cultural considerations in, 765
payment systems for, 115–117
personalized, 262–263
primary, 359
rationing in, 99
resource allocation and, 98–99
Health care *(Continued)*
trends in spending, 105–106, 105f, 106t
in United States, 46
Health Care and Education Reconciliation Act of 2010, government roles and, 198
Health care clinics, school-based, 784–785
Health care consumer, and health insurance, 113
Health care costs
chronic illness and, 107
corporate era, 103
demographics of, 106–107
factors influencing, 106–107
federal regulations contributing to, 108t
technology and intensity in, 107
Health care delivery
economics of, 91–120, 117b
models of
to children and adolescents of, 647
family-centered medical home and, 647
motivational interviewing and, 647
reform efforts, 56–58, 56b
Health care financing, 109–115
private support, 112–115
public health and, 112
public support, 109–112
Medicaid and, 111–112
Medicare and, 109–111
Health Care Financing Administration (HCFA), 198
Health care function, 579
Health care industry, environmental health threats from, 143
Health care insurance, social and family policy issue and, 599
Health care providers
communicating with, 944–945
postindustrial era, 102
Health care reform
advocacy and, 161
plan, 74
Health care spending, trends in, 105–106, 105f, 106t
Health care system, 73–75
challenges for the twenty-first century, 103–118
community health promotion and, 407
context of, 100–118, 101f
corporate era, 103
postindustrial era, 101–102
preindustrial era, 101
twenty-first century, 103–118
current, in United States, 48–50
access to, 49, 49b
cost of, 48–49
quality of, 49–50
evidence-based practice, 56b
factors influencing changes in, 53–56
natural disasters and, 84

Health care system (Continued)
new models for, 103
organization of, 50–53
primary focus of, 17
Health Care Without Harm (HCWH), 143
Health commodification, 71
Health determinants, 699–701, 699f
Health disparities, 396–397, 397b
cultural diversity and, 170–171
migrant and seasonal farmworkers and, 761
socioeconomic status and, 178–179
vulnerability and, 700–701
Health economics, 93
Health education, 414–436
for community groups, 427–433
examples of useful websites for, 424b
key points, 433
linking content to practice and, 416b
programs, develop, 420–421, 421b, 421f
Health educator
faith community nurse as, 997–998, 998f
school nurses as, 934
Health equity, 396–397, 697–699
Health fair, 421b
in faith communities, 997–998, 998f
Health for All by the Year 2000 (HFA2000), 63
Health for All in the 21st century (HFA21), 63
Health Impact Assessment (HIA), 381t
Health in All Policies (HiAP), 358
Health indicators, 377
Health inequities, 698
Health information technology (HIT), 48
case management and, 555
Health insurance, 105
evolution of, 112–113
migrant farmworkers and, 764
Netherlands and, 73
rural families and, 719
Health Insurance Portability and Accountability Act (HIPAA), 712, 917, 932, 939
evidence-based practice model and, 448–449
teen birth control services and, 774
trends in government roles and, 198
and workers health insurance coverage, 114
Health Insurance Prospective Payment System (HIPPS), 110
Health insurance reform, 1016
Health literacy, 179, 424
Health maintenance, 399–400
Health Maintenance Organization Act, 114
Health maintenance organizations (HMOs)
care management strategies and, 548–549
managed care and, 114
Medicare and, 109–111
primary care and, 50
utilization review and, 533–534
Health ministries, 994
Health Ministries Association (HMA), 991, 992–993
Health Ministry Documentation and Reporting System, 1002
Health-oriented perspective, 400
Health outcomes, 438
Health policy, definition of, 197
Health problem
of childhood, 642–647
acute illnesses of, 642
chronic health conditions of, 643–644, 644b
environmental tobacco smoke and, 646–647
oral health and, 643
in community
assessment of, 277b
quantification of, 275b
less developed countries and, 64, 65f
screening and, 282–284
Health professional shortage area (HPSA), 721
Health professionals, 103
Health program planning, 503
Health promotion, 409, 409b
community, 357–369
community trials and, 292
definition of, 359, 399–400
disabled population and, 688–689
disease oriented *versus* process and environmentally oriented, 400
healthy communities movement and, 359
historical perspectives on, 397
key points, 368
of migrant farmworkers, 766
models and frameworks of, 403–404
primary health care and, 45–46
primary prevention and, 280–281, 399, 399b
structure in the community for, 365–366
Health Promotion and Disease Prevention, 442
Health protection, 398
Health Resources and Services Administration (HRSA), 260, 441
Health risk, 608
assessment
behavioral (lifestyle), 615
biological, 612
environmental and occupational, 723–725
family, concepts in, 607–609
family health concepts and, 607–608, 607b
Health risk (Continued)
and nursing interventions, 609–615
reduction, 608
Health risk appraisal, 608
family, 609–615, 610b
Health screenings, 666
Health Security Act of 1993, 198
Health services
access to, resource allocation and, 98–99
community systems and, 385–386
delivery of, components of, 100–101, 101f
reorienting, 358
Health Services Pyramid, 5–6, 5f
Health status, vulnerability and, 701–702
Health status indicators, 376–377, 377t, 378t, 657–659
definition of, 657
morbidity as, 658
mortality as, 658–659
Health teaching, 241t, 244, 245b, 249
Health/wealth gradient, 700, 700f
Healthcare-associated infections (HAIs), 327–328
Healthy, Hunger-Free Kids Act, 932
Healthy Chico Kids 2000 community-wide initiative, 364
Healthy Cities Indiana, 358–359, 363
Healthy Cities movement, 66, 67b
Healthy communities and cities (HCC), 357–358
around the world, 361
in Bartholomew County, 364
definition of terms in, 359
development of, 361–365, 362f
evidence-based practice, 363b
of Henry County, 363–364
history of, 357–359
levels of prevention for, 367b
linking content to practice and, 367b
models for developing, 365–368, 365f, 366b
nurses in, 367
organize a community meeting about, 368b
process of, 358, 359
role of nurse and health professionals in, 367
in the United States, 360
work with, 367b
Healthy community, 362b
Healthy Eating and Exercising to Reduce Diabetes (HEED), 406
Healthy families, 585, 585b
Healthy Islands, 359
Healthy Municipalities and Cities, designing interventions and evaluating results of, 366b
Healthy Municipalities and Communities, 359
in PAHO, 359
Healthy outcomes, working with families, 590–598
in community for, 575–603
Healthy People
core public health functions and, 12
goal comparison and, 200, 200b
vulnerable populations and, 701
Healthy People 2000, 13, 13b, 200, 200b
vulnerable populations and, 701
Healthy People 2010
public health nursing specialist and, 12
vulnerable populations and, 701
Healthy People 2020, 55–56, 200, 200b, 377
access to care, objectives related to, 100b
case management strategies for, 548b
communicable disease and, 334b
competencies and, 157, 157b
different cultures and, 168
document related to occupational health, 972
environmental health objectives and, 124, 124b
epidemiologic objectives and, 271b
evidence-based practice and, 227, 227b
faith communities and, 1003, 1004b
family health objectives, 607b
family health promotion and, 609
forensic nursing and, 977
goal of improving access to comprehensive, high-quality health care and, 526b
goals, 1019
goals and objectives of, 37
health access goals for poor and, 748b
health care coverage for children and, 628
health education, objectives for, 415–416, 415b
healthy community and, 400b
framework of, 401–404
selected goals that pertain to, 359b
process of, 359
history of development of, 37–38b
increasing immunization coverage and, 631
infant mortality rates and, 628–629
infectious disease and, 302b
influenza immunization and, 318
lead poisoning goal and, 646
lifestyle components and, 615
measurable national health objective and, 512b
national health objectives and, 918, 918b
nurse-led health centers and, 439b

Healthy People 2020 (Continued)
obesity and, 634b
objectives, 512b
to family nursing, 576b
focused on children and adolescents and, 648–649b
for mental health and mental disorders and, 800, 801b
for migrant farmworker populations and, 768b
to reduce repeat teen pregnancy and, 782–783
related to adolescent reproductive health, 775b, 776
relevant to health issues and chronic disease of adults and, 658b
to strengthening public health infrastructure, 56, 56b
persons with disabilities and, 689–690, 689b
pertaining to injury and, 978b
program planning goals for, 509b
related to four overarching goals and, 888b
resource allocation and, 99
rural health objectives and, 730, 730b
school nurses and, 937
objectives, 937b
selected national health objectives related to the public health infrastructure and, 1019b
selected objectives that apply to global health care, 64b
social determinants of health and, 700
surveillance objectives and, 486b
tick-borne diseases and, 323
tobacco use and, 399b
substance use, 399b
TQM/CQI in community and public health and, 531
on vaccine-preventable diseases, 315
vulnerable populations and, 701
wellness centers and, 442
Wheel interventions and, 247–248, 248b
Healthy People 2030, vulnerable populations and, 701, 701b
Healthy People in Healthy Communities: A Community Planning Guide Using Healthy People, 359
Healthy public policy, 361
Healthy Villages, 359
Heart disease, 660–661
Help Americans Vote Act, 693–694
Hemolytic uremic syndrome (HUS), 321
Hemorrhagic colitis, 321
Henry Ford Macomb Faith Community Nursing, 1002
Henry Street Settlement, 18, 931t
Henry Street Visiting Nurse Service, 439
Hepatitis
hepatitis A virus as, 344–345
hepatitis B virus as, 345
hepatitis C virus as, 345–346
introduction to, 344–346, 344t
non-ABC, 346
Hepatitis A virus (HAV), 344–345, 345b
Hepatitis B surface antigen (HBsAg), 345
Hepatitis B virus, 345
OSHA regulations and, 345
Hepatitis C virus (HCV), 345–346
Herd immunity, 303
Heroic phase, 469
Herpes simplex virus, 343, 343f
Hewlett Foundation, 71
High-risk behaviors, adolescent, 773
High-risk population, homelessness and, 740–741
Highly active antiretroviral therapy (HAART), 334
AIDS in community and, 334
Hill, Wade, 128
HIPAA *see* Health Insurance Portability and Accountability Act
HIPAA Privacy Rule, adolescent clients and, 774
Hippocrates, 272
Hispanic Americans
children in poverty and, 627
cohabitation and, 582
fertility rates, 582
mental health and, 806
race and, 583
HIT *see* Health information technology
HIV antibody test, 337–338
rapid, 337
HIV infection *see* Human immunodeficiency virus (HIV) infection
HMA *see* Health Ministries Association
HMOs *see* Health maintenance organizations
Holistic approach, to care, 439
Holistic care, 995
Holistic health, 400
Holistic health care, 1000–1001
Holistic health centers, 990–991
Holocaust, 85
Holoendemic, 490
Home care and hospice services, 208
Home health, 672–673
agencies, 902f
evolution of, 901
levels of prevention of, 901b
palliative care, and hospice
accountability and quality management and, 914–915
evolution of, 903
legal, ethical, and financial issues, 917
Omaha system and, 907–910, 908f
Home health (Continued)
practice guidelines for, 910–911, 911b
practice models of, 900
professional development and collaboration, 915–917
scope and standards of practice for, 907
trends and opportunities and, 918–920
population-focused home care models, 900
Home health agencies, 873, 901
Home health aides, home health/hospice collaboration and, 917
Home health care, 901–903
Home Health Care Management and Practice, 918
Home Health Care Services Quarterly, 918
Home health nursing, 902
Home Health Nursing Scope and Standard, 916
Home Healthcare Nurse, 918
Home visits
advantages and disadvantages of, 615
nursing approaches to family health risk reduction and, 615–618
phases and activities of, 616t
process of, 615–618
purpose of, 615
reasons for, 617b
Homebound children, 950
Homeland Security Act of 2002, 457
Homeland Security Exercise and Evaluation Program (HSEEP), 464
Homeland Security Presidential Directive 5 (HSPD-5), 457
Homeland Security Presidential Directive 8 (HSPD-8), 457
Homeland Security Presidential Directive (HSPD) 21: Public Health and Medical Preparedness, 457
Homeless people
federal programs for, 748
health care for, 747–748
health problems of, 752
number of, 743
Homelessness, 735–755
in America, 751–752b
concept of, 742–745, 752
perceptions of homelessness and, 742–745
in United States, 743–745
definition of, 742
health effects of, 746–747
federal programs for, 748
high-risk populations and, 740–741
levels of prevention of, 750b
linking content to practice and, 751–752b
poverty and, 743
preventive services for, 748–750
Homelessness (Continued)
quality and safety education for, 742b
reason for, 744
role of nurse and, 750–752, 751–752b, 751b
trends in, 744
vulnerability and, 702, 702f, 713–714
Homicide, 839
Honeymoon phase, 469
Hong Kong bird flu *see* Avian influenza A (H5N1)
Honor Society of Nursing, 223b
Horizontal integration, 103
Horizontal transmission, 304
Hormonal birth control methods, for teenagers, 777t
Horsens, Denmark, 361
Hospice, 672
Hospice and Palliative Nurses Association (HPNA), 916
Hospice approach, to care in any setting, 905b
Hospice Association of America (HAA), 918
Hospice care, 903–905
evolution of, 903
home care of dying children and, 905
Hospice Foundation of America, 918
Hospice Nurses Association, 918
Hospice provider, Medicare-certified, 905
Hospital, psychiatric, 793
Hospital care visits, from faith community nurse, 997–998, 998f
Hospital Compare, 50
Hospital Insurance Trust Fund, 110
Hospital nursing, reimbursement of, 116
Hospitals, rapid growth of, 102
Host, 127, 962–963
in communicable disease transmission, 302–303, 303f
epidemiologic triangle and, 278, 279b, 279f
Host factor, 303
House calls programs, 442
Household structures, 580b
Housing, migrant farmworkers and, 758
"Housing First," 745
How To
apply care ethics decision process, 156b
apply deontological ethics decision process, 154b
apply feminist ethics decision process, 156b
apply principlism ethics decision process, 154b
apply telehealth interventions, 556b
apply utilitarian ethics decision process, 154b

How To *(Continued)*
- apply virtue ethics decision process, 155b
- assess health problems in a community, 277b
- assess members of vulnerable population groups, 709–710b
- be an effective communicator, 209b
- conduct a sentinel evaluation, 535b
- cost-effectiveness analysis (CEA), 97b
- develop a program plan, 508b
- distinguish chickenpox from smallpox, 312b
- do program evaluation, 513b
- educate nurses for roles in public health: curriculum objectives for public health nursing, 1017b
- ensure high-quality care, 557b
- evaluate the concept of homelessness, 751b
- help families complete a health history, 264b
- intervene with vulnerable populations, 712b
- label photos, 979b
- organize a community meeting about Healthy Communities, 368b
- participate as public health nurse, in essential services of public health, 5b
- plan for pandemic flu, 494b
- promote appropriate use of asthma medications by children, 690b
- provide for information exchange between nurse and client, 562b
- quantify a health problem in community, 275b
- recognize indicators of mental health issues, 801b
- recognize the signs and symptoms of pesticide exposure, 761b
- stay current about global health, 81b
- teach young children in school, 938b
- test values and beliefs about poverty, 742b
- use case management in working with vulnerable populations, 713b
- use evidence to determine interventions, 1014b

Howard Association of New Orleans, Louisiana, 26

Human capital, 96, 701
- primary care and, 100

Human ecology theory, 630

Human genome, and public health, 255–256

Human Genome Project (HGP), 256
- DNA testing and, 258–259

Human immunodeficiency virus (HIV) infection, 78–79, 340–341t
- adolescent and, 773
- adult health concerns and, 663
- antibodies, 334
- case management and, 558
- emergent diseases and, 307
- geographic distribution of, 337, 337f
- HIV surveillance and, 337
- introduction to, 335b, 336t, 338t
- levels of prevention for, 79b
- migrant farmworkers and, 763–764
- natural history of, 334–335
- opportunistic infections and, 327
- perinatal and pediatric HIV infection and, 338
- posttest counseling for, 351–352, 352b
- resources for, 339
- school children with, 949
- series testing for, 284
- stage 3 (AIDS) in community and, 338–339
- surveillance of, 337
- testing, 337–338
- transmission of, 335
- tuberculosis and, 78

Human-made disaster, 455, 455b

Human papillomavirus (HPV) infection, 340–341t, 343–344

Human rabies immunoglobulin (RIG), 325

Human trafficking, 840–842
- attitudes, 841
- pornography, 841–842
- victim or survivor, 842

Humanitarian Reform, 793

Hurricane Katrina, 83–84

Hurricanes, 84

Hyperendemic, 490

Hypertension
- homelessness and, 746
- older adults and, 661

Hypothermia, homelessness and, 746

Hypothetical death rate, 286

I

"I PREPARE," 131, 131b

Identification, genetic/genomic knowledge for, 264

Illness care, 408
- obesity and, 408–409

Illness prevention, 399
- of migrant farmworkers, 766

Illuminating values, in systematic problem solving, 563

Immigrant children, 627–628

Immigrants, 174–175

Immigration, 174–175

Immunizations, 175, 175b, 631–632
- barriers to, 631
- contraindications for, 632
- legislation and, 632, 632b
- measles and, 314–315
- and prevention of communicable diseases, 76–77
- public health nurse and, 1015, 1015f
- recommendations for, 632
- routine childhood schedule for, 314
- theory of, 631–632

Impact, 512

Impact evaluation, 499

Implementation, 391–392
- organizational competencies and, 892–893
- program planning and, 506

Implementing phase, 506

Impoverished adult, health disparities, 671

Improving Diagnosis in Health Care, 881

Improving Health in the Community: A Role for Performance Monitoring, 6

In-home phase, 617–618

In home supportive services (IHSS), 685

Inactive formulating, 503–505

Incest, 847

Incidence
- comparing prevalence and, 277
- comparison groups and, 286
- measures of, 275–276
- proportion of, 275–276
- rate of, 275–276
- sexually transmitted diseases and, 339

Incident Command System (ICS), 466, 466f

Incident commander, 1021, 1022f

Income inequality, 703

Incubation, 304, 334

Independent practice, 871

India, Bhopal gas tragedy in, 84

Indian Health Service, Intervention Wheel adoption and, 246, 246f

Indiana Public Health Association, 363

Indiana University School of Nursing, 363

Indirect adjusted rate, of age, 286

Indirect cultural encounters, 183

Individual education plan (IEP), 946

Individual health promotion models, 403

Individual-level practice, 236, 241

Individual racism, 185

Individualized education plans (IEPs), 693, 931

Individualized emergency plan, 941

Individualized family service plan (IFSP), 693

Individualized health plans (IHPs), 931

Individuals
- with disabilities, 683–685
  - abuse/neglect and, 687–688, 688b, 688f
- health insurance and, 114

Individuals with Disabilities Education Act (IDEA), 630–631, 931
- basic rights under, 693
- disabled children in community and, 686, 686b
- federal legislation and, 693

Individuals with Disabilities Education Improvement Act (IDEIA), 694, 931

Indonesia, tsunami in, 83–84

Indoor air quality (IAQ), 133
- checklist, 948f

Industrial Hygiene Hierarchy of Controls, 139–140, 139b

Industrial nursing, 958

Industrial Revolution, 26

Industry/occupational health, 872

"Inerts," 130

Infant care, pregnant teen and, 782

Infant mortality
- mortality rates and, less developed countries and, 64
- rates, 629
- status of children and, 628–629
- in United Kingdom, 74

Infant mortality rate (IMR), 278, 287
- adjustment of, 287

Infants
- developmental considerations and, 638
- with disabilities, 684, 686
- very-low-birth-weight, 275b

Infection, 304
- prevention, home health and, 914

Infectious disease, 333–356, 334b
- burden and financial impact of, 302
- history of, 300–302
- prevention and control of, 299–311, 334

Infectiousness, 303

Infectivity, 490

Inflation, 93

Influential multilevel community studies, 402–403

Influenza, 317–319
- antiviral drugs, 317–318
- immunization program, 940
- vaccine, 317–318

Informal groups, 427
- small, 421b

Informal pew-side consultations, 997–998, 998f

Informatics
- definition of, 18b
- home health/hospice nursing and, 919–920

Information, government health care functions and, 199–200, 199t

Information competencies, 894

Information exchange process, 561, 562t

Information management, Omaha system and, 907, 908f
Informing, in process of advocacy, 561–562
Inhalants, 815b
Inhalational anthrax, 311–312
Initiation phase, 616
Injection drug users
communicable disease, community outreach and, 350–351
HIV transmission and, 336
influence of place on, 287
Injuries, 637–641, 637f
child maltreatment and, 640
of childhood, prevention, 938
developmental consideration for adolescents and, 638
prevention, 640–641, 642b, 977
reducing gun violence and, 640–641
safe playgrounds and, 641, 642f
Insecticide-treated bed nets (ITNs), 79
Inshuti Mu Buzima (IMB), 69
Institut Pasteur, 71
Institute of Medicine (IOM)
community health and, 398–399
on defining public health, 270
definition of quality by, 522
Division of Health Promotion and Disease Prevention and, 606–607
Future of Public Health and, 270
Future of the Public's Health in the 21st Century and, 270–271
health care quality and, 49
medical errors and, 49
population health and, 396
priorities for public health, 1012
public health core functions and, 3–4
Institutional level interventions, 191
Institutional model, of faith community nursing, 1000
Institutional racism, 185
Institutional settings, 871–872
Institutional visits, from faith community nurse, 997–998
Institutionalization, 793
Instructive district nursing, 28
Instrumental activities of daily living (IADL), 682
Insurance plans, private, 50
Integrated Model of Forensic Nursing, 979–980
Integrated systems, definition of, 17
Integrative model
application of, 408–409
for community health promotion, 407–408
Integrative outcomes, 564
Integrative review, 224
Integrity, 156–157
Intensity, 100–101
health care spending and, 107
Intensive case management (ICM), 559–560
models for, 797
Interactive formulating, 503–505
Interagency Council on the Homeless (ICH), 748
Interagency team plan, in vulnerable populations, 712
Intermediate goals, selection of interventions and, 249
Intermittent source, 490
Internal consultant, 887
Internal locus of control, 702
Internal Revenue Service (IRS), 440b
International Association of Forensic Nurses (IAFN), 977, 980
International Classification of Diseases (ICD), 287–288
International Classification of Functioning, Disability and Health (ICF), 680
International Congress of Nursing, forensic nursing history and, 979
International cooperation, 359
International Council of Nurses (ICN)
Code of Ethics and, 261
global health and, 63
International Journal of Palliative Nursing, 918
International organizations, United Nations and, 201
International Parish Nurse Resource Center, 991
International Red Cross, 70–71
International Society of Nurses in Genetics (ISONG), 261
Internet
corporate era, 103
evidence data, 227
as tool for health education, 427
Interoperability, 919
Interpersonal competencies, 890–892
appraisal and coaching and, 891
communication and, 890, 890b
creating motivating workplace and, 891
promoting diversity and, 891–892
supervision and, 891
team building and, 891
Interpersonal health promotion models, 403–404
Interpersonal relationship, among employees and coworkers, 966
Interpreter, 177, 177–178b
Interprofessional collaboration, 900
Interprofessional community health assessment models, 381t
Interprofessional health team, 458, 916f
Interstate Nurse Licensure Compact, 207
Intervention, description of, 225
Intervention studies, 291–292
Intervention Wheel, 1017–1018
adoption of, 245–247
assumptions of, 234–239
Intervention Wheel *(Continued)*
components of, 239–245
levels of practice and, 240–241
population based model and, 240
public health interventions and, 241–245
evidence-based practice and, 228
linking content to practice and, 252b
model, case management and, 548
origins and evolution of, 232–234
population-based public health nursing practice and, 231–254, 232f, 245b
public health nursing, using of, 239
underlying assumptions of, 234–239
wedges of, 238f, 239
Interventions
communicable diseases and
community education and, 351
community outreach and, 350–351
drug use and, 350
evaluation, 351
introduction to, 349
sexual behavior, 349–350
community-based pregnant teens and, 784–785, 784b
definition of, 236–239
family systems theory and, 588
home-based pregnant teens and, 783–784, 783f
secondary level of prevention and, 281
Wheel assumptions and, 236–239
Wheel model and, 241–245
Intestinal parasitic infections, 326–327
Intimate partner violence (IPV), 843, 847–849
batterer's interventions, 849
intimate partner sexual abuse, 849
partnering with the community, 849
as process, 848
safety planning, 849
screening, 849
signs, 848
teen pregnancy and, 780
Intuition, 981
Investigation, disease
data display for, 492–494, 492f, 493f, 493t
steps in, 491–492, 491b, 492t
when to, 491, 491b
Involuntary contributions, 94
IOM *see* Institute of Medicine
IPV *see* Intimate partner violence
Irish Potato Famine, 85
Irish Sisters of Charity, 26
Iron deficiency, 82–83
pregnant teen and, 782
Isoniazid, 78

J

Japan, Fukushima meltdown, 84
John Hancock Life Insurance Companies, 35
Johnson, President Lyndon Baines, 35
Johnson & Johnson Company, 71
Joint Commission on Accreditation of Healthcare Organizations (JCAHO), 526
Joint Committee on Prepayment, 35
Journal of Community Health Nursing, 918
Journal of Forensic Nursing, 982
Journal of Hospice and Palliative Nursing, 918
Journal of Pediatric Oncology Nursing, 918
Journal of the American Medical Association, 220
Judicial branch, 197
Judicial law, 206
Juran trilogy, 525
"Just say no" approach, 813, 820
Justice, 568, 981

K

Kaiser Family Foundation, 78–79
Karns, Logan, 261
Kercheval: The Storefront That Did Not Burn, 36
Kernel estimation, 285–286
Kerner Commission, 738
Key informants, 377, 378b
Kitzman, Harriet, 906
Koplik's spots, 314
Kübler-Ross, Dr. Elisabeth, 903

L

Lactose intolerance, in ethnic groups, 171
Ladies' Benevolent Society of Charleston, South Carolina, 26
LANA the Iguana, 250, 250f
Land, 134
Landmark health promotion/disease prevention initiatives, 397b
Last Child in the Woods, 132
Latency, syphilis and, 342
Latex allergy, 349–350
Law
definition of, 197
enforcement, 599
health care and, 205–206
constitutional law and, 206
judicial and common law, 206
legislation and regulation, 206
scope of practice and, 206–207
professional negligence, 207
Lawful permanent residents, 175–178
Lead-based paint poisoning, 128
Lead exposure, 139
Lead poisoning, 122, 123f, 646
Leadership, 882
definition of, 429
examples of behaviors, 430b

Leadership competencies, 888–890
  critical thinking and, 890
  decision making and, 890
  delegation and, 888–889, 889b
  empowerment and, 888
League of Nations, 69–70
Learning
  barriers, 423–425
    educator-related types, 423–424
    learner-related, 424–425
  discussions and, 416
  formats for, 421b
  how people learn and, 416–417
  nature of, 416–417
  organizations, 883–884
Legal citations, case management and, 567
Legal immigrants, 175–178
Legal issues
  in case management, 567–569
  in faith community nursing practice, 1002
  health care practices and, 207–208
    correctional health and, 208
    home care and hospice, 208
    school and family health, 208
  home health/hospice nurses and, 917
  older adult care and, 656–657
Legal nurse consultants, 979
Legionnaire's disease, 300
Legislation
  federal
    affecting school nursing, 931–932, 932t
    civil rights for persons with mental disorders and, 795
    for people with disabilities, 691–694, 692b
    Statute Law and, 206
  health, 2
    process of, 209, 210f
  public health nurses, 1019
  related to occupational health, 972–974
  for vulnerable population groups, 709
Legislative action, 209–211, 211b
Legislative branch, 197
Legislative staff, 209
Lesbian, gay, bisexual, transgendered, and queer/questioning (LGBTQ) families, 622–623, 622–623b
Lesbian/gay/bisexual (LGB), 670
Less developed countries, 64
  diarrhea and, 79
  infant mortality and, 64
  iron deficiency in, 82–83
  nurses and, 67, 68f
  tuberculosis and, 78
"Let's Move!" campaign, 634
Leukemia, childhood, 122
Level of practice, Wheel model and, 232–233, 232f, 240–241
Levels of prevention, 266b
  cardiovascular disease and, 281b, 662b
  case management and, 564b
  childhood obesity and, 646b
  community, disaster response and, 476b
  community health education, 415b
  community mental health and, 796–797, 797b
  economic prevention strategies, 99b
  epidemiology and, 280–282, 281b
  ethics and, 159b
  global health care, 79b
  Healthy Communities, 367b
  intentional injury and, 978b
  interventions applied to definition of prevention, 236b
  lead-based paint exposure and, 140b
  migrant and farmworker health issues and, 767b
  nursing center application, 444b
  physically compromised clients and, 689b
  poverty/homelessness and, 750b
  program planning and evaluation, 512b
  public health nursing and, 1022b
  quality management and, 540b
  related to public health care system, 52b
  related to vulnerable populations, 709, 709b
  rural health care and, 727b
  in schools, 937–950, 937f
  strategies applied to families, 620b
  surveillance activities and, 493b
  teen pregnancy and, 779b
LGBTQ families *see* Lesbian, gay, bisexual, transgendered, and queer/questioning (LGBTQ) families
Liability
  case management and, 567
  insurance, professional, 207
Liberal democratic, 155t
Libertarian, 154
Liberty Mutual Insurance Company, 558
Licensure, 206–207, 208, 527
Life care planning, 557
Life-event risks, 610
Life expectancy, 107, 658, 659f, 660f
Lifespan, disability health care across, 678–696
Lifestyle
  health of nation and, 606–607
  healthy communities and, 395–396
  of migrant farmworkers, 757–758
  and primary prevention, 99
  rural populations and, 725
Limited services client, 578–579
Linguistically appropriate health care, 707
Lipid screening, guidelines for, 283
Literacy, low level of, 424–425, 425b
Literacy scale, 424
Liverpool Relief Society, 27
Living will, 656–657
Local advocacy organizations, 377t
Local education agency (LEA), 932t
Local public health agency, 1011, 1011b
Local system, 53
Locality development model, 360
Logical Observation Identifiers, Names, and Codes (LOINC), 919
Long-acting reversible contraception (LARC), 776
Long-Term Budget Outlook, 106
Long-term care facilities, 673, 872
Long-term evaluation, 426
Los Angeles County Department of Health Services, Intervention Wheel adoption and, 245–246
Low-birth-weight infants, 780
  teen pregnancy and, 780
Low health literacy, 562
Low-income housing, 749
Low-income populations, disabilities in, 687, 687f
Lutheran General Hospital, 991
Lyme disease, 300, 322–323
Lynch, Virginia, 979–980

M

Macroeconomic theory, 96
Macrosystems, 590
Mad cow disease, 300, 319
Magnetic wave sources, 134
Mainstream smoke, 817
Maintenance functions, 428
Maintenance norms, 429
Making appointment with the family, 591b
Malaria, 79
  diseases of travelers and, 324
  GIS and, 285–286
Malathion, 79
Malnutrition
  impact of, 83
  measles and, 314
Malpractice, 207
Malpractice litigation, 537
Man-made disasters, 84
Managed care, 524
  arrangements, 114
  defined, 50
  focus on, 8
  mental health care and, 800
  model, 50
  and rationing, 99
Managed care organizations (MCOs), 523
  nurse leaders and, 881
  utilization review and, 533–534
Managed competition, 114
Management planning, 501–502
Manager roles, 884–885
Managing care, liability for, 567
MAP-IT, 401
Maps, in community assessments, 380
Marburg virus, 300–301, 306–307
Marginalization, 85, 701, 703
Marine Hospital Service, 26, 109
Market, 95
Market justice, 160, 160t
Marriage, 581–582
Maryknoll Missionaries, 71
Masking, 291
Massachusetts Association of Public Health Nurses, Intervention Wheel adoption and, 246
Massachusetts Sanitary Commission, 26
Maternal and Child Health Bureau (MCHB), children with special health care needs and, 680
Maternal health, 81–82
Maternal-infant health, 721–722
McIver, Pearl, 32
McKesson Corporation, 548
MDGs *see* Millennium development goals
Meaningful use, 919
Means testing, 107
Measles, 314–315
  outbreaks, 1013
Measurable objective, 507
Médecins sans Frontières (MSF), 71, 83
  Plumpy' nut, 83
Mediator, 560
Medicaid, 98, 109
  children's health insurance and, 628
  disabled adults and, 685
  expenditures of, 111
  federally qualified health centers and, 441
  government role in health care and, 197–198
  Great Recession and, 49
  health care and, 599
  HIV and, 334
  home health services and, 901
  hospice care reimbursement and, 903
  low reimbursement in, 99
  Medicare *versus,* 109t
  mental health care and, 799–800
  migrant farmworkers and, 759
  poverty income levels and, 111
  public support and, 111–112
  Social Security Act of 1965, 36, 102
  status of children and, 628
  vulnerable populations and, 706
  waiver in, 111
Medical College of Virginia (Richmond), African-American nurses and, 31
Medical Expenditure Panel Survey (MEPS), 107
Medical home, 647
  see also Family-centered medical home

Medical model of disability, 679
Medical Reserve Corps (MRC), 461–462
Medical savings accounts (MSAs)
health insurance and, 115
Medicare and, 109–111
Medical technology, 100–101
Medically underserved areas, 731
Medicare
baby boomer population and, 49
demographics and, 46
federally qualified health centers and, 441
government role in health care and, 197–198
health care and, 599
HIV and, 334
home health services and, 901
hospice care reimbursement and, 903
Medicare *versus,* 109t
mental health care and, 799–800
out-of-pocket expenses in, 111
prescription plan in, 107
public support and, 109–111
Social Security Act of 1965, 36, 102
total expenses of, 110f
Medicare-certified home health services, 902
Medicare part A, 110
Medicare part B, 110
Medicare part C, 109–111
Medication, prescription, abuse, 629
MEDPAC, 209
Mendel, Gregor, 256
Menopause, 665
Men's health, 666
concerns of, 666–669, 667b
depression and, 669
erectile dysfunction and, 669
prostate cancer and, 668
testicular cancer and, 668–669
Mental disabilities, adults with, 670–671
Mental disorder, civil rights legislation for persons with, 795
Mental health
funding for, 792
Healthy People 2020, definition of, 790
HIV and, 339
older adults and, 662
problems, 944–945
rural communities and, 722–723
Mental Health: A Report of the Surgeon General, 800
Mental health care, 792–793
current and future perspectives in, 799–800
managed care and, 792
services and, 792–793
Mental health global action program (mhGAP), 790
Mental health issues, 789–810
conceptual frameworks for community mental health, 796–797
Mental health issues *(Continued)*
current and future perspectives of, 799–800
deinstitutionalization and, 794–796
linking content to practice, 803b
national objectives for services for, 800–807, 801b
role of the nurse in, 797–799
scope of mental illness in United States and, 790–792
systems of community mental health care and, 792–793
Mental Health Parity Act, 795
Mental Health Parity and Addiction Equity Act (MHPAEA), 795
Mental health service
and Medicare Part B, 110
national objectives for, 800–807, 801b
adults and, 802–803
children/adolescents and, 801–802
cultural diversity and, 805–807
older adults and, 804–805, 804b, 805b
state systems for, 795
Mental illness, 790–792
advocacy efforts and, 795–796
consumer advocacy and, 791
deinstitutionalization, 745, 794–796
disabilities and, 683
factors in care for, 789
neurobiology of, 791–792
scope of, 790–792
Mercury, 132, 644
Merit-based Incentive Payment System (MIPS), 919
Mesosystems, 590
Meta-analysis, 223–224
Metabolic syndrome, 791–792
Methicillin-resistant *Staphylococcus aureus* (MRSA), 300, 1016
Methylmercury, 143
Metropolitan area, 717–718
Metropolitan Life Insurance Company, 31
Mexican National Academy of Medicine, 66
Mexico
health care systems in, 73
NAFTA and, 66
MI *see* Motivational interviewing
Mi-yuk kook (seaweed soup), 177f
Microeconomic theory, 94–95
Micropolitan area, 717–718
Microsystems, 590, 884
Middle Eastern Respiratory Syndrome Coronavirus (MERS-CoV), 301
Migrant and seasonal farmworkers (MSFWs), 756
Migrant Clinicians Network (MCN), 759
TB tracking program of, 763
Migrant Education Program, 765
Migrant farmworkers
children and youth of, 764–765, 764f
common health problems of, 761–764
cultural considerations in health care, 765
definition of, 756–757
health care of, 759–760
health beliefs and practices and, 766
health values and, 765–766
nurse-client relationship in, 765–766, 766b
health promotion and illness prevention for, 766
health risks to, 723–724t
lifestyle of, 757–758
housing for, 758
occupational and environmental health problems of, 760–761
role of nurse and, 766–768, 767b, 768b
working in fields, 758f
Migrant Head Start Program, 765
Migrant Health Act, 759
Migrant health centers, 759
Migrant health issues, 756–771
Migrant lifestyle, 757–758
Milbank Memorial Fund, 71
Milio, Nancy, 36
Millennium development goals (MDGs), 65, 65b
maternal health and, 81
tuberculosis and, 77–78
vaccination and, 76–77
Millennium Report, 65
Mine Safety and Health Act of 1968, 972
Ministry of Public Health (China), 74
Minorities
health of, 723
poverty and, 739–740
toxic stress and, 741
Misuse of service, 525
Mitigation, 458–459
Mixed outbreak, 490
Mobilizing for Action through Planning and Partnerships (MAPP), 373, 381t, 514t, 515–517, 516f
Moderation Management, 816
Monitoring, 142
Mood, Lillian, 294
Moral distress, 151b, 153
Moral leadership, 157
Morality, 151b, 155–156
Morbidity, 389
adult health and, 658
Morbidity and Mortality Weekly Report, 305–306, 481–482
Morbidity/mortality measures, 274–278
attack rate and, 277
measures of incidence and, 275–276
mortality rates and, 276t, 277–278
Morbidity/mortality measures *(Continued)*
prevalence and incidence comparison in, 277
prevalence proportion and, 276–277
proportions, rates and risk in, 274–275
Mortality, 389
adult health and, 658
cause-specific, 278
maternal, 81
risk factors for, 82
rate, 276t, 277–278
health disparities and, 702
statistics
GBD and, 75–76
Mosquitoes
and communicable diseases, 79
malaria and, 324
West Nile virus and, 307
Motivating workplace, 891
Motivation, 425
Motivational interviewing (MI), 419–420, 647, 647f
Motor Voter Act, 694
Moulder, Betty, 958
Multi-attribute utility technique (MAUT), 514, 514t, 515b
Multidimensional poverty, 736–737
Multidisciplinary practice with interprofessional collaborative practice, 441t
Multidrug resistance, and tuberculosis, 78
Multifactorial disorders, 261b, 266b
Multigenerational poverty, 739
Multilateral organizations, 69
Multilevel interventions, 402
nurse-led health centers and, 439
Multisectoral cooperation, 359
Mutagen, 258
Mutations, genetic, 257–258
Mutual aid agreement, 465
Mycobacterium tuberculosis, 77–78

N

NAAL *see* National Assessment of Adult Literacy
Nairobi Global Conference on Health Promotion, 66
Naloxone (Narcan), 827b
Narrative review, 224
NASN *see* National Association of School Nurses
Nation, health of, 606–607
National Academy of Medicine (NAM)
recommendations for public health, 1012
National Advisory Council for Nursing Education and Practice (NACNEP), 202
National Agricultural Workers Survey (NAWS), 757
National Alliance for the Mentally Ill (NAMI), 795–796
National Assessment of Adult Literacy (NAAL), 424

National Association for Home Care & Hospice (NAHC), 918
National Association of Colored Graduate Nurses, 35
National Association of Local Boards of Health, 7
National Association of School Nurses (NASN)
  educational credentials for, 933
  standards of practice, 933
National Association of State Public Health Veterinarians, Inc., 325
National Campaign to Prevent Teen and Unplanned Pregnancy, 784
National Cancer Institute (NCI), 262
National Center for Health Statistics, 285–286, 377t
National Center for Injury Prevention and Control, 977
National Center for Nursing Research (NCNR), 37
National Center on Birth Defects and Developmental Disabilities, CDC and, 680
National Childhood Vaccine Injury Act, 632
National Civic League, 361–362
National Coalition for the Homeless, 747–748
National Coalition of Health Professional Education in Genetics (NCHPEG), 263
National Committee for Mental Hygiene, 793
National Committee for Quality Assurance (NCQA), 447
National Council of State Boards of Nursing, 207
National Depression Screening Day, 796
National Disaster Medical System (NDMS), 461–462
National Electronic Disease Surveillance System, 488
National Environmental Education Act, 141–142b
National Environmental Policy Act (NEPA), 141–142b
National Exercise Program (NEP), 464
National Health and Nutrition Examination Survey, 125
National Health Board, 109
National Health Circle for Colored People, 31
National health objectives, 363, 918
  faith communities and, 1003–1004
  public health nursing and, 1018–1019
National Health Planning and Resources Development Act, 499–501
National Health Security Strategy (NHSS), 457, 464
National Health Services Corps, 441
National health spending, 48
National Health Survey of 1935-1936, 33–34
National Healthcare Safety Network (NHSN), 328
National Heart, Lung and Blood Institute, faith-based toolkit from, 1003, 1003b
National Highway Traffic Safety Administration, 637
National Hospice and Palliative Care Organization, 918
National Human Genome Research Institute (NHGRI), 263
National Incident Management System (NIMS), 457
National Institute for Occupational Safety and Health (NIOSH), 973, 973b
  history of, 958–959
  occupational health and safety education and, 959–960
National Institute of Mental Health (NIMH), 683, 794
  Community Support Program of, 791
National Institute of Nursing Research (NINR)
  federal health agencies and, 203f
  financing and, 199
  public health nursing and, 37
National Institutes of Health (NIH), 197–198, 203, 260, 654
National League for Nursing (NLN), 35, 527
National League of Cities, 363
National Level Exercise, 464
National Library of Medicine (NLM)
  chemical information and, 127
  WISER and, 460, 461b
National Network of Public Health Institutes, 7
National Notifiable Diseases Surveillance System (NNDSS), 305–306, 486
National Nursing Centers Consortium (NNCC), 446
National Occupational Research Agenda (NORA), 973, 973b
National Office of Vital Statistics, 481–482
National Organization for Public Health Nursing (NOPHN)
  forensic nursing history and, 979
  funding public health nursing and, 35
  history of nursing and, 29–30
  professional nursing education and, 35–36
National Outbreak Reporting System (NORS), 322
National Preparedness Guidelines (NPG), 457
National Prevention, Health Promotion, and Public Health Council, 105
National Prevention Strategy (NPS), 398, 398f
National Public Health Performance Standards Program, 7, 1014–1015
National Quality Forum (2014), 915
National Response Framework (NRF), 457
National Response Plan (NRP), 457
National School Lunch or Breakfast Program, 932
National Syndromic Surveillance Program, 489
National Violent Death Reporting System (NVDRS), 842–843, 981
National Voter Registration Act of 1993, 694
Native Alaskans
  health disparities with, 287
  health risks to, 723–724t
Native American Genocide, 85
Native Americans, health risks to, 723–724t
Natural disasters, 83–87, 455, 455b, 455f
  aftermath of, 84
Natural experiment, 272
Natural history of disease, 280
Natural immunity, 303
Nature deficit disorder, 132
Near poverty, 719
Needs assessment, 418, 418b, 504, 504f
  tools of, 503t
Negative predictive value, 284
Neglect, definition of, 656
Negligent referrals, 567
Negotiation, 564, 886
  aftermath of, 565
  stages of, 564
Neighborhood poverty, 735
Nestlé, 71
Net positive value, 97
Netherlands, health care system in, 73
Neuman Systems Model, 372–373, 607
  five interacting variables and, 608
Neurobiology, of mental illness, 791–792
New Castle Healthy City community assessment, 363
New Perspective on the Health of Canadians, 397
New York City Mission, 27
NFP *see* Nurse-Family Partnership
Ngudo Nga Zwinepe (NNZ) Learning through Photos projects, 407
NIC *see* Nursing Interventions Classification (NIC) system
Nightingale, Florence
  disaster response and, 482
  environmental health history and, 124–125
  ethics and morality of, 150
  evidence-based quality and, 914
  history of nursing and, 26–27
NIH Revitalization Act of 1993, 654
NLN Accrediting Commission (NLNAC), 527
No Child Left Behind Act of 2001, 693, 932
Noddings, Nel, 155–156
Non-core areas, 718
Non-farm residency, 717, 717b
Non-gonococcal urethritis (NGU), 342
Non-native language session, 421b
Non-normative event, 611
Non-point sources, 132
Noncontingency contract, 618–619
Nongovernmental organizations (NGOs), 69
Nonhealthy families, 585
Nonimmigrants, 176
Nonjudgmental approach, 190
Nonmaleficence, 154, 154b, 568, 983–984
Nonverbal communication, cultural competence and, 172–173
NOPHN *see* National Organization for Public Health Nursing
Normative event, 611
Norms, 428
North American Free Trade Agreement (NAFTA), 66
North American Industry Classification System (NAICS), 970
North American Nursing Diagnosis Association (NANDA), 391
Nothing But Nets, 79
Nuclear magnetic resonance (NMR), 791–792
Numerator, 274
Nurse(s), 985b
  AIDS in the community and, 336
  caring for poor and, 752
  change in the childhood obesity rates and, 636–637
  climate change and, 129
  communicable disease prevention and, 347–353
  cultural competence of, 167
  definition of, 23
  definition of health and, 399–400
  disaster planning and management, 973–974b
  environmental health and, 144–145
  focus on quality and safety education for, 64b, 226b, 358b, 389b, 409b, 417b, 448–449b, 599–600b
  genomic competencies for, 263
  global health and, 66
  in Healthy Communities, 367
  healthy community and, 401–404
  HIV transmission and, 336
  in home health, palliative care, and hospice, 899–927, 901f, 921b
  home health/hospice and, 915–916
  identify HIV trends and, 336

Nurse(s) *(Continued)*
in infectious disease prevention, 310–311
legislation and regulations for, 206
in less developed countries, 67, 68f
as life care planners, 557
microeconomic and macroeconomic issues and, 96
occupational health, 958–959
population-centered health care and, 524t
population health and, 66–67
postindustrial era, 102
preventive care for communicable disease and, 347–353
primary prevention, 281
quality and safety education for, 41b
role of
in community, 374, 374b
in community mental health and, 797–799, 798b, 799b, 799f
in policy process and, 208–214, 209b
in rural communities, 732
in school, 928–956, 943b
assessing and screening children at, 942–943
controversies in, 950
educational and licensure credentials of, 933–934
ethics in, 950–951
federal legislation affecting, 931–932
functions of, 934–935
future trends in, 951–952
giving medication in, 942–943
Healthy People 2020 and, 937, 937b
history of, 929–931, 931t
linking content to practice, 952b
online resources for, 951t
roles and functions of, 934–935
school health services and, 935–937
standards of practice for, 933
screening and, 282–283
teamwork and collaboration in, 104b
teen pregnancy and, 783–785, 784b
in training, 102
tuberculin skin test, 347
in vulnerable populations, 712
websites providing education and training opportunities, 461b
working in community, 373
working with families
in community, 576–579
definition of family and, 577
uninsured, underinsured, and limited services and, 578–579
Nurse advocate, 1002
Nurse attorney, 979
Nurse case manager, 558
core values of, 548
historical evidence, in evidence-based examples and, 557–558
Nurse-Family Partnership (NFP), 442, 442f, 906, 1019–1020
Nurse leader
in community, 880–898, 887b
competencies for, 887–894
consultation and, 885–888
definitions for, 882–883
future of, 894–895
introduction of, 881
leadership and management applied to, 883–885, 884t
linking content to practice, 895b
major trends and issues of, 881–882
developing population of, 17
Nurse-led health center, 437–453, 444b
business aspects, 445–447
clinical aspects, 447, 447t
definition of, 438–440, 438b
director of, 443–444
education, 449
educators in, 444
health and community orientation of, 439
key points, 451–452
linking content to practice, 443b
logic model as framework, 449–450, 450f
nurse-led models of care and, 440–443
other members in, 444
overview of, 438–440
research, 449
researchers in, 444
students in, 444
team of, 443
types of, 440b
Nurse Licensure Compact Administrators (NLCA), 527
Nurse Life Care Planners Standards of Practice with Interpretive Statements (2012b), 557
Nurse-Managed Wellness Centers: Developing and Maintaining Your Center, a National Nursing Center Consortium Guide and Toolkit, 446
Nurse practice act, 206
scope of practice and, 206–207
Nurse practitioners (NPs), 440, 443, 864
Medicare part B and, 116
postindustrial era, 102
Nurses for National Defense, 33
Nurses' Settlement in Orange, New Jersey, 28
Nursing
advocacy process and, 562t
approaches to community care, 706–709
boards of, 206
care of working populations, 967–972
Nursing *(Continued)*
in China, 68
constitutional law and, 206
culturally competent principles for, 167
definition of, 270
in disasters, 86b
education
21st century and, 104–105
system of, in China, 74–75
epidemiology application in, 293–295, 294b
global health and, 67–69, 68f
government health functions/structures and, 205
Health and Environment, 124b
human genome and, 256
interprofessional application to, 408
the law and, 205–206
population-centered history of, 22–23
postindustrial era, 102
reimbursement for, 116–117
roles in vulnerable population group, 708b
in rural communities, 726–729
Nursing advocacy, 213–214, 213b
Nursing and Health Care Ethics: A Legacy and a Vision, 151
Nursing care
of community as client, 371–372
for emergencies in school, 940–941, 940b
in rural environments
nurse preparation for, 728–729
research needs in, 728
theory, research, and practice and, 726–728, 726b, 728f
of working populations, 967–972
workplace assessment, 970–972
Nursing centers, 871
establishment of, 446
overview of, 438
staff for
data manager program coordinator, 444
director/nurse executive as, 443–444
educators, 444
operations manager, 444
researchers, 444
students, 444
technology specialist, 444
Nursing Child Assessment Satellite Training Project (NCAST), 219
Nursing Code of Ethics, 158–159
Nursing for the Future, 35
Nursing interventions, major family health risks and, 609–615
Nursing Interventions Classification (NIC) system, in faith community nursing, 994b, 1002
Nursing models of care, 438
Nursing practice, 206
the law and, 205–206
laws specific to, 206
Omaha system and, 907, 908f
Nursing process, 907
application in practice and, 241t, 248
for care of poor and homeless, 751–752b
community level application and, 249–251
individual/family application level and, 248–249
Intervention Wheel assumptions and, 236, 236–237t
linked to preparedness, 485t
program planning and, 507t
systems level of practice scenario, application of, 251–252
Nursing science, perspectives of, 400
Nursing specialists, in problem definition at aggregate level, 11
Nursing theory, 726
Nursing's Social Policy Statement, 568
Nutrition
in cultural variations, 173–174
persons with disabilities and, 689
teen pregnancy and, 780–782, 781t
and world health, 82–83
Nutrition assessment, childhood obesity and, 634
Nutrition education, 364
Nutritional deficiencies, and diarrhea, 80
Nutting, Mary Adelaide, 30

O

OASIS-C2, 912, 913b
Obesity, 632–634, 633f
adult health concerns and, 664
community assessment and, 249–250
epidemic of, 271–272
illness care and, 408–409
built environment, 408–409, 408t
health promotion and, 408–409
illness/disease prevention and, 409
prevention, 634
Objectives, 418
program planning and, 507–509, 508b
Observational studies, 291–292
Occupational and environmental health nursing, 958
care of working populations, 967–972
disaster planning and management, 973–974b
Healthy People 2020, 972b
legislation and, 972–974
workers as population aggregate, 960–962
Occupational health
hazards, 960–961, 970
history, 968, 969f
migrant farmworkers and, 760–761
nurse in, 957–975

Occupational health *(Continued)*
risks, migrant workers and, 760, 763f
rural community risks and, 723–725
and safety programs, on-site, 966–967, 967b
Occupational health nursing
definition and scope of, 958
history and evolution of, 958–959
roles and professionalism in, 959–960
Occupational Safety and Health Act of 1970
occupational health and, 972–973
worksite nurses and, 958–959
Occupational Safety and Health Administration (OSHA), 141–142b, 201, 958–959, 972b, 973b
environmental and occupational health risks and, 723–724t, 723–725
hepatitis B virus regulation, 345
pesticide exposure and, 760–761
Occupational Safety and Health Education and Research Centers, 959–960
Occupational therapist, 917
"Off-time" transitions, 589
Office of Chief of Public Health Practice, CDC, 7
Office of Minority Health, 287
Office of Occupational Health Nursing, 958–959
Office on Women's Health, 664
Office within the Department of Homeland Security, 205
Official health agency, 32
Older Adult Health, 995b
Older adults
cohabitation and, 581
and Medicare payments, 110
mental health objectives for, 804–805, 804b, 805b
Older Americans Act (OAA), 655
Olds, Dr. David, 442, 906
Omaha system, 389–391, 907–910
description of, 907–910
informatics and, 919
Omaha System Intervention Scheme, 908–909, 909b, 910b
Omaha System Problem Classification Scheme, 908, 909b
Omaha System Problem Rating Scale for Outcomes, 909–910, 910t
Omnibus Reconciliation Act, 116
On Death and Dying (Kübler-Ross), 903
"On-time" transitions, 589
One Health, 467–469
One-stop services, 706
Online faith-based resources, example of, 1003b
Ontario (Canada) Healthy Communities Coalition, 361
Operational indicator, 508
Operations manager, 444
Opioids, 818–819, 819f
Opportunistic infection
AIDS-related, 334
parasitic, 327
Oral rehydration therapy (ORT), 281
Orange wedge, 238f, 239
Organization phase, of cultural assessment, 190–191
Organizational competencies, 892–893
implementing and coordinating and, 892–893
monitoring, evaluating, improving and, 893
organizing and, 892
planning and, 892
Organizational framework, of nurse-led centers, 443
Organizational partners, as nurse-led health center staff, 444
Organizational structure, nurse-led health centers and, 440
Organizations and agencies, influencing health, 201–205
federal health agencies and, 201–204
federal non-health agencies and, 204
international organizations and, 201
state/local health departments and, 204–205
Organophosphate pesticides, 760
OSHA *see* Occupational Safety and Health Administration
Osteoporosis, 666
SSRIs and, 791–792
Ottawa Charter for Health Promotion, 399–400
Outbreak, 490
detection, 490
investigation, 481–497
Outcome(s), 225
data, 482
distributive, 564
evaluation of, 517
evaluative studies and, 535
health status indicators, 249
integrative, 564
model, 912f
model CQI program and, 539
nurse-led health centers and, 438
Outcome and Assessment Information Set (OASIS), 912
Outcome-Based Quality Improvement (OBQI), 915
Outrage factors, 140, 140b
Outreach
definition of, 244
levels of intervention and, 241t
migrant farmworkers and, 766
vulnerable populations and, 708
Overt intentional prejudice/racism, 186b
Overt unintentional prejudice/racism, 186b
Overuse of service, 525
Overweight, CDC definition, 632–633
Oxfam, 69, 71
Oxycodone, 819, 824

P

Pacific Islander Americans, mental health and, 806
PAHO *see* Pan American Health Organization
Palliative care, 672, 903–905
and hospice, 899–905, 901f, 921b
Pan American Health Organization (PAHO)
international organizations and, 201
multilateral agencies and, 70
region, Healthy Municipalities and Communities in, 359, 361
Pandemic and All-Hazards Preparedness Act (PAHPA), 205
Pandemic and All Hazards Preparedness Reauthorization Act (PAHPRA), 457
Pandemic novel influenza A (H1N1), 318
Pandemics, 84, 304, 455, 490
PAPM *see* Precaution adoption process model
Paradigm shift, 220–221
Parasitic diseases, 325–327, 326t
control and prevention of, 327
foodborne/waterborne, 327
intestinal, 326–327
neglected, 326
opportunistic, 327
Parent organization, 446
Parenting
abusive, 782
family demographics and, 583–584
teen pregnancy and, 777
Parents As Teachers, 441–442
Parish, 993
Parish nurses, 990, 991f, 993
Parish nursing, 990
Parishioners, 1001
Parity, 792
Park Ridge Center for Health, Faith, and Ethics, 1003
Participant observation, 378
Participatory development framework, 361
consolidation phase of, 361
initial phase of, 361
planning process of, 361
Partner notification, 348
Partner pressure, 776
Partnerships, 373b, 524
approach, 360
in faith community nursing, 992
models of, 732
nurse leader in, 881
principles of, 1009, 1010b
Partnerships*(Continued)*
professional-community-client in rural settings, 365, 373, 373b, 730–732, 731b
public health and, 1009
rural community health care and, 722
Pasadena, California, 364
Passive immunization, 303
Passive neglect, 846
Passive participation, 373
Passive surveillance, 284
Passive system, as surveillance systems, 488
Pastoral care staff, 998–999
Paternalism, 983
Paternalistic intervention, 983
Paternity, 777–779
Pathfinder Fund, 71
Pathogenicity, 490
Pathologies of Power (2005), 64–65
Patient-centered medical home (PCMH), 672
Patient engagement, 555
Patient oriented evidence that matters (POEM), 224–225
Patient Protection and Affordable Care Act, 93, 656, 792
donut hole and, 107
employer incentives and, 95
government role in health care and, 197–198
health care barriers and, 99
nurse-led health centers and, 438, 438b
public health and, 1–2
rationing and, 99
Patient Safety Act of 1997, 209
Patient Self-Determination Act, 656–657
Patriarchal leadership, 430
Paying health care organizations, and health care payment systems, 115
Payment systems
for health care, 115–117
paying health care organizations, 115
paying health care practitioners and, 116–117
reimbursement for nursing services, 116–117
Pedagogy, 422
Pediatric advanced life support (PALS), 941
Pediatric health care, 648b
Pediatric HIV infection, 338
Pediculosis (lice), screening children for, 943–944
Pedigree, 264–266, 265f
Peer pressure, 776
Peer Review Improvement Act (PL 97-248), 534–535
Peer Review Organization (PRO), 526
Pelvic inflammatory disease (PID), 339
Pennsylvania Hospital, 23

People, in community, 371, 383–384
People who inject drugs, 825
Perceptivity, 981
Perinatal HIV transmission, 338
Permit, 141
Permitting, 141
Persistent bioaccumulative toxins (PBTs), 143
Persistent diarrhea, 80
Persistent organic pollutants (POPs), 143
Person, descriptive epidemiology and, 286–287
Person First Movement, 680–681
Person-time, 277–278
Personal beliefs, concepts of poverty and, 736–740
Personal preparedness, disaster management cycle, 459–460, 459–460b, 459f
Personal protective equipment (PPE), 460
Personal Responsibility and Work Opportunity Reconciliation Act, 656
Personal safety, 616–617
Personalized Health Care Initiative, 262–263
Perspective, program management and, 504
Pertussis, 316–317
 quality and safety education for, 317b
Pesticide exposure, 760–761
 to children, 137b
Pew Charitable Trusts, 750
Pew Internet & American Life Project, 418
Phaneuf's nursing audit method, 526
Pharmacy Act, 207
PHC *see* Primary health care
Philanthropic organizations, 70, 71
Photo elicitation, 379
Photography, 379
Photovoice, 379, 406–407
 process of, 379
Physical abuse, 844
Physical activity
 behavioral risk and, 614
 built environment and, 635, 636t
 women and, 659–660
Physical Activity and Neighborhood Resources in High School Girls study, 406
Physical agents, 965
Physical disabilities, adults with, 670–671
Physical environment, community systems and, 386, 386f
Physical limitations, rural community and, 720–721
Physical neglect, 846–847
Physical therapist, 917
Physician, home health/hospice collaboration with, 917
Physician leaders, 17
Physician Payment Review Commission, 116
Piaget, Jean, 630
"PICOT" format, 222
Pima County Health Department, 911
Pinel, Philippe, 793
Pinworm (Enterobiasis), 326–327
Pioneering Healthy Communities, 360
PL 111-148, 114
Place
 community systems in, 383, 384–387, 387f, 388b
 descriptive epidemiology and, 287
 geographic location of community as, 371
Plague, 300, 313
Plan
 evaluation of, 598
 for family assessment, 591b
Plan, Implement, and Evaluate a Health Fair, 419b
Plan-do-study-act (PDCA) model, 538, 538b, 538f
Planning, defined, 499
Planning approach to community health (PATCH), 514–515, 514t
Planning frameworks, common elements of, 375b
Planning process, 503–509, 504t
 nursing process and, 507t
 program management and, 504t
 program planning model and, 503–506
Plasmodium falciparum, 79
Plasmodium sporozoites, 79
Plasticizers, 644
Playgrounds, 641, 642f, 938
Plumpy' nut, 83
Point epidemic, 288
Point source, 132, 490
Points of dispensing (POD), 458–459
Police power, 197, 206
Policy
 definition of, 197
 development, 372
  case management and, 552
  core function and, 4f, 13, 18b
  definition of, 3–4, 19, 245
  ethics and, 157
  levels of intervention and, 241t
  public health nursing process and, 251
  shifting, 17–18
 enforcement, 241t, 245
 family health care and, 605
 makers, information based data for, 366
 setting, 200
Polio, eradication of, 310
Political advocates, 768
Political skills, 881–882
Politics
 community systems and, 385
 definition of, 197
Polity, 1001
Pollution, and communicable diseases, 77
Pollution Prevention Act (PPA), 141–142b
Polysubstance use or abuse, 821
Poor, economic risk and, 612
Popular epidemiology, 294–295
Population
 aging, 106
 changes in, 106
 characteristics of, 718–719
 definition of, 10–11, 19, 234
 disease patterns and, 274–275
 educational issues and, 421
 epidemiologic methods and, 272
 foreign-born, 46
 health of, role of, 66–67
 high-risk, definition of, 275
 Intervention Wheel assumptions and, 234
 linking content to practice and, 271b
 needs assessment, 502–503, 503t
Population at risk, 275
 definition of, 234
Population-based outcomes, 444
Population-centered nursing practice
 constitutional law and, 206
 ethics and core functions of, 156–157
 evidence-based practice methods for, 226–227
 in rural and urban environments, 716–734
  historic overview of, 716–717
Population-centered practice, 372
Population continuum, health on, 372f
Population-focused intervention, 869, 869b
Population-focused practice
 definition of, 10–11, 19
 developing population health nurse leaders, 17
 versus practice focused on individuals of, 10–11
 public health nursing and, 14f
Population-focused programs, 725–726
Population health, 438, 906–907
 definition of, 396–397, 397b, 698–699
 determinants of, 280f, 398f, 399f
 practice, 698t
Population management, 547
Population manager, 548
Population of interest, 234
Population replacement level, 46
Portfolios, 874–875, 1001
Positive predictive value, 284
Positive stress, vulnerability and, 703
Positron emission tomography (PET), 791–792
Post-visit phase, 618
Posttraumatic stress disorder (PTSD), 840
Potential lives lost, 97
Poverty, 735–755, 737f
 cohabitation and, 582
 concept of, 736–740
 defining and understanding, 736–740, 752
 and diarrhea, 80
 health effects of, 741, 752
  on children, 739, 741b
  on community, 745
  on older adults, 747–748, 747f
  on women, 739
 historical views of, 737–738, 738f
 levels of prevention for, 750b
 linking content to practice and, 751–752b
 neglected diseases of, 326
 quality and safety education for, 742b
 rates, by ethnic groups, 178t
 role of nurse and, 750–752, 751–752b, 751b
 status of children, 627, 627f
 teen pregnancy and, 780
 vulnerability and, 703–704, 713
Poverty income levels, 99
 Medicaid and, 111
Poverty Threshold Guidelines, 736, 736t
Power dynamics, 892
Practice focused on individuals, population-focused practice *versus*, 10–11
Practice guidelines, 532
Practice linkages, 911–914
 medication management of, 913–914
 outcome and assessment information, 912
 outcome-based quality improvement, 915
Practice models
 population-focused home care and, 900
 practice linkages and, 911–914
 transitional care and, 906, 906b
Practice setting, 900
Pre-existing conditions, 73
Pre-visit phase, 616–617, 616b
Preactive formulating, 503–505
Precaution adoption process model (PAPM), 403
Precautionary principle, 138–139
Precedent, 206
Preconceptual counseling, 664
Precontemplation, 403
Preferred provider organizations (PPOs), primary care and, 50
Pregnancy
 counseling for, 779
 homelessness and, 746
 migrant farmworker and, 761, 762b
 repeat, 782–783
 rural outcomes for, 721–722
 testing for, 779
 toxic exposures during, 137–138
Pregnancy prevention programs, 784

Pregnant teenagers, in school nursing, 950
Prejudice, 184–185
types of, 186b
Prematurity, 782
Premium competition, 113
Prenatal care, 780
initiation of, 780
Preparation for home visit: pre-visit phase, 616b
Preparedness, disaster management
disaster and mass casualty exercises and, 464–465, 465b
National Health Security Strategy and, 464
personal preparedness and, 459–460, 459–460b, 459f
professional preparedness and, 460–462
role of public health nurse in, 459–462
Preparedness, disaster management cycle, community preparedness and, 462–464, 463b, 463f
Preparing Registered Nurses for Enhanced Roles in Primary Care, 55
Preschoolers, developmental considerations and, 638
Prescriptive authority, 868
Presence, 981
Presentation, learning formats and, 421b
Presidential Policy Directive 8: National Preparedness (PPD-8), 457
President's Cancer Panel, 122
President's New Freedom Commission on Mental Health, 800
Preterm delivery, 780
Prevalence
comparison groups and, 286
comparison of incidence and, 277
cross-sectional studies and, 291
epidemiology of HIV/AIDS and, 336
Prevalence proportion, 276–277
Prevention
definition of, 235
focus on, vulnerable populations and, 711
hepatitis B virus and, 345
hepatitis C virus as, 346
Intervention Wheel assumptions and, 235–236
levels of, public health nursing and, 11b
of tuberculosis, 348b
Prevention-effectiveness analysis (PEAs), 100
Preventive interventions
intervention spectrum and, 282, 282f
levels of, 280–282, 281b
primary, 280–281
secondary, 281
tertiary, 281
Primary care case management (PCCM), 114
Primary care providers, 729
Primary caregiver, public health nurse as, 1020
Primary data, 285, 374
using of, 380
Primary health care (PHC), 54–55, 55b, 865, 870–871
barriers to integration, 54
concept of, 45
defined, 50, 359
and global health, 67
nurse-led health centers and, 440–441
quality and safety education for, 58b
Primary health care systems
integration of, 54
organization of, 50
quality and safety education for, 58b
Primary prevention, 99–100, 266b
communicable disease and, 348–351
assessment, 348–349
intervention, 349
community-level practice and, 236
definition of, 236b
epidemiology and, 280–281
health promotion and, 399
homelessness and, 749
infectious disease and, 310, 310b
mental illness and, 796
nursing care of working populations, 967
public health nursing practice and, 235–236
in school nursing, 937f, 938–940
Primary syphilis, 342
Principles of Bioethics, 154–156
Principles of Environmental Health for Nursing Practice, American Nurses Association's, 123b
Principlism, 151b, 154, 154b
Prioritizing, of data, 389
Privacy Rule, guidelines for, 448
Private contributions, 94
Private support, 112–115
employers and, 113–114
evolution of health insurance and, 112–113
health-specific savings accounts and, 115
individuals, 114
managed care arrangements and, 114
Private voluntary organizations (PVOs), 70
Problem/event, magnitude of, 490
Problem priority criteria, 391b
Problem-purpose-expansion method, of systematic problem solving, 563
Problem solving
generating alternatives and, 563
illuminating values and, 563
processes for, 152
systematic, 563
Process
evaluative studies and, 535
model CQI program and, 538–539
of regulation, 212–213
in structure-process-outcome evaluation, 517
Process data, 482
Process evaluation, 426, 499
Process model consultation, 885
Professional appraisal, 1001
Professional isolation, 875
Professional issues, in faith community nursing practice, 1001
Professional negligence, 207
Professional Standards Review Organization (PSRO), 526
Program, definition of, 499
Program effectiveness, 499
Program evaluation, 449, 509–512
aspects of, 511–512
benefits of, 509
definition of, 499
evaluation process and, planning for, 509–510, 510f
process of, 510–511, 510f
sources of, 511–512
Program management, 498–520
advanced planning methods and evaluation models and, 513–517
assessment of need and, 502–503, 502b
benefits of program planning and, 501–502
definitions and goals for, 499
historical overview of, 499–501, 500t
linking content to practice, 518b
planning process for, 503–509, 504t
program evaluation for, 509–512
program funding and, 517–518
Program management/supervisory level, 681b
Program planning, 391–392
Program planning method (PPM), 513–514, 514t
Program records, 509
Program resources, 504–505
Progress, 512
Prohibition, 812
Project BioShield, 466–467
Project DARE (Drug Abuse Resistance Education), 821–822
Project Hope, 69
Project Mosquito Net, 79
Projects, definition of, 499
Projects of National Significance, 693–694
Promote infection prevention standards, 914b
Promoting Health/Preventing Disease: Objectives for the Nation, 12
Propagated outbreak, 490
Proportion, 274
Proportionate mortality ratio (PMR), 278
Prospective cohort studies, 288–290, 289t
Prospective payment system (PPS), 110
Prospective reimbursement, 115
Prospective utilization review, 533–534
Prostate cancer, 668
Protected Health Information (PHI), 448
Protection and Advocacy Agencies (P&As), 693
Protection and Advocacy for Individuals with Mental Illness Act, 795
Protein, 82
Protestant women, nurses from, 990
Protocols, 868
Provident Hospital School of Nursing (Chicago), 29
Provider service records, 540
Provision of education, genetic/genomic knowledge for, 264
Psychiatric disorders, 75–76
Psychoactive drugs, 814, 815–819, 815b
alcohol, 815–816, 816b, 816f, 817t
cannabis (marijuana), 818, 818b
opioids, 818–819, 819f
tobacco, 816–818, 817t
Psychomotor domain, 417
Psychopharmacology, 791–792
Psychosocial agents, 965–966
Psychosocial development, 630
Psychosocial environment, 965–966
Psychosocial support, disaster recovery and, 475–476
PTSD *see* Posttraumatic stress disorder
Public Broadcasting Newshour, 562
Public good, 157
Public health, 1013–1014
community approach to, 1009–1010
core competencies of professionals, 7, 7b
core functions of, 5–7, 374
cost-effectiveness and, 97–98
definition, 3–5, 270–271
economics of, 93
essential services of, 4f, 5b
finance, 93
goal of, 93–94
of free-living, 14
health care financing and, 112
Healthy People 2020 and, 13b
history of, 22–44, 40b
1960s and nursing and, 36
from 1970s into twenty-first century, 37–38
during America's colonial period across new Republic, 23–26, 26f
change in, 23
community organization and, 36–37

Public health (Continued)
declining financial support for practice and professional organizations, 34–35, 35f
economic depression and rise of hospitals, 32
evidence-based practice and, 34b
federal action and, 32–33
health agencies and, 30–31
inadequate funding, for nurses in, 31
Industrial Revolution, 26–27
milestones in, 24–25t
Nightingale and origins of trained nursing in, 26–27
nursing education and, 35–36, 36b
profession comes of age and, 29–30
professional change and, 36–37
rise of chronic illness, 33–34
school nursing in America, 29
trained nurses and, 27–29
World War I and, 30–31
World War II and, 33
human genome and, 255–256
importance of, 5–6
integration of, 54
interprofessional application to, 408
investment in, 92
nursing specialization in, 9–13
policy, 196–217, 213b, 214b
quality and safety education for, 58b
quality improvement efforts in, 7
role of, 2
screening and, 282–284
support, Affordable Care Act and, 112
surveillance, 481–497
Public Health Accreditation Board (PHAB), 528, 915, 1012, 1015
Public Health and Professional Nurse Traineeships, 33
Public Health Code of Ethics, 157, 159b
Public health departments, 873
Public Health Foundation, 7
Public Health Information Network (PHIN), 466–467
Public health infrastructure, strengthening, objectives pertaining to, 56b
Public Health Institute, 364
Public Health Leadership Society (PHLS), Skills for the Ethical Practice of Public Health and, 160
Public health nurse (PHN), 371
climate change and, 129
community as client and, 372
comprehensive primary health care centers and, 440
future of genetics/genomics and, 266–267
Intervention Wheel and, 232, 232f
levels of practice and, 236
Public health nurse (Continued)
role in disaster response and, 470–474, 471t
sickle cell anemia case example and, 259
in the twenty-first century, 104
in vulnerable population group, 709
Public health nursing, 37–38
as area of specialization, 9–13
barriers to specializing in, 16–17
community, models and frameworks of, 401–403
community-based nursing *versus,* 14–15, 14f
community-based participatory research and, 401–403
competencies for disaster, 460–461, 461b
core functions of, 12–13, 156, 228t
cornerstones of, 239b
definition of, 15b, 1013–1014
determinants of health and, 234–235
developing population health nurse leaders in, 17
disaster management cycle and, 454–480
DNA and, 257–259
educational preparation for, 10, 10b
evidence-based practice to, 228
as foundation for healthy, for populations and communities, 2–9, 4f, 5b
future challenges in, 16–18
genomics in, 255–268
Intervention Wheel assumptions and, 234–239
levels of, 236
linking content to practice and, 40b
local, state, national levels of, 1009–1025, 1011b, 1023b
education and knowledge requirements for, 1018, 1018b
functions of nurses in, 1019–1023, 1020f
history and trends in, 1012–1013
issues and trend in, 1016–1017
models of practice for, 1017–1018
national health objectives for, 1018–1019
roles of, 1010–1012
scopes, standards, roles of, 1013–1016, 1014b, 1016b
policy development and, 13
population-focused practice, *versus* practice focused on individuals, 10–11
populations and, 18b
practice of, 270–271
principles of, 11b
process of, 236–237t, 241t, 248
Public health nursing (Continued)
resources for, 6b
roles in, 15–16
shifting public health practice and, 17–18
specialists in, 12–13
values and beliefs in, 239
Public Health Nursing: Population-Centered Health Care in the Community, 438
Public Health Nursing: Scope and Standards of Practice, 159–160, 239
Public Health Nursing Competencies, 375
Public health nursing process
application of, at community level of practice scenario, 249–251
at community level scenario
action plan and, 250
assessment and, 249–250
classroom activities and, 250
diagnosis and, 250
evaluation and, 251
family involvement and, 250
implementation plan and, 250
menu changes and, 250
diagnosis, 248–249
evaluation of, 249
family assessment, 248
implementation of, 249
planning, 249
systems level of practice scenario, application of, 251–252
assessment and, 251
diagnosis and, 251
evaluation and, 252
implementation and, 251–252
planning and, 251
Public Health Nursing Section, of APHA, 30
Public health nursing specialists
in defining problems, 11
evidence-based practice for, 12–13b
Public health programs, 1009
Public health protection, 481–482
Public Health Security and Bioterrorism Preparedness and Response Act (US Law 2002 PL 107-188), 198
Public Health Service (PHS), government roles and, 197–198
Public health surge, 455
Public health systems, 93
organization of, 50
public health nurse, 1009, 1010f
Public Health Threats and Emergencies Act (PL 106-505), 198
Public law, 116
Public policy, definition of, 197
Public protection, government health care functions and, 200
Public support
health care financing and, 109–112
other, 112
PulseNet, 320, 489
Purified protein derivative (PPD) test, 347

Q

Quad Council of Public Health Nursing Organizations, 124b, 375
cultural competency and, 189b
genetics/genomics and, 266b
history of, 39
migrant farmworkers and, 767b
population health concepts and, 271b
principles of public health nursing and, 1014, 1014b
public health nurses and, 9–10
Public Health Nursing Competencies and, 39
rural health settings and, 731b
vulnerable populations and, 708b
Quadruple Aim, 440
Quality, evaluating evidence and, 224
Quality assurance (QA), 509, 525
evaluation of outcome and, 539
measures, 539t
using QA/QI, 532, 532t
Quality health indicators, 447
Quality improvement, 522–523
general approaches to, 527–528
specific approaches to, 528–530
using QA/QI, 532, 532t
Quality improvement organization (QIO), 526
Quality management, 521–545, 530b
approaches to quality improvement and, 526–530
commonly used abbreviations in, 522t
definitions and goals for, 524–526
historical development of, 526
linking content to, 541b
Quality of adjusted life-years (QALYs), 97
Quality of care, cultural competence and, 168
Quality program, approaches to, 525
Quality review, professional review organizations and, 534–535
Quantity, evaluating evidence and, 224
Quinine, 79
Quintile, 47

R

Rabies (hydrophobia), 325
Race, 170, 170f, 583
mortality rates by, 287
Racism, 185, 738
types of, 186b
Radiation poisoning, 85
Radon, 133
Randomization, 225, 292
Randomized controlled trial (RCT), 221

Rape, 840
"Rape" kit collection, forensic nurse, 979–980
Rape trauma syndrome, 979–980
Rapid needs assessment, nursing role in, 471
Rapid re-housing, 745
Rate, 274–275
adjustment, 286
Rathbone, William, 27
Rationing, of health care, 98
REACH U.S., 360
Reactive formulating, 503–505
Readmission, reducing the rate of, 558
Reagan, President Ronald, 501
Reality norms, 429
Recognition, 528
Recombinant bovine growth hormone (rBGH), 134
Reconstruction phase, 469
Records, 540–541
community and public health agency, 540–541
previous, pre-encounter data collection, 591
Recovery
after disaster, 474–476
role of public health nurse, 475–476
in mental health, 797
Recreation, community systems and, 385
Red Cross Rural Nursing Service, 716–717
Red wedge, 238f, 239
Referral
and follow-up, 241t, 244, 245b, 249, 251
genetic/genomic nursing assessment and, 264
public health nurses and, 1020
source, 590–591
Refugees, 176
Regional Program for Nursing Research Development (WICHEN), 219
Registered nurses (RN), 206
genetic/genomic knowledge of, 263–264
role in primary care, 55
Regulations, 206
Medicare-certified agencies and, 902–903
Regulatory action, 211–212, 212f
Rehabilitation, 673
Rehabilitation Act of 1973, 692
Section 504 of, 931
Reimbursement
for home health, palliative care, and hospice, 917
systems, nurse-led health centers and, 440
"Reinstitutionalization," 795
Relapse management, 797
Relational health, 737
Relationship-based practice, 439
Relative risk, 275–276
Relevance, 511
Reliability, 283
Relief Nursing Service, 32
Religiosity, 990
Religious care, 995
Religious organizations, 71
Religious symbols, 994f
Remarriage, 590
Repeat pregnancy, 782–783
Report cards, 523
Reproductive age, workplace hazards to women of, 137t
Reproductive function, 579
Reproductive health
adolescent and, 774
women's health concerns and, 664–665
Request for proposals (RFP), 446
Required home visit, 617
Requisite variety of rules of transformation, 611
Research utilization, 219
Researcher, 870, 870b
as nurse-led health centers staff, 444
role of school nurse as, 935
Resilience, 701
Resistance, 303
Resource-based relative value scale (RBRVS), 116
Resource Center, for faith community nursing, 991
Resource Conservation and Recovery Act (RCRA), 141–142b
Resources, allocation of, and health care, 98–99
Respect, vulnerable populations and, 710
Respect for autonomy, 154, 154b
Respite care, 672
Respondeat superior, 207
Response, disaster, 465–474
to biological incidents, 466–467
National Incident Management System and, 465–466, 466f
National Response Framework and, 465
psychological stress of, workers in, 474
role of public health nurse in, 470–474, 471t
Retail clinics, 871
Retrospective audit, 533–534
Retrospective cohort studies, 289t, 290
Retrospective reimbursement, 115
Retrospective utilization review, 533–534
Rewards, 439
Ribonucleic acid (RNA), 257
Richmond (Virginia) Nurses ' Settlement, 28
Rifampin, 78
Right to know
environmental health and, 135
nurses and, 130
Risk, 439
appraisals of, 402–403
definition of, 140, 140b, 275, 698
health of nation and, 607
measure of incidence and, 275–276
ratio and, 276
vulnerability and, 701, 713
Risk assessment, of environmental health, 135
Risk-based plans, and managed care, 114
Risk communication, 140–141, 471
Risk management, 139
traditional quality assurance and, 534
Robert T. Stafford Disaster Relief and Emergency Assistance Act, 465
Robert Wood Johnson Foundation (RWJF), 376–377
Center to Advance Palliative Care and, 903
health care for homeless and, 750
Rockefeller Foundation, 71
Rockefeller Sanitary Commission, 30
Rocky Mountain spotted fever (RMSF), 323
Rogers, Lina, 29
Role structure, 429, 429b
Root, Frances, 27
Rotavirus, 80
Route of exposure, 140
Rubella, 315–316
Rules of transformation, 611
Rural communities
availability and access of health care in, 721
care delivery and barriers to health care in, 725–726, 725b
chronic illness in, 719–720, 720b
current perspectives in, 718–725
definition of terms for, 717
demographics of, 718, 730
environmental and occupational health risks in, 723–725
future perspectives for
Healthy People 2020 objectives and, 730
scarce resources and, 729, 729b
health care in, issues and barriers to care of, 725–726, 725b
health of children in, 722
health of minorities in, 723
health status in, 719–725, 733
historic overview of, 716–717
homelessness in, 743, 752
linking content to practice and, 731b
maternal-infant health in, 721–722
mental health in, 722–723
nursing care in, 726–729
patterns of health service use in, 721, 721b
perceived health status in, 719
Rural communities *(Continued)*
physical limitations and, 720–721
professional-community-client partnerships in, 730–732, 731b
Rural Healthy People 2010: A Companion Document to Healthy People, 730
Rural practice setting, 728–729
Rural-urban continuum, 717–718
Rural-urban residency, 718f
Rurality, 717
Rush, Benjamin, 793
Rwandan genocide, 85
Ryan White HIV/AIDS Treatment Extension Act of 2009, 334

S

Sackett, David, 219
Safe Cosmetics databases, 130, 130f
Safe Drinking Water Act (SDWA), 141–142b
Safe Routes to Schools initiative, 405–406
Safety
community systems and, 384–385
concepts in forensic nursing and, 981–982
definition of, 18b
home visits and, 591–592
Safety net, 741–742
Safety net providers, 99, 438
vulnerable populations and, 707
Saliva, rabies transmission, 325
Salmon, Marla, 201
Salmonellosis, 321
Sample selection, 225
Sample size, 225
"Sandwich generation," 686
SANE-A, 983
SANE-P, 983
Santa Cruz County, snapshot of, 389, 390f
Saunders, Dame Cicely, 903
Scaling factor, 277–278
School, 873
built environment and, 635
migrant children and, 765
pregnant teens and, 783
School-age children, developmental considerations and, 638
School for Deaconesses, 26–27
School Health Policies and Practices Study, 936–937
School health services, 935–937, 935b
federal school health programs and, 936, 936f
school-based health programs and, 936–937
school health policies and practices study 2016 and, 936–937
School nurse practitioner program, 931t
School nursing, 928–956, 943b
assessing and screening children at, 942–943

School nursing *(Continued)*
controversies in, 950
definition of, 933
educational and licensure credentials of, 933–934
ethics in, 950–951
federal legislation affecting, 931–932
functions of, 934–935
future trends in, 951–952
giving medication in, 942–943
Healthy People 2020 and, 937, 937b
history of, 29, 929–931, 931t
linking content to practice, 952b
online resources for, 951t
roles and functions of, 934–935
school health services and, 935–937
standards of practice for, 933
School-based health centers (SBHCs), 936–937
Scope and Standards of Practice, in faith community nursing, 993, 994
Scope and Standards of Public Health Nursing Practice, 9–10
Screening
definition of, 244
epidemiology and, 282–284
programs for, 282b
reliability of, 283
school nursing and, 241t, 244b
sensitivity of, 283–284
specificity of, 283–284
validity of, 283–284, 284t
Seamless system of care, 881–882
Seasonal farmworker, 756–757
Secondary data, 285, 374, 502
Secondary prevention, 266b
communicable diseases and, 351
definition of, 236b
epidemiology and, 281
homelessness and, 749
infectious disease and, 310, 310b
mental illness and, 796
nursing care of working populations, 968
PHN intervention and, 236
school nursing and, 937f, 940–946
screening and, 282
Secondary syphilis, 342
Section 504 of the Rehabilitation Act, 931
Secular trends, 287–288
Seguro Popular program, 73
Selected membership group, 431
Selection bias, 293
Selective survival, 288–289
Self-actualization, Maslow's theory of, 981
Self-insure, and employers, 113–114
Self-pay, as income source, 446
Senior center, as community care setting, 672
Senior management/executive level, 681b
Sensitivity, 283–284
Sentinel method, 535
Sentinel surveillance system, 284, 485
Series testing, 284
Serious mental illness, 790
Service animals, 694
Service delivery networks, 881–882
Service to others, 157
Settlement houses, 28
Seven "A's," 387–388, 388b
Severe acute respiratory syndrome (SARS)
in China, 74–75
history of, 301
Severe mental disorders, 789
Sex, mortality rates by, 287
Sexual abstinence, 349–350
Sexual abuse, 844
child, 847
teen pregnancy and, 776–777
Sexual activity, teens and, 776
Sexual assault nurse examiners (SANEs), 842, 977, 983
Sexual behavior, 349–350
adolescents and, 774–775
Sexual debut, 776
Sexual history, 348, 349b
Sexual practices, 349
Sexual risk assessment, 348–349
Sexual victimization, 776–777
Sexually transmitted diseases (STDs), 335b, 339–344, 340–341t, 840
adolescents and, 774, 774b
adult health concerns and, 663
chlamydia and, 342–343
cohabitation and, 582
gonorrhea and, 339–342
herpes simplex virus and, 343
human papillomavirus infection and, 343–344
prevention of, 663b
syphilis and, 342
Shattuck Report, 26
Shelter Plus Care, 749
Sheltering, nursing role in, 473–474
Sheppard-Towner Act, 31
policy setting and, 200
Shiga toxin-producing *E. coli* (STEC), 321
Shiprock Service Unit of the Indian Health Service, Intervention Wheel adoption and, 246
Short course chemotherapy, 78
Short-term evaluation, 426
Sickle cell anemia, case example on, 259
Sidestream smoke, 817
Single-photon emission computed tomography (SPECT), 791–792
Single-room-occupancy (SRO), 742–743
Sister Mary Augustine, 26
Sisters of Charity, Roman Catholic, 26
Skill development, for nurse advocate, 563
Skilled nursing facility (SNF), 110
Skilled nursing service, 902
Skin diseases, 760
Skinner, B.F., 405–406
Sleet, Jessie (Scales), 29
Sliding-fee, 446
"Small" communities, 717, 717b
Smallpox, 76, 312–313, 312b
SNOMED CT, 919
Social action model, 360
Social cognitive theory (SCT), 403–404
Social determinants of health (SDOH), 405–406, 405b, 735
nursing models of care and, 438
vulnerability and, 699–700
Social-ecological model, 372, 404, 705–706t, 705f
Social epidemiology, 279–280
Social exclusion, 737
Social interconnection, 737
Social justice, 154, 160, 372
market justice *versus,* 160t
vulnerable populations and, 701
Social mandate, 548
Social marketing, 241t, 245, 250
Social media, 418, 635–636
Social model of disability, 679
Social networking, 644
Social planning model, 360
Social policy, 599
Social risks, 612
Social Security Act (PL 92-603), 526, 534–535
Social Security Act of 1935, 102
government role in health care and, 197–198
vulnerable populations and, 706
Social Security Act of 1965
increased Medicare costs and, 110
Medicaid program and, 628
national health insurance and, 36
Title XIX of, 111
Title XVIII of, 109–111
Social Security Administration (SSA)
disability and, 679
models of disability and, 679
Social service models, for case management, 558
Social services, community systems and, 385–386
Social supports, for vulnerable populations, 713
Social workers, 443
collaboration and, 917
Socialization function, 579
Society for Women's Research, 654
Socioeconomic factors, maternal-infant health and, 722
Socioeconomic status, health disparities and, 178–179, 700
Soil, 134
Sound wave sources, 134
Sovereign immunity, 207
Spatial data, 379–380
Special care centers, 441–442
Special populations, disabilities in, 687
Special systems, as surveillance system, 489–490, 489b
Specialization, in faith community nursing, 992–993
Specialty case management, 549
Specific protection, 399
primary prevention and, 280–281
Specificity, 283–284
Spiritual care, 994
Spirituality, 174, 990
Sporadic problems, 490
Sports injuries, 638–640, 639f, 639t
Sports specialization, 639
Spouse abuse, 847–849
St. Mary's Hospital, 557–558
St. Paul-Ramsey County (MN) Department of Health, Intervention Wheel adoption and, 247, 247f
Staff public health nurses, 15
Staff review committee, 533
Stages of change (SOC), 403
Stakeholders, 377, 439
Standard population, 286
Standard precautions, 942
communicable diseases and, 353
Standardized mortality ratio (SMR), 286
Standards for Community Health Nursing Practice, 526
Standards of Occupational and Environmental Health Nursing Practice, 959
Standards of practice
advocacy and, 159–160
for forensic nurses, 982
for school nursing, 933
Standards of Practice for Case Management, 549, 568
State Cancer Profile, 377t
State Child Health Improvement Act (SCHIP) of 1997, 198
State Comprehensive Mental Health Services Plan Act of, 795
State Councils on Developmental Disabilities (SCDD), 693
State Health Access Data Assistance Center (SHADAC), 377t
State health commissioner, 1011
State health department, 206
State public health agency, 1011
State system, 52
States, case management and, 558
Statistical analysis, 225
Statistical associations, causality and, 292–293
Statutory rape, 776–777
STDs *see* Sexually transmitted diseases
Step 0, 222
Steps Communities, 360
Stereotyping, 184
Stewart, Ada Mayo, 29, 958
Stewart B. McKinney Homeless Assistance Act of, 748

Stewart Machine Co. v. Davis, 197
Stimulants, 815, 815b
Stop TB partnership, 78
Strategic Alliances for Health Communities, 360
Strategic National Stockpile (SNS), 458–459, 466–467
Strategic plan, nursing centers and, 439–440, 446
Strategic planning, definition of, 501
Streptococcus pyogenes, 300
Stress
 health burden of, 791
 mental health in adults and, 802
 migrant farmworkers and, 763
 vulnerability and, 703
 work-related and, 965–966
Stress reaction
 in community, disaster and, 468–469, 470f
 in individuals, disaster and, 467–468, 467b, 468b, 468f, 469f
Stressors, multiple, 710
Stroke, adult health concerns and, 661
Structure
 evaluation of, 517
 evaluative studies and, 535
 model CQI program and, 538
Structure-process-outcome evaluation, 517
Students, as nurse-led health centers staff, 444
Stunting, and poor nutrition, 82
Sub-Saharan Africa, maternal and women's health in, 81
Subpopulations, 10–11, 12f
Substance abuse, 814
 prevention education, 938–939
Substantial gainful activity (SGA), 679
Suburbs, 717b, 718
Sudden infant death syndrome (SIDS), 642–643
Sudden unexpected infant death (SUID), 642–643
 investigations, 981
Sudden Unexplained Infant Death Investigation program, 977
Suffering in Silence: A Report on the Health of California's Agricultural Workers, 759
Suicide, 842–843
 adolescent mental health and, 802
 case-control studies and, 290
 prevention of, 945
Summative evaluation, 499
Superfund Amendments and Reauthorization Act (SARA), 141–142b, 973–974b
Superfund sites, 134
Supervision, 891
Supplemental Security Income (SSI)
 migrant farmworkers and, 759
 older adults and, 753
Supply and demand, 95, 95b, 95f
Support, genetic/genomic knowledge for, 264
Support staff, 444
Supporting, in advocacy process, 562
Supportive housing, 749
Surveillance
 of communicable diseases, 304–306
 definition of, 241
 elements of, 304–306, 305b
 epidemiology and, 284
 HIV of, 337
 nursing role in, disaster and, 471
 public health
  case definitions and, 488
  collaboration in, 483–484
  data sources for, 485–486, 486b
  definitions of, 482
  features of, 482
  Healthy People 2020 and, 486b
  investigation and, 490–492
  notifiable disease and, 486–488, 487b
  nurse competencies in, 484–485
  nursing process and, 241t, 252
  purposes of, 483
 systems
  active system as, 489
  linking content to practice and, 494b
  passive system as, 488
  sentinel systems as, 489
  special systems as, 489–490, 489b
  types of, 488–490
Survey of Income and Program Participation (SIPP), disability determination and, 679
Survivor, in mental health, 801
Survivors, 842
Sustainability, 512
 for nursing centers, 450
Syndromic surveillance systems, 305, 489
Syphilis, 340–341t, 342
System-focused models, for case management, 558
Systematic review, 222
Systems-level practice, 236, 240–241
Systems theory
 community mental health and, 796
 for family, 588
Systems thinking, 884

T

Tanzania Nurse Initiative, 69–70
Targeted competency, 632b
Task Force on Community Preventive Services, 223b
 Centers for Disease Control and, 6
Task function, 428
Task norm, 428
Tax credit, 73
TEACH mnemonic, 418–419
Teamwork
 case management and, 565–567
 definition of, 18b
Technical intervention, 525
Techniques, to quality program, 525
Technology
 corporate era, 103
 definition of, 104
 health care spending and, 107
 introduction to less developed countries, 72
 medical, 100–101
 postindustrial era, 102
 preindustrial era, 101
 rural health practice and, 728–729
Technology specialist, 444
Teen pregnancy, 772–788
 see also Adolescents
 background factors for, 775–777
  other factors of, 776–777
  peer pressure and partner pressure and, 776
  sexual activity and use of birth control and, 776
 early identification of, 779–780
 nurse and
  community-based interventions and, 784
  home-based interventions and, 783–784, 783f
 prenatal care and, 780
 prevention of, 599, 784
 special issues in caring for, 780–783
 young men and paternity, 777–779, 778f
Teenage mother, in school nursing, 950
Telehealth
 home health/hospice nursing and, 920
 rural health practice and, 728–729
 technology and, 920
Telehomecare, 620–621
Telemedicine, 728–729
Telemonitoring, 920
Telephone-based collaborative care, 558
Temporary Assistance to Needy Families (TANF), 656
 homeless families and, 748
 poverty and, 737
Ten essential public health services, 372
"Ten Essential Services of Public Health"
 Intervention Wheel assumptions and, 239
Termination, 598
Termination phase, 618
Tertiary prevention, 235, 236b, 266b
 communicable diseases and, 352–353
 epidemiology and, 281
Tertiary prevention *(Continued)*
 health promotion and, 399–400
 homelessness and, 749
 infectious disease and, 310, 310b
 school nursing, 937f, 946–950, 946b
  children with asthma and, 947
  children with autism, ADHD and, 947–949
  children with diabetes mellitus and, 947
  children with DNAR orders, 950
  children with special needs, 949–950
  homebound children, 950
  pregnant teenagers and teenage mothers at school, 950
 in working populations, 968
Tertiary syphilis, 342
Test tube baby, 102
Testicular cancer, 668–669
The Community Guide, 360
The Community Guide: What Works to Promote Health, 6
The Joint Commission, 102
 accreditation and, 915
 disease management and, 557
 sexual assault victim protocol and, 979–980
"The new federalism", 501
Theory-based family nursing, 587f
Therapeutic question, 592
Third-party payers
 financing from, 109
 prospective reimbursement and, 115
 system, 113
Third-party reimbursement, 864–865
Thymine, 257
Ticks
 prevention and control of diseases from, 323
 vector-borne diseases and, 322
Time, descriptive epidemiology and, 287–288
Time perception, cultural competence and, 172
Title protection, 211
Title VI, 32
To Err Is Human, 881
To Err Is Human: Building a Safer Health System, 49
Tobacco, 816–818, 817t
Toddlers
 developmental considerations and, 638
 in migrant camp, 757b
Tolerable stress, vulnerability and, 703
Tolerance, 816–817
Tools for community action, 360
Tools for Schools, 133
Toronto, Healthy Cities movement and, 66, 67b
Total quality management (TQM), definition of, 531–535, 531t

Town and Country Nursing Service, 29
Toxic shock syndrome, 300
Toxic stress, 740–742
 vulnerability and, 703
Toxic Substances Control Act (TSCA), 141–142b
Toxic waste activists, 295
Toxicants, 136
Toxicology, 125–127, 126t
TOXNET, 143–144
Toxoplasma gondii, 327
ToxTown, 130
Tracer method, 517, 535
Tracers, 517
Traditional beliefs and practices, 765
 migrants and, 765
Traditional quality assurance, 532–535
 risk management and, 534
 staff review committee and, 533
 utilization review and, 533–534
Trans-Indiana National Road Heritage Trail (NRHT), 363–364, 364f
Transcultural nursing, 166
Transitional care
 faith community nurse and, 993b
 practice models and, 906, 906b
Transitional care home visits, 442
Transitional Care Model, 906
 in faith community nursing, 991–992
Transitions, 610
 of care, 577–578
Transmission mode, of infectious diseases, 304
Transportation, community systems and, 384–385
Transtheoretical model (TTM), 403, 425
Trauma, homelessness and, 744–745
Travelers, diseases of, 323–324
 diarrheal, 324
 foodborne and waterborne, 324
 malaria and, 324
Triage, 470–471, 472f
True negatives, 283
True positives, 283
Trust, vulnerable populations and, 710
Trust for America's Health (TFAH), 97–98
 bioterrorism and public health preparedness, 462b
Trust plans, U.K. health care system, 74
Truth, 982
Truth telling, 160b
Tsunamis, 83–84
TTM *see* Transtheoretical model
Tuberculin skin test (TST), 347, 347b
Tuberculosis (TB), 77–78
 African-American population and, 29
 diagnosis and treatment of, 347
 directly observed therapy programs for, 352–353
 epidemiology of, 346–347
Tuberculosis *(Continued)*
 human immunodeficiency virus and, 78
 introduction to, 346–347, 347t
 migrant farmworkers and, 763
 millennium development goals and, 77–78
 multidrug resistance of, 78
 transmission of, 964
 Working Group on, 77–78
Tularemia, 311
Tuskegee syphilis study, 185

U

Uganda, health care systems in, 73
Ukraine, Chernobyl meltdown, 84
UN Commission on the Status of Women, 201
Unauthorized immigrants, 176
Underinsured
 client, 577–578
 families in community and, 578–579
Underuse of service, 525
UNICEF *see* United Nations Children's Fund
Uninsured
 access to health care and, 49
 adult, health disparities, 671
 families in community and, 578–579
 resource allocation and, 98
Unintended pregnancy, 664
Unintentional injuries, 637–638, 638t
United Kingdom, health care systems in, 74
United Nations (UN), 201
 genocide and, 85
United Nations Children's Fund (UNICEF), international health organizations, 70
 children under 5 and, 70
 less developed countries and, 81
 women's health and, 81
United States
 health care cost and, 93
 healthy communities and cities in, 360
 NAFTA and, 66
Universal health care, 74
Universal precautions, 328
University Centers for Excellence in Developmental Disabilities-Education, Research and Services (UCEDD), 693
University of Colorado, nurse practitioner movement and, 36
University of Kentucky' s College of Nursing, 13
University of Tennessee Health Science Center, 980
Unsheltered homeless, 743
Urban communities, 717
 homelessness in, 745–750
U.S. Agency for International Development (USAID), 70
U.S. Census, 377t
 population data and, 285
U.S. Constitution, 206
 Article I, Section 8, 197
U.S. Consumer Product Safety Commission
 guidelines for playground safety and, 641
 lead in toys, steps to minimize, 646b
U.S. Department of Health and Human Services (USDHHS), 51, 51f, 52f, 52t, 53b, 109
 agencies of, 201–202
 Bureau of Primary Health Care (BPHC) and, 441
 disabilities and, 683
 federal poverty guideline and, 703
 government role in health care and, 197–200
 local and state influence of, 1002 1010
 Personalized Health Care Initiative and, 262–263
 primary prevention and, 100
U.S. Department of Homeland Security (USDHS), 52
U.S. Department of Housing and Urban Development, 748
U.S. Department of Justice, Guide to Disability Rights Law by, 691–692
U.S. Environmental Protection Agency (EPA), waterborne disease outbreaks and, 322
U.S. Preventive Services Task Force (USPSTF), 360
 evidence-based practice resources and, 223b
 Recommendations for Primary Care Practice, 100
 screening guidelines of, 283
U.S. Public Health Service (USPHS), 51–52, 109, 872
 African American nurses and, 31
 establishment of, 26
 injury prevention and, 977
 Nursing Council on National Defense and, 33
 Pearl McIver and, 32
 on Tuskegee Syphilis Study, 185
 World War I, 30–31
U.S. Public Health Services Advisory Committee on Immunization Practices (ACIP), 632
U.S. Public Health Services Task Force on Women's Health Issues, 654
U.S. Surgeon General
 communicable disease surveillance and, 304
 violence as health care issue and, 979–980
USDHHS *see* U.S. Department of Health and Human Services
USPHS *see* U.S. Public Health Service (USPHS)
USPTSF *see* U.S. Preventive Services Task Force
Usual, customary, and reasonable (UCR) charges, 116
Utilitarian framework, 473
Utilitarianism, 151b, 153–154, 372, 984
Utilization management, 548
Utilization review, 533–534

V

Vaccination
 animals and, 325
 event-related clusters and, 288
 for hepatitis A infection, 344
 for hepatitis B infection, 345
 and millennium development goals, 76
 for schoolchildren, 939–940
Vaccine Adverse Event Reporting System (VAERS), 632
Vaccine information statements (VIS), 632
Vaccines for Children (VFC), 631
Vaccinia vaccine, 312
Valid results, 283
Validity, 283–284, 284t
Value-based health care, 547
Values, 151b
 subgroups and, 717b, 718–719
Vancomycin-resistant *Staphylococcus aureus* (VRSA), 300
Variance analysis, 893
Variant Creutzfeldt-Jakob disease (vCJD), 300
Variation of service, 525
Vector-borne diseases, 322–323
 Lyme disease and, 322–323
 Rocky Mountain spotted fever and, 323
 tick-borne disease prevention/control and, 323
 zoonoses and, 324–325
Vectors, 304
Veil of ignorance, 155t
Veracity, 568
Verbal communication, cultural competence and, 172–173
Verifying, 562
Vermont Marble Company, 29
Vertical integration, 103, 881–882
Vertical transmission, 304
Veterans, 659
Viable community health model, rationale for health community nursing, 991–992
Viagra, 107
Vibrio cholerae, 80
Victim, of violence, 979, 982b
Victimization, 982
Violence, 836–862, 837b
 definition, 837
 family violence and abuse, 843–851
  development of abusive patterns, 843–844
  types of intimate partner and family violence, 844–851, 845b, 848b
 against individuals or oneself, 839–843
  assault, 839–840
  homicide, 839
  human trafficking, 840–842

Violence *(Continued)*
rape, 840
suicide, 842–843
nursing interventions, 851–858, 852b
primary prevention, 851–852, 851b
secondary prevention, 852–854, 853f, 854b
tertiary prevention, therapeutic intervention with abusive families, 854–858, 855b
pregnant teen and, 780
prevention, 981, 982b
at school, 945–946
social and community factors influencing, 837–839, 837b, 838f
community, 838
individual, 837
relationship, 837
societal, 838–839
in workplace, 966
Virtue ethics, 155
application of, 160b
Virtues, 155
Virulence, 490
Visiting nurse
education of, 30
history of nursing and, 28
Visiting Nurse Association (VNA), 28, 36f, 540
Visiting Nurse Association of America, 918
Visiting Nurse Association of Omaha, 907
Visiting Nurse Quarterly, 29–30
Visiting Nurse Service of New York, 28, 28f, 902
Visiting Nurse Society of Philadelphia, 33
Visiting Nursing in the United States, 29
Vital records, 285
Vitamin A, 82
Volcanic eruptions, 84
Voluntary home visit, 617
Volunteers, opportunities in disaster work, 462b
Voting Accessibility for the Elderly and the Handicapped Act of 1984, 694
Vulnerability
definition of, 701–704
health disparities and, 701–704
outcomes of, 704–709
risk factors and, 701
Vulnerable population group, 701–702, 713
assessment issues and, 709–713
check your practice and, 708b
ethical dilemmas with, 707, 708b
examples of, 701–702
linking content to practice and, 708b
nursing approaches to care and, 706–709
nursing roles in, 708b
planning and implementing care for, 710–713
case study on, 711b
Vulnerable population group *(Continued)*
public policies affecting, 704–706
quality and safety education for, 707b
trend in caring for, 706
Vulnerable populations, 397, 697–715
public health nursing and, 1015–1016
teenage parent families at risk, 621b

W

Waivers, and Medicaid, 111
Wakefield, Mary, 161
Wald, Florence, 903
Wald, Lillian, 706
environmental health history and, 124–125
Henry Street Settlement and, 18
nursing centers and, 438
nursing history and, 28
school nursing and, 929
Walking trail, 364f
War on Poverty, 738–739
Wars, and global health, 65
Washington v Harper(1990), 983
Water, 133–134
potable, 324
sources, contamination of, 63, 77
Waterborne disease and outbreak (WBDOs), 322
Waterborne Disease and Outbreaks Surveillance System, 322
Waterborne diseases
infectious disease prevention and, 319–322
outbreaks and pathogens of, 321–322
parasitic infections and, 327
travelers and, 324
Waters, Yssabella, 29
Watson, James, 256
Web of causality, 278–279
Web of causation model, vulnerable population group and, 701–702
Weight, control of, 663–664
Weight gain, during pregnancy, 781, 781t
Welfare reform, 1016
Wellness centers, 442–443
Wellness committee, 995
Wellness recovery action plan, 804
West Nile virus (WNV), 300, 307
Westberg, Granger, 990–991
Westberg Institute, 991, 999
Whelan, Linda Tarr, 201
White blood cell count, CD4, 334
Whites, viewing cohabitation, 582
WHO *see* World Health Organization
Whole-cell vaccine, 316
Whole person care, 995
Whooping cough *see* Pertussis
Wife abuse, 847–849
Wilburn, Susan, 143
Williams, Dr. Carolyn, 201
Windshield survey, 131–132, 381, 383t
Wingspread Statement on the Precautionary Principle, 138, 138b
Winslow, C.E.A., definition of public health and, 270
Wisconsin Department of Health, Intervention Wheel adoption and, 246
WISER-Wireless information system for emergency responders, 460, 461b
Withdrawal, 814
W.K. Kellogg Foundation, 71, 363
Women
with disabilities, 687–688
health effects of poverty on, 739
homeless, 746–747
and human immunodeficiency virus, 81
in workforce, 960
Women, Infants, and Children (WIC) program, 200, 736
economic risk and, 612
homeless families and, 748
Women for Sobriety, 831
Women's health, 654
breast cancer and, 666
cardiovascular disease and, 660–661
concerns of, 664–666
historical perspective of, 654
iron deficiency and, 82–83
maternal health and, 81–82
menopause and, 665
osteoporosis and, 666
Work, characteristics of, 960–961
Work-health interactions, 958, 961–962, 962f
Work-related health problem, 959
Worker assessment, 968–970
Worker health and safety, organizational and public efforts to promote, 966–967
Workers' Compensation, 973
migrant farmworkers and, 759
Workforce
characteristics of, 960, 961f
competencies and, 157
health care providers as, 102
population aggregate and, 960
women and, 960
Working Group on Tuberculosis, 77–78
Working poor, 719, 733
Working population, nursing care of, 967–972
Workplace
assessment, 970–972
changes in, 960
exposure, of worker, 968–970
hazards, 960–961
Works Progress Administration (WPA), 32
Worksite assessment guide, 971f
Worksite walk-through, 970
World Association for Disaster and Emergency Medicine (WADEM), 458
World Bank, as international health organization, 70
World Health Assembly (WHA), 63, 201
World Health Organization (WHO)
Alcohol, Smoking, and Substance Involvement Screening Test (ASSIST), 822
China and, 74
definition of health and, 270, 396
definition of mental health by, 790
diarrhea and, 80
environmental sanitation and, 77
Expanded Program on Immunization, 76–77
factors that affect health and, 699–700
forensic nursing history and, 978
functional disability and, 680
global burden of disease and, 75–76
as global health organization, 69–70
Global Outbreak Alert and Response Network and, 86
Global Tuberculosis Program (GTB) and, 78
Health Assembly, 55
health definition and, 371
health promotion definition and, 399–400
Healthy Cities program, 373
HFA21 and, 66
injury prevention and, 977
international organizations and, 201
malaria and, 324
maternal mortality and, 81
Ottawa charter of, 358
primary health care and, 67
smallpox and, 76
social determinants of health and, 405
tuberculosis and, 77–78
vaccines against childhood diseases and, 77
women's health and, 81
World Bank and, 70
worldwide disability and, 681
World Health Report, 201
World Health Statistics Annual, 55
World Resources Institute, 83–84
World War I, nursing history and, 30–31
World War II
and health insurance, 113
industrial nursing and, 958–959
mental illness and, 793
nursing history and, 33
UNICEF and, 70
Wrap-around services, vulnerable populations and, 706

Y

Yellow wedge, 238f, 239
Youth Risk Behavior Surveillance System, 773

Z

Zambia, community health nursing in, 68–69b
Zika virus, pregnancy and, 323b
Zinc, 83
Zoonoses, 324–325